Hip Joint Restoration

Joseph C. McCarthy • Philip C. Noble
Richard N. Villar
Editors

Hip Joint Restoration

Worldwide Advances in Arthroscopy, Arthroplasty, Osteotomy and Joint Preservation Surgery

Springer

Editors
Joseph C. McCarthy, MD
Orthopedic Surgery
Hip Joint Arthroplasty
Hip Arthroscopy Massachusetts General Hospital
Boston, MA, USA

Chief of Joint Surgery
Director Kaplan Joint Center
Newton-Wellesley Hospital
Newton, MA, USA

Richard N. Villar, MSc(Hons), MA, FRCS
Consultant Orthopedic Surgeon Orthopedics
The Villar Bajwa Practice
Spire Cambridge Lea Hospital
Cambridge, UK

Philip C. Noble, BE, MEngSci, PhD
Director of Research
Institute of Orthopedic Research and Education
Houston, TX, USA

Orthopedic Research
Joseph Barnhart Department of Orthopedic Surgery
Baylor College of Medicine
Houston, TX, USA

ISBN 978-1-4614-0693-8 ISBN 978-1-4614-0694-5 (eBook)
DOI 10.1007/978-1-4614-0694-5

Library of Congress Control Number: 2016937008

Printed on acid-free paper

This Springer imprint is published by Springer Nature
The registered company is Springer Science+Business Media LLC
The registered company address is: 233 Spring Street, New York, NY 10013, U.S.A.

Preface

Those of us who treat patients with hip pain know that the surgical treatment of hip disease has undergone tremendous growth during the last decade. Prior books on the hip have either addressed arthroplasty, in providing prosthetic solutions for end-stage hip arthritis, or focused on minimally invasive arthroscopy of the hip. Many of them were technical treatises. Yet hip surgery has moved on greatly from the days when all that might be offered was fracture fixation or arthroplasty and, for the younger patient, the instruction to wait until they had reached sufficient age to justify a prosthesis. The thrust of most surgeons in the twenty-first century is to achieve as much benefit as possible for the patient while keeping surgical trauma to a minimum. Fulfillment of this ambition requires an understanding of new concepts and new procedures, as well as new training to accompany them.

The authors of this book believe that hip disease presents as a spectrum of symptoms and pathology, and so any comprehensive text must include the accurate diagnosis and treatment of both the biologic and the prosthetic hip. With the explosion of information on hip disease in the literature, particularly in the treatment of younger patients, the authors felt that it was time for a comprehensive treatise on this subject. Arthroscopy of the Hip, according to many, is the fastest growing specialty area within orthopedics. Accordingly, an extensive amount of this book is devoted to determining proper surgical indications as well as knowledge of surgical techniques and outcomes for the expanding number of surgical procedures in this area.

This book is divided into 16 parts. Pathology within the hip is best understood in contradistinction to normal growth and development. Early chapters also focus on discerning extra-articular from intra-articular etiologies of hip pain. Digital imaging, including CT, MRI, and ultrasound, has immensely increased our diagnostic understanding of the joint and the periarticular soft tissues. At times, MR imaging may disclose combined issues in pathology such as intra-articular loose bodies in combination with osteonecrosis of the hip or, similarly, an acetabular labral tear in combination with abductor muscle attenuation.

The spectrum of treatment of hip disease importantly includes hip osteotomies, whether of the femur or the acetabulum, or in combination. Knowledge of these procedures and their indications is a critical prerequisite for successful outcomes, especially in young patients. However, some young patients do require total hip arthroplasty, typically secondary to osteonecrosis, tumors, trauma, or collagen disease. Several chapters are devoted to the latest evidence-based information on bearing surfaces, and implant selection as well as surgical techniques.

A critically important area for increased understanding is patient outcomes following hip arthroscopy, osteotomy, or total joint replacement. Importantly, world experts in validated outcome measures and quality of life indicators are authors of chapters in this book. Another unique feature of this volume is a section describing the growth and development of hip arthroscopic surgery in each of the world's continents, authored by experts in each of these geographical areas. Finally, there is an entire section devoted to research and future developments. The robustness of the information as well as the development in these areas adds significantly to the depth of knowledge contained within this book.

There has never been such an exciting time to be a specialist in hip surgery, nor such a time to feel so proud. This book brings together a large number of specialists in the field, each of whom has given up valuable hours to prepare their text. As editors we are enormously grateful to them. Our authors are excellent clinicians, respected practitioners, but, more than anything, good personal friends. So join us on the tidal wave of surgical development shown on these pages, the tidal wave in the surgical treatment of hip disease.

In conclusion, this book has been a truly collaborative effort but would never have been possible without the tireless efforts of Connie Walsh, Miranda Finch and Kristopher Spring at Springer whose expertise, patience, and attention to detail have been vital. We also profusely thank our colleagues and fellow members of ISHA (The International Society of Hip Arthroscopy) who have pitched in as authors and section editors to share their knowledge and understanding of hip disease in making this work an important treatise. And finally, we thank our spouses and families for their support and understanding during this extensive endeavor.

Newton, MA, USA — Joseph C. McCarthy, MD
Houston, TX, USA — Philip C. Noble, PhD
Impington, UK — Richard N. Villar, BSc(Hons), MA, FRCS

Abbreviations

ADL	Activities of daily living
AIIS	Anterior inferior iliac spine
ASIS	Anterior superior iliac spine
AVN	Avascular necrosis
BMP	Bone morphogenic proteins
BW	Body weight
CMI	Core muscle injury
COPD	Chronic obstructive pulmonary disease
CT	Computerized tomography
DEXRIT	Dynamic external rotatory impingement test
DGS	Deep gluteal syndrome
DHS	Dynamic hip screw
DIRI	Dynamic internal rotatory impingement test
EMG	Electromyography
FABER	Flexion, abduction, external rotation
FADDIR	Flexion adduction internal rotation test
FAI	Femoroacetabular impingement
GRF	Ground reaction force(s)
HHS	Harris hip score
HHSm	Modified Harris hip score
HPI	History of present illness
iHOT	international hip outcome tool
IPI	Iliopsoas impingement
ITB	Iliotibial band
L	Left
MAHORN	Multicenter arthroscopy of the hip outcomes research network
MFCA	Medial femoral circumflex artery
MRI	Magnetic resonance imaging
NAHS	Nonarthritic hip score
NSAIDS	Nonsteroidal anti-inflammatory drugs
OA	Osteoarthritis
ON	Osteonecrosis
ONFH	Osteonecrosis of the femoral head
PRP	Platelet rich plasma
R	Right
ROM	Range of motion
SCFE	Slipped capital femoral epiphysis
SI	Sacroiliac

TFL	Tensor fasciae latae
THA	Total hip arthroplasty
VAS	Visual Analog Pain Scale
WOMAC	Western Ontario and McMaster University

Contents

Contributors

Marco Acuña, MD Department of Adult Joint Reconstruction, National Rehabilitation Institute of Mexico, Mexico City, Mexico

Miguel Akkari, MD, PhD Department of Orthopedic Surgery and Traumatology, Pediatric Orthopaedics, Faculdade de Ciências Médicas da Santa Casa de São Paulo, São Paulo, Brazil

Jason D. Alder, MD Department of Orthopaedic Surgery, Houston Methodist Hospital, Houston, TX, USA

João E.D. Amadera, MD, PhD Faculty of Medicine, Spine Center, University of São Paulo, São Paulo, Brazil

A J.M.D. (Tony) Andrade, MSc, FRCS(Tr&Orth) Department of Trauma and Orthopaedics, Royal Berkshire NHS Foundation Trust, Reading Orthopaedic Centre,, Reading, Berkshire, UK

Jean-Noel Argenson, MD Department of Orthopedic Surgery, Institute for Locomotion, Sainte-Marguerite Hospital, Aix-Marseille University, Marseille, France

Samik Banerjee, MD Rubin Institute for Advanced Orthopedics, Center for Joint Preservation and Replacement, Sinai Hospital of Baltimore, Baltimore, MD, USA

Marcus J.K. Bankes, BSc, FRCS(Orth) Department of Orthopaedics, Guy's Hospital, London, UK

Samuel J. Barke, MBBS The Elective Orthopaedic Centre, Surrey, UK

Brian T. Barlow, MD Orthopaedic Surgery, Adult Reconstruction and Joint Replacement, Naval Medical Center San Diego, San Diego, CA, USA

Paul E. Beaulé, MD, FRCSC Orthopaedic Surgery Division, Surgery Department, The Ottawa Hospital, University of Ottawa, Ottawa, ON, Canada

Hany Bedair, MD Department of Orthopaedic Surgery, Massachusetts General Hospital/ Newton Wellesley Hospital, Boston, MA, USA

Asheesh Bedi, MD Division of Sports Medicine, Department of Orthopaedic Surgery, University of Michigan Hospital and Health Systems, Ann Arbor, MI, USA

Carl C. Berasi IV , MD Riverside Methodist Hospital, Columbus, OH, USA

Christopher Betz, DO Division of Sports Medicine, Department of Orthopaedics, University of Massachusetts, Worcester, MA, USA

Amit Bhargava, MD Advanced Pain and Sports Medical, Owings Mills, MD, USA

Patrick M. Birmingham, MD Division of Sports Medicine, Department of Orthopaedic Surgery, Northshore University Health System Chicago, Chicago, IL, USA

Catalina Larrain Birrell, MD Department of Orthopedic Surgery, Clinica Las Condes, Santiago, Región Metropolitana, Chile

Caroline Blakey, MBChB, MRCS, MD(res) Department of Orthopaedics, Sheffield Teaching Hospitals NHS Trust, Sheffield, South Yorkshire, UK

Thierry Boyer, MD Rheumatology, IAL Nollet Paris, Paris, France

Collin D. Bray, MD Department of Radiology, Musculoskeletal Imaging, Baylor College of Medicine, Houston, TX, USA

Edward D.R. Bray, MBBS, BSc (Hons) The EOC, Epsom General Hospital, Surrey, UK

Miriam A. Bredella, MD Department of Radiology, Musculoskeletal Imaging and Interventions, Massachusetts General Hospital, Harvard Medical School, Boston, MA, USA

Jason Brockwell, FRCSEdOrth, FHKAMOrth Orthopaedics Department, Hip and Pelvic Surgery, Asia Medical Specialists, Hong Kong, People's Republic of China

William D. Bugbee, MD Division of Orthopaedics, Scripps Clinic, University of California, San Diego, La Jolla, CA, USA

Brian D. Busconi, MD Division of Sports Medicine, Department of Orthopedics, University of Massachusetts Memorial Medical Center, Worcester, MA, USA

J.W. Thomas Byrd, MD Nashville Sports Medicine Foundation, Nashville, TN, USA

Department of Orthopaedic Surgery and Rehabilitation, Vanderbilt University, Nashville, TN, USA

Josip Nenad Cakic, MD, PhD, FSC(SA)Orth, MMed(Orth), WITS Orthopaedic Surgery, Private Practice, Life Fourways Hospital, Johannesburg, South Africa

Vikram Chatrath, MS, MCh(Ortho) Orthopedics Department, Adult Reconstruction and Trauma Surgery, Halifax Infirmary, Dalhousie University, Halifax, NS, Canada

Antonia F. Chen, MD, MBA Department of Orthopaedics, University of Pittsburgh, Pittsburgh, PA, USA

Anthony W.M. Cheng, PhD (Deceased) Department of Orthopaedic Surgery, Center for Cellular and Molecular Engineering, University of Pittsburgh, Pittsburgh, PA, USA

Jeffrey J. Cherian, DO Rubin Institute for Advanced Orthopedics, Center for Joint Preservation and Replacement, Sinai Hospital of Baltimore, Baltimore, MD, USA

Steven S. Chua, MD, PhD Department of Radiology, Baylor College of Medicine, Houston, TX, USA

John C. Clohisy, MD Orthopaedics Department, Adult Reconstruction and Hip Preservation, Washington University School of Medicine, St. Louis, MO, USA

Jeffrey C. Cowley, MS School of Kinesiology and Recreation, Illinois State University, Normal, IL, USA

Sachin Daivajna, MBBS, FRCS (Orth) The Villar Bajwa Practice, Spire Cambridge Lea Hospital, Cambridge, UK

Michael J. Decker, PhD Center of Orthopaedic Biomechanics, Mechanical and Materials Engineering Department, Felix Ritchie School of Engineering and Computer Science, University of Denver, Denver, CO, USA

Brian M. Devitt, MD, FRCSI Center for Outcomes-based Orthopaedic Research, The Steadman Philippon Research Institute, Vail, CO, USA

Alexandra Dimitrakopoulou, MD The London Hip Arthroscopy Center, Orthopaedics, The Wellington Hospital and Leeds Metropolitan University, London, UK

Leeds Metropolitan University, Leeds, UK

Fintan Doyle, MBBCh, BAO, MSc, FRCS(Orth) Princess Elizabeth Orthopaedic Centre, Royal Devon and Exeter NHS Foundation Trust, Exeter, UK

Stephen T. Duncan, MD Orthopaedics Department, Adult Reconstruction and Hip Preservation, Washington University School of Medicine, St. Louis, MO, USA

Maureen K. Dwyer, PhD, ATC Department of Orthopedics, Kaplan Joint Center, Newton Wellesley Hospital, Newton, MA, USA

Department of Orthopedics, Massachusetts General Hospital, Boston, MA, USA

Omar El Abd, MD Newton Wellesley Interventional Spine, Wellesley, MA, USA

Internal Medicine, PM&R, Newton Wellesley Hospital, Wellesley, MA, USA

Leah Elson, BSc Harris Laboratory, Department of Orthopedics, Massachusetts General Hospital, Boston, MA, USA

Keelan R. Enseki, MS, PT, ATC, OCS, SCS, CSCS Centers for Rehab Services, University of Pittsburgh Center for Sports Medicine, Pittsburgh, PA, USA

Department of Physical Therapy, University of Pittsburgh School of Health and Rehabilitation Sciences, Pittsburgh, PA, USA

Andrew E. Federer, BS Department of Orthopedic Surgery, Hip Preservation Center, Section of Sports Medicine, Rush Medical College of Rush University, Chicago, IL, USA

George Feldman, DMD, PhD Orthopaedic Research, Jefferson Medical College, Philadelphia, PA, USA

Fernando Portilho Ferro, MD Steadman Philippon Research Institute, Hospital de Acidentados, Goiânia, Goiás, Brazil

Richard E. Field, PhD, FRCS, FRCS(Orth) St. George's University of London, Research, The South West London Elective Orthopaedic Centre, Epsom and St. Helier NHS Trust, London, UK

Michael A. Flaherty, MD Department of Orthopedic Surgery, Albany Medical College, Albany, NY, USA

Xavier Flecher, MD Department of Orthopedic Surgery, Institute for Locomotion, Sainte-Marguerite Hospital, Aix-Marseille University, Marseille, France

Andrea Fontana, MD Ortopedia, COF Lanzo Hospital, Como, Italy

Ryan Freedman, BS, MS Department of Orthopedic Surgery, Hip Preservation Center, Section of Sports Medicine, Rush Medical College of Rush University, Chicago, IL, USA

Katherine E. Garrett, BA Institute of Orthopedic Research and Education, University of Texas School of Public Health, Houston, TX, USA

Paul Genever, BSc, PhD Department of Biology, University of York, York, UK

Sunit Ghosh, BSc, MBBS, FRCA, FFICM Anaesthesia, Papworth Hospital, Cambridge, UK

Philip J. Glassner, MD Hunterdon Orthopaedic Institute, Flemington, NJ, USA

Ioannis Gliatis, MD, PhD Department of Orthopaedics, University Hospital of Patras, Patras, Greece

Siôn Glyn-Jones, MA(Cantab), MBBS, FRCS(Orth), DPhil(Oxon) Nuffield Department of Orthopaedics, Rheumatology and Musculoskeletal Sciences, Medical Sciences, University of Oxford, Oxford, UK

Nuffield Orthopaedic Centre, Oxford, UK

Aaron Glynn, MCh, FRCS Adult Lower Limb Reconstruction, Rothman Institute, Thomas Jefferson University Hospital, Philadelphia, PA, USA

Mohammed S. Gobba, MD Department of Orthopedics and Traumatology, Cairo University, Cairo, Egypt

Stephanie L. Gold, BA Magnetic Resonance Imaging Division, Department of Radiology, Hospital for Special Surgery, New York, NY, USA

Victor M. Goldberg†, MD Department of Orthopaedic Surgery, University Hospitals Case Western Medical Center, Cleveland, OH, USA

Peter Goljan, MD Center for Outcomes-Based Orthopaedic Research, The Steadman Philippon Research Institute, Vail, CO, USA

Simon Görtz, MD Division of Sports Medicine, Department of Orthopaedic Surgery, University of California, San Diego, San Diego, CA, USA

Division of Sports Medicine, Department of Orthopaedic Surgery, Washington University in St. Louis, Chesterfield, MO, USA

Timothy Bryan Griffith, MD Division of Sports Medicine, Department of Orthopaedic Surgery, Peachtree Orthopaedic Clinic, Atlanta, GA, USA

Carlos A. Guanche, MD Southern California Orthopedic Institute, Van Nuys, CA, USA

Joshua D. Harris, MD Department of Orthopaedics and Sports Medicine, Houston Methodist Hospital, Houston, TX, USA

Clinical Orthopaedics, Weill Cornell Medical College, New York, NY, USA

Munif Hatem, MD Hip Preservation Center, Baylor University Medical Center, Dallas, TX, USA

Jaclyn F. Hill, MD Department of Pediatric Orthopaedic Surgery, Texas Children's Hospital, Houston, TX, USA

Department of Orthopaedic Surgery, Baylor College of Medicine, Houston, TX, USA

Michael G. Hogen, BA Institute of Orthopedic Research and Education, Houston, TX, USA

Tom Hogervorst, MD, PhD Orthopaedics, Haga, Den Haag, The Netherlands

Per Hölmich, DMSc Sports Orthopedic Research Center—Copenhagen, Arthroscopic Center Amager, Copenhagen University Hospital, Copenhagen, Denmark

Sports Groin Pain Center, Aspetar—Orthopedic and Sports Medicine Hospital, Doha, Qatar

Lissete Horna, MD Orthopedic and Traumatology Department, Hip Unit, University Hospital Infanta Leonor, Madrid, Spain

Elizabeth A. Howse, MD Department of Emergency Medicine, Hofstra North Shore-LIJ School of Medicine, Long Island Jewish Medical Center, New Hyde Park, NY, USA

Ugo N. Ihekweazu, MD, BS Department of Orthopaedic Surgery, Baylor College of Medicine, Houston, TX, USA

Victor M. Ilizaliturri Jr, MD Department of Adult Joint Reconstruction, National Rehabilitation Institute of Mexico, Mexico D.F., Mexico

Kimona Issa, MD Rubin Institute for Advanced Orthopedics, Center for Joint Preservation and Replacement, Sinai Hospital of Baltimore, Baltimore, MD, USA

Todd C. Johnson, MD Division of Sports Medicine, Department of Orthopaedics, Wake Forest University, Winston-Salem, NC, USA

Atul F. Kamath, MD Department of Orthopedic Surgery, Mayo Clinic, Rochester, MN, USA

Bhaveen H. Kapadia, MD Department of Orthopaedic Surgery and Rehabilitation Medicine, State University of New York (SUNY) Downstate Medical Center, Brooklyn, NY, USA

Rubin Institute for Advanced Orthopedics, Center for Joint Preservation and Replacement, Sinai Hospital of Baltimore, Baltimore, MD, USA

Mahalingam Karuppiah, MBBS, FRCS Consultant Orthopaedic Surgeon, Cork, Ireland

David Keeley, PhD Department of Human Performance Dance and Recreation, New Mexico State University, Las Cruces, NM, USA

Thomas W. Kernozek, FACSM, PhD Health Professions Department, Physical Therapy Program, University of Wisconsin-La Crosse, La Crosse, WI, USA

M. Munir Khan, MBBS, MRCS, PhD Division of Orthopaedics, Department of Trauma and Orthopaedics, Freeman Hospital, Sunderland, Tyne and Wear, UK

Karl-Philipp Kienle, MD Department of Orthopedic Surgery, University Bern, Bern, Switzerland

Young-Jo Kim, MD, PhD Department of Orthopaedics, Child and Adult Hip Program, Harvard School of Medicine, Children's Hospital Boston, Boston, MA, USA

Scott King, DO Division of Sports Medicine, Department of Orthopaedics, University of Massachusetts, Worcester, MA, USA

Benjamin R. Kivlan, PT, OCS, SCS, CSCS John G Rangos Sr School of Health Sciences, Duquesne University, Pittsburgh, PA, USA

Christopher M. Larson, MD Minnesota Orthopedic Sports Medicine Institute at Twin Cities Orthopedics, Edina, MN, USA

Cara Beth Lee, MD Department of Orthopaedics, Center for Hip Preservation, Virginia Mason Medical Center, Seattle, WA, USA

Joann Lee, MS Department of Orthopedics, Newton Wellesley Hospital, Newton, MA, USA

Virginie Legre-Boyer, MD Rheumatology, IAL Nollet Paris, Paris, France

Rheumatology, American Hospital of Paris, Paris, France

Neuilly Sur Seine, Neuilly, France

Scott S. Lenobel, MD Department of Radiology, Musculoskeletal Imaging and Interventions, Massachusetts General Hospital, Harvard Medical School, Boston, MA, USA

David G. Lewallen, MD Department of Orthopedic Surgery, Mayo Clinic, Rochester, MN, USA

Alexander Bent Tomic Loftkjaer, MD Orthopedic Surgery, Hip Surgery, Clinica Las Condes, Santiago, Chile

Orthopedic Surgery, Hip Surgery, Hospital Militar de Santiago, Santiago, Chile

Adolph V. Lombardi Jr , MD, FACS Joint Implant Surgeons, Inc., Columbus, OH, USA

Mount Carmel Health System, Columbus, OH, USA

Department of Orthopaedics, The Ohio State University, Columbus, OH, USA

Krissett A. Loya-Bodiford, MPH, BS Clinical Division, Orthopedic Department, Institute of Orthopedic Research and Education, Houston, TX, USA

Brett Lurie, BSc(Med), MBBS(Hons1) Magnetic Resonance Imaging Division, Department of Radiology, Hospital for Special Surgery, New York, NY, USA

Francesc Malagelada, MD Department of Orthopaedics, South West London Elective Orthopaedic Centre, Surrey, UK

Rodrigo Mardones, MD Tissue Engineering Lab, Orthopedics Department, Clinica Las Condes, Santiago, Chile

Oliver Marín-Peña, MD Orthopedic Surgery and Traumatology, Hip and Knee Orthopedic Surgery, University Hospital Infanta Leonor, Madrid, Spain

Hal David Martin, DO Hip Preservation Center, Baylor University Medical Center, Dallas, TX, USA

RobRoy L. Martin, PhD, PT, CSCS Department of Physical Therapy, UPMC—Center for Sports Medicine, Duquesne University, Pittsburgh, PA, USA

Scott D. Martin, MD Division of Sports Medicine, Department of Orthopedic Surgery, Brigham and Women's Hospital/Harvard Medical School, Boston, MA, USA

Richard C. Mather III , MD Department of Orthopaedic Surgery, Duke University Medical Center, Durham, NC, USA

Sean Mc Millan, DO Orthopedic Sports Medicine, Lourdes Medical Associates, Burlington, NJ, USA

Andrew W. McCaskie, MB ChB, MMus, MD, FRCS, FRCS(T&O) Division of Trauma and Orthopaedic Surgery, Department of Surgery, University of Cambridge, Cambridge University Hospitals NHS Foundation Trust, Cambridge, Cambridgeshire, UK

Frank McCormick, MD Department of Orthopedic Surgery, Sports Medicine, Rush University, Chicago, IL, USA

Morteza Meftah, MD Orthopaedic Surgery, New York University School of Medicine, Hospital for Joint Disease, New York, NY, USA

Omer Mei-Dan, MD Department of Orthopaedics, University of Colorado, Boulder, CO, USA

Nicholas G.H. Mohtadi, MD, MSc, FRCSC Division of Orthopaedics, Department of Surgery, Peter Longheed Centre, University of Calgary, Calgary, AB, Canada

Michael A. Mont, MD Rubin Institute for Advanced Orthopedics, Center for Joint Preservation and Replacement, Sinai Hospital of Baltimore, Baltimore, MD, USA

Nicole I. Montgomery, MD Department of Orthopedic Surgery, Baylor College of Medicine, Houston, TX, USA

Jeffrey F. Murray, DO Division of Sports Medicine, Department of Orthopedics, University of Massachusetts Memorial Medical Center, Worcester, MA, USA

Donald Anthony Neumann, PT, PhD, FAPTA Department of Physical Therapy, Marquette University, Milwaukee, WI, USA

Michael L. Nguyen, MD Division of Sports Medicine, Department of Orthopedic Surgery, Stanford University Medical Center, Redwood City, CA, USA

Shane J. Nho, MD, MS Department of Orthopedic Surgery, Hip Preservation Center, Section of Sports Medicine, Rush Medical College of Rush University, Chicago, IL, USA

Takashi Nishii, MD, PhD Department of Orthopaedic Medical Engineering, Osaka University Graduate School of Medicine, Suita, Japan

Catherine A. Nosal, BS University of Michigan, Ann Arbor, MI, USA

John M. O'Donnell, MBBS, FRACS, FAOrthA Hip Arthroscopy Australia, St. Vincents Private Hospital, Richmond, VIC, Australia

John N. O'Hara, FRCS, FRCSI, MCh The Birmingham Hip Clinic, Birmingham, UK

Amo Oduro, MBBS, FRCA, FRCP Anaesthesia, Papworth Hospital, Cambridge, UK

Adriana M.L. Oliveira, MD Department of Radiology, Musculoskeletal Imaging and Interventions, Massachusetts General Hospital, Harvard Medical School, Boston, MA, USA

George Chukwuka Ozoude, MD Division of Sports Medicine, Department of Orthopaedic Surgery, University of Texas Health Science Center at Houston, Houston, TX, USA

Andrew R. Palisch, MD Department of Radiology, Baylor College of Medicine, Houston, TX, USA

Ian James Palmer, PhD Hip Preservation Center, Baylor University Medical Center, Dallas, TX, USA

William E. Palmer, MD Division of Musculoskeletal Imaging, Department of Radiology, Massachusetts General Hospital, Boston, MA, USA

Athanasios V. Papavasileiou, BSc, MD, PhD Department of Physical Education and Sports Science, Aristotle University of Thessaloniki, Thessaloniki, Greece

Sports Injuries Lab, St. Lukes General Hospital, Thessaloniki, Greece

Sebastien Paratte, MD Department of Orthopedic Surgery, Institute for Locomotion, Sainte-Marguerite Hospital, Aix-Marseille University, Marseille, France

Caroline N. Park, BA Division of Clinical Research, Department of Orthopaedic Surgery, Hospital for Special Surgery, New York, NY, USA

Javad Parvizi, MD, FRCS Adult Lower Limb Reconstruction, Rothman Institute, Thomas Jefferson University Hospital, Philadelphia, PA, USA

Cecilia Pascual-Garrido, MD Hip Preservation, Sports Medicine, University of Colorado, Boulder, CO, USA

Lourenço P. Peixoto, MD Center for Outcomes-Based Orthopaedic Research, The Steadman Philippon Research Institute, Vail, CO, USA

Marc J. Philippon, MD The Steadman Clinic, Vail, CO, USA

Department of Surgery, Faculty of Health Sciences, McMaster University, Hamilton, ON, Canada

Department of Orthopaedic Surgery, University of Pittsburgh School of Medicine, Pittsburgh, PA, USA

Daniel Camargo Pimentel, MD, PhD Department of Orthopedics and Traumatology, University of Sao Paulo, School of Medicine, Spine Center, Sao Paulo, Brazil

Giancarlo C. Polesello, PhD Department of Orthopedic Surgery and Traumatology, Hip Group, Faculdade de Ciências Médicas da Santa Casa de São Paulo, São Paulo, Brazil

Tom Pollard, MD, FRCS(Tr&Orth), BSc(Hons) Department of Orthopaedics, Royal Berkshire Hospital, Reading, UK

Matthew A. Popa, MD Department of Orthopaedic Surgery, University Hospitals Case Medical Center, Cleveland, OH, USA

Hollis G. Potter, MD MRI Research, Magnetic Resonance Imaging, Hospital for Special Surgery, New York, NY, USA

Department of Radiology, Weill Medical College of Cornell University, New York, NY, USA

Hernan A. Prieto, MD Department of Orthopedic Surgery, Mayo Clinic, Rochester, MN, USA

Michael George Pritchard, BMedSci, MBBS(Hons), FRACS(Orth) Wellington Orthopaedics, University of Tasmania, Calvary Hospital Hobart, Hobart, TAS, Australia

David M. Privitera, MD Division of Sports Medicine, Department of Orthopedic Surgery, Rochester Regional Health System, Rochester, NY, USA

Marcelo C. Queiroz, MD Department of Orthopedic Surgery and Traumatology, Hip Group, Faculdade de Ciências Médicas da Santa Casa de São Paulo, São Paulo, Brazil

Narendra Ramisetty, MBBS, AFRCS, FRCS (Orth) The Villar Bajwa Practice, Spire Cambridge Lea Hospital, Cambridge, UK

Anil S. Ranawat, MD Division of Sports Medicine and Joint Preservation, Hospital for Special Surgery, New York, NY, USA

James B. Richardson, MBChB, FRCS, MD Department of Orthopaedics, Keele University, Oswestry, UK

Craig M. Roberto, DO Division of Sports Medicine, Department of Orthopaedics, University of Massachusetts, Worcester, MA, USA

Scott A. Rodeo, MD Department of Orthopedic Surgery, Weill Medical College of Cornell University, New York, NY, USA

Orthopedics Department, Sports Medicine and Shoulder Service, The Hospital for Special Surgery, New York, NY, USA

New York Giants Football, New York, NY, USA

Scott B. Rosenfeld, MD Department of Pediatric Orthopaedic Surgery, Texas Children's Hospital, Houston, TX, USA

Department of Orthopaedic Surgery, Baylor College of Medicine, Houston, TX, USA

Ardavan Ariel Saadat, BS, MD Institute of Orthopedic Research and Education, Baylor College of Medicine, Houston, TX, USA

Department of Orthopaedic Surgery, University of Illinois College of Medicine at Chicago, Chicago, IL, USA

Hassan Sadri, MD Department of Orthopaedic Surgery, Clinique Bois-Cerf, Lausanne, Switzerland

Marc R. Safran, MD Division of Sports Medicine, Department of Orthopaedic Surgery, Stanford University, Redwood City, CA, USA

Hatem Galal Said, MD, FRCSI Orthopaedics & Traumatology, Arthroscopy, Assiut University Hospital, Assiut, Egypt

Michael J. Salata, MD Department of Orthopaedic Surgery, Center for Joint Preservation and Cartilage Restoration, University Hospitals Case Medical Center, Case Western Reserve University, Cleveland, OH, USA

Matías Salineros, MD Orthopaedic Department, Joint Reconstruction, Clinica Las Condes, Santiago, Chile

Orthopaedic Department, Universidad de los Andes, Santiago, Chile

Srihari C. Sampath, MD, PhD, MPhil Division of Musculoskeletal Imaging and Intervention, Department of Radiology, Massachusetts General Hospital, Boston, MA, USA

Srinath C. Sampath, MD, PhD, MPhil Division of Musculoskeletal Imaging and Intervention, Department of Radiology, Massachusetts General Hospital, Boston, MA, USA

Thomas G. Sampson, MD Hip Arthroscopy, Post Street Surgery, Post Street Orthopaedics and Sports Medicine, San Francisco, CA, USA

Richard F. Santore, MD Orthopaedic Surgery, Sharp Memorial Hospital, San Diego, CA, USA

Orthopaedic Surgery, University of California San Diego, San Diego, CA, USA

Hind Sawan, BS Department of Orthopaedic Research, The Rothman Institute at Thomas Jefferson University, Philadelphia, PA, USA

Ernest Schilders, MD, FRCS, FFSEM The London Hip Arthroscopy Center, Orthopaedics, The Wellington Hospital, London, UK

Leeds Metropolitan University, Leeds, UK

Kevin Shelburne, PhD Department of Mechanical and Materials Engineering, The University of Denver, Denver, CO, USA

Vijay D. Shetty, MS(Orth) Orthopaedic Division, Hiranandani Orthopaedic Medical Education (HOME), Dr. L. H. Hiranandani Hospital, Mumbai, Maharashtra, India

Sangmin Ryan Shin, MD Department of Orthopaedic Surgery, Southeast Permanente Med Group, Atlanta, GA, USA

Amardeep Singh, MBBS, MS Division of Orthopaedic Surgery, University of Ottawa, Ottawa, ON, Canada

Orthopaedic Surgery, The Ottawa Hospital, Ottawa, ON, Canada

Parminder J. Singh, MBBS, MRCS, FRCS(Tr&Orth), MS, FRACS Department of Orthopaedics, Maroondah Hospital, Monash University, Monash, VIC, Australia

Daniel L. Skinner, MBChB, BSc (Hons) Orthopaedic Department, Research Division, Elective Orthopaedic Centre, Epsom General Hospital, Surrey, England

Kjeld Søballe, MD, DMSc Department of Orthopaedics, Section for Hip Surgery, Aarhus University Hospital, Aarhus, Denmark

Giles H. Stafford, MBBS, BSc (Hons), FRCS The EOC, Epsom General Hospital, Surrey, UK

Rebecca M. Stone, MS, ATC Minnesota Orthopedic Sports Medicine Institute at Twin Cities Orthopedics, Edina, MN, USA

Francesco Strambi, MD Research Unit, South West London Elective Orthopaedic Centre, Surrey, UK

Allston J. Stubbs, MD, MBA Division of Sports Medicine, Department of Orthopaedic Surgery, Wake Forest University, Winston-Salem, NC, USA

S. David Stulberg, MD Department of Orthopaedic Surgery, Northwestern University Feinberg School of Medicine, Chicago, IL, USA

Carlos Suarez-Ahedo, MD Department of Adult Joint Reconstruction, National Rehabilitation Institute of Mexico, Mexico D.F., Mexico

Nobuhiko Sugano, MD, PhD Department of Orthopaedic Medical Engineering, Osaka University Graduate School of Medicine, Suita, Japan

Jaron P. Sullivan, MD Division of Sports Medicine, Department of Orthopaedic Surgery, Vanderbilt University, Nashville, TN, USA

Moritz Tannast, MD Department of Orthopaedic Surgery, University of Bern, Inselspital, Bern, Switzerland

Kristian Thorborg, PhD Sports Orthopedic Research Center—Copenhagen, Arthroscopic Center Amager, Copenhagen University Hospital, Copenhagen, Denmark

Andrew John Timperley, MBChB, FRCS, DPhil(Oxon) Centre for Hip Surgery (Exeter), Princess Elizabeth Orthopaedic Hospital, Royal Devon and Exeter Hospital NHS Foundation Trust, Exeter, UK

Michael R. Torry, PhD Biomechanics Division, College of Applied Science and Technology, Illinois State University, Normal, IL, USA

Anders Troelsen, MD, PhD, DMSc Clinical Orthopaedic Research Hvidovre and Department of Orthopaedics, Section for Hip and Knee Surgery, Copenhagen University Hospital, Hvidovre, Copenhagen, Denmark

Rocky S. Tuan, PhD Department of Orthopaedic Surgery, Center for Cellular and Molecular Engineering, University of Pittsburgh, Pittsburgh, PA, USA

Joshua A. Tuck, DO, MS Division of Sports Medicine, Department of Orthopaedic Surgery, University of Massachusetts Medical School, University of Massachusetts Memorial Medical Center, Worcester, MA, USA

Veronica Ulici, MD, PhD Department of Orthopaedic Surgery, Center for Cellular and Molecular Engineering, University of Pittsburgh, Pittsburgh, PA, USA

Stephen Webb, MBBCh, FRCA, FFICM Anaesthesia, Papworth Hospital, Cambridge, UK

Glenn D. Wera, MD Department of Orthopaedic Surgery, University Hospitals Case Medical Center, Cleveland, OH, USA

Sarah L. Whitehouse, PhD Institute of Health and Biomedical Innovation, Queensland University of Technology, Brisbane, QLD, Australia

Paul Whittingham-Jones, MBBS, FRCS Trauma and Orthopaedics, Surgery, West Hertfordshire Hospitals NHS Trust, Watford and St. Albans City Hospital, Herts, UK

Matthew J. Wilson, FRCS(Eng), FRCS(Tr&Orth) Exeter Hip Unit, Princess Elizabeth Orthopaedic Centre, Exeter, UK

David A. Young, FRACS Melbourne Orthopaedic Group, Melbourne, Australia

Simon W. Young, FRACS Division of Sports Medicine, Department of Orthopaedic Surgery, Stanford University, Redwood City, CA, USA

About the Authors

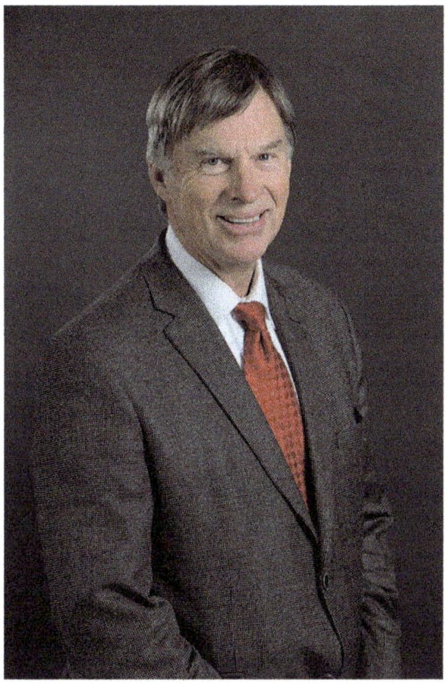

Joseph C. McCarthy, MD is the chief of Reconstructive Hip and Knee Joint Surgery at Newton Wellesley Hospital, a member of the joint arthroplasty staff at Massachusetts General Hospital, and Associate professor of Orthopedic Surgery at Harvard University, part-time. He is also a clinical professor of Orthopedic Surgery at Tufts University for the past 20 years. He has had a long-standing interest in hip joint preservation and, along with Dr. James Glick, pioneered hip arthroscopy in the United States. This focus included published work on hip anatomy and morphology as well as minimally invasive surgical approaches, development of a dedicated hip distractor and instruments solely for use in hip arthroscopic procedures.

Dr. McCarthy completed his undergraduate education at the University of Notre Dame, during which time he played on the varsity hockey and baseball teams. He then matriculated to Georgetown University medical school. Following a medical internship at Georgetown University Hospital, he completed surgical and orthopedic training at Tufts University in Boston. After residency, he completed a fellowship in hip and knee reconstructive joint surgery at Massachusetts General Hospital under the direction of Dr. William Harris and Hugh Chandler. Subsequently his entire practice career has been in Boston.

During his career he has served the American Academy of Orthopedic Surgeons as a member of the Committee on the Hip, program chair for the Hip Society, and has been on the board of directors for both the AAOS and the orthopedic research and education foundation (OREF). He has also been the chair of the board of specialty societies of the AAOS and chairman of the Shands Society of OREF. He is a founding member of the International Society of Hip Arthroscopy. He is also past president of the American Association of Hip and Knee Surgeons and the International Society of Hip Arthroscopy.

For his research he has received both the Otto Aufranc Award and the Frank Stinchfield Award from the Hip Society and the AAOS. Both of these awards were for work on understanding the acetabular labrum and, when injured, its relationship to degenerative arthritis of the hip joint. Dr. McCarthy has been Director of the biologic hip portion of the Harvard hip/knee course for the past 8 years and has been co-chairman of the AAOS Learning Center hip arthroscopy course for the past 12 years.

Dr. McCarthy has been committed to scholarship in the field of hip preservation, publishing the first validated hip outcomes scoring system for the native hip, as well as been an active member of MAHORN (Multi-center Arthroscopic Hip Outcomes Research Network). Most recently he has authored work on hip joint lubrication and EMG muscle effects associated with acetabular labral tears. Dr. McCarthy has authored over 175 peer-reviewed articles, posters, book chapters, and books.

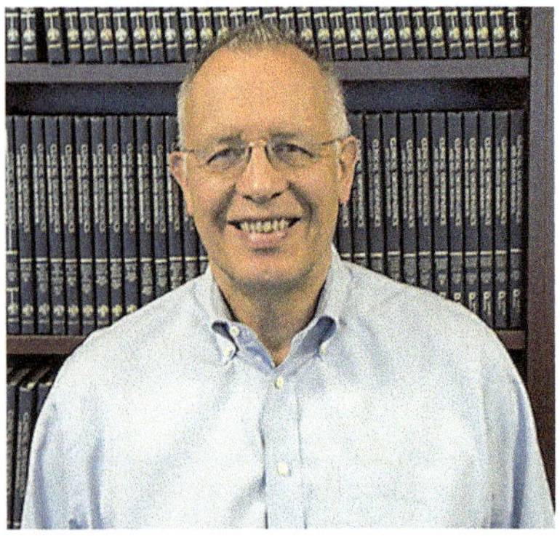

Philip C. Noble, BE MEngSci PhD was educated in Australia in diverse subjects including Engineering, the Physical Sciences, and Classical Philosophy. After being awarded a Winston Churchill Fellowship in 1979, he traveled throughout Europe, the United Kingdom, and North America and eventually returned to Houston to work in the Texas Medical Center. He was awarded his PhD from the University of Strathclyde in Glasgow, Scotland, where he studied the biomechanics of the hip and hip replacement under the direction of Professor John Paul. He now serves as the Director of Research in the Institute of Orthopedic Research and Education and holds the rank of Professor in the Department of Orthopaedic Surgery at Baylor College of Medicine.

Phil Noble's research interests include the biomechanics of the hip and knee joints and their replacements, the morphometry of human bones, the biology and biomechanics of cartilage, tendon, and ligaments, and the quantitative assessment of clinical outcomes. He has numerous publications related to the hip and is a frequent speaker at national and international conferences. He is also a member of The Hip Society, The Knee Society, The International Hip Society, and The American Academy of Orthopedic Surgeons. Dr. Noble is internationally renowned as a designer and innovator and is the holder of numerous patents. He has participated in the development of more than 20 designs of total hip and knee replacements and associated instrumentation.

Dr. Noble is active in philanthropic activities and is particularly interested in issues related to diversity and underrepresented minorities. He is also committed to mentorship and has been instrumental in the training and development of over 150 postgraduates interested in careers in orthopedic surgery and related research. His recreational interests include foreign travel, gardening, and ornamental glass.

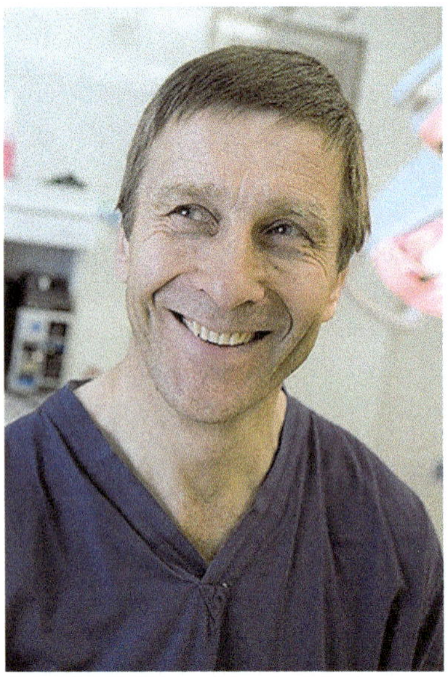

Richard N. Villar, BSc (Hons) MA MS FRCS qualified in medicine at St. Thomas's Hospital in London (UK) before joining the military as the Regimental Medical Officer to the SAS. After leaving the Army he completed his surgical studies in Southampton and Cambridge, joining the consultant staff of Addenbrooke's Hospital (Cambridge) in 1988. It was there that he developed his interest in conservative hip surgery and now has one of the largest experiences of hip arthroscopic (keyhole) procedures in the world.

Now in independent practice, Richard is a Founding Member, and first President, of the International Society for Hip Arthroscopy. He has served as a member of Council of the British Orthopaedic Association, is an assessor for the General Medical Council, and is a member of the United Kingdom's Disaster Emergency Response Team.

In this latter capacity he was operational in the aftermaths of the Kashmir, Java, and Haiti earthquakes. Richard regards orthopedic surgery as both his profession and hobby.

When not dealing with problematic hips and knees, he can be found either playing his classical guitar or on a mountainside, maintaining his skills as an International Mountain Leader.

Part I

Structure and Function of the Tissues of the Hip (Normal and Diseased)

Richard E. Field

Development of the Hip: Phylogeny and Ontogeny

1

Tom Hogervorst, Karl-Philipp Kienle, and Moritz Tannast

Introduction

The human hip is a conceptually simple ball and socket joint, but functions as part of a complex anatomic unit consisting of the femur, the pelvis and the lumbosacral spine. This unit is highly variable between different species of animals. Human hip evolution is characterized by obligate bipedal gait and encephalization (development of a disproportionately enlarged brain). This makes the female pelvis the only skeletal element that conveys information about these two most peculiar traits of human evolution. It shows both the adaptations that occurred to facilitate a permanent bipedal gait and, at the same time, the adaptations to accommodate the birth of a large-brained baby.

Human hip morphogenesis can deviate from its normal pathway by developmental hip disorders. Common developmental hip disorders such as developmental dysplasia of the hip, slipped capital femoral epiphysis (SCFE) but also femoroacetabular impingement can be explained from an evolutionary perspective. Below, we review relevant aspects of evolution (phylogeny) and human hip morphogenesis (ontogeny) that are relevant to the understanding of hip morphotypes and related hip disorders.

T. Hogervorst, MD, PhD (✉)
Haga Ziekenhuis, Lokatie Sportlaan,
Sportlaan 600, Den Haag 2566MJ, the Netherlands
e-mail: thogervorst@gmail.com

K.-P. Kienle, MD
Department of Orthopedic Surgery, University Bern,
Bern, Switzerland
e-mail: philipp.kienle@gmail.com

M. Tannast, MD
Department of Orthopaedic Surgery, University of Bern,
Inselspital, Murtenstrasse, Bern 3010, Switzerland
e-mail: moritz.tannast@insel.ch

Evolution of Bone and Locomotion

Mineralized tissues (enamel, dentine and bone) were a major breakthrough in evolution. Calcium carbonate ($CaCo_3$), the common constituent of rock, was always present in ocean water and started being used as reinforcement in organisms about half a billion years ago in the Cambrian era [1]. Since then, fossils demonstrate the calcified remains of life's evolution. But the fossil record will, by definition, always remain incomplete, and it is genetic studies that have revolutionized our understanding of the early stages in evolution of mineralized tissues. For example, a related family of genes that likely arose from a common ancestor produces the mineralized tissues for teeth (enamel, dentine) and skeletons (bone extracellular matrix) [2]. Teeth-like structures probably evolved first, allowing new forms of predation, followed by a dermal exoskeleton of dentine, enamel and bone [3]. Teeth produced big changes in feeding and predation while development of endo- and exoskeletons allowed radical changes in locomotion. Bone likely appeared as an attachment to dentine in scales [2] in exoskeletons. The stunning fossils from the Cambrian era document an explosion in the possible basic structures of bodies (body plans) [4, 5]. The vast majority of these have long gone extinct and the remaining body plans (i.e. at phylum and subphylum level) now show striking *invariability*, for which genetic explanations have been suggested recently [6]. In contrast, within phyla, a spectacular variety in animal form has developed. On the phylum level, the existence of an endo- versus an exoskeleton (e.g. Arthropodae) imparts major differences in function. An exoskeleton affords strength and allows limbs to be longer which enhances both protection and locomotion. An endoskeleton has the advantage over exoskeletons that it frees the skin to function as sensory and thermoregulatory organ.

Already in lobe-finned fishes such as the *Eusthenopteron* (Devonian period [415–375 million years ago]), we find the primordial tetrapod body structure consisting of a longitudinal body axis with four perpendicular appendages. Indeed, their paired breast and pelvic fins have the pattern of our

J.C. McCarthy et al. (eds.), *Hip Joint Restoration*, DOI 10.1007/978-1-4614-0694-5_1

limbs today: one proximal (femur and humerus) and two distal bones (tibia/fibula and radius/ulna, Fig. 1.1). Their pelvic fins had what can be interpreted as a proto-femur. Once "on land" a suite of further developments improved locomotion, both in endurance and speed.

Evolution of Tetrapod Gait

The development of terrestrial life forms hinged on the evolution of limbs from paired fins, limbs that, eventually, could bear the animal's weight against gravity (Fig. 1.2). Molecular genetic studies now show the fin to limb transformation can be made by subtle changes in a relatively small number of genetic switches [7], i.e. without the need for extraordinary processes or genetic mechanisms. Amphibians started walking with a sprawling gait, with the limbs still perpendicular to the long axis of the body—as with the paired fins in fish. But on land this requires permanent elevation of the body above the plane of the appendages to prevent contact between the trunk and the ground (Fig. 1.3).

Much heavier loads can be carried by limbs that are vertical than those that are horizontal, and so, vertical limb alignment allowed dinosaurs to grow to a huge size. The emergence of vertical limb positions and rounding of the hip joint also enabled increased stride length, while adoption of an erect posture decoupled walking from breathing. This increased stamina, as running no longer counteracted breathing [8].

Mammalian Hip Types

Mammals display large variation in hip morphology. Conceptually, two types of hip can be distinguished, *coxa recta* and *coxa rotunda* [9, 10], based on differences in *proximal femoral concavity* [11]. Concavity is a compound measure, influenced by the relative dimensions of the femoral head and neck (*head-neck ratio*), the roundness of the femoral head (*sphericity*) and the position of the femoral head relative to the neck [12]. Concavity thus determines the potential for femoral impingement (the acetabular parameters are depth and sphericity). Concavity can be quantified by angular measurements, e.g. alpha [13], beta, gamma and delta angles [12] and linear measurements (offset) or ratios. Coxa recta and rotunda relate to the ossification pattern of the proximal femur [14] and locomotor categories. Specifically, a single coalescence of the proximal femur is seen in coxa recta, whereas separation of the trochanteric and capital epiphysis is seen in coxa rotunda. Typically, coxa recta is seen in runners and jumpers, rotunda in climbers, amphibians and swimmers (Fig. 1.4. horse/walrus). In humans (and in the nonhuman apes), the two epiphyses of the proximal femur separate, i.e. a coxa rotunda ossification pattern. However, some morphotypes of the human hip appear to mimic the normal morphology of species with "coalesced" epiphyses [14], i.e. a coxa recta or "cam-type" hip [15].

Locomotion in the Nonhuman Apes

The nonhuman apes have a varied repertoire of locomotion including arm slinging, climbing, quadrupedal knuckle walking and bipedal walking. The nonhuman apes (chimpanzee, bonobo, gorilla, gibbon, orangutan) do not run bipedally [16], and their bipedal walking is not the true upright walking seen in modern humans. Due to a stiff spine [17], bipedal walking in the nonhuman apes requires flexion in both hips and knees to position the trunk over the feet (Fig. 1.5). Bipedal walking in the nonhuman apes therefore requires constant activity of hip extensors (hamstrings) and

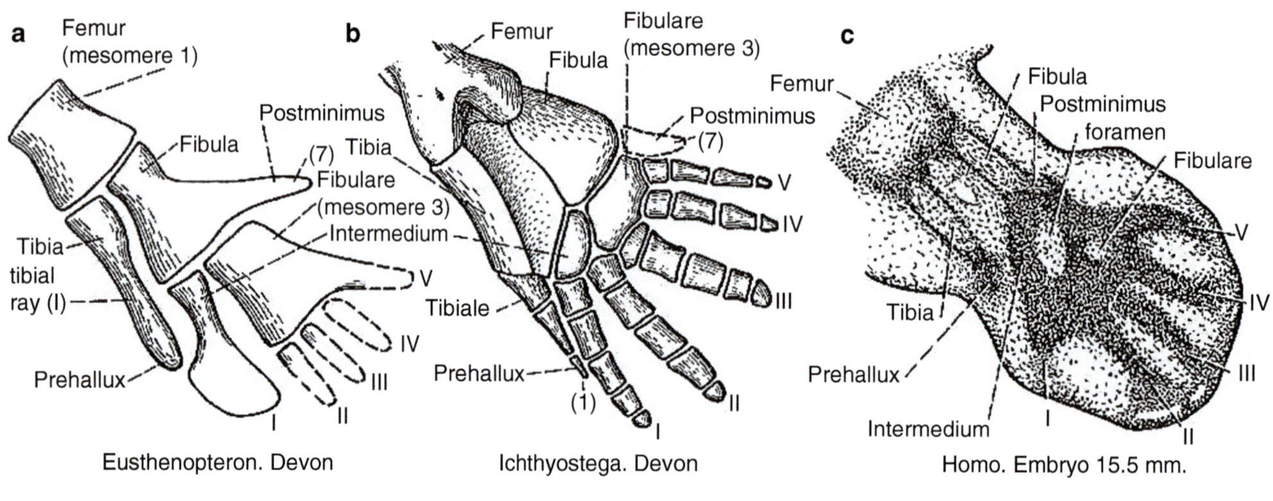

Fig. 1.1 The ancient building plan of (hind) limbs. Eusthenopteron is a lobe-finned fish, Ichtyostega is a *fishapod,* comparable to Acanthostega (Fig. 1.2) From [81] and Hogervorst T, Bouma HW, de Vos J. Evolution of the hip and pelvis. Acta Orthop Suppl. 2009 Aug;80(336):1–39. Reprinted with permission from Informa Healthcare

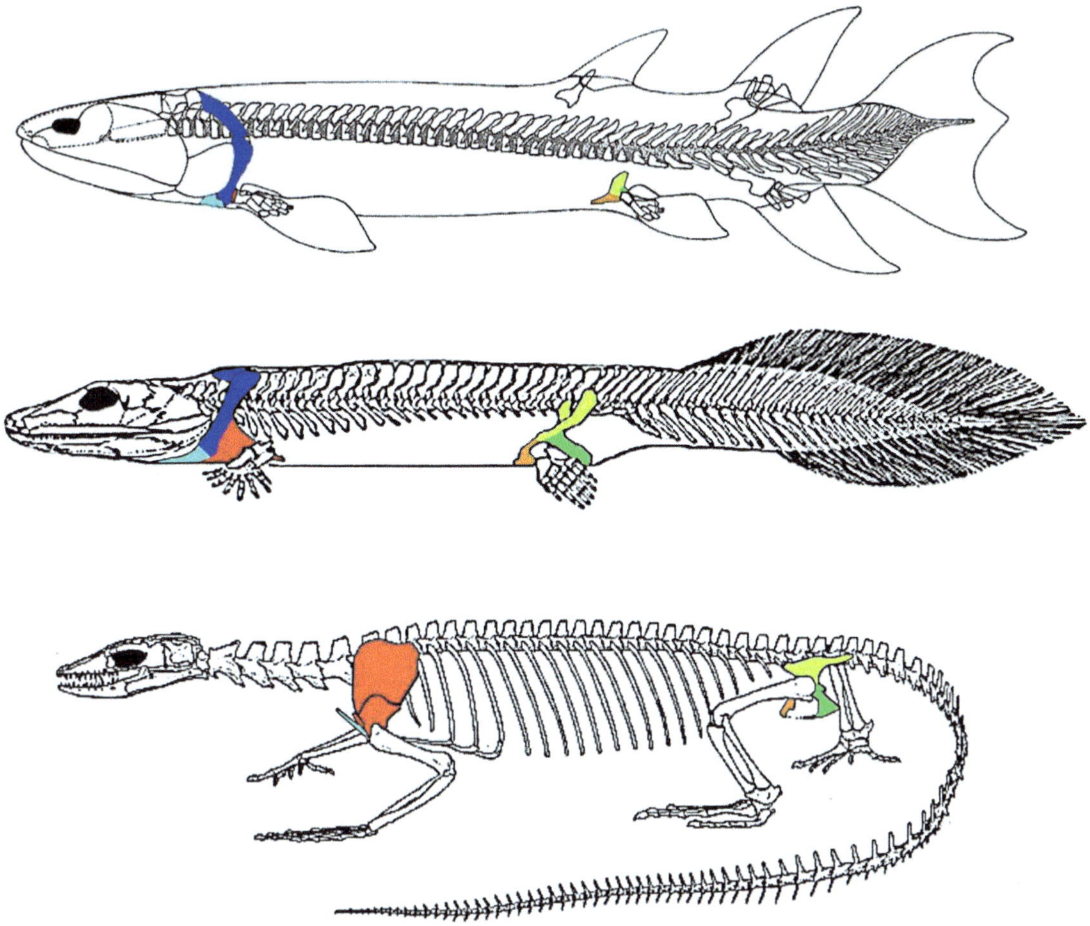

Fig. 1.2 *Eusthenopteron* (*top*), a fossil lobe-finned fish of approx. 380 million years ago, is thought to represent the beginning of the transition to land-life. It has no neck and a bony connection of the pectoral girdle (with its pectoral fins) to the skull. The pelvic bone (*yellow*, *green*, *orange*), however, is not attached to the spine. *Acanthostega* (a fossil *fishapod*, *middle*) can be seen as the other end of the transition to land-life, and the time elapsed between these two fossils is about 15 million years. The scapulocoracoid (*red*) has increased in size, and the pectoral girdle is no longer attached to the cranium. The pelvis has enlarged markedly and is now attached to the spine by ligaments and muscles. *Varanus* (*bottom*), an extant lizard, has its clavicle (*light blue*) not attached to the spine, allowing movement between the scapulocoracoid and the spine to increase stride length. The pelvis has a bony connection to the spine through the sacroiliac joints. From Hogervorst T, Bouma HW, de Vos J. Evolution of the hip and pelvis. Acta Orthop Suppl. 2009 Aug;80(336):1–39. Reprinted with permission from Informa Healthcare

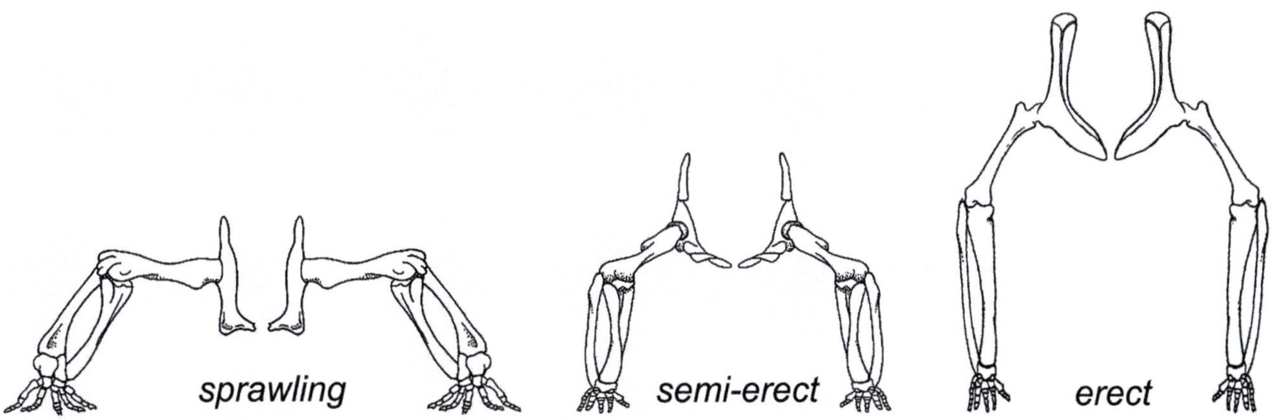

Fig. 1.3 Posture types: sprawling (e.g. reptiles), semi-erect and erect (e.g. cursorial mammals)

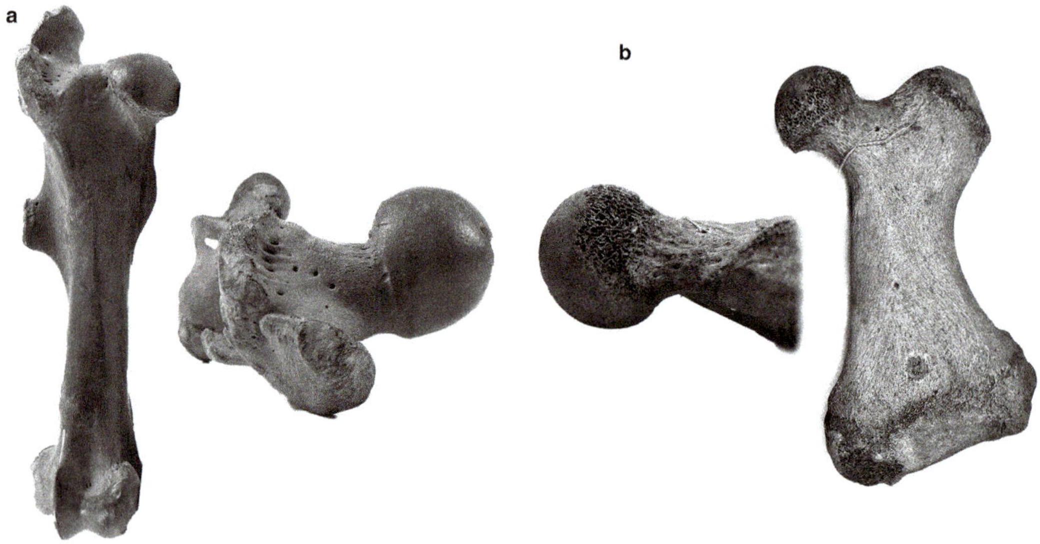

Fig 1.4 Femora of a horse (**a**), a cursorial (an animal adapted for running) with coxa recta (*left*) and a walrus (**b**), a swimmer with coxa rotunda (*right*)

knee extensors (quadriceps). Further, in the nonhuman apes, the orientation of the pelvic ala coincides with the coronal plane. Consequently, the gluteus medius and minimus continue to function as hip extensors rather than abductors (Fig. 1.6), and so nonhuman apes tend to walk with less lateral balance control [18].

Early Human Hips: Ancestors

DNA studies date the shared ancestor of chimpanzees and humans to approx. six to seven million years [19], which makes this a recent event, in evolutionary terms. Many quadrupedal mammals can also walk upright (e.g. bears, apes), but for modern humans, upright walking quickly became the *only* gait type. Many adaptations in lumbosacro-pelvic morphology occurred within a relatively short time span to enable this (for review see [17]). Spectacular fossil finds of the last 50 years [10] show that obligate and exclusive bipedal gait was established within 2–3 million years of early human evolution [20]. Human bipedal gait is highly efficient compared to that of the other large apes. Little muscle activity is required to maintain human upright posture [21]. Compared to the extensive changes in lumbosacral spine and pelvis, the changes in the early human hip joint can be considered minor. When comparing with the nonhuman apes, the changes in the proximal femur reflect the increased loading of bipedal gait and running (nonhuman apes do not run bipedally). The human hip has a thicker femoral neck (decreased head-neck ratio, Fig. 1.7) and reduced concavity compared to the nonhuman apes (Figs. 1.8 and 1.9).

Comparison of Human and Ape Hip Morphology

A comprehensive study of cadaveric femora of 375 North Americans (divided equally between males and females and blacks and whites) found considerable variability in the concavity of the femoral head-neck junction, both superiorly (gamma angle) and anteriorly (alpha angle) [12]. Epidemiology studies in predominantly white populations concur, with a prevalence of approx. 8–20 % of the coxa recta morphotype [13, 22–27]. Coxa profunda (defined as a lateral CE angle >39° or a posterior wall sign) appears to have comparable prevalence although this has been less extensively studied, and gender differences are conflicting [23, 27].

However, it appears that considerable differences in human hip morphology exist between different ethnic populations. Although studies comparable to Toogood et al. are as yet lacking, low concavity of the proximal femur appears to be rare in many [28–32], if not all [33, 34], Asian populations. Thus, it has been speculated that the lower incidence of osteoarthritis in the "Asian hip" [35, 36] is related to this higher concavity and decreased FAI [28, 37]. In contrast, the nonhuman apes share a much more uniform hip morphotype, with no important differences in concavity, either between species or between the sexes. In 210 cadaveric great ape femora (chimpanzee/bonobo and gorilla) examined using the exact methods of Toogood et al., much lower variability in concavity was found [38]. The nonhuman apes have coxa rotunda (Figs. 1.7 and 1.9), allowing a large range of motion, advantageous for a locomotion generalist and particularly so for climbing. Perhaps, increasing the loading history during

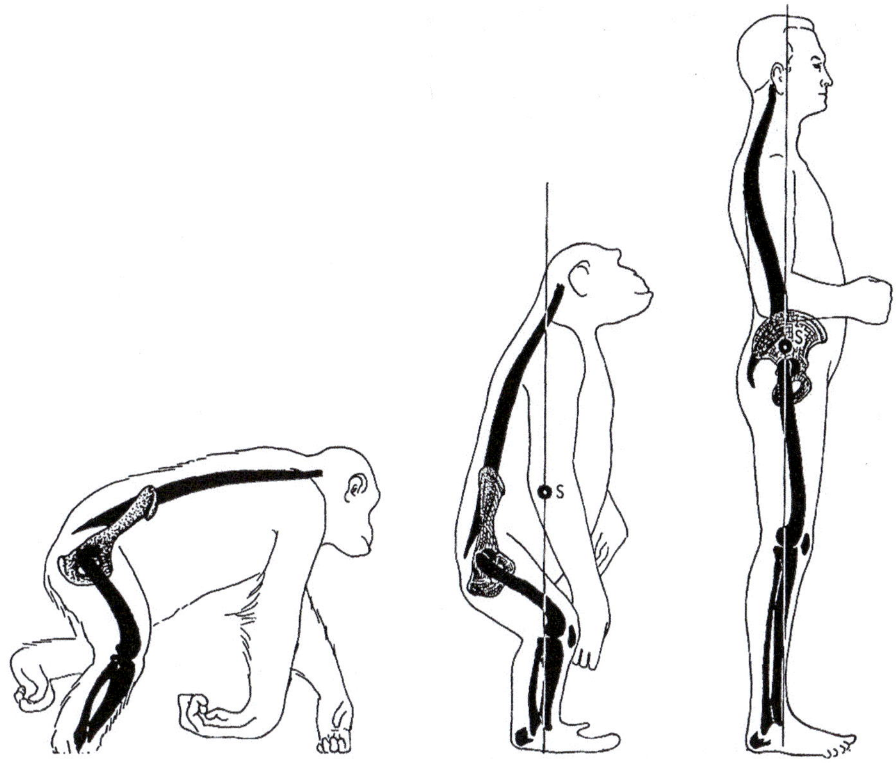

Fig. 1.5 Chimpanzee bent hip—bent knee gait has about the same position of the femur in the acetabulum as when knuckle walking, which is in its mid-range. From [82] Kummer B. Biomechanik: Form und Funktion des Bewegungsapparates. Dt. Ärzte-Verlag 2004. Reprinted with permission from German Ärzte-Verlag GmbH

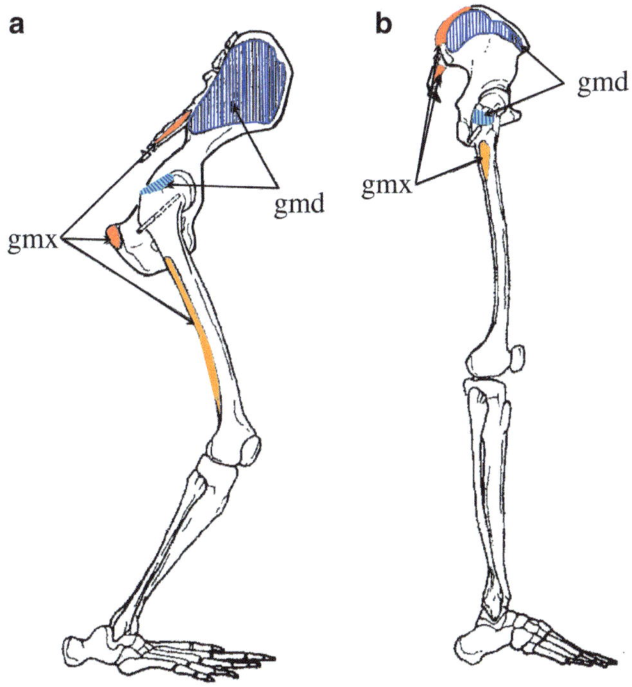

Fig. 1.6 Rearrangement of gluteal origins and insertions. A gorilla, B human. (*Red*) gluteus maximus origin, orange insertion. (*Blue*) gluteus medius origin, cyan insertion. *Gmx* gluteus maximus, *gmd* gluteus medius. From [83] Hogervorst T, Vereecke E. Evolution of the human hip. Part 2: muscling the double extension. J Hip Preserv Surg. 2015;2:3–14. Reprinted with permission from Oxford Journals

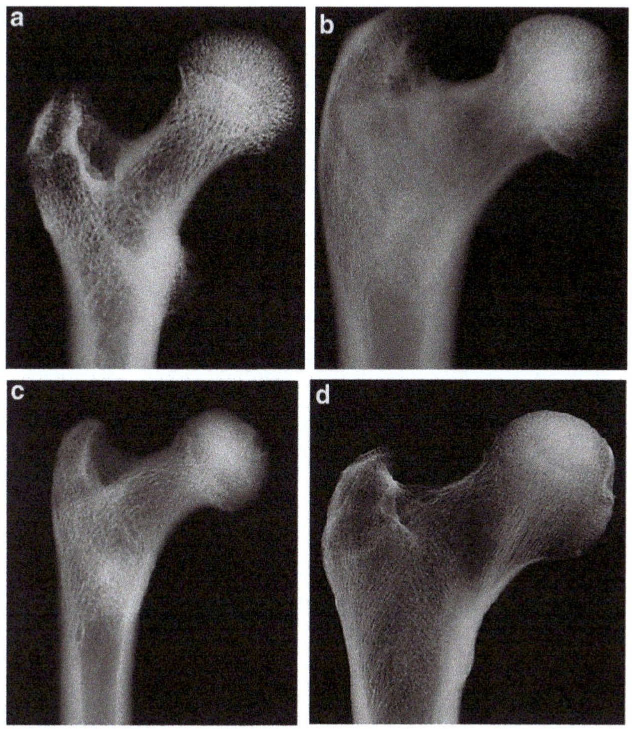

Fig. 1.7 Radiographs of hominid hips with head-neck ratios (head largest diameter divided by smallest neck width). The human hip has the thickest neck, decreasing offset and impingement-free motion. Also note thicker cortical bone in the superior femoral neck of the apes (from Lovejoy 2005 [15], with permission). (**a**) Orangutan (1.8) (**b**) Gorilla (1.5) (**c**) Chimpanzee (1.5) (**d**) Homo (1.35). AP view, not to scale

growth induces morphotype changes in macaques [39], as it may in humans (see below).

Thus, modern human hip morphology appears more variable than in the nonhuman apes. This variability currently has no full explanation, yet is important, as certain hip morphotypes are associated with development of OA. Both genetics and biomechanics (loading history) play a role in the development of hip morphotypes (ontogeny) [40].

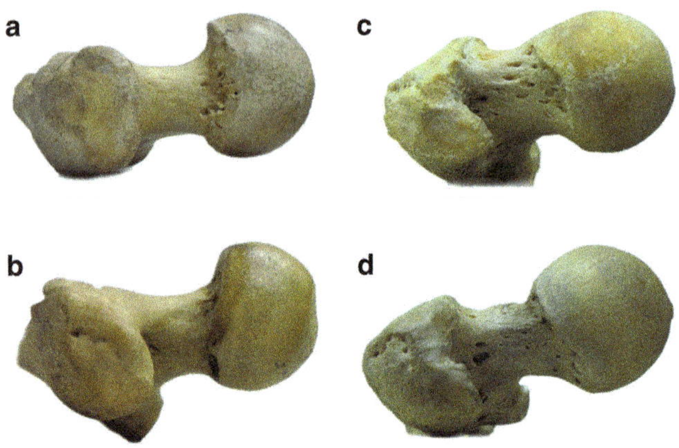

Fig. 1.8 Concavity in nonhuman apes and humans. (**a**) Gorilla, (**b**) chimpanzee, (**c**, **d**) human. The nonhuman apes uniformly have large concavity and more so anteriorly than posteriorly. Some humans (**c**) have only small concavity anteriorly, and others have larger anterior concavity (**d**), but virtually all humans have large concavity posteriorly (**c**, **d**). View is perpendicular to the superior femoral neck. From Fikkers JT, et al. What Ape Proximal Femora Tell Us About Femoroacetabular Impingement: A Comparison. Clin Orthop Relat Res. 2014 Jul 1. Reprinted with permission from Springer

Ontogeny: Growth and Development of the Human Hip

The evolutionary perspective outlined above can serve to better understand several phenomena of human hip growth and development. Quadrupedal mammals have a horizontal spine and the abdomen and uterus hang under it like a hammock. But the human foetus is positioned in an upright mother. It has a very large head and long legs, and, in the last trimester, the uterus wall tends to hyperflex the human hip, levering the long femur against the prominent anterosuperior iliac spine [41, 42]. (The nonhuman apes have no prominent anterior iliac spines, smaller heads and shorter legs; dysplasia is all but unknown.) The human hyperflexed position may be a mechanical factor to explain the decrease in relative acetabular depth [43, 44] and increase in femoral anteversion [44–47] with increasing gestation, producing a neonatal/infant hip dysplasia [41].

After birth, the human hip extends and more varied hip positions may explain the consistent finding in normal growth and development of postnatal femoral detorsion and relative deepening of the acetabulum [48]. Remarkably, for the rest of the hip's lifespan, most of its loading will occur near the limit of hip extension. Walking humans extend their hip approximately 5° at toe-off, and active prone extension is only 10°–20° [49, 50]. Active hip flexion is 120°, 35° when walking and 50° when running [51]. Thus, the human weight-bearing range of hip motion shifts close to its extension limit during bipedal gait development. Quadrupeds bear weight closer to

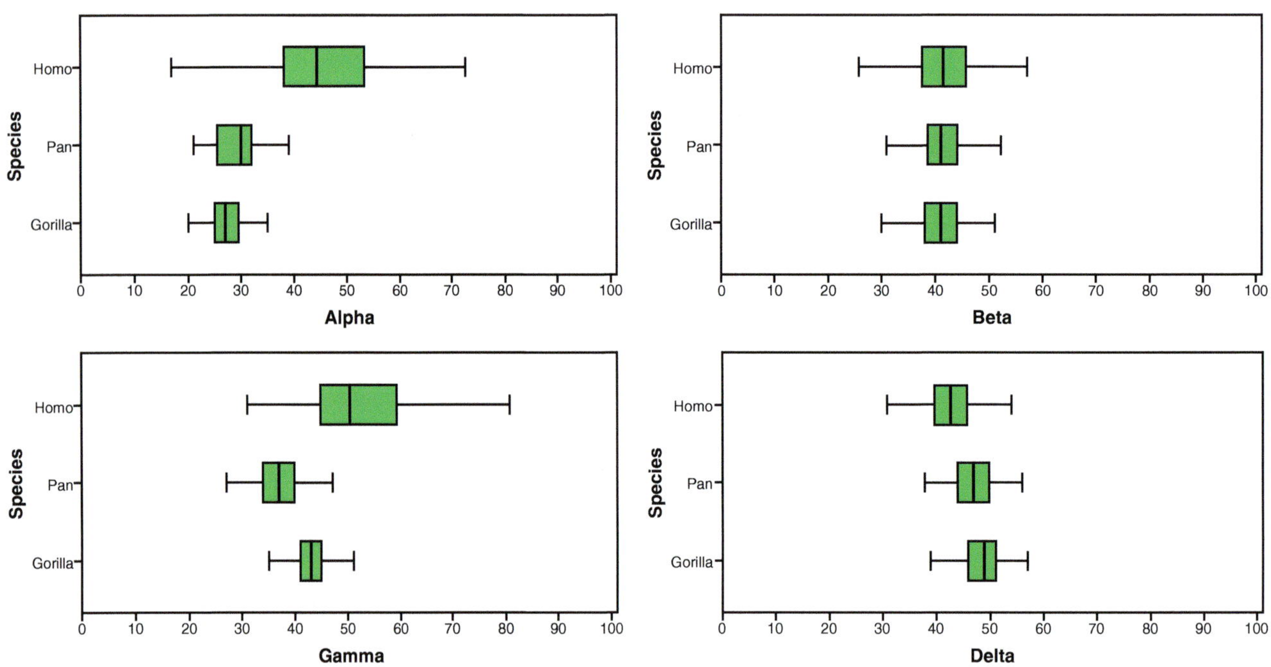

Fig. 1.9 Variable concavity measurements in humans, uniform in the nonhuman apes. From Fikkers JT, et al. What Ape Proximal Femora Tell Us About Femoroacetabular Impingement: A Comparison. Clin Orthop Relat Res. 2014 Jul 1. Reprinted with permission from Springer

mid-range hip flexion [52]. In this position femoral neck anteversion aligns the capital physis more perpendicular to the vertical gait forces [53]. The human (extended) hip position increases shear forces on the capital physis. During adolescence, the peripheral epiphysis extends towards the femoral neck (Fig. 1.10). Prospective MRI studies of children and adolescents (9–17 years) now show that in normal development, this extension is almost similar at each position of the femoral head, which means the epiphyseal torsion angle does not change (Figs. 1.10 and 1.11 [54, 55]).

Due to their specialized bipedal gait, humans have much higher peak hip forces than quadrupeds of similar weight, and these forces increase markedly with running or sports [56, 57]. These factors can summate to a loading history of high, perhaps excessive, loads on the growing hip, particularly because human growth and development is 5–6 years longer compared with chimpanzees [58, 59].

Thus, human hip ontogeny is characterized by specific mechanical factors that can be interpreted to explain neonatal/infant hip dysplasia, to increase shear forces on the capital epiphysis that may induce SCFE or subclinical slippage and to summate to a loading history that may induce morphologic changes in the growing hip [40].

Developmental Hip Disorders

During normal growth and development, the human femoral head is spherical in childhood [48], but aspherical femoral head morphology (coxa recta with alpha angle >60°) has already been shown in boys 12 years of age (Figs. 1.12 and 1.13) [60]. Asymmetric changes in physeal extension can reduce concavity at head-neck junction, creating a coxa recta. Siebenrock et al. found increased extension of the physeal scar in the anterosuperior head quadrant of FAI patients and suggested a growth abnormality of the physis can explain the differences in femoral head-neck offset between FAI patients and controls [61]. Alternatively, "subclinical" slippage of the epiphysis during adolescence has been proposed to explain the proximal femoral morphology of FAI, based on observations of epiphyseal tilt in cadaver femora, radiographs and recently MRI [11, 62, 63].

There are no longitudinal studies demonstrating the effect of loading on hip morphology in children or adolescents. But two cross-sectional studies in European populations found reduced concavity may develop with exposure of the hip to repetitive exercise through intense sports training during adolescence [60, 64]. Intriguingly, these differences were more pronounced in athletes with a closed capital physis, indicating ongoing effect of load history after physeal closure. Thus, high-intensity sports during adolescence may be associated with a higher prevalence of coxa recta morphotype, at least in European populations. As indicated above, comparable studies have not been undertaken in Asian populations. However, since coxa recta may be rare in Asian populations, the explanation that coxa recta exclusively occurs as an adaptive response to a high loading history appears not entirely sufficient [40]. Perhaps genetic differences explain varying responses to a given loading history. Research linking genes to hip morphotypes has begun to unravel the genetic basis of different hip morphotypes [65, 66] and has revealed that the majority of genes imparting OA susceptibility appear to be involved in skeletogenesis and/or homeostasis of bone and cartilage [40].

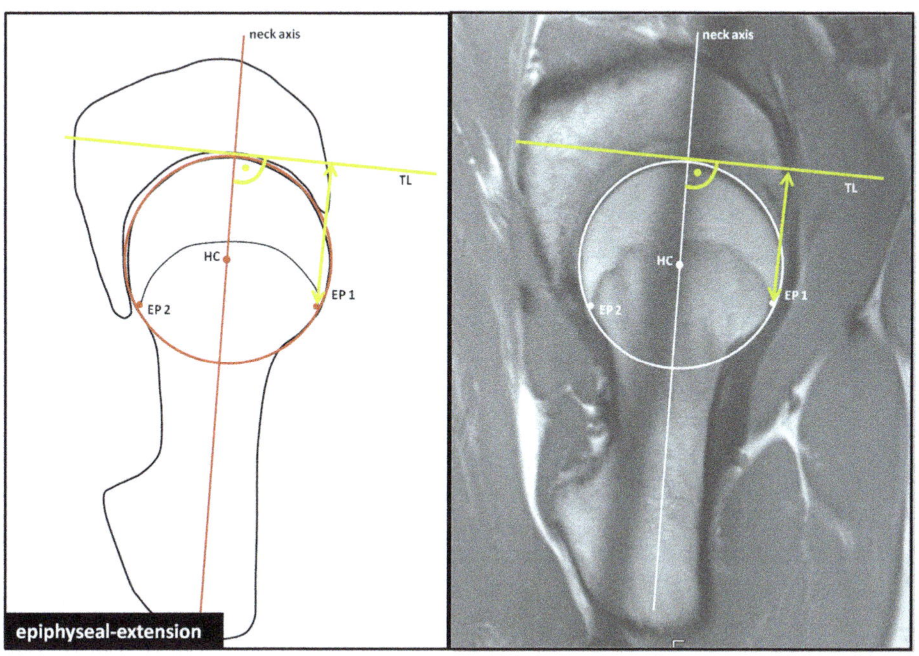

Fig. 1.10 Epiphyseal extension, defined as the distance from a orthogonal straight line on the femoral neck axis to EP1 (point with largest epiphyseal extension)

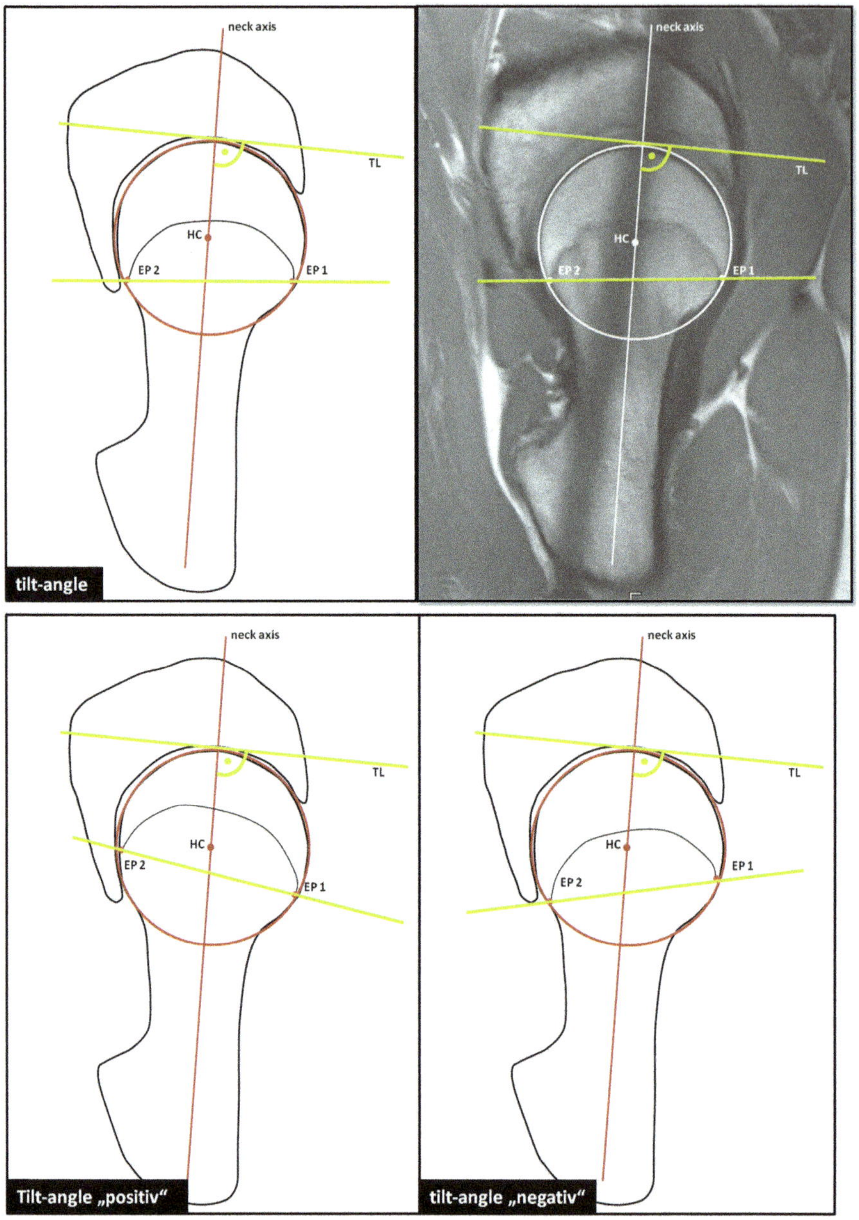

Fig. 1.11 The epiphyseal torsion angle is defined by two lines: one line is orthogonal to the femoral neck axis, and the other line connects EP1 and EP2, the points at the largest epiphyseal extension

In normal growth and development, the apical parts of the human acetabulum are retroverted in childhood, but become progressively anteverted during maturation, according to prospective MRI studies (Fig. 1.14). CT studies in normal adults report anteversion at the mid-level of the acetabulum of about 22°–24° in male and 19°–25° in females [67, 68]. The prevalence of retroversion is approx. 5 % in the general population, but 20 % in patients with osteoarthritis [69, 70].

Acetabular depth and anteversion determine the femoral head coverage and range of hip motion (Fig. 1.13). Reduced coverage in developmental dysplasia and overcoverage, either locally (retroversion) or globally (coxa profunda), can both produce local cumulative mechanical overload that can damage joint structures and lead to OA. In all, five parameters influence whether femoroacetabular impingement will occur: acetabular coverage and version, femoral head sphericity and version and neck shaft angle. Each of these five parameters has a reciprocal interaction with the others; for example, a shallow acetabulum delays impingement of the femoral head with the acetabular rim. New parameters are being developed that visualize and quantify this interaction of the proximal femur and acetabulum [71].

Population studies show small or no differences in the prevalence of both undercoverage (DDH) [23, 72] and overcoverage (coxa profunda) in males and females [23, 27]. In contrast, such differences do exist between different ethnic populations, with Asian populations having higher prevalence of DDH [37, 73, 74] and European or North American populations having more overcoverage [37].

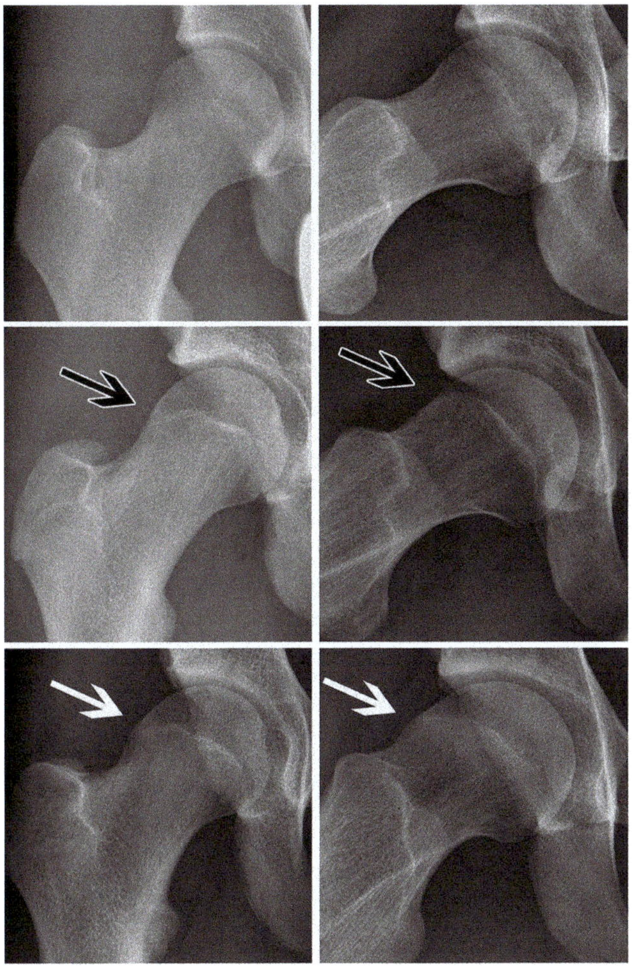

Fig. 1.12 Anteroposterior pelvic and frog leg lateral radiographs (*left*) in human adolescents illustrating normal (*top row*) and coxa recta (*middle* and *bottom rows*). From Agricola R, Bessems JH, Ginai AZ, Heijboer MP, van der Heijden RA, Verhaar JA, et al. The Development of Cam-Type Deformity in Adolescent and Young Male Soccer Players. Am J Sports Med. 2012 Mar 13;40(5):1099–106. Reprinted with permission from SAGE Publications

Perhaps the intrauterine mechanical factors outlined above help explain neonatal DDH (but clearly not its ethnic disparities). After birth, mechanical factors, such as prolonged extended hip positions used with the swaddling of babies, influence whether neonatal hip dysplasia corrects or not [75]. For DDH of later onset however, we lack prospective MRI studies documenting the causative changes. Ontogeny is characterized by reciprocal development of the femur and acetabulum and indeed extends to the entire innominate bone [76]. Cultures that keep the hips of infants extended during most of the time (i.e. through swaddling) have a much higher incidence of hip dysplasia than cultures in which the hips are held apart (and therefore in a centred position) during carrying (i.e. in a back sling) [73].

The origin of coxa profunda is unproven due to the same lack of prospective MRI studies. This limits explanations to speculation, with factors cited including the efficiency of the abductor muscles [77], obstetric factors [78] and sex hormones [79, 80] or a combination of these.

Summary

Reviewing human hip phylogeny, and comparing our hip to other mammals and the great apes, helps us recognize the peculiar features of the human hip. The hip joint sees a marked shift in the default loading position from a hyperflexed position in utero, to close to its extension limit in later life. The hip also has a remarkably long period of growth and development and is often exposed to large loads with its physes still open.

Prospective MRI studies that are now appearing may confirm earlier suggestions that a high loading history may determine a hip's eventual morphotype. Conversely, an emerging body of evidence attests to an interplay between

Fig. 1.13 Development of coxa recta in a highly active adolescent basketball player within 3 years

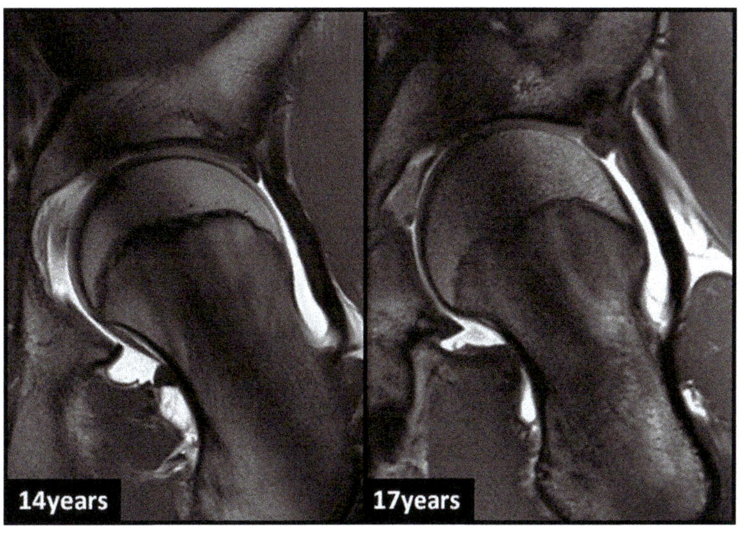

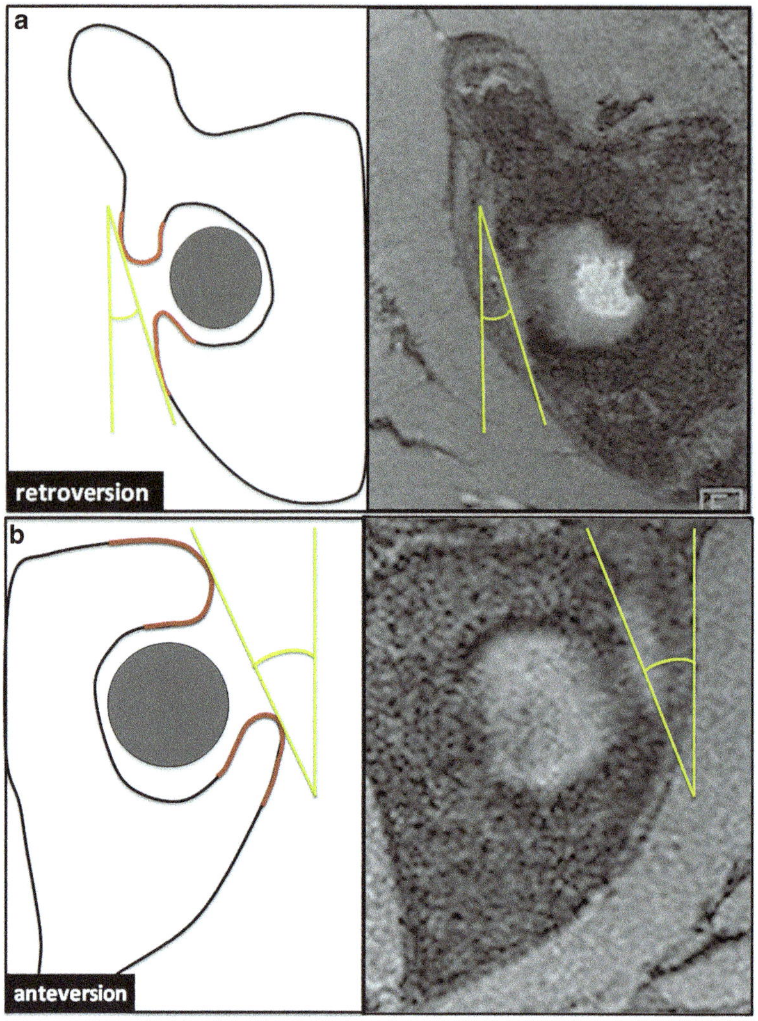

Fig. 1.14 Acetabular version in the apical part of the joint; measured between a straight sagittal line and a line connecting the anterior and posterior acetabular edge. *Top diagram* (**a**) and MR image depict the hip of a 7-year-old; the *bottom* (**b**) diagram and MR image depict the hip of a 15-year-old

genetic and mechanical factors in the development of the hip morphotype.

Genes orchestrate hip morphogenesis, but their influence most likely acts through several or numerous genes, each with modest effect sizes. Presently therefore, we do not know whether hip morphogenesis is primarily determined by genetic or mechanical factors.

Whether a given hip morphotype will lead to progressive OA is, again, influenced by mechanical factors, such as its loading history, but appears influenced also by an intrinsic ability of its cartilage to withstand mechanical stress.

References

1. Wagner DO, Aspenberg P. Where did bone come from? Acta Orthop. 2011;82(4):393–8.
2. Kawasaki K, Weiss KM. Mineralized tissue and vertebrate evolution: the secretory calcium-binding phosphoprotein gene cluster. Proc Natl Acad Sci U S A. 2003;100(7):4060–5.
3. Smith MM, Hall BK. Development and evolutionary origins of vertebrate skeletogenic and odontogenic tissues. Biol Rev Camb Philos Soc. 1990;65(3):277–373.
4. Briggs DEG, Erwin DH, Collier FJ. The fossils of the Burgess Shale. Washington: Smithsonian Institution Press; 1994.
5. Gould SJ. Wonderful life: the Burgess Shale and the nature of history. London: Vintage; 2000.
6. Davidson EH, Erwin DH. Evolutionary innovation and stability in animal gene networks. J Exp Zool B Mol Dev Evol. 2010;314(3):182–6.
7. Davis MC, Dahn RD, Shubin NH. An autopodial-like pattern of Hox expression in the fins of a basal actinopterygian fish. Nature. 2007;447(7143):473–6.
8. Carrier DR. The evolution of locomotor stamina in tetrapods: circumventing a mechanical constraint. Paleobiology. 1987;13:326–41.
9. Bouma HW, de Boer SF, de Vos J, van Kampen PM, Hogervorst T. Mammal hip morphology and function: coxa recta and coxa rotunda. Anat Rec. 2013;296(2):250–6.
10. Hogervorst T, Bouma HW, de Vos J. Evolution of the hip and pelvis. Acta Orthop Suppl. 2009;80(336):1–39.
11. Goodman DA, Feighan JE, Smith AD, Latimer B, Buly RL, Cooperman DR. Subclinical slipped capital femoral epiphysis. Relationship to osteoarthrosis of the hip. J Bone Joint Surg Am. 1997;79(10):1489–97.
12. Toogood PA, Skalak A, Cooperman DR. Proximal femoral anatomy in the normal human population. Clin Orthop Relat Res. 2009;467(4):876–85.
13. Nötzli HP, Wyss TF, Stoecklin CH, Schmid MR, Treiber K, Hodler J. The contour of the femoral head-neck junction as a predictor for

the risk of anterior impingement. J Bone Joint Surg Br. 2002;84(4):556–60.
14. Serrat MA, Reno PL, McCollum MA, Meindl RS, Lovejoy CO. Variation in mammalian proximal femoral development: comparative analysis of two distinct ossification patterns. J Anat. 2007;210(3):249–58.
15. Ganz R, Parvizi J, Beck M, Leunig M, Notzli H, Siebenrock KA. Femoroacetabular impingement: a cause for osteoarthritis of the hip. Clin Orthop Relat Res. 2003;417:112–20.
16. Doran DM. Ontogeny of locomotion in mountain gorillas and chimpanzees. J Hum Evol. 1997;32(4):323–44.
17. Lovejoy CO. The natural history of human gait and posture. Part 1. Spine and pelvis. Gait Posture. 2005;21(1):95–112.
18. Robinson JT, Freeman L, Sigmon BA. Some aspects of pongid and hominid bipedality. J Hum Evol. 1972;1:361–9.
19. Sibley CG, Ahlquist JE. DNA hybridization evidence of hominoid phylogeny: results from an expanded data set. J Mol Evol. 1987;26(1–2):99–121.
20. Lovejoy CO. The natural history of human gait and posture. Part 2. Hip and thigh. Gait Posture. 2005;21(1):113–24.
21. Pontzer H, Raichlen DA, Sockol MD. The metabolic cost of walking in humans, chimpanzees, and early hominins. J Hum Evol. 2009;56(1):43–54.
22. Murray RO. The aetiology of primary osteoarthritis of the hip. Br J Radiol. 1965;38(455):810–24.
23. Gosvig KK, Jacobsen S, Sonne-Holm S, Palm H, Troelsen A. Prevalence of malformations of the hip joint and their relationship to sex, groin pain, and risk of osteoarthritis: a population-based survey. J Bone Joint Surg Am. 2010;92(5):1162–9.
24. Reichenbach S, Juni P, Werlen S, et al. Prevalence of cam-type deformity on hip magnetic resonance imaging in young males: a cross-sectional study. Arthritis Care Res (Hoboken). 2010;62(9):1319–27.
25. Hack K, Di Primio G, Rakhra K, Beaule PE. Prevalence of cam-type femoroacetabular impingement morphology in asymptomatic volunteers. J Bone Joint Surg Am. 2010;92(14):2436–44.
26. Pollard TC, Villar RN, Norton MR, et al. Femoroacetabular impingement and classification of the cam deformity: the reference interval in normal hips. Acta Orthop. 2010;81(1):134–41.
27. Laborie LB, Lehmann TG, Engesaeter IO, Eastwood DM, Engesaeter LB, Rosendahl K. Prevalence of radiographic findings thought to be associated with femoroacetabular impingement in a population-based cohort of 2081 healthy young adults. Radiology. 2011;260(2):494–502.
28. Kim YH. Relationship between the sphericity of femoral head-acetabulum and the low incidence of primary osteoarthritis of the hip joint in Koreans. Yonsei Med J. 1989;30(3):280–7.
29. Takeyama A, Naito M, Shiramizu K, Kiyama T. Prevalence of femoroacetabular impingement in Asian patients with osteoarthritis of the hip. Int Orthop. 2009;33(5):1229–32.
30. Dudda M, Kim YJ, Zhang Y, et al. Morphologic differences between the hips of Chinese women and white women: could they account for the ethnic difference in the prevalence of hip osteoarthritis? Arthritis Rheum. 2011;63(10):2992–9.
31. Hoaglund FT, Shiba R, Newberg AH, Leung KY. Diseases of the hip. A comparative study of Japanese Oriental and American white patients. J Bone Joint Surg Am. 1985;67(9):1376–83.
32. Maini L, Palanisamy Y, Shetty V, Kasture S, Shetty V. Hip impingement in the Indian population: hip anthropometry measurements in 100 hips. Hip Int. 2012;22(3):335–8.
33. Malhotra R, Kannan A, Kancherla R, Khatri D, Kumar V. Femoral head-neck offset in the Indian population: a CT based study. Indian J Orthop. 2012;46(2):212–5.
34. Nakahara I, Takao M, Sakai T, Nishii T, Yoshikawa H, Sugano N. Gender differences in 3D morphology and bony impingement of human hips. J Orthop Res. 2011;29(3):333–9.
35. Nevitt MC, Xu L, Zhang Y, et al. Very low prevalence of hip osteoarthritis among Chinese elderly in Beijing, China, compared with whites in the United States: the Beijing osteoarthritis study. Arthritis Rheum. 2002;46(7):1773–9.
36. Lau EM, Lin F, Lam D, Silman A, Croft P. Hip osteoarthritis and dysplasia in Chinese men. Ann Rheum Dis. 1995;54(12):965–9.
37. Dudda M, Kim YJ, Zhang Y, et al. Morphological differences between Chinese and Caucasian female hips: could they account for the ethnic difference in hip osteoarthritis? Arthritis Rheum. 2011;63(10):2992–9.
38. Fikkers JT, Bouma HW, de Boer SF, Toogood PA, van Kampen PM, Hogervorst T. What ape proximal femora tell us about femoroacetabular impingement: a comparison. Clin Orthop Relat Res. 2015;473(4):1204–11.
39. Nakatsukasa M, Hayama S, Preuschoft H. Postcranial skeleton of a macaque trained for bipedal standing and walking and implications for functional adaptation. Folia Primatol (Basel). 1995; 64(1–2):1–29.
40. Hogervorst T, Eilander W, Fikkers JT, Meulenbelt I. Hip ontogenesis: how evolution, genes, and load history shape hip morphotype and cartilotype. Clin Orthop Relat Res. 2012;470(12):3284–96.
41. Le Damany P. La Luxation Congenitale de la Hanche, French: the congenital hip dislocation. Paris: Masson; 1923.
42. Browne D. Congenital deformities of mechanical origin: (section for the study of disease in children). Proc R Soc Med. 1936;29(11):1409–31.
43. Walker JM. Histological study of the fetal development of the human acetabulum and labrum: significance in congenital hip disease. Yale J Biol Med. 1981;54(4):255–63.
44. Ralis Z, McKibbin B. Changes in shape of the human hip joint during its development and their relation to its stability. J Bone Joint Surg Br. 1973;55(4):780–5.
45. Walker JM, Goldsmith CH. Morphometric study of the fetal development of the human hip joint: significance for congenital hip disease. Yale J Biol Med. 1981;54(6):411–37.
46. Jouve JL, Glard Y, Garron E, et al. Anatomical study of the proximal femur in the fetus. J Pediatr Orthop B. 2005;14(2):105–10.
47. Bonneau N, Simonis C, Seringe R, Tardieu C. Study of femoral torsion during prenatal growth: interpretations associated with the effects of intrauterine pressure. Am J Phys Anthropol. 2011; 145(3):438–45.
48. Ogden JA. Development and growth of the hip. In: Katz JF, Siffert RS, editors. Management of hip disorders in children. Philadelphia: J.B. Lippincott; 1983. p. 1–32.
49. Roaas A, Andersson GB. Normal range of motion of the hip, knee and ankle joints in male subjects, 30-40 years of age. Acta Orthop Scand. 1982;53(2):205–8.
50. Roach KE, Miles TP. Normal hip and knee active range of motion: the relationship to age. Phys Ther. 1991;71(9):656–65.
51. Novacheck TF. Walking, running, and sprinting: a three-dimensional analysis of kinematics and kinetics. Instr Course Lect. 1995;44:497–506.
52. Back W, Schamhardt HC, Savelberg HH, et al. How the horse moves: 2. Significance of graphical representations of equine hind limb kinematics. Equine Vet J. 1995;27(1):39–45.
53. Tayton E. Femoral anteversion: a necessary angle or an evolutionary vestige? J Bone Joint Surg Br. 2007;89(10):1283–8.
54. Bixby SD, Kienle K-P, Nasreddine A, Zurakowski D, Kim Y-J, Yen Y-M. Reference values for proximal femoral anatomy in adolescents based on sex, physis, and imaging plane. Am J Sports Med. 2013;41(9):2074–82.
55. Kienle KP, Keck J, Werlen S, Kim YJ, Siebenrock KA, Mamisch TC. Femoral morphology and epiphyseal growth plate changes of the hip during maturation: MR assessments in a 1-year follow-up on a cross-sectional asymptomatic cohort in the age range of 9-17 years. Skeletal Radiol. 2012;41(11):1381–90.

56. Bergmann G, Graichen F, Rohlmann A. Hip joint loading during walking and running, measured in two patients. J Biomech. 1993;26(8):969–90.
57. Bergmann G, Graichen F, Rohlmann A. Hip joint forces in sheep. J Biomech. 1999;32(8):769–77.
58. Shea BT. Allometry and heterochrony in the African apes. Am J Phys Anthropol. 1983;62(3):275–89.
59. Tardieu C. Short adolescence in early hominids: infantile and adolescent growth of the human femur. Am J Phys Anthropol. 1998;107(2):163–78.
60. Agricola R, Bessems JH, Ginai AZ, et al. The development of Cam-type deformity in adolescent and young male soccer players. Am J Sports Med. 2012;40(5):1099–106.
61. Siebenrock KA, Wahab KH, Werlen S, Kalhor M, Leunig M, Ganz R. Abnormal extension of the femoral head epiphysis as a cause of cam impingement. Clin Orthop Relat Res. 2004;418:54–60.
62. Schaeffeler C, Eiber M, Holzapfel K, Gollwitzer H, Rummeny EJ, Woertler K. The epiphyseal torsion angle in MR arthrography of the hip: diagnostic utility in patients with femoroacetabular impingement syndrome. AJR Am J Roentgenol. 2012;198(3): W237–43.
63. Stulberg SD, Cordell LD, Harris WH (1975) Unrecognized childhood hip disease: a major cause of idiopathic osteoarthritis of the hip. The hip. Proceedings of the Third Meeting of The Hip Society, Saint Louis, C.V. Mosby Company.
64. Siebenrock KA, Ferner F, Noble PC, Santore RF, Werlen S, Mamisch TC. The Cam-type deformity of the proximal femur arises in childhood in response to vigorous sporting activity. Clin Orthop Relat Res. 2011;469:3229–40.
65. Baker-Lepain JC, Lynch JA, Parimi N, et al. Variant alleles of the WNT antagonist FRZB are determinants of hip shape and modify the relationship between hip shape and osteoarthritis. Arthritis Rheum. 2012;64(5):1457–65.
66. Waarsing JH, Kloppenburg M, Slagboom PE, et al. Osteoarthritis susceptibility genes influence the association between hip morphology and osteoarthritis. Arthritis Rheum. 2011;63(5):1349–54.
67. Stem ES, O'Connor MI, Kransdorf MJ, Crook J. Computed tomography analysis of acetabular anteversion and abduction. Skeletal Radiol. 2006;35(6):385–9.
68. Murtha PE, Hafez MA, Jaramaz B, DiGioia AM. Variations in acetabular anatomy with reference to total hip replacement. J Bone Joint Surg Br. 2008;90(3):308–13.
69. Ezoe M, Naito M, Inoue T. The prevalence of acetabular retroversion among various disorders of the hip. J Bone Joint Surg Am. 2006;88(2):372–9.
70. Giori NJ, Trousdale RT. Acetabular retroversion is associated with osteoarthritis of the hip. Clin Orthop Relat Res. 2003;417:263–9.
71. Bouma HW, Hogervorst T, Audenaert E, Krekel P, van Kampen PM. Can combining femoral and acetabular morphology parameters improve the characterization of femoroacetabular impingement? Clin Orthop Relat Res. 2015;473(4):1396–403.
72. Jacobsen S, Sonne-Holm S, Soballe K, Gebuhr P, Lund B. Radiographic case definitions and prevalence of osteoarthrosis of the hip: a survey of 4 151 subjects in the Osteoarthritis Substudy of the Copenhagen City Heart Study. Acta Orthop Scand. 2004;75(6):713–20.
73. Inoue K, Wicart P, Kawasaki T, et al. Prevalence of hip osteoarthritis and acetabular dysplasia in french and Japanese adults. Rheumatology (Oxford). 2000;39(7):745–8.
74. Yoshimura N, Campbell L, Hashimoto T, et al. Acetabular dysplasia and hip osteoarthritis in Britain and Japan. Br J Rheumatol. 1998;37(11):1193–7.
75. Mahan ST, Kasser JR. Does swaddling influence developmental dysplasia of the hip? Pediatrics. 2008;121(1):177–8.
76. Tannast M, Pfannebecker P, Schwab JM, Albers CE, Siebenrock KA, Buchler L. Pelvic morphology differs in rotation and obliquity between developmental dysplasia of the hip and retroversion. Clin Orthop Relat Res. 2012;470(12):3297–305.
77. Hogervorst T, Bouma H, de Boer SF, de Vos J. Human hip impingement morphology: an evolutionary explanation. J Bone Joint Surg Br. 2011;93(6):769–76.
78. Ridley M. Brief communication: pelvic sexual dimorphism and relative neonatal brain size really are related. Am J Phys Anthropol. 1995;97(2):197–200.
79. Bernstein P, Crelin ES. Bony pelvic sexual dimorphism in the rat. Anat Rec. 1967;157(3):517–25.
80. Berdnikovs S, Bernstein M, Metzler A, German RZ. Pelvic growth: ontogeny of size and shape sexual dimorphism in rat pelves. J Morphol. 2007;268(1):12–22.
81. Jarvik E. Basic structure and evolution of vertebrates. London: Academic; 1980.
82. Kummer B. Biomechanik: Form und Funktion des Bewegungsapparates. Köln: Dt. Ärzte-Verlag; 2004.
83. Hogervorst T, Vereecke E. Evolution of the human hip. Part 2: muscling the double extension. J Hip Preserv Surg. 2015;2:3–14.

Anatomy: Cartilage

2

Veronica Ulici, Antonia F. Chen, Anthony W.M. Cheng†,
and Rocky S. Tuan

Introduction

The articular cartilage is a highly hydrated, avascular, aneural, and alymphatic tissue that provides a gliding surface for smooth articular motion and allows load distribution and reversible deformation in response to mechanical stimulation. Its complex organization and composition, including specific orientation of collagen fibers and chondrocytes within the different cartilage layers, contribute to these unique properties. Chondrocytes dynamically remodel their surrounding extracellular matrix and receive signaling cues from the matrix, communication that is essential for cartilage homeostasis. This unique cell type has multiple functions, from cartilage development to the mature functions of the articular cartilage. Chondrocytes are involved in growth plate development during the growth of the long bones, in the formation of articulations during joint development, and in the maintenance of the mature articular cartilage throughout life. During joint development it is believed that articular chondrocytes are derived from the interzone's outer layer; however, this is still a controversial topic, and more recent studies suggest that these cells may originate from an early chondrocyte subpopulation that arises at the same time as interzone formation. Due to its avascular nature, cartilage nutrition and waste product removal are dependent on processes such as diffusion and fluid flow. This complex, unique tissue is regulated by multiple mechanisms from mechanical to growth factor stimulation. Functional and structural dysregulations occurring early in development may lead to diseases such as chondrodysplasia, while later in life dysregulation during cartilage maintenance may lead to osteoarthritis (OA). In this chapter, we will discuss the macroscopic and microscopic features of cartilage and will describe the developmental mechanisms that contribute to its final form. In addition, we will briefly present a number of structural and biological changes in the cartilage that occur in joint diseases, such as OA.

V. Ulici, MD, PhD • A.W.M. Cheng, PhD (Deceased)
R.S. Tuan, PhD (✉)
Center for Cellular and Molecular Engineering,
Department of Orthopaedic Surgery, University of Pittsburgh
School of Medicine, Pittsburgh, PA, USA
e-mail: rst13@pitt.edu

A.F. Chen, MD, MBA
Center for Cellular and Molecular Engineering, Department of
Orthopaedic Surgery, University of Pittsburgh School of Medicine,
Pittsburgh, PA, USA

Department of Orthopaedics, Rothman Institute,
Philadelphia, PA, USA

Gross Anatomy of the Hip Cartilage

While the bony anatomy of the hip joint consists of the femoral head and the acetabulum, the soft tissue components of the hip are comprised of cartilage, ligaments, capsule, and synovium. The two main types of cartilage within the hip are articular hyaline cartilage on the femoral head and acetabulum and fibrocartilage that comprises the labrum.

The hyaline cartilage is the smooth, white tissue that covers 60–70 % of the spherical femoral head. All areas of the femoral head that articulate with the acetabulum are covered in hyaline cartilage, which extends past the equator of the femoral head. There is only one small, uncovered central area on the femoral head known as the fovea capitis, where the ligamentum teres inserts (Fig. 2.1).

The thickness of the articular cartilage varies throughout the femoral head (range 0.8–3.8 mm [1–3]) and acetabulum (range 1.2–4.8 mm [2, 3]). As expected, the thickness of the articular cartilage has been shown to be highest in the superolateral quadrant for both the femoral head and acetabulum. The thinnest region for the femoral head is medial to the fovea, whereas the area closest to the acetabular fossa is the thinnest for the acetabulum. The cartilage thickness decreases concentrically as one goes from the thickest to the thinnest cartilage point [4].

The function of the hyaline cartilage is to provide a nearly frictionless surface (coefficient of friction = 0.001) where the femoral head can move within the acetabular socket [5] and

J.C. McCarthy et al. (eds.), *Hip Joint Restoration*, DOI 10.1007/978-1-4614-0694-5_2

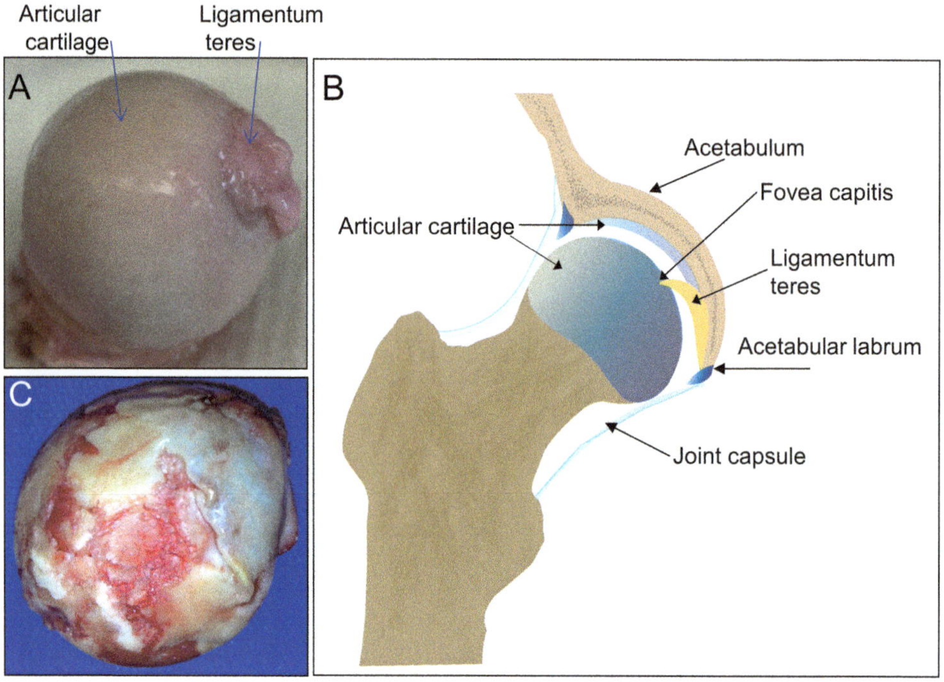

Fig. 2.1 The hip joint. (**a**) Appearance of the normal healthy cartilage surface of the spherical femoral head. (**b**) Hip joint schematic depicting the main components of the joint: femoral head and acetabulum covered by the articular cartilage, ligamentum teres, fovea capitis, acetabular labrum, and the joint capsule. (**c**) Cartilage degeneration manifests as fibrillations, cartilage loss, and deformations in the smooth cartilage structure

to support and distribute mechanical load [6]. Due to its viscoelastic properties, healthy articular cartilage can restore its original shape after deformation in response to mechanical stimuli [7, 8].

In the presence of osteoarthritis (OA), the frictional coefficient of the articulating surfaces increases in direct proportion to the severity of cartilage degeneration due to the increase in surface roughness of the tissue [9]. Grossly, this manifests as fibrillations and deformations in the smooth cartilage structure, which may lead to femoral head collapse (Fig. 2.1c). This loss of the cartilage also reduces the shock-absorbing capacity of the hyaline cartilage and leads to further cartilage degeneration.

Synovial Joint Formation

Developmental Skeletogenesis and Synovial Joint Formation

The process of limb development begins when mesenchymal cells from the lateral plate mesoderm condense at the future place of skeletal elements and form the skeletal blastema [10–13] (Fig. 2.2a). The cells in the center of these condensations then differentiate into chondrocytes (Fig. 2.2b.1), which deposit an extracellular matrix rich in collagen type II and proteoglycans (PG) [10, 14]. Members of the SOX family of transcription factors are required for this chondrogenic differentiation [15, 16]. At the periphery of the condensations, cells flatten and elongate to form the perichondrium and later differentiate into preosteoblasts (Fig. 2.2b.2) [17].

In the hind limb, these mesenchymal condensations start as uninterrupted Y-shaped structures with the proximal arm of the Y corresponding to the future femur and the two arms of the Y corresponding to the tibia and fibula [10, 13]. Once the shape of the future bones is defined, joint formation is initiated at the site of the future articulation, with the establishment of a region of high mesenchymal cell density called the interzone (Fig. 2.2b.3) [18]. This area can be differentiated from the neighboring cells histologically and also by the expression of specific markers such as growth differentiation factor 5, GDF5, a member of the transforming growth factor β (TGF-β) superfamily [19, 20]. The interzone is subdivided into three layers (Fig. 2.2c.1, 3): a central layer, the intermediate lamina (which will break down (Fig. 2.2d.1) and eventually form the joint cavity), and two layers of high cell density on either side of the intermediate lamina that eventually become two regions of articular chondrocytes separated from each other by the fluid-filled joint cavity (Fig. 2.2e.1, 2) [21]. The origin of the articular chondrocytes is still a controversial issue, and while a number of studies suggest that they are derived from interzone cells that redifferentiate into chondrocytes, more recent cell lineage tracing studies suggest that they may also originate from a subpopulation of early chondrocytes [19].

Human Hip Joint Development

In this section we will present a few selected stages of hip joint development as a guideline; however, the time lines of human embryonic joint development are quite variable, as described by many authors [22–24]. The interzone of the hip in a 13 mm

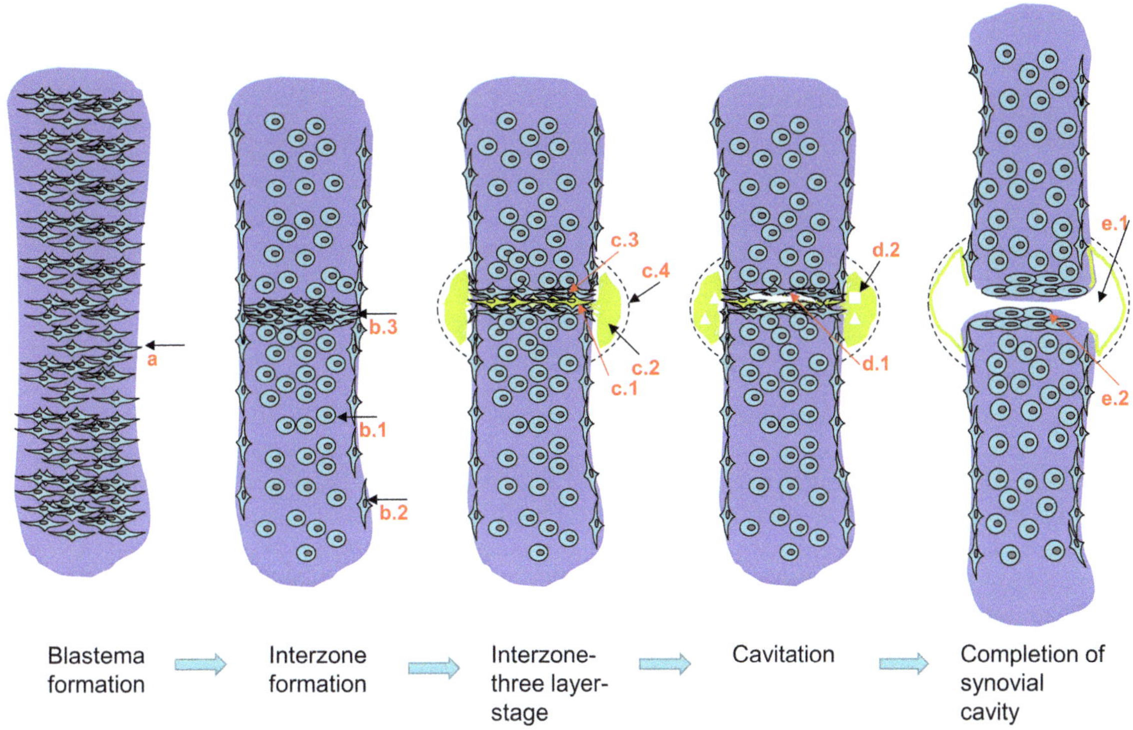

Fig. 2.2 Synovial joint formation. A schematic of a general synovial joint. (**a**) Condensation of mesenchymal cells at the location of future skeletal elements; (**b.1**) differentiation of mesenchymal cells into chondrocytes; (**b.2**) formation of the perichondrium; (**b.3**) establishment of the interzone. With further development, three layers of the interzone form: a central layer (**c.1**) and two outer layers of high cell density (**c.3**) that will eventually become two regions of articular chondrocytes (**e.2**). Within the general mesenchyme, the future fibrous capsule can be observed as condensations (**c.4**). In the next stages the central interzone layer (**c.1**) and the synovial mesenchyme (**c.2**) will start to break down (**d.1**, **d.2**) in order to form the joint cavity. After the cavitation process, the two future articulating bones (e.g., femur and acetabulum) will be separated from each other by a fluid-filled cavity (**e.1**)

embryo is continuous with the cartilage on either side of the joint and with the perichondrium peripherally. By 14 mm the shape of articular surfaces resembles their future final appearance. Both the joint fibrous capsule (Fig. 2.2c.4) and the synovial mesenchyme (Fig. 2.2c.2) (which lies between the capsule and the extracapsular perichondrium) are derived from the general mesenchyme in the vicinity of the joint [22]. It is believed that the intra-capsular structures, such as the ligamentum teres, are formed from condensations of the synovial mesenchyme. At ~16 mm, interzones are still continuous with the perichondrium, and no capsular structures can be yet identified at the hip [22]. Gardner and Gray [23] noticed a cellular condensation between the coxal bone and the femur as the first indication of the future capsule. By 30 mm the three layers of the interzone can be observed with the middle zone being differentiated from the other two zones by a difference in density of histological staining (Fig. 2.2c.1) [22–24].

The labrum and the ligamentum teres appear as cellular condensations when the human embryo is around 22–25 mm [23]. The central interzone layer is connected in the joint periphery with the synovial mesenchyme, while the two interzone chondrogenic layers are continuous with the intra-capsular perichondrium [22]. At ~30 mm the middle layer of the interzone and the interior part of the synovial mesenchyme are starting to break down (Fig. 2.2d.1, 2), in order to give rise to joint cavities by the process of liquefaction [22, 23]. Some of the cells from these regions will be destroyed, but the majority of them will actually attach to the wall of the joint cavity and become part of the joint lining [22–24]. At 34 mm the first appearance of the hip joint cavity has been reported by some investigators [23], though more advanced stages have been reported by others, e.g., Haines described a cavity that already surrounds the head of the femur, and ligamentum teres could also be identified within the synovium mesenchyme at this stage [22]. Haines [22] also observed the complete separation (dehiscence) (Fig. 2.2e.1, 2) of the two hip articular surfaces before the embryo reached 45 mm.

Structure and Composition of the Articular Cartilage

Cartilage Constituents

The articular cartilage is a hypocellular, avascular, aneural, and alymphatic tissue [25]. The mature articular cartilage is maintained by chondrocytes that are the only resident cell type (with the exception of a stem cell progenitor population [26, 27]) and represent only ~5 % of the wet weight of the tissue [28].

Fluid within this highly hydrated tissue is responsible for 60–80 % of its wet weight and contains water and dissolved gases, small proteins, metabolites, and ions [8, 11, 29]. Structural macromolecules make up the remaining 20–40 % of the wet weight, represented by collagens (15–22 %; mainly collagen type II, but also types IX and XI), proteoglycans (4–7 %), and other non-collagenous proteins [11, 30].

The collagen network is principally responsible for the tensile strength of the cartilage tissue, while the proteoglycans provide the cartilage with elastic resistance to compressive forces [7, 31]. The collagen network interacts intimately with proteoglycan aggregates which are highly sulfated and consist of a protein core (i.e., aggrecan), hyaluronic acid, and sulfated glycosaminoglycan (GAG) side chains made up of chondroitin sulfate, heparan sulfate, and dermatan sulfate [7, 28, 30].

Zonal Structure

The composition, organization, mechanical properties, cell morphology, and cell function of the articular cartilage vary with the depth from the joint surface. Four different zones have been identified, located from the articular surface to subchondral bone: superficial zone, transitional (middle) zone, deep zone, and the calcified cartilage zone [29].

The superficial zone is the thinnest cartilage zone (10–20 % of the articular cartilage thickness) [32, 33] and consists of two layers: the first layer, closest to the articular surface, is acellular and is comprised of a sheet of fine fibrous material; the second layer consists of flat chondrocytes with their long axis parallel to the cartilage surface. Their matrix is rich in collagen, fibronectin, and water, but is poor in proteoglycans [29], which can be seen with decreased staining with Safranin O (Fig. 2.3). The collagen fibers are also aligned parallel to the joint surface.

The transitional (middle) zone (40–60 %) [32, 33] has spheroidal-shaped chondrocytes and a matrix consisting of larger and less organized collagen fibers, with increased proteoglycan concentration and decreased collagen and water concentration relative to the superficial zone [29]. The deep zone (30–40 %) [32, 33] also has round chondrocytes that tend to organize in columns perpendicular to the articular surface (Fig. 2.3). Among all zones, the deep zone is the least hydrated and has the largest collagen fibers, which are oriented perpendicular to the articular surface, and the highest concentration of proteoglycan [29].

A wavy tidemark of basophilic matrix separates the deep zone from the final zone: the calcified cartilage zone. Collagen fibers lengthen from the middle zone to the calcified cartilage passing through the tidemark (Fig. 2.3). Mechanically, this region transfers joint forces from the cartilage to the underlying subchondral bone via vertically oriented collagen fibrils [34]. Chondrocytes in this zone are surrounded by a calcified matrix and have a small volume and a small amount of intracellular organelles. Overall, the calcified zone marks the transition from the soft cartilage to stiff subchondral bone and is important for connecting non-calcified cartilage to bone [29, 35].

The subchondral bone is interdigitated with calcified cartilage, except that the fibers do not extend from the calcified zone to the bone. The cortical portion of the subchondral bone is localized underneath the calcified cartilage and exhibits low porosity and vascularity, while the subchondral trabecular bone is positioned distally from the cortical bone (Fig. 2.3) and contains trabeculae oriented perpendicular to the cortical subchondral plate [36]. This physical linkage between the cartilage and bone is a critical component in the pathogenesis of degenerative diseases such as OA [34].

Extracellular Structure

The composition and organization of the extracellular matrix also change with the distance from the cell and can be divided in three regions: the pericellular, territorial, and interterritorial matrices [29]. The chondrocyte and its pericellular matrix form the chondron that is the basic cellular structural unit of the cartilage [37, 38]. The chondrocyte cell membrane appears to attach to the surrounding pericellular matrix, which is rich in proteoglycans (derived from aggrecan, perlecan, and biglycan), collagen (a non-fibrillar collagen type VI, which is specific to the pericellular matrix), and small amounts of collagen types II and IX), hyaluronan, and fibronectin [39, 40]. It is well established that the interactions between the extracellular matrix and chondrocytes are vital for normal cartilage function. The close contact of the pericellular matrix with the chondrocyte membrane suggests that cellular activities are critically regulated by these cell-matrix interactions [29, 40, 41].

The next region is the territorial matrix that surrounds the pericellular matrix of individual chondrocytes or a group of chondrocytes in some areas (e.g., the chondrocyte column in the deep zone) [29, 32]. This region contains thin collagen fibers that appear to adhere to the pericellular

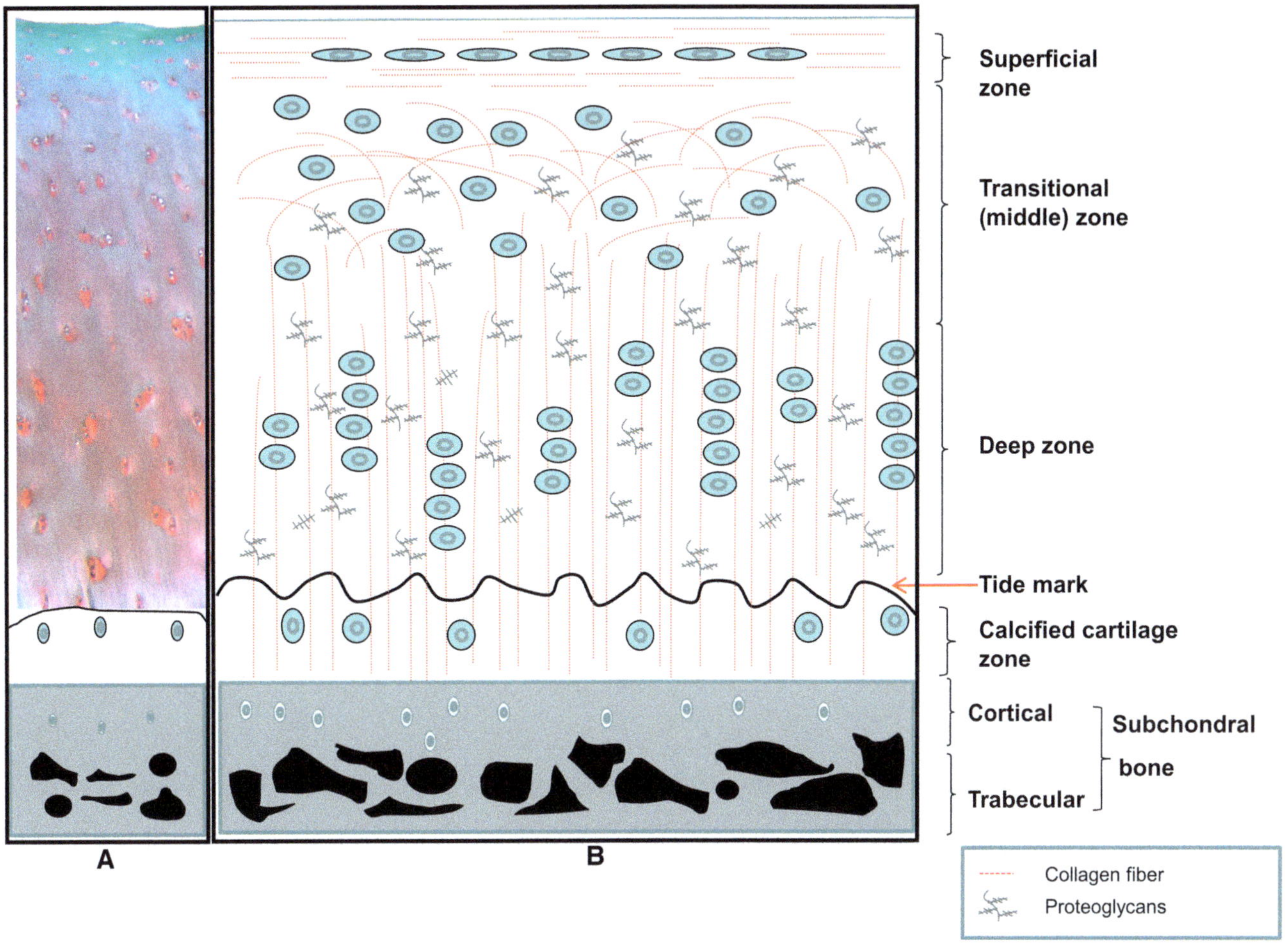

Fig. 2.3 The articular cartilage structure. Safranin O staining of femoral head cartilage from a 34-year-old woman (**a**); schematic of the articular cartilage (**b**). The articular cartilage consists of four different zones from articular surface to subchondral bone: superficial zone, transitional (middle) zone, deep zone, and the calcified cartilage zone. The superficial zone is rich in collagen, fibronectin, and water, but is poor in proteoglycans [29] which can be seen with decreased Safranin O stain (**a**). A wavy tidemark separates the deep zone from the calcified cartilage zone. Collagen fibers lengthen from the middle zone to calcified cartilage passing through the tidemark, but do not extend to the subchondral bone

matrix. These fibers intersect at different angles, at some distance from the cell, to form a fibrillar network around each chondrocyte [29].

The majority of the chondrocyte matrix is represented by the interterritorial matrix, which is the furthest away from the cell and contains thick collagen fibers. The orientation of these fibers is different than that in the territorial matrix, as they do not surround the chondrocytes but are angled differently in the distinct cartilage zones, changing their orientation from parallel to the articular surface in the superficial zone to perpendicular in the deep zone [29].

Chondrocyte-Matrix Interaction

Dynamic cell-matrix interactions are essential for the biological functions of the cartilage. Chondrocytes constantly remodel their matrix in response to different stimuli, such as physical and chemical changes in the neighboring environment [42]. The stimuli that can trigger anabolic or catabolic responses from chondrocytes include mechanical forces (e.g., exercise), biomolecules (e.g., cytokines, local growth factors, hormones), and matrix composition [28].

The matrix not only protects the chondrocytes from mechanical insults but also provides the cells with signaling cues that regulate gene expression. There is a direct interaction between the extracellular matrix molecules and chondrocytes through cell surface receptors such as the integrins, a family of dimeric transmembrane adhesion receptors consisting of α and β subunits [43, 44].

Integrins play an essential role in the attachment of cells to their extracellular matrix, but also in chondrocyte differentiation, survival and matrix regulation, and in mediating the response of chondrocytes to numerous signals, including mechanical loading. These receptors are known to interact with pericellular matrix proteins, such as collagen type VI and fibronectin, the latter interacting with α5β1 integrin as its primary receptor in chondrocytes [40, 44, 45].

In addition to integrins, a number of other transmembrane receptors mediate the interaction between chondrocytes and their matrix, such as annexins (annexin V or anchorin II-binds collagen type II) and the hyaluronan receptor, CD44.

Under physiological conditions, cells respond to the received signals by maintaining a regulated balance between matrix synthesis and degradation, which is required for the proper function of the articular cartilage [31, 41, 46]. The normal proteolytic turnover of proteoglycans in the articular cartilage is maintained by matrix metalloproteinases (MMPs), such as MMP-3, and aggrecanases, such as ADAMTS5. The collagen type II network is very stable, and the factors responsible for its destabilization are collagenases, such as MMP-1 and MMP-13 [31].

Cartilage Metabolism

Mature chondrocytes have lower rates of metabolism and proliferation compared to growth plate chondrocytes, but they are still dynamic cells that produce a highly organized cartilaginous matrix to give rise to the unique properties of the cartilage, such as reversible deformation in response to mechanical load [7, 41].

Being avascular, transport of nutrients and oxygen from synovial fluid and metabolic waste products to the synovial fluid must occur through diffusion and fluid flow (convection) [28, 30, 41]. It is believed that small molecules can travel via diffusion and larger solutes are transported by convection [30].

Intermittent mechanical loading is critical for chondrocyte nutrition. Cellular and tissue metabolites are driven out of the matrix during joint compression and are drawn back into the matrix upon load reversal [28]. Mechanical loading also has an effect on chondrocyte behavior by stimulating mechano-transduction pathways that regulate chondrocyte gene expression. Dynamic loading is in general thought to increase cartilage matrix synthesis, while static pressure can result in a reduction in synthesis of certain matrix components [28, 46].

Oxygen consumption is much lower in the cartilage than in other tissues; chondrocytes live in a hypoxic environment from ~6 % O_2 tension at the articular surface to ~2 % in the deep zone. All the enzymes necessary for anaerobic metabolism are present in the cartilage [24]. Chondrocytes do not only survive in this low O_2 environment, but they increase the expression of cartilage markers, such as SOX-9, collagen type II, and aggrecan at 5 % O_2 compared to 21 % O_2 [45, 47].

Consequently, glycolysis is the primary bioenergetic pathway utilized by chondrocytes. However, it has been recently shown that mitochondrial pathways also play an important role [45, 48]. Although fewer in number in mature chondrocytes compared to other cell types, the mitochondria still have important functions in cartilage homeostasis and are involved in production of reactive oxygen species (ROS), Ca^{2+} uptake, and cell death/survival [45, 48].

The articular cartilage has higher intrinsic tissue osmolality compared to other tissues (350–450 mOsm/kg, compared to ~300 mOsm/kg in synovial fluid) owing to the presence of highly negatively charged sulfated GAGs which attract cations (Na^+, K^+, H^+) and thereby water, associated with the hydration shell. This increased tissue osmotic pressure also contributes to the ability of the cartilage to sustain high compressive forces [45].

Metabolic Changes in Cartilage Degeneration

During cartilage degeneration, the homeostatic balance tilts toward catabolism. An increase in proteolytic activity is regulated by pro-inflammatory cytokines, such as interleukin-1β (IL-1β) and tumor necrosis factor α (TNF-α), which have been shown to increase the expression of MMPs, such as MMP-13, and decrease collagen type II and aggrecan synthesis [28, 29, 49, 50]. ROS have also been implicated in the degradation of matrix constituents [29, 41]. On the other hand, growth factors such as TGF-β and insulin-like growth factor 1 (IGF-1) increase the synthetic activity of the cells to produce more abundant cartilage matrix [28, 31, 41]. These factors also act on receptors on the chondrocyte surface and trigger cell signaling cascades that further regulate gene expression [28]. Finally, among the metabolic changes implicated in cartilage pathology, dysregulation of mitochondrial pathways also plays an important role [45, 50].

Conclusions

Despite a general misconception, the cartilage is not a static tissue; the interaction of its unique cells with their matrix manifests as a dynamic process. Tissue remodeling plays an important role in cartilage homeostasis and is more active during skeletal development and then in cartilage diseases such as OA. It is particularly noteworthy that these remodeling activities in the cartilage take place in a low oxygen environment without vascular and nerve input. The extracellular matrix synthesized by chondrocytes gives the cartilage its smooth appearance and near-frictionless characteristics and directly contributes to the unique, viscoelastic material properties that allow this tissue to sustain important mechanical forces and joint movement without damage or pain. Maintenance of the articular cartilage homeostasis depends on the proper balance between matrix synthesis and degradation, and its restoration is critical for the development of successful therapies for degenerative joint diseases, such as OA.

Acknowledgment Supported in part by Arthritis Foundation Postdoctoral Fellowship (VU), Orthopaedic Research and Education Foundation Resident Clinician Training Grant (AFC), Commonwealth of Pennsylvania Department of Health, National Institutes of Health (1U18 TR000532), and the US Department of Defense (W81XWH-08-2-0032, W81XWH-10-1-0850, and W81XWH-14-2-0003). This chapter is dedicated to the memory of our colleague, Anthony W. M. Cheng.

References

1. Armstrong CG, Gardner DL. Thickness and distribution of human femoral head articular cartilage. Changes with age. Ann Rheum Dis. 1977;36(5):407–12.
2. Shepherd DE, Seedhom BB. Thickness of human articular cartilage in joints of the lower limb. Ann Rheum Dis. 1999;58(1):27–34.
3. Wyler A, et al. Hyaline cartilage thickness in radiographically normal cadaveric hips: comparison of spiral CT arthrographic and macroscopic measurements. Radiology. 2007;242(2):441–9.
4. Kurrat HJ, Oberlander W. The thickness of the cartilage in the hip joint. J Anat. 1978;126(Pt 1):145–55.
5. Seror J, et al. Articular cartilage proteoglycans as boundary lubricants: structure and frictional interaction of surface-attached hyaluronan and hyaluronan—aggrecan complexes. Biomacromolecules. 2011;12(10):3432–43.
6. Boschetti F, et al. Biomechanical properties of human articular cartilage under compressive loads. Biorheology. 2004;41(3–4):159–66.
7. McDevitt CA. Biochemistry of articular cartilage. Nature of proteoglycans and collagen of articular cartilage and their role in ageing and in osteoarthrosis. Ann Rheum Dis. 1973;32(4):364–78.
8. James CB, Uhl TL. A review of articular cartilage pathology and the use of glucosamine sulfate. J Athl Train. 2001;36(4):413–9.
9. Lee SS, et al. Frictional response of normal and osteoarthritic articular cartilage in human femoral head. Proc Inst Mech Eng. 2013;227(2):129–37.
10. Shum L, et al. Morphogenesis and dysmorphogenesis of the appendicular skeleton. Birth Defects Res C Embryo Today. 2003;69(2):102–22.
11. Las Heras F, Gahunia HK, Pritzker KP. Articular cartilage development: a molecular perspective. Orthop Clin North Am. 2012;43(2):155–71. v.
12. Cohen Jr MM. Merging the old skeletal biology with the new. I. Intramembranous ossification, endochondral ossification, ectopic bone, secondary cartilage, and pathologic considerations. J Craniofac Genet Dev Biol. 2000;20(2):84–93.
13. Pacifici M, Koyama E, Iwamoto M. Mechanisms of synovial joint and articular cartilage formation: recent advances, but many lingering mysteries. Birth Defects Res C Embryo Today. 2005;75(3):237–48.
14. Archer CW, Rooney P, Wolpert L. Cell shape and cartilage differentiation of early chick limb bud cells in culture. Cell Differ. 1982;11(4):245–51.
15. DeLise AM, Fischer L, Tuan RS. Cellular interactions and signaling in cartilage development. Osteoarthritis Cartilage. 2000;8(5):309–34.
16. de Crombrugghe B, Lefebvre V, Nakashima K. Regulatory mechanisms in the pathways of cartilage and bone formation. Curr Opin Cell Biol. 2001;13(6):721–7.
17. Horton WA. Skeletal development: insights from targeting the mouse genome. Lancet. 2003;362(9383):560–9.
18. Murphy JM, et al. Distribution of cartilage molecules in the developing mouse joint. Matrix Biol. 1999;18(5):487–97.
19. Hyde G, et al. Lineage tracing using matrilin-1 gene expression reveals that articular chondrocytes exist as the joint interzone forms. Dev Biol. 2007;304(2):825–33.
20. Storm EE, et al. Limb alterations in brachypodism mice due to mutations in a new member of the TGF beta-superfamily. Nature. 1994;368(6472):639–43.
21. Karsenty G, Wagner EF. Reaching a genetic and molecular understanding of skeletal development. Dev Cell. 2002;2(4):389–406.
22. Haines RW. The development of joints. J Anat. 1947;81(1):33–55.
23. Gardner E, Gray DJ. Prenatal development of the human hip joint. Am J Anat. 1950;87(2):163–211.
24. Brower TD, Hsu WY. Normal articular cartilage. Clin Orthop Relat Res. 1969;64:9–17.
25. Bora Jr FW, Miller G. Joint physiology, cartilage metabolism, and the etiology of osteoarthritis. Hand Clin. 1987;3(3):325–36.
26. Dowthwaite GP, et al. The surface of articular cartilage contains a progenitor cell population. J Cell Sci. 2004;117(Pt 6):889–97.
27. Lafont JE. Lack of oxygen in articular cartilage: consequences for chondrocyte biology. Int J Exp Pathol. 2010;91(2):99–106.
28. Ulrich-Vinther M, et al. Articular cartilage biology. J Am Acad Orthop Surg. 2003;11(6):421–30.
29. Buckwalter JA, Mankin HJ, Grodzinsky AJ. Articular cartilage and osteoarthritis. Instr Course Lect. 2005;54:465–80.
30. Jackson A, Gu W. Transport properties of cartilaginous tissues. Curr Rheumatol Rev. 2009;5(1):40.
31. Aigner T, Fan Z. Cartilage surgery and future perspectives. In: Hendrich C, Nöth U, Eulert J, editors. Cartilage surgery and future perspectives. Berlin: Springer; 2003. p. 3–7.
32. Sophia Fox AJ, Bedi A, Rodeo SA. The basic science of articular cartilage: structure, composition, and function. Sports Health. 2009;1(6):461–8.
33. Schuurman W, et al. Cartilage regeneration using zonal chondrocyte subpopulations: a promising approach or an overcomplicated strategy? J Tissue Eng Regen Med. 2015;9(6):669–78.
34. Yang PJ, Temenoff JS. Engineering orthopedic tissue interfaces. Tissue Eng Part B Rev. 2009;15(2):127–41.
35. Keeney M, Pandit A. The osteochondral junction and its repair via bi-phasic tissue engineering scaffolds. Tissue Eng Part B Rev. 2009;15(1):55–73.
36. Kinney JH, et al. An orientation distribution function for trabecular bone. Bone. 2005;36(2):193–201.
37. Hall BK. Bones and cartilage: developmental and evolutionary skeletal biology. San Diego: Academic Press; 2005.
38. Poole CA. Articular cartilage chondrons: form, function and failure. J Anat. 1997;191(Pt 1):1–13.
39. Lee GM, Loeser RF. Interactions of the chondrocyte with its pericellular matrix. Cells Mater. 1998;8:135–49.
40. Guilak F, et al. The pericellular matrix as a transducer of biomechanical and biochemical signals in articular cartilage. Ann N Y Acad Sci. 2006;1068:498–512.
41. Huber M, Trattnig S, Lintner F. Anatomy, biochemistry, and physiology of articular cartilage. Invest Radiol. 2000;35(10):573–80.
42. Treadwell BV, Mankin HJ. The synthetic processes of articular cartilage. Clin Orthop Relat Res. 1986;213:50–61.
43. van der Kraan PM, et al. Interaction of chondrocytes, extracellular matrix and growth factors: relevance for articular cartilage tissue engineering. Osteoarthritis Cartilage. 2002;10(8):631–7.
44. Loeser RF. Integrins and cell signaling in chondrocytes. Biorheology. 2002;39(1–2):119–24.
45. Milner PI, Wilkins RJ, Gibson JS. Cellular physiology of articular cartilage in health and disease. In: Rothschild DBM, editor.

Principles of osteoarthritis—its definition, character, derivation and modality-related recognition. Croatia: InTech; 2012.

46. Hering TM. Regulation of chondrocyte gene expression. Front Biosci. 1999;4:D743–61.
47. Mathy-Hartert M, et al. Influence of oxygen tension on nitric oxide and prostaglandin E2 synthesis by bovine chondrocytes. Osteoarthritis Cartilage. 2005;13(1):74–9.
48. Terkeltaub R, et al. Invited review: the mitochondrion in osteoarthritis. Mitochondrion. 2002;1(4):301–19.
49. Kobayashi M, et al. Role of interleukin-1 and tumor necrosis factor alpha in matrix degradation of human osteoarthritic cartilage. Arthritis Rheum. 2005;52(1):128–35.
50. Tchetina EV. Developmental mechanisms in articular cartilage degradation in osteoarthritis. Arthritis. 2011;2011:683970.

Anatomy: Labrum

3

Michael L. Nguyen and Marc R. Safran

Introduction

The role and importance of the acetabular labrum has been debated for many years. However, recent research has suggested the labrum serves many functions in the hip—from (1) stabilizing the hip by helping deepen the socket and (2) helping maintain negative intra-articular pressure to (3) helping reduce cartilage deformation and distributing loads while also (4) reducing friction by maintaining joint fluid in the central compartment between the articular surfaces to (5) serving a neural role of providing proprioceptive input in addition to pain sensation and (6) helping maintain joint fluid in the central compartment to assist chondral nutrition [1]. These many functions are the result of the anatomic structure of the labrum.

Additionally, labral tears of the hip are a common cause of intra-articular hip pain and one of the most common indications for hip arthroscopy. Recent literature has detailed the gross and histologic anatomy of the labrum. This chapter will review the current status of what is known about the anatomy of the labrum.

Embryology

The acetabular labrum attaches to a bony margin that is derived from three bones: the pubis, ilium, and ischium. Centers of ossification of these three bones begin around the eighth week of gestation. The epiphysis of the pubis forms the anterior wall of the acetabulum, while the epiphysis of the ilium forms a good part of the superior wall, and the epiphysis of the ischium forms the posterior wall. During growth, these bones expand toward the periphery and thus contribute to the depth of the acetabulum. Interstitial growth within the triradiate part of the acetabular cartilage complex causes the hip acetabulum to expand during growth. The concavity of the acetabulum develops in response to the presence of the spherical femoral head [2].

Each of the three bones that form the acetabulum has a secondary rim epiphysis to which the labrum is attached. The labrum bridges the natural undulations of the bony rim.

Cashin and colleagues [3] microscopically studied the fetal hip and found differences between the anterior and posterior labra. The anterior labral-chondral junction had a marginal attachment to the acetabular articular cartilage and demonstrated an intra-articular labral projection. This projection appeared to form a recess between the articular surface of the acetabulum and the labrum. Additionally, the acetabular labrum had a sharp transition between the labrum and articular cartilage of the acetabulum and histologically demonstrated collagen fibers parallel to this labral-chondral junction. Posteriorly, however, the labrum was in continuity with the articular cartilage of the posterior acetabulum and had no labral projection into the articulation, while also showing a gradual transition between the articular cartilage and labrum, with perpendicular fibers that interdigitated the two structures [3].

Anatomy

The acetabular labrum is a horseshoe-shaped fibrocartilaginous structure attached to the periphery of the acetabulum (Fig. 3.1). The anterior and posterior horns are connected inferiorly by the transverse acetabular ligament, which bridges the inferior margin of the cotyloid fossa. In cross section the labrum is triangular, similar to the knee meniscus (Fig. 3.2). It is widest in the anterior half and thickest in the superior (lateral) third [4]. The labrum is continuous

M.L. Nguyen, MD
Division of Sports Medicine, Department of Orthopedic Surgery, Stanford University Medical Center, Redwood City, CA, USA

M.R. Safran, MD (✉)
Division of Sports Medicine, Department of Orthopaedic Surgery, Stanford University, 450 Broadway St, M/C 6342, Redwood City, CA 94063, USA
e-mail: msafran@stanford.edu

J.C. McCarthy et al. (eds.), *Hip Joint Restoration*, DOI 10.1007/978-1-4614-0694-5_3

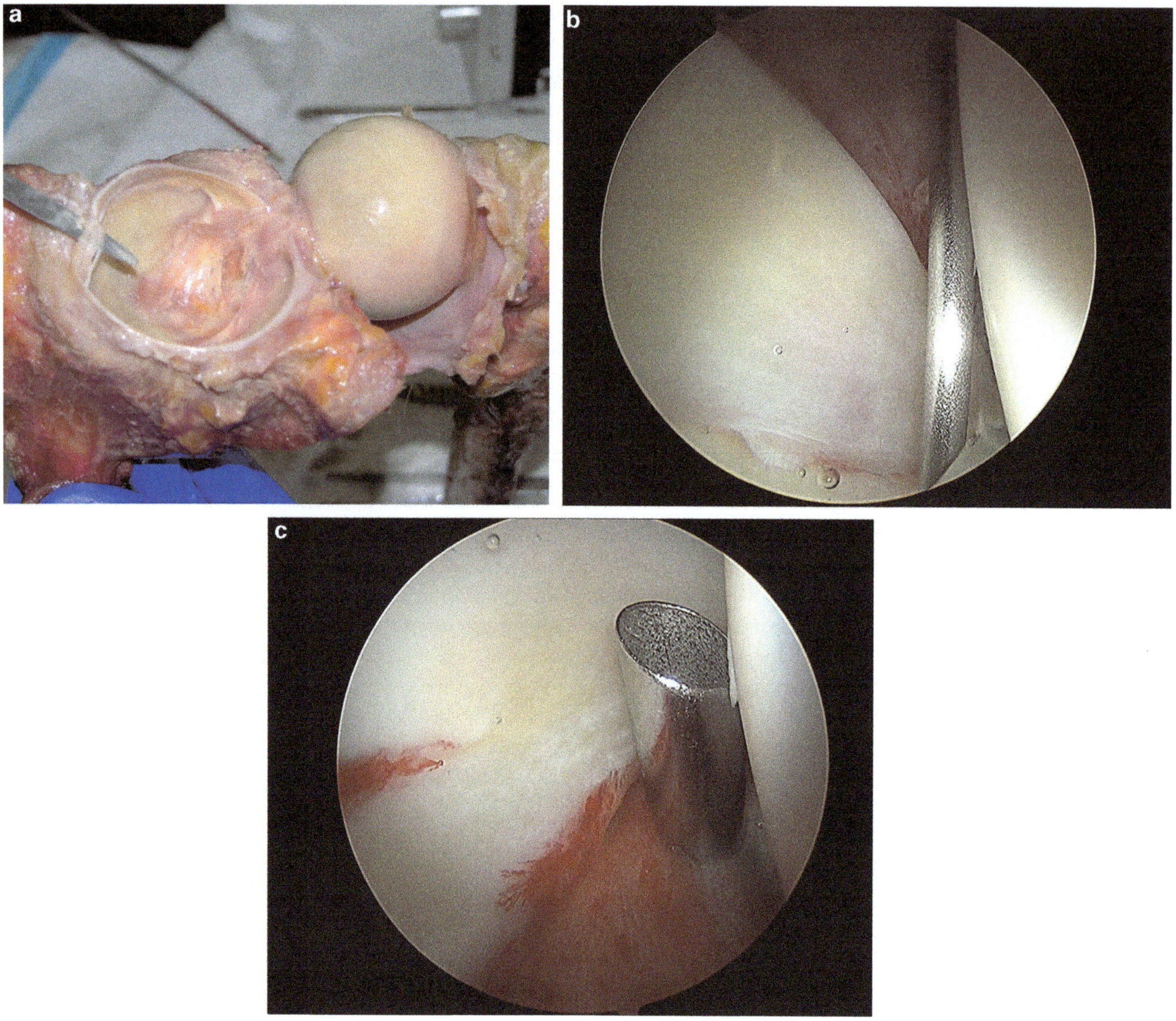

Fig. 3.1 (a) Cadaveric specimen of the labrum with a degenerative anterior-superior tear. (b) Arthroscopic view of the anterior labrum through an anterior portal. (c) Arthroscopic view of the posterior labrum through an anterior portal. Courtesy of Marc R. Safran, Redwood City, California

with the articular cartilage of the acetabulum; however, there are differences in the transition between the anterior and posterior transition zones. The anterior labral-chondral transition is sharp and abrupt with minimal interdigitation of fibers, while the posterior labral-chondral transition is smooth and gradual. This is due to differences in the orientation of collagen fibers of the labrum; the anterior fibers are parallel to the labral-chondral junction, while the posterior fibers are oriented perpendicularly, as mentioned above [3]. Some authors feel it is this variation in transition zones may account for the relative increased prevalence of anterior labral tears (as compared with posterior labral tears).

Under light microscopy, the labrum is divided into the capsular and articular regions. The capsular region is composed of types I and III collagen, and the articular region is composed mainly of fibrocartilage containing type I, II, and III collagen [5]. Using scanning electron microscopy, the labrum can be divided into three separate layers. The most superficial layer of the labrum is a 10-μm wide network of collagen fibrils without a distinct orientation. Beneath the superficial layer is a 40-μm wide lamellar layer consisting of collagen fibrils that intersect at various angles, but in a more organized fashion than the superficial layer. The final layer contains the majority of collagen fibrils, which are arranged in a circular, circumferential orientation. This layer measures 200–300 μm [5].

The osseous rim of the acetabulum inserts into the labrum at the articular region (Fig. 3.3) through a zone of calcified cartilage with a tidemark. On the capsular side, the labrum is attached to the acetabulum but without a zone of calcified cartilage or a tidemark. The hip capsule inserts directly onto

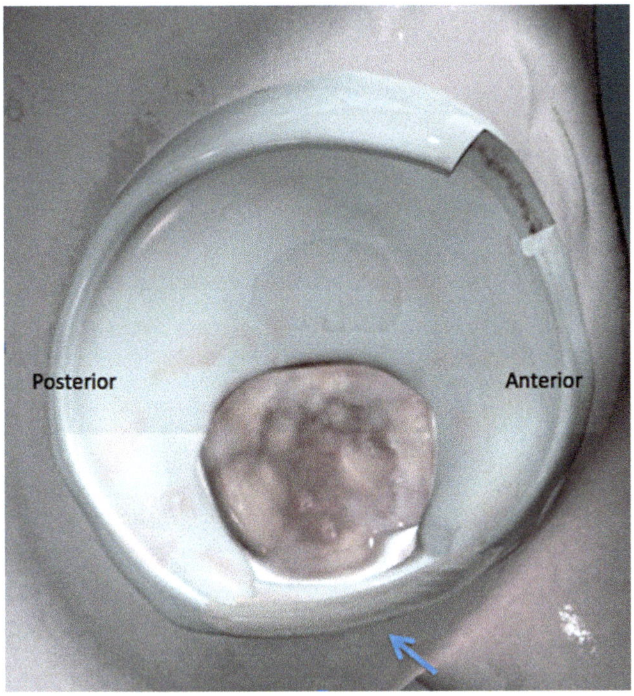

Fig. 3.2 Schematic of the acetabular labrum. The *arrow* points toward the transverse acetabular ligament, which connects the anterior and posterior horns of the labrum. The resected portion shows the triangular shape of the labrum. Courtesy of Marc R. Safran, Redwood City, California

the acetabulum just proximal to the labrum. This creates a capsulolabral recess that ranges from 6.6 mm anteroinferiorly to 7.9 mm posteroinferiorly [4]. It consists of vascularized connective tissue and fat. This recess may be important in allowing for hip motion, as it has been shown that scarring between the capsule and labrum may be a source of pain and limited motion in the postoperative hip arthroscopy patient [6].

Vascularity

The vascular supply to the acetabular labrum is provided by branches of the superior and inferior gluteal arteries, the medial and lateral circumflex arteries, and the intrapelvic vascular system [7, 8]. The major blood supply appears to come from the connective tissue that lies between the capsule and the capsular region of the labrum [5, 9] (Fig. 3.3). In consequence, the capsular region of the labrum is significantly more vascular than the articular side (Fig. 3.4).

The bone adjacent to the labrum also appears to be a significant source of vascular supply. An immunohistochemical study has shown vascular channels originating from the bony acetabulum crossing into the labrum [10]. These vessels

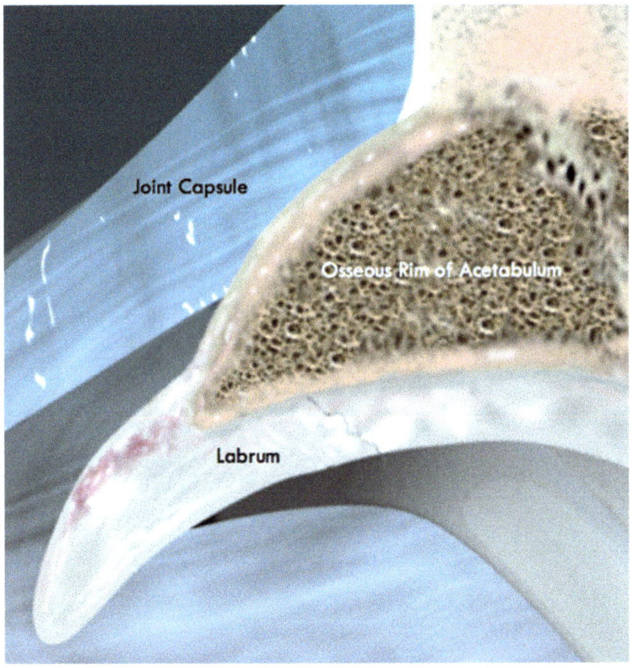

Fig. 3.3 Schematic representation of a cross section of the labrum and acetabulum. The osseous rim of the acetabulum juts into the labrum. Between the joint capsule and labrum lies connective tissue that provides blood supply to the capsular region of the labrum. Courtesy of Marc R. Safran, Redwood City, California

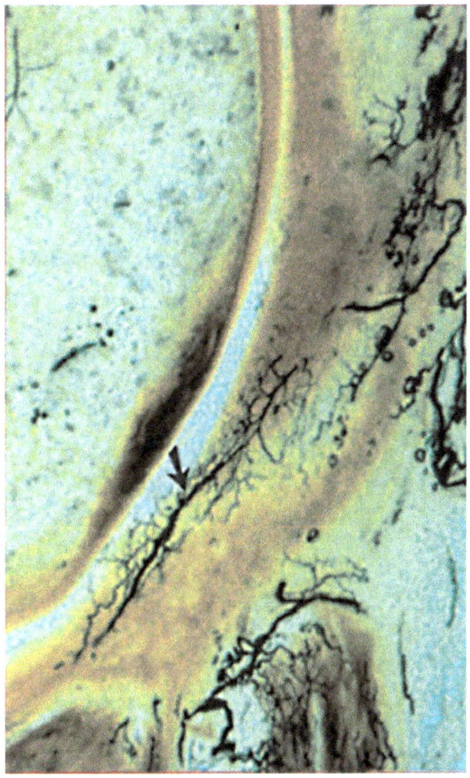

Fig. 3.4 High-power sagittal section of an India ink vascularity study of the labrum showing the capsular blood supply of the labrum. From Kelly BT et al. Vascularity of the Hip Labrum: A Cadaveric Investigation. Arthroscopy 2005 Jan;21 (1):3–11. Reprinted with permission from Elsevier

appear to travel circumferentially around the bony insertion to the labrum [4]. This gives the labral tissue adjacent to the bone a greater vascularity than the peripheral labrum [9]. This vascular anatomy, again, has important implications with regard to healing of labral tears and repairs.

Innervation

There are many nerves that contribute to the innervation of the labro-capsular complex including the sciatic nerve, the inferior gluteal nerve, and the femoral nerve [8]. However, the major contributor to labral innervation originates from branches of the nerve to the quadratus femoris and the obturator nerve [8]. There have been multiple different sensory end organs found in the hip labrum, including Vater-Pacini, Golgi-Mazzoni, Ruffini, and Krause corpuscles and free nerve endings [11]. Vater-Pacini, Golgi-Mazzoni, and Ruffini corpuscles are mechanoreceptors that aid in proprioception. Krause corpuscles are temperature receptors. Free nerve endings are involved in pain, tactile, and temperature sensations. Most of the sensory receptors were found on the articular side of the labrum (86 %) with a greater quantity of free nerve endings and mechanoreceptors found in the anterior-superior portion of the labrum near the chondrolabral junction [11, 12]. The presence of these neural structures suggests an important role of the labrum in pain sensation, as well as proprioceptive function.

Summary

The labrum has a complex architecture with limited blood supply. This architecture is important for the many functions of the labrum. The limited blood supply has implications for labral healing and labral repair, while the abundant innervation suggests additional important functions of the labrum, in addition to being a source of pain when injured.

References

1. Safran MR. The acetabular labrum: anatomic and functional characteristics and rational for surgical intervention. J Am Acad Orthop Surg. 2010;18:338–45.
2. Ponseti IV. Growth and development of the acetabulum in the normal child. Anatomical, histological, and roentgenographic studies. J Bone Joint Surg Am. 1978;60(5):575–85.
3. Cashin M, Uhthoff H, O'Neill M, Beaule PE. Embryology of the acetabular labral-chondral complex. J Bone Joint Surg Br. 2008;90(8):1019–24.
4. Seldes RM, Tan V, Hunt J, Katz M, Winiarsky R, Fitzgerald Jr RH. Anatomy, histologic features, and vascularity of the adult acetabular labrum. Clin Orthop Relat Res. 2001;382:232–40.
5. Petersen W, Petersen F, Tillmann B. Structure and vascularization of the acetabular labrum with regard to the pathogenesis and healing of labral lesions. Arch Orthop Trauma Surg. 2003;123(6):283–8.
6. Philippon MJ, Schenker ML, Briggs KK, Kuppersmith DA, Maxwell RB, Stubbs AJ. Revision hip arthroscopy. Am J Sports Med. 2007;35(11):1918–21.
7. Kalhor M, Horowitz K, Beck M, Nazparvar B, Ganz R. Vascular supply to the acetabular labrum. J Bone Joint Surg Am. 2010;92(15):2570–5.
8. Putz R, Schrank C. Anatomy of the labro-capsular complex [German]. Orthopade. 1998;21(10):675–80.
9. Kelly BT, Shapiro GS, Digiovanni CW, Buly RL, Potter HG, Hannafin JA. Vascularity of the hip labrum: a cadaveric investigation. Arthroscopy. 2005;21(1):3–11.
10. McCarthy J, Noble P, Aluisio FV, Schuck M, Wright J, Lee JA. Anatomy, pathologic features, and treatment of acetabular labral tears. Clin Orthop Relat Res. 2003;406:38–47.
11. Kim YT, Azuma H. The nerve endings of the acetabular labrum. Clin Orthop Relat Res. 1995;320:176–81.
12. Gerhardt M, Johnson K, Atkinson R, Snow B, Shaw C, Brown A, Vangsness Jr CT. Characterisation and classification of the neural anatomy of the human hip joint. Hip Int. 2012;22(1):75–81.

Anatomy: Capsule and Synovium

4

Richard E. Field, Caroline Blakey, and Francesc Malagelada

Introduction

The hip joint is encapsulated by a thick, cylindrical, fibrous sleeve. It arises from the outer margin of the acetabulum and inserts into the metaphyseal region of the proximal femur. Reinforced by distinct ligaments, taught at extremes of motion, the capsule functions to constrain the hip joint [1–3] and helps maintain joint congruence [3–5]. A synovial membrane lines the articular surface, and loose connective tissue surrounds the exterior, supporting its vascular supply [6]. Known to have mechanical, proprioceptive and nociceptive properties, recent work suggests that the capsule also contributes to the stability of the femoral head within the acetabulum [3] and plays an integral role in circulation of synovial fluid within the joint [7].

As joint-preserving hip surgery and hip arthroscopy develop, interventions on the femoral neck, the acetabular rim and the subspinous region are being undertaken with increasing frequency. Such interventions are facilitated by mobilisation or resection of the capsular structures. As with joint replacement surgery, surgical management of the capsule is a topic that is hotly debated with a spectrum of opinions regarding the need to repair or reconstruct breaches to the capsule structures. Knowledge of the anatomy of the capsule, its reinforcements, vascular supply and innervation is essential to understand these discussions and hopefully, minimise iatrogenic damage.

R.E. Field, PhD, FRCS, FRCS(Orth) (✉)
The South West London Elective Orthopaedic Centre, Dorking Road, Epsom, Surrey KT18 7EG, UK
e-mail: richardefield@aol.com

C. Blakey, MBChB, MRCS, MD(res)
Department of Orthopaedics, Sheffield Teaching Hospitals NHS Trust, Sheffield, South Yorkshire, UK
e-mail: cblakey4121@hotmail.com

F. Malagelada, MD
Department of Orthopaedics, South West London Elective Orthopaedic Centre, Epsom, Surrey, UK
e-mail: fmalagelada@gmail.com

Capsular Attachments

Embracing the margins of the acetabulum, the hip capsule inserts proximally, both anteriorly and posteriorly, just proximal to the acetabular labrum (Fig. 4.1).

It surrounds the femoral neck as a sleeve, with its distal attachment running along the intertrochanteric line anteriorly before reflecting upwards, to blend with the periosteum [6]. At its posterior aspect, the capsule only partially covers the femoral neck (Fig. 4.2).

Circular fibres of the zona orbicularis form a free arched border, running just over a centimetre higher than the anterior insertion [8] (Fig. 4.3).

Within the reflected capsular tissue, two synovial folds appear at the superior and inferior femoral neck (retinacula of Weitbrecht) and overlie the retinacular branches of the femoral circumflex artery, giving blood supply to the femoral capital epiphyses [8] (Fig. 4.4).

The Capsular Ligaments

Longitudinal fibres form the capsular ligaments, distinct bands extending across the joint. Appearing as thickenings of the joint capsule, each of the capsular ligaments arises from a constituent bone of the acetabulum and acts in conjunction with the bone to constrain the hip [1, 2]. With respect to the anatomical position, the capsular ligaments run in a medial to lateral direction, from the pelvis to the femur, reflecting evolution to upright posture [9]. Both the capsule and its ligaments consist of a proximal bone insertion, ligament or capsular substance and a distal bone insertion and both contain nerves that may sense joint motion and displacement.

The capsuloligamentous complex is dominated anterosuperiorly by the vertical fibres of the iliofemoral ligament [10]. The anterior capsule is reinforced inferiorly by the pubofemoral ligament, which blends with the fibres of the

J.C. McCarthy et al. (eds.), *Hip Joint Restoration*, DOI 10.1007/978-1-4614-0694-5_4

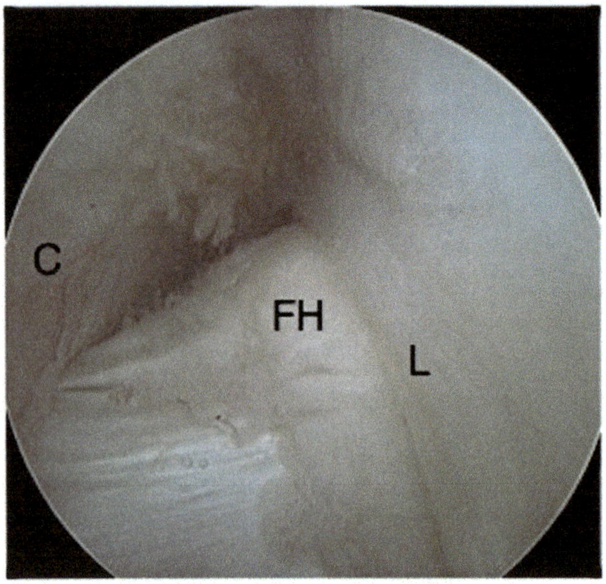

Fig. 4.1 Arthroscopic view of the central compartment of the hip demonstrating the femoral head (FH), labrum (L) and hip capsule (C)

iliofemoral ligament at its lateral insertion. Posteriorly, the capsule is capacious and lax. It is comprised of the thinner fibres of the ischiofemoral ligament, except distally where the zona orbicularis dominates and is more substantial. At their distal insertion points, the ischiofemoral ligament and the iliofemoral ligament are separated by thin capsular tissue and do not blend into each other. At the acetabular notch, capsular fibres blend with the transverse ligament [6, 8].

The anatomy of the hip capsule often described in terms of a clock face with 3 o'clock corresponding to the anterior capsule, 6 o'clock corresponding to the inferior capsule (acetabular notch) and 9 o'clock and 12 o'clock corresponding to the posterior and superior capsules, respectively.

The Iliofemoral Ligament

The iliofemoral ligament is the strongest ligament of the body. It lies anteriorly, in line with the femoral neck, and is stretched with extension of the femur beyond the trunk. The ligament originates between the anterior inferior iliac spine and the acetabular margin, around three centimetres from the acetabular rim [11]. It extends across the front of the joint as a fan of fibres, dividing distinctly into lateral and medial bands as an inverted Y, approximately five centimetres distal to the most superior aspect of the proximal attachment [11]. The lateral or superior band crosses the joint obliquely and can be seen to insert into the crest of greater trochanter, just superior to origin of intertrochanteric line. The medial or inferior band travels vertically and inserts more distally, marked by a subtle prominence on the anterior femur, at level of lesser trochanter [11]. At the level of insertion along the intertrochanteric line, the two bands of the iliofemoral ligament lie between 2 and 3 cm apart but remain connected by thin capsular tissue [2, 11] (Fig. 4.5).

Since the centre of gravity of the trunk lies behind the centre of rotation of the hip joints, the iliofemoral ligaments provide passive support to maintain an erect posture and reduce the requirement for an active muscular contribution. In dynamic movement the iliofemoral ligaments are seen to restrict extension of the joint beyond neutral and external rotation [1, 2, 8].

The Pubofemoral Ligament

The pubofemoral ligament reinforces the anterior and inferior capsule, resisting external rotation and abduction particularly in extension. Its medial insertion lies between the pubic portion of the acetabular rim, the obturator crest and the superior ramus of the pubis. The ligament runs outside the capsule before it reaches the acetabulum [8]. At the acetabular rim, fibres of the pubofemoral ligament blend with the proximal ischiofemoral ligament to reinforce the inferior capsule before it passes anteriorly within the capsule. The ligament has a 'hammock' appearance, running perpendicular to the zona orbicularis before blending with inferior fibres of the iliofemoral ligament at its lateral insertion [2] (Fig. 4.6). The pubofemoral ligament is sometimes described as lacking bony attachment since the capsular portion of the ligament has no singular bony insertion.

The Ischiofemoral Ligament

The ischiofemoral ligament lies posterior to the joint but is less well defined than either the iliofemoral or pubofemoral ligaments. It is spiral in shape, extending from the ischial rim of the acetabulum to the posterior part of the femoral neck at the base of the greater trochanter. The ligament has a broad triangular origin on the ischial acetabular margin near the root of the ischial ramus [11]. Two distinct bands of the ischiofemoral ligament have been described, both extending laterally from the ligament origin [8, 12] (Fig. 4.7).

The superior band courses upwards to insert at the base of the greater trochanter, while the inferior band travels in a downward direction blending with the inferior fibres of the zona orbicularis [8]. The ischiofemoral ligament serves to restrict internal rotation and adduction of the hip, most significantly in flexion [1, 2].

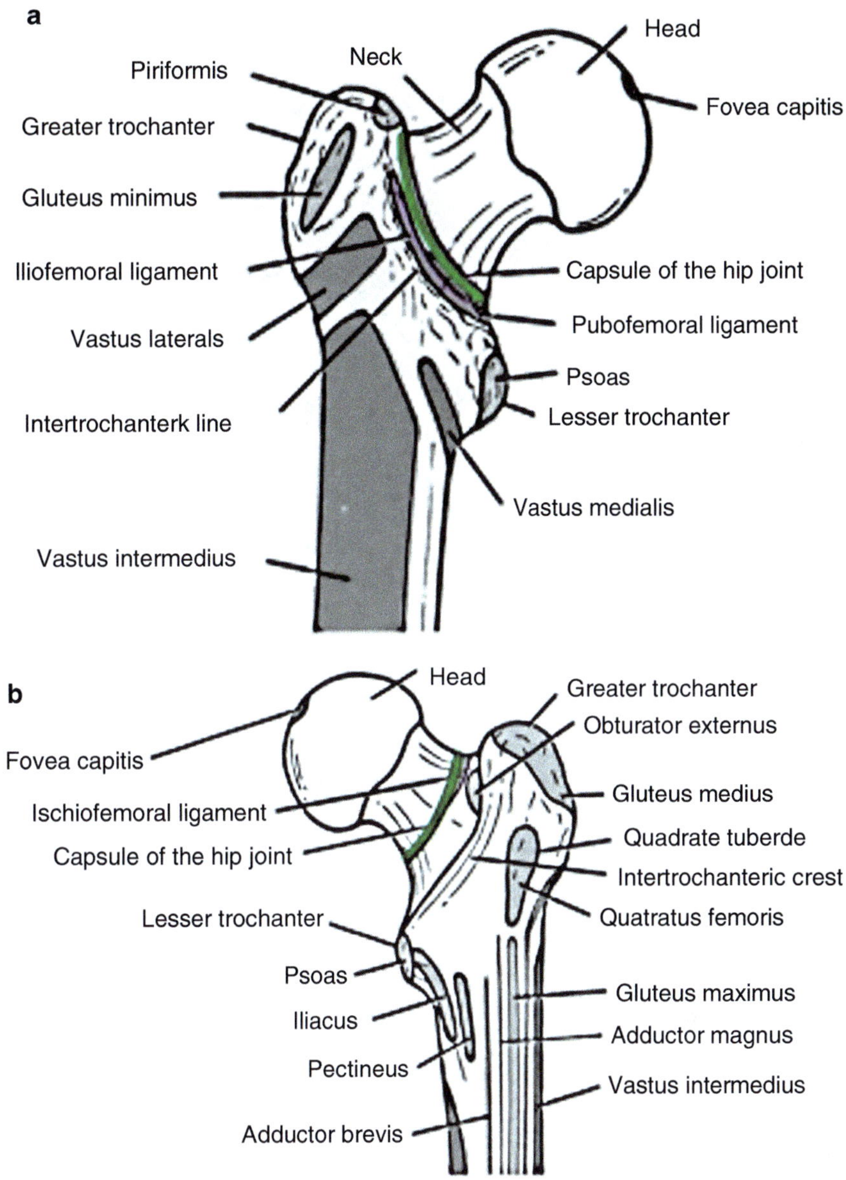

Fig. 4.2 (**a**) Anterior aspect of the proximal femur with the site of attachment of the hip capsule highlighted in *green*. (**b**) The posterior aspect of the proximal femur with the site of attachment of the hip capsule highlighted in *green*. Adapted from Clinical Anatomy, 2nd edition by Richard Snell. Little, Brown and Company (Inc) 1986

The Zona Orbicularis

The zona orbicularis (ZO), often described as a sling or collar around the neck of the femur, constitutes the narrowest area within the capsule (Fig. 4.8). Most substantial posteriorly and inferiorly, this condensed group of circular fibres acts a retaining ring, resisting distraction of the hip [3]. The ZO is easily visualised from within the peripheral compartment, making it a useful landmark at arthroscopy.

The term orbicularis derives from the Latin 'orbis', denoting a circular or disc-shaped structure. Traditionally, authors have described the ZO as a circular structure, wrapping around the femoral neck and acting as a ring that prevents the bigger femoral head slipping out of its position within the acetabulum. Thus, the capsule may be visualised as an hourglass with the ZO forming the isthmus.

Despite descriptions in classic textbooks of anatomy [6, 13–15], our understanding of the zona orbicularis' anatomy and function remains limited. Ito has suggested that the ZO contributes to hip stability and is the principal restraint to joint distraction [3]. More recently, it has been proposed that the ZO also has a role in synovial fluid circulation within the joint. It has been hypothesised that the ZO functions as a bellow-like mechanism to force synovial fluid from the peripheral compartment to the central compartment in a unidirectional flow [7]. When performing hip arthroscopy in the peripheral compartment, the ZO provides a landmark for arthroscope and instrument guidance and orientation [3, 16].

The circular fibres of the zona orbicularis run perpendicular to the axis of the joint as a sling around the femoral neck, just distal to the femoral head. Anteriorly fibres blend with the deep surface of the iliofemoral ligament [6, 8], but the zona orbicularis

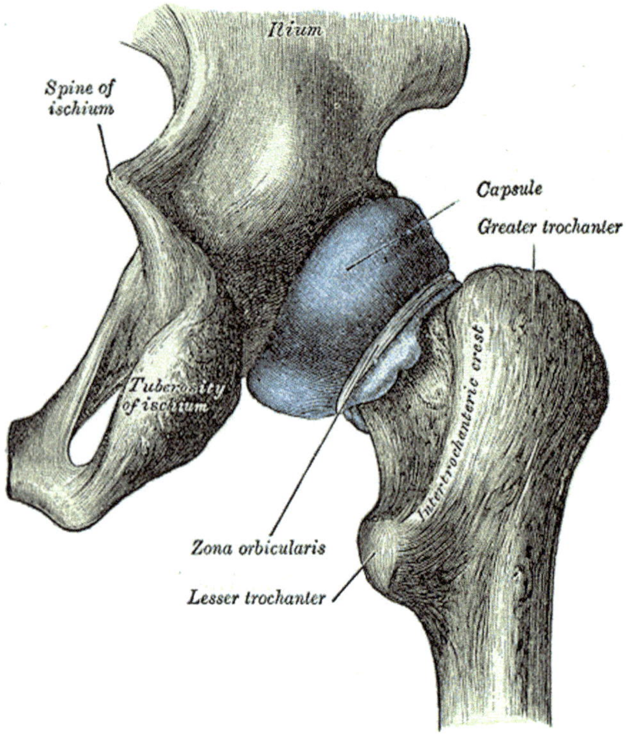

Fig. 4.3 The capsule of the hip and the zona orbicularis as seen from posterior aspect. From Gray, Henry. Anatomy of the Human Body. Philadelphia: Lea & Febiger, 1918; Bartleby.com, 2000. www.bartleby.com/107/. Reprinted with permission

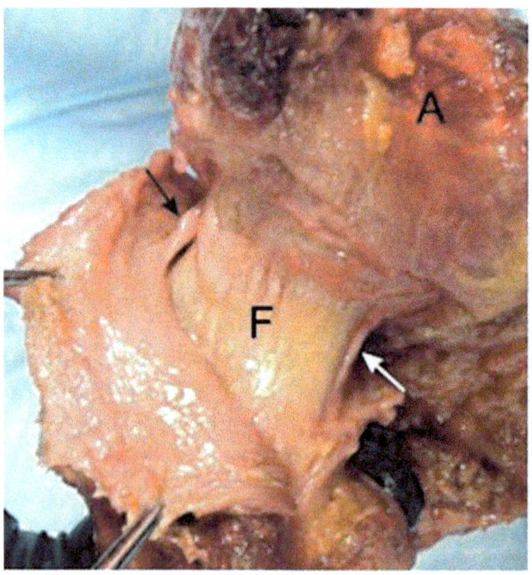

Fig. 4.4 Superior (*black arrow*) and inferior (*white arrow*) retinacular folds (retinacula of Weitbrecht). *A* acetabulum, *F* femur

is largely a posterior and inferior structure. At its superior aspect, its fibres are attached to the femur at the base of the greater trochanter, where they also blend with the distal insertion of the superior band of the ischiofemoral ligament. The zona orbicularis then runs across the back of the femoral neck, forming the

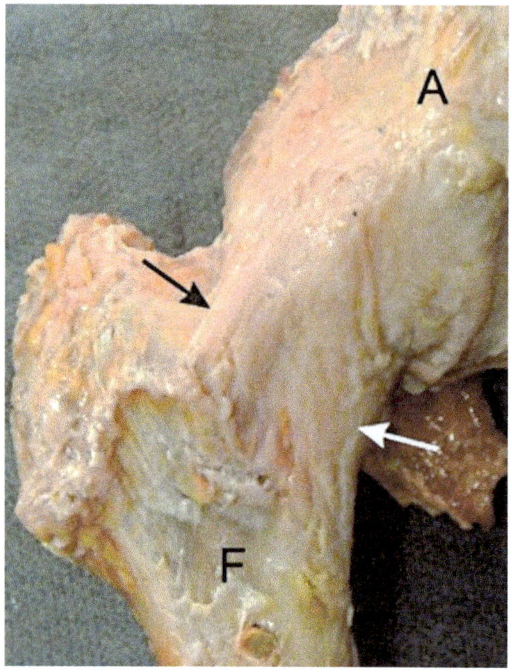

Fig. 4.5 Anterior view of the iliofemoral ligament demonstrating the superior (*black arrow*) and inferior bands (*white arrow*). *A* acetabulum, *F* femur. From Wagner et al. Capsular ligaments of the hip. Anatomic, histologic and positional study in cadaveric specimens with MR arthrography. Radiology 2012;263(1):189–198. Reprinted with permission from Radiology Society of North America

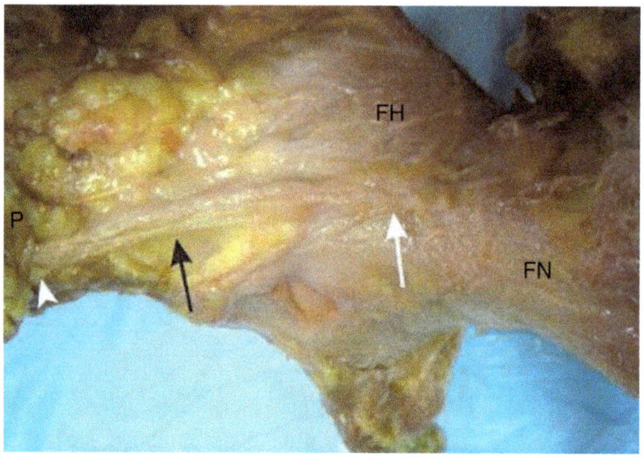

Fig. 4.6 The pubofemoral ligament. The ligament originates extracapsularly (*arrowhead*), in obturator crest of the pubis (P). It traverses the acetabulum (*black arrow*) and along the inferior portion of the articular capsule (*white arrow*). *FH* femoral head, *FN* femoral neck. From Wagner et al. Capsular ligaments of the hip. Anatomic, histologic and positional study in cadaveric specimens with MR arthrography. Radiology 2012;263(1):189–198. Reprinted with permission from Radiology Society of North America

free border of the posterior capsule, before blending with the fibres of the anteroinferior capsule [8]. In a recent study of MR arthrograms of normal hip joints, we observed that the ZO had a horseshoe shape in 18 of 25 cases (72%) and was absent anteriorly. In a further 5 of 25 cases (20%), the zona formed a full circle but was very thin anteriorly and in only 2 of 25 cases (8%) was it a full homogeneous circle.

Vascular Supply

The vascular supply of the capsule of the hip is derived from four main vessels, which enter the capsule peripherally and superficially [17]. Direct capsular branches of the medial femoral circumflex artery (MFCA) and the lateral femoral circumflex artery (LFCA) enter from the femoral aspect of the capsule and run on its superficial surface circumferentially, from distal to proximal. The superior gluteal artery (SGA) and the inferior gluteal artery (IGA) each give off corresponding supra-acetabular and acetabular branches that terminate as capsular vessels and run from proximal to distal [6, 17]. The gluteal arteries contribute largely to the vascular supply of the posterior capsule. Variable anastomosis can be found between the two systems, running beneath the gluteus minimus and the short external rotator muscles [17]. Further branches of the femoral vessels perforate the capsule to run as retinacular arteries and supply the femoral head.

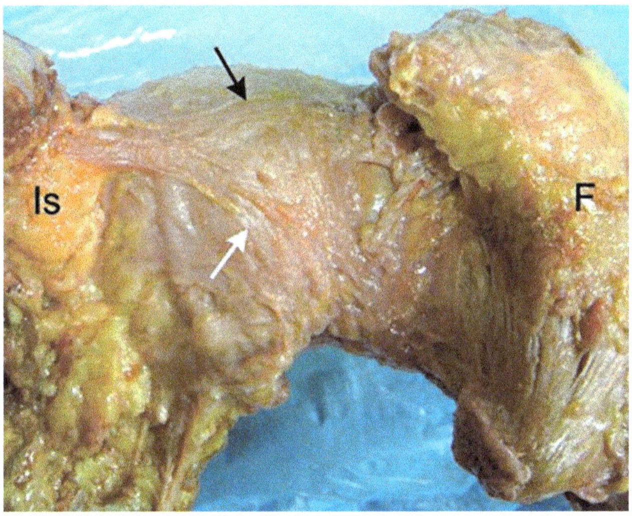

Fig. 4.7 Posterior view of the articular capsule. The ischiofemoral ligament can be seen to divide into superior (*black arrow*) and inferior bands (*white arrow*). *F* femur, *Is* ischium. From Wagner et al. Capsular ligaments of the hip. Anatomic, histologic and positional study in cadaveric specimens with MR arthrography. Radiology 2012;263(1):189–198. Reprinted with permission from Radiology Society of North America

Innervation of the Hip Capsule

Although anatomical description can vary, the capsule of the hip is generally thought to be innervated by branches of the obturator nerve and the nerve to quadratus femoris, with variable contributions from the femoral, sciatic and superior gluteal nerves, and the accessory obturator nerve [18]. Three primary articular nerves are described: the posterior articular nerves, giving the most prolific supply to the hip joint, the medial articular nerve, and the nerve to ligamentum capitus femoris.

The posterior articular nerves arise from the nerve to quadratus femoris, before its termination in its corresponding muscle belly [19]. These short articular branches from lateral aspect of the main nerve trunk run beneath the obturator internus and the gemelli muscles before entering the posterior capsule along the extent of its acetabular attachment. Superior, middle and inferior branches supply the posterior and posteroinferior capsule, respectively, including supply to the ischiofemoral ligament [19].

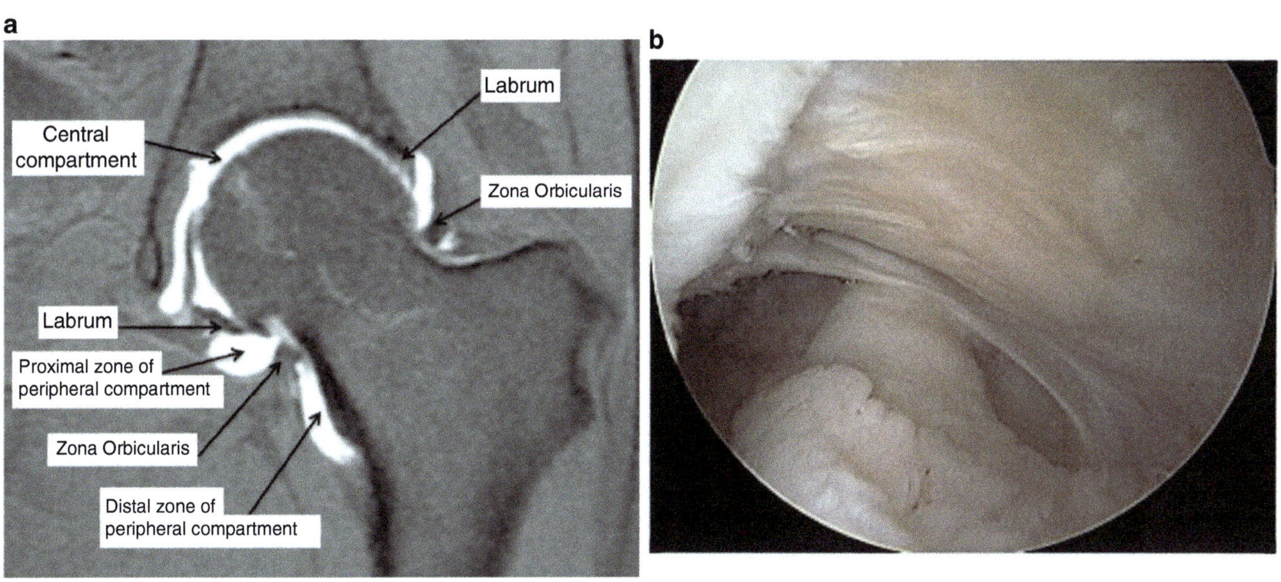

Fig. 4.8 MR arthogram. (**a**) Coronal view of the hip joint demonstrating fluid compartments. (**b**) Arthroscopic view of the zona obicularis

A single articular branch from the obturator nerve constitutes the medial articular nerve. It is occasionally given off from the main nerve within the obturator canal, but more commonly the articular nerve arises from the lateral branch of the anterior division as it leaves the obturator foramen. The medial articular nerve divides into two terminal branches, eventually supplying the antero-medial and inferior joint capsule [19]. Accessory articular nerves supply smaller portions of the capsule, the majority of these branches arising from the femoral nerve but also from the superior gluteal nerve and accessory femoral or obturator nerves [18].

The Arthroscopic Perspective

The capsular ligaments of the hip cannot be clearly identified from within the joint, but the orientation of the capsular ligaments from the perspective of the arthroscope has been described (Fig. 4.9) [11, 20].

Using the clock face system, the iliofemoral ligament, before diverging into its medial and lateral bands, runs from 12:45 to 3 o'clock. Within the central compartment, both the anterolateral and anterior portals pierce the iliofemoral ligament just within its lateral and medial borders, respectively [11, 20]. In the peripheral compartment, the location of the iliofemoral ligament can be identified in relation to the medial and lateral synovial folds [20]. The lateral border of the ligament runs anterior to the lateral synovial fold at the head-neck junction and the medial border of the ligament lateral to the medial synovial fold at the level of the zona orbicularis.

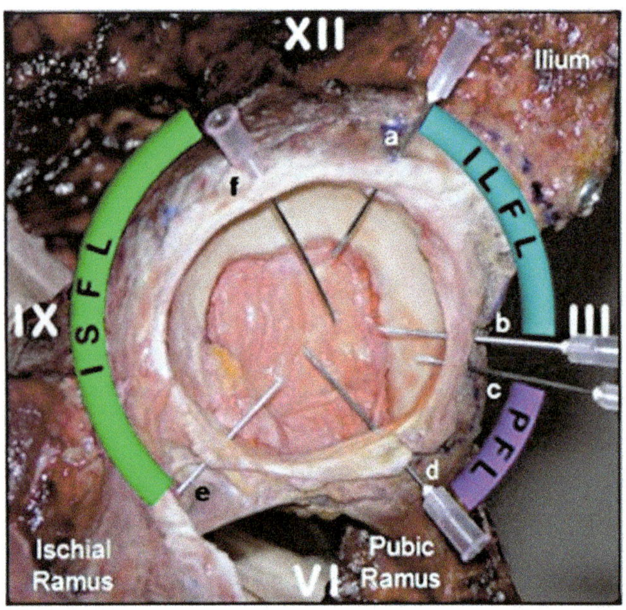

Fig. 4.9 The acetabular socket with locations of origin of the capsular ligaments (Reproduced with kind permission of Marc R. Safran)

The pubofemoral ligament runs from approximately 3:30 to 5:30 [11]. The lateral border of this ligament runs just anterior to the acetabular recess accommodating the psoas tendon. The medial border is found where the cotyloid fossa meets the anteroinferior acetabulum. In the peripheral compartment, the lateral border of the pubofemoral ligament lies lateral to the medial synovial fold at the level of the zona orbicularis [20].

The ischiofemoral ligament is pierced by the posterolateral arthroscopy portal at its superior/lateral border, which can be seen just posterior to the lateral synovial fold in the peripheral compartment. The ligament typically runs from 7:45 to 10:30 so that the inferior/medial border is found at the most posteroinferior aspect of the acetabulum.

The adoption of upright posture and bipedal gait has resulted in extension of the pelvis on the femoral head and has left the anterior portion of the femoral head relatively uncovered and unsupported. The exposed anterior femoral head is encased and supported by the joint capsule and the iliofemoral ligaments. Outside the capsule are the iliocapsularis muscle and the iliopsoas tendon. Babst et al. [21] has reported that the iliocapsularis is hypertrophied in individuals with hip dysplasia suggesting that the anterior soft tissue structures are of increasing importance to hip stability as the bony constraints diminish. Blakey et al. [22] identified that individuals with chronic capsular injury lose the normal elastic recoil seen on external rotation of the joint and used MR to demonstrate thinning at the lateral insertion of the ligament, attenuation of the iliofemoral ligament (most noticeably on maximum external rotation (60°) and the appearance of laxity despite full external rotation. A number of strategies have been described to tighten the hip capsule in cases of laxity. These include thermal shrinkage [23] and suture plication [24–26]. Clinical studies of capsular augmentation procedures are ongoing.

References

1. Hewitt JD, Glisson RR, Guilak F, Vail TP. The mechanical properties of the human hip capsule ligaments. J Arthroplasty. 2002;17(1):82–9.
2. Martin HD, Savage A, Braly BA, Palmer IJ, Beall DP, Kelly B. The function of the hip capsular ligaments: a quantitative report. Arthroscopy. 2008;24(2):188–95.
3. Ito H, Song Y, Lindsey DP, Safran MR, Giori NJ. The proximal hip joint capsule and the zona orbicularis contribute to hip joint stability in distraction. J Orthop Res. 2009;27(8):989–95.
4. Myers CA, Register BC, Lertwanich P, Ejnisman L, Pennington WW, Giphart JE, et al. Role of the acetabular labrum and the iliofemoral ligament in hip stability: an in vitro biplane fluoroscopy study. Am J Sports Med. 2011;39(Suppl):85S–91.
5. Crawford MJ, Dy CJ, Alexander JW, Thompson M, Schroder SJ, Vega CE, et al. The 2007 Frank Stinchfield Award. The biomechanics of the hip labrum and the stability of the hip. Clin Orthop Relat Res. 2007;465:16–22.

6. Gray H. Gray's anatomy. 20th ed. Lewis WH, editor. Philadelphia: Lea & Febinger; 1918.
7. Field RE, Rajakulendran K. The Labro-acetabular complex. J Bone Joint Surg Am. 2011;93 Suppl 2:22–7.
8. Wagner FV, Negrão JR, Campos J, Ward SR, Haghighi P, Trudell DJ, et al. Capsular ligaments of the hip: anatomic, histologic, and positional study in cadaveric specimens with MR arthrography. Radiology. 2012;263(1):189–98.
9. Aiello L, Dean C. The Hominoid Pelvis. An Introd. to Hum. Evol. Anat. 1st ed. London: Academic Press; 1990. p. 429–256.
10. Philippon MJ, Schenker ML. Athletic hip injuries and capsular laxity. Oper Tech Orthop. 2005;15(3):261–6.
11. Shu B, Safran MR. Hip instability: anatomic and clinical considerations of traumatic and atraumatic instability. Clin Sports Med. 2011;30(2):349–67.
12. Fuss FK, Bacher A. New aspects of the morphology and function of the human hip joint ligaments. Am J Anat. 1991;192(1):1–13.
13. Latarjet M, Ruiz Liard A. Coxofemoral joint. In: Human anatomy (spanish edition). 4th ed. Buenos Aires: Medica Panamericana; 2004. p. 706–45.
14. Rouviere H, Delmas A. Pelvic girdle joint. In: Human anatomy-descriptive, topographic and functional (spanish edition). 11th ed. Barcelona: Masson; 2005. p. 361–72.
15. Kapandji IA, ed. The hip. In: The physiology of the joints: lower limb annotated diagrams. of the mechanics of the human joints—lower limb. 5th ed. vol 2. Edinburgh: Elsevier; 1987. p. 24–33.
16. Byrd JW. Hip arthroscopy. J Am Acad Orthop Surg. 2006; 14:433–44.
17. Kalhor M, Beck M, Huff TW, Ganz R. Capsular and pericapsular contributions to acetabular and femoral head perfusion. J Bone Joint Surg Am. 2009;91(2):409–18.
18. Kampa RJ, Prasthofer A, Lawrence-Watt DJ, Pattison RM. The internervous safe zone for incision of the capsule of the hip. A cadaver study. J Bone Joint Surg Br. 2007;89(7):971–6.
19. Dee R. Structure and function of hip joint innervation. Ann R Coll Surg Engl. 1969;45(6):357–74.
20. Telleria JJM, Lindsey DP, Giori NJ, Safran MR. An anatomic arthroscopic description of the hip capsular ligaments for the hip arthroscopist. Arthroscopy. 2011;27(5):628–36.
21. Babst D, Steppacher SD, Ganz R, Siebenrock KA, Tannast M. The iliocapsularis muscle: an important stabilizer in the dysplastic hip. Clin Orthop Relat Res. 2011;469(6):1728–34. doi:10.1007/s11999-010-1705-x. Epub 2010 Dec 3.
22. Blakey CM, Field MH, Singh PJ, Tayar R, Field RE. Secondary capsular laxity of the hip. Hip Int. 2010;20(4):497–504.
23. Philippon MJ. The role of arthroscopic thermal capsulorrhaphy in the hip. Clin Sports Med. 2001;20:817–29.
24. Philippon MJ, Zehms CT, Briggs KK, Manchester DJ, Kuppersmith DA. Hip and pelvic problems in athletes. Oper Techn Sports Med. 2007;15(4):189–94.
25. Ranawat AS, McClincy M, Sekiya JK. Anterior dislocation of the hip after arthroscopy in a patient with capsular laxity of the hip. A case report. J Bone Joint Surg Am. 2009;91(1):192–7.
26. Domb BG, Giordano BD, Philippon MJ. Arthroscopic capsulotomy, capsular repair, and capsular plication of the hip: relation to atraumatic instability. Arthroscopy. 2013;29(1):162–73.

Fundamental and Clinical Considerations of the Muscles of the Hip

5

Donald Anthony Neumann

Introduction

This chapter will provide an overview of the actions of hip muscles, with a focus on understanding a muscle's action based on its line-of-force. Discussions will highlight on how the position of the hip at a given time affects the torque and ultimate action of certain hip muscles. Other mechanical aspects of hip muscle function will be discussed, such as how the forces generated by muscle contraction affect the stress on the hip and its periarticular tissues. This chapter should serve as a foundation for physicians and rehabilitation specialists who direct and provide care for patients following hip arthroscopic surgery.

Fundamentals of Hip Muscle Function

Describing a Muscle's Action at the Hip

The hip joint allows movement in three degrees of freedom. Virtually all muscles that cross the hip are capable of, at least to limited degrees, rotating the femur (and/or the pelvis) through a unique path that cuts through all three cardinal planes of motion. To simplify and standardize these kinematic descriptions, it is customary to describe the rotary *direction* of a muscle's action separately for each of the three movement planes [1]. For each plane, a muscle's rotary action is defined based on the orientation of its *line-of-force* relative to the joint's axis of rotation. These axes at the hip are defined as being medial-lateral for sagittal plane motions of flexion and extension, anterior-posterior for frontal plane motions of abduction and adduction, and vertical [longitudinal] for horizontal plane motions of internal and external rotation. Figure 5.1 illustrates the line-of-force for several muscles acting within the sagittal plane. This figure is based on a study by Dostal et al. using a straight-line model of muscle action [2, 3], a method used by several investigators [4–6]. Observe in Fig. 5.1 that a muscle's line-of-force that passes *anterior* to the joint's medial-lateral axis of rotation is a potential flexor (such as the highlighted rectus femoris); conversely, a muscle's line-of-force that passes *posterior* to the same axis, such as the gluteus maximus, is a potential extensor. The roles of other muscles can be also viewed in a similar way for the frontal plane (as abductors or adductors) and for the horizontal plane (as internal or external rotators).

This graphical representation depicted in Fig. 5.1 illustrates a muscle's potential action and, equally important, indicates the muscle's relative moment arm length (leverage) available to generate the torque for the particular action. The original data used to generate Fig. 5.1 are listed in Table 5.1 [3]. This table shows, for example, that the gluteus maximus has a 4.6 cm moment arm for extension, a 2.1 cm moment arm for external rotation, and 0.7 cm moment arm for adduction. It is important to realize that the lines-of-force and moment arms depicted in Fig. 5.1 apply *only* to the anatomic position. Once the hip is moved out the anatomic position, factors that influence a muscle's action as well as torque can vary considerably. These variations partially explain why maximal-effort strength measurements and, in some cases, even the muscle's action change as a function of hip position—a point discussed in greater detail later in this chapter.

Based on data published in the literature and observations made on cadaver and skeletal models, the muscles of the hip are designated as being primary or secondary for a given action (Table 5.2) [1]. Some muscles possess only a marginal ability to produce a particular action, due to variables such as small cross-sectional area or moment arm length, or a line-of-force that is nearly parallel with (versus strongly intersecting) a given axis of rotation.

D.A. Neumann, PT, PhD, FAPTA (✉)
Department of Physical Therapy, Marquette University, Schroeder Health Complex, PO Box 1881, Milwaukee, WI 53210-3319, USA
e-mail: Donald.Neumann@marquette.edu

J.C. McCarthy et al. (eds.), *Hip Joint Restoration*, DOI 10.1007/978-1-4614-0694-5_5

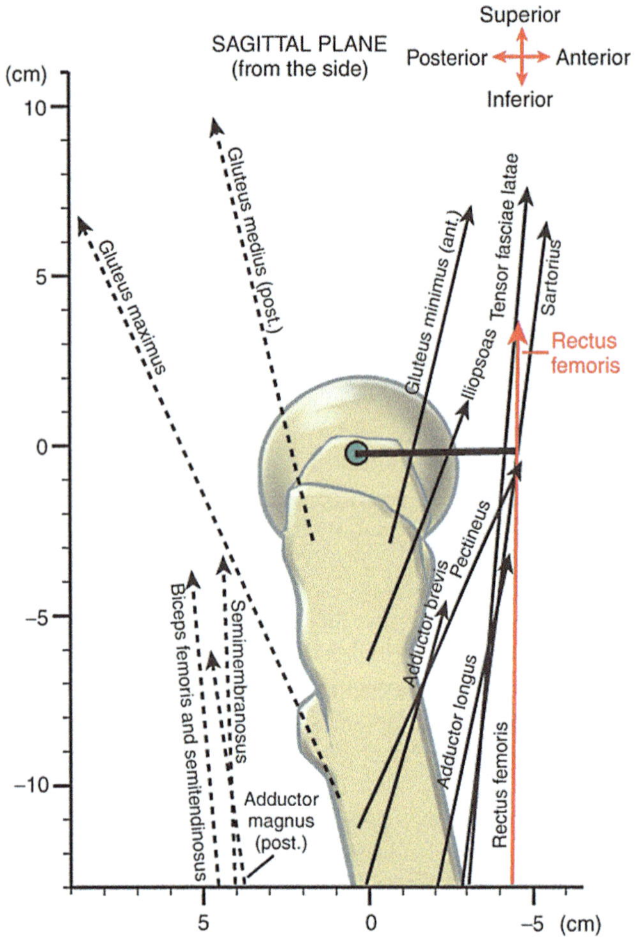

Fig. 5.1 A lateral view shows the sagittal plane line-of-force of several hip muscles. The axis of rotation (*green circle*) is directed in the medial-lateral direction through the femoral head. The flexors are indicated by *solid arrows* and the extensors by *dashed arrows*. The internal moment arm used by the rectus femoris is shown as a thick *black line*, originating at the axis of rotation. (For clarity, not all muscles are shown.) The lines-of-force are not drawn to scale and, therefore, do not indicate a muscle's relative force potential. From Neumann DA: Kinesiology of the Musculoskeletal System: Foundations for Physical Rehabilitation, second edition, 2010. Reprinted with permission from Elsevier Limited

Hip Muscle's Action Versus Torque Generation

Although the representation of muscles shown in Fig. 5.1 is useful for assessing a muscle's potential action within a given plane, it lacks information to authoritatively rank the muscle's relative *torque* potential within a given plane. While a muscle action describes the potential rotary direction of the joint following its activation by the nervous system, a muscle torque describes the "strength" of the action. Torque, or moment, is the rotary expression of a force. A muscle torque can be estimated by the product of the muscle force (in newtons or pounds) within a plane of interest *and* the muscle's associated moment arm length (in cm or inches). Both variables of force and moment arm are equally important when estimating the potential torque output, or strength, of a muscle. Although Fig. 5.1 is constructed to appreciate a muscle's likely action and relative moment arm length, it does *not* indicate the muscle's actual *force* potential. The arrows used in the figure are not vectors and are not drawn to scale. The orientation of the arrows represents only the assumed linear direction of a contractile pull, not its amplitude. Estimating a muscle's force requires other information, such as its cross-sectional area, pennation angle, and relative neural activation [7].

Many examples offered throughout this chapter show how diagrams of lines-of-force of muscles in the anatomical position, limited to the three cardinal planes, can provide a framework with which the clinician can make valuable inferences about the function of the muscles at the hip. Consider, for instance, how the relative torque potential of a hip muscle might be postulated primarily from the position and distance of its line-of-force from the hip joint. This can be visualized in any plane with knowledge of the location of the hip joint (i.e., the location of the axis of rotation) as well as the attachments of the muscle. For example, Fig. 5.2a shows actions of the piriformis and obturator externus in the horizontal plane with the hip in the anatomic position. Both of these muscles are typically characterized as external rotators of the hip. In the anatomic position, the piriformis is well positioned to externally rotate the femur. The obturator externus however, by passing directly through the axis of rotation, would lack a moment arm and therefore could not produce rotation. Figure 5.2a further reveals that, in the situation depicted, activity of the obturator externus would mainly compress the hip joint.

Figure 5.2b further illustrates this reasoning by assessing the potential for the middle fibers of the gluteus medius to rotate the femur in the horizontal plane about a vertical axis of rotation (depicted as a blue pin). Because this component of the muscle's overall force acts essentially *parallel* with the vertical axis of rotation, it is incapable of generating torque in the horizontal plane. Moving the femur away from the anatomic position however can dramatically alter the biomechanics. Flexing the hip to 100°, for example, creates a near perpendicular intersection between the muscle and the axis of rotation (which "followed" the flexed position of femoral shaft). In a flexed position, it is likely that the muscle fibers of the gluteus medius could, indeed, internally rotate the femur. Analyzing a muscle's action *outside* the anatomic position is a very useful way to fully appreciate a muscle's functional potential. This topic is a recurring theme throughout this chapter.

Table 5.1 Moment arm data (cm) for muscles of the hip, organized by their actions in the sagittal, horizontal, and frontal planes. Muscles are presented in alphabetical order

Muscle	Sagittal plane	Horizontal plane	Frontal plane
Adductor brevis	F: 2.1	IR: 0.5	Ad: 7.6
Adductor longus	F: 4.1	IR: 0.7	Ad: 7.1
Adductor magnus [anterior head]	E: 1.5	ER: 0.2	Ad: 6.9
Adductor magnus [posterior head]	E: 5.8	IR: 0.4	Ad: 3.4
Biceps femoris	E: 5.4	ER: 0.6	Ad: 1.9
Gemellus inferior	E: 0.4	ER: 3.3	Ad: 0.9
Gemellus superior	E: 0.3	ER: 3.1	Ab: 0.1
Gluteus maximus	E: 4.6	ER: 2.1	Ad: 0.7
Gluteus medius [anterior fibers]	E: 0.8	IR: 2.3	Ab: 6.7
Gluteus medius [middle fibers]	E: 1.4	IR: 0.1	Ab: 6.0
Gluteus medius [posterior fibers]	E: 1.9	ER: 2.4	Ab: 4.3
Gluteus minimus [anterior fibers	F: 1.0	IR: 1.7	Ab: 5.8
Gluteus minimus [middle fibers]	F: 0.2	ER: 0.3	Ab: 5.3
Gluteus minimus [posterior fibers]	E: 0.3	ER: 1.4	Ab:3.9
Gracilis	F: 1.3	ER: 0.3	Ad: 7.1
Iliopsoas	F: 1.8	IR: 0.5	Ab: 0.7
Obturator externus	F: 0.7	ER: 0.4	Ad: 2.4
Obturator internus	E: 0.3	ER: 3.2	Ad: 0.7
Pectineus	F: 3.6	IR: 1.0	Ad: 3.2
Piriformis	E: 0.1	ER: 3.1	Ab: 2.1
Quadratus femoris	E: 0.2	ER: 3.4	Ad: 4.4
Rectus femoris	F: 4.3	ER: 0.2	Ab: 2.3
Sartorius	F: 4.0	ER: 0.3	Ab: 3.7
Semimembranosus	E: 4.6	IR: 0.3	Ad: 0.4
Semitendinosus	E: 5.6	IR: 0.5	Ad: 0.9
Tensor fascia latae	F: 3.9	0.0	Ab: 5.2

Data are based on a male cadaver specimen being oriented in the anatomic position; data originally from Dostal et al. [3]

F flexion, *E* extension, *IR* internal rotation, *ER* external rotation, *Ab* abduction, *Ad* adduction

Table 5.2 Six muscle groups of the hip, listed according to their primary or secondary actions[a]

Flexors	Extensors	External rotators	Internal rotator	Adductors	Abductors
Primary					
Iliopsoas	Gluteus maximus	Gluteus maximus	**Not applicable**	Pectineus	Gluteus medius [all fibers]
Sartorius	Adductor magnus [posterior head]	Piriformis		Adductor longus	Gluteus minimus [all fibers]
Tensor fasciae latae	Biceps femoris [long head]	Obturator internus		Gracilis	Tensor fasciae latae
Rectus femoris	Semitendinosus	Gemellus superior		Adductor brevis	
Adductor longus	Semimembranosus	Gemellus inferior		Adductor magnus [anterior and posterior heads]	
Pectineus		Quadratus femoris			
Secondary					
Adductor brevis	Gluteus medius [middle and posterior fibers]	Gluteus medius [posterior fibers]	Gluteus minimus [anterior fibers]	Biceps femoris	Piriformis
Gracilis	Adductor magnus [anterior head]	Gluteus minimus [posterior fibers]	Gluteus medius [anterior fibers]	[long head]	Sartorius
Gluteus minimus [anterior fibers]		Obturator externus	Tensor fasciae latae	Gluteus maximus [posterior fibers]	Rectus femoris
		Sartorius	Adductor longus	Quadratus femoris	
		Biceps femoris [long head]	Adductor brevis	Obturator externus	
			Pectineus		
			Adductor magnus [posterior head]		

[a]Each action assumes a muscle is contracting from the anatomic position. Several of these muscles may have a different action when they are activated outside of the anatomic position

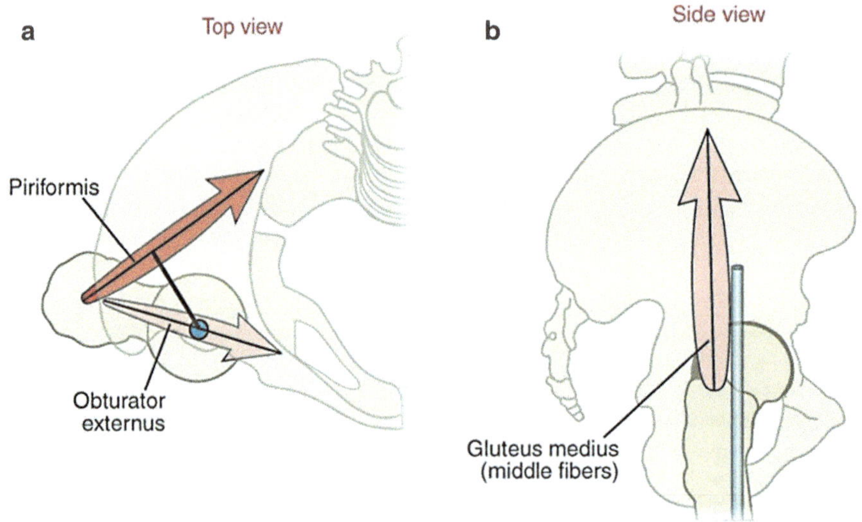

Fig. 5.2 Three muscle-produced forces are depicted as *large arrows*, each being considered for its ability to rotate the femur externally in the horizontal plane. The axes of rotation are shown in *blue*, and moment arm as a thick *dark line*, originating at the axis of rotation. (**a**) Shows a *top view* of an assumed line-of-force of the piriformis and the obturator externus. (**b**) Shows a side view of the middle fibers of the gluteus medius. As described, only the piriformis has a moment arm [shown as a thick *dark line*] to produce an external rotation torque. From Neumann DA: Kinesiology of the Musculoskeletal System: Foundations for Physical Rehabilitation, second edition, 2010. Reprinted with permission from Elsevier Limited

Functional Considerations of the Actions of Hip Muscles

Muscular Interactions Involving Hip Flexion

The hip flexor muscles have the dual role of advancing the lower limb during walking, running, and climbing, as well as flexing and stabilizing the sagittal plane orientation of the entire trunk-and-pelvis relative to the thighs. The latter typically more demanding "reverse action" of the hip flexor muscles is often underrated. Consider, for instance, a healthy person sitting erect on a backless stool while resisting a vigorous push from the front that would potentially topple the upper body uncontrollably into extension. The primary muscular resistance against such a mishap is strong activation of the hip flexor muscles, perhaps most notably the iliopsoas, contracting from a fixed pair of femurs. Certainly the abdominal muscles contract to help stabilize the upper body from such a perturbation, but these muscles only exert a flexion torque between the upper trunk and the pelvis. Because the abdominal muscles do not attach to the femurs, they do *not* flex the hip.

The large demand placed on the hip flexor muscles likely accounts for their relatively large torque potential. Of the six muscle groups of the hip (3 planes of movement × 2 directions per plane), only the hip extensor muscles generate greater torque than the flexors. The most potent or kinetically influential hip flexor muscle is the iliopsoas, a thick, 2-part muscle consisting of the iliacus and psoas major. During walking the iliopsoas is most active during the swing phase, as it produces force across the hips, sacroiliac joints, lumbosacral junction, and all joints within the lumbar spine. During the swing phase the iliopsoas is most responsible for the joint contact force imparted to the anterior aspect of the femoral head [8].

The large psoas major is ideal for providing vertical stability to the trunk as a whole [9]. More specifically, the muscle's dominant role in stabilizing the lumbar spine is supported by a study by Hu et al., who analyzed the bilateral fine-wire EMG activity of the iliacus and psoas major during a unilateral (right-sided) resisted, straight-leg raise in 17 healthy persons [10]. Results showed strong ipsilateral activation of the right iliacus (as expected), whereas the psoas major showed strong and consistent *bilateral* activation. The right psoas muscle, in this scenario, contributed directly to flexing the hip, while the left muscle presumably prevented the lumbar spine from laterally flexing to the right.

The iliopsoas crosses anterior and slightly medial to the femoral head, ultimately attaching to the lesser trochanter. In the course of this path, the muscle is deflected posteriorly 35°–40° as it passes over the junction of the superior pubic and illiopubic rami. The rami thus provide an overhang to distance the distal part of the iliopsoas from the femoral head, thereby increasing the muscle's leverage for flexion when in a fully extended position. As the hip flexes to 90°, the moment arm increases even further, which may compensate for the muscle's loss in force after it is significantly shortened [11]. Interestingly, a cadaver study by Neumann and

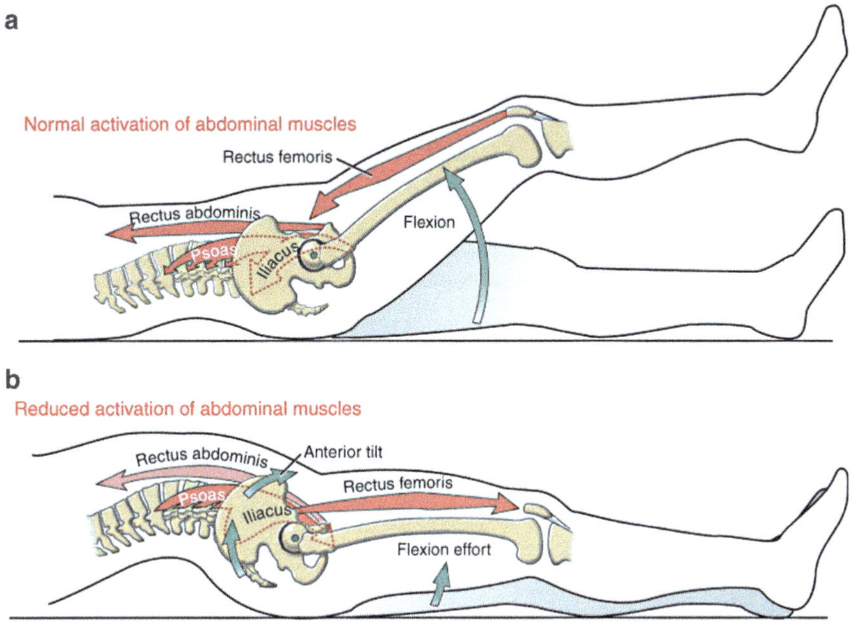

Fig. 5.3 The synergistic action between a representative abdominal muscle [rectus abdominis] and the iliopsoas and rectus femoris is illustrated while performing a straight-leg raise. (**a**) Sufficient activation of the abdominal muscles opposes the strong downward pull of the hip flexor muscles, preventing an anterior tilt of the pelvis. (**b**) With reduced activation of the abdominal muscles, contraction of the hip flexor muscles is shown producing a marked anterior tilt of the pelvis—increasing the lumbar lordosis. The reduced activation in the abdominal muscle is indicated by the lighter red color. From Neumann DA: Kinesiology of the Musculoskeletal System: Foundations for Physical Rehabilitation, second edition, 2010. Reprinted with permission from Elsevier Limited

Garceau suggests that the distal attachment of the psoas minor into iliac fascia may help control and thereby stabilize the relative position of the distal part of the iliopsoas relative to the hip joint [12].

The specific anatomy of the distal attachment of the iliopsoas has important clinical and surgical implications, especially when the tendon is associated with "internal snapping hip" syndrome [13]. En route to its femoral attachment, the iliopsoas forms a broad musculotendinous unit (MTU) lying anterior to the lateral aspect of the junction of the superior pubic and illiopubic rami. The medial part of the MTU is typically tendinous whereas the lateral part is muscular. Gross dissection clearly shows some of the muscle fibers blending with the anterior capsule of the hip joint. These muscle fibers may represent a distinct muscle which has been described as the iliocapsularis [14, 15]. Although the MTU attaches primarily to the lesser trochanter, a significant percentage of fibers from the lateral aspect of the iliacus remains muscular and inserts on the anterior aspects of the lesser trochanter as well as slightly below it [16]. Blomberg et al. showed that at the level of the lesser trochanter, the MTU consists of 60 % tendon and 40 % muscle fibers [17]. A tenotomy performed to release the iliopsoas tendon at this level would thus still spare 40 % of the integrity of the distal attachment of this muscle. This anatomical arrangement may explain why a tenotomy performed at the level of the lesser trochanter often produces excellent results in athletes. The source of the frictional impingement is reduced while sparing sufficient muscular fibers to prevent long-term weakness of hip flexion.

A complete discussion of the actions of the hip flexor muscles must include a discussion of the pelvic stabilization function of the abdominal muscles. Normally the abdominal muscles are strongly activated during a moderate to high-power hip flexion effort. This muscle synergy is easily demonstrated by performing a straight-leg-raise movement. The more superficial abdominal muscles (rectus abdominis, external and internal oblique) must generate a *posterior* pelvic tilt force of enough magnitude to counterbalance the strong potential for the hip flexor muscles to anteriorly tilt the pelvis.[1] This muscular relationship is shown between representative abdominal muscles and hip flexor muscles in Fig. 5.3a. The degree to which the abdominal muscles prevent an anterior pelvic tilt is dependent on the rigor of the activity (e.g., lifting one or both legs) and the relative forces produced by the activated muscles [18]. In addition to stabilizing the pelvis, the abdominal muscles help stabilize the entire lumbopelvic region by increasing intra-abdominal

[1] *Pelvic tilt* is defined as a short-arc (sagittal plane) rotation of the pelvis relative to both femoral heads. The direction of the tilt is named based on the direction of movement of a point on the iliac crest.

pressure and increasing the tension within the thoracolumbar fascia [19, 20].

Without sufficient stabilization of the pelvis by the abdominal muscles, contraction of the hip flexor muscles can unintentionally tilt the pelvis *anteriorly* (i.e., short-arc hip flexion) about the femoral heads (Fig. 5.3b). An excessive anterior pelvic tilt typically accentuates the lumbar lordosis. This might create an especially undesirable situation for someone with anterior femoral-acetabular impingement, or with a low back problem such as anterior spondylolisthesis or degenerated lumbar apophyseal joints. The abdominal weakness in Fig. 5.3b, if chronic, might lead to contracture of hip flexors. Muscles vulnerable to this impairment are not limited to the iliopsoas and rectus femoris shown in the illustration. Contracture of *any* hip flexor (primary or secondary) could contribute to excessive anterior pelvic tilt and exaggerated lumbar lordosis.

Muscular Interactions Involving Hip Extension

The hip extensor muscles produce the greatest isometric torque at the hip compared to all other muscle groups [21, 22]. With the hip in the anatomic position, the posterior head of the adductor magnus has the greatest moment arm to produce hip extension torque [3]. The gluteus maximus and adductor magnus have the greatest cross-sectional areas of all the primary extensors, strongly suggesting that these muscles have the potential to produce the largest peak extension forces across the hip [23].

Hip extensors best display their capability if the hip is flexed, as when a person starts to rise from a chair or from a deep squat. The muscles are elongated when the hip is flexed and can thus generate considerable force [5, 24, 25]. Furthermore, as will be described, with the hip significantly flexed, many of the adductor muscles produce an extension torque, thereby assisting the primary hip extensors.

Many functional movements of the lower limb incorporate forces generated *simultaneously* by the hip and knee extensor muscles. Consider, for example, the extension phase of jumping, climbing up a hill, or sprinting as depicted in Fig. 5.4. Combined hip and knee extension is controlled, in part, through a synergy among monoarticular and polyarticular muscles at both joints. Figure 5.4 shows a sample of muscular interactions involving the monoarticular gluteus maximus and the biarticular semitendinosus (representing the hamstrings) and quadriceps muscles. The active knee extension torque generated by the contracting quadriceps extends the knee and, by necessity, stretches the activated hamstrings. As implied by the classic force-velocity curve of muscle, forcefully elongating (or stretching) a muscle that is simultaneously being driven to contract naturally augments its force per level of effort [7]. The combined hip-and-knee extension motion shown in Fig. 5.4 therefore naturally enhances the *hip extension* potential of the semitendinosus. Furthermore, the actively contracting gluteus maximus extends the hip and thereby stretches the active rectus femoris, thereby enhancing its ability to assist the vasti muscles in extending the knee. A dynamic kinetic linkage is formed between several extensor muscles of the hip *and* knee. Due to the functional interdependence among these muscles, weakness in any one muscle may yield a global functional weakness of the combined motion. Consider, for example, the combined movement of hip-and-knee extension required to stand from a seated position. Weakness of the quadriceps could be expressed as weakened hip extension, whereas weakness of the gluteus maximus (or adductor magnus) could be expressed as weakened knee extension. From a

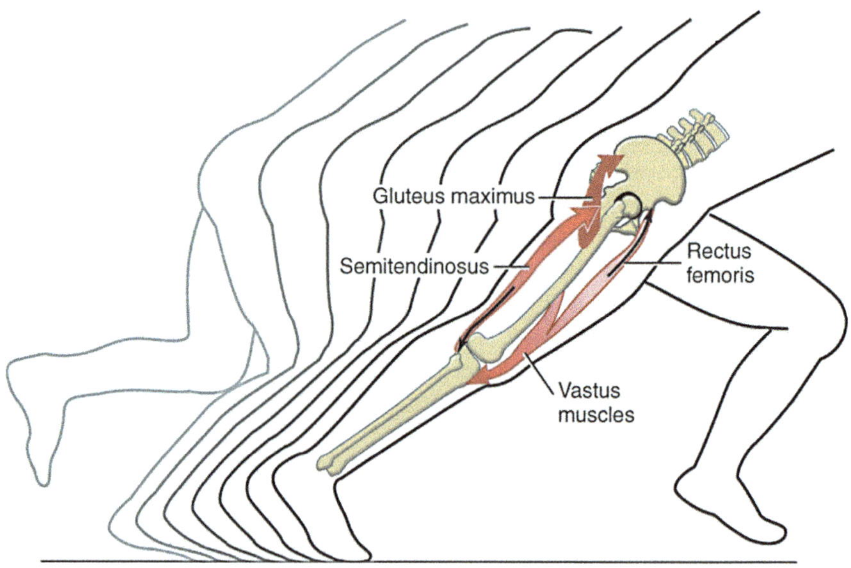

Fig. 5.4 The action of selected monoarticular and biarticular muscles at the hip and knee are depicted as they are simultaneously activated to extend the hip and knee during the start of a sprint. The stretched biarticular muscles are depicted by thin *black arrows*. From Neumann DA: Kinesiology of the Musculoskeletal System: Foundations for Physical Rehabilitation, second edition, 2010. Reprinted with permission from Elsevier Limited

physical therapy perspective, it is often logical to incorporate creative strengthening exercises that provide simultaneous resistance against both the hip and knee extensors. Furthermore, encouraging the patient to activate their hip extensor muscles to aid with knee extension may reduce the demands placed on the quadriceps. This strategy may be useful in cases where it is prudent to reduce quadriceps-based compression forces across a painful patellofemoral joint.

The relationships described above reinforce the importance of respecting the large natural strength potential of monoarticular muscles such as the gluteus maximus and adductor magnus. During a forceful hip-and-knee extension movement, the aforementioned hip extensor muscles must produce a hip extensor torque *that greatly exceeds* the hip flexion torque produced by activated rectus femoris. The functional net hip extensor torque is the *difference* between the hip extension torque and hip flexion torque generated by the active rectus femoris. A weakened gluteus maximus, for example, would reduce hip extension torque directly, but also indirectly by failing to adequately oppose the hip flexion torque produced by the rectus femoris. This relationship reinforces the functional importance of the extensor muscles being the strongest muscles at the hip.

With the trunk held relatively stationary, contraction of the hip extensor and abdominal muscles function as a force-couple to posteriorly tilt the pelvis (Fig. 5.5). As described earlier, a posterior tilting motion of the pelvis is actually a short-arc, bilateral [pelvic-on-femoral] *hip extension* movement. Assuming the trunk remains upright during this action, the lumbar spine must reverse its sagittal plane curvature slightly, thereby reducing its natural lordotic curve.

While standing upright over stationary thighs, a full posterior pelvic tilt increases the tension in most of the hip's capsular ligaments and hip flexor muscles. These tissues, if tightened, can restrict the end-range of a posterior pelvic tilt. Contraction of the abdominal muscles (acting as short-arc hip extensors as depicted in Fig. 5.5) can theoretically assist other hip extensor muscles in elongating (stretching) a tightened hip capsule or hip flexor muscle. Consider, for example, the classic method for stretching a tightened rectus femoris. The basis of the stretch, manually pulling the hip into full extension while holding the knee flexed, is transformed into a more effective stretch by including a strong co-activation of the abdominal *and* gluteus maximus muscles. Perhaps the maximal-effort volitional activation of the hip extensor muscles (including the abdominal muscles) may help relax or inhibit the antagonistic (and tightened) hip flexor muscle.

Achieving near full extension of the hips has important functional and perhaps physiologic benefits, such as increasing the muscular efficiency of upright standing. Full or nearly full hip extension allows a person's line-of-gravity to pass slightly *posterior* to the medial-lateral axis of rotation

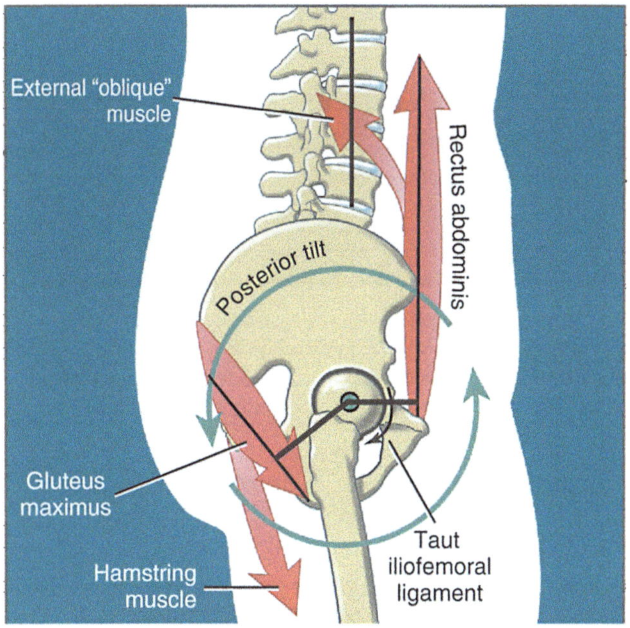

Fig. 5.5 The force-couple between representative hip extensors (gluteus maximus and hamstrings) and abdominal muscles (rectus abdominis and external oblique abdominis) is shown posteriorly tilting the pelvis while standing upright. The moment arms for each muscle group are indicated by the *dark black lines*. Note the resulting reduced lordosis at the lumbar spine. The extension at the hip stretches the iliofemoral ligament (shown as a short, *curved arrow* just anterior to the femoral head). From Neumann DA: Kinesiology of the Musculoskeletal System: Foundations for Physical Rehabilitation, second edition, 2010. Reprinted with permission from Elsevier Limited

joint's longitudinal (or vertical) axis of rotation.[2] The lines-of-force of these muscles are illustrated in Fig. 5.6. Clinical strength testing studies indicate that the maximal-effort torque produced by the internal and external rotators ranks relatively low compared with other muscles at the hip, about 55 % less than the dominant flexor-extensor group and 35 % less than the abductor and adductor group [21]. Given the minimal effect of gravity on the movement of a vertically oriented body with a relatively low moment of inertia in the horizontal plane, the internal and external rotators apparently do not need to be as strong as other hip muscles.

The primary *external rotators* of the hip are the gluteus maximus and five of the six "short" external rotators (Table 5.2). The obturator externus is relegated to a secondary rotator because, as indicated in Fig. 5.6, its line-of-force lies close to the longitudinal axis of rotation, therefore possessing limited leverage. The most dominant external rotator is the gluteus maximus, possessing about 16 % of the total cross-sectional area of all hip musculature [23]. With the

[2]The longitudinal axis of rotation at the hip is defined as running from femoral head to the center of the knee. Because of the neck-shaft angle and the slight forward bowing of the femur, much of this axis runs slightly posterior to the shaft of the femur

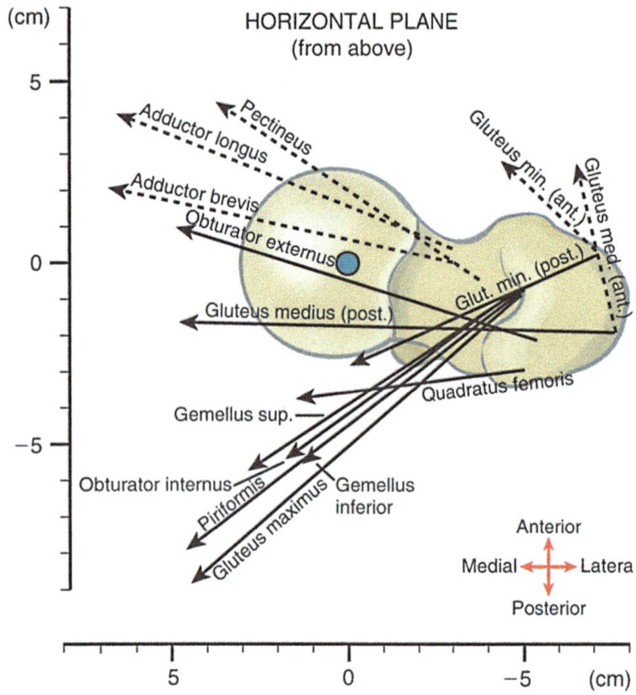

Fig. 5.6 A superior view depicts the horizontal plane line-of-force of several muscles that cross the hip. The longitudinal axis of rotation [*blue circle*] passes through the femoral head in a superior-inferior direction. The external rotators are indicated by *solid arrows* and the internal rotators by *dashed arrows*. For clarity, not all muscles are shown. The lines-of-force are not drawn to scale and, therefore, do not indicate a muscle's relative force potential. From Neumann DA: Kinesiology of the Musculoskeletal System: Foundations for Physical Rehabilitation, second edition, 2010. Reprinted with permission from Elsevier Limited

gluteus maximus directed some 45° from the frontal plane in the anatomic position, about 71 % (sin 45°) of its force is within the horizontal plane and therefore contributes strongly to an external rotation torque.

With the slight exception of the piriformis, the remaining short external rotators possess a near horizontal line-of-force. See, for example, the line-of-force of the quadratus femoris in Fig. 5.8. This orientation provides effective transfer of a contractile force to an external rotation torque. Furthermore, in a manner generally similar to the horizontally-oriented infraspinatus and teres minor at the glenohumeral joint, the short external rotators of the hip likely provide an important element of posterior stability to the hip. Interestingly, the posterior surgical approach to a total hip arthroplasty necessarily cuts through at least part the hip's posterior capsule, potentially disrupting several of the short external rotator tendons. Studies have indicated a significant reduction in the incidence of posterior hip dislocation following a posterior approach to the arthroplasty when careful repair of the posterior capsule and external rotator tendons is ensured [26–29]. The apparent surgical importance of these muscles has stimulated recent detailed anatomical dissection studies on these muscles [30, 31].

The functional potential of the external rotator muscles of the hip is well expressed through rotational activities of the trunk-and-pelvis relative to a fixed lower limb. With the right femur kept relatively fixed under the load of body weight, for example, contraction of the right external rotators would rotate the anterior side of the pelvis and attached trunk to the *left*—in a direction *contralateral* to the fixed right femur. Planting the limb and "cutting" to the opposite side (external rotation of the weight-bearing hip) is a natural way to abruptly change direction while running. The gluteus maximus, a potent extensor *and* external rotator, appears uniquely designed to perform this potentially powerful and useful activity.

Unlike the external rotators, muscles that *internally rotate* the hip run more vertically than horizontally and are thus poorly situated to purely rotate the hip about the longitudinal axis of rotation. Thus Table 5.2 lists only secondary internal rotators, including anterior fibers of the gluteus minimus and gluteus medius, along with the tensor fasciae latae, adductor longus, pectineus, adductor brevis, and posterior head of the adductor magnus [3, 32]. Although no single muscle among these can produce a very effective internal rotation on its own, their combined effort can generate the internal rotation torque at the hip needed for everyday purposes. During the stance phase of gait, for example, the internal rotators rotate the pelvis [relative to the femur] in the horizontal plane. Pelvic rotation about the right hip, for instance, is evident by the forward rotation of the *left* iliac crest. The right internal rotator muscles, therefore, provide some of the kinetic drive to the contralateral (left) swinging limb. During brisk walking, a greater demand is placed on the internal rotator muscles to increase the step length of the contralateral lower limb. It is interesting that many of internal rotator muscles also function as *abductors*, such as the gluteus minimus, gluteus medius, and tensor fasciae latae. From a pelvic-on-femoral perspective, these muscles produce torques for at least two different purposes: to drive part of the pelvic-on-femoral rotation just described and to furnish frontal plane stability during the single-limb support phase of walking.

Although the tensor fasciae latae is usually described as an internal rotator of the hip [33, 34], Table 5.1 reveals that this muscle has no moment arm for rotation in the horizontal plane [3]. But Table 5.1 is limited to the anatomic position, which corresponds to a near vertical alignment of the muscle. If the hip is externally rotated from anatomic position into what would be a more functionally meaningful posture, the tensor fasciae latae is twisted into a more oblique orientation that affords at least some moment arm for internal rotation. One should thus be careful of assessing *any* muscle's action strictly from the anatomic position. Some muscles possess a minimal potential for a given action in the anatomic position, but a near maximal potential when the hip is moved well outside the anatomic position.

Computer modeling and biomechanical studies suggest that the position of the hip in the sagittal plane can significantly alter and, in some cases, "reverse" the horizontal plane actions of entire (or parts of) certain hip rotator muscles. Consider the phenomenon for muscles such as the piriformis, posterior fibers of the gluteus minimus, and the more anterior fibers of the gluteus maximus. Different lines of research provide evidence that these "external rotators" reverse their rotary action and become *internal* rotators as the hip is significantly flexed [3, 6, 32]. The more extreme hip position shifts parts of the muscle's line-of-force to the "internal rotation" side of the hip's longitudinal axis of rotation. This concept can be visualized for the piriformis with the aid of a skeleton model and piece of string designed to mimic the line-of-force of the muscle. Delp et al. reported that the piriformis possesses an *external rotation* moment arm of 2.9 cm in 0 degrees of flexion, but a 1.4 cm *internal rotation* moment arm at 90 degrees of flexion [32]. The conjectured reversal in rotation of the piriformis at joint angles greater than 90 degrees of flexion may help justify the traditional practice of stretching this muscle by combining full hip flexion *with external rotation*. If the piriformis is actually an internal rotator in near full flexion, passive external rotation would indeed be a logical approach to effectively stretch this muscle.

Biomechanical studies have also analyzed the influence of hip position on the internal rotator muscles. Although the position of hip flexion has not been shown to actually reverse the action of any of the internal rotator muscles (as the case for parts of the external rotators), the position does significantly increase the moment arm of these muscles to produce internal rotation torque [3, 32, 35]. Delp and coworkers have looked specifically at the internal rotation moment arms of selected sets of fibers of the *gluteus medius* as the hip is flexed from 0° to 90° [32]. As depicted in Fig. 5.7a, the *anterior* fibers are only marginal internal rotators at 0 degrees of flexion, but show an eightfold increase in internal rotation leverage by 90 degrees of flexion. Such a dramatic increase in leverage would not be expected to translate into equally large increases in actual internal rotation torque production. The overly shortened length of many of the internal rotator muscles at 90° of hip flexion would likely physiologically reduce the muscles' overall force generation potential. Nevertheless, clinical strength testing studies on healthy subjects have reported that maximal-effort internal rotation torques are 33–50% greater with the hip flexed as a compared to extended [36–38]. This increased internal rotation torque with flexion may be caused by the increased leverage of some of the internal rotator muscles (such as the anterior fibers of the gluteus medius as depicted in Fig. 5.7a), or due to a reversal of rotary action of some of the traditional external rotators, such as the piriformis, or, as depicted in Fig. 5.7b, the posterior fibers of the gluteus medius.

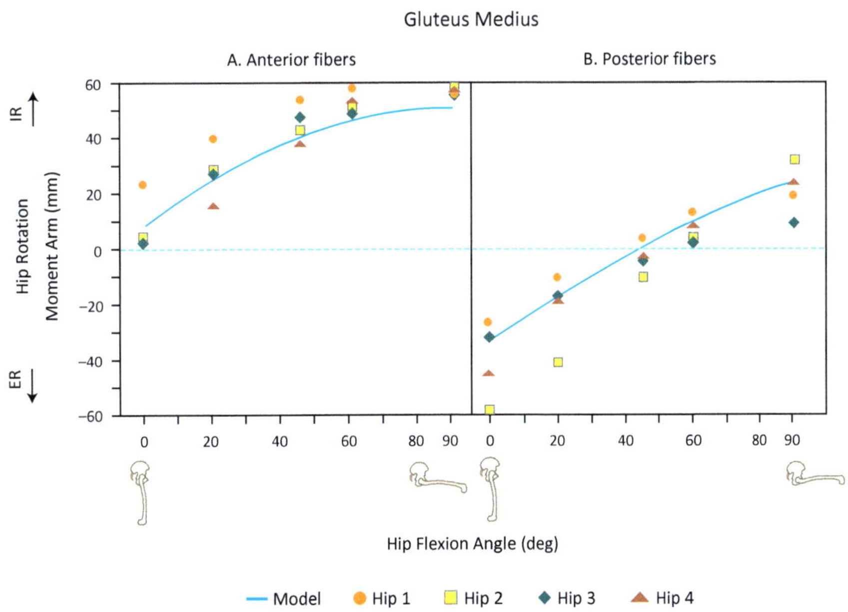

Fig. 5.7 Horizontal plane rotational moment arms [in mm] for two sets of fibers of the gluteus medius; (**a**) anterior fibers; (**b**) posterior fibers, plotted as a function of flexion (in degrees) of the hip. (*IR* internal rotation moment arm, *ER* external rotation moment arm.) The 0° flexion angle on the horizontal axis marks the anatomic [neutral] position of the hip. From Neumann DA: Kinesiology of the Hip: A Focus on Muscular Actions. J Orthop Sports Phys Ther. 2010, 40: 82–94, reprinted with permission from the Journal of Orthopaedic & Sports Physical Therapy. Data originally published by Delp et al., using four hip specimens and a computer model [32]

Regardless of the precise mechanism, sufficient evidence exists to conclude that flexing the hip increases internal rotation torque production at the hip. The clinical significance of an internal rotation torque bias with greater hip flexion has been described in the literature related to the excessively internally rotated and flexed ("crouched") gait pattern observed in some persons with cerebral palsy [32, 39]. With poor control or weakness of hip extensor muscles, the typically flexed posture of the hip amplifies the internal rotation torque potential of many muscles of the hip [32, 40, 41]. This gait pattern may be better controlled by greater activation of the hip extensor muscles.

Subtle and unexplained weakness of the external rotator muscles has been described in neurologically healthy persons, often combined with relative weakness of the hip abductors. Such weakness may be associated with the pathomechanics of chronic anterior knee pain, specifically involving the patellofemoral joint in adolescent females [42–47]. An underlying premise of this association is that reduced strength or control of the external rotator and abductor muscles of the hip during weight-bearing activities favors excessive valgus posturing at the knee. Such posturing may contribute to abnormal alignment of the patella relative to the femur, or vice versa [48].

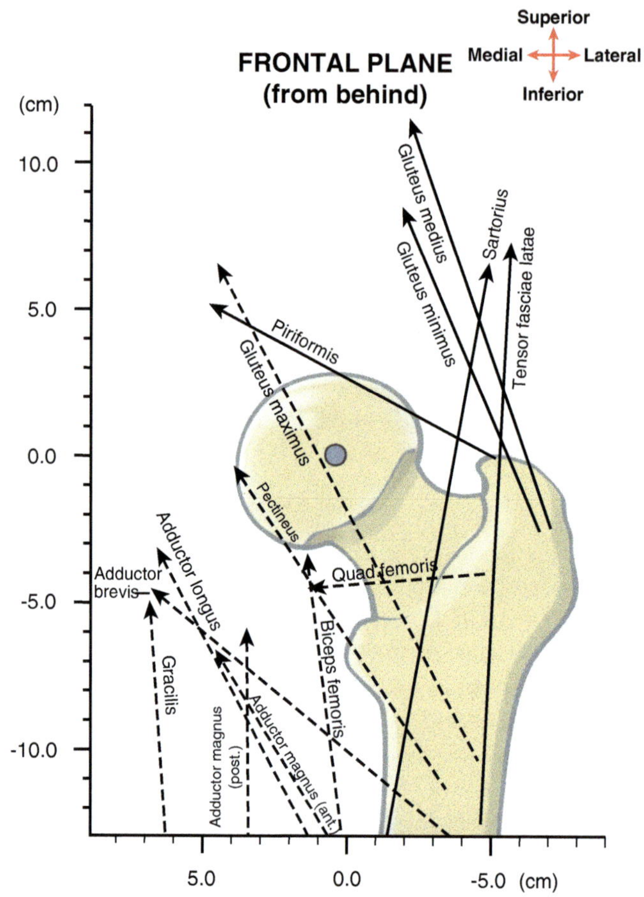

Fig. 5.8 A posterior view depicts the frontal plane line-of-force of several muscles that cross the hip. The axis of rotation (*purple circle*) is directed in the anterior-posterior direction through the femoral head. The abductors are indicated by solid arrows and the adductors by dashed arrows. For clarity, not all muscles are shown. The lines-of-force are not drawn to scale and, therefore, do not indicate a muscle's relative force potential. From Neumann DA: Kinesiology of the Musculoskeletal System: Foundations for Physical Rehabilitation, second edition, 2010. Reprinted with permission from Elsevier Limited

Utilitarian Function of the Adductor Muscles

The pectineus, adductor longus, gracilis, adductor brevis, and adductor magnus (both anterior and posterior heads), as primary adductors of the hip, have considerable leverage in the anatomic position, averaging almost 6 cm (Table 5.1) [3]. The line-of-forces of the primary adductors are illustrated in Fig. 5.8. With maximal effort, hip adduction torque exceeds abduction torque by only 4–7 % in healthy persons [49, 50]. Although the strength capacities of these two muscle groups are similar, the functional demands placed on them are very different.

Global function of the adductor muscles as a group is complex and not fully appreciated. The muscles obviously do much more than draw the femur closer to the midline of the body. These muscles are often active bilaterally to control multiplanar motions of the hip, typically involving the pelvis moving on the femur and at other times in a converse fashion. Consider, for example, a female soccer player firmly planting her left leg as she kicks a ball left-of-center using the right leg (Fig. 5.9). To varying degrees, the contracting right adductor muscles are capable of flexing, adducting, and internally rotating the right hip (femur relative to the pelvis) in order to accelerate the ball in the desired direction. As part of this kicking action, the left adductor muscles are shown contracting in a manner to pull the pelvis [on a fixed femur] in a direction toward hip adduction and internal rotation. Although such a pelvic-on-femoral motion can be driven by contraction of the left adductors, additional control of the motion may be accomplished by eccentric activation (braking effort) of the left hip abductors. Weakness of the hip abductors during a soccer kick may place greater valgus strain on the planted knee, which has been theorized to increase the risk of noncontact injury to the anterior cruciate ligament [51].

In addition to the more obvious frontal plane action of the hip adductors, these muscles also function in the sagittal plane as flexors *or* extensors, depending on the angle of the hip [3, 52]. Regardless of hip position, the adductor magnus, especially the posterior head, is a dominant extensor of the hip, similar to the hamstring muscles. In the rather extended anatomic position, however, most other adductors perform flexion (Table 5.1). If the hip is significantly flexed, however, lines-of-force of most of the adductors [except the adductor

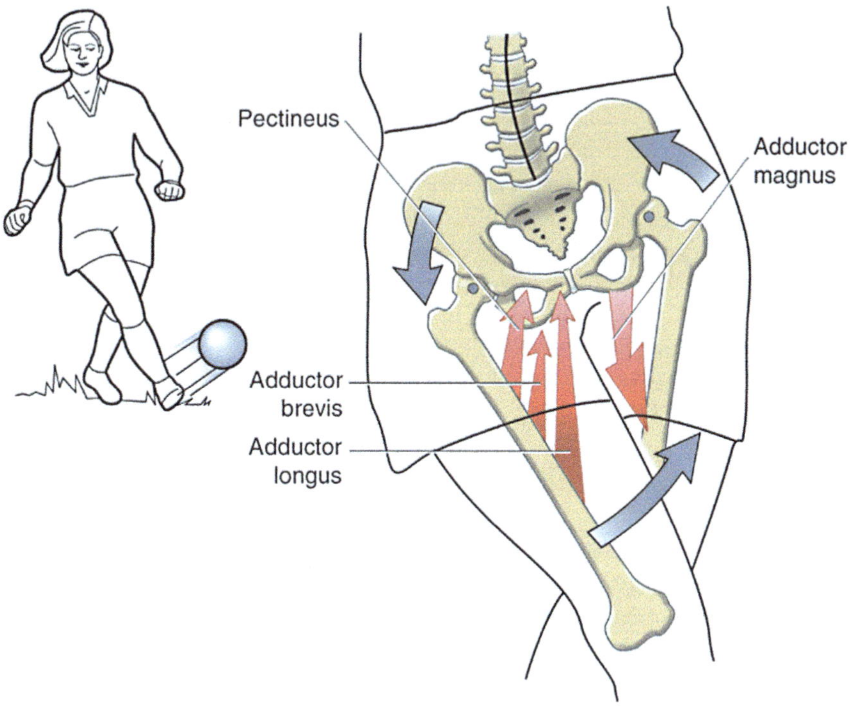

Fig. 5.9 The bilateral action of selected adductor muscles while kicking a soccer ball. The left adductor magnus is shown actively producing pelvic-on-femoral (hip) adduction. Several right adductor muscles are shown actively producing femoral-on-pelvic (hip) adduction torque, needed to accelerate the ball. From Neumann DA: Kinesiology of the Musculoskeletal System: Foundations for Physical Rehabilitation, second edition, 2010. Reprinted with permission from Elsevier Limited

magnus] appear to cross to the extensor (posterior) side of the medial-lateral axis of rotation of the hip, thereby gaining leverage as hip extensors.

Because each adductor muscle's line-of-force differs from that of the other adductors in the sagittal plane, no specific angle at the hip can be identified as a *single* point of reversal in flexor versus extensor action; this transition in function might rather be specified as a range, covering between 40° and 90° of sagittal plane motion [2, 3, 5, 6]. A reversal in sagittal plane action of any one adductor muscle (except the magnus) can be roughly estimated by observing a skeleton model from the side while using a piece of string that represents a particular adductor's line-of-force. Observations when employing this method for the *adductor brevis*, for example, suggest to this author that the muscle's line-of-force would intersect the medial-lateral axis of rotation at about 40 degrees of flexion. At this point the adductor brevis would have zero leverage to flex or extend at this point. At hip angles greater or less than 40° however, the muscle would gain leverage to rotate the femur *back to* the 40° position—its "neutral" point for producing sagittal plane torque. Functionally, the bidirectional sagittal plane torque potential of most of the adductor muscles is useful for powering cyclic activities such as sprinting, bicycling, or descending into and rising from a deep squat. When the hip is significantly flexed, the adductor muscles appear mechanically prepared to augment the other extensor muscles. Conversely when the hip is closer to full extension, these same adductors are mechanically prepared to reinforce other hip flexors. Further research like that published by Delp et al. [32] and Arnold et al. [24, 40, 53] is needed to more carefully define the flexion and extension leverage of the adductors throughout the sagittal plane.

Bidirectional action of the adductors in the sagittal plane also helps explain how the extremes of hip flexion and extension can each affect tightness of these muscles. Among many possible examples, consider the typically undesired, rounded low back posture that often accompanies the cross-legged sitting used in yoga. The bilateral abduction component of this position can place significant passive tension in the adductor muscles, especially if they are naturally tight. Because cross-legged sitting also requires considerable hip flexion, the increased passive tension in the stretched adductor muscles creates a passive hip *extension* torque at the hips, typically leading to a flexed lumbar spine and posteriorly tilted pelvis. Recall that a posterior tilt of the pelvis is fundamentally hip extension relative to the femurs. Sitting on a few pillows in the cross-legged position can *reduce* hip flexion which, in turn, decreases the passive extensor component of the adductors. This simple adjustment allows the lumbar spine to be less rounded, or more lordotic, in cross-legged sitting.

Finally, consider how the adductors act as secondary rotators of the hip. These muscles attach to the linea aspera on the *posterior* aspect of the femur and run medially and upward to attach to the inferior aspect of the pelvis. At first look, one might expect the adductors to assist in *externally* rotating the hip if the joint is in the anatomic position. Consider, though, that the shaft of the femur bows forward far enough to bring the linea aspera *anterior* to the vertical axis of rotation about the hip joint. The horizontal components of the adductor forces should thus *internally* rotate the hip. Studies have, in fact, shown most of the adductors to be positioned to produce modest internal rotation torque when the hip is in or near the anatomic position [3, 35, 54].

In summary, one of the most striking functional features of the adductor muscles is their ability to generate torques in all three planes, through both concentric and eccentric activations. The nearly constant biomechanical demand placed on these muscles often throughout a wide range of femoral and pelvic motions may partially explain their relatively high susceptibility to strain injury.

Hip Abductor Mechanism

Based primarily on combined size and moment arm length, the primary hip abductor muscles are the gluteus medius, gluteus minimus, and tensor fasciae latae [2, 55]. Several secondary abductor muscles are listed in Table 5.2. The gluteus medius and gluteus minimus possess the most substantial leverage to abduct the hip, based predominately on their laterally displaced attachments on the greater trochanter (Fig. 5.8).

The tendon of the *gluteus medius* consists of three distinguishable parts, the largest posterior part attaches to the superior-posterior facet on the greater trochanter [56]. Based on anatomic and EMG studies, the belly of the gluteus medius has been subdivided into three functional sets of fibers: anterior, middle, and posterior, each with a different moment arm to abduct the hip (Table 5.1) [3, 57]. Whereas all fibers contribute to abduction, in the anatomic position the anterior fibers also produce slight internal rotation and the posterior fibers produce extension and external rotation. As described earlier in this chapter, the strength and even the role of the gluteus medius as a rotator in the horizontal plane changes according to how much the hip is flexed or extended in the sagittal plane [24].

The tendon of the *gluteus minimus* can be divided into lateral and medial parts, with the main lateral part attaching to the lateral aspect of the anterior facet on the greater trochanter [56]. A smaller, medial part of the tendon attaches to the anterior and superior capsule of the hip [56, 58, 59]. This secondary tendinous attachment may retract the capsule from the joint at the extremes of hip motion, thereby preventing capsular impingement.

As with the gluteus medius, the fan-shaped belly of the gluteus minimus has been described as possessing three functionally different sets of fibers [3, 32]. All fibers produce abduction, while the more anterior fibers contribute to internal rotation, especially when the hip is flexed. Some studies report that the posterior fibers of the gluteus minimus function as a secondary external rotator [3, 57].

At 40° of hip abduction, close to the end-range of the joint, the hip abductors can produce only one third of the torque that they can generate at 10° of adduction, where the muscles are close to being fully lengthened [60]. Traditional manual muscle testing procedures specify full abduction for testing the "strength" of the hip abductors, a debatable proposition not only because the abductors are at such a disadvantage but also because there is little functional need to possess large abduction strength in this extreme position. At 10° of hip adduction, on the other hand, these muscles must strongly operate at the most critical point in gait. The slightly adducted position corresponds generally to the position when the body is in its single-limb support phase of gait, the time when these muscles are maximally challenged to generate frontal plane stability across the hip. At this point in the gait cycle, the external (gravitational) *adduction* torque about a given hip dramatically increases within the frontal plane as the contralateral limb leaves the ground [61]. The hip abductors respond by generating an abduction torque about the stance hip that stabilizes the pelvis relative to the femur. This stabilization function of the abductor muscles during single-limb support is an essential component of normal and efficient gait. Because the pelvis on the swing limb drops slightly throughout most of the single-limb support phase of gait, the hip abductors are active *eccentrically* during most of their critical period of activation.

The force produced by the hip abductor muscles during the stance phase of gait accounts for most of the compressive force generated between the acetabulum and femoral head. Compression produced by the gluteus medius during stance phase is directed superiorly and slightly anterior-medially within the acetabulum [8]. This happens to be the area of the acetabulum covered with the thickest articular cartilage [62].

The importance of the hip abductors in the stance phase of walking can be well appreciated by understanding the simple mechanics of a seesaw (Fig. 5.10) [7, 63]. In Fig. 5.10, the moment arm (D) of right hip abductor force (HAF) is about half the length of the moment arm (D_1) associated with body weight (BW) [64]. This requires the hip abductors to produce a force about *twice* superincumbent body weight to achieve frontal plane stability while in unilateral stance. The acetabulum is pulled down against the femoral head not only by the force of the activated hip abductor muscles but also by the gravitational pull of body weight. As shown in Fig. 5.10, the sum of these two forces equals about 2.5 times full body weight. Note that some 2/3 of this joint force is created by the hip abductors. To achieve static equilibrium while standing on one limb, these generally downward-directed forces are counteracted by a joint reaction force (JRF in Fig. 5.10) of equal magnitude, but oriented in a direction nearly opposite to the muscle force. According to early classic work by Inman, the JRF is directed about 15° from vertical, at an angle strongly influenced by the lines-of-force of the hip abductors [65].

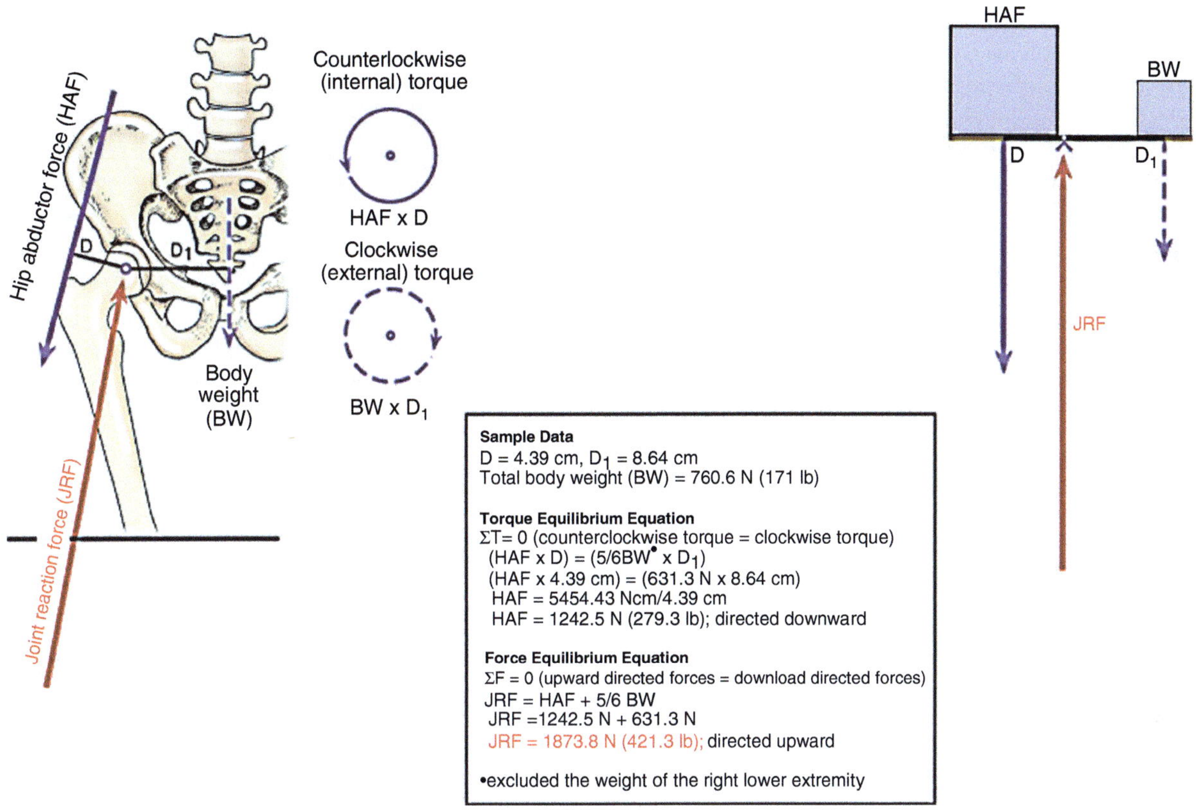

Fig. 5.10 A frontal plane diagram shows the hip abductor force (HAF) demands to stand on one limb only. The illustration on the left assumes that the pelvis and trunk are in static equilibrium about the right hip. The *counterclockwise* [*internal*] *torque* (*solid circle*) is the product of the HAF times its moment arm (D); the clockwise (*external*) *torque* (*dashed circle*) is the product of body weight (BW) times its moment arm (D_1). Because the system is assumed to be in equilibrium, the torques are equal in magnitude and opposite in direction: $HAF \times D = BW \times D_1$. The seesaw model (*right*) further simplifies the major kinetic events. A joint reaction force (JRF) is directed through the fulcrum of the seesaw (hip joint). The sample data in the box are used in the torque and force equilibrium equations. These equations allow an estimate of the approximate magnitude of the HAF and JRF needed to stand on one limb. To simplify the mathematics, the calculations assume that all forces are acting in a vertical direction. This assumption introduces modest error in the results. From Neumann DA: Kinesiology of the Musculoskeletal System: Foundations for Physical Rehabilitation, second edition, 2010. Reprinted with permission from Elsevier Limited

The logic described in Fig. 5.10 assumes a person is standing motionless on one limb. During the dynamic motions of gait, the JRF becomes higher than that estimated in Fig. 5.10 because ground reaction forces are higher and the abductors must decelerate pelvic rotation relative to the femoral head. Hip joint compression in fact reaches 3–5 times body weight in walking, attributable overwhelmingly to hip abductor activation [7, 66–68]. This joint force can increase to six times body weight in running or in ascent and descent of stairs [69].

In the healthy hip, the muscular-based compressive forces described above serve important physiologic functions, such as stabilizing the femoral head within the acetabulum and providing a stimulus for normal growth and ultimate shape of the hip in the growing child. Compression is usually well tolerated in most hips throughout a lifetime, thanks to damping characteristics inherent in healthy articular cartilage, congruent joint surfaces, and the yielding nature of trabecular bone.

Even though the fit of the healthy hip joint may appear relatively close and congruous on a roentgenogram, only about 35 % of the total acetabular cartilaginous surface makes contact with the femoral head during walking [70]. Consequently, the naturally large compression forces that cross the hip can potentially generate large joint *stress* (force per unit area). A hip with degenerative arthritis would likely have an acetabular cartilaginous contact area even less than 35 %, thereby potentially creating very large and damaging stress to the subchondral bone. Such a scenario can accelerate the overall degenerative process of hip osteoarthritis.

In an unstable, painful, or degenerating hip, reducing force generated by the hip abductors becomes paramount. Surgical and other therapeutic efforts typically take into account the rationale explained in Fig. 5.10. In surgery, for example, maintaining a long moment arm of the abductors would be important. An obese person with a painful hip would have a biomechanical reason to lose body weight. The reason for an antalgic ("Trendelenberg") gait might be better understood [60]. The biomechanics associated with Fig. 5.10

can further serve as a guide for many "joint protection" principles taught to patients to reduce hip joint forces while still allowing the performance of routine daily activities [71, 72]. For example, if a unilateral hand-held load (such as a weighted bucket) must be carried while walking, the load should be carried *ipsilateral* to the affected hip [73]. A cane can reduce abductor [and hence hip joint] forces when used in the hand *contralateral* to the affected hip [74, 75]. This can be made apparent in Fig. 5.10 if a cane force passing upward through the subject's *left* (contralateral) hand were added. The force of the cane would possess a sizable moment arm to produce a significant *counterclockwise* torque about the right (stance) hip. Since this cane-produced torque would act in the same rotary direction as that naturally produced by the right hip abductors to provide frontal plane support, torque from the contralateral cane would partially substitute for the abductor torque; with its long moment arm, a modest cane force can thus effectively reduce abductor activation and hence total JRF [76]. Measurements have shown that a "moderate and comfortable" cane force of 10 % of body weight reduces the EMG level of the hip abductor muscles by 31 % in persons during the stance phase of walking after a total hip replacement [75].

Following arthroscopic hip surgery, the status of the gluteus medius and other hip abductors is of both long-term and short-term concern. *In the long term*, persistent hip abductor weakness following hip arthroscopy can give rise to secondary problems. If postoperative exercises fail to elicit strong and functional hip abductor activity, walking becomes labored and inefficient due to poor control of frontal plane hip mechanics. Furthermore, weakened or poorly controlled hip abductors have been associated with excessive valgus loading on the knee [77–80], which may lead to further problems such as noncontact ACL injury or patellofemoral joint pain, particularly in females [51, 81–83]. *In the short term*, hip abductor activity can directly affect postoperative stresses on articular cartilage, labrum, capsule, proximal femur, etc. To help establish safe and effective protocols for the progression of hip abductor exercises, Philippon and colleagues used fine-wire EMG electrodes to record the activation levels of the gluteus medius in ten healthy subjects as they performed 13 common exercises [84]. Figure 5.11 shows a subset of the results of this study, highlighting the continuum of gluteus medius EMG activation [both peak and average magnitudes] across all exercises. The original paper provides additional valuable detail that cannot be adequately covered here. One important point is that the gluteus medius clearly participates strongly in movements other than hip abduction, such as resisted hip extension and the prone heel squeeze (hip external rotation). Also of clinical interest is the striking difference in demand placed on the gluteus medius (and underlying joint) for double and single-leg bridge exer-

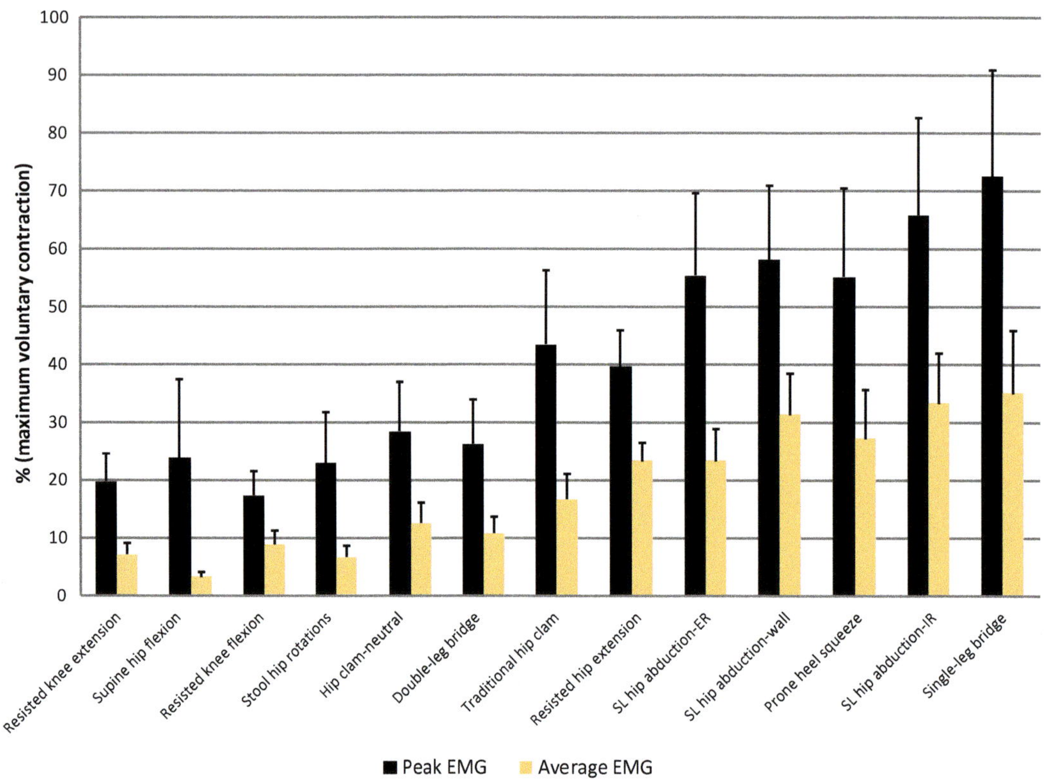

Fig. 5.11 Peak and average electromyography (EMG) amplitude (% maximum voluntary contraction) and standard errors from the gluteus medius during 13 hip rehabilitation exercises. Data from concentric contractions from ten healthy subjects. (*ER* external rotation, *ext* extension, *IR* internal rotation, *SL* sidelying). Data replotted from work of Philippon MJ et al. [9]

cises. The data set graphed in Fig. 5.11 was used in conjunction with other information to assign the 13 exercises to one of three phases of rehabilitation. This material can serve as a valuable guide for physicians and rehabilitation specialists who design postoperative exercise routines for the hip abductor muscles.

Closing Comments

Many muscles of the hip act in concert to control both the movement and stability of this important region of the body. The potential action of a single muscle can be understood by considering the muscle's line-of-force relative to the axes of rotation at the hip. Examples for each of the three cardinal planes of motion have been considered. Using a mechanical approach to assessing muscle function can help explain why the actions and torque potential of many hip muscles change based on the position of the hip. Understanding the kinematic and kinetic consequences of a hip muscle contraction both in and out of the anatomic position is an essential element in directing the course of rehabilitation following hip arthroscopy.

Acknowledgment The author wishes to thank Paul Andrew, Lauren Miller, Luke Garceau, and Martha Jerme for their careful review or other technical or research assistance in the preparation of this chapter.

References

1. Neumann DA. Kinesiology of the hip: a focus on muscular actions. J Orthop Sports Phys Ther. 2010;40:82–94.
2. Dostal WF, Andrews JG. A three-dimensional biomechanical model of hip musculature. J Biomech. 1981;14:803–12.
3. Dostal WF, Soderberg GL, Andrews JG. Actions of hip muscles. Phys Ther. 1986;66:351–61.
4. Brand RA, Crowninshield RD, Wittstock CE, Pedersen DR, Clark CR, van Krieken FM. A model of lower extremity muscular anatomy. J Biomech Eng. 1982;104:304–10.
5. Hoy MG, Zajac FE, Gordon ME. A musculoskeletal model of the human lower extremity: the effect of muscle, tendon, and moment arm on the moment-angle relationship of musculotendon actuators at the hip, knee, and ankle. J Biomech. 1990;23:157–69.
6. Pressel T, Lengsfeld M. Functions of hip joint muscles. Med Eng Phys. 1998;20(1):50–6.
7. Neumann DA. Kinesiology of the musculoskeletal system: foundations for physical rehabilitation. 2nd ed. St Louis: Elsevier; 2010.
8. Correa TA, Crossley KM, Kim HJ, Pandy MG. Contributions of individual muscles to hip joint contact force in normal walking. J Biomech. 2010;43(8):1618–22.
9. Park RJ, Tsao H, Cresswell AG, Hodges PW. Differential activity of regions of the psoas major and quadratus lumborum during submaximal isometric trunk efforts. J Orthop Res. 2012;30(2):311–8.
10. Hu H, Meijer OG, van Dieen JH, Hodges PW, Bruijn SM, Strijers RL, et al. Is the psoas a hip flexor in the active straight leg raise? Eur Spine J. 2011;20(5):759–65.
11. Blemker SS, Delp SL. Three-dimensional representation of complex muscle architectures and geometries. Ann Biomed Eng. 2005;33:661–73.
12. Neumann DA, Garceau LR. A proposed novel function of the psoas minor revealed through cadaver dissection. Clin Anat. 2015;28(2):243–52. doi:10.1002/ca.22467.
13. Contreras ME, Dani WS, Endges WK, De Araujo LC, Berral FJ. Arthroscopic treatment of the snapping iliopsoas tendon through the central compartment of the hip: a pilot study. J Bone Joint Surg Br. 2010;92(6):777–80.
14. Babst D, Steppacher SD, Ganz R, Siebenrock KA, Tannast M. The iliocapsularis muscle: an important stabilizer in the dysplastic hip. Clin Orthop Relat Res. 2011;469(6):1728–34.
15. Ward WT, Fleisch ID, Ganz R. Anatomy of the iliocapsularis muscle. Relevance to surgery of the hip. Clin Orthop Relat Res. 2000;374:278–85.
16. Tatu L, Parratte B, Vuillier F, Diop M, Monnier G. Descriptive anatomy of the femoral portion of the iliopsoas muscle. Anatomical basis of anterior snapping of the hip. Surg Radiol Anat. 2001; 23(6):371–4.
17. Blomberg JR, Zellner BS, Keene JS. Cross-sectional analysis of iliopsoas muscle-tendon units at the sites of arthroscopic tenotomies: an anatomic study. Am J Sports Med. 2011;39(Suppl):58S–63.
18. Dewberry MJ, Bohannon RW, Tiberio D, Murray R, Zannotti CM. Pelvic and femoral contributions to bilateral hip flexion by subjects suspended from a bar. Clin Biomech. 2003;18:494–9.
19. Hodges PW, Eriksson AE, Shirley D, Gandevia SC. Intra-abdominal pressure increases stiffness of the lumbar spine. J Biomech. 2005;38:1873–80.
20. Urquhart DM, Hodges PW, Story IH. Postural activity of the abdominal muscles varies between regions of these muscles and between body positions. Gait Posture. 2005;22:295–301.
21. Cahalan TD, Johnson ME, Liu S, Chao EY. Quantitative measurements of hip strength in different age groups. Clin Orthop Relat Res. 1989;246:136–45.
22. Magalhaes E, Fukuda TY, Sacramento SN, Forgas A, Cohen M, Abdalla RJ. A comparison of hip strength between sedentary females with and without patellofemoral pain syndrome. J Orthop Sports Phys Ther. 2010;40(10):641–7.
23. Winter DA. Biomechanics and motor control of human movement. Hoboken: Wiley; 2005.
24. Arnold AS, Delp SL. Rotational moment arms of the medial hamstrings and adductors vary with femoral geometry and limb position: implications for the treatment of internally rotated gait. J Biomech. 2001;34:437–47.
25. Samuel D, Rowe PJ. Effect of ageing on isometric strength through joint range at knee and hip joints in three age groups of older adults. Gerontology. 2009;55(6):621–9.
26. Dixon MC, Scott RD, Schai PA, Stamos V. A simple capsulorrhaphy in a posterior approach for total hip arthroplasty. J Arthroplasty. 2004;19:373–6.
27. Khan RJ, Yao F, Li M, Nivbrant B, Wood D. Capsular-enhanced repair of the short external rotators after total hip arthroplasty. J Arthroplasty. 2007;22:840–3.
28. Mihalko WM, Whiteside LA. Hip mechanics after posterior structure repair in total hip arthroplasty. Clin Orthop Relat Res. 2004;(420):194–8.
29. White RE, Jr, Forness TJ, Allman JK, Junick DW. Effect of posterior capsular repair on early dislocation in primary total hip replacement. Clin Orthop Relat Res. 2001;(393):163–7.
30. Pine J, Binns M, Wright P, Soames R. Piriformis and obturator internus morphology: a cadaveric study. Clin Anat. 2011; 24(1):70–6.
31. Solomon LB, Lee YC, Callary SA, Beck M, Howie DW. Anatomy of piriformis, obturator internus and obturator externus: implications

for the posterior surgical approach to the hip. J Bone Joint Surg Br. 2010;92(9):1317–24.
32. Delp SL, Hess WE, Hungerford DS, Jones LC. Variation of rotation moment arms with hip flexion. J Biomech. 1999;32:493–501.
33. Kendall FP, McCreary AK, Provance PG. Muscles: testing and function. 4th ed. Baltimore: Williams & Wilkins; 1993.
34. Stahelin T, Drittenbass L, Hersche O et al. Failure of capsular enhanced short external rotator repair after total hip replacement. Clin Orthop Relat Res. 2004;(420):199–204.
35. Mansour JM, Pereira JM. Quantitative functional anatomy of the lower limb with application to human gait. J Biomech. 1987;20:51–8.
36. Jarvis DK. Relative strength of the hip internal rotator muscles. Phys Ther Rev. 1952;32:500–3.
37. Johnson S, Hoffman M. Isometric hip-rotator torque production at varying degrees of hip flexion. J Sport Rehab. 2010;19(1):12–20.
38. Lindsay DM, Maitland ME, Lowe RC. Comparison of isokinetic internal and external hip rotation torques using different testing positions. J Orthop Sports Phys Ther. 1992;16:43–50.
39. Hicks JL, Schwartz MH, Arnold AS, Delp SL. Crouched postures reduce the capacity of muscles to extend the hip and knee during the single-limb stance phase of gait. J Biomech. 2008;41:960–7.
40. Arnold AS, Asakawa DJ, Delp SL. Do the hamstrings and adductors contribute to excessive internal rotation of the hip in persons with cerebral palsy? Gait Posture. 2000;11:181–90.
41. Arnold AS, Anderson FC, Pandy MG, Delp SL. Muscular contributions to hip and knee extension during the single limb stance phase of normal gait: a framework for investigating the causes of crouch gait. J Biomech. 2005;38:2181–9.
42. Baldon RM, Lobato DF, Carvalho LP, Santiago PR, Benze BG, Serrao FV. Relationship between eccentric hip torque and lower-limb kinematics: gender differences. J App Biomech. 2011;27(3):223–32.
43. Fukuda TY, Melo WP, Zaffalon BM, Rossetto FM, Magalhaes E, Bryk FF, et al. Hip posterolateral musculature strengthening in sedentary women with patellofemoral pain syndrome: a randomized controlled clinical trial with 1-year follow-up. J Orthop Sports Phys Ther. 2012;42(10):823–30.
44. Lawrence III RK, Kernozek TW, Miller EJ, Torry MR, Reuteman P. Influences of hip external rotation strength on knee mechanics during single-leg drop landings in females. Clin Biomech. 2008;23(6):806–13.
45. Noehren B, Pohl MB, Sanchez Z, Cunningham T, Lattermann C. Proximal and distal kinematics in female runners with patellofemoral pain. Clin Biomech. 2012;27(4):366–71.
46. Souza RB, Powers CM. Differences in hip kinematics, muscle strength, and muscle activation between subjects with and without patellofemoral pain. J Orthop Sports Phys Ther. 2009;39(1):12–9.
47. Willson JD, Davis IS. Lower extremity mechanics of females with and without patellofemoral pain across activities with progressively greater task demands. Clin Biomech. 2008;23:203–11.
48. Powers CM, Ward SR, Fredericson M, Guillet M, Shellock FG. Patellofemoral kinematics during weight-bearing and non-weight-bearing knee extension in persons with lateral subluxation of the patella: a preliminary study. J Orthop Sports Phys Ther. 2003;33(11):677–85.
49. Murray MP, Sepic SB. Maximum isometric torque of hip abductor and adductor muscles. Phys Ther. 1968;48(12):1327–35.
50. Thorborg K, Serner A, Petersen J, Madsen TM, Magnusson P, Holmich P. Hip adduction and abduction strength profiles in elite soccer players: implications for clinical evaluation of hip adductor muscle recovery after injury. Am J Sports Med. 2011;39(1):121–6.
51. Brophy RH, Backus S, Kraszewski AP, Steele BC, Ma Y, Osei D, et al. Differences between sexes in lower extremity alignment and muscle activation during soccer kick. J Bone Joint Surg Am. 2010;92(11):2050–8.
52. Nemeth G, Ohlsen H. Moment arms of the hip abductor and adductor muscles measured in vivo by computed tomography. Clin Biomech. 1989;4:133–6.
53. Arnold AS, Salinas S, Asakawa DJ, et al. Accuracy of muscle moment arms estimated from MRI-based musculoskeletal models of the lower extremity. Comput Aided Surg. 2000;5:108–19.
54. Lengsfeld M, Pressel T, Stammberger U. Lengths and lever arms of hip joint muscles: geometrical analyses using a human multibody model. Gait Posture. 1997;6:18–26.
55. Clark JM, Haynor DR. Anatomy of the abductor muscles of the hip as studied by computed tomography. J Bone Joint Surg Am. 1987;69:1021–31.
56. Hoffmann A, Pfirrmann CWA. The hip abductors at MI Imaging. Eur J Radio. 2010. doi:10.1016/j.ejrad.2010.03.002.
57. Soderberg GL, Dostal WF. Electromyographic study of three parts of the gluteus medius muscle during functional activities. Phys Ther. 1978;58:691–6.
58. Beck M, Sledge JB, Gautier E, Dora CF, Ganz R. The anatomy and function of the gluteus minimus muscle. J Bone Joint Surg Br. 2000;82:358–63.
59. Walters J, Solomons M, Davies J. Gluteus minimus: observations on its insertion. J Anat. 2001;198:239–42.
60. Neumann DA. Biomechanical analysis of selected principles of hip joint protection. Arthritis Care Res. 1989;2:146–55.
61. Hurwitz DE, Foucher KC, Andriacchi TP. A new parametric approach for modeling hip forces during gait. J Biomech. 2003;36:113–9.
62. Kurrat HJ, Oberlander W. The thickness of the cartilage in the hip joint. J Anat. 1978;126(1):145–55.
63. Debevec H, Pedersen DR, Iglic A, Daniel M. One-legged stance as a representative static body position for calculation of hip contact stress distribution in clinical studies. J Appl Biomech. 2010; 26(4):522–5.
64. Neumann DA, Soderberg GL, Cook TM. Comparison of maximal isometric hip torques between hip sides. Phys Ther. 1988;68: 496–502.
65. Inman VT. Functional aspects of the abductor muscles of the hip. J Bone Joint Surg Am. 1947;29:607–19.
66. Bergmann G, Graichen F, Rohlmann A. Hip joint loading during walking and running, measured in two patients. J Biomech. 1993;26:969–90.
67. Fraysse F, Dumas R, Cheze L, Wang X. Comparison of global and joint-to-joint methods for estimating the hip joint load and the muscle forces during walking. J Biomech. 2009;42(14):2357–62.
68. Hodge WA, Carlson KL, Fijan RS, Burgess RG, Riley PO, Harris WH, et al. Contact pressures from an instrumented hip endoprosthesis. J Bone Joint Surg Am. 1989;71:1378–86.
69. Stansfield BW, Nicol AC. Hip joint contact forces in normal subjects and subjects with total hip prostheses: walking and stair and ramp negotiation. Clin Biomech. 2002;17:130–9.
70. Harris MD, Anderson AE, Henak CR, Ellis BJ, Peters CL, Weiss JA. Finite element prediction of cartilage contact stresses in normal human hips. J Orthop Res. 2012;30(7):1133–9.
71. Krebs DE, Elbaum L, Riley PO, Hodge WA. Exercise and gait effects on in vivo hip contact pressures. Phys Ther. 1991; 71:301–9.
72. Neumann DA. An electromyographic study of the hip abductor muscles as subjects with a hip prosthesis walked with different methods of using a cane and carrying a load. Phys Ther. 1999; 79:1163–73.
73. Neumann DA. Hip abductor muscle activity in persons with a hip prosthesis while carrying loads in one hand. Phys Ther. 1996; 76:1320–30.

74. McGibbon CA, Krebs DE, Mann RW. In vivo hip pressures during cane and load-carrying gait. Arthritis Care Res. 1997;10(5):300–7.
75. Neumann DA. Hip abductor muscle activity as subjects with hip prostheses walk with different methods of using a cane. Phys Ther. 1998;78:490–501.
76. Ajemian S, Thon D, Clare P, Kaul L, Zernicke RF, Loitz-Ramage B. Cane-assisted gait biomechanics and electromyography after total hip arthroplasty. Arch Phys Med Rehabil. 2004;85:1966–71.
77. Claiborne TL, Armstrong CW, Gandhi V, Pincivero DM. Relationship between hip and knee strength and knee valgus during a single leg squat. J Appl Biomech. 2006;22:41–50.
78. Ford KR, Myer GD, Smith RL, Vianello RM, Seiwert SL, Hewett TE. A comparison of dynamic coronal plane excursion between matched male and female athletes when performing single leg landings. Clin Biomech. 2006;21:33–40.
79. Geiser CF, O'Connor KM, Earl JE. The effects of isolated hip abductor fatigue on frontal plane knee mechanics. Med Sci Sports Exerc. 2010;42:535–45.
80. Prins MR, van der Wurff P. Females with patellofemoral pain syndrome have weak hip muscles: a systematic review. Aust J Physiother. 2009;55:9–15.
81. Alentorn-Geli E, Myer GD, Silvers HJ, Samitier G, Romero D, Lazaro-Haro C, et al. Prevention of non-contact anterior cruciate ligament injuries in soccer players. Part 1: mechanisms of injury and underlying risk factors. Knee Surg Sports Traumatol Arthrosc. 2009;17:705–29.
82. Bolgla LA, Malone TR, Umberger BR, Uhl TL. Hip strength and hip and knee kinematics during stair descent in females with and without patellofemoral pain syndrome. J Orthop Sports Phys Ther. 2008;38:12–8.
83. Hewett TE, Myer GD, Ford KR, Heidt Jr RS, Colosimo AJ, McLean SG, et al. Biomechanical measures of neuromuscular control and valgus loading of the knee predict anterior cruciate ligament injury risk in female athletes: a prospective study. Am J Sports Med. 2005;33:492–501.
84. Philippon MJ, Decker MJ, Giphart JE, Torry MR, Wahoff MS, LaPrade RF. Rehabilitation exercise progression for the gluteus medius muscle with consideration for iliopsoas tendinitis: an in vivo electromyography study. Am J Sports Med. 2011; 39(8):1777–85.

Ligamentum Teres: Anatomy, Structure and Function

6

Alexandra Dimitrakopoulou and Richard N. Villar

Introduction

The ligamentum capitis femoris, generally called the ligamentum teres or round ligament, is well recognised as a source of hip pain [1, 2]. The awareness of ligamentum pathology has increased in recent years, alongside improvements in surgical techniques and imaging modalities. Yet its contribution to the role in the anatomy, biomechanics and mechanism of injury is not well known and remains debatable.

Anatomy and Embryology

The ligamentum teres develops when the embryo is aged 55–60 days with a crown-rump length of 20–25 mm. The ligament appears as an area of increased density within the region of the interzone, the position it will occupy in the fully formed joint. It consists of primitive fibroblasts cells with ovoid nuclei that merge with those of the transverse ligament inferiorly. The ligament increases in length and width and becomes more adducted as the femur grows [3]. During the last 4 months of intrauterine life, the composition of the ligament changes from a predominantly cellular structure to mature fibrous tissue.

The ligamentum teres is a flat, pyramidal band of fibres that arises from the posteroinferior margin of the acetabular fossa, blends with the transverse ligament and is attached posteroinferiorly to the centre of the femoral head (fovea capitis). The acetabular attachment consists of two bundles of fibres that gently transitions into a round ligament as it approaches and inserts into the fovea capitis.

A tubular sheath of synovium surrounds the ligament, which also enfolds an anterior branch of the obturator artery to the femoral head and adipose tissue. The synovium broadens across the floor of the acetabular fossa and extends under the transverse ligament [4]. Therefore, the ligament is considered as extrasynovial although it is intracapsular (Fig. 6.1). Its overall length in the adult is 30–35 mm. Walker [5] found, after dissecting 140 normal human foetuses between 12 weeks and term, that the shape of the ligament was variable; the predominant shape was that of a linear structure with length exceeding width. He noticed that the length of the ligamentum teres was the fastest-growing variable of hip joint development during the foetal period, increasing five-fold from 12 weeks to term. Also with increasing age, the ligament becomes a more robust structure. From imaging measurements [6], the average width of the intact ligamentum teres was 4.38 mm in its proximal third, 3.5 mm in the middle third and 2.7 mm distally. The overall length was 27.7 mm. It was most common for the ligamentum to have two bundles in its proximal portion.

Meanwhile, in developmental dysplasia of the hip (DDH), the ligamentum teres has been described as elongated and hypertrophied [7].

Histology and Structure

The ligamentum is composed of thick, well-organised, parallel fibres of types I, III and V collagen. Immunohistochemical analysis of the ligamentum has revealed free nerve endings (type IVa) for transmitting information about pain and inflammation (Fig. 6.2); it also has a possible role in nociception and proprioception of the hip [8]. Quantitative measurements on the incidence of free nerve endings have shown that there is no correlation with age [8]. Because of its special structure, a giant-cell tumour of the ligamentum has been described [9].

A. Dimitrakopoulou, MD
The London Hip Arthroscopy Center, Orthopaedics, The Wellington Hospital and Leeds Metropolitan University, Wellington Place, St. Johns Wood, London NW8 9LE, UK
e-mail: alexdimitr@yahoo.gr

R.N. Villar, MS, FRCS (✉)
Villar Bajwa Practice, Spire Cambridge Lea Hospital, 30 New Road, Impington, Cambridge CB24 9EL, UK
e-mail: rnv1000@aol.com

J.C. McCarthy et al. (eds.), *Hip Joint Restoration*, DOI 10.1007/978-1-4614-0694-5_6

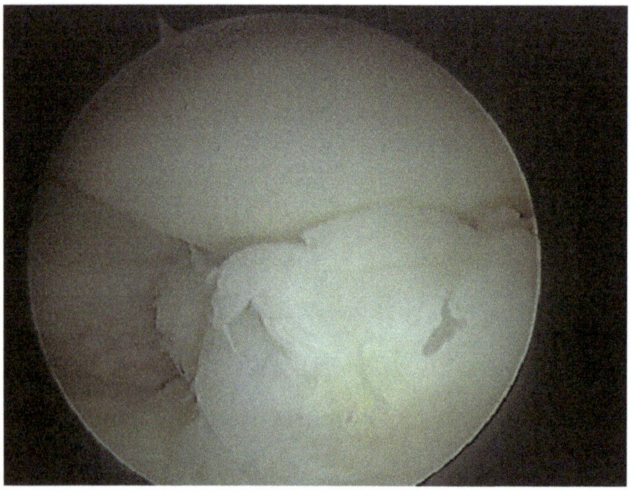

Fig. 6.1 Ganglion of the ligamentum teres

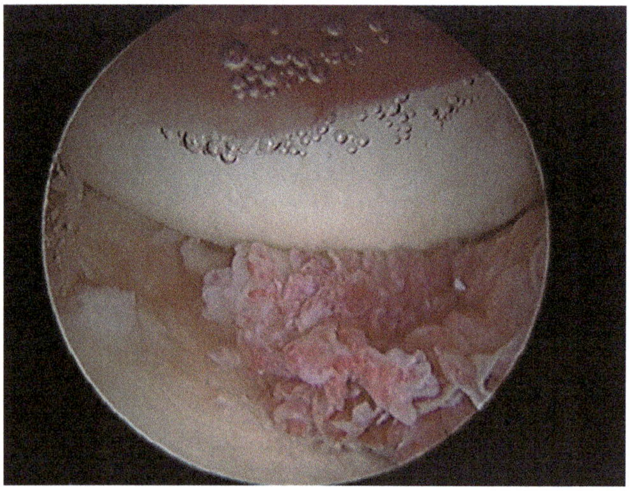

Fig. 6.2 Synovitis in cotyloid fossa

The Function and Role of the Ligamentum Teres

The exact function of the ligamentum teres remains unknown. Traditionally, it is believed to be a vestigial remnant with no important biomechanical function and an ambiguous vascular contribution. However, recently more studies have attempted to clarify its role.

It certainly provides a vascular supply, which contributes to the vascularisation of the femoral head proximally. It has also been proposed that the ligamentum may act as a "windshield wiper," spreading the synovial fluid into the joint during movements [1].

The ligamentum teres is tense in adduction, flexion and external rotation (Fig. 6.3) but lax in abduction and flexion [10]. Walker [5] tested the mobility of the hip in foetuses,

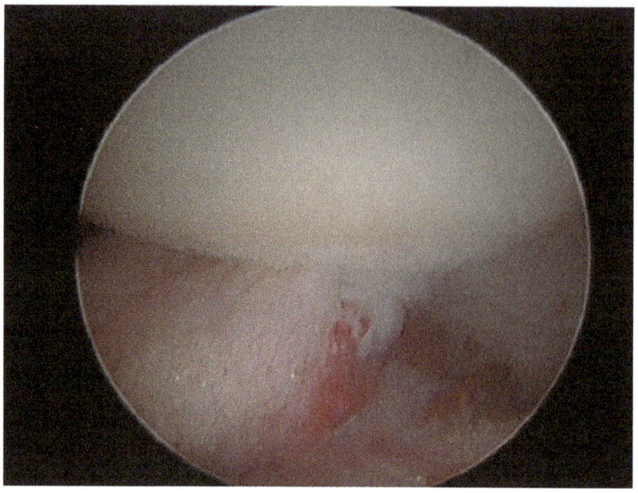

Fig. 6.3 Arthroscopic image showing the ligamentum teres to be tense with the leg in adduction, flexion and external rotation

and he found that the length of the ligamentum did not permit the femoral head to be displaced beyond the posterior rim of the acetabulum. Maximum movement of the ligamentum occurred in flexion, adduction and external rotation of the hip. Martin et al. [11] investigated the role of the ligamentum in hip stability using a biomechanical model. They found that external rotation in 90° flexion (squatting position) and internal rotation in 20° extension (crossing one leg behind the other while standing) placed the ligamentum under the greatest tension. They suggested that it may play a role in hip stability in individuals with inferior acetabular insufficiency when squatting or when crossing the legs while standing.

Kivlan et al. [12] tested the function of the ligamentum during simulated squatting in human cadavers. They concluded that the ligamentum teres functions as a sling, preventing the femoral head from inferior subluxation during flexion and abduction. It may also provide stability to the hip joint when the capsuloligamentous structures are insufficient [12]. It may serve as a co-stabiliser in extension while the capsular ligaments are under tension and as the primary stabiliser in flexion and external rotation when these ligaments are lax [11]. In relation to the femoral head, the ligamentum is found to limit movement in hip abduction, adduction and internal and external rotation and acts as a ball and string model [13].

The preservation and transfer of the ligamentum teres to act as a stabiliser in paediatric hip dislocation and redislocation after open surgical reduction appeared to provide additional stability and prevented a repeat dislocation [14].

The senior author has encountered many patients with ligamentum teres pathology after major trauma, sporting activities, dysplasia and femoroacetabular impingement while lifting a heavy object or even shopping. The mechanism of injury to the majority of the patients was while the extended hip was externally rotated. The ligament tightens in this position and it is placed at risk. It is very possible that acts as a sling and provides stability to the hip joint when the capsuloligamentous structures are lax as very often seen in dysplastic hips and ballet dancers.

Conclusion

The awareness of ligamentum teres role has increased in recent years due to advances in hip arthroscopy. It is well recognised as a persistent source of hip pain and mechanical symptoms. It contributes to the vascularisation of the femoral head proximally and provides proprioception and possible nociception senses. It is considered a strong structure as a result of its collagen-type fibres and has been demonstrated to play a role in hip stability acting as a sling when osseous deficiency (inferior acetabular insufficiency, dysplasia) or ligamentous instability (ligamentous laxity) is present.

Yet our knowledge is still limited and more studies on the anatomy, biomechanics and mechanism of injury should be undertaken.

References

1. Bardakos NV, Villar RN. The ligamentum teres of the adult hip. J Bone Joint Surg Br. 2009;91-B:8–15.
2. Byrd JWT, Jones KS. Traumatic rupture of the ligamentum teres as a source of hip pain. Arthroscopy. 2004;20:385–91.
3. Rooker GD. The embryological congruity of the human hip joint. Ann R Coll Surg Engl. 1979;6:357–61.
4. Villar RN, Santori N. Arthroscopic anatomy of the hip. In: Byrd TJW, editor. Operative hip arthroscopy. 2nd ed. New York: Springer; 2005. p. 117–28.
5. Walker JM. Growth characteristics of the fatal ligament of the head of femur: significance in congenital hip disease. Yale J Biol Med. 1980;53:307–16.
6. Blankenbaker DG, De Smet AA, Keene JS, Munoz del Rio A. Imaging appearance of the normal and partially torn ligamentum teres on hip MR arthrography. AJR Am J Roentgenol. 2012; 199:1093–8.
7. Byrd JWT, Jones KS. Hip arthroscopy in the presence of dysplasia. Arthroscopy. 2003;19:1055–60.
8. Leunig M, Beck M, Stauffer E, Hertel R, Ganz R. Free nerve endings in the ligamentum capitis femoris. Acta Orthop Scand. 2000;71:452–4.
9. Singh PJ, Constable L, O'Donnell J. Arthroscopic excision of a giant-cell tumour of the ligamentum teres. J Bone Joint Surg Br. 2009;91-B:809–11.
10. Gray AJ, Villar RN. The ligamentum teres of the hip: an arthroscopic classification of its pathology. Arthroscopy. 1997;13:575–8.
11. Martin RL, Palmer I, Martin HD. Ligamentum teres: a functional description and potential clinical relevance. Knee Surg Sports Traumatol Arthrosc. 2012;20:1209–14.
12. Kivlan BR, Clemente FR, Martin RL, Martin HD. Function of the ligamentum teres during multi-planar movement of the hip joint. Knee Surg Sports Traumatol Arthrosc. 2013;21(7):1664–8.
13. Martin RL, Kivlan BR, Clemente FR. A cadaveric model for ligamentum teres function: a pilot study. Knee Surg Sports Traumatol Arthrosc. 2013;21(7):1689–93.
14. Wenger DR, Mubarak SJ, Henderson PC, Miyanji F. Ligamentum teres maintenance and transfer as a stabilizer in open reduction for pediatric hip dislocation: surgical technique and early clinical results. J Child Orthop. 2008;2:177–85.

Functional Mechanics of the Human Hip

7

Philip C. Noble, Maureen K. Dwyer,
Mohammed S. Gobba, and Joshua D. Harris

Introduction

The hip joint provides an articulation that allows relative angulation between the upper body and the lower limbs. This is critical for achieving both an upright posture and normal ambulation. Most of the weight of the body is supported by the hip joint, especially in single leg support, and the muscles controlling the hip act relatively close to the center of the joint. Thus, the forces acting on the femoral head and the acetabulum are considerable and have significant consequences in terms of skeletal health and musculoskeletal function [1, 2]. Over the last hundred years, this has led to the emergence of a formal field of study, Musculoskeletal Biomechanics, which has made valuable contributions to our understanding of the hip. These have included new methods for evaluating joint function and understanding pathologic conditions, alternative surgical approaches for hip preservation and reconstruction, and the development of methods for measuring joint forces and moments developed in vivo. The application of scientific principles to the study of the hip has also provided insight into morphologic factors compromising hip motion, including acquired abnormalities (e.g., post-traumatic deformities, Perthes disease, slipped capital femoral epiphysis [SCFE]), developmental pathologies (e.g., congenital dislocation of the hip [CDH] and developmental dysplasia of the hip [DDH]), and abnormalities of unknown origin (e.g., cam deformity of the femoral head-neck junction and pincer deformities of the acetabular margin). Ongoing investigations of the biomechanics of the capsule, labrum, and femoroacetabular impingement (FAI) should further reduce the proportion of patients that are labeled as having "idiopathic" coxarthrosis.

Much of our recent knowledge derived from clinical and radiographic studies has confirmed that hip symptoms and even joint degeneration are not automatically predestined by abnormalities of anatomy or bony morphology [3–6]. Indeed, detailed analysis of cadaveric specimens confirms that dysmorphic conditions and soft tissue lesions are far more common than symptomatic impairment of hip function [7–9]. This observation leads us to study the interaction between the demands that function places on the hip, whether through sport, vocation, or lifestyle, and the capacity of the joint to function asymptomatically. In this chapter we will discuss the external demands placed upon the hip during function and the mechanisms for dissipating the loads developed across the joint, in both the normal joint and in the presence of structural and pathological abnormalities.

Forces Acting Across the Hip Joint

During functional activities, the magnitude and direction of the contact force developed between the head of the femur and the weight-bearing surface of the acetabulum is primar-

P.C. Noble, PhD (✉)
Director of Research, Institute of Orthopedic Research and Education, 6550 Fannin Street, Suite 2501, Houston, TX 77030, USA

Director of Research, Institute of Orthopedic Research and Education, Houston, TX 77030, USA
e-mail: pnoble@bcm.edu

M.K. Dwyer, PhD, ATC
Department of Orthopedics, Kaplan Joint Center, Newton Wellesley Hospital, 2014 Washington Street, Suite 361, Newton, MA 02462, USA

Department of Orthopedics, Massachusetts General Hospital, Boston, MA, USA
e-mail: mkdwyer@partners.org

M.S. Gobba, MD
Department of Orthopedics and Traumatology, Cairo University, Cairo, Egypt
e-mail: msgobba@houstonmethodist.org

J.D. Harris, MD
Department of Orthopedics and Sports Medicine, Houston Methodist Hospital, 6550 Fannin Street, Suite 2500, Houston, TX 77030, USA

Weill Cornell Medical College, Houston, TX, USA
e-mail: Jharris6@houstonmethodist.org

J.C. McCarthy et al. (eds.), *Hip Joint Restoration*, DOI 10.1007/978-1-4614-0694-5_7

ily dictated by the muscle forces needed to stabilize the hip and generate motion. Data collected using instrumented hip prostheses show that hip joint forces vary extensively, ranging from 2.1 to 4.3 times body weight (BW) during gait [10–13] and 2.3–5.5 BW during stair-climbing [10–12], to values in excess of 8 BW during accidental incidents of stumbling (Figs. 7.1 and 7.2) (Table 7.1) [11, 14].

The net (resultant) force applied to the head of the femur is directed both laterally and inferiorly during the stance phase of the gait cycle and changes direction from posterior at heel strike to anterior at toe off. Although the predominant component of the joint reaction force is directed down the shaft of the femur during gait, with peak values ranging from 1.4 to 4.1 BW, substantial forces are also observed in both the mediolateral (0.4–1.7 BW) and anterior-posterior directions (0.2–1.0 BW), especially at points of greatest flexion during the gait cycle or during the transitions between single- and double-limb support. The torsional and shear forces

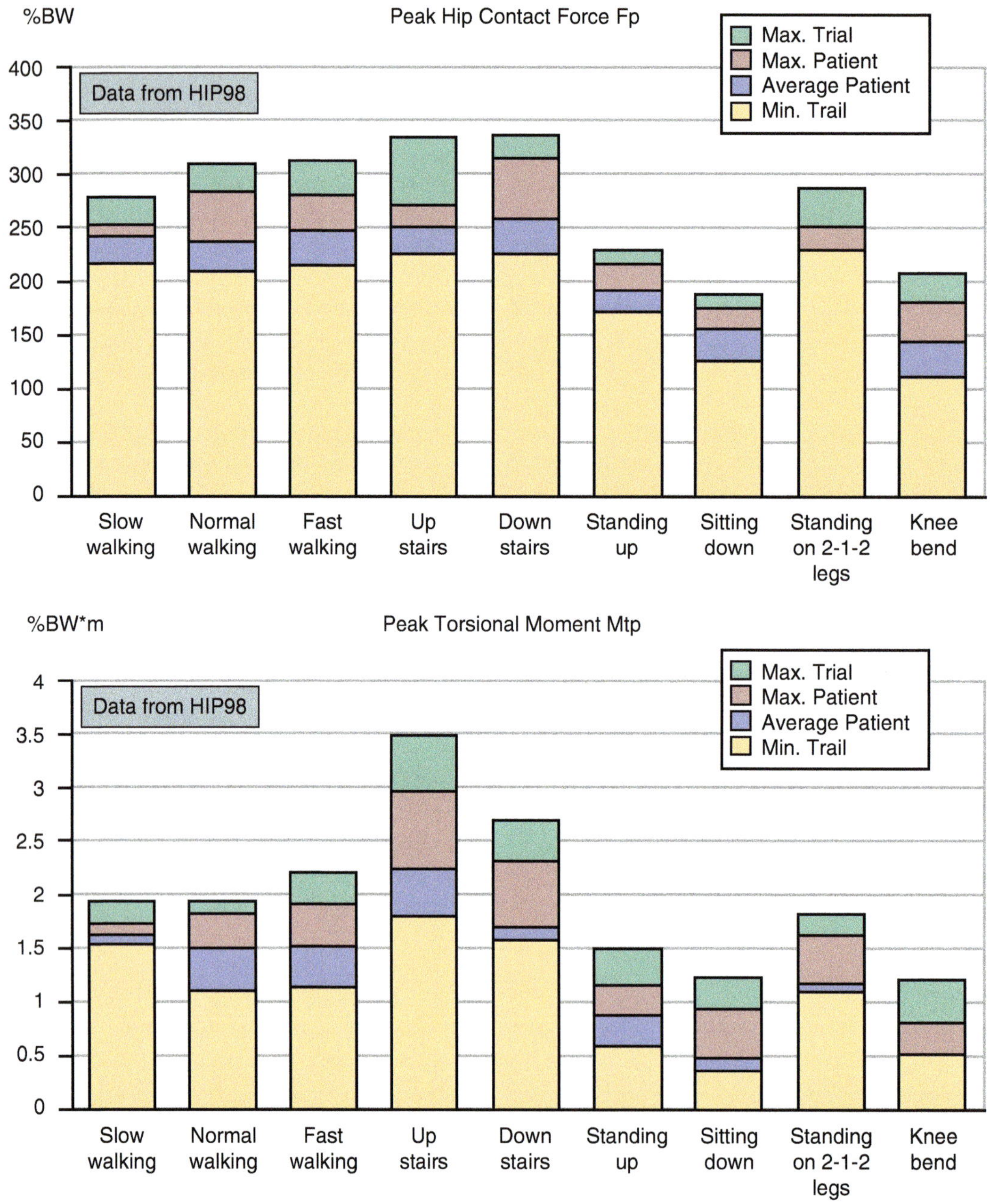

Fig. 7.1 Hip contact force data (*top*) and torsional moments (*bottom*) for a range of nine different activities recorded using instrumented hip prostheses. Hip forces are plotted in units of percentage of body weight (%BW), while moments are plotted in units of %BW × height of each subject in meters [%BW.m]. From Stal et al., Biomechanics of the Natural Hip Joint, In: Surgery of the Hip, D.J. Berry and J.R. Lieberman, eds. Volume 2. 2013, pp 5–13. Copyright Elsevier 2013, reprinted with permission

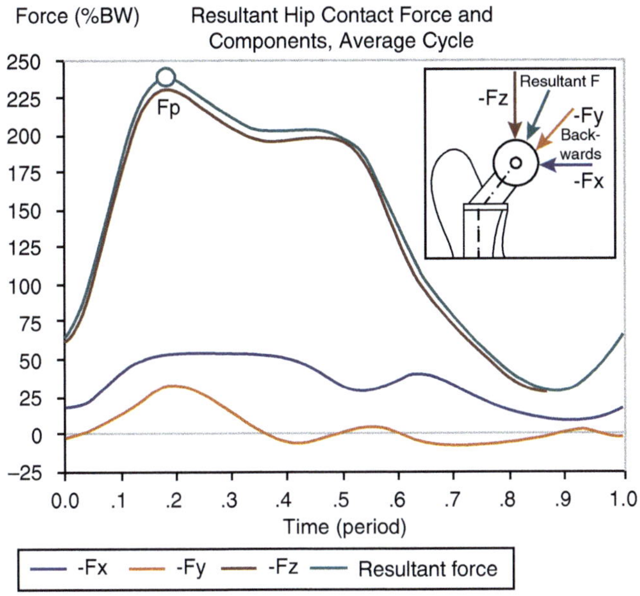

Fig. 7.2 Typical variation in the hip contact force and its components during an average gait cycle, commencing with heel strike. From Stal et al., Biomechanics of the Natural Hip Joint, In: Surgery of the Hip, D.J. Berry and J.R. Lieberman, eds. Volume 2. 2013, pp 5–13. Copyright Elsevier 2013, reprinted with permission

Table 7.1 Summary of values of the peak joint reaction force reported by Bergmann and coworkers during different investigations using instrumented hip prostheses

Activity	Typical peak force (BW)	Number of patients	Months post-op	References
Walking, slow	1.6–4.1	9	1–30	[10, 11]
Walking, normal	2.1–3.3	6	1–31	[10]
Walking, fast	1.8–4.3	7	2–30	[10, 11]
Jogging/running	4.3–5.0	2	6–30	[10, 11, 21]
Ascending stairs	1.5–5.5	8	6–33	[11]
Descending stairs	1.6–5.1	7	6–30	[11]
Standing up	1.8–2.2	4	11–31	[10]
Sitting down	1.5–2.0	4	11–31	[10]
Standing/2-1-1 legs	2.2–3.7	3	11–14	[10]
Knee bend	1.2–1.8	3	11–14	[10]
Stumbling	7.2–8.7	2	4–18	[12]

generated within the proximal femur during many routine functional activities are also significant and vary with activity [11–13, 15, 16]. For example, during stair-climbing the anterior-posterior component of the joint force reaches 20–25 % of the frontal plane load [12], whereas, the peak twisting moment and first peak contact force are decreased by 18 % and 14 %, respectively [16]. In contrast, the axial torques recorded during descending stairs and walking are of similar magnitude [11, 12, 17].

The magnitude of the joint reaction force and its direction with respect to the skeleton is affected by numerous factors, including the specific activity, the age, gender, height, body weight and gait velocity of the individual subject [17–21], and environmental factors such as the nature of any footwear and the surface upon which the activity is performed [22, 23]. In this chapter we will present a summary of the latest information on the mechanical environment of the hip joint, the kinematics of the joint during normal function, the role of tissues controlling joint motion, and the mechanics of pathological conditions, such as FAI, hip dysplasia, and chronic hip laxity.

Load Transfer Across the Hip Joint

The congruency of the joint surfaces allows for more even distribution of contact forces during loading [24, 25]. Under light loads, contact between the joint surfaces is limited to the anterior and posterior lunate surfaces. Increasing load results in a greater contact which extends to the superior, anterior, and posterior regions of the joint [25, 26]. Studies have shown that the area of joint contact varies greatly between individuals and changes in response to joint angle and load [24–26]. During gait, contact area is least during flexion when the joint load is low, as observed during terminal swing and heel strike. The area of joint contact increases as the hip moves through the stance phase of gait, peaking at terminal extension [24]. Maximum acetabular pressures of 3.3 MPa occur during midstance of gait and are located on the superior and posterior lateral roof. Activities which require higher ranges of motion reduce the amount of contact area and result in greater acetabular pressures. The greatest pressures occur during standing and sitting where pressures of 9–15 MPa have been recorded over the apex of the femoral head and the superior and posterior aspects of the acetabulum, which are sites of degenerative changes commonly reported in cadaveric studies [26, 27].

The Kinematics of the Normal Hip

The hip joint is a multiaxial joint formed by the articulation between the concave acetabulum and convex femoral head. Despite its sturdy joint capsule which limits extreme motion and prevents frank dislocation, the hip joint allows a great deal of mobility [28]. Joint motion is greatest in the sagittal plane, as the femur flexes and extends around a left-right axis [29]. Active hip flexion is greatest with the knee flexed (110°–120°) rather than extended (90°), due to the effects of hamstring tension [2, 29–31]. For Caucasian populations, typical values for single-plane motions are 120° for flexion, 20° for extension, 45° for abduction, 30° for adduction, and 40° for internal and external rotation [32–35] (Tables 7.2 and 7.3). In non-Western subjects accustomed to squatting for

Table 7.2 Difference in mean active range of motion (in degrees) for ages 25–39 years compared with ages 60–74 years by sex-race groups

Motion	All subjects	White men	White women	Black men	Black women
Hip flexion					
Ages 25–39 years	122°	123°	123°	115°	116°
Ages 60–74 years	118°	118°	119°	118°	106°
Hip extension					
Ages 25–39 years	22°	22°	22°	19°	17°
Ages 60–74 years	17°	17°	16°	16°	12°
Hip abduction					
Ages 25–39 years	44°	46°	44°	41°	38°
Ages 60–74 years	39°	39°	40°	38°	37°
Hip internal rotation					
Ages 25–39 years	33°	34°	33°	32°	27°
Ages 60–74 years	30°	31°	29°	27°	25°
Hip external rotation					
Ages 25–39 years	34°	33°	36°	32°	32°
Ages 60–74 years	29°	27°	32°	27°	28°

From Roach et al. [34]

Table 7.3 Range of motion of the hip during functional activities

Motion	Squatting (heels down)	Squatting (heels up)	Kneeling (dorsiflexed)	Kneeling (plantar-flexed)	Sitting cross-legged
Flexion	95.4±26.2	91.3±17.1	73.9±29.4	58.8±9.7	85.4±34.2
Abduction	28.2±13.9	31.7±11.2	25.3±15.3	27.6±12.5	36.5±15
External rotation	25.7±11.8	33.7±12.7	28.1±12.8	34±14.9	40.3±18.4

All values are expressed as the average±standard deviation; units are degrees. From Hemmerich et al. [36]

long periods, 130° of hip flexion is observed during a full squat and 90°–100° in a cross-legged position; hip external rotation has ranged from 5° to 36° for a full squat and 35°–60° while sitting cross-legged, and hip abduction has ranged from 10 to 30° for a full squat and 40°–45° while sitting cross-legged [36–39].

Tissues Controlling the Range of Motion of the Hip Joint

The limits of three-dimensional joint motion are determined by a complex interplay of impingement between the osseous and soft tissues of the joint and the passive restraint of structures connecting the femur to the pelvis [40]. The capsular ligaments of the hip make the largest contribution in limiting the range of motion of the hip, with a secondary contribution from the acetabular labrum. The muscles surrounding the joint contribute to the passive restraint of motion [40]. Computer modeling suggests that osseous impingement (e.g., abutting of the anterolateral head-neck junction against the acetabular rim) contributes primarily to restricting flexion, adduction, flexion combined with adduction, and flexion combined with adduction and internal rotation. Soft tissue impingement restricts abduction and abduction combined with flexion, while soft tissue restraint restricts extension and adduction through the midrange of joint flexion [41].

The Articular Surfaces

The osseocartilaginous surfaces of the femoral head and acetabulum are often thought of as being truly spherical, while in reality, both are more elongated in the direction of the neck axis, leading to an "egg-shaped" morphology (often termed "conchoidal") [28]. The femoral head forms two-thirds of a sphere, becoming flatter where the acetabulum applies its largest load [42, 43], while the acetabulum possesses a slightly smaller diameter than the femoral head [44]. The acetabulum covers approximately 170° of the femoral head, being incomplete in the inferior portion [45]. The lack of a truly congruent articulation permits rolling and gliding between the joints surfaces, allowing for a great deal of mobility while maintaining the inherent stability of the joint [28]. This morphologic configuration also allows the lower extremity to be placed in positions requiring simultaneous flexion-extension, abduction-adduction, and internal-external rotation.

The Hip Capsule and Ligaments

During abduction and adduction, the stability of the joint is maintained by the passive restraint of the hip capsule (the capsular ligaments and the zona orbicularis) which also keeps the hip from dislocating when loaded at the extremes of motion [41, 46, 47]. The capsule is a complex structure formed by three discrete ligaments: the iliofemoral, femoral arcuate (pubofemoral), and ischiofemoral ligaments. The iliofemoral ligament, also known as the "Y" ligament of Bigelow, is located anteriorly and restricts extension and external rotation of the joint [48–51]. The femoral arcuate ligament helps to limit abduction and external rotation. Lastly, the ischiofemoral ligament acts during flexion to limit internal rotation and adduction [48, 49]. The ischiofemoral ligament is the weakest of the capsular ligaments, which makes the joint susceptible to posterior dislocation [52]. Additionally, the zona orbicularis plays a role in preventing frank dislocation by stabilizing the axial position of the femur in the socket. The zona orbicularis is a circular condensation of the capsule which surrounds the femoral neck and appears to prevent distraction of the femoral head out of the joint [53, 54].

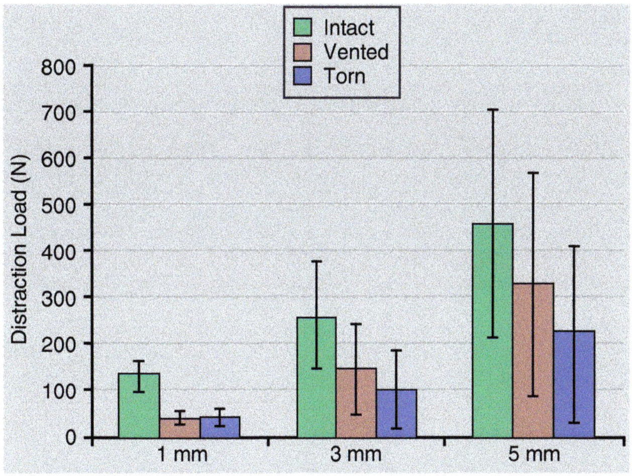

Fig. 7.3 Average load required to generate distraction of the femur with respect to the acetabular margin by distances of 1, 3, and 5 mm with the labrum intact, vented, and incised to simulate a full-thickness tear. From Stal et al., Biomechanics of the Natural Hip Joint, In: Surgery of the Hip, D.J. Berry and J.R. Lieberman, eds. Volume 2. 2013, pp 5–13. Copyright Elsevier 2013, reprinted with permission

The Acetabular Labrum

The acetabular labrum is a fibrocartilaginous extension of the bony edge of the acetabular rim with specialized structural properties, deepening the effective depth of the acetabular socket and dramatically increasing the resistance of the joint to dislocation. In mechanical terms, labral tissue is highly anisotropic, with a preferential stiffness in the circumferential direction [55] and significant variation as a function of gender, anatomic location, and the degenerative state of the hip [56, 57].

In the normal hip, the labrum only makes a small contribution to direct mechanical support of the femoral head; though with increasing degrees of acetabular dysplasia, weight is shifted more peripherally on the articular surface and the contributions of the labrum and capsule become far more significant [58, 59]. Studies performed over the past decade strongly suggest that the primary function of the labrum is not to increase the weight-bearing surface of the hip, but rather to form a compliant seal with the articular surface of the femoral head [60, 61, 62]. The ability of the labrum to seal off the central compartment of the hip is easily seen intraoperatively during distraction or dislocation of the hip (Fig. 7.3). Moreover, laboratory studies have shown that this suction phenomenon increases joint stability and allows the joint load to be distributed more uniformly over the articulating surfaces (Figs. 7.4 and 7.5) [63–65]. Computer simulations and in vitro experiments [62, 64, 66] have shown that the labrum controls the rate of egress of synovial fluid during weight-bearing which allows retention of a layer of synovial fluid between the femur and the acetabulum, thus preventing direct contact of the articulating surfaces during dynamic loading. If the labrum fails to perform this function, strains within the cartilage matrix are substantially increased. The rate of consolidation of cartilage under load, with displacement of internal synovial fluid, has been shown to increase by up to 40 % following excision of the labrum [62]. This leads to a dramatic rise in the internal stresses within the cartilage layers and subchondral shear stresses at the bone-cartilage junction, increasing the risk of delamination [62].

Damage to the labrum through injury or pathology can compromise its sealing function, leading to displacement of the head from its normal physiologic position. This leads to increase in peak articular stresses with a shift of loading to the acetabular rim, potentially leading to accelerated erosion of cartilage and early onset of osteoarthritis. Through the combination of these factors, labral tears occur predominantly in the anterior quadrant, leading to hip instability, as well as watershed labral lesions, which ultimately can lead to degenerative joint disease [60, 61, 67, 68].

In middle-aged to elderly individuals, labral pathology arises primarily through degenerative changes accompanying aging, as evidenced by the high incidence of lesions observed in cadaveric specimens [68, 69]. In younger individuals, primarily those engaged in sporting activities, labral pathology has been attributed to repetitive microtrauma, especially during high impact sports or those involving loading of the extremity at the extremes of the motion arc [70–72]. A common observation in patients with labral injury is enlargement of the anterior junction of the femoral head-neck junction, leading to cam-type FAI [73–75]. In these cases, it has been hypothesized that the mechanism of injury is forced passage of the enlarged area of the anterior head-neck junction beneath the labrum at the extremes of the natural range of joint motion. Repetition of the abnormal loading

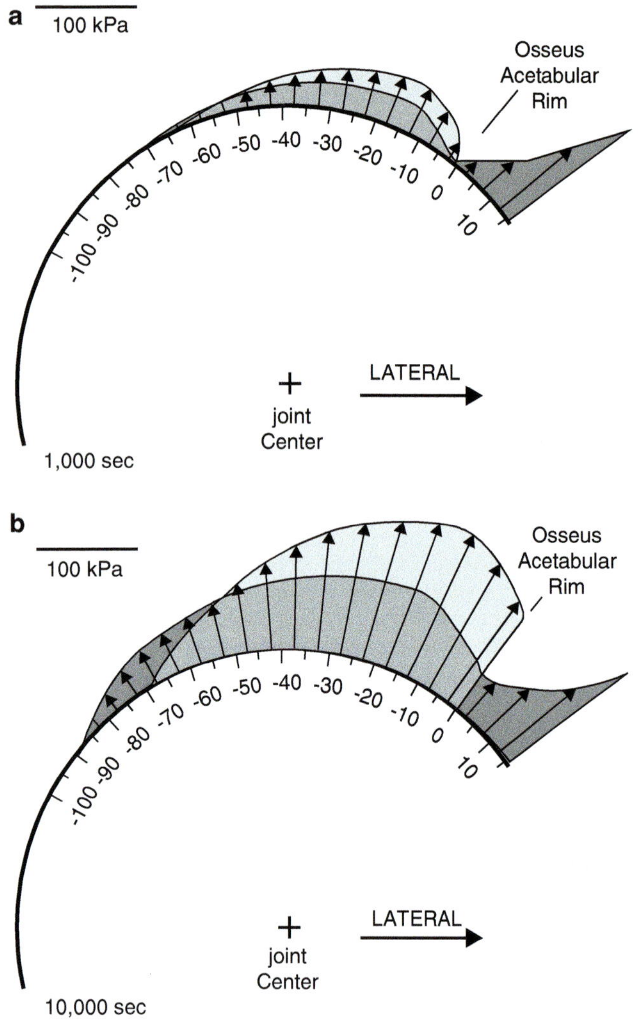

Fig. 7.4 Predicted distribution of cartilage contact stresses (solid on solid) at 1000 and 10,000 s after application of load to the hip joint in the presence of an intact labrum (*dark gray*) and without a labrum (*light gray*). From Ferguson SJ, et al. The influence of the acetabular labrum on hip joint cartilage consolidation: a poroelastic finite element model. Journal of Biomechanics. 2000; 33(8):953–960. Reprinted with permission from Elsevier

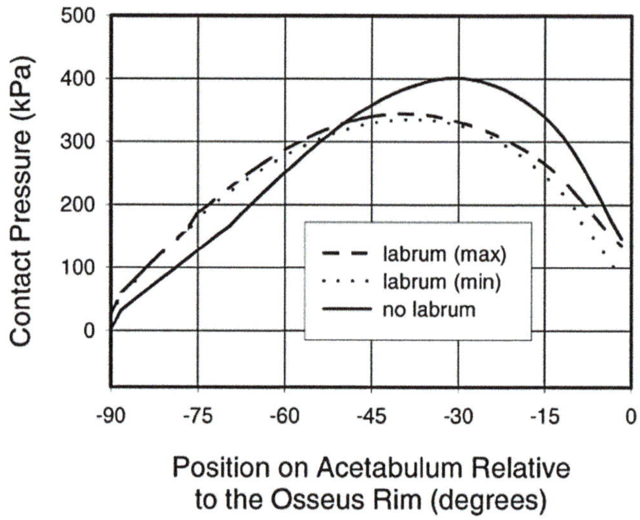

Fig. 7.5 Predicted variation in total contact pressure (interstitial fluid pressure plus solid contact stress) at 10,000 s after application of load to the hip joint, with and without an intact labrum. The *dashed* and *dotted lines* depict the maximum and minimum values of contact pressure corresponding to the extremes in assumed mechanical properties of the labrum within the finite element model. From Ferguson SJ, et al. The influence of the acetabular labrum on hip joint cartilage consolidation: a poroelastic finite element model. Journal of Biomechanics. 2000; 33(8):953–960. Reprinted with permission from Elsevier

caused by this event is thought to lead to tensile loading of the chondro-labral junction and formation of a "watershed" lesion.

An alternate hypothesis arises from the work of Dy et al. [76] who showed that substantial tensile strains can be developed within the anterior labrum without the occurrence of impingement. In this novel combination of experimental loading and finite element analysis, maximum strains were predicted at the junction between the labrum and the acetabular rim during activities involving twisting or pivoting of the hip with tightening of the joint capsule.

Labral injury may also occur secondary to compression and shear forces imposed by the iliopsoas tendon [77]. In this situation, the site of injury is often located more anteromedially than is seen in cases of femoroacetabular impingement [78]. Recognition of iliopsoas impingement has prompted hip preservation surgeons to repair these non-femoroacetabular impingement-induced labral injuries and to address the inciting cause, either the iliopsoas tendon or anterior inferior iliac spine and psoas groove [77, 79].

The Ligamentum Teres

The potential role of the ligamentum teres in stabilizing the hip remains a topic of debate [80, 81]. Anecdotal reports indicate that some patients obtain relief of hip symptoms following repair of acute ruptures of the ligamentum teres, although scientific data corroborating the role of this structure in enhancing hip stability is scarce [82]. It is known that the ligamentum teres is taut during hip adduction, flexion, and external rotation, positions in which the joint is least stable, which demonstrates the potential contribution of the ligamentum teres to hip stability [83, 84] (Figs. 7.6 and 7.7). In patients with developmental hip dysplasia and low lateral head coverage (lateral center-edge angle—acetabular inclination), the risk of ligamentum teres tears is significantly increased. Thus, tears of the ligamentum teres may occur secondary to subtle instability induced by acetabular undercoverage. In patients with atraumatic microinstability (e.g. ligamentous laxity due to hypermobility syndrome[s]), the ligamentum teres may be at increased risk of tear [85].

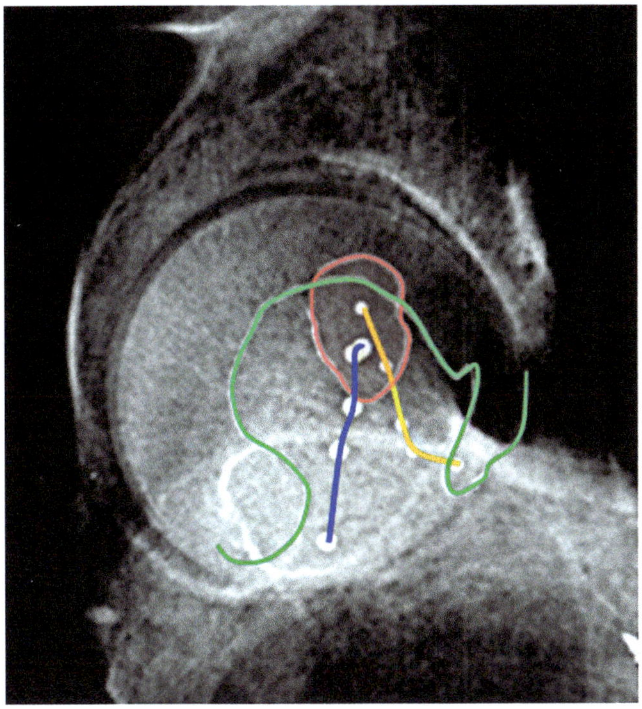

Fig. 7.6 Experimental radiograph of a hip joint in which radiopaque spheres have been implanted in the anterior and posterior bundles of the ligamentum teres. Implanted wires also define the inner edge of the articular surface of the acetabulum (*green*) and the fovea of the femoral head (*red*). In this case the hip has been placed in maximum external rotation in 90 degrees of flexion causing the posterior bundle to be loaded in tension

However, additionally, a tear of the ligamentum teres may also induce microinstability. Surgical treatment of ligamentum teres pathology includes both debridement and reconstruction [86–88]. Both techniques may be performed arthroscopically, with short-term clinical outcomes demonstrating success via improved pain, function, and return to sport [87, 88]. Further clinical and biomechanical studies are needed to conclusively demonstrate the magnitude of the stabilizing effect of the ligamentum teres in adults.

Pathological Impediments to Joint Motion

Femoroacetabular Impingement

Like any other joint, the hip is free to rotate in any direction (i.e., abduction-adduction, flexion-extension, and internal-external rotation) until constrained by either:

- Tightening of soft tissues crossing the joint (primarily the joint capsule and extracapsular ligaments, but also the surrounding musculature)
- Direct contact between the opposing articular surfaces (i.e. of the femur and the pelvis).

In the normal hip, the relative contributions of these limiting factors vary with the relative position of the femur and the pelvis. However, for most motions, joint motion is primarily determined by the laxity of the joint capsule and comes to an end once the ligamentous structures become taut [48, 89]. With some motions, for example, flexion and internal rotation, resistance to motion occurs before ligamentous tightness becomes significant. In these motions, contact either occurs between the bony surfaces (i.e., through bone-on-bone impingement) or the motion arc brings the femoral head to the edge of its spherical surface where the radius of curvature increases causing a cam braking effect if further rotation is attempted.

While these interactions are important for understanding the kinematics of the normal hip, they are of critical importance to our understanding of the role of pathologic bony morphology on chondro-labral degeneration and the development of osteoarthrosis. Characteristic deformities of the hip joint that are known to affect joint motion, especially flexion and internal rotation, include SCFE in the pediatric hip [90]; asphericity of the femoral head, with a flattening or extension of the articular surface at the anterolateral head-neck junction ("pistol grip deformity" [91]); and the presence of a deep acetabulum with overgrowth of the acetabular margin. It has long been appreciated that the mechanism of reduced flexion/internal rotation in patients with SCFE is posterior displacement ("slip") of the femoral head with respect to the neck leading to reduced offset at the anterior head-neck junction. This brings the femoral neck closer to the anterior rim of the acetabulum during flexion and further away during extension, leading to a shift in the functional motion arc and damage to the acetabular margin with repetitive impingement [92, 93].

In hips with morphologic changes in the shape of the head or the depth of the acetabulum, two distinctly different forms of FAI have been popularized, respectively termed "cam-type" and "pincer-type" impingement [53] (Figs. 7.8, 7.9, and 7.10). The first form ("cam-type") occurs when the femoral head rotates within the acetabulum until the point that an enlarged portion of at the head-neck junction encounters the acetabular rim and is forced beneath the labrum [94–96]. The forced expansion of the labrum causes a stress concentration at the chondro-labral junction where the relatively stiff subchondral plate with its overlaying cartilage surface meets the more flexible labrum. With repetitive engagement of the oversized cross-section of the head and head-neck junction with the anterior acetabulum, pathological changes may occur, including subchondral para-acetabular cysts, fibrillation and splitting of the chondral surface, and delamination of cartilage from underling bone [97]. Ultimately cysts may also develop within the femoral head or the head-neck junction.

The reduction in the functional range of hip motion arising from the abnormalities of the head-neck junction present

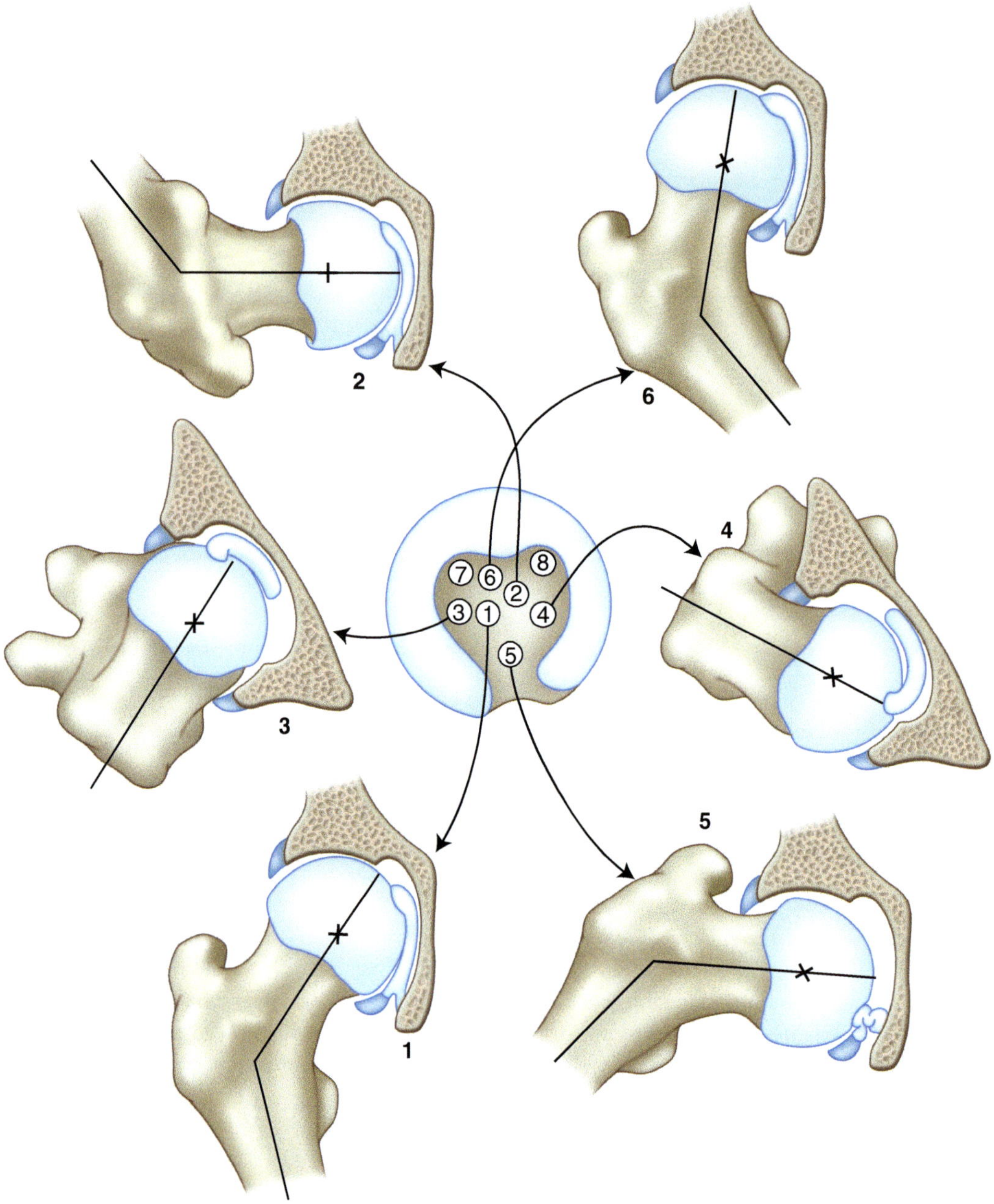

Fig. 7.7 Diagrammatic representation of the relative positions of the femur, ligamentum teres, and the floor of the acetabulum with placement of the hip joint in eight different positions encompassing the range of motion of the joint

in FAI has been extensively studied by Kubiak-Langer et al. [98], using computer simulation of hip motion. Using patient-specific models of the hip derived from CT reconstructions, significant loss of hip motion was demonstrated in FAI cases during flexion, abduction, and internal rotation in 90 degrees of flexion (Table 7.4). The pathomechanics of FAI at the tissue level has been investigated by Ferguson and coworkers using three-dimensional computational models of normal and pathological joints incorporating morphologic variations in the head-neck junction (alpha angle) and femoral head coverage (center-edge angle) [99] (Figs. 7.11 and 7.12). In this study, the effect of functional loading of the hip on stresses developed within the soft tissues of the joint was modeled for walking and sit-to-stand activities. Quite different stress distributions were predicted as a function of activity. During walking, von Mises stresses within the joint cartilage increased gradually as the center-edge angle decreased, but were not affected by the presence of a Cam-FAI (Fig. 7.12). Moreover, peak stresses only exceeded 4 MPa in simulations with a CE angle of less than 23°. Conversely, during a stand-to-sit activity, peak stresses in the normal hip were less than 2.5 MPa and changed little with

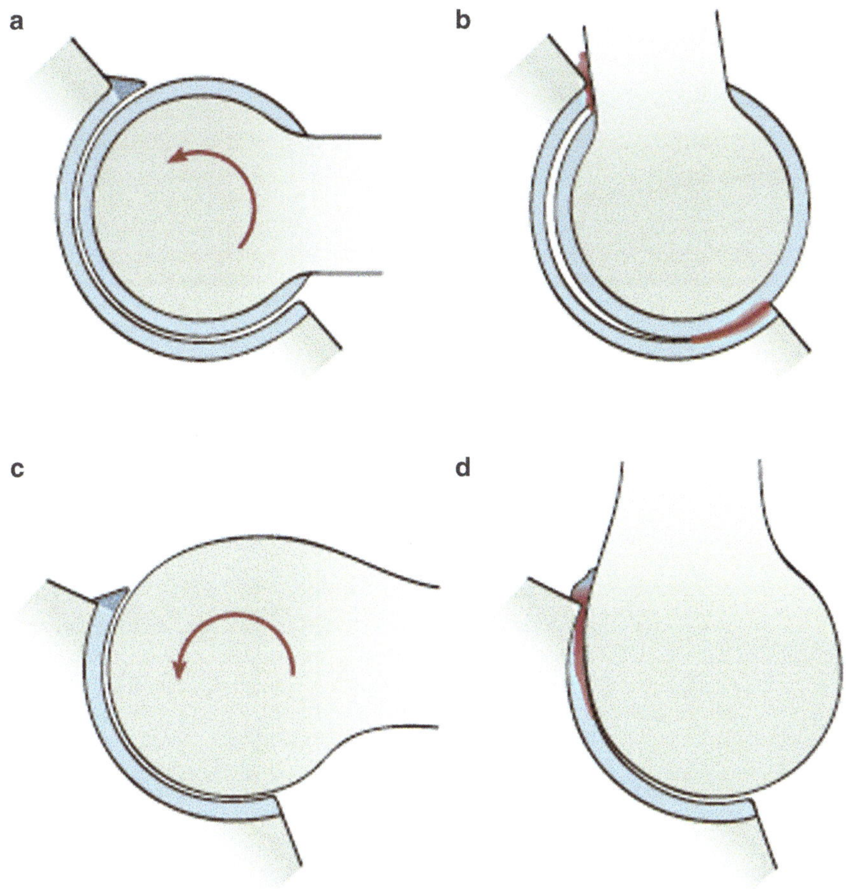

Fig. 7.8 Diagrammatic representation of the pathomechanics of joint damage associated with femoroacetabular impingement, as proposed by Ganz and coworkers [71, 90, 92–95]. "Pincer impingement" (**a**, **b**) is observed in cases over "over-coverage" of the femoral head by the acetabular margin, leading to direct impact at the extremes of motion and labral and articular damage. "Cam impingement" (**c**, **d**) occurs when an enlarged area of the femoral head at the head-neck junction is too large to fit into the acetabulum, typically during flexion and internal rotation. Attempts to force the hip to flex or rotate further cause overstuffing of the acetabulum and chondro-labral separation [92]. From Stal et al., Biomechanics of the Natural Hip Joint, In: Surgery of the Hip, D.J. Berry and J.R. Lieberman, eds. Volume 2. 2013, pp 5–13. Copyright Elsevier 2013, reprinted with permission

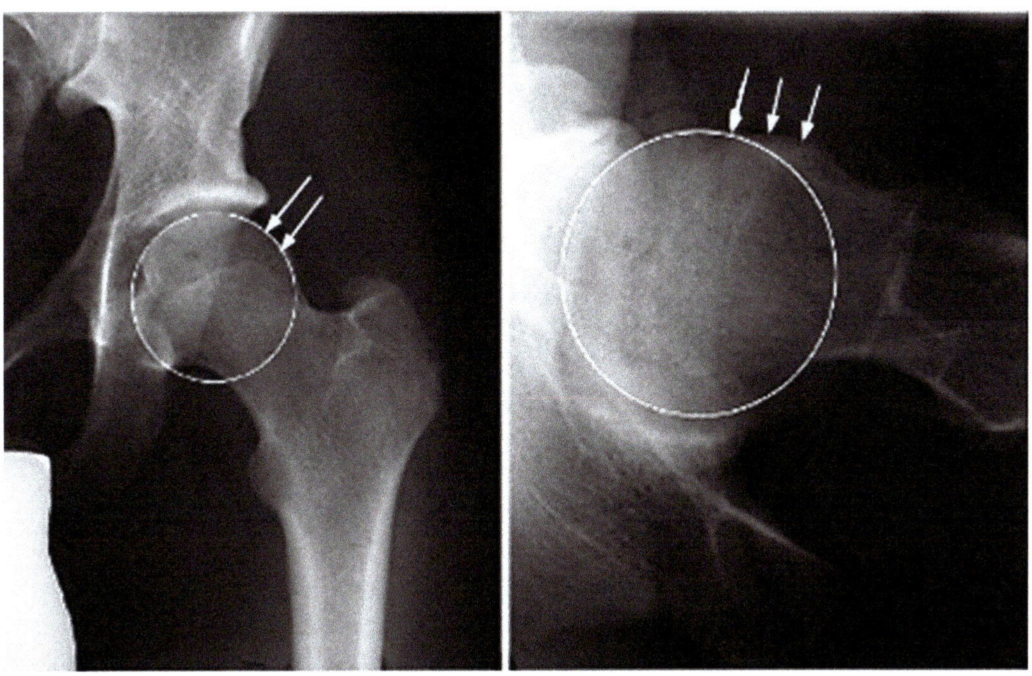

Fig. 7.9 Radiographic appearance of a cam-impinging hip with a "pistol grip" appearance. An aspherical section of the femoral head is seen extending beyond the circle of best fit to the head profile on both the AP and lateral radiographs (see *arrows*). From Stal et al., Biomechanics of the Natural Hip Joint, In: Surgery of the Hip, D.J. Berry and J.R. Lieberman, eds. Volume 2. 2013, pp 5–13. Copyright Elsevier 2013, reprinted with permission

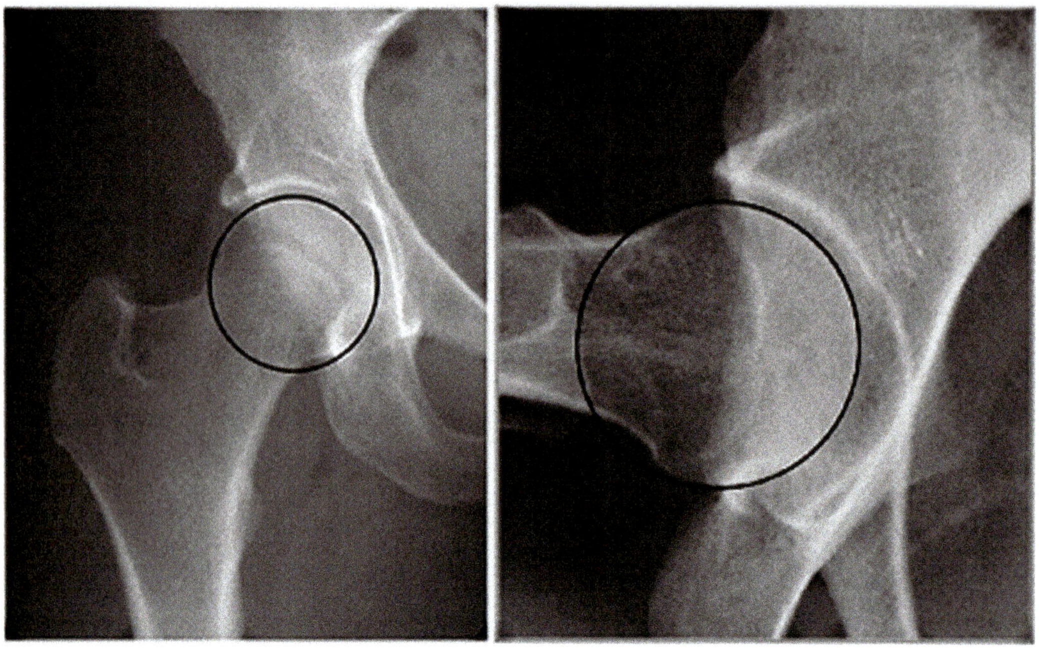

Fig. 7.10 Radiographic appearance of a hip with coxa profunda combined with pincer impinging appearance secondary to ossification of the acetabular labrum. The femoral head is spherical in both the AP and lateral views. From Stal et al., Biomechanics of the Natural Hip Joint, In: Surgery of the Hip, D.J. Berry and J.R. Lieberman, eds. Volume 2. 2013, pp 5–13. Copyright Elsevier 2013, reprinted with permission

Table 7.4 Hip motion (in degrees) predicted by computer simulation for a population of normals compared to patients with femoroacetabular impingement, before and after osteochondroplasty

Parameter	Normal hips	FAI hips (pre-op)	p value (normal vs. FAI)	FAI hips (post-osteoplasty)	p value (pre vs. post)
Flexion	122.0°±16.3°	105.2°±12.2°	<0.0001	125.4°±9.7°	<0.0001
Extension	56.5°±20.1°	61.1°±31.8°	0.751	71.1°±26.4°	0.051
Abduction	63.3°±10.9°	51.7°±12.2°	<0.0001	63.6°±7.5°	0.0001
Adduction	32.7°±12.3°	34.6°±12.3°	0.927	35.8°±15.3°	0.262
Internal rotation (90° flexion)	35.2°±6.9°	11.1°±6.9°	<0.001	35.8°±15.3°	0.002
External rotation (90° flexion)	102.5°±14.2°	83.0°±33.7°	0.194	93.9°±32.7°	0.327

All values are expressed as the average±standard deviation. From Kubiak-Langer et al. [98]

CE angle, except in cases of extreme femoral containment (CE angle=40°). Much higher stresses were calculated for the FAI cases, where peak values exceeding 5 MPa were predicted whenever the sum of the alpha and CE angles exceeded 90°, with stresses exceeding 10 MPa in almost all simulations with a CE angle of 30° or greater. These predictions correlate well with the clinical observations seen during the progression of joint degeneration in the face of FAI, including the development of chondral defects at the acetabular margin, full-thickness delamination of the acetabular cartilage, and detachment of the labrum at the chondro-labral junction [100] (Fig. 7.11).

Femoral and Acetabular Dysplasia

Finite element analysis has shown that subtle variations in the morphology and orientation of the femur and acetabulum may generate substantial perturbations in the distribution of load between the bony, cartilaginous, and soft tissues. This could explain the occurrence of secondary remodeling, deviations in joint kinematics, "microinstability," and, ultimately, osteoarthritis [101]. This patho-mechanical progression is exemplified by the dysplastic hip, in which the shallow acetabulum provides reduced coverage of the femoral head, combined with a more vertically inclined weight-bearing

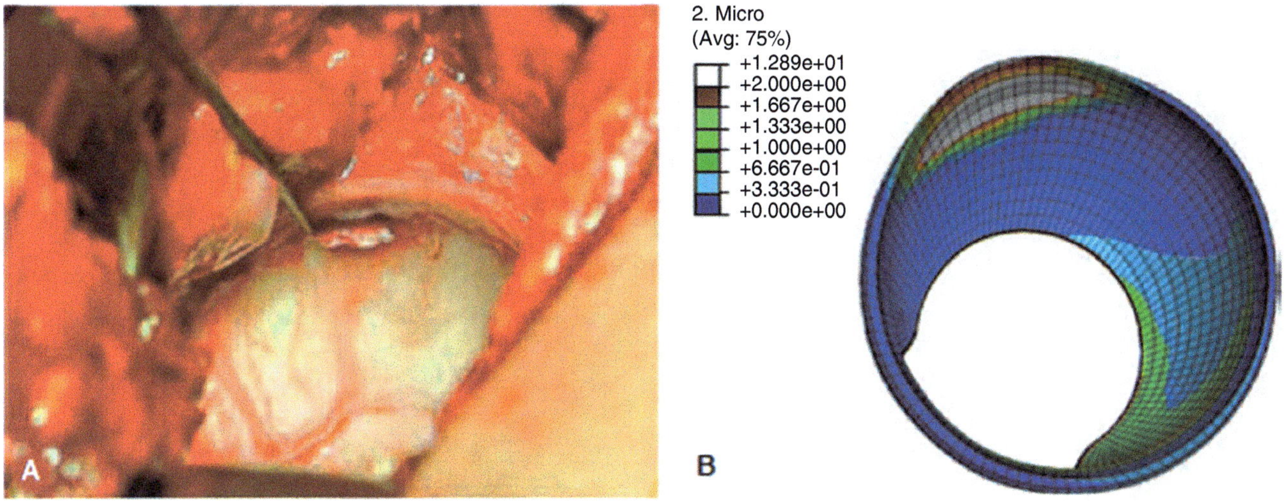

Fig. 7.11 (**a**) Intraoperative appearance of an anterior-superior labral tear in cases of cam impingement. (**b**) Distribution of von Mises stresses at the acetabular rim predicted by computer modeling of a severe cam-impinging joint ($\alpha = 80°$) during deep flexion (standing to sitting, anterior = *left*). From Chegini, S., et al. The effects of impingement and dysplasia on stress distributions in the hip joint during sitting and walking: a finite element analysis. J Orthop Res, 2009. 27(2): p. 195–201. Reprinted with permission from John Wiley and Sons

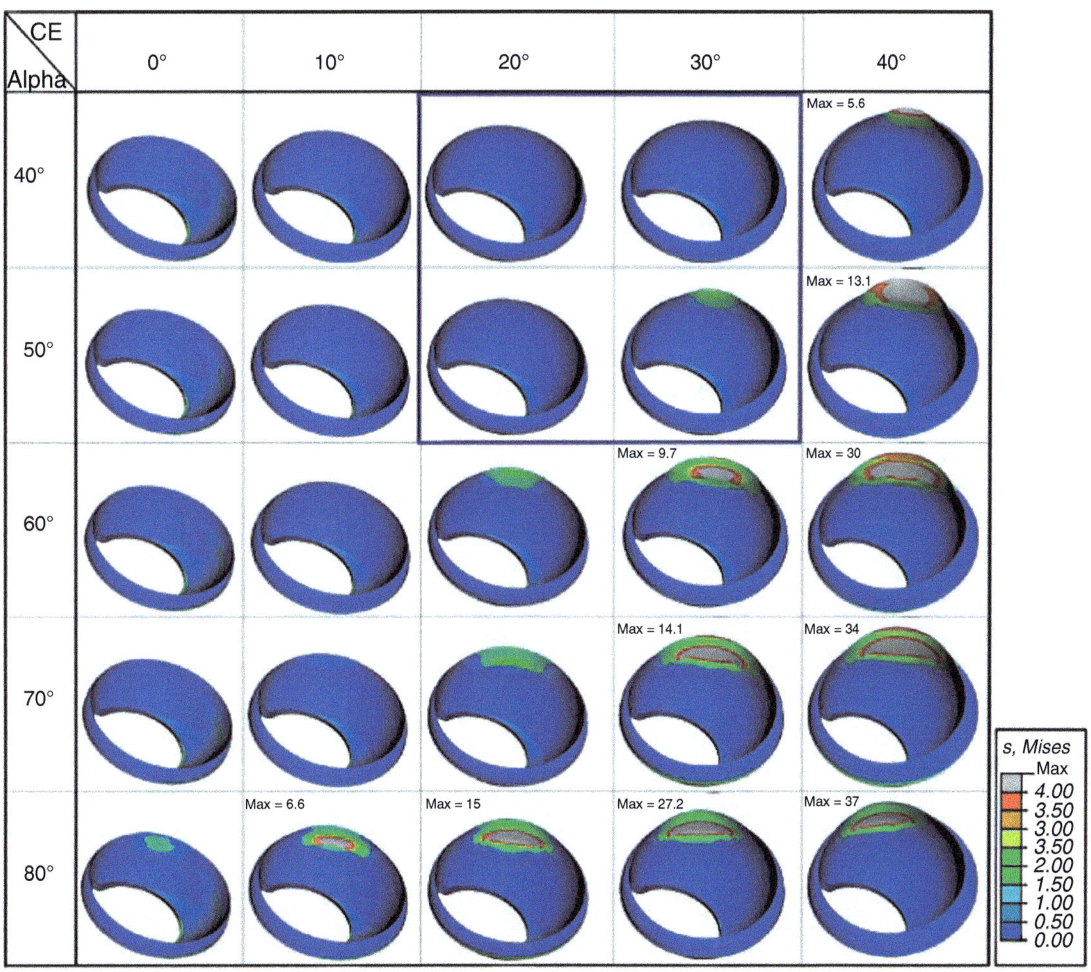

Fig. 7.12 Distribution of von Mises stresses (MPa) within the acetabular cartilage during standing to sitting for all simulated joint geometries. The joints considered normal are surrounded by the blue rectangle. From Chegini, S., et al. The effects of impingement and dysplasia on stress distributions in the hip joint during sitting and walking: a finite element analysis. J Orthop Res, 2009. 27(2): p. 195–201. Reprinted with permission from John Wiley and Sons

surface. This results in high contact stresses, overloading of the labrum and hip capsule, and premature joint degeneration [100, 102, 103].

The influence of acetabular dysplasia on contact pressure has been studied using a variety of computer simulation and experimental methods. One approach, presented by Genda and coworkers [19], utilized a 3D parametric model of the hip joint to explore the impact of classic anatomic parameters on the calculated value of the hip joint reaction force. These parameters included the center-edge (CE) angle, the Sharp angle, the head diameter, the direction of pull of the abductors, and the greater trochanter and the femoral head center. An interesting finding was that under conditions typical of the dysplastic hip (i.e., low CE angle), the model predicted that peak articular pressures would exceed 6 MPa when the abductor line of action was within 10° of vertical. This corresponds to four times peak pressures predicted for the normal female hip using the same method of analysis. Similar results were reported by Tsumura et al. [104] using patient-specific CT reconstructions. In this case, peak pressures of 2.5 MPa were predicted at the acetabular rim of normal hips, compared to 5.3 MPa for dysplastic cases.

Other authors, including Hadley et al. [105] and Russell et al. [102], have studied the effect on articular cartilage of cumulative pressure exposure over a simulated lifetime of loading. Substantial differences in cumulative pressure were demonstrated between normal and dysplastic hips, suggesting a patho-mechanical mechanism for cartilage degeneration in osteoarthritis based on chronic overload. Russell and coworkers [102] also highlighted that, beyond gross morphological differences, small bone irregularities can cause localized pressure elevations. Subsequent computational models have provided further insight into the relationship between joint morphology, daily loading, and cartilage contact pressures and stresses [106–108] (Figs. 7.13 and 7.14).

Soft tissue damage and degeneration are unavoidable consequences of the focal overload of the acetabular rim that occurs as part of the natural history of hip dysplasia [92, 94, 103]. As luxation of the femoral head progresses, high shearing and tensile stresses develop within the labrum as this peripheral structure takes over some of the load-bearing function of the acetabulum, leading to hyperplasia and ultimately damage to the labrum, typically within the anterior-superior quadrant [103], as predicted by computer models [98]. Clinical observations have provided confirmation of the causal link between focal overload of the acetabular rim and cartilage degeneration and labral rupture [103, 109, 110]. Thinning of the anterior cartilage has been observed in 80% of dysplasia patients, in association with forward and upward displacement of the femoral head [111]. Ultimately, the peripheral soft tissues of the joint are an inadequate substitute for the stability afforded by a congruent acetabulum with good lateral coverage; hence, acetabular reorientation surgery is often performed in an attempt to increase the longevity of the dysplastic hip [112, 113].

Microinstability

Some patients with radiographically normal hips and increased range-of-motion experience a sensation of joint instability without radiographic evidence of femoroacetabular impingement. In these cases, hypermobility of the joints is common syndrome with elevated Beighton and/or Brighton scores [114, 115]. Dancers, ballet dancers, figure skaters, yogi and yogini, cheerleaders, martial artists, and gymnasts

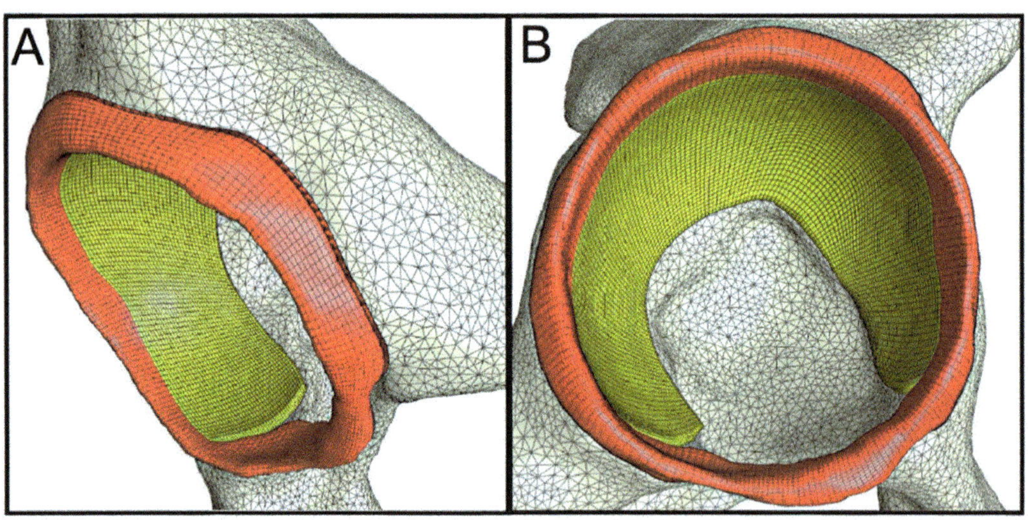

Fig. 7.13 The finite element mesh used by Henak and coworkers [107] to simulate load transfer across the hip joint in the presence of varying degrees of hip dysplasia and FAI morphology. The bony hemipelvis (*white*), the acetabular cartilage (*yellow*), and the labrum (*red*) are each represented. From Henak, C. R., et al. Role of the acetabular labrum in load support across the hip joint. Journal of Biomechanics, 2011;*44*(12):2201–2206. Reprinted with permission from Elsevier

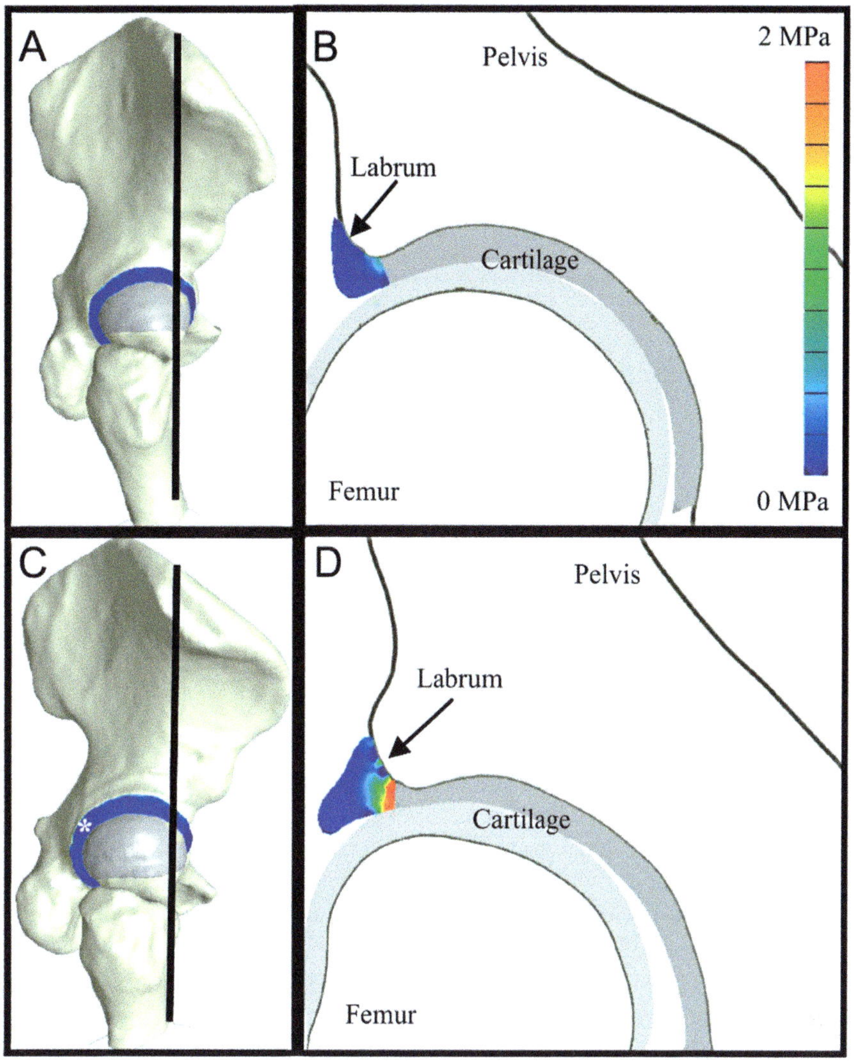

Fig. 7.14 Predicted values of internals stresses within the anterosuperior labrum developed in response to load transfer during walking (heel strike). This analysis was performed for the normal hip (**a**, **b**) and the dysplastic hip (**c**, **d**). The stresses depicted in the (**b**, **d**) were calculated for the vertical planes taken along the black lines in (**a**, **c**) corresponding to the approximate location of maximum deflection of the labrum. From Henak, C. R., et al. Role of the acetabular labrum in load support across the hip joint. Journal of Biomechanics, 2011;*44*(12):2201–2206. Reprinted with permission from Elsevier

may have a high prevalence of increased motion and potential microinstability, often prerequisite to the activity performed [116]. In a cohort of 59 professional ballet dancers, only one hip had evidence of a cam deformity, while several other abnormalities were identified on magnetic resonance imaging due to a dynamic "pincer" mechanism from the extreme motion involved with their dance activities [116]. Further, while in the "splits" position, all hips subluxed (mean: 2.1 mm). In comparison to a control group, the musculoskeletal abnormalities in the ballet group included a higher incidence of acetabular cartilage lesions (mostly superior), labral tears (mostly posterosuperior to anterosuperior), and a larger number of herniation pits in the superior femoral neck. Despite the relatively low incidence of bony deformities, 60 % of dancers reported groin pain, but only when dancing [117]. Further, when each dancer assumed the most demanding positions of classical ballet, the mean translation of the femoral head within the acetabulum ranged from 0.93 to 6.35 mm [118].

Iatrogenic microinstability may be induced in patients who have undergone hip arthroscopy with capsulotomy without capsular closure [119, 120]. This conclusion is consistent with the findings of four cadaveric biomechanical studies (Table 7.5) demonstrating the importance of the iliofemoral ligament to the structural integrity of normal hip joint mechanics. In each of these studies, sectioning the iliofemoral ligament increased external rotation, extension, and anterior translation of the hip with no difference between the intact and repaired state. Discrete frank hip dislocation is at the end of the microinstability spectrum. In the postoperative setting, instability may occur along this spectrum to variable degrees. Nine cases of post-arthroscopic iatrogenic hip dislocation have been presented in the literature [121–128]. Due to publication bias, this is likely a significant underestimate of the true incidence of instability following hip arthroscopy. Thus, to avoid micro- or macro-instability during hip preservation surgery, most authors recommend avoiding the following: extended capsulectomy without repair, labral

Table 7.5 Cadaveric studies examining the effect of the ligaments of the hip capsule on the stability and range of motion of the hip

Study	Study design	Role
Bayne et.al. (2014)[128]	Cadaveric biomechanical—motion tracking	• After capsulotomy, in neutral, increased distal, lateral, and anterior translation • After capsulotomy, in flexion, increased distal, medial, and posterior translation • After capsulotomy, more translation in neutral, more rotation in flexion • In maximal flexion, hips with capsulotomy rotated more than intact capsules
Myers et al., (2011) [50]	Cadaveric biomechanical—fluoroscopy	• Increased external rotation with IFL sectioning (increased 12.9°) ($p<.0001$) • Increased anterior translation with IFL sectioning (increased 1.8 mm) ($p<.001$) • No difference in external rotation or anterior translation between intact/repaired state
Martin et al. (2008) [48]	Cadaveric biomechanical—motion tracking	• Release of medial, lateral arms IFL gave greatest increase of external rotation • Lateral arm release provides more motion in flexion and neutral • Lateral arm release also provides more internal rotation, primarily in extension
Hewitt et al. (2002) [46]	Cadaveric biomechanical—load to failure	• IFL much stronger than the ischiofemoral ligaments • IFL greater stiffness than ischiofemoral ligaments • IFL greater tensile load to failure than ischiofemoral ligaments

resection (versus repair or refixation), aggressive acetabuloplasty (rim resection) in dysplastic configurations, and overall capsular laxity.

The presence of microinstability does not automatically preclude other concomitant intra- and extra-articular disorders. In fact, it is likely that subtle instability increases the loading of some of the structures of the hip including the labrum, the articular cartilage and underlying subchondral bone, the ligamentum teres, the iliopsoas tendon, the iliotibial band, the hip abductors, and the remaining normal capsule. Even patients with traditional femoroacetabular impingement may have subtle underlying microinstability due to preclusion of true ball-and-socket mechanics, thus causing anterior levering over the rim (fulcrum) with subsequent posterior instability. Further:

- Excessive acetabular anteversion can result in anterior hip instability and posterior acetabular rim impingement.
- Excessive acetabular retroversion can result in anterior impingement and posterior instability.
- Excessive femoral anteversion can result in anterior hip instability and posterior acetabular rim impingement.
- Excessive femoral retroversion can result in anterior impingement and posterior instability.

Conclusions

We believe that this chapter demonstrates how much Musculoskeletal Biomechanics has contributed to our understanding of the hip over the past half-century. The progress we have documented in this work has now delivered us to the dawn of Translational Biomechanics. This transformation has been made possible through the intersection of many advances in computing and imaging technology, combined with a deepening understanding of hip pathology. The focus of this field has shifted from academic predictions of hip joint forces to their direct measurement and from speculation as to possible relevance of stresses to OA to the prediction of tissue stresses in individual hips using patient-specific finite element models.

Meanwhile, the intense investigation by clinicians and scientists of common conditions affecting the health of the joint, most notably FAI, has led to the utilization of research tools in the study of the pathomechanics of hip degeneration and strategies for joint preservation. This approach has the potential for use in creating individual treatment plans in much the same manner as Medical Physics transformed the practice of radiotherapy in decades past.

The next steps in the emergence of "Translational Biomechanics" are already in motion. These include:

Patient- and activity-specific modeling of the mechanical response of the hip

Prediction of the risk of individual patients in developing hip OA on the basis of biomechanical risk factors

The role of instability and tissue laxity in the etiology of osteoarthritis of the hip.

The interaction of hard and soft tissues as determinants of joint stability and their effect on the mechano-biology of joint health and degeneration

The authors invite every reader to participate in this journey and contribute to its ultimate success!

References

1. Callaghan J, Rosenberg A, Rubash H. The adult hip. In: Hurwitz D, Andriacchi T, editors. Biomechanics of the hip, vol. 1. Philadelphia: Lippincott-Raven; 1998. p. 11.
2. Perry J, editor. Gait analysis: normal and pathological function. Thorofare: Slack; 1992.

3. Hack K, Di Primio G, Rakhra K, Beaulé PE. Prevalence of cam-type femoroacetabular impingement morphology in asymptomatic volunteers. J Bone Joint Surg Am. 2010;92(14):2436–44.
4. Register B, Pennock AT, Ho CP, Strickland CD, Lawand A, Philippon MJ. Prevalence of abnormal hip findings in asymptomatic participants: a prospective, blinded study. Am J Sports Med. 2012;40(12):2720–4.
5. Allen D, Beaulé PE, Ramadan O, Doucette S. Prevalence of associated deformities and hip pain in patients with cam-type femoroacetabular impingement. J Bone Joint Surg Br. 2009;91(5):589–94.
6. Wilson MG, Michet Jr CJ, Ilstrup DM, Melton Iii LJ. Idiopathic symptomatic osteoarthritis of the hip and knee: a population-based incidence study. Mayo Clin Proc. 1990;65(9):1214–21.
7. Seldes RM, Tan V, Hunt J, Katz M, Winiarsky R, Fitzgerald Jr RH. Anatomy, histologic features, and vascularity of the adult acetabular labrum. Clin Orthop Relat Res. 2001;382:232–40.
8. Baber YF, Robinson AHN, Villar RN. Is diagnostic arthroscopy of the hip worthwhile? A prospective review of 328 adults investigated for hip pain. J Bone Joint Surg Br. 1999;81(4):600–3.
9. Cotten A, Boutry N, Demondion X, Paret C, Dewatre F, Liesse A, Chastanet P, Fontaine C. Acetabular labrum: MRI in asymptomatic volunteers. J Comput Assist Tomogr. 1998;22(1):1–7.
10. Rydell NW. Forces acting on the femoral head-prosthesis: a study on strain gauge supplied prostheses in living persons. Acta Orthop. 1966;37(S88):1–132.
11. Bergmann G, et al. Hip contact forces and gait patterns from routine activities. J Biomech. 2001;34(7):859–71.
12. Bergmann G, Graichen F, Rohlmann A. Is staircase walking a risk for the fixation of hip implants? J Biomech. 1995;28(5):535–53.
13. Bergmann G, Graichen F, Rohlmann A. Hip joint contact forces during stumbling. Langenbecks Arch Surg. 2004;389(1):53–9.
14. Bergmann G, et al. Realistic loads for testing hip implants. Biomed Mater Eng. 2010;20(2):65–75.
15. Tackson SJ, Krebs DE, Harris BA. Acetabular pressures during hip arthritis exercises. Arthritis Care Res. 1997;10(5):308–19.
16. Foucher KC, Hurwitz DE, Wimmer MA. Do gait adaptations during stair climbing result in changes in implant forces in subjects with total hip replacements compared to normal subjects? Clin Biomech (Bristol, Avon). 2008;23(6):754–61.
17. Stansfield BW, Nicol AC. Hip joint contact forces in normal subjects and subjects with total hip prostheses: walking and stair and ramp negotiation. Clin Biomech (Bristol, Avon). 2002;17:130–9.
18. Duda GN, Schneider E, Chao EY. Internal forces and moments in the femur during walking. J Biomech. 1997;30:933–41.
19. Genda E, Iwasaki N, Li G, MacWilliams BA, Barrance PJ, Chao E. Normal hip joint contact pressure distribution in single-leg standing—effect of gender and anatomic parameters. J Biomech. 2001;34(7):895–905.
20. Lenaerts G, Bartels W, Gelaude F, Mulier M, Spaepen A, Van der Perre G, Jonkers I. Subject-specific hip geometry and hip joint centre location affects calculated contact forces at the hip during gait. J Biomech. 2009;42(9):1246–51.
21. Recnik G, Kralj-Iglič V, Iglič A, Antolič V, Kramberger S, Rigler I, Pompe B, Vengust R. The role of obesity, biomechanical constitution of the pelvis and contact joint stress in progression of hip osteoarthritis. Osteoarthritis Cartilage. 2009;17(7):879–82.
22. Bergmann G, Kniggendorf H, Graichen F, Rohlmann A. Influence of shoes and heel strike on the loading of the hip joint. J Biomech. 1995;28(7):817–27.
23. Hardin EC, van den Bogert AJ, Hamill J. Kinematic adaptations during running: effects of footwear, surface, and duration. Med Sci Sports Exerc. 2004;36(5):838–44.
24. Gu D, Hu F, Wei J, Dai K, Chen Y. Contributions of non-spherical hip joint cartilage surface to hip joint contact stress. In: Annual international conference of the IEEE, Boston; 2011. p. 8166–9.
25. Afoke N, Byers P, Hutton W. The incongruous hip joint—a casting study. J Bone Joint Surg Br. 1980;62B(4):511–4.
26. Greenwald A, Haynes D. Weight-bearing areas in the human hip joint. J Bone Joint Surg Br. 1972;54B(1):157–63.
27. Yoshida H, Faust A, Wilkcens J, Kitagawa M, Fetto J, Chao EYS. Three-dimensional dynamics hip contact area and pressure distribution during activities of daily living. J Biomech. 2006;39:1996–2004.
28. Menschik F. The hip joint as a conchoid shape. J Biomech. 1997;30(9):971–3.
29. Magee D. Orthopedic physical assessment. 4th ed. Pennsylvania: Saunders; 2002.
30. Fagerson TL, editor. The hip handbook. Woburn: Butterworth-Heinemann; 1998.
31. Frankel VH, Nordin M, editors. Basic biomechanics of the skeletal system, vol. 15. Philadelphia: Lea & Febiger; 1980. p. 303.
32. Reese N, Bandy W, editors. Joint range of motion and muscle length testing. Philadelphia: W.B. Saunders; 2002.
33. Pua YH, et al. Intrarater test-retest reliability of hip range of motion and hip muscle strength measurements in persons with hip osteoarthritis. Arch Phys Med Rehabil. 2008;89(6):1146–54.
34. Roach K, Miles T. Normal hip and knee active range of motion: the relationship to age. Phys Ther. 1991;71:656–65.
35. Moreside JM, McGill SM. Quantifying normal 3D hip ROM in healthy young adult males with clinical and laboratory tools: hip mobility restrictions appear to be plane-specific. Clin Biomech (Bristol, Avon). 2011;26(8):824–9.
36. Hemmerich A, et al. Hip, knee, and ankle kinematics of high range of motion activities of daily living. J Orthop Res. 2006;24:770–81.
37. Ahlberg A, Moussa M, Al-Nahdi M. On geographical variations in the normal range of joint motion. Clin Orthop Relat Res. 1988;(234):229–31.
38. Hoaglund FT, Yau AC, Wong WL. Osteoarthritis of the hip and other joints in southern Chinese in Hong Kong. J Bone Joint Surg Am. 1973;55:545–57.
39. Mulholland SJ, Wyss UP. Activities of daily living in non-Western cultures: range of motion requirements for hip and knee joint implants. Int J Rehabil Res. 2001;24:191–8.
40. Turley G, Williams M, Wellings R, Griffin D. Evaluation of range of motion restriction within the hip joint. Med Biol Eng Comput. 2013;51(4):467–77.
41. Smith M, Costic R, Allaire R, Schilling P, Sekiya J. A biomechanical analysis of the soft tissue and osseous constraints of the hip joint. Knee Surg Sports Traumatol Arthrosc. 2014;22(4):946–52.
42. Shindle MK, Ranawat A, Kelly B. Diagnosis and management of traumatic and atraumatic instability in the athletic patient. Clin Sports Med. 2006;25:309–26.
43. Kelly B, Williams RJ, Philippon M. Hip arthroscopy: current indications, treatment options, and management issues. Am J Sports Med. 2003;31(6):1020–37.
44. Konrath GA, Hamel AJ, Olson SA, Bay B, Sharkey NA. The role of the acetabular labrum and the transverse acetabular ligament in load transmission in the hip. J Bone Joint Surg Am. 1998;80-A(12):1781–8.
45. Bharam S. Labral tears, extra-articular injuries, and hip arthroscopy in the athlete. Clin Sports Med. 2006;25:279–92.
46. Hewitt JD, et al. The mechanical properties of the human hip capsule ligaments. J Arthroplasty. 2002;17(1):82–9.
47. Stewart KJ, et al. Spatial distribution of hip capsule structural and material properties. J Biomech. 2002;35(11):1491–8.
48. Martin HD, Savage A, Braly B, Palmer I, Beall DP, Kelly BT. The function of the hip capsular ligaments: a quantitative report. Arthroscopy. 2008;24(2):188–95.

49. Wagner F, Negrao J, Campos J, et al. Capsular ligaments of the hip: anatomic, histologic, and positional study in cadaveric specimens with MR arthrography. Radiology. 2012;263(1):189–98.
50. Myers CA, Register BC, Lertwanich P, et al. Role of the acetabular labrum and the iliofemoral ligament in hip stability: an in vitro biplane fluoroscopy study. Am J Sports Med. 2011;39:85S–91.
51. Domb B, Philipon M, Giordano B. Arthroscopic capsulotomy, capsular repair, and capsular plication of the hip: relation to atraumatic instability. Arthroscopy. 2013;29(1):162–73.
52. Offierski CM. Traumatic dislocation of the hip in children. J Bone Joint Surg Br. 1981;63-B(2):194–7.
53. Ito K, et al. Femoroacetabular impingement and the cam-effect. A MRI-based quantitative anatomical study of the femoral head-neck offset. J Bone Joint Surg Br. 2001;83(2):171–6.
54. Malagelada F, Tayar R, Barke S, Stafford G, Field RE. Anatomy of the zona orbicularis of the hip: a magnetic resonance study. Surg Radiol Anat. 2015;37(1):11–8.
55. Ferguson SJ, Bryant JT, Ito K. The material properties of the bovine acetabular labrum. J Orthop Res. 2001;19(5):887–96.
56. Ishiko T, Naito M, Moriyama S. Tensile properties of the human acetabular labrum-the first report. J Orthop Res. 2005; 23(6):1448–53.
57. Smith CD, et al. A biomechanical basis for tears of the human acetabular labrum. Br J Sports Med. 2009;43(8):574–8.
58. Konrath GA, et al. The role of the acetabular labrum and the transverse acetabular ligament in load transmission in the hip. J Bone Joint Surg Am. 1998;80(12):1781–8.
59. Lohe F, Eckstein F, Sauer T, Putz R. Structure, strain and function of the transverse acetabular ligament. Acta Anat. 1996;157:315–23.
60. Beaule PE, O'Neill M, Rakhra K. Acetabular labral tears. J Bone Joint Surg Am. 2009;91(3):701–10.
61. Crawford MJ, Dy CJ, Alexander JW, et al. The biomechanics of the hip labrum and the stability of the hip. Clin Orthop Relat Res. 2007;465:16–22.
62. Ferguson SJ, Bryant JT, Ganz R, Ito K. The influence of the acetabular labrum on hip joint cartilage consolidation: a poroelastic finite element model. J Biomech. 2000;33(8):953–60.
63. Eijer HL. Cross-table lateral radiographs for screening of anterior femoral head-neck offset in patients with femoro-acetabular impingement. Hip Int. 2001;11:37–41.
64. Ferguson SJ, Bryant JT, Ganz R, Ito K. An in vitro investigation of the acetabular labral seal in hip joint mechanics. J Biomech. 2003;36(2):171–8.
65. Takechi H, Nagashima H, Ito S. Intra-articular pressure of the hip joint outside and inside the limbus. Nippon Seikeigeka Gakkai Zasshi. 1982;56(6):529–36.
66. Ferguson SJ, et al. The acetabular labrum seal: a poroelastic finite element model. Clin Biomech (Bristol, Avon). 2000;15(6): 463–8.
67. McCarthy JC, et al. The watershed labral lesion: its relationship to early arthritis of the hip. J Arthroplasty. 2001;16(8 Suppl 1): 81–7.
68. Cashin M, et al. Embryology of the acetabular labral-chondral complex. J Bone Joint Surg Br. 2008;90(8):1019–24.
69. McCarthy JC, et al. The Otto E. Aufranc Award: the role of labral lesions to development of early degenerative hip disease. Clin Orthop Relat Res. 2001;393:25–37.
70. Groh MM, Herrera J. A comprehensive review of hip labral tears. Curr Rev Musculoskelet Med. 2009;2(2):105–17.
71. Beck M, Kalhor M, Leunig M, Ganz R. Hip morphology influences the pattern of damage to the acetabular cartilage femoroacetabular impingement as a cause of early osteoarthritis of the hip. J Bone Joint Surg Br. 2005;87(7):1012–8.
72. Ikeda T, Awaya G, Suzuki S, Okada Y, Tada H. Torn acetabular labrum in young patients. Arthroscopic diagnosis and management. J Bone Joint Surg Br. 1988;70(1):13–6.
73. Wenger DE, Kendell KR, Miner MR, Trousdale RT. Acetabular labral tears rarely occur in the absence of bony abnormalities. Clin Orthop Relat Res. 2004;426:145–50.
74. Tanzer M, Noiseux N. Osseous abnormalities and early osteoarthritis: the role of hip impingement. Clin Orthop Relat Res. 2004;429:170–7.
75. Dolan MM, Heyworth BE, Bedi A, Duke G, Kelly BT. CT reveals a high incidence of osseous abnormalities in hips with labral tears. Clin Orthop Relat Res. 2011;469(3):831–8.
76. Dy CJ, et al. Tensile strain in the anterior part of the acetabular labrum during provocative maneuvering of the normal hip. J Bone Joint Surg Am. 2008;90(7):1464–72.
77. Domb BG, Shindle MK, McArthur B, Voos JE, Magennis EM, Kelly BT. Iliopsoas impingement: a newly identified cause of labral pathology in the hip. HSS J. 2012;7:145–50.
78. Blankenbaker DG, Tuite MJ, Keene JS, Del Rio AM. Labral injuries due to iliopsoas impingement: can they be diagnosed on MR arthrography? AJR Am J Roentgenol. 2012;199:894–900.
79. Cascio BM, King D, Yen YM. Psoas impingement causing labrum tear: a series from three tertiary hip arthroscopy centers. J La State Med Soc. 2013;165:88–93.
80. Bardakos NV, Villar RN. The ligamentum teres of the adult hip. J Bone Joint Surg Br. 2009;91(1):8–15.
81. Martin RL, Palmer I, Martin HD. Ligamentum teres: a functional description and potential clinical relevance. Knee Surg Sports Traumatol Arthrosc. 2012;20(6):1209–14.
82. Wenger D, Miyanji F, Mahar A, Oka R. The mechanical properties of the ligamentum teres: a pilot study to assess its potential for improving stability in children's hip surgery. J Pediatr Orthop. 2007;27(4):408–10.
83. Kivlan BR, Clemente FR, Martin RL, Martin HD. Function of the ligamentum teres during multi-planar movement of the hip joint. Knee Surg Sports Traumatol Arthrosc. 2013;21(7):1664–8.
84. Martin RL, Kivlan BR, Clemente FR. A cadaveric model for ligamentum teres function: a pilot study. Knee Surg Sports Traumatol Arthrosc. 2013;21(7):1689–93.
85. Domb BG, Martin DE, Botser IB. Risk factors for ligamentum teres tears. Arthroscopy. 2013;29:64–73.
86. Simpson JM, Field RE, Villar RN. Arthroscopic reconstruction of the ligamentum teres. Arthroscopy. 2011;27(3):436–41.
87. Haviv B, O'Donnell J. Arthroscopic debridement of the isolated ligamentum teres rupture. Knee Surg Sports Traumatol Arthrosc. 2011;19:1510–3.
88. Amenabar T, O'Donnell J. Successful treatment of isolated, partial thickness ligamentum teres (LT) tears with debridement and capsulorrhaphy. Hip Int. 2013.
89. Bowman Jr KF, Fox J, Sekiya JK. A clinically relevant review of hip biomechanics. Arthroscopy. 2010;26(8):1118–29.
90. Leunig M, Casillas MM, Hamlet M, Hersche O, Nötzli H, Slongo T, Ganz R. Slipped capital femoral epiphysis: early mechanical damage to the acetabular cartilage by a prominent femoral metaphysis. Acta Orthop. 2000;71(4):370–5.
91. Stulberg SD, Cordell LD, Harris WH, Ramsey PL, MacEwen GD. Unrecognized childhood hip disease: a major cause of idiopathic osteoarthritis of the hip. In: The hip: Proceedings of the third open scientific meeting of the Hip Society. St Louis: CV Mosby; 1975. p. 212–28.
92. Leunig M, et al. Acetabular rim degeneration: a constant finding in the aged hip. Clin Orthop Relat Res. 2003;413:201–7.
93. Tannast M, et al. Hip damage occurs at the zone of femoroacetabular impingement. Clin Orthop Relat Res. 2008;466(2):273–80.
94. Ganz R, et al. The etiology of osteoarthritis of the hip: an integrated mechanical concept. Clin Orthop Relat Res. 2008;466(2): 264–72.
95. Ganz R, et al. Femoroacetabular impingement (FAI): a cause for osteoarthritis of the hip. Clin Orthop Relat Res. 2003;417:112–20.

96. Bardakos NV, Villar RN. Predictors of progression of osteoarthritis in Femoroacetabular impingement (FAI): a radiological study with a minimum of ten years follow-up. J Bone Joint Surg Br. 2009;91(2):162–9.
97. Parvizi J, Leunig M, Ganz R. Femoroacetabular impingement. J Am Acad Orthop Surg. 2007;15(9):561–70.
98. Kubiak-Langer M, Tannast M, Murphy SB, Siebenrock KA, Langlotz F. Range of motion in anterior femoroacetabular impingement. Clin Orthop Relat Res. 2007;458:117–24.
99. Chegini S, Beck M, Ferguson SJ. The effects of impingement and dysplasia on stress distributions in the hip joint during sitting and walking: a finite element analysis. J Orthop Res. 2009;27(2):195–201.
100. Johnston TL, Schenker ML, Briggs KK, Philippon MJ. Relationship between offset angle alpha and hip chondral injury in femoroacetabular impingement. Arthroscopy. 2008;24(6):669–75.
101. Brandt KD, Dieppe P, Radin EL. Etiopathogenesis of osteoarthritis. Rheum Dis Clin North Am. 2008;34(3):531–59.
102. Russell ME, et al. Cartilage contact pressure elevations in dysplastic hips: a chronic overload model. J Orthop Surg Res. 2006;1:6.
103. Noguchi Y, et al. Cartilage and labrum degeneration in the dysplastic hip generally originates in the anterosuperior weight-bearing area: an arthroscopic observation. Arthroscopy. 1999;15(5):496–506.
104. Tsumura H, Miura H, Iwamoto Y. Three-dimensional pressure distribution of the human hip joint—comparison between normal hips and dysplastic hips. Fukuoka Igaku Zasshi. 1998;89(4):109–18.
105. Hadley NA, Brown TD, Weinstein SL. The effects of contact pressure elevations and aseptic necrosis on the long-term outcome of congenital hip dislocation. J Orthop Res. 1990;8(4):504–13.
106. Anderson AE, Ellis BJ, Maas SA, Peters CL, Weiss JA. Validation of finite element predictions of cartilage contact pressure in the human hip joint. J Biomech Eng. 2008;130(5):051008.
107. Henak CR, Ellis BJ, Harris MD, Anderson AE, Peters CL, Weiss JA. Role of the acetabular labrum in load support across the hip joint. J Biomech. 2011;44(12):2201–6.
108. Anderson AE, Ellis BJ, Maas SA, Weiss JA. Effects of idealized joint geometry on finite element predictions of cartilage contact stresses in the hip. J Biomech. 2010;43(7):1351–7.
109. Klaue K, Durnin CW, Ganz R. The acetabular rim syndrome. A clinical presentation of dysplasia of the hip. J Bone Joint Surg Br. 1991;73(3):423–9.
110. Haene RA, Bradley M, Villar RN. Hip dysplasia and the torn acetabular labrum: an inexact relationship. J Bone Joint Surg Br. 2007;89(10):1289–92.
111. Kawabe K, Konishi N. Three-dimensional modeling of cartilage thickness in hip dysplasia. Clin Orthop Relat Res. 1993;289:180–5.
112. Clohisy JC, Barrett SE, Gordon JE, Delgado ED, Schoenecker PL. Periacetabular osteotomy for the treatment of severe acetabular dysplasia. J Bone Joint Surg Am. 2005;87(2):254–9.
113. Millis MB, Kim YJ. Rationale of osteotomy and related procedures for hip preservation: a review. Clin Orthop Relat Res. 2002;405:108–21.
114. Beighton P, Horan F. Orthopaedic aspects of the Ehlers-Danlos syndrome. J Bone Joint Surg Br. 1969;51(3):444–53.
115. Grahame R, Bird HA, Child A. The revised (Brighton 1998) criteria for the diagnosis of benign joint hypermobility syndrome (BJHS). J Rheumatol. 2000;27(7):1777–9.
116. Nawabi DH, Bedi A, Tibor LM, Magennis E, Kelly BT. The demographic characteristics of high-level and recreational athletes undergoing hip arthroscopy for Femoroacetabular impingement (FAI): a sports-specific analysis. Arthroscopy. 2014;30:398–405.
117. Duthon VB, Charbonnier C, Kolo FC, Magnenat-Thalmann N, Becker CD, Bouvet C, Coppens E, Hoffmeyer P, Menetrey J. Correlation of clinical and magnetic resonance imaging findings in hips of elite female ballet dancers. Arthroscopy. 2013;29(3):411–9.
118. Charbonnier C, Kolo FC, Duthon VB, et al. Assessment of congruence and impingement of the hip joint in professional ballet dancers: a motion capture study. Am J Sports Med. 2011;39:557–66.
119. Harris J, Slikker W, Gupta A, Abrams G, Nho S. Routine complete capsular closure during hip arthroscopy. Arthrosc Tech. 2013;2:e89–94.
120. McCormick F, Slikker III W, Harris JD, et al. Evidence of capsular defect following hip arthroscopy. Knee Surg Sports Traumatol Arthrosc. 2014;22(4):902–5.
121. Ranawat AS, McClincy M, Sekiya JK. Anterior dislocation of the hip after arthroscopy in a patient with capsular laxity of the hip. A case report. J Bone Joint Surg Am. 2009;91(1):192–7.
122. Benali Y, Katthagen BD. Hip subluxation as a complication of arthroscopic debridement. Arthroscopy. 2009;25(4):405–7.
123. Ilizaliturri Jr VM. Complications of arthroscopic femoroacetabular impingement treatment: a review. Clin Orthop Relat Res. 2009;467(3):760–8.
124. Matsuda DK. Acute iatrogenic dislocation following hip impingement arthroscopic surgery. Arthroscopy. 2009;25(4):400–4.
125. Mei-Dan O, McConkey MO, Brick M. Catastrophic failure of hip arthroscopy due to iatrogenic instability: can partial division of the ligamentum teres and iliofemoral ligament cause subluxation? Arthroscopy. 2012;28(3):440–5.
126. Sansone M, Ahlden M, Jonasson P, Sward L, Eriksson T, Karlsson J. Total dislocation of the hip joint after arthroscopy and ileopsoas tenotomy. Knee Surg Sports Traumatol Arthrosc. 2013;21(2):420–3.
127. Souza BG, Dani WS, Honda EK, Ricioli Jr W, Guimaraes RP, Ono NK, et al. Do complications in hip arthroscopy change with experience? Arthroscopy. 2010;26(8):1053–7.
128. Bayne CO, Stanley R, Simon P, Espinoza-Orias A, Salata MJ, Bush-Joseph CA, Nho SJ. Effect of capsulotomy on hip stability-a consideration during hip arthroscopy. Am J Orthop (Belle Mead NJ). 2014;43(4):160–5.

Part II

Clinical Evaluation of Hip Function

Allston J. Stubbs

Function of the Normal Hip

8

Michael R. Torry, Michael J. Decker, Jeffrey C. Cowley, David Keeley, Thomas W. Kernozek, and Kevin B. Shelburne

Introduction

The hip joint is both characterized and constrained by the osseous, ligamentous, and musculotendinous anatomical structures of the region. The purpose of this chapter is to review the literature examining the function of these osseous and ligamentous structures supporting the hip and the neuromuscular control strategies associated with hip function. We will also focus on the neuromuscular control related to hip stability and mobility during walking since the investigations related to gait represent the largest body of knowledge regarding hip function. Further, this chapter will describe the kinematics and kinetics of several sporting activities that are often associated with hip injury in an active population.

M.R. Torry, PhD (✉)
Illinois State University, School of Kinesiology, Campus Box 5120, Normal, IL 61790-5120, USA
e-mail: mtorry@ilstu.edu

M.J. Decker, PhD
Center of Orthopaedic Biomechanics, Mechanical and Materials Engineering Department, Felix Ritchie School of Engineering and Computer Science, University of Denver, Denver, CO, USA

J.C. Cowley, MS
School of Kinesiology and Recreation, Illinois State University, Normal, IL, USA

D. Keeley, PhD
Department of Human Performance Dance and Recreation, New Mexico State University, Las Cruces, NM, USA

T.W. Kernozek, FACSM, PhD
Health Professions Department, Physical Therapy Program, University of Wisconsin-La Crosse, La Crosse, WI, USA

K.B. Shelburne, PhD
Department of Mechanical and Materials Engineering, The University of Denver, Denver, CO, USA

Osseous Structures Contributing to Hip Stabilization

The adult hip is a ball and socket type of diarthrodial joint comprised by the femur and the acetabulum of the coxae bone. The boney congruency of this joint conveys much of its characteristic stability. Three aspects of these osseous structures are important to hip joint stability and the preservation of the labrum and articular cartilage: (1) appropriate femoral head-neck offset, (2) acetabular and femoral anteversion, and (3) acetabular coverage of the femoral head.

Proper function of the hip requires that the femoral head be offset from the femoral neck to allow a full range of joint motion without an impingement between the femur and the acetabulum. A reduction in this offset has been conferred as a cause for femoroacetabular impingement [1]. Likewise, excessive hip flexion [with or without external femoral rotation] may cause the femoral head-neck junction to contact the labrum also resulting in impingement [1–3]. Osseous abnormalities such as a large femoral head can serve to compensate for this reduced offset at the head-neck junction and aid joint stability [4].

Considerable disparities exist in the ranges of acetabular anteversion and femoral anteversion, and these ranges change within an individual from the time of birth through skeletal maturity. Normal anteversion of the acetabulum is essential to maintaining a normal relationship with the femoral head and range from 15° to 42° with a recommended range of 15°–20° using measurements employed by Murray (1993) [5–8]. Anteversion of the femur is also important in maintaining proper mechanics in the hip joint, and the degree of femoral anteversion diminishes with age. Infants demonstrate an average femoral anteversion of 31° which will likely decrease by ~5° by 8 years of age and further decrease 5°–10° by late adolescence [9]. As both joint stability and femoral head coverage depend upon the relative orientation of the femur and acetabulum, the combined effect of femoral and acetabular anteversion is important to consider. The McKibbin instability index is based on the sum of the angles

J.C. McCarthy et al. (eds.), *Hip Joint Restoration*, DOI 10.1007/978-1-4614-0694-5_8

of the femoral and acetabular anteversion [10]. This index predicts clinically high joint instability for summed angles of >60° and low instability for angles of less than 20°. Femoral head coverage provided by the acetabulum can also be measured radiographically. Normal center-edge angle is reported to be ~30° [11–14]. Dysplasia has been associated with early onset of osteoarthritis, and center-edge angles of less than ~20° correlate with abnormal orientation of the acetabulum, poor head coverage, and atypical intra-articular load transfer [11–18].

Hip Stabilization via Ligamentous Structures

The hip capsule is comprised of a series of ligaments divided into various functional and anatomical components. The five primary ligaments of the hip are the iliofemoral (includes both the lateral and the medial bundles), pubofemoral, ischiofemoral, the ligamentum teres femoris, and the ligamentum orbicularis [19–21].

The mechanical influence that these ligaments have on hip mechanics during dynamic [or even static] activities is scarce due to technological limitations in obtaining in vivo strain measures. However, as technology advances more information is becoming available on the synergistic roles that these ligaments play in limiting rotations as well as translations in concert with other structures of the hip. This has been investigated in a cadaveric study by Myers et al. [19] which showed that the iliofemoral ligament had an important role in limiting both external rotation and anterior translation of the femur, while the acetabular labrum provided a secondary stabilizing role.

Hip Stabilization via Neuromechanics

Maintaining appropriate femoral head positioning and load-bearing areas within the acetabulum is the principal feature of normal hip function. To accomplish this and acting in synergy with the ligamentous structures, muscles crossing the hip act as force modulators by regulating their intrinsic stiffness properties across a wide range of joint motions available at the hip joint. These neuromuscular control strategies begin with the activation of the single fiber and progress to altering the mechanical properties of the entire muscle. These underlying mechanisms are based on temporal/spatial summation of motor unit firing, fiber recruitment, muscle active-passive physiological composition, active-passive length-tension, and force-velocity properties as well as the intra- and extrafusal fiber feedback loops within the muscle [22–28]. Of these, the physical arrangement of the muscle fibers within a specific muscle (i.e., the skeletal muscle architecture) is of substantial mechanical importance at the hip given the large, pennated muscles that cross this joint. This is because the force-generating capacity of a muscle is proportional to its physiological cross-sectional area (PCSA), and its total excursion is determined by its fiber length. The mechanical properties of many of the larger muscles surrounding the hip have been well characterized as reviewed by Torry et al. [29].

Estimates of Individual Hip Muscular Contributions to Gait and Hip Joint Kinetics

Traditional gait analysis techniques allow the hip to be studied across a myriad of pathologies and yield in vivo hip joint forces and net muscle moments. Figures 8.1 and 8.2 provide the typical hip joint reaction forces and hip joint moments during the gait cycle of young, healthy males. On average, the hip experiences a bimodal vertical joint reaction force-loading pattern characterized by two distinct peaks ranging from 4 to 8 body weights (BW) occurring just after heel strike and again just prior to toe off [30]. Figure 8.2 shows the typical external hip moment profile during gait for the sagittal (flexion-extension) and frontal (adduction-abduction) planes. Excluding immediately after heel strike, the frontal plane hip moment is dominated by an external adduction torque exhibiting a bimodal pattern with peak magnitudes of 3–4 % BW*height (%BW*ht). The sagittal plane moment exhibits an external flexor torque peaking just after heel strike (5–6 %BW*ht) and continuing until 50 % midstance (foot flat) before transitioning to an external extensor torque reaching its peak just prior to toe off [30].

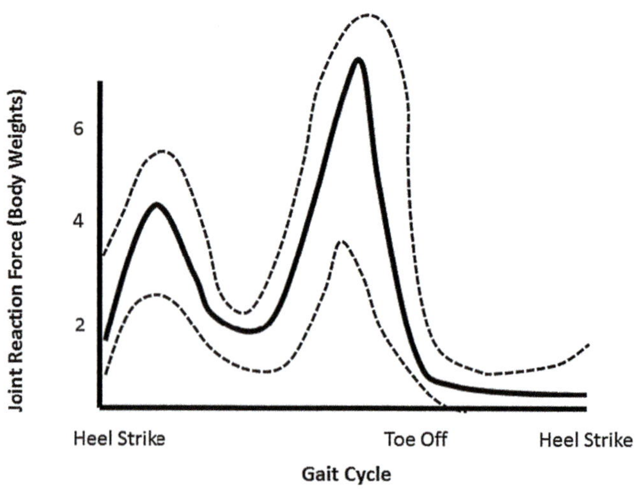

Fig 8.1 Time-normalized vertical hip joint reaction force curve of 12 healthy, college-aged males walking at self-selected speeds. Graph derived from data taken from Mathew P and Torry MR (2014). The Effects of Opedix (TM) Knee Support System on Lower Extremity Biomechanics During Walking and Jogging, Master's Thesis, Illinois State University [30]

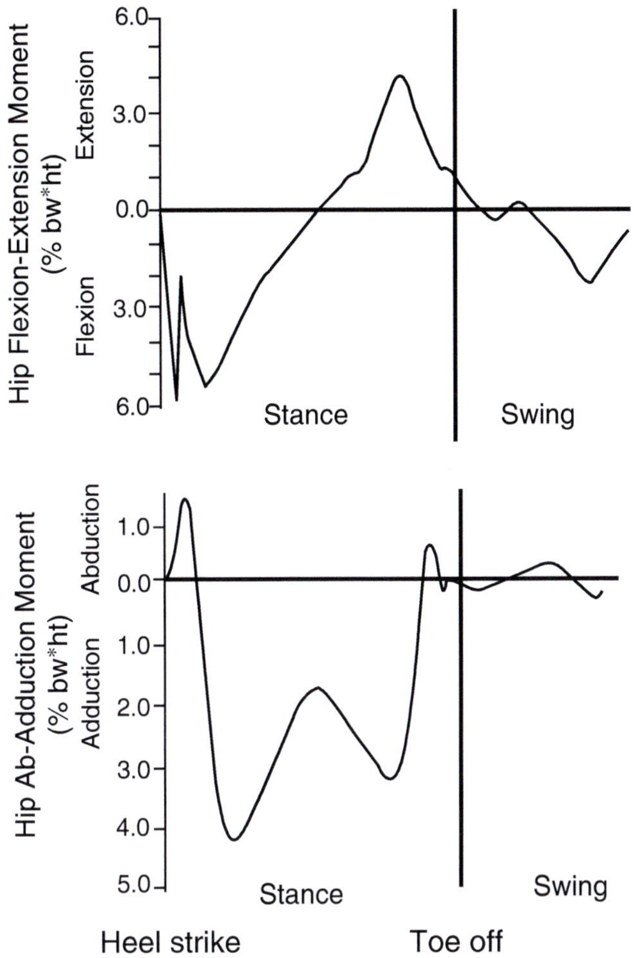

Fig 8.2 Time-normalized external hip moment profiles during gait for the sagittal (flexion-extension) and frontal (adduction-abduction) planes of 12 healthy, college-aged males walking at self-selected speeds. Graph derived from data taken from Mathew P and Torry MR (2014). The Effects of Opedix (TM) Knee Support System on Lower Extremity Biomechanics During Walking and Jogging, Master's Thesis, Illinois State University [30]

These moments, however, cannot be decomposed into individual muscle contributions to the motion or in determining joint loads without appropriate assumptions that obtain an equal number of unknowns and equations or by employing an optimization scheme. Optimization methods assume that the force distribution among the muscles is made by applying an objective function (usually based on a physical property of a muscle such as PCSA). Sophisticated models have employed more precise muscle paths through "wrapping functions" to better reflect the muscles' path around anatomic structures and more specific fiber length parameters for individual muscle bundles within the complex geometry of the entire muscle [31–35].

Anderson and Pandy (2003) developed a muscle model that included select hip musculature to analyze a complete gait cycle [36]. This model contained 54 independent muscles, and their results estimated each muscle's contribution to the support phase of gait. A muscle's potential for generating support was described by its contribution to the vertical ground reaction force per unit of muscle force. Of the hip muscles, the gluteus medius, maximus, and minimus provided the majority of the force in first 0 to 30 % of stance (Figs. 8.3a–c and 8.4). From foot flat to just after contralateral toe off (e.g., 10–50 % of stance), the gluteus maximus and posterior medius/minimus contributed significantly to the vertical ground reaction force. With assistance from skeletal structures against gravity, the anterior and posterior gluteus medius/minimus generated nearly all the force during midstance. Posterior gluteus medius/minimus provided force throughout midstance, while the anterior gluteus medius/minimus contributed only at the end of midstance (Fig. 8.4). This indicates that the role of the gluteus medius and minimus depends strongly on body position [36].

More recently, Correa and Pandy [34] described the hip intra-articular joint-loading profiles and relative contributions of individual muscle forces, gravitational forces, and centrifugal forces (i.e., forces arising from joint velocities) from the ipsilateral and contralateral hip joints during walking. Their results showed that (in the healthy, non-injured hip) the muscles were the major contributors to the hip contact force, with gravitational and centrifugal forces combining to contribute less than 5 % of the total contact force (Fig. 8.5). The four muscles spanning the hip, gluteus medius, gluteus maximus, iliopsoas, and hamstrings, contributed most to the hip contact force (Fig. 8.6).

Articular cartilage is uniquely characterized by its ability to receive and dissipate the contact loads across a joint. Harris et al. (2012) estimated the acetabular cartilage contact locations, contact stresses, and contact areas during five discrete time points during a complete walking cycle as well as during stair ascent and stair descent activities (Fig. 8.7) [37]. Peak stress ranged from 7.5 ± 2 MPa for heel strike during walking to 8.6 ± 3 MPa for heel strike during descending stairs (Fig. 8.7) [37]. Average contact area across all activities was 34 % of the surface area of the acetabular cartilage. While these authors demonstrated that although the contact location was different among activities, the average contact areas on the acetabular cartilage were similar during each activity for each individual. While the data also suggest that relatively small incongruences in femoral and acetabular cartilage have a very large effect on the contact stresses, it also demonstrates that there is a large diversity in cartilage contact stresses in healthy hips during activities of daily living across individuals; yet, any single person demonstrated remarkably low variability in cartilage loading across a rather wide variety of motions and external load demands [37].

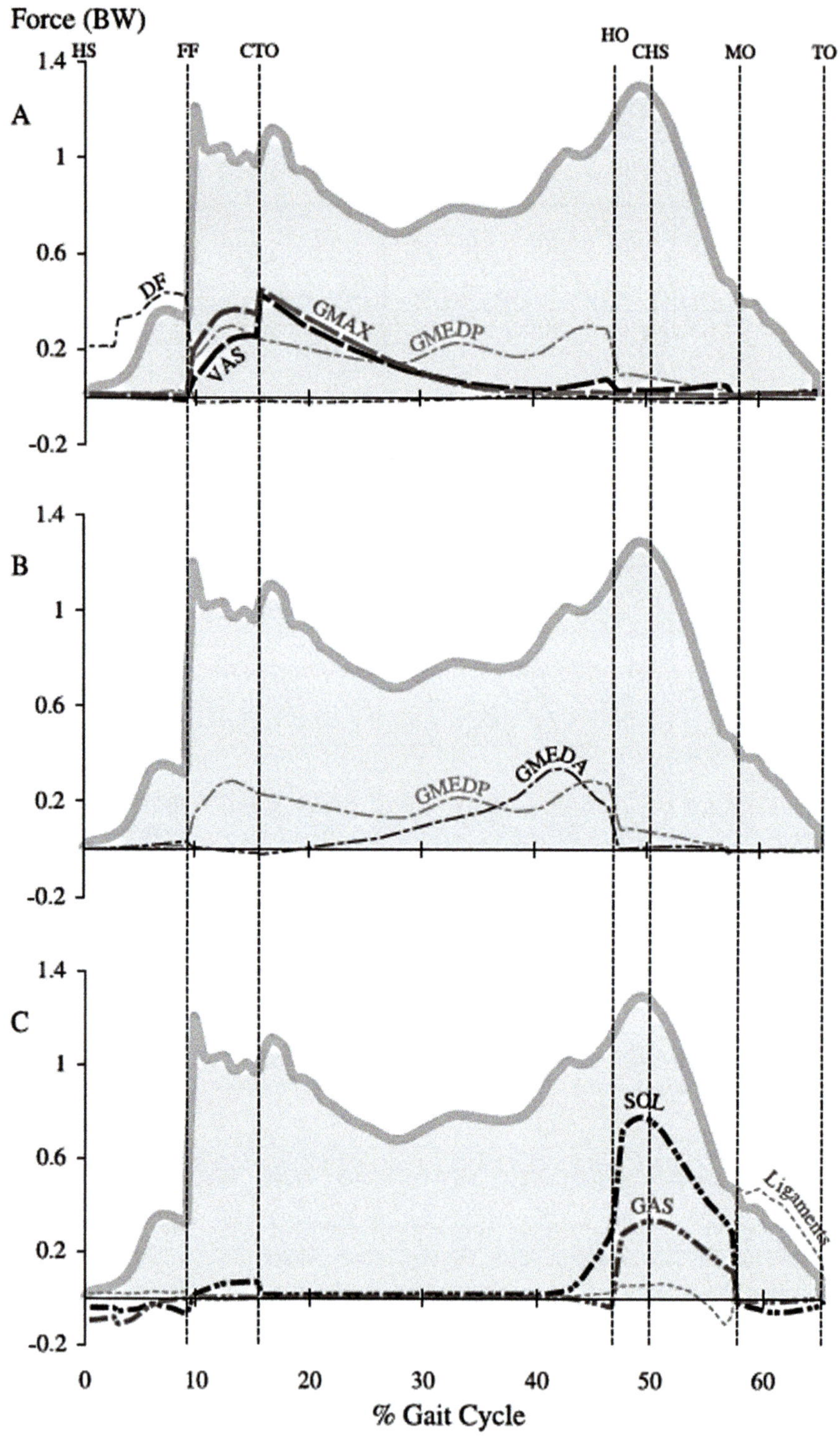

Fig. 8.3 (a–c) Individual muscle contributions to support during gait from heel strike (HS) to toe off (TO). Support is represented by the shaded *gray area* which is the vertical ground reaction force. *Symbols* used to represent muscles in the figure are *DF* ankle dorsiflexors, *GMAX* medial and lateral portions of the gluteus maximus, *VAS* vasti, *GMEDA* anterior gluteus medius/minimus, *GMEDP* posterior gluteus medius/minimus, *SOL* soleus, and *GAS* gastrocnemius. The gluteus maximus contributes the most muscle force to support in early stance; the posterior gluteus medius/minimus contributes notable force throughout the stance phase. In later stance, the anterior gluteus medius/minimus is most effective at maintaining support during gait. The passive resistance of the skeleton to the force of gravity was less than 50% of body weight throughout stance, suggesting that muscles are the most important parameter to support the body during gait. Of these muscles, the hip gluteus maximus contributed the most force to support, followed by the vasti, gluteus medius/minimus, and soleus/gastrocnemius of the body compared to all other muscles during gait. Unfortunately, the mechanical roles of the smaller hip muscles such as the pectineus, piriformis, superior and inferior gemellus, and obturator internus and externus were not included in this model. From Anderson, F. C. and M. G. Pandy (2003). Individual muscle contributions to support in normal walking. *Gait & Posture* 17(2): 159–69. Reprinted with permission from Elsevier

Electromyography of Hip Musculature

Electromyography (EMG) is a technique often utilized to measure the electrical input (excitation) of the muscle. There is considerable literature reporting the EMG activation of the hip muscles for walking, climbing stairs, and various sporting motions. Due to space limitations and the completeness of data content, only the EMG of hip muscles during gait is presented below. While EMG studies are valuable in determining *which* and *when* individual muscles are active, it is important to note that EMG cannot denote the amount of

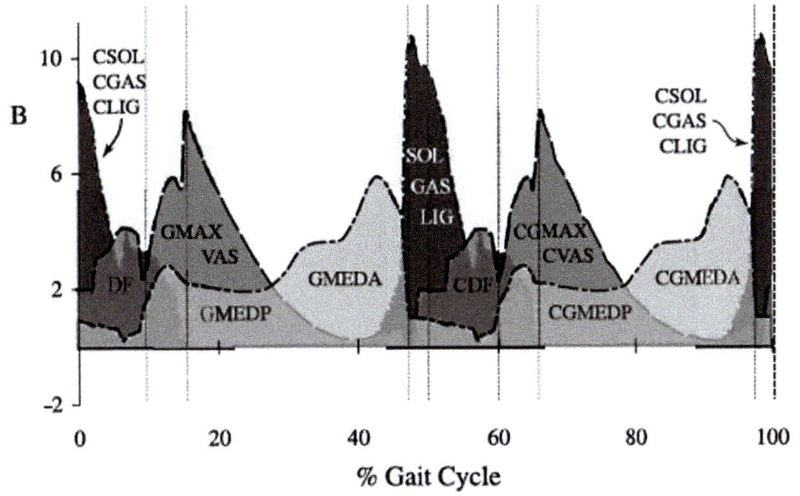

Fig. 8.4 Contributions of individual muscle groups to the net vertical acceleration of the center of mass of the walking model. Muscle symbols used are *CDF* dorsiflexors of the contralateral limb, *CSOL* soleus of contralateral limb, *CGAS* contralateral gastrocnemius, *CLIG* ligaments of contralateral limb, *CGMAX* contralateral gluteus maximus, *CGMEDA* contralateral anterior gluteus medius/minimus, *CGMEDP* contralateral posterior gluteus medius/minimus, *GMAX* medial and lateral portions of the gluteus maximus, *VAS* vasti, *GMEDA* anterior gluteus medius/minimus, *GMEDP* posterior gluteus medius/minimus, *SOL* soleus, and *GAS* gastrocnemius. Only muscles on the limb in contact with the ground contributed to the vertical acceleration of the center of mass. From Anderson, F. C. and M. G. Pandy (2003). Individual muscle contributions to support in normal walking. *Gait & Posture* 17(2): 159–69. Reprinted with permission from Elsevier

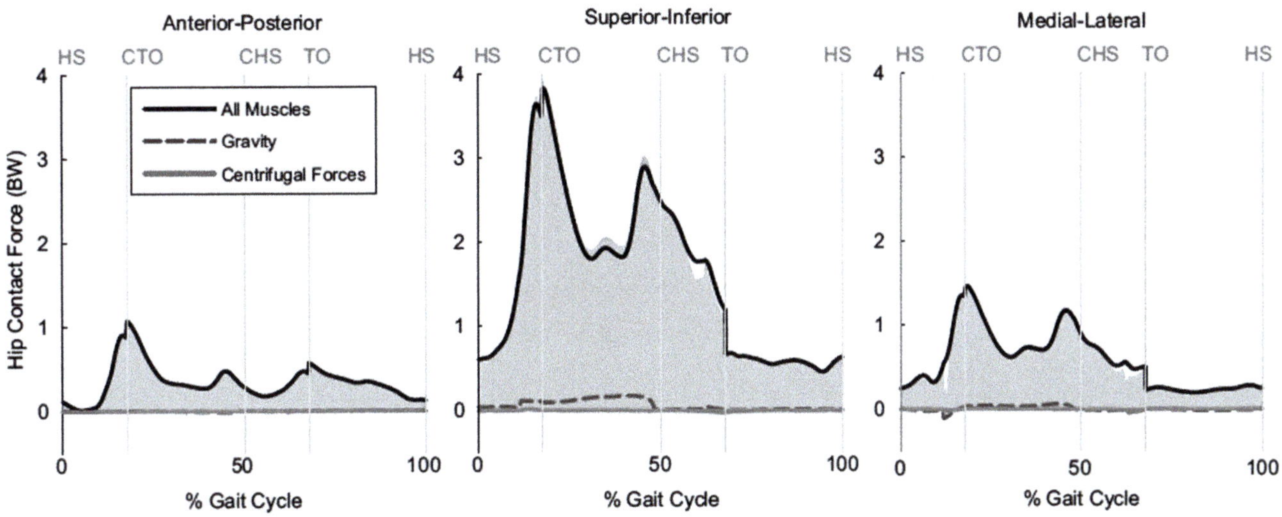

Fig. 8.5 Contributions of muscle gravitational forces and centrifugal forces to the three components of the hip contact force (in body weights) acting on the acetabulum with positive forces directed anteriorly, superiorly, and medially. The gait cycle is divided into phases starting at ipsilateral heel strike and includes contralateral toe off (CTO) and contralateral heel strike (CHS) demarcations and continues on to subsequent ipsilateral heel strike. The gray area represents the total (resultant) contact force. The data shows that the hip muscles were the major contributors to hip contact force, with gravitational and centrifugal forces combined contributing less than 5% of the total contact force. From Correa TA et al. Contributions of individual muscles to hip joint contact force in normal walking. J Biomech. 2010 May 28;43(8):1618–22. Reprinted with permission from Elsevier

force a muscle is producing. This limitation largely underscores the importance of computer modeling techniques to better understand the hip mechanics during functional activities, the mechanics associated with hip stabilization, the influence of bony geometry, and the actual muscle forces needed to stabilize the hip joint. Yet, the use of EMG is vital to provide these models with the appropriate onset and offset of muscle activation patterns such that these models identify and "recruit" the correct order and number of muscles within their optimization routine.

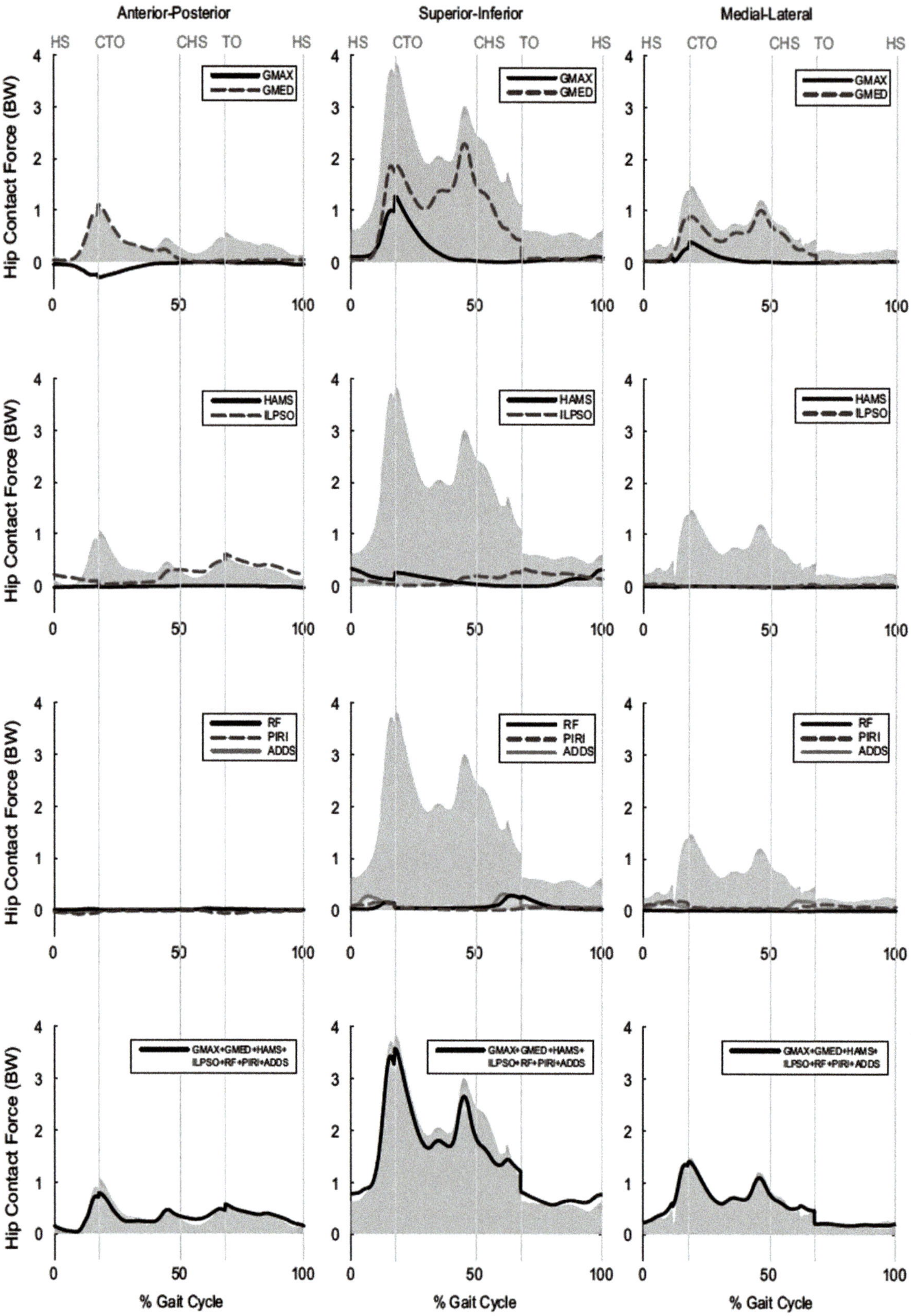

Fig. 8.6 Contributions of major hip muscles to the joint contact force. The *gray area* represents the total (resultant) contact force with the three components of the hip contact force (in body weights) acting on the acetabulum with positive forces directed anteriorly, superiorly, and medially. *HAMS* medial and lateral hamstring muscles, *GMAX* gluteus maximus, *GMED* gluteus medius and minimus combined, *ILPSO* iliacus and psoas combined, *RF* rectus femoris, *PIRI* piriformis, *ADDS* adductor magnus, longus, and brevis combined. From Correa TA et al. Contributions of individual muscles to hip joint contact force in normal walking. J Biomech. 2010 May 28;43(8):1618–22. Reprinted with permission from Elsevier

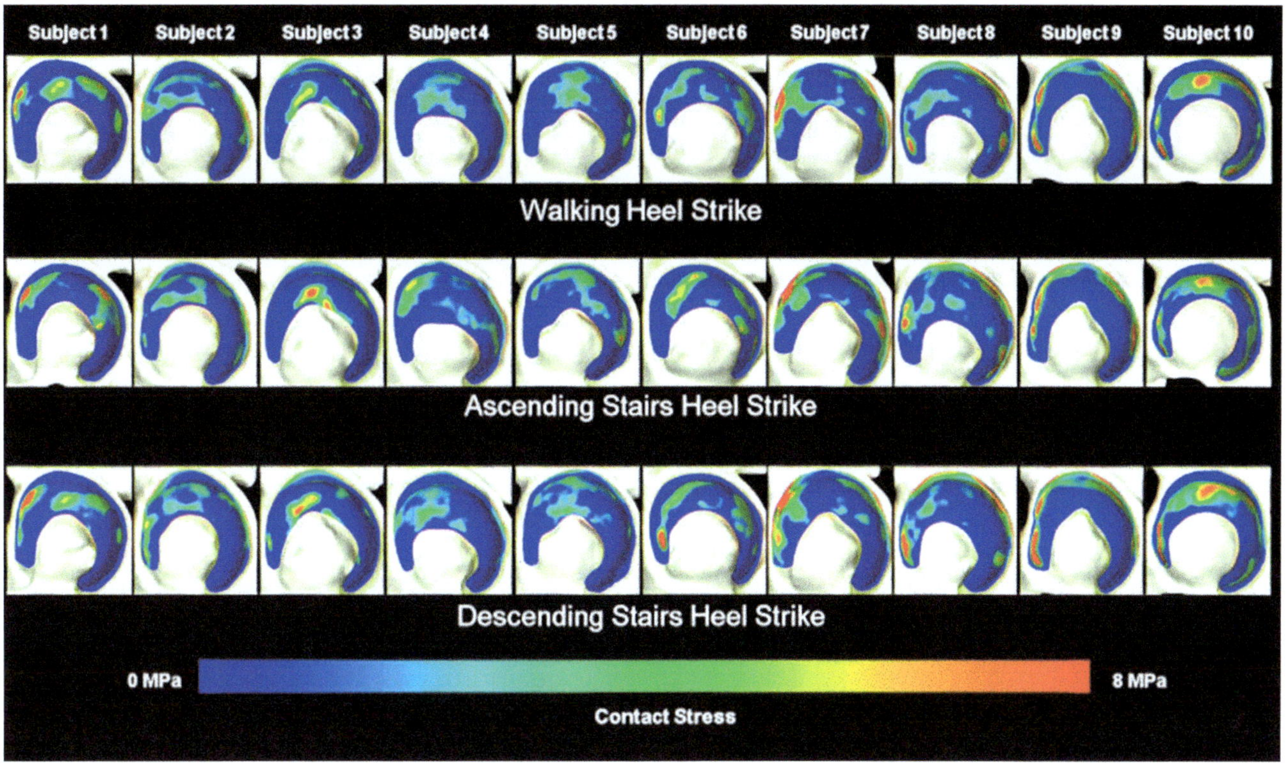

Fig. 8.7 Contact locations and stresses on the acetabular cartilage for ten subjects during walking, ascending stairs, and descending stairs. *Left* is anterior. The location of the peak stress tended to be similar for a particular subject across all activities (compare locations of and magnitudes of stresses for each subject down each column). Generally, the peak stresses increased slightly as the joint reaction force increased among activities. Variations in stresses across persons demonstrated high variability. From Harris MD, Anderson AE, Henak CR, Ellis BJ, Peters CL, and Weiss JA. Finite element prediction of cartilage contact stresses in normal human hips. J Orthop Res. 2012 Jul;30(7):1133–9. Reprinted with permission from John Wiley and Sons

The Deep Hip Muscles

Studies of the muscles of the hip joint have typically neglected the roles of the deeper musculature (pectineus, piriformis, superior and inferior gemellus, and obturator internus and externus) because of their inaccessibility [38, 39]. These muscles are often coined as "rotator cuff" muscles for the hip, and many studies in canine models have supported their roles in "fine-tuning" hip motions [40]. However, unlike the glenohumeral joint, the human hip is considered a more stable joint via its bony geometry requiring less muscular stabilization. To this end, many authors have suggested that the small PCSA of these deep muscles combined with their small moment arms (e.g., pectineus moment arms during gait has been estimated at less than 9 mm for stance phase of gait) are trivial in providing any "meaningful" forces for maintaining hip stability. Nevertheless, clinical views of the function of the pectineus make this muscle's role in hip function more important than one would ascertain from its rather small size and moment arm. The results of computational studies correspond well with EMG profiles measured in healthy persons during gait [41]. The pectineus is moderately active at mid-heel strike to mid-toe off, functioning to limit the amount of femoral abduction while contributing to femoral medial rotation. Some minor activity of this muscle is also present during the swing phase [42].

Shelburne et al. measured piriformis EMG activity during a squat exercise and determined its activation level to be less than 25 % of MVC throughout the motion. This activation data corresponded well with subsequent calculations of piriformis force during the same exercise which was less than 25 % of maximal capacity [43].

Iliopsoas

The iliopsoas has two major portions (the iliacus and the psoas) with separate innervations making selective activation of each portion feasible for any given movement. Recently, Philippon et al. determined that iliopsoas activation was increased for some hip strengthening/rehabilitation exercises and therefore may potentially aggravate hip flexor tendinitis [44]. Specifically, peak iliopsoas muscle activity ranged from 3 to 48 % MVC, while average iliopsoas activity ranged from 1 to 18% MVC. Supine hip flexion, side-lying hip abduction performed against the wall, side-lying hip abduction with external rotation, and hip clamshell exercises demonstrated moderate iliopsoas muscle activation (20%). All other exercises measured demonstrated minimal iliopsoas muscle activity [44].

Only a few studies have attempted to define and differentiate between the functional roles of the iliacus and psoas [45, 46]. Thus, there is some disagreement in the EMG information of this muscle, partly resulting from different techniques and the difficulty in measuring EMG in this muscle largely due to its location and pennation. Andersson et al. noted that both muscles are active during maximal thigh abduction; but no activity is noted for either psoas or iliacus during standing at ease or with the whole trunk flexed 30° forward at the hip. Andersson et al. concluded that the iliacus primarily stabilizes the hip and pelvis; whereas, the psoas assists in stabilizing the lumbar spine in the frontal plane when a heavy load is applied to the contralateral side [45].

Iliacus

Attempts to measure EMG of the iliacus have shown notable activity throughout flexion of the hip during the "sit-up in the supine position" [46]. LaBan et al. however, reported that there was little or no activity in the iliacus during the first 30° of hip flexion; but, these authors noted activity during a sit-up from the "hook-lying" position [47].

Psoas Major

Direct recordings from the psoas muscle are generally similar to those measured from the iliacus. There is slight activation during relaxed standing and strong activity during flexed postures [45]. Also, slight-to-moderate activity in abduction and lateral rotation is present (depending on the amount of hip flexion), with no activity during most medial rotation positions and little additional activity during most other positions involving the thigh [45, 46]. Nachemson concluded that the psoas has a significant role in maintaining upright postures [48].

Gluteus Maximus

Karlsson and Jonsson concluded that the gluteus maximus was active with hip extension, lateral rotation, abduction against a heavy resistance when the thigh is flexed to 90°, and with adduction against resistance while keeping the thigh abducted [49]. Joseph and Williams showed that the gluteus maximus is not an important postural muscle but exhibits moderate activity when bending forward and when straightening up from the toe-touch position [50].

Gluteus Medius and Minimus

The finding of Joseph and Williams that indicated that the gluteus medius and minimus are quiescent during relaxed standing serves to confirm that these abductors prevent the Trendelenburg sign, during abduction of the thigh and with medial rotation [51]. These roles of gluteus medius and minimus in medial rotation were confirmed by Greenlaw who reported triphasic activity for gluteus medius and biphasic activity for gluteus minimus during each cycle of walking [51]. Shelburne et al. measured EMG of the gluteus medius during the squat and determined the activation level to be less than 25% of MVC throughout the motion [43]. This activation largely corresponded well with the estimates of gluteus medius force being less than 25% of its maximal capacity during the same exercise [43, 52].

Philippon et al. measured gluteus medius activity using indwelling EMG during 13 rehabilitation exercises reporting peak gluteus medius muscle activity ranging from 16 to 73% MVC and average gluteus medius muscle activity from 3 to 35% MVC [44]. The single-leg bridge, the prone heel squeeze, and side-lying hip abduction whether performed with internal hip rotation, against a wall, or with external hip rotation had the highest peak gluteus medius activation (50% MVC). All other exercises demonstrated moderate gluteus medius activation (21–50% MVC) except for the resisted knee flexion and terminal knee extension exercises, which demonstrated minimal activation (<20% MVC) [44].

Tensor Fasciae Latae

Wheatley and Jahnke [53], Carlsoo and Fohlin [54], and Goto et al. [55] reported moderate muscle activity during hip flexion, medial rotation, and abduction. Greenlaw indicated that the muscle was active biphasically during each stride during gait [51]. This muscle has been shown to be active during bicycling, showing the greatest activity during the pedal's "upstroke" defined largely by hip flexion [56].

Adductors of the Hip Joint

Greenlaw examined EMG during both fast and slow movements, with various postures, and types of locomotion [51]. When in single-leg standing, the adductors on the stance leg remained silent, while the medial thigh rotation activated the hip adductors. During walking, there is a marked difference between the two parts of the adductors magnus; the upper portion possesses a pure adductor role and was active throughout the gait cycle, while adductor brevis and longus showed triphasic periods with the main peaks occurring at toe off [51].

Hip Strength Assessment

Objective assessments of hip strength are typically performed using one of two methods: using handheld dynamometry or with the use of an isokinetic dynamometer. Handheld dynamometry is an inexpensive and clinically feasible method for measuring hip strength. Many studies using isometric strength have implemented various dynamometer stabilization techniques to yield more reproducible data [57, 58]. Isokinetic machines can be also used to assess hip strength where the individual is largely constrained by the machine into a specific test position while allowing for specific joint motion.

Isometric hip flexion strength has been shown to decrease from nearly 25° to 130° of hip flexion and experiences the greatest strength near anatomical position [59, 60]. The hip extensors produce larger amounts of peak torque compared to other planes from isokinetic testing done in a standing position. The hip abductors and adductors produced less torque than the flexors and extensors. Murray and Sepic demonstrated that when the hip is abducted the abductor strength is reduced compared to the adductors [61]. Based on computed tomography measures, the hip abductors have about a 25 % reduction in muscle cross-sectional area in comparison to the knee extensors but produce considerable force due to their larger moment arms and better angle of pull [62]. Hip internal and external rotators are most often tested in a position where the hip and knee are flexed to 90°. In this test position the medial hip rotators have been shown to generate more force than the lateral hip rotators [63, 64].

Hip strength appears to be different based on gender and age. Young adults appear to have a greater ability to withstand fatigue than older adults and males appear to be stronger than females [61, 65]. Studies of hip strength asymmetry have largely been inconclusive where some investigations have shown differences, while others have not [66, 67]. Some of these studies have implicated strength asymmetry in injury in athletic populations [68].

Sport-Specific Motions of the Hip

A number of recent studies have applied different approaches to the study of hip biomechanics, particularly with respect to total hip replacements [69–71]. However, there is clearly a void in the literature relating to the function and pathology of the normal or injured, non-arthritic hip. Thus, the remaining chapter will offer our understanding as to how these injuries may affect the function of the hip in athletes by providing basic information relating to hip biomechanics during specific sports. For comparisons, Table 8.1 provides values for men during common activities of daily living. It is important to keep in mind that a majority of athletes undergoing hip arthroscopy have a complex injury pattern, with damage to the acetabular labrum, capsular structure, and cartilage surfaces. In order to ascertain the specific injury sequence and pattern(s) of cause and effect, additional research in performance assessment is still needed.

Table 8.1 Three-dimensional hip kinematics for common activities of daily living

	Sagittal	Frontal	Transverse
Squatting	122°	28°	26°
Ascending stairs	67°	16°	18°
Rising from chair	104°	20°	17°

Mean data from 33 healthy men [100]

Golf

During the downswing of a golfer, the trail limb's hip is forced into external rotation with axial loading. This movement tends to push the femoral head anteriorly and over time may lead to anterior capsular laxity with compromise of the iliofemoral ligament [29]. This may lead to increased translation of the femoral head within the acetabulum and result in instability. Labral tears, particularly in the anterosuperior weight-bearing region of the acetabulum, may follow [72]. As the labrum functions as a physiological seal, maintaining a negative pressure within the joint and stabilizing the femoral head in the acetabulum, further propagation of the labral injury may compromise the sealing function, further increasing translation of the femoral head under load [73, 74].

Taekwondo

In martial arts, particularly taekwondo, a good kick can be performed well above an athlete's head. Also, a proper taekwondo sidekick places the stance leg in 90° of external rotation. The stance leg must sustain significant loads, while the opposite leg performs the kick. Kim et al. measured the effects of target distance on the planted (pivot) hip, trunk, and pelvis in Taekwondo roundhouse kicks [75]. They reported that posterior pelvic tilt, peak pelvic rotation, peak hip hyperextension, and peak internal rotation increased as the "target distances" were increased in height. Similar to the mechanism in golfers, the forced external rotation and axial loading in the stance leg (non-kicking leg) may cause anterior capsular laxity and elongation of the iliofemoral ligament. It is hypothesized that the increased translation of the femoral head within the acetabulum leads to labral and chondral injuries.

Ballet

Elite ballet dancers and figure skaters often subject the hip to the extremes in rotational movement during their routines. Some athletes excel at these sports due to their instability secondary to repeated hip rotation and focal capsular laxity. A very common finding in ballet dancers (and figure skaters) undergoing hip arthroscopic surgery is capsular laxity with an associated labral tear [76].

Running

Although most cases of hip instability occur in sports requiring excessive axial rotational movements, runners may also present with subtle anterior hip instability [77]. The repeated hip hyperextension may stretch the anterior capsule and iliofemoral ligament in elite distance runners. This resulting microinstability may subtly increase femoral head translation and, with repeated insults, result in labral and chondral injury. During running, when the foot contacts the ground, the femur is in an abducted position in relation to the pelvis, causing eccentric loading of the gluteus medius and tensor fasciae latae [78]. As the support phase of running progresses, contraction of these muscles is necessary to keep the hip in adduction. Thus, it is believed that gluteus medius weakness may lead to decreased control of the thigh manifesting in increased hip abduction and internal femoral rotation. These changes may predispose the runner to several pathological conditions including iliotibial band syndrome as well as patellofemoral pain [78–80].

Jumping and Landing

The interest in landing mechanics largely stems from the interest in the etiology of noncontact injuries of the anterior cruciate ligament. Chaudhari and Andriacchi used a model of the hip to show that the stiffness of the hip influenced the valgus excursion of the knee in single-leg landing [81].

Baseball and Softball

For baseball pitchers, an understanding of the movement patterns of the hips is vital, as the force generated in throwing the ball is developed as the body unwinds, starting with the lower extremity. During pitching, a primary function of the lumbopelvic hip complex is to help generate a maximum energy transfer to the throwing arm via the trunk. As a result, high repetitive lower extremity may potentially lead to both degeneration of the hip joint and labral injuries [82–85]. Factors shown to impact the integrity of the hip joint during these actions include age, hip range of motion, physical loading levels, and body mass index [85–87]. During pitching, contraction of the adductors of the trailing leg also stabilizes the pelvis and lengthens the stride. Adequate peak hip abductor activity may contribute to the longer stride and reduce the risk of injury [88]. Unfortunately, weakness of hip abductors may result in a dysfunction in the kinetic chain, which can lead to increases in loading [89, 90] to hip structures [91]. Additionally, weakness and/or inflexibility in the trailing hip may affect the entire kinetic chain, leading to increased low back lordosis and excessive motion of the shoulder [91, 92]. Passive hip range of motion in the coronal and transverse planes appears to be related to ball velocity and aberrant trunk and pelvis motion.

Hip Function in Winter Sports

The identification of mechanisms which cause injury is important to injury treatment and prevention in any sport, but the playing surfaces and environments of winter sports have significantly impeded the acquisition of kinematic and, more specifically, kinetic data. As a result, limited normative data is available describing hip function during winter sports. However, the need for improved understanding, advances in synthetic ice, and enhanced data collection technology have improved our understanding in recent years [93, 94].

Ice Skating and Ice Hockey

Ice skating has been associated with several characteristic overuse injuries of the hip. Hockey players in particular sustain high rates of femoroacetabular impingement syndrome [93]. The susceptibility of skaters to impingement injuries is thought to be due to the combination of hip extension, abduction, and external rotation at the end of the push phase or a large degree of flexion and internal rotation of the hip during the swing phase. Additionally, the rapid abduction and extension of the hip during push-off have been identified as a potential cause of acute and chronic groin injuries. The prevalence of groin injuries among hockey players has led some to use the term "hockey hernia" [95]. However, caution should be exercised in this diagnosis as the early stages of femoroacetabular impingement syndrome may be mistaken for a groin injury, and care may be mismanaged [95].

Cross-Country Skiing

A high prevalence of overuse injuries of the hip has not been noted among cross-country skiers, and a reported two thirds of hip overuse injuries among cross-country skiers were a result of other forms of training [96]. Still the push techniques used in cross-country skiing involve forceful hip extension, abduction, and external rotation which may contribute to overuse injuries. Trochanteric bursitis was found to be among the most common overuse injuries seen in cross-country skiers [96]. Additionally, the attachment of a ski to the leg creates a large torsional moment arm which can contribute to rotational injuries particularly when unexpected situations are encountered. Acute rotational trauma to the hip is somewhat common in cross-country and alpine skiing [97]. Cross-country skiing may be considered an appropriate activity for patients of total hip replacement [98]. However, this conclusion is based on a comparison of vertical joint forces in walking, and it should be stressed that these results likely only reflect skiing under normal conditions. Unexpected situations may subject the hip to very different forces. Frontal and transverse plane kinematics of cross-country skiing are not well documented. Neither have mediolateral nor anteroposterior forces at the hip been accounted for. Data for skiers may also be difficult to generalize due to the significant contribution of the arms in cross-country skiing and the large variety of skiing techniques utilized [99]. Still three-dimensional kinematic and kinetic skiing data would be beneficial to understanding injury mechanisms in vivo.

Conclusions

The hip is one of the most stable but mobile joints in the lower extremity. It relies on complex interaction of osseous, ligamentous, and muscular control strategies during movement where it is often influenced by both trunk and lower limb positioning during functional and sporting tasks. The muscular contribution to support during weight-bearing movements is critical to the function of the hip resulting in large loads and stress to both cartilage and soft tissue structures. Loads posed by sporting movements are thought to pose an even greater risk of injury due to the larger magnitudes of loading coupled with more extremes in positioning. Despite advances in technology, differences in describing the motions of the hip in vivo across laboratories are apparent which makes generalizing outcomes from motion studies very difficult. Engineering-based research and data to support and/or to establish common, reliable, and valid standards for measuring, describing, and reporting 3D hip motions in vivo are still needed.

References

1. Lavigne M, Parvizi J, Beck M, Siebenrock KA, Ganz R, Leunig M. Anterior femoroacetabular impingement: part I. Techniques of joint preserving surgery. Clin Orthop Relat Res. 2004;418:61–6.
2. Ito K, Minka II MA, Leunig M, Werlen S, Ganz R. Femoroacetabular impingement and the cam-effect. A MRI-based quantitative anatomical study of the femoral head-neck offset. J Bone Joint Surg Br. 2001;83(2):171–6.
3. Notzli HP, Wyss TF, Stoecklin CH, Schmid MR, Treiber K, Hodler J. The contour of the femoral head-neck junction as a predictor for the risk of anterior impingement. J Bone Joint Surg Br. 2002;84(4):556–60.
4. Crowninshield RD, Maloney WJ, Wentz DH, Humphrey SM, Blanchard CR. Biomechanics of large femoral heads: what they do and don't do. Clin Orthop Relat Res. 2004;429:102–7.
5. Murray DW. The definition and measurement of acetabular orientation. J Bone Joint Surg Br. 1993;75(2):228–32.
6. Siebenrock KA, Schoeniger R, Ganz R. Anterior femoroacetabular impingement due to acetabular retroversion. Treatment with periacetabular osteotomy. J Bone Joint Surg Am. 2003;85-A(2):278–86.
7. Siebenrock KA, Wahab KH, Werlen S, Kalhor M, Leunig M, Ganz R. Abnormal extension of the femoral head epiphysis as a cause of cam impingement. Clin Orthop Relat Res. 2004;418:54–60.
8. Nordin JY, Attia D. [Fractures of the upper end of the femur in adults. Etiology, mechanism, diagnosis, development, prognosis, treatment]. Rev Prat. 1993;43(2):223–8.
9. Fabry G, Cheng LX, Molenaers G. Normal and abnormal torsional development in children. Clin Orthop Relat Res. 1994;302:22–6.
10. Hapa O, Yuksel HY, Muratli HH, Aksahin E, Gulcek S, Celebi L, et al. Axial plane coverage and torsion measurements in primary osteoarthritis of the hip with good frontal plane coverage and spherical femoral head. Arch Orthop Trauma Surg. 2010;130(10):1305–10.
11. Anda S, Terjesen T, Kvistad KA. Computed tomography measurements of the acetabulum in adult dysplastic hips: which level is appropriate? Skeletal Radiol. 1991;20(4):267–71.
12. Anda S, Terjesen T, Kvistad KA, Svenningsen S. Acetabular angles and femoral anteversion in dysplastic hips in adults: CT investigation. J Comput Assist Tomogr. 1991;15(1):115–20.
13. Fredensborg N. The CE, angle of normal hips. Acta Orthop Scand. 1976;47(4):403–5.
14. Goodman SB. Comparison of radiographic parameters for analysis of normal and dysplastic hips in the adult. Contemp Orthop. 1990;20(5):505–11.
15. Felson DT. Epidemiology of hip and knee osteoarthritis. Epidemiol Rev. 1988;10:1–28.
16. Lievense AM, Bierma-Zeinstra SM, Verhagen AP, Verhaar JA, Koes BW. Influence of hip dysplasia on the development of osteoarthritis of the hip. Ann Rheum Dis. 2004;63(6):621–6.
17. McCarthy JC, Noble PC, Schuck MR, Wright J, The LJ, Otto E. Aufranc Award: the role of labral lesions to development of early degenerative hip disease. Clin Orthop Relat Res. 2001; 393:25–37.
18. Reijman M, Hazes JM, Pols HA, Koes BW, Bierma-Zeinstra SM. Acetabular dysplasia predicts incident osteoarthritis of the hip: the Rotterdam study. Arthritis Rheum. 2005;52(3):787–93.
19. Myers CA, Register BC, Lertwanich P, Ejnisman L, Pennington WW, Giphart JE, et al. Role of the acetabular labrum and the iliofemoral ligament in hip stability: an in vitro biplane fluoroscopy study. Am J Sports Med. 2011;39 Suppl:85S–91.

20. Fuss FK, Bacher A. New aspects of the morphology and function of the human hip joint ligaments. Am J Anat. 1991;192(1):1–13.
21. Wasielewski R. The hip. 1998.
22. Gordon AM, Huxley AF, Julian FJ. The variation in isometric tension with sarcomere length in vertebrate muscle fibres. J Physiol. 1966;184(1):170–92.
23. Hill A. First and last experiments in skeletal muscle mechanics. London: Cambridge University Press; 1970.
24. Hoffer JA, O'Donovan MJ, Pratt CA, Loeb GE. Discharge patterns of hindlimb motoneurons during normal cat locomotion. Science. 1981;213(4506):466–7.
25. Horowits R, Podolsky RJ. The positional stability of thick filaments in activated skeletal muscle depends on sarcomere length: evidence for the role of titin filaments. J Cell Biol. 1987;105(5):2217–23.
26. Lieber RL, Brown CC. Quantitative method for comparison of skeletal muscle architectural properties. J Biomech. 1992;25(5): 557–60.
27. Moritani T, deVries HA. Neural factors versus hypertrophy in the time course of muscle strength gain. Am J Phys Med. 1979; 58(3):115–30.
28. Zajac FE. How musculotendon architecture and joint geometry affect the capacity of muscles to move and exert force on objects: a review with application to arm and forearm tendon transfer design. J Hand Surg Am. 1992;17(5):799–804.
29. Torry MR, Schenker ML, Martin HD, Hogoboom D, Philippon MJ. Neuromuscular hip biomechanics and pathology in the athlete. Clin Sports Med. 2006;25(2):179–97. vii.
30. Mathew P, Torry MR. The effects of Opedix (TM) knee support system on lower extremity biomechanics during walking and jogging. Master's Thesis, Illinois State University; 2014.
31. Anderson FC, Pandy MG. Dynamic optimization of human walking. J Biomech Eng. 2001;34:153–61.
32. Arnold AS, Salinas S, Asakawa DJ, Delp SL. Accuracy of muscle moment arms estimated from MRI-based musculoskeletal models of the lower extremity. Comput Aided Surg. 2000;5(2):108–19.
33. Correa TA, Baker R, Graham HK, Pandy MG. Accuracy of generic musculoskeletal models in predicting the functional roles of muscles in human gait. J Biomech. 2011;44(11):2096–105.
34. Correa TA, Crossley KM, Kim HJ, Pandy MG. Contributions of individual muscles to hip joint contact force in normal walking. J Biomech. 2010;43(8):1618–22.
35. Correa TA, Pandy MG. On the potential of lower limb muscles to accelerate the body's centre of mass during walking. Comput Methods Biomech Biomed Engin. 2013;16(9):1013–21.
36. Anderson FC, Pandy MG. Individual muscle contributions to support in normal walking. Gait Posture. 2003;17(2):159–69.
37. Harris MD, Anderson AE, Henak CR, Ellis BJ, Peters CL, Weiss JA. Finite element prediction of cartilage contact stresses in normal human hips. J Orthop Res. 2012;30(7):1133–9.
38. Wells C. Ancient lesions of the hip joint. Med Biol Illus. 1976;26(3):171–7.
39. Woodburne RT. The accessory obturator nerve and the innervation of the pectineus muscle. Anat Rec. 1960;136:367–9.
40. Lust G, Craig PH, Ross Jr GE, Geary JC. Studies on pectineus muscles in canine hip dysplasia. Cornell Vet. 1972;62(4):628–45.
41. Decker M, Krong J, Peterson D, Torry M, Philippon M. Deep hip muscle function during gait. In: 56th annual meeting of the Orthopedic Research Society, New Orleans, LA, 6–9 Mar 2010.
42. Takebe K, Vitti M, Basmajian JV. Electromyography of pectineus muscle. Anat Rec. 1974;180(2):281–3.
43. Shelburne K, Decker M, Philippon M, Torry M. Muscle forces at the hip during squatting exercise. In: 56th annual meeting of the Orthopedic Research Society, New Orleans, LA, 6–9 Mar 2010.
44. Philippon MJ, Decker MJ, Giphart JE, Torry MR, Wahoff MS, LaPrade RF. Rehabilitation exercise progression for the gluteus medius muscle with consideration for iliopsoas tendinitis: an in vivo electromyography study. Am J Sports Med. 2011;39(8):1777–85.
45. Andersson E, Oddsson L, Grundstrom H, Thorstensson A. The role of the psoas and iliacus muscles for stability and movement of the lumbar spine, pelvis and hip. Scand J Med Sci Sports. 1995;5(1):10–6.
46. Basmajian J, Greenlaw RK. EMG of iliacus and psoas with inserted fine-wire electrodes. Anat Rec. 1968;160:310–1.
47. LaBan MM, Raptou AD, Johnson EW. Electromyographic study of function of iliopsoas muscle. Arch Phys Med Rehabil. 1965;46(10):676–9.
48. Nachemson A. Electromyographic studies on the vertebral portion of the psoas muscle; with special reference to its stabilizing function of the lumbar spine. Acta Orthop Scand. 1966;37(2):177–90.
49. Karlsson E, Jonsson B. Function of the gluteus maximus muscle. An electromyographic study. Acta Morphol Neerl Scand. 1965;6:161–9.
50. Joseph J, Williams PL. Electromyography of certain hip muscles. J Anat. 1957;91(2):286–94.
51. Greenlaw RK. Function of the muscles about the hip during normal and level walking. Queen's University, Canada; 1973.
52. Shelburne K, Decker M, Philippon M, Torry M. A musculoskeletal model of the hip for the calculation of muscle and joint loads during physical activity. In: 56th annual meeting of the Orthopedic Research Society, New Orleans, LA, 6–9 Mar 2010.
53. Wheatley MD, Jahnke WD. Electromyographic study of the superficial thigh and hip muscles in normal individuals. Arch Phys Med Rehabil. 1951;32(8):508–15.
54. Carlsoo S, Fohlin L. The mechanics of the two-joint muscles rectus femoris, sartorius and tensor fasciae latae in relation to their activity. Scand J Rehabil Med. 1969;1(3):107–11.
55. Goto Y, Kumamoto M, Okamoto T. Electromyographic study of the function of the muscles participating in thigh elevation in various planes. Res J Phys Educ. 1974;18:269–76.
56. Houtz SJ, Fischer FJ. An analysis of muscle action and joint excursion during exercise on a stationary bicycle. J Bone Joint Surg Am. 1959;41-A(1):123–31.
57. Heinert BL, Kernozek TW, Greany JF, Fater DC. Hip abductor weakness and lower extremity kinematics during running. J Sport Rehabil. 2008;17(3):243–56.
58. Leetun DT, Ireland ML, Willson JD, Ballantyne BT, Davis IM. Core stability measures as risk factors for lower extremity injury in athletes. Med Sci Sports Exerc. 2004;36(6):926–34.
59. Jensen RH, Smidt GL, Johnston RC. A technique for obtaining measurements of force generated by hip muscles. Arch Phys Med Rehabil. 1971;52(5):207–15.
60. Kulig K, Andrews JG, Hay JG. Human strength curves. Exerc Sport Sci Rev. 1984;12:417–66.
61. Murray MP, Sepic SB. Maximum isometric torque of hip abductor and adductor muscles. Phys Ther. 1968;48(12):1327–35.
62. Clark JM, Haynor DR. Anatomy of the abductor muscles of the hip as studied by computed tomography. J Bone Joint Surg Am. 1987;69(7):1021–31.
63. Thorborg K, Petersen J, Magnusson SP, Holmich P. Clinical assessment of hip strength using a hand-held dynamometer is reliable. Scand J Med Sci Sports. 2010;20(3):493–501.
64. Lindsay DM, Maitland M, Lowe RC, Kane TJ. Comparison of isokinetic internal and external hip rotation torques using different testing positions. J Orthop Sports Phys Ther. 1992;16(1):43–50.
65. Lindle RS, Metter EJ, Lynch NA, Fleg JL, Fozard JL, Tobin J, et al. Age and gender comparisons of muscle strength in 654 women and men aged 20-93 yr. J Appl Physiol. 1997;83(5):1581–7.
66. May WW. Relative isometric force of the hip abductor and adductor muscles. Phys Ther. 1968;48(8):845–51.

67. Neumann DA, Soderberg GL, Cook TM. Comparison of maximal isometric hip abductor muscle torques between hip sides. Phys Ther. 1988;68(4):496–502.
68. Brophy RH, Chiaia TA, Maschi R, Dodson CC, Oh LS, Lyman S, et al. The core and hip in soccer athletes compared by gender. Int J Sports Med. 2009;30(9):663–7.
69. Freter SH, Fruchter N. Relationship between timed 'up and go' and gait time in an elderly orthopaedic rehabilitation population. Clin Rehabil. 2000;14(1):96–101.
70. Stryla W, Pogorzala AM, Rogala P, Nowakowski A. Algorithm of physical therapy exercises following total hip arthroplasty. Pol Orthop Traumatol. 2013;78:33–9.
71. Vaz MD, Kramer JF, Rorabeck CH, Bourne RB. Isometric hip abductor strength following total hip replacement and its relationship to functional assessments. J Orthop Sports Phys Ther. 1993;18(4):526–31.
72. Philippon MJ. New frontiers in hip arthroscopy: the role of arthroscopic hip labral repair and capsulorrhaphy in the treatment of hip disorders. Instr Course Lect. 2006;55:309–16.
73. Ferguson SJ, Bryant JT, Ganz R, Ito K. The acetabular labrum seal: a poroelastic finite element model. Clin Biomech (Bristol, Avon). 2000;15(6):463–8.
74. Ferguson SJ, Bryant JT, Ganz R, Ito K. An in vitro investigation of the acetabular labral seal in hip joint mechanics. J Biomech. 2003;36(2):171–8.
75. Kim JW, Kwon MS, Yenuga SS, Kwon YH. The effects of target distance on pivot hip, trunk, pelvis, and kicking leg kinematics in Taekwondo roundhouse kicks. Sports Biomech. 2010;9(2):98–114.
76. Philippon MJ. The role of arthroscopic thermal capsulorrhaphy in the hip. Clin Sports Med. 2001;20(4):817–29.
77. Guanche CA, Sikka RS. Acetabular labral tears with underlying chondromalacia: a possible association with high-level running. Arthroscopy. 2005;21(5):580–5.
78. Fredericson M, Cookingham CL, Chaudhari AM, Dowdell BC, Oestreicher N, Sahrmann SA. Hip abductor weakness in distance runners with iliotibial band syndrome. Clin J Sport Med. 2000;10(3):169–75.
79. Fredericson M, White JJ, Macmahon JM, Andriacchi TP. Quantitative analysis of the relative effectiveness of 3 iliotibial band stretches. Arch Phys Med Rehabil. 2002;83(5):589–92.
80. Powers CM. The influence of altered lower-extremity kinematics on patellofemoral joint dysfunction: a theoretical perspective. J Orthop Sports Phys Ther. 2003;33(11):639–46.
81. Chaudhari AM, Andriacchi TP. The mechanical consequences of dynamic frontal plane limb alignment for non-contact ACL injury. J Biomech. 2006;39(2):330–8.
82. Byrd JW, Jones KS. Hip arthroscopy in athletes. Clin Sports Med. 2001;20(4):749–61.
83. L'Hermette M, Polle G, Tourny-Chollet C, Dujardin F. Hip passive range of motion and frequency of radiographic hip osteoarthritis in former elite handball players. Br J Sports Med. 2006;40(1):45–9. Discussion-9.
84. Roach KE, Miles TP. Normal hip and knee active range of motion: the relationship to age. Phys Ther. 1991;71(9):656–65.
85. Spector TD, Harris PA, Hart DJ, Cicuttini FM, Nandra D, Etherington J, et al. Risk of osteoarthritis associated with long-term weight-bearing sports: a radiologic survey of the hips and knees in female ex-athletes and population controls. Arthritis Rheum. 1996;39(6):988–95.
86. Kettunen JA, Kujala UM, Raty H, Videman T, Sarna S, Impivaara O, et al. Factors associated with hip joint rotation in former elite athletes. Br J Sports Med. 2000;34(1):44–8.
87. Reid DC, Burnham RS, Saboe LA, Kushner SF. Lower extremity flexibility patterns in classical ballet dancers and their correlation to lateral hip and knee injuries. Am J Sports Med. 1987;15(4):347–52.
88. Yamanouchi T. EMG analysis of the lower extremities during pitching in high-school baseball. Kurume Med J. 1998;45(1):21–5.
89. Fleisig GS, Barrentine SW, Escamilla RF, Andrews JR. Biomechanics of overhand throwing with implications for injuries. Sports Med. 1996;21(6):421–37.
90. Wilk KE, Meister K, Fleisig G, Andrews JR. Biomechanics of the overhead throwing motion. Sports Med Arthrosc Rev. 2000;8:124–34.
91. Burkhart SS, Morgan CD, Kibler WB. The disabled throwing shoulder: spectrum of pathology part III: the SICK scapula, scapular dyskinesis, the kinetic chain, and rehabilitation. Arthroscopy. 2003;19(6):641–61.
92. Sisto DJ, Jobe FW. The operative treatment of scapulothoracic bursitis in professional pitchers. Am J Sports Med. 1986;14(3):192–4.
93. Stull JD, Philippon MJ, LaPrade RF. "At-risk" positioning and hip biomechanics of the Peewee ice hockey sprint start. Am J Sports Med. 2011;39(Suppl):29S–35.
94. Chang R, Turcotte R, Pearsall D. Hip adductor muscle function in forward skating. Sports Biomech. 2009;8(3):212–22.
95. Keogh MJ, Batt ME. A review of femoroacetabular impingement in athletes. Sports Med. 2008;38(10):863–78.
96. Orava S, Jaroma H, Hulkko A. Overuse injuries in cross-country skiing. Br J Sports Med. 1985;19(3):158–60.
97. Anderson K, Strickland SM, Warren R. Hip and groin injuries in athletes. Am J Sports Med. 2001;29(4):521–33.
98. van den Bogert AJ, Read L, Nigg BM. An analysis of hip joint loading during walking, running, and skiing. Med Sci Sports Exerc. 1999;31(1):131–42.
99. Holmberg HC, Lindinger S, Stoggl T, Eitzlmair E, Muller E. Biomechanical analysis of double poling in elite cross-country skiers. Med Sci Sports Exerc. 2005;37(5):807–18.
100. Johnston RC, Smidt GL. Measurement of hip-joint motion during walking. Evaluation of an electrogoniometric method. J Bone Joint Surg Am. 1969;51(6):1082–94.
101. Paul JP. Biomechanics. The biomechanics of the hip-joint and its clinical relevance. Proc R Soc Med. 1966;59(10):943–8.
102. Andriacchi TP, Ogle JA, Galante JO. Walking speed as a basis for normal and abnormal gait measurements. J Biomech. 1977;10(4):261–8.

9 Outcome Instruments for Assessment of Hip Function

Simon W. Young and Marc R. Safran

Introduction

Until recently, patients with osteoarthritis (OA) were the main focus of diagnosis and treatment in adult orthopedics. Outcome measures for the hip were therefore developed (and in some cases validated, usually in retrospect) for this primarily elderly patient group. These include the Harris hip score (HHS, commonly used in the United States) [1], the Merle d'Aubigné and Postel hip score (common in Europe) [2], the hip disability and osteoarthritis outcome score (HOOS) [3, 4], and the Oxford hip score (OHS) [5]. These tools were primarily designed to assess clinical outcome following total hip replacement (THR). In addition, more general measures of health such as the short form 36 (SF-36) [6] and disease-specific measures such as the Western Ontario and McMaster Universities Osteoarthritis Index (WOMAC) function score [7] have been commonly used.

As diagnostic methods have advanced, nonarthritic disorders such as femoroacetabular impingement (FAI) have increasingly been recognized in a younger population group, and this has coincided with the rapid development of arthroscopic techniques aimed at treating these conditions. This has led to growing interest in hip pathology that primarily affects active young and middle-aged adults. As a result, there is increasing interest in newer scoring systems which aim to more accurately reflect and communicate the functional status of these patients both prior to and after nonsurgical or surgical treatments. One of the first points of importance is to have a questionnaire developed and validated in the same patient group as it is intended to study. That is, questionnaires designed to measure the outcomes of young active patients with nonarthritic hip problems need to be developed and validated in this group prospectively. Applying arthritic hip scores that were developed to measure the functional status of older patients with hip arthritis or following hip arthroplasty is not scientifically valid and may misrepresent outcomes.

In a 2010 review, Safran and Hariri [8] noted at least 41 hip outcome scores (HOSs) reported in the literature, only 18 of which had undergone formal psychometric testing for reliability, validity, and responsiveness. More recently, five patient-reported outcome (PRO) questionnaires were evaluated in patients with a mean age of less than 50 years: the modified Harris hip score (mHHS) [9], the HOOS, the nonarthritic hip score (NHS) [10], the Copenhagen hip and groin outcome score (HAGOS) [11], and the international hip outcome tool (iHOT) [12]. While the HOS and NHS were validated in young, active patients with nonarthritic hip problems, the questions were derived from other questionnaires and clinician experience and expertise. The HAGOS and iHOT outcome tools were prospectively designed for the young patient with nonarthritic hip problems using the most scientifically rigorous methodology, including patient input.

Clinician-Based Versus Patient-Based Outcome Tools

The first outcome assessment scores were developed without standardized methodology and were clinician generated and clinician based. Relative weighting of symptom groups or clinical assessment parameters was therefore subject to the creator's bias in determining which items or clinical measurements were included, and therefore the content was not directly linked to what is important to patients. Martin surveyed 150 patients with hip pathology in addition to surveying their surgeons and enquired as to which factors they

S.W. Young, FRACS
Division of Sports Medicine, Department of Orthopaedic Surgery, Stanford University, Redwood City, CA, USA

M.R. Safran, MD (✉)
Division of Sports Medicine, Department of Orthopaedic Surgery, Stanford University, 450 Broadway St, M/C 6342, Redwood City, CA 94063, USA
e-mail: msafran@stanford.edu

J.C. McCarthy et al. (eds.), *Hip Joint Restoration*, DOI 10.1007/978-1-4614-0694-5_9

considered important related to their hip pain and function [13]. He found significant discrepancies in how patients and their surgeons rated the importance of different items related to symptoms, functional limitations, and occupation. Similarly, a physician's assessment of a patient's pain and physical status with regard to nonarthritic hip pain can differ widely from the patient's own opinion, particularly when the patient's overall satisfaction is low [14]. Clinician-based assessment tools may therefore not accurately reflect the patient's perceptions of outcome following treatment.

PRO questionnaires are now accepted as the gold standard in the assessment of musculoskeletal conditions, where the patient's perspective and health-related quality of life are paramount [15]. The development and validation of PRO questionnaires involve substantial psychometric testing, and the COSMIN (Consensus-based standards for the selection of health measurement instruments) initiative has established guidelines [15–17]. In general, a number of measurement properties are assessed across three domains: reliability, validity, and responsiveness [15]. *Reliability* refers to the extent to which scores for patients whose status has not changed are reproducible, and this can be tested under several conditions: retesting using different sets of items from the same questionnaire (internal consistency), over time (test-retest), by different examiners on the same occasion (interobserver) and by the same examiner on different occasions (intra-observer).

Validity refers to the degree to which an instrument measures what it sets out to measure. There are several forms of validity that are commonly evaluated, including content validity (extent to which the domain of interest is comprehensively sampled by the items in the questionnaire), construct validity (how well scores relate to other measures in a manner consistent with theoretical hypotheses), criterion validity (how well scores relate to a "gold standard"), and cross-cultural validity (how well a translated or adapted version reflects the performance of the original questionnaire). Finally, *responsiveness* refers to the ability of a questionnaire to detect clinically important changes over time.

Modern outcome instruments therefore focus on PRO data to capture the patient's own assessment of his or her pain and functional status. Ideally, these instruments consist of items that evaluate factors known to be most important to patients [12]. The relative importance of these factors will differ between patient groups; therefore the psychometric properties of a PRO instrument can only be related to a specific target population and the context in which it has been administered [18]. These instruments typically have the added advantage that they do not require a trained healthcare worker to administer (questionnaires administered by healthcare workers may introduce bias). In addition, floor and ceiling effects (the number of respondents who achieve the lowest or highest possible score) will differ depending on the average functional status of the target population. It is therefore logical to use different assessment tools following procedures in older patients (typically undergoing hip arthroplasty) to those in younger patients (more often undergoing hip arthroscopy).

Common Hip Outcome Scores in Older Patients

The Harris Hip Score

Available at: www.orthopaedicscores.com

The HHS was introduced in 1969 in a study of traumatic arthritis [1]. This is a clinician-based questionnaire covering the domains of pain (one item, 0–44 points), function (seven items, 0–47 points), absence of deformity (one item, 4 points), and range of motion (two items, 5 points), giving a total score out of 100. A total score of <70 is considered a poor result; 70–80 a fair result, 80–90 a good result, and 90–100 an excellent result [19]. It is the most widely used hip outcome measure in the United States [8]. The original publication describes the logic in formulating the score but did not use any validated outcome methodologies. Pain and functional capacity were considered the most important indicators for surgery and therefore received the heaviest weighting (91 of 100 points). The HHS is designed to be administered by a healthcare professional. The HHS demonstrates high validity and reliability in studying the outcomes of THA and also has a strong correlation with the WOMAC and the SF-36 pain and function domains [20, 21]. The HHS has also been correlated with both the original Merle d'Aubigné-Postel score and a later modification of this score by Matta et al. [22, 23]. Ceiling effects remain a concern with the HHS, particularly in younger, more active patients. That is to say, many of the young patients had high scores, as their function is greater or at the top of what the score measures, even though it may not be as great as the patient may want. Wamper reviewed all papers using the HHS in a single year [24] and reported unacceptable ceiling effects in 31 of 59 studies. Pooled data across the studies included ($n = 6667$ patients) suggested ceiling effects of 20 %, significantly limiting its validity. The main strength of the HHS is its widespread use throughout the orthopedic literature allowing comparison between studies.

The Merle d'Aubigné-Postel Score

Available at: www.ncbi.nlm.nih.gov/pmc/articles/PMC2600978

In 1954 d'Aubigné and Postel [2] reported a clinician-based outcome instrument to assess the outcome of a group of patients undergoing hip arthroplasty. Individual scores from 0 to 6 for the domains pain, walking ability, and range of motion are given. The scores for pain and ability to walk are added and then classified into the grades very good, good, medium, fair, and poor. These grades are often then adjusted 1–2 grades less for the mobility score to give the final clinical grade. Others have converted this to a total numeric score, giving equal weighting to the three domains [23]. A later modification proposed in 1986 for use following acetabular fractures is based on the same components as the original and individual scores, but with slight differences in language and grading [22]. As with the HHS, the main strength of the d'Aubigné-Postel score is its widespread use (mainly in Europe). It has been shown to offer a correlated but slightly more pessimistic assessment of outcome than the HHS [25] and also suffers from the same difficulties in regard to ceiling effects [23, 26].

Oxford Hip Score

Available at: phi.uhce.ox.ac.uk/ox_scores.php

The OHS was introduced in 1996 [27] and its scoring system slightly modified in 2007 [5]. The OHS covers two domains: pain (six items) and function (six items) of the hip in relation to daily activities such as walking, dressing, and sleeping. Questions were developed from patient interviews of patients with hip osteoarthritis. Each question is scored from 0 to 4 (worst to best), giving an overall score between 0 and 48 where 48 represents the best possible outcome. The OHS has shown high correlation with the HHS [28] and greater responsiveness to change than both the SF-36 and WOMAC [19, 29–31]. Its suitability for use as a postal questionnaire has led to its widespread use in large registry studies [32–34].

The Hip Dysfunction and Osteoarthritis Score

Available at: www.koos.nu

The HOOS was introduced in 2003 [3, 4] and consists of 40 items covering five domains: pain (ten items), symptoms (five items), activities of daily living (ADL) (17 items), sport/recreation function (four items), and hip-related quality of life (four items). A shorter questionnaire focusing on physical function, the HOOS-PS, was introduced in 2008 [35]. This questionnaire was developed for middle-aged and older adults with hip disorders and includes the WOMAC questions in their complete and original format allowing this score to also be calculated. Additional items were chosen after literature search and patient interviews [3] to increase its relevance to the hip and also its relevance to more active patients. Each item consists of a Likert scale and a normalized score from 0 (worst) to 100 (best) is calculated for each of the five subscales. Floor effects have been reported in the sports subscale after administration to hip OA patients [19], and ceiling effects have been reported in multiple subscales in patients 6 months post THR [3]. Validity has been adequate in comparisons to the OHS and SF-36, and the HOOS is reported to be both reliable and responsive to change in osteoarthritic patients [3, 4, 36, 37].

Common Hip Outcome Scores in Younger Patients

Modified Harris Hip Score

Available at: www.isha.net/education-training (Appendix 1)

In 2000, Byrd and Jones proposed a modified, patient self-reported HHS (mHHS) with the aim of better assessing hip arthroscopy patients and reducing ceiling effects [19]. The mHHS contains eight questions covering three domains, pain, function, and ADL, and like the original form gives a score from 0 (extreme symptoms) to 100 (no symptoms) [20]. found that the mHSS correlates well with short form 36 (SF-36) scores in patients undergoing arthroscopic labral debridement of the hip. However the mHHS derives from an arthritis hip score, and its authors acknowledge it is an "imperfect instrument" [19] for assessing the hip arthroscopy population. Consensus for its use in this population remains lacking [7]. Nonetheless, it is the most commonly reported outcome score following hip arthroscopy.

The Nonarthritic Hip Score

Available at: www.isha.net/education-training (Appendix 2)

Introduced in 2003, the 100-point, 20-question NHS is designed to discriminate between high levels of activity in younger patients with hip pain but no obvious pathology on plain radiographs [10]. It covers four domains: pain, mechanical symptoms (e.g., catching/locking), physical function, and level of activity (focusing on higher-demand activities such as jogging and cutting or pivoting sports). This is a patient self-administered questionnaire, with ten NHS questions measuring pain and function taken directly from the WOMAC index and the remaining ten developed on the basis of patient interviews and input from healthcare providers. The use of questions derived from an arthritic assessment questionnaire has been criticized [8]. Christensen correlated the NHS to the SF-12 and the HHS in 108 patients without radiographic evidence of arthritis and found it was reproducible and internally consistent [10], and it has been widely used in outcome studies for hip arthroscopy [38].

Hip Outcome Score

Available at: www.isha.net/education-training (Appendix 3)

The HOS was developed to assess the treatment effect of hip arthroscopy on labral tears in young, active patients and was introduced in 2006 [39]. It consists of 28 Likert-style items generated by physicians and physical therapists, covering two functional domains: ADL (19 items) and sport (9 items). ADL includes putting on socks and shoes, stairs, as well as more demanding activities like squatting and twisting/pivoting on the involved leg. The sports subscale assesses the ability to perform specific activities such as running 1 mile, starting and stopping quickly, and cutting/lateral movements. The HOS is self-administered and generates a total score for each subscale, ranging from 0 to 100, with a higher score indicating a higher level of function. It also allows the respondent to record "not applicable" if the activity questioned is limited by another pathology (e.g., back pain), eliminating a common deficiency of other outcome instruments. The HOS has been validated in individuals undergoing hip arthroscopy and for those with labral tears (with or without arthroscopy) [39, 40]. It correlates with the SF-36 score in physical function and appears reliable and responsive in describing the outcomes of hip arthroscopy for several indications [41].

The Copenhagen Hip and Groin Outcome Score

Available at: www.koos.nu (Appendix 4)

The HAGOS was introduced in 2011 [11] and consists of 37 questions covering six domains: pain, symptoms, physical function in daily living, physical function in sport and recreation, participation in physical activities, and hip- and/or groin-related quality of life. This instrument was developed for younger patients with hip pain, using content from the HOOS and HOS, which was then modified after expert and patient interviews. Each question is answered on a Likert scale, and each subscale is scored separately from 0 (worst) to 100 (best). The HAGOS was evaluated in a clinical study of 101 patients in Denmark; validity, reliability, and responsiveness were assessed according to the COSMIN guidelines and found to be adequate [11].

International Hip Outcome Tool

Available at: www.isha.net/education-training (Appendices 5 and 6)

The iHOT-33 was introduced in 2012 as a collaborative effort of the Multicenter Arthroscopic Hip Outcomes Research Network (MAHORN). It consists of 33 items covering four domains: symptoms and functional limitations, sports and recreational activities, job-related concerns, and social, emotional, and lifestyle concerns [12]. This instrument was developed for younger, active patients with hip disorders; questions were generated from an iterative process where patients ranked the relative importance of various factors, to ensure their content reflected patient concerns. Each question is answered on a visual analogue scale and a total score is calculated, ranging from 0 (worst) to 100 (best). The iHOT-33 has been shown to be reliable, with content and construct validity, and seems highly responsive to clinical change [12]. A condensed form, the 12-item iHOT-12, has also been shown to have similar characteristics in terms of validity, reliability, and responsiveness, despite its much shorter length [42]. However patients with certain diagnoses tend to score similarly within similar domains but different from other diagnoses with the 33-item questionnaire, and as a result both versions have utility. Ongoing research continues to examine whether the iHOT-33 can be used to aid diagnosis in patients with hip or groin pain [8].

Choice of Instrument

The selection of a particular instrument for a given clinical situation depends on a number of factors, including the demographics of the study population, the disease process, and the outcome domain(s) of interest (Table 9.1). Patient-based instruments tend to be easier to use as they typically do not require trained personnel to administer; however older clinician-based instruments continue to have wide use in the literature as they simplify comparisons to other studies. In 2008 Riddle reviewed 85 randomized trials in hip patients published since 2000 and found at least 20 different hip outcome measures were used [43]. Among trials measuring the outcome of THR, 52 % of investigators employed the HHS, 13 % the WOMAC, 12 % the d'Aubigné-Postel score, 6 % the SF-36, and 4 % the OHS. In 2013 Hetaimish reviewed 29 studies of patients treated for into FAI and found that 45 % used the mHHS, 28 % the NHS, 14 % the WOMAC, and 10 % each the HHS, HOS, and SF-12 [38].

This variability in outcome measure usage makes comparisons between studies difficult, and a number of recent literature reviews have compared different instruments and made recommendations as to their use. In 2010 Thorborg et al. reviewed the literature on a total of 12 hip PRO questionnaires for both arthritic and nonarthritic conditions [11]. They concluded that the HOOS was the recommended tool for evaluating patients with hip OA undergoing surgical or nonsurgical treatment, and the HOS was recommended for evaluating patients undergoing hip arthroscopy. In 2011 Lodhia compared the clinometric evidence for PRO instruments in FAI and labral hip pathology, comparing the HOS, NHS, and WOMAC [44]. They concluded the HOS was

Table 9.1 Commonly reported hip outcome measurements

Instrument	Target population	Advantages	Disadvantages
Harris hip score (HHS)	Arthritic hip patients	Widely used in literature High validity and reliability in studying outcomes hip arthroplasty	Clinician based Requires healthcare professional to administer Ceiling effects, particularly in younger patients
Merle d'Aubigné-Postel score	Hip arthroplasty patients	Widely used in literature, particularly in Europe	Clinician based Ceiling effects
Oxford hip score (OHS)	Arthritic hip patients	Simple to administer Widely used in registries Responsive to change	Ceiling effects
Hip dysfunction and osteoarthritis score (HOOS)	Arthritic hip patients	Includes WOMAC questions Reliable and responsive to change in arthritic patients	Floor and ceiling effects in younger patients
Modified Harris hip score (mHHS)	Younger patients with hip disorders	Most commonly reported score following hip arthroscopy	Derives from arthritic hip score Validity not proven
Nonarthritic hip score (NHS)	Younger patients with hip disorders	Reproducible and internally consistent	50 % of questions derive from arthritic hip score
Hip outcome score (HOS)	Younger patients with hip disorders	Validated in hip arthroscopy population Can exclude non-applicable questions	Not widely used
Copenhagen hip and groin outcome score (HAGOS)	Younger patients with hip disorders	Validity, reliability, and responsiveness confirmed in target population	Not widely used outside Europe
International hip outcome tool (iHOT)	Younger patients with hip disorders	Robust process for question development Validity, reliability, and responsiveness confirmed in target population Broad support among hip arthroscopy specialists	Not yet widely used

currently the most proven instrument in this population. In the same year, Tijssen reviewed the psychometric evidence for PRO instruments in hip arthroscopy patients, comparing the mHHS, NHS, and HOS [45]. They concluded there was no definitive evidence favoring one instrument over another and recommended a combination of the NHS and HOS be used. It should be noted however that these reviews predate the introduction of both the HAGOS and iHOT scores, both of which went through a more rigorous development process aiming to maximize their utility in this patient population. In particular, the development of iHOT by a broad network of international arthroscopic specialists (MAHORN) seems likely to ensure its widespread acceptance in assessment of younger patients with hip pathology. More usage of these more rigorously developed and validated outcome scores and comparison with other scores will determine which may be the best outcome tool to use in the long run. Short form scores (e.g., iHOT-12) offer obvious advantages for busy clinicians who want to measure their patients' outcome, while longer instruments (e.g., the iHOT-33) are suited to research applications where greater insight into the causes of patients' deficits is being sought. In patients with OA, the dominance of the HHS is likely to ensure its continued use, although this will likely be in combination with a patient-focused PRO with superior psychometric properties such as the HOOS.

Conflict of Interest All ICMJE Conflict of Interest Forms for authors and Clinical Orthopaedics and Related Research editors and board members are on file with the publication and can be viewed on request.

Appendix 1

Name______________________________ **Date**__________________

MODIFIED HARRIS HIP SCORE

Please answer the following questions as they pertain to your hip:

Pain:
☐None/Able to ignore it
☐Slight, occasional, no compromise in activity
☐Mild, no effect on ordinary activity, pain after usual activity, use aspirin/ibuprofen/Tylenol
☐Moderate, tolerable, makes concessions, occasional narcotic
☐Marked, serious limitations
☐Totally disabled

Function: Gait

Limp
☐None
☐Slight
☐Moderate
☐Severe
☐Unable to walk

Support
☐None
☐Cane for long walks
☐Cane all the time
☐Crutch
☐2 canes
☐2 crutches
☐Unable to walk

Distance Walked
☐Unlimited
☐6 blocks
☐2-3 blocks
☐Indoors only
☐Bed and chair

Functional Activities

Stairs
☐ ☐Can go up/down normally
☐ ☐Can go up/down normally with banister
☐ ☐Any method
☐ ☐Unable

Socks/Shoes
☐☐With ease
☐☐With difficulty
☐☐Unable

Sitting
☐☐Any chair, 1 hour
☐☐High chair, ½ hour
☐☐Unable to sit, ½ hour, any chair

Public Transportation
☐☐Able to enter public transportation
☐☐Unable to use public transportation (such as bus, or airport transportation)

For Internal Use:

Score__________
Initials_________

Appendix 2

NONARTHRITIC HIP SCORE

INSTRUCTIONS: The following 5 questions concern the amount of pain you are currently experiencing in the hip that you are having evaluated today. For each situation, please cir- cle the response that most accurately reflects the amount of pain experienced in the past 48 hours. Please circle one answer that best describes your situation.

QUESTION: How much pain do you have-

1. Walking on a flat surface? 4□none 3□mild 2 □ moderate 1 □ severe 0 □ extreme
2. Going up or down stairs? 4□none 3□mild 2 □ moderate 1 □ severe 0 □ extreme
3. At night while in bed? 4 □ none 3 □ mild 2 □ moderate 1 □ severe 0 □ extreme
4. Sitting or lying? 4□none 3□mild 2 □ moderate 1 □ severe 0 □ extreme
5. Standing upright? 4□none 3□mild 2 □ moderate 1 □ severe 0 □ extreme

INSTRUCTIONS: The following 4 questions concern the symptoms that you are cur- rently experiencing in the hip that you are having evaluated today. For each situation, please circle the response that most accurately reflects the symptoms experienced in the past 48 hours. Please circle one answer that best describes your situation.

QUESTION: How much trouble do you have with-

1. Catching or locking of your hip? 4□none 3□mild 2 □ moderate 1 □ severe 0 □ extreme
2. Your hip giving out on you? 4□none 3□mild 2 □ moderate 1 □ severe 0 □ extreme
3. Stiffness in your hip? 4□none 3□mild 2 □ moderate 1 □ severe 0 □ extreme
4. Decreased motion in your hip? 4□none 3□mild 2 □ moderate 1 □ severe 0 □ extreme

INSTRUCTIONS: The following 5 questions concern your physical function. For each of the following activities, please circle the response that most accurately reflects the diffi- culty that you have experienced in the past 48 hours because of your hip pain. Please circle one answer that best describes your situation.

QUESTION: What degree of difficulty do you have with-

1. Descending stairs? 4 □ none 3 □ mild 2 □ moderate 1 □ severe 0 □ extreme
2. Ascending stairs? 4 □ none 3 □ mild 2 □ moderate 1 □ severe 0 □ extreme
3. Rising from sitting? 4 □ none 3 □ mild 2 □ moderate 1 □ severe 0 □ extreme
4. Putting on socks/stockings? 4□none 3□mild 2 □ moderate 1 □ severe 0 □ extreme
5. Rising from bed? 4□none 3□mild 2 □ moderate 1 □ severe 0 □ extreme

INSTRUCTIONS: The following 6 questions concern your ability to participate in cer- tain types of activities. For each of the following activities, please circle the response that most accurately reflects the difficulty that you have experienced in the past month because of your hip pain. If you do not participate in a certain type of activity, please estimate how much trouble your hip would cause you if you had to perform that type of activity. Please circle one answer that best describes your situation.

QUESTION: How much trouble does your hip cause you when you participate in-

1. High demand sports involving sprinting or cutting (for example, football, basketball, tennis, and exercise aerobics) 4 □ none 3 □ mild 2 □ moderate 1 □ severe 0 □ extreme
2. Low demand sports (for example, golfing and bowling) 4 □ none 3 □ mild 2 □ moderate 1 □ severe 0 □ extreme
3. Jogging for exercise? 4 □ none 3□mild 2 □ moderate 1 □ severe 0 □ extreme
4. Walking for exercise? 4□none 3□mild 2 □ moderate 1 □ severe 0 □ extreme

Christensen, C. P., Althausen, P. L., Mittleman, M. A., Lee, J.-A., & McCarthy, J. C. (2003). The nonarthritic hip score: reliable and validated. *Clinical Orthopaedics and Related Research*, (406), 75–83.

Appendix 3

Hip Outcome Score (HOS)
Activity of Daily Living Scale

Please answer **every question** with one response that most closely describes to your condition within the past week.
If the activity in question is limited by something other than your hip mark not applicable (N/A).

	No difficulty at all	Slight difficulty	Moderate difficulty	Extreme difficulty	Unable to do	N/A
Standing for 15 minutes	□	□	□	□	□	□
Getting into and out of an average car	□	□	□	□	□	□
Putting on socks and shoes	□	□	□	□	□	□
Walking up steep hills	□	□	□	□	□	□
Walking down steep hills	□	□	□	□	□	□
Going up 1 flight of stairs	□	□	□	□	□	□
Going down 1 flight of stairs	□	□	□	□	□	□
Stepping up and down curbs	□	□	□	□	□	□
Deep squatting	□	□	□	□	□	□
Getting into and out of a bath tub	□	□	□	□	□	□
Sitting for 15 minutes	□	□	□	□	□	□
Walking initially	□	□	□	□	□	□
Walking approximately 10 minutes	□	□	□	□	□	□
Walking 15 minutes or greater	□	□	□	□	□	□

Appendix 4

Because of your hip how much difficulty do you have with:

	No difficulty at all	Slight difficulty	Moderate difficulty	Extreme difficulty	Unable to do	N/A
Twisting/pivoting on involved leg	□	□	□	□	□	□
Rolling over in bed	□	□	□	□	□	□
Light to moderate work (standing, walking)	□	□	□	□	□	□
Heavy work (push/pulling, climbing, carrying)	□	□	□	□	□	□
Recreational activities	□	□	□	□	□	□

How would you rate your current level of function during your usual activities of daily living from 0 to 100 with 100 being your level of function prior to your hip problem and 0 being the inability to perform any of your usual daily activities?

□□□.0 %

Appendix 5

Hip Outcome Score (HOS)
Sports Scale

Because of your hip how much difficulty do you have with:

	No difficulty at all	Slight difficulty	Moderate difficulty	Extreme difficulty	Unable to do	N/A
Running one mile	☐	☐	☐	☐	☐	☐
Jumping	☐	☐	☐	☐	☐	☐
Swinging objects like a golf club	☐	☐	☐	☐	☐	☐
Landing	☐	☐	☐	☐	☐	☐
Starting and stopping quickly	☐	☐	☐	☐	☐	☐
Cutting/lateral movements	☐	☐	☐	☐	☐	☐
Low impact activities like fast walking	☐	☐	☐	☐	☐	☐
Ability to perform activity with your normal technique	☐	☐	☐	☐	☐	☐
Ability to participate in your desired sport as long as you would like	☐	☐	☐	☐	☐	☐

How would you rate your current level of function during your sports related activities from 0 to 100 with 100 being your level of function prior to your hip problem and 0 being the inability to perform any of your usual daily activities?

☐☐☐.0 %

How would you rate your current level of function?

☐ Normal ☐ Nearly normal ☐ Abnormal ☐ Severely abnormal

Appendix 6

HAGOS

Questionnaire concerning hip and/or groin problems

Today's date: _____/______/______ Date of birth: _____/______/________

Name: ____

INSTRUCTIONS: This questionnaire asks for your view about your hip and/or groin problem. The questions should be answered considering your hip and/or groin function during the **past week**.This information will help us keep track of how you feel, and how well you are able to do your usual activities.

Answer **every** question by ticking the appropriate box. Tick only one box for each question. If a question does not pertain to you or you have not experienced it in the past week please make your "best guess" as to which response would be the most accurate.

Symptoms

These questions should be answered considering your hip and/or groin **symptoms** and difficulties during the **past week**.

S1 Do you feel discomfort in your hip and/or groin?

Never	Rarely	Sometimes	Often	Always
☐	☐	☐	☐	☐

S2 Do you hear clicking or any other type of noise from your hip and/or groin?

Never	Rarely	Sometimes	Often	All the time
☐	☐	☐	☐	☐

S3 Do you have difficulties stretching your legs far out to the side?

None	Mild	Moderate	Severe	Extreme
☐	☐	☐	☐	☐

S4 Do you have difficulties taking full strides when you walk?

None	Mild	Moderate	Severe	Extreme
☐	☐	☐	☐	☐

S5 Do you experience sudden twinging/stabbing sensations in your hip and/or groin?

Never	Rarely	Sometimes	Often	All the time
☐	☐	☐	☐	☐

Stiffness

The following questions concern the amount of stiffness you have experienced during the **past week** in your hip and/or groin. Stiffness is a sensation of restriction or slowness in the ease with which you move your hip and/or groin.

S6 How severe is your hip and/or groin stiffness after first awakening in the morning?

None	Mild	Moderate	Severe	Extreme
□	□	□	□	□

S7 How severe is your hip and/or groin stiffness after sitting, lying or resting **later in the day**?

None	Mild	Moderate	Severe	Extreme
□	□	□	□	□

Pain

P1 How often is your hip and/or groin painful?

Never	Monthly	Weekly	Daily	Always
□	□	□	□	□

P2 How often do you have pain in areas other than your hip and/or groin that you think may be related to your hip and/or groin problem?

Never	Monthly	Weekly	Daily	Always
□	□	□	□	□

The following questions concern the amount of pain you have experienced during the **past week** in your hip and/or groin. **What amount of hip and/or groin pain have you experienced during the following activities?**

P3 Straightening your hip fully

None	Mild	Moderate	Severe	Extreme
□	□	□	□	□

P4 Bending your hip fully

None	Mild	Moderate	Severe	Extreme
□	□	□	□	□

P5 Walking up or down stairs

None	Mild	Moderate	Severe	Extreme
□	□	□	□	□

P6 At night while in bed (pain that disturbs your sleep)

None	Mild	Moderate	Severe	Extreme
□	□	□	□	□

P7 Sitting or lying

None	Mild	Moderate	Severe	Extreme
□	□	□	□	□

The following questions concern the amount of pain you have experienced during the **past week** in your hip and/or groin. **What amount of hip and/or groin pain have you experienced during the following activities?**

P8 Standing upright

None	Mild	Moderate	Severe	Extreme
☐	☐	☐	☐	☐

P9 Walking on a hard surface (asphalt, concrete, etc.)

None	Mild	Moderate	Severe	Extreme
☐	☐	☐	☐	☐

P10 Walking on an uneven surface

None	Mild	Moderate	Severe	Extreme
☐	☐	☐	☐	☐

Physical function, daily living

The following questions concern your physical function. **For each of the following activities please indicate the degree of difficulty you have experienced in the past week due to your hip and/or groin problem.**

A1 Walking up stairs

None	Mild	Moderate	Severe	Extreme
☐	☐	☐	☐	☐

A2 Bending down, e.g. to pick something up from the floor

None	Mild	Moderate	Severe	Extreme
☐	☐	☐	☐	☐

A3 Getting in/out of car

None	Mild	Moderate	Severe	Extreme
☐	☐	☐	☐	☐

A4 Lying in bed (turning over or maintaining the same hip position for a long time)

None	Mild	Moderate	Severe	Extreme
☐	☐	☐	☐	☐

A5 Heavy domestic duties (scrubbing floors, vacuuming, moving heavy boxes etc)

None	Mild	Moderate	Severe	Extreme
☐	☐	☐	☐	☐

Function, sports and recreational activities

The following questions concern your physical function when participating in higher-level activities. Answer **every** question by ticking the appropriate box. If a question does not pertain to you or you have not experienced it in the past week please make your "best guess" as to which response would be the most accurate. **The questions should be answered considering what degree of difficulty you have experienced during the following activities in the past week due to problems with your hip and/or groin.**

SP1 Squatting

None	Mild	Moderate	Severe	Extreme
☐	☐	☐	☐	☐

SP2 Running

None	Mild	Moderate	Severe	Extreme
☐	☐	☐	☐	☐

SP3 Twisting/pivoting on a weight bearing leg

None	Mild	Moderate	Severe	Extreme
☐	☐	☐	☐	☐

SP4 Walking on an uneven surface

None	Mild	Moderate	Severe	Extreme
☐	☐	☐	☐	☐

SP5 Running as fast as you can

None	Mild	Moderate	Severe	Extreme
☐	☐	☐	☐	☐

SP6 Bringing the leg forcefully forward and/or out to the side, such as in kicking, skating etc.

None	Mild	Moderate	Severe	Extreme
☐	☐	☐	☐	☐

SP7 Sudden explosive movements that involve quick footwork, such as accelerations, decelerations, change of directions etc.

None	Mild	Moderate	Severe	Extreme
☐	☐	☐	☐	☐

SP8 Situations where the leg is stretched into an outer position (such as when the leg is placed as far away from the body as possible)

None	Mild	Moderate	Severe	Extreme
☐	☐	☐	☐	☐

Participation in physical activities

The following questions are about your ability to participate in your preferred physical activities. Physical activities include sporting activities as well as all other forms of activity where you become slightly out of breath. **When you answer these questions consider to what degree your ability to participate in physical activities during the past week has been affected by your hip and/or groin problem.**

PA1 Are you able to participate in your preferred physical activities for as long as you would like?

Always	Often	Sometimes	Rarely	Never
☐	☐	☐	☐	☐

PA2 Are you able to participate in your preferred physical activities at your normal performance level?

Always	Often	Sometimes	Rarely	Never
☐	☐	☐	☐	☐

Quality of Life

Q1 How often are you aware of your hip and/or groin problem?

Never	Monthly	Weekly	Daily	Constantly
☐	☐	☐	☐	☐

Q2 Have you modified your life style to avoid activities potentially damaging to your hip and/or groin?

Not at all	Mildly	Moderately	Severely	Totally
☐	☐	☐	☐	☐

Q3 In general, how much difficulty do you have with your hip and/or groin?

None	Mild	Moderate	Severe	Extreme
☐	☐	☐	☐	☐

Q4 Does your hip and/or groin problem affect your mood in a negative way?

Not at all	Rarely	Sometimes	Often	All the time
☐	☐	☐	☐	☐

Q5 Do you feel restricted due to your hip and/or groin problem?

Not at all	Rarely	Sometimes	Often	All the time
☐	☐	☐	☐	☐

Thank you very much for completing all the questions in this questionnaire.

APPENDIX 1

International Hip Outcome Tool (iHOT-33).

iHOT[33]

INTERNATIONAL HIP OUTCOME TOOL

NAME

DATE OF BIRTH

TODAY'S DATE

WHICH HIP IS THIS SURVEY ABOUT?
If we've asked you to tell us about one hip in particular, tick that. Otherwise, tick the one which causes most trouble.

○ **Left**

○ **Right**

QUALITY OF LIFE QUESTIONNAIRE FOR YOUNG, ACTIVE PEOPLE WITH HIP PROBLEMS

INSTRUCTIONS

- These questions ask about the problems you may be experiencing in your hip, how these problems affect your life, and the emotions you may feel because of these problems.
- Please indicate the severity by marking the line below each question with a slash.
  - » If you put a mark on the far **left**, it means that you **feel you are significantly impaired**. For example:

    SIGNIFICANTLY IMPAIRED /______________________________ NO PROBLEMS AT ALL

  - » If you put a mark on the far **right**, it means that you **do not think that you have any problems** with your hip. For example:

    SIGNIFICANTLY IMPAIRED ______________________________/ NO PROBLEMS AT ALL

  - » If the mark is placed in the middle of the line, this indicates that you are moderately disabled, or in other words, between the extremes of 'significantly impaired' and 'no problems at all'. It is important to put your mark at either end of the line if the extreme descriptions accurately reflect your situation.

TIP If you don't do an activity, imagine how your hip would feel if you had to try it.

- Please let your answers describe the typical situation in the last **month**.

SECTION 1 | SYMPTOMS AND FUNCTIONAL LIMITATIONS

The following questions ask about symptoms that you may experience in your hip and about the function of your hip with respect to daily activities. Please think about how you have felt most of the time over the past month and answer accordingly.

Q01 How often does your hip/groin ache?

CONSTANTLY ______________________________ NEVER

Q02 How stiff is your hip as a result of sitting/resting during the day?

EXTREMELY STIFF ______________________________ NOT STIFF AT ALL

Q03 How difficult is it for you to walk long distances?

EXTREMELY DIFFICULT ______________________ NOT DIFFICULT AT ALL

Q04 How much pain do you have in your hip while sitting?

EXTREME PAIN ______________________ NO PAIN AT ALL

Q05 How much trouble do you have standing on your feet for long periods of time?

SEVERE TROUBLE ______________________ NO TROUBLE AT ALL

Q06 How difficult is it for you to get up and down off the floor/ground?

EXTREMELY DIFFICULT ______________________ NOT DIFFICULT AT ALL

Q07 How difficult is it for you to walk on uneven surfaces?

EXTREMELY DIFFICULT ______________________ NOT DIFFICULT AT ALL

Q08 How difficult is it for you to lie on your affected hip side?

EXTREMELY DIFFICULT ______________________ NOT DIFFICULT AT ALL

Q09 How much trouble do you have with stepping over obstacles?

SEVERE TROUBLE ______________________ NO TROUBLE AT ALL

Q10 How much trouble do you have with climbing up/down stairs?

SEVERE TROUBLE ______________________ NO TROUBLE AT ALL

Q11 How much trouble do you have with rising from a sitting position?

SEVERE TROUBLE ______________________ NO TROUBLE AT ALL

Q12 How much discomfort do you have with taking long strides?

EXTREME DISCOMFORT ______________________ NO DISCOMFORT AT ALL

Q13 How much difficulty do you have with getting into and/or out of a car?

EXTREME DIFFICULTY ________________ NO DIFFICULTY AT ALL

Q14 How much trouble do you have with grinding, catching or clicking in your hip?

SEVERE TROUBLE ________________ NO TROUBLE AT ALL

Q15 How much difficulty do you have with putting on/taking off socks, stockings or shoes?

EXTREME DIFFICULTY ________________ NO DIFFICULTY AT ALL

Q16 Overall, how much pain do you have in your hip/groin?

EXTREME PAIN ________________ NO PAIN AT ALL

SECTION 2 | SPORTS AND RECREATIONAL ACTIVITIES

The following questions ask about your **hip** when you participate in sports and recreational activities. Please think about how you have felt most of the time over the past **month** and answer accordingly.

Q17 How concerned are you about your ability to maintain your desired fitness level?

EXTREMELY CONCERNED ________________ NOT CONCERNED AT ALL

Q18 How much pain do you experience in your hip after activity?

EXTREME PAIN ________________ NO PAIN AT ALL

Q19 How concerned are you that the pain in your hip will increase if you participate in sports or recreational activities?

EXTREMELY CONCERNED ________________ NOT CONCERNED AT ALL

Q20 How much has your quality of life deteriorated because you cannot participate in sport/recreational activities?

EXTREMELY DETERIORATED ________________ NOT DETERIORATED AT ALL

Q21 How concerned are you about cutting/changing directions during your sport or recreational activities?

☐ I do not do this action in my activities

EXTREMELY CONCERNED ________________________ NOT CONCERNED AT ALL

Q22 How much has your performance level decreased in your sport or recreational activities?

EXTREMELY DECREASED ________________________ NOT DECREASED AT ALL

SECTION 3 | JOB RELATED CONCERNS

The following questions relate to your hip with respect to your current work. Please think about how you have felt most of the time over the past month and answer accordingly.

☐ I do not work because of my hip *(please skip section)*
☐ I do not work for reasons other than my hip *(please skip section)*

Q23 How much trouble do you have pushing, pulling, lifting or carrying heavy objects at work?

☐ I do not do these actions in my activities

SEVERE TROUBLE ________________________ NO TROUBLE AT ALL

Q24 How much trouble do you have with crouching/squatting?

SEVERE TROUBLE ________________________ NO TROUBLE AT ALL

Q25 How concerned are you that your job will make your hip worse?

EXTREMELY CONCERNED ________________________ NOT CONCERNED AT ALL

Q26 How much difficulty do you have at work because of reduced hip mobility?

EXTREME DIFFICULTY ________________________ NO DIFFICULTY AT ALL

SECTION 4 | SOCIAL, EMOTIONAL AND LIFESTYLE CONCERNS

The following questions ask about social, emotional and lifestyle concerns that you may feel with respect to your hip problem. Please think about how you have felt most of the time over the past month and answer accordingly.

Q27 How frustrated are you because of your hip problem?

EXTREMELY FRUSTRATED ________________________ NOT FRUSTRATED AT ALL

Q28 How much trouble do you have with sexual activity because of your hip?

☐ This is not relevant to me

SEVERE TROUBLE ________________________ NO TROUBLE AT ALL

Q29 How much of a distraction is your hip problem?

EXTREME DISTRACTION ________________________ NO DISTRACTION AT ALL

Q30 How difficult is it for you to release tension and stress because of your hip problem?

EXTREMELY DIFFICULT ________________________ NOT DIFFICULT AT ALL

Q31 How discouraged are you because of your hip problem?

EXTREMELY DISCOURAGED ________________________ NOT DISCOURAGED AT ALL

Q32 How concerned are you about picking up or carrying children because of your hip?

☐ I do not do this action in my activities

EXTREMELY CONCERNED ________________________ NOT CONCERNED AT ALL

Q33 How much of the time are you aware of the disability in your hip?

CONSTANTLY AWARE ________________________ NOT AWARE AT ALL

APPENDIX

iHOT[12]

INTERNATIONAL HIP OUTCOME TOOL

NAME

DATE OF BIRTH

TODAY'S DATE

WHICH HIP IS THIS SURVEY ABOUT?

If we've asked you to tell us about one hip in particular, tick that. Otherwise, tick the one which causes most trouble.

○ Left

○ Right

QUALITY OF LIFE QUESTIONNAIRE FOR YOUNG, ACTIVE PEOPLE WITH HIP PROBLEMS

INSTRUCTIONS

- These questions ask about the problems you may be experiencing in your hip, how these problems affect your life, and the emotions you may feel because of these problems.
- Please indicate the severity by marking the line below each question with a slash.
  - » If you put a mark on the far **left**, it means that you **feel you are significantly impaired**. For example:

    SIGNIFICANTLY IMPAIRED /________________________________ NO PROBLEMS AT ALL

  - » If you put a mark on the far **right**, it means that you **do not think that you have any problems** with your hip. For example:

    SIGNIFICANTLY IMPAIRED ________________________________/ NO PROBLEMS AT ALL

  - » If the mark is placed in the middle of the line, this indicates that you are moderately disabled, or in other words, between the extremes of 'significantly impaired' and 'no problems at all'. It is important to put your mark at either end of the line if the extreme descriptions accurately reflect your situation.

    TIP If you don't do an activity, imagine how your hip would feel if you had to try it.
- Please let your answers describe the typical situation in the last **month**.

Q1 Overall, how much pain do you have in your hip/groin?

EXTREME PAIN ________________________________ NO PAIN AT ALL

Q2 How difficult is it for you to get up and down off the floor/ground?

EXTREMELY DIFFICULT ________________________________ NOT DIFFICULT AT ALL

Q3 How difficult is it for you to walk long distances?

EXTREMELY DIFFICULT ________________________________ NOT DIFFICULT AT ALL

Q4 How much trouble do you have with grinding, catching or clicking in your hip?

SEVERE TROUBLE ______________________________ NO TROUBLE AT ALL

Q5 How much trouble do you have pushing, pulling, lifting or carrying heavy objects?

SEVERE TROUBLE ______________________________ NO TROUBLE AT ALL

Q6 How concerned are you about cutting/changing directions during your sport or recreational activities?

EXTREMELY CONCERNED ______________________________ NOT CONCERNED AT ALL

Q7 How much pain do you experience in your hip *after* activity?

EXTREME PAIN ______________________________ NO PAIN AT ALL

Q8 How concerned are you about picking up or carrying children because of your hip?

EXTREMELY CONCERNED ______________________________ NOT CONCERNED AT ALL

Q9 How much trouble do you have with sexual activity because of your hip?

☐ This is not relevant to me

SEVERE TROUBLE ______________________________ NO TROUBLE AT ALL

Q10 How much of the time are you aware of the disability in your hip?

CONSTANTLY AWARE ______________________________ NOT AWARE AT ALL

Q11 How concerned are you about your ability to maintain your desired fitness level?

EXTREMELY CONCERNED ______________________________ NOT CONCERNED AT ALL

Q12 How much of a distraction is your hip problem?

EXTREME DISTRACTION ______________________________ NO DISTRACTION AT ALL

References

1. Harris WH. Traumatic arthritis of the hip after dislocation and acetabular fractures: treatment by mold arthroplasty. An end-result study using a new method of result evaluation. J Bone Joint Surg Am. 1969;51:737–55.
2. D'Aubigne RM, Postel M. Functional results of hip arthroplasty with acrylic prosthesis. J Bone Joint Surg Am. 1954;36-A: 451–75.
3. Nilsdotter AK, Lohmander LS, Klässbo M, Roos EM. Hip disability and osteoarthritis outcome score (HOOS)—validity and responsiveness in total hip replacement. BMC Musculoskelet Disord. 2003;4:10.
4. Klässbo M, Larsson E, Mannevik E. Hip disability and osteoarthritis outcome score. An extension of the Western Ontario and McMaster Universities Osteoarthritis Index. Scand J Rheumatol. 2003;32:46–51.
5. Murray DW, Fitzpatrick R, Rogers K, Pandit H, Beard DJ, Carr AJ, et al. The use of the Oxford hip and knee scores. J Bone Joint Surg Br. 2007;89:1010–4.
6. Söderman P, Malchau H. Validity and reliability of Swedish WOMAC osteoarthritis index: a self-administered disease-specific questionnaire (WOMAC) versus generic instruments (SF-36 and NHP). Acta Orthop Scand. 2000;71:39–46.
7. Stucki G, Sangha O, Stucki S, Michel BA, Tyndall A, Dick W, et al. Comparison of the WOMAC (Western Ontario and McMaster Universities) osteoarthritis index and a self-report format of the self-administered Lequesne-Algofunctional index in patients with knee and hip osteoarthritis. Osteoarthritis Cartilage. 1998;6: 79–86.
8. Safran MR, Hariri S. Hip arthroscopy assessment tools and outcomes. Oper Tech Orthop. 2010;20(4):264–77.
9. Byrd JW, Jones KS. Prospective analysis of hip arthroscopy with 2-year follow-up. Arthroscopy. 2000;16:578–87.
10. Christensen CP, Althausen PL, Mittleman MA, Lee J-A, McCarthy JC. The nonarthritic hip score: reliable and validated. Clin Orthop Relat Res. 2003;(406):75–83.
11. Thorborg K, Holmich P, Christensen R, Petersen J, Roos EM. The Copenhagen Hip and Groin Outcome Score (HAGOS): development and validation according to the COSMIN checklist. Br J Sports Med. 2011;45:478–91.
12. Mohtadi NGH, Griffin DR, Pedersen ME, Chan D, Safran MR, Parsons N, et al. The development and validation of a self-administered quality-of-life outcome measure for young, active patients with symptomatic hip disease: the International Hip Outcome Tool (iHOT-33). Arthroscopy. 2012;28:595–605. quiz 606–10.e1.
13. Martin RL, Mohtadi NG, Safran MR, Leunig M, Martin HD, McCarthy J, et al. Differences in physician and patient ratings of items used to assess hip disorders. Am J Sports Med. 2009;37: 1508–12.
14. Lieberman JR, Dorey F, Shekelle P, Schumacher L, Thomas BJ, Kilgus DJ, et al. Differences between patients "and physicians" evaluations of outcome after total hip arthroplasty. J Bone Joint Surg Am. 1996;78:835–8.
15. Mokkink LB, Terwee CB, Patrick DL, Alonso J, Stratford PW, Knol DL, et al. The COSMIN study reached international consensus on taxonomy, terminology, and definitions of measurement properties for health-related patient-reported outcomes. J Clin Epidemiol. 2010;63:737–45.
16. Terwee CB, Bot SDM, de Boer MR, van der Windt DA, Knol DL, Dekker J, et al. Quality criteria were proposed for measurement properties of health status questionnaires. J Clin Epidemiol. 2007;60:34–42.
17. Terwee CB, Mokkink LB, Knol DL, Ostelo RW, Bouter LM, de Vet HC. Rating the methodological quality in systematic reviews of studies on measurement properties: a scoring system for the COSMIN checklist. Qual Life Res. 2012;21:651–7.
18. Thorborg K, Roos EM, Bartels EM, Petersen J, Holmich P. Validity, reliability and responsiveness of patient-reported outcome questionnaires when assessing hip and groin disability: a systematic review. Br J Sports Med. 2010;44:1186–96.
19. Nilsdotter A, Bremander A. Measures of hip function and symptoms: Harris Hip Score (HHS), Hip Disability and Osteoarthritis Outcome Score (HOOS), Oxford Hip Score (OHS), Lequesne Index of Severity for Osteoarthritis of the Hip (LISOH), and American Academy of Orthopedic Surgeons (AAOS) Hip and Knee Questionnaire. Arthritis Care Res (Hoboken). 2011;63 Suppl 11:S200–7.
20. Söderman P, Malchau H. Is the Harris hip score system useful to study the outcome of total hip replacement? Clin Orthop Relat Res. 2001;384:189–97.
21. Söderman P, Malchau H, Herberts P. Outcome of total hip replacement: a comparison of different measurement methods. Clin Orthop Relat Res. 2001;390:163–72.
22. Matta JM, Mehne DK, Roffi R. Fractures of the acetabulum. Early results of a prospective study. Clin Orthop Relat Res. 1986;205: 241–50.
23. Øvre S, Sandvik L, Madsen JE, Røise O. Comparison of distribution, agreement and correlation between the original and modified Merle d'Aubigné-Postel Score and the Harris Hip Score after acetabular fracture treatment: moderate agreement, high ceiling effect and excellent correlation in 450 patients. Acta Orthop. 2005;76:796–802.
24. Wamper KE, Sierevelt IN, Poolman RW, Bhandari M, Haverkamp D. The Harris hip score: do ceiling effects limit its usefulness in orthopedics? Acta Orthop. 2010;81:703–7.
25. Callaghan JJ, Dysart SH, Savory CF, Hopkinson WJ. Assessing the results of hip replacement. A comparison of five different rating systems. J Bone Joint Surg Br. 1990;72-B:1008–9.
26. Kirmit L, Karatosun V, Unver B, Bakirhan S, Sen A, Gocen Z. The reliability of hip scoring systems for total hip arthroplasty candidates: assessment by physical therapists. Clin Rehabil. 2005;19:659–61.
27. Dawson J, Fitzpatrick R, Carr A. Questionnaire on the perception of patients about shoulder surgery. J Bone Joint Surg Br. 1996;78-B:593–600.
28. Kalairajah Y, Azurza K, Hulme C, Molloy S, Drabu KJ. Health outcome measures in the evaluation of total hip arthroplasties—a comparison between the Harris hip score and the Oxford hip score. J Arthroplasty. 2005;20:1037–41.
29. Garbuz DS, Xu M, Sayre EC. Patients' outcome after total hip arthroplasty: a comparison between the Western Ontario and McMaster Universities index and the Oxford 12-item hip score. J Arthroplasty. 2006;21:998–1004.
30. Ostendorf M, van Stel HF, Buskens E, Schrijvers AJP, Marting LN, Verbout AJ, et al. Patient-reported outcome in total hip replacement. A comparison of five instruments of health status. J Bone Joint Surg Br. 2004;86:801–8.
31. Dawson J, Fitzpatrick R, Frost S, Gundle R, McLardy-Smith P, Murray D. Evidence for the validity of a patient-based instrument for assessment of outcome after revision hip replacement. J Bone Joint Surg Br. 2001;83:1125–9.
32. Baker PN, van der Meulen JH, Lewsey J, Gregg PJ, National Joint Registry for England and Wales. The role of pain and function in determining patient satisfaction after total knee replacement. Data from the National Joint Registry for England and Wales. J Bone Joint Surg Br. 2007;89:893–900.
33. Dunbar MJ, Robertsson O, Ryd L, Lidgren L. Appropriate questionnaires for knee arthroplasty. Results of a survey of 3600 patients from The Swedish Knee Arthroplasty Registry. J Bone Joint Surg Br. 2001;83:339–44.
34. Rothwell AG, Hooper GJ, Hobbs A, Frampton CM. An analysis of the Oxford hip and knee scores and their relationship to early joint

revision in the New Zealand Joint Registry. J Bone Joint Surg Br. 2010;92:413–8.
35. Davis AM, Perruccio AV, Canizares M, Tennant A, Hawker GA, Conaghan PG, et al. The development of a short measure of physical function for hip OA HOOS-Physical Function Shortform (HOOS-PS): an OARSI/OMERACT initiative. Osteoarthritis Cartilage. 2008;16:551–9.
36. Ornetti P, Parratte S, Gossec L, Tavernier C, Argenson J-N, Roos EM, et al. Cross-cultural adaptation and validation of the French version of the Hip disability and Osteoarthritis Outcome Score (HOOS) in hip osteoarthritis patients. Osteoarthritis Cartilage. 2010;18:522–9.
37. de Groot IB, Reijman M, Terwee CB, Bierma-Zeinstra SMA, Favejee M, Roos EM, et al. Validation of the Dutch version of the Hip disability and Osteoarthritis Outcome Score. Osteoarthritis Cartilage. 2007;15:104–9.
38. Hetaimish BM, Khan M, Crouch S, Simunovic N, Bedi A, Mohtadi N, et al. Consistency of reported outcomes after arthroscopic management of femoroacetabular impingement. Arthroscopy. 2013;29(4):780–7. doi:10.1016/j.arthro.2012.11.011.
39. Martin R, Kelly BT, Philippon MJ. Evidence of validity for the hip outcome score. Arthroscopy. 2006;22(12):1304–11.
40. Martin RL, Philippon MJ. Evidence of validity for the hip outcome score in hip arthroscopy. Arthroscopy. 2007;23:822–6.
41. Martin RL, Philippon MJ. Evidence of reliability and responsiveness for the hip outcome score. Arthroscopy. 2008;24:676–82.
42. Griffin DR, Parsons N, Mohtadi NGH, Safran MR, Multicenter Arthroscopy of the Hip Outcomes Research Network. A short version of the International Hip Outcome Tool (iHOT-12) for use in routine clinical practice. Arthroscopy. 2012;28:611–6. quiz 616–8.
43. Riddle DL, Stratford PW, Bowman DH. Findings of extensive variation in the types of outcome measures used in hip and knee replacement clinical trials: a systematic review. Arthritis Rheum. 2008;59:876–83.
44. Lodhia P, Slobogean GP, Noonan VK, Gilbart MK. Patient-reported outcome instruments for femoroacetabular impingement and hip labral pathology: a systematic review of the clinimetric evidence. Arthroscopy. 2011;27:279–86.
45. Tijssen M, van Cingel R, van Melick N, de Visser E. Patient-Reported Outcome questionnaires for hip arthroscopy: a systematic review of the psychometric evidence. BMC Musculoskelet Disord. 2011;12:117.

Gait Analysis

10

Maureen K. Dwyer

Introduction

The fundamental goal of gait analysis is to assess an individual's functional capabilities and identify the presence and impact of impairments due to injury or disease processes on joint function. A comprehensive evaluation of the hip joint during gait should include measures of joint motion, joint forces, and neuromuscular function. Kinematics involves the study of the angular or translational motions of joints during gait and is measured through the use of 3-D motion analysis systems. Kinetics is the measure of the forces and moments acting upon the joints to create motion. The forces encountered during gait include those due to gravity, muscle contraction, and the passive tension created by the static structures of the joint. It is not possible to measure directly the forces acting upon the intact joint; therefore, forces are often estimated using mathematical analyses based upon foot/ground forces measured with load platforms combined with anatomical estimates of muscle size, shape, and activation patterns measured during gait. Electromyography (EMG) is employed to measure the myoelectric signals generating muscle contraction and can provide information on both the magnitude and timing of activation of individual muscles. Measurement of joint kinematic and kinetic parameters along with neuromuscular function assists in detecting impairments which are not identifiable through clinical tests. Data obtained from these analyses can be used to develop targeted treatment strategies and guide appropriate rehabilitation programs to address persistent impairments. Advancing our knowledge of biomechanical and neuromuscular function of the hip joint will lead to continued improvements in both the diagnosis and treatment of pathological conditions of the joint.

M.K. Dwyer (✉)
Newton Wellesley Hospital,
2000 Washington Street, Green Building, Ste 361, Newton, MA 02462, USA
e-mail: mkdwyer@partners.org

The Gait Cycle

The gait cycle encompasses the time from when one foot contacts the ground until that same foot makes contact with the ground again and includes both the stance and swing phases. Walking gait includes periods of both double-limb and single-limb support, with single-limb support accounting for 80 % of stance phase. The time spent in double-limb support decreases as gait speed increases [1]. The stance phase begins at initial foot contact and makes up 60 % of the gait cycle, while the swing phase is initiated at toe off of the weight-bearing limb. In order to better isolate and identify movement and force patterns, the gait cycle can be further broken down into eight distinct phases—initial contact, loading response, midstance, terminal stance, preswing, initial swing, midswing, and terminal swing (Fig. 10.1) [1–3].

Initial contact constitutes the weight acceptance phase of gait and makes up the first 10 % of the gait cycle. Loading response and midstance represent the single-limb stance phase of gait and occur from 10 to 50 % of the gait cycle, while the weight unloading phase, consisting of terminal stance and preswing, makes up the last 10 % of the stance phase (50–60 % of the gait cycle) [2, 3]. The weight acceptance and weight unloading phases represent the two double-limb support phases of gait. The latter 40 % of the gait cycle constitutes the swing phase of gait, during which time the limb is propelled forward. In initial swing (62–75 % of gait cycle), the limb is accelerated forward, while during terminal swing (87–100 % of gait cycle), deceleration of the limb occurs to prepare for initial limb contact with the ground [3].

Measurement of the timing and space parameters of gait can provide a quantifiable assessment of walking function. Parameters that are commonly reported include step length, stride length, cadence, gait velocity, and time spent in single-limb support. Step length is defined as the distance from initial contact of one foot to initial contact of the opposite foot, while stride length is the distance from initial contact of one foot to subsequent contact of the same foot [2, 3]. Cadence is the number of steps taken in a given period of time.

J.C. McCarthy et al. (eds.), *Hip Joint Restoration*, DOI 10.1007/978-1-4614-0694-5_10

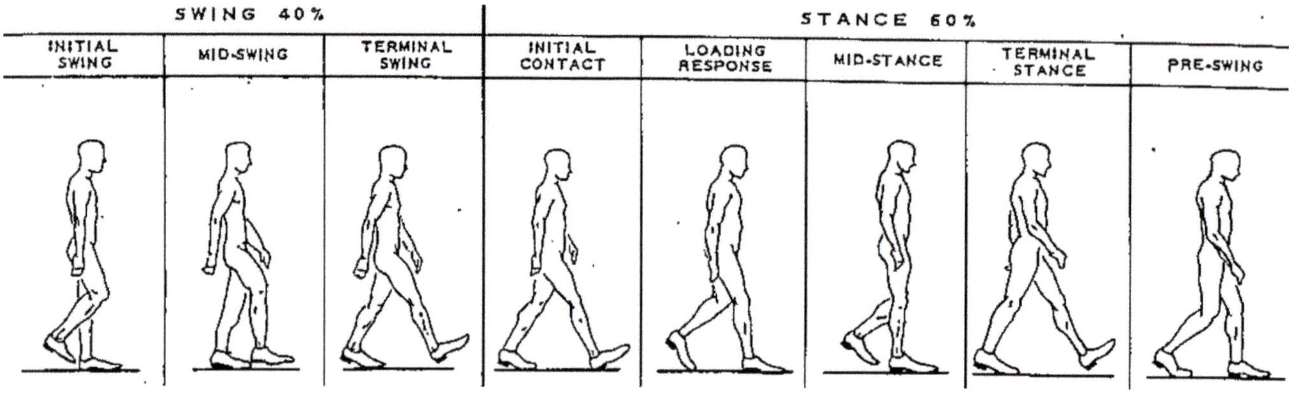

Fig. 10.1 Normal gait cycle. From Orthopedic Physical Assessment, 2nd Ed., Magee D, Chapter 14: Gait Assessment, p564–565. Reprinted with permission from Elsevier Ltd

Gait velocity is a measure of stride length divided by the amount of time to complete the stride, expressed as meters per second or miles per hour [1]. Quantification of the spatiotemporal characteristics of gait can provide important information regarding the impact of hip joint pathology on normal function.

Kinematics

A comprehensive kinematic analysis of hip joint motion during gait includes measurements of joint rotations in all three cardinal planes. The greatest arc of motion occurs in the sagittal plane and serves to move the limb forward during gait. The hip rotates through 40° of total sagittal plane motion during the gait cycle from approximately 10° of extension to 30° of flexion [1–3]. Maximum hip flexion (30°–35°) is attained during the swing phase, around 85% of the gait cycle. The thigh is flexed approximately 20° at initial contact and begins movement of the hip into extension, reaching neutral sagittal plane motion at 27% of the gait cycle [3]. Maximum hip extension (10°) occurs at the end of stance phase, just prior to toe off.

Total motion in both the frontal and transverse planes is minimal throughout the gait cycle. In both these planes, the hip joint is positioned in neutral at initial contact, then moving into adduction and internal rotation during stance phase, reaching maximum values of both motions (5°–10°) at the end of the loading response [3, 4]. After this point, the hip begins to rotate into abduction and external rotation, reaching peak of both motions (3°–5°) at the start of swing phase [2, 3]. Total transverse plane motion is roughly 8°–10° during the entire gait cycle [3, 4]. Motion in these planes assists with stability of the limb and absorption of external forces applied to the joint during walking.

Kinetics

The forces encountered by the native hip joint during the performance of functional activities play an important role in the health and longevity of the joint. Measurements of hip joint reaction forces have been provided by endoprostheses instrumented with strain gauges. During gait, peak forces of 200–480% of body weight (BW) have been reported, with higher values being observed at increased gait velocities [5–8]. The majority of the peak joint contact force occurs in the superior direction and exhibits two peaks during each gait cycle (Fig. 10.2) [3]. The first peak occurs at approximately 15% of the gait cycle at the transition between the loading response and midstance when the contralateral foot leaves the ground, while the second peak occurs at late terminal stance, just prior to contralateral heel strike. The relative magnitude of the two peaks varies extensively, depending on walking speed, the activity of the plantarflexors, the type of footwear worn, and the nature of the walking surface, but is classically depicted as being equal with one study reporting peak loads of 240% BW for the first resultant peak and 237% BW for the second resultant peak [9]. As virtually all of the direct measurement of hip joint forces during gait has been performed in arthritic patients after implantation of hip prostheses, the relevance of these measurements to the normal or pre-arthritic hip is not fully established; nonetheless, instrumented prostheses can provide a basis for validation of analytical models using data derived from gait analysis studies.

Computational models can be used to estimate joint forces during dynamic activities using measurements obtained through motion analysis such as joint position, ground reaction forces (GRFs), segment mass, muscle geometry, and inertial properties [10]. GRFs are those forces which act upon the body during the stance phase of gait [1]. The GRF

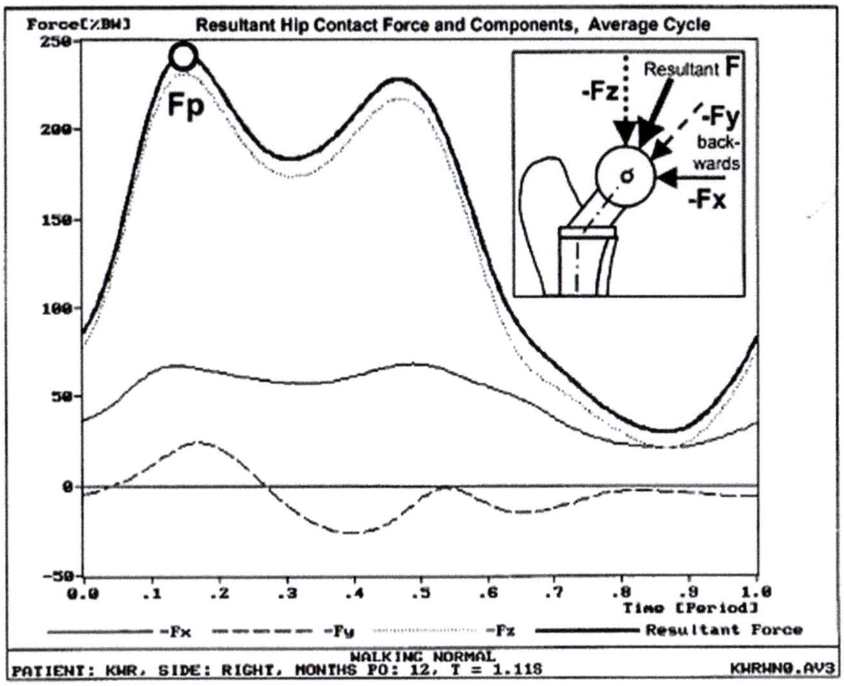

Fig. 10.2 Individual average of hip contact force F in % BW and its components $-F_x$, $-F_y$, and $-F_z$. The highest value is the peak force F_p. From Journal of Biomechanics, 34, Bergmann G, Deuretzbacher G, Heller M, Graichen F, Rohlmann A, Strauss J, Duda G, Hip contact forces and gait patterns from routine activities, 859–871, 2001. Reprinted with permission from Elsevier Ltd

can be broken down into vertical and shear forces, with those forces applied in the mediolateral and anteroposterior directions accounting for the shear forces. The dynamic optimization gait analysis describes GRF according to the specific contributions from muscle force, gravitational force, and centrifugal forces [11–13]. Based on these models, muscle contraction makes the major contributor to hip joint contact force and contributes 50–95% of the joint reactive force during stance, with minimal contribution from ground reaction and centrifugal forces (Fig. 10.3) [11]. The iliopsoas was the major contributor to the anteroposterior component of the joint force, while the gluteus medius made the largest contribution to both the superior and medial components. Examination of the vertical GRF revealed primary contributions from the hip extensors and abductors to limb support during gait [12]. The actions of the gluteal and hamstring muscles accounted for most of the first resultant peak force, while, of the hip muscles, the gluteus medius made the primary contribution to the second resultant peak. Using estimates derived from computational models, the peak joint contact forces were estimated to range from 200 to 430% BW, which is similar in magnitude to those measured in vivo [11, 14].

Muscle Activity

Muscle contraction propels the limb forward, provides stability, and counteracts the external forces encountered by the limb during gait. Limb acceleration occurs during swing phase, with primary contributions from the hip flexor muscles to help propel the limb forward [3]. As described above, muscles provide the primary contribution to support during the stance phase [12], with the greatest input provided by the hip extensor and abductor muscles [3, 12, 15]. Contraction of the muscles contributing to hip extension is initiated during late swing phase. The long head of the biceps femoris muscle, adductor magnus, and lower portion of the gluteus maximus muscles reach peak EMG muscle activation during initial foot contact and early in the loading response phase and cease activity around 10% of the gait cycle [3, 15]. The activation of these muscles assists deceleration of hip flexion as the limb begins move into extension; it also provides support of the hip joint during load acceptance [15].

A similar pattern of activation has been observed during gait for the hip abductors [3, 15–17]. These muscles are activated at terminal swing, with peak EMG amplitudes of the gluteus medius, gluteus minimus, and upper gluteus maximus muscles occurring during the loading response [3, 15–17]. Intramuscular EMG analysis of the individual segments of the gluteus medius and gluteus minimus muscles has revealed biphasic activity during gait, with an initial burst during the first 20% of the gait cycle and a second burst in the interval between 20 and 60% [16, 17]. All three segments of the gluteus medius muscle demonstrated similar intensity of activation during the two bursts; however, the timing of peak muscle activation occurred earlier for the posterior and middle segments of the muscle when compared to the anterior segment [17]. Conversely, differences in peak activation levels between the two segments of the gluteus

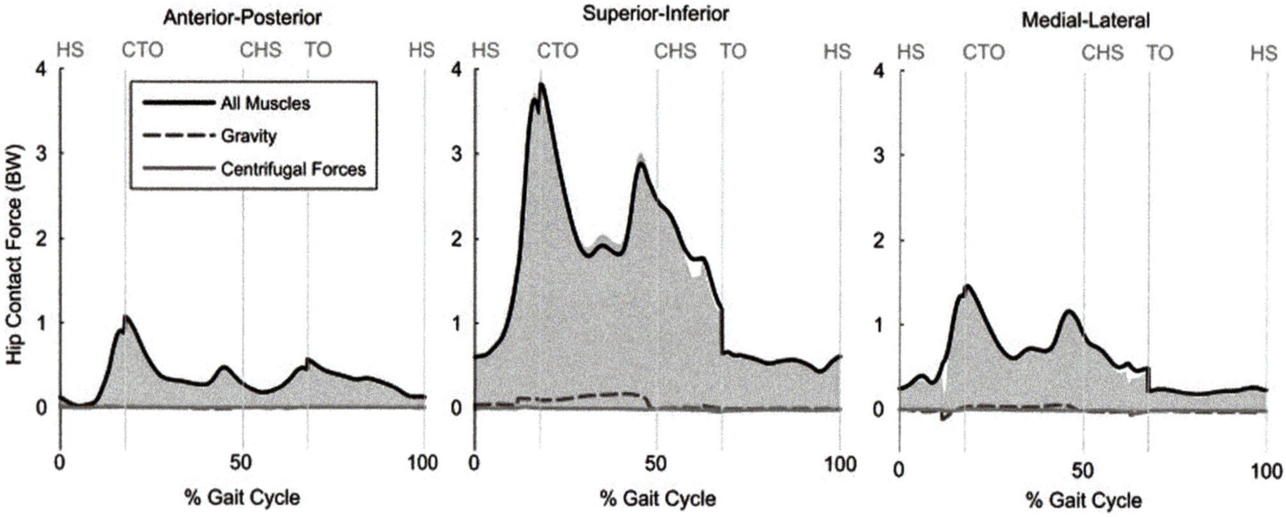

Fig. 10.3 Contributions of muscle forces, gravitational forces, and centrifugal forces to the three components of the hip contact force calculated in the model. Forces shown are the forces acting on the acetabulum in the model. The shaded areas represent the total contact forces acting along the three coordinate directions. All contact forces are specified in the femoral reference frame and are normalized by body weight (BW). Centrifugal forces and ligaments (not shown) made minimal contributions to the total contact force. The following gait cycle landmarks are demarcated by thin vertical lines: heel strike (HS), contralateral toe off (CTO), contralateral heel strike (CHS), and toe off (TO). Positive forces are directed anteriorly, superiorly, and medially; negative forces are directed posteriorly, inferiorly, and laterally. From Journal of Biomechanics, 43(8), Correa TA, Crossley KM, Kim HJ, Pandy MG, Contributions of individual muscles to hip joint contact force in normal walking, 1618–1622, 2010. Reprinted with permission from Elsevier Ltd

minimus were observed, with the posterior segment producing higher activation levels than the anterior segment during the first burst. The timing of the onset of activation of the anterior segment also occurred later than the posterior segment for both bursts for the minimus muscle [16]. The phasic activity of these prime abductors suggests that these muscles perform separate, complimentary functions during gait. These activation patterns, combined with the anatomical orientation of each muscle, suggest that gluteus minimus and the posterior segment of gluteus medius function primarily to stabilize the femoral head in the acetabulum during single-limb support, while the middle and anterior portions of the gluteus medius function to provide coronal plane hip and pelvic stability [16–18].

Gait Alterations Associated with Hip Joint Pathology

Preoperative Gait

Comprehensive biomechanical and neuromuscular examinations of gait in patients with intra-articular hip pathology are lacking and are limited to a handful of analyses in patients with femoroacetabular impingement (FAI). Gait velocity and cadence were found to be decreased in patients with FAI when compared to control subjects; however, step length remained unchanged for these patients during gait [19]. The most commonly observed change in the gait patterns of these patients is the presence of a hip flexion angle reversal during the stance phase of gait (Fig. 10.4) [19, 20]. Instead of the normal smooth transition from flexion at the start of stance phase to extension at the end of stance, individuals with FAI exhibit a reversal in which knee flexion increases by an average of 1.5° as the gait cycle progresses [20]. The reversal pattern of sagittal plane motion was found to be present in 45 % of patients during 30 % of gait trials [20]. A similar pattern of motion discontinuity has been observed in the sagittal plane during the stance phase of gait in patients with hip joint osteoarthritis (OA) [21]. Fifty-three percent of patients with OA demonstrated hip flexion reversals, which occurred during 65 % of trials with an average magnitude of 1.3° [21]. The existence of such a pattern was found to associate with both the presence and severity of joint disease in this cohort. These findings suggest that there may be a link between kinematic function, joint morphology, and joint disease, but the exact nature of this relationship requires further analyses.

A reduction in hip motion during gait has been reported in both sagittal and frontal planes for patients with FAI when compared to control subjects [19, 22]. The greatest change in sagittal plane motion was observed in hip extension near terminal stance (Fig. 10.5) [19, 22]. Patients with FAI reached an average of 5° less hip extension during terminal stance when compared to control subjects (7.4° ± 6.7° vs. 12.0° ± 7.2°, respectively) [19]. Musculoskeletal modeling has shown that the anterior component of the peak hip force occurs around 50 % of the gait cycle at the point of

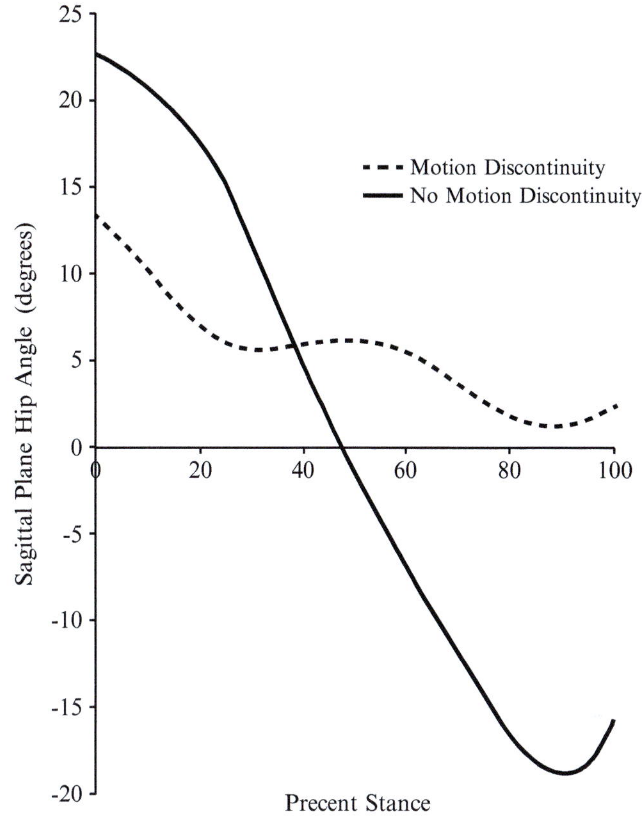

Fig. 10.4 Sagittal plane hip motion (hip flexion is positive; extension is negative) over time during walking in two representative subjects from the hip OA group studied. From Journal of Biomechanics, 45(8), Foucher KC, Schlink BR, Shakoor N, Wimmer MA, Sagittal plane hip motion reversals during walking are associated with disease severity and poorer function in subjects with hip osteoarthritis, 1360–1365, 2012. Reprinted with permission from Elsevier Ltd

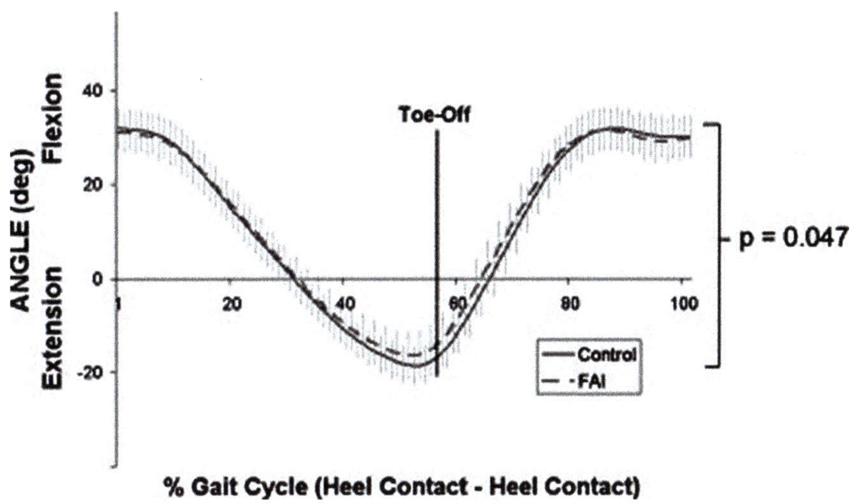

Fig. 10.5 Graph of mean (±standard deviation) sagittal hip angles of the FAI and control groups during level gait. The FAI group showed a trend of decreased total sagittal hip ROM ($p=0.047$). From Gait & Posture, 30(1), Kennedy MJ, Lamontagne M, Beaulé PE, Femoroacetabular impingement alters hip and pelvic biomechanics during gait: Walking biomechanics of FAI, 41–44, 2009. Reprinted with permission from Elsevier Ltd

maximum hip extension [13]. Increases in maximum hip extension were associated with larger values of the anterior component of the joint reaction force, with an increase of only 2° of maximum hip extension generating a 24 % increase in the anterior component of the joint reaction force [13]. The muscles providing the greatest contribution to the AP component of the hip force at peak hip extension were the anterior portion of the gluteus medius muscle, the iliacus, and the psoas major. However, it is unknown whether FAI alters the activation levels of these muscles during gait. Therefore, while the reduction in hip extension during gait observed for patients with FAI may be a compensatory strategy to unload the anterior hip joint, a more comprehensive analysis of the interplay between joint motion, joint forces, and neuromuscular function at the hip joint during gait is required to fully understand this relationship.

Conflicting results exist regarding alterations in frontal plane hip joint motion during gait for individuals with FAI. Kennedy et al. reported reductions in total hip motion in the frontal plane during gait [22], with a decrease in peak hip

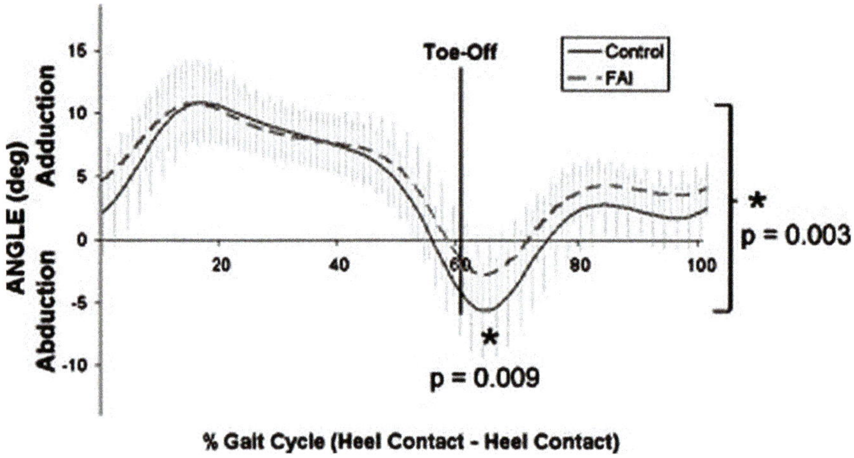

Fig. 10.6 Graph of mean (±standard deviation) frontal hip angles of the FAI and control groups during level gait. The FAI group had decreased peak hip abduction ($p=0.009$) and decreased total frontal hip ROM ($p=0.003$) *indicates location of statistically significant differences. From Gait & Posture, 30(1), Kennedy MJ, Lamontagne M, Beaulé PE, Femoroacetabular impingement alters hip and pelvic biomechanics during gait: Walking biomechanics of FAI, 41–44, 2009. Reprinted with permission from Elsevier Ltd

abduction at the initiation of swing phase and the affected limb remaining in a more adducted position throughout the swing phase (Fig. 10.6). In contrast, Hunt and colleagues observed a reduction in the peak hip adduction angle during the stance phase of gait, with the hip joint remaining in a more abducted position throughout the stance phase [19]. The lack of agreement between the two studies may be the result of different populations tested. Kennedy et al. examined only patients with cam-type FAI, whereas Hunt and colleagues tested patients with both cam-type and pincer-type FAI, as well as combined type FAI. It remains to be seen if and how the different types of morphological changes to the joint structures contribute to altered joint function. While reductions in hip abduction range of motion have been established for patients with FAI [23, 24], the observed peak hip abduction angles measured during gait (2°–5°) [22] are far below the reported maximum ranges of active abduction range of motion for these patients, approximately 50° [23, 24]. Therefore, it is unlikely that the reductions in frontal plane motion observed for patients with FAI are the result of bony impingement. As such, the decreases in motion are most likely the result of altered neuromuscular contributions to gait; however, without concomitant EMG data, specific contributions to altered frontal plane motion cannot be determined.

Alterations in hip joint kinetics during gait have also been reported for patients with FAI. While Kennedy et al. reported FAI has no effect on peak joint moments in any direction during gait [22], Hunt and colleagues observed reductions in peak external joint moments both for flexion moment during early stance phase and external rotation moment at terminal stance [19]. External joint moments require equal internal joint moments in the opposite direction to produce equilibrium. As such, the reduction in peak flexion moments and external rotation moments suggests a compensatory strategy which would limit the required internal rotation and extension muscle contributions. Given that the primary contributor to the AP component of the joint reaction force is the anterior portion of the gluteus medius muscle and the iliopsoas muscle, both active during internal rotation, a reduction in the external peak external rotation moment at terminal stance may, again, be a compensatory pattern to reduce the anterior hip joint force. Without evidence of altered muscle activation patterns through the collection of EMG during gait, the exact cause of the reduced external joint moments cannot be determined.

Postoperative Gait

Changes in biomechanical measures of gait have been reported for patients with FAI following surgical intervention [20, 25]. For the vast majority of patients, hip flexion reversals during the stance phase of gait were absent after surgery [20]. The motion discontinuity did persist in two patients; however, the prevalence and magnitude of the reversals was reduced for these patients [20]. Conflicting evidence exists regarding specific changes in motion patterns during gait after surgical intervention compared to presurgical values for patients with FAI. While no differences in frontal or sagittal plane hip motion have been observed for patients tested at an average of 21-month postsurgery [25], small increases in total sagittal plane hip motion were reported for FAI patients at 1-year postsurgery [20]. The increase in total sagittal plane motion was the result of an increase in peak hip flexion angle compared to preoperative values (22.7° vs. 19.9°) [20]. Maximum hip flexion values in the study by Brisson et al. were greater than 30° preoperatively, which falls within the normal range of peak hip flexion during gait and may be the reason for the lack of change following surgery [25]. The large discrepancy in peak hip flexion angles between the two studies may be the result of different populations studied. While Brisson and colleagues examined patients with isolated cam-FAI [25], Rylander et al. tested patients with pincer-type and combined type FAI [20]. Despite no changes in peak hip flexion motion after surgery compared to presurgical values, Brisson and colleagues did note the continued presence of reduced total sagittal plane motion when compared to control subjects [25]. Similar to the presurgical findings of Kennedy et al., the majority of the reduction in total sagittal plane motion occurred as a decrease in peak hip extension angles. Total frontal plane motion during gait remained unchanged following surgery in patients with FAI when compared to preoperative measures [20, 25], with range of motion remaining reduced compared to control subjects [25]. The lack of improvement in kinematic variables during gait postoperatively in patients with FAI suggests a persistence of compensatory strategies developed preoperatively to reduce pain. Given that a suggested link between joint kinematics, joint morphology, and joint disease exists for these patients, appropriate postoperative rehabilitation programs which focus on correcting pre- and postoperative impairments are needed to protect the health of the joint.

No differences in peak hip joint moments were observed during gait for patients with FAI when compared to presurgical values [20, 25]; however, significant reductions in peak abduction moment and internal rotation moment were present postsurgery when compared to control subjects [25]. The peak hip abduction and internal rotation moments occurred at approximately 10% of the gait cycle, which corresponds to contralateral limb toe off. This abrupt unloading of the contralateral limb shifts the body weight force vector medial to the hip joint center [3], requiring the generation of an abduction moment to stabilize the pelvis. The reduction in frontal plane hip motion observed for these patients may thus be a strategy to reduce the force required by the hip abductors to counteract body weight force by lowering the muscle's moment arm. Impaired hip abduction muscle strength has been reported for patients with FAI [26], and the altered frontal plane kinematic and kinetic variables during gait observed in postsurgical patients may suggest continued weakness in this muscle group. However, without concomitant muscle EMG and strength measures in postsurgical patients, this remains speculation.

While knowledge regarding gait biomechanics in patients with intra-articular hip pathology is growing, the current body of evidence only provides limited information for patients with FAI. Future work needs to expand biomechanical and neuromuscular analyses of the hip joint during gait to include populations with non-morphologically induced hip pain and injuries. In addition, while identification of altered kinematic patterns is important to our understanding of the biomechanics of injury, knowledge of the neuromuscular changes associated with these kinematic alterations is imperative to develop appropriate treatment programs to return normal gait patterns. Given that the alterations observed during gait for patients with FAI have also been observed in patients with advanced hip joint disease, addressing functional impairments both pre- and postsurgery may be protective for these patients.

References

1. Dicharry J. Kinematics and kinetics of gait: from lab to clinic. Clin Sports Med. 2010;29(3):347–64.
2. Magee D. Orthopedic physical assessment. 4th ed. Pennsylvania: Saunders; 2002. 614 p.
3. Perry J. Gait analysis: normal and pathological function. Thorofare: Slack; 1992. xxxii, 524 p.
4. Krebs DE, Robbins CE, Lavine L, Mann RW. Hip biomechanics during gait. J Orthop Sports Phys Ther. 1998;28(1):51–9.
5. Bergmann G, Deuretzbacher G, Heller M, Graichen F, Rohlmann A, Strauss J, et al. Hip contact forces and gait patterns from routine activities. J Biomech. 2001;34:859–71.
6. Bergmann G, Graichen F, Rohlmann A. Hip joint loading during walking and running, measured in two patients. J Biomech. 1993; 26(8):969–90.
7. Bergmann G, Graichen F, Rohlmann A. Hip joint contact forces during stumbling. Langenbecks Arch Surg. 2004;389(1):53–9.
8. Stansfield BW, Nicol AC, Paul JP, Kelly IG, Graichen F, Bergmann G. Direct comparison of calculated hip joint contact forces with those measured using instrumented implants. An evaluation of a three-dimensional mathematical model of the lower limb. J Biomech. 2003;36(7):929–36.
9. Damm P, Schwachmeyer V, Dymke J, Bender A, Bergmann G. In vivo hip joint loads during three methods of walking with forearm crutches. Clin Biomech. 2013;28(5):530–5.
10. Crowninshield RD, Johnston RC, Andrews JG, Brand RA. A biomechanical investigation of the human hip. J Biomech. 1978; 11(1–2):75–85.
11. Correa TA, Crossley KM, Kim HJ, Pandy MG. Contributions of individual muscles to hip joint contact force in normal walking. J Biomech. 2010;43(8):1618–22.
12. Anderson FC, Pandy MG. Individual muscle contributions to support in normal walking. Gait Posture. 2003;17:159–69.
13. Lewis CL, Sahrmann SA, Moran DW. Effect of hip angle on anterior hip joint force during gait. Gait Posture. 2010;32(4):603–7.
14. Hashimoto N, Ando M, Yayama T, Uchida K, Kobayashi S, Negoro K, et al. Dynamic analysis of the resultant force acting on the hip joint during level walking. Artif Organs. 2005;29(5):387–92.
15. Lyons K, Perry J, Gronley JK, Barnes L, Antonelli D. Timing and relative intensity of hip extensor and abductor muscle action during level and stair ambulation. Phys Ther. 1983;63(10):1597–605.
16. Semciw AI, Green RA, Murley GS, Pizzari T. Gluteus minimus: an intramuscular EMG investigation of anterior and posterior segments during gait. Gait Posture. 2014;39(2):822–6.
17. Semciw AI, Pizzari T, Murley GS, Green RA. Gluteus medius: an intramuscular EMG investigation of anterior, middle and posterior segments during gait. J Electromyogr Kinesiol. 2013;23(4): 858–64.
18. Gottschalk F, Kourosh S, Leveau B. The functional anatomy of tensor fasciae latae and gluteus medius and minimus. J Anat. 1989;166:179–89.

19. Hunt MA, Guenther JR, Gilbart MK. Kinematic and kinetic differences during walking in patients with and without symptomatic femoroacetabular impingement. Clin Biomech. 2013;28(5):519–23.
20. Rylander JH, Shu B, Andriacchi TP, Safran MR. Preoperative and postoperative sagittal plane hip kinematics in patients with femoroacetabular impingement during level walking. Am J Sports Med. 2011;39(Suppl):36S–42.
21. Foucher KC, Schlink BR, Shakoor N, Wimmer MA. Sagittal plane hip motion reversals during walking are associated with disease severity and poorer function in subjects with hip osteoarthritis. J Biomech. 2012;45(8):1360–5.
22. Kennedy MJ, Lamontagne M, Beaulé PE. Femoroacetabular impingement alters hip and pelvic biomechanics during gait Walking biomechanics of FAI. Gait Posture. 2009;30(1):41–4.
23. Tannast M, Kubiak-Langer M, Langlotz F, Puls M, Murphy SB, Siebenrock KA. Noninvasive three-dimensional assessment of femoroacetabular impingement. J Orthop Res. 2007;25(1):122–31.
24. Kubiak-Langer M, Tannast M, Murphy SB, Siebenrock KA, Langlotz F. Range of motion in anterior femoroacetabular impingement. Clin Orthop Relat Res. 2007;458:117–24.
25. Brisson N, Lamontagne M, Kennedy MJ, Beaule PE. The effects of cam femoroacetabular impingement corrective surgery on lower-extremity gait biomechanics. Gait Posture. 2013;37(2):258–63.
26. Casartelli NC, Maffiuletti NA, Item-Glatthorn JF, Staehli S, Bizzini M, Impellizzeri FM, et al. Hip muscle weakness in patients with symptomatic femoroacetabular impingement. Osteoarthritis Cartilage. 2011;19(7):816–21.

Evaluation of the Painful Hip

11

Joshua A. Tuck, Michael A. Flaherty, and Brian D. Busconi

Introduction

Examination of the hip is one of the most difficult clinical exams for the musculoskeletal specialist. Clinical presentation of hip pathology can be varied and confusing. It takes even the best clinicians a detailed history and thorough physical examination in order to devise an accurate differential diagnosis. Despite this degree of difficulty, if a thoughtful approach is combined with detailed examination, most hip pathologies can be reliably identified. Many hip pathologies such as femoroacetabular impingement (FAI), slipped capital femoral epiphysis (SCFE), hip dysplasia, and labral tears have been identified as precursors for hip arthritis [1–5]. Thus, the importance of early identification of these at-risk patients cannot be overstated.

A myriad of pathologies can manifest as hip pain. It is a challenge to determine whether the underlying pathology comes from within the central compartment of the hip joint or from the peripheral compartment, symphyseal structures, surrounding ligaments or muscles, low back, knee, sacroiliac joint, genitourinary system, or lower abdomen. It is therefore imperative, as part of a comprehensive hip examination, to include screening of the hips, back [6], thighs, knees, and abdomen.

J.A. Tuck, DO, MS
Division of Sports Medicine, Department of Orthopaedic Surgery, University of Massachusetts Medical School, University of Massachusetts Memorial Medical Center, Worcester, MA, USA
e-mail: jtuck@mchl.org; physh22@yahoo.com

M.A. Flaherty, MD
Department of Orthopaedic Surgery, Albany Medical College, Albany, NY, USA
e-mail: mflaherty@caportho.com

B.D. Busconi, MD (✉)
Division of Sports Medicine, Department of Orthopaedics, UMASS Memorial, 281 Lincoln St., Worcester, MA 01605, USA
e-mail: Brian.Busconi@umassmemorial.org

Some hip conditions remain undiscovered for prolonged periods of time. This may cause the patient to acquire compensatory adaptations. These adaptations include altered posture and gait, as well as pelvic or spine obliquity, and should always alert the clinician of a possible hip etiology.

History

A detailed history is crucial in the evaluation of hip pathology [7]. The onset of symptoms should be explored and any trauma should be recorded. It is important to make it simple for the patient to locate the pain as the differential diagnosis changes considerably according to the region of pain. One useful way of dividing the potential pathologies into regions is **anterior groin** (mostly intra-articular pathologies), **anterior midline** (symphysis, pubalgia, and adductors), **lateral** (mostly peripheral compartment), and **posterior** hip pain (Fig. 11.1).

Anterior hip pain in the groin is typical for hip joint pathology as well as problems in the muscles anterior to the hip. Intra-articular causes may include degenerative processes, labral tears, acetabular chondral flap lesions, impingement, effusion, avascular necrosis, loose bodies, synovial chondromatosis, intracapsular malignancies, and synovial pathologies. Pain is typically worse with twisting activities and ascending or descending stairs or inclines [8]. Painful catching in the hip, particularly when going from positions of flexion to extension (such as rising from a seated position), is also common [8]. In the case of FAI, a slow onset of initially intermittent groin pain after a minor trauma, which exacerbates with athletic activity or prolonged walking, is the typical presentation [9].

Other causes of anterior groin pain are iliopsoas snapping, hip flexor strains, and stress fractures in the anterior pelvis and proximal femur. Pain with active contraction or passive stretch may indicate a muscle tear or tendinopathy. History of recent increase in training routine, such as in military recruits, has been implicated in femoral neck stress frac-

J.C. McCarthy et al. (eds.), *Hip Joint Restoration*, DOI 10.1007/978-1-4614-0694-5_11

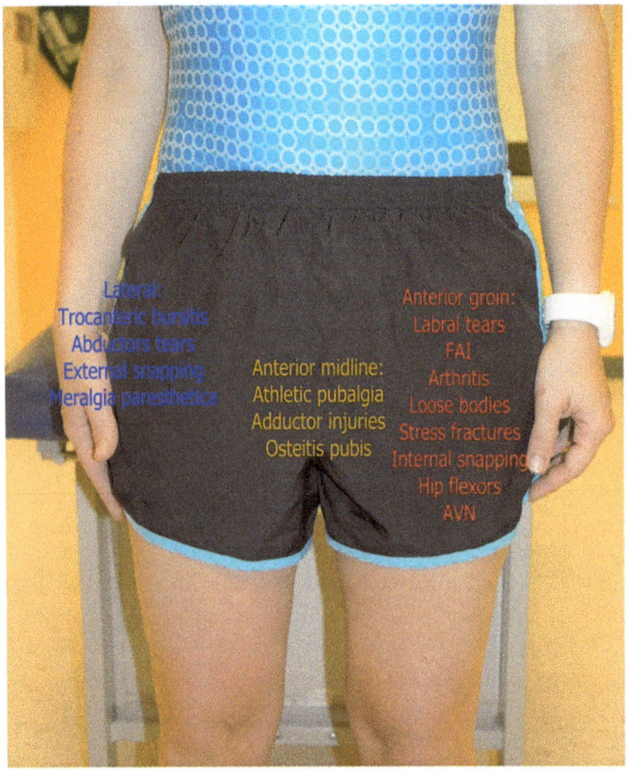

Fig. 11.1 Common causes of pain by location

tures [10, 11], whereas stress fractures of the anterior pelvic ring are usually associated with bony fragility most commonly seen in osteoporosis, rheumatoid arthritis, chronic renal failure, and other metabolic bone diseases [12].

Lateral hip pain can occur secondary to pathology around the greater trochanter such as bursitis, abductor tendon tears, iliotibial (IT) band problems, and neurologic conditions like meralgia paresthetica [13]. Abductor muscle fatigue related to underlying developmental dysplasia and structural instability may also occur representing a case of intra-articular pathology manifesting as lateral hip pain and weakness.

Posterior hip pain can be due to hip pathology although it is often generated by structures outside the gluteal region, including the lumbosacral spine and the sacroiliac joint [14]. It is important to inquire if there is associated low back pain, as pain rarely radiates cephalad from a hip pathology. If there is low back pain, a full neurologic examination should be carried out with special attention to dermatomal pattern of pain, as well as any motor and sensory loss. The quality of the pain would also help in this situation. Diffuse or vague pain, as opposed to focal and specific pain, is more likely referred from elsewhere. Posterior pain over the ischial tuberosity is most likely related to proximal hamstring tendinopathy or ischial bursitis. If this pain is associated with a traumatic event and ecchymosis is present, a proximal hamstring tear should be suspected [15]. Other local conditions that can cause posterior hip pain are gluteus maximus strains, ischiofemoral impingement, and piriformis syndrome.

Asking questions such as "when does it hurt?" may help to identify static versus dynamic problems, as well as any postural associations. Discomfort on hip flexion and with prolonged sitting is typically indicative of anterior FAI. Frequency of symptoms is important as well as intensity and any exacerbating and alleviating factors. Radiation of pain can be very revealing as some hip pathology can radiate in specific patterns, such as that felt distally toward the knee secondary to irritation of the anterior branch of the obturator nerve [16]. The presence of a limp, groin pain, or limited hip internal rotation predicts the diagnosis of a true hip disorder as opposed to one originating from the spine [17].

By the time the clinician examines the patient, he or she may have already initiated treatment for the condition. Thus, a thorough discussion of all attempted modalities of treatment is important. Patients are encouraged to recall if previous treatments were efficacious and to what extent. A patient may have tried ice, heat, stretching exercises, oral medications, physical therapy, or injections. In the case of injections, it is important to inquire as to who administered them, their composition, location, technique, and response.

Social history should be reviewed to determine current or prior use of alcohol, steroids, and tobacco, which might place the patient at risk for osteonecrosis [18]. Assessment of the patient's particular lifestyle needs and hobbies will help to identify risk factors and ultimate expectations. Different priorities, such as labor demands or sports participation, can make the same condition in different patients require different treatment plans.

A comprehensive review of systems can be of great value, particularly those of the gastrointestinal (GI), renal, genitourinary (GU), gynecologic, and neurologic systems. Other symptoms such as fevers, chills, night sweats, and unintentional weight loss may point toward malignancy or infection. Patients should specifically be asked about systemic illnesses such as malignancy, coagulopathies, and inflammatory disorders as well as any family history of these conditions. Various coagulation and metabolic disorders have been shown to impede vascular supply to the femoral head [19].

To better assess the impact that a hip condition has on a patient, several assessment tools have been developed. These tools assess the ability to return to an active life, subjective measures of symptoms, emotional health, and social needs. Questionnaires for hip pathologies such as the Harris hip score were developed for patients with hip fractures and those following hip arthroplasty [20, 21]. These outcome instruments have been described as having a ceiling effect [22] which may not be suitable for assessing younger individuals. For these reasons, the Multicenter Arthroscopy of the Hip Outcomes Research Network (MAHORN) developed a newer assessment tool named the International Hip Outcome Tool-33 (iHOT-33) [23], which is geared toward the young, active patients with hip pathology. This same group (MAHORN) also validated a simpler version of this tool called the iHOT-12, which demonstrated to be valid and reliable, with one third of the length [24] (Fig. 11.2).

Finally, it is important to acknowledge that there are many non-orthopedic conditions that can present with hip pain, including hernia, metastatic tumor, testicular neoplasm, ureteral colic, urinary tract infections (UTI), hydrocele, varicocele, ovarian cyst, pelvic inflammatory disease (PID), endometriosis, colorectal neoplasm, inflammatory bowel disease (IBD), and diverticulitis.

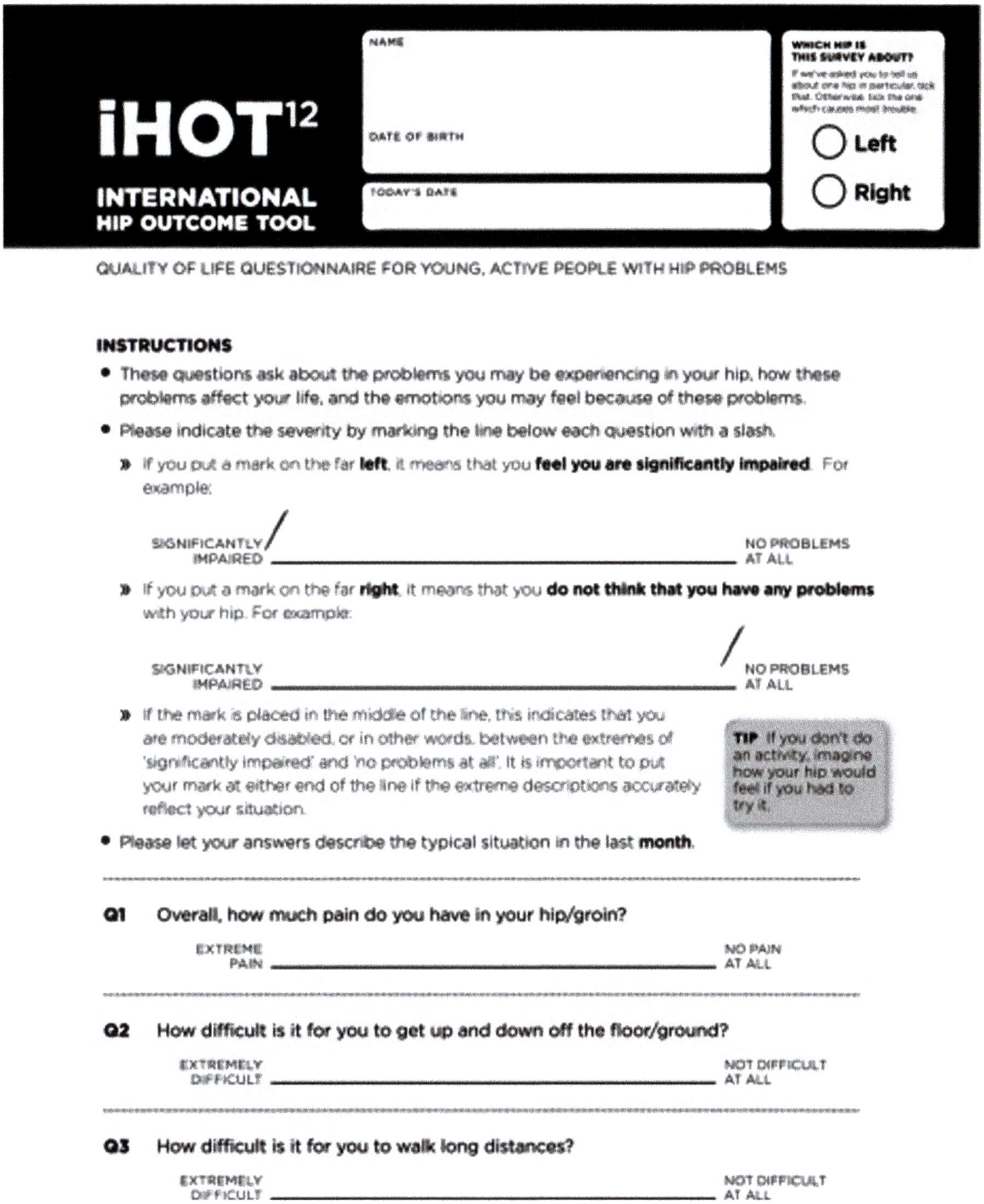

iHOT12

INTERNATIONAL HIP OUTCOME TOOL

NAME

DATE OF BIRTH

TODAY'S DATE

WHICH HIP IS THIS SURVEY ABOUT?

If we've asked you to tell us about one hip in particular, tick that. Otherwise, tick the one which causes most trouble.

○ Left

○ Right

QUALITY OF LIFE QUESTIONNAIRE FOR YOUNG, ACTIVE PEOPLE WITH HIP PROBLEMS

INSTRUCTIONS

- These questions ask about the problems you may be experiencing in your hip, how these problems affect your life, and the emotions you may feel because of these problems.
- Please indicate the severity by marking the line below each question with a slash.
  - » If you put a mark on the far **left**, it means that you **feel you are significantly impaired**. For example:

    SIGNIFICANTLY IMPAIRED / ______ NO PROBLEMS AT ALL
  - » If you put a mark on the far **right**, it means that you **do not think that you have any problems** with your hip. For example:

    SIGNIFICANTLY IMPAIRED ______ / NO PROBLEMS AT ALL
  - » If the mark is placed in the middle of the line, this indicates that you are moderately disabled, or in other words, between the extremes of 'significantly impaired' and 'no problems at all'. It is important to put your mark at either end of the line if the extreme descriptions accurately reflect your situation.

    TIP If you don't do an activity, imagine how your hip would feel if you had to try it.
- Please let your answers describe the typical situation in the last **month**.

Q1 Overall, how much pain do you have in your hip/groin?

EXTREME PAIN ______ NO PAIN AT ALL

Q2 How difficult is it for you to get up and down off the floor/ground?

EXTREMELY DIFFICULT ______ NOT DIFFICULT AT ALL

Q3 How difficult is it for you to walk long distances?

EXTREMELY DIFFICULT ______ NOT DIFFICULT AT ALL

Fig. 11.2 International Hip Outcome Tool-12 (iHOT-12) developed by the MAHORN group

Q4 How much trouble do you have with grinding, catching or clicking in your hip?

SEVERE TROUBLE ______________________________ NO TROUBLE AT ALL

Q5 How much trouble do you have pushing, pulling, lifting or carrying heavy objects?

SEVERE TROUBLE ______________________________ NO TROUBLE AT ALL

Q6 How concerned are you about cutting/changing directions during your sport or recreational activities?

EXTREMELY CONCERNED ______________________________ NOT CONCERNED AT ALL

Q7 How much pain do you experience in your hip *after* activity?

EXTREME PAIN ______________________________ NO PAIN AT ALL

Q8 How concerned are you about picking up or carrying children because of your hip?

EXTREMELY CONCERNED ______________________________ NOT CONCERNED AT ALL

Q9 How much trouble do you have with sexual activity because of your hip?

☐ This is not relevant to me

SEVERE TROUBLE ______________________________ NO TROUBLE AT ALL

Q10 How much of the time are you aware of the disability in your hip?

CONSTANTLY AWARE ______________________________ NOT AWARE AT ALL

Q11 How concerned are you about your ability to maintain your desired fitness level?

EXTREMELY CONCERNED ______________________________ NOT CONCERNED AT ALL

Q12 How much of a distraction is your hip problem?

EXTREME DISTRACTION ______________________________ NO DISTRACTION AT ALL

Fig. 11.2 (continued)

Physical Examination

Physical examination of the hip should be structured and comprehensive. As for every clinical encounter, vital signs are first obtained. The presence of fever in a patient with acute hip pain should warrant further investigation to rule out infection, particularly in the pediatric population [25]. Vital signs should then be followed by gait analysis, inspection, palpation, and evaluation of range of motion and strength, finishing with special tests. Musculoskeletal examination should always include the joint proximal and distal to the

Table 11.1 Commonly examined areas in different positions

Standing	Supine	Lateral	Prone
Gait	Palpation	Palpation	Palpation
Pelvic and spine alignment	ROM	Ober's test	ROM
Body habitus	Log roll (PSRT)	Lateral rim impingement	Femoral anteversion
Trendelenburg test	Leg length	FADDIR	Strength
Palpation	FADDIR	Active piriformis test	Ely's test
Strength	DEXRIT/DIRIT	Strength	
	FABER		
	Post rim impingement		
	SLR		
	SLRAR		
	Thomas test		
	Drehmann sign		
	Strength		
	Symphysis area		
	Lower abdomen		

DEXRIT dynamic external rotatory impingement test, *DIRIT* dynamic internal rotatory impingement test, *FABER* flexion abduction internal rotation, *FADDIR* flexion adduction internal rotation, *PSRT* passive supine rotation test, *ROM* range of motion, *SLR* straight leg raise, *SLRAR* straight leg raise against resistance

symptomatic one; therefore, a complete low back and knee examination is imperative [26]. Proper patient clothing should be used in order to provide good access for unimpeded physical examination, with appropriate patient comfort and unrestricted ROM. Following a standardized sequence will avoid having the patient go back and forth into a position (standing, supine, etc.), which may result in unnecessary discomfort for the patient and time loss for the clinician. Table 11.1 below lists the most commonly performed tests in their different positions.

Many tests exist in the physical examination of the hip. The experienced clinician will focus on those tests that are pertinent to the differential diagnoses, devised from obtaining a thorough history. Most often, a set of basic tests will be performed on every patient initially, followed by more specific tests to further delineate a suspected diagnosis.

Standing Examination

Gait testing is performed in a hallway so that at least 3–4 stride lengths can be viewed from both the front and back of the patient [27]. Antalgic gait is characterized by a decreased time in the stance phase on the affected limb. The affected limb is placed on the ground just long enough to quickly swing the unaffected limb to stance. This gait allows the patient to diminish pain by minimizing the weight-bearing time on that limb. Patients with hip pain present with a characteristic coxalgic gait [28]. This gait is characterized by shifting of the upper torso toward the painful hip during the single-limb stance phase on the affected hip (Fig. 11.3a). By shifting the torso over the painful hip, joint reaction forces are decreased, thus decreasing pain (Fig. 11.4). A Trendelenburg gait pattern (Fig. 11.3b) can result secondary to abductor weakness. Clinically, the gluteus medius and minimus are not strong enough to keep the pelvis level, and as a result, the pelvis will drop on the contralateral side during the stance phase of gait. As opposed to the coxalgic gait which typically keeps the pelvis leveled, the Trendelenburg gait is characterized by a contralateral hemipelvis drop.

This is an appropriate time to test single-leg stance and examine core body mechanics as well as lower extremity strength. The patient stands with the feet shoulder-width apart and then lifts the unaffected leg forward to 45° of hip flexion and 45° of knee flexion and holds this position for 6 s. Assessment of the overall conditioning and balance can be made.

Patients that walk slowly in a stooped gait with shortened stride and the lumbar spine bent forward are more likely suffering from lumbar spinal stenosis. The stooped gait observed in spinal stenosis is thought to be an adaptive mechanism to minimize lumbar epidural pressure that occurs during ambulation [29].

Limb length discrepancy (LLD) causes pelvic obliquity in the frontal plane [30–32]. Friberg [33] suggested that LLD may lead to hip arthrosis by placing the hip on the longer side into varus and therefore decreasing the load-bearing area of the femoral head. Rothenberg [34] also studied limb length inequality and suggested that sciatica occurred more often on the longer side while trochanteric bursitis occurred more frequently on the shorter side. There are multiple ways of assessing LLD. One technique that is pertinent to the hip

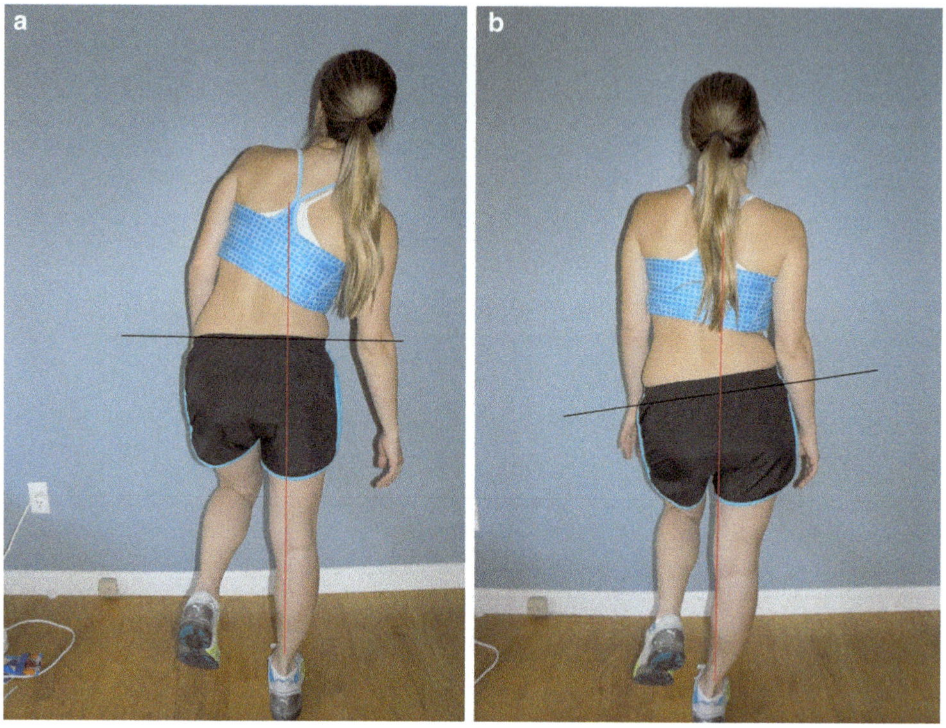

Fig. 11.3 (**a**) Coxalgic gait—patient shifts their upper body weight toward the affected right hip (*red line*) in order to decrease joint reaction forces (JRFs). The pelvis stays aligned (*black line*). (**b**) Trendelenburg gait—weak right abductors—the unaffected left hemipelvis drops resulting in pelvic obliquity (*black line*)

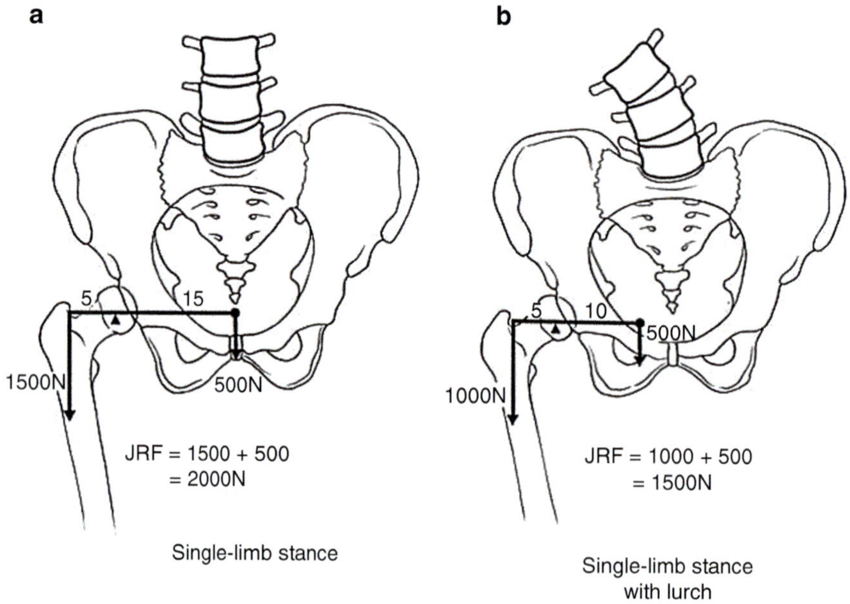

Fig. 11.4 Free-body diagram of the hip in single-limb stance. (**a**) Assume that the distance from the hip to the abductors is 5 cm and that the distance from the hip to the body center of gravity is 15 cm. If the weight of the body is 500 N, the abductors must exert 1500 N of force to maintain the static equilibrium. (The sum of the moments about the hip fulcrum must equal to zero, i.e., 1500 N × 5 cm = 500 N × 15 cm.) In this case, the JRF is the sum of the abductor force and the body weight, totaling 2000 N. (**b**) When the upper body is lurched toward the affected hip, the body center of gravity is effectively shifted in the same direction. Thus, if the distance from the hip to the body center of gravity is decreased to 10 cm, the abductors need to exert only 1000 N to maintain static equilibrium: 1000 N × 5 cm = 500 N × 10 cm. Therefore, the lurch reduces the JRF to 1500 N. From Lim MR, Huang RC, Wu A et al. Evaluation of the Elderly Patient with an Abnormal Gait. © 2007 American Academy of Orthopaedic Surgeons. Reprinted from the Journal of the American Academy of Orthopaedic Surgeons, Volume 15(2), pp. 107–117 with permission

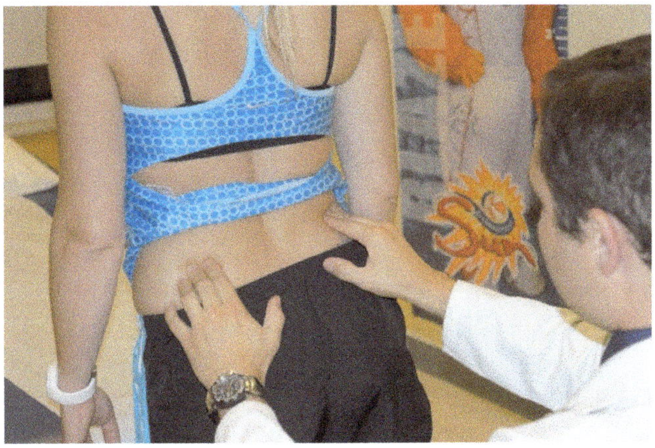

Fig. 11.5 Assessing pelvic obliquity

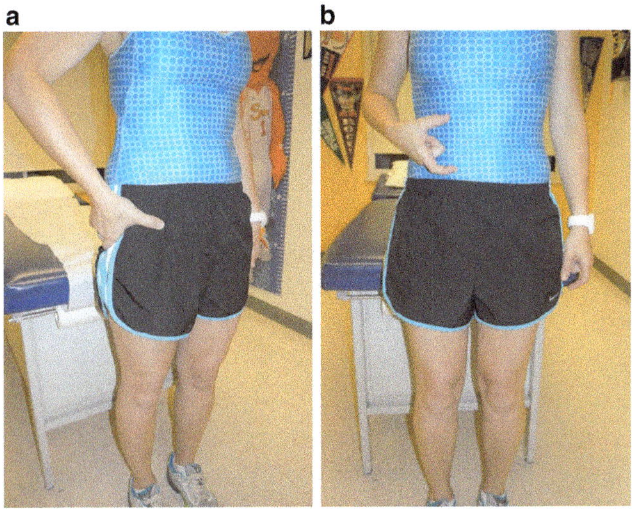

Fig. 11.6 C-sign was described by Byrd who noticed that some patients with intra-articular hip pathology (a) hold their hip with (b) their hand in a position that resembles the letter "C" when asked to localize the site of pain

examination and is carried out in the standing position is that of measuring the pelvic obliquity [35, 36]. Pelvic obliquity is measured by assessing the iliac crest height, which should be equal in both sides (Fig. 11.5). A line is drawn from one iliac crest to the other (this line should be parallel to the floor); a level tool can be used for this purpose. Blocks or boards of a known diameter are placed under the shorter leg in order to level the pelvic obliquity and assess the amount of LLD.

C-sign (Fig. 11.6) was first described by Byrd [37] who noticed that patients with intra-articular pathology consistently pointed to their hip making a "C" with their hand when asked to point toward the painful site. The hand is cupped over the greater trochanter gripping from the posterolateral hip all the way around anteriorly toward deep in the groin.

Standing examination will then conclude with a careful inspection for masses, scars, lesions, signs of trauma or previous surgery, muscle bulk, and symmetry of the hip and knee. Palpation is usually revealing for extra-articular source of hip symptoms (Fig. 11.7). All bony prominences should be palpated as well as the lumbar spine and sacroiliac joint. A table with the most common pathologies associated with bony prominence palpation has been provided (Table 11.2).

Assessing Range of Motion

Normal hip ROM for reference is highly variable secondary to several factors including age, gender, and BMI [50–52]. Multiple authors have reported on "normal" ROM values, but these reports are highly variable and usually lack appropriate documentation of age, gender, and other variables. The following ranges will be provided for reference only and should not be taken as absolute values: flexion = 120°–135°, extension = 10°–30°, internal rotation at 90° = 25°–40°, external rotation at 90° = 40°–60°, abduction at 0° = 45°, and adduction at 0° = 25°. In addition to assessing range of motion, the clinician must also assess for the presence of pain or mechanical blocking at the extremes of motion. When evaluating hip ROM, the examiner must always stabilize the lumbar spine and the pelvis.

Internal and external rotation can be measured in the prone position or with the hip flexed to 90° in either supine or seated position with the legs hanging from the edge of the table [53] (Fig. 11.8). Simoneau et al. [51] demonstrated that when measurements are performed in different positions (prone vs. seated), the results are different; therefore, the position in which the measurements were obtained should be recorded. If future measurements are going to be performed in order to assess any progress or response to therapy, they should be performed in the same position. An advantage of the seated position is that the pelvis is stabilized with both ischia square with the table while the hips and knees are flexed at 90°.

Extension is best evaluated with the patient in the prone position, again making sure that the pelvis and anterior superior iliac spines are stabilized on the examination table (Fig. 11.8c). Flexion of the hip is more readily measured in the supine position (Fig. 11.9), making sure that both sides of the pelvis and low back are fixed to the table.

The use of manual goniometers in the measurement of hip ROM was recently studied by Nussbaumer and colleagues [54], who found that goniometers overestimate hip ROM when compared to an electromagnetic tracking system. This may be due to the inadvertent measurement of multiple other segments, including lower back and pelvic motions. Nevertheless, the authors concluded that the use of manual goniometers was a practical instrument for the clinical evaluation of hip ROM.

Audenaert and colleagues [55] recently published a series comparing the hip ROM of three groups of patients. One group included asymptomatic patients with normal radiographic

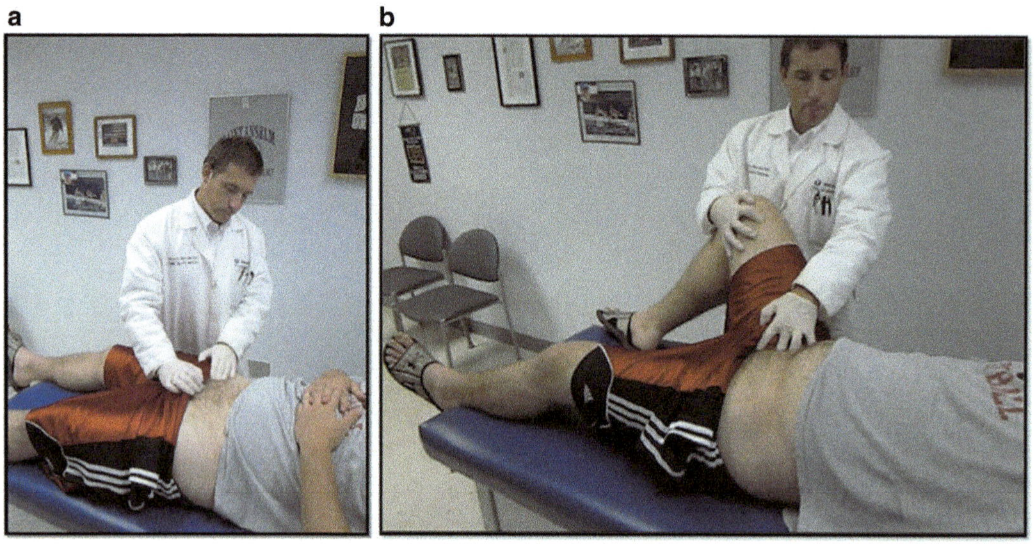

Fig. 11.7 (**a**) Symphysis pubis palpated in a 35-year-old hockey player with osteitis pubis. (**b**) Hip adductors are also examined at this time

Table 11.2 Differential diagnosis of pain to palpation

Palpation site	Keys to diagnosis	Most likely diagnosis
Greater trochanter (GT)	Female > male	Greater trochanter bursitis with/without abductor tear [38]
	May have abductor weakness	
ASIS	Adolescent runners, batters	Sartorius or iliotibial band avulsion [39]
	Acute-onset pain	
Just medial to ASIS	Anterolateral thigh pain, numbness, paresthesia	Meralgia paresthetica (LFCN) [40]
Iliac crest	Acute pain, ecchymosis	Hip pointer [41]
AIIS	Skeletally immature	Rectus femoris apophyseal avulsion [42]
	Skeletally mature	Subspinous impingement
Pubic symphysis (Fig. 11.6)	Males > females	Osteitis pubis [43]
	Soccer, hockey, rugby	
Sacroiliac (SI) joint	Sacrum base pressure test	Poor predictive value for SI joint dysfunction [44]
Ischial tuberosity	Adult acute injury	Proximal hamstring tears [45]
	Pain without acute injury	Ischiogluteal bursitis [46]
	4–12 years old, chronic	Osteochondrosis (Van Neck dz) [47]
	Adolescent acute onset	Ischial tuberosity apophyseal avulsion [48]
Posterior to GT	Pain increased with muscle contraction and prolonged sitting, sciatica symptoms	Piriformis syndrome [49]

ASIS anterior superior iliac spine, *AIIS* anterior inferior iliac spine, *LFCN* lateral femoral cutaneous nerve

studies (A), the second group were also asymptomatic but had radiologic features of FAI (B), and the third group consisted of symptomatic individuals with FAI and corresponding radiologic findings (C). These researchers found that there was a statistically significant difference in the internal rotation (IR) among the three groups. Group A (asymptomatic, normal imaging) had 27.9° IR. Group B (asymptomatic, FAI imaging) had 21.1° IR. Group 3 (symptomatic with FAI imaging) had 12.3° IR. Another study by Kubiak-Langer et al. [56] compared the hip ROMs of patients with documented FAI with those of asymptomatic individuals using a 3-D CT scan. They found that hips with FAI had significantly decreased ROM in flexion, adduction, and internal rotation.

Strength Testing

All plains of ROM of the hip should be also evaluated for strength. A scale from 1 to 5 has been classically used [57] although subtle weakness may be noticed when comparing

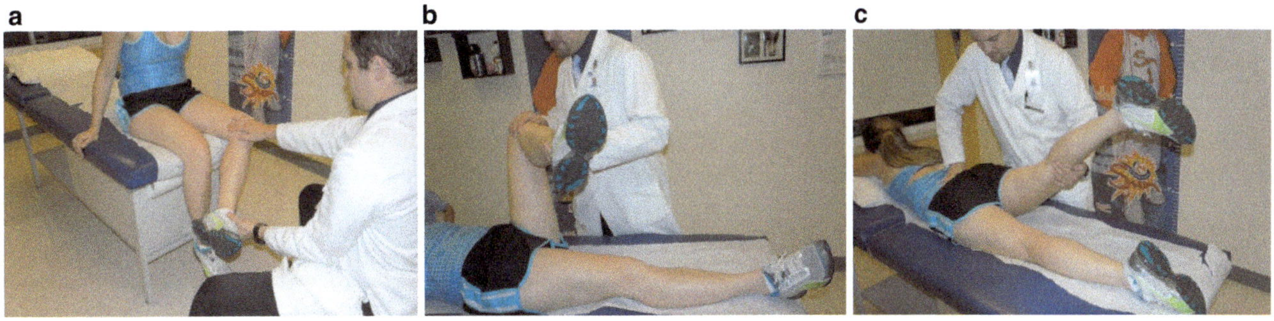

Fig. 11.8 ROM measuring can be performed in multiple positions as long as the pelvis and low back are well stabilized. (**a**) Seating—both ischium must lie flat against the table. (**b**) Supine—examiner's hand can go under the patient's lower back to assess lower back and pelvis alignment. (**c**) Prone position—the pelvis is stabilized to the table by making sure both ASIS are touching equally

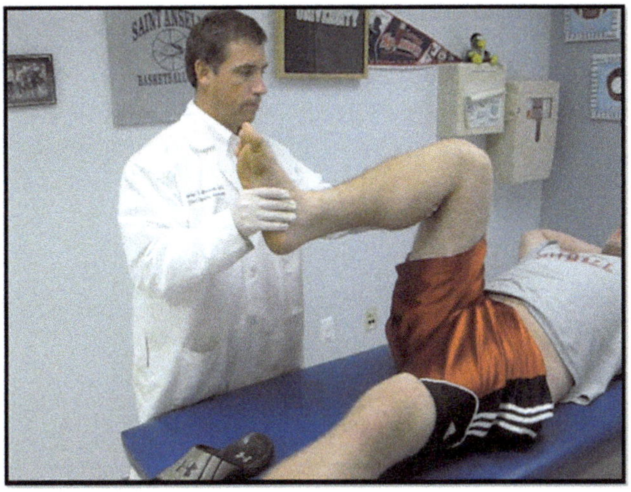

Fig. 11.9 Flexion examined in the supine position with the pelvis and low back flat against the table

with the contralateral side. These tests can be performed in different positions. Supine is usually best for flexion and adduction strength testing, whereas the lateral position is best for assessing abductors. Proper isolation of the examined muscle is essential in order to have an appropriate diagnosis. For example, in the lateral position, the gluteus medius can be isolated from the tensor fascia lata (TFL) by flexing the knee. This will be illustrated later when describing the Ober's test. Hip extensor strength is better evaluated in the prone position. Strength testing will also reproduce pain in the tested muscle group after an injury.

Provocative Tests

As previously stated, there are many physical examination maneuvers in the evaluation of the hip. Martin et al. designed a study with a panel of six expert hip surgeons in order to evaluate which tests were consistently performed by them [27]. They found that 18 tests were frequently performed (>40 %) by the examiners, 3 standing, 11 supine, 3 lateral, and 1 prone. Some of these tests such as ROM, gait analysis, and pelvic alignment have already been discussed. The following discussion will include some of the most commonly performed provocative maneuvers.

The **log roll examination**, also known as supine passive rotation test (SPRT), is performed in the supine position [58]. Although no strong data is available, it is generally considered to have weak sensitivity and good specificity for intra-articular hip pathology. With the hip in neutral flexion/extension and neutral abduction/adduction, the lower extremity is internally and externally rotated in a rolling maneuver (Fig. 11.10). It has been suggested that the basis for its specificity stems on the fact that log rolling moves only the femoral head in relation to the acetabulum and the surrounding capsule [59].

Straight leg raise (SLR), also known as Lasègue's sign, has long been used in attempts to screen for lumbar radiculopathy. It was studied by van der Windt et al. [60] in a Cochrane Database Systematic Review, where the authors noted that in a pooled population with high incidence of lumbar herniations, the SLR test had good sensitivity but with varied specificity. It has been generally considered to have poor sensitivity and specificity in the general population. The SLR is performed with the patient in the supine position and the examiner passively elevating the leg with the knee in extension. The test is considered positive if the patient experiences sciatic-type pain during the maneuver (Fig. 11.11).

Straight leg raise against resistance (SLRAR) is used for challenging hip flexors against resistance. Also known as Stinchfield test, the patient is positioned similar to that for a SLR test, but at 45° of hip flexion, the examiner's hand is placed over the patient's lower extremity to create resistance. The test is considered positive if hip flexor weakness is noted or if pain is recreated. It is theorized that pain can arise from pathology in the hip flexors or from the psoas rubbing against the anterior labrum. This exam can also elicit hip pain from intra-articular etiology, because this maneuver generates several times the normal body weight across the articular surfaces [59].

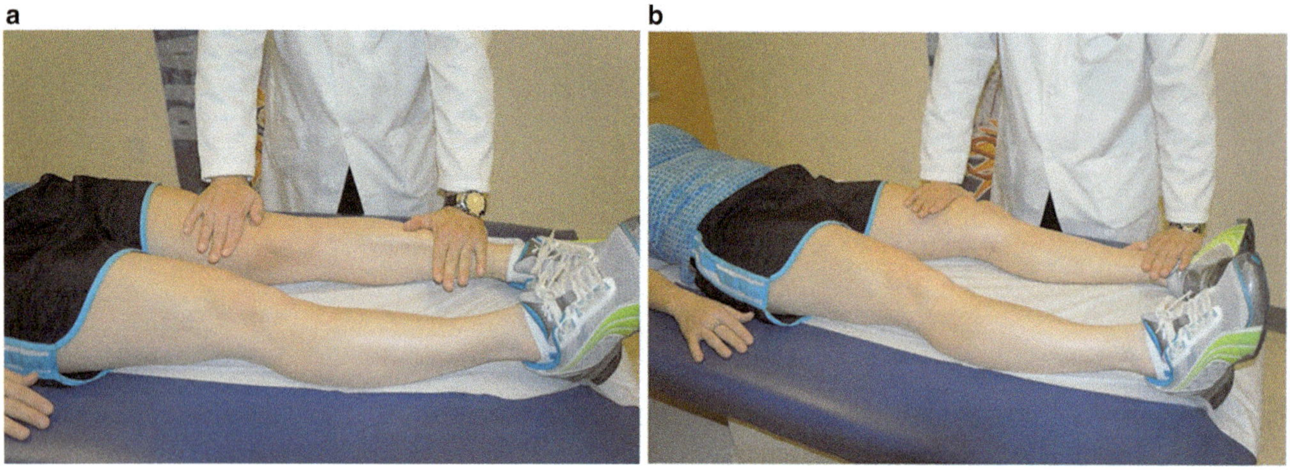

Fig. 11.10 Log roll maneuver. The patient is supine with the hip in neutral flexion. The entire extremity is log rolled back and forth to internal (**a**) and external rotation (**b**)

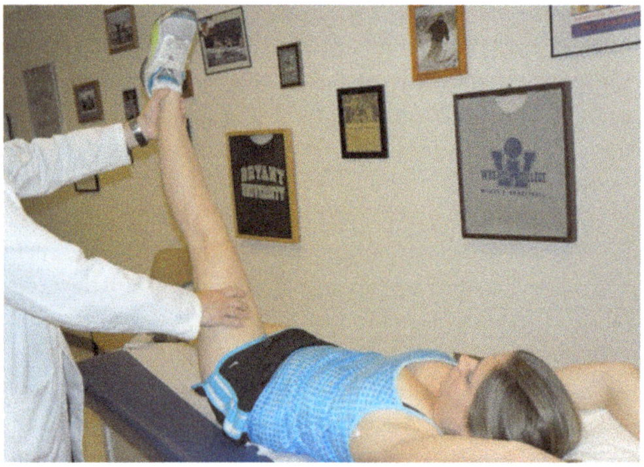

Fig. 11.11 Straight leg raise. The examiner should ask for sciatica-type symptoms. Although not intended originally with this maneuver, the examiner can also assess hamstring tightness

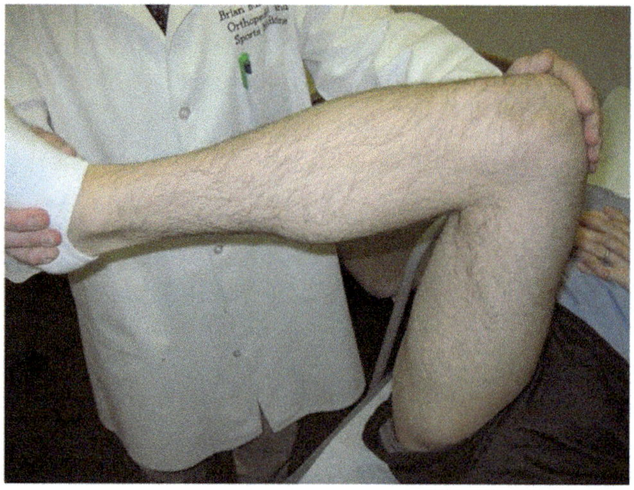

Fig. 11.12 Flexion, adduction, and internal rotation (FADDIR) also known as impingement test

Flexion, adduction, and internal rotation (FADDIR) test, also known as impingement test, can be performed in the supine or lateral position. The hip is flexed to 90°; adduction is then performed followed by internal rotation (Fig. 11.12). With this test, the reproduction of pain is recorded as well as the degree of internal rotation obtained. This test was originally described for hip dysplasia [4] but has more commonly been used for the diagnosis of FAI, labral tears, and other intra-articular pathologies. The **dynamic internal rotation impingement test** (DIRIT) [61] is similarly performed with the hip in flexion while dynamically taking it through a large range of internal rotation and adduction. A **McCarthy sign** [62] is positive when a painful click is noted when performing this examination in conjunction with dynamic hip extension from a flexed internally rotated position or flexed externally rotated position.

Snapping of the hip is usually an incidental finding. When it becomes recurrent and painful, however, it can be pathologic. Two types of snapping are commonly described, internal and external. In the case of internal snapping, the differentiation between iliopsoas snapping and true intra-articular pathology can be difficult. The recommended test for **internal snapping** is to provoke the iliopsoas tendon to transiently lodge on the anterior aspect of the hip capsule or pectineal eminence by bringing the hip from flexion, abduction, and external rotation (FABER) into extension and internal rotation (Fig. 11.13) [4]. Commonly, the patient is more readily able to recreate this snapping by performing his own particular movement.

External snapping hip has been described as happening at the confluence of the iliotibial band (ITB) and gluteus maximus over the greater trochanter [63]. This lateral and

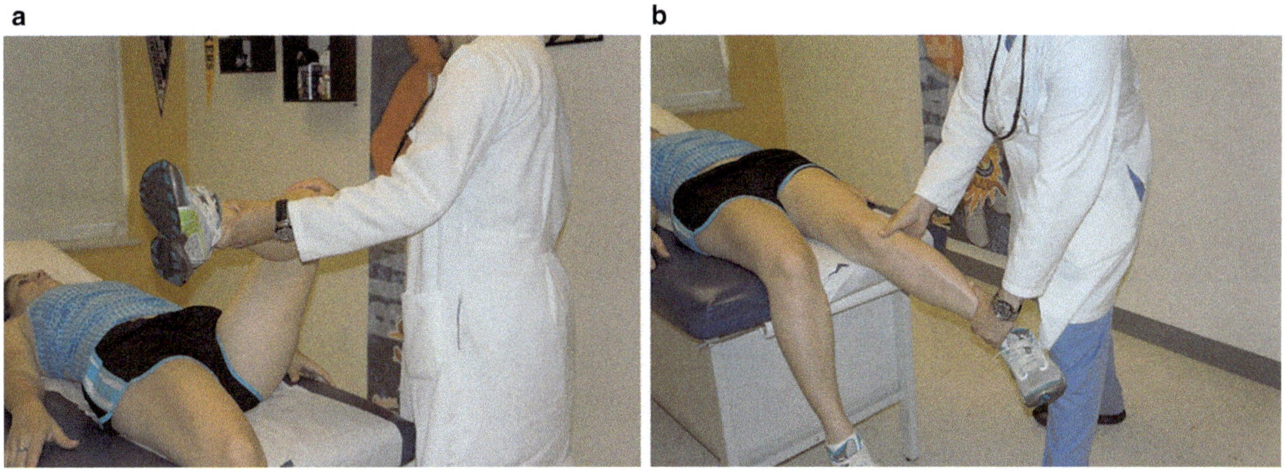

Fig. 11.13 Internal (iliopsoas) snapping can be elicited by taking the hip from (**a**) FABER to (**b**) extension and internal rotation in a dynamic maneuver

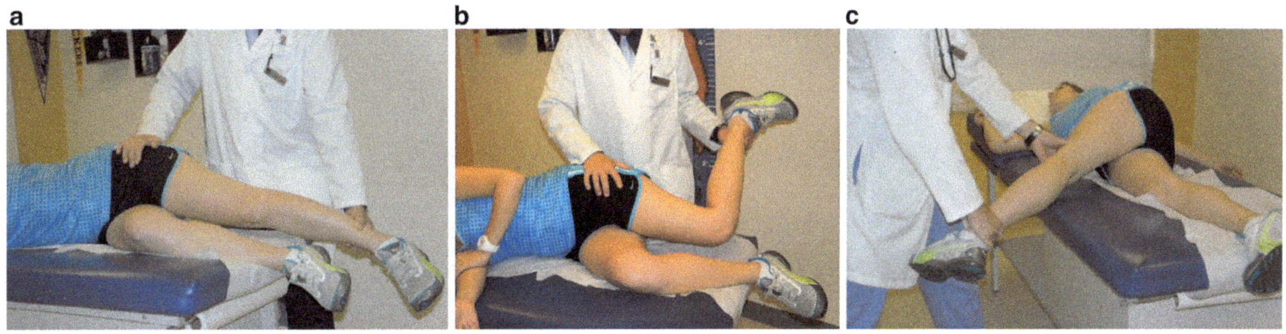

Fig. 11.14 Passive adduction test. (**a**) ITB is examined with the hip and knee extended. (**b**) Gluteus medius is examined with the knee flexed 90° in order to release the ITB. (**c**) Gluteus maximus is examined with the shoulder blades rotated toward the table with the hips flexed and knee extended

more superficial location may make external snapping hip easier to distinguish from intra-articular etiology. While the patient often describes the hip as subluxing or feeling "unstable," when asked to perform the characteristic maneuver, the ITB can be seen or felt snapping over the greater trochanter. The maneuver usually involves flexion and extension with a component of rotation. Other patients can reproduce the snapping by rotating the affected hip while tilting the pelvis in a standing position. A common teaching aphorism in snapping hip is "if you can hear it across the room, it's usually internal (iliopsoas) snapping, if you can see it from across the room, its external (ITB) snapping."

Hip adduction testing is similar to the **Ober's test**. It is performed in the lateral decubitus position with the affected extremity up. The contralateral hip is flexed in order to clear the space for the examined extremity to adduct. The examined leg should adduct until the extremity touches the table. Any restrictions or tightness should be recorded. This test should be performed in three positions in order to test TFL, gluteus medius, and gluteus maximus (Fig. 11.14) [27]. First, the test is performed with the knee and hip in extension in order to test the TFL. Next, the hip is extended and the knee flexed to 90° to test the gluteus medius (knee flexion will release the ITB and contract the gluteus medius). Finally, the patient is positioned with the shoulders rotated back toward the table and with the hip in flexion and knee in extension while taking the hip into adduction to stretch the gluteus maximus.

Flexion, abduction, and external rotation (FABER) test), or Patrick test, was originally used to localize pain to the sacroiliac joint. Nevertheless, this test has also been linked to intra-articular pathologies such as acetabular labral tears, particularly when the pain produced is anterior [64, 65]. With the patient in the supine position, the hip is flexed 45°, followed by abduction and external rotation, bringing the ankle toward the level of the contralateral knee (Fig. 11.15). The test is positive when posterior hip pain is noticed. Again, the amount of motion can also give a general sense for contractures and/or mechanical blocks.

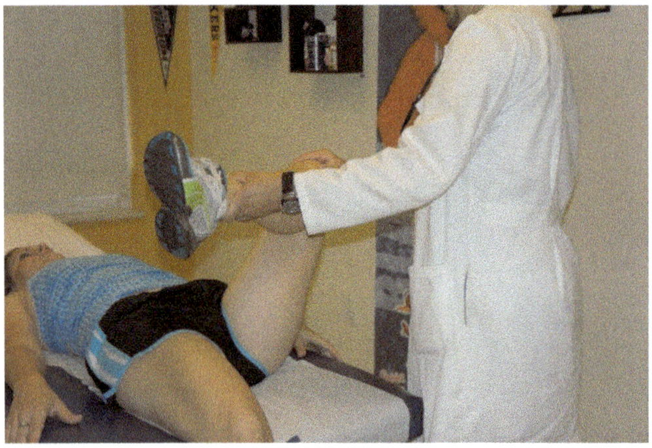

Fig. 11.15 Flexion, abduction, and external rotation (FABER). This position is also obtained when performing hip flexion in patients with SCFE that exhibit a Drehmann sign (obligatory external rotation with hip flexion)

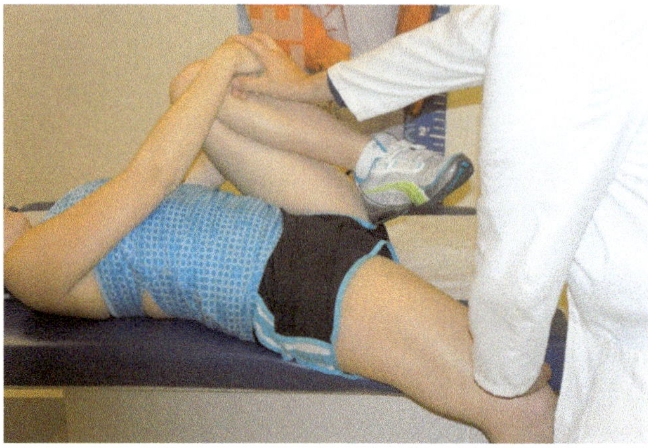

Fig. 11.16 Thomas test performed in the right knee. The clinician can check with his hand that the lumbar spine and pelvis are flat against the table avoiding lumbar lordosis

McCarthy sign—the patient is placed supine and, as with a Thomas sign, both hips are flexed to eliminate pelvic lordosis. While the unaffected hip remains flexed, the symptomatic hip is fully extended, first in external rotation then in internal rotation. A positive sign will elicit pain, a catching feeling, reproducing their symptoms or a locking event.

Drehmann sign has long been associated with SCFE [66, 67]. SCFE supposes a change in the proximal femur morphology and the Drehmann sign describes the obligatory external rotation that occurs with flexion of the hip [68]. It is noticed when flexing the hip while in the supine position as depicted in Fig. 11.14. SCFE has also been recognized as a cause for cam-type FAI. Kamegaya et al. [69] studied the finding of a Drehmann sign in patients with FAI after having suffered SCFE. They found that after SCFE, patients that demonstrated a positive Drehmann sign had an average alpha angle of 85.6° versus 63° in patients with a negative Drehmann sign, suggesting a worse prognosis in these patients.

Thomas test is used to rule out hip flexion contracture [70]. Tightness of the hip flexors can have multiple etiologies but is most likely due to spastic neurologic problems. The patient lies supine with the hips in the edge of the table. One knee is brought up and the patient holds it against his abdomen while the examined leg is extended (Fig. 11.16). The test is considered abnormal if the examined hip flexes without knee extension (tight iliopsoas), the hip abducts (tight TFL), or the knee extends (tight rectus femoris). This test can be confused with **Gaenslen's test** which was described by Gaenslen in 1927 [71] for sacroiliac joint pathology. This test is performed in a similar manner (supine, edge of table, one hip flexed, and the examined hip extended hanging off the edge of the table). Posterior hip pain is correlated with sacroiliac joint pathology.

In a similar fashion, the **posterior rim impingement** (PRI) **test** is also performed with the patient supine in the edge of the table, but this time both hips are extended (hanging freely from the edge of the table) (Fig. 11.17). By taking the hips into extension, the PRI test assesses the congruency of the posterior acetabular wall and femoral neck, and the test is considered to be abnormal if pain symptoms are reproduced or mechanical symptoms such as catching are noticed.

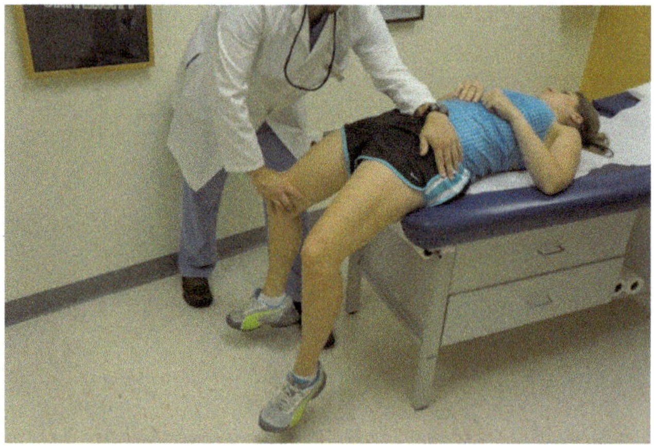

Fig. 11.17 Posterior rim test. Attention is taken to avoid lumbar lordosis and to stabilize the pelvis against table

Another type of hip impingement has been recently described as **ischiofemoral impingement** [72]. This entity was first described in patients after hip arthroplasty but has recently been identified in young individuals without previous surgery [73]. It has been noted that some patients with atypical posterior buttock and groin pain have an abnormal contact between the lesser trochanter and the ischium. The quadratus femoris occupies the space between the lesser trochanter and the ischium and may be compressed between these structures. Clinically, the symptoms of impingement can be reproduced by a combination of **extension, adduction, and external rotation** of the hip as described originally by Johnson in patients after hip arthroplasty (Fig. 11.18) [74].

Hip instability can be the sequel of a traumatic event or due to developmental deformities or soft tissue laxity [75]. Certain sports can place participants at higher risk of traumatic dislocations. After a traumatic dislocation, patients should be followed long term in order to assess for symptoms of instability. Medical and family histories should be investigated for connective tissue disorders. These patients also should be evaluated for **signs of generalized ligamentous laxity**, including the ability to bring the thumb to the radial aspect of the forearm, knee recurvatum, hyperextension of the elbows and metacarpophalangeal joints, and the ability to voluntarily dislocate or subluxate the shoulder. To assess for symptoms of anterior hip instability, the **dial test** can be performed [76]. The patient lies supine in neutral flexion/extension, and the examiner internally rotates the affected limb. The limb is then released and allowed to externally rotate. The test is positive when the patient's limb passively rotates >45° from vertical in the axial plane and lacks a mechanical end point. The contralateral limb is tested for comparison.

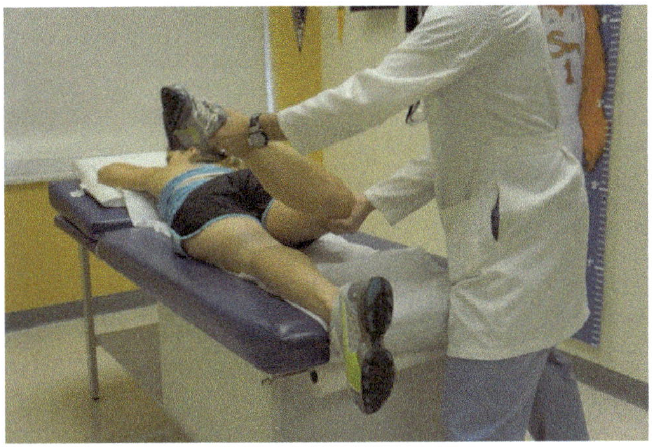

Fig. 11.18 Ischiofemoral impingement. The space between the lesser trochanter and ischium occupied by the quadratus femoris is challenged with extension, adduction, and external rotation

Most patients with **athletic pubalgia** have no symptoms while resting [77–79] and usually do not present with a palpable hernia [80]. Thus, provocative maneuvers are essential for obtaining the diagnosis. The pain associated with athletic pubalgia may radiate into the adductor region, perineum, rectus muscles, inguinal ligament, or testicular area. One provocative maneuver commonly employed involves having the patient perform a sit-up while the examiner applies pressure to the distal rectus abdominis insertion (Fig. 11.19). Pain elicited directly under the examiner's fingers is indicative of a positive test.

The physical exam of the hip should conclude with a **lower extremity vascular and neurologic examination**. Aortoiliac vascular occlusive disease (Leriche's syndrome) [81] is the triad of claudication, impotence, and decreased pulses due to aortoiliac occlusion. Patients may complain of buttock, hip, and thigh claudication. Pain is usually described as aching and may be associated with weakness and delayed wound healing. Starting at the groin, pulses can be diminished bilaterally and bruits are occasionally heard over the iliac or femoral arteries. Ankle-brachial index is an inexpensive test that can help assess vascular status. The lower extremity neurologic examination can be initiated with the SLR described previously and should include full motor and sensory evaluation, as well as deep tendon reflexes. **Sensation over the anterolateral thigh** is tested for loss or heightened sensation (dysesthesia, hyperesthesia), which may occur in cases of lateral femoral cutaneous nerve entrapment, commonly known as **meralgia paresthetica** [13].

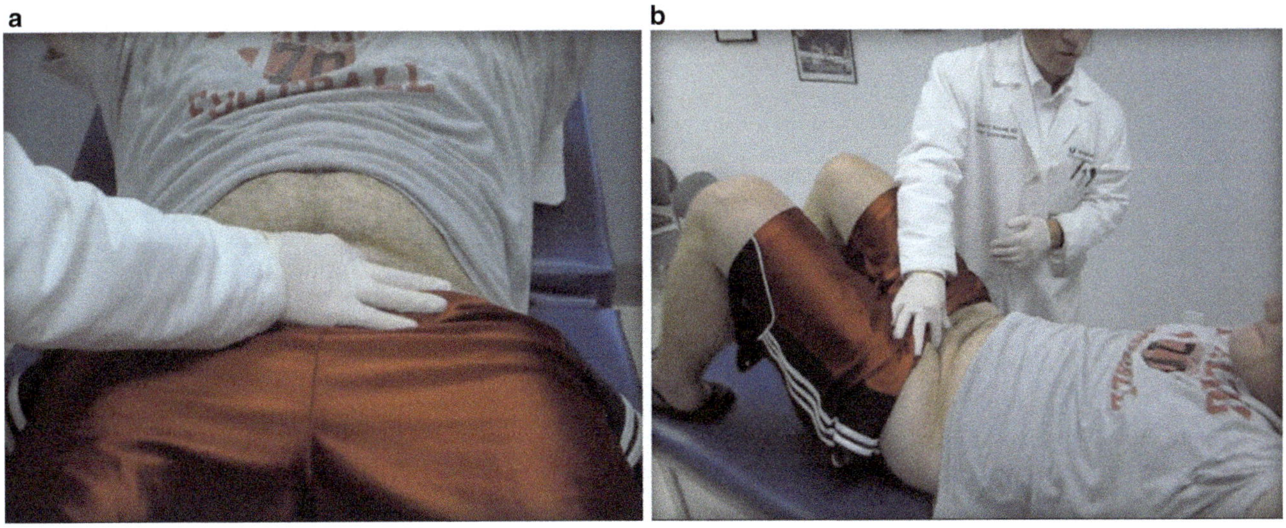

Fig. 11.19 (**a**) Sit-up while (**b**) applying pressure to the rectus abdominis distal insertion

Summary

Despite the advances in medical imaging, most of the decision making involved in hip pathology is based on a detailed history and physical examination. Using a thoughtful and methodical approach, an accurate differential diagnosis can most often occur. Pathologies originating from the hip, low back, lower abdomen, thigh, and knee can have similar presenting symptoms; therefore a thorough history and physical exam are essential.

References

1. Ganz R, Parvizi J, Beck M, et al. Femoroacetabular impingement: a cause for osteoarthritis of the hip. Clin Orthop Relat Res. 2003;417:112–20.
2. Leunig M, Ganz R. Femoroacetabular impingement. A common cause of hip complaints leading to arthrosis. Unfallchirurg. 2005;108(1):9–10. 12–7.
3. Jessel RH, Zurakowski D, Zilkens C, et al. Radiographic and patient factors associated with pre-radiographic osteoarthritis in hip dysplasia. J Bone Joint Surg Am. 2009;91(5):1120–9.
4. Klaue K, Durnin CW, Ganz R. The acetabular rim syndrome. A clinical presentation of dysplasia of the hip. J Bone Joint Surg Br. 1991;73(3):423–9.
5. Leunig M, Fraitzl CR, Ganz R. Early damage to the acetabular cartilage in slipped capital femoral epiphysis. Therapeutic consequences. Orthopade. 2002;31(9):894–9.
6. Brown MD, Gomez-Marin O, Brookfield KF, Li PS. Differential diagnosis of hip disease versus spine disease. Clin Orthop Relat Res. 2004;419:280–4.
7. Clohisy JC, Beaulé PE, O'Malley A, et al. AOA symposium: hip disease in the young adult. Current concepts of etiology and surgical treatment. J Bone Joint Surg Am. 2008;90(10):2267–81.
8. Byrd JW, Jones KS. Diagnostic accuracy of clinical assessment, magnetic resonance imaging, magnetic resonance arthrography, and intra-articular injection in hip arthroscopy patients. Am J Sports Med. 2004;32(7):668–74.
9. Javeri FM, Parvizi J. Hip pain in young adults: femoroacetabular impingement. J Arthroplasty. 2007;22(7 Suppl 3):37–42.
10. Talbot JC, Cox G, Townend M, et al. Femoral neck stress fractures in military personnel—a case series. J R Army Med Corps. 2008;154(1):47–50.
11. Ross RA, Allsopp A. Stress fractures in Royal Marines recruits. Mil Med. 2002;167(7):560–5.
12. Schapira D, Militeanu D, Israel O, Scharf Y. Insufficiency fractures of the pubic ramus. Semin Arthritis Rheum. 1996;25(6):373–82.
13. Patijn J, Mekhail N, Hayek S. Meralgia paresthetica. Pain Pract. 2011;11(3):302–8.
14. Vasudevan JM, Smuck M, Fredericson M. Evaluation of the athlete with hip pain. Curr Sports Med Rep. 2012;11(1):35–42.
15. Cohen S, Bradley J. Acute proximal hamstring rupture. J Am Acad Orthop Surg. 2007;15(6):350–5.
16. Yilmaz AE, Atalar H, Tag T. Knee joint pain may be an indicator for a hip joint problem in children: a case report. Malays J Med Sci. 2011;18(1):79–82.
17. Swezey RL. Overdiagnosed sciatica and stenosis, underdiagnosed hip arthritis. Orthopedics. 2003;26(2):173–4.
18. DeAngelis NA, Busconi BD. Assessment and differential diagnosis of the painful hip. Clin Orthop Relat Res. 2003;406:11–8.
19. Petrigliano FA, Lieberman JR. Osteonecrosis of the hip: novel approaches to evaluation and treatment. Clin Orthop Relat Res. 2007;465:53–62.
20. Callaghan JJ, Dysart SH, Savory CF, Hopkinson WJ. Assessing the results of hip replacement: a comparison of five different rating systems. J Bone Joint Surg Br. 1990;72:1008–9.
21. Unver B, Karatosun V, Gunal I. Assessing the results of thrust plate prosthesis: a comparison of four different rating systems. Clin Rehabil. 2005;19(6):654–8.
22. Wamper KE, Sierevelt IN, Poolman RW. The Harris hip score: do ceiling effects limit its usefulness in orthopedics? Acta Orthop. 2010;81(6):703–7.
23. Mohtadi NGH, Griffin DR, Pedersen ME, et al. The development and validation of a self-administered quality-of-life outcome measure for young, active patients with symptomatic hip disease: the International Hip Outcome Tool (iHOT-33). Arthroscopy. 2012;28(5):595–610.
24. Griffin DR, Parsons N, Mohtadi NG, Safran MR, Multicenter Arthroscopy of the Hip Outcomes Research Network. A short version of the International Hip Outcome Tool (iHOT-12) for use in routine clinical practice. Arthroscopy. 2012;28(5):611–6. quiz 616–8.
25. Kocher MS, Zurakowski D, Kasser JR. Differentiating between septic arthritis and transient synovitis of the hip in children: an evidence-based clinical prediction algorithm. J Bone Joint Surg Am. 1999;81(12):1662–70.
26. Wilson CH. The musculoskeletal examination. In: Walker HK, Hall WD, Hurst JW, editors. Clinical methods: the history, physical, and laboratory examinations. 3rd ed. Boston: Butterworths; 1990.
27. Martin HD, Kelly BT, Leunig M, et al. The pattern and technique in the clinical evaluation of the adult hip: the common physical examination tests of hip specialists. Arthroscopy. 2010;26(2):161–72.
28. Lim MR, Huang RC, Wu A, et al. Evaluation of the elderly patient with an abnormal gait. J Am Acad Orthop Surg. 2007;15(2): 107–17.
29. Suda Y, Saitou M, Shibasaki K, et al. Gait analysis of patients with neurogenic intermittent claudication. Spine. 2002;27:2509–13.
30. Young RS, Andrew PD, Cummings GS. Effect of simulating leg length inequality on pelvic torsion and trunk mobility. Gait Posture. 2000;11:217–23.
31. D'Amico M. Scoliosis and leg asymmetries: a reliable approach to assess wedge solutions efficacy. Stud Health Technol Inform. 2002;88:285–9.
32. Stricker SJ, Hunt T. Evaluation of leg discrepancy in children. Int Pediatr. 2004;19:134–42.
33. Friberg O. Clinical symptoms and biomechanics of lumbar spine and hip joint in leg length inequality. Spine. 1983;8(6):643–51.
34. Rothenberg RJ. Rheumatic disease aspects of leg length inequality. Semin Arthritis Rheum. 1988;17(3):196–205.
35. Woerman A, Binder-Macleod S. Leg length discrepancy assessment: accuracy and precision in five clinical methods of evaluation. J Orthop Sports Phys Ther. 1984;5:230–9.
36. Lampe HI, Swierstra BA, Diepstraten AF. Measurement of limb length inequality. Comparison of clinical methods with orthoradiography in 190 children. Acta Orthop Scand. 1996;67(3):242–4.
37. Byrd JWT. Physical examination. In: Byrd JWT, editor. Operative hip arthroscopy. 2nd ed. New York: Springer; 2005. p. 36–50.
38. Segal NA, Felson DT, Torner JC, et al. Greater trochanteric pain syndrome: epidemiology and associated factors. Arch Phys Med Rehabil. 2007;88(8):988–92.
39. White KK, Williams SK, Mubarak SJ. Definition of two types of anterior inferior iliac spine avulsion fractures. J Pediatr Orthop. 2002;22(5):578–82.
40. Grossman MG, Ducey SA, Nadler SS, Levy AS. Meralgia paresthetica: diagnosis and treatment. J Am Acad Orthop Surg. 2001;9(5):336–44.

41. Blazina ME. The "hip-pointer", a term to describe a specific kind of athletic injury. Calif Med. 1967;106(6):450.
42. Metzmaker JN, Pappas AM. Avulsion fractures of the pelvis. Am J Sports Med. 1985;13(5):349–58.
43. Hiti CJ, et al. Athletic osteitis pubis. Sports Med. 2011;41(5): 361–76.
44. Mitchell TD, Urli KE, Breitenbach J, Yelverton C. The predictive value of the sacral base pressure test in detecting specific types of sacroiliac dysfunction. J Chiropr Med. 2007;6(2):45–55.
45. Klingele KE, Sallay PI. Surgical repair of complete proximal hamstring tendon rupture. Am J Sports Med. 2002;30(5):742–7.
46. Cho KH, Lee SM, Lee YH, et al. Non-infectious ischiogluteal bursitis: MRI findings. Korean J Radiol. 2004;5(4):280–6.
47. Wait A, Gaskill T, Sarwar Z, Busch M. Van neck disease: osteochondrosis of the osteopubic synchondrosis. J Pediatr Orthop. 2011;31(5):520–4.
48. Gidwani S, Jagiello J, Bircher M. Avulsion fracture of the ischial tuberosity in adolescents—an easily missed diagnosis. BMJ. 2004;329(7457):99–100.
49. Parziale JR, Hudgins TH, Fishman LM. The piriformis syndrome. Am J Orthop (Belle Mead NJ). 1996;25(12):819–23.
50. Kouyoumdjian P, Coulomb R, Sanchez T, Asencio G. Clinical evaluation of hip joint rotation range of motion in adults. Orthop Traumatol Surg Res. 2012;98(1):17–23.
51. Simoneau GG, Hoenig KJ, Lepley JE, Papanek PE. Influence of hip position and gender on active hip internal and external rotation. J Orthop Sports Phys Ther. 1998;28(3):158–64.
52. James B, Parker AW. Active and passive mobility of the lower limb joints in elderly men and women. Am J Phys Med Rehabil. 1989;68(4):162–7.
53. American Academy of Orthopedic Surgeons. Joint motion: method of measuring and recording. Chicago: American Academy of Orthopedic Surgeons; 1965.
54. Nussbaumer S, Leunig M, Glatthorn JF, et al. Validity and test-retest reliability of manual goniometers for measuring passive hip range of motion in femoroacetabular impingement patients. BMC Musculoskelet Disord. 2010;11:194.
55. Audenaert EA, Peeters I, Vigneron L. Hip morphological characteristics and range of internal rotation in femoroacetabular impingement. Am J Sports Med. 2012;40(6):1329–36.
56. Kubiak-Langer M, Tannast M, Murphy SB, et al. Range of motion in anterior femoroacetabular impingement. Clin Orthop Relat Res. 2007;458:117–24.
57. Medical Research Council Scale. Aids to examination of the peripheral nervous system. Memorandum no. 45. London: Her Majesty's Stationery Office; 1976.
58. Philippon MJ, Schenker ML. Athletic hip injuries and capsular laxity. Oper Tech Orthop. 2005;15:261–6.
59. Byrd JWT. Evaluation of the hip: history and physical examination. N Am J Sports Phys Ther. 2007;2(4):231–40.
60. Van der Windt DA, Simons E, Riphagen II. Physical examination for lumbar radiculopathy due to disc herniation in patients with low-back pain. Cochrane Database Syst Rev. 2010;2: CD007431.
61. McCarthy JC, Busconi BD, Owens BD. Assessment of the painful hip. In: McCarthy JC, editor. Early hip disorders. New York: Springer; 2003. p. 3–6.
62. McCarthy JC, Busconi B. The role of hip arthroscopy in the diagnosis and treatment of hip disease. Orthopedics. 1995;18:753–6.
63. Ilizaliturri VM, Camacho-Galindo J. Endoscopic treatment of snapping hips, iliotibial band, and iliopsoas tendon. Sports Med Arthrosc. 2010;18(2):120–7.
64. Wang WE, Yue DB, Zhang NF, et al. Clinical diagnosis and arthroscopic treatment of acetabular labral tears. Orthop Surg. 2011;3(1):28–34.
65. Maslowski E, Sullivan W, Harwood JF, et al. The diagnostic validity of hip provocation maneuvers to detect intra-articular hip pathology. PM R. 2010;2(3):174–81.
66. Rab GT. The geometry of slipped capital femoral epiphysis: Implications for movement, impingement, and corrective osteotomy. J Pediatr Orthop. 1999;19:419–24.
67. Leunig M, Casillas MM, Hamlet AD, et al. Slipped capital femoral epiphysis: early mechanical damage to the acetabular cartilage by a prominent femoral metaphysis. Acta Orthop Scand. 2000;71:370–5.
68. Drehmann F. Drehmann's sign. A clinical examination method in epiphysiolysis (slipping of the upper femoral epiphysis). Description of signs, aetiopathogenetic considerations, clinical experience (author's transl). Z Orthop Ihre Grenzgeb. 1979;117(3):333–44.
69. Kamegaya M, Saisu T, Nakamura J, et al. Drehmann sign and femoro-acetabular impingement in SCFE. J Pediatr Orthop. 2011;31(8):853–7.
70. Harvey D. Assessment of the flexibility of athletes using the modified Thomas test. Br J Sports Med. 1998;32:68–70.
71. Gaenslen FJ. Sacro-iliac arthrodesis: indications, author's technique and end-results. JAMA. 1927;89(24):2031–5.
72. Stafford GH, Villar RN. Ischiofemoral impingement. J Bone Joint Surg Br. 2011;93(10):1300–2.
73. Patti JW, Ouellette H, Bredella MA, Torriani M. Impingement of lesser trochanter on ischium as a potential cause for hip pain. Skeletal Radiol. 2008;37:939–41.
74. Johnson KA. Impingement of the lesser trochanter on the ischial ramus after total hip arthroplasty: report of three cases. J Bone Joint Surg Am. 1977;59-A:268–9.
75. Boykin RE, Anz AW, Bushnell BD, et al. Hip instability. J Am Acad Orthop Surg. 2011;19(6):340–9.
76. Philippon MJ, Zehms CT, Briggs KK, et al. Hip instability in the athlete. Oper Tech Sports Med. 2007;15:189–94.
77. Hackney RG. The sports hernia: a cause of chronic groin pain. Br J Sports Med. 1993;27:58–62.
78. Larson CM, Lohnes JH. Surgical management of athletic pubalgia. Oper Tech Sports Med. 2002;10:228–32.
79. Farber AJ, Wilckens JH. Sports hernia: diagnosis and therapeutic approach. J Am Acad Orthop Surg. 2007;15(8):507–14.
80. Ahumada LA, Ashruf S, Espinosade-los-Monteros A, et al. Athletic pubalgia: definition and surgical treatment. Ann Plast Surg. 2005;55:393–6.
81. Leriche R, Morel A. The syndrome of thrombotic obliteration of the aortic bifurcation. Ann Surg. 1943;127(2).

12 Clinical Evaluation of Hip Function: Essential Features in the History

Allston J. Stubbs and Elizabeth A. Howse

Introduction

The success of hip surgery depends upon selecting the proper patient [1]. In determining the best possible outcome for the patient, one relies on delineating an adequate history, performing a physical exam focused on the hip, and obtaining the proper imaging [1]. Only then can the orthopedic surgeon determine what type of surgical intervention is best suited for his/her patient. As surgical and technological advances are made, these principles that guide appropriate patient selection will remain the foundation of the orthopedic practice [1]. The purpose of this chapter is to define the critical role a proper history plays in successful patient management.

Chief Complaint

Defining the chief complaint and attaining a thorough history of present illness are essential in evaluating the patient presenting with hip pain [1]. The chief complaint may be as straightforward as hip pain or may include other descriptions, for example, groin pain, buttock pain, or lower extremity pain [1]. The chief complaint should specify the right versus the left hip, or on occasion may refer to bilateral symptoms [1]. Ultimately, all future investigations regarding the patient's history, physical examination, imaging, and specialist consultations are guided by the chief complaint [1].

A.J. Stubbs, MD, MBA
Division of Sports Medicine, Department of Orthopaedic Surgery, Wake Forest University, Winston-Salem, NC, USA
e-mail: astubbs@wakehealth.edu

E.A. Howse, MD (✉)
Department of Emergency Medicine, Hofstra North Shore-LIJ School of Medicine, 270-05 76th Ave., New Hyde Park, NY 11040, USA
e-mail: howseea@gmail.com

History of Present Illness

The history of present illness captures the essence of a patient's journey into the specialist's office. It defines the age of the patient, determines if trauma has occurred, specifies the duration and localization of symptoms, and elicits if there are any associated activities [1]. An appropriate history will guide the physical examination, imaging tests, and ultimately decision making.

Patient's Age

The age of the patient determines the likelihood of skeletal maturity as well as the probability of an osteoarthritic condition; symptomatic physeal irritation is more likely in pediatric patients (i.e., iliac apophysitis) or injury (ASIS avulsion), whereas osteoarthritis is much more likely to be the presenting etiology of an older patient's symptoms [1]. "The orthopaedic adage of evaluating 'a joint above and a joint below' is a good starting point for even the most basic hip evaluation" [1]. This maxim, while always important, is particularly significant when faced with the extremes of age. Remembering that children have difficulty with the localization of their symptoms is evident in the classic presentation of SCFE or Legg–Calvé–Perthes as knee pain. Obviously, when faced with a pediatric patient, one should consider pediatric orthopedic disorders involving the hip and surrounding structures. Conversely, the greater the age of the patient, the more likely they are to have lumbar pathology associated with hip pathology [1].

Localization of Symptoms

Anterior hip pain has classically been associated with true hip joint pathology, whereas lateral or posterior hip pains have been associated with extra-articular sources [1].

J.C. McCarthy et al. (eds.), *Hip Joint Restoration*, DOI 10.1007/978-1-4614-0694-5_12

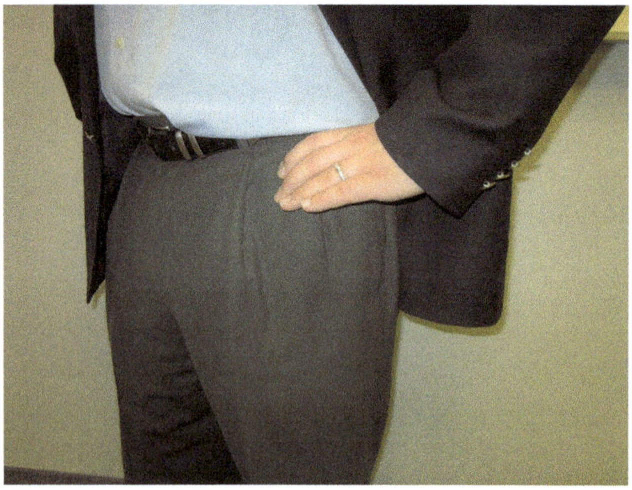

Fig. 12.1 C-sign photo. Hand demonstrating location of pain in the shape of a "C" with the thumb posterior and the fingers anterior

Table 12.1 Causes of pain around the hip joint [5]

Intra-articular	Extra-articular	Hip mimickers
Labral tears	Iliopsoas tendonitis	Athletic pubalgia
Loose bodies	Iliotibial band	Sports hernia
Femoroacetabular impingement	Gluteus medius or minimus	Osteitis pubis
Capsular laxity	Greater trochanteric bursitis	Endometriosis
Ligamentum teres rupture	Stress fracture	Cryptorchidism
Chondral damage	Adductor strain	Testicular torsion
Adhesive capsulitis	Piriformis syndrome	Inguinal hernia
Septic joint	Sacroiliac joint pathology	Core muscle injury
Pigmented villonodular synovitis	Slipped capital femoral epiphysis	Pubalgia syndrome
Osteoarthritis	–	Spondylolysis
Avascular necrosis	–	–
Legg–Calvé–Perthes	–	–

However, atypical hip pain patterns are common. According to Hilton's law [2], synovial joints share innervation with surrounding tissues [1, 3]. As such, intra-articular sources may present with atypical pain patterns, for example, lateral hip pain (i.e., trochanteric bursitis) or posterior hip pain (i.e., sacroiliitis) [1]. Other patterns may be secondary to primary joint pathology; groin pain maybe referred from the obturator nerve, thigh pain from the femoral nerve, and buttock pain from the sciatic nerve [1, 3]. More recently, the "C-sign" has been described as a presenting sign of intra-articular pathology. This is displayed by the patient placing his or her hand in the shape of the letter "C" about the outer circumference of the hemipelvis when describing the location of pain [1, 4] Fig. 12.1.

Familiarity with the presentation of pathologies, both orthopedic and non-orthopedic alike, which can be interpreted as "hip" pain, helps the examiner to guide the work-up and determine true intra-articular pathology from an impersonator (Table 12.1). Specifically, it is important for the surgeon to inquire about the presence of lower back pain and radicular complaints into the ipsilateral calf or foot. In order to clarify whether additional investigation about the lumbar spine is warranted, one should determine the relatedness of the lower back and radicular symptoms to the symptoms about the hemipelvis [1].

Onset of Symptoms

In our experience, most patients with hip pain fail to report a defining injury, but rather confirm a more insidious onset of symptoms over the course of months or years (see Textbox 12.1) [1]. When the patient presents with a history of hip injury, it should be specified as high or low energy as well as what type of event that occurred [1]. Low-energy events usually comprise twisting events during athletic competition, which can result in labral tears, acetabular chondral flap lesions, and loose bodies [5, 6]. Higher-energy events such as dislocations have a higher chance of an associated fracture or development of avascular necrosis of the femoral head [1].

Textbox 12.1: The Hip at Risk: Causes of Chondrolabral Dysfunction

Abnormal femoral torsion
Acetabular osteotomy
Adult dysplasia
Age
Femoroacetabular impingement
Dislocation/subluxation
Iatrogenic hardware
Iliopsoas impingement
Legg–Calvé–Perthes disease
Post-collapse avascular necrosis
Slipped capital femoral epiphysis

While activity is not a direct causative factor in the development of hip pathology, certain activities are correlated with a greater chance of intra-articular pathology in the setting of hip pain symptoms [1]. Obtaining a thorough history of patient activities which includes type of sports/activities that are played by the patient, as well as the extent to which they are performed (competitiveness, number of years), the examiner will gain additional insight to the type of stresses that the hip has endured. Athletes subject their bodies to extreme forces particularly around the hip joint [7, 8]. Furthermore, the extent of recurring microtrauma with continued repetition of that activity can result in overuse injuries [7, 9]. The orthopedic surgeon should be suspicious of an intra-articular source based on patients with a history of high-demand activities and hip pain symptoms [1]. Familiarity with the type of activities, how they are performed, and how they place excess force and rotation of the hip identifies trauma to the hip and surrounding structures not acknowledged by the patient. For example, running and jumping can cause forces greater than five times the patient's body weight [8, 10]. Additionally, running on banked surfaces has been associated with extra-articular sources of pain such as trochanteric bursitis [11]. Symptomatic hip impingement may develop in athletes who participate in contact sports, such as ice hockey, martial arts, American football, and baseball.

Most patients seek medical treatment due to pain. Some patients may have additional complaints of mechanical symptoms described as catching, locking, or snapping [1]. Mechanical symptoms alone do not require surgical (or even medical) intervention, but should be further investigated when concomitant with pain. The provoking painful activity, for example, active hip circumduction, and any additional symptoms such as audibility should be documented and raise suspicion for iliopsoas, iliotibial band, and ligamentum teres pathology as well as bursitis [1, 10, 12]. Finally, stiffness about the hip may be suggestive of osteoarthritis [3].

Inciting Activities

The examiner should then proceed in defining what specific activities incite the patient's symptoms [1]. We recommend documenting activities of daily living with questions such as whether the pain occurs with sitting, riding in a car, walking, running, or at night [1]. More pain with sitting than walking may suggest the presence of a prearthritic condition, such as femoroacetabular impingement, whereas osteoarthritis may present with the patient experiencing more pain when walking than with sitting [1]. Difficulty crossing one's legs or pivoting may be representative of an unstable labral cartilage tear or articular cartilage flap [1]. Symptoms associated with a specific impact activity may suggest the presence of a stress fracture [1]. Night pain symptoms may be indicative of advanced arthritic disease or more serious pathology such as a tumor [1]. Obviously, determination of when the patient experiences symptoms facilitates the examiner to narrow down the differential and clarify what additional diagnostic testing should be performed. Therefore, the aforementioned questions should be specifically asked of each patient. Additionally, as with all medical interviews, it is necessary to ask an open-ended question such as "When do you experience pain?" or "When does your hip bother you the most?" While these questions may be of limited diagnostic value, they are important, not simply because they allow the patient to feel heard but help to distinguish the patient's ultimate goals with intervention. This often presents as activity-related pain; it should be clarified and documented if the patient's activity level is affected [1]. This fact may be recorded as citing the specific activities that the patient cannot perform because of hip pain [1]. These complaints are vital in addressing patient satisfaction, as they help direct the conversation regarding realistic expectations involving post-operative recovery and the ability to return to play.

Special Considerations

The history of present illness should end with feathering out the mimickers of hip pain. Pain worsening with a Valsalva maneuver should raise suspicion for classic or atypical hernias about the anterior pelvis [1]. In male patients it is important to address gonadal pathology such as cryptorchidism, which increases the risk of testicular cancer [1]. For female patients, the orthopedic surgeon should investigate whether or not symptoms fluctuate with menses, as this is a sign of endometriosis [1]. A female whose history comprises the elements of the female athlete triad (amenorrhea, poor diet, and decreased bone density) should raise suspicion and investigation of a stress fracture [1].

Past History

The HPI is not complete without gathering information on previous treatments that the patient has undergone to treat his/her hip. Soliciting this information at the end of the HPI allows for a natural progression of the interview to discussing additional past medical and surgical history (which may or may not be relevant) to the patients' symptomatology and operative risk.

Prior Nonoperative Treatment

Prior to visiting an orthopedic surgeon, many patients have received treatment for their hip pain by other medical professionals. A detailed history of prior treatment and the patient's response to these interventions should be carefully documented [1]. Common nonoperative treatments to be explored include: anti-inflammatories, narcotics, injections, and therapy [1]. Many patients will have undergone physical therapy, chiropractic treatment, and massage therapy as a means of alleviating hip pain before seeking a surgical option [1]. The orthopedic surgeon should note the effect these treatments had on the patient's hip pain symptoms, as these can provide insight to intra-articular hip pathology. For example, aggressive stretching or strengthening programs will worsen a cartilage tear [1].

The location, intra-articular versus extra-articular, and the specific medications of hip injections should be thoroughly documented, and early and late term results determined. The patient should also be questioned as to whether the joint injection was performed under fluoroscopic or ultrasound guidance [1]. Injections about the hemipelvis, while potentially providing symptomatic relief, when investigated appropriately may also act as a diagnostic aid [1]. A patient with chronic hip pain will often present after several steroid-containing injections to various anatomical regions: the greater trochanteric bursa region, the lower lumbar spine, or ipsilateral sacroiliac joint [1]. Given the variable presentations of hip pathology, referred pain, and occasionally coexisting surrounding pathology (which may result in additional injury due to compensation), understanding the response to these injections is quite complex. Kivlan et al. have shown that patients with chondral damage obtain greater relief than patients without chondral damage, whereas pathology that is labral in nature yielded little therapeutic value from an injection. Furthermore, the existence of extra-articular pathology in their study did not alter the response to an intra-articular injection [13].

Prior Operative Treatment

As the chief complaint may not always immediately direct the clinician to hip pathology, it is important to document prior interventions to address the pain. In the native hip, previous operations may have been performed to address "hip mimickers." When these surgeries result in minimal or no improvement to the presenting complaint, the index of suspicion should be raised of true hip pathology, especially when "hip" symptoms began before the intervention occurred. For example, dyspareunia or "coxa amora" involving hip pain with intercourse may not be gonadal in origin, but rather attributed to intra-articular cartilage pathology [1]. Occasionally, a female patient's hip pain may have been attributed to gynecological in origin (endometriosis) and thereby unsuccessfully treated with oophorectomy or hysterectomy, resulting in no relief of symptoms [1]. Other times failure to obtain desired results after surgical correction may be due to only partially addressing the cause of pain. An example of this may be seen in patients presenting after surgical correction of pain from "athletic pubalgia" or core muscle injury (CMI). Both CMI and femoroacetabular impingement are related to recurring microtrauma, specifically from repetitive kicking, as well as twisting, and turning at high speeds. While these pathologies can occur individually, they often coexist [8, 14, 15]. Partial reduction in symptoms would therefore imply that the patient initially presents with the "sports hip triad," which consists of a labral tear, adductor strain, and rectus strain [8].

In the postoperative hip, differentiating an intra-articular source from a mimicker as the cause of pain is often complex. Sequelae of pediatric disease resulting in abnormal anatomy, loose bodies resulting from trauma not addressed by DHS, or failure of prior operative management to (fully) address the patient's symptoms all can indicate the need for an additional or revision operation. The type and severity of pathology as well as the expectations of the patient direct the examiner to determine what future intervention (arthroscopy versus replacement) is appropriate.

Past Medical and Social History

The past medical history provides more information than simply overall perioperative risks. This is true for many hip pathologies, but is perhaps most evident in osteonecrosis. Asthma and COPD, for example, not only pose intubation risks but also are commonly treated with steroids, thereby increasing the risk of developing AVN. Osteonecrosis should be considered when patients take steroids for medical as well as vanity reasons; it is also often seen as a complication of hemoglobinopathies such as sickle cell disease. Excessive alcohol intake has also been attributed to causing AVN and is relevant in all patients undergoing hip surgery, as it can be predictive of postoperative noncompliance associated with failure [3].

Family History

Finally, the patient's history should end with an investigation related to family-specific findings [1]. Occasionally, patients will report a first-degree relative who required a hip replacement at an early age [1]. While currently the genetics of hip osteoarthritis are poorly understood, this may not always be the case [1]. The orthopedic surgeon should appreciate that genetic risk factors may play a role in the onset of prearthritic hip disease [1]. Often the family history will not provide much insight to the examiner; however, when the patient discloses a family member who carries the diagnosis of a collagen disorder such as Ehlers–Danlos syndrome, this may explain why a patient is complaining of hip instability.

Conclusion

Obtaining a thorough history is important in the presurgical evaluation of the hip. The patient's history along with a detailed physical examination and dedicated imaging studies determines the appropriate surgical intervention or need for additional consultation. We recommend optimizing the history-taking process with patient-directed hip outcome measures.

References

1. Stubbs AJ. Patient selection for hip arthroscopy. In: Byrd JWT, Puddu G, Panni EAS, editors. Hip arthroscopy: indications and technique—surgical techniques in orthopaedics and traumatology. Rome: CIC Edizione Internationali; 2011. p. 1–8.
2. Hilton J. Rest and pain. London: Bell; 1863.
3. Purvis SA, Leopold SS. History and physical examination. In: Callaghan JJ, Rosenberg AG, Rubash HE, editors. The adult hip. 2nd ed. Philadelphia: Lippincott Williams & Willkins; 2007. p. 343–8.
4. Byrd JWT. Physical examination. In: Byrd JWT, editor. Operative hip arthroscopy. 2nd ed. New York: Springer; 2005. p. 36–50.
5. Tibor LM, Sekiya JK. Differential diagnosis of pain around the hip joint. Arthroscopy. 2008;24:1407–21.
6. Byrd JWT, Jones KS. Traumatic rupture of the ligamentum teres as a source of hip pain. Arthroscopy. 2004;20(4):385–91.
7. Kelly BT, Williams RJ, Philippon MJ. Hip arthroscopy: current indications, treatment options, and management issues. Am J Sports Med. 2006;31(6):1020–37.
8. Hammoud S, Bedi A, Magennis E, Meyers WC, Kelly BT. High incidence of athletic pubalgia symptoms in professional athletes with symptomatic femoroacetabular impingement. Arthroscopy. 2012;28(10):1388–95.
9. Micheli L, Fehlandt AF. Overuse injuries to tendons and apophyses in children and adolescents. Clin Sports Med. 1992;11(4):713–26.
10. Shah A, Busconi B. Hip and pelvis. In: DeLee JC, Drez D, Miller MD, editors. Orthopaedic sports medicine. 3rd ed. Philadelphia: Saunders Elsevier; 2010. p. 1451–76.
11. Baumfeld JA, Hart JA, Miller MD. Sports medicine. In: Miller MD, editor. Review of orthopaedics. 5th ed. Philadelphia: Saunders Elsevier; 2008. p. 266–7.
12. Singh PJ, O'Donnell JM. Arthroscopic surgery of the hip a justification. In: ISHA 2008: Proceedings of the first international society of hip arthroscopy conference, Paris, France, 10 Oct 2008.
13. Kivlan BR, Martin RL, Sekiya JK. Response to diagnostic injection in patients with femoroacetabular impingement, labral tears, chondral lesions and extra-articular pathology. Arthroscopy. 2011;27: 619–27.
14. Bedi A, Dolan M, Leunig M, Kelly BT. Static and dynamic mechanical causes of hip pain. Arthroscopy. 2007;27(2):235–51.
15. Kachingwe AF, Grech S. Proposed algorithm for the management of athletes with athletic pubalgia (sports hernia): a case series. J Orthop Sports Phys Ther. 2008;38(12):768–81.

13 Essential Findings in the Clinical Exam

Hal David Martin, Ian James Palmer, and Munif Hatem

Introduction

The physical examination continues to evolve as our understanding of the normal and pathologic hip advances. Asymptomatic patients often present hip imaging studies with abnormal findings, of which the significance is determined by history and physical examination. A structured physical examination will lead to a more accurate and specific diagnosis by evaluating all four layers of the hip: the osseous, capsulolabral, musculotendinous, and neurovascular [1]. The role of the fifth layer, the kinematic chain, is important for the appropriate treatment recommendations, since it represents the link between the hip and other musculoskeletal structures. Terminology of the examination needs to be consistent so that international variances can be eliminated. The following chapter is a description of a standardized approach to the clinical evaluation of the hip, which will provide the background on which to cast the shadow of hip pathology.

History

A comprehensive history of the patient is obtained prior to the physical examination of the hip. The present condition is documented including the date of onset, presence or absence of trauma, and mechanisms of injury. The pain features and presence or absence of popping will aid in the determination of intra-articular versus extra-articular causes. It is also necessary to identify related symptoms of the spine, abdomen, and lower extremity, primarily referred as knee pain. The following items must additionally be addressed: previous consultations, surgical interventions, past injuries, childhood or adolescent hip disease, ipsilateral knee disease, suggestive history of inflammatory arthritis, and risk factors for osteonecrosis. Treatments to date must be clearly defined and current limitations are detailed.

Participation in sports and other activities is documented and can help not only determine the type of injury but also guide the treatment considering the patient's goals and expectations. Final outcome is dependent upon the effects of treatment which should consider the mental and spiritual aspects of the patient. This assessment has proven useful in heart and cancer treatment and is required in complex hip pathology evaluation due to the critical role the hip plays in all activities of daily life.

The hip pain and function can be scored utilizing one or more of the following questionnaires: Harris Hip Score (HHS); modified HHS; or preferably one of the following validated, activity measuring scores: the Western Ontario and McMaster University (WOMAC) osteoarthritis index, nonarthritic hip score (NAHS), international hip outcome tool (iHOT)-33, and iHOT-12. A complete review of the history is given in Table 13.1.

The Physical Examination of the Hip

Access for exposure and patient comfort with loose-fitting clothes about the waist is helpful. A consistent hip examination provides the background to screen the hip, back, abdominal, neurovascular, and neurologic systems quickly and efficiently and to find the comorbidities that coexist with complex hip pathology. An assistant to record the examination on a standardized written form aids in accurate documentation and thoroughness, especially when first starting a comprehensive hip evaluation. Each examination or physical evaluation has a specific method of being performed, although the technique of physical examination is dependent on the examiner's experience and efficiency. The MAHORN (Multicenter Arthroscopy of the Hip Outcomes

H.D. Martin, DO (✉) • I.J. Palmer, PhD • M. Hatem, MD
Hip Preservation Center, Baylor University Medical Center,
411 N Washington Avenue, Suite 7300, Dallas, TX 75246, USA
e-mail: haldavidmartin@yahoo.com; ianjamespalmer@gmail.com; munifhatem@gmail.com

J.C. McCarthy et al. (eds.), *Hip Joint Restoration*, DOI 10.1007/978-1-4614-0694-5_13

Table 13.1 Complete review of patient history

Recorded by an assistant. *VAS* **visual analog pain scale,** *AVN* **avascular necrosis of the femoral head,** *ONFH* **osteonecrosis of the femoral head,** *ADL* **activities of daily living**

NAME: ____________________ **DATE:** __________ **AGE:** ______
DUTIES: ____________________ **REFERRED BY:** ____________________
CHIEF COMPLAINT: **L HIP** **R HIP** **OTHER:** ____________________
HISTORY OF PRESENT ILLNESS:

- Date of onset ________
- Pain location ________
- Traumatic/nontraumatic
- Mechanism of injury ______
- Popping/locking ______
- Knee pain ____ Back pain ____
- Pain at Rest (VAS 0-10) ______
- Pain With Activity(VAS 0-10) ____
- Pain a.m. / p.m.______
- Pain increased with ______
- Pain decreased with ______
- Have you ever been diagnosed with AVN/ONFH ? ____________
  Alcohol use____ Tobacco use ____Steroid use____ Other ______
- Suggestive history of inflammatory arthritis____________

TREATMENT TO DATE

Rest Ice Heat NSAIDS______
Physiotherapy______
Surgery__________
Chiropractic tx________
Injections__________
Support (cane, crutch)______
Orthotics__________

TESTS AND EVALUATIONS:

MRI MRI Arthrogram X-rays Lab Biometrics Consults________

PAST INJURIES: ____________________

LIMITATIONS:

- Sitting
- Getting in or out of tub
- Getting in or out of car
- Jogging

Length of time able to sit
Sports
Stairs
Work

ADL's
Household activities

FUNCTION:

HHS m________iHOT-33________

ASSOCIATED

- Spine sacroiliac affection
- Night pain awakening

Knee pathology
Genitourinary complaints

Numbness
Abdominal Pain

SPORTS AND ACTIVITIES: ____________________
GOAL IN TREATMENT:____________________
REVIEW OF SYSTEMS:

Research Network) group common tests form the core of a multilayered hip evaluation [2].

Standardization enhances the physical examination reliability [3], and the most efficient order of examination begins with standing tests followed by seated, supine, and lateral tests, ending with prone tests [4] (Table 13.2).

Standing Examination

In a standing position, a general point of pain is noted with one finger and can usually help direct the examination. The groin region directs a suspicion of intra-articular problem. Lateral-based pain may be associated with intra- or

Table 13.2 Physical examination of the hip—intake form

Height: ____ Weight: _____ Temperature: _____ Breath rate: _____ Pulse : _____ Blood pressure: ______

Standing Examination:

- Shoulder height: Equal Not equal
- Iliac crest height: Equal Not equal
- Active forward bend: _______degrees of lumbar flexion
- Spine: straight
  scoliosis: structural non-structural
- Lordosis : normal increased paravertebral muscle spasms
- Laxity tests: little fingers thumbs elbows knees spine
- Gait: normal antalgic/short stance phase abductor deficient (Trendelenburg)
  pelvic wink abnormal arm swing short stride length
  Foot progression angle: normal excessive external rotation internal rotation
- Single leg stance phase test (Trendelenburg test): R ____ L ____

Seated Examination:

- Circulation: Dorsalis pedis _____ Posterior tibial ______________
- Skin Inspection: ______________________________
- Lymphatic: lymphedema no lymphedema pitting edema: 1+ 2+
- Neurologic Findings:
  Sensory: _______

Motor: _______ DTR: Achilles _______ Patellar________

- Straight Leg Raise: R _____ L ______
- Range of Motion: Internal Rotation: R______ L_____ External Rotation: R_____ L_____
- Posterior pain tests:
  Pain on palpation: lateral to ischial tuberosity (IT) hamstring origin medial to IT
  Seated piriformis stretch test __________
  Active Knee flexion test against resistance; 30 degrees_________ 90 degrees

Supine Examination:

- Leg lengths: R____cm L____cm equal/not equal
- Palpation:

Abdomen:	Tender	Non-tender
Palpation pubic symphysis/ Adductor	Tender	Non-tender
Adductor Tubercle:	Tender	Non-tender

- ROM:

	Right Hip	Left Hip
Abduction:	10 20 30 45 50	10 20 30 45 50
Adduction:	0 10 20 30	0 10 20 30
Flexion:	80 100 110 120 130 140	80 100 110 120 130 140

• Hip flexion contracture test (Thomas test):	R + -	L + -
• FABER (Patrick test) :	R + -	L + -
• DIRI:	R + -	L + -
• DEXRIT:	R + -	L + -
Posterior rim impingement test:	R + -	L + -
Apprehension sign:	R + -	L + -
• Heel strike:	R + -	L + -
• Straight leg raise against resistance (Stitchfield test):	R + -	L + -
• Passive supine rotation test (log roll test):	R + -	L + -
• Dial test	R + -	L + -

Table 13.2 (continued)

Lateral Examination

- Palpation:

Supra SI area	Tender	Non-tender	Piriformis	Tender	Non-tender
SI joint	Tender	Non-tender	Sciatic nerve	Tender	Non-tender
G. Max origin	Tender	Non-tender	TFL	Tender	Non-tender
Greater trochanter	Tender	Non-tender			

- Abductor strength: Straight leg ______ Gluteus max______ Gluteus medius______
- Tensor fascia lata contracture test: Grade(1-3)______
- Gluteus medius contracture test: Grade(1-3)______
- Gluteus maximus contracture test: Grade(1-3)______
- FADDIR test: R + - L + -
- Lateral rim impingement test: R + - L + -
- Apprehension test R + - L + -
- Posterior pain tests:
  Active piriformis test ____________ Ischiofemoral impingement test __________

Prone Examination:

- Lumbar hyperextension test
- Femoral Anteversion Test:_____ estimated degrees of anteversion
- Rectus Contracture Test (Ely's Test): R + - L + -

Hip Snapping Tests

External snapping tests Snapping Iliopsoas tendon tests

extra-articular aspects, which can coexist. A characteristic sign of patients with intra-articular hip pain is the "C sign" [5]. The patient will hold his or her hand in the shape of a C and place it above the greater trochanter, with the thumb positioned posterior to the trochanter and fingers extending into the groin. Posterior-superior pain requires a thorough evaluation in differentiating hip and back pain. The shoulder height and iliac crest heights are noted to evaluate leg length discrepancies (Fig. 13.1a, b). Incremental wooden blocks placed under the short side foot help in orthotic considerations. Side and forward bending of the trunk are performed to evaluate the lumbar spine and to differentiate structural from nonstructural scoliosis, recording the degree of trunk flexion (Fig. 13.1c, d). General body habitus and joint laxity are assessed (Fig. 13.1e).

Gait abnormalities often help detect hip pathology. The patient is taken into the hallway to observe a full gait of six to eight stride lengths. Key points of gait evaluation include foot progression angle, pelvic rotation, stance phase, and stride length. The following abnormal gait patterns can be associated with hip pathologies: winking gait (excessive pelvic rotation in the axial plane), abductor deficient gait (Trendelenburg gait or abductor lurch), antalgic gait with a shortened stance phase on the painful side, and short leg gait with dropping of the shoulder in the direction of the short leg.

In addition to body habitus and gait evaluation, the single-leg stance phase test (Trendelenburg test) is performed during the standing evaluation of the hip. The single-leg stance phase test is performed bilaterally, with the non-affected leg examined first, to establish a baseline (Fig. 13.1f). If the abductor musculature is weak or the neural loop of proprioception is disrupted on the bearing side, the pelvis will drop toward the nonbearing side or shift more than 2 cm toward the bearing (affected) side. Trunk inclination for the bearing (affected) side is also noted in a positive single-leg stance test. In an athletic population, this assessment can be performed in a dynamic fashion.

Seated Examination

The seated hip examination consists of a thorough vascular, lymphatic, and neurologic examination. The need to check the basics is obvious, even in apparently healthy individuals. The posterior tibial pulse is checked first, any swelling of the extremity is noted, and inspection of the skin is performed at this time. Neurologic evaluation includes the assessment of sensation, motor function, and patellar and Achilles deep tendon reflexes. A straight leg raise test is then performed by passively extending the knee into full extension, in order to detect radicular symptoms.

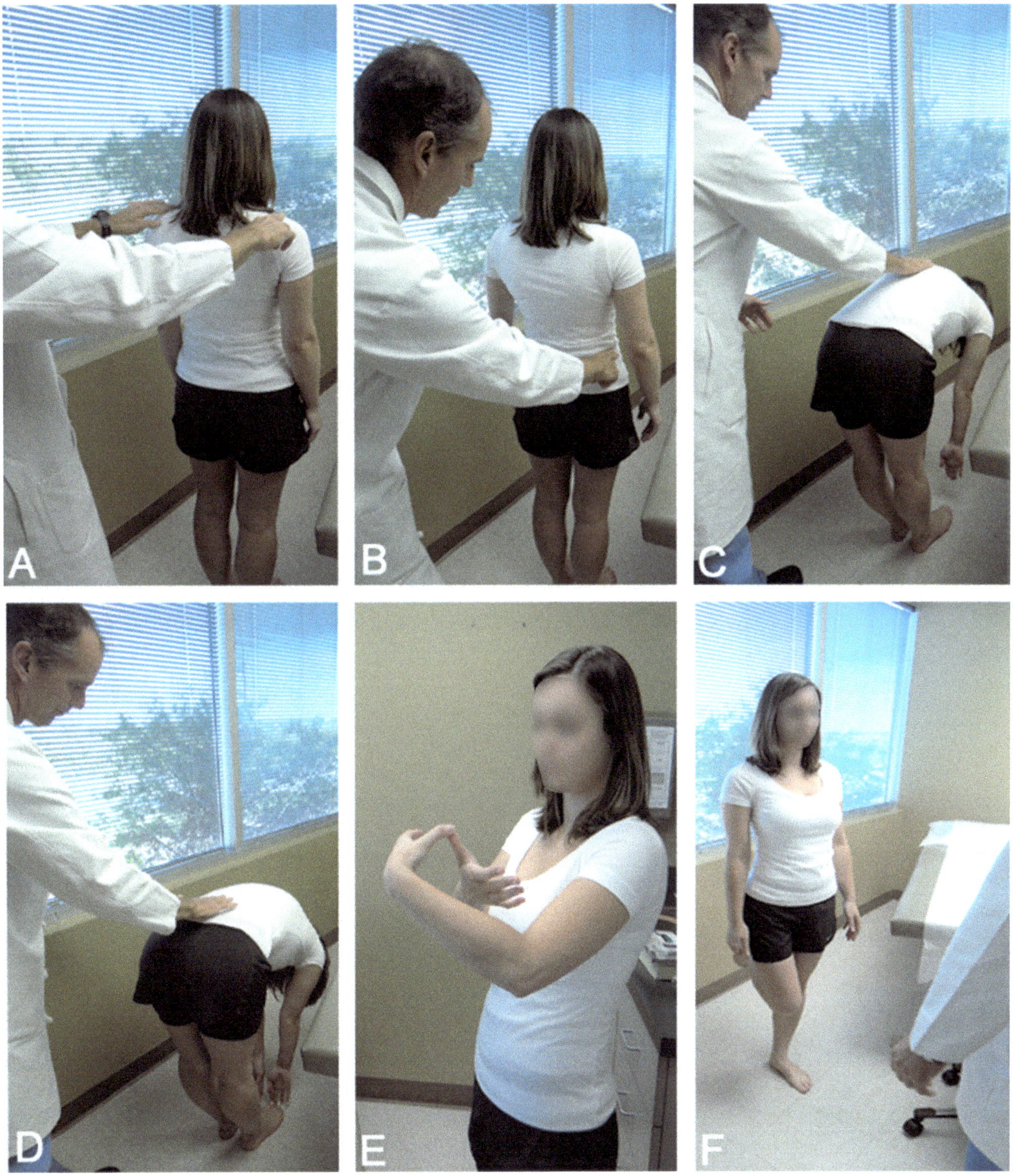

Fig. 13.1 Standing evaluation. (**a**, **b**) Shoulder and iliac crest heights are examined with the patient with dynamic loading of the hip joint in the standing position. (**c**) As the patient bends forward at the trunk, spinal alignment is palpated. (**d**) The degree of trunk flexion is noted in full flexion. (**e**) Laxity of the thumb. (**f**) The single-leg stance phase test is performed bilaterally and observed from behind and in front of the patient. The patient flexes the hip and knee at 45° and holds this position for 6 s

The seated position is utilized to assess the hip rotations (Fig. 13.2a, b). The ligamentous function, pelvic position, and methodology of measurement can cause differences up to 10° in the values of hip rotation measured in different positions (seated, prone, supine). Joint mobility also varies from race to race and decreases with age. Sufficient internal

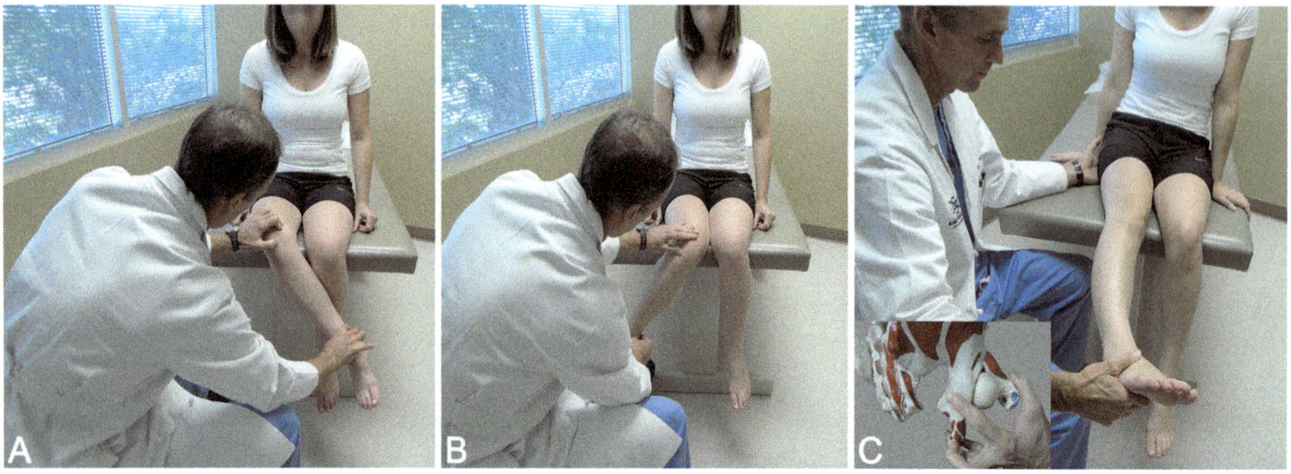

Fig. 13.2 Seated rotation range of motion and piriformis stretch test. Seated external (**a**) and internal (**b**) rotation range of motion. Passive internal and external rotation testing is compared from side to side. In the seated position, the ischium is square to the table, thus providing sufficient stability at 90° of hip flexion. The seated position offers the most reproducible platform for the accurate rotational measurement. (**c**) Piriformis stretch test. The patient is in the seated position with the knee in extension, and the examiner passively moves the 90° flexed hip into adduction with internal rotation while palpating 1 cm lateral to the ischium and proximally at the sciatic notch (index finger)

Table 13.3 Normal hip range of motion

Range of motion assessment	Range (degrees)	Abnormal (degrees)
Seated internal rotation	20–35	<20
Seated external rotation	30–45	<30
Extended internal rotation	20–35	<20
Extended external rotation	30–45	<30
Supine hip flexion	100–110	<100
Adduction	20–30	<20
Abduction	45	<45

rotation is important for proper hip function, and there should be at least 10 degrees of internal rotation at the midstance phase of normal gait [6], but less than 20° is abnormal (see Table 13.3 for normal ROM). An increased internal rotation combined with a decreased external rotation may indicate excessive femoral anteversion. Conversely increased external rotation combined with decreased internal rotation may indicate excessive femoral retroversion.

In patients presenting with extra-articular posterior hip pain, some tests are performed in a seated position. The ischial tuberosity should be utilized as reference on palpation. Pain superolateral to the ischium at the sciatic notch suggests deep gluteal syndrome [7]; lateral to the ischium, ischial tunnel syndrome is considered; at the ischium, hamstring tendon pathologies are probable; and medial to the ischium, pudendal nerve entrapment is considered. The seated piriformis stretch test is performed with the hip flexed to 90° [8] (Fig. 13.2c). A positive test is the re-creation of the posterior pain at the level of the piriformis or external rotators, indicating sciatic nerve entrapment. The combination of the seated piriformis stretch test with the piriformis active test (lateral examination) has a sensitivity of 91 % and specificity of 80 % for the endoscopic finding of sciatic nerve entrapment [8]. An active knee flexion test against resistance, with 30 degrees versus 90 degrees of knee flexion, is utilized to evaluate the proximal hamstring tendons.

Supine Examination

The supine examination begins with the assessment of leg lengths. Next, palpation of the abdomen is performed and any tenderness is documented. Palpation of the adductor tubercle with active testing will detect adductor tendinitis. Sports hernia/athletic pubalgia is an occult and poorly recognized hernia and should be differentiated from isolated adductor tendinitis.

The supine position is also utilized for passive range of motion assessment. Passive abduction and adduction range of motion are evaluated with the hip in extension. After that, both knees are brought up to the chest and the degree of flexion is recorded (Fig. 13.3a). It is important to note the pelvic position because the hip may stop early in flexion, with the end range of motion being predominately pelvic rotation. From this position, the hip flexion contracture test (Thomas test) [9] is performed (Fig. 13.3b). A false-negative result can be found in patients with hyperlaxity or lumbar spine hyperlordosis.

The flexion, abduction, external rotation (FABER) test, conventionally known as the Patrick test [9], is helpful in determining hip versus sacroiliac complaints (Fig. 13.3c). Ipsilateral or contralateral sacroiliac discomfort can be felt. Re-creation of hip pain can be associated with posterior femoroacetabular impingement, ligamentous injury, or trochanteric pathologies.

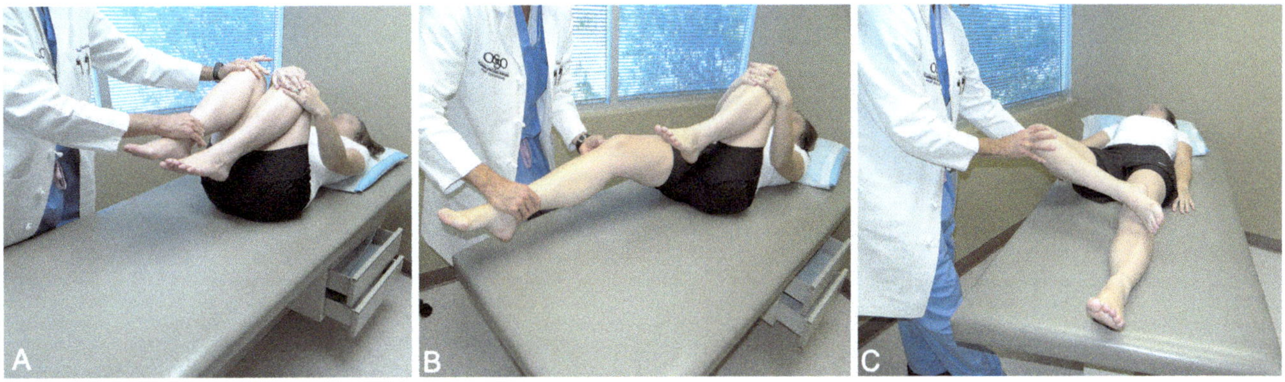

Fig. 13.3 Supine examination starting position, hip flexion contracture test, and FABER test. (**a**) Starting position. Zero set point of the pelvis is achieved by having the patient hold the contralateral leg in full flexion, thus establishing neutral pelvic inclination. (**b**) Hip flexion contracture test. With the patient holding the contralateral leg in full flexion (zero set point for the lumbar spine), the examined hip is passively extended toward the (lack of terminal hip extension) this demonstrates a hip flexion contracture. (**c**) Flexion, abduction, external rotation (FABER) test. The examiner brings the leg into 90 degrees flexion and externally rotates and abducts it so that the ipsilateral ankle rests distal to the knee of the contralateral leg

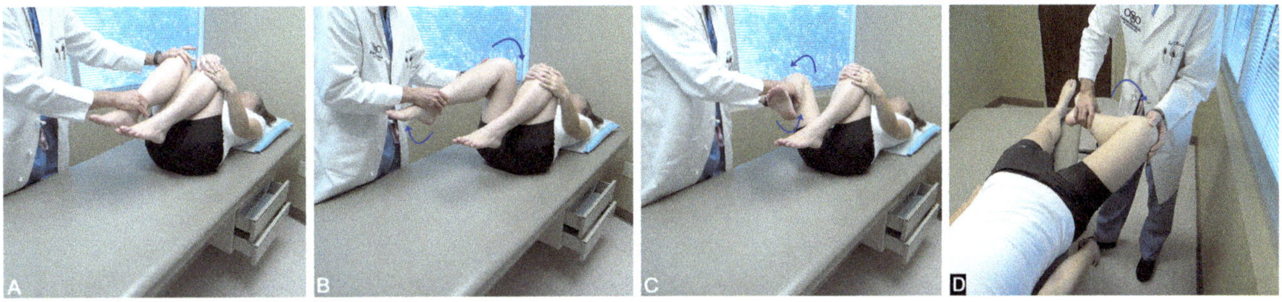

Fig. 13.4 Femoroacetabular congruence tests in the supine position. (**a**) Patient is in the supine position and instructed to hold the non-affected leg in flexion beyond 90°, thus establishing a zero pelvic set point and eliminating lumbar lordosis. (**b**) DIRI: the examined hip is brought into 90° flexion or beyond and is passively taken through a wide arc of adduction and internal rotation. (**c**) DEXRIT: the hip is then brought into 90 degrees flexion or beyond and dynamically taken through a wide arc of abduction and external rotation. (**d**) Posterior rim impingement test. The patient rests at the edge of the examining table, with the affected leg hanging freely at the hip while holding the contralateral leg in full flexion. The examined leg is then brought into full hip extension, abducted, and externally rotated

The femoroacetabular congruence is assessed using a variety of tests, aiming to detect femoroacetabular impingement, instability, or intra-articular pathology. This assessment was traditionally performed with flexion, adduction, and internal rotation [10]. McCarthy described the dynamic assessment of the femoroacetabular congruence and relationship to the labrum [11].

For the dynamic internal rotatory impingement test (DIRI) [2], the hip is dynamically taken in a wide arc of adduction internal rotation to test the anterior femoroacetabular congruence (Fig. 13.4a, b). The degree of flexion that causes the femoroacetabular impingement depends on the pelvic tilt and femoral version. A positive result is noted with re-creation of the complaint pain and can also be seen in posterior hip instability.

The dynamic external rotatory impingement test (DEXRIT [2]) includes a wide arc movement of passive abduction and external rotation (Fig. 13.4c). The DEXRIT reproduces superolateral and posterior femoroacetabular impingement, but may also be positive in cases of anteroinferior hip instability, anteroinferior acetabular hypoplasia, torn teres ligament, and capsular laxity. A positive result is noted with re-creation of pain or feeling of instability. DEXRIT and DIRI can be performed intraoperatively for femoroacetabular congruence assessment.

The posterior rim impingement test is performed to assess the congruence between the posterior wall and femoral neck (Fig. 13.4d). It takes the hip into extension, abduction, and external rotation and assesses the congruence of the posterior acetabular wall and femoral neck. The symptoms can be recreated by posterior impingement or anterior instability.

Other useful tests may be performed in the supine position: the heel strike test for occult fracture (Fig. 13.5a), the straight leg raise against resistance or Stinchfield test [9] for psoas impingement (Fig. 13.5b), and the passive supine rotation log roll (Fig. 13.5c). The dial test is a modification of the log roll test aiming to assess iliofemoral ligament laxity. It includes passive internal rotation of the leg, followed by releasing the

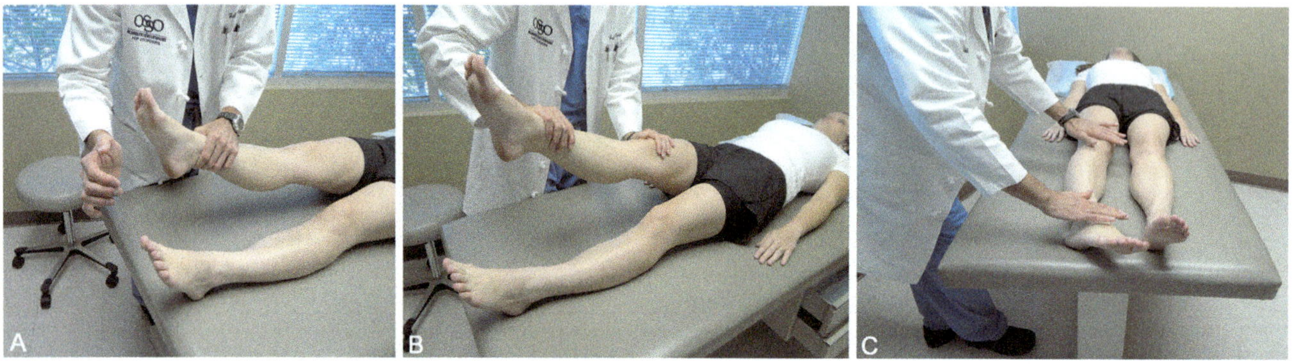

Fig. 13.5 Additional tests in the supine position. (**a**) The heel strike is performed by striking the heel abruptly and is used in trauma or stress fracture. (**b**) Straight leg raise against resistance, used for assessment of hip flexor and psoas strength. It is also useful for evaluation of psoas impingement and intra-articular irritation, as the psoas places pressure on the labrum. (**c**) The passive supine rotation test involves passive internal rotation (shown) and external rotation of the femur, with the leg lying in an extended position. Both limbs are examined for comparison, assessing capsular laxity, synovitis, or joint effusion

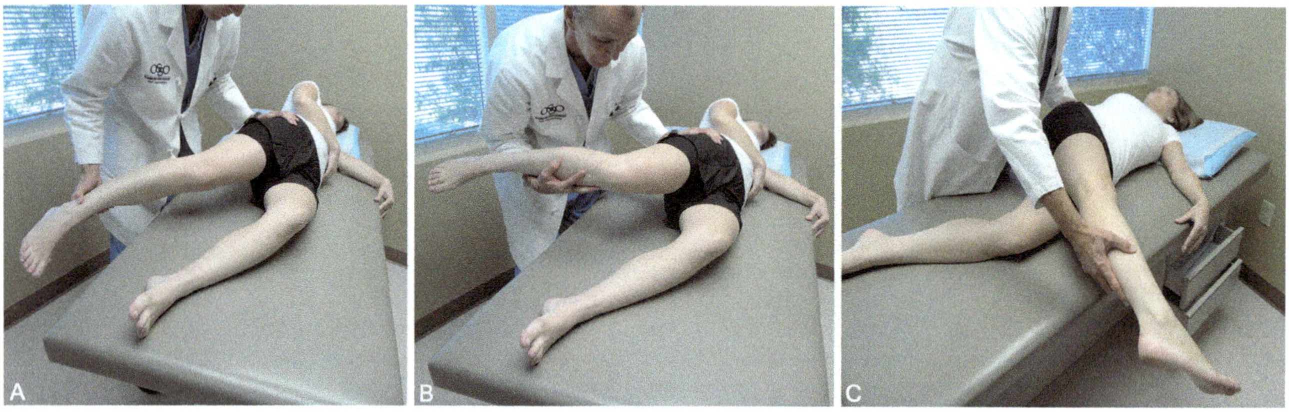

Fig. 13.6 Passive adduction tests. (**a**) The tensor fascia lata contracture test: with the knee in extension, the examiner passively brings the hip into extension then adduction. (**b**) Gluteus medius contracture test is performed with knee flexion, thus excluding the gluteus maximus contribution for the iliotibial band. The examiner passively adducts the hip toward the examination table. (**c**) The gluteus maximus contracture test is performed with the ipsilateral shoulder rotated toward the examination table. With the examined leg held in knee extension, the examiner passively brings the hip into flexion then adduction

leg and allowing it to external rotate. If the external rotation is more than 45° in relation to the vertical, the test is considered positive [12].

Lateral Examination

The lateral examination begins with the patient on the contralateral side and palpating the areas of the suprasacroiliac area, sacroiliac (SI) joint, gluteus maximus origin, piriformis muscle, and sciatic nerve. The greater trochanter is palpated on its facets: anterior, lateral, supero-posterior, and posterior. The gluteus minimus insertion is at the greater trochanteric anterior facet, the gluteus medius at the greater trochanteric supero-posterior and lateral facets, and the trochanteric bursa is at the posterior facet.

Strength is assessed with any type of lateral-based hip complaint. The tests are performed in lateral decubitus with the patient actively abducting the hip against resistance. The gluteus medius strength test is performed with the knee in flexion to release the gluteus maximus contribution for the iliotibial band. The overall abductor strength is evaluated with the knee in extension, and the gluteus maximus is tested asking the patient to abduct and extend the hip.

A set of passive adduction tests (similar to Ober's test [9]) is performed with the leg in three positions—extension (tensor fascia lata contracture test) (Fig. 13.6a), neutral (gluteus medius contracture test) (Fig. 13.6b), and flexion (gluteus maximus contracture test) (Fig. 13.6c).

The lateral decubitus is also utilized for femoroacetabular congruence evaluation. The passive flexion adduction internal rotation (FADDIR) test is performed in a dynamic

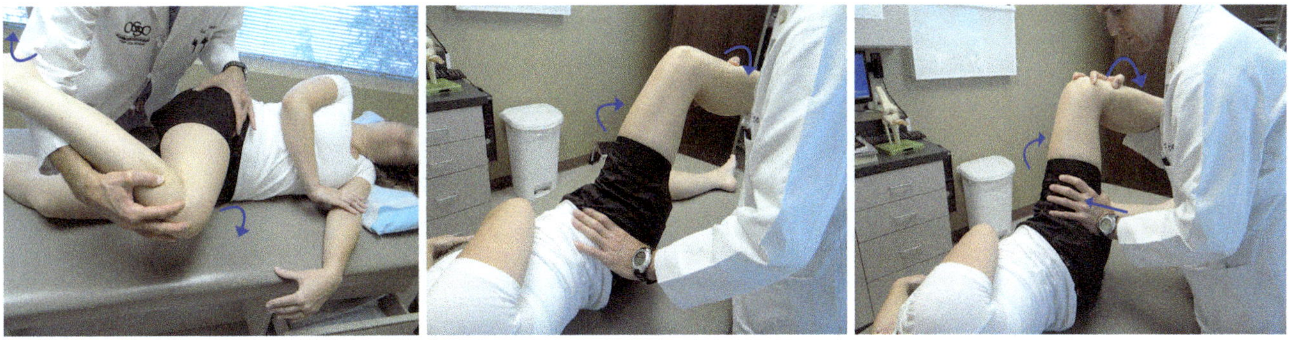

Fig. 13.7 Femoroacetabular congruence tests in the lateral position. (**a**) Flexion, adduction, internal rotation (FADDIR). In the lateral position, the examiner dynamically brings the examined hip into flexion, adduction, and internal rotation while monitoring the superior aspect of the hip. (**b**) Lateral rim impingement test. The examiner cradles the patient's lower leg with one arm and monitors the hip joint with the opposing hand. The affected hip is passively brought through a wide arc from flexion to extension in continuous abduction while externally rotating the hip. (**c**) Apprehension test. The examiner brings the hip from flexion to extension in external rotation and abduction. With the opposite hand, the examiner forces forward the proximal femur to provoke anterior-inferior subluxation of the femoral head

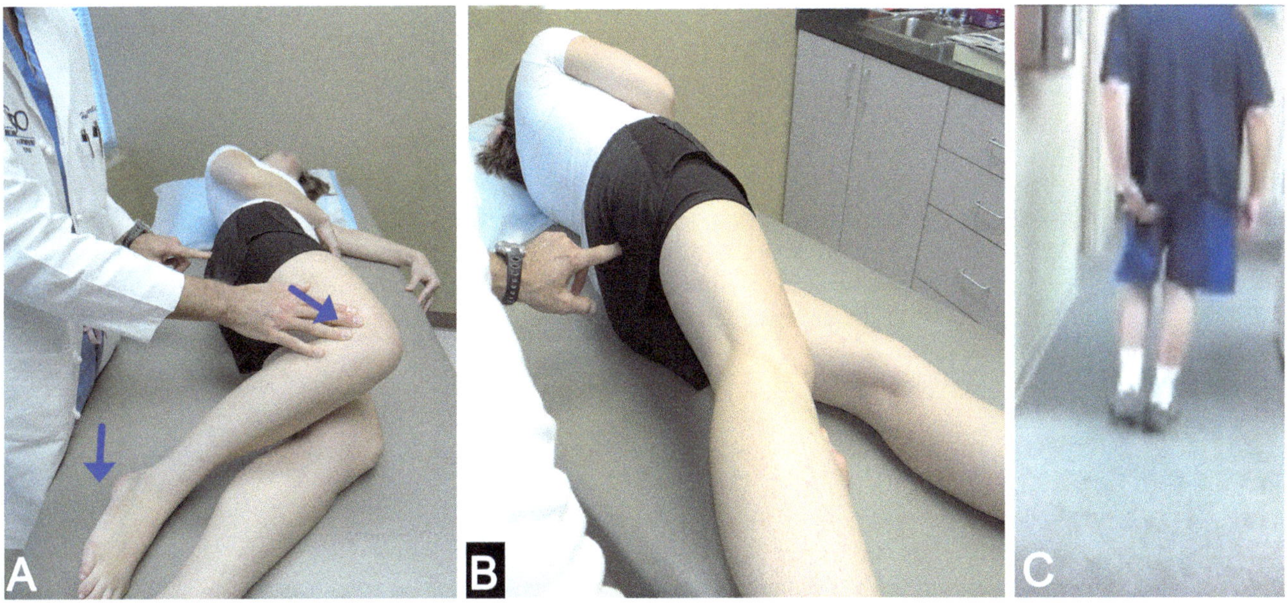

Fig. 13.8 Assessment of posterior extra-articular hip pain in the lateral position. (**a**) Active piriformis test. With the patient in the lateral position, the examiner palpates the piriformis. The patient drives the heel into the examining table, thus initiating external hip rotation while actively abducting and externally rotating against resistance (*arrows*), while the examiner monitors the piriformis. (**b**) Passive hip extension and adduction to provoke impingement between the lesser trochanter and ischium. (**c**) Patient with ischiofemoral impingement grabbing the posterior hip during long-stride walking

manner (Fig. 13.7a). Any reproduction of the patient's complaint and the degree of femoroacetabular impingement are noted. FADDIR is traditionally performed as part of the supine assessment.

The lateral rim impingement test is performed with the hip passively abducted and externally rotated (Fig. 13.7b). Reproduction of the patient's pain is scored positive and can be caused by anterior instability or posterior impingement. If the feeling of guarding or anterior pain is present, the test is positive for instability. An apprehension test with a provocative maneuver is also executed in the lateral position (Fig. 13.7c), including a forward force to test anteroinferior instability [13]. Beyond the capsular and teres ligament, this test is also useful to detect acetabular anteroinferior hypoplasia.

Assessment of the posterior extra-articular hip pain is also performed in the lateral decubitus. For the investigation of sciatic nerve entrapment, an active piriformis test is performed [8] (Fig. 13.8a). The active piriformis test recreates the pain as the affected nerve is compressed during the contraction of the piriformis and obturator internus/gemelli complex. Impingement between the lesser trochanter and

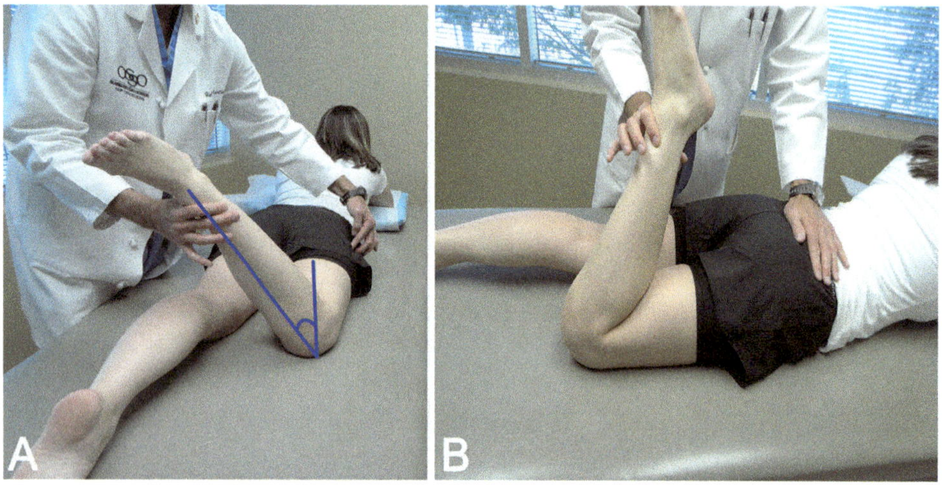

Fig. 13.9 Femoral anteversion and rectus contracture tests. (**a**) Femoral anteversion test. The knee is flexed to 90° and the examiner manually rotates the leg while palpating the greater trochanter. The examiner positions the greater trochanter so that it protrudes most laterally, noting the angle between the axis of the tibia and an imaginary vertical line. (**b**) Rectus contracture test. The lower extremity is flexed toward the gluteus maximus. Any raise of the pelvis or restriction of knee flexion motion is indicative of rectus femoris contracture

ischium can cause posterior pain and is assessed by passive extension of the hip, reproducing the patient's symptoms with the hip adducted and obtaining relief in extension with abduction (Fig. 13.8b, c). These findings are also seen in the ischiofemoral impingement gait, with the patient grabbing the posterior hip lateral to the ischium during long-stride walking, while relieved with short strides.

Prone Examination

The femoral anteversion test, traditionally known as Craig's test [9], will give the examiner an idea of femoral anteversion and retroversion (Fig. 13.9a). Normally, femoral anteversion is between 10° and 20°. In the prone position is also performed the rectus contracture test (also known as Ely test [9]) (Fig. 13.9b).

Hip Snapping Tests

Snapping iliopsoas tendon tests—a fan test (the patient circumducts and rotates the hip in a rotatory fashion)—can help delineate the presence of the snapping iliopsoas tendon over the femoral head or the innominate. Often, this diminishes with an abdominal contraction. A FABER maneuver, followed by extension, can be also performed in assessing the snapping of the iliopsoas tendon over the iliopectineal eminence.

Hip external snapping tests—a hula hoop maneuver, in which the patient stands and twists, or a bicycle test [14] (performed in the lateral position)—can help distinguish the pop internally from the external pop of coxa saltans externus caused by the subluxing iliotibial band over the greater trochanter. The bicycle test is performed with the patient in the lateral position. The motion of a bicycle pedaling pattern is recreated as the examiner monitors the iliotibial band for the detection of coxa saltans externus.

Conclusion

As our understanding of anatomy and biomechanics evolve, the structured physical examination of the hip allows for an assessment of the osseous, capsulolabral, musculotendinous, and neurovascular layers of the hip in the patients who present with hip pain [1]. All layers of the hip are assessed by this battery of tests with 16 assessing the osteochondral layer, 13 the capsulolabral layer, 11 the musculotendinous layer, 7 the neurovascular layer, and 5 the kinematic chain. Sixteen maneuvers or group of maneuvers evaluate more than one layer. A 5-layer diagnosis on each patient should be considered in order to be thorough and comprehensive in organizing diagnostic and treatment strategies.

References

1. Draovitch P, Edelstein J, Kelly BT. The layer concept: utilization in determining the pain generators, pathology and how structure determines treatment. Curr Rev Musculoskelet Med. 2012; 5(1):1–8.

2. Martin HD, Kelly BT, Leunig M, et al. The pattern and technique in the clinical evaluation of the adult hip: the common physical examination tests of hip specialists. Arthroscopy. 2010;26(2):161–72.
3. Cibere J, Thorne A, Bellamy N, et al. Reliability of the hip examination in osteoarthritis: effect of standardization. Arthritis Rheum. 2008;59(3):373–81.
4. Martin HD. Clinical examination of the hip. Oper Tech Orthop. 2005;15:177–81.
5. Byrd JW. Operative hip arthroscopy. New York: Springer; 2005. p. 78–83.
6. Perry J. Gait analysis normal and pathological function. Thorofare: SLACK; 1992.
7. Martin HD, Hatem MA, Champlin K, Palmer IJ. The endoscopic treatment of sciatic nerve entrapment/deep gluteal syndrome. Tech Orthop. 2012;27(3):172–83.
8. Martin HD, Kivlan BR, Palmer IJ, Martin RL. Diagnostic accuracy of clinical tests for sciatic nerve entrapment in the gluteal region. Knee Surg Sports Traumatol Arthrosc. 2014;22(4):882–8.
9. Reider B, Martel J. Pelvis, hip and thigh. In: Reider B, Martel J, editors. The orthopedic physical examination. Philadelphia: WB Saunders; 1999. p. 159–99.
10. Ganz R, Parvizi J, Beck M, Leunig M, Notzli H, Siebenrock KA. Femoroacetabular impingement: a cause for osteoarthritis of the hip. Clin Orthop Relat Res. 2003;417:112–20.
11. McCarthy JC, Busconi BD, Owens BD. Assessment of the painful hip. In: McCarthy JC, editor. Early hip disorders. New York: Springer; 2003. p. 3–6.
12. Philippon M, Zehms C, Briggs K, Manchester D, Kuppersmith D. Hip instability in the athlete. Oper Tech Sports Med. 2007;15:189–94.
13. Martin RL, Palmer I, Martin HD. Ligamentum teres: a functional description and potential clinical relevance. Knee Surg Sports Traumatol Arthrosc. 2012;20(6):1209–14.
14. Plante M, Wallace R, Busconi BD. Clinical diagnosis of hip pain. Clin Sports Med. 2011;30(2):225–38.

Part III

Hip Pathology

Brian D. Busconi

Osteoarthritis of the Hip

14

Matthew A. Popa, Victor M. Goldberg†,
and Glenn D. Wera

Introduction

The concept of primary osteoarthritis (OA) of the hip has undergone a dramatic evolution over the past 50 years, developing into a dynamic field of study encompassing areas of genetics, biology, epidemiology, and anatomy. Historically, primary or idiopathic hip OA develops in adult life, rarely before age 40. This is believed to be due to an undetermined abnormality of the cartilage or subchondral bone, which is abnormally superimposed on grossly normal growth and development of the hip [1]. The disease process is characterized clinically by hyaline cartilage fibrillation and loss, synovial inflammation, ligament laxity, muscle weakness, and periarticular changes in the bone [2]. Originally considered an inevitably progressive, degenerative disease process, primary hip OA is now believed to involve a dynamic process of repair with heterogeneous results, including long periods of minimal change to tissue structure.

The known causes of hip arthrosis are myriad, encompassing primary osteoarthritis and inflammatory arthritides, as well as degeneration brought about secondary to other conditions (Textbox 14.1). In addition, an interplay between avascular necrosis (AVN) and OA can be difficult to distinguish in some cases. Primary hip OA is a diagnosis of exclusion made once other causes have been ruled out. It is characterized by the degeneration of hip articular cartilage with concomitant changes seen in other tissues of the hip joint in the absence of other obvious influences. Most cases of hip arthritis seen in individuals greater than 55 years of age are classified as "primary" or "idiopathic" OA, as there is no gross anatomical abnormality nor any associated comorbidity. Predominant risk factors for the development of hip OA are age, genetic history, and female gender [3]. Increased bone density, obesity, and joint laxity may also play a role in OA [3, 4]. Certain individuals may have a particular hip anatomy that predisposes them to develop hip OA. Subtle morphological differences have been seen in many individuals with degenerative disease of the hip that may actually be the engine of the disease process in that person. One such morphological variation includes femoroacetabular impingement (FAI). FAI indicates that many cases of "idiopathic" OA are actually secondary to subtle changes in hip anatomy. Additionally, increasing evidence of the large influence of genetic factors in the heritability of hip disease in largely European-based populations alludes to hip OA as a distinct entity in comparison to the arthritic degeneration of other joints [5]. The purpose of this chapter is to describe the epidemiology, genetics, pathoanatomy, and biologic factors associated with primary osteoarthritis of the hip.

Textbox 14.1: Common Causes of Hip Arthritis

- Primary idiopathic osteoarthritis
- Inflammatory arthritis (e.g., rheumatoid arthritis, psoriatic arthritis, lupus)
- Crystalline arthropathy (e.g., gout, pseudogout)
- Trauma
- Osteonecrosis
- Sepsis
- Developmental dysplasia
- Skeletal dysplasias (multiple epiphyseal dysplasia, spondyloepiphyseal dysplasia)
- Enzymatic disorders (Gaucher's disease)
- Neuropathic arthropathy (Charcot arthropathy)
- Childhood hip disorders (e.g., SCFE, Legg–Calve–Perthes)
- Paget's disease
- Hemochromatosis
- Dysbarism

M.A. Popa, MD • V.M. Goldberg†, MD • G.D. Wera, MD (✉)
Department of Orthopaedic Surgery, University Hospitals Case Medical Center, 11100 Euclid Ave., Cleveland, OH 44106, USA
e-mail: vmgoldbg@aol.com; matt.popa@gmail.com; gwera@yahoo.com

J.C. McCarthy et al. (eds.), *Hip Joint Restoration*, DOI 10.1007/978-1-4614-0694-5_14

Textbox 14.2: Kellgren–Lawrence Grading Scale

Grade	Radiographic features
0	No features of osteoarthritis
1	Doubtful: questionable osteophytes or questionable joint space narrowing
2	Minimal: definitive small osteophytes, little or mild joint space narrowing
3	Moderate: definitive moderate osteophytes, joint space narrowing >50 %
4	Severe: joint space impaired severely, cysts and sclerosis of subchondral bone

Epidemiology and Economic Burden

The difficulty in determining the true prevalence of hip OA in a population lies in the general problem of identifying the presence of arthritis in an individual due to the discrepancy between clinical presentation and radiographic evidence. Several studies have attempted to quantify the prevalence of hip OA, but there are no standard criteria that are used. The radiographic definition involves a radiographic scoring system of some form; the system most commonly used is the Kellgren–Lawrence scale [6] (Textbox 14.2).

Self-reported criteria utilize patients reporting a prior diagnosis of OA to an investigator. The symptomatic definition of OA considers patients with joint-related symptoms in addition to radiographic evidence. A systematic review by Pereira et al. to understand the differences in prevalence and incidence estimates of OA in the knee, hand, and hip found a higher prevalence of OA when a radiographic definition was used [7]. Osteoarthritis prevalence determined by self-reported criteria or by a symptomatic definition yielded similar estimates.

Considerable variability exists in comparison of the prevalence of hip osteoarthritis between countries. A higher prevalence is seen in many European countries or in those countries with a large European influence in the population such as the United States. Distinctly lower rates of hip OA are seen in many African and Asian countries. Radiographic surveys have shown rates of primary hip OA of 0.4 % in Hong Kong, 0.5 % in South Africa, and 0.1 % in India [5]. A prevalence of 1 % was seen in Japan [8] and China [9] when a radiographic definition was used. Comparatively, 7.0 % of patients in the United Kingdom had radiographic evidence of hip OA with another study showing an overall rate of 4.0 % in European patients [5]. This rate is double that is seen in Jamaican [10], black African, and American Indian populations (2 %) [5]. Using the symptomatic definition, a low percentage of hip OA has been found in Turkey (1 %) [11], Greece (0.9 %) [12], and Italy (1.6 %) [13].

Combining symptomatic criteria with radiographic evidence, studies have found an estimated prevalence of hip OA of 3 % in the United States [14], 5 % in France [15], and 7.4 % in Spain [16]. A prevalence of 9.7 % was seen in the Netherlands when self-reported criteria were used [17]. These numbers are not seen in individuals of non-European descent living in the United States. In comparison to whites of European ancestry, those of Chinese, African, Japanese, or Hispanic descent living in the United States have low rates of hip arthroplasty for primary hip OA, but comparable rates of hip replacement for other causes of hip disease. Osteonecrosis is much more frequent in Asian and African populations [18, 19], and developmental dysplasia is the most common cause of hip OA in the Japanese population [20]. While racial differences may be seen, significant differences in the prevalence of hip OA between men and women do not appear to exist [21].

Hip osteoarthritis as a disease process poses a huge economic burden on the societies in which it is prevalent. In the United States alone, the number of older adults with arthritis or other chronic musculoskeletal joint symptoms is projected to almost double from 21.4 million in 2005 to 41.1 million by 2030 [22]. As the elderly population in many developed countries assumes a greater percentage of the overall census, the medical costs attributable to hip osteoarthritis are expected to increase accordingly. In 2009, Bitton estimated the direct medical costs of hip osteoarthritis may exceed $100 billion dollars per year, with indirect costs possibly 1.5 times greater than the direct costs [23]. The US Centers for Disease Control and Prevention's National Hospital Discharge Database shows that over 330,000 primary total hip arthroplasties were performed in the United States in 2010. By 2030, that number is projected to reach 572,000 procedures [24]. As the total direct healthcare costs of total hip arthroplasty (THA) currently approach $100,000 per patient [25], it is readily apparent that the economic impact of hip OA treatment will continue to have a profound effect on the healthcare system.

Genetic Influence of Hip Osteoarthritis

Hip osteoarthritis appears to be significantly influenced by genetic factors. Family and twin studies have demonstrated an estimated heritability for primary OA of 50–60 % [26]. These results are similar to heritability rates of radiological knee and hand OA which have been estimated between 39 and 65 % following a study on British female twins [27]. The genetic influence on cartilage volume, increased relative risk for hip OA, and the need for THA in siblings have been demonstrated in a number of studies [28, 29].

A genetic basis for the multifactorial etiology of osteoarthritis, at least in part, has been well established, but the identification of the causative genes is an ongoing process. Two genes, deiodinase iodothyronine type 2 (*DIO2*) and growth differentiation factor 5 (*GDF5*), have been found to be consistently associated with hip OA [30–32]. More specifically, a single nucleotide polymorphism (SNP) associated with each gene has demonstrated an increased odds ratio for the development of hip OA. *DIO2* is associated with an increased risk in Caucasians, while *GDF5* is linked with hip OA development in Asian populations [31]. Candidate gene association studies have identified a number of other potential OA-associated genes including asporin (*ASPN*), *FRZB*, and *PTGS2* [31]. Some of these genes including *GDF5* and *ASPN* are involved in the bone morphogenetic protein signaling pathway. *DIO2* encodes an intracellular enzyme in the thyroid pathway, and it has been associated with a specific hip shape, causing nonoptimal hip geometry [33].

Pathoanatomy

The theory of FAI had its earliest foundation laid in the 1960s with the work of Murray. He initially suggested that the development of OA of the hip was related to either a previously unrecognized acetabular dysplasia or a rather subtle deformity of the proximal femur, which he termed the "tilt deformity" [34]. In patients with hip OA, he identified a 37 % incidence of dysplasia in women and a 74 % incidence of femoral head tilt in men [34]. He concluded that 90 % of hip OA was secondary to these deformities [35]. His theory was picked up and extended by Solomon in South Africa and Harris in the United States. Harris felt that the majority of cases thought to be primary or idiopathic hip OA were actually secondary to mild developmental abnormalities [1]. With further characterization provided by Ganz and others recently, FAI has gained notable credence as a theory for the development of primary hip OA in many individuals.

Severe deformity has long been recognized as a cause of the development of hip OA. "Obvious" deformities, such as those secondary to severe trauma, slipped capital femoral epiphysis, Legg–Calve–Perthes disease, developmental dysplasia, as well as other causes of secondary OA (e.g., inflammatory disease, infection, osteonecrosis), are excluded from the theory of FAI. Significant deformity causes focal overloading of hip cartilage secondary to reduced contact area. This increased contact stress leads to subsequent degeneration. Murray's work suggested that hip OA could develop secondary to subtle, sometimes previously unrecognized deformities that occurred before skeletal maturation. This subtle deformity maintains a congruent joint which implies a different arthritic process. Postmortem studies confirm that certain femoral geometries correlate with acetabular wear and arthritis of the hip [36].

The morphological subtleties described in FAI occur on both the acetabular and the femoral side of the hip joint. The process is termed "pincer" FAI when the acetabulum is involved, whereas "cam" FAI describes femoral involvement. Purely pincer or purely cam impingement may exist, but more commonly there is a mixed deformity in which each aspect of the joint is slightly abnormal. Acetabular deformity is more common in women, while femoral changes predominate in men. Pincer deformity typically develops and manifests later in life than cam FAI does, and it mainly affects women between the ages of 30 and 40 [35]. Active men in the third decade tend to experience cam FAI [35].

As pathologic hip deformity can be subtle in impingement, the anatomical nuances that produce FAI went largely unnoticed for years. Defining "normal" and "abnormal" anatomy as seen on radiographs is critical. The most commonly utilized views when evaluating a hip for impingement are an AP (anteroposterior) pelvis, a frog-leg lateral of the hip, and a cross-table lateral of the hip. Additionally, a 45° or 90° Dunn view and a false-profile view may be helpful. The Dunn view is performed with the patient supine on the x-ray table, and the symptomatic hip is flexed to either 45° or 90° and abducted 20° while being maintained in a position of neutral rotation [37] (Fig. 14.1).

The radiographic evaluation of femoral anatomy for FAI predominantly assesses the sphericity of the femoral head. A femoral head that is nonspherical at the anterosuperior head–neck junction is the most common anatomical variant in cam impingement. Anterosuperior femoral head nonsphericity is quantified by the measurement of the alpha angle. This angle is formed by two lines: (1) a line between the center of the femoral head and the center of the femoral neck and (2) the line between the center of the femoral head and the point at the femoral head–neck contour where the radius of the femoral head diverges from the femoral neck [38] (Fig. 14.2). Studies using both radiographs and MRI to measure the alpha angle have shown a consistent increase in symptomatic patients with signs of FAI. FAI patients generally have alpha angles greater than 70°, whereas the angle is reliably 50° or less in control patients [38, 39]. Based on these consistent results, an alpha angle of 55° has been proposed to be diagnostic of FAI. Beaule demonstrated that patients with cam-type FAI and an alpha angle of 65° or more are at increased risk of significant acetabular cartilage damage [40]. Alpha angle is an independent predictor of the risk for progression to THA. A long-term case control over 20 years demonstrated that patients with THA had a higher prevalence of cam deformity (median alpha angle 62.4°) than did control patients (median alpha angle 45.8°) [41]. In patients with cam FAI, the alpha angle of the anterosuperior aspect of the femoral head is reliably the greatest, and the posteroinferior aspect of the femoral head measures the least [42]. The Dunn view in 45° or 90° of flexion and a cross-table hip radiograph in internal rotation are the best radiographs to assess femoral head–neck asphericity [39].

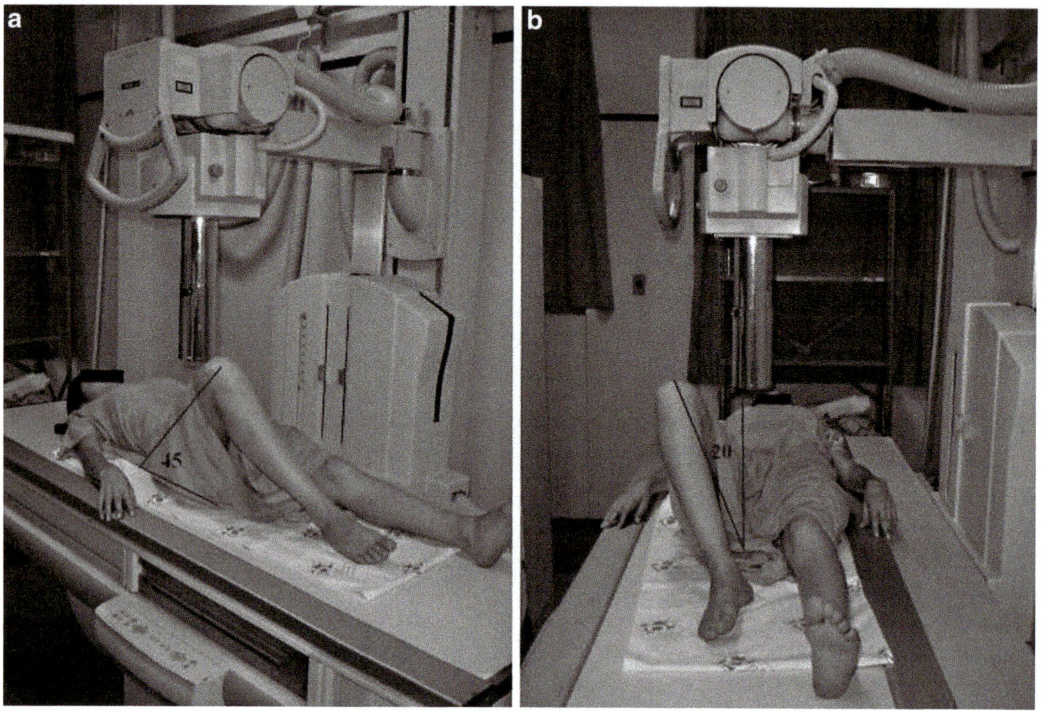

Fig. 14.1 (**a**, **b**) Dunn radiographic view is performed with the symptomatic hip at either 45° or 90° of flexion with 20° abduction and neutral rotation. The beam is centered on the hip. From Barros HJM et al. Femoral head–neck junction deformity is related to osteoarthritis of the hip. Clin Orthop Relat Res 2010;468:1923. Reprinted with permission from Springer

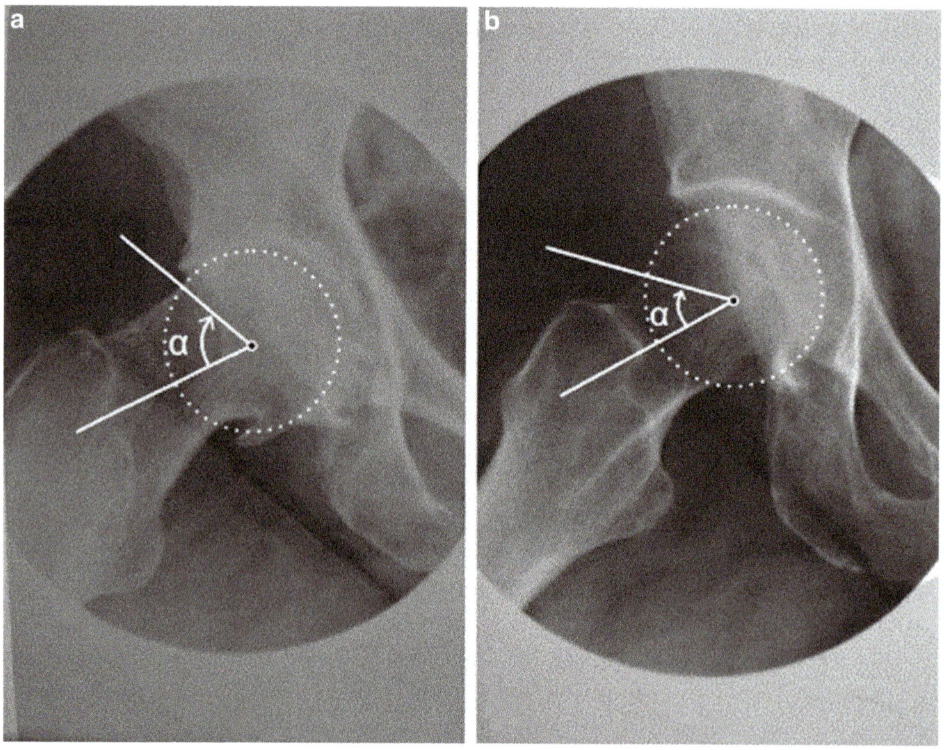

Fig. 14.2 The alpha angle is determined by the angle between the neck axis and a line connecting the center of the femoral head with the point at which the femoral head–neck junction exits an ideally spherical femoral head. (**a**) A right hip with severe OA, with an increased alpha angle, and (**b**) a right hip without OA, with a normal alpha angle, are shown. From Barros HJM et al. Femoral head–neck junction deformity is related to osteoarthritis of the hip. Clin Orthop Relat Res 2010;468:1923. Reprinted with permission from Springer

Determination of acetabular morphology is integral to the diagnosis and treatment of FAI. The predominant acetabular variations that produce impingement are acetabular retroversion, coxa profunda, or coxa protrusio. Acetabular retroversion, particularly cranial acetabular retroversion, indicates that the anterior acetabular rim is more lateral than the posterior rim in the superior portion of the acetabulum. In coxa profunda, the floor of the acetabulum touches or overlaps the

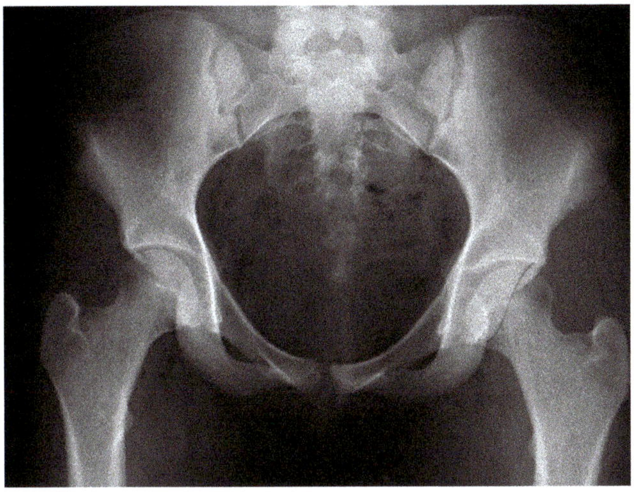

Fig. 14.3 A well-centered anteroposterior radiograph of the pelvis is shown, demonstrating a crossover sign with the anterior wall of the acetabulum (*dotted line*) meeting the posterior wall (*solid line*) in the middle of the acetabulum instead of meeting at the superolateral margin of the acetabulum. This relationship of the anterior and posterior acetabular margins is suggestive of acetabular retroversion. From Grissom L, Harcke HT, Thacker M. Imaging in the surgical management of developmental dislocation of the hip. Clin Orthop Relat Res 2008;466:793. Reprinted with permission from Springer

ilioischial line on a normal AP pelvis radiograph. Protrusio refers to overlapping of the ilioischial line by the femoral head. Assessment of the acetabulum can be difficult on a standard AP pelvis radiograph due to its complex three-dimensional structure. Computed tomography is the most accurate method to measure acetabular version. On an AP radiograph, acetabular version can be estimated by the presence of the "crossover sign." The crossover sign occurs when the most proximal anterior acetabular rim appears lateral to the posterior rim, creating a figure eight and suggesting acetabular retroversion above this level [43] (Fig. 14.3). The crossover sign has been shown to reliably predict a cranial acetabular version of less than 4° [44].

Pincer impingement is produced when there is either local (e.g., acetabular retroversion) or global (e.g., coxa profunda or protrusio) overcoverage of the femoral head by the acetabulum (Fig. 14.4a, b). This abnormal coverage leads to linear impact of the acetabular rim against the femoral head–neck junction with certain movements of the hip. With prolonged impact of the acetabular rim, the first substance to fail is the labrum [45]. Intrasubstance fissuring and ganglion formation are initially seen [35]. Labral damage is the initial cause of pain in pincer FAI as it is a well-innervated structure. This damage is likely the reason for more pronounced symptoms seen with pincer FAI than the cam variety. Over time, a contrecoup mechanism develops with the femur levering off of the acetabular overcoverage leading to the development of posteroinferior or central OA [35]. Posteroinferior cartilage lesions are a characteristic finding on MR arthrograms of patients with pincer FAI [42].

A nonspherical extension of the femoral head is the deformity found in cam FAI (Fig. 14.4c, d). This nonsphericity is most commonly seen in the anterolateral aspect of the head–neck junction. Often it is not visible on a routine AP x-ray of the pelvis. It has been shown that the deformity is most commonly an abnormality of the capital femoral epiphysis [45]. Long-term studies have demonstrated that several etiologies for a cam lesion exist, namely, mild SCFE, Perthes disease, multiple epiphyseal dysplasia, and spondyloepiphyseal dysplasia [1, 35, 46–48]. The process of cam impingement occurs differently from the pincer variety. The femoral lesion impacts into the acetabular cartilage and the labrum is largely untouched in the early stages. The diminished labral involvement causes symptoms to be less pronounced, but the process is more destructive than its pincer counterpart. Tannast et al. demonstrated that the typical location of early chondrolabral damage is located in the anterosuperior quadrant of the acetabulum [49]. Eventually, the cartilage and subchondral bone in this area degenerate, which may lead to labral tear or avulsion.

Significant uncertainty remains as to whether FAI is the dominant cause of primary hip OA. The genetics and epidemiology of hip impingement seem to mirror that of hip OA, as siblings of patients with FAI have an increased prevalence of the same pathology. Populations that have lower rates of primary hip OA, such as Japanese and Chinese patients, also report lower rates of FAI [20]. The causative nature of FAI in the disease process is still being questioned. Several studies have demonstrated that the prevalence of FAI does not necessarily correlate with an increased rate of coxarthrosis in the same subpopulation. A long-term study of middle-aged Greek patients found that only 18 % of those with FAI developed hip OA after 19-year follow-up [50]. Japanese persons overall have a significantly smaller center-edge angle than British persons as well as a much higher incidence of dysplasia [8], but the rate of primary OA is much lower in Japan. Similarly, black and Polynesian populations with a higher incidence of SCFE do not display the same rate of primary OA as Caucasian populations [51].

Biology of Hip Osteoarthritis

The osteoarthritic process is no longer viewed from the purely mechanistic standpoint of unrelenting progressive "wear and tear" of the cartilage leading to a degenerative joint. Biological and biochemical processes in the bone, cartilage, and other periarticular tissues play an important role in the development of OA. Significant focus has been given to uncovering these molecular processes associated with primary OA.

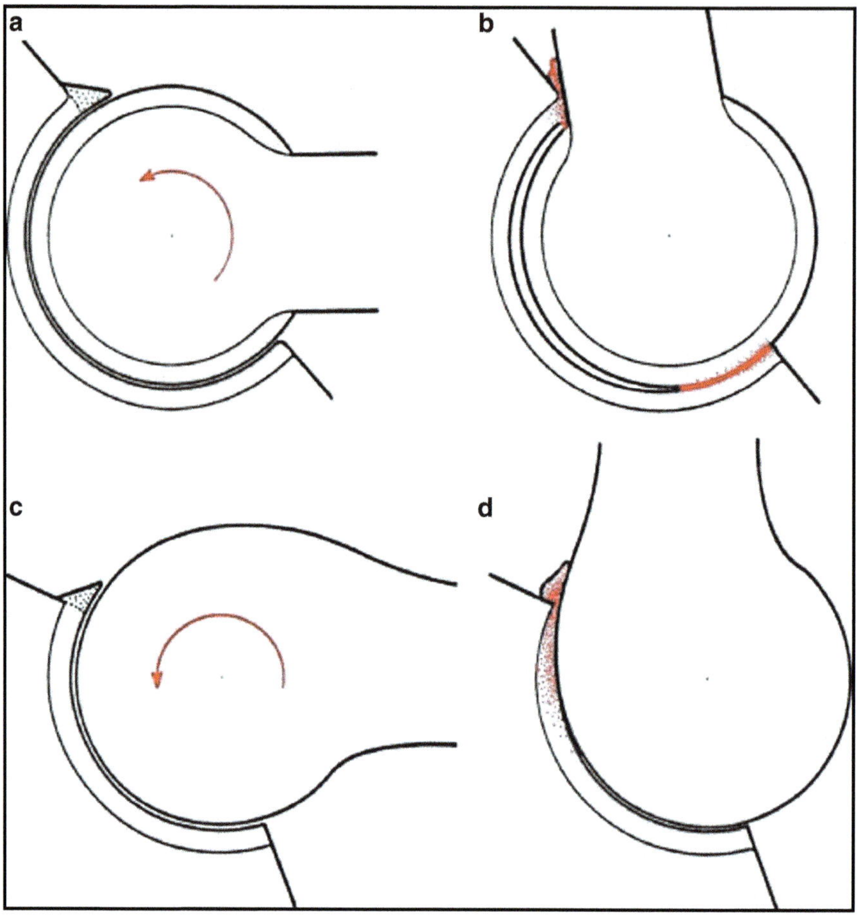

Fig. 14.4 Diagrams illustrate the proposed mechanisms of joint damage in FAI. (**a**) Acetabular overcoverage of the femoral head leads to linear impact of the acetabular rim against the femoral head–neck junction, often leading to early labral damage. The persistent abutment with chronic leverage of the head in the acetabulum sometimes results in chondral injury to the "contrecoup" region of the posteroinferior acetabulum. (**b**) In cam FAI, a nonspherical femoral head (**c**) is forced into the acetabulum with flexion and internal rotation of the hip (**d**). The early damage occurs to the acetabular cartilage with the labrum often spared initially. From Ganz R et al. The etiology of osteoarthritis of the hip: an integrated mechanical concept. Clin Orthop Relat Res 2008;466(2):268. Reprinted with permission from Springer

Articular Cartilage Biology

The degenerative changes seen in articular cartilage are partially driven by the activation of chondrocytes [52], initially at the layers closest to the joint surface where shear stress is the greatest [53]. Mechanical and inflammatory factors induce chondrocyte activation through the stimulation of the nuclear factor kappa-light-chain-enhancer of activated B cells (NF-κB) and stress-induced and mitogen-activated protein kinase (MAPK) pathways [54]. This activation leads to increased cell proliferation as well as increased production of matrix proteins and matrix-degrading enzymes. Mechanical stimulation on the cartilage and subchondral bone induces signals for the production of degradative enzymes. These enzymes include matrix metalloproteinases (MMPs) and ADAMTS (a disintegrin and metalloproteinase with thrombospondin motifs, also known as aggrecanases) proteases, which can lead to irreversible collagen matrix degradation [54]. In a mouse surgical model, ADAMTS-5-knockout mice were protected against OA progression, indicating the importance of matrix proteoglycan degradation and depletion [55].

The importance of the wingless mouse mammary tumor virus integration (Wnt) pathway has been demonstrated to influence the contribution from the cartilage and bone on OA development. Wnt proteins are important components in the embryonic development and maintenance of both bone and cartilage tissue. This protein family also appears to play an important role in OA progression. Activation of Wnt signaling through Frizzled receptors may lead to matrix destruction, whereas inhibitors of Wnt activation may have a protective effect [54]. Overexpression of Wnt-induced signaling protein-1 (WISP-1) induced an increased expression of MMPs and aggrecanases, leading to extracellular cartilage matrix damage in a murine knee joint model [56].

Bone Biology

While OA is often considered to be a disease primarily of articular cartilage, the alteration of the cartilage matrix may actually be secondary to changes in the bony microenvironment with a complex interplay of multiple growth factors and signaling molecules. Bone changes in OA are often seen prior to changes in cartilage as the bone has a more rapid capacity for alteration in response to stress [54]. As the arthritic process develops, the subchondral cortical bone becomes sclerotic early on, with increased mechanical stress. This bony response may be responsible for a downregulation of sclerostin, a protein which acts as an inhibitor of the Wnt signaling pathway [57]. The end result of this process appears to be that the sclerotic subchondral bone actually causes diminished bone mineral density in the underlying trabecular bone [58].

Molecular regulation in bone-forming osteoblasts influences bone mass, structure, and function, and it may contribute to the pathological process in OA. Growth factors, such as insulin-like growth factor-1 (IGF-1), that increase osteoblastic activity and lead to increased bone mass may stimulate osteophyte formation [59]. The effect of these growth factors may explain the higher bone mineral density that has been shown around arthritic joints [2]. This abnormal osteoblastic activity appears to negatively impact bony remodeling as well maintenance of normal cartilage matrix. Altered levels of expression are seen in numerous proteins including RANK ligand, osteoprotegerin, cathepsin K, and matrix metalloproteinase 9, which can have detrimental effects on both bone and cartilage homeostasis [60]. When co-incubated with cartilage cultures, osteoblasts from the bone of patients with OA have the ability to modulate cartilage metabolism in a manner not seen with osteoblasts from patients who do not have joint disease [61].

The Wnt and tissue growth factor beta (TFG-β) pathways are two signaling pathways that are currently areas of intense research. Wnt-related molecules have been shown to be critically involved in OA development, as differential Wnt expression correlates with cartilage destruction [62]. Additionally, increased Wnt signaling induces the expression of MMPs which promote cartilage catabolism [63]. Wnt molecules also affect bone tissue and may be related to bony sclerosis and the formation of osteophytes seen around arthritic joints [2].

At least four Wnt signaling pathways exist. The Wnt/β-catenin pathway is defined by the cytoplasmic accumulation of β-catenin, which then translocates to the nucleus of the cell where it activates a number of transcription factors [64]. This pathway is the most studied of the Wnt protein family, and it appears to be particularly important to bone biology. The altered expression of Wnt-related proteins likely has implications for the altered bone remodeling and the production of degradative enzymes seen in hip OA [2, 64]. The TGF-β signaling pathway has a significant role in the development and function of the osteoblast, and differential expression of TGF-β molecules has also been found in the bone of OA patients [65]. The production of TGF-β, bone morphogenetic protein 2 (BMP-2), and other growth factors has been implicated in osteophyte formation [66, 67]. The complete functional role of these pathways is still unknown, but the molecules involved offer promising targets for therapy aimed at the treatment and possible prevention of OA.

Synovium Biology

Inflammation of the synovium is found in joints affected by inflammatory arthritis as well as osteoarthritis. Synovitis may be seen in the early stages of OA, but its prevalence increases as the disease process advances [68, 69]. Synovitis has been shown to strongly correlate with symptomatic joint pain [68, 70, 71]. Ample evidence exists to suggest the influence of synovial inflammation on OA progression. In a study of 514 patients with knee pain but lacking radiographic evidence of knee OA, the presence of an effusion and synovitis was associated with the development of cartilage erosion based on MRI findings [72]. The degeneration of the articular extracellular matrix in OA appears to exacerbate synovitis through activation of various pro-inflammatory mechanisms, including Toll-like receptors and the complement cascade [73]. These pathways as well as the chemokines and cytokines associated with joint inflammation are the subjects of intense research as potential targets for OA treatment.

Conclusion

Osteoarthritis of the hip is now understood to be a multifaceted disease composed of a complex interplay of biological, genetic, and anatomic factors. As our understanding of this dynamic process increases, so too does the realization that our functional knowledge of the role of each component remains incomplete. Continuing investigations into the surgical treatment of FAI indicate the possibility of joint preservation if appropriately addressed, but greater long-term studies are needed. Pharmaceutical therapy targeted at specific genes or molecular signaling pathways are not yet available. Currently, the only definitive treatment for hip OA is joint arthroplasty, which occurs long after the disease has developed. The paradigm from treatment of hip osteoarthritis to its prevention continues to shift as we uncover new information about this complex disease.

References

1. Harris WH. Etiology of osteoarthritis of the hip. Clin Orthop Relat Res. 1986;213:20–33.
2. Kumarasinghe DD, Hopwood B, Kuliwaba JS, Atkins GJ, Fazzalari NL. An update on primary hip osteoarthritis including altered Wnt and TGF-β associated gene expression from the bony component of the disease. Rheumatology (Oxford). 2011;50(12):2166–75.

3. Buckwalter JA, Saltzman C, Brown T. The impact of osteoarthritis: implications for research. Clin Orthop Relat Res. 2004; (427 Suppl):S6–15.
4. Cooper C, Snow S, McAlindon TE, Kellingray S, Stuart B, Coggon D, et al. Risk factors for the incidence and progression of radiographic knee osteoarthritis. Arthritis Rheum. 2000;43(5): 995–1000.
5. Hoaglund FT. Primary osteoarthritis of the hip: a genetic disease caused by European genetic variants. J Bone Joint Surg Am. 2013;95(5):463–8.
6. Reijman M, Hazes JM, Koes BW, Verhagen AP, Bierma-Zeinstra SM. Validity, reliability, and applicability of seven definitions of hip osteoarthritis used in epidemiological studies: a systematic appraisal. Ann Rheum Dis. 2004;63(3):226–32.
7. Pereira D, Peleteiro B, Araújo J, Branco J, Santos RA, Ramos E. The effect of osteoarthritis definition on prevalence and incidence estimates: a systematic review. Osteoarthritis Cartilage. 2011;19(11):1270–85.
8. Yoshimura N, Campbell L, Hashimoto T, Kinoshita H, Okayasu T, Wilman C, et al. Acetabular dysplasia and hip osteoarthritis in Britain and Japan. Br J Rheumatol. 1998;37(11):1193–7.
9. Nevitt MC, Xu L, Zhang Y, Lui LY, Yu W, Lane NE, et al. Very low prevalence of hip osteoarthritis among Chinese elderly in Beijing, China, compared with whites in the United States: the Beijing osteoarthritis study. Arthritis Rheum. 2002;46(7):1773–9.
10. Bremner JM, Lawrence JS, Miall WE. Degenerative joint disease in a Jamaican rural population. Ann Rheum Dis. 1968;27(4): 326–32.
11. Yeşil H, Hepgüler S, Öztürk C, Çapacı K, Yeşil M. Prevalence of symptomatic knee, hand and hip osteoarthritis among individuals 40 years or older: a study conducted in İzmir city. Acta Orthop Traumatol Turc. 2013;47(4):231–5.
12. Andrianakos AA, Kontelis LK, Karamitsos DG, Aslanidis SI, Georgountzos AI, Kaziolas GO, et al. Prevalence of symptomatic knee, hand, and hip osteoarthritis in Greece. The ESORDIG study. J Rheumatol. 2006;33(12):2507–13.
13. Salaffi F, Carotti M, Stancati A, Grassi W. Health-related quality of life in older adults with symptomatic hip and knee osteoarthritis: a comparison with matched healthy controls. Aging Clin Exp Res. 2005;17(4):255–63.
14. Felson DT, Lawrence RC, Dieppe PA, Hirsch R, Helmick CG, Jordan JM, et al. Osteoarthritis: new insights. Part 1: the disease and its risk factors. Ann Intern Med. 2000;133(8):635–46.
15. Roux CH, Saraux A, Mazieres B, Pouchot J, Morvan J, Fautrel B, et al. Screening for hip and knee osteoarthritis in the general population: predictive value of a questionnaire and prevalence estimates. Ann Rheum Dis. 2008;67(10):1406–11.
16. Quintana JM, Arostegui I, Escobar A, Azkarate J, Goenaga JI, Lafuente I. Prevalence of knee and hip osteoarthritis and the appropriateness of joint replacement in an older population. Arch Intern Med. 2008;168(14):1576–84.
17. Nho SJ, Kymes SM, Callaghan JJ, Felson DT. The burden of hip osteoarthritis in the United States: epidemiologic and economic considerations. J Am Acad Orthop Surg. 2013;21 Suppl 1:S1–6.
18. Kang JS, Park S, Song JH, Jung YY, Cho MR, Rhyu KH. Prevalence of osteonecrosis of the femoral head: a nationwide epidemiologic analysis in Korea. J Arthroplasty. 2009;24(8):1178–83.
19. Lubega N, Mkandawire NC, Sibande GC, Norrish AR, Harrison WJ. Joint replacement in Malawi: establishment of a National Joint Registry. J Bone Joint Surg Br. 2009;91(3):341–3.
20. Takeyama A, Naito M, Shiramizu K, Kiyama T. Prevalence of femoroacetabular impingement in Asian patients with osteoarthritis of the hip. Int Orthop. 2009;33(5):1229–32.
21. Lawrence RC, Felson DT, Helmick CG, Arnold LM, Choi H, Deyo RA, et al. Estimates of the prevalence of arthritis and other rheumatic conditions in the United States. Part II. Arthritis Rheum. 2008;58(1):26–35.
22. Leveille SG. Musculoskeletal aging. Curr Opin Rheumatol. 2004;16(2):114–8.
23. Bitton R. The economic burden of osteoarthritis. Am J Manag Care. 2009;15(8 Suppl):S230–5.
24. Kurtz S, Ong K, Lau E, Mowat F, Halpern M. Projections of primary and revision hip and knee arthroplasty in the United States from 2005 to 2030. J Bone Joint Surg Am. 2007;89(4):780–5.
25. Lovald ST, Ong KL, Lau EC, Schmier JK, Bozic KJ, Kurtz SM. Mortality, cost, and downstream disease of total hip arthroplasty patients in the medicare population. J Arthroplasty. 2014;29(1):242–6.
26. Spector TD, MacGregor AJ. Risk factors for osteoarthritis: genetics. Osteoarthritis Cartilage. 2004;12 Suppl A:S39–44.
27. Spector TD, Cicuttini F, Baker J, Loughlin J, Hart D. Genetic influences on osteoarthritis in women: a twin study. BMJ. 1996; 312(7036):940–3.
28. Hunter DJ, Snieder H, March L, Sambrook PN. Genetic contribution to cartilage volume in women: a classical twin study. Rheumatology (Oxford). 2003;42(12):1495–500.
29. Chitnavis J, Sinsheimer JS, Clipsham K, Loughlin J, Sykes B, Burge PD, et al. Genetic influences in end-stage osteoarthritis. Sibling risks of hip and knee replacement for idiopathic osteoarthritis. J Bone Joint Surg Br. 1997;79(4):660–4.
30. Meulenbelt I, Min JL, Bos S, Riyazi N, Houwing-Duistermaat JJ, van der Wijk HJ, et al. Identification of DIO2 as a new susceptibility locus for symptomatic osteoarthritis. Hum Mol Genet. 2008;17(12):1867–75.
31. Chapman K, Valdes AM. Genetic factors in OA pathogenesis. Bone. 2012;51(2):258–64.
32. Kerkhof HJ, Lories RJ, Meulenbelt I, Jonsdottir I, Valdes AM, Arp P, et al. A genome-wide association study identifies an osteoarthritis susceptibility locus on chromosome 7q22. Arthritis Rheum. 2010; 62(2):499–510.
33. Waarsing JH, Kloppenburg M, Slagboom PE, Kroon HM, Houwing-Duistermaat JJ, Weinans H, et al. Osteoarthritis susceptibility genes influence the association between hip morphology and osteoarthritis. Arthritis Rheum. 2011;63(5):1349–54.
34. Murray RO. The aetiology of primary osteoarthritis of the hip. Br J Radiol. 1965;38(455):810–24.
35. Ganz R, Leunig M, Leunig-Ganz K, Harris WH. The etiology of osteoarthritis of the hip: an integrated mechanical concept. Clin Orthop Relat Res. 2008;466(2):264–72.
36. Streit JJ, Levine A, Barrett IJ, Cooperman DR, Goldberg V. The shape of the proximal femur influences acetabular wear patterns over time. Clin Orthop Relat Res. 2013;471(2):478–85.
37. Clohisy JC, Carlisle JC, Beaulé PE, Kim YJ, Trousdale RT, Sierra RJ, et al. A systematic approach to the plain radiographic evaluation of the young adult hip. J Bone Joint Surg Am. 2008;90 Suppl 4:47–66.
38. Nötzli HP, Wyss TF, Stoecklin CH, Schmid MR, Treiber K, Hodler J. The contour of the femoral head-neck junction as a predictor for the risk of anterior impingement. J Bone Joint Surg Br. 2002;84(4): 556–60.
39. Meyer DC, Beck M, Ellis T, Ganz R, Leunig M. Comparison of six radiographic projections to assess femoral head/neck asphericity. Clin Orthop Relat Res. 2006;445:181–5.
40. Beaulé PE, Hynes K, Parker G, Kemp KA. Can the alpha angle assessment of cam impingement predict acetabular cartilage delamination? Clin Orthop Relat Res. 2012;470(12):3361–7.
41. Nicholls AS, Kiran A, Pollard TC, Hart DJ, Arden CP, Spector T, et al. The association between hip morphology parameters and nineteen-year risk of end-stage osteoarthritis of the hip: a nested case-control study. Arthritis Rheum. 2011;63(11):3392–400.

42. Pfirrmann CW, Mengiardi B, Dora C, Kalberer F, Zanetti M, Hodler J. Cam and pincer femoroacetabular impingement: characteristic MR arthrographic findings in 50 patients. Radiology. 2006;240(3):778–85.
43. Reynolds D, Lucas J, Klaue K. Retroversion of the acetabulum. A cause of hip pain. J Bone Joint Surg Br. 1999;81(2):281–8.
44. Jamali AA, Mladenov K, Meyer DC, Martinez A, Beck M, Ganz R, et al. Anteroposterior pelvic radiographs to assess acetabular retroversion: high validity of the "cross-over-sign". J Orthop Res. 2007;25(6):758–65.
45. Ganz R, Parvizi J, Beck M, Leunig M, Nötzli H, Siebenrock KA. Femoroacetabular impingement: a cause for osteoarthritis of the hip. Clin Orthop Relat Res. 2003;417:112–20.
46. Solomon L. Patterns of osteoarthritis of the hip. J Bone Joint Surg Br. 1976;58(2):176–83.
47. Harris WH, Bourne RB, Oh I. Intra-articular acetabular labrum: a possible etiological factor in certain cases of osteoarthritis of the hip. J Bone Joint Surg Am. 1979;61(4):510–4.
48. Solomon L. Geographical and anatomical patterns of osteoarthritis. Br J Rheumatol. 1984;23(3):177–80.
49. Tannast M, Goricki D, Beck M, Murphy SB, Siebenrock KA. Hip damage occurs at the zone of femoroacetabular impingement. Clin Orthop Relat Res. 2008;466(2):273–80.
50. Hartofilakidis G, Bardakos NV, Babis GC, Georgiades G. An examination of the association between different morphotypes of femoroacetabular impingement in asymptomatic subjects and the development of osteoarthritis of the hip. J Bone Joint Surg Br. 2011;93(5):580–6.
51. Hoaglund FT, Steinbach LS. Primary osteoarthritis of the hip: etiology and epidemiology. J Am Acad Orthop Surg. 2001;9(5):320–7.
52. Goldring MB, Marcu KB. Cartilage homeostasis in health and rheumatic diseases. Arthritis Res Ther. 2009;11(3):224.
53. Andriacchi TP, Mündermann A, Smith RL, Alexander EJ, Dyrby CO, Koo S. A framework for the in vivo pathomechanics of osteoarthritis at the knee. Ann Biomed Eng. 2004;32(3):447–57.
54. Loeser RF, Goldring SR, Scanzello CR, Goldring MB. Osteoarthritis: a disease of the joint as an organ. Arthritis Rheum. 2012;64(6):1697–707.
55. Glasson SS, Askew R, Sheppard B, Carito B, Blanchet T, Ma HL, et al. Deletion of active ADAMTS5 prevents cartilage degradation in a murine model of osteoarthritis. Nature. 2005;434(7033):644–8.
56. Blom AB, Brockbank SM, van Lent PL, van Beuningen HM, Geurts J, Takahashi N, et al. Involvement of the Wnt signaling pathway in experimental and human osteoarthritis: prominent role of Wnt-induced signaling protein 1. Arthritis Rheum. 2009;60(2):501–12.
57. Chan BY, Fuller ES, Russell AK, Smith SM, Smith MM, Jackson MT, et al. Increased chondrocyte sclerostin may protect against cartilage degradation in osteoarthritis. Osteoarthritis Cartilage. 2011;19(7):874–85.
58. Karvonen RL, Miller PR, Nelson DA, Granda JL, Fernández-Madrid F. Periarticular osteoporosis in osteoarthritis of the knee. J Rheumatol. 1998;25(11):2187–94.
59. Massicotte F, Fernandes JC, Martel-Pelletier J, Pelletier JP, Lajeunesse D. Modulation of insulin-like growth factor 1 levels in human osteoarthritic subchondral bone osteoblasts. Bone. 2006;38(3):333–41.
60. Logar DB, Komadina R, Prezelj J, Ostanek B, Trost Z, Marc J. Expression of bone resorption genes in osteoarthritis and in osteoporosis. J Bone Miner Metab. 2007;25(4):219–25.
61. Westacott C. Interactions between subchondral bone and cartilage in OA. Cells from osteoarthritic bone can alter cartilage metabolism. J Musculoskelet Neuronal Interact. 2002;2(6):507–9.
62. Chun JS, Oh H, Yang S, Park M. Wnt signaling in cartilage development and degeneration. BMB Rep. 2008;41(7):485–94.
63. Velasco J, Zarrabeitia MT, Prieto JR, Perez-Castrillon JL, Perez-Aguilar MD, Perez-Nuñez MI, et al. Wnt pathway genes in osteoporosis and osteoarthritis: differential expression and genetic association study. Osteoporos Int. 2010;21(1):109–18.
64. Krishnan V, Bryant HU, Macdougald OA. Regulation of bone mass by Wnt signaling. J Clin Invest. 2006;116(5):1202–9.
65. Hopwood B, Tsykin A, Findlay DM, Fazzalari NL. Microarray gene expression profiling of osteoarthritic bone suggests altered bone remodelling, WNT and transforming growth factor-beta/bone morphogenic protein signalling. Arthritis Res Ther. 2007;9(5):R100.
66. Zoricic S, Maric I, Bobinac D, Vukicevic S. Expression of bone morphogenetic proteins and cartilage-derived morphogenetic proteins during osteophyte formation in humans. J Anat. 2003;202(Pt 3):269–77.
67. Blaney Davidson EN, van der Kraan PM, van den Berg WB. TGF-beta and osteoarthritis. Osteoarthritis Cartilage. 2007;15(6):597–604.
68. Scanzello CR, McKeon B, Swaim BH, DiCarlo E, Asomugha EU, Kanda V, et al. Synovial inflammation in patients undergoing arthroscopic meniscectomy: molecular characterization and relationship to symptoms. Arthritis Rheum. 2011;63(2):391–400.
69. Krasnokutsky S, Belitskaya-Lévy I, Bencardino J, Samuels J, Attur M, Regatte R, et al. Quantitative magnetic resonance imaging evidence of synovial proliferation is associated with radiographic severity of knee osteoarthritis. Arthritis Rheum. 2011;63(10):2983–91.
70. Hill CL, Hunter DJ, Niu J, Clancy M, Guermazi A, Genant H, et al. Synovitis detected on magnetic resonance imaging and its relation to pain and cartilage loss in knee osteoarthritis. Ann Rheum Dis. 2007;66(12):1599–603.
71. Torres L, Dunlop DD, Peterfy C, Guermazi A, Prasad P, Hayes KW, et al. The relationship between specific tissue lesions and pain severity in persons with knee osteoarthritis. Osteoarthritis Cartilage. 2006;14(10):1033–40.
72. Roemer FW, Guermazi A, Felson DT, Niu J, Nevitt MC, Crema MD, et al. Presence of MRI-detected joint effusion and synovitis increases the risk of cartilage loss in knees without osteoarthritis at 30-month follow-up: the MOST study. Ann Rheum Dis. 2011;70(10):1804–9.
73. Scanzello CR, Goldring SR. The role of synovitis in osteoarthritis pathogenesis. Bone. 2012;51(2):249–57.

Hip Disease Etiologies: FAI and Dysmorphias

15

Xavier Flecher, Sebastien Parratte, and Jean-Noel Argenson

Introduction

In the early 1980s, the poor long-term results of THA in the young adult led to development of joint preservation procedures, with promising early results [1, 2]. With the more recent advancements of total hip arthroplasty, conservative treatment appeared more controversial since the introduction of modern hip arthroscopy or mini-invasive approaches. It is thus actually more crucial than ever that the orthopedic surgeon be aware of mechanical disorders that can affect the hip and lead to its degeneration, as most of those can be addressed surgically with success.

Developmental Dysplasia of the Hip

The clinical presentation of this disease is often evident. The majority of patients are young females who describe hip pain, instability, limping, or sometimes leg length discrepancy. The patient is frequently symptomatic with pain usually located in the groin, but can be occasionally over the greater trochanter, in the gluteal region, or around the knee. A nonsteroidal anti-inflammatory medication may be used for pain relief on an occasional basis, and the duration of symptoms is likely to exceed 1 year. The examiner must assess the lower limb range of motion. Internal rotation in extension and in flexion may be higher than normal (normal = 30°) in cases where excessive anteversion is present. However, in the painful hip, internal rotation and free flexion (maximum, 110°) typically appear restricted compared with that of the normal hip. Occasionally, a labral tear may be associated and felt by the patient as a mechanical snapping, popping, or locking. Thus, the impingement test is positive when hip flexion, adduction, and internal rotation elicit groin pain. However, the diagnosis is determined radiographically.

Anteroposterior Quantitative Measurements

The same radiographic assessment has to be performed for each patient. It includes an anteroposterior (AP) pelvis view, a false profile according to Lequesne and de Sèze [3], a surgical lateral view of the pelvis, and a dynamic AP view of the hip looking for the proper positioning of the hip by abduction of the lower limb.

These radiographs evaluate the deficiency of head coverage and its severity, the articular congruency, and the presence of osteoarthritis. A CT scan may also be performed in order to assess the femoral neck and acetabulum anteversion.

Additionally, MR arthrography may be added to rule out the presence of intra-articular disorders such as labral tears or minimal chondral disease [4, 5].

Structural Evaluation (Fig. 15.1)

Lateral Center Edge Angle

The angle formed between the two lines passing through the center of the femoral head, one of which extends to the lateral edge of sourcil (A) and the line perpendicular (B) to that joining the two teardrops. The normal angle of an adult is greater than 25°. Beyond 40° may indicate pincer impingement [6].

Tönnis Angle

The angle formed by the intersection of the so-called horizontal line (the line joining the two tear drops) passing through the femoral head center and the line that passes

X. Flecher, MD • S. Parratte, MD
Department of Orthopedic Surgery, Institute for Motion and Locomotion, Sainte-Marguerite Hospital, Aix-Marseille University, Marseille, France
e-mail: Xavier.FLECHER@ap-hm.fr

J.-N. Argenson, MD (✉)
Service de Chirurgie Orthopedique, Hopital Sainte-Marguerite, 270 Boulevard Sainte-Marguerite, Marseille 13009, France
e-mail: jean-noel.argenson@ap-hm.fr

J.C. McCarthy et al. (eds.), *Hip Joint Restoration*, DOI 10.1007/978-1-4614-0694-5_15

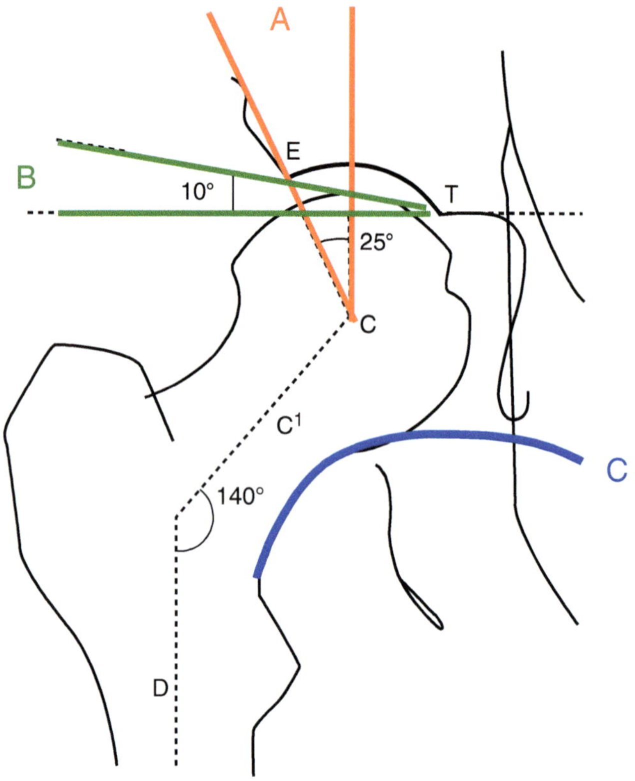

Fig. 15.1 Radiographic measurement of developmental dysplasia of the hip. *A*. LCE. *B*. Tönnis angle. *C*. Shenton's line

through medial edge of the sourcil. Normal is 0°–10°, less than 0° indicates risk of impingement, and higher than 10° indicates structural instability [7].

Break in Shenton's Line

There is an imaginary line connecting the medial aspect of the femoral neck to the superior pubic ramus. It is used to determine the relationship/alignment of the head of the femur to the acetabulum by observing the alignment of the femur and pelvis to determine if they align in an approximately smooth arc. If the curve is "broken" by more than 5 mm, then Shenton's line is said to have a break [8]. Interruption of the curve occurs with subluxation or dislocation of the hip.

Acetabulum Anteversion–Retroversion

It is routinely estimated through the AP view of the hip as described by Reynolds et al. [9] (Fig. 15.2). Three points are pointed out: "T" is the point on the external side of the acetabular roof, "B" the posterior horn, and "U" the teardrop. The anterior wall is figured by the "T-U" line and the posterior wall by the ""T-B" line. On a normal acetabulum, these two lines do not cross and figure a triangle. In cases of excessive anteversion, they figure an "O" shape, and in cases of excessive retroversion, an "X" shape or crossover sign.

False-Profile Quantitative Measurements: Anterior Center Edge Angle

Anterior center edge (ACE) angle allows assessing the anterior coverage of the femoral head and diagnosing arthritis affecting the anterior part of the joint (Fig. 15.3). The ACE angle is measured on images in the false-profile projection and is defined as the angle between an imagined vertical line and the line that extends from the center of the femoral head to the lateral edge of the sourcil. An ACE angle less than 20° is indicative for structural instability [10].

According to the Hip Study Group classification [11], hips were classified as average DDH when lateral center edge (LCE) or VCA (vertical center anterior) angles are between 25° and 21°, severe between 20° and 5°, and extreme below 5°.

Joint Congruity

The study of the articular congruency is conducted through the surgical profile, evaluating the S/FH ratio (S, projected acetabulum surface; FH, ½ projected femoral head surface) and recentering radiographs by abduction, classified as favorable, neutral, or unfavorable (Fig. 15.4).

Von Rosen visual scores [12] allow visual classification of joint congruency. It can be used both with images taken in the Von Rosen position and standard standing AP position.

- **Excellent**—if the curvature of the acetabulum and that of the femoral head is almost identical and the joint space is adequately maintained
- **Good**—if the curvature of the acetabulum and the femoral head is not identical but the joint space is adequately maintained
- **Fair**—if partial narrowing of the joint space has occurred
- **Poor**—if partial disappearance of joint space has occurred

Osteoarthritis Evaluation

Joint Space Width

It is defined as the smallest distance between the femoral head and the acetabulum [13]. The distance should normally be 3–5 mm. Smaller distance than 3 mm, or a distance that is smaller than that of the opposite hip, indicates radiological osteoarthritis.

Tönnis Classification

The presence of osteoarthritis is evaluated according to Tönnis classification [11] (grade 0 is represented by the absence of osteoarthritis, grade 1 by a widened sclerosis zone and minimal osteophytes, grade 2 by a moderate loss of joint width and cysts, and grade 3 by a joint space less than 1 mm).

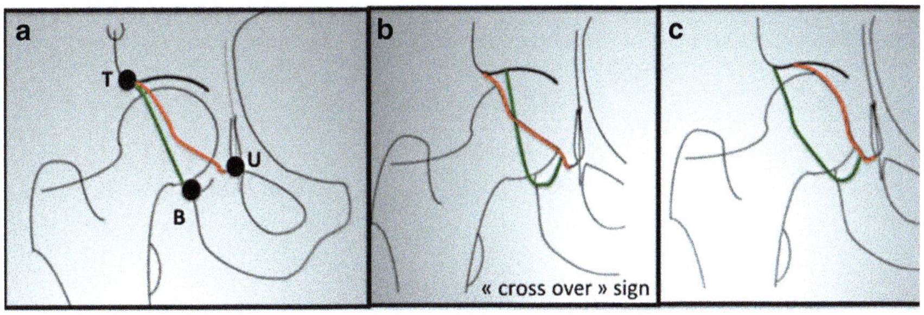

Fig. 15.2 Acetabular version evaluation on AP pelvic view and crossover sign

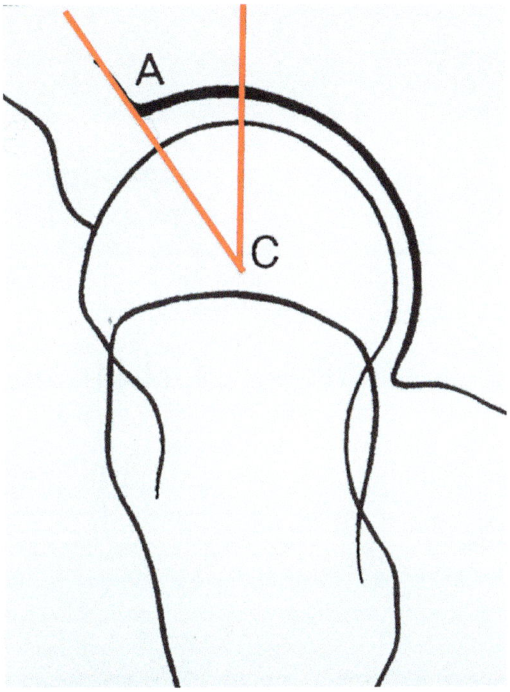

Fig. 15.3 Anterior center edge angle measured on a hip lateral view

Femoroacetabular Impingement

It was first described by Carlioz et al. [14] in 1968 and then identified by Ganz et al. [15] following excessive displacement of peri-acetabular osteotomies with excessive anterior and lateral correction. Reinhold Ganz defined it as "a repeated abnormal contact between the area of head/neck of femur and acetabular rim, resulting in damage to the labrum and cartilage," thus popularizing the concept of femoroacetabular impingement (FAI). This is probably one of the major diagnostic discoveries in understanding the development of hip osteoarthritis in the young. Responsibility for this particular anatomy in the genesis of premature osteoarthritis in young patients is now universally recognized. This disease causes hip pain in young adults and is a source of early degenerative arthritis. FAI may be responsible for the major causes of "primary" osteoarthritis in the hip according to Beck et al. [16] and Ganz et al. [17].

Clinical Diagnosis

Hip impingement is increasingly recognized as a common etiology of hip pain in athletes, adolescents, and adults. It injures the labrum and articular cartilage and can lead to osteoarthritis of the hip if left untreated. Patients with FAI often report anterolateral hip pain, especially in the groin, and less commonly laterally or in the buttock. Pain is usually gradual and progressive. They often cup the anterolateral hip with the thumb and forefinger in the shape of a "C," termed the C-sign [18]. Pain is sharp when turning or pivoting, especially toward the affected side. Common aggravating activities include prolonged sitting, leaning forward, getting in or out of a car, and pivoting in sports.

Anatomical predisposition is suspected when the hip is flexed 90° and concurrent hip internal rotation is less than 20°. The onset of pain during the maneuver of hip flexion, adduction, and internal rotation can help confirm the diagnosis. Nevertheless, it is a condition where the dynamic anatomical predispositions have to be combined with a patient involved in activities that repetitively irritate the hip joint and allow for the development of cartilage and labral pathology (Fig. 15.5). It is because of this that high-level athletes are of most concern.

Etiologies

FAI may be related to childhood hip disorders such as Legg–Calve–Perthes (LCP) disease, slipped capital femoral epiphysis (SCFE), or prior fractures of the pelvis or femur [19]. Despite those correlations, the majority of FAI cases are of unclear etiology [20]. It is theorized that physeal stresses placed on the femoral head and/or acetabulum during development may play a key role in the onset of FAI. Activities such as gymnastics, dancing, and rigorous sports during the development process are potential sources of FAI.

Legg–Calve–Perthes Disease

LCP syndrome is a form of osteochondritis of the hip joint, whereby there is a disruption of blood flow to the femoral head. This lack of blood flow may lead to some degree of

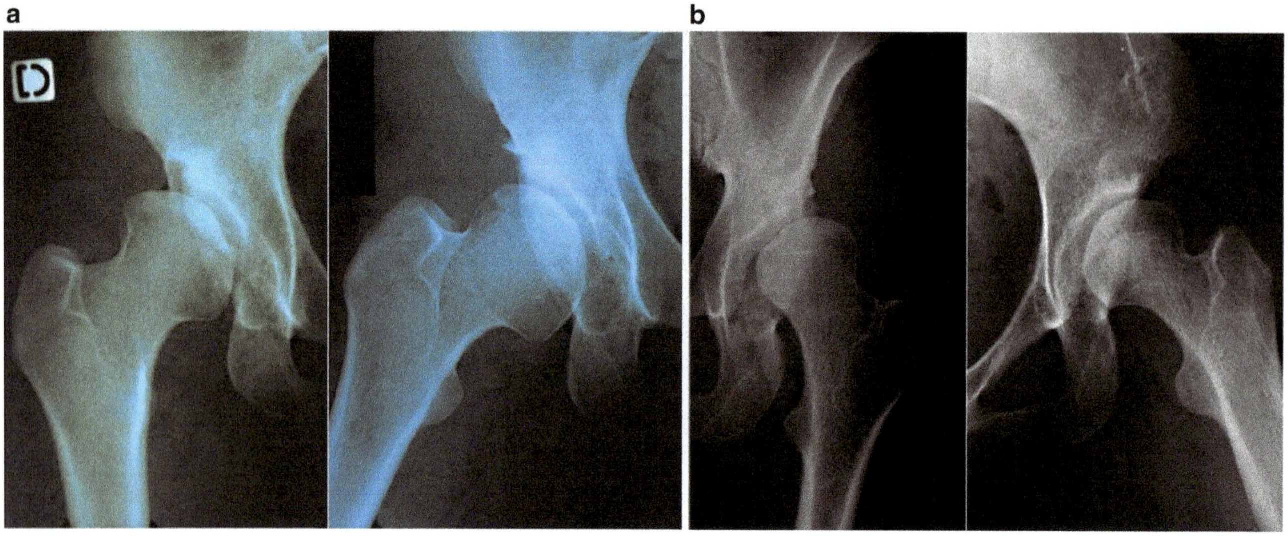

Fig. 15.4 Visual classification of joint congruency [(**a**) excellent, (**b**) fair]

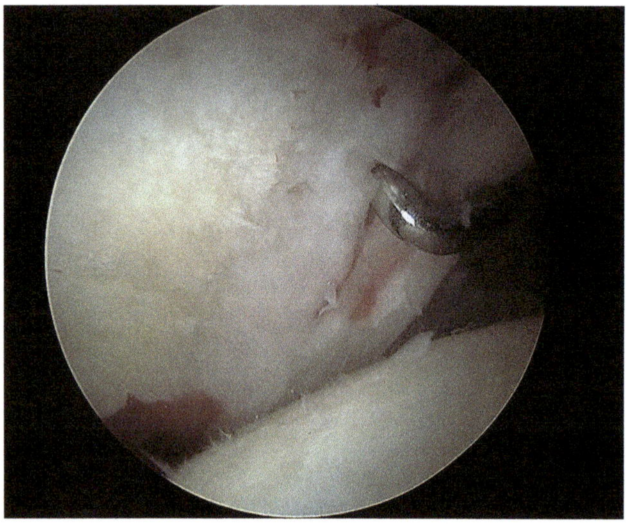

Fig. 15.5 Arthroscopic view of labral tear related to a Cam lesion

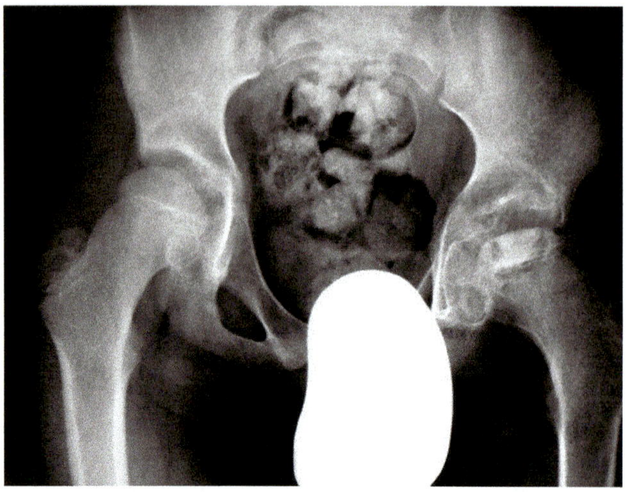

Fig. 15.6 Legg–Calve–Perthes disease (left hip)

collapse of the femoral head and possible secondary changes to the surface of the acetabulum (Fig. 15.6). It is characterized by idiopathic avascular osteonecrosis of the capital femoral epiphysis of the femoral head leading to an interruption of the blood supply of the head of the femur close to the hip joint. The disease is theorized to include the artery of ligamentum teres femoris being constricted or even blocked too early, not allowing for time when the medial circumflex femoral artery takes over. The medial femoral circumflex artery is the principle source of blood supply to the femoral head.

Although no one has identified the cause of Perthes disease, it is known that there is a reduction in blood flow to the joint. Currently, a number of factors have been implicated, including heredity, trauma, endocrine, inflammatory, nutritional, and altered circulatory hemodynamics [21]. Risk factors include, but are not limited to, impaired and disproportionate growth, low birth weight, delayed skeletal maturity, short stature, systemic hormonal changes, and low economic index [22]. Genetics do not appear to be a determining factor. It has been suggested, albeit not proven, that a deficiency of blood factors with anticoagulant properties that normally disperse blood clots may lead to blockages in the vessels supplying the joint. It has also been suggested that there is a deficiency of proteins C and S which also act as blood anticoagulants; if that were the case, it is possible that their deficiency could cause clot formation in the ligamentum teres femoris artery and hinder blood supply to the femoral head. However, there is no evidence of this; over the years many theories have been published, but none have stood up to professional research.

Slipped Capital Epiphysis

SCFE, also known as "slipped upper femoral epiphysis" (Fig. 15.7), refers to a fracture through the growth plate of the upper femur, which results in slippage of the overlying

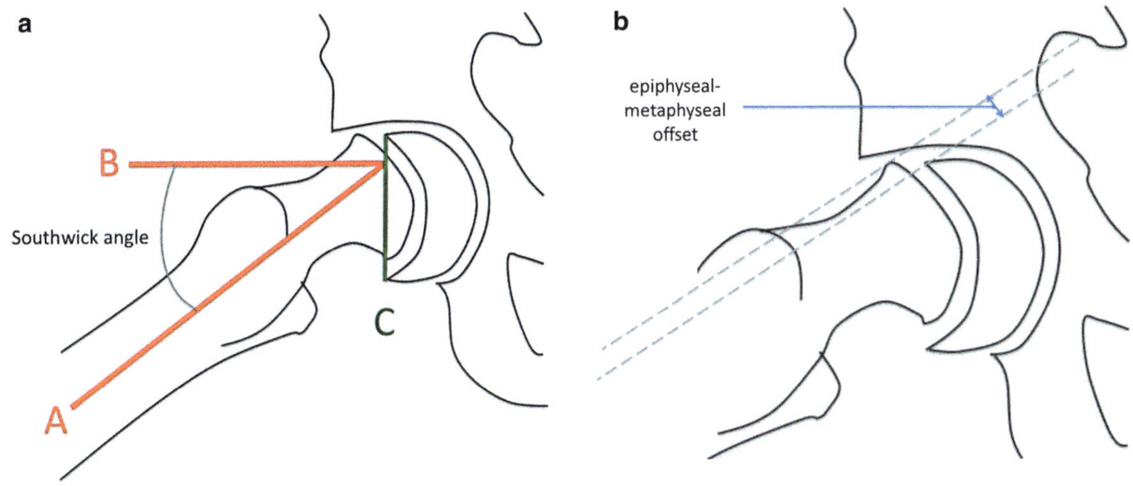

Fig. 15.7 Slipped capital femoral epiphysis with Southwick angle (**a**) and epiphyseal–metaphyseal offset (**b**)

epiphysis. SCFE occurs most of the time in growing children, usually between 8 years old to the late teenage years. It is the most common hip disorder in adolescence.

The diagnosis is a combination of clinical suspicion plus radiological investigation. 20–50 % of SCFE are missed or misdiagnosed on their first presentation to a medical facility [23]. This is because the common symptom is knee pain, which is referred from the hip. The knee can often be the initial joint investigated and is found to be normal. This disease warrants X-rays of the pelvis (AP and frog lateral). The appearance of the head of the femur in relation to the shaft likens that of a "melting ice cream cone." The severity of the disease can be measured using the Southwick angle [24].

The **Southwick angle** is of interest in determining the amount of correction required for SCFE cases. It is defined as the angle between lines A and B, where line A extends in the direction of the femoral shaft and line B is perpendicular to line C, which connects the edges of the slipped epiphysis [25].

The **epiphyseal–metaphyseal offset** is measured as the distance between a line drawn along the anterior edge of the epiphysis parallel to the femoral neck and a line drawn along the proximal–anterior edge of the metaphysis also parallel to the femoral neck [26].

Paraclinic Confirmation

Standard conventional radiographic imaging for FAI includes two radiographs: an anteroposterior pelvic view and a cross-table lateral view of the proximal femur [27]. An alternative to the cross-table lateral view, a Dunn/Rippstein view, preferably in 45° of flexion, can be obtained to reveal pathomorphologies of the anterior femoral head–neck junction [28]. For the anteroposterior pelvic radiograph, the patient is in the supine position with the legs 15° internally rotated to compensate for femoral anteversion and to provide better visualization of the contour of the lateral femoral head–neck junction [29]. The film-focus distance is 1.2 m; the central beam is directed to the midpoint between a line connecting both anterosuperior iliac spines and the superior border of the symphysis (Fig. 15.4). This can easily and reproducibly be palpated by the radiology technician [30, 31]. Accordingly, the cross-table lateral view of the proximal femur is taken with the leg internally rotated, with a film-focus distance of 1.2 m, and with the central beam directed to the inguinal fold [32]. If these prerequisites of correct positioning of the patient and accurate radiographic technique are not fulfilled, the radiographs must be interpreted with caution. The X-ray work-up can recognize anatomical anomalies, but fails to understand the labral or cartilage pathology. It should follow a strict and reproducible protocol to control pelvic tilt and rotation [33]. Distance between public symphysis and the tip of coccyx (i.e., pelvic tilt) should be 1–3 cm, and the tip of coccyx should be in line with public symphysis (i.e., pelvic rotation should be low).

Primary paraclinical investigation to look for femoral morphological abnormality with cam-type FAI must include specific radiographic projections of the hip from the following: cross-table lateral, frog leg, or Dunn (90° and 45° flexion). A frog-leg-type view with fixed angles can be obtained with the patient in a supine position, with the hip in 45° flexion abduction and 30° external rotation.

Femoral Side

A "Cam" lesion translates into an increase in the radius of curvature and a decrease in the anterior concavity (Fig. 15.8). During flexion, this anatomic predisposition leads to excessive

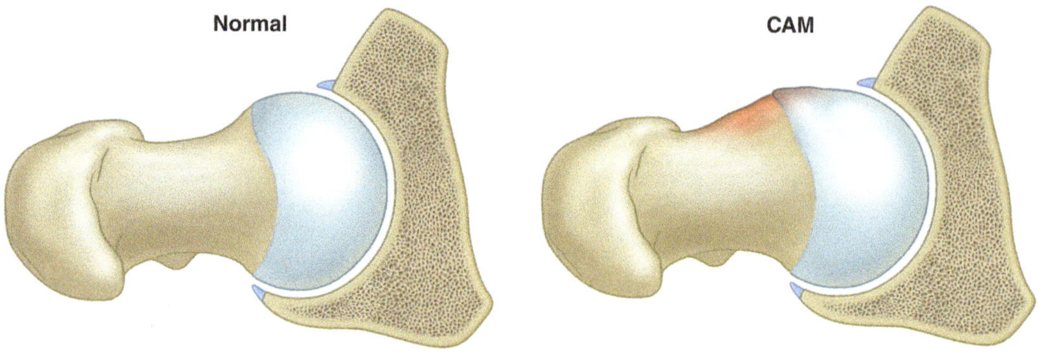

Fig. 15.8 Normal head–neck junction (*left*) and Cam effect (*right*)

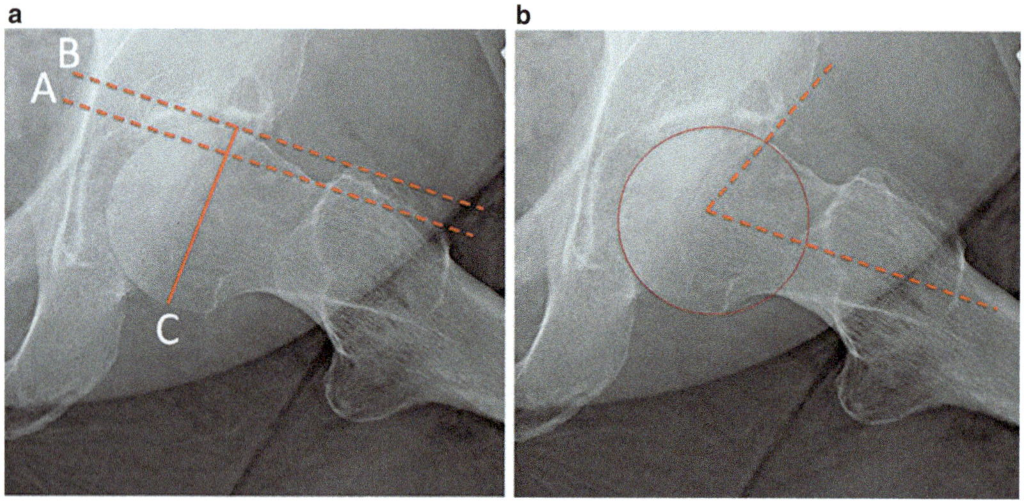

Fig. 15.9 Alpha angle (**a**) and head–neck ratio (b)

irritation to the anterolateral acetabulum, resulting in cartilage delamination and labral lesions (Fig. 15.5).

The hip deformation presents as a characteristic "pistol grip" [34] which reflects the prominent curvilinear nature of the head–neck junction responsible for the impingement. The head–neck junction deformity can be quantified via the alpha angle. This assessment must be completed by MR arthrography with radial reconstructions, as this is the gold standard by consensus.

Alpha Angle

The alpha angle (Fig. 15.9) is the angle between two lines originating in the center of the femoral head. One line extends out through the center of the femoral neck, and the other line extends out through the point where the radius of the head starts to increase compared to the central aspect (i.e., where the femoral head extends out of its boundary circle). An alpha angle beyond 55° indicates cam impingement [35].

Head–Neck Offset Ratio

The head–neck offset ratio (Fig. 15.9) is calculated as the distance between lines A and B, divided by the diameter of the femoral head, C. Line A extends through the anterior-most aspect of the femoral neck, while line B extends through the anterior-most aspect of the femoral head [36]. Both lines are parallel to the long axis of the femoral neck. An offset ratio that is less than 0.17 indicates that cam deformity is likely.

Acetabular Side

This over-coverage, more common in females, typically exists along the anterosuperior rim of the acetabulum, forming a "pincer" lesion, which results in the labrum being "pinched" between the rim and the anterior femoral head–neck junction. The pincer form of the impingement is typically secondary to: (1) acetabular retroversion (a turning back of the socket), (2) coxa profunda (a socket that is too deep), (3) and acetabular protrusion (a situation where the femoral head extends into the pelvis).

Crossover Sign

A hip with a normal pelvic inclination should have the anterior and posterior rims coincide at the edge of the acetabulum. If "Fig. 15.8" is noted, this is positive for a crossover sign. This is caused by the anterior wall projecting lateral to the posterior wall of the acetabulum (see Fig. 15.2) [9].

Ischial Spine Sign

Acetabular retroversion is reflected by the "ischial spine sign" [37]. In this radiographic finding, the ischial spine is prominently projected into the pelvic cavity, medial to Kohler's line.

Posterior Wall Sign

If the posterior wall of the acetabulum is medial to the center of the femoral head, then the hip is positive for "posterior wall sign".

Conclusion

While current results of modern conservative hip surgery make both the surgeon and the patient feel more confident about the procedures, it is becoming more crucial to extensively investigate hip pain without associated osteoarthritis in the young. Simple and reproducible clinical examination should be performed very early facing unrecognized groin, lateral hip, or buttock pain. This includes performing plain X-rays and, thus, aiding the ability to diagnose degenerative hip disease before osteoarthritis occurs. Finally, indications for conservative procedures depend on intra-articular imaging that assesses labral and cartilage pathology, the working knowledge of the orthopedic surgeon, and patient education.

References

1. Collis DK. Cemented total hip replacement in patients who are less than fifty years old. J Bone Joint Surg Am. 1984;66(3):353–9.
2. Boeree NR, Bannister GC. Cemented total hip arthroplasty in patients younger than 50 years of age. Ten- to 18-year results. Clin Orthop Relat Res. 1993;287:153–9.
3. Lequesne M, de Sèze S. Le faux profil du bassin. Nouvelle incidence radiographique pour l' étude de la hanche. Son utilitè dans les dysplasies et les differentes coxopathies. Rev Rhum Mal Osteoartic. 1961;28:643–52.
4. Klaue K, Durnin CW, Ganz R. The acetabular rim syndrome. J Bone Joint Surg Br. 1991;73:423–9.
5. Leunig M, Werlen S, Ungersböck A, Ito K, Ganz R. Evaluation of the acetabular labrum by MR arthrography. J Bone Joint Surg Br. 1997;79:230–4.
6. Wiberg G. Studies on dysplastic acetabula and congenital subluxation of the hip joint. Acta Chir Scand. 1939;58(Suppl):5–135.
7. Clohisy JC, et al. A systematic approach to the plain radiographic evaluation of the young adult hip. J Bone Joint Surg Am. 2008;90 Suppl 4:47–66.
8. Siebenrock KA, Kalbermatten DF, Ganz R. Effect of pelvic tilt on acetabular retroversion: a study of pelves from cadavers. Clin Orthop Relat Res. 2003;407:241–8.
9. Reynolds D, Lucas J, Klaue K. Retroversion of the acetabulum. A cause of hip pain. J Bone Joint Surg Br. 1999;81(2):281–8.
10. Lequesne MG, Laredo JD. The faux profil (oblique view) of the hip in the standing position. Contribution to the evaluation of osteoarthritis of the adult hip. Ann Rheum Dis. 1998;57(11):676–81.
11. Tonnis D. Congenital dysplasia and dislocation of the hip in children and adults. Springer; 1987. pp. 113–31, 65–71, 370–81.
12. Yasunaga Y, et al. Rotational acetabular osteotomy in patients forty-six years of age or older: comparison with younger patients. J Bone Joint Surg Am. 2003;85-A(2):266–72.
13. Fredensborg N, Nilsson BE. The joint space in normal hip radiographs. Radiology. 1978;126:325–6.
14. Carlioz H, Pous JG, Rey JC. Upper femoral epiphysiolysis. Rev Chir Orthop. 1968;54:387–491.
15. Ganz R, Parvizi J, Beck M, Leunig M, Notzli H, Siebenrock KA. Femoroacetabular impingement: a cause for osteoarthritis of the hip. Clin Orthop Relat Res. 2003;417:112–20.
16. Beck M, Kalhor M, Leunig M, Ganz R. Hip morphology influences the pattern of damage to the acetabular cartilage: femoroacetabular impingement as a cause of early osteoarthritis of the hip. J Bone Joint Surg Br. 2005;87:1012–8.
17. Ganz R, Leunig M, Leunig-Ganz K, Harris WH. The etiology of osteoarthritis of the hip: an integrated mechanical concept. Clin Orthop Relat Res. 2008;466:264–72.
18. Byrd JW. Physical examination. In: Operative hip arthroscopy. New York: Springer; 2005. p. 36–50.
19. Leunig M, et al. The concept of femoroacetabular impingement: current status and future perspectives. Clin Orthop Relat Res. 2009;467(3):616–22.
20. Philippon M, et al. Femoroacetabular impingement in 45 professional athletes: associated pathologies and return to sport following arthroscopic decompression. Knee Surg Sports Traumatol Arthrosc. 2007;15(7):908–14.
21. Yochum R. Essentials of skeletal radiology. Baltimore: Williams & Wilkins; 1987. p. 995.
22. Kim HK. Legg-Calvé-Perthes disease. J Am Acad Orthop Surg. 2010;18(11):676–86.
23. Green DW, Reynolds RA, Khan SN, Tolo V. The delay in diagnosis of slipped capital femoral epiphysis: a review of 102 patients. HSS J. 2005;1(1):103–6.
24. Damaceno FL, Santili C, Longui CA. Normal reference values of Southwick's anteroposterior angle in prepubertal and pubertal normal adolescents. J Pediatr Orthop B. 2007;16(6):389–92.
25. Southwick WO. Osteotomy through the lesser trochanter for slipped capital femoral epiphysis. J Bone Joint Surg Am. 1967; 49:807–35.
26. Leunig M, et al. In situ pinning with arthroscopic osteoplasty for mild SCFE. Clin Orthop Relat Res. 2010;468:3160–7.
27. Ganz R, Parvizi J, Beck M, Leunig M, Nötzli H, Siebenrock KA. Femoroacetabular impingement: a cause for osteoarthritis of the hip. Clin Orthop Relat Res. 2003;417:1–9.
28. Meyer DC, Beck M, Ellis T, Ganz R, Leunig M. Comparison of six radiographic projections to assess femoral head/neck asphericity. Clin Orthop Relat Res. 2006;445:181–5.
29. Tannast M, Murphy SB, Langlotz F, Anderson SE, Siebenrock KA. Estimation of pelvic tilt on anteroposterior X-rays: a comparison of six parameters. Skeletal Radiol. 2006;35:149–55.
30. Siebenrock KA, Kalbermatten DF, Ganz R. Effect of pelvic inclination on determination of acetabular retroversion: a study on cadaver pelves. Clin Orthop Relat Res. 2003;407:241–8.

31. Tannast M, Zheng G, Anderegg C, et al. Tilt and rotation correction of acetabular version on pelvic radiographs. Clin Orthop Relat Res. 2005;438:182–90.
32. Eijer H, Leunig M, Mahomed MN, Ganz R. Crosstable lateral radiograph for screening of anterior femoral head–neck offset in patients with femoro-acetabular impingement. Hip Int. 2001;11:37–41.
33. Siebenrock KA, Kalbermatten DF, Ganz R. Effect of pelvic tilt on acetabular retroversion: a study of pelves from cadavers. Clin Orthop Relat Res. 2003;407:241–8.
34. Stulberg SD, Cordell LD, Harris WH, et al. Unrecognized childhood hip disease: a major cause of idiopathic osteoarthritis of the hip. In: The hip. Proceedings of the third meeting of the Hip Society. Saint Louis: C.V. Mosby; 1975. pp. 212–28.
35. Notzli HP, et al. The contour of the femoral head-neck junction as a predictor for the risk of anterior impingement. J Bone Joint Surg Br. 2002;84(4):556–60.
36. Peelle MW, et al. Acetabular and femoral radiographic abnormalities associated with labral tears. Clin Orthop Relat Res. 2005;441: 327–33.
37. Kalberer F, Sierra RJ, Madan SS, Ganz R, Leunig M. Ischial spine projection into the pelvis :a new sign for acetabular retroversion. Clin Orthop Relat Res. 2008;466:677–83.

16 Synovial Pathology of the Hip

Thierry Boyer and Virginie Legre-Boyer

Synovial pathology within the hip joint varies substantially. Diagnosis and treatment are often difficult in some specific diseases.

Dystrophic Synovitis or Synovial Pseudotumors

Synovial Chondromatosis

This usually benign disorder is characterized by the formation of cartilaginous nodules (chondromas), which can ossify secondarily in a joint (osteochondromas) or, in rare cases, in a synovial sheath. They occur most commonly in the hip and the knee. Synovial chondromatosis can take on a typical primitive form or a secondary, more distinctive, form.

Primary Chondromatosis

Primary chondromatosis affects young adults, predominantly males, and occurs through metaplasia of a synovial membrane. This process leads to chondromas that can detach and transform into a pedicle, forming free loose bodies in the joint cavity. They can grow and ossify forming osteochondromatosis. The disease is most commonly monoarticular.

T. Boyer, MD (✉)
Rheumatology, IAL Nollet Paris, 23 rue Brochant, Paris 75017, France
e-mail: thierry.boyer13@wanadoo.fr

V. Legre-Boyer, MD
Rheumatology, IAL Nollet Paris, 23 rue Brochant, Paris, 75017, France

Rheumatology, American Hospital of Paris, Neuilly, France

Rheumatology, Hôpital Pitié-Salpétrière, Paris, France

Clinical Presentation

The disease progresses slowly and is initially asymptomatic, with clinical signs being reported in later stages. Chondromas tend to occupy joint recesses, where they may have few intermittent symptoms. Later mobilization of the bodies results in pain and limitation of joint motion. Characteristic symptoms are the following:

- Intermittent mechanical pain, sometimes accompanied by articular effusions. Aspiration of joint effusion (which may be performed via ultrasound) characteristically yields a leukocyte cell count less than 2000 cells/mL.
- A more common symptom is pain associated with "locking" of the joint with certain movements as a result of the interposition of cartilaginous loose bodies between the articular surfaces.
- In later phases, the chondromatosis (ossified bodies) leads to joint stiffness and loss of range of motion.
- Clinical examination often demonstrates anterior hip pain and limits in motion, particularly in flexion-adduction-internal rotation. In some cases, these clinical findings may display features similar to femoroacetabular impingement [1].

Paraclinical

- There is no biological abnormality.
- Diagnosis is easy in osteochondromatosis form, where chondromas are calcified or ossified.

Typically, plain radiographs show multiple radiopaque intra-articular bodies, often of comparable size (osteochondromas). However, radiographs can appear normal when chondromas are not ossified, making the diagnosis more difficult. In this case, other indirect signs may suggest the diagnosis including: enlargement of the coxofemoral joint space compared to the healthy side [2] or bone erosions in areas of synovial reflection [2]. An increase in periarticular density associated with numerous chondromas and synovial

J.C. McCarthy et al. (eds.), *Hip Joint Restoration*, DOI 10.1007/978-1-4614-0694-5_16

thickening can sometimes also be detected, usually with MRI scanning. In later stages, secondary osteoarthritis can be observed.

Diagnostic Imaging

- CT arthrogram (Fig. 16.1) is the best test for the diagnosis of chondromatosis and is often used to visualize loose bodies in the young patient with chronic mechanical hip pain in the presence of normal radiographs. CT arthrogram is able to locate free chondromas, surrounded by contrast, and guide the resulting therapeutic approach. Radiolucent bodies (purely cartilaginous) appear as oval or rounded polyhedral spaces in the contrast image. Partially ossified chondromas are seen as distinctive bodies with a radio-opaque center and a radiolucent cartilaginous peripheral shell. The synovial membrane, when active, appears thickened and irregular. At the initial stage of the disease process, prior to the release of chondromas into the joint cavity, diagnosis is more difficult because one can only observe the nonspecific hypertrophic synovitis. As the condition progresses, CT arthrogram may be utilized to follow the associated osteochondral degradation and to detect capsular retraction, thus assisting therapy. A simple CT showing no non-ossified chondromas is not sufficient to evaluate this disease.
- Bone scintigraphy contributes little over the course of chondromatosis due to a moderate, diffuse, and inconsistent uptake.
- MRI without arthrogram is difficult to interpret when chondromatosis exists as cartilaginous nodules since they have a signal similar to that of the synovial membrane and synovial fluid on both T1 and T2 scans [3].
- Noncalcified chondromas have an intermediate signal on T1 and the same signal than effusion (slightly higher signal) in T2. Overall, the heterogeneous appearance of the effusion can sometimes assist the diagnosis.
- Osteochondromas have a variable signal. If they are partially calcified, they can appear as punctuated nodules or as a rosette with a central hypointense signal on T1 and T2. If they are heavily ossified, nodules appear hypointense on T1 and T2 scans, edged with the highest synovial signal, especially in T2. At this stage, osteochondromas also appear visible on plain radiographs.
- The IV injection of gadolinium sometimes enables clinicians to observe a hypertrophic synovium (if it is active and well vascularized), which helps detection of the chondroma.
- In the case of free chondromas, loose bodies may become visible on the MR arthrogram once the contrast agent has diffused throughout the joint space revealing inverse images of the chondromas within the joint fluid.
- MRI highlights the presence of areas of bony erosion as well as the extent of the disease and permits detection of bone marrow expansion as a marker of the rare malignant transformation of the disease process.
- MR imaging however may be nondiagnostic or understate the extent of disease. Thus, hip arthroscopy, when indicated, remains the gold standard for accurate diagnosis and treatment of this disease.

Arthroscopy

Arthroscopy plays a diagnostic role in cases when CT arthrogram is inconclusive and can allow correction of a misdiagnosis. Chondromatosis is often an unexpected finding during arthroscopic exploration of cases of "mysterious" hip pain [4]. Arthroscopy allows an immediate diagnosis of this pathology by enabling visualization of the intra-articular chondromas (Figs. 16.2, 16.3, and 16.4), whether as free loose bodies within the joint, in the pedunculated form (Fig. 16.5) or

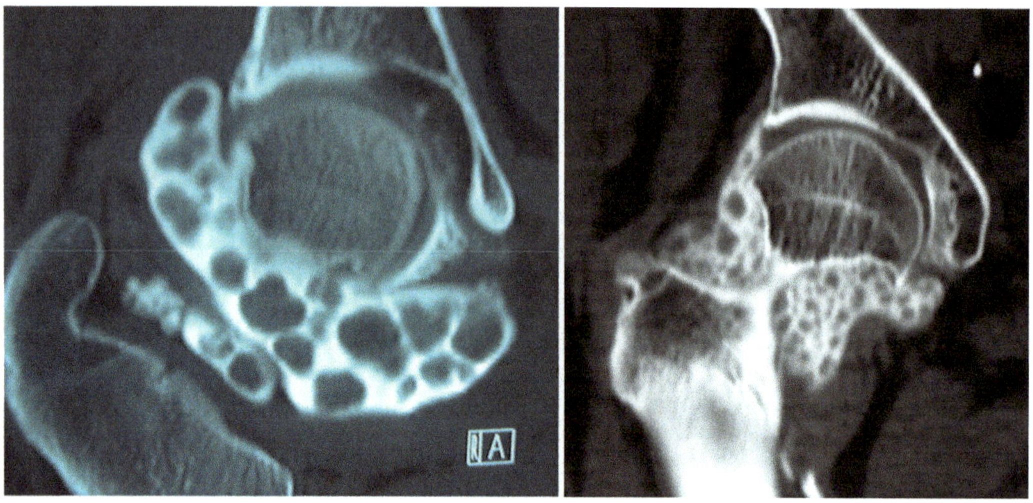

Fig. 16.1 Arthro-CT (Published with kind permission of ©Thierry Boyer 2015. All Rights Reserved)

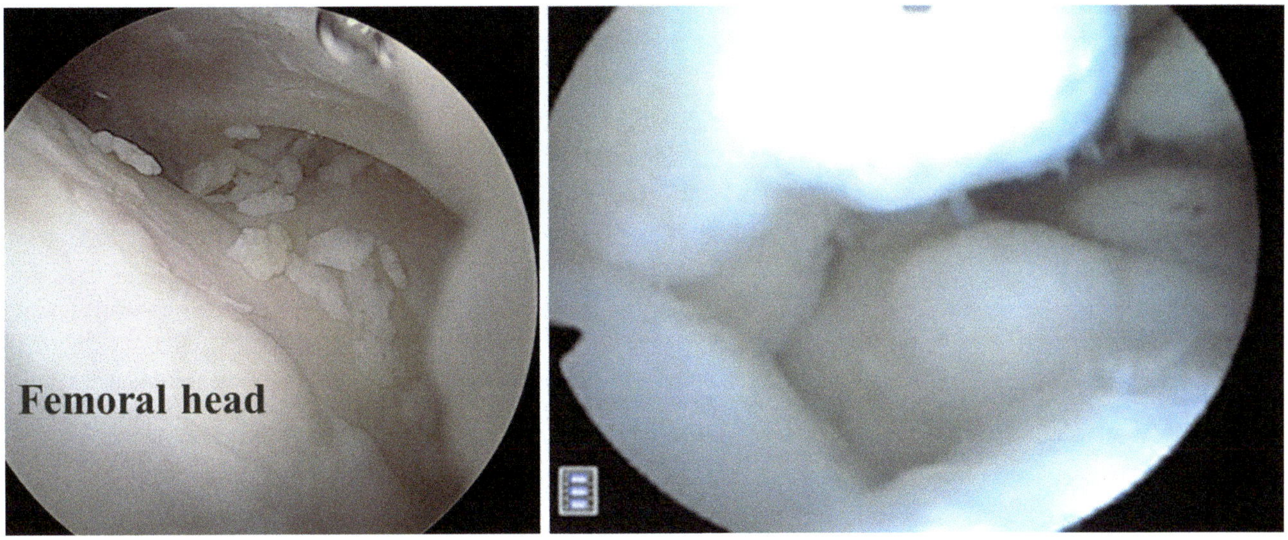

Fig. 16.2 Loose bodies peripheral compartment. (*Left*) Rice-like. (*Right*) Huge chondromas (Published with kind permission of ©Thierry Boyer 2015. All Rights Reserved)

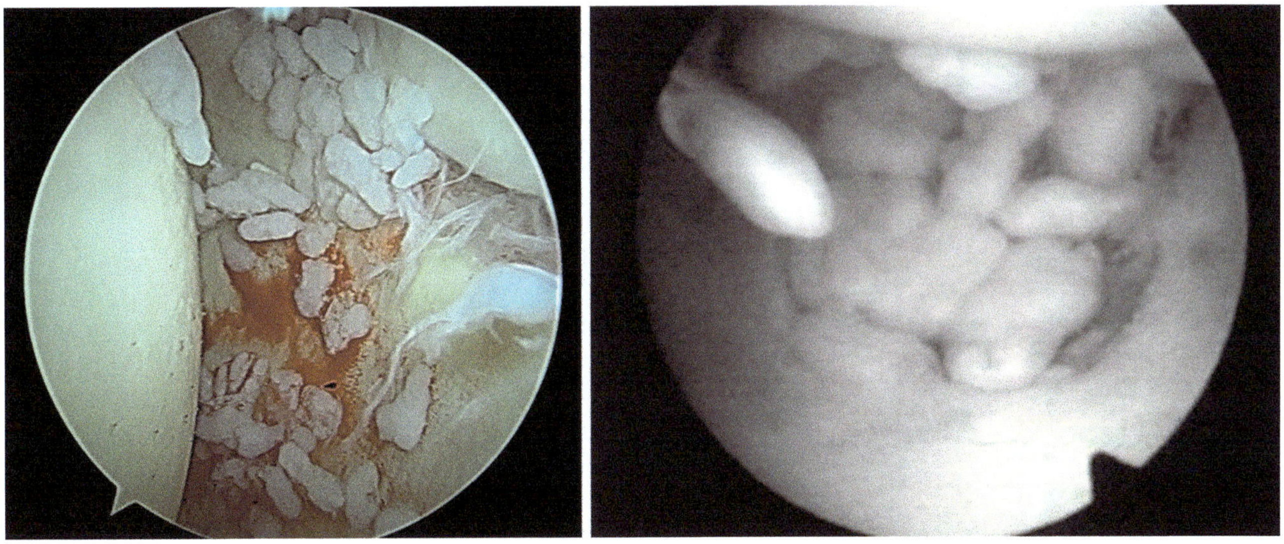

Fig. 16.3 Loose bodies (central compartment) (Published with kind permission of ©Thierry Boyer 2015. All Rights Reserved)

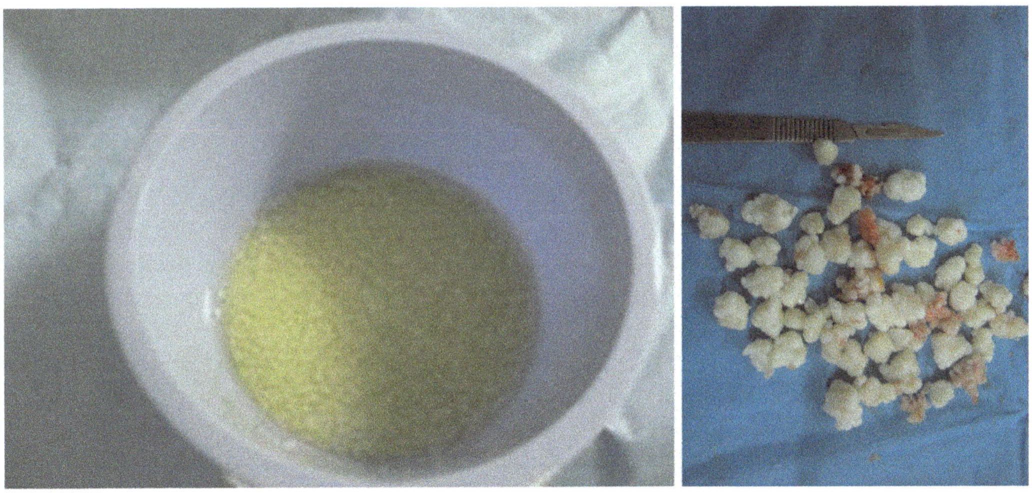

Fig. 16.4 Loose bodies after extraction (Published with kind permission of ©Thierry Boyer 2015. All Rights Reserved)

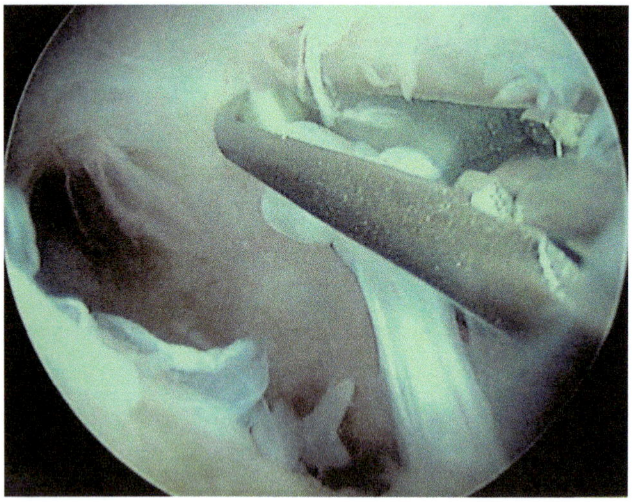

Fig. 16.5 Pedunculated chondroma (Published with kind permission of ©Thierry Boyer 2015. All Rights Reserved)

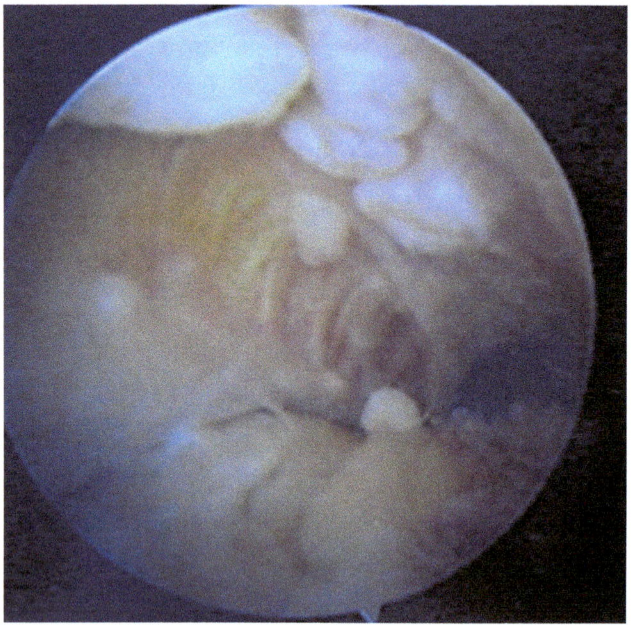

Fig. 16.6 Embedded chondromas (Published with kind permission of ©Thierry Boyer 2015. All Rights Reserved)

embedded form (Fig. 16.6). Furthermore, these three types of chondroma can coexist. Arthroscopy can also reveal a synovial hypertrophy, a clear indicator of the stage of the disease. Lastly, it allows the extraction of free loose bodies.

Pathology

The macroscopic appearance of the articular chondromas is very distinctive, often taking the form of multiple small cartilaginous beads consisting of active clusters of chondrocytes surrounded by a hyaline cartilaginous matrix. The histology of the active synovial membrane is indicative of chondroid metaplasia and consists of islands of chondrocytes immersed in chondroid ground substance. Between these metaplastic areas, the synovial membrane is normal. This demonstrates the importance of obtaining multiple samples using arthroscopy.

The synovial metaplasia develops in three progressive stages [5]:

- Subintimal proliferation of pseudofibroblastic cells that differentiate into chondroblasts capable of secreting chondromucine, the precursor of the ground substance of cartilage.
- As they mature, the chondroblasts form nodular masses of chondrocytes (chondromas).
- The chondromas can form synovial pedicles and detach inside the joint cavity. There is no associated synovial inflammation. Atypical cells are not uncommon in active chondroblasts, which sometimes causes difficulty for interpretation with chondrosarcoma.

Evolution

The clinical course of synovial chondromatosis is sporadic and results in a variable appearance at clinical presentation. The anatomical changes that are observed follow the three stages described by Milgram [5]:

- Stage I: Intrasynovial chondromas (embedded in the synovium), sessile or pedunculated
- Stage II: The emergence of free chondromas in combination with intrasynovial chondromas
- Stage III: Free chondromas in association with an inactive synovium

In the first two stages, the synovium is still productive, and there is a risk of recurrence after treatment. However, it seems that the production of synovial chondromas fades spontaneously. In stage III, the simple extraction of loose bodies usually helps healing. In later stages, the disease progresses to secondary osteoarthritis. Further study of synovial chondromatosis is justified by the possibility of late sarcomatous transformation [6].

Particular Forms of Chondromatosis

- A decalcifying form of chondromatosis has been observed at the hip, with a regional radiological demineralization of the femoral head, neck, and acetabulum [7]. Differentiation of this condition from complex regional pain syndrome (CRPS) is based on a longer evolution, no blurring of bone contours, little or no radionuclide uptake, and the absence of regional bone edema on MRI.
- A retractable form, mimicking capsulitis, has been reported at the hip [8]. The joint stiffness is severe and often refractory in this form, with small chondromas embedded in the synovium.

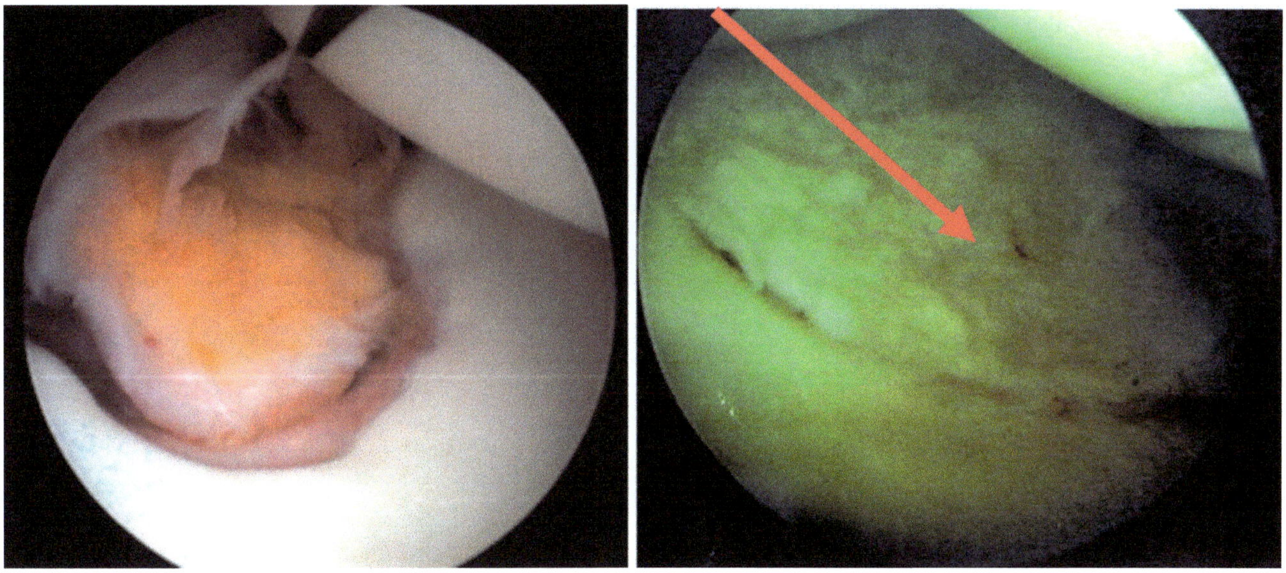

Fig 16.7 Pancake-like clump (fossae). (*Left*) Normal. (*Right*) Chondromatosis (Published with kind permission of ©Thierry Boyer 2015. All Rights Reserved)

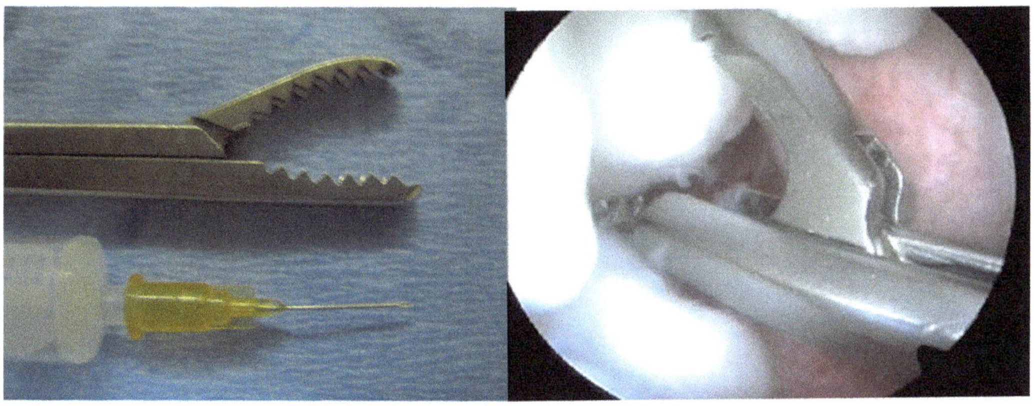

Fig. 16.8 Huge grasper (Published with kind permission of ©Thierry Boyer 2015. All Rights Reserved)

- An erosive pseudocystic form of chondromatosis exists in which large erosions are present in areas of synovial reflection (femoral neck). These erosions can mimic bone cysts and arise in response to the pressure developed between synovial metaplastic masses and the underlying bone. A stiffening form (Fig. 16.6) is also observed at the hip [8]. In this pattern, osteochondromas are embedded into the synovial membrane.
- A filling of the fovea: In this form, a conglomerate of osteochondromas ("pancake"-like) fills the fovea (Fig. 16.7). At the last stage, when the "pancake" is completely ossified, it becomes an osteophyte on imaging.

Treatment

The treatment depends on the clinical impact of the chondromatosis, the location of the chondromas, and the evolutionary stage of the disease. Treatment is not undertaken in the absence of symptoms.

In the symptomatic cases, the treatment consists of removal of chondroma, with or without synovectomy. The decision to perform a synovectomy in cases of active synovium (stages I and II) is controversial as it exposes the patient to the risk of developing joint stiffness.

Open surgical removal of osteochondromas is indicated when they are too large [4], extra-articular, or too embedded to be treated by arthroscopy.

The results of arthroscopic removal of chondromas and osteochondromas were analyzed in several publications [4, 9–12] including a personal study of 120 cases [13].

The arthroscopic technique consists of removing loose bodies using cannulas and large alligator graspers (Fig. 16.8). The peripheral approach without traction [14, 15] is always performed first. The arthroscope is introduced through the anterolateral portal. Loose bodies are extracted via a second (and sometimes a third) portal. These portal sites depend on the localization of the (osteo)chondromas on imaging. The use of arthroscopes with 30° and 70° lenses is recommended to make debridement of the articular cavity as complete as possible. The central approach is performed in all cases to remove loose bodies (if present on imaging) or to maintain the normality of the compartment.

Some pearls may facilitate the treatment: long and curve instrumentation [16] and the use of a flexible endotracheal cannula [17].

Partial synovectomy may be undertaken if chondromas remain embedded in the synovial membrane. The results of arthroscopic treatment of 111 patients are reported with a mean of 78 months [13]. The results are good or excellent in 56% of cases. At the time of review, 17% of patients had a total hip replacement [13].

Arthroscopy may be regarded as the basis for treatment of chondromatosis in the hip; however, the recurrence rate is high [11–13]. Eighteen patients in our cohort of 147 cases had at least one re-arthroscopy. Open synovectomy may have a lower recurrence rate [18, 19] but at the cost of higher morbidity and a higher rate of secondary arthroplasty.

Secondary Osteochondromatosis

Secondary osteochondromatosis develops in response to the release of cartilage or bone fragments from non-synovial osteoarticular areas. These fragments can ossify and grow in the synovial fluid and may be captured by the synovium [20]. Synovial histology differs from the primary osteochondromatosis in that the synovium can be inflammatory and exhibit a macrophage-type reaction around captured osteochondromas. However, in this condition the synovium does not produce chondromas and is not metaplastic.

Secondary and primary osteochondromatoses are very different. The secondary osteochondromatosis affects older patients, and the clinical symptoms depend of the original arthropathy. The loose bodies present within the joint are larger and fewer in number (generally no more than five) of variable shape and size and are usually ossified. The treatment depends on the stage of the arthropathy. The removal of the loose bodies in cases of advanced osteoarthritis is often ineffective.

Villonodular Synovitis (VNS)

This benign synovial proliferation develops classically from the synovial membrane of the joint. In terms of frequency, PVNS occurs most frequently in the knee, followed by the hip [21, 22]. It is almost always monoarticular. PVNS usually occurs in young adult patients. The annual incidence, all joints combined, is estimated at 1.8 cases per million [22] but could be higher due to improved detection using advanced imaging (i.e., MRI) [23–25]. There are two forms: diffuse and localized, which differ vastly in terms of clinical, imaging, and treatment.

Clinical Presentation

By rule, the evolution of PVNS is very slow, with symptoms appearing far in advance of definitive diagnosis. Clinical signs are generally mild and intermittent in the early stages and then gradually become enduring.

PVNS diagnosis must be considered in the case of progressive unilateral mechanical joint pain. Locking or catching is less frequent.

Clinical Forms

Some forms of PVNS have misleading clinical manifestations:

- Localized PVNS (tumorlike) can occur an articular mechanical disturb as pain, locking or catching when a pedunculated nodule behaves like a loose body.
- A pseudoseptic form of VNS has been described, with a highly inflammatory monoarthritis including fever, elevated ESR or high CRP levels, and purulent effusion. Aseptic fluid and synovial biopsy help to confirm a diagnosis of aseptic arthritis. This pseudoseptic form is probably due to an acute necrosis of a tumorlike lesion twisting its pedicle, as evidenced by histological analysis of necrotic fragments [22].

Paraclinical

- Biology appears normal without inflammatory syndrome (except in the case of a rare tumorlike lesion necrosis).
- Plain knee radiographs appear normal. Some signs can be detected in diffuse forms however. At advanced stages the destructive nature of the PVNS results in bone erosions or the formation of multiple or polycyclic bone lesions, often identifiable by a sclerotic border that can lie on the joint surfaces [23]. When they are located on the periphery of the joint in the reflection zones of the synovium (femoral neck), they are suggestive of synovial disease. This location also differentiates them from osteoarthritis lesions located in bearing zones. The joint space is often preserved and there is no intra-articular calcification or foreign substances. In a study of 58 hips with PVNS, radiographic osteoarticular lesions were observed in 95% of cases. In 62%, lesions were suggestive of PVNS (erosions, cysts). They were mimicking osteoarthritis in 16% (joint narrowing and osteophytes). In 14% they were mimicking a rheumatological disease (joint space narrowing and erosions) [23].
- CT arthrogram is of little value in the diagnosis of PVNS. One can observe an irregular and heterogeneous joint cavity, with multiple lacunar images related to villous proliferation, and/or the nodularity of the synovium; however, these signs are nonspecific. Bone erosions communicating with the joint cavity appear clearly. Spontaneous hyperdensity is observed on CT slices, in

connection with hemosiderin deposits. The absence of loose bodies should allow differentiation of PVNS from synovial chondromatosis, although villi can be confused with chondromas.

- MRI is the best imaging modality because it provides a good diagnostic approach as well as a better understanding of the expansion of the synovium. It also detects bone lesions not yet visible on plain radiographs. The combination of sequences T1, T2, and especially T1 with gadolinium is essential to allow thorough analysis of the pathological synovial membrane and to distinguish it from the neighboring synovial fluid [24]. Detection of hemosiderin deposits with inherent magnetic properties is a distinctive feature of the MR image which is pathognomonic for PVNS.

The appearance of typical diffuse articular PVNS suggests:

- Hyperplastic heterogeneous and hypervascular synovial lesions hypointense on T1, enhanced after gadolinium injection displays hyperintense on T2. On the T1 sequence after injection of gadolinium, the villi and areas of PVNS appear in contrast to the synovial fluid (which is not modified by gadolinium).
- On the T1 and T2 scans, hemosiderin deposits appear as small hypointense areas located in the synovial masses that are not enhanced by gadolinium. These deposits are even more visible on gradient echo sequences that enhance contrast. This aspect is very suggestive of PVNS. Differential diagnosis is calcium pyrophosphate dihydrate deposition (CPPD) deposits that would give the same signal, as well as chronic joint bleeding (hemophilia, synovial hemangioma).
- Hyperintense regions on the T1 and T2 scans may occur in association with synovial hyperplasia. It corresponds to the presence of foam cells (macrophages) [25].
- Bone erosions are detected by MRI at an early radiologic stage. Bone marrow edema can be seen around the erosions.
- The focal intra-articular forms of VNS (tumorlike lesion) present themselves as rounded masses that are isointense on T1, hypointense on fast spin echo (fibrosis), and hyperintense on T2, with less significant hypointense hemosiderin deposits than in diffuse forms. The tumorlike lesion is enhanced by the injection of gadolinium.

Arthroscopy shows the characteristic appearance of PVNS and enables histological confirmation:

- In diffuse forms, major synovial hypertrophy occurs which is villous and/or nodular. The synovium is ocher or brown in color (Fig. 16.9), often with a red/brown stain characteristic of hemorrhage. However, the extent of the lesions (especially posterior) cannot be well evaluated via arthroscopy.

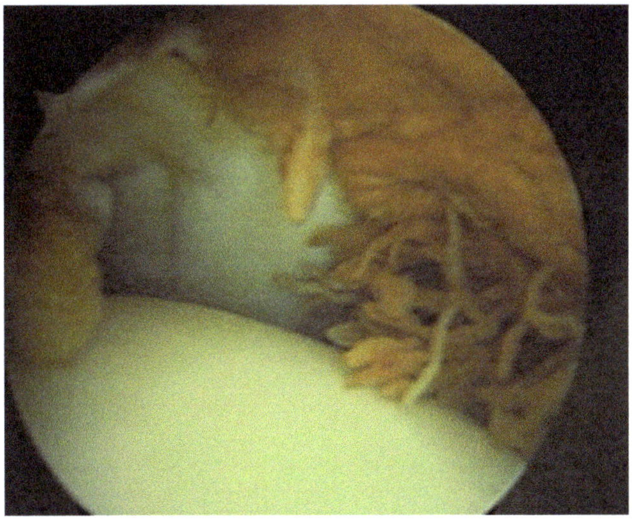

Fig. 16.9 VNS (diffuse) (Published with kind permission of ©Thierry Boyer 2015. All Rights Reserved)

- Localized PVNS (Fig. 16.10) takes the form of a typical ocher nodule of firm consistency, sessile or more often pedunculated, and sometimes vividly colored by hemorrhagic staining.
- These pathologic conditions can be diagnosed from a synovial biopsy which is taken arthroscopically. Examination via microscope reveals a villous hyperplasia and/or a richly vascularized nodular synovium, consisting of a cellular infiltrate of macrophages, foam cells (or xanthomatous), and the presence of multinucleated giant cells in varying numbers. Some cells contain vividly colored iron deposits (hemosiderin).

Pathophysiology

The pathologic etiology of PVNS is not clear.

- It has been suggested that the synovial proliferation associated with a chronic inflammation is due to a reaction to hemarthrosis and repeated trauma [26]. However, the synovitis observed in hemophilic arthropathy is dissimilar in that it does not contain foam cells or giant cells, and it also does not extend into the soft tissues. The concept of prior trauma is common (53 %) in the series of Myers and Masi [22] but exceptional (3 %) for Flipo et al. [23].
- A tumoral cell proliferation with locoregional destructive potential is also suspected. The discovery of chromosomal abnormalities (abnormal chromosome 1, trisomy 7) and monoclonality can be identified [27, 28].
- The potential role of metabolic factors is cited by some who note the presence of an abnormal local lipid metabolism in the presence of significant numbers of xanthomatous cells (foam) in association with synovial disease.

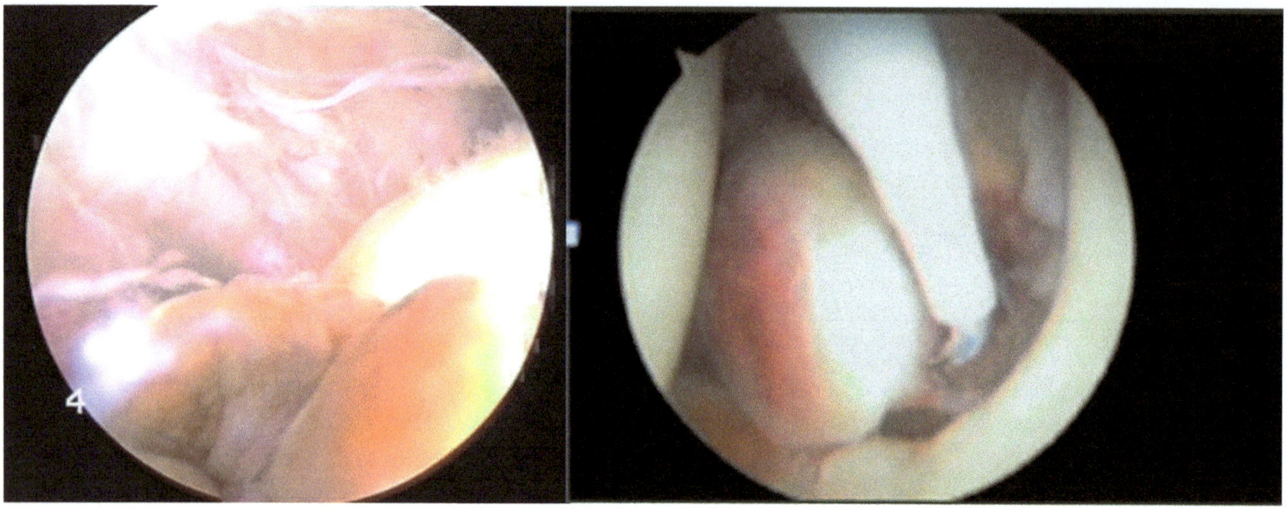

Fig. 16.10 Focal VNS. (*Left*) Peripheral. (*Right*) Central (Published with kind permission of ©Thierry Boyer 2015. All Rights Reserved)

Evolution

- PVNS evolves with slow diffusion of the synovitis and local destruction of bone (erosions, cysts).
- If left untreated, a localized PVNS can evolve into a diffuse form [29].
- If we refer to the same lesion at the knee [30], localized forms heal after complete resection, with almost no risk of recurrence.
- In up to 50 % of cases, the diffuse forms of PVNS recur after surgery, probably because of the difficulty of obtaining a complete synovectomy [29, 31]. Recurrences occur mainly in the first 4 years postoperatively, but sometimes even later, justifying a follow-up MRI [31, 32]. Diffuse articular PVNS gradually leads to bone and joint destruction in the long term and may require joint replacement in young patients.
- A malignant form of PVNS was recently uncovered, following the report of a few isolated cases. Its diagnosis is histological and the risk of recurrence and metastasis is high [27, 33].

Treatment

The treatment of PVNS consists of surgical removal of all affected tissue via a total synovectomy as a precaution to prevent recurrence. If possible, this is done via arthroscopy, to avoid the functional consequences of an open procedure. However, complete arthroscopic synovectomy is a very difficult challenge, and open synovectomy is often necessary. The additional course to low-dose radiation therapy is controversial [34, 35].

The localized VSN usually heals after the removal of the isolated nodule, which is performed arthroscopically, if possible. The risk of recurrence is minimal if resection is performed in a safe area (i.e., by wide resection of the pedicle). The value of an additional synovectomy has not yet been established.

Mechanical and Inflammatory Synovitis

Synovial Proliferation in Osteoarthritis

At the hip, mechanical synovial proliferation over the course of osteoarthritis sometimes takes a very unusual turn. Voluminous fringes of synovial tissue can become trapped between the articular surfaces, clinically explaining locking or catching. X-ray arthrogram CT imaging or MR arthrography may display villi of such a size that they can be confused with loose bodies (Fig. 16.11). Arthroscopic synovectomy has not been proved useful in this mechanical proliferation.

Mechanical Synovitis Around Pectinéo-Foveal (Medial) Fold

At the lower edge of the femoral neck, there exists a constant fibrous infolding within the synovium, known in France as "the Amantini pectinéo-foveal fold" and as the "medial fold" in Anglo-Saxon countries. The extra-articular iliopsoas tendon crosses the fold. A conflict may arise between the two structures with the appearance of a synovitis at their crossing (Fig. 16.12). Nonspecific pain is the lone symptom.

The diagnosis can never be made clinically and imaging of this fold is very difficult. May et al. [36] provides the results of arthroscopic resection of the fold. In a retrospective series of ten cases, he isolates a small homogeneous group of six cases of a painful hip in young athletic patients, with no previous hip symptoms. In each case, hip pain was

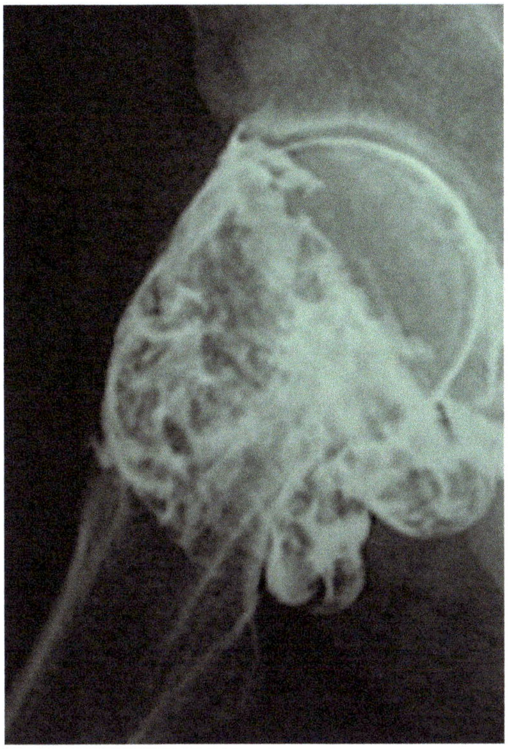

Fig. 16.11 Synovitis/chondromas (Published with kind permission of ©Thierry Boyer 2015. All Rights Reserved)

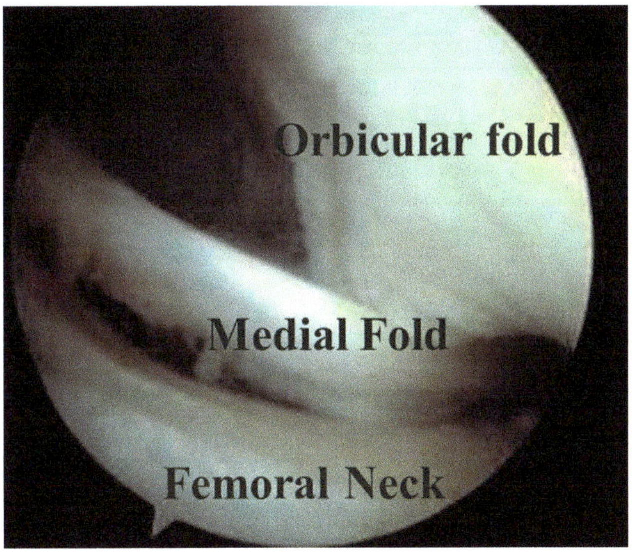

Fig. 16.12 Medial fold (Published with kind permission of ©Thierry Boyer 2015. All Rights Reserved)

aggravated by bending in association with rotational movements of the lower limb. Duration of symptoms before arthroscopy was 20 months on average. The conflict was always a discovery of arthroscopy which revealed no other abnormalities. The results of the resection of the fold were excellent in six cases, with a return to sport at the same pre-injury level. We obviously cannot draw solid conclusions from a retrospective series without long-term follow-up, but it is worth noting considering the disease has been relatively unknown until now.

Inflammatory Synovitis

The control of joints afflicted with inflammatory rheumatism achieved by new biologic therapies has made arthroscopic synovectomy exceptionally useful. One should, however, be familiar with the endoscopic appearance of inflammatory arthritis (Fig. 16.13) to perform a synovial biopsy whenever villi have a suspicious appearance. As in other joints, it is necessary to recognize fibrin masses and not to confuse them with other abnormalities found within the joint.

Malignant Synovial Tumors

Fortunately these tumors are rare and can occasionally cause hemarthrosis. MRI is the modality of choice for detecting the disease and guiding the collection of tissue biopsies.

Synovial Sarcoma

Synovial sarcoma accounts for 5–10 % of all soft tissue sarcomas and occurs at sites within the extremities in 90 % of cases, most frequently in the lower extremities [37]. It is rarely initiated within the joint cavity but usually develops in an area adjacent to the joint in contact with the capsule. Subsequent invasion of bone or joint may be made by contiguity.

Radiographs should indicate the presence of small calcifications, which are common (30 %) and evocative [25]. Bone erosions may occur later. CT scans show a heterogeneous soft tissue mass and track calcifications more easily. The MRI shows a tumor of heterogeneous appearance.

Chondrosarcoma

Chondrosarcoma is an exceptional finding. It can occur spontaneously or as a result of the malignant transformation of a synovial osteochondromatosis. Poorly differentiated chondrosarcomas present the appearance of a very indistinct heterogeneous tumor on MRI. In its differentiated form, its calcified cartilaginous nodules may be present, making the differential diagnosis difficult from synovial chondromatosis [38]. The histological criteria for differentiating chondrosarcomas from primitive chondromatoses are (i) the presence of large atypical cells with hyperchromic and sometimes multiple nuclei, (ii) disruption of the intra-tumoral architecture, and (iii) invasion of the bone and soft tissues [38].

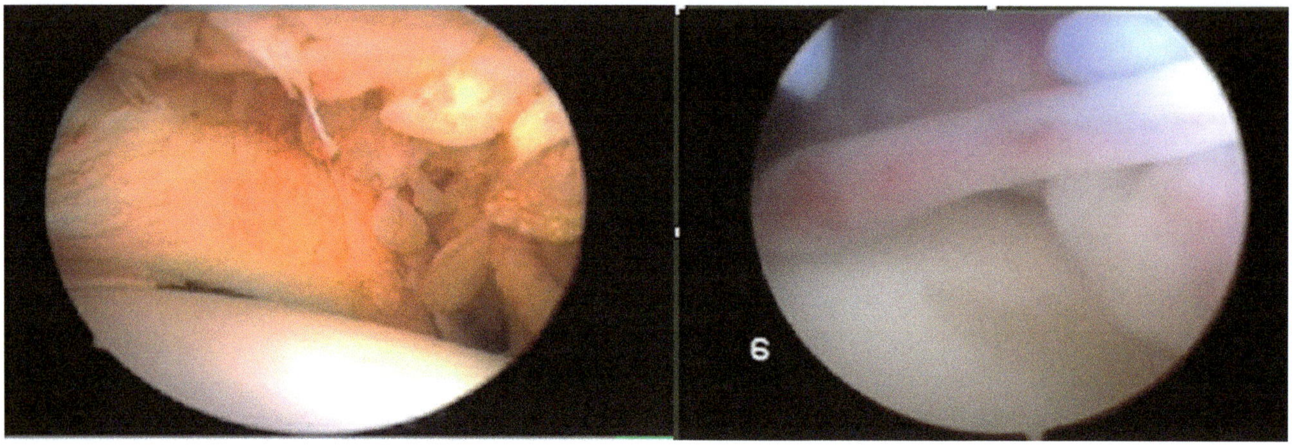

Fig. 16.13 Synovitis. (*Left*) Mechanical. (*Right*) Rheumatoid arthritis (Published with kind permission of ©Thierry Boyer 2015. All Rights Reserved)

Summary

Synovial conditions of the hip joint are more frequent than previously recognized. The clinical presentation can be subtle and confusing to the clinician. Advancements in imaging, especially MR scanning, have greatly improved diagnostic accuracy and facilitated treatment in these wide ranging conditions. A high index of suspicion, combined with a thorough clinical examination, is paramount to facilitate effective treatment of these diseases.

References

1. Abolghasemian M, Gharaizadeh K, Kuzyk P, Masdari Z, Fakharian M, Safir O. Hips with synovial chondromatosis may display the features of femoroacetabular impingement. J Bone Joint Surg Am. 2014;96(12).
2. Lequesne M, Mathieu P, Winkler P. La chondromatose synoviale de la hanche. Rev Rhum. 1999;66(Suppl):41–7.
3. Cotten A, Demondion X, Boutry N, Chastanet P, Delfaut E. Imagerie des affections synoviales, tumorales ou non. J Radiol. 2000;81:381–9.
4. Marchie A, Panuncialman I, McCarthy JC. Efficacy of hip arthroscopy in the management of synovial chondromatosis. Am J Sports Med. 2011;39(Suppl):126S–31.
5. Milgram JW. Synovial osteochondromatosis. A histopathological study of thirty cases. J Bone Joint Surg Am. 1977;59: 792–801.
6. Campanacci DA, Matera D, Franchi A, Capanna R. Synovial chondrosarcoma of the hip: report of two cases and literature review. Chir Organi Mov. 2008;3:139–44.
7. Lequesne M, Becker J, Bard M, Witvoet J, Postel M. Capsular constriction of the hip: arthrographic and clinical considerations. Skeletal Radiol. 1981;6:1–10.
8. Dorfmann H, De Bie B, Bonvarlet JP, Boyer T. Arthroscopic treatment of synovial chondromatosis of the knee. Arthroscopy. 1989;5:48–51.
9. Gilbert SR, Lachiewicz PF. Primary synovial osteochondromatosis of the hip: report of two cases with long-term follow-up after synovectomy and a review of the literature. Am J Orthop. 1997;26:555–60.
10. Lim SJ, Chung HW, Choi YL, Moon YW, Seo JG, Park YS. Operative treatment of primary osteochondromatosis of the hip. J Bone Joint Surg Am. 2006;88:256–64.
11. Lee JB, Kang C, Lee CH, Hwang DS. Arthroscopic treatment of synovial chondromatosis of the hip. Am J Sports Med. 2012;40(6):1412–8.
12. Zini R, Longo UG, deBenedetto M, Loppini M, Carraro A, Maffulli N, Denaro V. Arthroscopic management of primary synovial chondromatosis. Arthroscopy. 2013;29(3):420–6.
13. Boyer T, Dorfmann H. Arthroscopy in primary synovial chondromatosis of the hip: description and outcome of treatment. J Bone Joint Surg Br. 2008;90-B:314–8.
14. Dienst M, Godde S, Seil R, Hammer D, Kohn D. Hip arthroscopy without traction: in vivo anatomy of the peripheral hip joint cavity. Arthroscopy. 2001;17:924–31.
15. Dorfmann H, Boyer T, Henry P, De Bie B. A simple approach of hip arthroscopy. Arthroscopy. 1988;4(141).
16. Marchie A, Glassner PJ, Panuncialman I, McCarthy JC. Technical pearls for hip arthroscopy in the management of synovial chondromatosis. Am J Orthop (Belle Mead NJ). 2012;41(6):284–7.
17. Randelli F, Randelli P, Banci L, Arrigoni P. Intra-articular loose body removal during hip arthroscopy. Orthopedics. 2010;33(7):476.
18. Schoeniger R, Naudie DD, Siebenrock KA, Trousdale RT, Ganz R. Modified complete synovectomy prevents recurrence in synovial chondromatosis of the hip. Clin Orthop Relat Res. 2006;451: 195–200.
19. Nisar A, Gulhane S, Mahendra A, Meek RM, Patil S. Surgical dislocation of the hip for excision of benign tumours. J Orthop. 2014;11(1):28–36.
20. Villacin AB, Brigham LN, Bullough PG. Primary and secondary synovial chondrometaplasia. Histopathological and clinicoradiologic differences. Hum Pathol. 1979;10:439–51.
21. Durr HR, Stabler A, Maier M, Refior HJ. Pigmented villonodular synovitis. A review of 20 cases. J Rheumatol. 2001;28: 1620–30.
22. Myers BW, Masi AT. Pigmented villonodular synovitis and tenosynovitis: a clinical epidemiologic study of 166 cases and literature review. Medicine. 1989;59:223–38.

23. Flipo RM, Desvigne-Noulet MC, Cotten A, Fontaine C, Dusquenoy B, Lequesne M, Delcambre B. La synovite villo-nodulaire pigmentée de la hanche. Résultats d'une enquête nationale à propos de 58 observations. Rev Rhum. 1994;61:85–95.
24. Hughes TH, Sartoris DJ, Schweitzer ME, Resnick DL. Pigmented villonodular synovitis: MRI characteristics. Skeletal Radiol. 1995;24:7–12.
25. Cotten A, Dabbache C, Vieillard MH. Synovial tumors and pseudotumors. Rev Rhum. 2006;73:593–602.
26. Granowitz SP, D'antonio J, Mankin HL. The pathogenesis and long term end results of Pigmented villonodular synovitis. Clin Orthop. 1976;114:335–51.
27. Choong PF, Willen H, Nilbert M, Mertens F, Mandahl N, et al. Pigmented villonodular synovitis. Monoclonality and metastasis. A case for neoplastic origin? Acta Orthop Scand. 1995;66:64–8.
28. Ohjimi Y, Iwasaki H, Ishiguro M, et al. Short arm of chromosome 1 aberration recurrently found in pigmented villonodular synovitis. Cancer Genet Cytogenet. 1996;90:80–5.
29. Bouali H, Deppert EJ, Leventhal LJ, Reeves B, Pope T. Pigmented villonodular synovitis: a disease in evolution. J Rheumatol. 2004;31:1659–62.
30. Loriaut P, Djian P, Boyer T, Bonvarlet JP, Delin C, Makridis KG. Arthroscopic treatment of localized pigmented villonodular synovitis of the knee. Knee Surg Sports Traumatol Arthrosc. 2012;20(8):1550–3.
31. Rochwerger A, Groulier JP, Curvale G, Franceschi JP, Dufour M. Synovite villo-nodulaire pigmentée du genou: résultats des traitements à partir de 22 cas. Rev Chir Orthop. 1998;84:600–6.
32. Pinaroli A, Ait Si Selmi T, Servien E, Neyret P. Prise en charge de la synovite villo-nodulaire hémo-pigmentée du genou et de ses récidives. Rev Chir Orthop. 2006;92:437–47.
33. Bertoni F, Unni KK, Beabout JW, Sium FH. Malignant giant cell tumor of the tendon sheaths and joint (malignant pigmented villonodular synovitis). Am J Surg Pathol. 1997;21:153–63.
34. Shabat S, Kollender Y, Merimsky O, Isakov J, Flusser G, Nykska M, Meller I. The use of surgery and Yttrium 90 in the management of extensive and diffuse pigmented villonodular synovitis of large joints. Rheumaology (Oxford). 2002;41(10):1113–8.
35. Nicolas M, Biau D, Ayral X, Tomeno B, Anract P. Interet de la synoviorthèse adjuvante dans le traitement conservateur des synovites villonodulaires du genou, etude retrospective d'une série de 42 patients. Rev Chir Orthop. 2007;93:39–40.
36. May O, Boyer T, Dorfmann H. Pathologie du repli pectinéo-fovéal et traitement arthroscopique. Rev Chir Orthop. 2004;90:182.
37. Raney RB. Synovial sarcoma in young people: background, prognostic factors, and therapeutic questions. J Pediatr Hematol Oncol. 2005;27:207–11.
38. Anract P, Katabi M, Forest M, Benoit J, Witvoet J, Tomeno B. Chondromatose synoviale et chondrosarcome. Etude des rapports entre les deux affections. Rev Chir Orthop. 1996;82:216–23.

Hip Pathology: Overload Syndromes

17

Allston J. Stubbs and Elizabeth A. Howse

The object of such a distribution of the joints, in accurate association, is to insure mechanical and physiological consent between the external muscular, or moving force, and the vital endurance of the parts moved, namely, of the joints, thus securing in health a true balance of force and friction until deterioration occurs. [1]

—*John Hilton, F.R.S., F.R.C.S.*

Introduction

Repetitive impact or supraphysiologic loads placed on the musculoskeletal system overtime can result in the onset of pain without a notable injury, which is typically thought of as an overuse injury [2, 3]. An overuse injury is defined as the development of symptoms that can be as mild as causing a single day absence from ordinary training, to requiring the athlete to seek treatment from a medical practitioner [3]. Essentially, the stress placed on the bone exceeds its capacity for repair, as seen with stress fractures [3]. The purpose of this chapter is to demonstrate the various processes that alter the force and motion of the hip, ultimately overloading the hip joint, as well as show how compensation for these changes may result in additional pathology and ultimately symptomatology. This is perhaps most evident in the competitive athletes who test these limits when they push themselves to the extremes in range of motion.

A.J. Stubbs, MD, MBA (✉)
Division of Sports Medicine, Department of Orthopaedic Surgery, Wake Forest University, 131 Miller St., Winston Salem, NC 27103, USA
e-mail: astubbs@wakehealth.edu

E.A. Howse, MD
Department of Emergency Medicine, Hofstra North Shore-LIJ School of Medicine, Long Island Jewish Medical Center, New Hyde Park, NY, USA
e-mail: howseea@gmail.com

Instability

Instability has traditionally been characterized in the literature as either traumatic or atraumatic [4, 5]. Traumatic instability of the hip can present in a variety of different ways, the most obvious being the patient who has or gives a history of a clearly dislocated hip or acute injury. Atraumatic instability, however, is often attributed to congenital connective tissue disorders in which an underlying systemic process leads to the development of bony or soft tissue pathology [4, 5]. While these two definitions are distinct, they fall on either end of a spectrum of hip instability; therefore, the literature to date has been unclear as to how to classify the middle of the spectrum, essentially "overload instability" [4, 5]. Overload instability results from serial micro- and minor traumatic events that cannot be directly identified but cumulatively alter osseous and soft tissue anatomy ultimately overloading the joint consequently displaying disease that is normally attributed to major pathology [4–8]. This in turn can lead to the cyclical process of capsule-ligamentous attenuation pathology, as the ligaments and tendons compensate for the rotational instability afforded by a lax capsule and vice versa (Fig. 17.1) [6].

The labrum is believed to enhance stability of the hip joint by contributing to the negative intra-articular pressure [9]. When the labrum cannot dissipate the force placed on the joint during movement, the labrum tears, separating it from the acetabular cartilage [9]. Guanche theorized that the stride phase of running where the hip is repetitively placed in hyperextension ultimately causes stress to the cartilage-labral junction leading to subtle instability and potential

J.C. McCarthy et al. (eds.), *Hip Joint Restoration*, DOI 10.1007/978-1-4614-0694-5_17

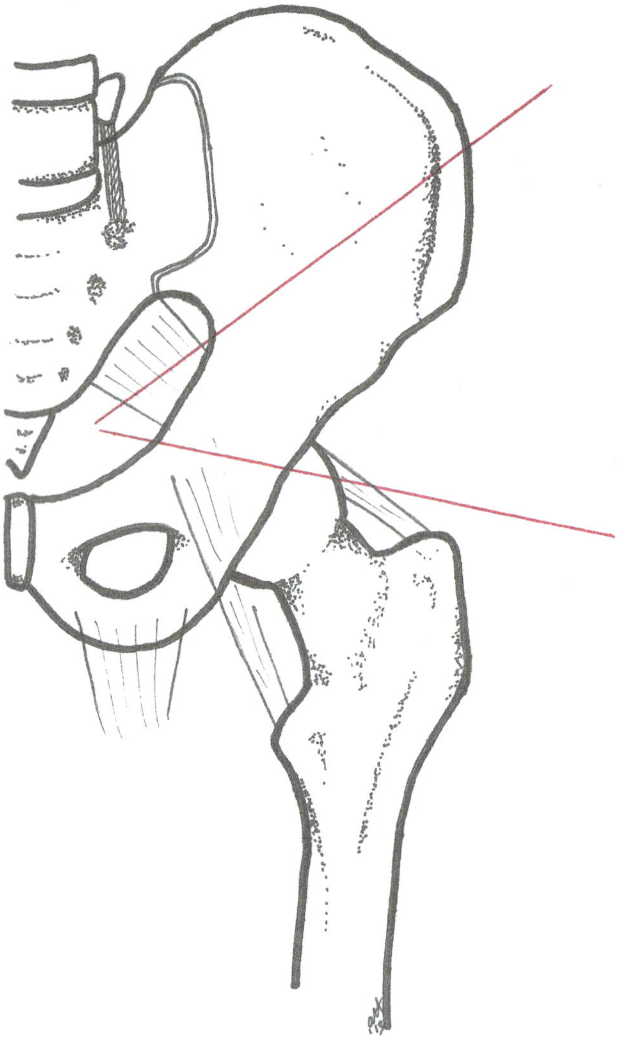

Fig. 17.1 Hemipelvis diagram depicting location of pathology. Anterior: core muscle injury, pubalgia, osteitis pubis, adductor tendonitis, genital radiculopathy. Lateral: femoroacetabular impingement, iliopsoas impingement, proximal hamstring rupture, piriformis syndrome, subspinal AIIS impingement, iliopsoas tendonitis, labral tear, ligamentous tear, avulsion of rectus femoris, capsuloligamentous attenuation, trochanteric bursitis. Posterior: lumbar radiculopathy, lumbar pain, sacroiliitis, pudendal neuralgia, pseudoradiculopathy, sciatica/non-discogenic sciatica

subluxation. Subtle differences in the morphology of the acetabulum will confound the potential for resultant pathology [9]. Stress fractures of the femoral neck are commonly seen in military recruits and endurance athletes who increase the intensity of or begin different forms of high-stress activities [2, 3]. In addition to changes in training, physiologic factors (i.e., female gender, nutritional deficiencies, bone mineral density) and underlying anatomy (coxa vara, femoroacetabular impingement (FAI), and acetabular retroversion) are proposed risk factors for the development of stress fractures around the hip [2, 3]. For example, Kuhn et al. showed that femoral neck stress fractures in military recruits are more common in patients with acetabular retroversion than in those without. It is theorized that acetabular retroversion alters the distribution of the load an athlete places on his/her hip, thereby increasing the amount of force placed across the proximal femur predisposing these individuals to a stress fracture [2, 6]. The additional force placed on the femur from acetabular retroversion in athletic competition can also be dispensed to other anatomically adjacent sites, such as the pubic rami.

While further investigation is warranted, this is the hypothesized development of injury in three collegiate level athletes who have presented to the senior author's clinic for evaluation of hip pain. Each had subsequently been diagnosed with pubic rami stress fractures, FAI bone morphology, and acetabular labral tears by MRI (Figs. 17.2 and 17.3). Two have been successfully treated with activity modification and the third is currently undergoing treatment. These stress fractures of the pubic ramus represent an extreme of anterior pelvis overuse injury, falling on the same spectrum as pain at the pubic symphysis, resulting from inflammation or instability known as osteitis pubis [10–13]. Verrall et al. performed a preliminary cohort study of 29 elite Australian football players to demonstrate that restriction of hip motion predisposes athletes to pubic bone stress injuries [10, 11]. It is hypothesized that the adductors and obturator externus, which originate from the pubis and insert on the femur, can cause a shearing injury by displacing force as the athlete attempts to overcome restriction in range of motion particularly with twisting of the hip [11, 12, 14, 15].

The ligamentum teres, while historically overlooked, is increasingly becoming recognized as a cause of persistent intra-articular hip pain when damaged [16]. Gray and Villar classified pathology of the ligamentum teres into three groups: complete rupture, partial rupture, and degenerative fraying [17]. While complete rupture was initially attributed to major trauma (dislocation or surgical intervention of the hip), recent literature has theorized that repetitive hyper-abduction stresses of the hip can result in an avulsion of the ligamentum teres without disruption to the capsule after subluxation with spontaneous reduction [16, 18–21]. In extreme abduction, the ligamentum teres normally becomes taut, with the addition of "superadded flexion," and in external rotation, the ligamentum teres is ruptured as impingement of the acetabular rim on the femoral neck levers the femoral head out of the acetabulum [20]. In many of the reported cases, the history was only suggestive of subluxation as the patient was unable to identify an acute injury. Furthermore, clinical examination failed to demonstrate signs of instability. For example, Kusma et al. postulated that repetitive hyper-abduction of the hip during horse riding resulted in occult subluxation of the hip and subsequently avulsion of the ligamentum teres [18]. It is plausible that in addition to the extent of the injury to the ligamentum teres, the location

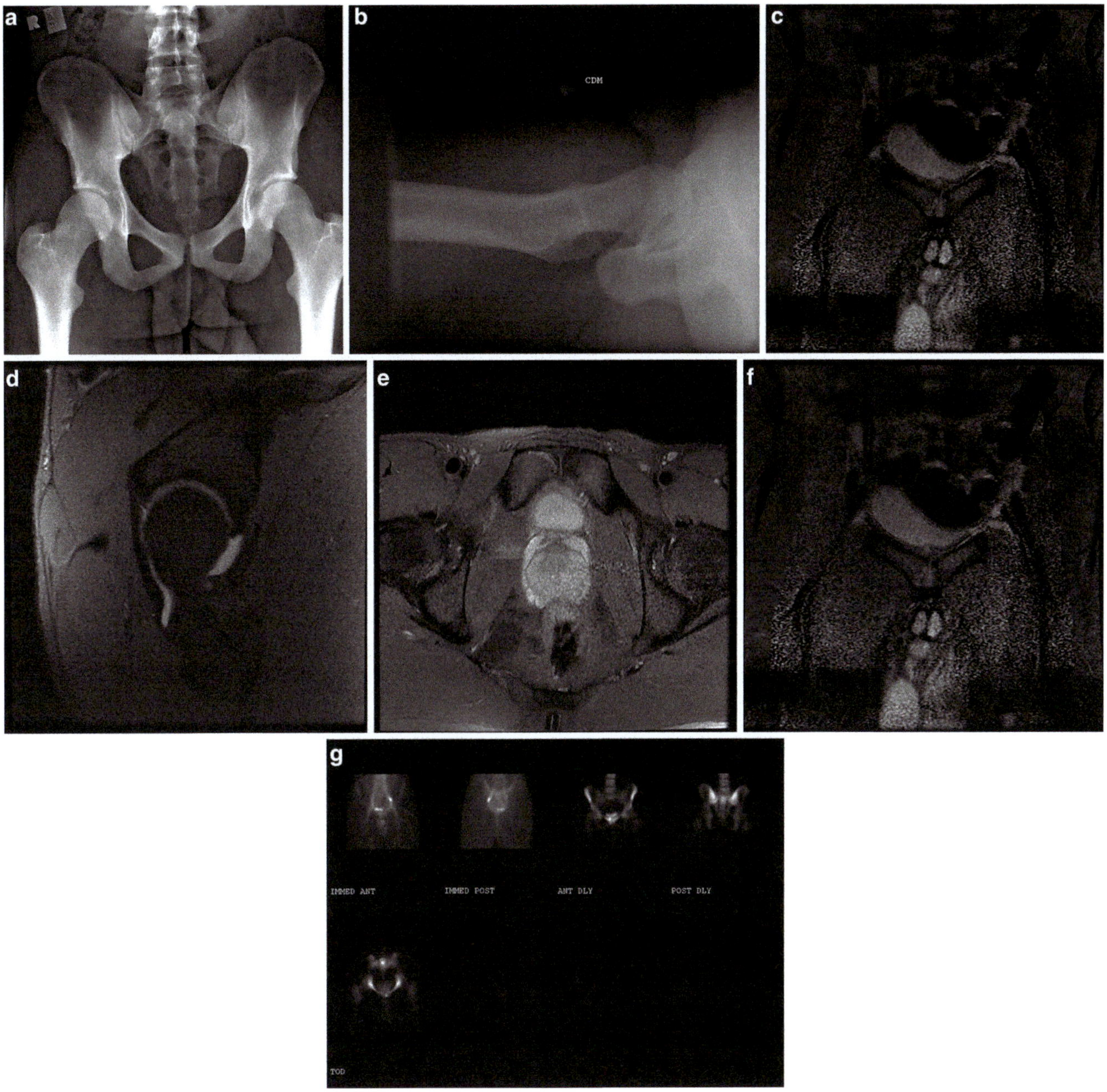

Fig. 17.2 Imaging of triad of FAI, acetabular labral tear, and pubic ramus stress fracture in right hip: (**a**) AP pelvis, (**b**) cross table lateral view, (**c**) anterior superior labral tear visualized in coronal plane of MRI arthrogram, (**d**) anterior superior labral tear visualized in oblique plane of MRI arthrogram, (**e**) axial view of T2-weighted MRI, (**f**) coronal view of T2-weighted MRI, (**g**) technetium-99m bone scintigraphy, *ANT* anterior, *Post* posterior, *IMMED* immediate, *DLY* delay, *TOD* tail-on-the-detector

may play a significant role regarding patient presentation. Barrett et al. reported a case in which a 5-year-old girl suffered an avulsion fracture of the ligamentum teres after a seemingly minor injury—stumbling down three stairs and landing on her feet [21]. Examination of the child immediately following the injury demonstrated generalized ligamentous laxity and widening of the joint space without evidence of fracture or dislocation [21]. Intraoperative findings showed an osteocartilaginous fragment attached to the ligamentum teres obstructing the complete reduction of the femoral head and thereby suggesting prior dislocation [21]. It is postulated that without the associated osteocartilaginous fragment, the femoral head would have returned to its normal position allowing the patient to bear weight without further symptoms.

Traumatic dislocation of the hip is classically described as following a high-energy injury (such as a motor vehicle collision or contact athletic competition) where the hip is in a flexed and adducted position and a significant force applied

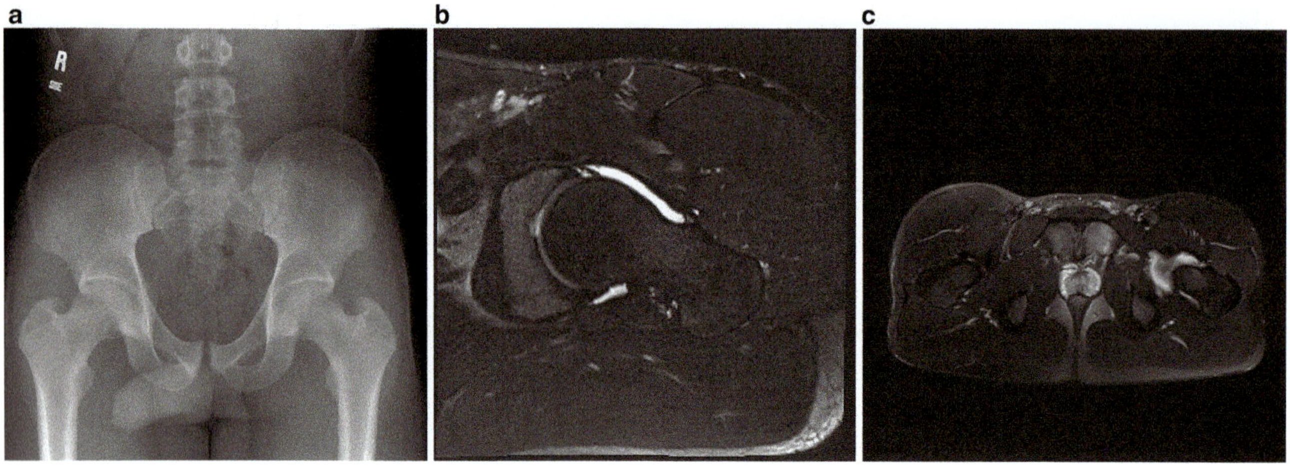

Fig. 17.3 Imaging of triad of FAI, acetabular labral tear, and pubic ramus stress fracture in left hip: (**a**) AP pelvis, (**b**) axial plane view of labral tear in T2-weighted MRI arthrogram, (**c**) ramus stress fracture in axial plane of T2-weighted MRI

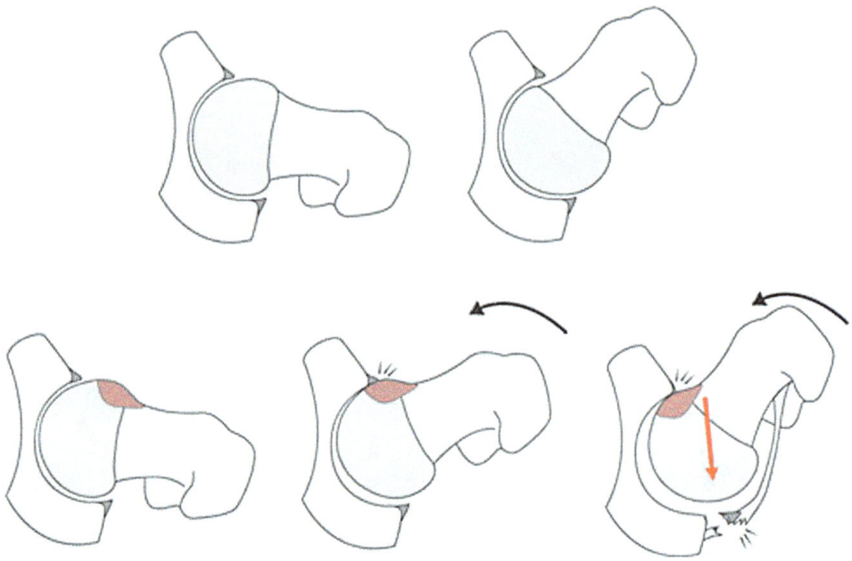

Fig. 17.4 Diagraph illustrates a theorized mechanism of injury for patients with FAI and posterior hip instability. *Top row*: with normal osseous hip anatomy, internal rotation is not impeded. *Bottom row*: in patients with cam-type FAI, internal rotation is limited. Attempts at achieving internal rotation cause anterior impingement and levering, which drives the femoral head posteriorly (*red arrow*). From Krych AJ, et al. Is Posterior Hip Instability Associated with Cam and Pincer Deformity? Clin Orthop Relat Res. 2012;470(12):3390–7. Reprinted with permission from Springer

distally displaces the femur posteriorly. In addition to dislocation of the joint, supplemental pathology has been documented such as fractures of the acetabulum, femoral head and neck, labral tears, chondral defects, and loose bodies [22]. These same intra-articular pathologies may be caused from lower-energy injuries where the hip is subluxated rather than dislocated. Recent literature has recognized occult subluxation of the hip as both a cause (i.e., avulsion of the ligamentum teres, capsule and labral tears, and osteochondral lesions) and effect (from pathologies such as posterior capsule instability and FAI) of hip pain in many young athletes [5, 20].

FAI is the condition in which the ROM of the hip is restricted as the proximal femur contacts the acetabulum due to abnormal bony morphology. FAI can be described as cam impingement in which the contact is attributed to an aspherical femoral head, pincer impingement in which there is over coverage of the acetabulum, or more commonly a combination between the two [23–26]. In pincer impingement, the labrum is compressed as the femoral neck abuts with the acetabulum. This contact over time results in degeneration and subsequently ossification of the labrum at the point of contact [24, 25]. The ossification of the labrum exacerbates the initial underlying deformity by further restricting hip flexion [24, 25]. As the athletes, over time, continue to push themselves in competition to their extremes of motion, impingement at the anterosuperior rim of the labrum forces the femoral head posteriorly (Fig. 17.4) [8, 24]. Consequently, chondral shear injuries and capsular redundancy theoretically develop as contrecoup injuries of the posterior-labral junction in chronic FAI, as the area of impingement serves as a lever [5, 24, 27–29]. Repeating the offending motion made by an athlete in competition makes seemingly innocuous movement a setup for damage normally attributed to major trauma, such as subluxation and/or dislocation of the hip [4, 5, 8, 22, 28]. As depicted in Fig. 17.4, the morphology that causes the impingement may serve as a lever, thereby creating enough force to allow posterior subluxation of the femoral head [5, 8, 19, 28].

The consequence of one form of pathology in relation to additional injuries is exemplified in the "sports hip triad" consisting of a labral tear, adductor strain, and rectus strain [11, 30, 31]. As an athlete attempts to overcome the restriction of terminal flexion and internal rotation caused by FAI, the athlete alters his/her motion, thereby placing abnormal stresses on the surrounding muscles (adductors, abductors, hip flexors, iliopsoas, and proximal hamstrings) of the hemipelvis [31, 32]. This notion has gained popularity, as FAI and athletic pubalgia/core muscle injuries are becoming concurrent diagnoses with increasing frequency [30–32]. Core muscle injury (CMI) is a term applied to pelvic injuries that involve the abdominal and pelvis musculature on either side of the pubic symphysis, outside of the hip joint [33]. Originally attributed to abdominal rectus weakness, the adductor muscles have gained increasing recognition to the development of CMI pathology [33]. It has been hypothesized that a muscular imbalance between strong hip flexor and adductor musculature, relative to a weaker abdominal rectus, produces a shearing force across the pubic symphysis [34]. Repetitive trauma as the athlete flexes, extends, abducts, and adducts his/her hip ultimately produces a shearing force causing inflammation at the symphysis resulting in osteitis pubis [6, 35, 36]. When the hip is forced into external rotation, the adductor longus undergoes the most strain as it has the least mechanical advantage on the hip [35]. While the treatment of FAI or CMI alone may result in a cessation of symptoms, many athletes only notice partial relief and require operative management of both conditions in order to return to their previous level of play [31, 37]. Additional investigation is warranted in order to better understand the relationship between FAI and CMI. In addition to strains of the core musculature, FAI may contribute to strains of the lower extremity muscles. Eccentric contraction in sports (backswing) places the athlete's hip into hyperextension (with the knee in flexion) and thereby produces significant tension that ultimately may result in a hip flexor strain or avulsion [11, 38]. Conversely, when the hip is suddenly forced into flexion with the knee in extension (hamstring contracted), a hamstring strain, or in more severe cases rupture of the hamstring tendon from the ischium, may occur [39–41]. Hammoud et al. further postulate hamstring tendinopathy to result from chronic shortening of the hamstring as a means to offset anterior impingement with a compensatory posterior pelvic tilt [11].

While bony impingement has been recognized since 1936, extra-articular causes of impingement such as from the anterior inferior iliac spine (AIIS) have only been recognized in the last few years [42–45]. The AIIS is just superior to the acetabular rim. When a patient has a prominent AIIS, it may abut against the femur, thereby limiting the patient's motion, much like acetabular retroversion or FAI [42–44]. A prominent AIIS may be developmental or may in itself be the consequence of an overuse injury [42–44]. Avulsion fractures of the AIIS can result from acute trauma or a product of repeated stresses that, as the athlete trains, weaken the cohesion of the epiphyseal plate and ultimately cause hypertrophy of the muscle and the apophysis [42–44, 46].

Tijssen et al., in a review of physical exam maneuvers used to diagnose FAI and labral pathology, found that the "Patrick sign" or flexion-abduction-external rotation (FABER) test is both highly sensitive and specific (0.90 or greater) in the diagnosis of anterior hip impingement [47]. The FABER maneuver is performed with the patient lying supine; the examined leg is put in the "Fig. 17.4" position (flexed, abducted, and externally rotated). FABER has classically been used in order to diagnose sacroiliac pathology by stressing the sacroiliac (SI) joint but has since been recognized to also assess the external rotation of the hip [47]. Loss of external rotation of the hip (where the knee of the examined leg remains floating in the air) implicates anterior impingement/labral pathology [47]. Tijssen et al. stated that it is important for the examiner to determine anterior versus posterior pain in order to distinguish hip from SI pathology.

In addition, we theorize that when the external rotation of the hip is decreased, this transfers an additional physiologic load onto the SI joint. The SI joint is a diarthrodial joint, which cannot move kinetically like the hip (a ball and socket joint). It therefore absorbs the increased energy caused from hip pathology (Fig. 17.5). This increased energy from overloading of the hip theoretically stresses the SI joint and results in sacroiliitis. This is demonstrated by the addition of posterior pain or low back pain as described by Vad et al. in a population of golfers [48]. They alleged that loss of range of motion in the lead hip was secondary to repetitive microtrauma resulting in capsular contracture, which ultimately manifested as low back pain [48]. Loss of internal and external rotation results in an increased distance of flexion-abduction-external rotation and extension of the hip, and the excess torque is thereby transmitted to the lumbar spine [48, 49]. Loss of lumbar extension was also noted in these patients, and while this may be a result of decreased flexibility, it is speculated that as a protective mechanism against the increased load on the spine the patient reflexively limits lumbar extension [48, 50]. Grimshaw and Burden further support the theory of limited range of motion of the hip resulting in low back pain in a case study of a 22-year-old professional golfer whose hip pain resolved after being coached to

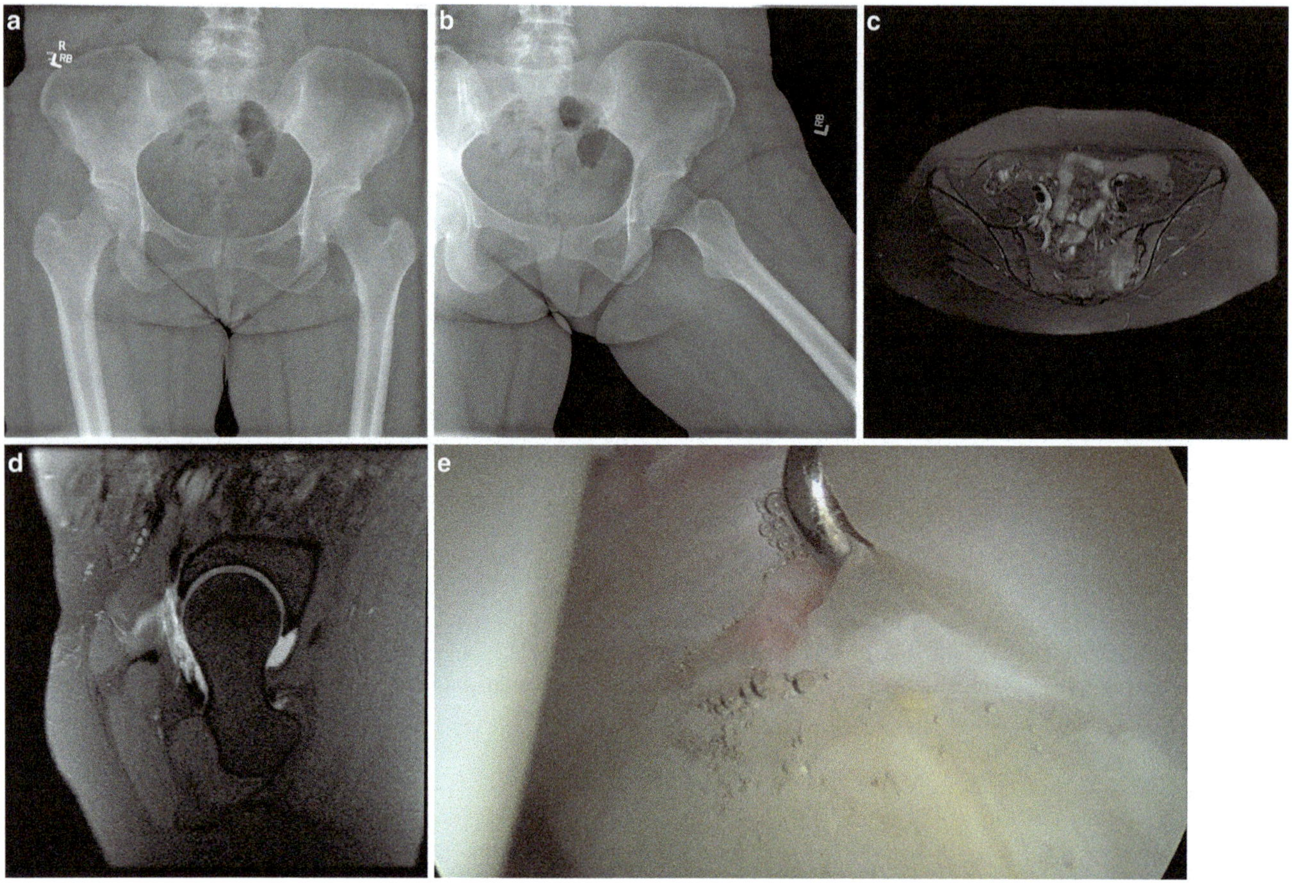

Fig. 17.5 (**a**) AP view of pelvis, (**b**) frog leg view of left hip, (**c**) T2-weighted axial view of MRI, (**d**) T2-weighted oblique MRI demonstrating left labral tear, (**e**) intraoperative photograph demonstrating labral tear

increase his hip (and shoulder) range of motion throughout his swing [48, 51].

Domb et al. in a retrospective review of 36 hips described overuse of the iliopsoas tendon resulting in labral tears in a condition they termed "iliopsoas impingement" (IPI) [11, 52]. In each of the hips, under arthroscopic visualization, the iliopsoas tendon appeared inflamed and overlaid an isolated injury of the labrum at the 3 o'clock (iliopsoas notch) position [52]. They speculated three forms of pathophysiology. The first being impingement of the anterior labrum by the iliopsoas while the hip is in extension, the second a repetitive traction injury from adherence of the tendon to the anterior capsule-labral complex, and the third described as traction causing a labral injury due to contractions of a hyperactive iliocapsularis muscle [52, 53]. Pathology of the iliopsoas tendon may additionally result in iliopsoas bursitis whereby activities involving hip flexion mechanically irritate the bursa [6].

Another cause of hip overload is secondary to a leg length discrepancy [54–57]. An individual with a leg length discrepancy has a vertically displaced center of gravity. This in turn causes additional compressive and tensile stresses applied to the lower extremity joints, secondary to altered weight distribution in stance and compensatory changes in movement during gait [54, 55]. For example, increasing the amount of hip adduction (or knee flexion) effectively minimizes the discrepancy and thus reduces the amount of energy expended [54, 55]. This change in hip positioning can result in microtrauma of the piriformis muscle since functionally it attributes to hip flexion, provides abduction while in flexion and external rotation when in extension, and helps to provide postural stability [57–59]. This is one of the theorized causes for the development of piriformis syndrome. Sun et al. recently presented a case describing a 22-year-old female with a congenital leg length discrepancy that developed piriformis syndrome in her longer leg as a consequence of postural compensation (increased hip flexion) [54]. Conversely, Dere et al. presented two cases in which piriformis syndrome occurred, also due to a leg length discrepancy. However, their patients developed piriformis syndrome in the contralateral (shorter) leg conceivably due to spasm from compensatory leg extension [56]. While there are many proposed methods of treatment for piriformis syndrome, correction of leg length inequality with an aid such as a shoe lift has shown to be both therapeutic and preventative [54, 55]. We further hypothesize that patients without leg length discrepancies may develop iatrogenic piriformis syndrome due to imposed differences in leg lengths when treating lower leg pathology. Two patients who presented to the senior author's clinic with pain at the piriformis after wearing a CAM boot orthosis support this theory.

Pathology associated with the piriformis muscle has furthermore been identified as one of the potential causes of non-discogenic sciatica or deep gluteal syndrome (DGS) defined by Martin et al. as gluteal and radicular pain experienced during hip movement which subsequently entraps the sciatic nerve [11, 59]. As the patient flexes his hip, the tendon impinges upon the sciatic nerve, thereby eliciting pain and paresthesias [59]. Anatomical variations of the sciatic nerve in relation to the piriformis muscle may also predispose the patient to developing symptoms (such as bifurcation of the nerve or a split piriformis tendon). Furthermore, the close anatomical associations of the hamstring, obturator internus, gemellus complex, or greater trochanteric bursa can result in DGS when diseased [59]. For example, Martin et al. found that 27 of 35 patients with DGS had an excessively thickened greater trochanteric bursa with fibrous scar bands appearing to extend near the sciatic nerve when examined endoscopically [59]. Greater trochanteric bursitis may result from overuse and thereby inflammation of the iliotibial band (ITB). The ITB, consisting of the tensor fascia lata and gluteus maximus, serves as a flexor, abductor, and medial rotator of the hip. It also provides lateral knee stability when standing. Dysfunction or tearing of the gluteals can cause the ITB to thicken/tighten, ultimately resulting in coxa saltans externa (snapping of the ITB) over the greater trochanter and thereby inflaming the bursa as the hip is flexed [6, 60]. An alternative formation of DGS may form when the nerve adheres to the hamstring tendons after an avulsion injury, preventing it from gliding during flexion [11, 59]. As the hip stabilizers become diseased, they encroach upon the surrounding nerves (altering proprioception) and vasculature (obstructing arterial supply and/or causing venous congestion), thereby resulting in a form of genital radiculopathy (pelvic, perineal and inguinal pain, in addition to sciatic pain) and ultimately sexual dysfunction [61].

Conclusion

While overload syndromes of the hip have only recently become recognized, and further investigation is necessary, it is important to keep in mind that the forms of presenting pathology are vast and manifest in a variety of ways. Intra-articular pathology can present as extra-articular problems, and conversely the surrounding extra-articular structures can result in intra-articular pathology. The surgeon must be aware of the relationship of the surrounding anatomy and how it can affect the hip, in order to alleviate symptoms and prevent recurrence.

References

1. Hilton J. Rest and pain. London: Bell; 1863.
2. Kuhn KM, Riccio AI, Saldua NS, Cassidy J. Acetabular retroversion in military recruits with femoral neck stress fractures. Clin Orthop Relat Res. 2010;468:846–51.
3. Rolf C. Overuse injuries of the lower extremity in runners. Scand J Med Sci Sports. 1995;5:181–90.
4. Boykin RE, Anz AW, Bushnell BD, Kocher MS, Stubbs AJ, Philippon MJ. Hip Instability. J Am Acad Orthop Surg. 2011;19:1–10.
5. Guanche CA. Hip instability. In: Byrd JWT, editor. Operative hip arthroscopy. 2nd ed. New York: Springer; 2005. p. 339–48.
6. Pappas GP, Safran MR. Hip injuries in the athlete. In: Margheritini F, Rossi R, editors. Orthopedic sports medicine: principles and practice. Milano: Springer; 2011. p. 275–99.
7. Bowman KF, Fox J, Sekiya JK. A clinically relevant review of hip biomechanics. Arthroscopy. 2010;26(8):1118–29.
8. Berkes MB, Cross MB, Shindle MK, Beedi A, Kelly BT. Traumatic posterior hip instability and femoroacetabular impingement in athletes. Am J Orthop. 2012;41(4):166–71.
9. Guanche CA, Sikka RS. Acetabular labral tears with underlying chondromalacia: a possible association with high-level running. Arthroscopy. 2005;21(5):580–5.
10. Verrall GM, Slavotinekc GTF. Incidence of pubic bone marrow oedema in Australian rules football players: relation to groin pain. Br J Sports Med. 2001;35:28–33.
11. Hammoud S, Magennis E, Voos JE, Bedi A, Kelly BT. Compensatory disorders around the hip. In: Byrd JWT, editor. Operative hip arthroscopy. 3rd ed. New York: Springer; 2013. p. 385–402.
12. Paajanen H, Hermunen H, Karonen J. Pubic magnetic resonance imaging findings in surgically and conservatively treated athletes with osteitis pubis compared to asymptomatic athletes during heavy training. Am J Sports Med. 2008;36:117–21.
13. Radic R, Annear P. Use of pubic symphysis curettage for treatment-resistant osteitis pubis in athletes. Am J Sports Med. 2008;36: 122–8.
14. Williams JG. Limitation of hip joint movement as a factor in traumatic osteitis pubis. Br J Sports Med. 1978;12:129–33.
15. Williams PR, Thomas DP, Downes EM. Osteitis pubis and instability of the pubic symphysis: when nonoperative measures fail. Am J Sports Med. 2000;28(3):350–5.
16. Byrd JWT, Jones KS. Traumatic rupture of the ligamentum teres as a source of hip pain. Arthroscopy. 2004;20(4):385–91.
17. Gray AJR, Villar RN. The ligamentum teres of the hip: an arthroscopic classification of its pathology. Arthroscopy. 1997; 13(5):575–8.
18. Kumsa M, Jung J, Dienst M, Goedde S, Kohn D, Seil R. Arthroscopic treatment of an avulsion fracture of the ligamentum teres of the hip in an 18-year-old horse rider. Arthroscopy. 2004;20(6):64–6.
19. Delcamp DD, Klaaren HE, Pompe van Meerdervoot HF. Traumatic avulsion of the ligamentum teres without dislocation of the hip. J Bone Joint Surg Am. 1988;70:933–5.
20. Oh KJ, Pandher DS, Lee SH. Arthroscopic management of acute painful hip following occult subluxation: evidence-based case report. Knee Surg Sports Traumatol Arthrosc. 2007;15:1370–4.
21. Barrett IR, Goldberg JA. Avulsion fracture of the ligamentum teres in a child. J Bone Joint Surg Am. 1989;71:438–9.

22. Philippon MJ, Kuppersmith DA, Wolff AB, Briggs KK. Arthroscopic findings following traumatic hip dislocation in 14 professional athletes. Arthroscopy. 2009;25(2):169–74.
23. Tibor LM, Sekiya JK. Differential diagnosis of pain around the hip joint. Arthroscopy. 2008;24:1407–21.
24. Beck M, Kalhor M, Leunig M, Ganz R. Hip morphology influence the pattern of damage to the acetabular cartilage: femoroacetabular impingement as a cause of early osteoarthritis of the hip. J Bone Joint Surg Br. 2005;87:1012–8.
25. Shindle MK, Voos JE, Heyworth BE, Mintz DN, Moya LE, Buly RL, Kelly BT. Hip arthroscopy in the athletic patient: current techniques and spectrum of disease. J Bone Joint Surg Am. 2007;89:29–43.
26. Clohisy JC, Knause ER, Hunt DM, Lesher JM, Harris-Hayes M, Prather H. Clinical presentation of patients with symptomatic anterior hip impingement. Clin Orthop Relat Res. 2009;467:638–44.
27. Bedi A, Galano G, Walsh C, Kelly BT. Capsular management during hip arthroscopy: from femoroacetabular impingement to instability. Arthroscopy. 2011;27(12):1720–31.
28. Krych AJ, Thompson M, Larson CM, Bryd JWT, Kelly BT. Is posterior hip instability associated with cam and pincer deformity? Clin Orthop Relat Res. 2012;470(12):3390–7.
29. Telleria JJM, Lindsey DP, Giori NJ, Safran MR. An anatomic description of the hip capsular ligaments for the hip arthroscopist. Arthroscopy. 2011;27(5):628–36.
30. Nepple JJ, Brophy RH, Matava MJ, Wright RW, Clohisy JC. Radiographic findings of femoroacetabular impingement in national football league combine athletes undergoing radiographs for previous hip or groin pain. Arthroscopy. 2012;28(10):1396–403.
31. Hammoud S, Bedi A, Magennis E, Meyers WC, Kelly BT. High incidence of athletic pubalgia symptoms in professional athletes with symptomatic femoroacetabular impingement. Arthroscopy. 2012;28(10):1388–95.
32. Bedi A, Dolan M, Leunig M, Kelly BT. Static and dynamic mechanical causes of hip pain. Arthroscopy. 2007;27(2):235–51.
33. Meyers WC, McKechnie A, Philippon MJ, Horner MA, Zoga AC, Devon ON. Experience with "sports hernia" spanning two decades. Ann Surg. 2008;248:656–65.
34. Kachingwe AF, Grech S. Proposed algorithm for the management of athletes with athletic pubalgia (sports hernia): a case series. J Orthop Sports Phys Ther. 2008;38(12):768–81.
35. Shah A, Busconi B. Hip and pelvis. In: DeLee JC, Drez Jr D, Miller MD, editors. DeLee & Drez's orthopaedic sports medicine. 3rd ed. Philadelphia: Saunders Elsevier; 2010. p. 1451–76.
36. Anderson K, Strickland SM, Warren R. Hip and groin injuries in athletes. Am J Sports Med. 2001;29(4):521–33.
37. Larson CM, Pierce BR, Giveans MR. Treatment of athletes with symptomatic intra-articular hip pathology and athletic pubalgia/sports hernia: a case series. Arthroscopy. 2011;27:768–75.
38. Hsu CJ, Fischer DA, Wright RW. Proximal rectus femoris avulsions in National Football League kickers: a report of two cases. Am J Sports Med. 2005;33(7):1085–7.
39. Miller SL, Webb GR. The proximal origin of the hamstrings and surrounding anatomy encountered during repair. J Bone Joint Surg. 2007;89-A:44–8.
40. Cohen S, Bradley J. Acute proximal hamstring rupture. J Am Acad Orthop Surg. 2007;15:350–5.
41. Clanton TO, Coupe KJ. Hamstring strains in athletes: diagnosis and treatment. J Am Acad Orthop Surg. 1998;6:237–48.
42. Pan HL, Kawanabe K, Akiyama H, Goto K, Onishi E, Nakamura T. Operative treatment of hip impingement caused by hypertrophy of the anterior iliac spine. J Bone Joint Surg Br. 2008;90-B:677–9.
43. Hestroni I, Larson CM, Torre KD, Zbeda RM, Magennis E, Kelly BT. Anterior inferior iliac spine deformity as an extra-articular source for hip impingement: a series of 10 patients treated with arthroscopic decompression. Arthroscopy. 2012;28(11):1644–53.
44. Larson CM, Kelly BT, Stone RM. Making a case for anterior inferior iliac spine/subspine hip impingement: three representative case reports and proposed concept. Arthroscopy. 2011;27(12):1732–7.
45. Smith-Petersen MN. Treatment of malum coxae senilis, old slipped upper femoral epiphysis, intrapelvic protrusion of the acetabulum, and coxa plana by means of acetabuloplasty. J Bone Joint Surg Am. 1936;18(4):869–80.
46. Rossi F, Dragoni S. Acute avulsion fractures of the pelvis in adolescent competitive athletes: prevalence, location and sports distribution of 203 cases collected. Skeletal Radiol. 2001;30:127–31.
47. Tijssen M, van Cingel R, Willemsen L, de Visser E. Diagnostics of femoroacetabular impingement and labral pathology of the hip: a systematic review of the accuracy and validity of physical tests. Arthroscopy. 2012;28(6):860–71.
48. Vad VB, Bhat AL, Basrai D, Gebeh A, Aspergen DD, Andrews JR. Low back pain in professional golfers: the role of associated hip and low back range-of-motion deficits. Am J Sports Med. 2004;32(2):494–7.
49. Barbee-Ellison J, Rose SJ, Sahrmann SA. Patterns of hip rotation range of motion: a comparison between healthy subjects and patients with low back pain. Phys Ther. 1990;70:537–41.
50. Lindsay D, Horton J. Comparison of spine motion in elite golfers with and without low back pain. J Sports Sci. 2002;20:599–605.
51. Grimshaw PN, Burden AM. Case report: reduction of low back pain in a professional golfer. Med Sci Sports Exerc. 2000; 32:1667–73.
52. Domb BG, Shindle MK, McArthur B, Voos JE, Magennis E, Kelly BT. Iliopsoas impingement: a newly identified cause of labral pathology in the hip. HSS J. 2011;7:1–6.
53. Delp SL, Hess WE, Hungerford DS, Jones LC. Variation of rotation of moment arms with hip flexion. J Biomech. 1999;32:493–501.
54. Sun CH, Lu SC, Wu YT, Chang ST. Development of unilateral piriformis syndrome in a female with congenital leg length discrepancy. Open J Orthop. 2012;2:135–7.
55. Golightly YM, Allen KD, Helmick CG, Renner JB, Jordan JM. Symptoms of the knee and hip in individuals with and without limb length inequality. Osteoarthritis Cartilage. 2009; 17:596–600.
56. Dere K, Akbas M, Luleci N. A rare cause of a piriformis syndrome. J Back Musculoskelet Rehabil. 2009;22:55–8.
57. Boyajian-O'Neill LA, McClain RL, Coleman MK, Thomas PP. Diagnosis and management of piriformis syndrome: an osteopathic approach. J Am Osteopath Assoc. 2008;108(11):657–64.
58. Cassidy L, Walters A, Bubb K, Shoja MM, Tubbs RS, Loukas M. Piriformis syndrome: implications of anatomical variations, diagnostic techniques, and treatment options. Surg Radiol Anat. 2012;34:479–86.
59. Martin HD, Shears SA, Johnson JC, Smathers AM, Palmer IJ. The endoscopic treatment of sciatic nerve entrapment/deep gluteal syndrome. Arthroscopy. 2011;27(2):172–81.
60. Stubbs AJ, Mason P. Iliotibial band release. In: Byrd JWT, editor. Operative hip arthroscopy. 3rd ed. New York: Springer; 2013. p. 291–8.
61. Cox JM, Bakkum BW. Possible generators of retrotrochanteric gluteal and thigh pain: the gemelli-obturator internus complex. J Manipulative Physiol Ther. 2005;28(7):534–8.

Hip Disease Etiologies: Trauma

18

Joshua A. Tuck, Scott King, Craig M. Roberto,
and Brian D. Busconi

Introduction

In this chapter, we will review traumatic injuries to the hip experienced usually by athletes. Traumatic instability cases and fractures involving the hip region are much less frequent in athletes than soft tissue or avulsion injuries, but are much more violent and dangerous to the athlete. This chapter will provide the general insight regarding the history and presentation of the injured athlete and will help the clinician determine the diagnosis and treatment.

Traumatic Hip Instability

Hip dislocations are uncommon in sports, with a reported incidence of approximately 2–5 % of all hip dislocations occurring in sporting activities [1, 2]. Dislocations of the hip, with or without associated fractures, have been reported in sports such as football, rugby, wrestling, soccer, gymnastics, snow/water skiing, volleyball, tennis, equestrian riding, and jogging [2–8]. Children may be more prone to this injury than adults because less force is required to dislocate the joint [2, 9].

Posterior hip dislocations occur more frequently than anterior dislocations in sports, just as in motor vehicle accidents [1, 2, 6]. The two most common mechanisms that lead to the injuries are either falling forward onto the knee with transmission of an axial load up the thigh into the hip or, similarly, falling down onto all four extremities, in the hand and knees position, again with axial loading of the femur [2]. Typically, the injured player falls under the weight of an opponent when the injury occurs, causing increased axial load to be supported by an adducted hip, leading to posterior dislocation [1, 2, 6]. Anterior dislocations occur when the hip is forced into abduction and external rotation, as if doing the splits, and are more commonly seen in sports such as gymnastics or track and field events [6]. Whether a simple dislocation occurs or a fracture-dislocation occurs depends on the amount of hip flexion and adduction at the time of the posterior dislocation [2]. A simple posterior dislocation is more likely with greater hip flexion and adduction [2].

Upon examination, the lower extremity is in a flexed, internally rotated, and adducted position with posterior dislocations and in an extended, externally rotated, and abducted position with anterior dislocations. As with any dislocation, prompt closed reduction, if possible, is paramount. The risk of osteonecrosis or sciatic-related nerve palsy increases with the length of the delay in achieving reduction. Check the neurovascular status of the ipsilateral extremity, evaluating for a foot drop that may have occurred with the posterior dislocation, as the peroneal division of the sciatic nerve can be involved. A complete evaluation of the ipsilateral knee is important, with particular attention to the extensor mechanism, as the injury usually involves a direct trauma to the anterior knee. In a series of 28 knees with ipsilateral hip dislocations, Schmidt et al. [10] reported that 21 (75 %) patients had pain, 25 (89 %) had visible soft tissue injury, and MR imaging of 27 of these cases revealed that almost all (93 %) had musculoskeletal abnormalities. Thirty-seven percent had knee effusion, 33 % had bone bruises, and 30 % had meniscal tears.

In terms of imaging, an AP radiograph of the pelvis, AP and lateral radiographs of the involved side, as well as Judet (45° rotation views to evaluate the acetabulum) views should

J.A. Tuck, DO, MS
Division of Sports Medicine, Department of Orthopaedic Surgery, University of Massachusetts Medical School, University of Massachusetts Memorial Medical Center, Worcester, MA, USA

S. King, DO • C.M. Roberto, DO
Division of Sports Medicine, Department of Orthopaedics, University of Massachusetts, Worcester, MA, USA

B.D. Busconi, MD (✉)
Division of Sports Medicine, Department of Orthopaedics, University of Massachusetts Memorial Medical Center, 281 Lincoln St., Worcester, MA 01605, USA
e-mail: Brian.Busconi@umassmemorial.org

J.C. McCarthy et al. (eds.), *Hip Joint Restoration*, DOI 10.1007/978-1-4614-0694-5_18

be obtained upon reduction of the hip. Concentric reduction should be confirmed from the radiographic images. If this is not present, an osteochondral fragment, possibly from an acetabular rim or femoral head fracture, may be incarcerated within the joint or soft tissue may be interposed between the joint surfaces. Nonconcentric reduction should be followed by urgent CT scan for preoperative planning of surgical correction. Moorman et al. [11] evaluated the MRI findings after a traumatic subluxation of the hip and described the triad of posterior acetabular lip fracture, iliofemoral ligament disruption, and hemarthrosis. In a series of 14 patients with MRI performed in the acute setting, Laorr and colleagues [12] noted femoral head bone contusions, acetabular lip fractures, intra-articular loose bodies, ligamentum teres entrapment, and ILFL injury.

Prompt reduction of the dislocated joint is imperative to minimize the risk of avascular necrosis (AVN) of the femoral head. Hougaard and Thomsen [13] noted a 4.8 % incidence of AVN for hips reduced within 6 hours of the dislocation versus a 52.9 % incidence in hips reduced after 6 hours. Reduction is performed under sedation or general anesthesia, and the surgeon must be ready and the patient consented for an open reduction if necessary. Again, a CT scan should be obtained if reduction is not completely concentric on standard radiographs. After reduction, the hip is dynamically examined for stability and smoothness of motion. If an acetabular rim fragment >25 % is not present and there are no incarcerated intra-articular loose bodies and no mechanical hip symptoms or an associated femoral head or neck fracture, nonsurgical management would be prescribed.

After a successful reduction of the hip joint, the patient should be warned of hip position precautions. The posterior dislocation patient should avoid flexion >90°, internal rotation >10°, and adduction. After an anterior dislocation, external rotation and extension past neutral should be avoided. Weight-bearing status after a simple dislocation is controversial. Originally no weight bearing was advocated for 4–6 weeks, but this has been challenged lately by good results with assisted early weight bearing. If an MRI is obtained in the acute setting and a large hemarthrosis is detected, acute aspiration is recommended [11]. MRI is the most sensitive study for detection of osteonecrosis, and its use after dislocation has been advocated as early as 6 weeks post injury [14]. Patients who have no signs of osteonecrosis on magnetic resonance imaging at 6 weeks may undergo a gradual return to play and sports activities as tolerated. Patients in whom osteonecrosis is diagnosed at 6 weeks are at risk for collapse and joint degeneration and should be advised against returning to sports.

Although most cases of femoral head osteonecrosis ultimately require surgical treatment, the decision between operative and nonoperative treatment is dependent on the clinical and pathologic staging of the osteonecrosis. Conservative medical treatment is effective only in the early stages of disease for symptomatic relief. Nonoperative treatment that has been utilized includes rest and activity modification, pharmacological therapy, extracorporeal shock-wave therapy, and electrical stimulation treatment.

Rehabilitation of a simple hip dislocation (no associated fracture) begins with early protected weight-bearing progressing to full weight bearing once pain and muscle spasm permit. The rehabilitation program should focus on pain control while achieving optimal ROM and strengthening surrounding musculature. As stated earlier, certain position restrictions will be recommended according to the direction of the dislocation. Cardiovascular fitness is maintained with upper extremity aerobic exercises. Gait training typically starts after 2 weeks. At 4 weeks, if the patient is comfortable with full weight bearing, functional weight-bearing exercises are initiated, such as shallow squats and standing dips with cord resistance. This should be followed by sports-specific training and overall core body strengthening. The patient can be discharged to return to competitive sports activity once painless joint function is achieved with symmetric lower extremity range of motion and strength.

Surgical intervention may be necessary to address residual symptomatic instability of the affected hip or for treatment of chondral lesions. Multiple joint preserving surgical options have been described for the treatment of osteochondral or chondral lesions of the hip. These include debridement, microfracture, osteochondral autograft transplantation (OATS) and mosaicplasty, autologous chondrocyte implantation, osteochondral allograft transplantation, and cartilage re-fixation utilizing suture techniques [15, 16].

Results of operative treatment of chondral lesions of the hip in athletes have been variable. Athletes should be cautioned that outcomes of return to their previous level of play are dependent on their intra-articular pathology present, specifically the extent of articular cartilage injury. Early diagnosis and treatment of acetabular labral tears is vital to minimize progressive degenerative changes of the hip [17]. Multiple studies have demonstrated a return to sport following surgical treatment of chondral lesions in athletes [17–19].

Byrd and Jones [18] evaluated 10-year outcomes of 15 athletes who underwent hip arthroscopy for a diagnosis of chondral damage, labral tear, arthritis, AVN, loose body, or synovitis. Thirteen patients (87 %) returned to their sport after treatment. All five athletes with radiographic hip osteoarthritis underwent total hip arthroplasty at an average of 6 years. Although good results have been reported following cartilage restoration procedures in limited case series, further studies with a control group and larger patient groups are required to build on the current available literature.

Labral repair in the acute setting is rarely indicated unless a displaced labral tear does not allow a concentric hip reduction. For patients with residual symptoms of instability upon physical activities, labral repair with capsular placation may be considered [20]. The importance of the iliofemoral ligament (ILFL) in providing hip stability cannot be overstated. A recent biomechanical study [21] has shown that the ILFL has a significant role in limiting external rotation and anterior translation of the femur, while the acetabular labrum provides a secondary stabilizing role for these motions, suggesting that, if injured, both these structures should be repaired in order to restore hip function.

Hip arthroscopy after a traumatic hip dislocation has been proven to be safe although the optimal timing between reduction and arthroscopy has not been clearly determined. Hip arthroscopy, following a traumatic dislocation, is indicated for removal of intra-articular loose bodies as well as an irreducible dislocation. It should also be considered following a hip dislocation if the athlete exhibits pain and/or mechanical symptoms that prohibit them from returning to their sport or even their previous level of play. Philippon et al. [22] and Ilizaliturri et al. [23] evaluated arthroscopic findings of symptomatic patients who sustained a hip dislocation.

Philippon and colleagues [22] reported on the findings of 14 professional athletes that underwent hip arthroscopy after a simple dislocation of the hip. Surgery was performed an average of 125 days (range 0–556 days) after the injury. The professional athletes were referred for arthroscopic evaluation if they could not return to their sport. Ilizaliturri and colleagues [23] also reported their findings on 17 patients that underwent hip arthroscopy after a traumatic hip dislocation due to continuance of mechanical hip symptoms. Average time between closed reduction and arthroscopy was 3 months. In both studies, a high prevalence of labral tears, chondral lesions, and osteochondral fragments was reported. Athletes in the middle of their season may want to wait until the end of their season to address their labral or chondral lesions, as well as their concomitant FAI, if present. Athletes returning to play with symptomatic hip pathology should perform core and pelvic stabilization exercises and stretching and minimize activities causing hip flexion greater than 90°, including deep squats. Arthroscopic treatment of the symptomatic chondral or labral pathology should be considered to decrease the risk of the development of osteoarthritis. Studies have demonstrated that most professional athletes can return to the professional level, if treatment is initiated before radiographic evidence of osteoarthritis [24].

As previously stated, all patients with hip dislocation were noted at arthroscopy to have articular cartilage lesions. This could be the prime reason for the occurrence of post-traumatic arthritis as one of the most common complications, up to 24%, after an episode of traumatic instability [25]. AVN is another potential devastating consequence, which, as stated earlier, is very well correlated with time to reduction. Heterotopic ossification has been seen more in the fracture-dislocation setting, and no clear recommendations for prophylaxis exist for patients with simple dislocations. Thromboembolism is another potentially catastrophic complication after high-energy trauma to the hip region. Virchow's triad of stasis, endothelial injury, and hypercoagulability occurs, placing the patient at high risk for deep venous thrombosis. Early ambulation is encouraged in the appropriate clinical setting. Pneumatic compression stockings as well as pharmacological prophylaxis are recommended.

A review of literature by Cornwall and Radomisli [26] reported a 10% nerve injury incidence in adults and 5% in children. The peroneal branch of the sciatic nerve was usually involved. The sciatic nerve can be acutely lacerated, stretched, or compressed, or later encased in heterotopic ossification. Careful physical examination and documentation in the acute setting is paramount. At least partial recovery of nerve function occurs in 60–70% of patients, with no clear correlation with injury or treatment type. Rehabilitation of these patients should include avoidance of equinus deformity of the foot via bracing and maintaining adequate ROM of the entire lower extremity. Nerve conduction studies can help to assess the extent of nerve injury.

Femoral Head Fractures

Femoral head fractures, almost always associated with hip fracture-dislocations, are exceedingly rare in sports, with only case reports in the literature [1]. Femoral head fractures occur secondary to a shearing effect as the head translates over the posterior rim of the acetabulum. With posterior dislocations, the anterior margin of the femoral head is typically involved, whereas, with anterior dislocations, the posterolateral aspect of the head is involved [27].

Since femoral head fractures are associated with hip dislocations, please refer to the dislocations section regarding the typical mechanism of injury, history/presentation, physical examination, imaging, and acute treatment (reduction of the dislocation).

The Pipkin classification is commonly used to describe the location of the femoral head fracture and any associated fractures. There is also the Brumback classification of femoral head fractures, which is more comprehensive, including the direction of the dislocation (posterior, anterior, central); in addition, it specifies the location of fracture on the femoral head, acetabular involvement, as well as describing the presence of any instability of the hip. Both classification systems have prognostic value; however, we will focus on using the Pipkin classification in terms of treatment [28].

In a Pipkin type I injury, the location of the fracture is inferior to the fovea centralis. Nonoperative management can be considered if the displacement of the fragments is less than 2 cm, there is no incarcerated fragment, and the hip joint is congruent and stable. Type I fractures involve the non-weight-bearing portion of the head; therefore, weight bearing may be allowed sooner than type II fractures.

A Pipkin type II injury involves a fracture that extends superior to the fovea centralis, involving the weight-bearing surface. Nonsurgical management can be considered for type II fractures that meet the same reduction criteria as type I fractures, however. Type II fractures typically involve a larger amount of the femoral head, which can render the hip joint unstable [29]. Therefore, most Pipkin type II fractures are treated with surgical reduction and fixation due to the typical large fragment size, as well as the weight-bearing location of the injury.

Pipkin type III and IV injuries involve a femoral head fracture, with an associated femoral neck fracture and acetabular fracture. These fractures almost always require surgical reduction and fixation. Both the posterior and anterior (Smith-Peterson) approaches can be used for femoral head fractures.

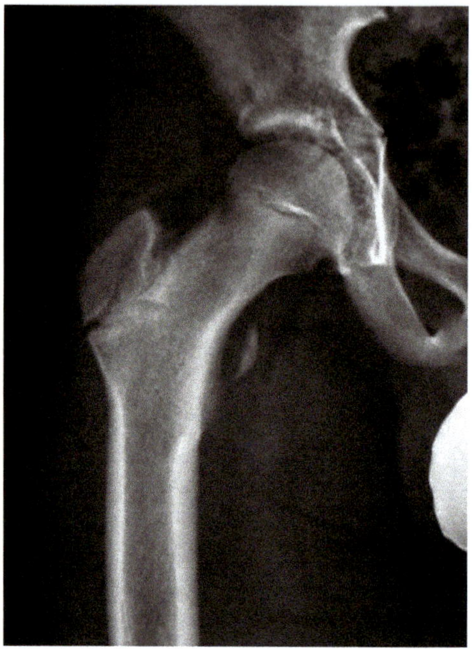

Fig. 18.1 A lesser trochanter apophyseal avulsion fracture with proximal displacement

Lesser Trochanteric Fractures

The lesser trochanter apophysis fuses between the ages of 15 and 17 [30]. The iliopsoas tendon inserts onto the lesser trochanter. Avulsions to this region typically occur from kicking or sprinting. The patient will usually complain of pain in the groin or proximal anteromedial thigh region and will hold the lower extremity in a slightly flexed position at the hip to reduce tension of the involved musculotendinous unit.

Physical examination will reveal localized tenderness to palpation over the anteromedial thigh and groin region. Attempts at active hip flexion or passive hip extension cause an increase in pain. Plain radiographs will typically demonstrate a superiorly displaced fracture fragment from the pull of the iliopsoas muscle (Fig. 18.1). A plain film of the involved side with slight external rotation will help better visualize the lesser trochanter. There is greater displacement of fracture fragments involving the ischial tuberosity, anterior superior iliac spine (ASIS), and lesser trochanter; this is due to less soft tissue attachments. In comparison, the iliac crest and anterior inferior iliac spine (AIIS) have limited displacement secondary to additional soft tissue attachments [31].

Like most apophyseal avulsion fractures, conservative management of this injury has been successful with most athletes. Generally, nonoperative treatment for apophyseal avulsion fractures provides great results for the majority of patients [30–33]. In a series of cases reported by Dimon et al., patients found the use of crutches helpful for an initial period of 2 weeks with weight bearing as tolerated [34]. By 3 months, most patients were able to return to competitive participation without restrictions and without any signs of lingering pain or weakness.

We did not find any surgical cases for the operative reduction and fixation of lesser trochanteric avulsion fractures, although indications can include a symptomatic nonunion.

Femoral Neck Stress Fractures

Femoral neck stress fractures (FNSFs) typically occur in young athletes and military recruits and have been associated with significant morbidity [35–38]. Several sports have been implicated, including long distance running, endurance athletes, ballet, and some aerobic exercises. These populations are exposed to a constant repetitive load and are more susceptible to stress fractures in which a dose-dependent relationship is present between the amount of training and the likelihood of injury [39, 40]. Genetic predisposition to such fractures has been recently studied by Korvala and colleagues [41] who examined eight genes involved in bone metabolism or pathology (COL1A1, COL1A2, OPG, ESR1, VDR, CTR, LRP5, IL-6) in 72 military recruits with femoral neck fractures and 120 healthy controls. They noticed individuals who lacked the allele CTR-C and/or the haplotype *VDR* C-A had a threefold increase in the risk of FNSF when compared to carriers of both. This suggests that genetic factors can play a role in the development of stress fractures in individuals subjected to heavy exercise and mechanical loading.

Fragility fractures of the femoral neck also occur in the older population with a low bone density. For the purpose of

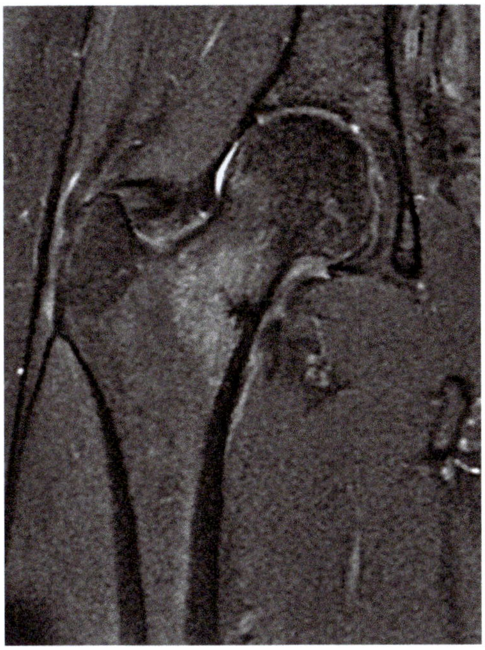

Fig. 18.2 MRI showing a compression type femoral neck stress fracture

this discussion, we will focus in the young athlete with an insufficiency fracture of an otherwise normal bone rather than a fragility fracture which supposes the presence of weak, pathologic bone [42]. The fracture is thought to be caused by repetitive submaximal stresses that occur with a frequency that exceeds the adaptive ability of the bone [42]. Female endurance athletes with amenorrhea have been noted to have decreased bone mineral density (BMD) when compared with eumenorrheic individuals [43]. In this population, both fragility and fatigue loading are present as they have weaker bones (fragility) that are subjected to excessive stress (fatigue). Pouilles et al. [44] measured the BMD of 41 military recruits that had suffered any type of stress fracture using dual photon absorptiometry and observed a 10% reduction in bone density in patients with a calcaneal or a femoral fracture when compared to controls.

FNSFs are typically divided into those occurring in the inferior aspect of the femoral neck (compression type) (Fig. 18.2), the superior aspect of femoral neck (tension type), or completely displaced [42]. The incidence of fracture displacement at the time of initial diagnosis ranges anywhere from 12 to 66% [45, 46]. A severity grading classification based on MRI findings will be discussed in the imaging section. The clinical presentation can be varied, and often the fracture is not diagnosed for long periods following the probable onset of the injury, which significantly increases the risk of displacement and further morbidity [35]. In one series, the diagnosis was delayed an average of 14 weeks from onset of symptoms [35], while on another, the average was 3.4 weeks [46]. In the case of military recruits, Joshi et al. [47] noticed that 74% occurred during the fourth to seventh week of intense training.

A high index of suspicion should be maintained with every high impact athlete who reports symptoms suggestive of stress fracture, making a detailed history and physical exam imperative. Patients typically complain of activity-related anterior groin pain. Many report pain which increases with weight-bearing activities and diminishes with rest. Antalgic gait may be occasionally present. There may be tenderness to palpation over the anterior groin and proximal thigh, as well as pain with resisted straight leg raise and log roll examination. Sometimes the presenting symptoms may be varied, such as lateral or even gluteal pain [48]; therefore, the need for a high index of suspicion cannot be overstated.

Plain radiographs are the first line of imaging for hip fractures although they can be normal in individuals with FNSF. AP views of the pelvis and dedicated views of the affected hip are performed. The AP radiograph should show the femoral neck in full profile by internally rotating the extremity sufficiently to eliminate the effect of femoral anteversion. In this view, a radiolucent fracture line can often be seen, and later callus formation can sometimes be noticed. If a FNSF is suspected and radiographs are normal, MRI or nuclear medicine bone scan is recommended.

MRI is the study of choice for FNSF. It can help classify these injuries in a scale from I to V [49, 50], being the grade I and II considered lower grade and the grade III and IV higher grade. Grade V was assigned to those demonstrating callus formation in the cortical bone. A typical early sign of a stress-related bone injury is endosteal marrow edema. This has been considered a nonspecific finding because it can also be present in infection, bone bruise, and malignancy [51]. In the appropriate clinical setting, lower grade fractures are diagnosed when there is an area of marrow edema even without a discrete fracture line. Edema is characterized by an area of high signal intensity on short tau inversion recovery (STIR) and T2-weighted images and low signal intensity on T1-weighted images. A fracture line is considered to be specific for a bone stress injury, appearing as an intramedullar low signal intensity in all pulse sequences; whereas callus appears as an intermediate cortical signal intensity. Coronal STIR views are optimal for visualization of a low intensity line specific for a stress fracture.

For patients in which MRI is contraindicated (e.g., cardiac pacemakers, brain aneurysm clips, middle ear prostheses, neurostimulators), nuclear medicine studies can be performed. These have been performed long before the advent of MRI for their high sensitivity to capture changes in bone metabolism. The most commonly used radiopharmaceuticals are 99mTcphosphate analogs. Pathological uptake can be seen within 6–72 hours of the bone stress injury [52].

A study by Bryant et al. [53] compared 38 patients that underwent planar scintigraphy with 39 patients that had undergone planar scintigraphy with SPECT (single-photon emission computed tomography) in order to assess the capacity of grading FNSFs into low grade and high grade. They noticed that planar scintigraphy with SPECT was more sensitive and accurate in assessing FNSF grade than planar scintigraphy alone. CT scans are also helpful to delineate the bony anatomy but have less sensitivity than MRI or bone scintigraphy [49].

Treatment options are based on the fracture pattern and location. Fractures that are located on the tension side of the femoral neck are at a higher risk of displacement than those on the compression side [45, 54], and therefore, internal fixation of tension-side fractures is recommended [55]. Shin and Gillingham [42] subdivided compression side fractures into grade 1 (no fracture line seen on MRI), grade 2 (fracture line less than 50 % of the femoral neck width), and grade 3 (fracture line ≥50 %). For grade 1 and 2 fractures (no fracture line or line <50 % of femoral neck width), nonsurgical management is recommended with non-weight bearing on crutches combined with close follow-up to detect any signs of progression. For grade 3 fractures (fracture line >50 % of femoral neck width) and fractures that progress when treated nonsurgically, the bony fragments should be stabilized with internal fixation.

Rehabilitation will be dictated by the type of fracture and whether or not surgery is performed. The patient may return to weight-bearing activities when full weight bearing is painless, there is no tenderness to palpation on physical examination, and imaging studies are consistent with a healed fracture. Core body strengthening, proprioception, and sports-specific activities are then resumed with complete lower extremity reconditioning.

Complications are most likely related to the fracture pattern [35]. A delay in diagnosis can become important as undisplaced fractures may become displaced in the interim. For displaced fractures, major factors contributing to the development of AVN have been identified as a prolonged time from displacement to surgical stabilization and the presence of varus alignment on the postoperative AP radiograph [46]. Other devastating complications are nonunion, varus malunion, and posttraumatic arthritis of the hip [35, 40].

Prevention is the best treatment in this type of injuries. Once a stress fracture has occurred, we know that the athlete is at increased risk of suffering another stress injury. As healthcare providers, we have the duty to assess for risk factors for low BMD such as poor nutrition, low calcium, vitamin D intake, excessive or inappropriate training, and hereditary factors. Counseling the patient in order to avoid other types of stress fractures should be part of the overall management of these largely preventable injuries.

Summary

Overuse injuries of the hip are increasing in prevalence and are diverse in their presentation. A thorough knowledge of the patients' history, exam, and appropriate imaging can facilitate a proper diagnosis and treatment program.

References

1. Yasin FN, Singh VA. Can posterior hip fracture-dislocation occur in indoor football (futsal)? A report of two cases. BMJ Case Rep. 2009. doi: 10.1136/bcr.12.2008.1317.
2. Chudik SC, Allen AA, Lopez V, Warren R. Hip dislocations in athletes. Sports Med Arthrosc Rev. 2002;10(2):123–33.
3. Giza E, Mithöfer K, Matthews H, Vrahas M. Hip fracture-dislocation in football: a report of two cases and review of the literature. Br J Sports Med. 2004;38(4):E17.
4. Venkatachalam S, Heidari N, Greer T. Traumatic fracture-dislocation of the hip following rugby tackle: a case report. Sports Med Arthrosc Rehabil Ther Technol. 2009;1:28.
5. Giannoudis PV, Zelle BA, Kamath RP, Pape HC. Posterior fracture-dislocation of the hip in sports. Eur J Trauma. 2003;29:399–402.
6. Pallia CS, Scott RE, Chao DJ. Traumatic hip dislocation in athletes. Curr Sports Med Rep. 2002;1:338–45.
7. Hawkins RD, Hulse MA, Wilkinson C, Hodson A, Gibson M. The Association Football Medical Research Programme: an audit of injuries in professional football. Br J Sports Med. 2001;35:43–7.
8. Nielsen AB, Yde J. Epidemiology and traumatology of injuries in soccer. Am J Sports Med. 1989;17(6):803–7.
9. Offierski CM. Traumatic dislocation of the hip in children. J Bone Joint Surg Br. 1981;63:194–7.
10. Schmidt GL, Sciulli R, Altman GT. Knee injury in patients experiencing a high-energy traumatic ipsilateral hip dislocation. J Bone Joint Surg Am. 2005;87(6):1200–4.
11. Moorman III CT, Warren RF, Hershman EB, et al. Traumatic posterior hip subluxation in American football. J Bone Joint Surg Am. 2003;85-A(7):1190–6.
12. Laorr A, Greenspan A, Anderson MW, et al. Traumatic hip dislocation: early MRI findings. Skeletal Radiol. 1995;24(4):239–45.
13. Hougaard K, Thomsen PB. Traumatic posterior dislocation of the hip—prognostic factors influencing the incidence of avascular necrosis of the femoral head. Arch Orthop Trauma Surg. 1986; 106(1):32–5.
14. Poggi JJ, Callaghan JJ, Spritzer CE, Roark T, Goldner RD. Changes on magnetic resonance images after traumatic hip dislocation. Clin Orthop Relat Res. 1995;319:249–59.
15. Crawford K, Philippon MJ, Sekiya JK, et al. Microfracture of the hip in athletes. Clin Sports Med. 2006;25:327–35.
16. Sekiya JK, Martin RL, Lesniak BP. Arthroscopic repair of delaminated acetabular articular cartilage in femoroacetabular impingement. Orthopedics. 2009;32:629.
17. McCarthy J, Barsoum W, Puri L, et al. The role of hip arthroscopy in the elite athlete. Clin Orthop Relat Res. 2003;(406):71–4.
18. Byrd JW, Jones KS. Hip arthroscopy in athletes: 10-year follow-up. Am J Sports Med. 2009;37:2140–3.
19. Singh PJ, O'Donnell JM. The outcome of hip arthroscopy in Australian football league players: a review of 27 hips. Arthroscopy. 2010;26:743–9.
20. Smith MV, Sekiya JK. Hip instability. Sports Med Arthrosc. 2010; 18(2):108–12.

21. Myers CA, Register BC, Lertwanich P. Role of the acetabular labrum and the iliofemoral ligament in hip stability: an in vitro biplane fluoroscopy study. Am J Sports Med. 2011;39(Suppl):85S–91.
22. Philippon MJ, Kuppersmith DA, Wolff AB, Briggs KK. Arthroscopic findings following traumatic hip dislocation in 14 professional athletes. Arthroscopy. 2009;25(2):169–74.
23. Ilizaliturri VM, Gonzalez-Gutierrez B, Gonzalez-Ugalde H, et al. Hip arthroscopy after traumatic hip dislocation. Am J Sports Med. 2011;39(Suppl):50S–7.
24. Ellis HB, Briggs KK, Philippon MJ. Innovation in hip arthroscopy: is hip arthritis preventable in the athlete? Br J Sports Med. 2011;45:253–8.
25. Upadhyay SS, Moulton A, Srikrishnamurthy K. An analysis of the late effects of traumatic posterior dislocation of the hip without fractures. J Bone Joint Surg Br. 1983;65(2):150–2.
26. Cornwall R, Radomisli TE. Nerve injury in traumatic dislocation of the hip. Clin Orthop Relat Res. 2000;377:84–91.
27. Blankenbaker DG, De Smet AA. Hip injuries in athletes. Radiol Clin North Am. 2010;48:1155–78.
28. Droll KP, Broekhuyse H, O'Brien P. Fracture of the femoral head. J Am Acad Orthop Surg. 2007;15:716–27.
29. Matsuda DK. A rare fracture, an even rarer treatment: the arthroscopic reduction and internal fixation of an isolated femoral head fracture. Arthroscopy. 2009;25(4):408–12.
30. Moeller JL. Pelvic and hip apophyseal avulsion injuries in young athletes. Curr Sports Med Rep. 2003;2:110–5.
31. Fernbach SK, Wilkinson RH. Avulsion injuries of the pelvis and proximal femur. AJR Am J Roentgenol. 1981;137:581–4.
32. Metzmaker JN, Pappas AM. Avulsion fractures of the pelvis. Am J Sports Med. 1985;13(5):349–58.
33. Rossi F, Dragoni S. Acute avulsion fractures of the pelvis in adolescent competitive athletes: prevalence, location and sports distribution of 203 cases collected. Skeletal Radiol. 2001;30:127–31.
34. Veselko M, Smrkolj V. Avulsion of the anterior superior iliac spine in athletes: case reports. J Trauma. 1994;36(3):444–6.
35. Johansson C, Ekenman I, Törnkvist H, Eriksson E. Stress fractures of the femoral neck in athletes. The consequence of a delay in diagnosis. Am J Sports Med. 1990;18(5):524.
36. Pihlajamäki HK, Ruohola JP, Kiuru MJ, Visuri TI. Displaced femoral neck fatigue fractures in military recruits. J Bone Joint Surg Am. 2006;88:1989–97.
37. Ha KI, Hahn SH, Chung MY, Yang BK, Yi SR. A clinical study of stress fractures in sports activities. Orthopedics. 1991;14:1089–95.
38. Sterling JC, Edelstein DW, Calvo RD, Webb R. Stress fractures in the athlete. Diagnosis and management. Sports Med. 1992;14:336–46.
39. Jones BH, Harris JM, Vinh TN, Rubin C. Exercise-induced stress fractures and stress reactions of bone: epidemiology, etiology, and classification. Exerc Sport Sci Rev. 1989;17:379–422.
40. Devas MB. Stress fractures of the femoral neck. J Bone Joint Surg Br. 1965;47:728–38.
41. Korvala J, Hartikka H, Pihlajamäki H, et al. Genetic predisposition for femoral neck stress fractures in military conscripts. BMC Genet. 2010;11:95.
42. Shin AY, Gillingham BL. Fatigue fractures of the femoral neck in athletes. J Am Acad Orthop Surg. 1997;5:293–302.
43. Drinkwater BL, Nilson K, Chesnut III CH, et al. Bone mineral content of amenorrheic and eumenorrheic athletes. N Engl J Med. 1984;311:277–81.
44. Pouilles JM, Bernard J, Tremollières F, Louvet JP, Ribot C. Femoral bone density in young male adults with stress fractures. Bone. 1989;10:105–8.
45. Fullerton LR, Snowdy HA. Femoral neck stress fractures. Am J Sports Med. 1988;16:365–77.
46. Lee CH, Huang GS, Chao KH, et al. Surgical treatment of displaced stress fractures of the femoral neck in military recruits: a report of 42 cases. Arch Orthop Trauma Surg. 2003;123:527–33.
47. Joshi A, Kc BR, Shah BC, et al. Femoral neck stress fractures in military personnel. JNMA J Nepal Med Assoc. 2009;48(174):99–102.
48. Scott MP, Finnoff JT, Davis BA. Femoral neck stress fracture presenting as gluteal pain in a marathon runner: case report. Arch Phys Med Rehabil. 1999;80(2):236–8.
49. Kiuru MJ, Pihlajamaki HK, Ahovuo JA. Bone stress injuries. Acta Radiol. 2004;45:317–26.
50. Kiuru MJ, Pihlajamaki HK, Perkio JP, Ahovuo JA. Dynamic contrast-enhanced MR imaging in symptomatic bone stress of the pelvis and the lower extremity. Acta Radiol. 2001;42:277–85.
51. Pathria MN, Issacs P. Magnetic resonance imaging of bone marrow. Curr Opin Radiol. 1992;4:21–31.
52. Greaney RB, Gerber FH, Laughlin RL, et al. Distribution and natural history of stress fractures in U.S. Marine recruits. Radiology. 1983;146:339–46.
53. Bryant LR, Song WS, Banks KP. Comparison of planar scintigraphy alone and with SPECT for the initial evaluation of femoral neck stress fracture. AJR Am J Roentgenol. 2008;191(4):1010–5.
54. DeFranco MJ, Recht M, Schils J, et al. Stress fractures of the femur in athletes. Clin Sports Med. 2006;25(1):89–103.
55. Egol KA, Koval KJ, Kummer F, et al. Stress fractures of the femoral neck. Clin Orthop Relat Res. 1998;348:72–8.

The Understanding of Hip Etiologies: Osteonecrosis of the Femoral Head

19

Bhaveen H. Kapadia, Kimona Issa, Samik Banerjee, and Michael A. Mont

Introduction

Osteonecrosis, also known as avascular necrosis (AVN), ischemic necrosis, atraumatic necrosis, or aseptic necrosis, is a devastating and debilitating pathologic condition that has a poorly understood pathogenesis [1, 2]. It primarily affects the femoral head of young adults in the third and fourth decades of life [3, 4]. The true incidence of this disease is not known; however, in the United States, it is estimated that 10,000–20,000 new cases are diagnosed every year, and this accounts for approximately 10% of all total hip arthroplasties annually, excluding obvious causes such as femoral neck fractures [5]. There are a wide range of etiologies, which can be classified as direct and indirect risk factors; however, the underlying cellular pathology of the disease is similar (Table 19.1) [6]. Therefore, the following chapter will describe the pathology, pathophysiology, and associated risk factors for this disease. Further discussion of treatment strategies will be described in a subsequent chapter.

B.H. Kapadia, MD (✉)
Department of Orthopaedic Surgery and Rehabilitation Medicine, State University of New York (SUNY) Downstate Medical Center, Brooklyn, NY, USA

Rubin Institute for Advanced Orthopedics, Center for Joint Preservation and Replacement, Sinai Hospital of Baltimore, Baltimore, MD, USA
e-mail: bhaveen.k@gmail.com

K. Issa, MD • S. Banerjee, MD • M.A. Mont, MD
Rubin Institute for Advanced Orthopedics, Center for Joint Preservation and Replacement, Sinai Hospital of Baltimore, Baltimore, MD, USA
e-mail: mmont@lifebridgehealth.org; Rhondamont@aol.com

Pathogenesis

The exact pathogenesis of atraumatic osteonecrosis of the femoral head is not entirely understood; however, multiple theories have been proposed. These include thromboembolic events, fat cell hypertrophy, and sickle cells, each of which results in increased bone marrow pressure, arteriolar obstruction, and obstruction of venous outflow.

In addition to the abovementioned risk factors, genetic variations may be a contributing factor in the pathophysiology of osteonecrosis. Specifically, genetic alterations in components of the coagulation cascade seen in thrombophilic disorders, such as protein C, protein S, and plasminogen activator inhibitor-1 gene, have been implicated as one of the most important etiological factors in this disease [7–9]. Additionally, genetic polymorphisms in the nitric oxide synthase gene, which is responsible for promoting bone formation, angiogenesis, and inhibiting platelet aggregation, have been shown to increase the risk of osteonecrosis in some studies [10]. Furthermore, studies have shown that variations in single nucleotide polymorphisms in the angiotensin I-converting enzyme (ACE) gene and sterol regulatory element-binding transcription protein-3 (IGFBP-3) have been associated with an increased chance of progression of osteonecrosis [7].

Most of these theories are not mutually exclusive. Therefore, osteonecrosis may not be considered to have a single association, but rather it may be more appropriate to consider it as a multifactorial, heterogeneous group of disorders that has a final common pathway leading to femoral head bone death.

Pathology

Although there are various associated or direct risk factors which contribute to osteonecrosis, ultimately this disease leads to one common pathway, disruption of the

J.C. McCarthy et al. (eds.), *Hip Joint Restoration*, DOI 10.1007/978-1-4614-0694-5_19

Table 19.1 Risk factors for hip osteonecrosis

Direct	Indirect
Trauma/dislocation	Alcohol abuse
Radiation	Chronic corticosteroids
Sickle cell disease	Coagulation disorders
Caisson disease (decompression sickness, diver's disease, or the bends)	HMG-CoA reductase inhibitors (statins)
Myeloproliferative disorders	Systemic lupus erythematosus (SLE)
	Human immunodeficiency virus (HIV)

microcirculation to the femoral head. The predominant mechanisms leading to vascular disruption are via direct compromise from trauma, occlusion of vasculature from thrombosis, or through extravascular compression of blood vessels from intraosseous hypertension. This disruption of perfusion to the femoral head leads to decreased oxygen delivery to osteocytes, which subsequently results in cell death within 2–3 h of ischemia.

Following the initial ischemic event of osteocytes, death of marrow elements also occurs. However, all cell types including osteocytes, hematopoietic cells, and adipocytes are affected in the osteonecrotic process. The adipocytes in these regions commonly have large cytoplasmic lipid vacuoles which remain unchanged with cell death. This causes the MRI signals to remain unchanged during the early stages of cell death. MRI changes begin to appear when cell membranes rupture and the lipid containing vacuoles undergo denaturation. During this phase, the cancellous bone structure remains unaffected causing radiographs to look normal (Ficat Arlet stage 0 and 1). A reparative process follows the necrotic event, which, unless the lesion involves less than 15 % of the femoral head, is usually ineffective and leads to femoral head collapse.

In early lesions, the histological changes seen are cellular necrosis, areas of hemorrhage, and fibrosis surrounded by areas of fatty marrow. The marrow adipocytes undergo microvesicular changes followed by marked necrosis of hematopoietic and fatty elements. The central region of the necrotic lesion remains acellular for many years; however, the peripheral zone reflects a flux between necrosis and repair. The trabecular bone is often devoid of osteocytes and consists of loose marrow fibrosis and may show increased vascularity. Additionally, the necrotic collagen products stimulate osteoclastic migration which resorbs dead trabeculae and leads to replacement by appositional new bone. Complete healing can occur; however, as stated above, this has been shown to be dependent on the size and location of the necrotic lesion.

In advanced lesions, there is often a large wedge-shaped area of completely dead bone of the femoral head. This region is composed of fatty tissue and disorganized trabeculae, which eventually undergoes replacement by reticular, granular, or amorphous tissue. Beneath this region, there is a repair zone made of thickened trabeculae and neovascularized fibrosis in marrow spaces. This area of bone resorption and formation appears as an increased density on radiographs. As part of an attempt to heal the lesion (referred to as creeping substitution), revascularization of dead segments is seen, perhaps in response to angiogenic factors. Additionally, byproducts of dead bone are postulated to recruit local mesenchymal cells followed by osteoclastic resorption of necrotic tissue and recruitment of osteoblasts to regions of osteogenesis.

The next phase of the repair process can damage the integrity of the bone mass. Thick fibrous scar tissue forms at the base of the necrotic bone and separates it from viable tissue and prevents penetration from the vasculature. This phase is irreversible and prevents additional episodes of necrosis from repair, leading to progression of the lesion. Throughout the course of this remodeling process, the necrotic bone reaches a point of weakened biomechanical integrity and may subsequently lead to collapse. Additionally, the cyclic loading on the hip can lead to stress-induced microfractures. When the mechanical stresses exceed the bone strength of the necrotic region, a subchondral fracture results. This leads to collapse of the overlying articular cartilage and deformity of the femoral head. Furthermore, following collapse this deformity leads to cartilage breakdown, articular incongruity, and degenerative joint disease.

Risk Factors

There are several risk factors that are postulated to be associated with hip osteonecrosis. Overall, these factors can be divided into direct and indirect causes.

Direct Risk Factors

Direct risk factors are those diseases or conditions that directly lead to mechanical obstruction of the blood flow resulting in ischemia or direct cell death. These include trauma/dislocation, sickle cell disease, Caisson disease, radiation necrosis, and myeloproliferative disorders. An example to understand is a traumatic event to the hip (especially to the femoral neck and medial femoral circumflex artery) that can directly limit blood flow to the hip and result in ischemia.

Sickle cell hemoglobinopathy is an autosomal recessive disorder with an estimated prevalence of 0.34 % in patients who are African-Americans [11]. In this disease, three mechanisms [12] may contribute to vessel occlusion, reduced nutrient delivery to bone, local ischemia, and ultimately osteonecrosis. The change in shape from a round and flexible cell to a sickle-shaped and inflexible cell incapable of properly flowing through capillary beds is exacerbated by a reduced blood oxygen level. Risk factors prompting a sickle cell crisis, therefore, include any situation that leads to low blood oxygen levels, including strenuous exercise, spending time at high altitude, or infection [13]. Also, the adhesion of red blood cells to the venular endothelium can also contribute to vessel occlusion. In addition, the rapid consumption of nitric oxide, a vasodilator, by hemoglobin released during hemolysis may cause local vasoconstriction. Microscopically, secondary osteonecrosis due to sickle cell disease exhibits a nonspecific inflammatory response involving lymphocytes without specific lesions of sepsis, inflammation, tumor cells, or advanced alteration. This absence of bacterial contamination is the salient difference from idiopathic osteonecrosis [14].

Radiation can potentially cause injury to vessel wall and result in vascular compromise. Furthermore, it is purported that radiation also negatively affects the function of osteoblasts and results in reduced bone matrix production and further contributes to osteoradionecrosis [15].

Caisson disease (decompression sickness, diver's disease, or the bends) can also directly cause osteonecrosis due to rapid pressure changes that result in the formation of nitrogen bubbles. These can cause intra- or extravascular nitrogen emboli and blockade of vessels and lead to permanent bone tissue injury through a mechanism also known as dysbaric osteonecrosis (DON). Other proposed mechanisms include fat emboli, osmotic gas effects, and increased coagulability from hemoconcentration [16, 17].

Myeloproliferative disorders are also known to be direct risk factors for osteonecrosis and have several known mechanisms of action. The excessive proliferation of lymphoblasts may overcrowd the bone marrow space and cause the death of adjacent blood cells. Additionally, rouleaux formation, which is characterized by red blood cell stacking, increases blood viscosity, decreases blood flow, and impairs nutrient delivery to the bone. Treatment of the disease may also exacerbate the necrotic process since chemotherapeutic agents are cytotoxic to rapidly dividing cells such as progenitor cells in bone marrow.

Indirect Risk Factors

The indirect risk factors are those which are known to be associated with osteonecrosis; however, their mechanism of action has not yet been fully elucidated. The most common factors include chronic corticosteroid use, alcohol consumption, tobacco smoking, and human immunodeficiency virus (HIV) infection. Other risk factors include inherited conditions such as coagulation abnormalities, which lead to thrombophilia and hypofibrinolysis.

The most common risk factor of osteonecrosis is chronic corticosteroid use. The overall incidence of corticosteroid-associated osteonecrosis ranges from 0.3 to 52% [18, 19]. It has been demonstrated in some studies that patients who receive a cumulative dose of greater than 2 grams were at higher risk for developing osteonecrosis [1, 2]. A study by Nakamura et al. evaluated 201 patients who had SLE and observed that the risk of developing osteonecrosis was associated with an increase in the cumulative dose of corticosteroids [20]. In this study, 15% of patients who required an increase in corticosteroid dose developed the disease. It is postulated that corticosteroid use may lead to adipocyte hypertrophy in the marrow of some individuals, which results in an increase in the marrow volume and intracortical pressure. This is thought to reduce blood flow through the retinacular arteries. However, this does not occur in all individuals, and some have suggested that this predisposition may be the result of abnormal lipid metabolism.

In genetically susceptible individuals, excess alcohol consumption has been shown to have a profound effect on fat metabolism, which may influence the blood supply and arterial perfusion to end organs such as the femoral head. Alcohol has been demonstrated to cause marrow fat cell hypertrophy and proliferation and thinning of trabeculae and hinder hematopoiesis [21]. Animal models have demonstrated that doses of 7.2–9.2 grams per kilogram body weight a day of ethanol induced osteonecrosis and caused disturbances in bone metabolism [22, 23]. However, the precise quantity necessary to induce osteonecrosis in humans is still unknown. A study by Hirota et al. proposed that an alcohol intake of >400 mL per week may increase the relative risk of osteonecrosis by approximately tenfold [24].

Tobacco smoking has also been implicated as a risk factor for osteonecrosis of the femoral head. The relative risk of this disease for current smokers may be increased by fourfold; however, a cumulative effect of smoking has also been reported with ≥20 pack-years of smoking [24–27]. Nicotine and carcinogens in cigarettes have been demonstrated to delay osteogenesis and disrupt revascularization [28, 29]. Furthermore, nicotine may cause vasoconstriction in the femoral head, leading to ischemia which may be the underlying pathophysiology of osteonecrosis [30].

Patients who have HIV may also be at an increased risk of osteonecrosis (60–100-fold) [31]. This was first described in 1990, with the appearance of several reports and studies subsequently in the literature [32, 33]. These findings suggest that the incidence of osteonecrosis may be increasing with the advent of antiretroviral therapy, potentially as a side effect of treatment [34]. A study by Reis et al. of 38 consecutive series of patients who had osteonecrosis of the femoral head was reviewed to determine the prevalence of HIV as a risk factor for this disease [35]. Of these patients, seven were HIV positive and 31 were HIV negative. It was reported by the authors that there was a significantly higher proportion of patients who had osteonecrosis in the HIV-positive cohort with no other known risk factors for this disease when compared to the HIV-negative cohort (57 % vs. 13 %; $p=0.0245$). It is not well documented whether the retrovirus or the antiretroviral therapy medications (especially protease inhibitors) used are the potential causes [36, 37]. Furthermore, it is not known whether the incidence of osteonecrosis increases with the duration of antiretroviral therapy, HIV infection, or possibly a combination of both [38].

Additional studies have described the development of osteonecrosis in patients with thrombophilic coagulation disorders, although the exact mechanism for how these disorders contribute to disease progression is not known. In 1993, there were reports of two patients who had idiopathic bilateral hip osteonecrosis who were also homozygous for hypofibrinolytic polymorphisms of the plasminogen activator inhibitor-1 (PAI-1) gene [39]. These patients were shown to have high levels of PAI-1 gene byproduct and hypofibrinolytic plasminogen activator inhibitor. It has been postulated that venous thrombosis in the femoral head, generally mediated by thrombophilia and hypofibrinolysis, leads to increased intraosseous pressure and subsequently impaired arterial blood flow followed by bone death [40]. A study by Glueck et al. compared measures of thrombophilia and hypofibrinolysis in patients who had idiopathic osteonecrosis (71 patients) to a cohort who had secondary osteonecrosis (62 patients) [41]. The authors found that heritable traits were significantly more common in patients with osteonecrosis than the control cohort, particularly with high levels of thrombophilic factor VIII ($p=0.0004$) and hypofibrinolytic lp(a) ($p=0.016$).

Summary

Osteonecrosis is associated with many etiological risk factors, and these can be classified as either direct or indirect. Although it is known that these factors influence the development and progression of osteonecrosis, the precise pathomechanism is still unknown. It is postulated, however, that the common pathway is disruption of the microcirculation to the femoral head. Genetic variations associated with heritable diseases and thrombophilic disorders have also been shown to play a role in the etiology of osteonecrosis. Osteonecrosis has a high prevalence of progression to symptomatic disease and femoral head collapse. Early diagnosis and treatment has been shown to markedly improve clinical outcomes. Therefore, further studies evaluating the underlying pathophysiology of this disease may contribute to a better understanding of and consequently may lead to more effective management of osteonecrosis.

References

1. Mont MA, Hungerford DS. Non-traumatic avascular necrosis of the femoral head. J Bone Joint Surg Am. 1995;77:459–74.
2. Mont MA, Jones LC, Hungerford DS. Nontraumatic osteonecrosis of the femoral head: ten years later. J Bone Joint Surg Am. 2006;88:1117–32.
3. Etienne G, Mont MA, Ragland PS. The diagnosis and treatment of nontraumatic osteonecrosis of the femoral head. Instr Course Lect. 2004;53:67–85.
4. Mont MA, Ragland PS, Etienne G. Core decompression of the femoral head for osteonecrosis using percutaneous multiple small-diameter drilling. Clin Orthop Relat Res. 2004;(429):131–8.
5. Babis GC, Sakellariou V, Parvizi J, Soucacos P. Osteonecrosis of the femoral head. Orthopedics. 2011;34:39.
6. Rajpura A, Wright AC, Board TN. Medical management of osteonecrosis of the hip: a review. Hip Int. 2011;21:385–92.
7. Hong JM, Kim TH, Kim HJ, Park EK, Yang EK, Kim SY. Genetic association of angiogenesis- and hypoxia-related gene polymorphisms with osteonecrosis of the femoral head. Exp Mol Med. 2010;42:376–85.
8. Akinyoola AL, Adediran IA, Asaleye CM, Bolarinwa AR. Risk factors for osteonecrosis of the femoral head in patients with sickle cell disease. Int Orthop. 2009;33:923–6.
9. Glueck CJ, Freiberg RA, Oghene J, Fontaine RN, Wang P. Association between the T-786C eNOS polymorphism and idiopathic osteonecrosis of the head of the femur. J Bone Joint Surg Am. 2007;89:2460–8.
10. Koo KH, Lee JS, Lee YJ, Kim KJ, Yoo JJ, Kim HJ. Endothelial nitric oxide synthase gene polymorphisms in patients with nontraumatic femoral head osteonecrosis. J Orthop Res. 2006;24:1722–8.
11. Motulsky AG. Frequency of sickling disorders in U.S. blacks. N Engl J Med. 1973;288:31–3.
12. Mack AK, Kato GJ. Sickle cell disease and nitric oxide: a paradigm shift? Int J Biochem Cell Biol. 2006;38:1237–43.
13. Addae S, Adzaku F, Mohammed S, Annobil S. Sickle cell disease in permanent residents of mountain and low altitudes in Saudi Arabia. Trop Geogr Med. 1990;42:342–8.
14. Mukisi-Mukaza M, Gomez-Brouchet A, Donkerwolcke M, Hinsenkamp M, Burny F. Histopathology of aseptic necrosis of the femoral head in sickle cell disease. Int Orthop. 2011;35:1145–50.
15. Mitchell MJ, Logan PM. Radiation-induced changes in bone. Radiographics. 1998;18:1125–36. quiz 242–3.
16. Coulthard A, Pooley J, Reed J, Walder D. Pathophysiology of dysbaric osteonecrosis: a magnetic resonance imaging study. Undersea Hyperb Med. 1996;23:119–20.
17. Wade CE, Hayashi EM, Cashman Jr TM, Beckman EL. Incidence of dysbaric osteonecrosis in Hawaii's diving fishermen. Undersea Biomed Res. 1978;5:137–47.
18. Kang JS, Park S, Song JH, Jung YY, Cho MR, Rhyu KH. Prevalence of osteonecrosis of the femoral head: a nationwide epidemiologic analysis in Korea. J Arthroplasty. 2009;24:1178–83.
19. Johnson AJ, Mont MA, Tsao AK, Jones LC. Treatment of femoral head osteonecrosis in the United States: 16-year analysis of the nationwide inpatient sample. Clin Orthop Relat Res. 2014; 472(2):617–23.
20. Nakamura J, Harada Y, Oinuma K, Iida S, Kishida S, Takahashi K. Spontaneous repair of asymptomatic osteonecrosis associated with

corticosteroid therapy in systemic lupus erythematosus: 10-year minimum follow-up with MRI. Lupus. 2010;19:1307–14.
21. Wang XS, Zhuang QY, Weng XS, Lin J, Jin J, Qian WW. Etiological and clinical analysis of osteonecrosis of the femoral head in Chinese patients. Chin Med J (Engl). 2013;126:290–5.
22. Wang Y, Yin L, Li Y, Liu P, Cui Q. Preventive effects of puerarin on alcohol-induced osteonecrosis. Clin Orthop Relat Res. 2008;466:1059–67.
23. Broulik PD, Vondrova J, Ruzicka P, Sedlacek R, Zima T. The effect of chronic alcohol administration on bone mineral content and bone strength in male rats. Physiol Res. 2010;59:599–604.
24. Hirota Y, Hirohata T, Fukuda K, et al. Association of alcohol intake, cigarette smoking, and occupational status with the risk of idiopathic osteonecrosis of the femoral head. Am J Epidemiol. 1993;137:530–8.
25. Matsuo K, Hirohata T, Sugioka Y, Ikeda M, Fukuda A. Influence of alcohol intake, cigarette smoking, and occupational status on idiopathic osteonecrosis of the femoral head. Clin Orthop Relat Res. 1988;(234):115–23.
26. Gullihorn L, Karpman R, Lippiello L. Differential effects of nicotine and smoke condensate on bone cell metabolic activity. J Orthop Trauma. 2005;19:17–22.
27. Glassman SD, Anagnost SC, Parker A, Burke D, Johnson JR, Dimar JR. The effect of cigarette smoking and smoking cessation on spinal fusion. Spine. 2000;25:2608–15.
28. Jorgensen LN, Kallehave F, Christensen E, Siana JE, Gottrup F. Less collagen production in smokers. Surgery. 1998;123:450–5.
29. Ma L, Sham MH, Zheng LW, Cheung LK. Influence of low-dose nicotine on bone healing. J Trauma. 2011;70:E117–21.
30. Wessel JH, Dodson TB, Zavras AI. Zoledronate, smoking, and obesity are strong risk factors for osteonecrosis of the jaw: a case-control study. J Oral Maxillofac Surg. 2008;66:625–31.
31. Morse CG, Mican JM, Jones EC, et al. The incidence and natural history of osteonecrosis in HIV-infected adults. Clin Infect Dis. 2007;44:739–48.
32. Goorney BP, Lacey H, Thurairajasingam S, Brown JD. Avascular necrosis of the hip in a man with HIV infection. Genitourin Med. 1990;66:451–2.
33. Goorney BP, Craske J, Turner AJ. Human immunodeficiency virus infection acquired in Thailand. J Infect. 1990;20:264–5.
34. Sighinolfi L, Carradori S, Ghinelli F. Avascular necrosis of the femoral head: a side effect of highly active antiretroviral therapy (HAART) in HIV patients? Infection. 2000;28:254–5.
35. Ries MD, Barcohana B, Davidson A, Jergesen HE, Paiement GD. Association between human immunodeficiency virus and osteonecrosis of the femoral head. J Arthroplasty. 2002;17:135–9.
36. Allison GT, Bostrom MP, Glesby MJ. Osteonecrosis in HIV disease: epidemiology, etiologies, and clinical management. AIDS. 2003;17:1–9.
37. Hasse B, Ledergerber B, Egger M, et al. Antiretroviral treatment and osteonecrosis in patients of the Swiss HIV Cohort Study: a nested case-control study. AIDS Res Hum Retroviruses. 2004;20:909–15.
38. Mary-Krause M, Billaud E, Poizot-Martin I, et al. Risk factors for osteonecrosis in HIV-infected patients: impact of treatment with combination antiretroviral therapy. AIDS. 2006;20:1627–35.
39. Glueck CJ, Glueck HI, Mieczkowski L, Tracy T, Speirs J, Stroop D. Familial high plasminogen activator inhibitor with hypofibrinolysis, a new pathophysiologic cause of osteonecrosis? Thromb Haemost. 1993;69:460–5.
40. Kubo T, Tsuji H, Yamamoto T, Nakahara H, Nakagawa M, Hirasawa Y. Antithrombin III deficiency in a patient with multifocal osteonecrosis. Clin Orthop Relat Res. 2000;(378):306–11.
41. Glueck CJ, Freiberg RA, Wang P. Heritable thrombophilia-hypofibrinolysis and osteonecrosis of the femoral head. Clin Orthop Relat Res. 2008;466:1034–40.

Part IV

Imaging Advances

Victor M. Ilizaliturri Jr

The Bony Morphology of Femoroacetabular Impingement

20

Paul Whittingham-Jones and Paul E. Beaulé

Introduction

Femoroacetabular impingement (FAI) is recognised as a cause of hip pain, labral chondral damage and early degenerative osteoarthritis in the young and active individual [1, 2]. The pathomechanism of FAI is thought to result from premature and/or abnormal contacts between the acetabular rim and femoral head/neck junction leading to premature failure of the labrum in cases of excessive acetabular overcoverage (pincer) and of the acetabular cartilage in cases of femoral asphericity/lack of offset (cam) [3]. However, what represents normality versus deformity versus pathological deformity is still evolving as we continue to study the dynamic nature of this pathology as well as defining the optimal treatment options [4].

One aspect in defining the spectrum of bony anatomy and its relationship to degenerative hip disease is understanding the genesis of that deformity. Although very little is known in regard to the genesis of the pincer deformity, the development of the cam deformity during childhood/adolescence has long been suspected and described using varying terminology including tilt deformity, pistol grip and subclinical slipped capital femoral epiphysis [5–8]. Murray first postulated an association between activity level and the development of femoral tilt deformity [5]. Supporting the concept that intense physical activity may influence upper femoral development are two recently published studies in the paediatric population, where young adolescents during high level impact activity were more likely to have a cam deformity [9, 10] as well as the high prevalence of the cam deformity (greater than 50 %) in competitive collegiate athletes [9, 10].

This chapter will deal with the bony patho-anatomy associated with FAI, as well as the current level of evidence in what are the current diagnostic criteria defining these pathologies.

P. Whittingham-Jones, MBBS, FRCS
Trauma and Orthopaedics, Surgery, West Hertfordshire Hospitals NHS Trust, Watford and St. Albans City Hospital, Watford, Herts, UK
e-mail: mrpaulwj@gmail.com

P.E. Beaulé, MD FRCSC (✉)
Orthopaedic Surgery Division, Surgery Department, University of Ottawa, The Ottawa Hospital, 501 Smyth Rd, Room W1646, Ottawa, ON, Canada K1H 8L6
e-mail: pbeaule@ottawahospital.on.ca

The Acetabulum-Pincer FAI

Pincer-type FAI results from focal or a generalised overcoverage of the femoral head/neck [1]. During the movements of flexion and often-internal rotation in particular, but also throughout a greater movement arc in more profound cases, there is a linear area of contact at the acetabular rim. This causes compression of the labrum with subsequent labral failure, tearing and cartilaginous lesions. “Contrecoup” injuries posteriorly are also seen. The contrecoup lesion is the result of abnormal contact posteriorly as the anterior lesion pushes the entire femoral head in that direction. The contrecoup may be on the posterior aspect of the femoral head or the posterior chondro-labral complex. In the original paper describing the cartilage damage associated with FAI, Beck et al. [3] described varying degrees of overcoverage associated with pincer deformity with protrusio being the most severe when the femoral head crossed the ilioischial line and focal overcoverage where only the cranial portion of the acetabulum is retroverted (Fig. 20.1). This anterior overcoverage may be associated with a deficient posterior wall and is visible as a crossover sign on the plain radiograph [11–13]. A crossover sign does not necessarily mean a deficient posterior wall; however, so care must be taken to appreciate the relationship between the posterior wall and the centre of rotation of the femoral head. The most lateral edge of posterior wall should lie lateral to the centre of rotation. The crossover sign is also present in patients with acetabular dysplasia in a third to one sixth of cases [14, 15] as well as after overcorrection of a pelvic osteotomy [3]; consequently, the

J.C. McCarthy et al. (eds.), *Hip Joint Restoration*, DOI 10.1007/978-1-4614-0694-5_20

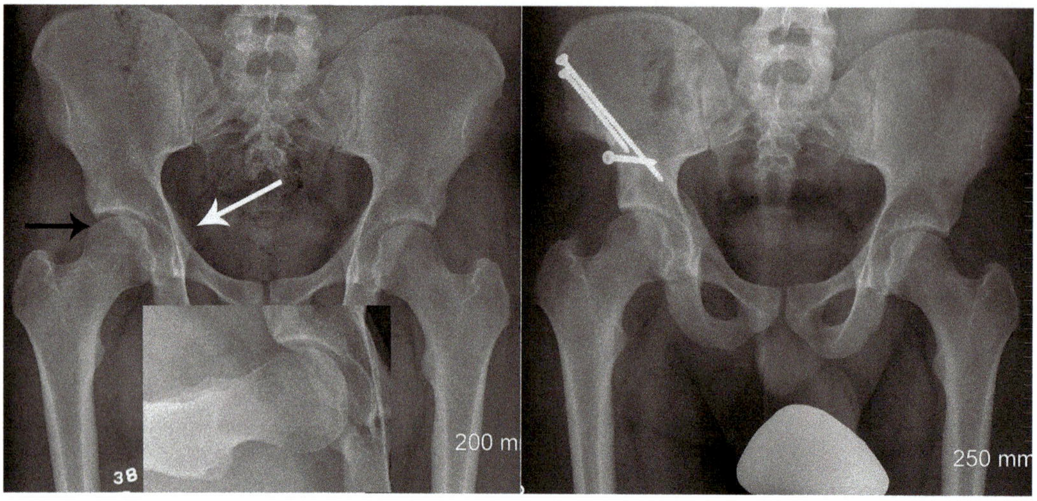

Fig. 20.1 Prominent ischial spine sign (*white arrow*) with crossover sign (*black arrow*) indicative of a retroverted acetabulum in a 26-year-old male. *Inset* shows normal head–neck offset. Postsurgical correction with a reverse peri-acetabular osteotomy

importance of overall pelvic orientation is critical prior to concluding that impinging causing acetabular retroversion is present. However, several recent papers have shown this radiographic feature of coxa profunda to be present in non-impinging as well as dysplastic hips [16–18]. A review of collegiate football players and patients undergoing hip preservation surgery revealed that coxa profunda existed in a wide spectrum of hips with lateral centre-edge angles between −18° and 60° [18]. Recent work from Nepple et al. [17] has confirmed that coxa profunda may be considered a normal finding; profunda was present in 76 % of asymptomatic hips and was more common in females (70 % cf 24 %), whilst other markers for overcoverage such as lateral centre-edge angle of >40° or acetabular inclination of <0° were present in only 22 % of hips with coxa profunda [17]. Similarly, Boone et al. [16] found a relatively poor specificity (62 %) for radiographic coxa profunda as a surrogate for global overcoverage.

Consequently, the initial report of Beck et al. [3] where 47 % cam impingement had associated pincer deformity which included coxa profunda has to be revisited with regard to how patients with hip pain associated with FAI are treated. When Allen et al. [19] looked at the risk of developing hip pain in patients with cam FAI, the presence of pincer deformity was not a significant risk factor for pincer impingement. Consequently, one has to approach the finding of pincer with caution with cranial retroversion in non-dysplastic hips as well as protrusion being the main structural abnormalities.

The Femur: Cam FAI

A loss of offset or concavity between head and neck of the femur is the leading cause of cam FAI. The antero-superior head–neck deformity, which is seen, may be caused by extension of the epiphysis during skeletal maturation and localised bony overgrowth. This may be the same phenomenon responsible for the well-described "pistol grip" deformity [8, 20]. A similar deformity with a prominence more distal in the metaphyseal region may be caused following slipped capital femoral epiphysis. Although the exact aetiology of the cam deformity is still unclear, genetic predisposition, high activity level, as well as mild slipped capital femoral epiphysis have been proposed [21–23]. Symptomatic, anteriorly based lesions may also be the result of malunion following femoral neck fracture [24] or developmental retroversion of the femoral neck, where both will also produce a relative loss of anterior offset, potentially giving rise to a cam-type deformity. This may be associated with coxa vara, which will further exacerbate the proximity of the anterior cam to the acetabulum and acetabular labrum when the affected hip is brought into flexion and internal rotation. Also described are conditions in which morphology of both sides of the hip joint results in FAI such as Legg–Calve–Perthes [25, 26]. In this condition, the developing femoral head (coxa magna) affects the development of the acetabulum. In the femur, a deformed coxa magna is seen with a high riding greater trochanter and resultant coxa vara. On the acetabular side in Legg–Calve–Perthes, there is under development (dysplasia), leading to relative femoral head under coverage and acetabular retroversion. A cam type of impingement is seen in lesser cases and a pincer impingement when the enlarged head fails to fit into the acetabulum in worse cases.

Far more unusual is a posteriorly based lesion on the femoral neck as a result of combined coxa valga with femoral antetorsion. In this instance, bringing the hip into external rotation and extension can give rise to postero-inferior femoroacetabular impingement. Also any neoplastic lesion on the anterior femoral neck may result in FAI.

Table 20.1 Summary of etiologies of FAI

Aetiology	Femoral side	Acetabular side	Extra-articular
SCFE	✓	x	x
Mal-united femoral neck fracture	✓	x	x
Femoral neck retroversion	✓	x	x
Femoral retrotorsion	✓	x	x
Femoral neck neoplasm	✓	x	x
Legg–Calve–Perthes	✓	✓	✓
Acetabular overcoverage—global/focal	X	✓	x
Acetabular retroversion—global/focal	X	✓	x
Developmental hip dysplasia	X	✓	x
Post pelvic osteotomy	X	✓	x
Greater/lesser trochanteric impingement	X	x	✓
Sub-anterior inferior iliac spine impingement	X	x	✓
Generalised ligamentous laxity	✓	✓	✓

Table 20.2 Summary of plain radiographic findings associated with FAI

Radiographic parameter	Appearance summary	Significance
Crossover sign	Line of the anterior rim crosses the posterior rim before reaching the sourcil	Acetabular retroversion
Prominence of ischial spine	Prominent extension of the ischial spine into the pelvis	Acetabular retroversion
Posterior wall sign	Posterior rim lies medial to the centre of rotation	Lack of posterior acetabular coverage
Lateral centre-edge angle	Angle subtended between a vertical axis up forms the centre of rotation and the line from the centre of rotation and the lateral aspect of the sourcil	<25° hip dysplasia >39° global acetabular over coverage
Anterior centre-edge angle	As above, using the false-profile projection	<20° suggests hip dysplasia
Tonnis angle	Angle subtended between a horizontal and the length of the sourcil	>10° hip dysplasia
Alpha angle	Angle subtended between a line up the centre of the femoral neck, from the centre of rotation and the first point from which an aspherical deformity is visible	>60° cam deformity

Other Types of FAI

A further type of FAI may also be encountered which is extra-articular impingement of both the greater and lesser trochanters [27–31]. Non-pathological morphology with FAI may exist in the presence of generalised ligamentous laxity and higher demands on the hip joint such as in high-impact sports or dancing; there is also an associated risk of FAI [3, 32]. Table 20.1 summarises the various etiologies of FAI.

Imaging of Femoroacetabular Impingement

Radiographic workup for a patient with presumed FAI will likely include conventional radiography with specialised lateral views as well as multiplanar imaging using MRI or computer tomography (CT). Bony abnormalities causing FAI are well visualised on well-oriented radiographs in two planes [33]: a well-centred anteroposterior view of the pelvis (anteroposterior pelvic view) [13], a cross-table lateral view [34], a 45° or 90° Dunn view [35, 36], a frog-lateral view [37] and a false-profile view to assess post articular wear [38]. Advanced imaging (MRI and 3D CT) is critical to rule out other pathologies such neoplasm or stress fracture as well as better identifying borderline deformities. Table 20.2 summarises the various radiographic findings associated with FAI.

Acetabular Morphology

For evaluation of acetabular version, an appropriate AP pelvic radiograph is required to allow appreciation of pelvic positioning, tilt and rotation. There are a number of specific radiographic signs to appreciate. The crossover sign has been shown to have a sensitivity and specificity of 96 % and 95 %, respectively, when assessing for acetabular retroversion in the cranial portion of the acetabulum [11]. Ischial spine projection into the pelvis [12] is described as a sign of acetabular retroversion with a sensitivity and specificity of 91 % and 98 %, respectively, and is known as the prominence of the ischial spine (PRIS) sign (Fig. 20.1). Unlike dysplasia where the lateral centre-edge angle provides a quantification of severity of disease, this is lacking for acetabular retroversion where surgical treatment is based on the mere presence or absence of the deformity. Recent work by Dandachli et al. using computer tomography showed that acetabular retroversion is not associated with increased total acetabular coverage but rather characterised by posterior deficiency with increased coverage anteriorly [39]. Consequently, when considering surgical management by means of arthroscopy, resection of the anterior acetabular rim could potentially decrease overall acetabular coverage, increasing contact pressures within the joint. In addition, it remains unclear as to how well a static radiograph assesses functional acetabular coverage although the frontal plane of the pelvis is likely very close to the standing position [40]; attempts have been made to correlate 2D imaging with 3D models for acetabular version [12, 41].

Because defining the appropriate amount of bone to be resected from the pincer impingement area to achieve correction remains to be validated [42], a reverse peri-acetabular osteotomy would provide reliable surgical technique to achieve appropriate correction without compromising total acetabular coverage. Arthroscopic resection of a pincer deformity remains a developing area.

Femoral Morphology

On the femoral side, there are several key parameters that need evaluation: femoral head sphericity, femoral head/neck offset, femoral neck-shaft angle and femoral torsion. The plain anteroposterior projection, the cross-table lateral, the Dunn view and the frog-lateral provide most information necessary.

Sphericity: To assess femoral sphericity, Notzli described the alpha angle on multiplanar MRI [43]. It is obtained by the angle subtended between a line from the centre of the femoral head to the point on the anterior or anterolateral aspect of the head–neck junction where the radius of the femoral head first becomes greater than the radius of the femoral head within the acetabulum and a line drawn through the centre of the femoral neck through the centre of the femoral head. The alpha angle has been determined to have different clinical cut-off points depending on which radial imaging plane is used. In looking at 200 asymptomatic volunteers, Hack et al. defined normative values for the alpha using multiplanar imaging [44], where the α-angle measured at the 3 o'clock position of a clock face is lower by on average 10° compared to the 1:30 position in the same individuals. Hence threshold values should take into account the area in which they are measured. This was confirmed by the paper of Sutter et al. where an alpha angle of 60° as a threshold will reduce false-positives whilst maintaining a sensitivity of 72–80 % for cam deformity [45].

Although originally described on multiplanar MRI, the alpha angle [43] has been validated on plain radiographs. Barton et al. [46] showed the Dunn view to have a positive predictive value of 93 % for diagnosing a cam deformity associated with FAI, and more recently, Nepple et al. showed the Dunn view as the most sensitive view to correlate with CT findings for a cam lesion [47]. For diagnostic and treatment purposes, a series of AP, frog-lateral and Dunn view radiographs will effectively characterise the femoral head–neck junction (Fig. 20.2).

Femoral head–neck offset: Femoral head–neck offset can also be assessed which is distinct from sphericity as it describes the region of the head–neck junction, rather than the shape of the head. This was originally described by Eijer using the cross-table lateral [34], where hips with symptomatic impingement had a mean ratio of 0.13 compared to 0.21 in normal hips. Looking at a larger group of patients, Beaulé et al. [48] found that an offset ratio $\leq$0.15 had a 9.5-fold increased relative risk of having an α-angle $\geq$50.5° consistent with the presence of a cam deformity.

Femoral torsion: Another important consideration when considering the femur in FAI is the overall femoral torsion leading to intra-articular hip pathology (Fig. 20.3). When reviewing 135 patients with proven labral pathology who had undergone three-dimensional computer tomography, Dolan et al. [49] found that 13 % of patients had a femoral version of less than 5° (i.e., femoral retrotorsion) and 16 % had excessive femoral anteversion (>25°). In another study,

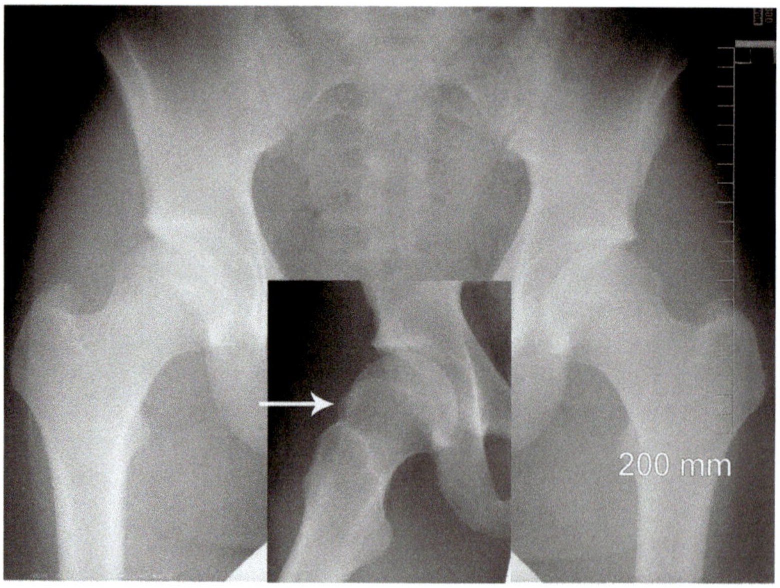

Fig. 20.2 Eighteen-year-old male with severe right hip pain secondary to cam FAI. *Inset* shows large deformity with convexity (*white arrow*)

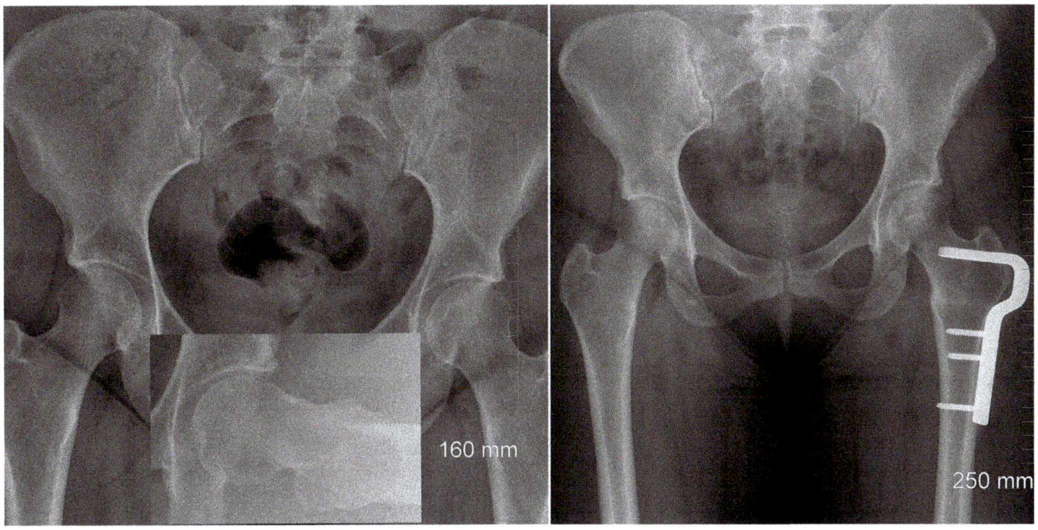

Fig. 20.3 Thirty-year-old female with bilateral hip pain. Anteroposterior (AP) pelvic radiograph shows normal acetabular coverage but absence of lesser trochanter on both hips suggestive of femoral retroversion. *Inset* shows lack of femoral anteversion. AP pelvis postsurgical correction by means of derotational osteotomy

Sutter et al. found a statistically significant association between high femoral antetorsion and pincer-type FAI with individuals with pincer FAI having also a significantly higher femoral version compared to those with cam FAI, perhaps indicative of a postero-inferior FAI [50]. Either MRI or CT offers reasonable solutions to the assessment of femoral torsion, provided images of the distal femur as reference for the proximal anatomy are obtained.

Three-Dimensional Imaging

The need for advanced 3D imaging in gaining a better understanding in the diagnosis and management of FAI is becoming more and more evident [49–52], as well as helping in defining complex and/or borderline deformities [53]. In addition, this can be helpful in planning surgical correction of the bony deformity as well as potentially identifying lack or insufficient correction post surgery. It is yet unclear if CT will become a standard due to the concerns of radiation especially in this young active population.

Conclusion

The understanding of FAI and its treatment is constantly evolving. An appreciation of the anatomy and the pathological processes are important. The surgeon must be keenly aware as knowledge increases and the complexity of possible surgical solutions evolve. Finally, the presence of bony morphological abnormalities is not in itself an indication for surgery as a careful history and physical examination remain the cornerstone for the treatment of patients.

References

1. Ganz R, Parvizi J, Leunig M, Siebenrock KA. Femoroacetabular impingement: a cause for osteoarthritis of the hip. Clin Orthop. 2003;417(417):112–20.
2. Agricola R, Heijboer MP, Bierma-Zeinstra SMA, Verhaar JA, Weinans H, Waarsing JH. Cam impingement causes osteoarthritis of the hip: a nationwide prospective cohort study (CHECK). Ann Rheum Dis. 2013;72(6):918–23.
3. Beck M, Kalhor M, Leunig M, Ganz R. Hip morphology influences the pattern of damage to the acetabular cartilage: femoroacetabular impingement as a cause of early osteoarthritis of the hip. J Bone Joint Surg Br. 2005;87B(7):1012–8.
4. Leunig M, Beaule PE, Ganz R. The concept of femoroacetabular impingement: current status and future perspectives. Clin Orthop Rel Res. 2009;467(3):616–22.
5. Murray RO, Duncan C. Athletic activity in adolescence as an etiological factor in degenerative hip disease. J Bone Joint Surg Br. 1971;53(3):406–19.
6. Stulberg SD, Cordell LD, Harris WH, Ramsey PL, MacEwen GD. Unrecognized childhood hip disease: a major cause of idiopathic osteoarthritis of the hip. In: Amstutz HC, editor. The hip, proceedings of the third open scientific meeting of the Hip Society. St. Louis: C.V. Mosby; 1975. p. 212–28.
7. Solomon L. Patterns of osteoarthritis of the hip. J Bone Joint Surg Br. 1976;58(3):176–83.
8. Goodman DA, Feighan JE, Smith AD, Latimer B, Buly RL, Cooperman DR. Subclinical slipped capital femoral epiphysis. J Bone Joint Surg Am. 1997;79A(10):1489–97.
9. Agricola R, Bessems JH, Ginai AZ, Heijboer MP, van der Heijden RA, Verhaar JA, et al. The development of Cam-type deformity in adolescent and young male soccer players. Am J Sports Med. 2012;40(5):1099–106.
10. Kapron AL, Anderson AE, Aoki SK, Phillips LG, Petron DJ, Toth R, et al. Radiographic prevalence of femoroacetabular impingement in collegiate football players: AAOS Exhibit Selection. J Bone Joint Surg Am. 2011;93(19). e111(1–10).

11. Kalberer F, Sierra RJ, Madan SS, Ganz R, Leunig M. Ischial spine projection into the pelvis: a new sign for acetabular retroversion. Clin Orthop Relat Res. 2008;466(3):677–83.
12. Werner CM, Copeland CE, Ruckstuhl T, Stromberg J, Turen CH, Kalberer F, et al. Radiographic markers of acetabular retroversion:correlation of the cross-over sign, ischial spine sign and posterior wall sign. Acta Orthop Belg. 2010;76(2):166–73.
13. Jamali AA, Maldenov K, Meyer DC, Martinez A, Beck M, Ganz R, et al. Anteroposterior pelvic radiographs to assess acetabular retroversion: high validity of the "cross-over-sign". J Orthop Res. 2007;25(6):758–65.
14. Li PL, Ganz R. Morphologic features of congenital acetabular dysplasia: one in six is retroverted. Clin Orthop Relat Res. 2003;416: 245–53.
15. Mast JW, Brunner RL, Zebrack J. Recognizing acetabular version in the radiographic presentation of hip dysplasia. Clin Orthop Relat Res. 2004;418(418):48–53.
16. Boone G, Pagnotto MR, Walker JR, Trousdale RT, Sierra RJ. Radiographic features associated with differing impinging hip morphologies with special attention to coxa profunda. Clin Orthop Relat Res. 2012;470(12):3414–20.
17. Nepple JJ, Lehmann CL, Ross JR, Schoenecker PL, Clohisy JC. Coxa profunda is not a useful radiographic parameter for diagnosing pincer-type femoroacetabular impingement. J Bone Joint Surg Am. 2013;95(5):417–23.
18. Anderson LA, Kapron AL, Aoki SK, Peters CL. Coxa profunda: is the deep acetabulum overcovered? Clin Orthop Relat Res. 2012;470(12):3467–9.
19. Allen DJ, Beaule PE, Ramadan O, Doucette S. Prevalence of associated deformities and hip pain in patients with cam type femoroacetabular impingement. J Bone Joint Surg Br. 2009;91B(5):589–94.
20. Harris WH. Etiology of osteoarthritis of the hip. Clin Orthop Relat Res. 1986;213:20–33.
21. Pollard TC, Batra RN, Judge A, Watkins B, McNally EG, Gill HS, et al. The hereditary predisposition to hip osteoarthritis and its association with abnormal joint morphology. Osteoarthritis Cartilage. 2013;21(2):314–21.
22. Pollard TC, Batra RN, Judge A, Watkins B, McNally EG, Gill HS, et al. Genetic predisposition to the presence and 5-year clinical progression of hip osteoarthritis. Osteoarthritis Cartilage. 2012; 20(5):368–75.
23. Siebenrock KA, Ferner F, Noble PC, Santore RF, Werlen S, Mamisch TC. The cam-type deformity of the proximal femur arises in childhood in response to vigorous sporting activity. Clin Orthop Relat Res. 2011;469(11):3229–40.
24. Strehl A, Ganz R. [Anterior femoroacetabular impingement after healed femoral neck fractures]. Unfallchirurg. 2005;108(4): 263–73.
25. Ross JR, Nepple JJ, Baca G, Schoenecker PL, Clohisy JC. Intraarticular abnormalities in residual Perthes and Perthes-like hip deformities. Clin Orthop Relat Res. 2012;470(11):2968–77.
26. Froberg L, Christensen F, Pedersen NW, Overgaard S. Radiographic changes in the hip joint in children suffering from Perthes disease. J Pediatr Orthop B. 2012;21(3):220–5.
27. Eijer H, Podeszwa DA, Ganz R, Leunig M. Evaluation and treatment of young adults with femoro-acetabular impingement secondary to Perthes' disease. Hip Int. 2006;16(4):273–80.
28. Ganz R, Huff TW, Leunig M. Extended retinacular soft-tissue flap for intra-articular hip surgery: surgical technique, indications, and results of application. Instr Course Lect. 2009;58:241–55.
29. Quain S, Catterall A. Hinge abduction of the hip. Diagnosis and treatment. J Bone Joint Surg Br. 1986;68(1):61–4.
30. Snow SW, Keret D, Scarangella S, Bowen JR. Anterior impingement of the femoral head: a late phenomenon of Legg-Calve-Perthes' disease. J Pediatr Orthop. 1993;13:286–9.
31. Wenger DR, Kishan S, Pring ME. Impingement and childhood hip disease. J Pediatr Orthop. 2006;15(4):233–43.
32. Anderson SE, Siebenrock KA, Tannast M. Femoroacetabular impingement: evidence of an established hip abnormality. Radiology. 2010;257(1):8–13.
33. Clohisy JC, Carlisle JC, Beaule PE, Kim Y-J, Trousdale RT, Sierra RJ, et al. A systematic approach to the plain radiographic evaluation of the young adult hip. J Bone Joint Surg Am. 2008;90A Suppl 4:47–66.
34. Eijer H, Leunig M, Mahomed N, Ganz R. Cross-table lateral radiographs for screening of anterior femoral head-neck offset in patients with femoro-acetabular impingement. Hip Int. 2001; 11(1):37–41.
35. Dunn DM. Anteversion of the neck of the femur; a method of measurement. J Bone Joint Surg Br. 1952;34:181–6.
36. Meyer DC, Beck M, Ellis T, Ganz R, Leunig M. Comparision of six radiographic projections to assess femoral head/asphericity. Clin Orthop. 2006;445(445):181–5.
37. Clohisy JC, Nunley RM, Otto RJ, Shoenecker PL. The frog-lateral radiograph accurately visualised hip cam impingement abnormalities. Clin Orthop Relat Res. 2007;462:115–21.
38. Lequesne M. The false profile view of the hip: role, interest, economic considerations. Joint Bone Spine. 2002;69:109–13.
39. Dandachli W, Ul Islam S, Liu M, Richards R, Hall-Craggs M, Witt J. Three-dimensional CT analysis to determine acetabular retroversion and the implications for the management of femoro-acetabular impingement. J Bone Joint Surg Br. 2009;91(B):1031–6.
40. Nishihara S, Sugaro N, Nishii T, et al. Measurement of pelvic flexion angle using three-dimensional computed tomography. Clin Orthop Relat Res. 2003;451:154–60.
41. Dandachli W, Kannan V, Richards R, et al. Analysis of cover of the femoral head in normal and dysplastic hips: new CT-based technique. J Bone Joint Surg Br. 2008;90(11):1428–34.
42. Gross C, Salata M, Manno K, Yelavarthi V, Barker J, Williams J, et al. New radiographic parameters to describe anterior acetabular rim trimming during hip arthroscopy. Arthroscopy. 2012; 28(10):1404–9.
43. Notzli HP, Wyss TF, Stoecklin CH, Schmid MR, Treiber K, Hodler J. The contour of the femoral head-neck junction as a predictor for the risk of anterior impingement. J Bone Joint Surg Br. 2002; 84(4):556–60.
44. Hack K, Diprimio G, Rakhra K, Beaule PE. Prevalence of CAM type femoroacetabular impingement in asymptomatic volunteers. J Bone Joint Surg Am. 2010;92A(14):2436–44.
45. Sutter R, Dietrich TJ, Zingg PO, Pfirrmann CW. How useful is the alpha angle for discriminating between symptomatic patients with cam-type femoroacetabular impingement and asymptomatic volunteers? Radiology. 2012;264(2):514–21.
46. Barton C, Salineros MJ, Rakhra KS, Beaule PE. Validity of the alpha angle measurement on plain radiographs in the evaluation of cam-type femoroacetabular impingement. Clin Orthop Relat Res. 2011;469(2):464–9.
47. Nepple JJ, Martell JM, Kim Y-J, Zaltz I, Clohisy JC. Do plain radiographs correlate with CT for imaging of cam-type femoroacetabular impingement? Clin Orthop Relat Res. 2012;470(12): 3313–20.
48. Beaule PE, Harvey N, Zaragoza EJ, LeDuff M, Dorey FJ. The femoral head/neck offset and hip resurfacing. J Bone Joint Surg Br. 2007;89(1):9–15.
49. Dolan MM, Heyworth BE, Bedi A, Duke G, Kelly BT. CT reveals a high incidence of osseous abnormalities in hips with labral tears. Clin Orthop Relat Res. 2011;469(3):831–8.
50. Sutter R, Dietrich T, Zingg PO, Pfirrmann C. Femoral antetorsion; comparing asymptomatic volunteers and patients with femoroacetabular impingement. Radiology. 2012;263(2):475–83.

51. Tannast M, Kubiak-Langer M, Langlotz F, Puls M, Murphy SB, Siebenrock KA. Noninvasive three-dimensional assessment of femoroacetabular impingement. J Orthop Res. 2007;25(1): 122–31.
52. Milone MT, Bedi A, Poultsides L, Magennis E, Byrd JW, Larson CM, et al. Novel CT-based three-dimensional software improves the characterization of cam morphology. Clin Orthop Relat Res. 2013;471(8):2484–91.
53. Beaule PE, Zaragoza EJ, Motamedic K, Copelan N, Dorey J. Three-dimensional computed Tomography of the hip in the assessment of femoro-acetabular impingement. J Orthop Res. 2005;23(4): 1286–92.

21 Imaging of Cartilage Patho-anatomy

Steven S. Chua, Jason D. Alder, Joshua D. Harris, Andrew R. Palisch, Collin D. Bray, and Philip C. Noble

Introduction

The integrity and health of the structures of the hip are vital for the proper initiation of movement and support. However, as articular cartilage is avascular, aneural, and alymphatic, its capacity for repair and regeneration is limited. Early cartilage injury may be both a biochemical and mechanical process. Inflammatory biochemical processes are present in early hip osteoarthritis, evident in synovial fluid and synovial tissue analysis. Mechanical processes are also present early in the disease, such as those frequently associated with femoroacetabular impingement (FAI). Early detection of degenerative changes is crucial to mitigate disease progression with both nonsurgical and surgical joint preservation interventions. Noninvasive imaging modalities, such as plain radiographs, magnetic resonance imaging (MRI), ultrasound, and computed tomography (CT), are the cornerstone of early detection of articular cartilage anatomy and patho-anatomy.

The ideal modality for imaging of articular cartilage would enable rapid acquisition of images, in addition to being inexpensive, noninvasive, and easy to perform, reproducible, sensitive, specific, reliable, and responsive. Any modality possessing these qualities would allow early detection of degenerative changes and permit monitoring of treatment interventions. Plain radiography is frequently the first modality utilized in hip joint evaluation. However, it is limited by its inability to directly image cartilage as significant cartilage damage may be present despite a normal joint space. Currently, MRI is the best imaging modality to characterize normal and abnormal hip articular cartilage and underlying subchondral bone because of good tissue contrast. Moreover, MRI surpasses surgical visualization in its ability to reveal the underlying femoral and acetabular anatomy of the hip. However, conventional MRI techniques are limited in their capacity to quantify the inherent integrity of cartilaginous tissue, including regions of softening and increased permeability, and the presence of fissures, fibrillation, and contained non-displaced delamination. Recent MRI techniques attempt to overcome these issues by better illustrating and characterizing hip hyaline cartilage ultrastructure via type II collagen and glycosaminoglycan content. In this chapter, we will discuss the current state of imaging of articular cartilage and the application of these techniques to the detection and monitoring of common pathological conditions threatening the longevity and function of the hip joint.

Cartilaginous Tissues: Basic Features

Hip joint articular cartilage is of the hyaline type, consisting predominantly (>90 %) of an extracellular matrix (water, type II collagen, proteoglycans, and non-collagen proteins) embedded with chondrocytes. As articular cartilage is avascular, aneural, and alymphatic, the diffusion of nutrients to chondrocytes is highly dependent on the flux of synovial

S.S. Chua, MD, PhD • A.R. Palisch, MD
Department of Radiology, Baylor College of Medicine, One Baylor Plaza, Houston, TX 77030, USA

J.D. Alder, MD
Department of Orthopaedics and Sports Medicine, Houston Methodist Hospital, 6550 Fannin St., Suite 2500, Houston, TX, 77030, USA
e-mail: jdalder@houstonmethodist.org

J.D. Harris, MD
Department of Orthopaedics and Sports Medicine, Houston Methodist Hospital, 6550 Fannin Street, Suite 2500, Houston, TX 77030, USA

Weill Cornell Medical College, Houston, TX 77030, USA
e-mail: Jharris6@houstonmethodist.org

C.D. Bray, MD
Department of Radiology, Musculoskeletal Imaging, Baylor College of Medicine, One Baylor Plaza, Houston, TX 77030, USA
e-mail: cbray@bcm.edu

P.C. Noble, PhD (✉)
Director of Research, Institute of Orthopedic Research and Education, 6550 Fannin Street, Suite 2501, Houston, TX 77030, USA

Director of Research, Institute of Orthopedic Research and Education, Houston, TX 77030, USA
e-mail: pnoble@bcm.edu

J.C. McCarthy et al. (eds.), *Hip Joint Restoration*, DOI 10.1007/978-1-4614-0694-5_21

fluid generated by cyclic compression and relaxation of cartilage during joint loading and movement. The high proportion of water within cartilage is responsible for its high signal intensity compared to bone when exposed to fluid-sensitive MRI sequences (e.g., T2, STIR [short-tau inversion recovery]) [1].

The thickness of the cartilage layer varies with the specific joint within the body, ranging from less than 1 mm in the small joints of the hand and foot, to 2–3 mm on the acetabulum and the femoral head, and up to 8 mm in the knee joint. Regardless of its thickness, articular cartilage consists of three zones: the superficial (tangential) zone, the middle (transitional) zone, and the deep (radial) zone [2]. The superficial zone consists of a low concentration of glycosaminoglycans (GAGs) in a dense network of fibers, mostly type II collagen and flattened chondrocytes orientated parallel to the joint surface. The acellular lamina splendens, which is approximately 5 μm in thickness, is the most superficial layer of the superficial zone. A transitional zone (at approximately 100 μm deep to the articular surface) within the superficial zone is likely the source of shear stress transmission that may herald the onset of degenerative changes that begin in this zone [3]. The middle transitional zone of articular cartilage has a higher GAG concentration with collagen fibers oriented oblique to the cartilage surface. The deep radial zone contains the highest concentration of GAGs with collagen fibers aligned perpendicular to the cartilage surface. The transition from noncalcified cartilage to the calcified cartilage zone is delineated by an undulating "tidemark", while the boundary between the calcified cartilage zone and the subchondral bone plate is delineated by the cement line [2].

In early osteoarthritis, the balance of homeostasis is shifted toward degradation over repair. Mild superficial damage to collagen and proteoglycans is present and occurs in concert with a relative increase in the hydrostatic pressure of water which leads to swelling of the cartilage surface. This level of tissue damage may be repaired by natural healing processes as chondrocytes synthesize new matrix [2]. However, with the progression of the degenerative process, the change in relative water content and the loss of the chondrocytes' ability to repair lead to fissures and fibrillations [2]. Focal full-thickness articular cartilage lesions with exposed bone are the precursors to more diffuse degenerative joint disease. Isolated defects can be imaged best with MRI. Osteoarthritis with joint space narrowing, osteophytes, subchondral sclerosis, and cyst formation can be visualized on plain radiographs, CT, MRI, and ultrasound, but only MRI can detect earlier changes of osteoarthritis.

Another form of cartilage, fibrocartilage, has a tougher and harder consistency than hyaline cartilage. In addition to having type II collagen, fibrocartilage also contains denser type I collagen. Because of its more robust properties, fibrocartilage is found in intervertebral disks, knee menisci, within the articulating disk of the pubic symphysis, and the labrum of the hip and shoulder. The labrum of the hip is an important structure necessary for normal joint function and prevention of degenerative arthritis. The imaging of the labrum of the hip will be discussed later in this chapter.

Imaging Modalities Utilized to Evaluate Cartilage Health

Conventional Radiography

Plain radiography is the initial screening tool for detection of osteoarthritis of the hip. Due to its indirect assessment of the status of the articular cartilage, plain radiography is of limited application in early osteoarthritis where joint space is maintained but cartilage damage has already occurred. It is more useful in advanced degenerative joint disease, where joint space narrowing and osteophyte formation can be seen. Many facets of joint disease, including pathologic abnormalities of the labrum, capsule, and musculotendinous and neurovascular structures are unable to be visualized on plain radiographs [3]. Nonetheless, clinicians utilize plain radiographs as the initial objective screening tool for hip pathology. In addition to osteoarthritis, several other diagnoses may be seen with x-ray including FAI, dysplasia, fracture, tumor, and infection, among others. In patients with joint disease, plain films have also been used as a follow-up tool to evaluate disease progression.

Ultrasonography

Another modality gaining popularity in the evaluation of joint morphology is ultrasonography, which allows evaluation of joint health through changes in the echotexture of articular cartilage [4, 5]. Advantages of ultrasonography include the lack of ionizing radiation, general acceptance by patients, multiplanar capability, and speed of imaging. However, it is widely recognized that this modality is also susceptible to artifacts and is dependent upon the skill and experience of the operator, factors that appear to be difficult to standardize. In addition, this modality can be limited by lack of a suitable acoustic window and an optimal insonation angle to allow adequate evaluation of the joint(s). For example, the hip joint is more difficult to evaluate than the knee or the hand. Nonetheless, ultrasonography has been used to a large extent in rheumatology in Europe for assessment of degenerative changes to articular cartilage secondary to arthritis and/or inflammatory conditions. This modality is superior to radiography in evaluating for surface changes in cartilage, quality of cartilage, and thickness and surface area [4]. A normal hyaline cartilage is visualized as a homogenous anechoic band [5] and blurring of cartilage edges, loss of homogeneity, focal and diffuse thinning, and/or complete absence can be evaluated and assessed in the various disease stages in osteoarthritis [4, 6, 7]. In crystal diseases, deposits of calcium pyrophosphate dihydrate (CPPD) can be imaged by ultrasound to be located within cartilage as opposed to crystals located along the cartilage border in gout [8]. In addition, the portability of ultrasound enables its use at the bedside or in the clinic setting where it may also be used to guide joint aspirations and delivery of drugs directly into the joint space [4, 6].

Computed Tomography (CT)

Although computed tomography (CT) of the hip has distinct advantages for visualizing two- and three-dimensional osseous morphology, it adds little to the evaluation of articular or labral cartilage [2, 7]. In the preoperative evaluation of FAI, CT allows the surgeon to formulate a surgical plan for bone resection based on cam and pincer morphology, femoral and acetabular version, head asphericity, tilt, offset, and neck-shaft angle. Another application is in CT arthrography, where cartilage damage may be evaluated after injection of a contrast agent into the joint prior to CT imaging [8].

MRI

MRI offers a better soft tissue assessment versus plain radiographs and CT and is thus the optimal method for evaluating not only articular cartilage damage but also the capsule, labrum, and the surrounding musculotendinous and neurovascular structures. However, several factors prevent conventional planar MR images from reliably depicting subtle signs of early musculoskeletal damage, including the spherical nature and oblique anatomical position of the hip joint and the thin and intimately apposed articular cartilage and labrum, in addition to chemical shift artefacts and partial volume averaging. For this reason, radial imaging has been suggested as a technique to circumvent some of these limitations [9].

Typical MRI sequences utilized in clinical radiology to image cartilage morphology include fluid-sensitive proton density (PD), T2 fat saturated, and T1. In addition, certain specialized sequences are commonly available, including three-dimensional spoiled-gradient (3D-SPGR) and fast low angle shot (FLASH) sequences [10]. In the research arena, the double-echo-steady state (DESS) [11] and 3D-SPGR sequences are thought to generate very high-resolution images with narrow slice thickness [12].

Early depletion of type II collagen and negatively charged glycosaminoglycans significantly alters matrix permeability and increases the relative water content [2, 13]. The apparent diffusion coefficient of water is low in normal cartilage but increases in damaged cartilage [2]. As such, a number of enhanced techniques that evaluate for changes in cartilage composition exploit this pathophysiology for detecting early articular cartilage injury before conventional MRI may demonstrate any changes [1, 2]. These methods include T2 and T2* mapping, dGEMRIC (delayed gadolinium-enhanced MRI of cartilage), T1 rho, sodium imaging, CEST (chemical exchange saturation transfer), diffusion, and ultrashort TE complement conventional imaging [2, 14]. A brief description of these specialized imaging techniques is presented in Table 21.1 and will be expanded upon in the Future Advances section of this book.

Challenges of MRI for Hip Articular Cartilage Defects

Magnetic resonance evaluation of articular cartilage lesions on both the femoral head and acetabulum is challenging. The image must delineate normal from abnormal articular cartilage, articular cartilage from joint synovial fluid, and articular cartilage from underlying subchondral bone. To minimize partial volume averaging effects, high spatial resolution is necessary, achievable with higher strength magnets (1.5 and 3.0 T), which improves signal-to-noise ratio (SNR) and subsequent spatial resolution and acquisition time. These effects occur when the voxel dimensions are larger than the structure or abnormality (e.g., fissure, fibrillation, and delamination). In addition, chemical shift artifacts occur due to misregistration of fat and water. On image sequences without fat suppression, the marrow fat and deep noncalcified cartilage misregister and may cause the subchondral bone plate to appear thicker and the articular cartilage thinner than in actuality.

MRI Versus MRA

In the hip, the addition of intra-articular contrast may enhance the visualization of chondrolabral pathology. However, the injection of contrast agent into the joint is frequently painful, with little to no actual anesthetic effect, despite the addition of a local anesthetic to the contrast agent. This precludes clinician evaluation of the possible anesthetic effect at the time of the injection (performed by radiologist), and may confound future intra-articular injections for therapeutic purposes. For this reason, most hip preservation surgeons do not utilize MRI or MRA for the evaluation of the labrum. However, common applications include the detection of subchondral bone abnormalities (e.g., edema, cysts), musculotendinous evaluation (e.g., hip abductor insertion, hip adductor insertion, pubic symphysis, iliopsoas tendon), and for eliminating uncommon causes of hip pain from the differential diagnosis (e.g., stress fracture, tumor, infection, or avascular necrosis).

Unfortunately, the literature is not replete with high-quality studies comparing MRI and MRA. For MRA, the

Table 21.1 A summary of the specialized techniques available for imaging cartilage, the physical basis of each technique and the characteristics of the images generated

T2 mapping	• T2 relaxation time is dependent upon hydration status, type II collagen content, and orientation
	• Any change in water or collagen content may alter T2 relaxation time
	• Zonal stratification: T2 values increase from deep (deep radial zone) to superficial (superficial tangential zone)
dGEMRIC	• Based upon fixed negative charge density of glycosaminoglycans in extracellular matrix
	• Intravenous gadolinium diethylenetriaminepentaacetic acid is negatively charged
	• Gadolinium reduces T1 relaxation time (and, to lesser extent, T2 and T2* relaxation time)
	• Gadolinium and glycosaminoglycans oppose one another
	• Thus, if increased gadolinium uptake, low glycosaminoglycan content
	• Thus, the lower the T1 relaxation time, the lower the glycosaminoglycan content
T1-rho	• Based upon spin-lattice relaxation time in the rotating frame
	• Related to T2 maps, but more sensitive to glycosaminoglycan content and less sensitive to collagen orientation
Sodium imaging	• Sodium is positively-charged cation (natural counter-ion to negative glycosaminoglycan)
	• High-field magnets and specialized hardware permits direct image production reflecting the fixed charge density in articular cartilage
GAG-CEST mapping	• Specifically maps regional cartilage glycosaminoglycan content
	• Relationship between water exchange between hydroxyl groups in free extracellular matrix water and glycosaminoglycans

interobserver reliability is reported as only fair (kappa 0.268) [15]. Further, the sensitivity and specificity for two radiologist reviewers are suboptimal (86 %/86 % and 75 %/50 %, respectively), which is not significantly different from non-arthrogram MRI. The negative predictive value is low (19 %/13 %), and the positive predictive value is high (99 %/98 %). The high positive predictive value is attributed to the high prevalence of labral tears within both the older population and subjects being evaluated for hip preservation surgery.

Imaging Specific Pathologic Conditions

Femoroacetabular Impingement

Patients with FAI often present with hip pain, associated symptoms, and osteoarthritis which arise from a mechanical conflict between the femoral head and the acetabular rim. Two distinct morphologic abnormalities underlie this condition: (i) the presence of a femoral head with an insufficient spherical portion to allow a normal range of motion of the hip (cam-type deformity) or (ii) where there is excessive coverage of the femoral head by the acetabular margin or the periacetabular bone (pincer-type deformity), or a combination of both [16, 17]. The presence of these deformities is often associated with damage to intra-articular structures (labrum and articular cartilage), especially in very active individuals [18, 19].

Although the primary deformity of the cam FAI femur is enlargement of the anterior head-neck junction, with loss of head-neck offset, this condition often occurs in association with a host of other components of bony deformity, including an aspherical femoral head, relative femoral retroversion, enlargement of the femoral neck, displacement of the neck on the femoral shaft, and changes in the neck-shaft angle (Fig. 21.1). Pincer morphology involves either global or focal acetabular pathology (Fig. 21.2). Simple overgrowth of the anterolateral edge of the acetabular (loss of cranial anteversion) accounts for focal pincer impingement. Acetabular retroversion most commonly leads to global pincer impingement. A prominent anterior inferior iliac spine (AIIS) may also lead to impingement (sub-spine impingement) further distal on the anterior femoral neck than traditional pincer impingement (Fig. 21.3). The iliopsoas may also impinge on the far anterior (3 o'clock position in right hip) acetabulum and cause labral injury in an atypical location (versus 12–2 o'clock in cam/pincer impingement). Trochanteric-pelvic impingement is an extra-articular form of impingement which occurs at the limit of hip abduction through contact between the tip of the greater trochanter and the lateral pelvic wall above the acetabular rim (Fig. 21.4). Extra-articular ischiofemoral impingement may also occur during external rotation of the hip in extension and external rotation leading to contact between the greater trochanter and the ischium.

Plain radiography is the initial evaluation of choice for patients with hip pain. Plain radiographs characterize femoral and acetabular morphology in both arthritic (joint space

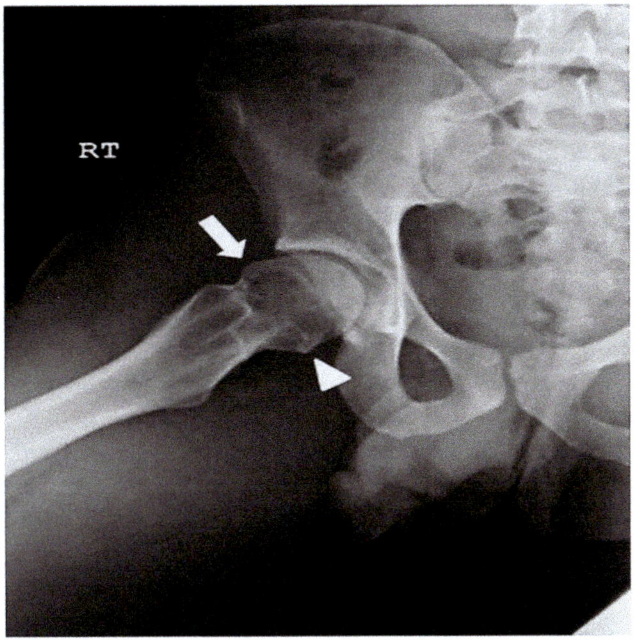

Fig. 21.1 Frog-leg lateral plain radiograph of a right hip in a skeletally mature male patient with femoral cam morphology. The cam is present from anterolateral (*arrowhead*) to inferomedial (*arrow*)

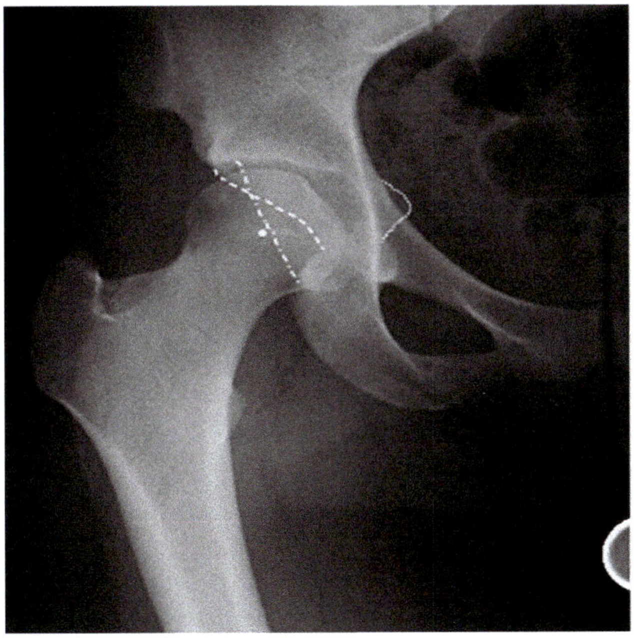

Fig. 21.2 Anteroposterior (AP) plain radiograph of 18 year old female with pincer FAI. Evidence of loss of cranial acetabular anteversion indicates focal pincer impingement (crossing of anterior and posterior walls of acetabulum—*hashed lines* crossing on this figure; the normal appearance indicates anterior and posterior walls meeting at the lateral sourcil). Global pincer impingement is evident with relative acetabular retroversion indicated by the posterior wall sign (posterior wall is medial to the center of the femoral head—*single dot* indicates the head center) and the ischial spine sign (*dotted line* medial to the iliopectineal line)

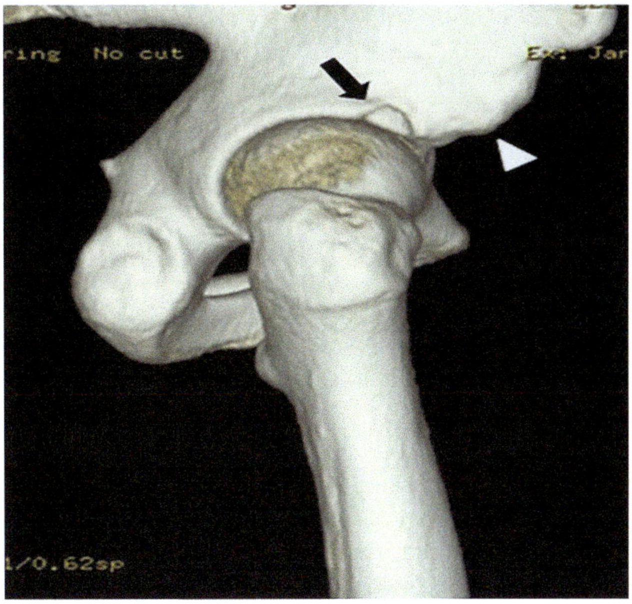

Fig. 21.3 Three-dimensional computed tomography lateral view of a right hip in a skeletally mature male patient with a prominent anterior inferior iliac spine (*white arrowhead*). Note the presence of an os acetabuli (superolateral acetabular rim fracture) (*black arrow*)

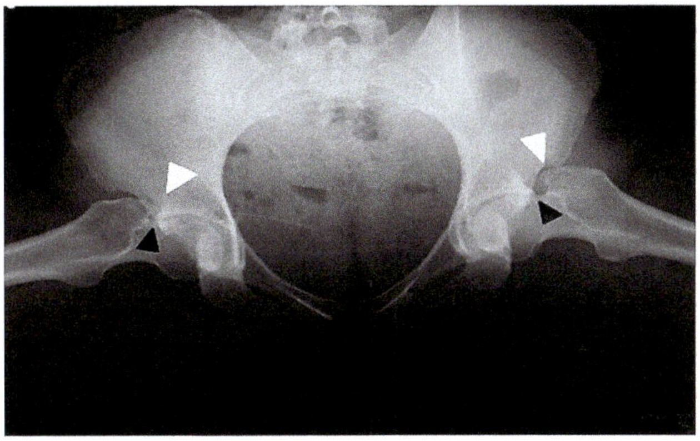

Fig. 21.4 Plain radiograph of skeletally mature female while performing the abduction splits maneuver. Trochanteric-pelvic impingement is evident (*white arrowheads*), in addition to pincer impingement (*black arrowheads*)

narrowing, subchondral sclerosis, and cysts, osteophytes) and non-arthritic (FAI) joints [20, 21]. A weight-bearing anteroposterior (AP) pelvis view is obtained with the legs internally rotated 15° and the x-ray beam directed to the midpoint between a line joining the ASIS and symphysis pubis [22, 23]. An adequate AP radiograph has symmetric obturator foramina and lesser trochanter profiles with the coccyx and pubic symphysis parallel. Typically, the tip of the coccyx will be located two centimeters above the most superior aspect of the symphysis. Various lateral views are used, according to clinician preference, including 45° and 90°

Dunn views, false profile, frog-leg lateral, Lauenstein lateral, and cross-table lateral. The 45° Dunn view has been shown to best profile the appearance of the most common location of cam morphology (anterior) [24].

The cam-type deformity has been described as a pistol grip deformity [25]. Although most commonly found at the anterior head-neck junction, the cam deformity may extend posterosuperiorly (between 10 and 12 o'clock on the right hip) or inferomedially (between 5 and 7 o'clock on the right hip). The parameters most commonly used to quantify the deformity are the alpha angle and the head-neck offset ratio [26].

- The **alpha angle** was originally described by Notzli et al. on an axial oblique MRI [26]. However, this method of measurement has been extrapolated to plain radiographs and is calculated as follows: A circle fitting the subchondral contour of the femoral head is superimposed on the image of the head and the center is marked. The point where the anterior contour of head deviates from the circle is also marked. A line is then drawn connecting the center of the femoral head to the point defining the limit of head sphericity. A second line is drawn along the axis of the femoral neck through the center of the head. The alpha angle is defined as the angle between these two lines. Given the large range of angles seen in control groups of multiple studies, there is significant disagreement regarding "normal" alpha angles. However, many authors agree that angles greater than 55°–63° are abnormal [21, 27, 28].
- The **head-neck offset (HNO or OSR) ratio** is the ratio between the projected diameter of the femoral head and the distance between two lines drawn parallel to the femoral neck axis and tangent to the anterolateral edge of the femoral head and the anterolateral edge of the femoral neck [29]. A normal HNO ratio of 0.17–0.19 has been proposed, with values less than 0.14–0.17 being suggestive of loss of offset and the presence of a cam morphology [24, 30, 31].

Radiographic evaluation of pincer-type deformity focuses on detecting retroversion and focal or global acetabular overcoverage [32]. Focal retroversion (loss of cranial acetabular anteversion) may be illustrated as a crossover sign on the AP pelvis [33]. The crossover sign is seen when the anterior wall projects lateral to the posterior wall before converging at the lateral acetabular sourcil. The posterior wall may be localized distally near the ischium and the anterior wall may be noted due to its more horizontal trajectory. However, a prominent AIIS may be responsible for the appearance of a crossover sign in the absence of acetabular retroversion [34]. An elevated lateral center edge angle (greater than 40°), and ischial spine sign and posterior wall sign may all be seen on the AP pelvis view and suggest acetabular retroversion. Pincer-type impingement may also occur with coxa profunda, wherein the medial acetabular fossa touches or projects medial to the ilioischial line, or protrusio acetabuli, wherein the medial femoral head protrudes medial to the ilioischial line. The AIIS may be a source of impingement with deep flexion (sub-spine impingement) and is best viewed on false-profile radiographs or 3D imaging [21, 35]. Measurements from plain radiography can also demonstrate the presence of acetabular dysplasia or under-coverage. Dysplastic parameters include a lateral center edge angle less than 20°, a Tonnis angle greater than 10°, an anterior center edge angle less than 20°, and a femoral head extrusion index greater than 25 %.

Osteoarthritis

Standard radiography is the first line of evaluation of hip osteoarthritis. An anteroposterior (AP) view is initially obtained and is used to grade hip osteoarthritis according to the Kellgren–Lawrence [36–40] and/or Joint Space Narrowing classifications [36–38]. These classifications are based on the radiographic features of osteophytes on the joint margins, cystic areas, sclerosis of subchondral bone, shape of the femoral head, and joint space narrowing and a radiographic atlas was developed from the original 1996 OARSI (Osteoarthritis Research Society International) atlas [39]. Kellegren and Lawrence described four grades of hip OA:

- Grade 1 (doubtful OA): Possible narrowing of the joint space medially and possible osteophytes around the femoral head.
- Grade 2 (mild OA): Definite narrowing of the joint space inferiorly, definite osteophytes, and slight sclerosis.
- Grade 3 (moderate OA): Marked narrowing of the joint space, slight osteophytes, some sclerosis and cyst formation, and deformity of the femoral head and acetabulum.
- Grade 4 (severe OA): Gross loss of joint space with sclerosis and cysts, marked deformity of the femoral head and acetabulum, and large osteophytes [40].

Although radiography is widely available and easily obtainable, its limitations lie in the inability to directly evaluate cartilage and soft tissues such as the labrum, joint capsule, and musculature. As it is important to detect any early degenerative changes in hip cartilage before morphological changes are evident using either standard MRI sequences and/or radiographs [1], special techniques have been developed. Typically, scans are taken using a 1.5 or 3 T magnet with a combination of a different array of cardiac coils, shoulder coils, and small field of view coils with a combination of fast spin echo T1 and fluid-sensitive sequences [1]. The oblique axial plane affords good visualization of the anterior and posterior acetabular cartilage and the labrum, the coronal plane, the general landscape of the superior labrum and cartilage, and the sagittal plane, the best imaging of the anterior labrum and labrochondral tears [1].

Because cartilage has a high percentage of water, proteoglycans, and collagen, it possesses a unique high signal characteristic when compared to bone during exposure to T1-weighted gradient echo sequences [1]. To reduce scan time and to evaluate partial-thickness chondral defects with high tissue contrast, an intermediate-weighted 2D non-fat-suppressed fast spine echo (FSE) sequence can be used [41]. Using this method, MR imaging may be used to detect focal cartilage fissures and full-thickness defects in cases where a normal joint space may still be present on plain radiographs [1]. For example, actively delaminating cartilage will show high signal due to the containment of fluid at the site of damage (i.e., the bone-cartilage interface) [1]. As a diagnostic modality, the merits of MRI include the ability to detect osteochondral separations from lesions within the underlying bone, including subchondral fractures, which is valuable for evaluating the "health" of articular cartilage, the viability of subchondral bone, and stability of the joint in the face of cartilage damage [1].

MRI arthrography allows evaluation of the thickness of the thin layer of articular cartilage lining the surfaces of the femoral head and the acetabulum. Normally, the articular cartilage of the femoral head thickens from the periphery to the center with maximal thickness at the attachment site of the ligamentum teres, while the articular cartilage of the acetabulum thickens from the center to the periphery [16]. Both CT and MRI arthrography have been used to measure cartilage thickness in the hip, with the most accurate measurements being derived from CT arthrography performed without a contrast agent or a diluted solution of iohexol (25 % vs. 50–75 % contrast) [42]. At the fovea capitis, the thickness of femoral head cartilage on coronal sections ranges from 1.5 to 3.8 mm by CT and 1.9 to 3.9 mm by MRI [16, 43]. However, it is believed that the absolute thickness is not as important as regional differences, which likely manifest as regions of early cartilage loss, and can be a harbinger of future osteoarthritis, especially in weight-bearing areas [44].

Pfirrmann and coworkers [41] have shown that identification of cartilage delamination is more specific when coronal T1-weighted imaging is used (90–95 %), compared to coronal T1 FS (fat saturation) intermediate-weighted imaging, though both sequences are only of intermediate sensitivity (35–52 % (coronal T1 weighted) versus 52–74 % (coronal T1 FS)).

An additional application of MR imaging is the assignment of "joint health" scores and detection of hips at risk. Roemer and coworkers [45] developed a 14-point osteoarthritis scale based on MRI imaging with strong association between findings seen in Kellgren–Lawrence grades of OA severity by radiographs versus MRI imaging. For example, the more radiographically severe the lesions, the more frequent bony lesions were detected by MRI. There is also a similar grading system for the knee, the MRI Osteoarthritis Knee Score (MOAKS) and hand, the Oslo Hand MRI Score (OSHA-MRI).

Labral Pathology

The gold standard evaluation of the labrum is surgical visualization. However, the best noninvasive imaging technique of the labrum, which is composed of fibrocartilage, is MRI [46]. The labrum displays low signal intensity at the acetabular margin and can be quite a variable structure based on age and sex [54]. The etiology of labral tears includes trauma, degenerative disease, and laxity of the capsule [1]. Using MRI, labral tears are suspected in areas of increased signal intensity with fluid signal between the labrum and acetabular articular cartilage [22, 47] and can often be associated with paralabral cysts, which can then lead to secondary erosion [1]. The prevalence of labral tears is quite high in asymptomatic athletes (from 40 to 90 %) [48, 49].

Though technically challenging, detection of small tears of the labrum is important as these findings may foreshadow further damage, though these findings are often seen in asymptomatic and/or normal individuals [22]. Petchprapa and coworkers [44] suggested that radial imaging, which is perpendicular to the hip joint, affords better visualization because this method goes through the center of the joint and mitigates the effect of "volume averaging" seen in the antero- and anterosuperior regions in the axial and superior regions in the sagittal planes. As the radial plane must be imaged perpendicular to the acetabular opening and en face, a double oblique orientation is necessary using image localizers [9].

Imaging of Other Components of the Hip

MRI can be utilized to evaluate damage to joint capsule consisting of the zona orbicularis and iliofemoral, pubofemoral, and ischiofemoral ligaments, which are damaged in traumatic fractures/dislocations and stress fractures of the femoral neck [50, 51]. Because of its superior soft tissue definition, MRI can be used to evaluate synovial folds, synovial fluid, bursae, and the acetabular fossa [16].

Additionally, MRI has the high sensitivity and specificity necessary to assess injuries of musculotendinous junctions of the hip musculature and the bony attachment sites of tendons and ligaments. For example, the finding of hypertrophy in the iliocapsularis (iliacus minor) muscle in hip dysplasia showed its importance in stabilizing the hip where other tissues are inadequate due to the inherent bony instability of the dysplastic joint. In hips with excessive over-coverage, there is fatty infiltration of the muscle that suggests atrophy [52]. Special attention should be made to evaluate for tendon pathology of the gluteus medius and minimus muscles in renal patients because these structures are often involved in renal patients with hip pain [53]. Furthermore, tendon tears of hip abductors and adductors in groin strain and sports hernia, osteitis pubis (pubalgia) can be imaged. Last but not least, intrapelvic pathology, including ovarian masses, colorectal cancer, iliac artery aneurysm, and other soft tissue masses, can be delineated by MR imaging.

Conclusion

The early detection of cartilage damage is essential to delay and ameliorate the progression of osteoarthritis changes. Plain film radiography offers a good first approximation of the baseline appearance of a joint but is insensitive for the detection of cartilage damage unless moderate to severe changes have already taken place. Ultrasonography is useful to evaluate for cartilage changes, but its widespread application is dependent upon the know-how and training needed, operator skill, and the type of joint to be evaluated—larger joints are more difficult to image than smaller ones because of lack of a proper acoustic window and overlapping structures. Though CT has good tissue contrast and allows good visualization of bone detail, its use for the evaluation of cartilage is limited. With CT arthrography, the sensitivity to detect for cartilage damage increases. At the present moment, MRI remains the most sensitive methodology to detect cartilage injury before manifestations of joint space narrowing are evident in radiography and its sensitivity is increased with the employment of contrast arthrography. However, direct contrast injection of the joint is not without its share of complications, including pain, risk of injection, patient discomfort, and injury. Thus, developing methods to better document cartilage change that is not invasive would be ideal. In summary, the ideal modality for imaging of cartilage is inexpensive, non-invasive, rapid, easy to perform, reproducible, sensitive, and specific. Any modality possessing these qualities would allow early detection of degenerative changes and monitoring of preventive therapies. Although none of the modalities currently available offers all of these attributes, MRI currently offers the greatest potential to provide earlier detection of cartilage degeneration which are certain to become even more sensitive as new and novel techniques become available in the future.

References

1. Gold SL, Burge AJ, Potter HG. MRI of hip cartilage: joint morphology, structure and composition. Clin Orthop Relat Res. 2012;470:3321–31.
2. Palmer AJ, Brown CP, McNally EG, Price AJ, Tracey I, Jezzard P, Carr AJ, Glyn-Jones S. Non-invasive imaging of cartilage in early osteoarthritis. Bone Joint J. 2013;95-B(6):738–46.
3. Buckley MR, Bonassar LJ, Cohen I. Localization of viscous behavior and shear energy dissipation in articular cartilage under dynamic shear loading. J Biomech Eng. 2013;135(3):31002.
4. Iagnocco A, Naredo E. Osteoarthritis: research update and clinical applications. Rheumatology. 2012;51:vii2–5.
5. Kane D, Balint PV, Sturrock R, Grassi W. Musculoskeletal ultrasound—a state of the art review in rheumatology. Part 1: current controversies and issues in the development of musculoskeletal ultrasound in rheumatology. Rheumatology. 2004;43:823–8.
6. Micu MC, Bogdan GD, Fodor D. Steroid injection for hip osteoarthritis: efficacy under ultrasound guidance. Rheumatology. 2010;49:1490–4.
7. Nicolaou S, Liang T, Murphy DT, et al. Dual-energy CT: a promising new technique for assessment of the musculoskeletal system. Am J Roentgenol. 2012;195:S78–86.
8. Driban JB, Tassinari A, Lo GH, et al. Bone marrow lesions are associated with altered trabecular morphometry. Osteoarthritis Cartilage. 2012;20:1519–26.
9. Kutty S, Schneider P, Faris P, Kiefer G, Frizell B, Park R, et al. Reliability and predictability of the centre-edge angle in the assessment of pincer femoroacetabular impingement. Int Orthop. 2012;36(3):505–10.
10. Gold GE, Burstein D, Dardzinski B, Lang P. MRI of articular cartilage in OA: novel pulse sequences and compositional/functional markers. Osteoarthritis Cartilage. 2006;14:A76–86.
11. Eckstein F, Guermazi A, Roemer FW. Quantitative MR imaging of cartilage and trabecular bone in osteoarthritis. Radiol Clin North Am. 2009;47:655–73.
12. Hani AF, Kumar D, Malik AS, Ahmad RM, Razak R, Kiflie A. Non-invasive and in vivo assessment of osteoarthritic articular cartilage: a review on MRI investigations. Rheumatol Int. 2015;35(1):1–16.
13. Mankin HJ, Dorfman H, Lippiello L, Zarins A. Biochemical and metabolic abnormalities in articular cartilage from osteo-arthritic human hips. II. Correlation of morphology with biochemical and metabolic data. J Bone Joint Surg Am. 1971;53-A:523–37.
14. Mosher TJ, Walker EA, Petscavage-Thomas J, Guermazi A. Osteoarthritis year 2013 in review: imaging. Osteoarthritis Cartilage. 2013;21:1425–35.
15. Reurink G, Jansen SP, Bisselink JM, Vincken PW, Weir A, Moen MH. Reliability and validity of diagnosing acetabular labral lesions with magnetic resonance arthrography. J Bone Joint Surg Am. 2012;94(18):1643–8.
16. Sutter R, Zanetti M, Pfirrmann CWA. New developments of hip imaging. Radiographics. 2012;264(3):651–67.
17. Cobb J, Logishetty K, Davda K, Iranpour F. Cams and pincer impingement are distinct, not mixed: the acetabular pathomorphology of femoroacetabular impingement. Clin Orthop Relat Res. 2010;468(8):2143–51.
18. Beck M, Kalhor M, Leunig M, Ganz R. Hip morphology influences the pattern of damage to the acetabular cartilage: femoroacetabular impingement as a cause of early osteoarthritis of the hip. J Bone Joint Surg Br. 2005;87(7):1012–8.
19. Siebenrock KA, Ferner F, Noble PC, Santore RF, Werlen S, Mamisch TC. The cam-type deformity of the proximal femur arises

in childhood in response to vigorous sporting activity. Clin Orthop Relat Res. 2011;469(11):3229–40.
20. Dudda M, Albers C, Mamisch TC, Werlen S, Beck M. Do normal radiographs exclude asphericity of the femoral head-neck junction? Clin Orthop Relat Res. 2009;467(3):651–9.
21. Nepple J, Prather H, Trousdale R, Clohisy J, Beaule P, Glyn-Jones S, Rakhra K, Kim Y. Diagnostic imaging of femoroacetabular impingement. J Am Acad Orthop Surg. 2013;21(Suppl):S20–6.
22. Schmitz MR, Campbell SE, Fajardo RS, Kadrmas WR. Identification of acetabular labral pathological changes in asymptomatic volunteers using optimized, noncontrast 1.5-T magnetic resonance imaging. Am J Sports Med. 2012;40(6):1337–41.
23. Tannast M, Zheng G, Anderegg C, Burckhardt K, Langlotz F, Ganz R, et al. Tilt and rotation correction of acetabular version on pelvic radiographs. Clin Orthop Relat Res. 2005;438:182–90.
24. Meyer DC, Beck M, Ellis T, Ganz R, Leunig M. Comparison of six radiographic projections to assess femoral head/neck asphericity. Clin Orthop Relat Res. 2006;445:181–5.
25. Harris WH. Etiology of osteoarthritis of the hip. Clin Orthop Relat Res. 1986;213:20–33.
26. Nötzli HP, Wyss TF, Stoecklin CH, Schmid MR, Treiber K, Hodler J. The contour of the femoral head-neck junction as a predictor for the risk of anterior impingement. J Bone Joint Surg Br. 2002;84(4):556–60.
27. Hack K, Di Primio G, Rakhra K, Beaule PE. Prevalence of cam-type femoroacetabular impingement morphology in asymptomatic volunteers. J Bone Joint Surg Am. 2010;2(14):2436–44.
28. Gosvig KK, Jacobsen S, Sonne-Holm S, Gebuhr P. The prevalence of cam-type deformity of the hip joint: a survey of 4151 subjects of the Copenhagen Osteoarthritis Study. Acta Radiol. 2008;49(4):436–41.
29. Eijer H, Leunig M, Mahomed N, Ganz R. Cross-table lateral radiographs for screening of anterior femoral head–neck offset in patients with femoroacetabular impingement. Hip Int. 2001;11:37–41.
30. Pollard TC, Villar RN, Norton MR, Fern ED, Williams MR, Simpson DJ, et al. Femoroacetabular impingement and classification of the cam deformity: the reference interval in normal hips. Acta Orthop. 2010;81(1):134–41.
31. Beaule PE, Harvey N, Zaragoza E, Le Duff MJ, Dorey FJ. The femoral head/neck offset and hip resurfacing. J Bone Joint Surg Br. 2007;89:9–15.
32. Clohisy JC, Carlisle JC, Beaulé PE, et al. A systematic approach to the plain radiographic evaluation of the young adult hip. J Bone Joint Surg Am. 2008;90 Suppl 4:47–66.
33. Reynolds D, Lucas J, Klaue K. Retroversion of the acetabulum: a cause of hip pain. J Bone Joint Surg Br. 1999;81(2):281–8.
34. Zaltz I, Kelly BT, Hetsroni I, Bedi A. The crossover sign overestimates acetabular retroversion. Clin Orthop Relat Res. 2013;471(8):2463–70.
35. Edwards DJ, Lomas D, Villar RN. Diagnosis of the painful hip by magnetic resonance imaging and arthroscopy. J Bone Joint Surg Br. 1995;77(3):374–6.
36. Altman RD, Fries JF, Bloch DA, Cartens J, Cooke TD, Genant H, et al. Radiographic assessment of progression in osteoarthritis. Arthritis Rheum. 1987;30:1214–25.
37. Spector TD, Hochberg MC. Methodological problems in the epidemiological study of osteoarthritis. Ann Rheum Dis. 1994;53:143–6.
38. Murphy Jr WA, Altman RD. Updated osteoarthritis reference standard. J Rheumatol. 1995;22 Suppl 43:56–9.
39. Altman RD, Gold GE. Atlas of individual radiographic features in osteoarthritis, revised. Osteoarthritis Cartilage. 2007;15:A1–56.
40. Kellegren JH, Lawrence JS. Radiological assessment of osteoarthrosis. Ann Rheum Dis. 1957;16:494–502.
41. Pfirrmann CW, Duc SR, Zanetti M, Dora C, Hodler J. MR arthrography of acetabular cartilage delamination in femoroacetabular cam impingement. Radiology. 2008;249:236–41.
42. Anderson AE, Ellis BJ, Peters CL, Weiss JA. Cartilage thickness: factors influencing multidetector CT measurements in a phantom study. Radiology. 2008;246(1):133–41.
43. Wyler A, Bousson V, Bergot C, Polivka M, Leveque E, Vicaut E, et al. Comparison of MR-arthrography and CT arthrography in hyaline cartilage-thickness measurement in radiographically normal cadaver hips with anatomy as gold standard. Osteoarthritis Cartilage. 2009;17(1):19–25.
44. Petchprapa CN, Dunham KS, Lattanzi R, Recht MP. Demystifying radial imaging of the hip. Radiographics. 2013;33:E97–112.
45. Roemer FW, Hunter DJ, Winterstein A, Li L, Kim YJ, Cibere J, et al. Hip Osteoarthritis MRI Scoring System (HOAMS): reliability and associations with radiographic and clinical findings. Osteoarthritis Cartilage. 2011;19(8):946–62.
46. Stoller DW, Sampson TG, Li AE, Bredella MA. The hip. In: Stollwer DW, editor. Magnetic resonance imaging in orthopedics and sports medicine. 3rd ed. Philadelphia: Lippincott Williams & Wilkins; 2007.
47. Philippon MJ, Ho CP, Briggs KK, Stull J, LaPrade RF. Prevalence of increased alpha angles as a measure of cam-type femoroacetabular impingement in youth ice hockey players. Am J Sports Med. 2013;41(6):1357–62.
48. Register B, Pennock AT, Ho CP, Strickland CD, Lawand A, Philippon MJ. Prevalence of abnormal hip findings in asymptomatic participants: a prospective, blinded study. Am J Sports Med. 2012;40(12):2720–4.
49. Kapron AL, Anderson AE, Aoki SK, Phillips LG, Petron DJ, Toth R, Peters CL. Radiographic prevalence of femoroacetabular impingement in collegiate football players: AAOS Exhibit Selection. J Bone Joint Surg Am. 2011;93(19):e111.1–10.
50. Telleria JJM, Lindsey DP, Giori NJ, Safran MR. An anatomic arthroscopic description of the hip capsular ligaments for the hip arthroscopist. Arthroscopy. 2011;27(5):628–36.
51. Hewitt JD, Glisson RR, Guilak F, Vail TP. The mechanical properties of the human hip capsule ligaments. J Arthroplasty. 2002;17(1):82–9.
52. Babst D, Steppacher SD, Ganz R, Siebenrock KA, Tannast M. The iliocapsularis muscle: an important stabilizer in the dysplastic hip. Clin Orthop Relat Res. 2011;469(6):1728–34.
53. Demant AW, Kocovic L, Henschkowski J, Siebenrock KA, Ferrari P, Steinbach LS, et al. Hip pain in renal transplant recipients: symptomatic gluteus minimus and gluteus medius tendon abnormality as an alternative MRI diagnosis to avascular necrosis. Am J Roentgenol. 2007;188(2):515–9.
54. Aydingoz U, Ozturk MH. MR imaging of the acetabular labrum: a comparative study of both hips in 180 asymptomatic volunteers. Eur Radiol. 2001;11:567–74.

Magnetic Resonance Imaging of the Hip Labrum, Capsule, and Synovium

22

Brett Lurie, Stephanie L. Gold, and Hollis G. Potter

Introduction

Magnetic resonance imaging (MRI) is the imaging modality of choice in the preoperative and postoperative assessment of patients undergoing hip arthroscopy. With advances in surgical technique, more versatile surgical instruments, and improvements in imaging [1], the list of indications for hip arthroscopies continues to grow.

MRI offers high soft tissue contrast, sensitivity to fluid, and direct multi-planar acquisition and avoids exposure to ionizing radiation. Imaging the hip is inherently challenging due to a variety of anatomic factors, including the location of the joint from the isocenter of the MRI scanner, the curvilinear contour of joint structures and the relatively thin articular cartilage. Despite these challenges, with attention to scan parameters, accurate and reproducible imaging can be obtained allowing for precise assessment of the labrum, capsule, synovium, and cartilage.

B. Lurie, BSc(Med), MBBS(Hons1) • S.L. Gold, BA
Magnetic Resonance Imaging Division, Department of Radiology, Hospital for Special Surgery, 535 E. 70th St., New York, NY 10021, USA
e-mail: lurieb@hss.edu; golds@hss.edu

H.G. Potter, MD (✉)
Magnetic Resonance Imaging Division, Department of Radiology, Hospital for Special Surgery, 535 E. 70th St., New York, NY 10021, USA

Department of Radiology, Weill Medical College of Cornell University, New York, NY, USA
e-mail: potterh@hss.edu

Labrum

Imaging Anatomy

Primarily composed of circumferential type I collagen fibers [2], the fibrocartilaginous labrum attaches to the acetabulum both directly and indirectly by merging with the hyaline cartilage of the acetabular dome [3] through a thin transition zone known as the chondrolabral junction. It is continuous inferiorly with the transverse acetabular ligament forming a labroligamentous sulcus. The normal cleft between the extra-articular portion of the labrum and the capsule [4] is referred to as the perilabral sulcus on MR arthrography studies. There are also variable reports of a sublabral sulcus between the labral base and the acetabulum [5–7] although the exact prevalence of this sulcus is unclear.

While classically described as triangular, the shape of the labrum can vary in asymptomatic individuals, appearing rounded or irregular with increasing age [8]. On conventional two-dimensional intermediate echo time fast spin echo (FSE) sequences, the labrum is uniformly low signal intensity, with the occasional identification of intermediate intensity signal within the substance of uninjured labra that is attributed to the presence of small fibrovascular bundles [4, 8]. The low signal intensity of the labrum is a reflection of the short T2 relaxation times encountered in fibrocartilage and tissues derived largely of type 1 collagen (Fig. 22.1). The labrum is largely avascular, deriving a minimal blood supply from the capsule [9].

By deepening the bony acetabulum, the labrum plays a role in stabilizing the femoral head and decreasing contact stresses through load sharing. It also functions as a joint seal helping to maintain synovial fluid pressure between the femoral head and acetabular dome. This layer of synovial fluid prevents direct contact between the chondral surfaces and aids in the even distribution of contact stresses within the joint [10, 11]. Loss of these myriad functions may partly

J.C. McCarthy et al. (eds.), *Hip Joint Restoration*, DOI 10.1007/978-1-4614-0694-5_22

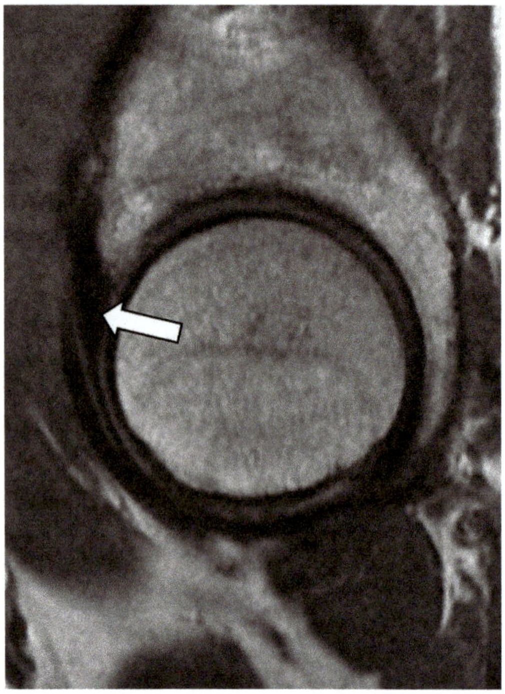

Fig. 22.1 Sagittal intermediate echo time fast spin echo (FSE) image demonstrates the normally triangular anterosuperior labrum (*arrow*). The uniformly low signal intensity of the labrum is a reflection of the short T2 relaxation times encountered in fibrocartilage and tissues derived largely of type 1 collagen

explain the association between labral injury and the development of osteoarthritis [12, 13], although recent studies have highlighted the role of osseous impingement as the common cause of both labral and chondral damage [14].

Imaging Techniques

MRI of the hip is ideally performed on a 1.5 or a 3 Tesla (T) magnet using either a dedicated hip or two-part shoulder coil. To ensure high in-plane resolution and adequate signal to noise, a small field of view wrap coil or multiple channel cardiac coil may be used. Large field of view body coils are not ideally suited to hip imaging because of significant phase wrap with the necessary in-plane resolution. For optimal tissue contrast, a moderate echo time FSE technique with effective echo times of 34 ms at 1.5 T and 28 ms at 3 T is suggested [15].

There is controversy in the literature regarding the optimum technique for imaging the labrum. Many advocate the use of MR arthrography citing a higher sensitivity and specificity for detecting labral tears [6, 16]. The accuracy of indirect arthrography, where contrast is administered intravenously and allowed to diffuse into the joint, is less well described and presents different diagnostic and logistical challenges [17]. A recent meta-analysis [7] of studies evaluating conventional MRI and direct MR arthrography for the evaluation of labral tears concluded that MR arthrography was superior to conventional MRI but that conventional MRI was more specific. A pooled analysis of the data yielded a sensitivity of 66 % and a specificity of 79 % for conventional MRI compared with a sensitivity of 87 % and specificity of 64 % for MR arthrography [7].

It is difficult to generalize the above results due to significant differences in MRI technique, patient populations, and varying levels of assessor experience across the evaluated studies. In our experience, the intermediate echo time FSE sequence with optimized parameters achieves excellent contrast between synovial fluid, hyaline cartilage, and fibrocartilage, facilitating visualization of the labrum and allowing for the diagnosis of labral tears with high sensitivity (96 %) and accuracy (94 %) with superior accuracy in the detection of articular cartilage lesions as well, with accuracy over the acetabulum of 88 % and over the femoral head of 87 % and weighted Kappa measures of reproducibility of 0.8 [18].

Conventional MRI also allows for the assessment of synovial conditions and patterns of synovial proliferation without the confounding factor of artificial joint distension and the overwhelming signal afforded by the presence of intra-articular gadolinium contrast. In addition, MR arthrography can be uncomfortable for patients and not without risk of synovitis or, rarely, infection. If the joint is accessed fluoroscopically, there is the added risk of ionizing radiation, although ultrasound may also be used for guidance and does not employ radiation. Close attention to conventional MRI scan protocols leads to improved spatial resolution and soft tissue contrast and obviates the need for arthrographic assessment [19], preserving MRI as a noninvasive diagnostic test.

An Approach to Interpreting the Hip MRI

Multiple planes of imaging are needed to completely and accurately assess the labrum. The anterior and posterior aspects of the labrum are seen to best effect on oblique axial images, the anterosuperior labrum is well seen in the sagittal plane, and the superior labrum is best evaluated with coronal imaging. A clockface description of the location of labral pathology has been advocated with 3:00 located anteriorly [20] regardless of laterality; however, as is the case in the shoulder, a descriptive system of localizing labral pathology may be less prone to misinterpretation.

Given the anatomic complexities of the hip joint and surrounding soft tissues, a logical structured approach to interpreting the hip MRI is recommended. Structures well seen on axial images include the cartilage of the anterior and posterior acetabular walls; the parafoveal femoral head cartilage; the ligamentum teres; the short external rotator muscles;

and the sciatic, femoral, and obturator nerves. Oblique axial imaging is also useful for assessing femoral head-neck junction offset, acetabular retroversion, and over-containment of the femoral head.

The coronal plane demonstrates the cartilage at the chondrolabral junction, the suprafoveal and superolateral femoral head cartilage, the iliofemoral ligament, the hip abductors, the psoas tendon, and the adductor and hamstring tendons.

Sagittal images are useful for further assessment of the cartilage of the acetabular dome and suprafoveal femoral head, the iliopsoas tendon, and the sciatic nerve.

A review of the fat-saturated, fluid-sensitive wide field of view coronal images may highlight occult fractures, avascular necrosis, and fluid within the various bursae around the hip. These images are also essential for disclosing clinically unsuspected pathology such as inflammatory sacroiliitis or bone neoplasms.

Evaluation of pelvic pathology is possible utilizing a wide field of view axial FSE sequence to examine the lower gastrointestinal tract, genitourinary structures, pelvic vessels, lymph nodes, and the inguinal regions for hernias. The sacroiliac joints and pubic symphysis should be assessed for the presence of pathology. Finally, an analysis of femoral version can be performed in combination with limited images through the distal femoral condyles to correct for the degree of distal femoral rotation.

Etiology of Labral Tears

MRI is a valuable tool not only for the detection of a labral tear but also for discerning an underlying cause or anatomic predisposition of the lesion. This is possible due to the excellent soft tissue contrast and multi-planar capabilities that MRI provides [21]. Trauma, femoroacetabular impingement (FAI), capsular or ligamentous laxity, hip dysplasia, and degenerative joint disease are the most common causes of labral tears [1].

While a history of trauma may precede the onset of hip symptoms, trauma alone is an uncommon cause of labral tears [1]. Traumatic labral tears may occur as a result of subluxation or dislocation events, or following a lateral impact [22] resulting in force transmission to the hip joint which commonly occurs in contact sports or other high-energy trauma. In addition to clinical history, the presence of soft tissue edema, ligamentous injury, bone marrow edema pattern, and coexisting chondral shear injuries are useful ancillary findings in determining whether a tear is likely to be posttraumatic. Unrecognized events of previous trauma may be seen as remodeling deformities of the acetabulum or old Pipkin fractures of the femoral head where there may be foci of proliferative bone formation or subchondral depression with subtle loss of femoral head sphericity.

A more common and increasingly recognized cause of labral tears and labral pathology is FAI. FAI is a pathomechanical process [23] that results from abnormal bony contact between the acetabulum and the femur either as a result of insufficient femoral head-neck offset (CAM type) or when there is functional over-containment of the femoral head due to acetabular retroversion or overhang of the acetabular rim (pincer type). Patients commonly present with a combination of both types [24] of FAI, occasionally with an element of hip dysplasia as well. The altered biomechanics that occur in FAI result in damage to the labrum causing labral degeneration, intralabral ossification, and labral tears.

Developmental hip dysplasia is seen as under-coverage of the femoral head due to a shallow acetabular fossa or dome, with resultant compensatory hypertrophy of the labrum. Hip dysplasia has been associated with an increased risk of labral tears due to several factors including abnormal motion of the unconstrained femoral head [25] and an increased role of the labrum in weight bearing [26].

Capsular laxity may be a part of general ligamentous laxity, an underlying connective tissue disorder or a result of repetitive trauma to the capsule from certain sports [27]. An inadequate repair of the iliofemoral ligament following hip arthroscopy may also lead to femoral head instability. Whatever the underlying cause, patients with laxity can develop subtle rotational instability or other forms of micro-instability of the hip [1] resulting in repetitive trauma to the labrum and cartilage.

Lastly, degeneration and chronic tearing of the labrum may coexist with osteoarthritis or other arthritides (Fig. 22.2). With appropriate spatial and through plane (slice thickness) resolution, conventional MRI is very sensitive for detecting chondral damage even in the absence of joint space narrowing on conventional radiography and correlates highly with grading of chondral damage at arthroscopy [18].

Classification of Labral Tears

The majority of labral tears are located anteriorly and anterosuperiorly [6, 7, 12, 18, 20, 28], which may relate to the prevalence of FAI or anteriorly directed torque forces an underlying cause of labral tears [29]. This region of the labrum may also be intrinsically susceptible to degeneration and injury due to its inferior mechanical properties compared with the remainder of the labrum [12]. Tears of the posterior labrum usually occur in the setting of trauma or degenerative joint disease.

There are several imaging and arthroscopic systems for classifying and describing labral tears. Lage et al. [28] developed a descriptive system based on arthroscopy, dividing labral tears into radial fibrillated, radial, longitudinal peripheral, and unstable. Radial fibrillated tears were defined as irregularity at

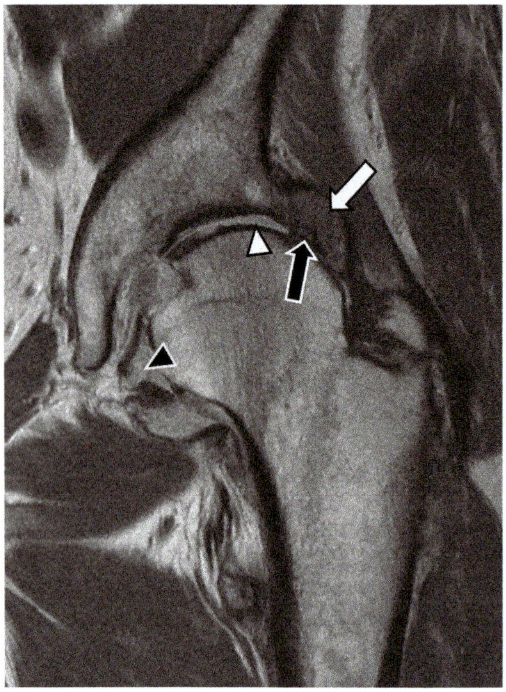

Fig. 22.2 Coronal intermediate weighted FSE image in a patient with osteoarthritis. A debris-filled ganglion cyst (*white arrow*) is seen superolateral to the labrum (*black arrow*), which is chronically degenerated and torn. Extensive full thickness cartilage loss over the femoral head (*white arrowhead*) and acetabular dome results in bone on bone apposition and a secondary synovitis (*black arrowhead*)

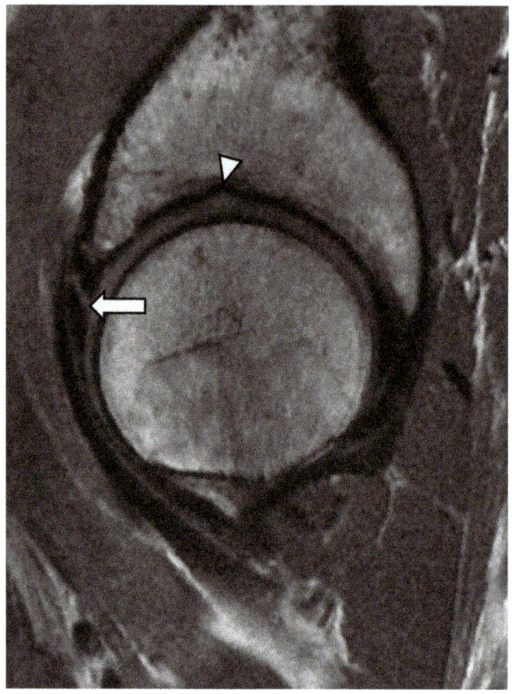

Fig. 22.3 Sagittal intermediate weighted FSE image demonstrates a tear (*arrow*) through the substance of the partially ossified anterosuperior labrum in a middle-aged patient with femoroacetabular impingement. Note the presence of the normal stellate crease (*arrowhead*)

the free edge of the labrum. Radial tears extended into the labral substance resulting in the formation of a flap. Longitudinal peripheral tears occurred at the base of the labrum at the attachment to the acetabulum. The diagnosis of an unstable tear was more on the basis of function than morphology, referring to subluxation of the labrum into the joint.

The Czerny et al. [6] MR arthrography-based classification system takes into account labral morphology, signal change, and the obliteration of the normal perilabral sulcus. The normal labrum is classified as type 0. Intralabral high signal not extending to the surface of the labrum is type IA. Type 1B is defined as intralabral high signal and globular labral morphology obliterating the perilabral sulcus. Type 2A and 2B are the correlates of a Lage radial tear, either with a triangular morphology (2A) or with globular morphology (2B). Type 3A and 3B are the correlates of a longitudinal peripheral tear in the Lage classification system, with and without globular labral morphology, respectively.

Abe et al. [8], in a study of asymptomatic individuals, described the labrum as triangular, round, irregular, or absent. Round labra were found in all age groups but with increasing frequency with age, which the authors ascribed to normal variation or normal aging. Labral signal was also taken into account, with uniform low signal defined as grade 1; intrasubstance intermediate signal intensity as grade 2A; intrasubstance high signal intensity as grade 2B; and signal intensity extending to the surface of the labrum as grade 3A and diffuse high signal intensity of the labrum as grade 3B. Cadaveric studies of the labrum suggest that intralabral high signal in the absence of a tear (type 2B) corresponds to eosinophilic, mucoid, mucoid cystic, vacuolar, or mixed degeneration histologically [4], whereas intermediate signal intensity (type 2A) may relate to the presence of fibrovascular bundles [8].

We advocate a descriptive approach to the reporting of labral damage similar to the approach of Beck et al. [14]. The labrum can be divided into anterior, anterosuperior, superior, posterosuperior, and posterior segments, roughly corresponding to 9:00–10:00, 10:00–11:00, 11:00–1:00, 1:00–2:00, and 2:00–3:00 positions on the clockface, respectively, based on the sagittal image with 3:00 anteriorly.

Focal or diffuse high signal intensity within the labrum is reported as degeneration regardless of morphology or hypertrophy. Undersurface or free edge fraying corresponding to the Lage radial fissure tear is reported as fissuring or irregularity. A tear is diagnosed when fluid signal intensity extends into the substance of the labrum (Fig. 22.3). Tears through the base of the labrum close to the chondrolabral junction corresponding to the Lage peripheral longitudinal tear is reported as a "tear through the base" with or without displacement [18]. The presence of intralabral ossification is included in the description and graded (Fig. 22.4).

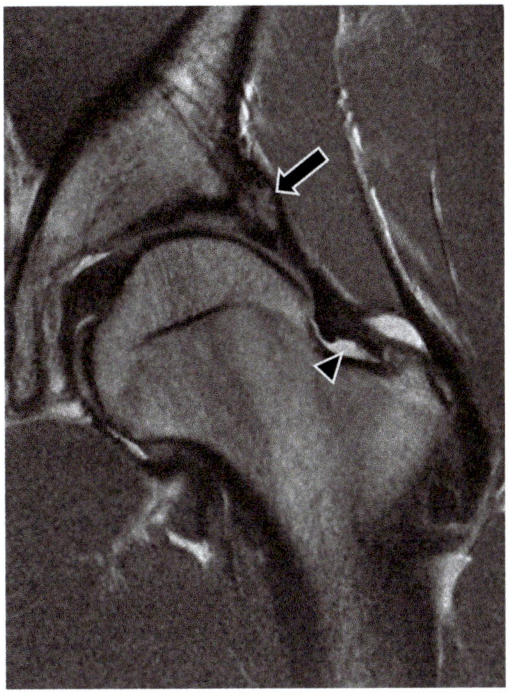

Fig. 22.4 Coronal intermediate weighted FSE image demonstrating marked intralabral ossification in a patient with femoroacetabular impingement (*arrow*). A mild synovitis is noted (*arrowhead*)

Paralabral or ganglion cysts are commonly seen in association with chronic labral tears and can be an indirect sign of labral pathology. Ganglion cysts are very common in the setting of developmental dysplasia of the hip, where large intraosseous ganglia are common in the anterior and lateral margins of the dome (Fig. 22.5). A large ganglion may dissect outside the capsule and present as a primary soft tissue mass on physical examination. Histologically, ganglion cysts are lined with connective tissue and do not communicate with the joint, whereas synovial cysts are lined by synovial cells and may or may not demonstrate a communication with the joint [30]. The terms are often used interchangeably. More globular areas of signal intensity associated with a linear tear can be assumed to represent incipient ganglion formation.

The identification of a labral tear, particularly in the setting of FAI, should prompt closer examination of the chondrolabral junction for the coexistence of chondral delamination (Fig. 22.6). The so-called "carpet lesion" [14] occurs when there is separation of the labrum from the adjacent hyaline cartilage and basilar delamination of a segment of cartilage from the subchondral bone, which can then move like a "carpet on slippery floor" when probed arthroscopically [31]. Basilar delamination is visualized as hyperinten-

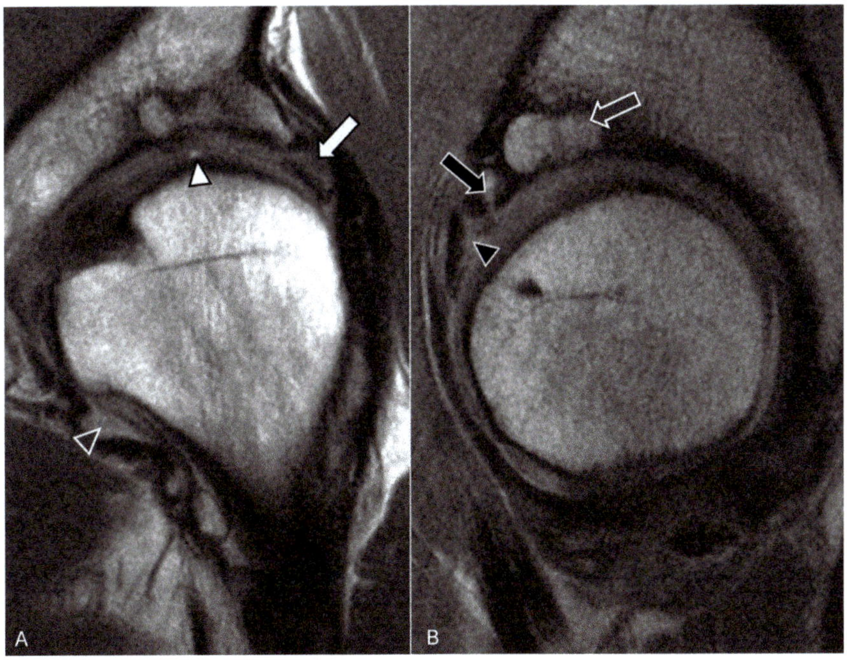

Fig. 22.5 (**a**) Coronal intermediate weighted FSE image in a patient with dysplasia and coxa valga shows hypertrophy and degeneration of the labrum (*white arrow*). The femoral head and acetabular cartilage are hyperintense and fibrillated with a focal full thickness chondral defect over the femoral head (*arrowhead*). A reactive synovitis is present (*gray arrowhead*). (**b**) Sagittal image from the same patient shows a tear through the base of the degenerated anterosuperior labrum (*black arrowhead*). A large ganglion cyst dissects secondarily into the acetabular dome (*gray arrow*) with its neck indicated by the *black arrow*

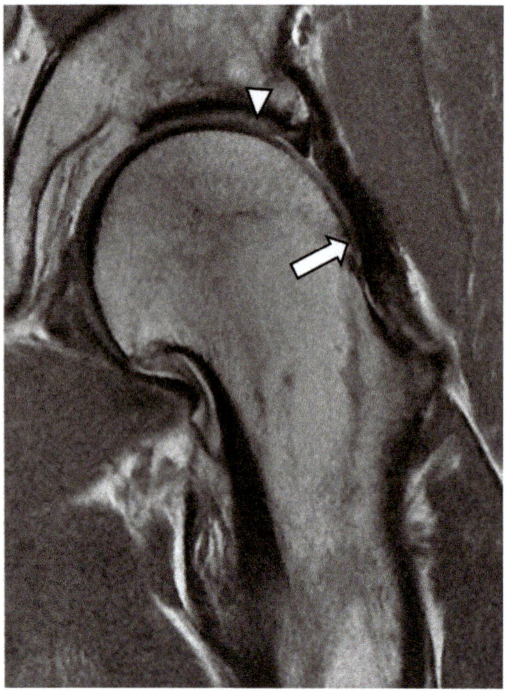

Fig. 22.6 Coronal intermediate weighted FSE image demonstrates insufficient femoral head-neck offset (*arrow*) in a patient with femoroacetabular impingement. Cartilage hyperintensity at the chondrolabral junction is indicative of basilar delamination (*arrowhead*)

sity paralleling the subchondral plate or tidemark where one would expect lower signal due to the highly organized nature of collagen in the basal chondral layers (Fig. 22.7).

Asymptomatic Labral Tears

Recently Register et al. conducted MRI examinations in 200 asymptomatic volunteers discovering labral tears in greater than 50 % of those imaged [29]. 85 % of patients under the age of 40 in their cohort had labral tears. This study highlights the importance of combining clinical history and examination findings with findings at MRI when deciding on the best course of treatment for patients identified as having a labral tear. One should also be vary of the so-called satisfaction of search when identifying a labral tear at MRI, to the exclusion of other clinically unsuspected intra-articular and extra-articular pathologies.

The Postoperative Labrum

Interpretation of the postoperative labrum should take into account the type of arthroscopic treatment that has been instituted. The partially debrided labrum may appear truncated or

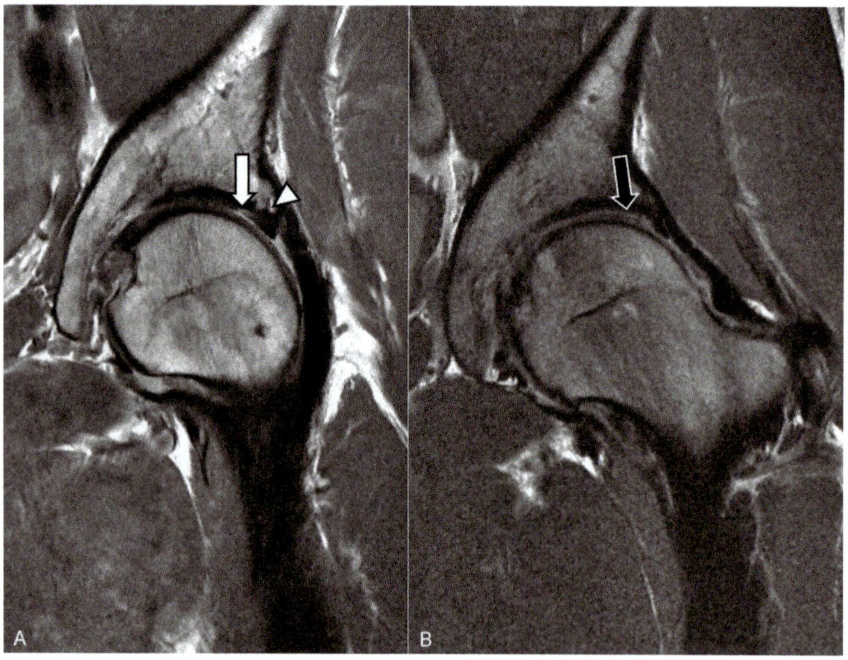

Fig. 22.7 Coronal intermediate weighted FSE images from two different patients with femoroacetabular impingement demonstrate cartilage damage at the chondrolabral junction. (**a**) A full thickness fissure is present with chondral flap formation (*white arrow*). Intralabral ossification is also seen (*white arrowhead*). (**b**) Marked chondral hyperintensity paralleling the tidemark is indicative of basilar delamination (*black arrow*)

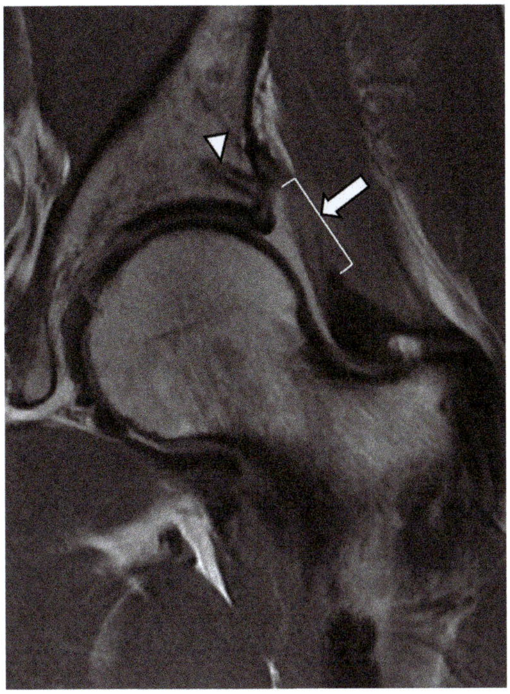

Fig. 22.8 Coronal intermediate weighted FSE MR image demonstrates a large gap in the iliofemoral ligament (*white arrow*) following arthroscopic labral repair (*arrowhead* indicating suture anchor). The patient presented with instability and repeated subluxation events. Subsequent repair of the defect required the use of soft tissue augmentation

slightly irregular in the absence of a re-tear, although excessive irregularity may be a sign of recurrent injury [32]. Suture anchors, visualized as low signal intensity linear foci radiating from the acetabular rim, are evidence of prior labral repair even in the absence of a detailed surgical history (Figs. 22.8 and 22.9).

In our experience, fluid imbibition into the labrum itself or between the labral repair and the acetabulum is the most specific sign of labral re-injury (Fig. 22.9). Distinguishing fluid imbibition from granulation tissue within a repair site requires the use of high spatial resolution and high contrast conventional MRI pulse sequences. Other useful findings in deciding on the presence of recurrent injury to the labrum include a detached or displaced fragment, a new paralabral cyst, or extension of the tear to a different location [32].

Capsule

Imaging Anatomy

The capsule is a strong fibrous structure composed primarily of type I collagen with a cylindrical sleevelike shape [22]. It attaches to the margin of the acetabulum and distally to the proximal femur encircling the femoral neck [27]. The capsule is thickest anterosuperiorly, varying between 2 and 6 mm in thickness [33]. The iliofemoral ligament, ischiofemoral ligament, pubofemoral ligament, and the zona orbicularis reinforce the capsule [34]. The capsule contributes to hip stability, particularly in the setting of hip dysplasia when there is deviation from normal osseous anatomy [1]. It is sensitive to stretch and may act as a mechanism for muscular feedback [27].

The iliofemoral ligament is well seen on MRI and assessment of the status of the ligament should be included as part of the standard hip MRI report. The ligament, also known as the "Y" ligament or the ligament of Bigelow, is fan-shaped composed of an inferior or medial band and a superior or lateral band [22, 34], which insert onto the greater trochanter. At the acetabulum, the ligament blends with the origin of the reflected head of the rectus femoris. The iliofemoral ligament can be assessed in all imaging planes but is best seen using the coronal and oblique axial sequences. The normal ligament should be uniformly low signal intensity.

The pubofemoral and ischiofemoral ligaments are less clearly distinguished on MRI. The pubofemoral ligament arises adjacent to the obturator foramen reinforcing the inferior portion of the capsule, blending with the inferior band of the iliofemoral ligament. The ischiofemoral ligament arises from the ischial portion of the acetabulum blending with the zona orbicularis to form a partial sling for the femoral neck [34] posteroinferiorly.

The zona orbicularis consists of compact fibers running perpendicular to the axis of the femoral neck forming the narrowest portion of the joint [34]. While not usually assessed independently, the zona orbicularis is well seen in all imaging planes.

The synovium is reflected at various locations on the femoral neck as retinacular folds known as the retinacula of Weitbrecht, which overlie the arterial branches supplying the femoral head [34]. Gojda and Bartoníček [35] described the variable existence of three retinacula from cadaveric dissection—the anterior, lateral (superior), and medial (inferior) retinacula. Blankenbaker et al. [36] described the presence of a pectinofoveal fold at the inferior aspect of the femoral neck in 95 % of MR arthrograms in their cohort. Additional plicae have been described adjacent to the labrum and the ligamentum teres which may be flat or villous in appearance [37] and are often visualized on MR arthrographic studies [38]. While there are few reports of plicae presenting with mechanical symptoms in the literature [39], the majority of plicae identified on imaging are asymptomatic [32].

Capsular and Ligamentous Injury

Injuries to the capsule can disturb the biomechanics of the hip resulting in instability and a decreased ability to absorb

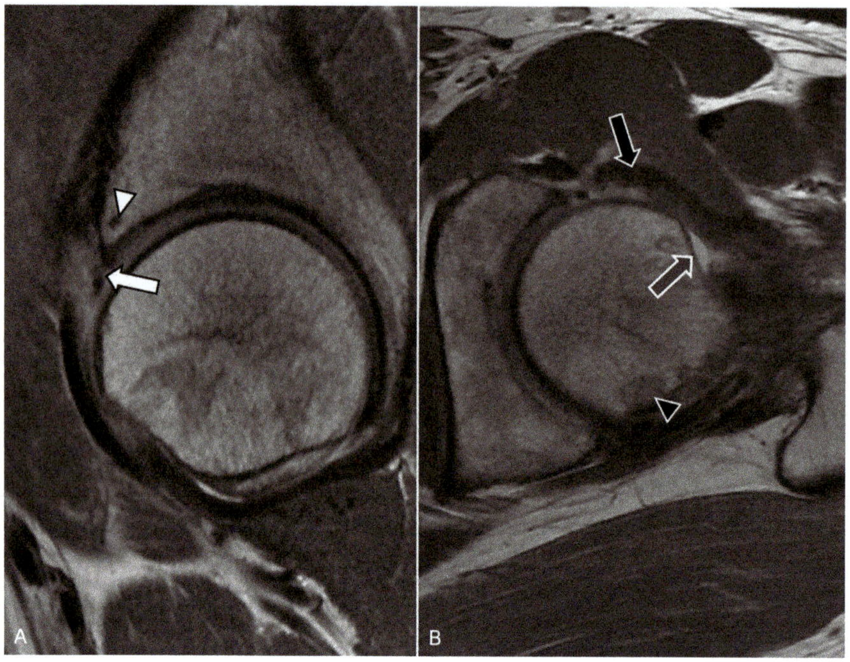

Fig. 22.9 Sagittal (**a**) and axial (**b**) intermediate weighted FSE MR images in a patient with a history of labral repair and anterior femoral neck debridement. The effects of a recent anterior subluxation event are seen. (**a**) The labral remnant (*white arrow*) is irregular secondary to impaction with a tear through the base of the repair. (**b**) The iliofemoral ligament (*black arrow*) is hyperintense reflecting interstitial injury and is torn at the acetabulum. Focal signal change at the posterior aspect of the femoral head is seen at the site of femoral head impaction (*black arrowhead*). Concavity of the anterior femoral neck (*gray arrow*) indicates prior osteochondroplasty

stress [1]. Hip instability may follow an acute dislocation or subluxation event resulting in damage to the labrum, capsule, and capsular supporting ligaments (Fig. 22.9). Nontraumatic hip instability may occur in patients with general ligamentous laxity, connective tissue disorders, and developmental hip dysplasia or relate to the repetitive microtrauma associated with certain sports and activities requiring hip flexibility [1, 22, 34]. Over time, repetitive external rotation may push the femoral head anteriorly, stretching the anterior capsule and the iliofemoral ligament [22, 34]. Iatrogenic injury to the capsule and the iliofemoral ligament with inadequate iliofemoral ligament repair has also been implicated in the development of hip instability and subsequent osteoarthritis (Fig. 22.9) [40].

On MRI, the iliofemoral ligament can appear thinned or stretched in patients with laxity. Scar remodeling as a response to a single traumatic event or repetitive injury can result in ligament thickening. Marked hyperintensity of an attenuated ligament is indicative of poor tissue quality or poor remodeling following injury. Finally, frank discontinuity of the ligament can be seen either off the acetabulum or at the distal insertions. Following arthroscopy, focal or diffuse thickening of the capsule and intra-articular adhesions can be seen [33].

Ancillary intra-articular and extra-articular findings, as well as an appropriate clinical history, may help narrow the differential diagnosis when an abnormality of the capsule or capsular ligaments is detected. An example is the triad of imaging findings observed in American football players with posterior dislocations, which consists of a tear of the iliofemoral ligament, posterior acetabular rim fracture, and hemarthrosis [41].

Hip instability can be a difficult disorder to diagnose clinically [1] and on imaging. With the advent of arthroscopic techniques for the treatment of capsular laxity including capsular plication and modification of collagen through thermal capsulorrhaphy [27], the recognition of the signs of instability on MRI is increasingly important in guiding surgical management.

Ligamentum Teres

The ligamentum teres is composed of collagen types 1, 3, and 4 and originates from the transverse acetabular ligament and the acetabular notch with a broad base to insert into the fovea on the medial aspect of the femoral head. It is covered with fat over which there is a layer of synovial epithelium [42].

While the exact function of the ligamentum teres is unknown, it appears to play a role in hip stability, proprioception, and nociception [43]. The ligament provides blood supply to the developing femoral head in utero, although its contribution to femoral head vascularity in adults is minimal or absent [42]. A "wind-screen" wiper mechanism has also been proposed whereby the ligament may act to distribute synovial fluid within the hip joint [44]. Injuries to the ligament are associated with an increased likelihood of developing microinstability and subsequent chondral or labral damage [43].

On MRI, the ligamentum teres can be partially torn, completely torn, or degenerated [42, 44]. A tear of the ligamentum teres is suggested when there is effacement of fat in the acetabular fossa, edema within or around the ligament, irregularity of the ligament, or a change in ligament thickness [38].

While dysfunction of the ligamentum teres can cause instability, the ligament can also be secondarily affected in patients with instability for other reasons. Hypertrophy of the ligament in the setting of hip dysplasia has been observed and may represent ligament recruitment to resist recurrent subluxation [42]. Less well described in the literature is the frequent observation of synovial scarring surrounding the ligamentum teres in patients with instability. In our experience, focal synovial scarring can be identified on conventional MRI as indistinct intermediate signal intensity material partially effacing the fat around an otherwise intact ligament (Fig. 22.10).

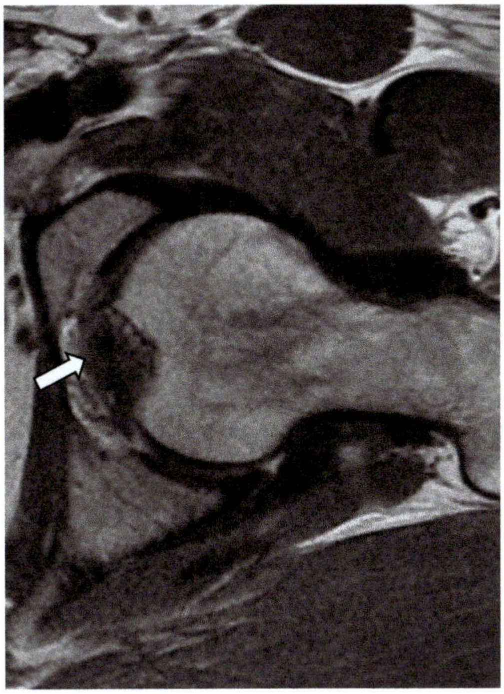

Fig. 22.10 Axial intermediate weighted FSE MR image demonstrates synovial scarring surrounding the ligamentum teres (*white arrow*) in an adolescent female dancer with microinstability

Adhesive Capsulitis

Adhesive capsulitis of the hip closely resembles the clinical presentation in the shoulder, although it is less common with only a few reported cases in the literature [45]. A capsular pattern of decreased motion is the most common clinical finding in patients presenting with the condition [1]. A history of injury is variable and not of any specific diagnostic value [45]. Patients typically have significant synovitis at the time of presentation and may respond to fluoroscopically guided intra-articular injection. In those who fail to respond, arthroscopic capsular release can be attempted with mixed results [1].

Imaging reports of adhesive capsulitis in joints other than the shoulder describe a common underlying pathology with global inflammation of the capsule eventually progressing to fibrosis and scarring [46]. On MRI, adhesive capsulitis of the shoulder is seen as global capsular thickening and hyperintensity which correlates with the clinical and histological stages of the disease process [47]. Marked thickening and increased capsular signal intensity similar to that of adjacent muscle are observed early on (Fig. 22.11). Eventually the hyperintensity resolves, leaving a thickened low signal capsule that remodels over time. A similar range of imaging appearances can be expected in this rare condition of the hip.

Synovial Conditions

Synovitis of the hip may present as nonspecific hip pain, with few clinical features to indicate a more specific diagnosis [15]. The differential for hip synovitis includes osteoarthritis, inflammatory arthritis, infection, and synovial proliferative disorders such as pigmented villonodular synovitis (PVNS) and synovial chondromatosis.

The identification of a joint effusion on a large field of view fluid-sensitive sequence should prompt closer examination of the pattern of synovial proliferation on high resolution surface coil images of the hip [15].

Arthritis

A reactive synovitis in commonly observed in patients with early and advanced osteoarthritis and may be accompanied

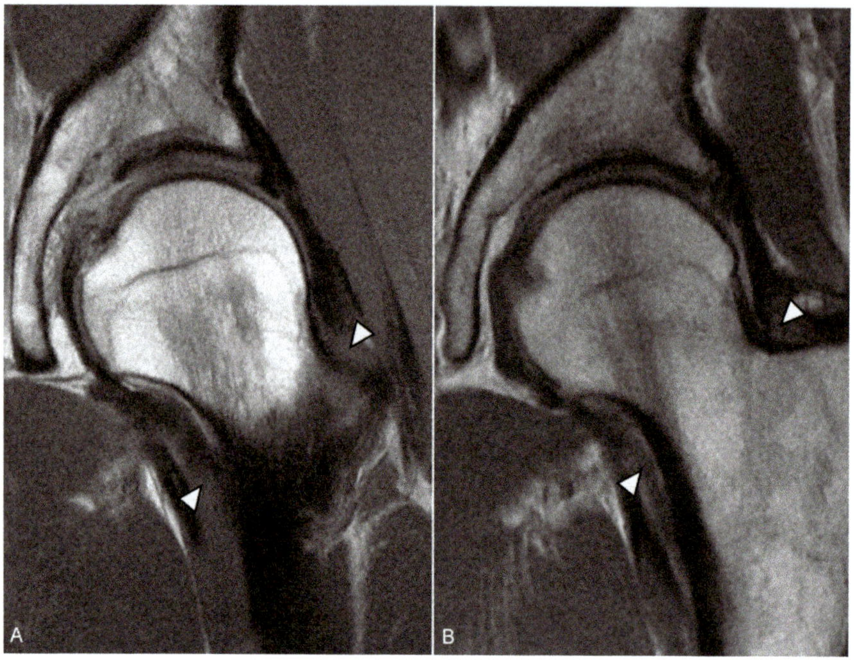

Fig. 22.11 Coronal intermediate weighted FSE MR images from two different patients (**a**, **b**) with reduced range of motion. Diffuse thickening and hyperintensity of the capsule (*arrowheads*) indicates adhesive capsulitis

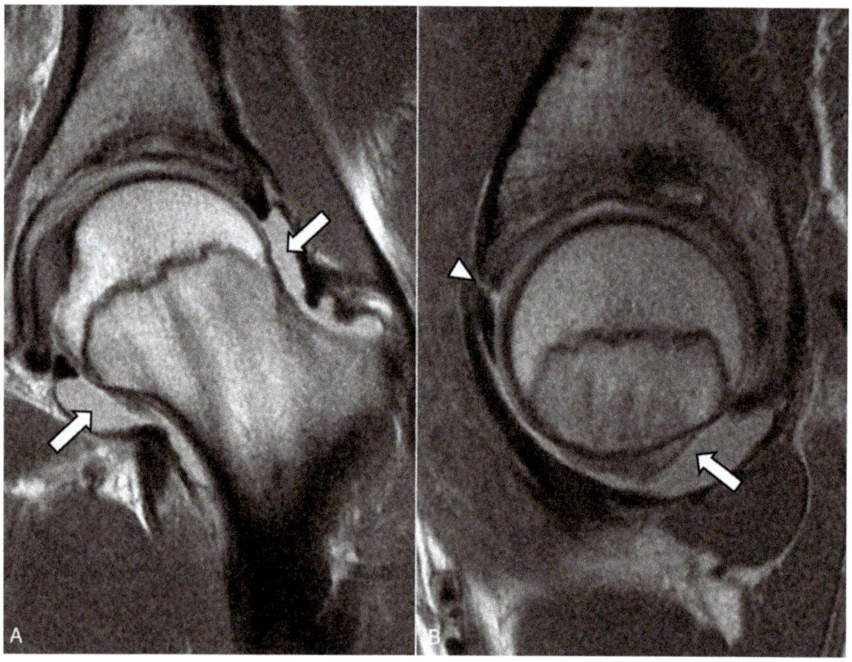

Fig. 22.12 Coronal (**a**) and axial (**b**) intermediate weighted FSE MR images in a skeletally immature patient with a seronegative spondyloarthropathy demonstrates marked synovitis (*arrows*). A tear through the base of the anterosuperior labrum is also well seen (*arrowhead*)

by the presence of loose intra-articular fragments and small chondral debris (Fig. 22.12). In patients with FAI the presence of synovitis is a useful indirect sign of early chondral damage and should alert the radiologist or surgeon to closely examine the cartilage of the hip, particularly at sites predisposed to early damage such as the chondrolabral junction and the posterosuperior aspect of the joint. The presence of synovitis on MRI often correlates to clinical features of night pain and a positive response to aspiration and intra-articular injection of anti-inflammatory agents.

MRI is sensitive for the detection of early inflammatory arthritis [48], demonstrating early synovial proliferation and radiographically occult bone erosions. The appearance of "rice bodies" on MRI is due to the sloughing of necrotic foci of proliferative synovium into the joint, which are seen as ill-defined, intermediate to hyperintense intra-articular foci.

Septic Arthritis

Septic arthritis of the hip presents as a joint effusion without any pathognomonic appearances on MRI. Findings described in the setting of joint infection not surprisingly include synovial thickening, perisynovial edema, and synovial enhancement [49], which may be seen in a variety of other diseases. Findings suggestive of osteomyelitis should be sought as well as any evidence of rapid joint destruction but are often absent.

A study of synovitis following knee arthroplasty has shown that when present, a "lamellated" appearance to the synovium has a high positive predictive value for infection as an isolated finding [50]. The positive predictive value of this finding is increased when combined with the additional findings of extracapsular soft tissue edema, extracapsular collections, and regional adenopathy [50]. However, the absence of a "lamellated" synovium does not exclude the presence of infection, and further study is required to determine the applicability of this finding to native joints.

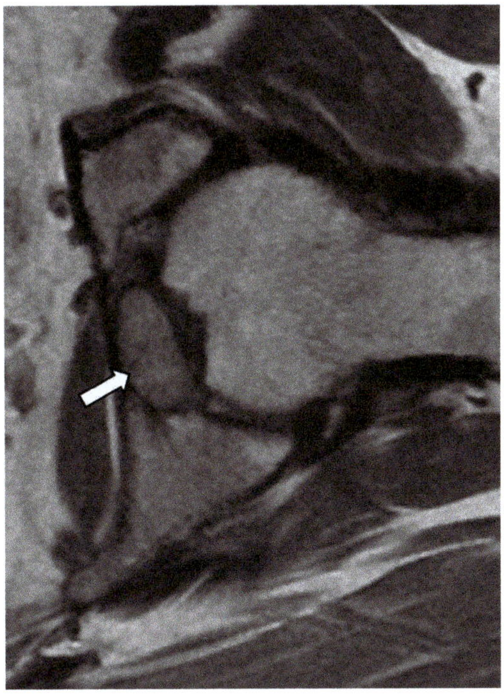

Fig. 22.13 Axial intermediate weighted FSE MR image demonstrates the focal form of pigmented villonodular synovitis (*arrow*). The low signal intensity relates to the presence of hemosiderin

Pigmented Villonodular Synovitis

PVNS is a monoarticular proliferative disease of the synovium which can be focal or diffuse [51]. Both intra-articular and extra-articular forms are recognized, with nodular PVNS involving a tendon also known as a giant cell tumor of tendon sheath. Histologically, PVNS is characterized by the presence of lipid-laden macrophages, multinucleated giant cells, stromal cell proliferation, and hemosiderin [52].

The nodular form of PVNS is seen on MRI as an intracapsular soft tissue mass of intermediate to low signal intensity (Fig. 22.13) [15]. PVNS in the acetabular bare area can be misinterpreted as the ligamentum teres or focal synovial scarring. A high index of suspicion is required to make the diagnosis. The diffuse form of PVNS appears as thickened low signal intensity synovium filling the capsular recesses of the hip and can be associated with pressure erosions of the acetabulum or femur, which are more common in the confined space of the hip joint (Fig. 22.14).

The characteristic low signal intensity of PVNS is due to the presence of hemosiderin and is particularly prominent on gradient echo sequences. Hemosiderin is paramagnetic causing local magnetic field inhomogeneity that results in rapid spin dephasing and loss of signal. Gradient echo sequences are particularly sensitive to these alterations in the local magnetic environment, as they do not employ a rephasing pulse in the generation of signal. On gradient echo, the signal loss associated with hemosiderin is larger than the actual size of the deposit, a phenomenon referred to as "blooming."

MRI clearly demonstrates the degree of intracapsular and extracapsular involvement as well as the effect on surrounding structures such as the neurovascular bundles. It is also useful for posttreatment follow-up to detect residual or recurrent disease.

Synovial Chondromatosis

Primary synovial chondromatosis was previously thought to represent synovial metaplasia although is currently classified as a benign neoplastic process. While commonly intra-articular, it can also involve tendon sheaths and bursae, known as tenosynovial and bursal chondromatosis, respectively. Histologically, the synovium is hyperplastic and there are numerous nodular projections of hyaline cartilage [53].

The MRI signal characteristics of synovial chondromatosis vary depending on the degree of mineralization or ossification that is present within the cartilage nodules [54]. Unmineralized foci are intermediate to high signal intensity (Fig. 22.15), mineralized bodies appear lower signal (Fig. 22.16) and ossified bodies show variable signal intensity depending on the amount of fatty marrow that is present. Multiple chondral bodies may be present in the joint space as individually distinguishable foci or give rise to a "cobblestone appearance." Over time, conglomeration of the individual bodies may lead to the formation of large masses (Fig. 22.17) [55].

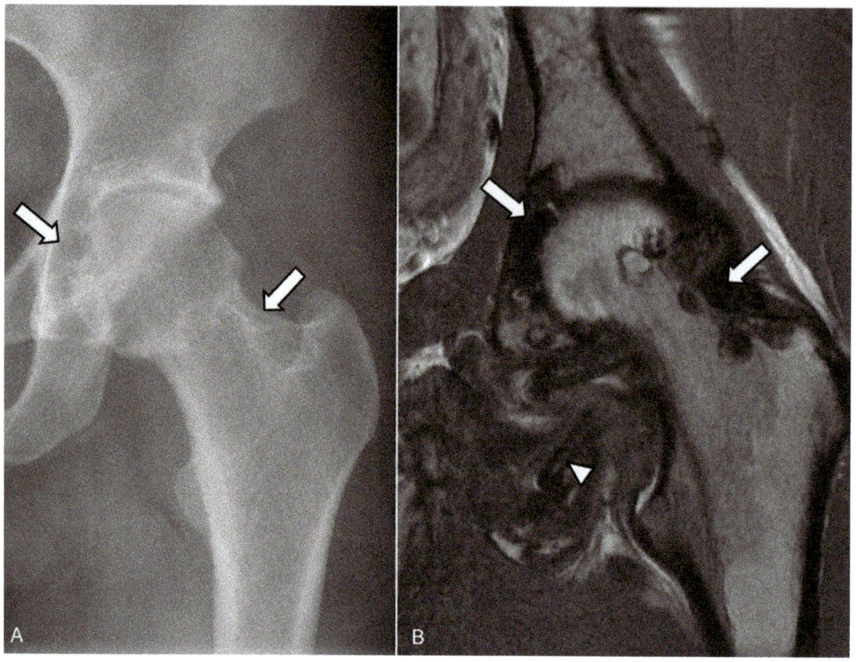

Fig. 22.14 Diffuse PVNS. (**a**) Plain radiograph demonstrating erosions of the acetabulum and femoral neck (*arrows*). (**b**) Intermediate weighted FSE MR image demonstrates the extent of bony (*arrows*) and surrounding soft tissue involvement (*white arrowhead*), with low signal intensity characteristic of PVNS

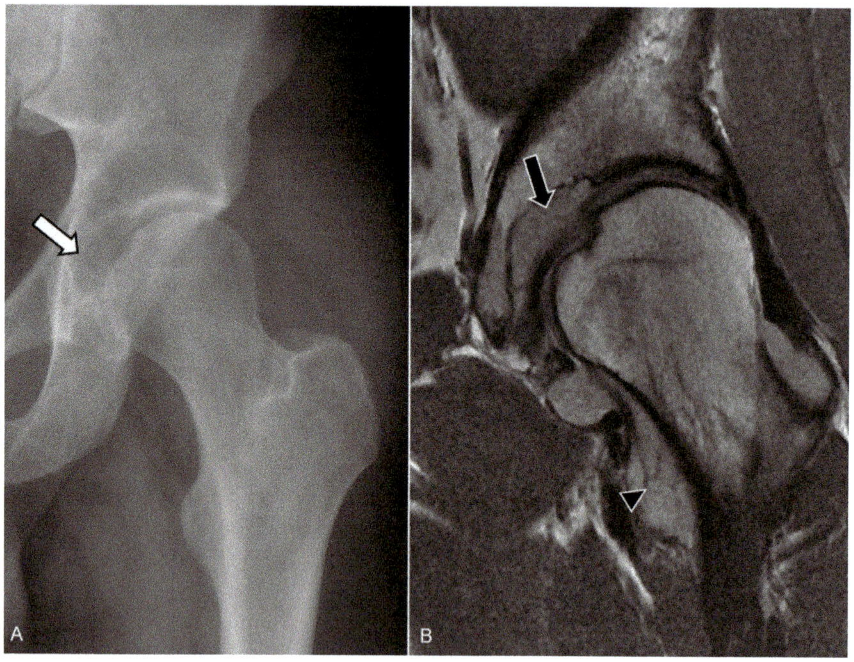

Fig. 22.15 Unmineralized synovial chondromatosis. (**a**) Plain radiograph demonstrating subtle erosion of the acetabulum. (**b**) Coronal intermediate weighted FSE MR image shows nodular synovial hypertrophy. Individual hyperintense nodules (*black arrowhead*) are still distinguishable but are starting to conglomerate. The acetabular erosion (*black arrow*) is well demonstrated on MRI

Conclusion

MRI is the modality of choice in the evaluation of patients with hip pain and hip pathology, providing valuable information for the treating clinician in both the preoperative and postoperative setting. Conventional MRI imaging offers reproducible, accurate assessment of bony and soft tissue anatomy around the hip including the labrum, capsule, and the synovium. Attention to image quality through optimized imaging parameters obviates the need for arthrographic assessment of the joint and preserves MRI as a noninvasive investigation. Finally, a close working relationship between the referring surgeon and his/her radiologist helps to ensure that surgically relevant information is being conveyed, generates opportunities for research and fosters an increased understanding of complicated disease processes.

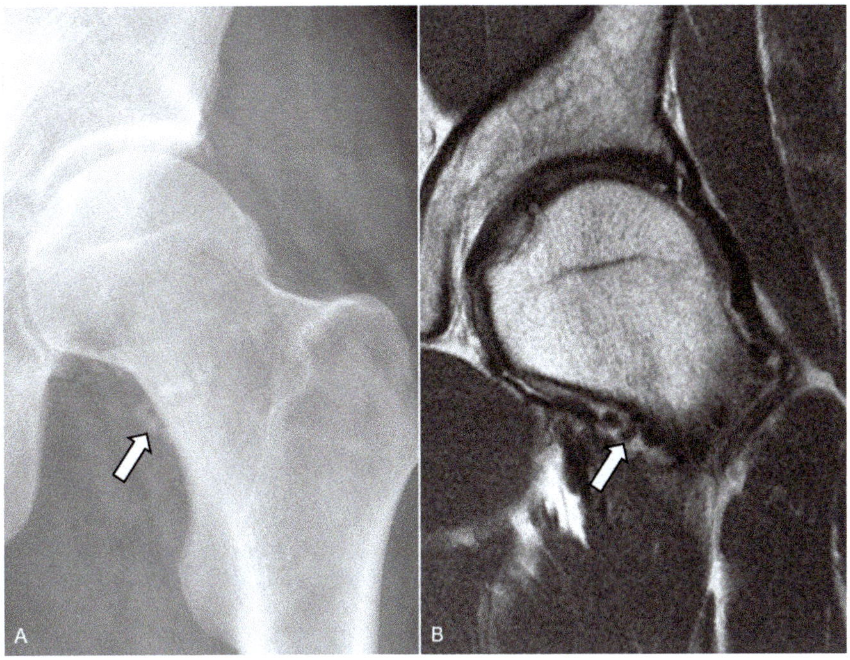

Fig. 22.16 Plain radiograph (**a**) and axial intermediate weighted FSE MR image (**b**) in a patient with synovial chondromatosis. The low signal intensity of the intra-articular bodies (*arrows*) reflects mineralization of the hyaline nodules

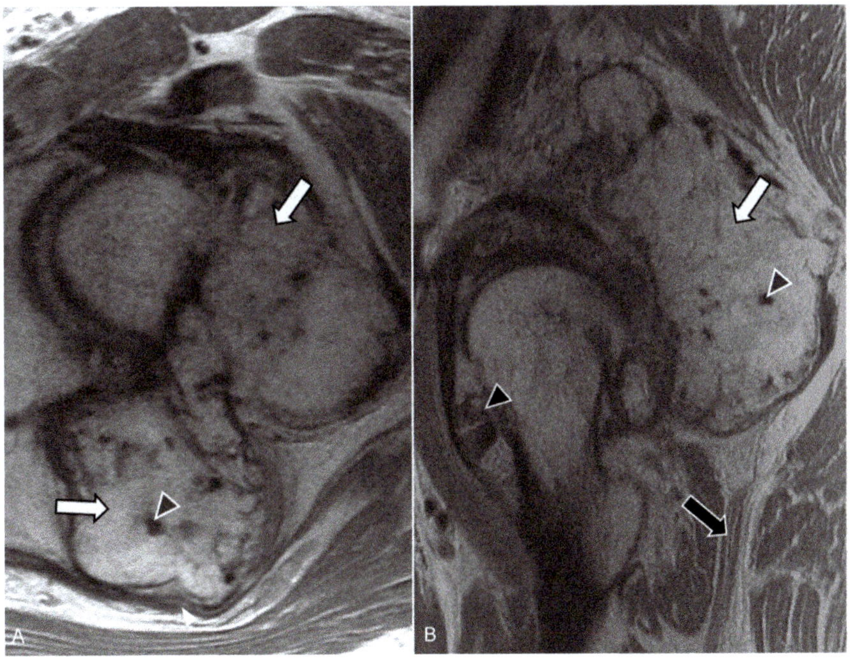

Fig. 22.17 Synovial chondromatosis. (**a**) Axial intermediate weighted FSE MR image demonstrates a conglomeration of ossified nodules (*white arrows*) above the femoral neck and extending into the posterior soft tissues. The piriformis muscle and tendon (*white arrowhead*) are secondarily deformed. A few non-ossified nodules are identified within the mass (*gray arrowhead*). (**b**) Sagittal MR image shows the extent of soft tissue involvement as well as the proximity to the sciatic nerve (*black arrow*). Additional mineralized intra-articular bodies are seen within the joint anteriorly (*black arrowhead*)

References

1. Kelly BT, Buly RL. Hip arthroscopy update. HSS J. 2005; 1(1):40–8.
2. Petersen W, Petersen F, Tillmann B. Structure and vascularization of the acetabular labrum with regard to the pathogenesis and healing of labral lesions. Arch Orthop Trauma Surg. 2003;123(6): 283–8.
3. Seldes RM, Tan V, Hunt J, Katz M, Winiarsky R, Fitzgerald RH. Anatomy, histologic features, and vascularity of the adult acetabular labrum. Clin Orthop Relat Res. 2001;382:232–40.
4. Hodler JJ, Yu JSJ, Goodwin DD, Haghighi PP, Trudell DD, Resnick DD. MR arthrography of the hip: improved imaging of the

acetabular labrum with histologic correlation in cadavers. AJR Am J Roentgenol. 1995;165(4):887–91.
5. Petersilge CA, Haque MA, Petersilge WJ, Lewin JS, Lieberman JM, Buly R. Acetabular labral tears: evaluation with MR arthrography. Radiology. 1996;200(1):231–5.
6. Czerny CC, Hofmann SS, Neuhold AA, Tschauner CC, Engel AA, Recht MPM, et al. Lesions of the acetabular labrum: accuracy of MR imaging and MR arthrography in detection and staging. Radiology. 1996;200(1):225–30.
7. Smith TO, Hilton G, Toms AP, Donell ST, Hing CB. The diagnostic accuracy of acetabular labral tears using magnetic resonance imaging and magnetic resonance arthrography: a meta-analysis. Eur Radiol. 2010;21(4):863–74.
8. Abe I, Harada Y, Oinuma K, Kamikawa K, Kitahara H, Morita F, et al. Acetabular labrum: abnormal findings at MR imaging in asymptomatic hips. Radiology. 2000;216(2):576–81.
9. Kelly BT, Shapiro GS, Digiovanni CW, Buly RL, Potter HG, Hannafin JA. Vascularity of the hip labrum: a cadaveric investigation. Arthroscopy. 2005;21(1):3–11.
10. Ferguson SJ, Bryant JT, Ganz R, Ito K. An in vitro investigation of the acetabular labral seal in hip joint mechanics. J Biomech. 2003;36(2):171–8.
11. Crawford MJ, Dy CJ, Alexander JW, Thompson M, Schroder SJ, Vega CE, et al. The 2007 Frank Stinchfield Award. The biomechanics of the hip labrum and the stability of the hip. Clin Orthop Relat Res. 2007;465:16–22.
12. McCarthy JC, Noble PC, Schuck MR, Wright J, Lee J. The watershed labral lesion: its relationship to early arthritis of the hip. J Arthroplasty. 2001;16(8 Suppl 1):81–7.
13. Ferguson SJS, Bryant JTJ, Ganz RR, Ito KK. The acetabular labrum seal: a poroelastic finite element model. Clin Biomech (Bristol, Avon). 2000;15(6):463–8.
14. Beck M, Kalhor M, Leunig M, Ganz R. Hip morphology influences the pattern of damage to the acetabular cartilage: femoroacetabular impingement as a cause of early osteoarthritis of the hip. J Bone Joint Surg Br. 2005;87(7):1012–8.
15. Potter HG, Schachar J. High resolution noncontrast MRI of the hip. J Magn Reson Imaging. 2010;31(2):268–78.
16. Byrd JWT. Diagnostic accuracy of clinical assessment, magnetic resonance imaging, magnetic resonance arthrography, and intra-articular injection in hip arthroscopy patients. Am J Sports Med. 2004;32(7):1668–74.
17. Zlatkin MB, Pevsner D, Sanders TG, Hancock CR, Ceballos CE, Herrera MF. Acetabular labral tears and cartilage lesions of the hip: indirect MR arthrographic correlation with arthroscopy—a preliminary study. AJR Am J Roentgenol. 2010;194(3):709–14.
18. Mintz DN, Hooper T, Connell D, Buly R, Padgett DE, Potter HG. Magnetic resonance imaging of the hip: detection of labral and chondral abnormalities using noncontrast imaging. Arthroscopy. 2005;21(4):385–93.
19. Rakhra KS, Lattanzio PJ, Cárdenas-Blanco A, Cameron IG, Beaule PE. Can T1-rho MRI detect acetabular cartilage degeneration in femoroacetabular impingement? A pilot study. J Bone Joint Surg Br. 2012;94(9):1187–92.
20. Blankenbaker DG, Smet AA, Keene JS, Fine JP. Classification and localization of acetabular labral tears. Skeletal Radiol. 2007; 36(5):391–7.
21. Gold SL, Burge AJ, Potter HG. MRI of hip cartilage: joint morphology, structure, and composition. Clin Orthop Relat Res. 2012;470(12):3321–31.
22. Braly BA, Palmer IJ, Beall DP, Kelly B. The function of the hip capsular ligaments: a quantitative report. Arthroscopy. 2008; 24(2):188–95.
23. Leunig M, Beaulé PE, Ganz R. The concept of femoroacetabular impingement: current status and future perspectives. Clin Orthop Relat Res. 2008;467(3):616–22.
24. Pfirrmann CWA, Mengiardi B, Dora C, Kalberer F, Zanetti M, Hodler J. Cam and pincer femoroacetabular impingement: characteristic MR arthrographic findings in 50 patients. Radiology. 2006;240(3):778–85.
25. Haene RAR, Bradley MM, Villar RNR. Hip dysplasia and the torn acetabular labrum: an inexact relationship. J Bone Joint Surg Br. 2007;89(10):1289–92.
26. Petersilge CA. Chronic adult hip pain: MR arthrography of the hip1. Radiographics. 2000;20 Suppl 1:S43–52.
27. Philippon MJM. The role of arthroscopic thermal capsulorrhaphy in the hip. Clin Sports Med. 2001;20(4):817–29.
28. Lage LA, Patel JV, Villar RN. The acetabular labral tear: an arthroscopic classification. Arthroscopy. 1996;12(3): 269–72.
29. Register B, Pennock AT, Ho CP, Strickland CD, Lawand A, Philippon MJ. Prevalence of abnormal hip findings in asymptomatic participants: a prospective, blinded study. Am J Sports Med. 2012;40(12):2720–4.
30. Magee T, Hinson G. Association of paralabral cysts with acetabular disorders. AJR Am J Roentgenol. 2000;174(5):1381–4.
31. Pfirrmann CWA, Duc SR, Zanetti M, Dora C, Hodler J. MR arthrography of acetabular cartilage delamination in femoroacetabular cam impingement 1. Radiology. 2008;249(1):236–41.
32. Blankenbaker DG, De Smet AA, Keene JS. MR arthrographic appearance of the postoperative acetabular labrum in patients with suspected recurrent labral tears. AJR Am J Roentgenol. 2011; 197(6):W1118–22.
33. Weidner J, Büchler L, Beck M. Hip capsule dimensions in patients with femoroacetabular impingement: a pilot study. Clin Orthop Relat Res. 2012;470(12):3306–12.
34. Wagner FV, Negrão JR, Campos J, Ward SR, Haghighi P, Trudell DJ, et al. Capsular ligaments of the hip: anatomic, histologic, and positional study in cadaveric specimens with MR arthrography. Radiology. 2012;263(1):189–98.
35. Gojda J, Bartoníček J. The retinacula of Weitbrecht in the adult hip. Surg Radiol Anat. 2012;34(1):31–8.
36. Blankenbaker DG, Davis KW, De Smet AA, Keene JS. MRI appearance of the pectinofoveal fold. AJR Am J Roentgenol. 2009;192(1):93–5.
37. Fu Z, Peng M, Peng Q. Anatomical study of the synovial plicae of the hip joint. Clin Anat. 1997;10(4):235–8.
38. Bencardino JT, Beltran J. MR imaging of the glenohumeral ligaments. Radiol Clin North Am. 2006;44(4):489–502.
39. Katz LD, Haims A, Medvecky M, McCallum J. Symptomatic hip plica: MR arthrographic and arthroscopic correlation. Skeletal Radiol. 2010;39(12):1255–8.
40. Mei-Dan O, McConkey MO, Brick M. Catastrophic failure of hip arthroscopy due to iatrogenic instability: can partial division of the ligamentum teres and iliofemoral ligament cause subluxation? Arthroscopy. 2012;28(3):440–5.
41. Moorman CT, Warren RF, Hershman EB, Crowe JF, Potter HG, Barnes R, et al. Traumatic posterior hip subluxation in American football. J Bone Joint Surg Am. 2003;85-A(7):1190–6.
42. Rao J, Zhou YX, Villar RN. Injury to the ligamentum teres. Mechanism, findings, and results of treatment. Clin Sports Med. 2001;20(4):791.
43. Cerezal L, Arnaiz J, Canga A, Piedra T, Altónaga JR, Munafo R, et al. Emerging topics on the hip: ligamentum teres and hip microinstability. Eur J Radiol. 2012;81(12):3745–54.
44. Gray AJ, Villar RN. The ligamentum teres of the hip: an arthroscopic classification of its pathology. Arthroscopy. 1997; 13(5):575–8.
45. Byrd JWT, Jones KS. Adhesive capsulitis of the hip. Arthroscopy. 2006;22(1):89–94.
46. Griffiths HJ, Utz R, Burke J, Bonfiglio T. Adhesive capsulitis of the hip and ankle. AJR Am J Roentgenol. 1985;144(1):101–5.

47. Sofka CM, Ciavarra GA, Hannafin JA, Cordasco FA, Potter HG. Magnetic resonance imaging of adhesive capsulitis: correlation with clinical staging. HSS J. 2008;4(2):164–9.
48. Tehranzadeh J, Ashikyan O, Dascalos J. Magnetic resonance imaging in early detection of rheumatoid arthritis. Semin Musculoskelet Radiol. 2003;7(2):79–94.
49. Karchevsky M, Schweitzer ME, Morrison WB, Parellada JA. MRI findings of septic arthritis and associated osteomyelitis in adults. AJR Am J Roentgenol. 2004;182(1):119–22.
50. Plodkowski AJ, Hayter CL, Miller TT, Nguyen JT, Potter HG. Lamellated hyperintense synovitis: potential MR imaging sign of an infected knee arthroplasty. Radiology. 2013;66(1):256–60.
51. Tyler WKW, Vidal AFA, Williams RJR, Healey JHJ. Pigmented villonodular synovitis. J Am Acad Orthop Surg. 2006;14(6):376–85.
52. Dorwart RH, Genant HK, Johnston WH, Morris JM. Pigmented villonodular synovitis of synovial joints: clinical, pathologic, and radiologic features. AJR Am J Roentgenol. 1984;143(4): 877–85.
53. Murphey MD, Rhee JH, Lewis RB, Fanburg-Smith JC, Flemming DJ,WalkerEA.FromthearchivesoftheAFIP@;DELIM@;continuing medical education: pigmented villonodular synovitis: radiologic-pathologic correlation1. Radiographics. 2008;28(5):1493–518.
54. Kramer J, Recht M, Deely DM, Schweitzer M, Pathria MN, Gentili A, et al. MR appearance of idiopathic synovial osteochondromatosis. J Comput Assist Tomogr. 1993;17(5):772–6.
55. Murphey MD, Vidal JA, Fanburg-Smith JC, Gajewski DA. Imaging of synovial chondromatosis with radiologic-pathologic correlation. Radiographics. 2007;27(5):1465–88.

Extra-articular Pathology of the Hip

23

Scott S. Lenobel, Adriana M.L. Oliveira,
and Miriam A. Bredella

Introduction

Hip pain is a common clinical problem and is often the result of soft tissue pathology around the hip joint. Knowledge of the anatomy in this region is important in correctly diagnosing the cause of pain. Diagnostic imaging plays an important role in the management of these patients due to the numerous potential causes of hip pain. In this chapter we review extra-articular hip anatomy as well as several common and uncommon extra-articular causes of hip pain.

Bursae and Bursitis

Bursitis is a common cause of hip pain. The three main bursae around the hip joint are the trochanteric bursa, the iliopsoas bursa, and the ischial bursa [1]. The gluteus medius and gluteus minimus tendons insert onto the greater trochanter of the femur. Four facets are identified on the greater trochanter: anterior, lateral, superoposterior, and posterior facets. The trochanteric bursal complex consists of three distinct components: the subgluteus maximus bursa, the subgluteus medius bursa, and the subgluteus minimus bursa. The subgluteus maximus bursa is the largest bursal component and is located deep to the gluteus maximus muscle and iliotibial band and overlies the posterior facet of the greater trochanter [2]. The subgluteus medius bursa is located between the undersurface of the gluteus medius tendon and the greater trochanteric lateral facet. The subgluteus minimus bursa is located between the undersurface of the gluteus minimus tendon and the greater trochanteric anterior facet.

Trochanteric bursitis is typically caused by chronic excessive friction of the iliotibial band and gluteal tendons against the underlying greater trochanter. The most common finding of trochanteric bursitis on MR imaging is a T1 hypointense and T2 hyperintense fluid collection. Peripheral enhancement can be seen following administration of intravenous contrast (Fig. 23.1a, b). Synovial thickening, internal debris, and/or septations within the bursal collection suggest inflammation. Fluid-fluid levels or T1 hyperintensity within the bursal collection suggests the presence of hemorrhage.

The iliopsoas bursa is the largest synovial bursa in humans [3, 4] and is located between the iliopsoas and the anterior hip joint capsule. It communicates with the hip joint in 10–15 % of adults [5]. Iliopsoas bursitis is most commonly caused by chronic excessive friction of the iliopsoas tendon against the anterior hip joint but can also be caused by a systemic inflammatory disease such as rheumatoid arthritis or infection. In addition the tendonitis can also occur as a by-product of excessive femoral anteversion. In the prosthetic hip, it may also be the resolute of an oversized acetabular or femoral component. The typical appearance of iliopsoas bursitis on MRI is T1 hypointense and T2 hyperintense (Fig. 23.1b, c) and the characteristic location of the bursa can help differentiate bursitis from a mass.

Ischial bursitis is an uncommon cause of buttock pain and can occur after an acute or repetitive injury to the ischial tuberosity. It is located inferomedial to the ischial tuberosity and is cystic in appearance [6, 7].

S.S. Lenobel, MD • A.M.L. Oliveira, MD
M.A. Bredella, MD (✉)
Department of Radiology, Musculoskeletal Imaging and Interventions, Massachusetts General Hospital, Harvard Medical School, Yawkey 6E, 55 Fruit Street, Boston, MA 02114, USA
e-mail: mbredella@partners.org

J.C. McCarthy et al. (eds.), *Hip Joint Restoration*, DOI 10.1007/978-1-4614-0694-5_23

Muscles and Tendons

Abnormalities of muscles and tendons can be grouped into three categories: tendinous avulsion, muscle contusion, and myotendinous strain. Acute tendinous avulsion can occur due to deceleration or eccentric muscle contraction leading to tensile overload [1]. Chronic avulsion is typically caused by repetitive stress or overuse. MR imaging is the preferred imaging modality for diagnosing tendinous avulsions when displaced bony fragments are not visible on radiographs. MR imaging allows direct visualization of the torn tendon and can accurately measure the degree of tendon retraction (Fig. 23.2). Associated findings in the setting of an acute tendinous avulsion include adjacent soft tissue hematoma as well as periosteal stripping and bone marrow edema at the site of tendon attachment. These findings are not typically present in the setting of a chronic tendinous avulsion injury. Instead, muscle atrophy and soft tissue scarring are usually present.

The myotendinous junction is the weakest point in the myotendinous unit and is susceptible to injury as tensile force generated by muscle fiber contraction is transmitted from the muscle through the myotendinous junction to the tendinous attachments. Three degrees of myotendinous injuries, or strains, exist [8]. In grade 1 strain, only minor disruption of fibers at the myotendinous junction occurs, producing a perifascicular feathery T2 hyperintense pattern on MR imaging secondary to interstitial edema and hemorrhage [8, 9]. In grade 2 strain, also described as a partial tear, partial disruption of myotendinous fibers occurs. Adjacent soft tissue edema and hemorrhage are more prominent and perifascicular edema is frequently seen. A hyperintense focal defect on fluid-sensitive MR sequences can be seen along with partial retraction of muscle fibers (Fig. 23.3). In grade 3 strain, or complete tear, full-thickness disruption of the myotendinous junction is often associated with tendon retraction and significant surrounding hemorrhage and edema. Third-degree myotendinous strain is usually clinically evident, but MR imaging can be useful in presurgical planning.

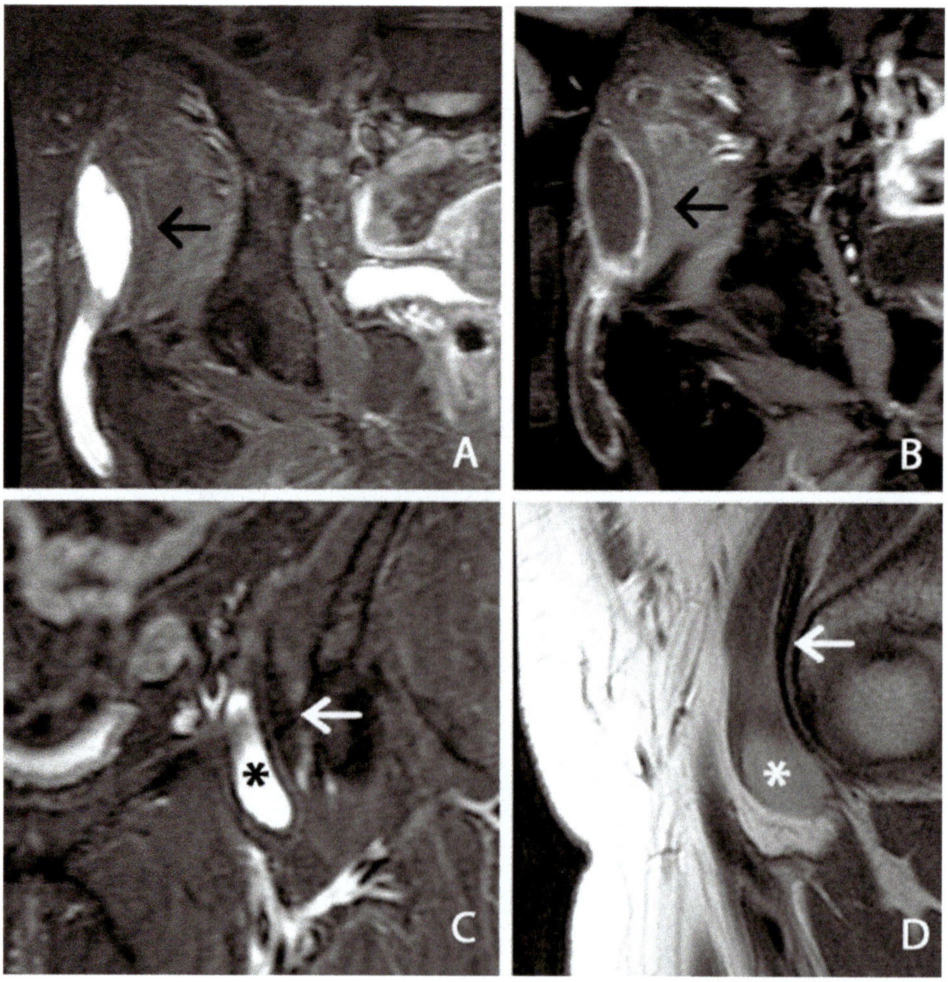

Fig. 23.1 Bursitis. (**a**) Coronal STIR and (**b**) coronal fat-suppressed post-gadolinium T1-weighted images demonstrate large amount of fluid in the greater trochanteric bursa with peripheral enhancement (*black arrows*). (**c**) Coronal fat-suppressed T2 and (**d**) sagittal proton density-weighted images show a fluid distended left iliopsoas bursa (*asterisks*). Note its relationship to the iliopsoas tendon (*white arrows*)

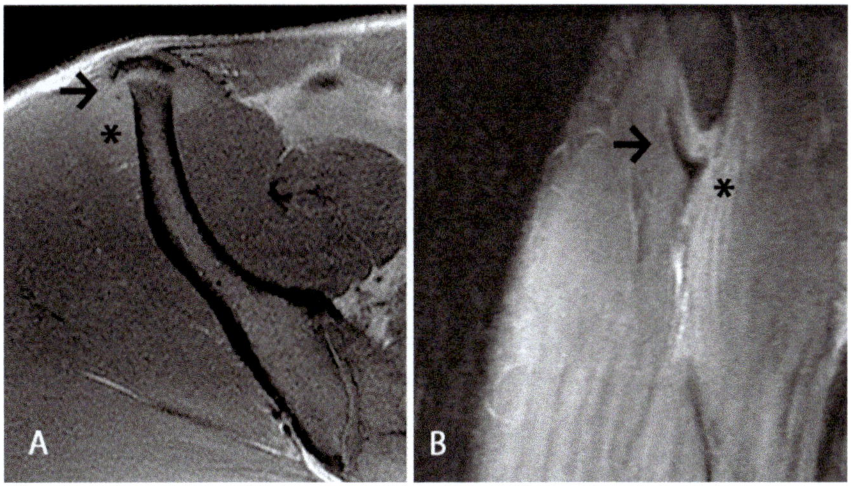

Fig. 23.2 Tendinous avulsion. (**a**) Axial and (**b**) coronal fat-suppressed T2-weighted images demonstrate avulsion injury of sartorius tendon from the anterior superior iliac spine (*black arrows*) with surrounding muscle edema (*asterisks*)

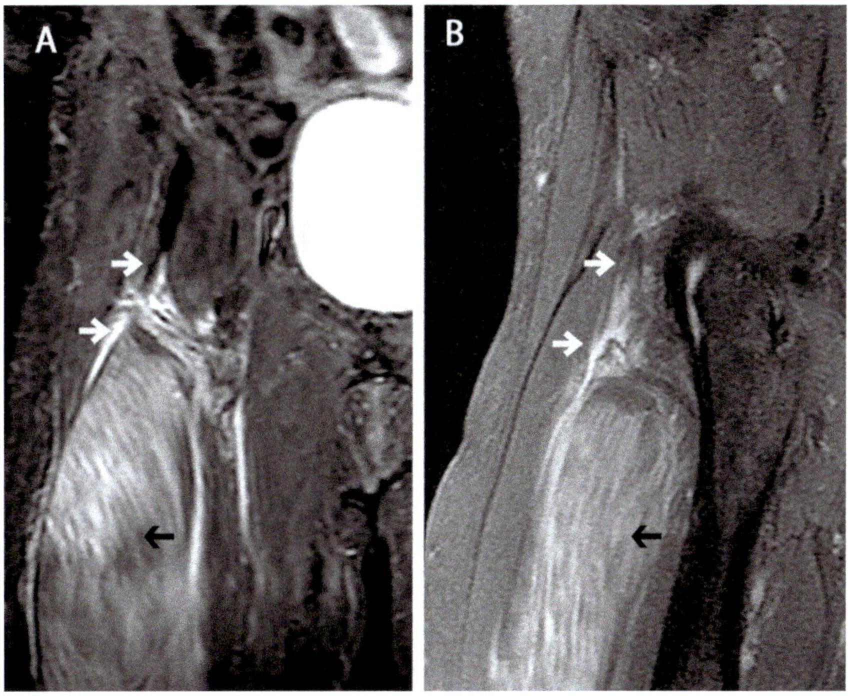

Fig. 23.3 Myotendinous injury. (**a**) Coronal and (**b**) sagittal fat-suppressed T2-weighted images demonstrate tear of the myotendinous junction of vastus lateralis with retraction of muscle belly (*white arrows*). Note feathery increased T2 signal in the muscle belly due to interstitial edema and hemorrhage (*black arrows*)

A muscle contusion is usually caused by blunt trauma. The most commonly contused muscle group around the hip joint is the gluteal musculature. In mild muscle contusion, edematous changes of the muscle fibers are characterized by a T2 hyperintense feathery appearance, similar to the appearance of grade 1 myotendinous strain. However, in muscle contusion, the muscle belly is typically involved and not the myotendinous junction. Intramuscular hematomas can develop in the setting of more severe trauma. On MR imaging, an intramuscular hematoma typically appears heterogeneous on both T1 and fluid-sensitive sequences (Fig. 23.4). On ultrasound, hematomas can present as irregular or circumscribed collections without significant internal vascularity. However, the imaging appearance of an intramuscular hematoma can vary, depending on chronicity and degree of hemoglobin oxidation. It is therefore important to differentiate a soft tissue sarcoma from a hematoma. On MR imaging, sarcomas typically are more homogeneous in signal intensity and hyperintense on fluid-sensitive sequences and contain nodular enhancing components, and show interval growth [10, 11]. MR imaging features that favor hematoma include T1 hyperintensity, absence of nodular enhancing components, and the presence of a low intensity hemosiderin rim. Since imaging characteristics of a sarcoma can vary, an intramuscular mass should be biopsied or followed to resolution with clinical examinations or imaging, particularly in the absence of significant trauma.

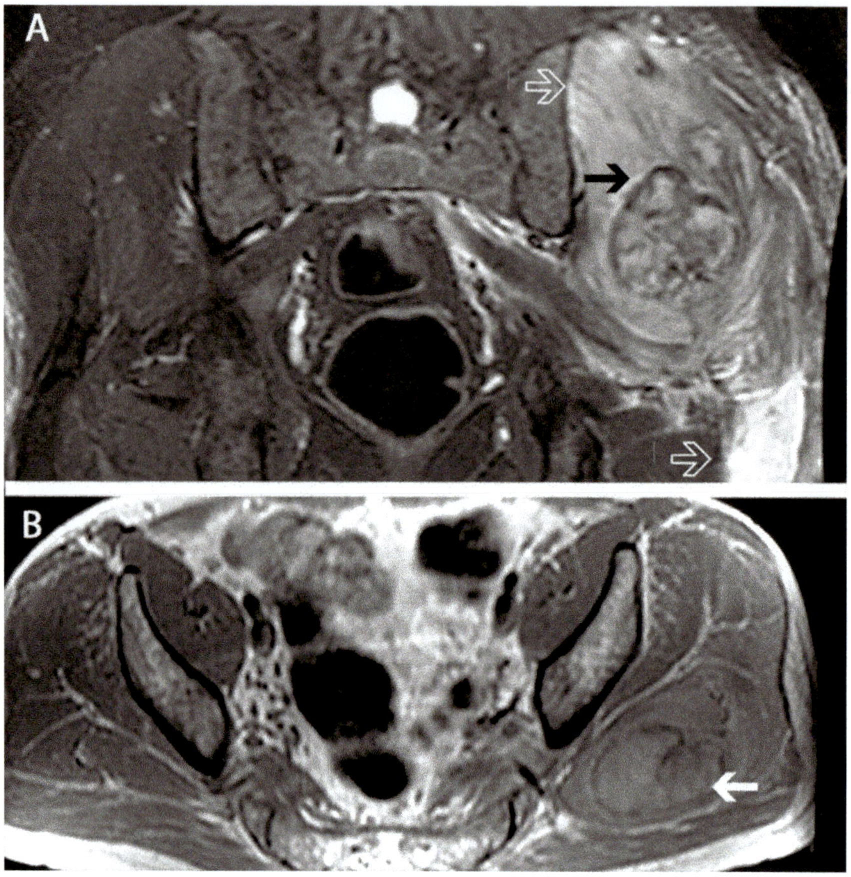

Fig. 23.4 Intramuscular hematoma. (**a**) Coronal STIR and (**b**) axial proton density-weighted images demonstrate a large hematoma centered in the left gluteus medius muscle. Hypointense rim (*black arrow* in (**a**)) and heterogeneous signal intensity (*white arrow* in (**b**)) are secondary to blood products in different stages. Marked associated edema of gluteus medius muscle (*open arrows* in (**a**)) is present

Additional types of injuries to tendons include tendinosis and calcific tendinitis. Tendinosis can develop from repetitive microtrauma, intrasubstance degeneration, or tendon weakening due a systemic process such as gout, diabetes, or collagen vascular disease [1]. On MR imaging, findings of tendinosis include tendon thickening and/or increased intrasubstance signal intensity within the tendon [12]. T2 hyperintensity representing edema can be seen in the peritendinous soft tissue. Calcific tendinitis is characterized by the deposition of amorphous hydroxyapatite crystals in the tendon, usually near the tendon insertion site, and can be associated with significant peritendinous inflammation.

Myositis Ossificans

Myositis ossificans is a benign, self-limiting process characterized by heterotopic ossification within skeletal muscle. It is often associated with trauma and specifically muscle contusions but can also occur in the absence of any reported trauma [13]. Activation of osteoprogenitor cells in the perimysial tissue is thought to play an important role in the development of myositis ossificans. However, the exact mechanism is unknown. Myositis ossificans typically presents with a peripheral rim of calcification and progressive centripetal ossification (Fig. 23.5). CT or radiographs best depict myositis ossification due to the ease of visualizing ossification. The MR imaging appearance of myositis ossificans can vary depending on the age of injury, degree of myonecrosis, maturity of ossification, and extent of the associated inflammatory reaction. It is important to differentiate myositis ossificans from a soft tissue sarcoma on imaging [8, 13]. If a diagnosis cannot be made, serial imaging is recommended, or alternatively percutaneous biopsy or surgical resection can be performed for definitive diagnosis.

Surgical excision should not be performed until the ossification process is quiescent. To prevent recurrence pre-op radiation or administration of Indocin is indicated.

Compartments of the Hip and Thigh

Muscle and tendon abnormalities can also be evaluated based on their anatomic compartment. The muscles and tendons of the hip and thigh can be divided into four compartments based on anatomic location and function: anterior, posterior, medial, and lateral [12].

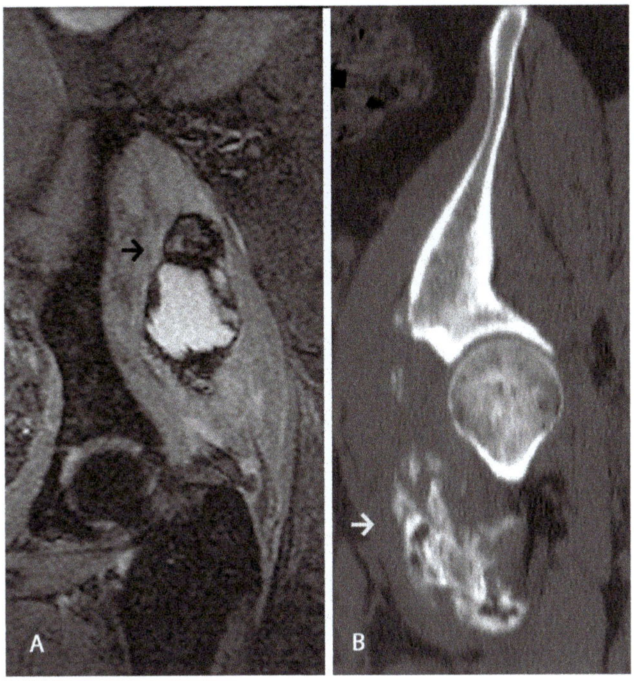

Fig. 23.5 Myositis ossificans. (**a**) Coronal gradient echo image shows a heterogeneous mass in the gluteus medius muscle with peripheral low signal intensity and blooming artifact (*black arrow*) from partial muscle ossification. (**b**) Sagittal CT in a different patient with palpable mass in the groin demonstrates ossification of the iliopsoas muscle (*white arrow*), consistent with myositis ossificans

Anterior Compartment

The anterior compartment consists of the hip flexors, which include the iliopsoas, sartorius, and quadriceps muscles and tendons. Pathology of the iliopsoas and quadriceps muscles will be discussed as injuries to these muscles, and tendons are much more commonly encountered. Pathology of the sartorius is rare and will not be discussed in this chapter.

Two tendons combine to form the iliopsoas: the iliacus and the psoas major [14, 15]. The psoas major muscle arises from the T12-L5 vertebral bodies and descends inferiorly. The iliacus muscle arises from the iliac fossa. As it descends inferiorly through the pelvis, some of its fibers cross medially and join the psoas major to form the iliopsoas tendon, which inserts onto the lesser trochanter of the femur. An anatomic variant is present in some patients in which the crossing iliacus fibers terminate at the level of the femoral neck. Below this level a thin intramuscular tendon in the medial aspect of the iliacus muscle runs parallel to the adjacent iliopsoas tendon. A fat plane separates the two tendons, which should not be confused with a longitudinal split tear of the iliopsoas tendon [15]. The remaining iliacus muscle fibers insert directly onto the proximal femoral diaphysis. The iliopsoas tendon is located in a bony groove between the anterior inferior iliac spine laterally and the iliopectineal eminence medially.

The severity of iliopsoas tendon injuries increases with age. In patients younger than 65 years, injuries are usually related to sports or other trauma and primarily consist of muscle strains and partial tendon tears. In patients older than 65 years, complete tears are more often seen and commonly result from chronic systemic disease, corticosteroid use, or complications from surgery [16–19]. Athletic injuries are less common. The most common location of an iliopsoas tendon tear is the tendon attachment to the lesser trochanter [16, 17]. Intramuscular hematoma can be seen in association with both partial and complete tendon tears. Avulsion fracture of the lesser trochanter of the femur at the iliopsoas tendon insertion site can be due to trauma in skeletally immature patients due to the relative weakness of the bone-apophysis interface [12, 19]. In adult patients, an avulsion fracture of the lesser tuberosity is more commonly caused by a pathologic fracture related to malignancy.

Snapping Hip Syndrome

Snapping hip syndrome is characterized by sudden, painful, and audible snapping of the hip [12, 20] and is typically seen in young, physically active adults. Symptoms can be reproduced with specific movements such as moving the hip from a frog-leg position to neutral. Snapping hip syndrome can be due to extra-articular or intra-articular causes, with extra-articular causes being further classified as internal or external. External extra-articular snapping hip syndrome involves lateral structures, typically the iliotibial band and gluteus maximus muscle. Snapping occurs as these structures pass over the greater trochanter during hip flexion and extension. Due to the easily reproducible symptoms with hip flexion and extension, this diagnosis is usually made clinically without imaging.

Internal hip snapping is the more common than external hip snapping and occurs when the iliopsoas tendon passes over the iliopectineal eminence and/or lesser trochanter [21]. Ultrasound is extremely useful in evaluating the iliopsoas tendon in hip snapping because it allows dynamic evaluation of the tendon during snapping and also allows evaluation of the tendon for pathology and associated bursitis [21–23]. Snapping can be induced by moving a flexed, abducted, and externally rotated hip into full extension and is seen on ultrasound as a sudden lateral-to-medial movement of the tendon as it passes over the iliopectineal eminence or the lesser trochanter. In addition to its diagnostic utility, ultrasound can also be used to guide injection of corticosteroid and/or local anesthetic into the iliopsoas bursa [24, 25]. Dynamic MR imaging can also demonstrate snapping of the iliopsoas tendon [12]. On MR imaging, the location and quality of the iliopsoas tendon can be easily evaluated and bursal fluid identified (Fig. 23.1b, c). Intra-articular hip snapping causes include labral tears, intra-articular bodies, synovial chondromatosis, synovial folds, and fracture fragments [12, 20].

Quadriceps

The quadriceps muscle group is comprised of the rectus femoris, vastus lateralis, vastus intermedius, and vastus medialis, with the rectus femoris being most commonly injured. Rectus femoris injuries most often occur when the hip is hyperextended and the knee is flexed [12, 26]. The rectus femoris origin consists of two components: the straight head, which arises from the anterior inferior iliac spine, and the reflected head, which arises posterolaterally adjacent to the acetabulum. Injuries to the straight head are more common. MR imaging is the modality of choice for imaging injuries to the rectus femoris, which often are associated with bone marrow edema of the anterior inferior iliac spine and peritendinous edema (Fig. 23.6). The reflected head shows similar findings on MR but the location is posterolateral to the anterior inferior iliac spine.

Posterior Compartment

The posterior compartment contains muscles that extend and externally rotate the hip [12, 26]. Injuries most commonly occur in the hamstring muscle complex, which is comprised of the semimembranosus, semitendinosus, and biceps femoris muscles. The hamstring tendon originates from the ischial tuberosity, with the semimembranosus arising from the superolateral facet and the semitendinosus and long head of the biceps femoris sharing a common origin from the medial facet. The short head of the biceps tendon arises from the linea aspera, lateral supracondylar line, and intermuscular septum. The semimembranosus tendon inserts distally onto the proximal medial tibia via five tendon attachment sites [12, 27]. The distal semitendinosus tendon inserts onto the proximal medial tibia as well. The distal biceps femoris tendon inserts onto the fibular head.

The hamstring complex primarily functions by eccentric contraction, which occurs when the muscles are passively stretched. Injuries typically occur when the hip is flexed and the knee is extended [28]. Hamstring injuries most often occur at the myotendinous junction and range from low-grade strains to complete tears. MR findings can range from peritendinous edema to full-thickness tendon disruption with retraction (Fig. 23.7). Avulsion injuries of the ischial tuberosity are also relatively common and can be associated with marrow edema within the ischial tuberosity on MR imaging fluid-sensitive sequences. Bony proliferative changes can be seen at the ischial tuberosity in cases of chronic tendon injuries.

Medial Compartment

The adductor muscles are located in the medial compartment and assist in adduction and flexion of the thigh. The adductor muscle group is comprised of the adductor longus, adductor brevis, adductor magnus, obturator externus, and quadratus femoris. The adductor longus originates from the anterior pubis and inserts onto the linea aspera. The adductor brevis originates from the inferior pubic ramus and also inserts onto the linea aspera. The adductor magnus originates from the ischial tuberosity and pubis and inserts onto the linea aspera, supracondylar femur, and adductor tubercle of the distal medial femur. The adductor tendons undergo similar injuries to the tendons in other compartments such as tendinopathy, calcific tendinitis, and partial and full-thickness tears (Fig. 23.8).

Adductor insertion avulsion syndrome is a painful condition affecting the femur at the insertion of the adductor muscles and is also known as thigh splints [29, 30]. Calcifications may be seen on radiographs along the posterior proximal

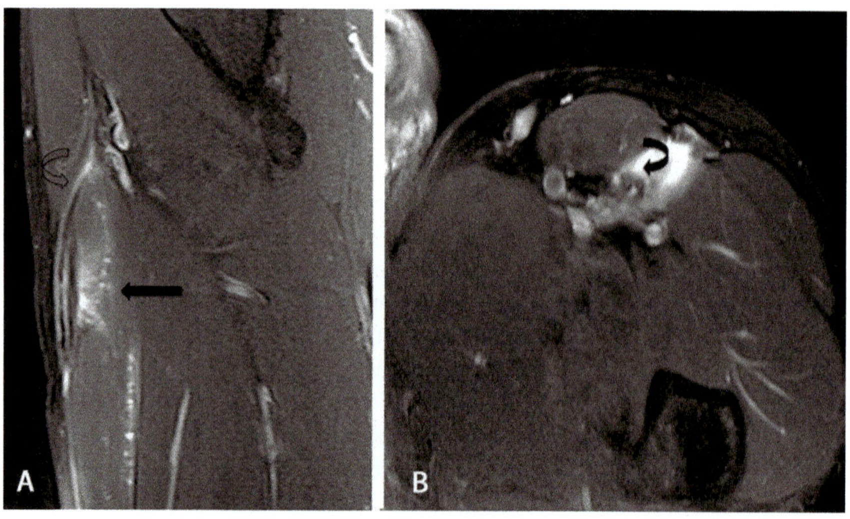

Fig. 23.6 Rectus femoris tear. (**a**) Sagittal and (**b**) axial fat-suppressed T2-weighted images show complete tear of the myotendinous junction of the rectus femoris which is thickened and retracted (*curved arrows*). There is associated interstitial edema and hemorrhage (*straight arrow* in (**a**))

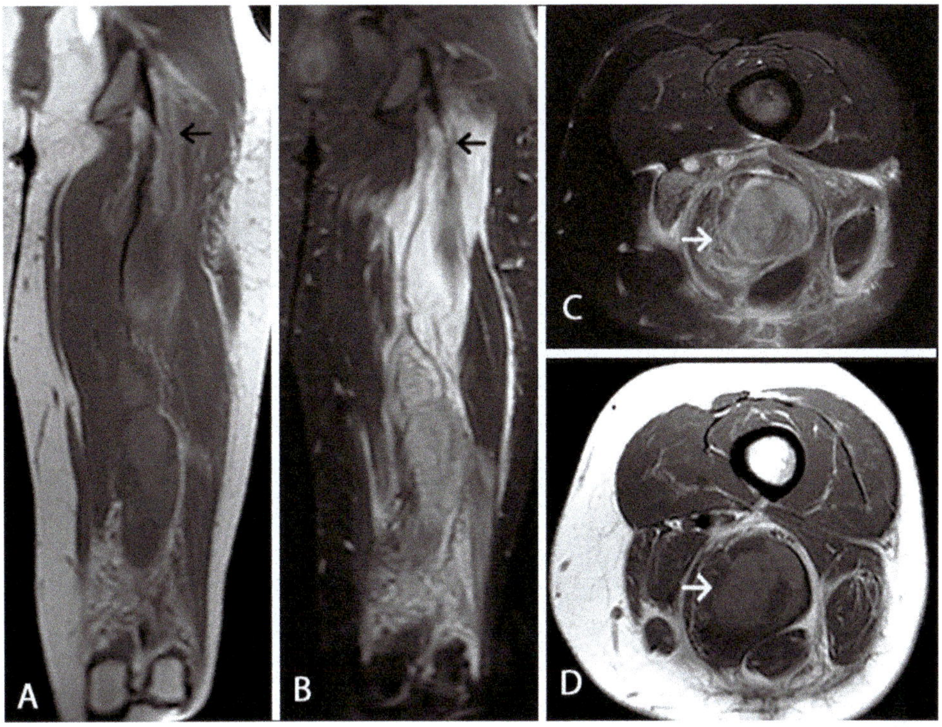

Fig. 23.7 Hamstring tear. (**a**) Coronal T1 and (**b**) coronal fat-suppressed T2-weighted images show high-grade tear of the proximal semimembranosus tendon (*black arrows*). (**c**) Axial fat-suppressed T2 and (**d**) axial T1-weighted images demonstrate large associated intramuscular hematoma (*white arrows*)

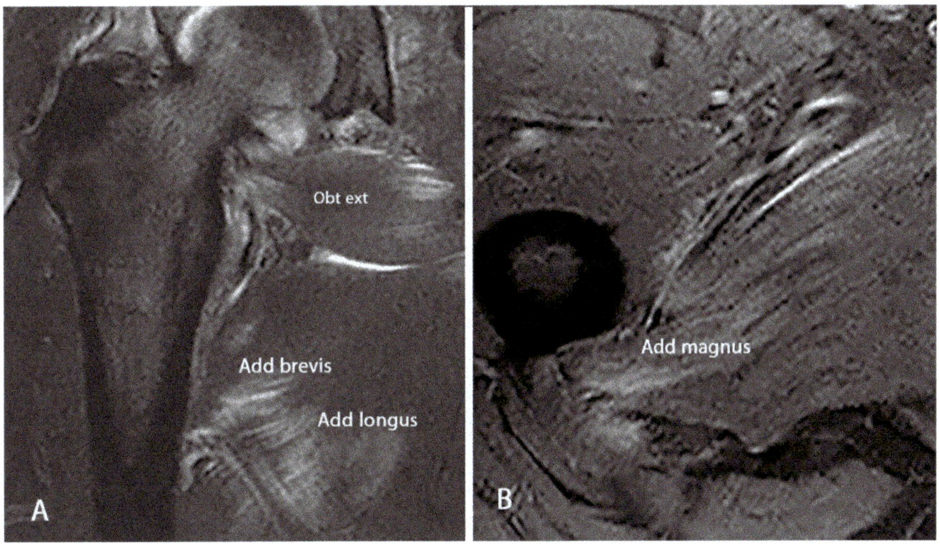

Fig. 23.8 Adductor strain. (**a**) Coronal and (**b**) axial fat-suppressed T2-weighted images demonstrate feathery edema from muscle strain in the adductor compartment (*Obt ext* obturator externus, *Add brevis* adductor brevis, *Add longus* adductor longus, *Add magnus* adductor magnus)

thigh secondary to chronic inflammation. On MR imaging, the adductor tendons are typically thickened and increased in T2 signal. Peritendinous edema can also be associated with adductor insertion avulsion.

The quadratus femoris muscle arises from the inferolateral ischial tuberosity, just anterior to the hamstring tendon origin, and inserts onto the quadrate tubercle of the posteromedial proximal femur. It is located posterior to the obturator externus and anterior to the sciatic nerve. The quadratus femoris can undergo strains or partial tears but is also subject to impingement between the ischial tuberosity and lesser trochanter of the femur. Impingement has been shown to be associated with an ischiofemoral distance of less than or equal to 17 mm and the space between the hamstring tendon origin and iliopsoas tendon insertion measuring less than or equal to 8 mm. This abnormality can cause hip pain which is not easily localized on clinical exam so is best assessed by MR imaging [31, 32]. On MR imaging, the quadratus femoris can be edematous, partially torn, and/or atrophied, depending on the chronicity of the impingement (Fig. 23.9). Associated hamstring tendon origin abnormalities also are commonly seen.

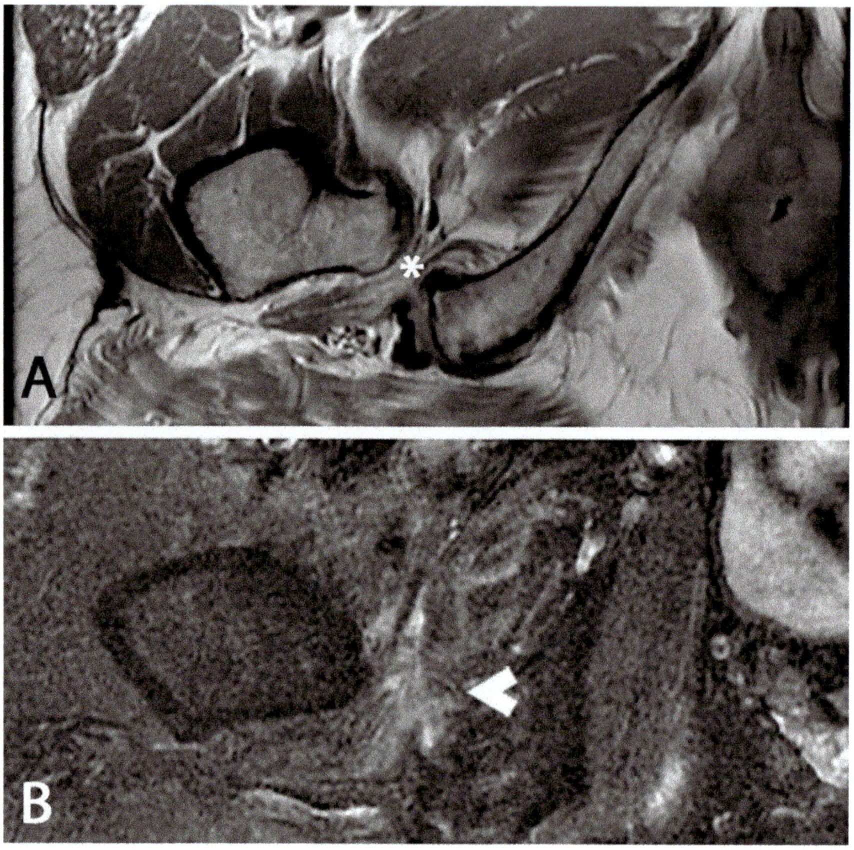

Fig. 23.9 Ischiofemoral impingement. (**a**) Axial proton density and (**b**) axial fat-suppressed T2-weighted images demonstrate narrowing of the right ischiofemoral space (*asterisk* in (**a**)) with associated edema of the quadratus femoris muscle (*arrowhead* in (**b**))

Lateral Compartment

The lateral compartment contains the abductors, which consist of the gluteus medius and gluteus minimus muscles. The greater trochanter is the primary attachment site for the abductors and has four facets: anterior, lateral, posterior superior, and posterior. The gluteus medius attaches onto the posterior superior and lateral facets, and a portion blends with the gluteus minimus tendon to insert onto the anterior facet. The gluteus minimus tendon inserts onto the anterior facet and the superior capsule of the hip joint. The gluteus maximus is not considered a hip abductor and is not discussed in this chapter.

Greater trochanteric pain syndrome is characterized by pain and tenderness over the lateral hip and greater trochanter. It is commonly associated with gluteal tendon abnormalities and greater trochanteric bursitis [33–35]. Peritendinous edema, tendinopathy, calcific tendinitis, and partial or complete tears can be seen as well as bursitis, bony proliferative changes, and muscular atrophy (Fig. 23.10). T2 hyperintense signal adjacent to the greater trochanter is nearly always present in greater trochanteric pain syndrome but is not a specific finding as it is also seen in many asymptomatic individuals [33].

Joint Capsule and Iliofemoral Ligament Injuries

The hip joint capsule is an important stabilizer of the hip joint and has several areas of focal thickening, referred to as capsular ligaments, which reinforce the capsule [36, 37]. The capsular ligaments include the pubofemoral, iliofemoral, and ischiofemoral ligaments and are composed of longitudinally oriented fibers with respect to the hip joint and femoral head/neck axis. The iliofemoral is the strongest capsular ligament and has an inferior band that restricts extension and a superior band that restricts external rotation. It is frequently injured in athletes who undergo repetitive twisting and pivoting of the hip [38] and can cause microinstability of the hip joint. On MR imaging, T2 hyperintense signal is seen around the ligament with partial or complete disruption of the ligament fibers. If MR arthrography is performed, contrast can transect the ligament.

Morel-Lavallée Lesion

A Morel-Lavallée lesion is a closed degloving injury of the proximal lateral thigh due to abrupt separation of the skin and subcutaneous fat from the underlying superficial muscu-

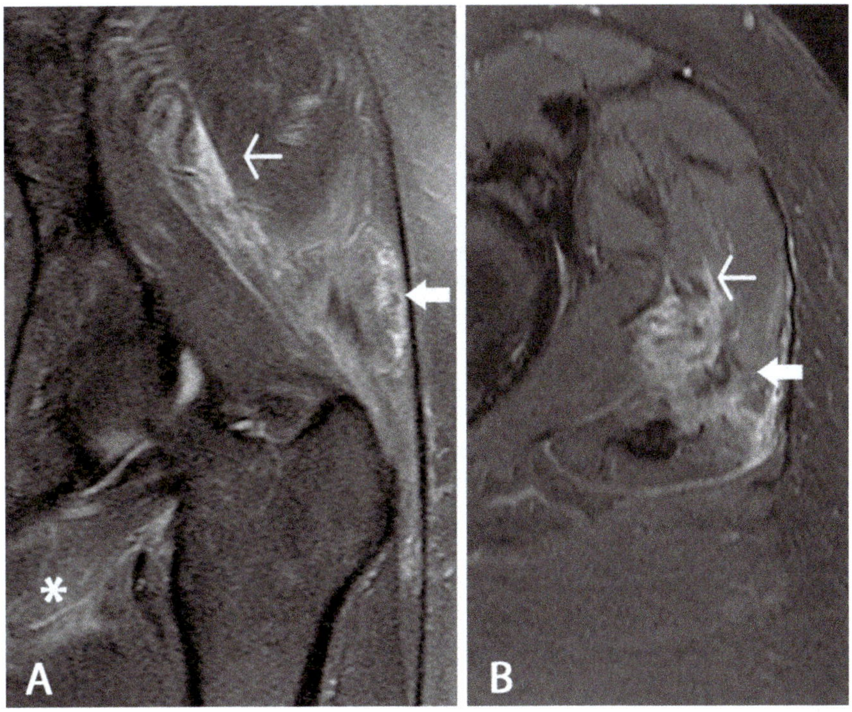

Fig. 23.10 Gluteal tears. (**a**) Coronal and (**b**) axial fat-suppressed T2-weighted images demonstrate tendinopathy and partial tear of gluteus minimus (*thin arrows*) and gluteus medius (*block arrows*). There is edema of the quadratus femoris (*asterisk* in (**a**))

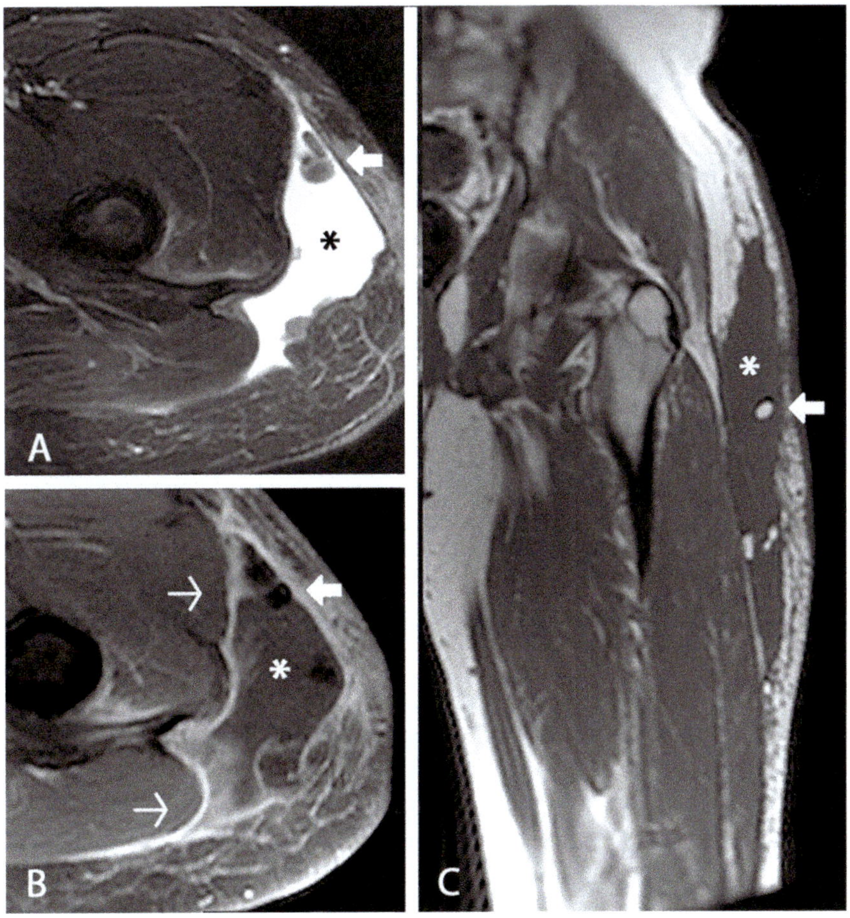

Fig. 23.11 Morel-Lavallée lesion. (**a**) Axial fat-suppressed T2, (**b**) axial fat-suppressed post-gadolinium T1, and (**c**) coronal T1-weighted images demonstrate a large fluid collection (*asterisks*) with rim enhancement (*thin arrows* in (**b**)) within the subcutaneous soft tissues of lateral thigh. Multiple foci of fat are visible within the lesion (*white block arrows*)

lar fascia. The injury is usually the result from a force vector of combined compression and shear causing avulsion of the subcutaneous fat off of the underlying fascia [39, 40]. Due to the extensive vascular supply of this region, leakage of blood and debris from disrupted capillaries into the perifascial plane forms a fluid collection. Inflammation leads to formation of a fibrous capsule. These lesions often slowly enlarge and can mimic soft tissue sarcomas. MR imaging is the diagnostic modality of choice to evaluate Morel-Lavallée lesions. MR imaging characteristics include T1 hypointense and T2 hyperintense signal with a peripheral hypointense ring (Fig. 23.11). Different stages of hemorrhage and evolving hematoma can lead to a variable appearance. These lesions can occasionally become infected [41].

Summary

The complex anatomy and physiology of the extra-articular hip structures create diagnostic challenges. Familiarity with anatomy and functional roles of the soft tissue structures around the hip is necessary for accurate interpretation of imaging findings.

References

1. Bencardino JT, Kassarjian A, Palmer WE. Magnetic resonance imaging of the hip: sports-related injuries. Top Magn Reson Imaging. 2003;14:145–60.
2. Pfirrmann CW, Chung CB, Theumann NH, Trudell DJ, Resnick D. Greater trochanter of the hip: attachment of the abductor mechanism and a complex of three bursae—MR imaging and MR bursography in cadavers and MR imaging in asymptomatic volunteers. Radiology. 2001;221:469–77.
3. Armstrong P, Saxton H. Ilio-psoas bursa. Br J Radiol. 1972;45:493–5.
4. Harper MC, Schaberg JE, Allen WC. Primary iliopsoas bursography in the diagnosis of disorders of the hip. Clin Orthop Relat Res. 1987;(221):238–41.
5. Steinbach LS, Schneider R, Goldman AB, Kazam E, Ranawat CS, Ghelman B. Bursae and abscess cavities communicating with the hip. Diagnosis using arthrography and CT. Radiology. 1985;156:303–7.
6. Cho KH, Lee SM, Lee YH, et al. Non-infectious ischiogluteal bursitis: MRI findings. Korean J Radiol. 2004;5:280–6.
7. Kim SM, Shin MJ, Kim KS, et al. Imaging features of ischial bursitis with an emphasis on ultrasonography. Skeletal Radiol. 2002;31:631–6.
8. Palmer WE, Kuong SJ, Elmadbouh HM. MR imaging of myotendinous strain. AJR Am J Roentgenol. 1999;173:703–9.
9. Steinbach LS, Fleckenstein JL, Mink JH. Magnetic resonance imaging of muscle injuries. Orthopedics. 1994;17:991–9.
10. Gomez P, Morcuende J. High-grade sarcomas mimicking traumatic intramuscular hematomas: a report of three cases. Iowa Orthop J. 2004;24:106–10.
11. Imaizumi S, Morita T, Ogose A, et al. Soft tissue sarcoma mimicking chronic hematoma: value of magnetic resonance imaging in differential diagnosis. J Orthop Sci. 2002;7:33–7.
12. Bancroft LW, Blankenbaker DG. Imaging of the tendons about the pelvis. AJR Am J Roentgenol. 2010;195:605–17.
13. Kneeland JB. MR imaging of sports injuries of the hip. Magn Reson Imaging Clin N Am. 1999;7:105–15. viii.
14. Blankenbaker DG, Tuite MJ. Iliopsoas musculotendinous unit. Semin Musculoskelet Radiol. 2008;12:13–27.
15. Polster JM, Elgabaly M, Lee H, Klika A, Drake R, Barsoum W. MRI and gross anatomy of the iliopsoas tendon complex. Skeletal Radiol. 2008;37:55–8.
16. Bui KL, Ilaslan H, Recht M, Sundaram M. Iliopsoas injury: an MRI study of patterns and prevalence correlated with clinical findings. Skeletal Radiol. 2008;37:245–9.
17. Bui KL, Sundaram M. Radiologic case study: iliopsoas tendon rupture. Orthopedics. 2008;31(10).
18. Lecouvet FE, Demondion X, Leemrijse T, Vande Berg BC, Devogelaer JP, Malghem J. Spontaneous rupture of the distal iliopsoas tendon: clinical and imaging findings, with anatomic correlations. Eur Radiol. 2005;15:2341–6.
19. Shabshin N, Rosenberg ZS, Cavalcanti CF. MR imaging of iliopsoas musculotendinous injuries. Magn Reson Imaging Clin N Am. 2005;13:705–16.
20. Deslandes M, Guillin R, Cardinal E, Hobden R, Bureau NJ. The snapping iliopsoas tendon: new mechanisms using dynamic sonography. AJR Am J Roentgenol. 2008;190:576–81.
21. Pelsser V, Cardinal E, Hobden R, Aubin B, Lafortune M. Extraarticular snapping hip: sonographic findings. AJR Am J Roentgenol. 2001;176:67–73.
22. Cardinal E, Buckwalter KA, Capello WN, Duval N. US of the snapping iliopsoas tendon. Radiology. 1996;198:521–2.
23. Vaccaro JP, Sauser DD, Beals RK. Iliopsoas bursa imaging: efficacy in depicting abnormal iliopsoas tendon motion in patients with internal snapping hip syndrome. Radiology. 1995; 197:853–6.
24. Idjadi J, Meislin R. Symptomatic snapping hip: targeted treatment for maximum pain relief. Phys Sportsmed. 2004;32:25–31.
25. Wahl CJ, Warren RF, Adler RS, Hannafin JA, Hansen B. Internal coxa saltans (snapping hip) as a result of overtraining: a report of 3 cases in professional athletes with a review of causes and the role of ultrasound in early diagnosis and management. Am J Sports Med. 2004;32:1302–9.
26. Chatha DS, Arora R. MR imaging of the normal hip. Magn Reson Imaging Clin N Am. 2005;13:605–15.
27. Koulouris G, Connell D. Hamstring muscle complex: an imaging review. Radiographics. 2005;25:571–86.
28. LaBan MM, McNeary L. An avulsion of the semitendinosus and biceps femoris conjoined tendons. Am J Phys Med Rehabil. 2008;87:168.
29. Anderson MW, Kaplan PA, Dussault RG. Adductor insertion avulsion syndrome (thigh splints): spectrum of MR imaging features. AJR Am J Roentgenol. 2001;177:673–5.
30. Tshering-Vogel D, Waldherr C, Schindera ST, Steinbach LS, Stauffer E, Anderson SE. Adductor insertion avulsion syndrome, "thigh splints": relevance of radiological follow-up. Skeletal Radiol. 2005;34:355–8.
31. Patti JW, Ouellette H, Bredella MA, Torriani M. Impingement of lesser trochanter on ischium as a potential cause for hip pain. Skeletal Radiol. 2008;37:939–41.
32. Torriani M, Souto SC, Thomas BJ, Ouellette H, Bredella MA. Ischiofemoral impingement syndrome: an entity with hip pain

and abnormalities of the quadratus femoris muscle. AJR Am J Roentgenol. 2009;193:186–90.
33. Blankenbaker DG, Ullrick SR, Davis KW, De Smet AA, Haaland B, Fine JP. Correlation of MRI findings with clinical findings of trochanteric pain syndrome. Skeletal Radiol. 2008;37:903–9.
34. Cvitanic O, Henzie G, Skezas N, Lyons J, Minter J. MRI diagnosis of tears of the hip abductor tendons (gluteus medius and gluteus minimus). AJR Am J Roentgenol. 2004;182:137–43.
35. Kong A, Van der Vliet A, Zadow S. MRI and US of gluteal tendinopathy in greater trochanteric pain syndrome. Eur Radiol. 2007;17:1772–83.
36. Ito H, Song Y, Lindsey DP, Safran MR, Giori NJ. The proximal hip joint capsule and the zona orbicularis contribute to hip joint stability in distraction. J Orthop Res. 2009;27:989–95.
37. Wagner FV, Negrao JR, Campos J, et al. Capsular ligaments of the hip: anatomic, histologic, and positional study in cadaveric specimens with MR arthrography. Radiology. 2012;263: 189–98.
38. Myers CA, Register BC, Lertwanich P, et al. Role of the acetabular labrum and the iliofemoral ligament in hip stability: an in vitro biplane fluoroscopy study. Am J Sports Med. 2011;39(Suppl):85S–91.
39. Mellado JM, Perez del Palomar L, Diaz L, Ramos A, Sauri A. Long-standing Morel-Lavallée lesions of the trochanteric region and proximal thigh: MRI features in five patients. AJR Am J Roentgenol. 2004;182:1289–94.
40. Mukherjee K, Perrin SM, Hughes PM. Morel-Lavallée lesion in an adolescent with ultrasound and MRI correlation. Skeletal Radiol. 2007;36 Suppl 1:S43–5.
41. Mellado JM, Bencardino JT. Morel-Lavallée lesion: review with emphasis on MR imaging. Magn Reson Imaging Clin N Am. 2005;13:775–82.

24 Magnetic Resonance Imaging of the Hip

Srinath C. Sampath, Srihari C. Sampath, and William E. Palmer

Introduction

The hip is a ball-and-socket joint comprised of four major bones plus several supporting soft tissue structures. Together these structures allow for multiaxial motion of the lower extremity while maintaining structural stability. Here we present an overview of current methods in hip imaging, focusing on evaluation by noncontrast magnetic resonance (MR) imaging and direct MR arthrography. Protocols and technical parameters for MR imaging of the hip are presented. Basic MR anatomy of the hip is reviewed, including normal arthrographic appearance of the intraarticular structures. Given that symptoms referable to the hip can be caused by disorders of both the hip itself or by abnormalities of other regional structures [1], both intra- and extraarticular pathologies are discussed, with emphasis on the range of possible imaging presentations. Finally, common pitfalls are illustrated, including those relevant to both noncontrast and arthrographic evaluation.

Arthrographic Technique

MR arthrography of the hip is performed for improved evaluation of the intraarticular structures, particularly the acetabular labrum and articular cartilage, ligamentum teres as well as of the hip capsule [2, 3]. Although a variety of needle placements have been described [4], at our institution, an anterolateral approach is commonly used for contrast injection. The location of the femoral vessels is first identified by palpation, and the fluoroscopic detector is rotated approximately 15° lateral, in order to decrease the probability of intravascular injection. With the leg in neutral position, a 3.5-in. 22-gauge spinal needle is advanced under fluoroscopic guidance to the superolateral head-neck junction (Fig. 24.1a). After access to the joint is confirmed, approximately 10 cm^3 of dilute gadolinium/iodinated contrast/lidocaine solution (consisting of 10 mL diluted gadolinium (0.4 mL of gadopentetate dimeglumine [Magnevist; Bayer Healthcare] in 50 mL of normal saline), 5 mL of iopamidol 41 % [Isovue-M-200; Bracco Diagnostics], and 5 mL of preservative-free lidocaine 1 %) is injected (Fig. 24.1b). Care is taken to avoid intramuscular injection, which can be distinguished on MRI by feathery increased intramuscular T1 and T2 signal (Fig. 24.1c, d).

Following intraarticular injection, MR imaging of the hip is performed with either a 1.5 Tesla (T) or 3 T magnet, utilizing a phased array surface coil. Routine noncontrast and arthrographic protocols are presented in Table 24.1 and include wide field-of-view (FOV) T2-weighted fat-saturated or short time inversion recovery (STIR) images of the entire pelvis, as well as multiplanar T1-, T2-, and PD-weighted imaging that targets the hip of interest. Wide FOV images are crucial for detection of extraarticular abnormalities, such as sacral insufficiency fracture, which may cause pain referred to the hip [5] (Tables 24.1, 24.2, and 24.3).

Relevant Imaging Anatomy

The bony hip is comprised of the acetabulum and proximal femur. The acetabulum itself is comprised of three bones (ilium, ischium, and pubis), which in skeletally immature patients are joined by the triradiate cartilage. The majority of the articular surface of the acetabulum is covered by articular cartilage (Fig. 24.2a, b). The coverage of the acetabulum is increased by the presence of a fibrocartilaginous labrum (Fig. 24.2a), which extends anteriorly, superiorly, and posteriorly. The labrum is incomplete inferiorly, where it merges with the transverse acetabular ligament (Fig. 24.2a, c). In most cross-sectional planes, the labrum demonstrates a

S.C. Sampath, MD, PhD, MPhil • S.C. Sampath, MD, PhD, MPhil
W.E. Palmer, MD (✉)
Division of Musculoskeletal Imaging and Intervention, Department of Radiology, Massachusetts General Hospital, 55 Fruit St., Yawkey Bldg. 6060, Suite 6E, Boston, MA 02114, USA
e-mail: srinathsc@gmail.com; sriharisc@gmail.com; wpalmer@partners.org

J.C. McCarthy et al. (eds.), *Hip Joint Restoration*, DOI 10.1007/978-1-4614-0694-5_24

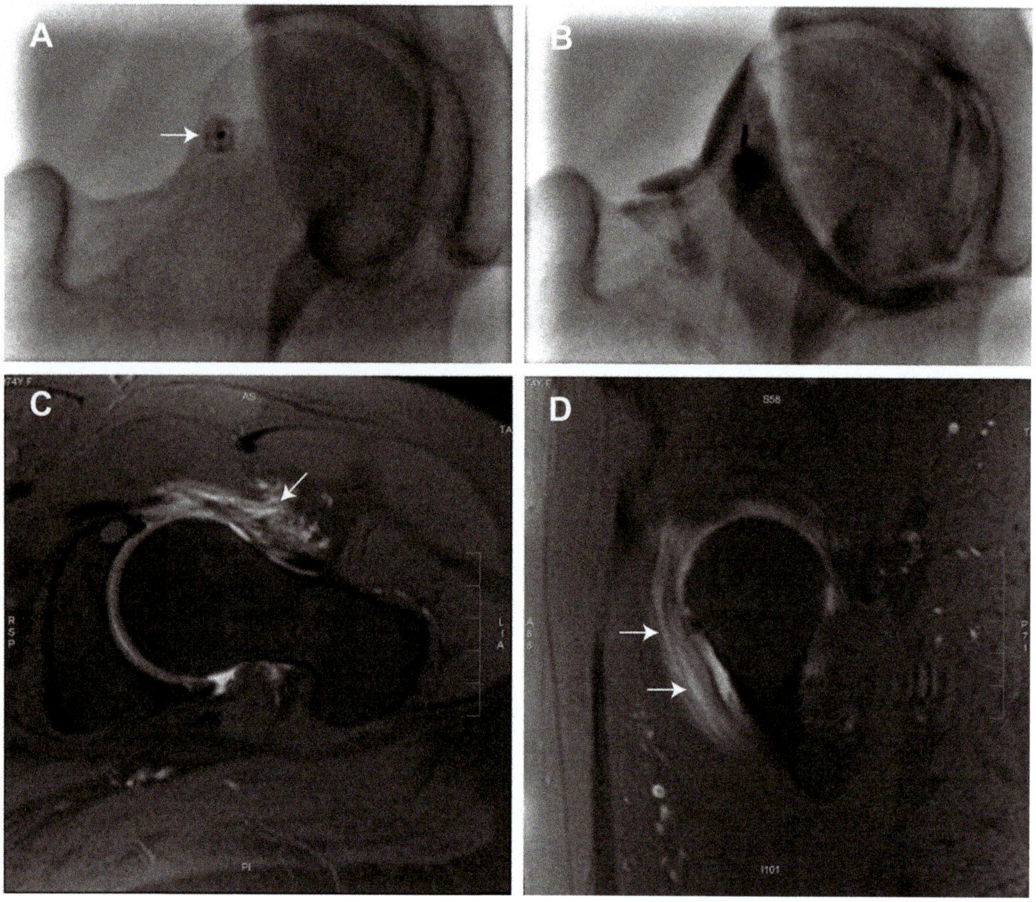

Fig. 24.1 MR arthrography. (**a**, **b**) Frontal fluoroscopic images demonstrating correct needle placement at the superolateral quadrant of the femoral head (*arrow*), and normal appearance of intraarticular contrast (**b**). (**c**, **d**) Axial T1-weighted (**c**) or coronal T2-weighted (**d**) fat-saturated arthrographic images demonstrating feathery hyperintensity following inadvertent intramuscular injection

Table 24.1 MR imaging parameters at 1.5-T

Sequence	TR	TE	TI	NEX	Matrix	ST×Sk	FOV	Flip angle
Cor FMPIR	3800	45	150	1	320×192	5×6	360	90
Axial PD	1933	27		2	320×256	4×5	180	90
Cor T1	483	10		1	384×224	4×5	200	90
Cor T2 FS	4150	76		1.5	320×224	4×5	200	90
Sag PD	2267	44		1	320×224	4×5	200	90
Obl ax PD FS	2583	35		1	512×256	4×5	180	90

Table 24.2 MR imaging parameters at 3-T

Sequence	TR	TE	TI	NEX	Matrix	ST×Sk	FOV	Flip angle
Cor FMPIR	4250	48	200	1	320×192	4×4.4	360	120
Axial PD	2730	9		1	256×256	4×4.4	200	140
Cor T1	931	15		2	384×307	4×4.6	199	140
Cor T2 FS	3070	60		1	256×256	4×5	200	150
Sag PD	3500	43		2	384×307	4×4.4	199	170
Obl ax PD FS	4000	69		2	256×154	3×3	200	150

triangular configuration, though a blunted morphology is also common (Fig. 24.2d) [4]. Normal sublabral sulci and other developmental variants have been described, particularly anterosuperiorly and posteroinferiorly [6, 7], which can be mistaken for a labral tear. Articular cartilage partially undercuts the medial boundary of the labrum near the acetabular attachment and can also be confused with a labral tear [8]. Moreover, while the acetabular labrum is usually

Table 24.3 MR arthrogram imaging parameters at 1.5-T

Sequence	TR	TE	NEX	Matrix	ST×Sk	FOV	Flip angle
Ax T2 FS	2250	53	3	320×192	4×4	160	180
Cor T1	660	14	2	320×192	4×4	160	180
Cor T1 FS	563	12	2	320×224	4×4	160	180
Cor T2 FS	2250	53	3	320×192	4×4	160	180
Sag T1 FS	550	11	2	320×192	3.5×3.5	160	180
Obl ax T1 FS	600	15	2	320×192	3.5×3.5	160	180

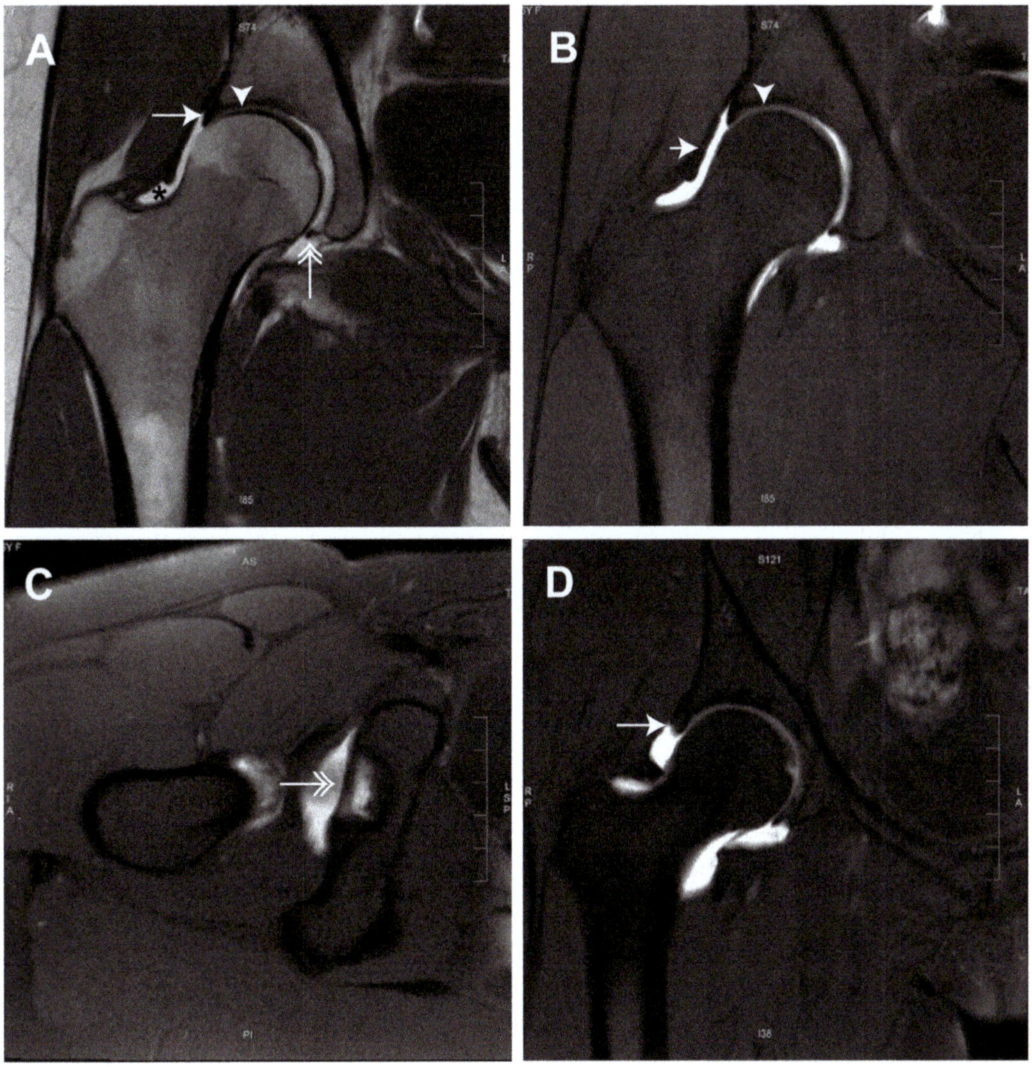

Fig. 24.2 Normal anatomy at MR arthrography. (**a**, **b**) Coronal T1-weighted arthrographic images demonstrating normal appearance of intraarticular contrast (*asterisk*), labrum (*arrow*), articular cartilage (*arrowhead*), and transverse ligament (*double arrowhead*) and hip capsule (*short arrow*). (**c**, **d**) Axial (**c**) or coronal (**d**) T2-weighted fat-saturated arthrographic images demonstrating normal appearance of the transverse ligament (*double arrowhead*) and a blunted but normal appearance of the labrum (*arrow*)

described as uniformly low in signal intensity on all pulse sequences, numerous variations have been described, which may represent age-related changes or artifact [9, 10].

A bony depression known as the acetabular fossa is normally visualized at the medial wall of the acetabulum (Fig. 24.3a) and is not covered by articular cartilage. The acetabular fossa may contain fibrofatty tissue and can fill variably on MR arthrography [11]. The ligamentum teres originates within the acetabular fossa and extends to the fovea of the femoral head and is an uncommon site of injury (Fig. 24.3a) [12]. In addition to the acetabular fossa, a variably cartilage lined, smoothly marginated supraacetabular fossa has been described [13], occurring at the acetabular roof near the 12 o'clock position (Fig. 24.3b).

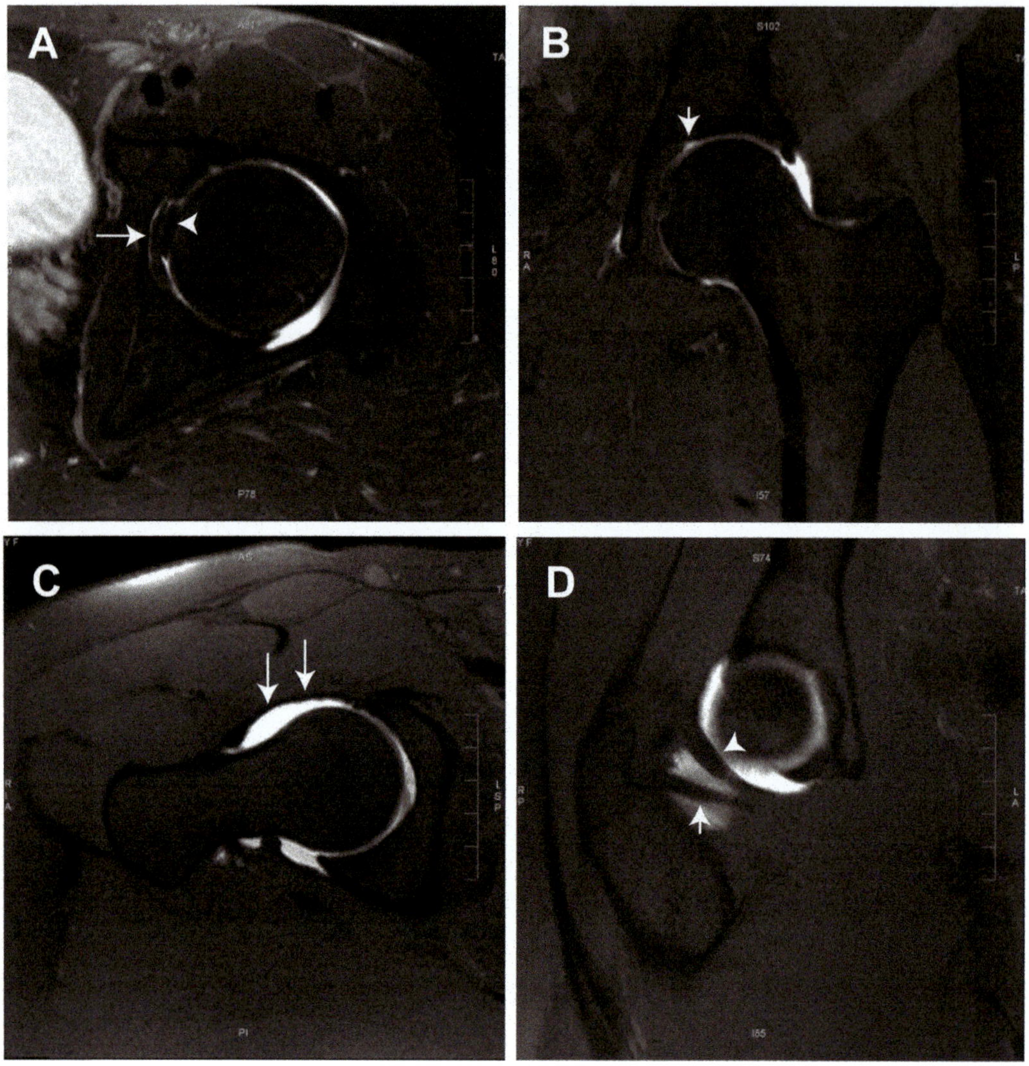

Fig. 24.3 Normal anatomy at MR arthrography. (**a**, **b**) Axial (**a**) or coronal (**b**) T2-weighted fat-saturated arthrographic images demonstrating normal appearance of the acetabular fossa (*arrow*), ligamentum teres (*arrowhead*), and supraacetabular fossa (*short arrow*). (**c**, **d**) Axial (**c**) or coronal (**d**) T2-weighted fat-saturated arthrographic image demonstrating normal appearance of the iliofemoral ligament (*arrowheads*), ischiofemoral ligament (*short arrow*), and zona orbicularis (*arrowhead*)

This is most often seen in the third and fourth decades and likely represents a developmental variant. A second entity known as the stellate crease is also variably appreciated on MR images adjacent to the supraacetabular fossa or acetabular notch [14] and may reflect normal development-associated scarring of the articular cartilage, possibly related to closing of the supraacetabular fossa.

The joint capsule of the hip is reinforced by the iliofemoral, pubofemoral, and ischiofemoral ligaments [15]. Of these the iliofemoral is the strongest ligament and is located anteriorly (Fig. 24.3c), extending in an inverted Y configuration from the lateral margin of the ilium to the anterior base of the femoral neck. The pubofemoral ligament originates anteriorly from the iliopubic eminence and superior ramus of the pubis and blends with the iliofemoral ligament and capsule as it passes inferolaterally, attaching to intertrochanteric line. Finally the ischiofemoral ligament originates posteriorly on the ischium and inserts onto the intertrochanteric line and zona orbicularis (Fig. 24.3d), a ringlike area of capsular thickening and tightening encircling the femoral neck.

As a result of the progressive fatty replacement of the normal erythropoietic marrow seen in childhood, normal bone marrow signal intensity varies by age and location within the femur. Yellow marrow is typically seen within the medullary space of the proximal femoral epiphysis and greater trochanter, which therefore demonstrate increased signal on nonfat-saturated T1-weighted images; the remainder of the proximal femur may contain red marrow and therefore demonstrate relatively decreased signal intensity on T1-weighted images [16]. A small amount of joint fluid can be seen within a normal joint on non-arthrographic MR images.

Pathological Disorders

Intraarticular

Intraarticular pathology includes abnormalities of the cartilage, labrum, proximal femur, and joint space.

Osteoarthritic change is extremely common in the hip and manifests as joint space narrowing (due to loss of articular cartilage over the superior joint space), subchondral sclerosis and/or cystic change, and osteophytosis (Fig. 24.4a, b). Subchondral bone marrow edema is a common associated finding in the setting of osteoarthritis.

The cartilage coverage of the hip is thin, usually only 1–2 mm [17], likely contributing to the lower than expected sensitivity of MR imaging for the detection of focal chondral defects [18, 19]. Focal osteochondral injuries may manifest on arthrographic images as T1 hyperintense contrast material undercutting the cartilage, indicating partial or full-thickness defects, delamination, flap formation, and fissuring (Fig. 24.4c, d). Focal cartilage lesions are most commonly encountered superolaterally within the acetabulum but can occur in all quadrants [2].

The multiplanar orientation of the labrum necessitates evaluation in all three planes of imaging, with the anterior and posterior labrum best assessed on oblique axial or sagittal images, and the superolateral labrum on oblique axial or coronal images. The oblique axial imaging plane has been advocated for improved labral visualization [20] and is routinely acquired at our institution. The labrum is most commonly torn superolaterally [6, 21], though an increased incidence of posterosuperior tear has been reported in younger patients and Eastern demographics. It has also been

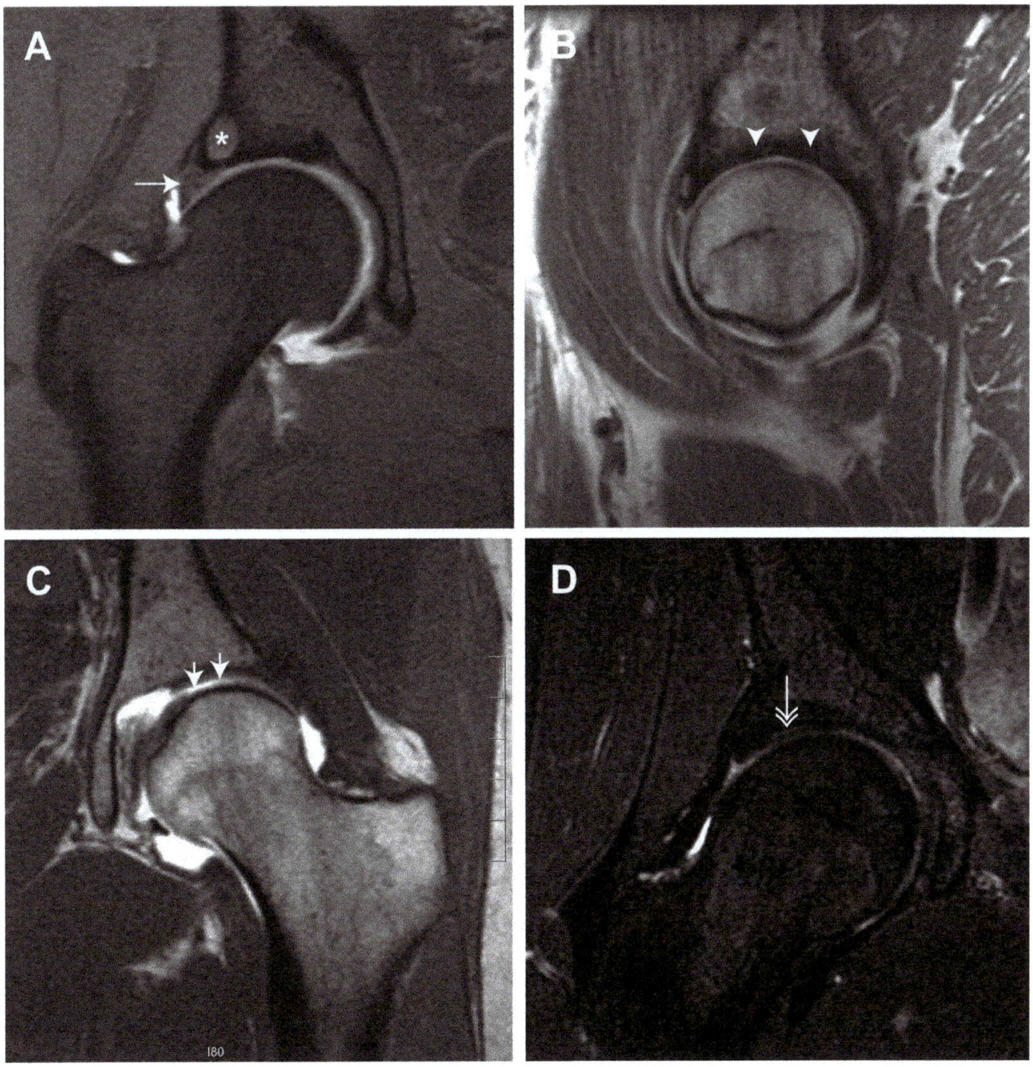

Fig. 24.4 Intraarticular pathology. (**a**) Coronal T1-weighted fat-saturated arthrographic image demonstrating degenerative change within the labrum (*arrow*) and cystic change at the superolateral acetabulum (*asterisk*). (**b**) Sagittal T1-weighted arthrographic image demonstrating subchondral sclerosis. (**c**) Coronal T1-weighted arthrographic image demonstrating full-thickness cartilage defect (*short arrows*). (**d**) Coronal T2-weighted fat-saturated arthrographic image demonstrating T2 hyperintense line indicative of cartilage delamination

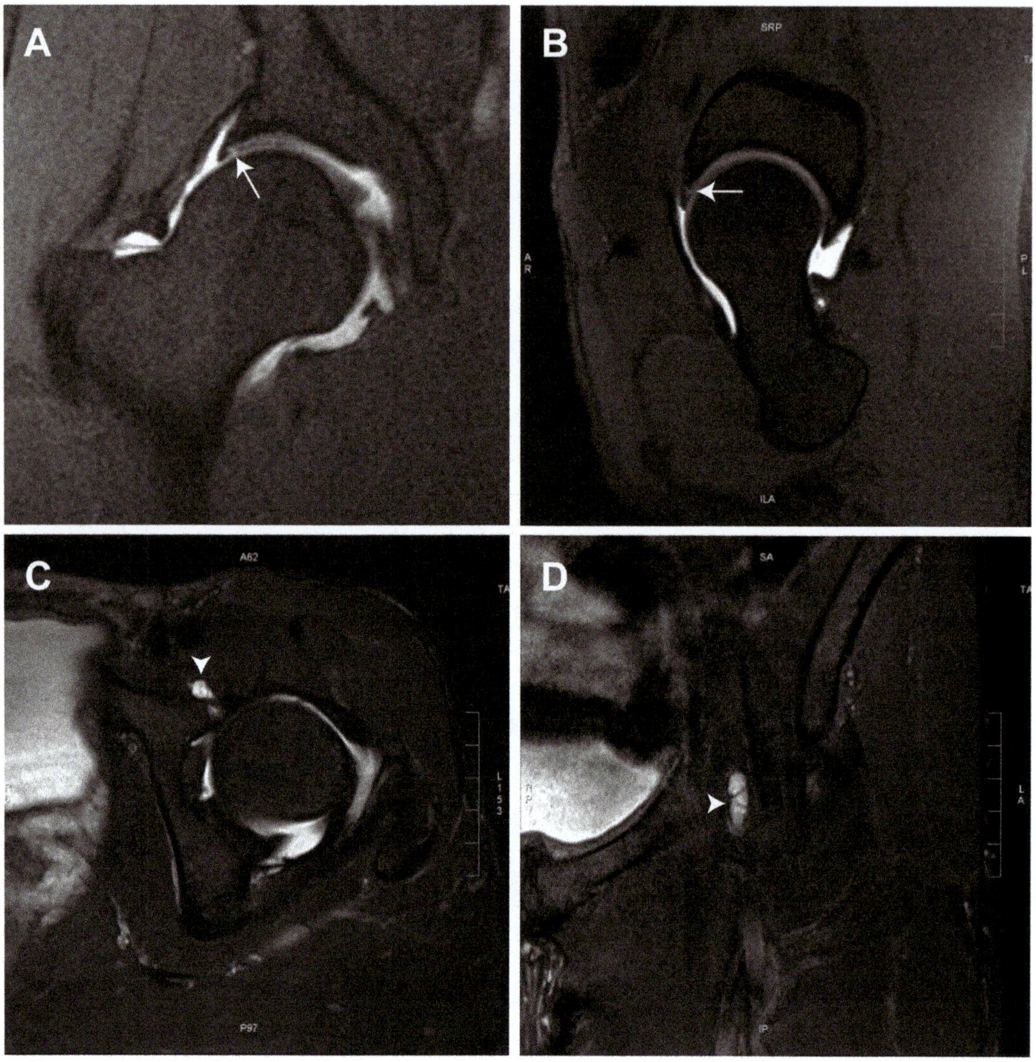

Fig. 24.5 Intraarticular pathology. (**a, b**) Coronal T1 (**a**)- or oblique axial T2 (**b**)-weighted fat-saturated arthrographic images demonstrating linear signal abnormality indicative of labral tear. (**c, d**) Axial (**c**) or coronal (**d**) T2-weighted fat-saturated arthrographic images demonstrating paralabral cyst (*arrowhead*)

recently reported that isolated anteromedial tears occur, more frequently in females. A labral tear manifests on noncontrast imaging by linear decreased (T1) or increased (T2) signal extending to the labral surface along the interface with articular cartilage (Fig. 24.5a, b). The presence of a paralabral cyst (Fig. 24.5c, d) should prompt close inspection for an associated labral tear. Like other fibrocartilaginous structures, the labrum is susceptible to degeneration without accompanying tear, which may be seen as increased intrasubstance signal (Fig. 24.4a) [9]. MR arthrography significantly increases the sensitivity and specificity for true labral tear [22], where tears can be seen as areas of abnormal increased T1 intensity extending to the labral surface.

MR arthrography also enhances detection of intraarticular filling defects, as can be seen in the setting of synovitis, synovial (osteo)chondromatosis, and pigmented villonodular synovitis (PVNS). Loose bodies are defined by the visualization of fluid (either joint fluid or contrast) surrounding a focal bony or cartilaginous structure. In the setting of synovial osteochondromatosis, multiple loose bodies of similar sizes are visualized (Fig. 24.6a, b), the signal intensity of which may vary based on their degree of mineralization [23]. These bodies may eventually give rise to osseous erosions involving the femur or acetabulum (Fig. 24.6b). PVNS is characterized by synovial proliferation causing focal or diffuse intraarticular soft tissue masses, which as a result of the accumulation of hemoglobin degradation products classically displays decreased signal intensity on most pulse sequences (Fig. 24.6c, d), particularly those susceptible to field inhomogeneity (i.e., gradient echo sequences) [24, 25].

Abnormalities of the femoral head or neck can lead to hip pain. Such abnormalities include degenerative changes as

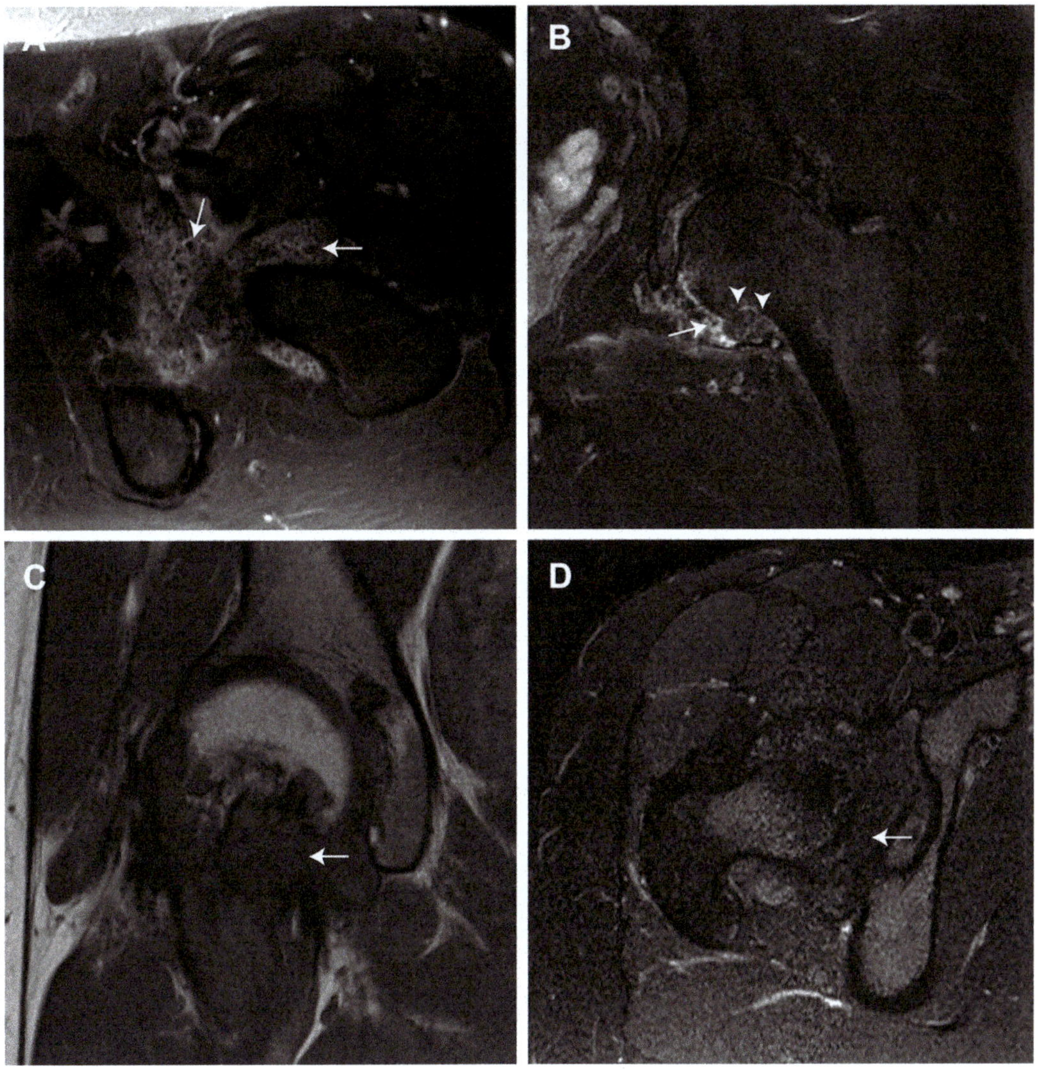

Fig. 24.6 Intraarticular pathology. (**a**, **b**) Axial (**a**) or coronal (**b**) T2-weighted fat-saturated arthrographic images demonstrating multiple small intraarticular loose bodies in the setting of synovial chondromatosis. Erosion at the femoral neck is also noted ((**b**), *arrowheads*). (**c**, **d**) Coronal T1- (**a**) or axial (**b**) T2-weighted fat-saturated arthrographic images demonstrating low-intensity intraarticular masses causing erosions (*arrows*) in the setting of PVNS

described above, stress reaction/fracture, subchondral fracture, and avascular necrosis. Bony fractures (both stress and traumatic) are often noted on T2-weighted fat-saturated images, where geographic bone marrow edema is seen. Stress reaction may be differentiated from stress fracture by the absence of a T1 and T2 hypointense line in the former (Fig. 24.7a, b). Stress fracture can be subdivided into fatigue fracture (abnormal stress on normal bone) and insufficiency fracture (normal stress on abnormal bone). In addition to intraarticular locations, such insufficiency fractures often can be seen within the sacrum (Fig. 24.7c). Subchondral fracture is distinguished by the presence of a distinct low-intensity fracture paralleling the cortical surface (Fig. 24.7d), with adjacent bone marrow edema.

Avascular necrosis of the femoral head classically manifests on MR in the form of a "double-line" sign, with apposing inner hyperintense and outer hypointense lines on T2-weighted images [26], which can be accompanied in later stages by collapse of the articular surface [27, 28]. In addition to stress reaction, bone marrow edema within the femur in the absence of a hypointense line can be seen in the setting of transient osteoporosis of the hip [29, 30], itself thought to represent a form of insufficiency injury or ischemic insult; this entity can further be distinguished from AVN by the absence of a subchondral distribution and the absence of risk factors for AVN [31].

Visualization of joint fluid outside of the articular space is diagnostic of a capsular defect. The identification of a capsular defect is aided by the distention of the joint capsule with intraarticular contrast (Fig. 24.8). Image registration between planes can help to pinpoint the area of capsular discontinuity.

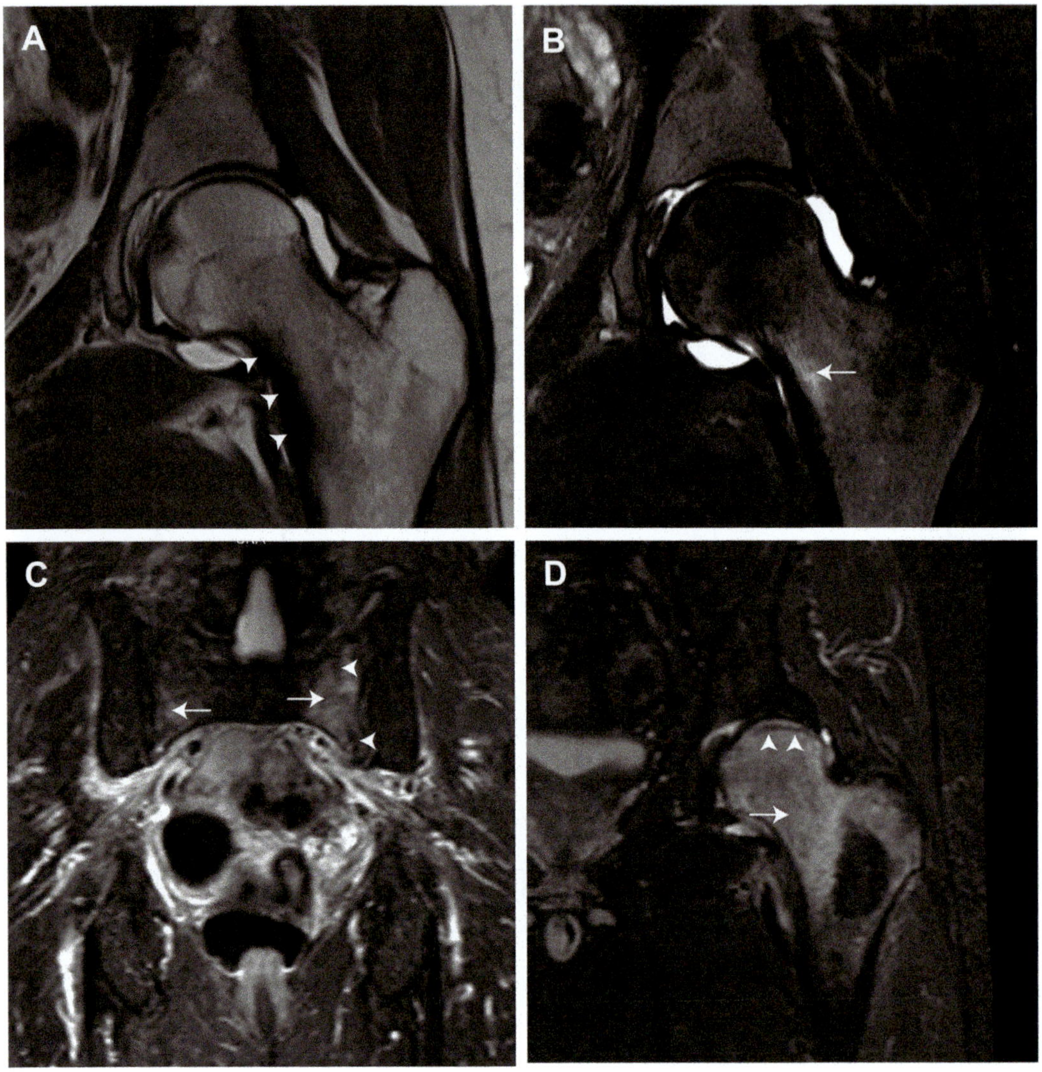

Fig. 24.7 Intraarticular pathology. (**a**, **b**) Coronal T1-weighted (**a**) or T2-weighted fat-saturated (**b**) arthrographic images demonstrating sclerosis (*arrowheads*) and mild edema (*arrow*) in the setting of stress reaction. (**c**) Coronal T2-weighted fat-saturated image demonstrating edema (*arrows*) and low-intensity line (*arrowheads*) indicative of stress fracture. (**d**) Coronal T2-weighted fat-saturated image demonstrating geographic bone marrow edema (*arrow*) and subchondral fracture (*arrowheads*)

Extraarticular

Extraarticular pathologies leading to hip pain include abnormalities of the bursae, regional tendons, and sacrum. Additionally, various forms of impingement have been described about the hip, some of which may contribute to hip pain in the young patient population.

MRI is highly sensitive for the detection of bursitis. Three main bursae are seen about the hip: the greater trochanteric, iliopsoas, and ischiogluteal bursae [32]. These are often collapsed and therefore not visible on MR imaging but can become visible when they accumulate T2-hyperintense fluid in the setting of repetitive trauma or inflammation (Fig. 24.9). Of note, approximately 15% of patients will demonstrate communication between the joint space and the iliopsoas bursa, a normal variant [33], and a distended iliopsoas bursal collection may extend into the pelvis (Fig. 24.9d). In addition to mechanical bursitis, bursal and/or intraarticular fluid collections (so-called pseudotumors) may be seen in setting of certain classes of hip arthroplasty [34], where they may display variable signal intensity and be associated with abnormal soft tissue components.

Close attention should be paid to the tendons about the hip to examine for the presence of tendinopathy or tearing; commonly injured tendons include those of the gluteus minimus/medius, iliopsoas, hamstrings, and rectus femoris [35]. Tendons are typically hypointense on both T1- and T2-weighted images, and tendinopathy is therefore visualized as focal thickening and/or increased signal intensity within a tendon, with partial or complete tear indicated by increased (near-fluid) signal intensity and varying degrees of fiber discontinuity or avulsion from the osseous attachment site (Fig. 24.10a, b).

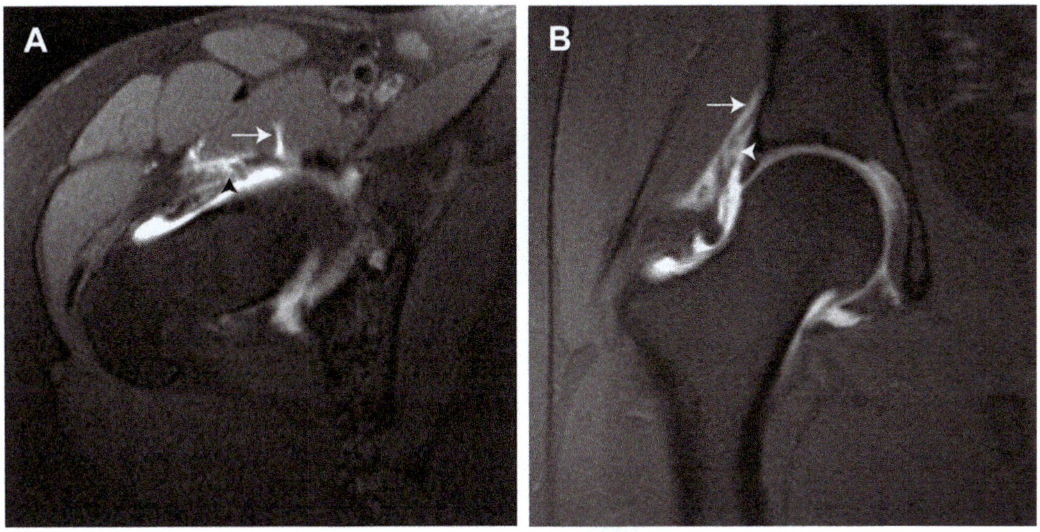

Fig. 24.8 Capsular defect. (**a**, **b**) Axial T2-weighted (**a**) or coronal T1-weighted (**b**) fat-saturated arthrographic images demonstrating capsular irregularity (*arrowhead*) and extraarticular contrast (*arrow*) indicative of capsular defect

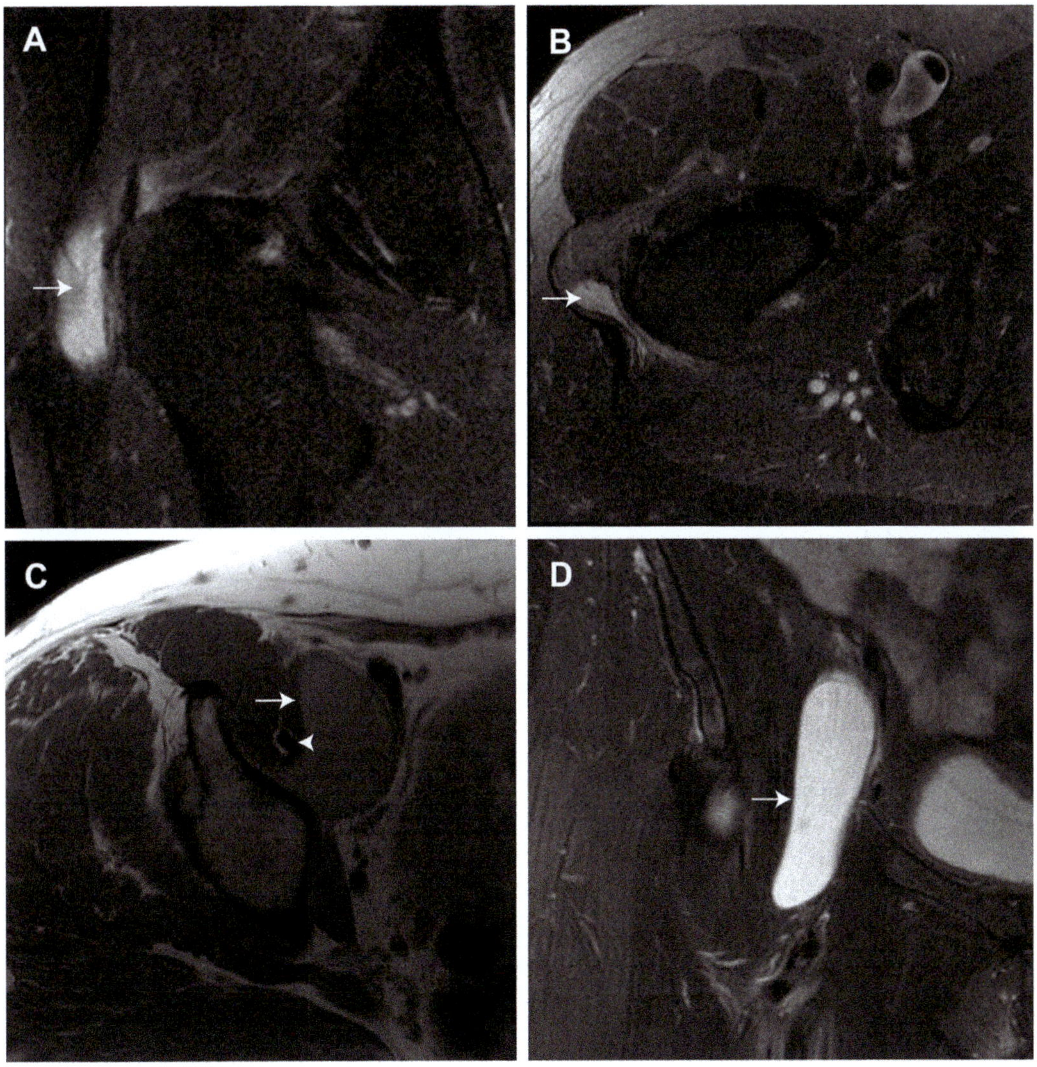

Fig. 24.9 Extraarticular pathology. (**a**, **b**) Axial (**a**) or coronal (**b**) T2-weighted fat-saturated images demonstrating abnormal trochanteric bursal fluid (*arrows*), indicative of bursitis. (**c**, **d**) Axial PD (**a**) or coronal T2-weighted fat-saturated (**b**) images demonstrating abnormal iliopsoas bursal fluid. *Arrowhead* indicated iliopsoas tendon

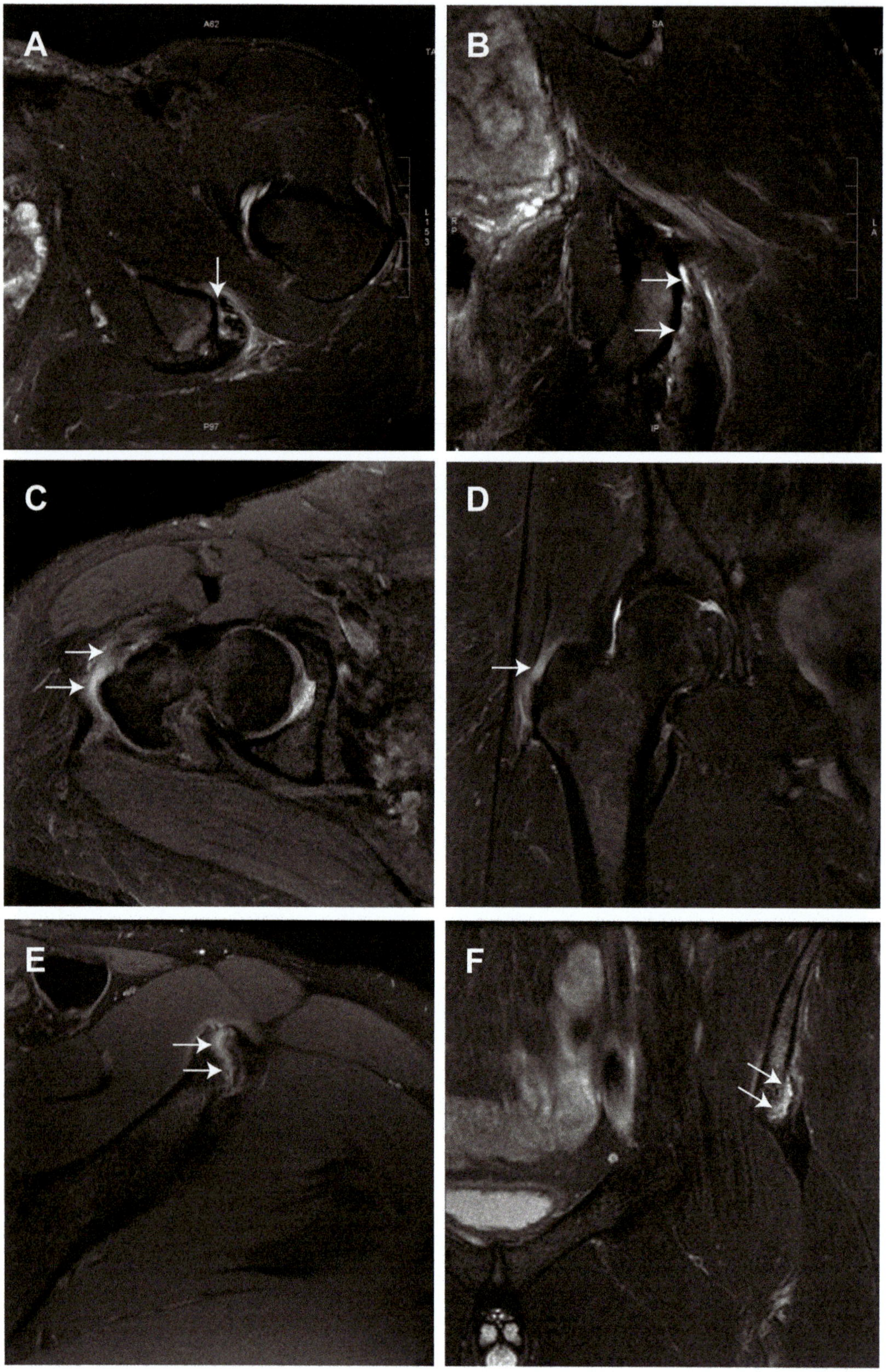

Fig. 24.10 Extraarticular pathology. (**a**, **b**) Axial (**a**) or coronal (**b**) T2-weighted fat-saturated images demonstrating fluid signal undercutting the common hamstrings insertion, consistent with partial tear. (**c**, **d**) Axial (**c**) or coronal (**d**) T2-weighted fat-saturated images demonstrating increased signal adjacent to the greater trochanter in the setting of gluteal tendon partial tear. (**e**, **f**) Axial (**e**) or coronal (**f**) T2-weighted fat-saturated images demonstrating fluid signal (*arrows*) undercutting the insertion of the direct head of the rectus femoris at the anterior inferior iliac spine, compatible with high-grade tear

Additional signs of abductor tendon injury include T2 hyperintensity superior or lateral to the greater trochanter (Fig. 24.10c, d) [36]. The origins of the rectus femoris at both the anterior inferior iliac spine (direct head; Fig. 24.10e, f) and acetabular rim (reflected head) should be carefully scrutinized. Care must be taken in interpretation of linear increased signal intensity within the iliopsoas tendon as a tear, as the prevalence of accessory iliacus tendons on MR arthrograms has been reported as high as 66 % [10].

As mentioned previously, it is crucial to inspect wide field-of-view images for evidence of fracture or other bone marrow abnormality outside of the hip proper, as insufficiency fracture commonly involves the superior acetabulum, sacrum (Fig. 24.6c), intertrochanteric region, or pubic rami [37]. However, areas of marrow edema associated with subcortical cysts or other sequela of degenerative osteoarthritis (for instance, adjacent to the sacroiliac joints) should not be mistaken for fractures.

Various forms of impingement have been described as causes of pain about the hip, including femoral acetabular impingement (FAI) and ischiofemoral impingement. As these entities have been discussed extensively in recent reviews [38, 39], they are only briefly mentioned here. FAI has been described as a cause of early onset osteoarthritis and has been divided into cam and pincer types, though these two forms most commonly coexist. Cam-type FAI is characterized by decreased osseous offset of the femoral head-neck junction, with resulting abnormal contact between the head-neck junction and acetabular rim. Pincer-type FAI is characterized by overcoverage of the femoral head by the acetabulum and can occur in the setting of acetabular retroversion or protrusio acetabuli. A variety of plain film and MRI signs have been described for both forms of FAI, which eventually result in abnormalities of the anterosuperior cartilage, labrum, and osseous head-neck junction [39].

Ischiofemoral impingement has been reported as a cause of hip pain and is defined by narrowing of the space between the ischial tuberosity and lesser trochanter [38]. Several anatomic parameters have been described to accompany these findings, including decreased ischiofemoral (≤17 mm) or quadratus femoris (≤8 mm) spaces [40]. Impingement between the ischium and lesser trochanter may result in injury to the quadratus femoris and hamstrings tendons, manifesting as increased T2 signal and/or fiber discontinuity (Fig. 24.11).

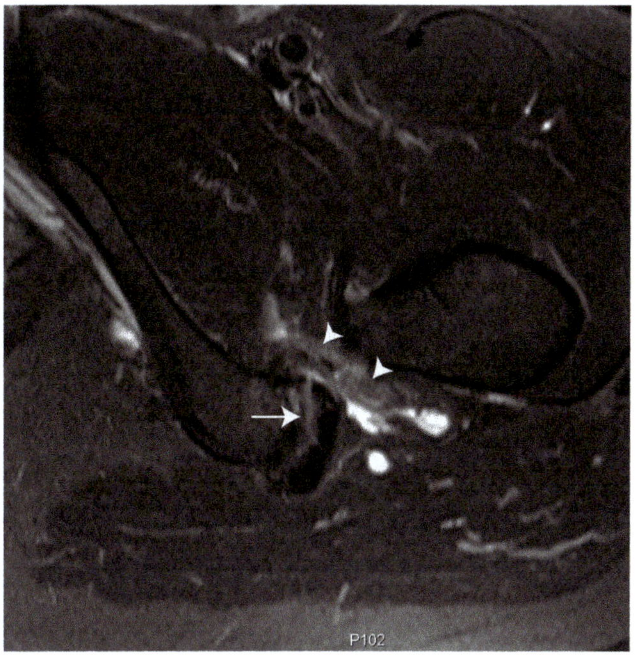

Fig. 24.11 Extraarticular pathology. Axial T2-weighted fat-saturated image demonstrating edema within the quadratus femoris (*arrowheads*) and partial tear of the common hamstrings tendon (*arrow*) in the setting of ischiofemoral impingement

Conclusion

Conventional and arthrographic MRI have proven useful in the evaluation of hip pain and the diagnosis of both intra- and extraarticular abnormalities. MR imaging can simultaneously evaluate bone marrow and soft tissues, enabling specific and cost-effective management of numerous musculoskeletal disorders.

References

1. Tibor LM, Sekiya JK. Differential diagnosis of pain around the hip joint. Arthroscopy. 2008;24(12):1407–21.
2. Schmid MR, Notzli HP, Zanetti M, Wyss TF, Hodler J. Cartilage lesions in the hip: diagnostic effectiveness of MR arthrography. Radiology. 2003;226(2):382–6.
3. Freedman BA, Potter BK, Dinauer PA, Giuliani JR, Kuklo TR, Murphy KP. Prognostic value of magnetic resonance arthrography for Czerny stage II and III acetabular labral tears. Arthroscopy. 2006;22(7):742–7.
4. Llopis E, Fernandez E, Cerezal L. MR and CT arthrography of the hip. Semin Musculoskelet Radiol. 2012;16(1):42–56 [Review].
5. Featherstone T. Magnetic resonance imaging in the diagnosis of sacral stress fracture. Br J Sports Med. 1999;33(4):276–7 [Case Reports].
6. Dinauer PA, Murphy KP, Carroll JF. Sublabral sulcus at the posteroinferior acetabulum: a potential pitfall in MR arthrography diagnosis of acetabular labral tears. AJR Am J Roentgenol. 2004;183(6):1745–53.
7. Studler U, Kalberer F, Leunig M, Zanetti M, Hodler J, Dora C, et al. MR arthrography of the hip: differentiation between an anterior sublabral recess as a normal variant and a labral tear. Radiology. 2008;249(3):947–54.
8. Czerny C, Hofmann S, Urban M, Tschauner C, Neuhold A, Pretterklieber M, et al. MR arthrography of the adult acetabular capsular-labral complex: correlation with surgery and anatomy. AJR Am J Roentgenol. 1999;173(2):345–9 [Comparative Study].
9. Abe I, Harada Y, Oinuma K, Kamikawa K, Kitahara H, Morita F, et al. Acetabular labrum: abnormal findings at MR imaging in asymptomatic hips. Radiology. 2000;216(2):576–81.
10. DuBois DF, Omar IM. MR imaging of the hip: normal anatomic variants and imaging pitfalls. Magn Reson Imaging Clin N Am. 2010;18(4):663–74 [Review].

11. Chang CY, Huang AJ. MR imaging of normal hip anatomy. Magn Reson Imaging Clin N Am. 2013;21(1):1–19.
12. Gray AJ, Villar RN. The ligamentum teres of the hip: an arthroscopic classification of its pathology. Arthroscopy. 1997;13(5):575–8.
13. Dietrich TJ, Suter A, Pfirrmann CW, Dora C, Fucentese SF, Zanetti M. Supraacetabular fossa (pseudodefect of acetabular cartilage): frequency at MR arthrography and comparison of findings at MR arthrography and arthroscopy. Radiology. 2012;263(2):484–91 [Comparative Study].
14. Keene GS, Villar RN. Arthroscopic anatomy of the hip: an in vivo study. Arthroscopy. 1994;10(4):392–9.
15. Wagner FV, Negrao JR, Campos J, Ward SR, Haghighi P, Trudell DJ, et al. Capsular ligaments of the hip: anatomic, histologic, and positional study in cadaveric specimens with MR arthrography. Radiology. 2012;263(1):189–98.
16. Chatha DS, Arora R. MR imaging of the normal hip. Magn Reson Imaging Clin N Am. 2005;13(4):605–15 [Review].
17. Hong RJ, Hughes TH, Gentili A, Chung CB. Magnetic resonance imaging of the hip. J Magn Reson Imaging. 2008;27(3):435–45 [Review].
18. Neumann G, Mendicuti AD, Zou KH, Minas T, Coblyn J, Winalski CS, et al. Prevalence of labral tears and cartilage loss in patients with mechanical symptoms of the hip: evaluation using MR arthrography. Osteoarthritis Cartilage. 2007;15(8):909–17.
19. Mintz DN, Hooper T, Connell D, Buly R, Padgett DE, Potter HG. Magnetic resonance imaging of the hip: detection of labral and chondral abnormalities using noncontrast imaging. Arthroscopy. 2005;21(4):385–93 [Comparative Study].
20. Ziegert AJ, Blankenbaker DG, De Smet AA, Keene JS, Shinki K, Fine JP. Comparison of standard hip MR arthrographic imaging planes and sequences for detection of arthroscopically proven labral tear. AJR Am J Roentgenol. 2009;192(5):1397–400 [Comparative Study].
21. Lage LA, Patel JV, Villar RN. The acetabular labral tear: an arthroscopic classification. Arthroscopy. 1996;12(3):269–72.
22. Toomayan GA, Holman WR, Major NM, Kozlowicz SM, Vail TP. Sensitivity of MR arthrography in the evaluation of acetabular labral tears. AJR Am J Roentgenol. 2006;186(2):449–53.
23. Murphey MD, Vidal JA, Fanburg-Smith JC, Gajewski DA. Imaging of synovial chondromatosis with radiologic-pathologic correlation. Radiographics. 2007;27(5):1465–88 [Review].
24. Hughes TH, Sartoris DJ, Schweitzer ME, Resnick DL. Pigmented villonodular synovitis: MRI characteristics. Skeletal Radiol. 1995;24(1):7–12.
25. Cotten A, Flipo RM, Chastanet P, Desvigne-Noulet MC, Duquesnoy B, Delcambre B. Pigmented villonodular synovitis of the hip: review of radiographic features in 58 patients. Skeletal Radiol. 1995;24(1):1–6 [Multicenter Study].
26. Mitchell DG, Joseph PM, Fallon M, Hickey W, Kressel HY, Rao VM, et al. Chemical-shift MR imaging of the femoral head: an in vitro study of normal hips and hips with avascular necrosis. AJR Am J Roentgenol. 1987;148(6):1159–64.
27. Mitchell DG, Rao VM, Dalinka MK, Spritzer CE, Alavi A, Steinberg ME, et al. Femoral head avascular necrosis: correlation of MR imaging, radiographic staging, radionuclide imaging, and clinical findings. Radiology. 1987;162(3):709–15 [Comparative Study].
28. Lafforgue P, Dahan E, Chagnaud C, Schiano A, Kasbarian M, Acquaviva PC. Early-stage avascular necrosis of the femoral head: MR imaging for prognosis in 31 cases with at least 2 years of follow-up. Radiology. 1993;187(1):199–204.
29. Vande Berg BC, Malghem JJ, Lecouvet FE, Jamart J, Maldague BE. Idiopathic bone marrow edema lesions of the femoral head: predictive value of MR imaging findings. Radiology. 1999;212(2): 527–35.
30. Hayes CW, Conway WF, Daniel WW. MR imaging of bone marrow edema pattern: transient osteoporosis, transient bone marrow edema syndrome, or osteonecrosis. Radiographics. 1993;13(5): 1001–11. [Review]; Discussion 12.
31. Guerra JJ, Steinberg ME. Distinguishing transient osteoporosis from avascular necrosis of the hip. J Bone Joint Surg Am. 1995;77(4):616–24 [Review].
32. Bencardino JT, Palmer WE. Imaging of hip disorders in athletes. Radiol Clin North Am. 2002;40(2):267–87. [Review]; vi–vii.
33. Petersilge CA. From the RSNA Refresher Courses. Radiological Society of North America. Chronic adult hip pain: MR arthrography of the hip. Radiographics. 2000;20 Spec No:S43–52.
34. Campe CB, Palmer WE. MR imaging of metal-on-metal hip prostheses. Magn Reson Imaging Clin N Am. 2013;21(1):155–68.
35. Petchprapa CN, Bencardino JT. Tendon injuries of the hip. Magn Reson Imaging Clin N Am. 2013;21(1):75–96.
36. Cvitanic O, Henzie G, Skezas N, Lyons J, Minter J. MRI diagnosis of tears of the hip abductor tendons (gluteus medius and gluteus minimus). AJR Am J Roentgenol. 2004;182(1):137–43 [Evaluation Studies].
37. Khoury NJ, Birjawi GA, Chaaya M, Hourani MH. Use of limited MR protocol (coronal STIR) in the evaluation of patients with hip pain. Skeletal Radiol. 2003;32(10):567–74 [Comparative Study Evaluation Studies].
38. Taneja AK, Bredella MA, Torriani M. Ischiofemoral impingement. Magn Reson Imaging Clin N Am. 2013;21(1):65–73.
39. Bredella MA, Ulbrich EJ, Stoller DW, Anderson SE. Femoroacetabular impingement. Magn Reson Imaging Clin N Am. 2013;21(1):45–64.
40. Torriani M, Souto SC, Thomas BJ, Ouellette H, Bredella MA. Ischiofemoral impingement syndrome: an entity with hip pain and abnormalities of the quadratus femoris muscle. AJR Am J Roentgenol. 2009;193(1):186–90.

Imaging the Previously Operated Hip

25

Philip J. Glassner and Joseph C. McCarthy

Introduction

The volume of arthroscopic surgery of the hip has increased dramatically over the past decade for multiple hip disorders, including labral tears, chondral damage, femoroacetabular impingement (FAI), synovial chondromatosis, loose bodies, foreign body removal, and crystalline hip arthropathy [1, 2]. For primary hip arthroscopies, in the absence of joint arthritic changes, patients generally have excellent outcomes with return to active lifestyles. Numerous papers have shown 90–93 % good to excellent results [3–6] with resolution of mechanical symptoms and improved modified Harris hip scores [7, 8]. Still, there are patients who never fully experience relief following surgery, or develop recurrent symptoms of hip pathology. This may be from a new injury or due to an inadequate surgical procedure. Further, studies have shown that patients with degenerative arthritis (more specifically Grade 3–4 cartilage wear on the Outerbridge classification) have significantly worse outcomes than those with isolated labral tears and/or only mild chondral pathology [9–11].

Long-term studies have demonstrated the condition of articular cartilage to be the most important factor related to long-term outcome [4]. Several studies have correlated the findings of magnetic resonance arthrography (MRA) with primary hip arthroscopy, demonstrating sensitivity of 71–100 % [12–17] and specificity of 44–100 % [15, 18, 19]. Byrd and colleagues demonstrated an improved sensitivity of MRA compared to MRI using arthroscopic hip findings as the gold standard, improving the rate of false-negative results from 42 % with MRI to 8 % with MRA [20]. Further, for other orthopedic diagnoses, studies have evaluated the utility of MRA compared to surgical findings at revision knee arthroscopy (evaluating menisci and chondral damage/repair) [21–24] and revision shoulder arthroscopy [25, 26] (evaluating rotator cuff and labral pathology), but there is limited data on the prognostic value of MRA before revision hip arthroscopy.

There have been some recent studies that evaluated the utility of MRA in the diagnosis and treatment of ongoing or recurrent symptoms in patients who have had a prior hip arthroscopy. There have also been some recent studies that evaluated the use of 3D Cat Scans (CT) and delayed gadolinium-enhanced magnetic resonance imaging of cartilage (dGEMRIC) scans for an attempt at more precise evaluation of bone and cartilage defects of the hip [27, 28]. This chapter will review this data and how it can be used to better care for hip arthroscopy patients.

Data from Imaging Studies

Following a thorough patient history and examination, standard AP and frog-lateral radiographs should be the initial evaluation of any patient who has recurrent or ongoing symptoms of hip pain after hip arthroscopy. At times a false profile view to assess anterior femoral head coverage can be useful. This is taken standing, with the affected hip against the cassette, the ipsilateral foot parallel to the cassette, and the pelvis rotated 65° from the plane of the cassette. Ideally, these images should be compared to any radiographs taken prior to the original hip arthroscopy to assess for any change. If there has been a substantial progression of degenerative joint disease, with narrowing of the joint space, osteophytes, or subchondral cysts, then no further imaging may be necessary. In these patients with worsening cartilage wear, it is at times

P.J. Glassner, MD (✉)
Hunterdon Orthopaedic Institute, 6 Sand Hill Rd., Suite 102, Flemington, NJ 08822, USA
e-mail: philip.glassner@gmail.com

J.C. McCarthy
Kaplan Joint Center, Newton-Wellesley Hospital, Green Bldg, Suite 361, 2000 Washington St., Newton, MA 02462, USA

Department of Orthopedic Surgery, Massachusetts General Hospital, Boston, MA, USA
e-mail: JCMCCARTHY1@PARTNERS.ORG; JCMCCARTHY1@mgh.harvard.edu

J.C. McCarthy et al. (eds.), *Hip Joint Restoration*, DOI 10.1007/978-1-4614-0694-5_25

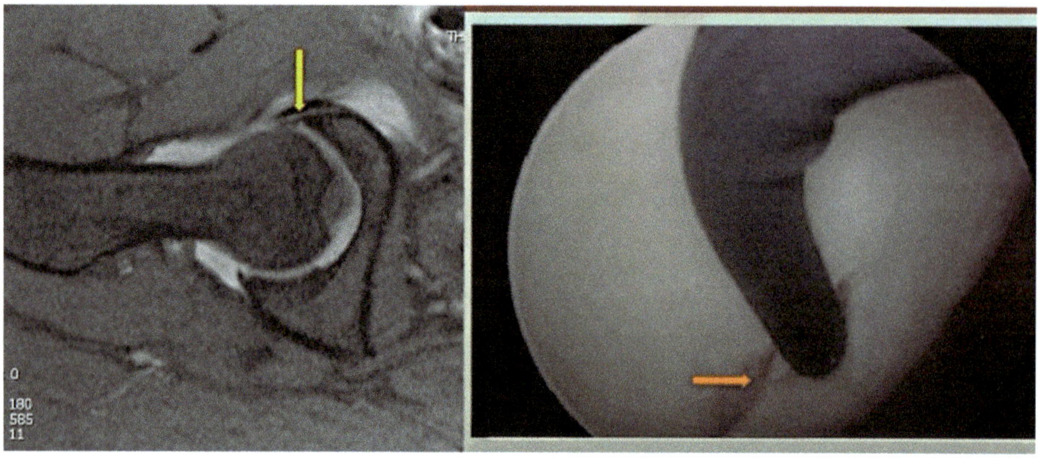

Fig. 25.1 An axial oblique T1 MRA image showing an anteromedial labral tear (*yellow arrow*), confirmed at the time of arthroscopy (*orange arrow*)

best to manage them with anti-inflammatory medications, exercises, activity modification, and injections with a discussion of a future total hip arthroplasty (THA) as an option. Further, it is always necessary to evaluate the patient for other sources of pain that could be hindering their recovery, such as the knee or spine, or at times an inguinal hernia [29]. When there is no apparent referred source of pain, and no obvious change on basic radiographs, then advanced imaging is necessary.

As noted earlier, plain MRI can be used for evaluation of the painful hip, but studies have shown MRA to increase sensitivity to assess labral and chondral injuries in patients who have not had prior hip surgery. An MRI can show basic muscle pathology in patients with suspected extra-articular pathology or to assess the bone in those patients where there is a concern for avascular necrosis (AVN) of the femoral head [30, 31]. If there is more of a clinical concern for intra-articular pathology, then MRA should be considered.

The standard MRA imaging protocol involves injecting a 15 cm^3 mixture of 0.9 % normal saline, Marcaine 0.5 % with epinephrine, and contrast (i.e., Isovue 300 and Prohance) into the hip joint space, followed by imaging with a 1.5 T, or higher, MR scanner. The following sequences are performed: coronal T1, coronal T1 with fat suppression, coronal T2 with fat suppression, coronal STIR, sagittal oblique T1 with fat suppression, axial proton density with fat suppression, and axial oblique T1 with fat suppression.

There are two recent studies that have assessed the utility of MRA to evaluate labral injury in patients who have had prior hip arthroscopy, and one of these also addressed chondral pathology. The study by Aprato et al. retrospectively reviewed the data on 60 patients who had undergone revision hip arthroscopy at a single center [32]. Patients were split into two groups: Group 1 was 40 patients who had undergone labral debridement or repair at the time of the index procedure; Group 2 was 20 patients (who served as the control) who did not have labral surgery at the time of the index procedure. They sought to determine the accuracy of MRA to identify labral tears at revision hip arthroscopy in Group 1. In regard to identifying labral pathology, they found that the sensitivity was only 53 % in Group 1 as compared to 71 % in Group 2 and that the specificity was 50 % for Group 1 and 92 % for Group 2. The positive predictive value (PPV) was quite similar in both groups, 81 % and 83 %, respectively. However, they found that the negative predictive value (NPV) was only 21 % for Group 1 versus 86 % for Group 2 and that the accuracy was also inferior in Group 1 (53 % as compared to 85 % for Group 2). They concluded that MRA was not a reliable tool for accurate diagnosis of new or recurrent labral tears in patients who have prior labral surgery. This was supported by the fact that of 21 patients who had an MRA read as a labral tear, 17 of these did truly have a labral tear at revision surgery, as compared to the 19 patients who had an MRA read as normal labrum, in which only 4 were actually intact at the time of surgery. In other words, of the 32 patients who had labral tears at the revision surgery, 19 (53 %) were read as normal labrum on MRA (Fig. 25.1).

In a similar study by Glassner and McCarthy, a retrospective review of 70 revision hip arthroscopies (62 patients) was performed to correlate MRA and intraoperative findings in regard to labral and chondral pathology at revision surgery [33]. The labral tears were identified based on location and the cartilage injuries based on location and Outerbridge grade [34]. In regard to labral pathology, the comparison of MRA and intraoperative findings revealed a sensitivity of 82 %, a specificity of 70 %, a PPV of 94 %, and an NPV of 39 %.

This study did show better sensitivity and specificity than the study by Aprato et al., but the positive, and more specifically the negative, predictive values were similar. The similarity in the NPV was demonstrated by 11 patients with an MRA interpretation of a normal labrum, who were all found to have a labral tear intraoperatively. This low NPV is consistent with studies on primary hip arthroscopy, with an NPV of only 13 % in a study by Keeney et al. [35], as compared to 21 and 39 % in the above studies. The reason for the low NPV in the studies of patients who had prior surgery may be due to the patient population of these studies; i.e. patients with a prolonged course of pain and prior hip surgery have a higher likelihood of having intra-articular pathology than the general population, making a true negative MRA result less likely.

In comparing the sensitivities and specificities between these two studies, the study by Aprato showed a sensitivity of only 53 % versus 82 % in the study by Glassner and a specificity of 50 % versus 70 %. The second study is comparable to past studies in evaluating the labrum at primary hip arthroscopy, which have shown a 71–100 % sensitivity [12–17]. Specificity has had a much broader range in prior studies, from 44 to 100 %, making the data comparable for both studies [15, 18, 19]. The reason for the difference in sensitivity is unclear, but could be related to different experience levels of the interpreting radiologists or simply the size and location of the tears, as larger tears would be easier to identify than small tears, and the size of the tear was not addressed in the studies.

In regard to the location of labral pathology, the second study was consistent with findings at primary hip arthroscopy, with 97 % of tears being located anterior versus 52–92 % in prior studies of primary hip arthroscopy [12, 15, 35–38]. Interestingly, they found that 53 % of these tears were more specifically anteromedial, a location that is difficult to assess with MRA and difficult to access arthroscopically. The authors felt that the discrepancy regarding the anteromedial lesions is that currently MRA cannot adequately distinguish a postsurgical change from a new injury. This is in agreement with the conclusion made by Aprato, but in contrast, largely due to the better sensitivity, the authors felt that MRA is a useful tool in the evaluation of patients with prior hip surgery.

In the evaluation of MRA to detect chondral pathology, they found a sensitivity of 65 %, specificity of 90 %, PPV of 94 %, and NPV of 50 %. Seventeen patients had an MRA read of normal articular cartilage, who in fact had chondral damage in at least one location at the time of arthroscopy.

This data is consistent with previous studies for primary hip arthroscopy. One of these, by Keeney et al., demonstrated the sensitivity, specificity, PPV, and NPV to be 47 %, 89 %, 84 %, and 59 %, respectively [35]. Another, by Schmid et al., found some variability between two interpreting radiologists, with specificities of 79 and 50 %, sensitivities of 77 and 84 %, PPV of 73 and 71 %, and NPV of 83 and 68 %, but overall similar results [39].

The study by Glassner et al. also found that MRA was more accurate in detection of chondral damage of the femoral head (20/21) and then in detection of acetabular chondral damage (36/65). Further, MRA was superior at detecting Grade III and IV acetabular chondral injuries (18/22) as compared to Grade I and II injuries (15/31, i.e., 52 % of these early lesions were not identified). The prior mentioned study by Keeney, on primary hip arthroscopies, also demonstrated the difficulty of MRA at detecting Grade I and II lesions, in which 22.8 % of these injuries were not identified.

In respect to the location of chondral injuries, they found that 78 % of acetabular chondral injuries were found in the anterior acetabulum at the time of surgery. This was similar to a prior study by McCarthy et al. of 457 primary hip arthroscopies, which showed chondral injuries in the anterior acetabulum in 59 % of the cases [40]. The authors concluded that there was utility for MRA before revision hip arthroscopy in regard to cartilage lesions, but with the abovementioned limitations.

These limitations have led other researchers to search for a superior imaging study for evaluating cartilage injuries. In one such study with a goal of improving the detection of cartilage lesions, the researchers added a cartilage-sensitive three-dimensional spoiled gradient-recalled echo (SPGR) sequence with iterative decomposition of water and fat with echo asymmetry and least-squares estimation (IDEAL) fat-water separation to the hip MR arthrography studies [41]. The study included 67 patients who underwent standard MRA followed by MRA with the additional IDEAL-SPGR sequence and subsequently had hip arthroscopy. They found that the IDEAL-SPGR had a similar sensitivity to traditional MRA, 74 % versus 70 %, but a lower specificity, 77 % versus 84 %. Importantly, the IDEAL-SPGR was more accurate at grading cartilage lesions, leading them to conclude that it could be a useful adjunct to traditional MRA. This could prove to be of benefit for patients who have had a prior hip arthroscopy, due to the limitations in identifying cartilage injuries previously mentioned.

Future studies, for more accurate detection of early chondral damage, could also include the use of dGEMRIC scans (which measure the biochemical integrity of cartilage by detecting changes in glycosaminoglycans). Recent studies have shown that a mean dGEMRIC index in morphologically normal hips is 570 ± 90 ms and that levels less than this correlated with pain in the hip [28]. There is also data on dGEMRIC scans in patients with hip dysplasia and pre-radiographic osteoarthritis that found that age (>30) and presence of a labral tear were independent risk factors for developing osteoarthritis, as these patients had significantly lower dGEMRIC index [42]. For patients who have had a prior hip arthroscopy, and have ongoing pain, but have had an MRA that did not detect a cartilage lesion, dGEMRIC scans may prove to be useful in identifying early cartilage lesions (Fig. 25.2).

Interest in improved imaging studies can be expected, as the number of clinical studies focusing on reasons for failure of hip arthroscopy is increasing. Separate studies by Heyworth, Philippon, and Aprato all focused on the reasons

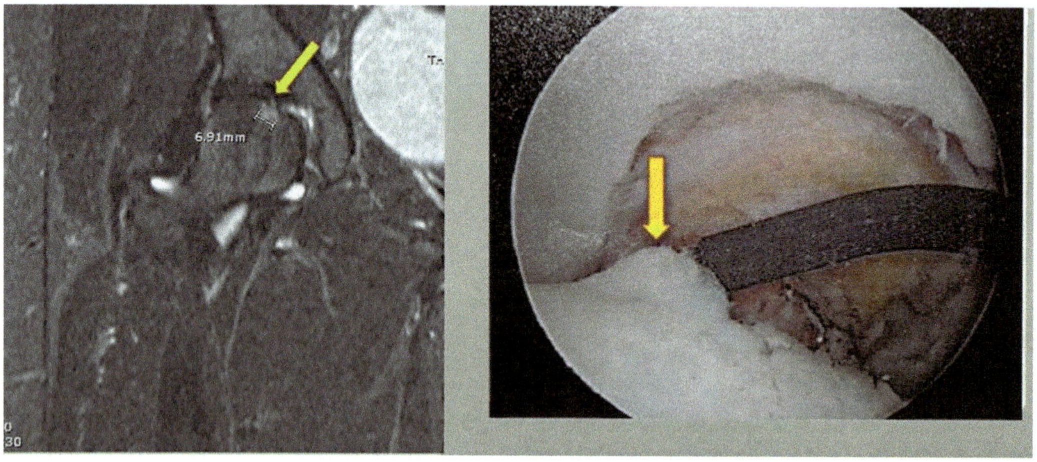

Fig. 25.2 A coronal STIR MRA image showing a superior femoral head cartilage lesion (*yellow arrow*), with underlying bone marrow edema (*cursor*), correlating with intraoperative findings of a chondral flap lesion of the superior femoral head (*orange arrow*) with Grade 2–3 wear

for revision, citing labral lesions and FAI that were not addressed, or inadequately addressed, at the initial surgery [43–45]. Recurrent symptoms from FAI ranged from 31 to 95 %, and recurrent symptoms from a persistent, or possibly new, labral tear were found in up to 92 % of cases. While the majority of patients in these studies had preoperative MRA or MRI, the authors did not specifically evaluate the accuracy of the imaging studies in these revision operations.

Conclusion

The evaluation of patients who have had a prior hip arthroscopy should start with a thorough clinical assessment, to determine if imaging of the hip is the next appropriate step. If so, one should begin with plain radiographs and progress to advanced imaging, such as MRA for further evaluation of the cartilage and labrum. The data on MRA of these patients is preliminary, but does show promise. Studies thus far have shown that MRA is superior at ruling in, rather than ruling out, a diagnosis, with PPV up to 94 % for labral and chondral pathology and an NPV of 21–39 % for labral tears, and 50 % for chondral damage. More conclusive data with larger sample sizes should become available as the number of primary and revision hip arthroscopies continue to increase. This, combined with innovative imaging techniques, should lead to a clearer understanding of the underlying pathology and aid surgeons in the diagnosis and treatment of these challenging and complex patients.

References

1. McCarthy JC, Lee J. Arthroscopic intervention in early hip disease. Clin Orthop Relat Res. 2004;429:157–62.
2. Yusaf MA, Hame SL. Arthroscopy of the hip. Curr Sports Med Rep. 2008;7(5):269–74.
3. Beaule PE, O'Neill M, Rakhra K. Current concepts review: acetabular labral tears. J Bone Joint Surg Am. 2009;91:701–10.
4. Byrd JW, Jones KS. Prospective analysis of hip arthroscopy with 2-year follow-up. Arthroscopy. 2000;16:578–87.
5. McCarthy J, Barsoum W, Puri L, et al. The role of hip arthroscopy in the elite athlete. Clin Orthop Relat Res. 2003;406:71–4.
6. Shindle MK, Voos JE, Nho SJ, et al. Arthroscopic management of labral tears in the hip. J Bone Joint Surg Am. 2008;90 Suppl 4:2–19.
7. O'Leary JA, Berend K, Vail TP. The relationship between diagnosis and outcome in arthroscopy of the hip. Arthroscopy. 2001;17:181–8.
8. Potter BK, Freedman BA, Andersen RC, et al. Correlation of short form-36 and disability status with outcomes of arthroscopic acetabular labral debridement. Am J Sports Med. 2005;33:864–70.
9. Farjo LA, Glick JM, Sampson TG. Hip arthroscopy for degenerative joint disease. Arthroscopy. 1998;14:435.
10. Margheritini F, Villar RN. The efficacy of arthroscopy in the treatment of hip osteoarthritis. Chir Organi Mov. 1999;84:257–61.
11. Walton NP, Jahromi I, Lewis PL. Chondral degeneration and therapeutic hip arthroscopy. Int Orthop. 2004;28:354–6.
12. Burnett RS, Della Rocca GJ, Prather H, et al. Clinical presentation of patients with tears of the acetabular labrum. J Bone Joint Surg Am. 2006;88:1448–57.
13. Chan YS, Lien LC, Hsu HL, et al. Evaluating hip labral tears using magnetic resonance arthrography: a prospective study comparing hip arthroscopy and magnetic resonance arthrography diagnosis. Arthroscopy. 2005;21:1250.
14. Czerny C, Hofmann S, Neuhold A, et al. Lesions of the acetabular labrum: accuracy of MR imaging and MR arthrography in detection and staging. Radiology. 1996;200:225–30.
15. Freedman BA, Potter BK, Dinauer PA, Giuliani JR, Kuklo TR, Murphy KP. Prognostic value of magnetic resonance arthrography for Czerny stage II and III acetabular labral tears. Arthroscopy. 2006;22:742–7.
16. Toomayan GA, Holman WR, Major NM, Kozlowicz SM, Vail TP. Sensitivity of MR arthrography in the evaluation of acetabular labral tears. AJR Am J Roentgenol. 2006;186:449–53.
17. Zeigert AJ, Blankenbaker DG, De Smet AA, et al. Comparison of standard hip MR arthrographic imaging planes and sequences for detection of arthroscopically proven labral tear. AJR Am J Roentgenol. 2009;192:1397–400.

18. Leunig M, Werlen S, Ungersböck A, et al. Evaluation of the acetabular labrum by MR arthrography. J Bone Joint Surg Br. 1997;79:230–4.
19. Mitchell B, McCrory P, Brukner P, et al. Hip joint pathology: clinical presentation and correlation between magnetic resonance arthrography, ultrasound, and arthroscopic findings in 25 consecutive cases. Clin J Sport Med. 2003;13(3):152–6.
20. Byrd JW, Jones KS. Diagnostic accuracy of clinical assessment, magnetic resonance imaging, magnetic resonance arthrography, and intra-articular injection in hip arthroscopy patients. Am J Sports Med. 2004;32:1668–74.
21. Cardello P, Gigli C, Ricci C, et al. Retears of postoperative knee meniscus: findings on magnetic resonance imaging (MRI) and magnetic resonance arthrography (MRA) by using low and high field magnets. Skeletal Radiol. 2009;38:149–56.
22. Gobbi A, Kon E, Berruto M, et al. Patellofemoral full-thickness chondral defects treated with hyalograft-C: a clinical, arthroscopic, and histologic review. Am J Sports Med. 2006;34:1763–73.
23. Magee T, Shapiro M, Rodriguez J, et al. MR arthrography of postoperative knee: for which patients is it useful? Radiology. 2003;229:159–63.
24. Makino A, Muscolo DL, Puigdevall M, et al. Arthroscopic fixation of osteochondritis dissecans of the knee: clinical, magnetic resonance imaging, and arthroscopic follow-up. Am J Sports Med. 2005;33:1499–504.
25. Magee TH, Gaenslen ES, et al. MR imaging of the shoulder after surgery. Am J Roentgenol. 1997;168(4):925–8.
26. Probyn L, White L, Salonen D, et al. Recurrent symptoms after shoulder instability repair: direct MR arthrographic assessment-correlation with second-look surgical evaluation. Radiology. 2007;245(3):814–23.
27. Heyworth BE, Dolan MM, Nguyen JT, et al. Preoperative three-dimensional CT predicts intraoperative findings in hip arthroscopy. Clin Orthop Relat Res. 2013;470:1950–7.
28. Kim YJ, Jaramillo D, Millis MB, et al. Assessment of early osteoarthritis in hip dysplasia with delayed gadolinium-enhanced magnetic resonance imaging of cartilage. J Bone Joint Surg Am. 2003;85:1987–92.
29. Tibor L, Sekiya J. Current concepts: differential diagnosis of pain around the hip joint. Arthroscopy. 2008;24(12):1407–21.
30. Jacobson JA, Bedi A, Sekiya JK, et al. Evaluation of the painful athletic hip: imaging options and imaging-guided injections. AJR Am J Roentgenol. 2012;199:516–24.
31. Robinson HJ, Hartleben PD, Lund G, et al. Evaluation of magnetic resonance imaging in the diagnosis of osteonecrosis of the femoral head. Accuracy compared with radiographs, core biopsy, and intraosseous pressure measurements. J Bone Joint Surg Am. 1989;71:650–63.
32. Aprato A, Jayasekera N, Villar RN. The accuracy of magnetic resonance arthrography in hip arthroscopic labral revision surgery. Hip Int. 2013;23(1):99–103.
33. Glassner PJ, Marchie A, Lee JA, McCarthy JC. MR imaging in patients with prior surgery: what are the limitations? In: 42nd annual Harvard arthroplasty course, Boston, MA; 2012.
34. Outerbridge R. The etiology of chondromalacia patellae. J Bone Joint Surg. 1961;43B:752–4.
35. Keeney J, Peele M, Jackson J, et al. Magnetic resonance arthrography versus arthroscopy in the evaluation of articular hip pathology. Clin Orthop Relat Res. 2004;429:163–9.
36. Fitzgerald Jr RH. Acetabular labrum tears: diagnosis and treatment. Clin Orthop Relat Res. 1995;31:60–8.
37. Lage LA, Patel JV, Villar RN. The acetabular labral tear: an arthroscopic classification. Arthroscopy. 1996;12:269–72.
38. McCarthy JC, Busconi B. The role of hip arthroscopy in the diagnosis and treatment of hip disease. Orthopedics. 1995;18:753–6.
39. Schmid M, Notzli H, Zanetti M, et al. Cartilage lesions in the hip: diagnostic effectiveness of MR. Arthrography. 2003;226(2):382–6.
40. McCarthy JC, Noble PC, Schuck MR, et al. The Otto E. Aufranc Award: the role of labral lesions to development of early degenerative hip disease. Clin Orthop Relat Res. 2001;393:25–37.
41. Blankenbaker DG, Ullrick SR, Kijowski R, et al. MR arthrography of the hip: comparison of IDEAL-SPGR volume sequence to standard MR sequences in the detection and grading of cartilage lesions. Radiology. 2011;261:863–71.
42. Jessel RH, Zurakowksi D, Zilkens C, et al. Radiographic and patient factors associated with pre-radiographic osteoarthritis in hip dysplasia. J Bone Joint Surg Am. 2009;91:1120–9.
43. Aprato A, Jayasekera N, Villar RN. Revision hip arthroscopic surgery: outcome at three years. Knee Surg Sports Traumatol Arthrosc. 2014;22(4):932–7.
44. Heyworth BE, Shindle MK, Voos JE, et al. Radiologic and intraoperative findings in revision hip arthroscopy. Arthroscopy. 2007;23:1295–302.
45. Philippon MJ, Schenker ML, Briggs KK, et al. Revision hip arthroscopy. Am J Sports Med. 2007;35:1918–21.

Advances in 2D and 3D Imaging for FAI Surgical Planning

26

Jaron P. Sullivan, Timothy Bryan Griffith, Caroline N. Park, and Anil S. Ranawat

Introduction

Femoral acetabular impingement (FAI) is a biomechanical entity arising from the presence of an osseous anatomical abnormality of the femur and/or acetabulum which presents with decreased range of motion (ROM) and pain [1]. It is characterized by repetitive contact, typically of the anterosuperior femoral head-neck junction and the acetabular rim during flexion and internal rotation of the hip, manifesting as pain and decreased ROM. This results in labral damage, chondral degeneration, and possibly secondary osteoarthritis of the hip joint [2]. Three distinct types of FAI have been described. On the femoral side, a misshapen femoral head-neck junction, typified by a loss of sphericity and a reduced femoral head-neck offset, causes "cam"-type impingement. On the acetabular side, an excessively deep or maloriented socket causes "pincer"-type impingement. A combination of these two abnormalities is known as "mixed" impingement. Due to the complex nature of the associated femoral and acetabular deformities in FAI, computed tomography (CT) scans are helpful to identify osseous abnormalities for surgical decision making in arthroscopic, open, or combined procedures.

Clinical studies have shown that surgical correction of the osseous abnormalities that cause impingement improves ROM and function and relieves pain [3–6]. As with other areas of joint preservation surgery, the surgical treatment of FAI has inevitably progressed toward the use of less-invasive techniques such as hip arthroscopy. This procedure remains technically demanding with a significant learning curve [7]. A common reason for failure of arthroscopic FAI surgery is inaccurate resection, either under- or overresection, which is perhaps not surprising as the surgeon has to treat complex 3D "cam" and "pincer" deformities through a 2D arthroscope [8, 9]. This problem has, in part, fueled the drive toward computer-assisted solutions.

This chapter will focus on imaging advances for preoperative planning. Section XVI discusses the computer-assisted techniques (CAS) and robotic implications of this planning. CAS and hip arthroscopy encompasses three broad categories: preoperative assessment tools, navigation programs, and robotic-assisted surgery. Preoperative tools provide the surgeon with a patient-specific reconstruction of osseous anatomy in three dimensions (3D). Depending on the software, a virtual bony resection can then be performed based on strict anatomic or kinematic parameters in order to minimize impingement and improve ROM. Navigation, on the other hand, allows the visualization of the surgeon's instruments in relation to a virtual reconstruction of the patient, which can then guide the surgeon intraoperatively in a precise manner. Navigation may or may not have a preoperative assessment tool and requires an intraoperative registration process. Robotic-assisted surgery moves one step beyond preoperative planning and navigation with even greater accuracy. It combines both preoperative and navigation tools with a "guided" intraoperative cutting device that is automated based on a preoperative plan.

J.P. Sullivan, MD
Division of Sports Medicine, Department of Orthopaedic Surgery, Vanderbilt University, 1215 21st Ave., South, Suite 4200 Medical Center East South Tower, Nashville, TN 37232-8774, USA
e-mail: jaron.sullivan@vanderbilt.edu

T.B. Griffith, MD
Division of Sports Medicine, Department of Orthopaedic Surgery, Peachtree Orthopaedic Clinic, Atlanta, GA, USA
e-mail: tgriffith@pocatlanta.com

C.N. Park, BA
Division of Clinical Research, Department of Orthopaedic Surgery, Hospital for Special Surgery, 535 East 70th St., 6th Floor, New York, NY 10021, USA
e-mail: caroline.park7@gmail.com

A.S. Ranawat, MD (✉)
Division of Sports Medicine and Joint Preservation, Hospital for Special Surgery, 535 East 70th St., 6th Floor, Suite 637, New York, NY 10021, USA
e-mail: ranawatanil@hss.edu; anilranawat1974@gmail.com

J.C. McCarthy et al. (eds.), *Hip Joint Restoration*, DOI 10.1007/978-1-4614-0694-5_26

This review outlines the various surgical techniques used to treat FAI and addresses their current limitations. It will focus on the evolution of CAS to address the limitations of both open as well as arthroscopic hip impingement surgery. The most current research and the latest technology of computer-assisted techniques for preoperative planning, intraoperative navigation, and surgical execution in impingement surgery will be presented.

Limitations of FAI Surgery

FAI surgery can be performed open or arthroscopically. Irrespective of the approach, there are multiple factors which contribute to a successful outcome from FAI surgery and therefore many areas where mistakes can be made. These include patient selection, patient expectations, indications for surgery, appropriate imaging, preoperative planning, patient positioning, visualization of the lesion, localization of the deformity, and treatment of primary bony abnormalities and secondary lesions. In addition, rehabilitation is incredibly important. Here we will discuss the limitations unique to both the open or arthroscopic approaches while focusing primarily on proper visualization and correction of osseous lesions and deformities.

Open surgical hip dislocation is the historical gold-standard treatment for FAI. Good to excellent results at midterm follow-up (2–12 years after arthroscopy) range between 70 and 80% [5, 6, 10, 11]. The open approach allows for circumferential visualization of the hip joint. Femoral, rim, and chondral pathologies can be treated and the zone of impingement can be assessed dynamically. Open surgical hip dislocation is currently the best option for the precise treatment of complex bony abnormalities including extra-articular impingement, global FAI, and femoral version anomalies. However, there are disadvantages with this technique, which include trochanteric nonunion and pain, potential risk of avascular necrosis, and increased inpatient hospital stays and rehabilitation periods. In an effort to minimize these disadvantages, mini-open approaches have been used, such as the Hueter approach, which provides good visualization of the anterior femoral head-neck junction without surgical dislocation [12]. However, the potential for assessment of lateral and posterior pathology as well as the chondral surfaces is limited. These limitations with open techniques coupled with new advances in hip arthroscopy marked a gradual shift among FAI surgeons to less-invasive arthroscopic techniques.

In the early days of hip arthroscopy, the technique provided an effective option to deal with intra-articular pathology, including chondral lesions, loose bodies, labral injury and degeneration, synovial lesions, and infection. With improvement in instrumentation and increased surgical experience, femoral osteochondroplasties, acetabular rim resections, and labral repairs can now be effectively performed [13]. Arthroscopy has the advantages of being minimally invasive, avoiding the morbidity of a surgical hip dislocation and trochanteric osteotomy, and allowing for faster rehabilitation [14]. Cadaveric studies have shown arthroscopic osteochondroplasties to be comparable in accuracy, safety, and precision to open techniques [15, 16]. Clinically, arthroscopic techniques have yielded equally significant improvements in modified Harris hip scores [14, 17] and comparable efficacy to open surgical dislocation in restoring head-neck offset and achieving a similar depth, arc, and length of resection for anterosuperior "cam"-type impingement [18]. The basic indications for arthroscopic hip surgery are actively symptomatic structural hip deformities such as "cam"- or "pincer"-type deformities.

Although arthroscopic hip surgery continues to increase in popularity, it has its own unique set of challenges. First, it remains technically demanding with a steep surgical learning curve [7, 14]. Second, a dynamic assessment of the zone of impingement is difficult to perform with the hip fixed in a traction device. Third, the relative inflexibility of small portals being used to maneuver instruments within a thick capsule limits visualization, which can cause iatrogenic injury and increases operative time. This can also increase the risk of neurovascular injuries from prolonged traction. In addition, the capsulotomy required for performing the bony resection can result in significant retroperitoneal fluid accumulation and hemodynamic consequences. Finally, poor visualization may make appropriate osseous resection difficult. Inadequate arthroscopic resection in FAI patients accounts for 78–90% of all failed arthroscopic hip surgeries [8, 9, 19]. Overresection on the other hand may lead to hip instability, dislocation, or a femoral neck fracture [20].

The intraoperative assessment of when an adequate "volume of resection" has been achieved is limited in both open and arthroscopic techniques, but especially for arthroscopic hip surgery. The open surgeon uses spherometer gauges and fluoroscopy for guidance, and the arthroscopic surgeon uses fluoroscopy as an adjunct. The problem remains that two-dimensional modalities are being utilized to define a three-dimensional morphology. Furthermore, the difficulty in deciding when you have done "enough" is compounded by the lack of appropriate preoperative planning tools. The combination of a complex decision-making process in defining a 3D problem using a technically demanding surgery has resulted in the recent research into computer-assisted preoperative planning solutions.

Role of the CT Scan in FAI Surgery

After a patient has been identified as having clinical signs and symptoms consistent with FAI, appropriate imaging is utilized to evaluate the extent of pathology. An appropriate imaging work-up starts with plain radiographs of the hip and

Table 26.1 Variables to measure with a CT scan for proper preoperative planning of a patient with FAI

Variable	Normal values	Abnormal values
CAM location		Lesion between 12 and 4 o'clock
Acetabular version 1 o'clock	5°	
Acetabular version 2 o'clock	10°	
Acetabular version 3 o'clock	15°	>30°
Neck-shaft angle	126°–139°	Coxa vara <126° Coxa valga >139°
Sagittal center-edge angle	31°	<20°
Coronal center-edge angle	41°	<20°
Alpha angle		>55°
AIIS width	1 cm	
Distal base of AIIS to acetabular rim	≥0.5 cm	<0.5 cm
Femoral version angle	15°–20°	>30°
McKibbin index	30°–60°	>60° or <30°

pelvis; however, two-dimensional imaging limits the ability of the surgeon to understand the extent of disease. CT scanning and 3D reconstruction techniques have become invaluable for evaluating the hip and pelvis. Surface rendering techniques also help better evaluate osseous impingement from the proximal femur or pelvis [21]. The goals of imaging are to identify the extent of pathology, to determine the need for surgery in the appropriately selected patient, and to determine the adequacy and extent of a surgical intervention. During the imaging work-up for FAI, it is important for the surgeon to look for cam impingement, pincer impingement, or a mixed pathology that involves both.

CT scanning and 3D reconstruction techniques are currently the gold standard to fulfill quantitative and qualitative disease assessment. Preoperative planning with a CT should have several variables measured to help tailor the operative approach (Table 26.1). Cam lesion location is commonly defined by using clock-face terminology. Typically, 12 o'clock represents the most superolateral aspect, 3 o'clock represents the most anterior aspect, and 6 o'clock represents the most inferomedial aspect of the femoral head-neck junction. The cam is most commonly found between 12 o'clock and 4 o'clock [22]. Cam lesions that are beyond 12 o'clock (i.e., 11 o'clock) toward the posterior aspect of the hip are difficult to address arthroscopically and may be more amenable to an open procedure. The alpha angle is measured at the maximal offset where the abnormal bony contour of the femoral head-neck junction extends beyond the spherical confines of the femoral head. The alpha angle can be measured in the coronal as well as the sagittal plane. The measurement is an angle from the central axis of the femoral neck to the point where the head-neck junction loses its spherical contour (Fig. 26.1) [23]. An alpha angle greater than 55° is considered to be abnormal.

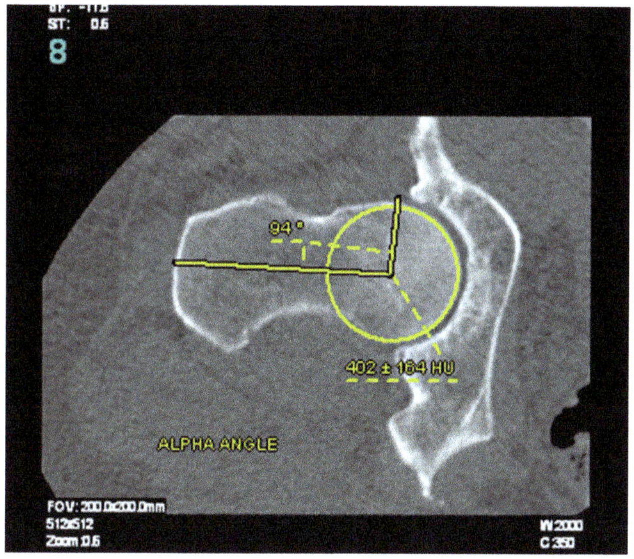

Fig. 26.1 Alpha angle determined by measuring the angle subtended between a line along the axis of the femoral neck and the point at which the femoral head loses its sphericity. An angle >55° is considered to be abnormal

The center-edge angle (CEA) can be measured on the sagittal or coronal views. The coronal CEA is measured by first drawing a line through the center of the femoral head perpendicular to the transverse pelvic axis. Next, a line is drawn through the center of the femoral head to the superolateral aspect of the acetabular roof. The angle between these lines defines the coronal CEA (Fig. 26.2a). This corresponds to the lateral CEA on radiographs [24], where a CEA<20° is considered to be abnormal. The sagittal CEA is measured by first drawing a vertical line through the center of the femoral head. Next, a line is drawn through the center of the femoral head to the most anterior aspect of the acetabular rim. The angle between these lines defines the sagittal CEA (Fig. 26.2b). This corresponds to the anterior CEA on radiographs [25], where a CEA<20° is considered to be abnormal. The CEA corresponds to the degree of coverage of the femoral head by the acetabulum. A higher CEA indicates a greater degree of coverage, whereas a lower CEA indicates a lesser degree of coverage. In patients with a CEA<20°, procedures such as a periacetabular osteotomy (PAO) may be indicated.

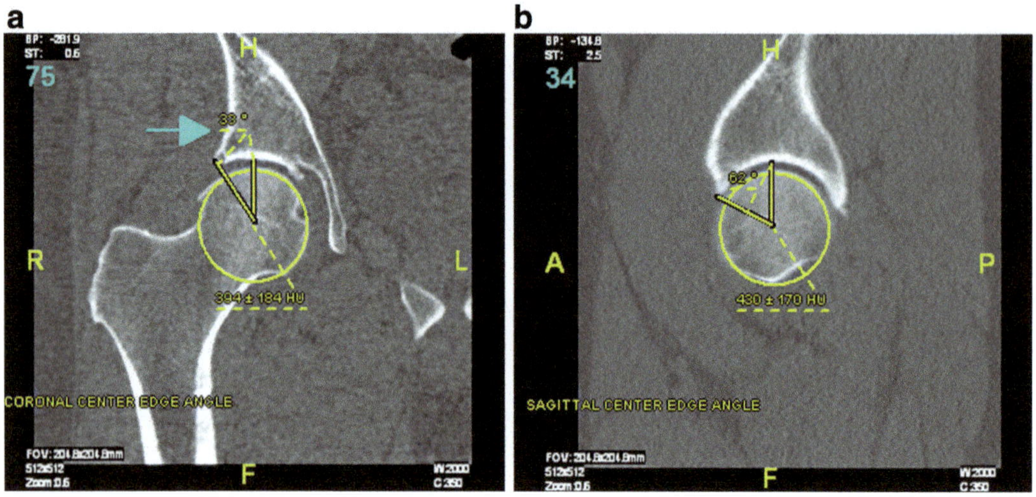

Fig. 26.2 (**a**) Coronal center-edge angle (*arrow*) and (**b**) sagittal center-edge angle. A center-edge angle <20° is considered to be abnormal

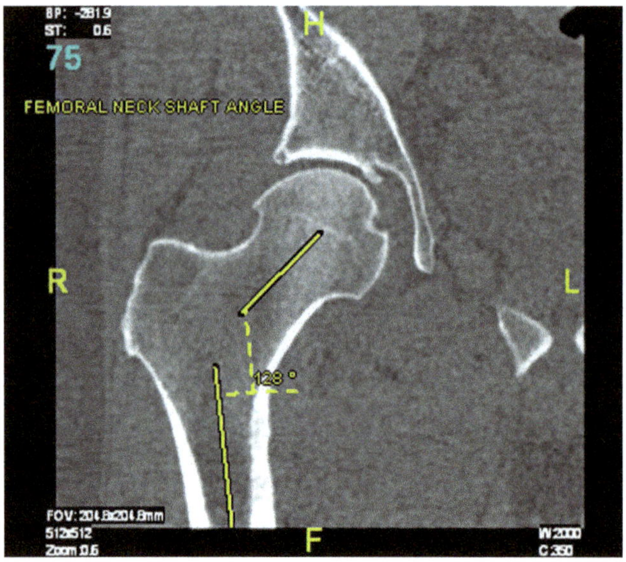

Fig. 26.3 Neck-shaft angle (*arrow*) is normally between 126° and 139°

The neck-shaft angle (NSA) is measured on the coronal view. This NSA angle is the angle subtended by the femoral neck and diaphyseal axes (Fig. 26.3). The neck axis is defined by the line connecting the center of the femoral head and the center of the femoral neck at its isthmus. The diaphyseal axis is defined by the line connecting the midpoint of two lines drawn perpendicularly across the diaphysis of the femur. A normal NSA is between 126° and 139°. Coxa vara is defined as a NSA< 126° and coxa valga is defined as NSA> 139° [26]. Acetabular version angle is formed by the intersection of the line perpendicular to the line between the posterior pelvic margins and the line connecting the anterior and posterior rim of the acetabulum (Fig. 26.4) [27]. This measurement is conducted at 1 o'clock, 2 o'clock, and 3 o'clock with normal being approximately 5°, 10°, and 15°, respectively. Larger acetabular anteversion angles >30° can predispose the patient to instability. Patients with retroverted acetabulums are associated with pincer-type FAI. During evaluation of the acetabular version, consideration also needs to be made to the version angle of the proximal femur, as well as the total limb version.

Total limb version is an important consideration in the evaluation of a patient with FAI. Total limb version is broken down into tibial and femoral components. The patient evaluation starts with a detailed physical exam which can then guide the surgeon to make appropriate radiographic inquiries. The physical exam has to be broken down into three components: total limb torsion, tibial torsion, and femoral version. Net limb torsion is quickly identified via the foot progression angle during gait. The foot progression angle is the direction the foot is pointed during normal gait, with neutral being parallel to the direction of travel. It is important to recognize that a normal foot progression angle does not necessarily mean that the patient has normal torsion of the femur and the tibia. Excessive external torsion of the tibia combined with increased femoral torsion (anteversion) can yield a net neutral foot progression angle during gait (compensatory). On the other hand, combining increased internal torsion of the tibia and increased anteversion of the femur can yield a severe in-toeing gait (non-compensatory) [26].

Several clinical exam tests help the clinician to localize the deformity components. Tibial torsion can be identified by using the thigh foot axis and the transmalleolar axis. The thigh foot axis is done by flexing the knee to 90° and evaluating the angle subtended by the longitudinal axis of the thigh and the foot. The transmalleolar axis is determined by comparing an imaginary line between the medial and lateral malleolus and a second line through the medial and lateral epicondyles of the distal femur. Femoral version can be evaluated via hip internal and external rotation with the hip at

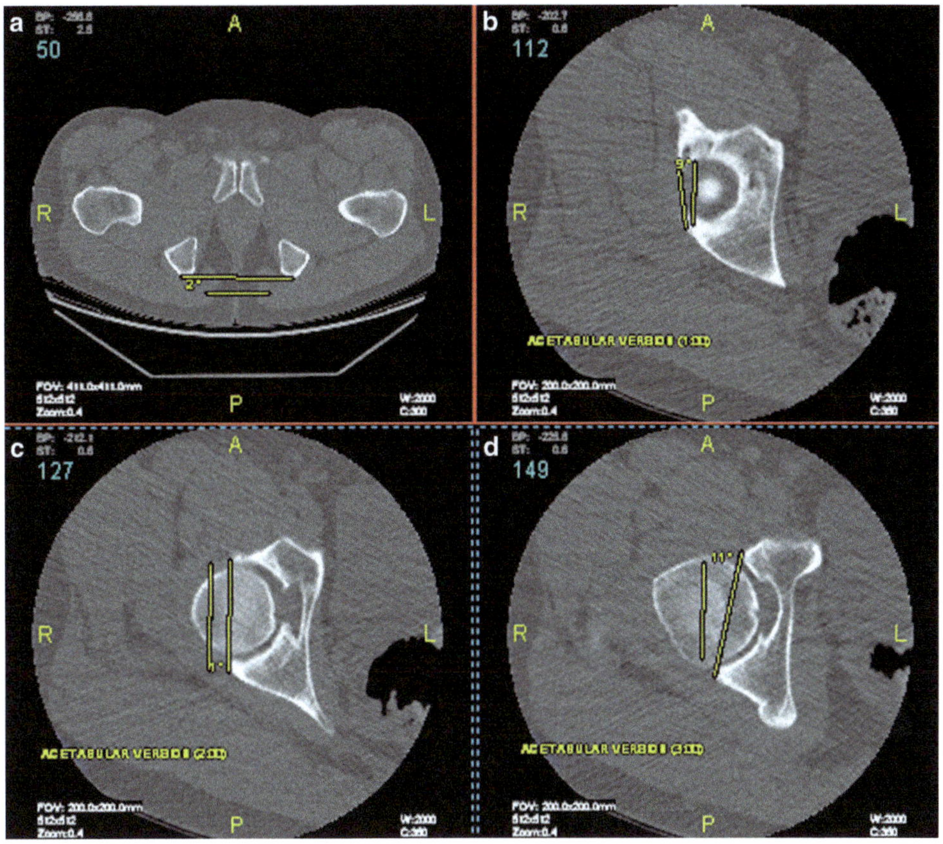

Fig. 26.4 Acetabular version. (**a**) Represents a line connecting the posterior pelvic margin and the angle it creates with the horizontal line of the image screen. This angle represents the amount of correction (2°) that will need to be added to the subsequent measurements in (**b–d**). (**b**) Represents the acetabular version at 1 o'clock measuring −7° (−9°+2° of correction). (**c**) Represents the acetabular version at 2 o'clock measuring 1° (1°+2° of correction). (**d**) Represents the acetabular version at 3 o'clock measuring 13° (11°+2° of correction). Acetabular version angle is normally 5°, 10°, and 15° at 1 o'clock, 2 o'clock, and 3 o'clock, respectively

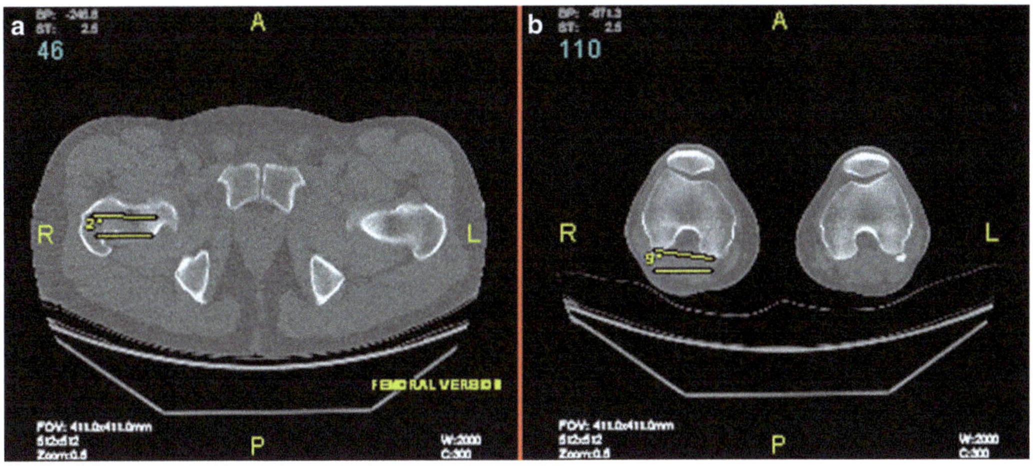

Fig. 26.5 Femoral version is measured by finding the angle between the femoral head and neck axis (*Left*) and the posterior condylar angle (*Right*). Normal femoral version angle ranges between 15 and 20° of anteversion

neutral and at 90° of flexion. Asymmetric or excessive motion should be noted and can point to underlying etiologies for symptoms. Once abnormalities are identified on physical examination, appropriate radiographic studies can further elucidate the deformity. The gold standard to evaluate rotational deformities is currently the CT scan; however, MRI and EOS imaging systems offer low radiation alternative options that should be further studied to evaluate comparative accuracy and precision.

Femoral version angle is measured by first taking limited CT cuts from the femoral head and neck down to the distal femur. The femoral head center image is then superimposed on the transcondylar knee image. The femoral version angle is the angle subtended between the femoral head and neck axis and the posterior condylar angle (Fig. 26.5) [28, 29]. A normal femoral version angle ranges between 15 and 20° of anteversion. Femoral anteversion >30° is consistent with instability. The femoral version angle is also important in determining the starting point of the anterolateral portal in hip arthroscopic procedures. More femoral retroversion should dictate a more anterior starting point for the anterolateral portal to avoid crowding with the greater trochanter. The bimalleolar method described by Goutallier et al. can be used to assess tibial version, which is measured as the angle between a long along the posterior contour of the proximal tibia and the intermalleolar axis [30].

Besides total limb torsion, another more critical index is the McKibbin instability index. This is the sum of the femoral version angle and the acetabular version angle measured at 3 o'clock. A normal McKibbin index ranges between 30° and 60°. A McKibbin index >60° predisposes the hip to instability, while a McKibbin index <30° predisposes the hip to impingement [26, 31]. In evaluating overall limb version, the patient is considered "compensated" if foot alignment remains neutral during the gait cycle. Those patients within the normal McKibbin range are treated arthroscopically. Patients with low or high McKibbin indexes that are uncompensated often require osteotomy during surgical management. Conversely, patients that are compensated with a low McKibbin index are often treated with arthroscopy only, while those compensated with a high McKibbin index may require arthroscopy and open surgery, or combined methods.

Preoperative Planning in FAI Surgery

The most commonly used measurements to evaluate FAI have been described above, but they are all two-dimensional metrics used in the evaluation of a three-dimensional disease. Continued advancements in 3D rendering of CT scans can further improve their usefulness in addressing hip pathology. While the mainstay of current treatment evaluation and planning involves the qualitative assessment of 3D reconstructions and 2D quantitative evaluations utilizing the measurements listed above, efforts are being made to more precisely evaluate and treat FAI using CAS.

CAS has been gaining popularity in FAI surgery to minimize the limitations outlined in the previous sections but specifically to address the issues of accurate and precise osseous resections. Preoperative planning software systems have been designed to perform a virtual bony resection to minimize impingement and improve ROM. The present limitations of preoperative planning software highlight many of the problems with FAI surgery in general, which include defining the depth and surface area of resection.

The gold-standard assessment of FAI cam impingement has been reduced anterior femoral head-neck offset defined by the alpha angle. The alpha angle does have its limitations. For instance, the head-neck offset may be present at different locations in different patients. The alpha angle also does not take into account the length of the "cam" lesion down the femoral neck. If the "bump" is long, the resection may have to be advanced into the intertrochanteric line. Clohisy et al. evaluated the alpha angle in patients with FAI and asymptomatic controls and found a comparable range of normal and abnormal alpha angles in the two groups [32]. They could not define an alpha angle threshold beyond which a pathological diagnosis can be considered. This brings us to question whether the alpha angle is an appropriate metric to define anatomy as normal or abnormal. A recent systematic review demonstrated that correction of the alpha angle resulted in significant improvements in ROM and patient visual analog scales, non-arthritic hip scores, Harris hip scores, and the short-form-12 [33].

Recent trends in anatomic planning software use a 3D alpha angle or volumetric measurement (Fig. 26.6). This concept takes into account continuous alpha angles circumferentially around the femoral head and neck as well as length and area so a true zone of impingement can be identified. In addition to identifying volumetric areas of impingement, efforts are being made to perform 3D kinematic evaluations to predict and correlate motion relative to the gross anatomy. Tannast et al. designed the first comprehensive preoperative assessment tools, utilizing "HipMotion" software (Bern, Switzerland) to perform a CT-based 3D kinematics analysis of the hip joint (Fig. 26.7) [34]. This software uses a kinematic plan to define zones of impingement and predict improvement in ROM after a virtual resection, addressing the need for an accurate kinematic preoperative plan while enhancing the visual guidance of the surgeon. Virtual postoperative ROM is simulated by reconstructing the hip joint using the recommended postresection parameters, allowing the surgeon to assess the efficacy of the planned procedure. This program utilizes the imageless BrainLAB (Feldkirchen, Germany) software, which was validated by comparing virtual with real ROM (Fig. 26.8). The accuracy of HipMotion was 0.7° ± 3.1° in a plastic bone setup and −5.0° ± 5.6° in a cadaveric setup. An encouraging aspect of HipMotion is that it calculates the volume of resection based on a desirable postoperative ROM rather than a postoperative alpha angle. One limitation of the program is that it assumes the hip joint has a perfect center of rotation, which is debated with more accurate models that have been proposed. HipMotion was also used in a clinical pilot study by the same authors to compare the ROM in 28 hips with anterior FAI to a control group of 33 normal hips [35]. The hips with FAI had decreased flexion, internal rotation, abduction, and internal rotation in 90° of flexion. The zones of impingement were found anterosuperiorly and were similar in the two groups. The virtual postoperative ROM improved in all subgroups of FAI, with the biggest improvement (15.7°) seen in mixed impingement.

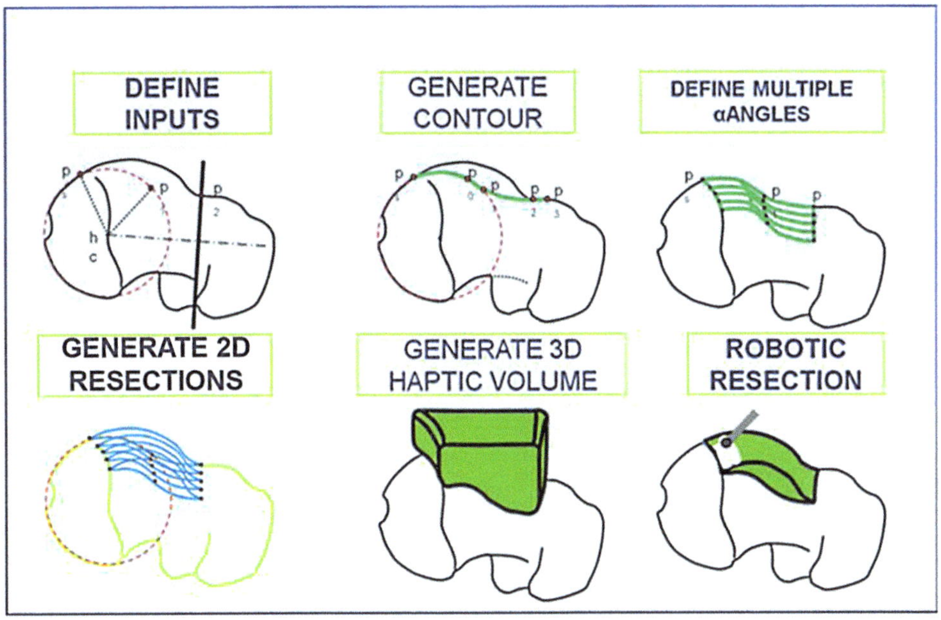

Fig. 26.6 Anatomic planning software that measures 3D alpha angle and planned robotic resection. From Caroline N. Park et al. Robotic-assisted femoral osteochondroplasty is more precise than a freehand technique in a Sawbone model J Hip Preserv Surg (2015) 2 (2): 136–144. Reprinted with permission

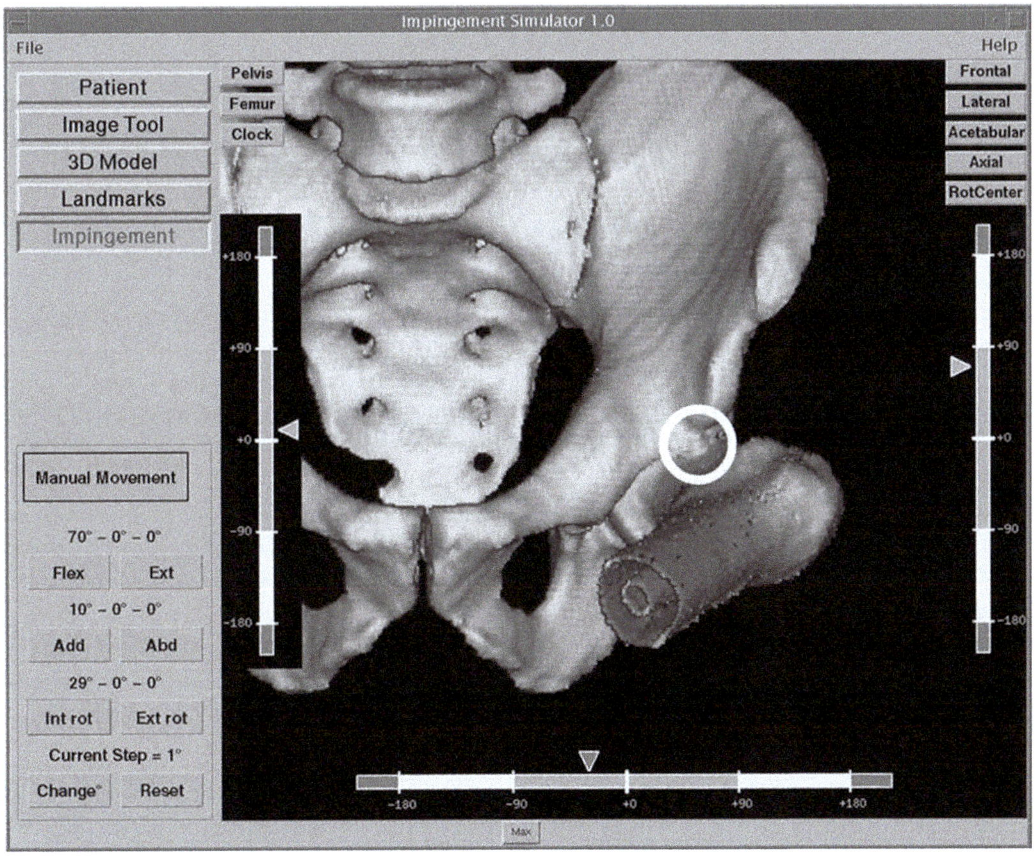

Fig. 26.7 "HipMotion" Software (Bern, Switzerland) utilized to perform a CT-based 3D kinematics analysis of the hip joint. From Kubiak-Langer M, et al. Range of motion in anterior femoroacetabular impingement. Clin Orthop Relat Res. 2007;458:117–124. Reprinted with permission from Wolters Kluwer Health

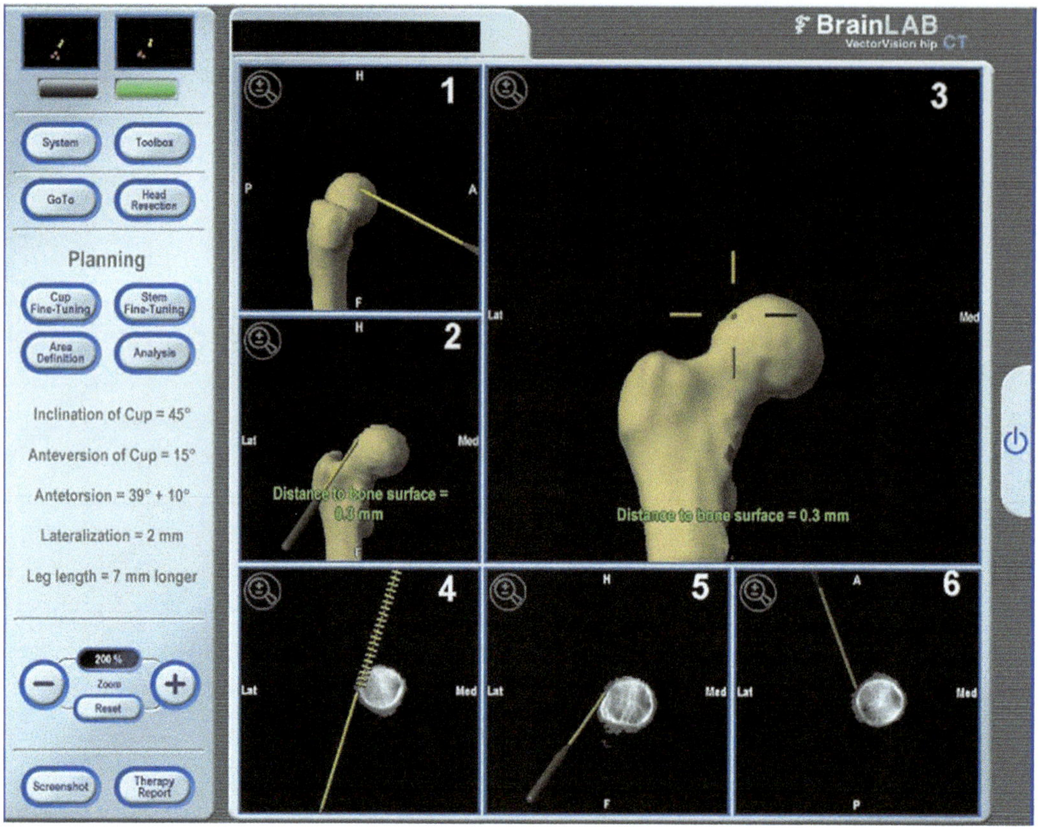

Fig. 26.8 BrainLAB (Feldkirchen, Germany) software showing the position of the surgical instrument in relation the femoral neck. From Brunner A, et al. Evaluation of a Computed Tomography-Based Navigation System Prototype for Hip Arthroscopy in the Treatment of Femoroacetabular Cam Impingement. Journal of Arthroscopy. 2009; 25(4): 382–391. Reprinted with permission from Elsevier Limited

Another company's imaging program, known as Dyonics Plan (formerly known as A3 surgical) (Smith and Nephew, Tennessee, USA), is producing innovative solutions that also use preoperative CT scans to plan impingement scenarios. They use an anatomic plan using alpha angles in various planes thus allowing for accurate resection in targeted areas. In a recent study, a prototype CT-based 3D analysis software program (A^2 Surgical, Saint-Pierre-d'Allevard, France) that uses an automated algorithm based on radial sequences to determine the maximum alpha angle and its location was used to compare software alpha angles with values obtained from plain radiographs and CT images, as well as to evaluate the size and location of cam deformities. The mean alpha angle determined by the software was 70.8° at 1:23 o'clock, and 60 % of maximum alpha angles were detected between 12:45 and 1:45. Plain radiographs and CT underestimated the alpha angle by 8.2° and 5.7°, respectively. The software-based location of alpha angle was anterosuperior to the mean CT and plain radiograph locations by 41 and 97 min, respectively. The ability of 3D analysis software to assess the femoral head-neck junction circumferentially gives value to its use as a preoperative planning tool for characterizing FAI [36].

Conclusion

Symptomatic FAI is a challenging pathology to treat in the hip, secondary to the complex three-dimensional anatomy that is buried in a soft tissue envelope. The appropriate treatment of FAI requires clinical acumen in order to correlate radiographic abnormalities with symptoms. Regardless of whether the surgical exposure methods are open or arthroscopic, there still remains the difficulty of knowing how much bone to resect in order to give the patient impingement-free physiologic ROM. Plain radiographs are used as an initial tool to evaluate the magnitude of pathology. Although plain radiographs are limited because they cannot project the three-dimensional nature of the disease, they still are invaluable tools for screening, intraoperative evaluation, and follow-up evaluations due to decreased cost, low radiation, and almost universal accessibility. The current gold standard to evaluate cam and pincer hip pathology is the 3D CT reconstruction. The 3D CT allows the surgeon to evaluate the full profile of the patient's anatomy. With the assistance of computer planning software and 3D CTs, the extent of the patient's pathology can be mapped and quantified. Using this principle, the ideal planning system would define preoperatively the zone of impingement and allow the surgeon to plan the bony resection based on a virtual impingement-free ROM. Methods to implement this plan are currently being developed that utilize CAS solutions that will be further discussed in Section XVI.

References

1. Leunig M, Beaule P, Ganz R. The concept of femoroacetabular impingement: current status and future perspectives. Clin Orthop Relat Res. 2009;467:616–22.
2. Ganz R, Parvizi J, Beck M, Leunig M, Notzli H, Siebenrock KA. Femoroacetabular impingement: a cause for osteoarthritis of the hip. Clin Orthop Relat Res. 2003;417:112–20.
3. Stahelin L, Stahelin T, Jolles BM, Herzog RF. Arthroscopic offset restoration in femoroacetabular cam impingement: accuracy and early clinical outcome. Arthroscopy. 2008;24(1):51–7.
4. Lavigne M, Parvizi J, Beck M, Siebenrock KA, Ganz R, Leunig M. Anterior femoroacetabular impingement: part I. Techniques of joint preserving surgery. Clin Orthop Relat Res. 2004;428:61–6.
5. Beck M, Leunig M, Parvizi J, Boutier V, Wyss D, Ganz R. Anterior femoroacetabular impingement: part II. Midterm results of surgical treatment. Clin Orthop Relat Res. 2004;418:67–73.
6. Beaule PE, Le Duff MJ, Zaragoza E. Quality of life following femoral head-neck osteochondroplasty for femoroacetabular impingement. J Bone Joint Surg Am. 2007;89:773–9.
7. Konan S, Rhee SJ, Haddad FS. Hip arthroscopy: analysis of a single surgeon's learning experience. J Bone Joint Surg Am. 2011;93 Suppl 2:52–6.
8. Philippon MJ, Schenker ML, Briggs KK, Kuppersmith DA, Maxwell RB, Stubbs AJ. Revision hip arthroscopy. Am J Sports Med. 2007;35:1918–21.
9. Heyworth BE, Shindle MK, Voos JE, Rudzki JR, Kelly BT. Radiologic and intraoperative findings in revision hip arthroscopy. Arthroscopy. 2007;23:1295–302.
10. Murphy S, Tannast M, Kim YJ, Buly R, Millis MB. Debridement of the adult hip for femoroacetabular impingement: indications and preliminary clinical results. Clin Orthop Relat Res. 2004;429: 178–81.
11. Peters CL, Erickson JA. Treatment of femoro-acetabular impingement with surgical dislocation and debridement in young adults. J Bone Joint Surg Am. 2006;88:1735–41.
12. Laude F, Sariali E, Nogier A. Femoroacetabular impingement treatment using arthroscopy and anterior approach. Clin Orthop Relat Res. 2009;467:747–52.
13. Byrd JW, Jones KS. Arthroscopic femoroplasty in the management of cam-type femoroacetabular impingement. Clin Orthop Relat Res. 2009;467:739–46.
14. Botser IB, Smith Jr TW, Nasser R, Domb BG. Open surgical dislocation versus arthroscopy for femoroacetabular impingement: a comparison of clinical outcomes. Arthroscopy. 2011;27(2):270–8.
15. Sussman PS, Ranawat AS, Lipman J, Lorich DG, Padgett DE, Kelly BT. Arthroscopic versus open osteoplasty of the head-neck junction: a cadaveric investigation. Arthroscopy. 2007;23:1257–64.
16. Sussmann PS, Ranawat AS, Shehaan M, Lorich D, Padgett DE, Kelly BT. Vascular preservation during arthroscopic osteoplasty of the femoral head-neck junction: a cadaveric investigation. Arthroscopy. 2007;23(7):738–43.
17. Larson CM, Giveans MR. Arthroscopic management of femoroacetabular impingement: early outcome measures. Arthroscopy. 2008;24:540–6.
18. Bedi A, Zaltz I, De La Torre K, Kelly BT. Radiographic comparison of surgical hip dislocation and hip arthroscopy for treatment of cam deformity in femoroacetabular impingement. Am J Sports Med. 2011;39(Suppl):20–8.
19. Zumstein M, Hahn F, Sukthankar A, et al. How accurately can the acetabular rim be trimmed in hip arthroscopy for pincer-type femoral acetabular impingement: a cadaveric investigation. Arthroscopy. 2009;25:164–8.
20. Matsuda DK. Acute iatrogenic dislocation following hip impingement arthroscopic surgery. Arthroscopy. 2009;25:400–4.
21. Kang RW, Yanke AB, Espinoza Orias AA, Inoue N, Nho SJ. Emerging ideas: novel 3-D quantification and classification of cam lesions in patients with femoroacetabular impingement. Clin Orthop Relat Res. 2013;471(2):358–62.
22. Bedi A, Dolan M, Magennis E, Lipman J, Buly R, Kelly BT. Computer-assisted modeling of osseous impingement and resection in femoroacetabular impingement. Arthroscopy. 2012;28(2):204–10.
23. Notzli HP, Wyss TF, Stoecklin CH, Schmid MR, Treiber K, Hodler J. The contour of the femoral head-neck junction as a predictor for the risk of anterior impingement. J Bone Joint Surg Br. 2002;84:556–60.
24. Wiberg G. Studies on dysplastic acetabula and congenital subluxation of the hip joint: with special reference to the complication of osteoarthritis. Acta Chir Scand Suppl. 1939;83 Suppl 58:1–135.
25. Crockarell JR, Trousdale RT, Guyton JL. The anterior centre-edge angle: a cadaver study. J Bone Joint Surg Br. 2000;82-B:532–4.
26. Tonnis D, Heinecke A. Acetabular and femoral anteversion: relationship with osteoarthritis of the hip. J Bone Joint Surg Am. 1999;81:1747–70.
27. Jacquemier M, Jouve JL, Bollini G, Panuel M, Migliani R. Acetabular anteversion in children. J Pediatr Orthop. 1992;12:373–5.
28. Murphy SB, Simon SR, Kijewski PK, Wilkinson RH, Griscom NT. Femoral anteversion. J Bone Joint Surg Am. 1987;69:1169–76.
29. Weiner DS, Cook AJ, Hoyt Jr WA, Oravec CE. Computed tomography in the measurement of femoral anteversion. Orthopedics. 1978;1:299–306.
30. Goutallier D, Van Driessche S, Manicom O, Sariali E, Bernageau J, Radier C. Influence of lower-limb torsion on long-term outcomes of tibial valgus osteotomy for medial compartment knee osteoarthritis. J Bone Joint Surg Am. 2006;88:2439–47.
31. Dorr LD, Malik A, Wan Z. Combined anteversion technique for total hip arthroplasty. Clin Orthop Relat Res. 2009;467(1):119–27.
32. Clohisy JC, Nunley RM, Otto RJ, Schoenecker PL. The frog-leg lateral radiograph accurately visualized hip cam impingement abnormalities. Clin Orthop Relat Res. 2007;462:115–21.
33. Brunner A, Horisberger M, Herzog RF. Evaluation of a computed tomography-based navigation system prototype for hip arthroscopy in the treatment of femoroacetabular cam impingement. Arthroscopy. 2009;25(4):382–91.
34. Tannast M, Kubiak-Langer M, Langlotz F, Puls M, Murphy SB, Siebenrock KA. Noninvasive three-dimensional assessment of femoroacetabular impingement. J Orthop Res. 2006;25(1): 122–31.
35. Kubiak-Langer M, Tannast M, Murphy SB, Siebenrock KA, Langlotz F. Range of motion in anterior femoroacetabular impingement. Clin Orthop Relat Res. 2007;458:117–24.
36. Milone MT, Bedi A, Poultsides L, Magennis E, Byrd KWT, Larson CM, Kelly BT. Novel CT-based three-dimensional software improves the characterization of cam morphology. Clin Orthop Relat Res. 2013;471:2484–91.

Part V

Non Arthroscopic Treatment of Hip Disease

Jason Brockwell

The Natural History of Untreated Osteoarthritis of the Hip

27

S. David Stulberg

Introduction

The etiology of primary osteoarthritis (OA) of the hip has been a topic of intense interest for many years [1–7]. The recognition that mechanical factors, such as hip dysplasia, may be associated with the occurrence of osteoarthritis in a large proportion of cases has generated hope that treatment of these factors may slow progression of the disease. The recent description of femoroacetabular impingement (FAI) as an additional mechanical cause of hip arthritis has led to the introduction of additional potential treatment options. The efficacy of any intervention designed to prevent or forestall the development of severe degenerative disease of the hip cannot be assessed unless the natural history of the disease is understood. The purpose of this chapter is to determine what we know about the natural history of osteoarthritis in hips that have not received treatment for a disease or deformity thought to be associated with the development of arthritis.

The natural history of hip arthritis will be considered separately for three groups: (1) patients without a history of childhood hip disease and without a recognizable developmental deformity of the hip, (2) untreated patients with a history of one of the three most common childhood hip diseases, and (3) patients with a deformity of the hip (e.g., the pistol-grip deformity or FAI) and no history of childhood hip disease.

As important as the knowledge of the natural history of hip arthritis is, it is essential to understand how difficult it is to obtain this information. The evidence for identifying prognostic variables that influence the progression of osteoarthritis is generally weak or inconclusive because of inconsistencies in the way in which data are collected and measured. The length of the follow-up periods of studies that are available varies [8, 9]. There are very few prospective studies, and most of these have relatively short follow-up. The composition of the study populations also varies. Studies vary in the way in which they define the existence, extent, and impact of the disease. Although radiographs are commonly used to measure progression of the disease, the way in which the radiographs are obtained and evaluated varies substantially among studies. Physicians providing care for hip conditions that may lead to arthritis should be aware of the limitations of the information currently available on the natural history of hip arthritis.

Progression of Osteoarthritis of the Hip in Patients Without a History of Childhood Hip Disease

Wright et al. [10] performed a systematic review of the evidence contained in prospective studies that examined prognostic variables associated with progression of osteoarthritis of the hip in patients with primary osteoarthritis. Primary osteoarthritis was defined to exist if either functional or radiographic signs of arthritis were present and not associated with any factor known to be associated with the development of hip degeneration. Patients with secondary osteoarthritis were carefully excluded. Many studies cited by Wright had suggested that mechanical and environmental factors, including age, sex, obesity, joint injury, excessive occupational joint load, and sports activities contributed to the rate of progression of the hip arthritis [11, 12]. However, Wright concluded that clinical findings were relatively unhelpful in predicting the course of hip arthritis. There was strong evidence (consistent findings in ≥2 high-quality cohort studies) for only three clinical variables that were predictive of progression of hip osteoarthritis: (1) age, (2) baseline hip pain, and (3) a Lequesne Index score ≥10. (Although the Lequesne Index includes a number of variables, the score is derived from the summation of the numerical values assigned to each variable.) The evidence for an association with

S.D. Stulberg, MD (✉)
Department of Orthopaedic Surgery,
Northwestern University Feinberg School of Medicine,
680 N. Lake Shore Dr., Suite 924, Chicago, IL 60611, USA
e-mail: jointsurg@gmail.com

J.C. McCarthy et al. (eds.), *Hip Joint Restoration*, DOI 10.1007/978-1-4614-0694-5_27

disease progression was considered weak (identified in only one high-quality study or consistent findings in ≥3 low-quality cohorts) for (1) a Kellgren-Lawrence (64) hip grade ≥2 together with hip pain, (2) a combination of radiographic grade 3 or 4 together with previous nonsteroidal anti-inflammatory drug use and global assessment of pain above the median, (3) functional impairment ≥2, (4) mean global patient assessment ≥47 over the first 6 months, (5) disability index score ≥5, and (6) restricted flexion. The use of nonsteroidal anti-inflammatory agents, even for prolonged periods of time, had a weak association with progression. In addition, a patient's sex, presence of night pain, a patient's assessment of change in symptoms, and a decrease in exercise tolerance provided inconclusive evidence of disease progression. The evidence that body mass index (BMI) influenced the progression of disease was also considered weak. Thus, only consistent hip pain and substantial decrease in function in older patients reliably predicted progression of hip arthritis.

Wright et al. [9, 10], as well as other investigators [12–18], have reported that arthritis progression could be more reliably predicted from radiographs. There was strong evidence that a joint space ≤2 mm, femoral head migration, femoral osteophytes, and a Kellgren-Lawrence hip grade of 3 were strongly predictive of progression of hip OA.

These observations were confirmed in a large, retrospective cohort study from Iceland that followed the x-rays of normal hips up to 28 years [19, 20]. However, these authors, as well as others, have emphasized that a significant proportion of patients (4 of 5 in the study from Iceland) having radiographic signs of hip OA may continue to function well enough to avoid total hip replacement surgery for decades.

Thus, in the absence of a history of childhood hip disease or significant developmental hip deformity, the rate of progression of hip OA is difficult to predict, even in the presence of mild to moderate (joint space >2 mm) radiographic disease [13, 21, 22].

Progression of Osteoarthritis of the Hips in Patients with a History of Untreated Childhood Hip Disease

Slipped Capital Femoral Epiphysis

There is strong agreement among those that have reported the long-term outcomes of untreated slipped capital femoral epiphysis (SCFE) that the risk of developing significant clinical dysfunction or moderate to severe radiographic degenerative joint disease is directly related to the severity and stability of the slip [9, 23–31]. Carney et al. [32] evaluated a group of 28 patients with a mean follow-up of 41 years and a mean age at follow-up of 54. The mean Iowa Hip Rating was 92 for mild slips, 87 for moderate slips, and 75 for severe slips. Hundred percent of patients with mild slips had an Iowa Hip Rating >80 at follow-up, whereas only 64 % of hips with moderate or severe slips had similar ratings. Thirty-six percent of hips with mild slips had no radiographic evidence of degenerative disease at follow-up. Hundred percent of hips with moderate or severe slips had radiographic evidence of degenerative arthritis. Other studies have confirmed the observation that the natural history of SCFE is favorable into the sixth decade if the slip is mild and stable [32]. These observations have been confirmed by reports of long-term treatment that consistently find that in situ pinning is associated with the best long-term functional and radiographic results, and that the best results of in situ pinning occur when the slip is mild. However, reports have suggested that patients with mild slips or pre-slips can develop symptoms suggestive of FAI [33, 34]. The natural history of the hips in these patients is not yet known. SCFE occurs at an age when the majority of acetabular development is complete. Therefore, there is very little opportunity for the acetabulum to remodel in response to the femoral deformity produced by the disease. If, moreover, avascular necrosis occurs as a consequence of an SCFE, it is invariably associated with a poor clinical and radiographic result in a comparatively short period of time. Authors have emphasized that the osteonecrosis that develops in patients with SCFE differs from that associated with other pediatric hip disorders (e.g., Perthes' disease).

A number of authors have observed that it is not uncommon for patients who have had unilateral SCFE to develop, without having had a history of a contralateral SCFE, a femoral head configuration in the unaffected hip that is suggestive of a slip. However, there are few long-term follow-up studies of the fate of this contralateral deformity in patients who are known to have had an SCFE [35]. Because the deformities that occur in the contralateral hip of patients with a history of unilateral SCFE most closely resemble mild slips, it is tempting to believe that most of these deformities are unlikely to be associated with significant clinical symptoms or radiographic evidence of degenerative joint disease at least into the sixth decade.

Developmental Dysplasia of the Hip

Of all of the childhood hip diseases associated with the subsequent development of degenerative arthritis, hip dysplasia has been the most extensively studied. Since Wiberg's classic publication in 1939 [36], it has been accepted that residual dysplasia of the hip predisposes to osteoarthritis [31, 37–50]. This association has been reinforced by observations that the presence of osteoarthritis in adults without a history of childhood hip disease is often associated with radiographic evidence of hip dysplasia. However, the frequency with which the arthritis develops in the presence of dysplasia and its rate of progression are topics of continued intense interest [22, 38, 39, 51–53]. A recent meta-analysis of published literature from 1975 to 2007 on the natural history of developmental dysplasia found that the level of evidence was not sufficient to determine that persisting mild dysplasia (i.e., a dysplastic hip with a stable, well-centered femoral) is a relevant etio-pathological factor for osteoarthritis of the hip [50]. This review emphasizes the widely held belief that the natural history of dysplasia without subluxation differs significantly from dysplasia with subluxation.

Jacobsen and coworkers [16, 22, 38] using the Copenhagen Osteoarthritis Sub-study of the Copenhagen City Heart Study have carried out the most extensive series of population-based studies of the relationship between hip dysplasia without subluxation and osteoarthritis of the hip. They found that the prevalence of hip dysplasia ranged from 5.4 to 12.6%, depending upon the radiographic index applied. Hips with dysplasia were more likely to be associated with the presence of osteoarthritis than non-dysplastic hip. The extent of the arthritis, as measured by joint space width, increased in postmenopausal women as they aged, but did not increase with age in men.

These investigators also performed a longitudinal study over 10 years of 81 subjects with mild or moderate hip dysplasia (dysplasia without subluxation) in whom no evidence of associated arthritis existed at the beginning of the evaluation. There was no tendency for radiological degeneration, measured by joint space narrowing, compared to 136 control subjects followed over the same period. There were also no differences in self-reported pain over the 10-year period.

In summary, hip dysplasia associated with radiographic subluxation invariably leads to degenerative arthritis. The rate of progression of the arthritis is directly related to the severity of the subluxation and the age of the patient. Hip dysplasia that is not associated with subluxation may be associated with an increased incidence of radiographic osteoarthritis, particularly in older, female patients. However, the rate of progression of the arthritis in this group is not predictable and does not vary from the progression in patients without dysplasia who have equivalent radiographic arthritis [51].

Perthes' Disease

There are relatively few long-term studies of Perthes' disease. In general, those with a follow-up of less than 40 years show that the majority of patients, even those with a deformed femoral head, are active and relatively asymptomatic [31, 54–68]. In studies with follow-ups, after first onset of symptoms, of 20–40 years, most patients (70–90%) are active and relatively pain-free [69]. Symptoms and a clinically relevant decrease in range of motion are likely to occur during this time period only in patients with flattened, irregular femoral heads. Recently, however, symptoms of FAI have been observed even in patients with less severe deformities [70]. Radiographic findings of osteoarthritis are likely to begin appearing in the fourth or fifth decade, even in patients with only moderate residual femoral deformities. The extent of the arthritis appears to be related to the degree to which the femoral head is congruous with the acetabulum.

However, follow-up studies beyond 40 years from onset of the disease show a substantial reduction in function and significant progression in radiographic osteoarthritis. In a follow-up study of patients an average of 48 years after onset of symptoms, McAndrew and Weinstein [58] found that only 40% of patients maintained an Iowa Hip Rating of greater than 80 points. Forty percent of the patients had had an arthroplasty and an additional 10% were suffering from disabling osteoarthritis. In contrast, an earlier report from Iowa on a similar group of patients followed an average of 36 years found that 93% of patients had an Iowa Hip Rating above 80 points. Eight per cent of the patients had had an arthroplasty. Mose observed a group of Perthes patients into their seventh decade and found that all patients with irregular femoral heads had radiographic evidence of significant arthritis [59]. Sixty-seven per cent of patients with relatively round femoral heads had at least moderate degenerative arthritis. None of these patients had had radiographic arthritis in their fourth decade.

Summary of the Natural History of the Three Most Common Childhood Hip Diseases

The ultimate deformities produced by each of the three diseases may appear radiographically similar. However, the natural history of these deformities is specific to the disease. The large majority (70–90%) of patients with mild deformities have very little functional limitation until the fifth decade. Patients with hip dysplasia not associated with subluxation, patients with mild slips, and Perthes' patients with congruous joints are very likely to remain highly functional and only mildly symptomatic into their sixth or seventh decade. Radiographic evidence of arthritis starts to appear in the fourth or fifth decade. The relationship between the deformity produced by each disease and the rate at which the arthritis progresses is variable and unpredictable. It is likely that deformity in conjunction with the patient's predisposition to developing arthritis, perhaps genetically based, determines the rate of disease progression.

The Natural History of Deformities Associated with Femoroacetabular Impingement

It has been long recognized that severe developmental or acquired deformities of the hip that occur in infancy or childhood are associated with the development, in mid- and late adulthood, of osteoarthritis of the hip. Murray [71], however, evaluated anteroposterior radiographs of the hip and suggested that hip osteoarthritis could develop secondary to a subtle, often previously unrecognized, femoral configuration that developed before skeletal maturity that was reminiscent of a mild slipped capital femoral epiphysis. He called this developmental configuration the "tilt" deformity. He quantified this deformity with a head-neck offset ratio. Stulberg, Cordell, Harris, and coworkers [2, 3, 47, 72] extended Murray's observations. They evaluated the anteroposterior, frog lateral, and true lateral radiographs of 75 patients with SCFE and 187 patients with Perthes' disease. They identified and characterized a deformity that resulted from mild cases of these childhood hip diseases and frequently occurred in the contralateral, apparently uninvolved, hip. They called this developmental configuration the "pistol-grip" deformity. They then examined the hips of 75 patients with "idiopathic" osteoarthritis. Forty percent of these patients were found to have a pistol-grip deformity. Moreover, the deformity frequently occurred in the contralateral, asymptomatic hip. An additional 39 % of the 75 patients were found to have acetabular dysplasia as determined by measurements that the authors had described in a previous study. Thus, the pistol-grip deformity and acetabular dysplasia occurred in 79 % of patients previously felt to have primary arthritis. Solomon et al. [73–76] made similar observations in Caucasians living in South Africa, reinforcing the concept that mechanical factors could be implicated in the etiology of a large proportion of patients with previously diagnosed idiopathic hip arthritis.

The underlying presumption in this association between subtle hip joint deformity and the development of arthritis was that even minor anatomic abnormalities resulted in changes in the joint contact area that increased contact pressures on the articular cartilage. This is the mechanism that is widely believed to be associated with the premature onset of arthritis in patients who have developed severe deformities as a consequence of known childhood hip diseases, such as dysplasia, SCFE, and Perthes'. The rationale for surgical treatment (e.g., pelvic osteotomies) of these significant childhood deformities is to broaden the contact area and reduce the contact pressure felt to be resulting from the deformities. It is widely believed that if a reduction in contact pressures can be achieved, the progression to degenerative arthritis in these hips with significant deformities will be slowed. However, Harris and collaborators did not feel that a major reduction in contact area would be a satisfactory explanation for the premature development of osteoarthritis in patients with subtle hip joint deformities [35].

In 2003, Ganz and coworkers [52] proposed an alternative mechanism linking subtle hip joint deformities to the premature development of degenerative arthritis: FAI. Defined as a clinical entity in which a pathologic mechanical process causes hip pain when morphologic abnormalities of the acetabulum and/or femur, combined with vigorous hip motion, lead to repetitive collisions that damage the soft-tissue structures within the joint, FAI contains five essential elements: (1) abnormal morphology of the femur and/or acetabulum, (2) abnormal contact between the femur and acetabulum, (3) especially vigorous supraphysiologic motion that results in such abnormal contact and collision, (4) repetitive motion resulting in the continuous insult, and (5) the presence of soft-tissue damage. The morphologic abnormalities of the femoral head and/or acetabulum result in abnormal contact between the femoral neck and head and the acetabular margin. This leads to abnormal stress that causes tearing of the labrum and avulsion of the underlying cartilage region. The continued abnormal contact results in further deterioration and wear of the articular cartilage, with the eventual onset of degenerative arthritis [34, 77–82].

This stimulating concept embraced the notion that subtle morphologic abnormalities of the hip were associated with the premature occurrence of arthritis [83–87]. However, this original FAI concept was based upon studies in elderly patients with existing OA [88]. The potential value of these studies was limited by the concern that it could be difficult to differentiate premorbid deformity from changes secondary to osteoarthritis (e.g., femoral neck osteophytes). The description of FAI, and its promise of offering treatment interventions that might delay or halt the degenerative process [89], has stimulated a number of large scale radiographic studies of asymptomatic young and middle-aged adults to determine the prevalence of FAI findings in asymptomatic individuals [62, 90–93]. These studies have tended to demonstrate a relatively high prevalence (25–50 %) of the morphologic abnormalities associated with FAI in individuals, particularly males, with minimal or no symptoms. These studies have been carried out predominately in regions of the world, mainly Europe and America, where osteoarthritis of the hip is relatively prevalent, raising the concern that factors in addition to FAI morphologic abnormalities (e.g., genetic, cultural, level, and type of activity) [94] are influencing the prevalence of the disease. Additional longitudinal studies have sought to establish the natural history of FAI deformities [95]. These studies seek to establish the likelihood that individuals with FAI deformities will develop significant arthritis and to determine the rate of progression of the arthritis. The studies have radiographically followed individuals with FAI deformities and little or no arthritis for up to 29 years. The conclusions from these and other studies make it clear that factors in addition to hip morphology play an important role in the evolution of arthritis of the hip.

A cam deformity of the femoral head is said to exist if, on an anteroposterior radiograph, there is excessive bone along the superior surface of the femoral neck. This excessive bone is characterized by abnormal asphericity at the anterolateral femoral head-neck junction. The magnitude of a cam deformity can be quantified by measuring the alpha angle and anterior offset ratio [70]. The term cam deformity is synonymous with the terms tilt deformity (described by Murray to often exist in the, unaffected, contralateral hip of patients known to have had a slipped capital femoral epiphysis [71]) and pistol-grip deformity (described by Stulberg et al. [64] as the deformity often occurring in the unaffected contralateral hip of patients known to have had hip dysplasia, Perthes disease, or slipped capital femoral epiphyses). However, the term cam implies the impingement mechanism felt to initiate the articular cartilage degenerative process. Cam deformities were common in males (17 %) in a large cross-sectional Danish study [55]. However, the authors found no significant relationship between the presence of hip joint arthritis and the deformity. Another review of 96 patients with radiological evidence of FAI followed an average of 18.5 years found that 82.3 % of hips remained free of arthritis [86]. Only the presence of significant arthritis in the contralateral hip at final follow-up was predictive of the development of arthritis in the FAI hip. In general, the longitudinal studies indicate that the overwhelming majority of hips with cam deformities do not develop osteoarthritis. Moreover, the studies suggest the progression of arthritis in those with mild to moderate FAI deformities is slow (>10 years) and is similar to that seen in hips with mild arthritis without the deformities. Nevertheless, a number of studies examining the relationship of the presence of a cam deformity and the presence of arthritis have noted that there appears to be a relationship between the severity of the cam deformity and the rate of progression of arthritis.

Conclusion

Osteoarthritis is a disorder of diverse etiologies. A multitude of factors, including genetic, mechanical, and biochemical, play a role in the cause of the disease. It is the interplay of these factors that determine the natural history of osteoarthritis of the hip [6, 60, 96–103].

There is significant evidence that genetics plays a pivotal role in the etiology of osteoarthritis of the hip [19, 20, 41, 104–110]. This genetic basis is well established in Europeans and those of European descent [106]. Primary osteoarthritis is virtually nonexistent in non-European-based populations [111], including those of India, China [112–114], Pakistan, Saudi Arabia, Korea [115], Kuwait, Iran, Malawi, Nigeria, Togo, Singapore, and Japan [116]. Although many studies suggest that mechanical and environmental factors, including age, sex [117], obesity [118, 119], joint injury, excessive occupational joint load, nonsteroidal medication [120], and sports activities [121], may contribute to the rate of progression of the disease, it is not known if or how genetic predisposition influences the impact of mechanical and environmental factors on the progression of osteoarthritis [122]. These mechanical and environmental factors are as prevalent in areas of the world in which osteoarthritis of the hip is virtually nonexistent as they are in Europe and America.

The importance of the interplay of the various etiologic factors of osteoarthritis of the hip on the natural history of the disease is particularly noteworthy when one attempts to relate the presence of morphologic features of the hip to the progression of arthritis [17]. There is general agreement that when a severe deformity results from one of the three most common childhood hip diseases, clinical and radiographic evidence of osteoarthritis will inevitably be present by the fourth or fifth decade. The cause for the development of this premature arthritis is generally felt to be based on the presence of abnormal load transmission on articular cartilage resulting from eccentric overload. However, even patients with significant deformities resulting from one of these childhood hip diseases develop the signs and symptoms of arthritis at highly variable rates, suggesting that factors, in addition to mechanical overload, play a role in the natural history of the arthritis even in presence of gross intra-articular deformities.

When the deformity resulting from one of the three most common childhood hip diseases is mild, the progression of arthritis is slow and unpredictable. Patients with hip dysplasia, a disease known to have both a genetic and mechanical basis (increased incidence of left hips, increased incidence in first born, increased incidence in babies swaddled with extended hips), appear to have no greater tendency for radiological degeneration, measured by joint space narrowing, compared to control subjects if no subluxation is present. This suggests that not only are factors other than abnormal joint mechanics important in determining the progression of arthritis, but that the genetic factors influencing its rate of development are separate from the genetic factors related to the occurrence of the dysplasia. The best predictor of arthritis progression in patients with mild deformities known to be secondary to a childhood hip disease appears to be the presence and progression of arthritis of the contralateral hip.

The natural history of arthritis in patients without a history of childhood hip disease whose hips have morphologic features suggestive of a mild childhood hip disease (e.g., the pistol-grip deformity) is uncertain. Although the occurrence of radiographic arthritis in these patients may be greater when they are over 50 [83], the rate of progression of arthritis does not appear to differ from the progression in patients with equivalent degrees of arthritis without the deformities. Because these deformities have been most exhaustively evaluated in Europe and America, locations where osteoarthritis of the hip is relatively prevalent and felt to be genetically based, their role in determining the natural history of the disease is difficult to establish. The deformities themselves may in many, perhaps most, cases be genetically based.

However, it is not known if the genetic basis for the deformity is related to a genetic predisposition for the development of arthritis.

There have been recent suggestions that strenuous physical activity in preadolescence may be associated with the development of abnormal morphologic features of the hip [121, 123, 124]. It is not known what the natural history of deformities produced by this mechanism is. Whether hips with these deformities will behave like the mild deformities following a known childhood hip disease or like deformities occurring without a history of childhood hip disease that may be genetically based is unknown.

The role of the mechanism of FAI on the natural history of arthritis is a topic generating intense interest [78]. The concept was originally described in patients without a history of childhood hip disease who had morphologic abnormalities of the femur or acetabulum that resulted in abnormal contact between the femoral neck and head and the acetabular margin. This led to abnormal stress that caused tearing of the labrum, avulsion of the underlying cartilage region, and the subsequent development of arthritis. The interaction of this mechanism with a genetic predisposition to hip arthritis is not known. Moreover, the relative importance of this mechanism in the development and progression of arthritis in patients with a mild hip deformity and a known history of childhood hip disease is not yet known [33].

In summary, it is apparent that just as multiple factors play a role in the etiology of osteoarthritis of the hip, many factors also influence its natural history. While there is a strong genetic impact on the occurrence of the disease [106], how this factor affects the progression of the disease is not understood. Similarly, mechanical factors, particularly significant joint deformity, play an undeniable and important role in the occurrence and progression of the disease. The prevention of these severe deformities has had a positive impact on slowing the progression of hip arthritis. The appropriate treatment of mild deformities and their associated effects on intra-articular pathology needs to be clarified. These deformities can cause significant symptoms, particularly in young, active patients. It remains to be clarified whether the treatment of these acute symptoms, even when effective, has an impact on the natural history of the involved joint.

What becomes very clear when one studies the natural history of osteoarthritis of the hip is that there is a need for well-conceived and designed prospective longitudinal long-term follow-up studies, particularly radiographic studies, of conditions that affect the hip. Physicians that care for children, adolescents, and young adults with hip disease should be strongly encouraged to put in place mechanisms that allow for this follow-up. Adult reconstructive surgeons should be encouraged to collaborate with their pediatric orthopedic colleagues that treat childhood hip diseases. The effort should be worldwide, especially in those regions where osteoarthritis of the hip is prevalent. Specialty organizations devoted to the study of hip disease should make such studies a priority. In an era when health care is increasingly evidence-based, the absence of longitudinal information about the natural history of osteoarthritis of the hip should not be acceptable. Current computer-based technologies make such follow-up more feasible than ever before. The job will only get done when it is approached with the same sense of urgency that is currently being given to the treatment regimens being promoted to prevent the progression of arthritis of the hip.

References

1. Elmslie RC. Aetiological factors in osteoarthritis of the hip. BMJ. 1933;1:1–3.
2. Gower WE, Johnson RC. Legg-Perthes disease. Long-term follow-up of thirty patients. J Bone Joint Surg Am. 1971;53A:759–68.
3. Hack K, DiPrimio G, Rakhra K, Beaule PE. Prevalence of cam-type femoroacetabular impingement morphology in asymptomatic volunteers. J Bone Joint Surg Am. 2010;92-A:2436–44.
4. Harris WH. Etiology of osteoarthritis of the hip. Clin Orthop Relat Res. 1986;213:20–33.
5. Hartofilakidis G, Bardakos NV, Babis GC, Georgiades G. An examination of the association between different morphotypes of femoroacetabular impingement in asymptomatic subjects and the development of osteoarthritis of the hip. J Bone Joint Surg Br. 2011;93(5):580–6.
6. Kelman A, Lui L, Yao W, Krumme A, Nevitt M, Lane NE. Association of higher levels of serum cartilage oligomeric matrix protein and N-Telopeptide crosslinks with the development of radiographic hip osteoarthritis in elderly women. Arthritis Rheum. 2006;54:236–43.
7. Nho SJ, Kymes SM, Callaghan JJ, Felson DT. The burden of hip osteoarthritis in the United States: epidemiologic and economic considerations. J Am Acad Orthop Surg. 2013;21 Suppl 1:S1–6.
8. Goker B, Sancak A, Haznedaroglu S. Radiographic hip osteoarthritis and acetabular dysplasia in Turkish men and women. Rheumatol Int. 2005;25(6):419–22.
9. Wemsaas A, Svenningsen S, Terjesen T. Long-term follow-up of slipped capital femoral epiphysis: a 38 year follow-up of 66 patients. J Child Orthop. 2011;5:75–82.
10. Wright AA, Cook C, Abbott JH. Variables associated with the progression of hip osteoarthritis: a systematic review. Arthritis Rheum. 2009;1(7):925–36.
11. Birrell F, Afzal C, Nahit E, Lunt M, Macfarlane GJ, Cooper C, et al. Predictors of hip joint replacement in new attenders in primary care with hip pain. Br J Gen Pract. 2004;53:26–30.
12. Dougados M, Gueguen A, Nguyen M, Berdayh L, Lequesne M, Mazieres B, et al. Radiological progression of hip osteoarthritis: definition, risk factors and correlations with clinical status. Ann Rheum Dis. 1996;55:356–62.
13. Conrozier T, Jousseaume CA, Mathieu P, Tron AM, Caton J, Bejui J, et al. Quantitative measurement of joint space narrowing progression in hip osteoarthritis: a longitudinal retrospective study of patients treated by total hip arthroplasty. Br J Rheumatol. 1998;37:961–8.

14. Dougados M, Gueguen A, Nguyen M, Berdah L, Lequesne M, Mazieres B, et al. Radiographic features predictive of radiographic progression of hip osteoarthritis. Rev Rhum Engl Ed. 1997;64:795–803.
15. Dougados M, Gueguen A, Nguyen M, Berdah L, Lequesne M, Mazieres B, et al. Requirement for total hip arthroplasty: an outcome measure of hip osteoarthritis? J Rheumatol. 1999;26:855–61.
16. Jacobsen S, Sonne-Holm S, Soballe K, Beguhr P, Lund B. The distribution and inter-relationships of radiologic features of osteoarthrosis of the hip: a survey of 4151 subjects of the Copenhagen City Heart Study. The Osteoarthrosis Substudy. Osteoarthritis Cartilage. 2004;12:704–10.
17. Macys JR, Bullough PG, Wilson Jr PD. Coxarthrosis: a study of the natural history based on a correlation of clinical, radiographic and pathologic findings. Semin Arthritis Rheum. 1980;10:66–80.
18. Reijman M, Hazes JM, Pols HA, Bernsen RM, Koes BW, Bierma-Zeinstra SM. Role of radiography in predicting progression of osteoarthritis of the hip: prospective cohort study. BMJ. 2005; 330:1183.
19. Ingvarsson T, Hagglund G, Lohmander LS. Prevalence of hip osteoarthritis in Iceland. Ann Rheum Dis. 1999;58:201–7.
20. Ingvarsson T. Prevalence and inheritance of hip osteoarthritis in Iceland. Acta Orthop Scand Suppl. 2000;298:1–46.
21. Jacobsen S, Sonne-Holm S, Soballe K, Beguhr P, Lund B. The relationship of hip joint space to self reported hip pain: a survey of 4,151 subjects of the Copenhagen City Heart Study. The Osteoarthritis Substudy. Osteoarthritis Cartilage. 2004;12:692–7.
22. Jacobsen S, Sonne-Holm S, Soballe K, Beguhr P, Lund B. Joint space width in dysplasia of the hip. A case-control study of 82 adults followed for 10 years. J Bone Joint Surg Br. 2005;87-B:471–7.
23. Aronsson DD, Loder RT, Breur GJ, Weinstein SL. Slipped capital femoral epiphysis: current concepts. J Am Acad Orthop Surg. 2006;14:666–79.
24. Boyer DW, Mickelson MR, Ponseti IV. Slipped capital femoral epiphysis: long-term follow-up and study of one hundred and twenty-one patients. J Bone Joint Surg Am. 1981;63A:85–95.
25. Jerre T. A study in slipped upper femoral epiphysis with special reference to late functional and roentgenological results and the value of closed reduction. Acta Orthop Scand. 1950;(Suppl): 6.
26. Jerre T. Physiolysis of the hip: epidemiology, diagnosis and long term follow-up. Thesis Geteborg; 1995.
27. Johnston RC, Larson CB. Results of treatment of hip disorders with cup arthroplasty. J Bone Joint Surg. 1969;51A:1461–79.
28. Kallio PE, Mah ET, Foster BK, Paterson DC, LeQuesne GW. Slipped capital femoral epiphysis: incidence and clinical assessment of physeal instability. J Bone Joint Surg Br. 1995;77-B:752–5.
29. Larson AN, Sierra RJ, Yu EM, Trousdale RT, Stans AA. Outcomes of slipped capital femoral epiphysis treated with in situ pinning. J Pediatr Orthop. 2012;32:125–30.
30. Ross PM, Lyne ED, Morawa LG. Slipped capital femoral epiphysis: long-term results after 1–38 years. Clin Orthop. 1979;141: 176–80.
31. Weinstein SL. Natural history and treatment outcomes of childhood hip disorders. Clin Orthop Relat Res. 1997;344:227–42.
32. Carney BT, Weinstein SL, Noble J. Long-term follow-up of slipped capital femoral epiphysis. J Bone Joint Surg Am. 1991;73A:667–74.
33. Dodds MK, McCormack D, Mulhall KJ. Femoroacetabular impingement after slipped capital femoral epiphysis: does slip severity predict clinical symptoms? J Pediatr Orthop. 2009;29:535–9.
34. Leunig M, Casillas MM, Hamlet M, Hersche O, Notzli H, Slongo T, Ganz R. Slipped capital femoral epiphysis: early mechanical damage to the acetabular cartilage by a prominent femoral metaphysis. Acta Orthop Scand. 2000;71:370–5.
35. Ganz R, Leunig M, Leunig-Ganz K, Harris WH. The etiology of osteoarthritis of the hip: an integrated mechanical concept. Clin Orthop Relat Res. 2008;466(2):264–72.
36. Wiberg G. Studies on dysplastic acetabulum and congenital subluxation of the hip joint with special reference to the complication of osteoarthritis. Acta Chir Scand. 1939;83(Suppl):58.
37. Inoue K, Wicart P, Kawasaki T, et al. Prevalence of hip osteoarthritis and acetabular dysplasia in French and Japanese adults. Rheumatology (Oxford). 2000;39:745–8.
38. Jacobsen S, Sonne-Holm S. Hip dysplasia: a significant risk factor for the development of hip osteoarthritis. A cross-sectional survey. Rheumatology. 2005;44:211–8.
39. Jacobsen S. Adult hip dysplasia and osteoarthritis: studies in radiology and clinical epidemiology. Acta Orthop Suppl. 2006;77: 1–37.
40. Lane NE, Lin P, Christiansen L, et al. Association of mild acetabular dysplasia with an increased risk of incident hip osteoarthritis in elderly white women: the study of osteoporotic fractures. Arthritis Rheum. 2000;43:400–4.
41. Lane NE, Nevitt MC, Hochberg MC, Hung Y, Palermo L. Progression of radiographic hip osteoarthritis over eight years in a community sample of elderly white women. Arthritis Rheum. 2004;50:1477–86.
42. Lievense AM, Bierma-Zeinstra SM, Berhagen AP, Verhaaar JA, Koes BW. Influence of hip dysplasia on the development of osteoarthritis of the hip. Ann Rheum Dis. 2004;63(6):621–6.
43. Lievense AM, Koes BW, Verhaar JA, Bohnen AM, Bierma-Zeinstra SM. Prognosis of hip pain in general practice: a prospective followup study. Arthritis Rheum. 2007;57:1368–74.
44. Malvitz TA, Weinstein SL. Closed reduction for congenital dysplasia of the hip. Functional and radiographic results after an average of 30 years. J Bone Joint Surg Am. 1994;76(12):1777–92.
45. Murphy SB, Ganz R, Muller ME. The prognosis in untreated dysplasia of the hip: a study of radiographic factors that predict the outcome. J Bone Joint Surg Am. 1995;77-A:985–9.
46. Reijman M, Hazes JM, Pols HA, Koes BW, Bierma-Zeinstra SM. Acetabular dysplasia predicts incident osteoarthritis of the hip: the Rotterdam study. Arthritis Rheum. 2005;52:787–93.
47. Stulberg SD. Acetabular dysplasia, development of osteoarthritis of the hip. In: Harris WH, editor. The hip: proceedings of the second open scientific session of the Hip Society. St Louis: CV Mosby; 1974. p. 82–93.
48. Wedge JH, Wasylenko MJ. The natural history of congenital disease of the hip. J Bone Joint Surg Br. 1979;61-B:334–8.
49. Yoshimura N, Campbell L, Hashimoto T, et al. Acetabular dysplasia and hip osteoarthritis in Britain and Japan. Br J Rheumatol. 1998;37(11):1193–7.
50. Ziegler J, Thielemann F, Mayer-Athenstaedt C, Gunther KP. The natural history of developmental dysplasia of the hip: a meta-analysis of the published literature. Orthopade. 2008;37:515–24.
51. Cooperman DR, Wallensten R, Stulberg SD. Acetabular dysplasia in the adult. Clin Orthop. 1983;175:79–85.
52. Ganz R, Parvizi J, Beck M, Leunig M, Notzli H, Siebenrock KA. Femoroacetabular impingement: a cause for osteoarthritis of the hip. Clin Orthop Relat Res. 2003;417:112–20.
53. Mladenov K, Dora C, Wicart P, Seringe R. Natural history of hips with borderline acetabular index and acetabular dysplasia in infants. J Pediatr Orthop. 2002;22:607–12.
54. Franklin J, Ingvarsson T, Englund M, Lohmander LS. Sex differences in the association between body mass index and total hip or knee joint replacement resulting from osteoarthritis. Ann Rheum Dis. 2009;68:536–40.
55. Gosvig KK, Jacobsen S, Sonne-Holm S, Gebuhr P. The prevalence of cam-type deformity of the hip joint: a survey of 4151 subjects of the Copenhagen Osteoarthritis Study. Acta Radiol. 2008;4:436–41.

56. Ippolito E, Tudisco C, Farsetti P. The long-term prognosis of unilateral Perthes' disease. J Bone Joint Surg Br. 1987;69B:243–50.
57. Kim HKW, Herring JA. Pathophysiology, classifications and natural history of Perthes disease. Orthop Clin North Am. 2011;42:285–95.
58. McAndrew MP, Weinstein SL. A long-term follow-up of Legg-Calve-Perthes disease. J Bone Joint Surg Am. 1984;66A:860–9.
59. Mose K, Hjorth L, Ulfeldt M, Christensen ER, Jensen A. Legg-Calve-Perthes disease. The late occurrence of coxarthrosis. Acta Orthop Scand Suppl. 1977;169:1–39.
60. Onishi E, Ikeda N, Ueo T. Degenerative osteoarthritis after Perthes' disease: a 36 year follow-up. Arch Orthop Trauma Surg. 2011;131(5):701–7.
61. Ratliff AHC. Perthes disease: a study of thirty-four hips observed for thirty years. J Bone Joint Surg Br. 1967;49B:102–7.
62. Reichenbach S, Juni P, Werlen S, et al. Prevalence of cam-type deformity on hip magnetic resonance imaging in young males: a cross-sectional study. Arthritis Care Res (Hoboken). 2010;62(9): 1319–27.
63. Specchiulli F, Cofano RE. Long-term follow-up of Perthes' disease in adolescence. Chir Organi Mov. 2001;86(1):7–13.
64. Stulberg SD, Cooperman DR, Wallensten R. The natural history of Legg-Calve-Perthes disease. J Bone Joint Surg Am. 1981;63A:1095–108.
65. Weinstein SL. Legg-Perthes disease. The results of long-term follow-up. In: Fitzgerald R, editor. The hip. Proceedings of the thirteenth open scientific meeting of the Hip Society. St. Louis: CV Mosby; 1985. p. 28–37.
66. Weinstein SL. Legg-Calve-Perthes disease. In: Morrissy RT, Weinstein SL, editors. Lovell and Winter's pediatric orthopaedics. Philadelphia: Lippincott Raven Press; 1996. p. 951–92.
67. Yrjonen T. Prognosis in Perthes' disease after non-containment treatment. 106 hips followed for 28-47 years. Acta Orthop Scand. 1992;63:523–6.
68. Zarzycka M, Zarzycki D, Kacki W, Jasiewicz B, Ridan T. Long-term results of conservative treatment in Perthes' disease. Ortop Traumatol Rehabil. 2004;6(5):595–603.
69. Larson AN, Sucato DJ, Herring JA, Adolfse SE, et al. A prospective multicenter study of Legg-Calve-Perthes disease. Functional and radiographic outcomes of nonoperative treatment at a mean follow-up of twenty years. J Bone Joint Surg Am. 2012;94: 584–92.
70. Eijer H, Podeszwa DA, Ganz R, Leunig M. Evaluation and treatment of young adults with femoro-acetabular impingement secondary to Perthes' disease. Hip Int. 2006;16:273–80.
71. Murray RO. The aetiology of primary osteoarthritis of the hip. Br J Radiol. 1965;38:810–24.
72. Stulberg SD. Unrecognized childhood hip disease: a major cause of idiopathic osteoarthritis of the hip. In: Cordell LD, Harris WH, Ramsey PL, MacEwen GD, editors. The hip: proceeding of the third open scientific meeting of the Hip Society. St Louis: MO Mosby; 1975. p. 212–28.
73. Solomon L. Patterns of osteoarthritis of the hip. J Bone Joint Surg Br. 1976;58:176–83.
74. Solomon L. Geographical and anatomical patterns of osteoarthritis. Br J Rheumatol. 1984;23:177–80.
75. Solomon L, Beighton P. Osteoarthrosis of the hip and its relationship to pre-existing in an African population. J Bone Joint Surg Br. 1973;55:216–7.
76. Solomon L, Schnitzler CM, Browett JP. Osteoarthritis of the hip: the patient behind the disease. Ann Rheum Dis. 1982;41:118–25.
77. Agricola R, Heijboer MP, Bierma-Zeinstra SM, et al. Cam impingement causes osteoarthritis of the hip: a nationwide prospective cohort study (CHECK). Ann Rheum Dis. 2013;72: 918–23.
78. Beck M, Kalhor M, Leunig M, Ganz R. Hip morphology influences the pattern of damage to the acetabular cartilage: femoroacetabular impingement as a cause of early osteoarthritis of the hip. J Bone Joint Surg Br. 2005;87:1012–8.
79. Lavigne M, Parvizi J, Beck M, Siebenrock KA, Ganz R, Leunig M. Anterior femoroacetabular impingement: part I. Techniques of joint preserving surgery. Clin Orthop Relat Res. 2004;418: 61–6.
80. Leunig M, Ganz R. The evolution and concepts of joint-preserving surgery of the hip. Bone Joint J. 2014;96-B(1):5–18.
81. Li PL, Ganz R. Morphologic features of congenital acetabular dysplasia: one in six is retroverted. Clin Orthop Relat Res. 2003;416:245–53.
82. Sankar WN, Nevitt M, Parvizi J, Felson DT, Agricola R, Leunig M. Femoroacetabular impingement: defining the condition and its role in the pathophysiology of osteoarthritis. J Am Acad Orthop Surg. 2013;21(Supp 1):S7–15.
83. Doherty M, Courtney P, Doherty S, et al. Nonspherical femoral head shape (pistol grip deformity), neck shaft angle, and risk of hip osteoarthritis: a case-control study. Arthritis Rheum. 2008;58(10):3172–82.
84. Ezoe M, Naito M, Inoue T. The prevalence of acetabular retroversion among various disorders of the hip. J Bone Joint Surg Am. 2006;88-A:372–9.
85. Froberg L, Christensen F, Pedersen NW, Overgaard S. Long-term follow-up of a patient cohort with Legg-Calve-Perthes disease. J Pediatr Orthop B. 2011;20(5):273–7.
86. Harris WH. Primary osteoarthritis of the hip: a vanishing diagnosis. J Rheumatol. 1983; Suppl 9: 64.
87. Wagner S, Hofstetter W, Chiquet M, et al. Early osteoarthritic changes of human femoral head cartilage subsequent to femoroacetabular impingement. Osteoarthritis Cartilage. 2003;11: 508–18.
88. Clohisy JC, Dobson MA, Robison JF, et al. Radiographic structural abnormalities associated with premature, natural hip-joint failure. J Bone Joint Surg Am. 2011;93 Suppl 2:3–9.
89. Clohisy JC, McClure JR. Treatment of anterior femoroacetabular impingement with combined hip arthroscopy and limited anterior decompression. Iowa Orthop J. 2005;25:164–71.
90. Goodman DA, Geighan JE, Smith AD, et al. Subclinical slipped capital femoral epiphysis: relationship to osteoarthritis of the hip. J Bone Joint Surg Am. 1997;79(10):1489–97.
91. Gossec L, Tubach F, Baron G, Ravaud P, Logeart I, Dougados M. Predictive factors of total hip replacement due to primary osteoarthritis: a prospective 2 year study of 505 patients. Ann Rheum Dis. 2005;64:1028–32.
92. Gosvig KK, Jacobsen S, Sonne-Holm S, Palm H, Troelsen A. Prevalence of malformations of the hip joint and their relationship to sex, groin pain, and risk of osteoarthritis: a population-based survey. J Bone Joint Surg Am. 2010;92-A:162–1169.
93. Leunig M, Juni P, Werlen S, Limacher A, et al. Prevalence of cam and pincer-type deformities on hip MRI in asymptomatic young Swiss female population: a cross-sectional study. Osteoarthritis Cartilage. 2013;21(4):544–50.
94. Pollard TC, Villar RN, Norton MR, Fern ED, Williams MR, Murray DW, Carr AJ. Genetic influences in the aetiology of femoroacetabular impingement: a sibling study. J Bone Joint Surg Br. 2010;92(2):209–16.
95. Bardakos NV, Villar RN. Predictors of progression of osteoarthritis in femoroacetabular impingement: a radiological study with a minimum of 10 years follow-up. J Bone Joint Surg Br. 2009;91(2):162–9.
96. Beattie MS, Lane NE, Hung Y, Nevitt MC. Association of statin use and development and progression of hip osteoarthritis in elderly women. J Rheumatol. 2005;32:106–10.

97. Chaganti RK, Kelman A, Lui L, Yao W, Javaid MK, Bauer D, et al. Change in serum measurements of cartilage oligomeric matrix protein and association with the development and worsening of radiographic hip osteoarthritis. Osteoarthritis Cartilage. 2008;16:566–71.
98. Felson DT. The course of osteoarthritis and factors that affect it. Rheum Dis Clin North Am. 1993;19:607–15.
99. Flugsrud GB, Nordsletten L, Espehaug B, Havelin LI, Meyer HE. Risk factors for total hip replacement due to primary osteoarthritis: a cohort study in 50,034 persons. Arthritis Rheum. 2002;46:675–82.
100. Flugsrud BB, Nordsletten L, Espehaug B, Havelin LI, Meyer HE. Weight change and the risk of total hip replacement. Epidemiology. 2003;14(5):578–84.
101. Flugsrud GB, Nordsletten L, Espehaug B, Havelin LI, Engeland A, Meyer HE. The impact of body mass index on later total hip arthroplasty for primary osteoarthritis: a cohort study in 1.2 million persons. Arthritis Rheum. 2006;54(3):802–7.
102. Hiagkund FT, Steinbach LS. Primary osteoarthritis of the hip: etiology and epidemiology. J Am Acad Orthop Surg. 2001;9:320–7.
103. Mazieres B, Garnero P, Gueguen A, Abbal M, Berdah L, Lequesne M, et al. Molecular markers of cartilage breakdown and synovitis at baseline as predictors of structural progression of hip osteoarthritis: the ECHODIAH cohort. Ann Rheum Dis. 2006;65:354–9.
104. Ali-Gombe A, Croft PR, Silman AJ. Osteoarthritis of the hip and acetabular dysplasia in Nigerian men. J Rheumatol. 1996;23(3): 512–5.
105. Botha-Scheepers SA, Watt I, Slagboom E, Meulenbelt I, Rosendaal FR, Breedveld FC, et al. Influence of familial factors on radiologic disease progression over 2 years in siblings with osteoarthritis at multiple sites: a prospective longitudinal cohort study. Arthritis Rheum. 2007;57:626–32.
106. Hoaglund FT. Primary osteoarthritis of the hip: a genetic disease caused by European genetic variants. J Bone Joint Surg Am. 2013;95:463–8.
107. Hochberg MC. Do risk factors for incident hip osteoarthritis (OA) differ from those for progression of hip OA? J Rheumatol Suppl. 2004;70:6–9.
108. Lane NE, Nevitt MC, Lui LY, de Leon P, Corr M, Study of Osteoporotic Fractures Research Group. Wnt signaling antagonists are potential prognostic biomarkers for the progression of radiographic hip osteoarthritis in elderly Caucasian women. Arthritis Rheum. 2007;56:3319–25.
109. Reijman M, Hazes JM, Bierma-Zeinstra SM, Koes BW, Christgau S, Christiansen C, et al. A new marker for osteoarthritis: cross-sectional and longitudinal approach. Arthritis Rheum. 2004;50:2471–8.
110. Shi D, Dai J, Zhu P, et al. Association of the D repeat polymorphism in the ASPN gene with developmental dysplasia of the hip: a case-control study in Han Chinese. Arthritis Res Ther. 2011;13(1):R27.
111. Oishi CS, Hoaglund FT, Gordon L, Ross PD. Total hip replacement rates are higher among Caucasians than Asians in Hawaii. Clin Orthop. 1998;353:166–74.
112. Dudda M, Kim YJ, Zhang Y, et al. Morphologic differences between the hips of Chinese women and white women: could they account for the ethnic difference in the prevalence of hip osteoarthritis? Arthritis Rheum. 2011;63(q10):2992–9.
113. Lau EM, Lin F, Lam D, Silman A, Croft P. Hip osteoarthritis and dysplasia in Chinese men. Ann Rheum Dis. 1995;54(12):965–9.
114. Nevitt MC, Xu L, Zhang Y, et al. Very low prevalence of hip osteoarthritis among Chinese elderly in Beijing, China compared with whites in the United States: The Beijing osteoarthritis study. Arthritis Rheum. 2002;46(7):1773–9.
115. Kim HA, Koh SH, Lee G, et al. Low rate of total hip replacement as reflected by a low prevalence of hip osteoarthritis in South Korea. Osteoarthritis Cartilage. 2008;16(12):1572–5.
116. Chung CY, Park MS, Lee KM, et al. Hip osteoarthritis and risk factors in elderly Korean population. Osteoarthritis Cartilage. 2010;18(3):312–6.
117. Maillefert JF, Gueguen A, Monreal M, Nguyen M, Berdah L, Lequesne M, et al. Sex differences in hip osteoarthritis: results of a longitudinal study in 508 patients. Ann Rheum Dis. 2003;62:931–4.
118. Lohmander LS, Gerhardsson de Verdier M, Rollof J, Nilsson PM, Enstrom G. Incidence of severe knee and hip osteoarthritis in relation to different measures of body mass: a population-based prospective cohort study. Ann Rheum Dis. 2009;68:490–6.
119. Reijman M, Pols HA, Bergink AP, Hazes JM, Belo JN, Lievense AM, et al. Body mass index associated with onset and progression of osteoarthritis of the knee but not of the hip: the Rotterdam Study. Ann Rheum Dis. 2007;66:158–62.
120. Reijman M, Bierma-Zeinstra SM, Pols HA, Koes BW, Stricker BH, Hazes JM. Is there an association between the use of different types of nonsteroidal anti-inflammatory drugs and radiologic progression of osteoarthritis? The Rotterdam Study. Arthritis Rheum. 2005;52:3137–42.
121. Lindberg H, Roos H, Gardsell P. Prevalence of coxarthrosis in former soccer players: 286 players compared with match controls. Acta Orthop Scand. 1993;64:165–7.
122. Ledingham J, Dawson S, Preston B, Milligan G, Doherty M. Radiographic progression of hospital referred osteoarthritis of the hip. Ann Rheum Dis. 1993;52:263–7.
123. Armfield DR, Towers JD, Roberston DD. Radiographic and MR imaging of the athletic hip. Clin Sports Med. 2006;25: 211–39. viii.
124. Siebenrock KA, Ferner F, Noble PC, Santore RF, Werlen S, Mamisch TC. The cam-type deformity of the proximal femur arises in childhood in response to vigorous sporting activity. Clin Orthop Relat Res. 2011;469(11):3229–40.

28 Nonsurgical Treatment (Indications, Limitations, Outcomes): Injections

Omar El Abd, João E.D. Amadera,
Daniel Camargo Pimentel, and Amit Bhargava

The need for management of chronic painful musculoskeletal conditions is on the rise; this is mostly due to the aging of the population and the active lifestyle of patients of all age groups. Local injections constitute currently one of the main forms of nonsurgical treatment for painful musculoskeletal conditions including the hip. Other forms of management include oral medications, physical therapy, and alternative medicine. Injections are often used for therapeutic and diagnostic purposes, and in many instances, therapeutic injections are used as a last resort to avoid or to delay surgical interventions. They can also be used to reduce pain and improve function in poor surgical candidates.

There are a significant number of causes of pain from the hip girdle area emanating from extra-articular and intra-articular structures. The accuracy in the identification of the cause of pain is obviously crucial for improving injections outcomes.

Clinically, the hip area pain is divided into two categories: pain originating from the hip girdle structures and pain referred to the hip area (Fig. 28.1).

O. El Abd, MD (✉)
Newton Wellesley Interventional Service,
378 Washington St., Wellesley, MA 02481, USA

Internal Medicine, PM&R, Newton Wellesley Hospital,
Wellesley, MA, USA
e-mail: oelabd@partners.org

J.E.D. Amadera, MD, PhD
Faculty of Medicine, Spine Center, University of São Paulo,
São Paulo, Brazil
e-mail: joaoamadera@gmail.com

D.C. Pimentel, MD, PhD
Department of Orthopedics and Traumatology, University of Sao Paulo, School of Medicine, Spine Center, Sao Paulo, Brazil
e-mail: daniel@spinecenter.med.br

A. Bhargava, MD
Advanced Pain and Sports Medical, Owings Mills, MD, USA

Pain from the hip girdle structures can be further divided into two groups: intra-articular (hip joint) and extra-articular [1, 2] (Table 28.1). Other causes of pain referral from the abdomen and pelvis are beyond the scope of this chapter.

Pain Originating in the Hip

Intra-articular

Differentiation of Intra-articular vs. Extra-articular Hip Pathologies with Injections

Several structures can produce pain in the hip area. For this reason, intra-articular joint injection of a local anesthetic can be used as a diagnostic tool. The main benefit from a diagnostic intra-articular injection is to differentiate the source of pain: intra-articular causes vs. extra-articular or referred pain causes. If the patient experiences significant relief after the diagnostic injection, it is more likely than not that the pain originates from the hip joint, and a therapeutic procedure can be performed such as steroid hip injection or surgery [3–5].

Hip Degenerative Joint Disease (Osteoarthritis)

Degenerative joint disease (DJD)/osteoarthritis (OA) is the most common type of arthritis, which affects over 27 million US adults [6]. It is described as a progressive degenerative process that starts with joint cartilage disruption, followed by changes in the subchondral bone, synovium, joint margins, and adjacent structures [7]. The hip joint is the second most commonly affected site of OA, after the knee, with an estimated lifetime risk around 19 % for men and 29 % for women [8]. It impacts directly daily activities, due to limitations in performing movements such as walking, standing, bending, or stooping [9].

Intra-articular injections are often used for diagnosis of painful hips and management of painful hip OA.

The most commonly used method of imaging guidance is live fluoroscopy, due to its enhanced precision in needle and contrast visualization [10]. Recently ultrasound guidance

J.C. McCarthy et al. (eds.), *Hip Joint Restoration*, DOI 10.1007/978-1-4614-0694-5_28

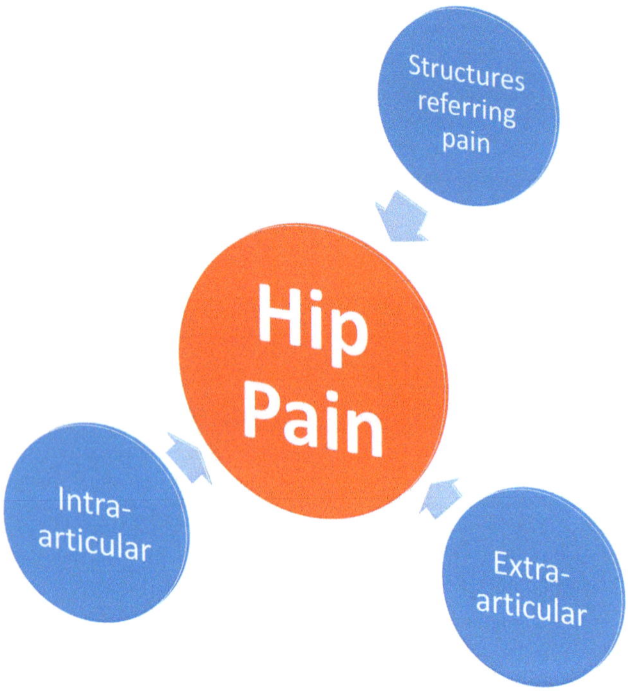

Fig. 28.1 Causes of hip pain can be intra-articular, extra-articular, and other structures referring pain to the hip

has been gaining popularity [11, 12]. Ultrasound can be advantageous in that it is potentially cheaper, it can be performed in the office, and there is no radiation exposure. There are no evidence-based studies comparing ultrasound vs. fluoroscopic guided hip injections. On the other hand, fluoroscopic guidance allows the visualization of an arthrogram when contrast is used, which may be useful in certain diagnoses, though there are no reports on this.

There has been debate over the necessity for image-guided (or image-confirmed) injections. Several groups have reported over 90 % accuracy without image guidance [13–18], whereas other groups have reported accuracy as low as 60 % [19–21].

The most common problem with nonimage-guided (or confirmed) hip injections is, if the injection does not relieve pain, the doctor faces the problem of deciding whether the injection was a false negative (injection intra-articular, but pain not relieved) or true negative (injection in the joint, but pathology outside the joint). If the injection relieves the pain, the possibilities are true positive (injection in the joint, pathology in the joint) or false positive (the injection was not in the joint, but the pain was relieved—probably because the pain generator was not in the joint—thought there are reports of extra-articular injections relieving pain believed to be of intra-articular origin). For these reasons, we prefer image-guided injection and confirmation that the injection is intra-articular if possible. However, if imaging guidance is not available, it is appropriate to offer the patient an unguided injection.

Agents injected for the treatment of hip OA are often a combination of a local anesthetic and steroid. The common steroids used are triamcinolone acetonide (Kenalog®), methylprednisolone (Depo-Medrol®), or a combination of betamethasone sodium phosphate and betamethasone acetate (Celestone Soluspan®) in volumes ranging from 3 mL but not exceeding 9 mL. We use in our practice 4 cm^3 of Celestone Soluspan® and 5 cm^3 of lidocaine 1 %. Our preference is to use Celestone Soluspan® due to the fact that it has both potent short-acting and long-acting components (Table 28.2) secondary to [22]:

- Inhibition of phospholipase A2 activity
- Prevention of degranulation of granulocytes, mast cells, and macrophages
- Suppression of macrophage migration inhibitory factor
- Stabilization of lysosomal and cell membranes

Synthetic steroids are more potent than endogenous cortisol and possess variable glucocorticoid and mineralocorticoid activity. Chemically engineered modifications have generated a variety of steroid compounds with different glucocorticoid and mineralocorticoid activity, enhanced potency, and longer duration of action (Table 28.2).

Systemically steroids have a potent anti-inflammatory and immunosuppressive action, which is accomplished mainly through their action on lymphocytes. By inhibiting lymphocyte mitotic activity and reducing IL-2 release through the inhibition of the movement of NF-κB, they decrease the blood lymphocyte count and profoundly alter the immune responses of lymphocytes. They reduce local inflammation through the upregulation of lipocortin, which inhibits the action of phospholipase A2. Ultimately the release of arachidonic acid from tissue phospholipids is impeded, and the formation of leukotrienes, thromboxanes, prostaglandins, and prostacyclins is reduced.

The outcomes of hip OA management with guided intra-articular steroid injections were evaluated in a few randomized controlled clinical trials vs. placebo and vs. anesthetics only injections [23].

Pain relief is unreliable and unpredictable, and patients must be warned that they may not benefit from injection. Pain relief varied from 2 weeks to 3 months. Range of motion, quality of life, and improvement in daily activities performance were also noted [24–29]. Randomized controlled trials evaluating the effects of intra-articular hip injections for OA treatment with longer follow-up periods are still needed to better understand this treatment modality.

There is a handful of reports of successful radiofrequency denervation of the hip joint, with pain relief lasting a few months [30–33]. This may be a useful technique for patients with pain which is not responsive to intra-articular injection or who are unable to undergo surgery.

Table 28.1 Select hip pain etiologies

Intra-articular	Extra-articular	Referred
Degenerative joint disease	Piriformis syndrome	Myofascial pain syndrome
Labral tears	Snapping hip syndrome	Osteitis pubis
Femoroacetabular impingement	Bursitis	Fractures
Inflammatory conditions	– Trochanteric	– Pubic ramus
– Rheumatoid arthritis	– Iliopsoas	– Sacral fracture
– Septic arthritis	– Gluteal	Spinal pathology
– Spondyloarthropathies	Tendinopathies	– Lumbar radicular pain
Bony pathologies	– Hamstrings	– Sacroiliac pain syndrome
– Avascular necrosis of femoral head	– Iliopsoas	– Lumbar disk herniation
– Tumors	– Gluteal muscles	– Lumbar facet pain
Deposition disease		
– Amyloid arthropathy		
Synovial abnormalities		
– Pigmented villonodular synovitis		
– Chondromatosis		

Table 28.2 Locally injectable steroids

	Hydrocortisone	Methylprednisolone (Depo-Medrol®)	Triamcinolone acetonide (Kenalog®)	Betamethasone sodium phosphate and acetate (Celestone Soluspan®)	Dexamethasone sodium phosphate (Decadron® phosphate)
Relative anti-inflammatory potency	1	5	5	25	25
PH	5.0–7.0	7–8	4.5–6.5	6.8–7.2	7–8.5
Onset	Fast	Slow	Moderate	Fast	Fast
Duration of action	Short	Intermediate	Intermediate	Long	Long
Concentration mg/mL	50	40–80	20	6	4 mg/mL
Relative mineralocorticoid activity	2+	0	0	0	0

Measures of Improvement

1. Hip pain reduction: A reduction of pain measured using Western Ontario and McMaster Universities (WOMAC) scale of 11.8 % [25, 28] to 49.2 % [25] in pain intensity in 67.7 % of patients [25] at 2 months after injection. At 3 months, the pain reduction was still observed in up to 58.1 % of patients [24, 25]. Pain reduction was also measured using visual analogue scale (VAS) with reduction of 21.4 % [26] to 68.8 % [29] in values at 2–3 weeks, and the benefit of the injection was still observed after 3 months with reduction of VAS scores of 16.5 % [26] to 35.2 % [29]. Pain on weight bearing was the most responsive, with an improvement of 75.5 % and 41.5 % in 3 weeks and 3 months, respectively [29]. SF-36 form was also used to assess pain in one study that showed an improvement of 61 % in "bodily pain" domain after 3 months of injection [25]. A study by Robinson et al. [28] indicated that after 3 months, the pain level was not different from the baseline level; however, their study had a major limitation with the absence of a control group. Similarly, an uncontrolled study by Plant et al. [26] that evaluated pain after 6 months showed no difference in VAS values as compared to baseline.
2. Stiffness: Kullenberg et al. [29] evaluated the hip range of motion 3 weeks after the steroid injection. An increase was found for flexion (8°), internal rotation (10°), and external rotation (11°). Stiffness was also measured using WOMAC questionnaire with an improvement of 16.6 % at 6 weeks [28]. At 3 months, the improvement ranged from 22 % [24] to 45 % [25].
3. Function: Improvements in physical functioning ranged from 9.05 % in 6 weeks [28] to 44.4 % in 3 months [25] using WOMAC questionnaire. SF-36 questionnaire also showed an improvement in "physical functioning" domain at 3 months of 61.8 % [25]. Kullenberg et al. also used the Katz and Akpom scale, a five-grade scale that measures function, and it demonstrated an improvement of 80 % and 45 % at 3 weeks and 3 months of the hip injection, respectively [29].

4. Social functioning and global assessment of health were also measured by Lambert et al. in the only randomized double-blinded placebo-controlled trial published to date [25]. Improvement in patients' global assessment of health was 31.2 % (WOMAC), and social functioning improved in 20.3 % (SF-36) at 3 months.

The relationship between the steroid dose and the duration of the response was evaluated [28]. Injection of 80 mg of methylprednisolone showed an improvement in stiffness and disability at 3 months after the injection compared to 40 mg of prednisolone with the effect only lasting for 6 weeks. It is important to note that there are no studies that we could identify that evaluated the effects of steroid hip injections for OA beyond 6 months.

New Hip OA Treatments

Viscosupplementation (VS)

Viscosupplementation (VS) is a known treatment option for knee OA, although its effectiveness is still not established, and can be an alternative in treating patients with painful hip OA. To date only few studies have indicated a promising role of this agent in pain control and mobility improvement of the hip for as long as 6 months [34–36].

Hyaluronic acid (HA) is a physiologic component of the synovial fluid which is reduced in OA joints. Therefore, intra-articular injection of HA, due to its viscoelastic properties and protective effect on articular cartilage and soft tissue surfaces of joints, can restore the articular homoeostasis. Viscosupplementation with different HA preparations (low and high molecular weight) can be considered after failure of conservative management or if the patient is intolerant to analgesics or NSAIDs [37].

There are six injectable forms of HA approved by the US FDA (Table 28.3). Each of these HA products differs in their method of production, molecular weight, dosing instructions, and biologic characteristics. Comparison of the efficacy of lower and higher molecular weight VS in the treatment of hip osteoarthritis failed to show any differences regarding outcomes between low and high molecular weight but with a positive intragroup effect in both formulation weights [38]. Studies that investigated at the effectiveness of HA for hip osteoarthritis are small and scarce with few controlled trials. Recently, Migliore et al. retrospectively evaluated total hip replacement (THR) rate in a cohort of 176 patients treated with intra-articular HA injections every 6 months [39]. In this study, six orthopedists independently assessed whether 176 patients with hip OA that were treated with intra-articular injections of sodium hyaluronate (MW 1500–2000 kDa) were candidates for THR)according to the clinical data and radiological exams collected at the first intra-articular sodium hyaluronate injection visit. In the group of 93 patients considered by the majority of the surgeons' candidates for THR, only 34 % had undergone THR after 48 months of treatment and 20 % more in the 2 years follow-up. On the contrary, in 2009 Richette et al. conducted a randomized placebo-controlled trial to evaluate the efficacy and tolerability of a single injection of HA for the treatment of hip OA in adult subjects [36]. In this study 85 subjects with symptomatic hip OA were randomized to receive fluoroscopic guided intra-articular HA injection or placebo injection. The responder rates were 33.3 % and 32.6 % in the HA and placebo groups, respectively ($p = 0.94$).

Platelet-Rich Plasma

Future perspectives also include the use of platelet-rich plasma (PRP) injected into the hip joint as a possible treatment for hip OA. PRP therapy has shown promising clinical results in the treatment of tendon and ligament pathologies [40]. The rationale for its use is the induction of chemokines, cytokines, and growth factors aiming to stimulate intrinsic repair mechanisms [41, 42].

In vitro, PRP was found to enhance hyaluronic acid and angiogenic growth factor secretion in human synovial cells [43–45]. PRP injections may stimulate collagen deposition in the ligaments, tendons, and capsules of osteoarthritic joints through starting and stimulating the healing cascade [40]. Additionally, platelets contain growth factors that induce tissue repair through stimulation of chemotaxis, cell migration, angiogenesis, proliferation, differentiation, and matrix production [46]. To formulate PRP and to release the growth factors, autologous whole blood is filtered to separate the platelet-rich plasma from the platelet-poor plasma and the red cells. The addition of citrate helps inhibit clotting, and the addition of calcium chloride or thrombin activates the PRP and releases the growth factors from the platelet granules [40] (Textbox 28.1).

Table 28.3 FDA-approved VS products and characteristics according to the manufacturer's full prescribing information

Product	Hyaluronic acid source	Dose per injection (mg)	Molecular weight ($\times 10^6$ Da) (human HA is 6×10^6 Da)	Number of injections
Sodium hyaluronate (Hyalgan®)	Avian	20	0.5–0.7	3–5
Hylan G-F 20 (Synvisc®)	Synthetic	16	6.0	3
Sodium hyaluronate (Supartz®)	Avian	25	0.6–1.2	3–5
High molecular weight hyaluronan (Orthovisc®)	Bacterial cells	30	1.0–2.9	3–4
1 % sodium hyaluronate (Euflexxa®)	Bacterial cells	20	2.4–3.6	3
Hylan G-F 20 (Synvisc-One®)	Synthetic	48	6.0	1

Textbox 28.1: Growth Factors in Platelet-Rich Plasma

Insulin-like growth factor-1 (IGF-1)
Transforming growth factor-ß (TGF-ß)
Platelet-derived growth factor (PDGF)
Vascular endothelial growth factor (VEGF)
Basic fibroblast growth factor (FGF)

Practices vary as to the frequency of treatment and the PRP preparation protocol. For OA PRP is performed with at least 2 months between treatments [33]. A recent comparison between hip injection with viscosupplements and PRP showed the two are equally efficacious in terms of functional improvement and pain reduction at 12-month follow-up [47].

Bone Marrow Mesenchymal Injection

Another technique that was recently introduced is the bone marrow mesenchymal cell injections for hip osteoarthritis. Hauser and Orlofsky reported a case series of three patients who received five hip injections with unfractionated whole bone marrow into their osteoarthritic joints in combination with hyperosmotic dextrose. No imaging guidance was noted. The results cannot be taken into consideration as there was simultaneous use of two different injectates, and results cannot be discerned as to how much is each contributing to the benefit [48]. There are various ongoing clinical trials investigating bone marrow mesenchymal injections at the time of preparation of this chapter.

Femoroacetabular Impingement Syndrome and Labral Tears

Femoroacetabular impingement syndrome is the painful impact of the acetabular rim and the femoral head-neck junction. It is a common etiology of hip pain in active patients [49]. If left untreated, this condition is now recognized as a common cause of prearthritic hip pain and secondary osteoarthritis [41, 50]. The acetabular labrum is a fibrocartilaginous structure that aids in stability against femoral head translation by deepening the joint [51, 52]. Investigators of several studies suggest that acetabular labral tears are a precursor to hip arthritis [53] and that surgical intervention is more favorable than conservative management of symptomatic labral tears [54–59].

Diagnostic hip intra-articular injection with local anesthetic and the performance of magnetic resonance arthrography have a 92 % sensitivity, 97 % specificity, and 90 % accuracy for diagnosis of an intra-articular disorder [60]. The absence of pain relief with the injection is a negative test for femoroacetabular impingement and suggests an extra-articular source of pain [61, 62].

There are no published studies of nonsurgical treatment of femoroacetabular impingement syndrome with injections. If the diagnostic injection is positive, a treatment with a therapeutic steroid injection can be performed. However, patients with refractory symptoms for longer than 6 weeks should be referred for consideration of arthroscopy.

Hunt et al. recently published the first study comparing surgery to nonsurgical treatment for prearthritic hip disorders [53]. After a course of nonoperative management, patients with continued pain, functionally limiting symptoms, and a surgically amenable lesion on an MR arthrography were offered surgical intervention vs. physical therapy, patient education, and steroid injections as a means of reducing pain to enhance participation in therapeutic exercise. In this study subjects were able to choose whether or not to have surgery. Forty-four percent of patients successfully improved their function and decreased their pain with nonoperative measures, and 56 % underwent surgery. The presence of subtle osseous abnormalities did not predict the failure of conservative treatment. All patients treated either with nonoperative treatment alone or with nonoperative treatment followed by surgery demonstrated significant improvement in pain and function from baseline to 1-year follow-up.

Diagnostic and Therapeutic Intra-articular Injection Technique

Anterior Approach

This is our preferred technique, as landmarks are easily identifiable; patients are comfortable lying in a supine position, and there is a lower risk of femoral artery penetration.

Positioning: In a supine position, the lower extremity is held in internal rotation approaching the anterior aspect of the hip obliquely from lateral to medial. An anteroposterior fluoroscopic view of the hip joint should visualize the intertrochanteric line and the femoral head.

Preparation: After sterile preparation of the skin and covering the area with sterile drapes, the skin is anesthetized with 0.5 cm^3 of lidocaine 1 % and a 22-gauge (G) spinal needle inserted and advanced toward the femoral head-neck junction (Fig. 28.2).

Technique: The entry point of the needle is the midpoint between the lesser and greater trochanters. The needle is advanced under fluoroscopic guidance reaching the capsule in the region of the head-neck junction. The needle is advanced to the femoral neck abutting the bone and slightly withdrawn and rotated to effectively penetrate the joint capsule. Intra-articular needle placement is : confirmed with an injection of 1–2 cm^3 of iopamidol 300. Contrast is necessary to confirm intra-articular injection, and without the use of contrast, extra-capsular injection can occur. Contrast is also necessary to avoid intravascular injections, as this is readily identifiable with fluoroscopy. If intra-articular injection is confirmed, medications are injected.

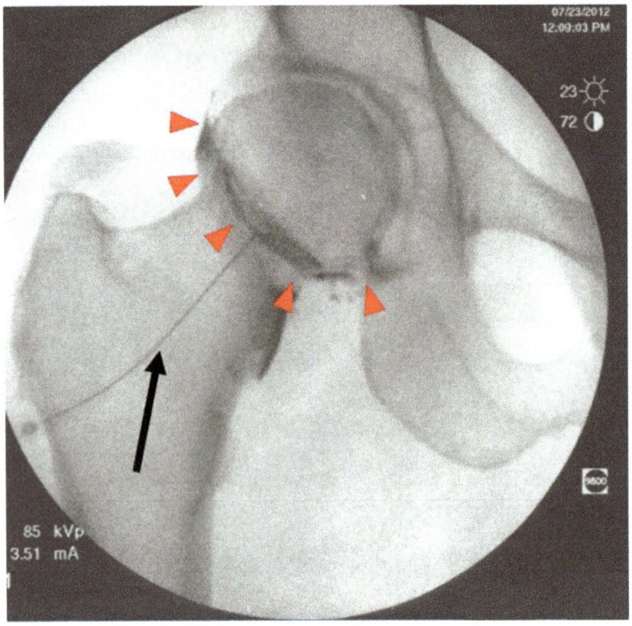

Fig. 28.2 Fluoroscopic guided right hip intra-articular injection. *Arrow*: needle. *Arrow heads*: contrast collecting cephalad to the zona orbicularis and outlining the acetabular labrum

Lateral Approach

Positioning: In a supine or lateral position, a lateral fluoroscopic view of the hip joint should visualize the greater trochanter and the femoral head.

Preparation: After sterile preparation and covering the area with sterile drapes, the skin is anesthetized with 0.5 cm^3 of lidocaine 1 %.

Technique: The entry point of the needle is the skin above the great trochanter. A 22-gauge (G) spinal needle is inserted and advanced toward the top of greater trochanter to confirm coronal alignment. The needle is then withdrawn and advanced under fluoroscopic guidance in the same coronal angle reaching the greater trochanter aiming for the head-neck junction. Intra-articular needle placement is confirmed with an injection of 1–2 cm^3 of iopamidol 300. If intra-articular injection is confirmed, medications are injected.

Medications: In our practice, for diagnostic injections, we use 4 cm^3 of lidocaine 2 %.

Testing the efficacy of an injection should be performed at 5 min by asking the patient to move the lower extremity and hip to reproduce pain usually external/internal rotation, sitting to standing or walking. If a significant improvement is obtained from the injection, the injection is considered positive for an intra-articular cause of pain.

For therapeutic injections: Positioning, preparation, and technique are the same as for diagnostic injections. We use 5 cm^3 of lidocaine 1 % and 4 cm^3 of Celestone Soluspan®. In patients who obtain short-term relief from local anesthetic infiltration but fail to experience long-term benefit from the corticosteroid, the possibility of a non-inflammatory contributor should be considered.

Recently the use of local anesthetics became controversial after reports of chondrotoxicity in joints after the use of local anesthetic pumps following arthroscopies [63, 64]. This was followed by a few studies on animals and in vitro also demonstrating chondrolysis even with a single dose [63–65]. The recent data support the use of ropivacaine as it was shown to be the safest on cartilage [63]. Up to the writing of this text, there are no studies that we are aware of on patients undergoing local anesthetic injections for diagnostic and therapeutic purposes showing evidence of chondrolysis. Due to the animal, in vitro and local anesthetic pump reports, interventional practices are switching to ropivacaine use. The major problem is that it is more expensive than other local anesthetics.

Complications

Serious complications of intra-articular hip injections are rarely reported. Most commonly patients experience temporary increase in pain after the local anesthetic wears off. The main medication complication of intra-articular hip injection is allergy. Allergy to nonionic contrast is immediate and requires immediate management with antihistamines and epinephrine if anaphylaxis occurs. The risk of anaphylaxis is reported to be 0.04 % [66]. Patients with known allergy to contrast may receive oral steroids and antihistamines prior to contrast injection. In our institution we use prednisone 50 mg 24 h, 12 h, and 1 h prior to the injection with oral diphenhydramine 50 mg 1 h prior to contrast injections. Patients with known anaphylaxis to contrast should avoid its use and gadolinium can be used instead. The use of new fluoroscopy equipment with digital subtraction technology allows adequate visualization of the intra-articular gadolinium injection. Gadolinium and contrast media should be avoided in renal insufficiency. There is no reported allergic reaction to local anesthetics in the amide group such as lidocaine, prilocaine, ropivacaine, and bupivacaine. We recommend their use in preservative-free preparations if possible. However, we caution about intravascular injection of local anesthetics. Large amounts (more than 10 cm^3 of bupivacaine or 40 cm^3 of lidocaine 1 %) intravascularly can lead to central nervous system toxicity followed by cardiac toxicity. These are much higher volumes than recommended for intra-articular injections, so the risk is probably small. Peak plasma concentration occurs within 10–20 min. It is proposed and widely accepted that the selective administration of steroids, such as in epidural, perineural, or intra-articular injections, produces high local concentration of the steroids without significant systemic absorption. The consensus is that systemic absorption after these procedures is insufficient to cause serious systemic side effects [67]. However, there is minute portion of the injectate that penetrates to the bloodstream [68, 69], and diabetics must be warned that their sugar control may be impaired for several days, or, occasionally, weeks. If injections are repeated frequently, adrenal cortical suppression, depression of osteoblastic activity [70–72], and hyperglycemia [73] may occur.

Adverse reactions to locally injected steroids are limited to temporary elevation of blood sugar, temporary increase on blood pressure, facial and chest flushing, low-grade fever, insomnia, occasional fluid retention, weight gain, and psychological changes that might last for few days. We recommend avoiding the use of steroids in patients with history of steroid psychosis. All patients should be warned of the risk of psychological disturbances, and pilots and other operators of commercial transport and machinery should not work for 48 h following injection.

Aseptic technique should always be used when performing any kind of intra-articular injections. Under aseptic conditions intra-articular steroid injections of the hip did not increase the risk of infection in patients undergoing total hip arthroplasty [74, 75].

The concern of cartilage degradation is usually raised on the repetitive use of steroid injections. Raynauld et al. [76] evaluated the safety and efficacy of long-term intra-articular steroid injections for knee pain related to osteoarthritis (OA) in 68 subjects. Injections were performed every 3 months for 2 years (placebo vs. triamcinolone acetonide) and found that the steroid injections were not associated with accelerated disease progression compared to placebo injections. Moreover, a reduction in stiffness and significant pain relief was associated with steroid injections.

Extra-articular

Greater Trochanteric Syndrome

Pain and tenderness in the region of the greater trochanter, buttock, or lateral thigh may be associated with myriad causes including gluteal tendinopathy and tears, bursitis, muscle tears, trigger points, iliotibial band disorders, and other general and localized pathology in surrounding tissues [77, 78].

Trochanteric bursitis affects patients of all ages with higher incidence in patients 40–60 years old. In total, four bursae were corroborated around the GT, with three being present in most individuals. These bursae serve to provide cushioning for the gluteus tendons, ITB, and tensor fascia lata muscles [79]. The trochanteric bursa is located between the insertion of the gluteus medius and the gluteus minimus in the lateral aspect of the greater trochanter.

Trochanteric bursae may get inflamed and often become painful because of repetitive motion. Bursitis is also noted in the presence of inflammatory arthritis such as rheumatoid arthritis. Pathologies of the gluteal tendons and the iliotibial tract can cause an inflammation to the adjacent tissues also causing inflammation of the trochanteric bursa. Traumatic bursitis and idiopathic bursitis are also described. Patients usually complain of pain during active hip abduction, and physical examination will show trochanteric pain on palpation. Ultrasound and magnetic resonance imaging may reveal tendon tears or fluid in the bursa.

The initial treatment is rest from the activities that cause pain. Physical therapy (consisting of hip and pelvic stabilization and iliotibial tract stretching) and NSAIDs are beneficial to some patients. Patients with high pain levels and those who fail conservative initial treatment may benefit from injections prior to engaging further in physical therapy. Corticosteroid injection for trochanteric bursitis is considered an effective treatment to reduce the inflammation [77, 80–83].

Corticosteroid injections can be done with or without image guiding. Fluoroscopy and ultrasound are the most common methods used to perform bursa injections. Ultrasound verifies needle positioning. Fluoroscopy confirms the bursal spread (bursogram) identifying that the injectate is in the area of pathology and that there is no vascular flow [84].

Most patients need only one corticosteroid injection, with or without anesthetics, to obtain pain relief, with studies showing that improvement ranges from 49 to 100 % of subjects [77, 80–83]. Benefits were demonstrated after 6 months for at least 60 % of patients [77, 82]. As for other soft tissue injections, adverse effects are very rare but include skin irritation, swelling, and temporary increase in local pain.

In our practice we use 2 cm^3 Depo-Medrol 40 mg, Kenalog, or 2 cm^3 Celestone 6 mg with additional 3–4 cm^3 of lidocaine 1 % [67].

Iliopsoas Bursitis and Tendinosis

Iliopsoas tendinosis and bursitis are a common cause of hip and groin pain, which is often seen in the setting of rheumatoid arthritis, acute trauma, overuse injury, or after total hip arthroplasty [68, 70, 71, 85–88]. Pain is increased with weight-bearing activities, forward flexion, or on transition from sitting to standing. Since rheumatoid arthritis is a risk factor for iliopsoas bursitis, blood tests may help in assessing for rheumatological disorders. Magnetic resonance imaging is the current imaging standard for evaluation of iliopsoas bursitis [72].

Injection of the iliopsoas bursa and iliopsoas tendon can be useful for both diagnostic and therapeutic purposes [71, 73]. In one study ultrasound-guided bursa injection was beneficial for 72.5 % of subjects with improvement lasting for up to 10 months. In another study 90 % of patients with iliopsoas-related symptoms after hip arthroplasty achieved significant relief with ultrasound-guided steroid injections without the need for surgical release or revision arthroplasty [71].

Piriformis Syndrome

Pain in the hip, buttock, and lower extremity caused by sciatic nerve entrapment while traveling through or deep to the piriformis muscle is called piriformis syndrome (PS) [89]. The piriformis muscle arises from the pedicles of S2 to S4 and adjacent bone and has fascial origin from the sacroiliac joint capsule and the sciatic nerve [90]. Causes of piriformis syndrome include anatomic variation in the piriformis muscle or the sciatic nerve, piriformis hypertrophy or spasm, and muscular fibrosis following trauma [91]. PS can be present in up to 8 % of patients complaining of low back pain [92].

There is a lack of consensus regarding piriformis syndrome work-up. Imaging is often not informative, and electrodiagnostic examination is of low specificity [90]. Therefore, the patient's history and physical examination are suggestive of the diagnosis. Pain is usually exacerbated by prolonged sitting on hard surfaces or with bowel movements and mitigated by walking as it releases the nerve compression. Tenderness on palpation of the piriformis muscle, the sciatic notch, or the greater trochanter area may be present in addition to neural tension maneuvers such as compressing the sciatic nerve by stretching the piriformis muscle flexion abduction and internal rotation (FAIR test) and Lasègue sign. The diagnosis of PS is confirmed through a guided piriformis muscle injection [91, 93]. We recommend thorough work-up and MRI imaging of the lumbar spine and the pelvis prior to diagnosing PS.

Piriformis muscle injection should always be done under guidance to improve accuracy, as the piriformis is a relatively small muscle in a deep location, close to important neurovascular structures [94]. The most practical method of piriformis muscle injection is using fluoroscopy with an electrical stimulator. For this method, the patient is placed in a prone position and the buttock area is prepped and draped in a sterile way. An AP view of the pelvis with inclusion of the acetabular region of the hip and the inferior aspect of the sacroiliac joint is obtained. The target point lies at one-third of the line between superior-lateral aspect of the acetabulum and the inferior aspect of the sacroiliac joint. The skin is anesthetized, and a 22-gauge insulated needle is introduced and advanced under fluoroscopic view with the electrical stimulator turned on to avoid contact with the sciatic nerve. At any sign of extremity paresthesias or contractions of the leg muscles innervated by the sciatic nerve and its main motor branches, the needle should be promptly repositioned. On contacting the posterior ilium, the needle is withdrawn 1–2 mm stopping inside the piriformis muscle. There should be a slight needle movement caused by the electrical stimulation, without evident gluteal contraction, confirming the piriformis intramuscular position of the needle. After anesthetic administration, needle movement should cease. Finally, a piriformis myogram is obtained after injecting 1 cm^3 of radiographic contrast [95]. The same technique as described above has been reported as accurate and safe without the use of an electric stimulator, being its use optional [94].

Other guidance methods for piriformis injection also described are the use of CT scan or MRI. Ultrasound guidance with or without motor stimulation is gaining popularity [96–98]. Electric stimulation guidance without using any image method is also used [99] although it should be discouraged due to its decreased accuracy.

Piriformis injections can be either diagnostic or therapeutic [91, 93]. We suggest an injection of 5 cm^3 of lidocaine 1 % (there are no studies that we are aware of on drug/doses of diagnostic injections). Fishman et al. [100] in a cohort uncontrolled study of 733 subjects that received 1.5 mL of lidocaine 2 % and 20 mg of triamcinolone acetonide demonstrated a subjective pain improvement of at least 50 % in 79 % of patients after a mean of 10.2 months follow-up. Some of their patients received a second injection after 6 weeks if partial benefit was achieved with the first injection. In another study Masala et al. [97] compared improvement in a group of patients with PS that received piriformis injection with 1 cm^3 of 40 mg of methylprednisone acetate and 10 mg of lidocaine and physical therapy, with a control group that received physical therapy only. A significant improvement in pain using VAS at 2 months (73.8 %) and 12 months (88.9 %) was noted in the injection group. Naja et al. [101] evaluated the injection of bupivacaine and clonidine in a randomized double-blind study. Eighty patients were divided into two groups: one that received an injection of 9 mL of bupivacaine 0.5 % and 1 mL of clonidine 150 μg/mL with a control group that received an injection of 9 mL of bupivacaine 0.5 % and 1 mL of saline. At 6 months, 92 % of patients in the clonidine group were pain-free, as compared to 22 % of patients who received saline. Patients in this study received up to four injections at 1-week intervals.

Another injectate that has been increasingly used for musculoskeletal pain conditions treatment is botulinum toxin (BTX). BTX acts at the neuromuscular junction inhibiting the presynaptic release of acetylcholine (ACh), paralyzing the muscle [102]. Its exact mechanism on pain remains unclear although it is accepted that when BTX relaxes the spastic muscles, it results in pain relief [102]. Currently, there are two types of . BTX in the market: type A and type B. Both inhibit ACh release, although through different ways and with different potencies. BTX type A is available as

Botox® (Allergan, Inc., Irvine, California) and Dysport® (Ipsen, Ltd., Berks, UK) and type B as Myobloc® (Solstice Neurosciences, San Francisco, California). BTX type A has an additional mechanism that may contribute to management of painful conditions: it affects motor and sensory pathways by inhibiting gamma motor neurons, thus blocking type Ia afferent signals at the muscle spindle level. Additionally, it was shown in vitro experiments that BTX type A can inhibit the release of substance P from nerve terminals of embryonic rat cells which may lead to an analgesic effect [103]. From studies using BTX type A to treat PS, the dose ranges from 100 to 200 U of Botox® and 150 U of Dysport®, and there is an improvement in pain scores in 65–77 % of patients in 1–12 weeks after the injection. The adverse events observed are flu-like symptoms, ecchymosis, worsening of pain, and numbness, which were all transient lasting less than 3 days. BTX type B was also evaluated for management of PS pain; doses used were from 5000 to 12,500 U with pain improvement noted in 75 % of patients at 3–16 weeks [104].

In another approach for management, Mullin et al. [105] investigated the caudal steroid injection using 60–80 mg of triamcinolone and 15 mL of bupivacaine 0.25 % for the treatment of PS in a retrospective study of only 12 subjects. A relief of 25–100 % of pain was found at 9 months to 2 years follow-up after the caudal block. The improvement reported was not only due to the sciatic nerve irritation relief but was also due to the release of the muscle spasm and pain of piriformis muscle contracture by blocking the innervation of the muscle itself.

Referred Hip Pain from Other Structures

Sacroiliac Pain Syndrome

Sacroiliac joint pain should be considered in the differential diagnosis of patients with posterior pelvic pain, groin pain, and low back pain. Pain from the sacroiliac joint (SIJ) is commonly caused by spondyloarthropathies, trauma, lifting, and torsional stresses [106]. It is also believed to occur spontaneously [107]. Pregnant women, athletes, and individuals sustaining regional trauma are considered more susceptible [108]. Ninety-four percent of patients with sacroiliac joint pain syndrome refer pain in the gluteal and posterior hip area [109]. There is no pathognomonic physical examination sign or imaging modality that unequivocally proves the diagnosis of SIJ pain [108, 110]. Three or more positive pain provocation SIJ tests have sensitivity and specificity of 91 % and 78 %, respectively [111]. Additionally, hip provocative physical examination maneuvers commonly reproduce pain from the SIJ; thus, it can greatly mimic hip joint pain. The gold standard of the diagnosis of SIJ syndrome is a positive response to a diagnostic SIJ injection with local anesthetic [112–114]. Bone scan has a reported sensitivity of 12–46 % and specificity of 90 % when compared to diagnostic SIJ diagnostic injections [115, 116].

We recommend the use of a small volume (usually 0.8 cm^3) of local anesthetic such as lidocaine 2 % as we have observed the use of large amounts of local anesthetics (exceeding 5 cm^3) may lead to inadvertent anesthetization of surrounding structures and can give false-positive results especially if the local anesthetic infiltrates the sciatic nerve. Interventional treatment modalities for management of SIJ pain include therapeutic steroid injections and radiofrequency (RF) ablation [117]. Significant pain relief is reported after one to three injections [118, 119] in about 66.7 % of patients [120], with the effects lasting from 1 month to 2 years [117].

We recommend imaging guidance in performing SIJ injections. The successful positioning of blind SIJ injections is extremely low, varying from 12 % [121] to 22 % [122]. Fluoroscopy is the traditional method, CT scan is also used, and recently ultrasound is gaining popularity [123].

Radiofrequency ablation of the SIJ was recently popularized for management of patients with temporary improvement of pain after steroid injections. Cohen initially showed more than 50 % pain relief at 9 months in 8 out of 9 patients [124]. Yin demonstrated more than 50 % relief in 64 % of his 14 patients at 6 months follow-up [125]. Patel et al. showed improvement in 59 % of patients in pain, disability, physical function, and quality of life for 9 months [126]. There are several methods of SIJ RF ablation techniques described [123]. The most common method used is the ablation of the L5 dorsal ramus and S1 to S3 lateral branches.

Recently interventionalists started injecting the SIJ with botulinum toxin A [127] and prolotherapy agents [128].

Lee et al. [127] evaluated the injection of botulinum toxin type A for the treatment of SIJ pain. Thirty-nine patients were randomly allocated into two groups to receive either 100 U of Dysport® botulinum toxin or 40 mg of triamcinolone with 2 mL of lidocaine 0.5 %. The outcome measures were pain using a numeric rating scale (NRS) and disability using the Oswestry Disability Index (ODI). At 1 month, there was no statistically significant difference between the two groups. At the second month, NRS decrease was 71.9 % and 39.3 %, and at the third month, NRS decrease was 70.3 % and 19.7 % for botulinum toxin and triamcinolone groups, respectively. ODI values decreased 65.8 % and 63.4 % in the botulinum toxin group and 28.2 % and 15.5 % in the triamcinolone group at the second and third months after injection, respectively. This is the only such study we are aware of and the sample size is small.

There is a scarcity of controlled studies, and there are many different prolotherapy solutions and treatment protocols. Cusi et al. [129] described the use of prolotherapy showing positive clinical outcomes for 76 % of the patients.

He performed three injections of hypertonic dextrose solution into the dorsal interosseous ligament of the affected SIJ of 25 patients, under CT guidance, in 6-week intervals. Kim et al. [128] compared intra-articular injection of dextrose to intra-articular injection of steroids in the SIJ of 48 subjects. The pain and disability scores were significantly improved from baseline in both groups at the 2-week follow-up, with no significant difference between them, but the long-term effect shown by the cumulative incidence of ≥50 % pain relief was 58.7 % in the prolotherapy group and only 10.2 % in the steroid group at 15 months. Even though results are promising, further controlled studies are needed to confirm the safety and efficacy of this procedure and to validate an appropriate injection protocol.

Fluoroscopy Diagnostic and Therapeutic Intra-articular SIJ Injection Technique

Position: The patient is placed in a prone position. An ipsilateral anteroposterior (AP) fluoroscopic view of the sacrum (with the beam generator positioned under the patient) should visualize the sacroiliac joint with two visible joint lines, the anterior and the posterior joint planes of the SIJ.

Preparation: After sterile preparation of the skin and covering the area with sterile drapes, the skin should be anesthetized. A 22-gauge (G) spinal needle is inserted and advanced toward the SIJ.

Technique: The fluoroscopy beam is rotated contralateral to the target joint to align the two visible joint planes until they overlap at the caudal portion of the joint. The entry point of the needle is medial to the most caudal third of the joint line (adjacent to the sacral cortical line). The needle is advanced under fluoroscopy, and intra-articular needle placement is confirmed with an injection of 0.5–1 cm^3 of contrast material. After a positive arthrogram, 0.5 cm^3 of lidocaine 2 % and 2 cm^3 of Celestone Soluspan® are injected. Lidocaine 2 % is injected only for diagnostic purposes (Fig. 28.3).

In patients who obtain short-term relief from local anesthetic infiltration, but fail to experience long-term benefit from the corticosteroid, radiofrequency ablation of the SIJ innervation is recommended.

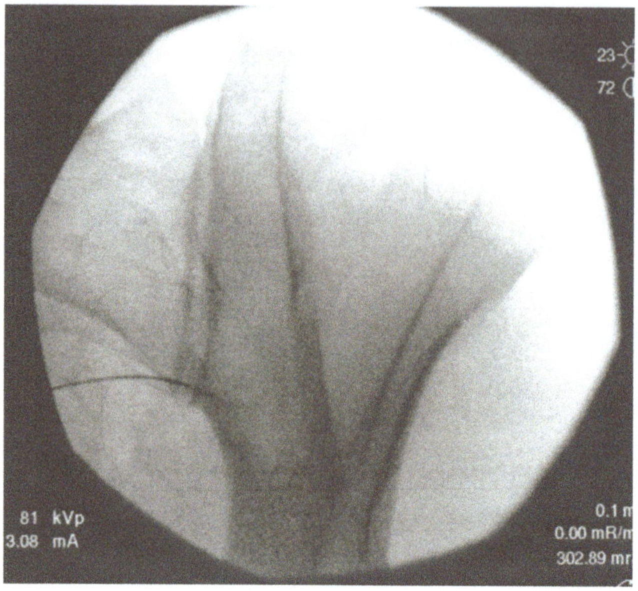

Fig. 28.3 Fluoroscopic guided sacroiliac joint intra-articular injection

Sacral Stress Fractures

Sacral stress fractures are divided into two major types, each of which tends to occur in a very different patient population. Insufficiency stress fractures occur when a bone of abnormally low density fractures under normal stress. These occur most commonly in the elderly population, especially those with osteoporosis. They also tend to occur more commonly in women and the mean age of occurrence is 71 years [130]. Conversely, fatigue stress fractures of the sacrum occur when a bone of normal density fractures under abnormally high stress. This is most commonly seen in young athletes, especially those who participate in repetitive weight-bearing exercises for prolonged periods of time, such as long-distance runners and military recruits. They tend to occur with equal frequency in females and males and tend to occur in a patient's third or fourth decade of life [131]. Patients with a sacral stress fracture will likely have low back, buttock, pelvic, and/or groin pain. Imaging with MRI is generally considered to be the diagnostic study of choice due to the high sensitivity and specificity it offers [131, 132]. Bone scans in conjunction with CT scanning provide accurate diagnosis as well. Plain radiographs provide poor visualization of sacral stress fractures and are used to rule out alternative diagnoses.

Recently, cement sacroplasty became an attractive alternative treatment option for patients with insufficiency stress fractures of the sacrum, primarily because it offers much more rapid relief of their symptoms. In a prospective observational cohort study of 37 patients by Frey et al. [133], patients experienced an improvement of almost 60 % in their pain after the procedure, with continued improvement through the end of the first year. Similarly, Butler et al. also found that most patients who undergo percutaneous sacroplasty for treatment of sacral insufficiency fractures experience significant relief within the first 48 h after the procedure [134]. Percutaneous sacroplasty is similar to the well-known procedure of vertebroplasty and involves the injection of polymethyl methacrylate (PMMA) cement into the bone. The procedure is performed in an outpatient setting, under fluoroscopic guidance with conscious sedation. Under an oblique view, aligning the entire sacroiliac joint, two 13-gauge bone trochars are positioned between the sacral foramina and the sacroiliac joint on the side of the fractured ala at a 45° angle in the direction of the sacroiliac joint. The needles are inserted approximately to the midpoint of the sacrum, under lateral view, maintaining the 45° angle under AP imaging, and 2–5 mL of PMMA is injected, monitoring the spread of the bone cement, to avoid medial extension toward the sacral nerve roots [133].

Lumbar Facet Pain

Pain emanating from the lumbar facet joints can be referred to the hip area [135]. The facet joints are constantly submitted to mechanical stress which leads to degenerative changes accompanied by mechanical stress and inflammation with subsequent pain [136]. Facet joint pain is very common and represents about 15–30 % of all chronic low back pain. To establish the diagnosis, as in the case of SIJ, the gold standard is the diagnostic fluoroscopically guided intra-articular facet block or diagnostic guided medial branch (nerve branches that innervate the facets) block [137].

Once the diagnosis is established, therapeutic intra-articular facet steroid injections are provided, and if these injections provide the patients with temporary improvement, then medial branch radiofrequency ablation (RFA) is performed [137, 138]. Both modalities have good outcomes in pain and functionality. RFA therapeutic effects usually last longer [138] than injections.

Facet injections or facet blocks with or without steroids are reported to reduce pain intensity more than 50 % and increase functional status more than 40 % in 85–90 % of patients over a minimum 2-year period. Over the course of the 2 years, 5–6 injections were necessary to achieve this outcome [139]. Facet blocks are a safe and effective treatment [140]. Complications may include intravascular injection, local bleeding, oozing, hematoma, and vasovagal reaction, which are all considered minor conditions [141].

RFA of the medial branches of the dorsal rami is the treatment modality if temporary improvement occurs with therapeutic facet joints injections [142]. Van Kleef reported more than 50 % improvement of pain intensity after a year in 67 % of his patients that underwent therapeutic lumbar RFA versus 12 % of subjects that underwent sham RFA [135]. Dreyfuss et al. reported that 60 % of their subjects had more than 90 % relief and 87 % had more than 60 % relief at 1 year [143].

Myofascial Pain Syndrome

Myofascial pain syndrome (MPS) can be responsible for persistent pain and functional disability in patients with hip osteoarthritis. Usually the presence of MPS is not assessed in OA patients and therefore not adequately treated [144]. MPS involves a muscle with a taut band and one or more trigger points (TrPs). The difference between a muscle causing MPS and simple spasm of muscles crossing a painful joint is the presence of a TrP. TrPs are tender points in the muscle that, when palpated, reproduce the subjects' pain, not necessarily at the muscle but also distally from the muscle as a referred pain.

Muscles that can radiate pain to the hip and lateral thigh are the quadratus lumborum, gluteus maximus, gluteus medius, gluteus minimus, tensor fasciae latae, piriformis, vastus lateralis, vastus intermedius, rectus femoris, pectineus, adductor longus, adductor magnus, sartorius, and biceps femoris [144, 145].

The best therapeutic effect after dry needling or lidocaine infiltration of muscle trigger point is related to the occurrence of local twitch response [146].

Diskogenic Pain

Back pain with referral to the groin is observed in patients with lumbar disk disease without nerve root compression. In a study we conducted using provocative lumbar diskography, we observed that approximately one-fifth of the patients (total 124 subjects were included) had abdominal and/or inguinal pain provoked during a positive lumbar diskogram [147]. While groin pain referral is not usually the presenting complaint in patients with lumbar degenerative disk disorders, it has been documented by several authors [148–151]. Although the cause of pain referral is not established, there is ample evidence that the lumbar sympathetic fibers play an important role in the transmission of pain in patients with diskogenic pain. Healthy lumbar intervertebral disks receive sensory supply into the annulus fibrosus. There are two extensively interconnected nerve plexuses: the anterior and posterior plexuses, both of which serve as the source of nerve endings within the lumbar intervertebral disks. The anterior plexus is formed from branches of both sympathetic trunks. Thus, the anterior part of the disk is innervated solely by sympathetic fibers [152, 153]. The sinuvertebral nerves constitute the vast majority of the posterior plexus. It is now widely accepted that the sinuvertebral nerve is the main nerve supply to all structures in the spinal canal. It gives off multiple ascending and descending branches, which eventually combine to form a plexus along the posterior longitudinal ligament [154, 155]. Transmission of referred pain occurs through the sinuvertebral nerve [156–158]. This can be explained using the convergence projection theory [159], which is based on the fact that somatic and visceral fibers have synapses in the common dorsal root ganglion [160]. Somatically referred pain occurs as a result of the stimulation of nerve endings in adult tissue derived from embryologic somites, as are intervertebral disks. The noxious sensation of pain results from misperception of the signal origin, which is transmitted to the brain by a convergent sensory pathway [161]. Just as pain can be referred from the visceral organs to the skin of the abdomen, chest, and back, diskogenic pain transmitted through afferent sympathetic fibers to the dermatomal area supplied by the corresponding dorsal root ganglion may result in groin pain.

Transforaminal Epidural Injections

The transforaminal approach can only be performed using fluoroscopic guidance. This injection approach aims for the disk and spinal nerve interface. This is performed through the introduction of the needle into a triangular space within the anterior-superior third of the neural foramen bounded by the pedicle superiorly, the exiting nerve inferior medially, and the lateral margin of the neural foramen laterally "the safe triangle" (Fig. 28.4). Once the needle is in position, efficient injection of the medicine into the lateral epidural space or around the emerging nerve root depending on needle position and bevel orientation becomes possible.

The administration of steroids at the level of the pathology is crucial to achieve effectiveness. With experienced hands, the transforaminal approach is safe and provides good outcomes. Transforaminal epidural steroid injection (TFESI) is currently becoming more popular than the interlaminar approach because it is more effective to administer the medicines at the spinal nerve/disk interface in the lateral epidural space rather than in the dorsal epidural space, which is separated from the lateral epidural space by the ligamentum flavum (Fig. 28.5).

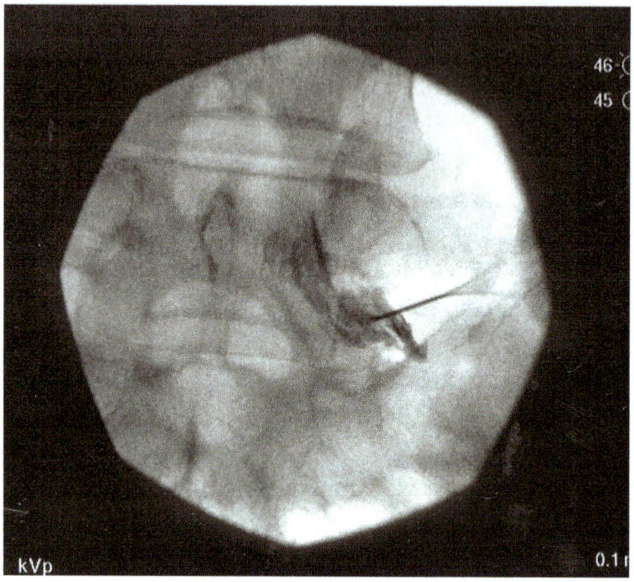

Fig. 28.5 Right L5 transforaminal epidural steroid injection with contrast flowing into the epidural space along the L5 nerve root

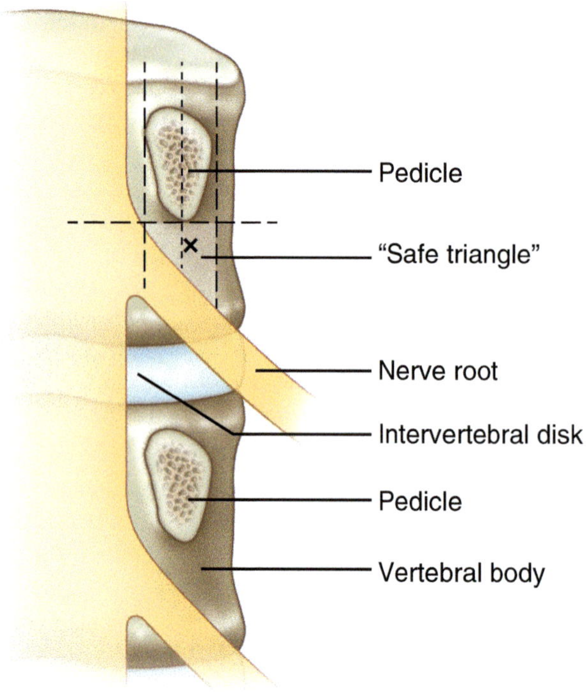

Fig. 28.4 The safe triangle

TFESI was found to achieve ventral flow in 100 % of injections [162]. Furthermore, vascular evacuation of the therapeutic medication occurs in 11 % of caudal epidural steroid injection (CESI) and interlaminar epidural steroid injection (ILESI) and in 2 % of TFESI [163, 164] preventing the therapeutic agent from reaching its target. Therefore, the instillation of therapeutic doses of corticosteroid into the anterior epidural space, hence maximally reaching the targeted intervertebral disk, is best accomplished by the transforaminal approach rather than the interlaminar or caudal techniques.

Summary

Musculoskeletal interventional procedures are on the rise and are becoming very popular with the new generation of spine/sports non-orthopedic specialists. The developments of new techniques and new products as well as establishing evidence-based interventional algorithms are a crucial task for this new generation of specialists. These techniques are an essential component of nonsurgical care and can also be a critical differentiator in determining appropriate surgical procedures in the persistently symptomatic patient.

References

1. Flannery O, Green C, Harmon D, Masterson E. Chronic painful conditions of the hip. Orthop Trauma. 2011;25:223–9.
2. Mengiardi B, Pfirrmann CW, Hodler J. Hip pain in adults: MR imaging appearance of common causes. Eur Radiol. 2007;17:1746–62.
3. Faraj AA, Kumaraguru P, Kosygan K. Intra-articular bupivacaine hip injection in differentiation of coxarthrosis from referred thigh pain: a 10 year study. Acta Orthop Belg. 2003;69:518–21.
4. Illgen Ii RL, Honkamp NJ, Weisman MH, Hagenauer ME, Heiner JP, Anderson PA. The diagnostic and predictive value of hip anesthetic arthrograms in selected patients before total hip arthroplasty. J Arthroplasty. 2006;21:724–30.
5. Pateder DB, Hungerford MW. Use of fluoroscopically guided intra-articular hip injection in differentiating the pain source in concomitant hip and lumbar spine arthritis. Am J Orthop (Belle Mead NJ). 2007;36:591–3.
6. Lawrence RC, Felson DT, Helmick CG, et al. Estimates of the prevalence of arthritis and other rheumatic conditions in the United States: part II. Arthritis Rheum. 2008;58:26–35.
7. Altman R, Alarcon G, Appelrouth D, et al. The American College of Rheumatology criteria for the classification and reporting of osteoarthritis of the hip. Arthritis Rheum. 1991;34:505–14.
8. Suri P, Morgenroth DC, Hunter DJ. Epidemiology of osteoarthritis and associated comorbidities. PM R. 2012;4:S10–9.
9. Murphy L, Helmick CG. The impact of osteoarthritis in the United States: a population-health perspective: a population-based review of the fourth most common cause of hospitalization in U.S. adults. Orthop Nurs. 2012;31:85–91.
10. Margules KR. Fluoroscopically directed steroid instillation in the treatment of hip osteoarthritis: safety and efficacy in 510 cases. Arthritis Rheum. 2001;44:2449–50.
11. Karim Z, Brown AK, Quinn M, et al. Ultrasound-guided steroid injections in the treatment of hip osteoarthritis: comment on the letter by Margules. Arthritis Rheum. 2004;50:338–9.
12. Pourbagher MA, Ozalay M, Pourbagher A. Accuracy and outcome of sonographically guided intra-articular sodium hyaluronate injections in patients with osteoarthritis of the hip. J Ultrasound Med. 2005;24:1391–5.
13. Masoud MA, Said HG. Intra-articular hip injection using anatomic surface landmarks. Arthrosc Tech. 2013;2:e147–9.
14. Mauffrey C, Pobbathy P. Hip joint injection technique using anatomic landmarks: are we accurate? A prospective study. Int J Orthop Surg. 2006;3:1.
15. McCarty D. A basic guide to arthrocentesis. Hosp Med. 1968;4:77–97.
16. Mei-Dan O, McConkey MO, Petersen B, McCarty E, Moreira B, Young DA. The anterior approach for a non-image-guided intra-articular hip injection. Arthroscopy. 2013;29:1025–33.
17. Singh J, Khan W, Marwah S, Wells G, Tannous D, Sharma H. Do we need radiological guidance for intra-articular hip injections? Open Orthop J. 2014;16:114–7.
18. Ziv YB, Kardosh R, Debi R, Backstein D, Safir O, Kosashvili Y. An inexpensive and accurate method for hip injections without the use of imaging. J Clin Rheumatol. 2009;15:103–5.
19. Leopold SS, Battista V, Oliverio JA. Safety and efficacy of intraarticular hip injection using anatomic landmarks. Clin Orthop Relat Res. 2001;(391):192–7.
20. Diracoglu D, Alptekin K, Dikici F, Balci HI, Ozcakar L, Aksoy C. Evaluation of needle positioning during blind intra-articular hip injections for osteoarthritis: fluoroscopy versus arthrography. Arch Phys Med Rehabil. 2009;90:2112–5.
21. Kurup H, Ward P. Do we need radiological guidance for hip joint injections? Acta Orthop Belg. 2010;76:205–7.
22. Hayashi N, Weinstein JN, Meller ST, Lee HM, Spratt KF, Gebhart GF. The effect of epidural injection of betamethasone or bupivacaine in a rat model of lumbar radiculopathy. Spine (Phila Pa 1976). 1998;23:877–85.
23. Flanagan J, Casale FF, Thomas TL, Desai KB. Intra-articular injection for pain relief in patients awaiting hip replacement. Ann R Coll Surg Engl. 1988;70:156–7.
24. Young R, Harding J, Kingsly A, Bradley M. Therapeutic hip injections: is the injection volume important? Clin Radiol. 2012;67:55–60.
25. Lambert RGW, Hutchings EJ, Grace MGA, Jhangri GS, Conner-Spady B, Maksymowych WP. Steroid injection for osteoarthritis of the hip: a randomized, double-blind, placebo-controlled trial. Arthritis Rheum. 2007;56:2278–87.
26. Plant MJ, Borg AA, Dziedzic K, Saklatvala J, Dawes PT. Radiographic patterns and response to corticosteroid hip injection. Ann Rheum Dis. 1997;56:476–80.
27. Jones A, Doherty M. Intra-articular corticosteroids are effective in osteoarthritis but there are no clinical predictors of response. Ann Rheum Dis. 1996;55:829–32.
28. Robinson P, Keenan AM, Conaghan PG. Clinical effectiveness and dose response of image-guided intra-articular corticosteroid injection for hip osteoarthritis. Rheumatology (Oxford). 2007;46:285–91.
29. Kullenberg B, Runesson R, Tuvhag R, Olsson C, Resch S. Intraarticular corticosteroid injection: pain relief in osteoarthritis of the hip? J Rheumatol. 2004;31:2265–8.
30. Gupta G, Radhakrishna M, Etheridge P, Besemann M, Finlayson RJ. Radiofrequency denervation of the hip joint for pain management: case report and literature review. US Army Med Dep J. 2014:41–51.
31. Kawaguchi M, Hashizume K, Iwata T, Furuya H. Percutaneous radiofrequency lesioning of sensory branches of the obturator and femoral nerves for the treatment of hip joint pain. Reg Anesth Pain Med. 2001;26:576–81.
32. Rivera F, Mariconda C, Annaratone G. Percutaneous radiofrequency denervation in patients with contraindications for total hip arthroplasty. Orthopedics. 2012;35:e302–5.
33. Wu H, Groner J. Pulsed radiofrequency treatment of articular branches of the obturator and femoral nerves for management of hip joint pain. Pain Pract. 2007;7:341–4.
34. Alberto M, Umberto M, Emanuele B, et al. Intra-articular injection of hyaluronic acid (MW 1,500–2,000 kDa; HyalOne®) in symptomatic osteoarthritis of the hip: a prospective cohort study. Arch Orthop Trauma Surg. 2011;131:1677–85.
35. Migliore A, Massafra U, Bizzi E, et al. Comparative, double-blind, controlled study of intra-articular hyaluronic acid (Hyalubrix) injections versus local anesthetic in osteoarthritis of the hip. Arthritis Res Ther. 2009;11:R183.
36. Richette P, Ravaud P, Conrozier T, et al. Effect of hyaluronic acid in symptomatic hip osteoarthritis: a multicenter, randomized, placebo-controlled trial. Arthritis Rheum. 2009;60:824–30.
37. Abate M, Pulcini D, Di Iorio A, Schiavone C. Viscosupplementation with intra-articular hyaluronic acid for treatment of osteoarthritis in the elderly. Curr Pharm Des. 2010;16:631–40.
38. Tikiz C, Unlu Z, Sener A, Efe M, Tuzun C. Comparison of the efficacy of lower and higher molecular weight viscosupplementation in the treatment of hip osteoarthritis. Clin Rheumatol. 2005;24:244–50.
39. Migliore A, Bella A, Bisignani M, et al. Total hip replacement rate in a cohort of patients affected by symptomatic hip osteoarthritis following intra-articular sodium hyaluronate (MW 1,500-2,000 kDa) ORTOBRIX study. Clin Rheumatol. 2012;31:1187–96.
40. Vora A, Borg-Stein J, Nguyen RT. Regenerative injection therapy for osteoarthritis: fundamental concepts and evidence-based review. PM R. 2012;4:S104–9.

41. Sanchez M, Guadilla J, Fiz N, Andia I. Ultrasound-guided platelet-rich plasma injections for the treatment of osteoarthritis of the hip. Rheumatology (Oxford). 2012;51:144–50.
42. Battaglia M, Guaraldi F, Vannini F, et al. Platelet-rich plasma (PRP) intra-articular ultrasound-guided injections as a possible treatment for hip osteoarthritis: a pilot study. Clin Exp Rheumatol. 2011;29:754.
43. van Buul GM, Koevoet WL, Kops N, et al. Platelet-rich plasma releasate inhibits inflammatory processes in osteoarthritic chondrocytes. Am J Sports Med. 2011;39:2362–70.
44. Anitua E, Sanchez M, Nurden AT, et al. Platelet-released growth factors enhance the secretion of hyaluronic acid and induce hepatocyte growth factor production by synovial fibroblasts from arthritic patients. Rheumatology (Oxford). 2007;46:1769–72.
45. Anitua E, Sanchez M, Zalduendo MM, et al. Fibroblastic response to treatment with different preparations rich in growth factors. Cell Prolif. 2009;42:162–70.
46. Nguyen RT, Borg-Stein J, McInnis K. Applications of platelet-rich plasma in musculoskeletal and sports medicine: an evidence-based approach. PM R. 2011;3:226–50.
47. Battaglia M, Guaraldi F, Vannini F, et al. Efficacy of ultrasound-guided intra-articular injections of platelet-rich plasma versus hyaluronic acid for hip osteoarthritis. Orthopedics. 2013;36: e1501–8.
48. Hauser RA, Orlofsky A. Regenerative injection therapy with whole bone marrow aspirate for degenerative joint disease: a case series. Clin Med Insights Arthritis Musculoskelet Disord. 2013;6: 65–72.
49. Cohen SB, Huang R, Ciccotti MG, Dodson CC, Parvizi J. Treatment of femoroacetabular impingement in athletes using a mini-direct anterior approach. Am J Sports Med. 2012;40: 1620–7.
50. Beck M, Kalhor M, Leunig M, Ganz R. Hip morphology influences the pattern of damage to the acetabular cartilage: femoroacetabular impingement as a cause of early osteoarthritis of the hip. J Bone Joint Surg Br. 2005;87:1012–8.
51. Groh MM, Herrera J. A comprehensive review of hip labral tears. Curr Rev Musculoskelet Med. 2009;2:105–17.
52. Bharam S. Labral tears, extra-articular injuries, and hip arthroscopy in the athlete. Clin Sports Med. 2006;25:279–92. ix.
53. Hunt D, Prather H, Harris Hayes M, Clohisy JC. Clinical outcomes analysis of conservative and surgical treatment of patients with clinical indications of prearthritic, intra-articular hip disorders. PM R. 2012;4:479–87.
54. Byrd JW. Hip arthroscopy: surgical indications. Arthroscopy. 2006;22:1260–2.
55. McCarthy J, Noble P, Aluisio FV, Schuck M, Wright J, Lee JA. Anatomy, pathologic features, and treatment of acetabular labral tears. Clin Orthop Relat Res. 2003;(406):38–47.
56. Robertson WJ, Kadrmas WR, Kelly BT. Arthroscopic management of labral tears in the hip: a systematic review of the literature. Clin Orthop Relat Res. 2007;455:88–92.
57. Hickman JM, Peters CL. Hip pain in the young adult: diagnosis and treatment of disorders of the acetabular labrum and acetabular dysplasia. Am J Orthop (Belle Mead NJ). 2001;30:459–67.
58. Kelly BT, Williams III RJ, Philippon MJ. Hip arthroscopy: current indications, treatment options, and management issues. Am J Sports Med. 2003;31:1020–37.
59. Safran MR. The acetabular labrum: anatomic and functional characteristics and rationale for surgical intervention. J Am Acad Orthop Surg. 2010;18:338–45.
60. Byrd JW, Jones KS. Diagnostic accuracy of clinical assessment, magnetic resonance imaging, magnetic resonance arthrography, and intra-articular injection in hip arthroscopy patients. Am J Sports Med. 2004;32:1668–74.
61. Martin RL, Irrgang JJ, Sekiya JK. The diagnostic accuracy of a clinical examination in determining intra-articular hip pain for potential hip arthroscopy candidates. Arthroscopy. 2008;24:1013–8.
62. Kivlan BR, Martin RL, Sekiya JK. Response to diagnostic injection in patients with femoroacetabular impingement, labral tears, chondral lesions, and extra-articular pathology. Arthroscopy. 2011;27:619–27.
63. Dragoo JL, Braun HJ, Kim HJ, Phan HD, Golish SR. The in vitro chondrotoxicity of single-dose local anesthetics. Am J Sports Med. 2012;40:794–9.
64. Kamath R, Strichartz G, Rosenthal D. Cartilage toxicity from local anesthetics. Skeletal Radiol. 2008;37:871–3.
65. Webb ST, Ghosh S. Intra-articular bupivacaine: potentially chondrotoxic? Br J Anaesth. 2009;102:439–41.
66. Katayama H, Yamaguchi K, Kozuka T, Takashima T, Seez P, Matsuura K. Adverse reactions to ionic and nonionic contrast media. A report from the Japanese Committee on the Safety of Contrast Media. Radiology. 1990;175:621–8.
67. El Abd O. Steroids in spine interventions. In: Slipman CWD, Derby R, Simeone FA, Mayer TG, editors. Interventional spine an algorithmic approach. Philadelphia: Saunders Elsevier; 2008. p. 153–60.
68. Taher RT, Power RA. Iliopsoas tendon dysfunction as a cause of pain after total hip arthroplasty relieved by surgical release. J Arthroplasty. 2003;18:387–8.
69. Habib GS. Systemic effects of intra-articular corticosteroids. Clin Rheumatol. 2009;28:749–56.
70. Johnston CA, Wiley JP, Lindsay DM, Wiseman DA. Iliopsoas bursitis and tendinitis. A review. Sports Med. 1998;25:271–83.
71. Adler RS, Buly R, Ambrose R, Sculco T. Diagnostic and therapeutic use of sonography-guided iliopsoas peritendinous injections. AJR Am J Roentgenol. 2005;185:940–3.
72. Parziale JR, O'Donnell CJ, Sandman DN. Iliopsoas bursitis. Am J Phys Med Rehabil. 2009;88:690–1.
73. Blankenbaker DG, De Smet AA, Keene JS. Sonography of the iliopsoas tendon and injection of the iliopsoas bursa for diagnosis and management of the painful snapping hip. Skeletal Radiol. 2006;35:565–71.
74. Meermans G, Corten K, Simon JP. Is the infection rate in primary THA increased after steroid injection? Clin Orthop Relat Res. 2012;470(11):3213–9.
75. Chitre AR, Fehily MJ, Bamford DJ. Total hip replacement after intra-articular injection of local anaesthetic and steroid. J Bone Joint Surg Br. 2007;89:166–8.
76. Raynauld J-P, Buckland-Wright C, Ward R, et al. Safety and efficacy of long-term intraarticular steroid injections in osteoarthritis of the knee: a randomized, double-blind, placebo-controlled trial. Arthritis Rheum. 2003;48:370–7.
77. Williams BS, Cohen SP. Greater trochanteric pain syndrome: a review of anatomy, diagnosis and treatment. Anesth Analg. 2009;108:1662–70.
78. Tortolani PJ, Carbone JJ, Quartararo LG. Greater trochanteric pain syndrome in patients referred to orthopedic spine specialists. Spine J. 2002;2:251–4.
79. Shbeeb MI, Matteson EL. Trochanteric bursitis (greater trochanter pain syndrome). Mayo Clin Proc. 1996;71:565–9.
80. Lustenberger DP, Ng VY, Best TM, Ellis TJ. Efficacy of treatment of trochanteric bursitis: a systematic review. Clin J Sport Med. 2011;21:447–53.
81. Brinks A, van Rijn RM, Willemsen SP, et al. Corticosteroid injections for greater trochanteric pain syndrome: a randomized controlled trial in primary care. Ann Fam Med. 2011;9:226–34.
82. Rowand M, Chambliss ML, Mackler L. Clinical inquiries. How should you treat trochanteric bursitis? J Fam Pract. 2009;58: 494–500.

83. Farmer KW, Jones LC, Brownson KE, Khanuja HS, Hungerford MW. Trochanteric bursitis after total hip arthroplasty: incidence and evaluation of response to treatment. J Arthroplasty. 2010;25:208–12.
84. Cohen SP, Narvaez JC, Lebovits AH, Stojanovic MP. Corticosteroid injections for trochanteric bursitis: is fluoroscopy necessary? A pilot study. Br J Anaesth. 2005;94:100–6.
85. Allen WC, Cope R. Coxa saltans: the snapping hip revisited. J Am Acad Orthop Surg. 1995;3:303–8.
86. Trousdale RT, Cabanela ME, Berry DJ. Anterior iliopsoas impingement after total hip arthroplasty. J Arthroplasty. 1995;10:546–9.
87. Taylor GR, Clarke NM. Surgical release of the 'snapping iliopsoas tendon'. J Bone Joint Surg Br. 1995;77:881–3.
88. Heaton K, Dorr LD. Surgical release of iliopsoas tendon for groin pain after total hip arthroplasty. J Arthroplasty. 2002;17:779–81.
89. Yeoman W. The relationship of arthritis of the sacro-iliac joint to sciatica. Lancet. 1928;2:1119–22.
90. McCrory P, Bell S. Nerve entrapment syndromes as a cause of pain in the hip, groin and buttock. Sports Med. 1999;27:261–74.
91. Tibor LM, Sekiya JK. Differential diagnosis of pain around the hip joint. Arthroscopy. 2008;24:1407–21.
92. Hallin RP. Sciatic pain and the piriformis muscle. Postgrad Med. 1983;74:69–72.
93. Windisch G, Braun E, Anderhuber F. Piriformis muscle: clinical anatomy and consideration of the piriformis syndrome. Surg Radiol Anat. 2007;29:37–45.
94. Gonzalez P, Pepper M, Sullivan W, Akuthota V. Confirmation of needle placement within the piriformis muscle of a cadaveric specimen using anatomic landmarks and fluoroscopic guidance. Pain Physician. 2008;11:327–31.
95. Betts A. Combined fluoroscopic and nerve stimulator technique for injection of the piriformis muscle. Pain Physician. 2004;7: 279–81.
96. Chen CP, Shen CY, Lew HL. Ultrasound-guided injection of the piriformis muscle. Am J Phys Med Rehabil. 2011;90:871–2.
97. Masala S, Crusco S, Meschini A, Taglieri A, Calabria E, Simonetti G. Piriformis syndrome: long-term follow-up in patients treated with percutaneous injection of anesthetic and corticosteroid under CT guidance. Cardiovasc Intervent Radiol. 2012;35:375–82.
98. Huerto AP, Yeo SN, Ho KY. Piriformis muscle injection using ultrasonography and motor stimulation—report of a technique. Pain Physician. 2007;10:687–90.
99. Hanania M. New technique for piriformis muscle injection using a nerve stimulator. Reg Anesth. 1997;22:200–2.
100. Fishman LM, Dombi GW, Michaelsen C, et al. Piriformis syndrome: diagnosis, treatment, and outcome—a 10-year study. Arch Phys Med Rehabil. 2002;83:295–301.
101. Naja Z, Al-Tannir M, El-Rajab M, et al. The effectiveness of clonidine-bupivacaine repeated nerve stimulator-guided injection in piriformis syndrome. Clin J Pain. 2009;25:199–205.
102. Monnier G, Tatu L, Michel F. New indications for botulinum toxin in rheumatology. Joint Bone Spine. 2006;73:667–71.
103. Aoki KR, Guyer B. Botulinum toxin type A and other botulinum toxin serotypes: a comparative review of biochemical and pharmacological actions. Eur J Neurol. 2001;8 Suppl 5:21–9.
104. Kirschner JS, Foye PM, Cole JL. Piriformis syndrome, diagnosis and treatment. Muscle Nerve. 2009;40:10–8.
105. Mullin V, de Rosayro M. Caudal steroid injection for treatment of piriformis syndrome. Anesth Analg. 1990;71:705–7.
106. Prather H, Hunt D. Conservative management of low back pain, part I. Sacroiliac joint pain. Dis Mon. 2004;50:670–83.
107. Chou LH, Slipman CW, Bhagia SM, et al. Inciting events initiating injection-proven sacroiliac joint syndrome. Pain Med. 2004;5:26–32.
108. Foley BS, Buschbacher RM. Sacroiliac joint pain: anatomy, biomechanics, diagnosis, and treatment. Am J Phys Med Rehabil. 2006;85:997–1006.
109. Vanelderen P, Szadek K, Cohen SP, et al. 13. Sacroiliac joint pain. Pain Pract. 2010;10:470–8.
110. Dreyfuss P, Michaelsen M, Pauza K, McLarty J, Bogduk N. The value of medical history and physical examination in diagnosing sacroiliac joint pain. Spine (Phila Pa 1976). 1996;21: 2594–602.
111. van der Wurff P, Buijs EJ, Groen GJ. A multitest regimen of pain provocation tests as an aid to reduce unnecessary minimally invasive sacroiliac joint procedures. Arch Phys Med Rehabil. 2006;87:10–4.
112. Cohen SP. Sacroiliac joint pain: a comprehensive review of anatomy, diagnosis, and treatment. Anesth Analg. 2005;101:1440–53.
113. Rupert MP, Lee M, Manchikanti L, Datta S, Cohen SP. Evaluation of sacroiliac joint interventions: a systematic appraisal of the literature. Pain Physician. 2009;12:399–418.
114. Hansen HC, McKenzie-Brown AM, Cohen SP, Swicegood JR, Colson JD, Manchikanti L. Sacroiliac joint interventions: a systematic review. Pain Physician. 2007;10:165–84.
115. Slipman CW, Sterenfeld EB, Chou LH, Herzog R, Vresilovic E. The value of radionuclide imaging in the diagnosis of sacroiliac joint syndrome. Spine (Phila Pa 1976). 1996;21:2251–4.
116. Maigne JY, Boulahdour H, Chatellier G. Value of quantitative radionuclide bone scanning in the diagnosis of sacroiliac joint syndrome in 32 patients with low back pain. Eur Spine J. 1998;7:328–31.
117. Stone JA, Bartynski WS. Treatment of facet and sacroiliac joint arthropathy: steroid injections and radiofrequency ablation. Tech Vasc Interv Radiol. 2009;12:22–32.
118. Hawkins J, Schofferman J. Serial therapeutic sacroiliac joint injections: a practice audit. Pain Med. 2009;10:850–3.
119. Chou R, Atlas SJ, Stanos SP, Rosenquist RW. Nonsurgical interventional therapies for low back pain: a review of the evidence for an American Pain Society clinical practice guideline. Spine (Phila Pa 1976). 2009;34:1078–93.
120. Liliang PC, Lu K, Weng HC, Liang CL, Tsai YD, Chen HJ. The therapeutic efficacy of sacroiliac joint blocks with triamcinolone acetonide in the treatment of sacroiliac joint dysfunction without spondyloarthropathy. Spine (Phila Pa 1976). 2009;34:896–900.
121. Hansen HC. Is fluoroscopy necessary for sacroiliac joint injections? Pain Physician. 2003;6:155–8.
122. Rosenberg JM, Quint TJ, de Rosayro AM. Computerized tomographic localization of clinically-guided sacroiliac joint injections. Clin J Pain. 2000;16:18–21.
123. Aydin SM, Gharibo CG, Mehnert M, Stitik TP. The role of radiofrequency ablation for sacroiliac joint pain: a meta-analysis. PM R. 2010;2:842–51.
124. Cohen SP, Abdi S. Lateral branch blocks as a treatment for sacroiliac joint pain: a pilot study. Reg Anesth Pain Med. 2003;28:113–9.
125. Yin W, Willard F, Carreiro J, Dreyfuss P. Sensory stimulation-guided sacroiliac joint radiofrequency neurotomy: technique based on neuroanatomy of the dorsal sacral plexus. Spine (Phila Pa 1976). 2003;28:2419–25.
126. Patel N, Gross A, Brown L, Gekht G. A randomized, placebo-controlled study to assess the efficacy of lateral branch neurotomy for chronic sacroiliac joint pain. Pain Med. 2012;13:383–98.
127. Lee JH, Lee S-H, Song SH. Clinical effectiveness of botulinum toxin a compared to a mixture of steroid and local anesthetics as a treatment for sacroiliac joint pain. Pain Med. 2010;11:692–700.
128. Kim WM, Lee HG, Jeong CW, Kim CM, Yoon MH. A randomized controlled trial of intra-articular prolotherapy versus steroid injection for sacroiliac joint pain. J Altern Complement Med. 2010;16:1285–90.

129. Cusi M, Saunders J, Hungerford B, Wisbey-Roth T, Lucas P, Wilson S. The use of prolotherapy in the sacroiliac joint. Br J Sports Med. 2010;44:100–4.
130. Weber M, Hasler P, Gerber H. Insufficiency fractures of the sacrum. Twenty cases and review of the literature. Spine (Phila Pa 1976). 1993;18:2507–12.
131. Zaman FM, Frey M, Slipman CW. Sacral stress fractures. Curr Sports Med Rep. 2006;5:37–43.
132. Featherstone T. Magnetic resonance imaging in the diagnosis of sacral stress fracture. Br J Sports Med. 1999;33:276–7.
133. Frey ME, DePalma MJ, Cifu DX, Bhagia SM, Daitch JS. Efficacy and safety of percutaneous sacroplasty for painful osteoporotic sacral insufficiency fractures: a prospective, multicenter trial. Spine (Phila Pa 1976). 2007;32:1635–40.
134. Butler CL, Given II CA, Michel SJ, Tibbs PA. Percutaneous sacroplasty for the treatment of sacral insufficiency fractures. AJR Am J Roentgenol. 2005;184:1956–9.
135. van Kleef M, Vanelderen P, Cohen SP, Lataster A, Van Zundert J, Mekhail N. 12. Pain originating from the lumbar facet joints. Pain Pract. 2010;10:459–69.
136. Kalichman L, Hunter DJ. Lumbar facet joint osteoarthritis: a review. Semin Arthritis Rheum. 2007;37:69–80.
137. Cohen SP, Raja SN. Pathogenesis, diagnosis, and treatment of lumbar zygapophysial (facet) joint pain. Anesthesiology. 2007; 106:591–614.
138. Civelek E, Cansever T, Kabatas S, et al. Comparison of effectiveness of facet joint injection and radiofrequency denervation in chronic low back pain. Turk Neurosurg. 2012;22:200–6.
139. Manchikanti L, Singh V, Falco FJ, Cash KA, Pampati V. Evaluation of lumbar facet joint nerve blocks in managing chronic low back pain: a randomized, double-blind, controlled trial with a 2-year follow-up. Int J Med Sci. 2010;7:124–35.
140. Schulte TL, Pietilä TA, Heidenreich J, Brock M, Stendel R. Injection therapy of lumbar facet syndrome: a prospective study. Acta Neurochir. 2006;148:1165–72.
141. Manchikanti L, Malla Y, Wargo BW, Cash KA, Pampati V, Fellows B. Complications of fluoroscopically directed facet joint nerve blocks: a prospective evaluation of 7,500 episodes with 43,000 nerve blocks. Pain Physician. 2012;15:E143–50.
142. Van Zundert J, Vanelderen P, Kessels A, van Kleef M. Radiofrequency treatment of facet-related pain: evidence and controversies. Curr Pain Headache Rep. 2012;16:19–25.
143. Dreyfuss P, Halbrook B, Pauza K, Joshi A, McLarty J, Bogduk N. Efficacy and validity of radiofrequency neurotomy for chronic lumbar zygapophysial joint pain. Spine (Phila Pa 1976). 2000;25:1270–7.
144. Travell JG, TSimons LS. Myofascial pain and dysfunction: the trigger point manual, vol. 2. The lower extremities. 2nd ed. Philadelphia: Lippincott Williams & Wilkins; 1993.
145. Kaziyama HHS, Souza LPM, Pimentel DC, Targino R, Hsing WT. A study of the chronic myofascial pain syndrome in patients with primary osteoarthritis of the hip. Acta Fisiatr. 2005;12:295.
146. Hong CZ. Lidocaine injection versus dry needling to myofascial trigger point. The importance of the local twitch response. Am J Phys Med Rehabil. 1994;73:256–63.
147. El Abd O. The Physiatric Association of Spine, Sports, and Occupational Rehabilitation research forum. In: AAPMR annual assembly, 2003, Chicago; 2003.
148. Ashton IK, Ashton BA, Gibson SJ, Polak JM, Jaffray DC, Eisenstein SM. Morphological basis for back pain: the demonstration of nerve fibers and neuropeptides in the lumbar facet joint capsule but not in ligamentum flavum. J Orthop Res. 1992;10:72–8.
149. Nakamura S, Takahashi K, Takahashi Y, Morinaga T, Shimada Y, Moriya H. Origin of nerves supplying the posterior portion of lumbar intervertebral discs in rats. Spine (Phila Pa 1976). 1996;21:917–24.
150. Saifuddin A, Emanuel R, White J, Renton P, Braithwaite I, Taylor BA. An analysis of radiating pain at lumbar discography. Eur Spine J. 1998;7:358–62.
151. Schwarzer AC, Aprill CN, Derby R, Fortin J, Kine G, Bogduk N. The prevalence and clinical features of internal disc disruption in patients with chronic low back pain. Spine (Phila Pa 1976). 1995;20:1878–83.
152. Bogduk N. The innervation of the lumbar spine. Spine (Phila Pa 1976). 1983;8:286–93.
153. Weinstein J, Claverie W, Gibson S. The pain of discography. Spine (Phila Pa 1976). 1988;13:1344–8.
154. Groen GJ, Baljet B, Drukker J. The innervation of the spinal dura mater: anatomy and clinical implications. Acta Neurochir (Wien). 1988;92:39–46.
155. Pedersen HE, Blunck CF, Gardner E. The anatomy of lumbosacral posterior rami and meningeal branches of spinal nerve (sinu-vertebral nerves); with an experimental study of their functions. J Bone Joint Surg Am. 1956;38-A:377–91.
156. Bogduk N, Tynan W, Wilson AS. The nerve supply to the human lumbar intervertebral discs. J Anat. 1981;132:39–56.
157. Wiberg G. Back pain in relation to the nerve supply of the intervertebral disc. Acta Orthop Scand. 1949;19:211–21. illust.
158. Slipman CW, Patel RK, Zhang L, et al. Side of symptomatic annular tear and site of low back pain: is there a correlation? Spine (Phila Pa 1976). 2001;26:E165–9.
159. Ruch T. The pathophysiology of pain. In: Fulton J, editor. A textbook of physiology. Philadelphia: WB Saunders; 1997. p. 358–76.
160. Cervero F, Tattersall JE. Cutaneous receptive fields of somatic and viscerosomatic neurones in the thoracic spinal cord of the cat. J Comp Neurol. 1985;237:325–32.
161. Bogduk N. Clinical anatomy of the lumbar spine and sacrum. New York: Churchill-Livingstone; 1997.
162. Botwin K, Natalicchio J, Brown LA. Epidurography contrast patterns with fluoroscopic guided lumbar transforaminal epidural injections: a prospective evaluation. Pain Physician. 2004;7: 211–5.
163. Sullivan WJ, Willick SE, Chira-Adisai W, et al. Incidence of intravascular uptake in lumbar spinal injection procedures. Spine (Phila Pa 1976). 2000;25:481–6.
164. Furman MB, O'Brien EM, Zgleszewski TM. Incidence of intravascular penetration in transforaminal lumbosacral epidural steroid injections. Spine (Phila Pa 1976). 2000;25:2628–32.

Groin Pain in Athletes: Assessment and Nonsurgical Treatment

29

Per Hölmich and Kristian Thorborg

Introduction

Descriptions of hip and groin injuries in athletes can be confusing because of the lack of common terminology between different specialists, particularly orthopaedic surgeons and general surgeons, and because of the rapidly evolving understanding of early hip disease brought about by advances in imaging and arthroscopy, which renders previous diagnoses questionable [1].

In soccer, characteristic activities causing pain include sprinting, cutting, kicking the ball, and making a sliding tackle. In many cases these injuries tend to be ignored by both athletes and trainers leading to the development of chronic conditions. Symptoms often seem to be contradictory and confusing in the athlete with long-standing groin pain. In the past, in about 25–35 % of the patients, multiple causes for the chronic groin pain could be found [2–4], but with recent improvements in understanding and assessment, we believe we can give each player a single 'clinical entity' diagnosis. The nonoperative treatment should be based on a systematic examination and an exact identification of the structures causing the pain. Muscle imbalances and biomechanical problems should be considered and treated.

P. Hölmich, DMSc (✉)
Sports Orthopedic Research Center-Copenhagen, Arthroscopic Center Amager, Copenhagen University Hospital, Amager-Hvidovre, Italiensvej 1, Copenhagen 2300, Denmark

Sports Groin Pain Center, Aspetar—Orthopedic and Sports Medicine Hospital, Doha, Qatar
e-mail: per.holmich@amh.regionh.dk

K. Thorborg, PhD
Sports Orthopedic Research Center-Copenhagen, Arthroscopic Center Amager, Copenhagen University Hospital, Amager-Hvidovre, Italiensvej 1, Copenhagen 2300, Denmark
e-mail: kristianthorborg@hotmail.com

Patient Evaluation and Diagnosis

In November 2014, 24 international experts from 14 different countries participated in a consensus meeting to develop a clinically based taxonomy of groin pain in athletes [5]. Systematic reviews were performed to give an up-to-date synthesis of the current evidence on major topics concerning groin pain in athletes. All members participated in a Delphi questionnaire prior to the meeting, and a unanimous agreement was reached on the following classification system in which groin pain in athletes is described under three major subheadings:

- Defined clinical entities for groin pain: adductor-related, iliopsoas-related, inguinal-related, and pubic-related groin pain
- Hip-related groin pain
- Other causes of groin pain in athletes

These definitions and terminology are based on history and physical examination to categorize athletes, making it simple and suitable for both clinical practice and research. The further development of this terminology seems very promising, and it is recommended to utilize this terminology for future scientific and clinical work.

The group also discussed a number of popular terms and chose not to recommend: adductor and iliopsoas tendinitis or tendinopathy, athletic groin pain, athletic pubalgia, biomechanical groin overload, Gilmore's groin, groin disruption, hockey goalie syndrome, hockey groin, osteitis pubis, sports groin, sportsman's groin, sports hernia, and sportsman's hernia.

This agreed terminology is in line with the 'clinical entity' approach for groin injuries in athletes that has proven very useful in differentiating the injuries and planning the appropriate treatment [2–4].

J.C. McCarthy et al. (eds.), *Hip Joint Restoration*, DOI 10.1007/978-1-4614-0694-5_29

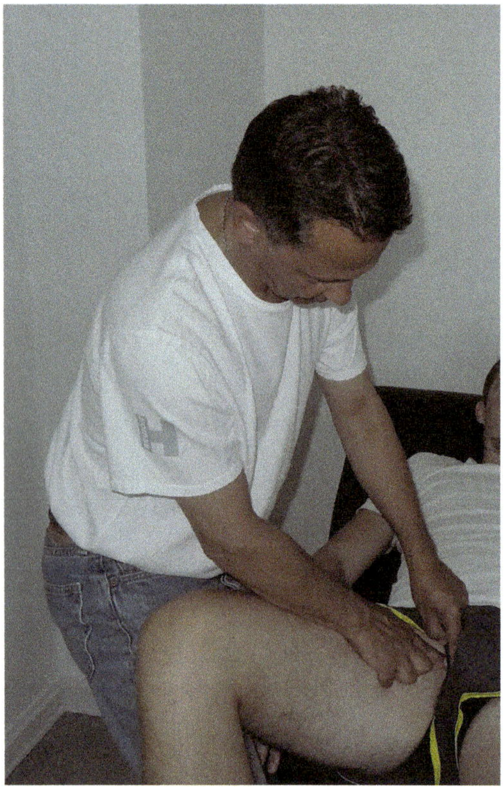

Fig. 29.1 Tenderness of the adductor tendons

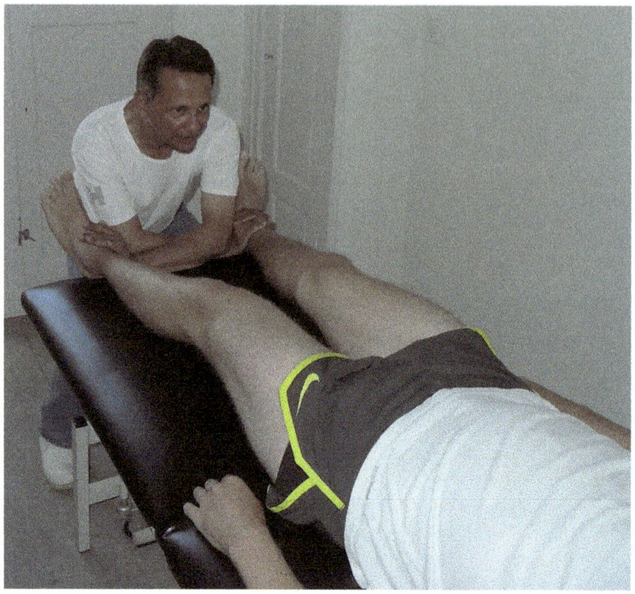

Fig. 29.2 Resisted hip adduction test

Adductor-Related Groin Pain

Adductor-related groin pain is localized medially in the groin and may radiate down along the adductor group on the medial side of the thigh. The clinical signs are defined as:

- Tenderness of the origin of the adductor longus and/or the gracilis at the inferior pubic ramus (Fig. 29.1)
- Pain at the proximal part of the adductors on resisted adduction (Fig. 29.2)

Iliopsoas-Related Groin Pain

Iliopsoas-related groin pain is localized in the anterior part of the proximal thigh more laterally than adductor-related groin pain. It sometimes radiates down the anterior thigh and may involve an element of lower abdominal pain lateral to the rectus abdominis muscle. In differentiating between the intra- and the extra-articular problems, it is very important to know that the anterior impingement test can cause pain through folding (flexion), twisting (adduction), and pulling (internal rotation) of a sore iliopsoas.

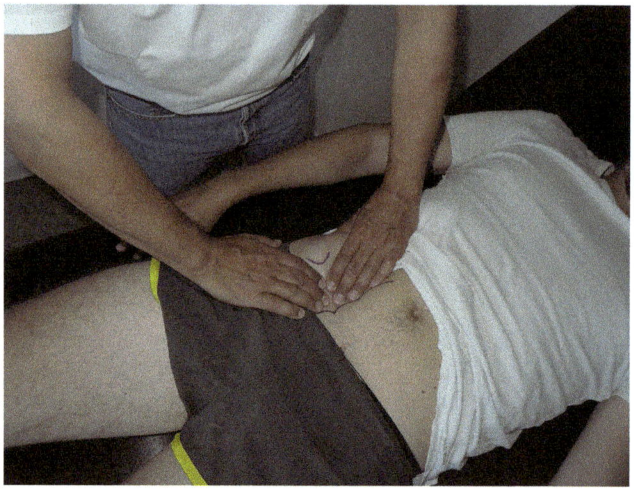

Fig. 29.3 Palpating the iliopsoas muscle through the abdominal wall

The clinical signs of iliopsoas-related groin pain are defined as:

- Pain when palpating the muscle through the lower abdominal wall and/or just below the inguinal ligament (Fig. 29.3)
- Pain at passive stretching of the muscle using the Thomas test position [4, 6] (Fig. 29.4)

Inguinal-Related Groin Pain

Inguinal-related groin pain can probably be attributed to a number of anatomical structures. The problem has been given numerous names in the literature such as sports hernia, sports-

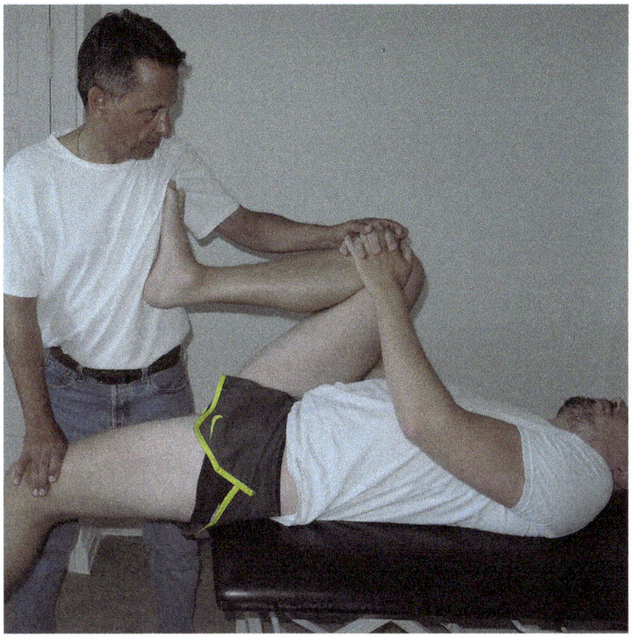

Fig. 29.4 The use of Thomas test for iliopsoas: If the patient is positioned near the end of the bed, the lumbar lordosis is flattened by flexion of the opposite hip, and the hip under test is extended by hanging over the end of the couch, thus stretching the iliopsoas muscle and tendon

man's hernia, incipient hernia, Gilmore's groin, pubic pain, athletic pubalgia, and others [7]. Within the literature, the underlying lesions are described as nonspecific, with large variations in the patho-anatomy. Inguinal-related groin pain is experienced 'deep' in the groin, slightly more proximal than the adductor-related pain. The pain tends to be diffuse with radiation along the inguinal ligament, the perineum, the rectus muscles, and the adductor muscles and sometimes also to the opposite side. Increased intra-abdominal pressure such as coughing or sneezing will usually cause increased pain.

The clinical signs of inguinal-related groin pain are defined as:

- Tenderness at the conjoint tendon towards the pubic tubercle
- Tenderness of the posterior wall in the external ring of the inguinal canal [4]

Related or Unusual Diagnoses Associated with Groin Pain

Other common diagnoses related to the muscles and tendon related to the hip and groin are the internal and external coxa saltans (snapping hip).

Nerve entrapment can occur when a peripheral nerve is entrapped by the neighbouring fascia, tendons, or muscles causing ischemia and nerve dysfunction. Nerves most commonly affected are the genitofemoral, ilioinguinal, and lateral femoral cutaneous nerves. The pain is usually experienced with hyperesthesia or hypoesthesia of the skin along the specific nerve's innervation area (Fig. 29.5). Localized tenderness at the site of penetration of the nerve through the fascia is considered to be the most pathognomonic finding. The characteristics of the pain may vary considerably. With the exception of the lateral femoral cutaneous nerve, with its discrete area of sensation and typical symptoms, nerve entrapments are a diagnostic challenge.

Neoplasms may present as a sports-related problem in seemingly otherwise healthy athletes and should be kept in mind as a possible cause of hip and groin pain. Osteosarcomas, chondrosarcomas, and other malignant tumours have been diagnosed often at a late stage, due to both patient's and doctor's delay. X-ray examination should always be included at an early stage in patients with groin pain, and, in patients with diffuse pain of uncertain diagnosis, MRI should also be performed early.

Treatment

The physician, the therapist, the trainer, and the athlete all need to be aware that, in most cases, the treatment will be lengthy. Therefore, supervision, encouragement, and patience are imperative to reach a good result. Most treatment modalities suggested in the literature are based on the experiences of clinical practice in the absence of randomized trials. It is important to be aware of all possible causes of groin pain when planning a treatment programme since multiple etiologies are often found in the same patient [2, 4, 8].

Acute Muscle-Tendinous Injuries

The acute treatment includes the rest, ice, compression, elevation, and mobilization (RICEM), as with other muscle injuries [7]. Mobilization including gentle movements towards outer positions can be commenced when the acute phase is over. Gentle isometric contractions precede more forceful contractions and contractions during lengthening [7]. Obtaining full isometric strength as compared to the other side is the first main goal of the treatment. Once this has been achieved, more forceful lengthening contractions can be included in the rehabilitation programme, and sports-specific drills such as running, accelerating, sprinting, kicking, and skating can be progressively commenced. Return to sport can be commenced when isometric and eccentric strength and ROM are normalized, and strenuous activities such as sprinting, changing direction, forceful skating strides, and kicking can be performed pain-free.

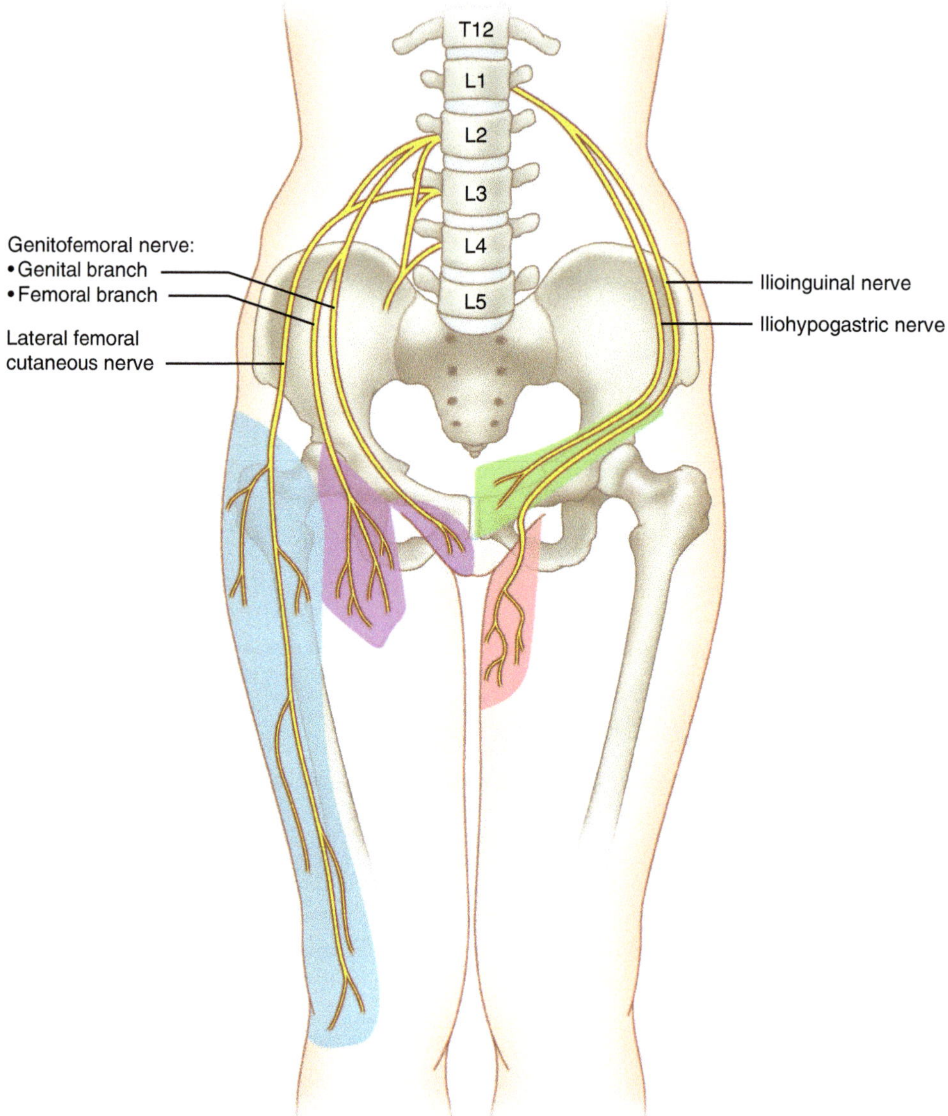

Fig. 29.5 Cutaneous innervation of groin region

Adductor-Related Groin Pain

A specific exercise programme has been shown to be highly effective in the treatment of adductor-related groin pain in a clinical randomized trial [9]. This programme consists of two modules: The first module consists of careful static and dynamic exercises to teach the patient to reactivate the adductor muscles. In most cases the athlete with adductor-related groin pain has difficulties activating these muscles, probably as a result of negative feedback caused by the pain.

In the second module, more demanding exercises are gradually added, including heavier resistance training as well as challenging balance and coordination exercises. This exercise programme is performed three times a week alternating with the exercises from module 1 on the days in between [9]. The total length of the exercise-training period is between 8 and 12 weeks. Sports activities are not allowed during the treatment period; however, bicycle riding is allowed if it can be performed without pain.

After 6 weeks of treatment, jogging is allowed as long as it does not provoke any groin pain. The exercise rehabilitation programme is successfully completed once the patient is able to jog and undergo their regular treatment without pain. At this point, athletes are allowed to gradually progress to demanding sports-specific training followed by sports participation. No stretching of the adductor muscles is allowed during this 2–3 month exercise-training period. However, stretching of the other lower extremity muscles, in particular the iliopsoas muscle, is recommended. Local injection of corticosteroids to treat athletes with adductor-related groin pain is not recommended, as, in our experience, there is no long-term beneficial effect. Moreover, if the injections affect the pain temporarily, it only makes it more difficult to monitor the training programme needed to cure the groin pain. Good studies to support adductor tenotomy are lacking, and it is the experience of the authors that this is only very rarely indicated.

Iliopsoas-Related Groin Pain

Though no evidence-based treatment has been published, the authors' preferred treatment of iliopsoas-related groin pain consists of systematic strengthening—including isometric, concentric, and eccentric contractions [10]—combined with a series of pelvic stabilization and balance exercises (Fig. 29.6).

Supplementary physiotherapy, including stretching, massage, and trigger point stimulation for symptomatic relief, might also be helpful. If the treatment regimen is not progressing satisfactorily, an ultrasound-guided local corticosteroid injection of the iliopsoas bursa may be considered to alleviate the pain and the tension of the muscle, thereby making it easier to exercise and strengthen the iliopsoas muscle.

In our experience, treatment of internal coxa saltans (snapping psoas) with a strengthening and stretching programme is effective in the vast majority of cases, though on rare occasions a partial release of the tendon at or close to the insertion may be performed with good results. The surgery can be performed as an open or arthroscopic/endoscopic procedure [11, 12].

Inguinal-Related Groin Pain

Surgery is an option that can be tempting to use, but the risk of complications and the lack of evidence call for caution. In these cases, the authors' preferred primary treatment (no evidence-based treatment has been published) is a training programme targeting pelvic stabilization by improving the strength, balance, and coordination of the involved muscles to give any abdominal wall lesion a chance to heal. This strategy allows simultaneous treatment of the other diagnostic entities causing groin pain that are often found at the same time as inguinal-related groin pain. If the exercise regimen fails, surgery can be appropriate to treat the underlying cause of the pain.

In our experience, the cause of symptoms in the vast majority of cases is weakness of the posterior wall. The probable connection between the decreased ROM caused by FAI and the overuse of the muscles and tendons related to the hip and the pelvis in connection with physical activity has been discussed in the literature [13, 14]. If the hip is irritable on testing and intra-articular injection of local anaesthetic significantly relieves symptoms, the same approach may be considered for treating the FAI. However, in most cases the primary surgical treatment should be directed at the weakness of the posterior wall.

The basic principles of the surgical procedure and the postoperative regime are identical to those for manifest hernias, apart from the fact that there is no hernia sac to invert or remove. A number of different procedures have been described both as open and as endoscopic surgery [15–17]. As with the exercise treatment, good controlled trials, examining the best treatment, are lacking.

External Snapping Hip

External snapping hip is caused by tight gluteus maximus muscles, but may be related to groin pain. The authors' preferred treatment (no evidence-based treatment has been published) consists of systematic strengthening of the gluteal muscles, including dynamic hip abduction exercises in the side-lying position with concentric, isometric, and eccentric contractions. This exercise has been proven effective in improving both isometric and eccentric strength of gluteus medius and the tensor fascia lata, including the iliotibial band [18]. Furthermore, the forward lunge is also a good exercise that incorporates balance and coordination of the hip and pelvis, combined with strengthening the hip extensors and external rotators. In resistant cases, good results may be achieved following surgical release of the iliotibial band at the level of the greater trochanter. The surgery can be performed as an open or arthroscopic/endoscopic procedure [19].

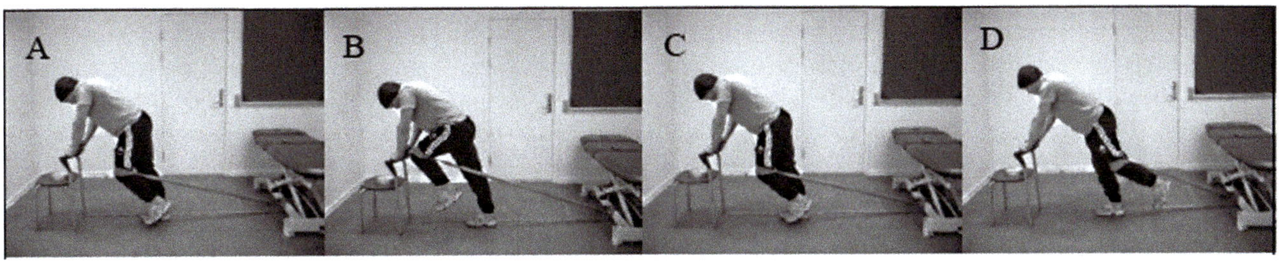

Fig. 29.6 Hip flexion strength training with elastic band

Outcome Assessment

Outcome measures used in the evaluation of patients with hip and groin pain should be reliable, valid, and responsive [20]. Various outcome scores for young patients with hip pain have been developed and used through the last 10 years. The 'first-generation' scores were modifications of existing hip scores designed for arthritis and hip arthroplasty patients. The 'modified Harris hip score' was one of the first measures aimed at younger patients with non-arthritic hip pathology, but this measure has never been sufficiently investigated for its measurement quality and validity in this patient group [21].

'Second-generation' scores, such as the Hip Outcome Score (HOS) [22], were developed specifically for younger patients with non-arthritic hip pathology and found reliable, valid, and responsive for patients undergoing hip arthroscopy. However, none of these measures are aimed at conditions such as muscle-tendinous injuries [20, 23]. Because of the limitations of these first- and second-generation outcome scores, new 'third-generation' scores have been developed, including the International Hip Outcome Tool (iHOT) [24] and the Copenhagen Hip And Groin Outcome Score (HAGOS) [25].

The HAGOS was developed specifically for younger patients with hip and groin pain, and it is not exclusively intended for patients undergoing hip arthroscopy, although they are covered as well [25]. This questionnaire refers to the patient's hip and/or groin pain and is therefore also useful in patients with musculoskeletal problems who are not candidates for hip arthroscopy, but are treated with exercises or other conservative interventions. HAGOS provides a quantitative measure of hip and/or groin function and associated problems according to the different levels of the International Classification of Functioning, Disability and Health (ICF) of the World Health Organization (WHO) [26]. The measure reflects the patient's assessment of their disability as well as their actual physical impairment. The HAGOS is a patient-reported outcome measure consisting of five-item Likert scales arranged in six subscales: pain, other symptoms, physical function in daily living, function in sport and recreation, participation in physical activities, and hip-related quality of life. The prior week is considered when answering the questions. Standardized answer options are given (five Likert boxes) and each question gets a score from 0 to 4. A normalized score (100 indicating no symptoms and 0 indicating extreme symptoms) is calculated for each subscale. The result can be plotted as an outcome profile.

The HAGOS can be used over both short and long time intervals and has been found to be reliable, valid, and responsive in younger patients with hip and groin pain [25]. This outcome instrument is self-explanatory and can be administered in the waiting room or used as a mailed survey. It has a user-friendly format and takes approximately 10 min to complete. It can be used to monitor the response of individual patients as well as groups of patients to treatment (medication, surgery, physical therapy) on an ongoing basis.

Preventing Injury and Reinjury

The introduction of a sports-specific prevention strategy to reduce the risk of groin injury in sport should include components of adequate and targeted rehabilitation for athletes with previous injury, as well as early identification of hip strength deficits. Furthermore, each athlete's total workload should be specifically addressed, with a reduction in activity during periods of hip and groin pain. In the off-season, athletes should be aware of continuing sports-specific activities and exercises including strength training, in order to stimulate musculotendinous health and repair.

Adequate Rehabilitation of Previous Injuries

Previous groin injury is a well-established risk factor for a new groin injury [27]. However, there are other related factors that are highly relevant and potentially modifiable. These factors may include:

- How the injured athlete was treated
- If there was specific treatment for the injury
- If the treatment addressed the functional demands of the athlete's sport
- If the athlete returned to the sport (including competition) with complete rehabilitation of this injury (i.e. full pain-free and functional ROM regained, full strength on resisted testing, concentric and eccentric muscle-specific function retrained)

It is important to use specific treatment methods that treat the dysfunction related to the specific structural damage that caused the groin pain as well as restoring associated pelvic muscular instability. This approach provides retraining of the muscles of the torso as well as the muscles of the hip and pelvis. It is not enough to treat a damaged tendon insertion with steroid injections and time off from the sport and then return to play when the pain is gone. Likewise, if treatment is limited to 'core stability' exercises to stimulate the abdominal and low back muscles [28] prior to return to sport, the damaged tendon insertion will not be healed, and recurrence of the groin injury will not be prevented.

To prevent recurrence of previous groin injuries, athletes should complete a programme consisting of treatment, exercise, and rehabilitation prior to returning to full participation in their sport. The treatment component, aimed at healing structural damage, should be combined with an exercise programme to reestablish the pelvic stability and a rehabilitation programme, which gradually incorporates the demands and skills needed to participate in the athlete's particular sport. Otherwise there is a risk that the factors that originally led to the structural damage will again 'take over' and combined with fatigue because of lack of sports-specific rehabilitation may eventually lead to groin reinjury and possibly to other injuries as well [27].

Strength Training

A study of ice hockey players has suggested that the ratio between adductors and abductors is an important risk factor for groin injury and that players with adductor/abductor strength ratio <80 % may benefit from preseason strength training of the adductor muscles in terms of the number of adductor-related groin injuries [29].

We examined the combination of strengthening of the adductors and the abductors and enhancing abdominal muscle recruitment in a randomized treatment study. Our treatment regimen included specific training of the adductor muscles (isometric, concentric, and eccentric), as well as exercises for the muscles related to the pelvis and torso including core stability principles. This study showed a highly significant effect in the treatment of adductor-related groin injuries [9].

Another randomized controlled trial including 1022 male soccer players examined the possible preventive value of an exercise programme consisted of:

- Isometric adduction exercises squeezing a soccer ball between the feet and between the knees in the supine position
- Dynamic adductor and abductor strengthening exercises (concentric and eccentric) performed with a partner
- Coordination of the hip joint-related muscles and the muscles of the pelvis and torso using a dynamic exercise combining sit-up, hip flexion, and adduction
- Dynamic proprioceptive exercises stimulating both concentric and eccentric strength utilizing the principles of core stability (i.e. including the muscles of the torso as well as the muscles of the lower extremities)
- Stretching exercises for the iliopsoas muscle, given the nature of secondary involvement of this muscle in the presence of groin pain [30]

The trial found that the incidence of groin injuries was 31 % less in the intervention group, compared to the control group, but the difference was not statistically significant. Despite the inconclusiveness of this study, if the 31 % reduction in the risk of groin injury were demonstrated in a larger and adequately powered study, this programme could be a valuable component of soccer training programmes in the future.

References

1. Nepple JJ, et al. Radiographic findings of femoroacetabular impingement in National Football League Combine athletes undergoing radiographs for previous hip or groin pain. Arthroscopy. 2012;28(10):1396–403.
2. Lovell G. The diagnosis of chronic groin pain in athletes: a review of 189 cases. Aust J Sci Med Sport. 1995;27(3):76–9.
3. Holmich P, et al. Incidence and clinical presentation of groin injuries in sub-elite male soccer. Br J Sports Med. 2014;48(16):1245–50.
4. Holmich P. Long-standing groin pain in sportspeople falls into three primary patterns, a "clinical entity" approach: a prospective study of 207 patients. Br J Sports Med. 2007;41(4):247–52. Discussion 252.
5. Weir A, Brukner P, Delahunt E, et al. Doha agreement meeting on terminology and definitions in groin pain in athletes. Br J Sports Med. 2015;49:768–74.
6. Holmich P, Holmich LR, Bjerg AM. Clinical examination of athletes with groin pain: an intraobserver and interobserver reliability study. Br J Sports Med. 2004;38(4):446–51.
7. Nicholas SJ, Tyler TF. Adductor muscle strains in sport. Sports Med. 2002;32(5):339–44.
8. Werner J, et al. UEFA injury study: a prospective study of hip and groin injuries in professional football over seven consecutive seasons. Br J Sports Med. 2009;43(13):1036–40.
9. Holmich P, et al. Effectiveness of active physical training as treatment for long-standing adductor-related groin pain in athletes: randomised trial. Lancet. 1999;353(9151):439–43.
10. Thorborg K, Bandholm T, Zebis M, Andersen LL, Jensen J, Holmich P. Large strengthening effect of a hip-flexor training programme: a randomized controlled trial. Knee Surg Sports Traumatol Arthrosc. 2015 Mar 22. [Epub ahead of print].
11. Ilizaliturri Jr VM, et al. Prospective randomized study of 2 different techniques for endoscopic iliopsoas tendon release in the treatment of internal snapping hip syndrome. Arthroscopy. 2009;25(2):159–63.
12. Flanum ME, et al. Arthroscopic treatment of the painful "internal" snapping hip: results of a new endoscopic technique and imaging protocol. Am J Sports Med. 2007;35(5):770–9.
13. Hölmich P. Adductor-related groin pain in athletes. Sports Med Arth Rev. 1998;5:285–91.
14. Larson CM, Pierce BR, Giveans MR. Treatment of athletes with symptomatic intra-articular hip pathology and athletic pubalgia/sports hernia: a case series. Arthroscopy. 2011;27(6):768–75.
15. Paajanen H, et al. Laparoscopic surgery for chronic groin pain in athletes is more effective than nonoperative treatment: a randomized clinical trial with magnetic resonance imaging of 60 patients with sportsman's hernia (athletic pubalgia). Surgery. 2011;150(1):99–107.
16. Muschaweck U, Berger L. Minimal Repair technique of sportsmen's groin: an innovative open-suture repair to treat chronic inguinal pain. Hernia. 2010;14(1):27–33.
17. Ekstrand J, Ringborg S. Surgery versus conservative treatment in soccer players with chronic groin pain: a prospective randomized study in soccer players. Eur J Sports Traumatol Relat Res. 2001;23:141–5.
18. Thorborg K, et al. Hip abduction strength training in the clinical setting: with or without external loading? Scand J Med Sci Sports. 2010;20 Suppl 2:70–7.

19. Ilizaliturri Jr VM, et al. Endoscopic iliotibial band release for external snapping hip syndrome. Arthroscopy. 2006;22(5): 505–10.
20. Thorborg K, et al. Validity, reliability and responsiveness of patient-reported outcome questionnaires when assessing hip and groin disability: a systematic review. Br J Sports Med. 2010;44(16): 1186–96.
21. Thorborg K, Tijssen M, Habets B, Bartels EM, Roos EM, Kemp J, Crossley KM, Holmich P. Patient-Reported Outcome (PRO) questionnaires for young to middle-aged adults with hip and groin disability: a systematic review of the clinimetric evidence. Br J Sports Med. 2015;49(12):812. doi:10.1136/bjsports-2014-094224. Epub 2015 Jan 13. Review.
22. Martin RL, Kelly BT, Philippon MJ. Evidence of validity for the hip outcome score. Arthroscopy. 2006;22(12):1304–11.
23. Thorborg K, et al. The iHOT-33: how valid is it? Arthroscopy. 2012;28(9):1194–5. Author reply 1195–6.
24. Mohtadi NG, et al. The development and validation of a self-administered quality-of-life outcome measure for young, active patients with symptomatic hip disease: the International Hip Outcome Tool (iHOT-33). Arthroscopy. 2012;28(5):595–605. Quiz 606–10.e1.
25. Thorborg K, et al. The Copenhagen Hip and Groin Outcome Score (HAGOS): development and validation according to the COSMIN checklist. Br J Sports Med. 2011;45(6):478–91.
26. WHO. International classification of functioning, disability and health; 2001.
27. Maffey L, Emery C. What are the risk factors for groin strain injury in sport? A systematic review of the literature. Sports Med. 2007;37(10):881–94.
28. Jansen JA, et al. Changes in abdominal muscle thickness measured by ultrasound are not associated with recovery in athletes with longstanding groin pain associated with resisted hip adduction. J Orthop Sports Phys Ther. 2009;39(10):724–32.
29. Tyler TF, et al. The effectiveness of a preseason exercise program to prevent adductor muscle strains in professional ice hockey players. Am J Sports Med. 2002;30(5):680–3.
30. Holmich P, et al. Exercise program for prevention of groin pain in football players: a cluster-randomized trial. Scand J Med Sci Sports. 2010;20(6):814–21.

30 The Painful Groin

Alexandra Dimitrakopoulou and Ernest Schilders

Introduction

Groin pain is a very common problem especially in sports such as soccer, rugby, football, running, ice hockey and Australian football [1–3] with an incidence of 5–18 % [1]. It constitutes a great challenge because the groin anatomy is complex and multiple pathologies with similar symptoms may co-exist. Moreover, lack of consensus in terminology for the different groin entities may further confuse and complicate the diagnosis as well as the treatment.

The definition of groin pain is broad and usually vague; it involves pathologies from the lower abdomen, inguinal region, proximal adductors, hip joint, upper anterior thigh and perineum. Detailed knowledge of the anatomy is paramount in order to better understand and manage the groin problems.

The most commonly seen musculoskeletal groin pathology of adductor-related, rectus abdominis and rectus femoris-related groin pain will be discussed.

Adductor Muscles Anatomy

The adductor muscles consist of the adductor longus, adductor magnus, adductor brevis, pectineus and gracilis and are located on the medial side of the thigh. Adductor longus and gracilis are mainly involved in adductor-related groin pain. They originate from the pubic bone and are innervated by the obturator nerve.

The origin [4], a fibrocartilaginous enthesis, of the adductor longus starts below the insertion of the inguinal ligament, and it decreases in size as the distance distally increases, and therefore the tendon/muscle ratio on a cross section decreases from proximal to distal [5]. The gracilis originates from the inferior ramus of the pubis and from the ramus of the ischium through a flat aponeurosis, and it is a very flat muscle.

Adductor Longus Injuries

Epidemiology

The most common musculoskeletal cause of groin pain is adductor longus injuries.

In a large cohort study [1] in professional soccer, they accounted for 23 % of all the muscle injuries resulting in 14 days of absence from sports. Strains (grade I, mild stretching; grade II, incomplete tearing) have the highest incidence in the age group between 22 and 30 years. Risk factors for adductor muscle injuries are previous injury and reduced adductor muscle strength [6–8]. The reinjury rate following adductor muscle injuries (either acute or chronic) has been reported as high as 18 % [1]. Adductor injuries are a common problem in contact-type sports that involve kicking and twisting movements with rapid changes of direction.

Mechanism of Injury

A common mechanism of injury is a forceful abduction with external rotation of the hip. The most common site of injury is the musculotendinous junction (Fig. 30.1) and less often at the origin (avulsion of enthesis) (Fig. 30.2).

Repetitive microtrauma or reinjury can result in chronic adductor-related groin pain (chronic adductor enthesopathy).

A. Dimitrakopoulou, MD, Orthopaedic Surgeon (✉)
• E. Schilders, MD, FRCS, FFSEM
The London Hip Arthroscopy Centre, Orthopaedics,
The Wellington Hospital, Wellington Place, St. Johns Wood,
London NW8 9LE,, UK

Leeds Beckett University, Leeds, UK
e-mail: alexdimitr@yahoo.gr; e.schilders@btopenworld.com

J.C. McCarthy et al. (eds.), *Hip Joint Restoration*, DOI 10.1007/978-1-4614-0694-5_30

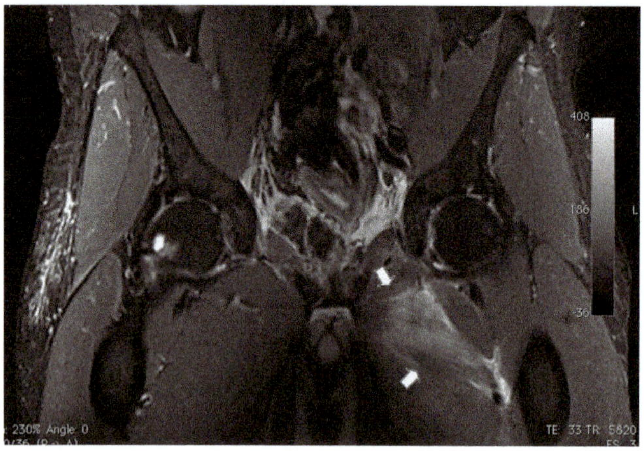

Fig. 30.1 MRI of an acute tear of the adductor longus at the proximal musculotendinous junction (*white arrows*). Published with kind permission of © E. Schilders 2015. All Rights Reserved

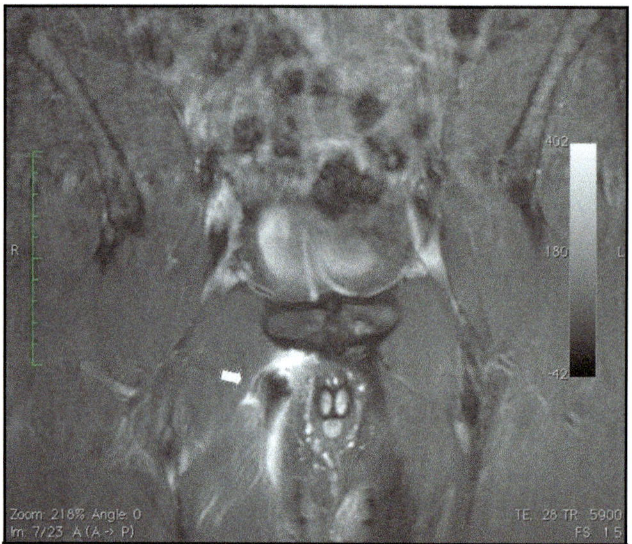

Fig. 30.2 Avulsion of the enthesis (*white arrow*) of the adductor longus in a professional soccer player. Note the retraction of the enthesis and the surrounding oedema/haematoma. Published with kind permission of © E. Schilders 2015. All Rights Reserved

Diagnosis of Adductor Longus Injuries

Clinical Presentation

The onset in adductor-related groin pain is insidious, and the athletes usually feel a "toothache-like pain" located deeply in the adductor area. Initially the symptoms are present after a game; gradually athletes get stiffness and pain in the morning and at the beginning of their activities which will be improved after warming-up, but they will end in pain making them unable to play. The pain may radiate to the inguinal region or lower abdomen (at the insertion of rectus abdominis). Sprinting, changing direction and kicking a ball are painful and they may experience pain at night.

Sometimes the athletes may report a sharp pain exacerbation of their long-standing (chronic) pain and this might be an acute tearing on the grounds of chronicity. In acute injuries athletes feel a sharp pain in adductor longus origin and are unable to play.

Physical Examination

Palpation of the origin of the adductor longus and gracilis can reproduce the pain, and in the case of an avulsed enthesis, a gap may be palpable [9, 10]. Resisted adduction of the hips can elicit pain. A detailed examination of the inguinal region and the rectus abdominis as well as the hip joint should also be included as there is a common association of adductor problems and sports hernia [11–13] or femoroacetabular impingement with often overlapping of symptoms [13].

Entheseal pubic cleft injection may be used as a diagnostic test for differentiation of adductor-related groin pain from hip-related groin pain or other pathologies present with groin pain from the lower abdomen, perineum, inguinal region and upper anterior thigh.

Radiographic Assessment

A specific groin study protocol [14] using gadolinium-enhanced MR imaging can reveal acute and chronic adductor problems. It consists of axial oblique T1-weighted turbo spin echo (TSE) and T2-weighted TSE fat-suppressed sequences and sagittal T1-weighted TSE and sagittal T2-weighted fat-suppressed sequences of 3 mm slice thickness [14].

Treatment

Proximal adductor longus avulsions require surgical refixation in athletes [10], while adductor strains at musculotendinous junction can be treated non-surgically.

Chronic adductor-related groin pain can be more challenging to treat. A strengthening programme for the adductors should be the cornerstone of the treatment [15]. Entheseal pubic cleft injections may employ as a short-term treatment in adductor-related groin pain as described by Schilders et al. [16, 17].

Surgical treatment is indicated for chronic adductor enthesopathy resistant to nonoperative management. Percutaneous nonselective adductor tenotomies have been performed in chronic cases with mixed results [12, 18, 19], and more recently a selective partial adductor longus release showed excellent pain relief with high rate of return to the preinjury level of sport [13].

Rectus Femoris

Anatomy

The rectus femoris is a fusiform and biarticular long muscle forming the most anterior part of the quadriceps muscle group. Its origin has two heads: a direct head or straight which arises from the anterior inferior iliac spine (AIIS) and forms the superficial tendon and an indirect or reflected which arises from the superior acetabular ridge [20] and forms the deep part of the rectus femoris. The two heads form the conjoined tendon and it is innervated by the femoral nerve. The muscle executes movements that require significant length change or high shortening velocity [21], and it stabilises the pelvis on the femur in weight-bearing[22, 23].

Rectus Femoris Injuries

Epidemiology

Quadriceps muscle injuries are common in sports that require repetitive kicking and sprinting such as soccer, basketball, American football and rugby [1, 2, 21, 23, 24]. In professional soccer they account for 19% of muscle injuries and usually the dominant leg is affected [1], whereas in National Football League (NFL), quadriceps strains are the fourth more common injury for kickers [25].

The rectus femoris is the most commonly affected muscle of the quadriceps group and causes more missed games in soccer than do the hamstrings [1] with the reinjury rate as high as 17% [1].

Although the most common site of injury is the myotendinous junction distally [21], proximally tears are located at the junction of the conjoined tendon with the muscle belly or at the deep musculotendinous junction of the indirect head [20, 26, 27]. The latter is the most common location of rectus femoris tendon tears in soccer (Fig. 30.3), associated with a significantly longer rehabilitation time [28], while the direct head and conjoined tendon are less likely to be injured [28, 29].

Mechanism of Injury

Rectus femoris injury occurs as a result of forceful stretching or violent contraction or may occur with eccentric loading while the knee is flexed and the hip extended during sprinting or kicking a ball [30, 31]. The injury is higher in sprinting during the acceleration and deceleration phases while in kicking during the backswing and wind-up phases for the kicking leg [21].

Diagnosis of Rectus Femoris Injuries

Clinical Presentation

In acute injuries the athlete reports pain and a tearing sensation in the anterior thigh stopping the athlete from playing.

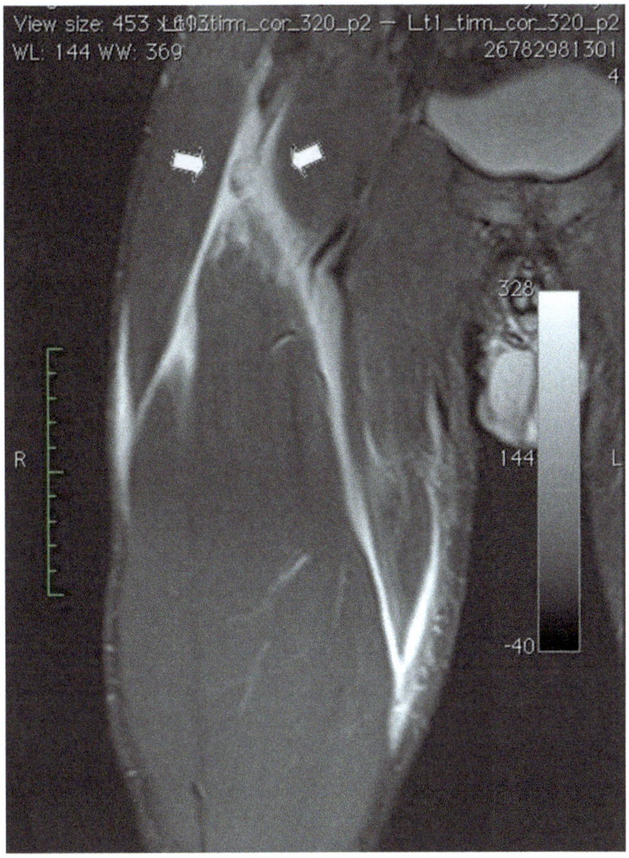

Fig. 30.3 MRI demonstrating acute tear of direct (straight) and indirect (reflected) heads of the rectus femoris in a professional soccer player. Note the retraction of the origin of the rectus femoris due to a complete tear of both heads. Published with kind permission of © E. Schilders 2015. All Rights Reserved

Tenderness may be present at the mid-anterior thigh. A gradual onset of pain during running and kicking can be present in subacute injuries. A mass-like effect has also been described when there is retraction upon activation after a complete tear of the indirect head of the rectus femoris [27].

Physical Examination

The diagnosis can be made clinically and with imaging. Athletes often present with minimal clinical symptoms but usually are not able to continue with their sport. The pain is localised at the anterior thigh proximally, and when a complete avulsion of the direct head of the rectus femoris is present, a gap can sometimes be felt, 8–10 cm below the AIIS. Resisted flexion of the hip can be painful.

Radiographic Assessment

MR imaging can be used for the exact anatomical location and the grading of the injury [1, 21, 29]. Grade I strains are demarcated by a high-intensity signal focally or diffusely, grade II acute partial tears are shown by interstitial feathery high-intensity signal (haematoma), but chronic injuries are shown by low signal (due to fibrosis or haemosiderin). Grade

III are complete tears with or without retraction and are shown by increased signal defined "bull's eye sign" [27, 32] and represent evolving stages of injury, but when it is associated with atrophy and fatty infiltration, this reflects an old injury. Occasionally a pseudocyst may also be present.

Ultrasound can be used for a dynamic assessment of the tear and for further follow-up during rehabilitation.

Plain radiographs may be important to rule out avulsion of the AIIS in the skeletally immature player.

Treatment

The optimal management of proximal rectus femoris tendon ruptures remains controversial; good outcomes and return to sport have been reported both with nonoperative [23] and operative management [21, 23, 24, 33]. The majority of tears can be treated nonoperatively, but when the athlete remains symptomatic or has debilitating symptoms preventing the return to sport, then surgical treatment should be considered [33].

In acute injuries reattachment of the avulsed head can be carried out to restore the anatomy and facilitate return to normal function/power [33], and in chronic cases, excision of the indirect head has been reported with fair to good outcomes [26].

Reinjury and complications can be responsible for persistent groin pain in the athletes. Flexibility and strengthening are important in the prevention of recurrence of these injuries [34, 35]. Complications described after proximal rectus femoris injuries are re-tear, adhesions, myositis ossificans and enthesophytes of the straight head of the rectus femoris. Large enthesophytes in soccer players often require surgical resection because of impinging during kicking activities [36]. If a resection of a myositis ossificans of the rectus femoris is planned, a bone scan should be done to exclude active bone formation of the lesion [36]. To avoid recurrence of spurs following resection, patients should receive indomethacin and, in persistent cases, radiotherapy.

Rectus Abdominis

Anatomy

The rectus abdominis is located on both sides of the linea alba and lies in the rectus sheath which is formed anteriorly by the aponeurosis of the external and internal obliques and transversus abdominis and posteriorly by the thin fascia transversalis. The sheath is inserted on the anterosuperior edge of the pubic bone and joins the fascia of the common adductors [37].

Rectus Abdominis Injuries

Rectus abdominis injuries can occur during sprinting and running with rapid changes of direction. The mechanism of injury has been described as eccentric overload followed by forced contraction of the contralateral (non-dominant) rectus abdominis during the cocking phase in tennis and baseball players [38, 39].

The pain is located at the suprapubic area (insertion of the rectus abdominis) and radiates at the adductor area (due to common aponeurosis). The pain is elicited when the patient lifts both legs straight from the examination table and is increased when the hips are flexed and abducted.

In soccer there is commonly an association between rectus abdominis problems and adductor-related groin pain [11, 40].

Treatment

The treatment is predominately nonoperative [39, 41], but surgical management ranging from release to reconstruction has also been reported with good outcomes [11, 42].

Differential Diagnosis of Painful Groin

Osteitis pubis (athletic pubalgia) is named every condition with pain over the pubic symphysis and surrounding structures [43–47]. Therefore, the clinical diagnosis should only be made when other conditions have been excluded. It is a diagnosis made predominately by imaging and is characterised by an increased uptake of signal in the pubic bone; resorption or sclerosis is the radiographic finding. It can be as a result of repetitive trauma during athletic activities such as kicking, running, jumping or twisting, a common feature in asymptomatic elite soccer players [44, 45, 48].

Nerve entrapments can manifest with groin pain. Obturator nerve entrapment is the fascial entrapment of its anterior branch and has a characteristic clinical pattern of exercise-induced medial thigh pain commencing in the region of the adductor muscle origin and radiating distally along the medial thigh [49]. Diagnosis can be supported by electromyography which can demonstrate denervation of the adductor muscle [50] or by the use of a diagnostic local anaesthetic under ultrasound guide.

Entrapment of the ilioinguinal nerve as a cause of groin pain has been described in hockey players, 51, 52].

Lateral cutaneous femoral nerve entrapment gives typical pain with a burning sensation and numbness over the anterolateral aspect of the thigh [53] and is probably the most common nerve entrapment around the groin area.

Fatigue fractures on the femoral neck or shaft [54–58], or on pubic rami [57–59], are well evident on MRI.

Residual or untreated paediatric conditions like slipped capital femoral epiphysis, Legg-Calvé-Perthes disease, DDH, etc. have to be recognised immediately, and therefore, radiographs of the hips remain a helpful imaging investigation.

Apophyseal injuries in adolescents are relatively common. Avulsion of the anterior superior iliac spine (sartorius muscle) and AIIS (direct head of the rectus femoris) is frequently seen during mid-adolescence and often coincides with periods of relatively rapid growth.

Other musculoskeletal pathologies like inguinal hernia (also known as sports hernia, sportsman's hernia or groin disruption) and iliopsoas pathology will be discussed in different chapters.

Conclusion

Groin pain is a common occurrence in sports. Because of the anatomical proximity of many structures in this area, diagnostic and treatment programmes may be imprecise. A thorough knowledge of the bony and neuromuscular anatomy and pathomechanics by the treating physician will greatly facilitate a correct healing programme.

References

1. Ekstrand J, Hagglund M, Walden M. Epidemiology of muscle injuries in professional football (soccer). Am J Sports Med. 2011;39:1226–32.
2. Kirkendall DT, Garrett Jr WE. Clinical perspectives regarding eccentric muscle injury. Clin Orthop Relat Res. 2002;403S:81–9.
3. Armfield DR, David Hyun-Min DK, Towers JD, Bradley JP, Robertson DD. Sports-related muscle injury in the lower extremity. Clin Sports Med. 2006;25:803–42.
4. Tuite DJ, Finegan PJ, Saliaris AP, Renstrom PA, Donne B, O'Brien M. Anatomy of the proximal musculotendinous junction of the adductor longus muscle. Knee Surg Sports Traumatol Arthrosc. 1998;6(2):134–7.
5. Strauss E, Campbell K, Bosco J. Analysis of the cross-sectional area of the adductor longus tendon: a descriptive anatomic study. Am J Sports Med. 2007;35:996–9.
6. Engebretsen A, Myklebust G, Holme I, et al. Prevention of injuries among male soccer players. A prospective, randomized intervention study targeting players with previous injuries or reduced function. Am J Sports Med. 2008;36:1052–60.
7. Engebretsen A, Myklebust G, Holme I, et al. Intrinsic risk factors for groin injuries among male soccer players: a prospective cohort study. Am J Sports Med. 2010;38:2051–7.
8. Tyler TF, Nicholas SJ, Campbell RJ, et al. The association of hip strength and flexibility with the incidence of adductor muscle strains in professional ice hockey players. Am J Sports Med. 2001;29:124–8.
9. Holmich P, Holmich LR, Bjerg AM. Clinical examination of athletes with groin pain: an intraobserver and interobserver reliability study. Br J Sports Med. 2004;38:446–51.
10. Dimitrakopoulou A, Schilders EMJ, Talbot JC, Bismil Q. Acute avulsion of the fibrocartilage origin of the adductor longus in professional soccer players: a report of two cases. Clin J Sport Med. 2008;18(2):167–9.
11. Martens M, Hansen L, Mulier JC. Adductor tendinitis and musculus rectus abdominis tendopathy. Am J Sports Med. 1987;15:353–6.
12. Robertson I, Curran C, McCaffrey N, et al. Adductor tenotomy in the management of groin pain in athletes. Int J Sports Med. 2011;32:45–8.
13. Schilders E, Dimitrakopoulou A, Cooke M, Bismil Q, Cooke C. Effectiveness of a selective partial adductor release for chronic adductor-related groin pain in professional athletes. Am J Sports Med. 2013;41(3):603–7.
14. Robinson P, Barron DA, Parsons W, Grainger AJ, Schilders EM, O'Connor PJ. Adductor-related groin pain in athletes: correlation of MR imaging with clinical findings. Skeletal Radiol. 2004;33:451–7.
15. Holmich P, Uhrskou P, Ulnits L, et al. Effectiveness of active physical training as treatment for long-standing adductor related groin pain in athletes: randomized trial. Lancet. 1999;353:439–43.
16. Schilders E, Bismil Q, Robinson P, et al. Adductor-related groin pain in competitive athletes. Role of adductor enthesis, magnetic resonance imaging, and entheseal pubic cleft injections. J Bone Joint Surg Am. 2007;89:2173–8.
17. Schilders E, Talbot JC, Robinson P, Dimitrakopoulou A, Gibbon WW, Bismil Q. Adductor-related groin pain in recreational athletes: role of adductor enthesis, magnetic resonance imaging, and entheseal pubic cleft injections. J Bone Joint Surg Am. 2009;91:2455–60.
18. Akermark C, Johansson C. Tenotomy of the adductor longus tendon in the treatment of chronic groin pain in athletes. Am J Sports Med. 1992;20:640–3.
19. Atkinson H, Parminder J, Falworth M, et al. Adductor tenotomy: its role in the management of sports-related chronic groin pain. Arch Orthop Trauma Surg. 2010;130:965–70.
20. Hasselman CT, Best T, Hughes C, Martinez S, Garrett W. An explanation for various rectus femoris strain injuries using previously undescribed muscle architecture. Am J Sports Med. 1995;23:493–9.
21. Mendiguchia J, Alentorn-Geli E, Idoate F, Myer G. Rectus femoris muscle injuries in football: a clinically relevant review of mechanisms of injury, risk factors and preventive strategies. Br J Sports Med. 2013;47(6):359–66.
22. Shu B, Safran MR. Hip instability: anatomic and clinical considerations of traumatic and atraumatic instability. Clin Sports Med. 2011;30:349–67.
23. Gamradt S, Brophy R, Barnes R, Warren R, Byrd T, Kelly B. Nonoperative treatment for proximal avulsion of the rectus femoris in professional American football. Am J Sports Med. 2009;37:1370–4.
24. Garcia V, Duhrkop D, Seijas R, Ares O, Cugat R. Surgical treatment of proximal ruptures of the rectus femoris in professional soccer players. Arch Orthop Trauma Surg. 2012;132(3):329–33.
25. Brophy R, Wright R, Powell J, et al. Injuries to kickers in American football: the National League experience. Am J Sports Med. 2010;38:1166–73.
26. Wittstein J, Klein S, Garrett WE. Chronic tears of the reflected head of the rectus femoris. Results of operative treatment. Am J Sports Med. 2011;39(9):1942–7.
27. Hughes IV C, Hasselman CT, Best TM, Martinez S, Garrett Jr WE. Incomplete, intrasubstance strain injuries of the rectus femoris muscle. Am J Sports Med. 1995;23(4):501–6.
28. Cross TM, Gibbs N, Houang MT, Cameron M. Acute quadriceps muscle strains: magnetic resonance imaging features and prognosis. Am J Sports Med. 2004;32(3):710–9.

29. Ouellette H, Thomas B, Nelson E, Torriani M. MR imaging of rectus femoris origin injuries. Skeletal Radiol. 2006;35(9):665–72.
30. Garrett WE. Muscle strain injuries. Am J Sports Med. 1996;24:S2–8.
31. Kellis E, Baltzopoulos V. Isokinetic eccentric exercise. Sports Med. 1995;19:202–22.
32. Gyftopoulos S, Rosenberg ZS, Schweitzer ME, et al. Normal anatomy and strains of the deep musculotendinous junction of the proximal rectus femoris: MRI features. AJR Am J Roentgenol. 2008;190:182–6.
33. Irmola T, Heikkila J, Orava S, Sarimo J. Total proximal tendon avulsion of the rectus femoris muscle. Scand J Med Sci Sports. 2007;17:378–82.
34. Witvrouw E, Danneels L, Asselman P, et al. Muscle flexibility as risk factor for developing muscle injuries in male professional soccer players. A prospective study. Am J Sports Med. 2003;31:41–6.
35. Fousekis K, Tsepis E, Poulmedis P, et al. Intrinsic risk factors of non-contact quadriceps and hamstring strains in soccer: a prospective study of 100 professional players. Br J Sports Med. 2011;45:709–14.
36. Dimitrakopoulou A, Schilders E, Bismil Q, Talbot JC, Kazakos K. An unusual case of enthesophyte formation following an adductor longus rupture in a high-level athlete. Knee Surg Sports Traumatol Arthrosc. 2010;18(5):691–3.
37. O'Brien M, Delaney M. The anatomy of the hip and groin. Sports Med Arthrosc Rev. 1997;5(4):252–67.
38. Conte SA, Thompson MM, Marks MA, Dines JS. Abdominal muscle strains in professional baseball: 1991-2010. Am J Sports Med. 2012;40(3):650–6.
39. Maquirriain J, Ghisi JP, Kokalj AM. Rectus abdominis muscle strains in tennis players. Br J Sports Med. 2007;41:842–8.
40. Atkins JM, Taylor JC, Kane SF. Acute and overuse injuries of the abdomen and groin in athletes. Curr Sports Med Rep. 2010;9(2):115–20.
41. Johnson R. Abdominal wall injuries: rectus abdominis strains, oblique strains, rectus sheath hematoma. Curr Sports Med Rep. 2006;5(2):99–103.
42. Biedert RM, Warnke K, Meyer S. Symphysis syndrome in athletes: surgical treatment for chronic lower abdominal, groin, and adductor pain in athletes. Clin J Sport Med. 2003;13(5):278–84.
43. Mandelbaum B, Mora SA. Osteitis pubis. Oper Tech Sports Med. 2005;13(1):62–7.
44. Beatty T. Osteitis pubis in athletes. Curr Sports Med Rep. 2012;11:96–8.
45. Mullens FE, Zoga AC, Morrison WB, et al. Review of MRI technique and imaging findings in athletic pubalgia and the "sports hernia". Eur J Radiol. 2012;81:3780–92.
46. Zoga AC, Kavanagh EC, Omar IM, et al. Athletic pubalgia and the "sports hernia": MR imaging findings. Radiology. 2008;247:797–807.
47. Omar IM, Zoga AC, Kavanagh EC, et al. Athletic pubalgia and "sports hernia": optimal MR imaging technique and findings. Radiographics. 2008;28:1415–38.
48. Lovell G. Osteitis pubis and assessment of bone marrow edema at the pubic symphysis with MRI in an elite junior male soccer squad. Clin J Sport Med. 2006;16(2):117–22.
49. Bradshaw C, McCrory P, Bell S, Brukner P. Obturator nerve entrapment. A cause of groin pain in athletes. Am J Sports Med. 1997;25(3):402–8.
50. Martinoli C, Miguel-Perez M, Padua L, Gandolfo N, Zicca A, Tagliafico A. Imaging of neuropathies about the hip. Eur J Radiol. 2013;82(1):17–26.
51. Irshad K, Feldman LS, Lavoie C, Lacroix VJ, Mulder DS, Brown RA. Operative management of "hockey groin syndrome": 12 years of experience in National Hockey League players. Surgery. 2001;130(4):759–64.
52. Holzheimer RG, Gresser U. Inguinal hernia vs. arthritis of the hip in sporting adolescent-case report and review of the literature. Eur J Med Res. 2007;12(7):314–9.
53. Cheatham SW, Kolber MJ, Salamh PA. Meralgia paresthetica: a review of the literature. Int J Sports Phys Ther. 2013;8(6):883–93.
54. Jacobs JM, Cameron KL, Bojescul JA. Lower extremity stress fractures in the military. Clin Sports Med. 2014;33(4):591–613.
55. Behrens SB, Deren ME, Matson A, Fadale PD, Monchik KO. Stress fractures of the pelvis and legs in athletes: a review. Sports Health. 2013;5(2):165–74.
56. Shin AY, Gillingham BL. Fatigue fractures of the femoral neck in athletes. J Am Acad Orthop Surg. 1997;5(6):293–302.
57. Iwamoto J, Takeda T. Stress fractures in athletes: review of 196 cases. J Orthop Sci. 2003;8(3):273–8.
58. Miller C, Major N, Toth A. Pelvic stress injuries in the athlete: management and prevention. Sports Med. 2003;33(13):1003–12.
59. Fredericson M, Jennings F, Beaulieu C, Matheson GO. Stress fractures in athletes. Top Magn Reson Imaging. 2006;17(5):309–25.

31 Limited Open Procedures

Aaron Glynn and Javad Parvizi

Introduction

Femoroacetabular impingement (FAI) has been described as an abutment conflict occurring between the proximal femur and anterior acetabular rim arising from morphological abnormalities affecting the acetabulum or the proximal femur or both [1]. Reduced anterolateral joint clearance arises from loss of the normal femoral head sphericity and leads to repetitive encroachment of damaged, hypertrophic bone on soft tissue with hip motion. The abnormal contact may result in a labral tear, chondral separation and eventual degenerative arthritis of the hip [2–6].

Predisposing factors for FAI include those which cause reduced joint clearance, either through prominence of the anterior acetabular rim (acetabular retroversion, protrusio acetabuli, post overcorrection from peri-acetabular osteotomy) or decreased femoral head-to-neck ratio (post slipped upper femoral epiphysis, previous Legg-Calve-Perthes disease or idiopathic development of the "cam" lesion on the antero-superior femoral neck).

Cam lesions are more commonly associated with athletic young male patients, while "pincer" impingement is more likely seen in middle-aged female patients [7]. In reality, the two processes are commonly seen together in patients with FAI [2].

A. Glynn, MCh, FRCS (✉)
Adult Lower Limb Reconstruction, Our Lady's Hospital, Navan, Co Meath, Ireland
e-mail: aaronaglynn@gmail.com

J. Parvizi, MD, FRCS
Adult Lower Limb Reconstruction, Rothman Institute, Thomas Jefferson University Hospital, 925 Chestnut St., 5th Floor, Philadelphia, PA 19107, USA
e-mail: parvj@aol.com

Surgical Treatment of Femoroacetabular Impingement

Successful surgical treatment of FAI involves removing the impingement lesion on the femoral neck and/or the anterior acetabular wall, stabilising the acetabular cartilage and restoring the labral seal of the hip joint. Failure to address any of these prevents a successful surgical outcome and return to full activity by the patient [5, 8].

Debridement of Cam Lesion

Femoral cam lesions were found in 100% of 293 hips undergoing surgical management for FAI in one study [9]. The lesion is typically covered by discoloured, frayed cartilage, which allows differentiation from adjacent normal, whitish hyaline cartilage [1]. The abnormal cartilage has been shown to be histologically similar to that seen in a degenerative hip [10].

Resection of the cam lesion restores the normal concavity of the antero-superior proximal femur and improves intraoperative flexion and internal rotation of the hip [11].

Resection of the Anterior Acetabular Wall

Resection of any osseous prominence of the anterior acetabular wall can be performed after temporary detachment and protection of the acetabular labrum. It is important not to remove so much bone as to cause instability and to ensure that a prominent anterior wall is not associated with acetabular retroversion and posterior acetabular undercoverage, and this may result in postoperative joint instability.

J.C. McCarthy et al. (eds.), *Hip Joint Restoration*, DOI 10.1007/978-1-4614-0694-5_31

Chondral Stabilisation

Delaminated, loose cartilage in the antero-superior aspect of the acetabulum has been reported in 64–87 % of hips treated surgically for FAI [9, 11, 12]. The cartilage damage can be treated according to surgeon's experience. Areas of denuded cartilage may be addressed using microfracture. There is a little evidence for long-term success of this procedure in the hip, but good early results have been reported [13]. The need for microfracture in full-thickness cartilage lesions, especially larger ones, has been associated with a poorer outcome [11].

Labral Fixation

Labral lesions have been reported to be present in 75–100 % of patients requiring surgical correction of FAI [9, 11, 12]. Labral retention, with repair of a damaged labrum if required, is preferable in almost all cases to labral resection [14, 15]. Most techniques for addressing FAI lesions allow repair of a damaged labrum through rim detachment, stabilisation of the tear, preparation of the bony acetabular rim and refixation with anchor sutures. Excision of a hypertrophic acetabular labrum, typically found in patients with acetabular dysplasia, can lead to accelerated joint degeneration and should be discouraged.

Options for Surgical Management of Femoroacetabular Impingement

Peri-acetabular Osteotomy

Peri-acetabular osteotomy (PAO) may be employed to address FAI arising from a retroverted acetabulum [16]. This is diagnosed radiologically on AP radiograph of the pelvis, where a crossover sign is seen in conjunction with a short posterior wall sign indicating inadequate coverage of the femoral head posteriorly [17]. The advantage of this technique is that it is the only method to reorient the acetabulum to address this undercoverage while removing the anterior source of impingement. The disadvantages are that is a major surgical undertaking, involving a significant learning curve, and, depending on the technique used, may require a prolonged period of restricted weight bearing postoperatively. Potential complications include delayed or nonunion of the osteotomy, risk of nerve injury, major intraoperative blood loss and heterotopic bone formation [18].

Surgical Dislocation

Surgical dislocation of the hip is a commonly employed technique for addressing FAI lesions [1, 19]. Good-to-excellent outcomes are reported [20, 21]. The hip is approached by performing a "trochanteric flip" osteotomy and a z-shaped capsulotomy which preserves the arterial supply to the femoral head. The advantages of this technique include 360° access to the femoral head and acetabulum, coupled with a low (negligible) risk of avascular necrosis, fracture or nerve injury. The disadvantages include a period of restricted weight bearing while the trochanteric osteotomy unites. Complications include trochanteric nonunion, sciatic neuropraxia, clinically relevant heterotopic ossification [19] and painful capsular scarring [21].

Arthroscopy

Hip arthroscopy is an effective method to treat FAI. The advantages are that it is minimally invasive, with negligible blood loss, can be performed as an outpatient operation and does not require trochanteric osteotomy. The disadvantage is that it is technically difficult, with a steep learning curve [22]. In particular, surgeons learning the technique may have difficulty performing an adequate femoroplasty. Iatrogenic damage to the femoral head is common [23]. The technique can potentially involve prolonged traction of the hip and carries potential for perineal nerve palsy.

Intertrochanteric Osteotomy

A rotational and/or valgus intertrochanteric osteotomy can improve joint clearance in patients with increased or decreased version or a varus position of the femoral neck [24]. It is possible to compensate for the impingement produced by reduced anteversion by performing a generous femoroplasty.

The advantage of this procedure is that it can properly correct abnormal version [25]. The disadvantages are the risk of nonunion inherent in any osteotomy, a period of reduced weight bearing and the possibility of complicating later total hip arthroplasty (THA).

Mini-Open Femoroacetabular Osteoplasty

The rationale for mini-open femoroacetabular osteoplasty (FAO) is that it allows sufficient access to the hip joint to address the majority of pathology associated with FAI, via a simple open approach which is familiar to most surgeons—there is only a very shallow learning curve. The procedure is minimally invasive, being performed through a small incision (<4 cm). It avoids the need for trochanteric osteotomy or muscular detachment, permitting faster rehabilitation. Because the capsular incision is smaller than that employed in surgical dislocation, we hypothesise that there may be less risk of postoperative scarring.

Successful outcomes using this technique have been reported. Smith-Petersen presented his early results of acetabuloplasty in 1936. He cautioned against femoroplasty, feeling that the femoral neck could not spare the bone [26]. Heyman et al. reported the good results of the "cervical osteoplasty" procedure Smith-Petersen cautioned against, though the approach was not described [27]. Ribas et al. reported significant improvements in Merle d'Aubigné-Postel and WOMAC scores in 105 patients following mini-open FAO, which were maintained at 3 years of follow-up in patients with Tönnis grade 0 and 1 degenerative change on radiographs [28]. Trevino-Garza also reported on 117 hips treated with mini-open FAO at minimum 2-year follow-up and found similar improvements in patients with no or mild arthritis [29]. Chiron et al. used a modified anterolateral approach to treat FAI lesions in 120 hips in 108 patients. They reported an overall significant improvement in the non-arthritic hip score (NAHS) by 32.5 points, internal rotation by 19.0° and the alpha angle by −24.9° at an average follow-up of 2.2 years (range 12–54 months). Four failures (3.5 %) were revised by arthroplasty [30].

Several authors have reported on the use of a limited open procedure combined with hip arthroscopy for FAI [31–33]. Laude et al. used a mini-open anterior Hueter approach with arthroscopic assistance. They found this technique gave good access to the femoral neck for cam resection, rim trimming and labral refixation, while avoiding surgical dislocation. Retrospective review of 91 patients (94 hips) with a minimum follow-up of 28.6 months (mean, 58.3 months) revealed the NAHS increased significantly from 54.5 ± 12 to 84.3 ± 16 points. One hip developed a femoral neck fracture and 11 hips developed osteoarthritis and required a THA [31]. Clohisy et al. retrospectively reviewed 35 patients treated for FAI with combined limited open osteochondroplasty and arthroscopy at a minimum follow-up of 2 years. The average modified Harris hip score improved from 63.8 points preoperatively to 87.4 points at the time of the last follow-up. The average alpha angle was reduced from 58.6° preoperatively to 37.1° at the time of follow-up. Minor complications included one superficial wound infection, one deep vein thrombosis and four cases of asymptomatic Brooker grade I heterotopic ossification. There were no femoral neck fractures or cases of femoral head osteonecrosis, and no hip was converted to an arthroplasty [33].

Indications for Mini-Open Femoroacetabular Osteoplasty

We generally consider surgical management in young adult patients who present with groin or buttock pain unresponsive to activity modification and NSAID therapy with appropriate clinical and radiological findings.

Clinical examination typically reveals decreased hip flexion and internal rotation, and a combination of these movements with adduction should reproduce pain (the "anterior impingement sign") [34]. Radiographs should include an AP view of the pelvis, not just a single hip, in order to demonstrate acetabular depth, and a cross-table lateral or Dunn view [35]. Radiological parameters for diagnosis include an alpha angle of >50.5° on AP, cross-table lateral, Dunn or frog-leg lateral x-ray [35–37] (Fig. 31.1). Tönnis grade 0 or 1 [38] is associated with a better outcome in FAI surgery [28, 29, 31], and only very young patients with Tönnis grade 2 hip arthritis, in whom a THA would be undesirable, would be considered for mini-open FAO. We perform an MR arthrogram in certain cases to look for evidence of labral pathology. If clinical findings are inconsistent, a diagnostic injection may be performed to confirm the hip is the source of the symptoms.

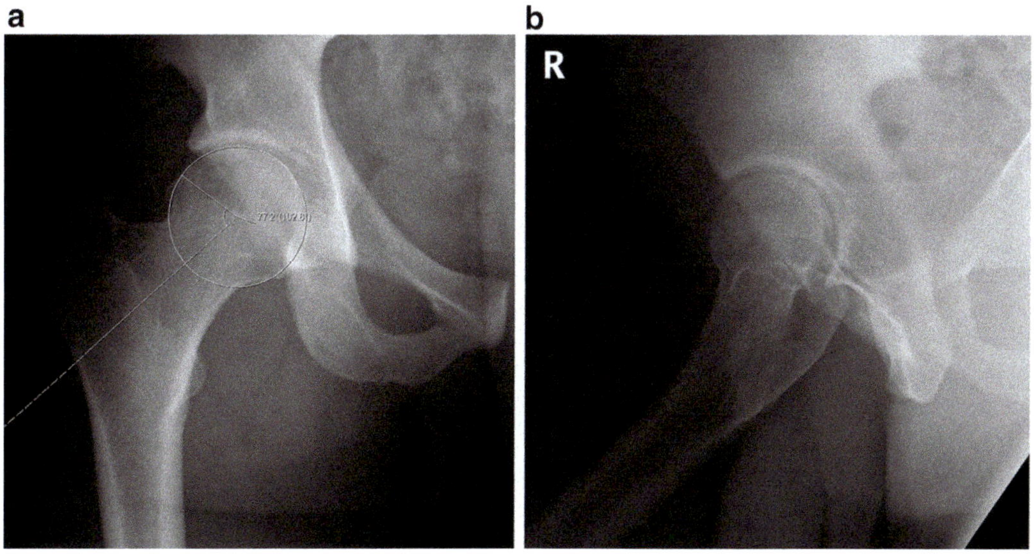

Fig. 31.1 AP and lateral radiographs of a right hip in a 35-year-old athlete showing obvious loss of sphericity of the femoral head

Patients are carefully counselled what to expect following surgical management. The presence of advanced degenerative changes, including joint space narrowing and cartilage loss, or prior resection of the labrum, is associated with poorer outcomes [9, 15, 20, 39, 40]. THA may be a better option for these patients. Patients with severe acetabular retroversion with deficient posterior wall and global overcoverage (i.e. protrusio) are not adequately treated with this approach, and this should be considered a contraindication.

Mini-Open Femoroacetabular Osteoplasty: The Senior Author's Preferred Surgical Technique

1. Muscle relaxation is necessary. Any form of anaesthesia which provides adequate muscle relaxation is suitable. We prefer spinal because it provides muscle relaxation intraoperatively, as well as superior pain control postoperatively.
2. The patient is placed in the supine position on a standard operating table.
3. The operative leg is draped free, and the skin is exposed from the umbilicus to the upper thigh.
4. A modified Hueter approach, as popularised by Smith-Petersen, is used. A 4 cm skin incision is made, starting at a point 2 cm lateral and inferior to the anterior superior iliac spine and extending distally and slightly laterally so as to overlie the belly of the tensor fasciae latae (TFL) muscle. The superficial fascia (Scarpa's fascia) is incised, and the TFL is identified. The perimysium overlying TFL is cut, and the muscle retracted laterally. The posterior perimysium is split to expose the rectus femoris muscle underneath: This manoeuvre avoids the true interval between TFL and the sartorius, in order to protect the lateral femoral cutaneous nerve (LFCN) by staying lateral to it. The LFCN runs from under the inguinal ligament, within 1 cm medial to the anterior superior iliac spine, and runs distally between the fascia lata and the sartorius muscle.
5. Once in the true interval, the superior aspect of the femoral neck is readily palpable. A blunt Hohmann retractor can be passed through the thin fascia posterior to TFL superior to the femoral neck. The rectus femoris muscle is retracted medially to expose the underlying capsule of the hip joint. The ascending branches of the lateral femoral circumflex artery should be identified and electrocoagulated at this point. The branches are variable in number and location, but they can routinely be found overlying the fascial layer of the rectus and TFL. Taking care to avoid the muscle bulk of the vastus intermedius, a second blunt Hohmann retractor can be placed around the femoral neck inferiorly. The first Hohmann retractor is now placed superolaterally.
6. The muscle belly of the rectus femoris is gently detached from the joint capsule with a Cobb elevator, and the remaining fascia or fat overlying the capsule is removed. A long-handled knife is used to make an I-shaped capsulotomy from the intertrochanteric line to the femoral head. When cutting towards the acetabular labrum, care is taken not to cut through it. Once the incision is made cephalad to the labrum, expand the top part of the "I" shape along anterior acetabular wall, gaining good anterior and posterior exposure. The labrum is exposed as widely as possible. Similarly, the base of the "I" along the intertrochanteric line is expended to improve access. The Hohmann retractors are placed inside the capsule around the femoral neck.
7. A sharp double-curved retractor with an attached light source is placed over the anterior acetabular wall, such that the tip rests at the upper part of the anterior inferior iliac spine, inferior and medial to the origin of the rectus femoris to retract this muscle medially. The hip is flexed after insertion of this retractor, to ensure it is not engaging the femoral head.
8. Abutment of the femoral cam lesion against the acetabular labrum can be directly visualised during this flexion manoeuvre.
9. If there is a labral tear which requires repair or if the procedure is being performed to remove an osseous prominence of the acetabular wall, the labrum must be detached. Later repair is facilitated by excising a thin rim of acetabular bone with the labrum: a curved osteotome is used to cut a thin (3 mm) rim of the bone from the anterior acetabular wall along the length of the labrum. Excise the inner portion of labrum if this is torn. A greater amount of bony rim may be removed if overcoverage is present anteriorly, but avoid excessive resection which could lead to instability.
10. Apply axial traction to the limb to sublux the hip. Pass a Cobb elevator into the interval between the femoral head and detached labrum. The Cobb elevator is gently advanced into the joint space, and the femoral head is held subluxed (Fig. 31.2). Torn or delaminated acetabular cartilage is often present anterosuperiorly and may be seen or palpated with the nerve root retractor. Insert the long-handled knife sideways under any delaminated cartilage to free it up, and remove it with a small pituitary forceps. A 90° pick can be used to create microfracture if full-thickness cartilage defects are present.
11. The femoral head is now reduced into the acetabulum and the labrum is repaired. The anterior acetabular wall is trimmed to expose bleeding bone. Three or four absorbable suture anchors are placed along the anterior wall, taking care not to penetrate the hip joint. Strong non-absorbable sutures are passed through the labrum, which is tied tightly against the anterior acetabular wall. Knots are tied outside the joint.

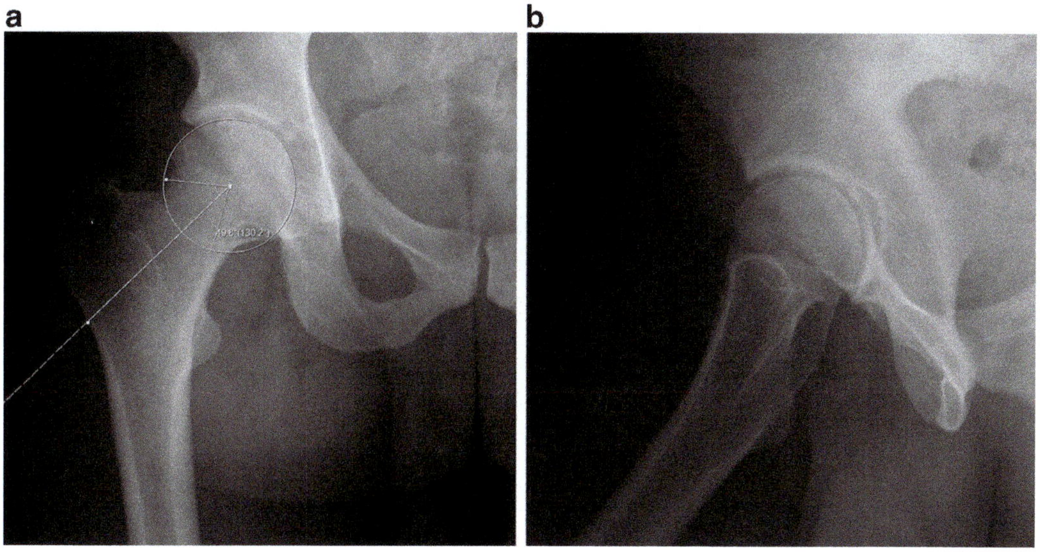

Fig. 31.2 Postoperative AP and lateral radiographs of the same patient as seen in Fig. 31.1. The cam lesion has been resected, showing restoration of normal femoral head sphericity

12. The cam lesion on the femoral neck is now addressed. The hip is held in neutral or slight extension. Use a curved osteotome to demarcate a line along the abnormal reddish cartilage approximately 15 mm from the labral edge. It is important not to hyperextend the hip, which would allow resection of too much of the femoral head, possibly creating iatrogenic instability. The surgical assistant internally rotates and adducts the leg to improve access to the lesion superiorly, while being careful to avoid the retinacular vessels. These are located just posterior to where the anterior aspect of the greater trochanter joins the femoral neck. The curved osteotome is used to mark a second line 5 mm distal to the first, and the intervening trough of cartilage is excised. A 5 mm high-speed burr is used to debride the cam lesion fully, to the full 5 mm depth of the burr. The leg may need to be placed in the figure-of-4 position to improve access to the postero-inferior aspect of the lesion. Although access to this part of the hip is limited, the cam lesion associated with FAI is most commonly located in the antero-superior aspect of the joint.
13. The hip is flexed to ensure restoration of normal joint clearance; care is taken not to crush the femoral nerve against the medial retractor while examining range of motion. There should no longer be abutment of femoral neck against the anterior acetabular wall. Digital examination ensures there is no impingement with flexion/internal rotation of the hip. Bone wax is placed over the raw bone.
14. The hip capsule is closed with two absorbable sutures. Haemostasis is obtained, checking particularly that there is no bleeding from perforating branches of ascending LFCA.
15. The perimysium is closed over the TFL—sartorius interval with absorbable sutures. The superficial fat and skin are closed with absorbable sutures.
16. Postoperative AP and lateral radiographs are checked before the patient is allowed to mobilise with protected weight bearing for a 6-week period.

Operative times for mini-open FAO have been reported as 64–115 min (mean = 75 min) and blood loss as 50–350 mL (mean = 120 mL) [12].

Results

Early surgical intervention in FAI is aimed not only at providing pain relief and improving function but also at delaying and/or preventing subsequent osteoarthritis. The senior author's experience with the mini-open FAO has been reported [9]. One hundred and forty-nine patients (156 hips) were included in the study. Thirty-six were Tönnis grade 0; 99 hips were Tönnis grade 1, and 21 hips were Tönnis grade 2.

There was a significant improvement in modified Harris hip scores from 58.3 preoperatively to 85.6 postoperatively ($P<0.001$) at a minimum follow-up of 2 years (range 2–4.2 years). WOMAC scores also demonstrated substantial improvement from 44.5 preoperatively to 10.7 postoperatively ($P<0.001$), and UCLA activity scores improved from 6.2 preoperatively to 7.9 postoperatively ($P<0.001$).

Range of motion improved on average from 89° of flexion and 8.6° of internal rotation to 118° of flexion and 39° of internal rotation ($P<0.001$). There were no intraoperative complications. Postoperative complications included one neuroma that required excision, one subtrochanteric hip fracture that required open reduction and internal fixation, one repeat labral tear that underwent arthroscopic debridement and one patient with persistent trochanteric bursitis that required iliotibial band lengthening and greater trochanteric bursa excision. Twelve hips underwent THA, due to degenerative joint disease at an average of 1.4 years postoperatively [9]. Although the numbers were too small to reach statistical significance, it was found that patients who required conversion to THA appeared to have more medical and psychological comorbidities, and a higher proportion had undergone previous surgery on the affected hip.

Summary

We believe the mini-open approach for surgical management of FAI is technically straightforward and allows the surgeon to satisfactorily and safely perform all of the procedures necessary for a successful surgical outcome. Outcomes are equivalent to other surgical modalities of treatment, and the procedure carries a low risk of morbidity.

Acknowledgement The authors wish to thank Dr Claudio Diaz Ledezma for his help in the preparation of this manuscript.

References

1. Lavigne M, Parvizi J, Beck M, Siebenrock KA, Ganz R, Leunig M. Anterior femoroacetabular impingement: part I. Techniques of joint preserving surgery. Clin Orthop Relat Res. 2004;(418):61–6.
2. Beck M, Kalhor M, Leunig M, Ganz R. Hip morphology influences the pattern of damage to the acetabular cartilage: femoroacetabular impingement as a cause of early osteoarthritis of the hip. J Bone Joint Surg Br. 2005;87:1012–8.
3. Johnston TL, Schenker ML, Briggs KK, Philippon MJ. Relationship between offset angle alpha and hip chondral injury in femoroacetabular impingement. Arthroscopy. 2008;24:669–75.
4. Tannast M, Goricki D, Beck M, Murphy SB, Siebenrock KA. Hip damage occurs at the zone of femoroacetabular impingement. Clin Orthop Relat Res. 2008;466:273–80.
5. Ganz R, Parvizi J, Beck M, Leunig M, Notzli H, Siebenrock KA. Femoroacetabular impingement: a cause for osteoarthritis of the hip. Clin Orthop Relat Res. 2003;(417):112–20.
6. Ito K, Minka 2nd MA, Leunig M, Werlen S, Ganz R. Femoroacetabular impingement and the cam-effect. A MRI-based quantitative anatomical study of the femoral head-neck offset. J Bone Joint Surg Br. 2001;83:171–6.
7. Zebala LP, Schoenecker PL, Clohisy JC. Anterior femoroacetabular impingement: a diverse disease with evolving treatment options. Iowa Orthop J. 2007;27:71–81.
8. Bardakos NV, Vasconcelos JC, Villar RN. Early outcome of hip arthroscopy for femoroacetabular impingement: the role of femoral osteoplasty in symptomatic improvement. J Bone Joint Surg Br. 2008;90:1570–5.
9. Parvizi J, Huang R, Diaz-Ledezma C, Og B. Mini-open femoroacetabular osteoplasty: how do these patients do? J Arthroplasty. 2012;27(8 Suppl):122–5.
10. Wagner S, Hofstetter W, Chiquet M, Mainil-Varlet P, Stauffer E, Ganz R, Siebenrock KA. Early osteoarthritic changes of human femoral head cartilage subsequent to femoro-acetabular impingement. Osteoarthritis Cartilage. 2003;11:508–18.
11. Naal FD, Miozzari HH, Schar M, Hesper T, Notzli HP. Midterm results of surgical hip dislocation for the treatment of femoroacetabular impingement. Am J Sports Med. 2012;40:1501–10.
12. Cohen SHR, Ciccotti M, Dodson C, Parvizi J. Treatment of femoroacetabular impingement in athletes using a mini-direct anterior approach. Am J Sports Med. 2012;40:1620–7.
13. Crawford K, Philippon MJ, Sekiya JK, Rodkey WG, Steadman JR. Microfracture of the hip in athletes. Clin Sports Med. 2006;25:327–35. x.
14. Larson CM, Guanche CA, Kelly BT, Clohisy JC, Ranawat AS. Advanced techniques in hip arthroscopy. Instr Course Lect. 2009;58:423–36.
15. Espinosa N, Beck M, Rothenfluh DA, Ganz R, Leunig M. Treatment of femoro-acetabular impingement: preliminary results of labral refixation. Surgical technique. J Bone Joint Surg Am. 2007;89 Suppl 2 Pt.1:36–53.
16. Siebenrock KA, Schoeniger R, Ganz R. Anterior femoro-acetabular impingement due to acetabular retroversion. Treatment with periacetabular osteotomy. J Bone Joint Surg Am. 2003;85-A:278–86.
17. Reynolds D, Lucas J, Klaue K. Retroversion of the acetabulum. A cause of hip pain. J Bone Joint Surg Br. 1999;81:281–8.
18. Biedermann R, Donnan L, Gabriel A, Wachter R, Krismer M, Behensky H. Complications and patient satisfaction after periacetabular pelvic osteotomy. Int Orthop. 2008;32:611–7.
19. Ganz R, Gill TJ, Gautier E, Ganz K, Krugel N, Berlemann U. Surgical dislocation of the adult hip a technique with full access to the femoral head and acetabulum without the risk of avascular necrosis. J Bone Joint Surg Br. 2001;83:1119–24.
20. Beaule PE, Le Duff MJ, Zaragoza E. Quality of life following femoral head-neck osteochondroplasty for femoroacetabular impingement. J Bone Joint Surg Am. 2007;89:773–9.
21. Beck M. Groin pain after open FAI surgery: the role of intraarticular adhesions. Clin Orthop Relat Res. 2009;467:769–74.
22. Konan S, Rhee SJ, Haddad FS. Hip arthroscopy: analysis of a single surgeon's learning experience. J Bone Joint Surg Am. 2011;93 Suppl 2:52–6.
23. Byrd JW. Hip arthroscopy. The supine position. Clin Sports Med. 2001;20:703–31.
24. Boos N, Krushell R, Ganz R, Muller ME. Total hip arthroplasty after previous proximal femoral osteotomy. J Bone Joint Surg Br. 1997;79:247–53.
25. Tonnis D, Heinecke A. Acetabular and femoral anteversion: relationship with osteoarthritis of the hip. J Bone Joint Surg Am. 1999;81:1747–70.
26. Smith-Petersen MN. Treatment of malum coxae senilis, old slipped upper capital femoral epiphysis, intrapelvic protrusion of the acetabulum, and coxae plana by means of acetabuloplasty. J Bone Joint Surg Am. 1936;18:869–80.
27. Heyman CH, Herndon CH, Strong JM. Slipped femoral epiphysis with severe displacement; a conservative operative treatment. J Bone Joint Surg Am. 1957;39-A:293–303.
28. Ribas M, Ledesma R, Cardenas C, Marin-Pena O, Toro J, Caceres E. Clinical results after anterior mini-open approach for femoroacetabular impingement in early degenerative stage. Hip Int. 2010;20 Suppl 7:36–42.
29. Trevino-Garza O, Rivas-Fernandez M, Marin-Pena O, Esteban-Ledezma R, Vilarubias-Guillament JM. [Treatment of femoroacetabular impingement by a minimally invasive approach. Results at 2 years follow-up]. Acta Ortop Mex. 2009;23:57–69.
30. Chiron P, Espie A, Reina N, Cavaignac E, Molinier F, Laffosse JM. Surgery for femoroacetabular impingement using a minimally invasive anterolateral approach: analysis of 118 cases at 2.2-year follow-up. Orthop Traumatol Surg Res. 2012;98:30–8.

31. Laude F, Sariali E. [Treatment of FAI via a minimally invasive ventral approach with arthroscopic assistance. Technique and midterm results]. Orthopade. 2009;38:419–28.
32. Barton C, Banga K, Beaule PE. Anterior Hueter approach in the treatment of femoro-acetabular impingement: rationale and technique. Orthop Clin North Am. 2009;40:389–95.
33. Clohisy JC, Zebala LP, Nepple JJ, Pashos G. Combined hip arthroscopy and limited open osteochondroplasty for anterior femoroacetabular impingement. J Bone Joint Surg Am. 2010;92:1697–706.
34. Ganz R, Leunig M, Leunig-Ganz K, Harris WH. The etiology of osteoarthritis of the hip: an integrated mechanical concept. Clin Orthop Relat Res. 2008;466:264–72.
35. Barton C, Salineros MJ, Rakhra KS, Beaule PE. Validity of the alpha angle measurement on plain radiographs in the evaluation of cam-type femoroacetabular impingement. Clin Orthop Relat Res. 2011;469:464–9.
36. Notzli HP, Wyss TF, Stoecklin CH, Schmid MR, Treiber K, Hodler J. The contour of the femoral head-neck junction as a predictor for the risk of anterior impingement. J Bone Joint Surg Br. 2002;84:556–60.
37. Meyer DC, Beck M, Ellis T, Ganz R, Leunig M. Comparison of six radiographic projections to assess femoral head/neck asphericity. Clin Orthop Relat Res. 2006;445:181–5.
38. Tonnis D. Normal values of the hip joint for the evaluation of X-rays in children and adults. Clin Orthop Relat Res. 1976;(119):39–47.
39. Beck M, Leunig M, Parvizi J, Boutier V, Wyss D, Ganz R. Anterior femoroacetabular impingement: part II. Midterm results of surgical treatment. Clin Orthop Relat Res. 2004;(418):67–73.
40. Murphy S, Tannast M, Kim YJ, Buly R, Millis MB. Debridement of the adult hip for femoroacetabular impingement: indications and preliminary clinical results. Clin Orthop Relat Res. 2004;(429): 178–81.

Limitations of Open and Arthroscopic Surgical Technique for the Treatment of Femoroacetabular Impingement

32

Sangmin Ryan Shin and Scott D. Martin

Introduction

Femoroacetabular impingement (FAI) has been implicated in producing hip pain in young, active adults, as well as in the development of osteoarthritis of the hip [1–3]. As our understanding of its pathoanatomy, pathomechanics, and natural history of the disease has advanced, our techniques in treating FAI have evolved exponentially.

Ganz introduced open surgical dislocation for treatment of FAI in the 1990s, and since then, it has gained popularity in treating proximal femur and acetabular osseous pathologies as well as labral pathology [2]. However, morbidity risk associated with an open technique cannot be underestimated [2].

In the past decade, hip arthroscopy has also gained popularity in treating FAI (Figs. 32.1 and 32.2). There has been an 18-fold increase in a number of hip arthroscopy cases performed by the American Orthopaedic board candidate members in the past 10 years [4]. In order to compliment the strengths and minimize limitations of both arthroscopic and open techniques in the treatment of FAI, a combination of arthroscopy with a limited anterior approach to the hip (mini-open technique) has been proposed [5]. Despite refinement in techniques and equipment, there is no gold standard operative intervention in the treatment of FAI. Every technique proposed has advantages, limitations, and complications.

S.R. Shin, MD
Department of Orthopaedic Surgery, Southeast Permanente Med Group, 20 Glenlake Parkway NE, Atlanta, GA 30328, USA
e-mail: sangmin.r.shin@kp.org

S.D. Martin, MD (✉)
Division of Sports Medicine, Department of Orthopedic Surgery, Brigham and Women's Hospital/Harvard Medical School, 75 Francis Street, Boston, MA 02115, USA
e-mail: sdmartin@partners.org

Surgical Dislocation of the Hip

Since Ganz introduced surgical dislocation of the adult hip with detailed vascular anatomy of the proximal femur for safe dislocation, it has gained popularity in treating FAI [2]. This technique allows complete circumferential visual evaluation of the acetabulum and proximal femur (Fig. 32.3). Osteoplasties of the acetabulum and proximal femur can be easily achieved, and the use of a femoral head template facilitates the procedure. Moreover, Ganz speculates that this technique can be used for cartilage restorative procedures [2].

Limitations

In order to prevent devastating vascular injury to the femoral head, open surgical dislocation requires extensive but meticulous soft tissue dissection with trochanteric osteotomy. Ganz reported in his series of 213 surgical dislocations, an average estimated blood loss of 300 mL [2]. In one patient, Peters reported an estimated blood loss up to 1500 mL [6]. There are no reports of osteonecrosis of the femoral head to date [2, 6–11]. This may be due to anatomic variation of the medial femoral circumflex artery penetration of the femoral head via an average of 4 retinacular vessels [12].

Commonly reported complications are related to trochanteric osteotomy. Beck and Buchler reported 46 % of the patients experienced pain over the greater trochanter at rest, and 24 % of the patients experienced activity related pain at 1-year follow-up [7]. Ganz reported three failures of trochanteric fixation requiring reoperation in his series of 213 surgical dislocations [2]. Peters reported two trochanteric complications (one early loss of fixation and one nonunion) requiring reoperation in his series of 94 patients at minimum of 18-month follow-up [6]. Beaule et al. reported one patient with early failure of trochanteric fixation requiring reoperation and nine patients with hardware pain from a trochanteric

J.C. McCarthy et al. (eds.), *Hip Joint Restoration*, DOI 10.1007/978-1-4614-0694-5_32

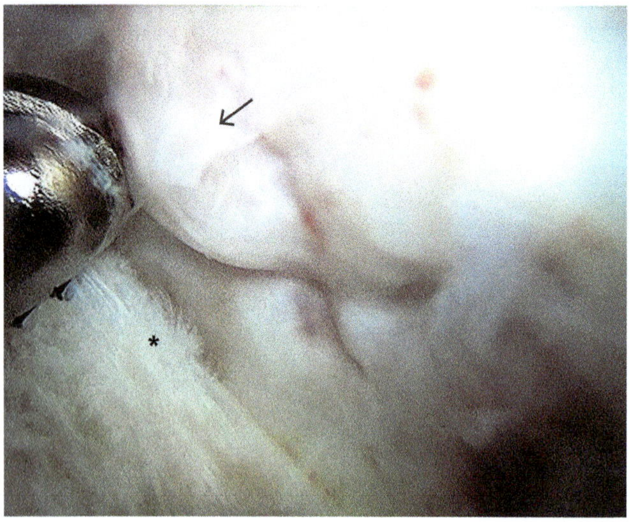

Fig. 32.1 Cam lesion (*arrow*) with labral fraying (*asterisk*). Scott D. Martin, MD ©2013. All Rights Reserved

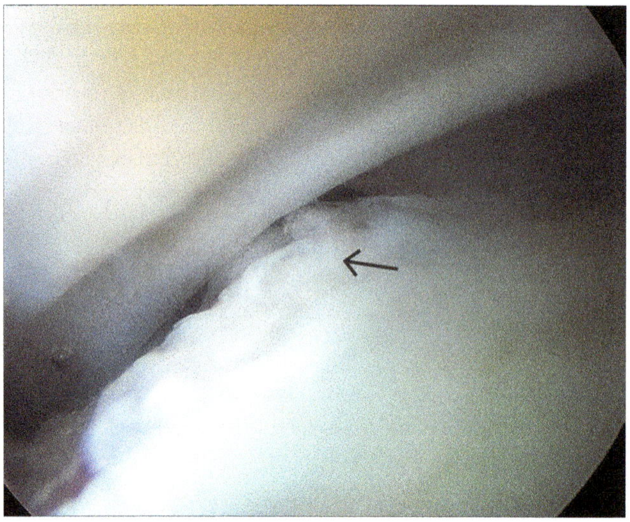

Fig. 32.2 Cam (*arrow*) impingement with hip flexion and internal rotation. Scott D. Martin, MD ©2013. All Rights Reserved

internal fixation device requiring removal of hardware at an average of 8 months postoperatively [8]. Graves and Mast reported two patients with pain resulting from trochanteric hardware requiring hardware removal [9]. In one study, hardware removal was not considered a complication despite requiring additional surgery; 80 % of the patients underwent hardware removal, and it was considered routine postoperative course [10]. In a multicenter study of 355 surgical dislocations of the hip, Sink et al. reported an overall incidence of 9 % complication rate with six trochanteric nonunions requiring additional surgeries [11]. Neither trochanteric pain nor hardware removal was routinely reported as a complication or limitation.

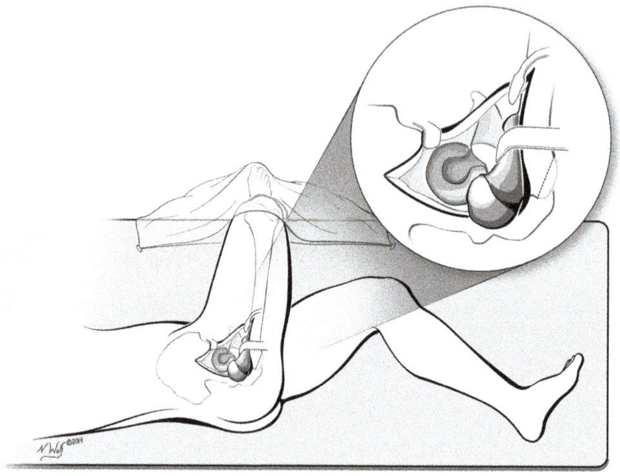

Fig. 32.3 Surgical dislocation of the hip. Nicole Wolf ©2014. All Rights Reserved

Heterotopic ossification (HO) has been associated with surgical dislocation of the hip. In a series of 213 patients, Ganz reported 79 hips with varying degree of HO with an incidence of 37 % at 1-year follow-up [2]. Beaule et al. reported, in their series of 37 hips at an average follow-up of 3.1 years, one patient with Brooker grade IV HO requiring surgical resection at 10 months postoperatively [8]. In a multicenter report of complication after surgical dislocation, Sink et al. reported 18 hips with Brooker grade I or II heterotopic ossification, which accounts for 60 % of all complications [11].

Beck hypothesized that persistent postoperative groin pain can be caused by intra-articular adhesions that can form between the joint capsule and labrum and between the joint capsule and prior osteoplasty site [13]. Beck theorized that an adhesion in a prior osteoplasty site can lead to labral impingement during range of motion [13]. Moreover, an adhesion can function as an intra-articular loose body causing articular cartilage damage to both the acetabulum and femoral head. This leads to persistent groin pain and impingement signs in 10–15 % of patients after surgical dislocation of the hip [13]. Treatment for symptomatic intra-articular adhesions is hip arthroscopy.

Trochanteric osteotomy fixation requires protected postoperative rehabilitation; patients are instructed to be partial weight bearing for 6 weeks [2, 6–11]. Some authors promote soft splint or brace as a part of postoperative rehabilitation protocol [2, 11].

Inpatient hospital stays with a need for postoperative anticoagulation is routine for surgical dislocation of the hip. Ganz reported an average of a 5-hospital-day stay with 8 weeks of anticoagulation [2]; Peters reported an average of a 3-hospital-day stay with 6 weeks of anticoagulation [6]. The impact on healthcare cost, day loss in wages, and opportunistic cost has not been elucidated in any of the studies.

Comparison to Hip Arthroscopy

Hip arthroscopy is minimally invasive in nature. Advances in techniques and equipment have spurred a debate between utility of surgical dislocation to that of hip arthroscopy. Domb et al. prospectively reviewed a matched cohort of 30 patients (ten patients in surgical dislocation group and 20 patients in hip arthroscopy group) with 25-month follow-up [10]. The hip arthroscopy group had significant improvement in the Hip Outcome Score and Non-arthritic Hip Score [10]. Two patients in the surgical dislocation group underwent revision hip arthroscopy; one patient underwent microfracture of the femoral head, and the other underwent labral debridement, chondroplasty, and lysis of adhesion [10]. One patient in the hip arthroscopy group underwent iliopsoas release 18 months postoperatively [10]. Eight of ten patients (80 %) in the surgical dislocation group underwent hardware removal, but were not considered complications, since it is a routine procedure [10].

Botser et al. reported, in a systemic review of 26 articles, that the arthroscopy group had greater improvement in modified Harris hip scores compared to the surgical dislocation group [14]. The hip arthroscopy group had an overall complication rate of 1.7 %. The surgical dislocation group, on the other hand, had an overall complication rate of 9.2 % [14]. The most common complication in the hip arthroscopy group was heterotopic ossification, while trochanteric osteotomy related complications were most common in the surgical dislocation group [14]. Clohisy et al. conducted a systemic review of 11 surgical dislocation studies; they reported 0–18 % complication rate with symptomatic hardware being the most common complication [15]. Krueger et al. reported revision hip arthroscopy after surgical dislocation for the treatment of FAI in 16 patients; all 16 patients had intra-articular adhesions requiring arthroscopic release [16].

Although patients who have arthroscopic labral repair may require protected weight bearing up to 6 weeks, this is only a subset of hip arthroscopy patients. It is an outpatient procedure and does not require prolonged anticoagulation.

A major advantage of hip arthroscopy is the accessibility of the intra-articular and peripheral compartments. It allows 270° access to the intra-articular (Fig. 32.4) and peripheral compartments (Fig. 32.5) but with inaccessibility to the inferior-medial region of both compartments (Figs. 32.6, 32.7, 32.8, 32.9, 32.10, 32.11, and 32.12).

To date, there is no level I study comparing hip arthroscopy to surgical dislocation of the hip. One level II study is included in systematic review but most are level IV [15]. Moreover, there is no study in comparing hospital stay, rehabilitation, return to work status, healthcare cost, and opportunistic cost between hip arthroscopy and surgical dislocation of the hip.

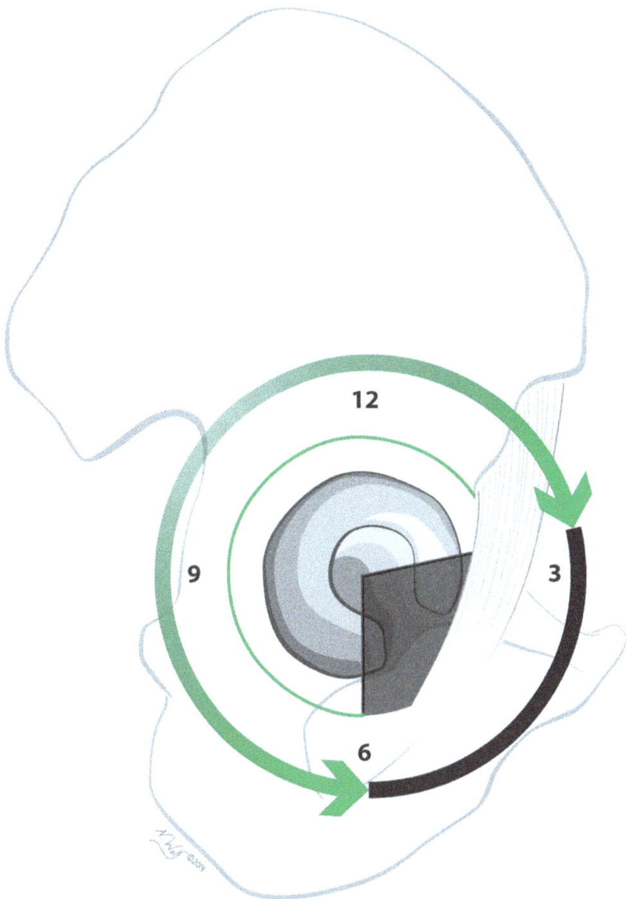

Fig. 32.4 Central compartment. *Shaded area* inaccessible to viewing arthroscopically. Nicole Wolf ©2014. All Rights Reserved

Combined Hip Arthroscopy and Limited Anterior Open Decompression

Clohisy and McClure, Laud et al., and Lincoln et al. independently recognized morbidity associated with the surgical dislocation of the hip; a consistent pathologic osseous lesion was noted over the anterolateral aspect of the head-neck junction of the proximal femur. Therefore, the authors proposed combined hip arthroscopy with limited open decompression to maximize benefits and minimize risks of both procedures [5, 17, 18]. Arthroscopy was used as a diagnostic tool and to address any acetabular and/or labral pathology, and the limited open technique was used through the Smith-Petersen approach with arthrotomy of the hip joint to address any proximal femoral pathology (Fig. 32.13).

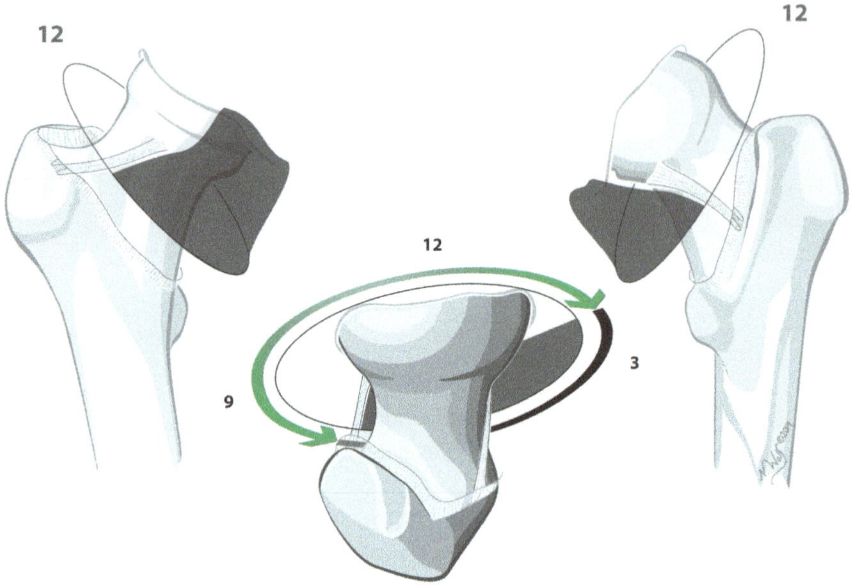

Fig. 32.5 Peripheral compartment. *Shaded area* inaccessible to viewing arthroscopically. Nicole Wolf ©2014. All Rights Reserved

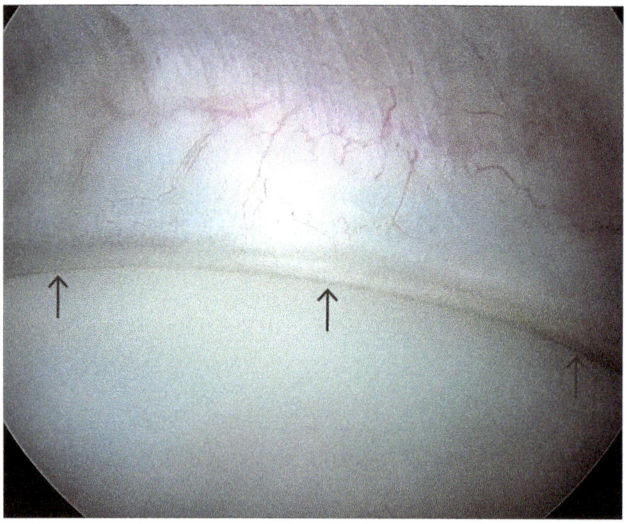

Fig. 32.6 View of labral seal (*arrows*) from the peripheral compartment. Scott D. Martin, MD ©2013. All Rights Reserved

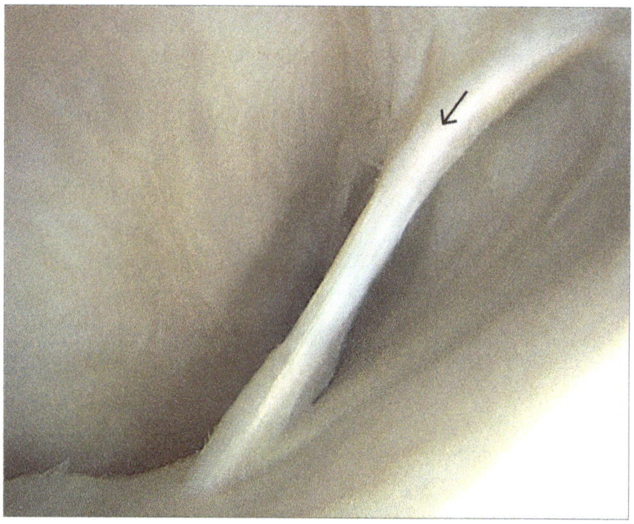

Fig. 32.8 View of lateral synovial fold (*arrow*) and lateral gutter from the anterior portal. Scott D. Martin, MD ©2013. All Rights Reserved

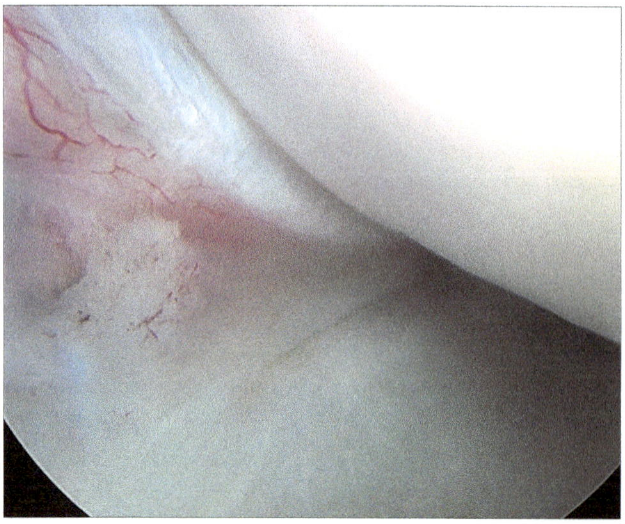

Fig. 32.7 Posterior lateral recess. Scott D. Martin, MD ©2013. All Rights Reserved

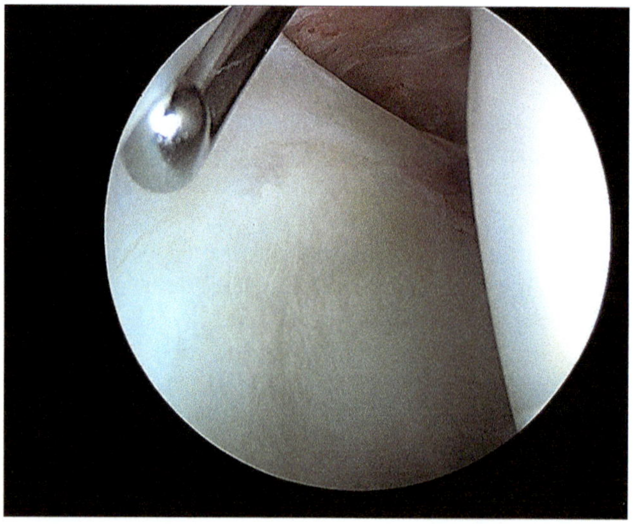

Fig. 32.9 Central compartment view of the anterior superior labrum from 11 (probe) to 2 o'clock. Scott D. Martin, MD ©2013. All Rights Reserved

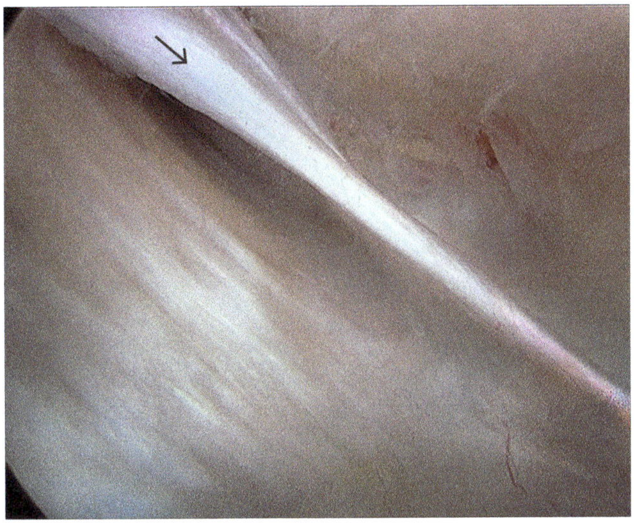

Fig. 32.10 Medial synovial fold (*arrow*) looking into the gutter. Scott D. Martin, MD ©2013. All Rights Reserved

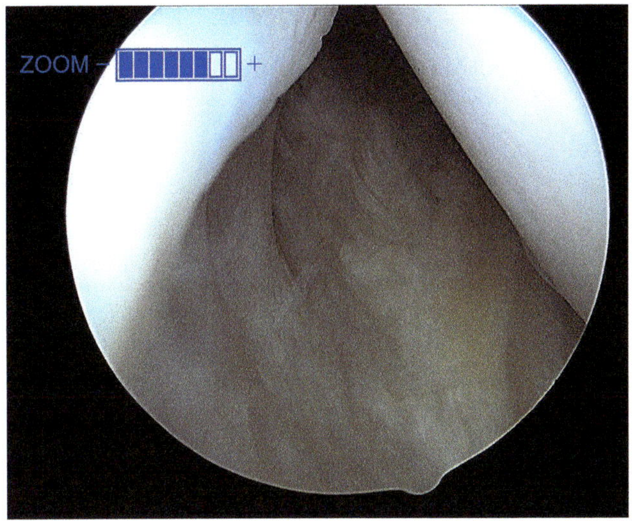

Fig. 32.12 View of inferior recess (6 o'clock) from the central compartment. Scott D. Martin, MD ©2013. All Rights Reserved

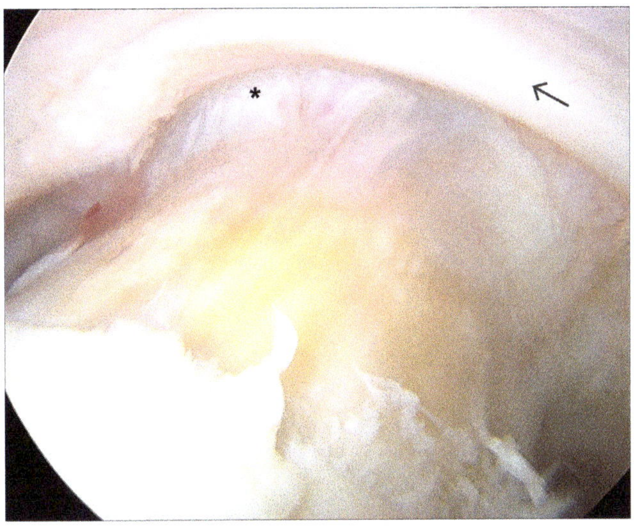

Fig. 32.11 Zona orbicularis (*arrow*), both gutters, capsular reflection (*asterisk*). Scott D. Martin, MD ©2013. All Rights Reserved

Limitations

The limited open decompression requires surgical dissection of proximal hip musculature, which includes detaching and reattaching of the direct and reflected head of the rectus and arthrotomy to expose the pathology [5]. To protect the repair of rectus heads, Clohisy and McClure did not allow active flexion until 6 weeks postoperatively [5]. Lincoln et al. described an anterior approach in which the reflected head of the rectus was transected [18].

Protection of the lateral femoral cutaneous nerve (LFCN) is greatly emphasized with the Smith-Petersen approach. Lincoln et al. reported six patients (38 %) with transient paresthesia of the LFCN which resolved in all patients at 3 months [17]. Ribas et al. noted of 35 hips, six patients (17 %) experienced LFCN paresthesia; one patient had persistent symptoms at 29-month follow-up [19].

Although the authors described the Hueter technique as minimally invasive, studies suggest otherwise. Patients are admitted for observation after the procedure [5, 19]. Clohisy reported that patients are observed overnight and five were started on an anticoagulation and HO prophylaxis for 6 weeks [5]. In another study, patients had a mean hospital stay of 2.6 days [19].

Laude et al. reported in 94 hips, 13 patients with persistent pain requiring revision surgery [17]. Eight of the 13 patients were noted to have failure of labral fixation with labral damage, and six patients underwent revision femoral osteoplasties for inadequate resection [17]. One patient had femoral neck fracture at 3 weeks postoperatively, two patients developed a deep infection requiring surgical debridement with prolonged course of antibiotics, and one patient developed Brooker grade 2 HO requiring surgical resection [17]. Lincoln et al. reported one patient with recurrent mechanical symptoms at 1.5 years postoperatively requiring revision arthroscopy [18].

Comparison to Hip Arthroscopy

Boster et al. reported in a systemic review of 1462 hips with treatment for FAI, a mixture of both the combined approach and hip arthroscopy alone. The overall complication rate was 16 % for the combined group and 1.7 % for the hip arthroscopy group [14]. Interestingly, the combined group had the highest overall complication rate of all of the surgical techniques [14].

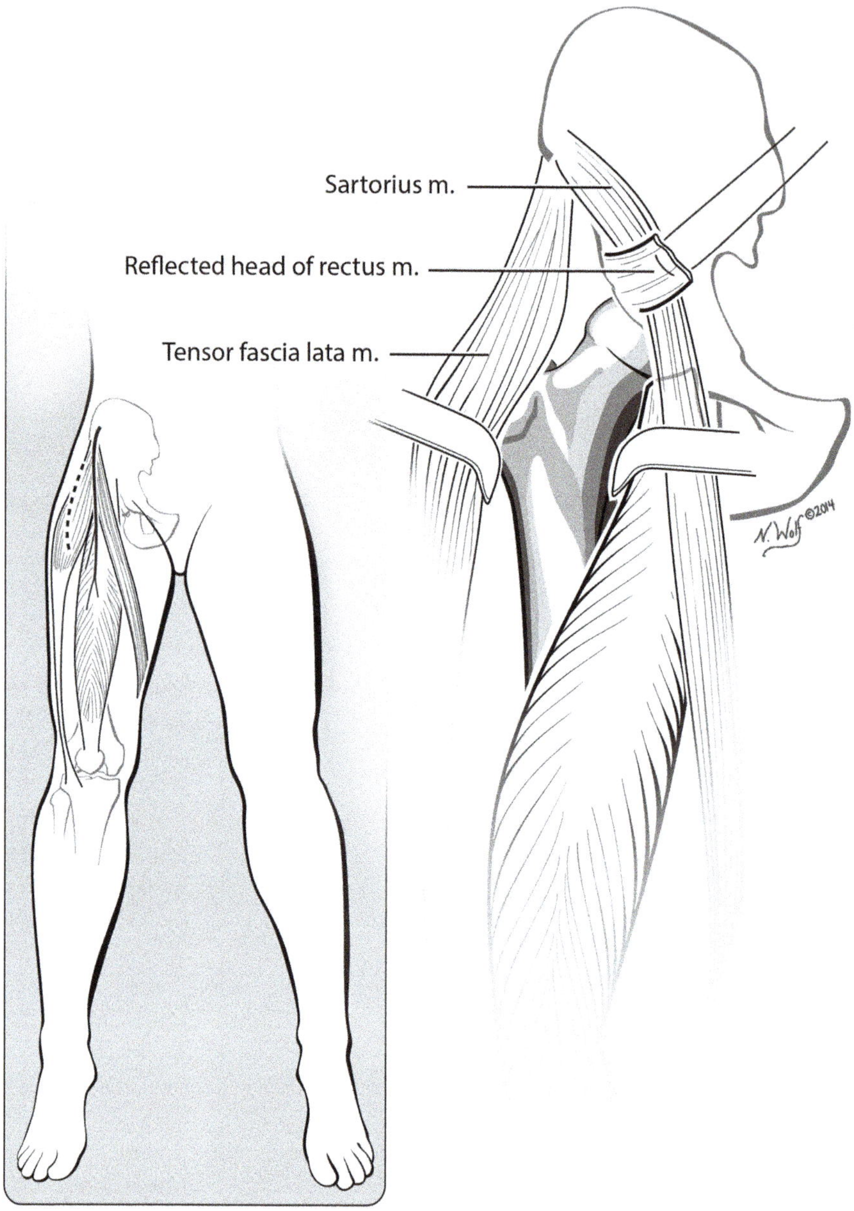

Fig. 32.13 Limited anterior approach to address proximal femoral pathology. Nicole Wolf ©2014. All Rights Reserved

In another systematic review of comparison between surgical treatments of FAI, four combined approach studies were compared to eight arthroscopic approach studies [20]. Both groups showed comparable outcomes and conversion rate to total hip arthroplasty; however, the arthroscopy group showed much lower complication rate than the combined approach group [20]. Unfortunately, there is no level I study to date that compares the combined approach group to the arthroscopy group.

Arthroscopy of Total Hip Replacement [21–25]

Advanced degenerative changes, including chondral damage, may occur after untreated symptomatic FAI. This may lead to total hip replacement or resurfacing arthroplasty in selected patients. Continued pain after total joint replacement may require hip arthroscopy for evaluation and treatment [24]. Hip arthroscopy can be useful for palliative irrigation and debridement of infected hips and iliopsoas recession in total hips with oversized or anteriorly proud cups, when component revision is not feasible. It can also be useful for secondary iliopsoas impingement and for the removal of loose third-body wear, including loose cement.

Technique

The anterolateral portal is established first. Location of portals is equivalent to native primary hips but does present certain challenges. For example, a thick scarred capsule can lead to nitinol wire breakage during portal placement

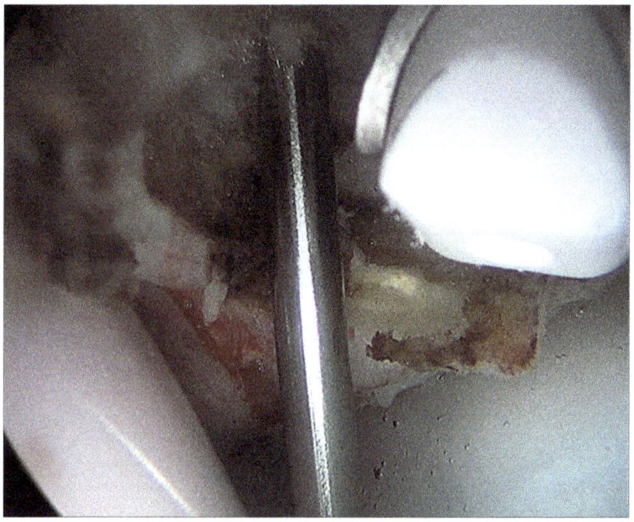

Fig. 32.14 When placing portals in a patient with a THR, the nitinol wire can break easily. Scott D. Martin, MD ©2013. All Rights Reserved

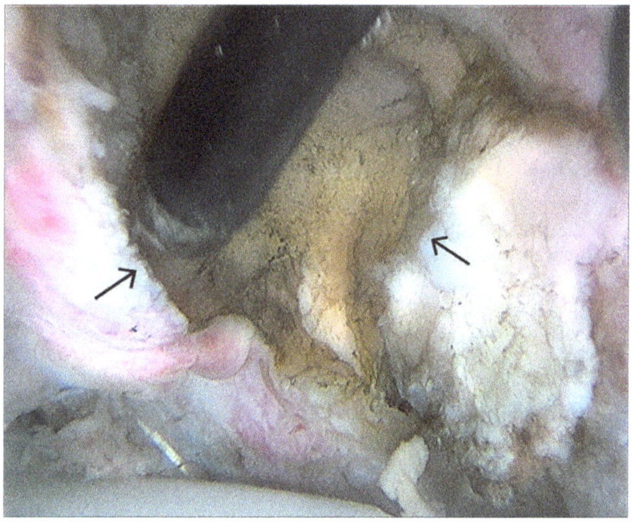

Fig. 32.15 Iliopsoas tendon edge (*arrows*) after recession. Underlying iliacus is exposed. Scott D. Martin, MD ©2013. All Rights Reserved

(Fig. 32.14). Great care should be taken to advance the cannula and obturator slowly, staying collinear with the wire. Do not apply a direct linear force; use a twisting motion while advancing the cannula and be careful not to diverge the obturator. Establish a second utility portal anteriorly, and alternate the shaver with radioablation until an ample window of viewing is achieved. The thick overlying capsule of most total hips can lead to breakage of instruments during levering, so care should be taken to perform capsulotomy of the portals to ease freedom of instrument maneuverability.

Recession of the iliopsoas tendon is completed just off the acetabular rim, leaving the underlying iliacus tendon exposed during release (Fig. 32.15). Be careful not to release the reflected head of the rectus, which can lead to additional hip flexion weakness.

Excessive traction is not required, since hip subluxation is not necessary to access most regions around the hip joint. Care is taken not to scuff the polyethylene liner and/or femoral head during arthroscopy.

Arthroscopy of a total hip arthroplasty can be performed safely, as a day surgical procedure, with immediate mobilization without restrictions. These advantages make it a sound choice in treating some complications after hip replacement surgery.

Conclusion

As our understanding of femoroacetabular impingement expands, various treatment options are explored. Each treatment offers advantages and limitations (Table 32.1). To date, there is no level I study in comparing different treatment options. Open treatment of the hip offers great visualization, template-assisted osteoplasty, and 360° access to the hip joint at the cost of surgical morbidity. It is indicated in patients requiring concomitant acetabular or femoral osteotomy for hip dysplasia, global retroversion, coxa protrusion, or inaccessible hip joint with maximal traction.

Table 32.1 A comparison

Open	Hip arthroscopy
View	
360°	270°
Hospital stay	
3–5 days	Day surgery
Anticoagulation	
Exposure	
Hip dislocation with possible violation of blood supply to femoral head	Minimal trauma to the soft tissue envelope of the hip
Procedure	
Guides for reproducible resection of CAM lesion	Reproducible excellent outcomes with proper patient selection
Ability to perform concomitant osteotomy	
Known complications	
Heterotopic ossification	Residual cam lesions
Intra-articular adhesions	Over and under resection of cam and pincer lesions
Painful hardware	Traction injuries
	Iatrogenic osteochondral injuries
	Results greatly contingent upon experience and expertise of surgeon
Recovery	
Significant days lost from work	
Painful hardware	
Economics	
Disadvantage to the patient and healthcare system	Advantage to the patient and healthcare system

A combined approach offers the advantages of hip arthroscopy and open treatment of the hip, but at the risk of multiplying the complications of both techniques. With advances in techniques and equipment, hip arthroscopy can be a valuable alternative outpatient treatment option with limited morbidity in experienced hands, making it an attractive procedure in a cost conscience era of healthcare.

References

1. Ganz R, Parvizi J, Beck M, Leunig M, Notzli H, Siebenrock KA. Femoroacetabular impingement: a cause for osteoarthritis of the hip. Clin Orthop Relat Res. 2003;417:112–20.
2. Ganz R, Gill TJ, Gautier E, Ganz K, Krugel N, Berlemann U. Surgical dislocation of the adult hip a technique with full access to the femoral head and acetabulum without the risk of avascular necrosis. J Bone Joint Surg Br. 2001;83:1119–24.
3. Clohisy JC, Knaus ER, Hunt DM, Lesher JM, Harris-Hayes M, Prather H. Clinical presentation of patients with symptomatic anterior hip impingement. Clin Orthop Relat Res. 2009;467(3): 638–44.
4. Colvin AC, Harrast J, Harner C. Trends in hip arthroscopy. J Bone Joint Surg Am. 2012;94(4):e23.
5. Clohisy JC, McClure JT. Treatment of anterior femoroacetabular impingement with combined hip arthroscopy and limited anterior decompression. Iowa Orthop J. 2005;25:164–71.
6. Peters CL, Erickson JA. Treatment of femoro-acetabular impingement with surgical dislocation and debridement in young adults. J Bone Joint Surg Am. 2006;88(8):1735–41.
7. Beck M, Buchler L. Prevalence and impact of pain at the greater trochanter after open surgery for the treatment of femoroacetabular impingement. J Bone Joint Surg Am. 2011;93 Suppl 2:66–9.
8. Beaule PE, Le Duff MJ, Zaragoza E. Quality of life following femoral head-neck osteochondroplasty for femoroacetabular impingement. J Bone Joint Surg Am. 2007;89(4):773–9.
9. Graves ML, Mast JW. Femoroacetabular impingement do outcomes reliably improve with surgical dislocations? Clin Orthop Relat Res. 2009;467:717–23.
10. Domb BG, Stake CE, Botser IB, Jackson TJ. Surgical dislocation of the hip versus arthroscopic treatment of femoroacetabular impingement: a prospective matched pair study with average 2 year follow up. Arthroscopy. 2013;29(9):1506–13.
11. Sink EL, Beaule PE, Sucato D, et al. Multicenter study of complications following surgical dislocation of the hip. J Bone Joint Surg Am. 2011;93(12):1132–6.
12. McCormick F, Kleweno CP, Kim YJ, Martin SD. Vascular safe zones in hip arthroscopy. Am J Sports Med. 2011;39 Suppl:64S–71.
13. Beck M. Groin pain after open FAI surgery: the role of intraarticular adhesions. Clin Orthop Relat Res. 2009;467(3):769–74.
14. Botser IB, Smith TW, Nasser R, Domb BG. Open surgical dislocation versus arthroscopy for femoroacetabular impingement: a comparison of clinical outcomes. Arthroscopy. 2011;27(2):270–8.
15. Clohisy JC, St Johon LC, Schutz AL. Surgical treatment of femoroacetabular impingement a systemic review of the literature. Clin Orthop Relat Res. 2009;468:555–64.
16. Krueger A, Leunig M, Siebenrock KA, Beck M. Hip arthroscopy after previous surgical hip dislocation for femoroacetabular impingement. Arthroscopy. 2007;23(12):1285–9.
17. Laude F, Sariali E, Nogier A. Femoroacetabular impingement treatment using arthroscopy and anterior approach. Clin Orthop Relat Res. 2009;467(3):747–52.
18. Lincoln M, Johnston K, Muldoon M, Santore R. Combined arthroscopic and modified open approach for cam femoroacetabular impingement: a preliminary experience. Arthroscopy. 2009;25(4):392–9.
19. Ribas M, Marin-Pena OR, Regenbrecht B, De La Torre B, Vilarrubias JM. Hip osteoplasty by an anterior minimally invasive approach for active patients with femoroacetabular impingement. Hip Int. 2007;17:91–8.
20. Matsuda DK, Carlisle JC, Arthurs SC, Wierks CH, Philippon MJ. Comparative systematic review of the open dislocation mini-open, and arthroscopic surgeries for femoroacetabular impingement. Arthroscopy. 2011;27(2):252–69.
21. Whitehouse MR, Duncan CP. Arthroscopy as a diagnostic tool for painful trunnion corrosion after hip arthroplasty. Knee Surg Sports Traumatol Arthrosc. 2015;23(9):2601–4.
22. Lahner M, von Schulze Pellengahr C, Lichtinger TK, Vetter G, Pesendorfer SH, Hagen M, Daniilidis K, von Engelhardt LV, Teske W. The role of arthroscopy in patients with persistent hip pain after total hip arthroplasty. Technol Health Care. 2013;21(6):599–606.
23. Khanduja V, Villar RN. The role of arthroscopy in resurfacing arthroplasty of the hip. Arthroscopy. 2008;24(1):122.e1–3. doi: 10.1016/j.arthro.2006.
24. McCarthy JC, Jibodh SR, Lee JA. The role of arthroscopy in evaluation of painful hip arthroplasty. Clin Orthop Relat Res. 2009;467(1):174–80.
25. Pattyn C, Verdonk R, Audenaert E. Hip arthroscopy in patients with painful hip following resurfacing arthroplasty. Knee Surg Sports Traumatol Arthrosc. 2011;19(9):1514–20. doi:10.1007/s00167-011-1463-7. Epub 2011 Mar 16.

Open Surgical Treatment: Advantages and Potential Complications of Modern Surgical Approaches

33

Hany Bedair

Introduction

Although the arthroscopic treatment of hip diseases has experienced enormous popularity with an explosion in surgical techniques and instruments to treat a vast array of pathologies, there are limitations to hip arthroscopy. There are certain conditions that are better addressed through open approaches and certainly many procedures where arthroscopy is not an option, like open reduction and internal fixation of pelvic fracture or total hip arthroplasty (THA). Many open approaches to the hip exist and hip surgeons should be facile with most, if not all, of these approaches. Certain surgical procedures demand the use of a specific approach, for example, the sliding trochanteric osteotomy for surgical dislocation of the hip or a posterior approach for the fixation of a posterior column fracture, but for most procedures, more than one approach can safely and effectively be used. There are specific approaches that are almost exclusively used for pediatric patients and pediatric diseases, such as the Ludloff and Ferguson approaches, that will not specifically be addressed in this chapter. The choice of approach is often based on surgeon comfort level, experience, the need for an extensile approach, or perceived benefits of one approach over another. As most of the reports of complications regarding various approaches to the hip have been reported in relation to THA, data presented in the chapter will necessarily be biased toward hip arthroplasty, but fundamentally similar for any surgery performed through a specific approach.

The zeal for potential benefits of different open approaches can sometimes overshadow the potential complications. In THA, for example, the two-incision approach was touted as a muscle sparing, minimally invasive approach for total hip replacement that resulted in early recovery, reduced pain, and high levels of patient satisfaction. As many surgeons began to adopt this technique and it was critically studied [1], it became clear that these advantages were most likely due to the perioperative management protocols rather than the surgical approach itself and that this approach was associated with higher rates of complications compared to other approaches [2]. Potential complications of a surgical approach should be clearly understood from the etiology to rates of occurrence so that the surgeon may make the optimal choice of approach for each individual patient.

H. Bedair, MD (✉)
Department of Orthopaedic Surgery, Massachusetts General Hospital/Newton Wellesley Hospital, 55 Fruit Street, Boston, MA 02114, USA
e-mail: HBEDAIR@mgh.harvard.edu; hbedair@partners.org

Direct Anterior

The anterior approach was described by Smith-Petersen in 1917 [3] and then later in 1949 for the mold arthroplasty. It has been and can be used for multiple procedures including the reduction of congenital hip dislocation, debridement of a septic joint, labral repair and osteoplasty, as well as THA. The direct anterior approach to the hip recently has gained popularity for THA with the development of specialized retractors, instruments, and traction tables and more resembles the approach described by Hueter in 1883 [4].

This approach takes advantage of the intermuscular and internervous planes superficially between the sartorius (femoral nerve) and tensor fascia lata (superior gluteal nerve) and deep between the rectus femoris (femoral nerve) and the gluteus medius (superior gluteal nerve), providing excellent exposure to the acetabulum and a limited exposure to the proximal femur. The patient is positioned supine.

Anatomic Consideration

There are several potential complications to this approach, the most common being injury to the lateral femoral cutaneous nerve (LFCN) which lies on the sartorius muscle. Incising the fascia over the TFL more laterally to the interval

J.C. McCarthy et al. (eds.), *Hip Joint Restoration*, DOI 10.1007/978-1-4614-0694-5_33

between the sartorius and TFL can best mitigate this complication by avoiding the LFCN and keeping it medial to the plane of dissection along with the sartorius. The TFL is retracted laterally and the deep fascia overlying the hip joint accessed. Another common complication is inadvertent injury to the ascending branches of the lateral circumflex vessels of the hip. If dissection is needed far enough distally to encounter these vessels, they should be identified and either ligated or cauterized as they can be a significant source of intraoperative bleeding. The release of the reflected head of the rectus femoris is required to obtain adequate exposure, but the clinical significance of this is unknown. Other potential complications are related to suboptimal access to the proximal femur, particularly in muscular males, which may hinder completion of the preparation of the femur in THA. This can result in undersized stems, malposition of components, femoral fracture, perforation of the lateral or posterior cortex, and inadvertent cutting or fracture of the greater trochanter. Unfortunately, due to the limited possibility to extend this approach, addressing these complications can be difficult, if not impossible. Increased surgical time and complications related to traction tables, including pudendal nerve injuries, ankle fractures, and medial collateral ligament injuries of the knee, have all been reported [5].

Clinical Considerations

The direct anterior approach is best suited for those patients with low BMI who are flexible and nonmuscular and who have no significant femoral deformity or retained hardware. The concern with this approach in larger patients may be related to large abdominal pannus that may overhang onto the incision resulting in wound healing problems [6]. Advocates of this approach claim that due to the relative lack of subcutaneous adipose tissue anteriorly compared to laterally and posteriorly, this approach may be easier than others in large patients. Roue et al. [7] prospectively compared patients with BMI <25 and >25 and observed longer operative times, increased blood loss, incision extension, and abrasions in the larger patients with the anterior approach. Component positioning and infection rates were not different. Restrepo et al. [8] compared patients with BMI <30 undergoing THA through a direct anterior vs. a direct lateral approach and found no differences in complication rates and modest short-term improvement (<2 years) in patient-reported outcome measures in the direct anterior group. Barrett et al. [9] reported on a prospective randomized trial of direct anterior THA vs. posterior THA. These authors reported only minimal improvement in function in the direct anterior group that did not exceed 6 weeks postoperatively for most measures and no difference in any measure beyond 3 months. There were no differences in complication rates. The most common complication, injury to the LFCN, was reported on by Goulding et al. [10] with 81 % of patients reporting symptoms of neurapraxia after THA using the direct anterior approach and only 6 % having complete resolution at 1 year. Barton et al. [5] reviewed reported complication rates after direct anterior THA including femoral canal perforation in 0.5 %, femoral fracture of up to 2.2 %, and dislocation rates ranging between 0.6 and 1.5 %. As with the adoption of any new surgical technique or approach, challenges may be expected. Many authors have reported on the "learning curve" associated with the use of the direct anterior approach to the hip for THA during which time complications including increased operative time and femoral fractures have been reported at higher rates, particularly during the first 100 cases [11].

Watson-Jones

Often referred to as the anterolateral approach to the hip, this approach, popularized by Watson-Jones [12] and modified later by others such as Charnley, Muller, and Harris, is primarily used for THA and open reduction and internal fixation of femoral neck fractures. This approach utilizes the intermuscular, intranervous plane between the tensor fascia lata (superior gluteal nerve) and the gluteus medius (superior gluteal nerve). Traditionally combined with a trochanteric osteotomy or the release of the abductor musculature from the greater trochanter, the use of specialized surgical tables, instruments, and variations in surgical technique allows total hip replacement through this approach without disruption of the abductor complex. The patient can be positioned supine or lateral for this approach.

Anatomic Considerations

The most common complications are problems associated with the abductor muscle complex. Nonunion and malunion of the trochanteric osteotomy, if performed, can occur. Prominent fixation devices used for the osteotomy may cause pain. Limping or, in severe cases, hip instability can occur from failure to reconstitute the abductor complex, whether from failed fixation of osteotomy or failed repair of the abductor muscle tendons to the greater trochanter [13]. Other complications relate to neurapraxias of the femoral nerve due to aggressive retraction. Injury to the superior gluteal vessels and nerve may also occur if this approach is extended proximally into the tensor fascia lata. The ability to convert this approach to a more extensile one is quite limited [14].

Clinical Considerations

Early encouraging reports for this approach for THA are related to its abductor sparing approach and early postoperative function. In a multicenter prospective randomized clinical trial of this approach for THA compared to direct lateral or posterior [15], there was no difference in patient-reported quality of life or satisfaction. However, the complications related to femoral-sided fracture and subsidence were significantly higher in the Watson-Jones group compared to the others, and the authors of this study have abandoned this technique. Other authors have also reported problems related to femoral component malalignment [16], with no difference in clinical outcomes in terms of gait [17] or patient-reported outcome measures [18].

Direct Lateral

The direct lateral approach, often referred to as the Hardinge approach due to his popularization of it [19], is an extensile approach used largely for hip arthroplasty. This approach uses an intramuscular, intranervous plane through the gluteus medius (superior gluteal nerve) superiorly and the vastus lateralis (femoral nerve) distally. The tendinous insertion of the gluteus medius onto the greater trochanter is partially elevated anteriorly (usually the anterior one third), while the muscles of the gluteus medius and vastus lateralis are split in line with their muscle fibers to create a large anterior-based sleeve of tissue. The patient is most often positioned laterally for this approach but can also be positioned supine.

Anatomic Considerations

Potential complications with this approach include injury to the superior gluteal nerve, which innervates the gluteus medius proximal to the greater trochanter in line with the dissection [20]. Care must be taken not to carry the dissection too far proximally (3–5 cm) as denervation of the abductor complex may lead to limp and hip instability. These problems may also arise if the abductor tendon repair fails to heal or trochanteric fracture occurs through drill holes often made through the trochanter and used to repair the tendon [21]. The transverse branch of the lateral circumflex artery of the thigh is also at risk of injury as the vastus lateralis is split and should be cauterized to avoid excessive bleeding. This approach can be extended distally if needed, but proximal extension is limited by the superior gluteal nerve.

Clinical Considerations

One of the main potential advantages of the direct lateral approach is a lower dislocation rate reported in various studies. Krenzel et al. [22] reported a 0.37 % dislocation rate with this approach compared to 3.6 % in the posterior approach to the hip after THA. Many studies have reported on these types of findings; however, in a thorough literature review using criteria set forth though the Cochrane review database, Jolles et al. [23] found no evidence to support the claim that this approach lowered the rate of postoperative dislocation compared to the posterior approach. Moreover these authors reported that the only difference between the direct lateral and the posterior approach was a higher rate of nerve injury in the direct lateral group as well as restricted motion in the direct lateral group, specifically internal rotation in extension. Using electrophysiological testing, Ramesh et al. [20] reported on 81 patients undergoing THA using the direct lateral approach and found that 23 % showed evidence of superior gluteal nerve damage 2 weeks after surgery and that a stunning 11 % (9/81) showed no evidence of recovery at 1 year. Demos et al. [24] reported an 11.6 % rate of moderate to severe limp and a 2.5 % rate of heterotopic ossification after direct lateral THA at a minimum of 1 year after surgery. Harwin et al. [25] reported a 14.8 % rate of heterotopic ossification after this approach. Iorio et al. [26] reported a 4.9 % rate of lateral trochanteric pain after lateral approach for THA compared to 1.2 % after posterior approach.

Posterior

The posterior approach to the hip is the most widely used approach and can be used for hip arthroplasty, open reduction and internal fixation of posterior acetabular fractures, and hip irrigation and drainage for sepsis. It was first described by Langenbeck for drainage of infection in 1874 [27]. It has since acquired a variety of names, including "posterolateral," "Southern" (for the point of the compass), Kocher-Langenbeck, and Moore. This approach uses an intranervous, intramuscular plane through the gluteus maximus (inferior gluteal nerve) superficially. The deep dissection is carried out posterior to the abductor muscle complex and requires the release of the short external rotators of the hip. Patients are usually positioned laterally.

Anatomic Considerations

Complications from this approach are usually related to injury of the sciatic nerve. Though relatively rarely encountered in this approach, the sciatic nerve can be compressed by errant retraction or failure to release the gluteus maximus tendon which can compress the sciatic nerve as it travels below the tendon in the posterior thigh, particularly when the leg is rotated for femoral preparation in hip arthroplasty [28]. Other complications related to the posterior approach are those of hip instability, particularly if the procedure is performed without repair of the posterior capsule. This approach is extensile both proximally and distally and considered the workhorse approach for revision hip surgery.

Clinical Considerations

The most commonly perceived complication after THA through a posterior approach is dislocation. This has been studied extensively and most authors have reported dislocation rates that are slightly higher, but comparable to those with other approaches, particularly with modern implants that appropriately restore offset and have larger heads and if a posterior capsular repair is performed [29–31]. As mentioned above, a Cochrane systematic review did not find any difference in dislocation rates between the posterior and direct lateral approaches to the hip [23].

However, uncommonly, the repair of the short external rotators may fail, despite adequate suturing, leading to frank instability, a fluid collection continuous with the joint, or subtle symptoms of weakness or discomfort. A good quality MRI may demonstrate the problem [32].

Multiple authors have investigated the rate of nerve palsy (particularly sciatic nerve) after posterior approach to the hip. In a large series of 1000 patients, Navarro et al. [33] reported a 0.6 % rate of nerve injury. The authors of this study concluded that the most likely factor contributing to nerve injury after hip surgery was not the approach but rather the complexity of the surgical procedure. Hurd et al. reduced their rate of sciatic nerve injury to zero by releasing the gluteus maximus tendon [28]. Similarly Weale et al. [34] reported that although not clinically appreciated, subclinical nerve injuries may be detected by electrophysiology.

Though reported to be abductor and muscle sparing, muscle damage, as measured by serum creatinine kinase levels, appears to be greater with this approach compared to the direct anterior, but overall markers of systemic inflammation are no different [35]. Component positioning, one of the most important factors for long-term survival of any arthroplasty, is reported to be most accurate with the posterior approach compared to the direct lateral and two-incision THA [36].

Conclusion

Open approaches to the hip continue to be necessary for the vast majority of treatments for diseases of the hip. Owing to its large size and multiple muscle and tissue planes, there exist many different modern surgical approaches. While in some cases the disease pathology dictates only one approach, many procedures can be safely accomplished through several different approaches. While each approach may have certain advantages and disadvantages, it is critical that the surgeon understand all of these in order to provide safe surgical care while optimizing clinical outcomes.

References

1. Della Valle CJ, et al. A prospective randomized trial of mini-incision posterior and two-incision total hip arthroplasty. Clin Orthop Relat Res. 2010;468(12):3348–54.
2. Bal BS, et al. Early complications of primary total hip replacement performed with a two-incision minimally invasive technique. J Bone Joint Surg Am. 2005;87(11):2432–8.
3. Smith-Petersen MN. A new supra-articular subperiosteal approach to the hip joint. J Bone Joint Surg Am. 1917;215(8):592–5.
4. Rachbauer F, Kain MS, Leunig M. The history of the anterior approach to the hip. Orthop Clin North Am. 2009;40(3):311–20.
5. Barton C, Kim PR. Complications of the direct anterior approach for total hip arthroplasty. Orthop Clin North Am. 2009;40(3):371–5.
6. Christensen CP, Karthikeyan T, Jacobs CA. Greater prevalence of wound complications requiring reoperation with direct anterior approach total hip arthroplasty. J Arthroplasty. 2014;29(9):1839–41.
7. Roue J, et al. [Influence of body mass index on outcome of total hip arthroplasty via a minimally invasive anterior approach]. Rev Chir Orthop Reparatrice Appar Mot. 2007;93(2):165–70.
8. Restrepo C, et al. Prospective randomized study of two surgical approaches for total hip arthroplasty. J Arthroplasty. 2010;25(5):671–9. e1.
9. Barrett WP, Turner SE, Leopold JP. Prospective randomized study of direct anterior vs postero-lateral approach for total hip arthroplasty. J Arthroplasty. 2013;28(9):1634–8.
10. Goulding K, et al. Incidence of lateral femoral cutaneous nerve neuropraxia after anterior approach hip arthroplasty. Clin Orthop Relat Res. 2010;468(9):2397–404.
11. Masonis J, Thompson C, Odum S. Safe and accurate: learning the direct anterior total hip arthroplasty. Orthopedics. 2008; 31(12 Suppl 2).
12. Watson-Jones R, Robinson WC. Arthrodesis of the osteoarthritic hip joint. J Bone Joint Surg Br. 1956;38-B(1):353–77.
13. Glassman AH. Complications of trochanteric osteotomy. Orthop Clin North Am. 1992;23(2):321–33.
14. Laffosse JM, et al. Learning curve for a modified Watson-Jones minimally invasive approach in primary total hip replacement: analysis of complications and early results versus the standard-incision posterior approach. Acta Orthop Belg. 2006;72(6):693–701.
15. Greidanus NV, et al. Outcomes of minimally invasive anterolateral THA are not superior to those of minimally invasive direct lateral and posterolateral THA. Clin Orthop Relat Res. 2013;471(2):463–71.
16. Bernasek TL, et al. Minimally invasive primary THA: anterolateral intermuscular approach versus lateral transmuscular approach. Arch Orthop Trauma Surg. 2010;130(11):1349–54.
17. Pospischill M, et al. Minimally invasive compared with traditional transgluteal approach for total hip arthroplasty: a comparative gait analysis. J Bone Joint Surg Am. 2010;92(2):328–37.
18. Inaba Y, et al. Little clinical advantage of modified Watson-Jones approach over modified mini-incision direct lateral approach in primary total hip arthroplasty. J Arthroplasty. 2011;26(7):1117–22.
19. Hardinge K. The direct lateral approach to the hip. J Bone Joint Surg Br. 1982;64(1):17–9.
20. Ramesh M, et al. Damage to the superior gluteal nerve after the Hardinge approach to the hip. J Bone Joint Surg Br. 1996;78(6):903–6.
21. Mulliken BD, et al. A modified direct lateral approach in total hip arthroplasty: a comprehensive review. J Arthroplasty. 1998;13(7):737–47.

22. Krenzel BA, et al. High preoperative range of motion is a significant risk factor for dislocation in primary total hip arthroplasty. J Arthroplasty. 2010;25(6 Suppl):31–5.
23. Jolles BM, Bogoch ER. Posterior versus lateral surgical approach for total hip arthroplasty in adults with osteoarthritis. Cochrane Database Syst Rev. 2004;1:CD003828.
24. Demos HA, et al. Instability in primary total hip arthroplasty with the direct lateral approach. Clin Orthop Relat Res. 2001;393: 168–80.
25. Harwin SF. Trochanteric heterotopic ossification after total hip arthroplasty performed using a direct lateral approach. J Arthroplasty. 2005;20(4):467–72.
26. Iorio R, et al. Lateral trochanteric pain following primary total hip arthroplasty. J Arthroplasty. 2006;21(2):233–6.
27. Gibson A. Posterior exposure of the hip joint. J Bone Joint Surg Br. 1950;32-B(2):183–6.
28. Hurd JL, et al. Sciatic nerve palsy after primary total hip arthroplasty: a new perspective. J Arthroplasty. 2006;21(6):796–802.
29. Berry DJ, et al. Effect of femoral head diameter and operative approach on risk of dislocation after primary total hip arthroplasty. J Bone Joint Surg Am. 2005;87(11):2456–63.
30. Pellicci PM, Bostrom M, Poss R. Posterior approach to total hip replacement using enhanced posterior soft tissue repair. Clin Orthop Relat Res. 1998;355:224–8.
31. Lachiewicz PF, Soileau ES. Dislocation of primary total hip arthroplasty with 36 and 40-mm femoral heads. Clin Orthop Relat Res. 2006;453:153–5.
32. Pellicci PM, et al. MRI shows biologic restoration of posterior soft tissue repairs after THA. Clin Orthop Relat Res. 2009;467(4): 940–5.
33. Navarro RA, et al. Surgical approach and nerve palsy in total hip arthroplasty. J Arthroplasty. 1995;10(1):1–5.
34. Weale AE, et al. Nerve injury after posterior and direct lateral approaches for hip replacement. A clinical and electrophysiological study. J Bone Joint Surg Br. 1996;78(6):899–902.
35. Bergin PF, et al. Comparison of minimally invasive direct anterior versus posterior total hip arthroplasty based on inflammation and muscle damage markers. J Bone Joint Surg Am. 2011;93(15): 1392–8.
36. Callanan MC, et al. The John Charnley Award: risk factors for cup malpositioning: quality improvement through a joint registry at a tertiary hospital. Clin Orthop Relat Res. 2011;469(2):319–29.

Part VI

Arthroscopic Treatment of Hip Disease

Michael J. Salata

The History of Hip Arthroscopy

34

Sachin Daivajna, Richard N. Villar, and Narendra Ramisetty

Introduction

Hip arthroscopy is a unique specialty, which has its roots in the early part of the nineteenth century. The last decade has seen an exponential rise in the number of hip arthroscopies performed, and it is now a well-recognized and accepted procedure [1]. Orthopedic surgery has come a long way from the hip arthroscope's early use for diagnostic purposes, to its current use in delivering stem cells for managing joint arthritis. The ideology and aspiration of joint preservation through a minimal approach drives the ever-changing field of hip arthroscopy.

The First Endoscope

One of the earliest pioneers of endoscopy was Philipp Bozzini, who presented a device called the "Lichtleiter" or light conductor to the Josephinum, the surgical military academy in Vienna in 1806 [2]. This was a very crude invention, which used candlelight and some mirrors to illuminate a hollow tube. The use of this endoscope was limited by poor lighting until Thomas Edison invented the incandescent light bulb in 1880. Later the Zeiss company in 1907 produced a combination of lenses, which enabled an image to be seen the right way up (not inverted as in early cameras) [3].

Endoscopes were mainly used to examine bladders until Severin Nordentoft first reported a homemade "trokart-endoscope" being used to examine human joints [4]. He coined the term "arthroscopy" in the literature and described the handling of the instrument. During this period, Professor Hans Christian Jacobaeus from Stockholm developed an endoscope to examine abdominal and thoracic cavities in 1913 [5]. His invention was popularly known as the "Jacobaeus endoscope," and he is considered the founder of human laparoscopy and thoracoscopy.

In 1918, Professor Kenji Takagi from Tokyo used a cystoscope to examine knee joints [6]. Takagi developed a 3.5 mm knee arthroscope and eventually 12 different arthroscopes with varying viewing angles. On the other side of the world, Dr. Eugene Bircher from Switzerland was independently examining knee joints using an endoscope. He published his work on 60 knee arthroscopies using a Jacobaeus endoscope and named this procedure as "arthroendoscopy" [7]. However, Bircher eventually decided that arthroscopy was inadequate and returned to the use of arthrography as a diagnostic procedure.

The Birth of Hip Arthroscopy

Michael Burman was responsible for first describing hip arthroscopy, albeit in cadavers [8]. A year earlier he had visited Berlin in order to study endoscopy and then returned to his native USA to further develop the technique. His device comprised a 4 mm trocar and a 3 mm arthroscope. In 1931, Burman used this to examine different joints in more than 90 cadavers, of which 20 were hip joints. He then stated "it is manifestly impossible to insert a needle between the head of the femur and acetabulum." He never inspected the central compartment of the hip as all his specimens were examined without traction. His preferred portal was "anterior paratrochanteric," a portal used commonly today. In this way, Burman might be regarded as laying down the foundation of hip arthroscopy.

Later, Takagi in 1939 reported the first clinical application of hip arthroscopy in four patients: two with Charcot's joint, one with tuberculosis, and one with septic arthritis [9]. World War II delayed further advances in hip arthroscopy, and it took more than 30 years for its next clinical use to appear in the literature.

S. Daivajna, MBBS, FRCS (Orth) • R.N. Villar, MS, FRCS (✉)
N. Ramisetty, MBBS, AFRCS, FRCS (Orth)
Villar Bajwa Practice, Spire Cambridge Lea Hospital,
30 New Road, Impington, Cambridge CB24 9EL, UK
e-mail: sachin.daivajna@gmail.com; rnv1000@aol.com

J.C. McCarthy et al. (eds.), *Hip Joint Restoration*, DOI 10.1007/978-1-4614-0694-5_34

The Development of Fiber Optics (Post-War Era)

Watanabe, who had worked under Takagi in Japan, carried forward his superior's work in developing arthroscopy. He used electronics and optics to improve light management and soon established himself as the founder of modern arthroscopy [10]. In 1959, Watanabe no. 21 arthroscope appeared, which gained popularity in the Western world. Its main drawback was an occasional shattering of the light bulb in the joint because of a short circuit. This matter was resolved by Professor Harold Hopkins from the UK, who developed the "Hopkins-rod lens" endoscope in 1965. This used cold light fiber optics and made arthroscopy safer. Indeed, this technology is still used in modern, rigid arthroscopes.

Although the developments of arthroscopy were surging forward in Japan, it was not widely popular in the Western world. Dr. Robert W. Jackson, a surgeon working in Toronto, visited Watanabe in 1964 during the Summer Olympic Games [11]. Following his visit, Jackson started practicing knee arthroscopy in Toronto and subsequently presented his results to the American Academy of Orthopedic Surgeons (AAOS) in 1968 [12]. His colleagues in the USA soon embraced this technique, and arthroscopy was frequently used to treat knee disorders. In 1974, David Dandy, after working with Robert Jackson in Toronto brought this skill to the UK. The next few years experienced rapid progress in the field of arthroscopy.

The senior author (RNV) has long classified the history of hip arthroscopy into four periods, as follows:

- Introductory (up to 1990)
- Consolidation (1990–2000)
- Expansion (2000–2010)
- Diversification (2010–today)

The Introductory Period (Up to 1990)

Since Tagaki, hip arthroscopy was almost abandoned due to the difficult visualization of structures and tedious nature of surgery. This remained until Aignan first presented his work on diagnostic hip arthroscopy and synovial biopsy in 50 patients at the International Arthroscopy Association meeting in Copenhagen in 1975 [13]. Two years later, Richard Gross from the USA published his results of hip arthroscopy in the English literature, on children with slipped upper femoral epiphysis [14]. This was followed by Holgersson et al., who reported on the role of arthroscopy in assessing 15 hips in 13 children with juvenile chronic arthritis in 1981 [15]. Between these two clinical series, there were two separate case reports by Shifrin and Reis and Vakili, Salvati, and Warren regarding the removal of foreign bodies from total hip replacements [16, 17].

In 1982, Eriksson and Sebik published their observations regarding the choice of either gas or fluid within the hip joint during arthroscopy. They felt that gas was superior in terms of identifying articular changes and also described the suction seal of the hip joint [18].

Hip arthroscopy was commonly performed in the supine position until Glick and Sampson developed the technique in the lateral position; this was said to be simpler for obese patients. Glick also designed a specialist hip distractor system that was in due course manufactured by Arthronix (Arthronix, New City, NY, USA) in 1986 [19].

Subsequently McCarthy developed a hip-specific distractor with superior mechanical advantage, particularly for addressing pathology in the central compartment of the hip (Innomed Corp., Savannah, Georgia, USA). This distractor provided superior protection of the perineum and the ankle joint during distraction and minimized complications to these structures.

The 70° arthroscope started to become widely used for hip arthroscopy as it provided a wider field of view than its 30° equivalent and improved the identification of the structures in the hip. However, a key feature of this era of hip arthroscopy was that the procedure was frequently solely diagnostic rather than the therapeutic procedure that is so often the case in the modern era. By the end of this introductory period of hip arthroscopy, the number of procedures performed was still small, although a diversity of conditions were being treated, different techniques were being described, while most agreed that hip arthroscopy was a technically demanding operation.

The forces involved in hip distraction can be tremendous, a feature noted by Eriksson and Arvidsson in 1986 [20]. They found that a hip held in distraction could generate forces as high as 900 N when awake compared with 300 N when anesthetized.

The Consolidation Period (1990–2000)

During this period hip arthroscopy was increasingly used for therapeutic procedures such as removal of loose bodies, synovectomy, and biopsy. Interest in hip arthroscopy was greatly increased by the development of gadolinium arthrogram MRI scanning of the joint, developed by McCarthy and Palmer at MGH in Boston. This imaging procedure remarkably increased resolution of joint pathologies, including labral tears and loose bodies. In the early 1990s, Dr. Amo Oduro-Dominah, an anesthetist, and Colin Dunling, an operating department assistant, proposed that that arthroscopic access to the hip joint could be made simpler by using a guide wire. This suggestion was based on the use of a guide wire for microdiscectomy in those days. In 1990, Dvorak, Duncan, and Day published a paper on the arthroscopic anatomy of the hip, albeit in cadavers [21]. This was followed by an in vivo anatomy publication from Keene and Villar in 1994 [22]. In 1995 McCarthy, Busconi, and Day described the principal access portals for hip arthroscopy in the *Journal of the American Academy of Orthopedic Surgeons*. A year later, Byrd, Pappas, and Pedley described the relationships between portals and neurovascular structures in a cadaver study [23].

In 1992, Richard Villar from Cambridge (UK) published the first textbook on hip arthroscopy, based on his experience of the operation since his first procedure in 1988. Anatomical knowledge gathered momentum with the publication in 1994 by Byrd of his results for 20 patients operated in the supine position [24]. He found that orientation of anatomical structures was easier for surgeons and staff in the supine position. A separation of hip arthroscopic surgeons into those who favored the lateral position and those who favored the supine began at about this time.

In 1996, Dorfmann and Boyer, both rheumatologists in Paris, described the hip joint as comprising two compartments—central and peripheral [25]. They had actually undertaken their first peripheral compartment hip arthroscopy in a hospital at Aulnay-sous-Bois in the environs of Paris in 1984. The central compartment comprised intra-articular structures medial to and including the labrum, while the peripheral compartment was the intracapsular part of the joint outside the labrum. This was subsequently reinforced by Dienst, Godde, and Seil who in 2001 described the technique of entering the peripheral compartment without traction [26]. This consolidation period also saw the introduction of angled shaver blades to improve access to structures within the hip.

By this time hip arthroscopy had established itself to be a complex, albeit a low-risk procedure. Although complications were rare, some reports had appeared, mainly relating to neurological compromise. The most common was a pudendal nerve neuropraxia, which was presented by Rodeo, Forster, and Weiland and Lyon et al. in 1993 [27, 28]. Funke and Munzinger reported complications related to traction and fluid extravasation in 3 out of 19 patients in 1996 [29]. In 1999, Griffin and Villar reported an overall complication rate of 1.6% with no long-term sequelae in a cohort of 640 patients [30]. Clarke, Arora, and Villar later described a complication rate of 1.4% after reviewing 1054 hip arthroscopy cases in 2003 [31]. Rarer complications such as avascular necrosis, femoral neck fracture, deep vein thrombosis, and pulmonary embolism were reported as case reports elsewhere in the literature.

During this consolidation period, the number of procedures, patients, and surgeons involved with hip arthroscopy began to increase dramatically. Special instrumentation started to appear, research picked up speed, and complications were being quantified. Meanwhile industry began to show some degree of interest, although this was highly variable. Certainly, during this period, therapeutic hip arthroscopy as opposed to the diagnostic variety began to develop further.

The Expansion Period (2000–2010)

The expansion period was perhaps when hip arthroscopy could be regarded as truly beginning to make its mark on orthopedic surgery worldwide. Following McCarthy and Glick's initial development of hip-specific instrumentation in the 1980s (Arthrex Corp., Naples, FL, USA), more specialist instrumentation began to appear, particularly the slotted cannula, which allowed safe introduction of curved instruments and easier removal of loose bodies [32]. Power instrumentation was widely used then, as it is now, but the arrival of radiofrequency devices revolutionized hip arthroscopy. A brief phase of laser surgery was of interest but never established itself widely in the field of hip arthroscopy. Radiofrequency probes gave the surgeon the opportunity to reach structures around the fovea and cotyloid fossa. Suture anchors were introduced to repair labral tears and knotless anchors helped simplify the procedure.

In 2001, Ito et al. published a dynamic MRI, which postulated that the loss of the head-neck offset might cause impingement between the femoral head and acetabular margin, causing labral tears [33]. They called this the "cam-effect" and introduced the concept of femoroacetabular impingement (FAI). This single diagnosis did much to popularize hip arthroscopy both for surgeons and for patients.

In 2003, Ganz et al. published a review of more than 600 non-dysplastic patients who had a surgical dislocation for the treatment of FAI and suggested that it could be a precursor for osteoarthritis. Open surgical dislocation was considered a standard approach for treatment of FAI at this time [34]. By 2005, this concept was embraced by the hip arthroscopy fraternity, and arthroscopic treatments of FAI were being used [35]. Reports by Guanche and Bare, and Sampson, suggested that arthroscopic surgery showed favorable results compared with open surgery [36, 37]. During this expansion period, huge numbers of hip arthroscopic procedures, numbering into the multiple thousands, were being undertaken in some units around the world. It became routine for surgeons to arthroscope both the peripheral and central compartments as part of most hip arthroscopic procedures. The indications for surgery expanded, results began to appear in the literature instead of isolated cases reports, and descriptions of technique alone became less of a feature. Major hip arthroscopic units around the world were often in continuous touch with each other, helped by the creation of the International Society for Hip Arthroscopy, founded in Paris in 2008. Education developed alongside this, as it was realized that in order to arthroscope a hip joint, often a different set of surgical skills was required when compared with open surgery or even when compared with arthroscopy of other joints. Industry now began to develop an intense interest in hip arthroscopic surgery and made a major contribution to its development. Governments also showed interest with, for example, the UK's National Institute for Health and Care Excellence (NICE) producing a report in March 2007 which concluded that "current evidence on the safety and efficacy of arthroscopic femoro-acetabular surgery for hip impingement syndrome does not appear adequate for this procedure to be used without special arrangements for consent and for audit or research" [38].

Larson and Giveans in 2008 reported midterm results of arthroscopic treatment for FAI. They reported good to excellent results in 75% of patients [39]. In the same year, Bardakos, Vasconcelos, and Villar demonstrated the importance of cam excision in combination with labral debridement in order to improve results [40]. Byrd and Jones published their 10-year results in athletes in 2009 and reported good results but concluded that preexisting arthritis affected the final outcome [41].

The Diversification Period (2010–Today)

Hip arthroscopy continues to develop enormously. There has been an increasing acceptance that it has now earned its place in modern orthopedic surgery and most realize that there is still plenty more development to occur. The NICE follow-up report of September 2011 says much, when it concludes: "Current evidence on the efficacy of arthroscopic femoro-acetabular surgery for hip impingement syndrome is adequate in terms of symptom relief in the short and medium term. With regard to safety there are well-recognized complications [42]. Therefore the procedure may be used provided that normal arrangements are in place for clinical governance, consent and audit with local review of outcomes."

Not only is hip arthroscopy being used to treat labral tears and chondral damage, it is now also a tool in the management of problematic hip arthroplasties [43].

Apart from intra-articular pathology, hip arthroscopy has been used to treat pathology affecting the iliopsoas tendon, trochanteric bursa, iliotibial band, sciatic nerve, and periarticular bursae [44, 45]. The management of hip instability is also forming part of the hip arthroscopic repertoire. Indeed, the ligamentum teres was once considered a vestigial structure, but now there is much interest in its function [46]. Ligamentum teres reconstruction has even been performed arthroscopically [47]. Meanwhile arthroscopic grafting of bone cysts has also been described, while the use of fibrin glue to seal areas of chondral damage has shown good short-term results [48].

More than a decade after its popularization, FAI continues to dominate hip arthroscopy although there appears no true consensus on the ideal management of labral tears. Larson and Giveans addressed this in 2012 by publishing their results from 94 hips that had either labral debridement or re-fixation. Their cohort of patients with labral re-fixation had a better outcome compared with those who underwent labral debridement at a mean of 3.5 years [49]. Matsuda et al. and Botser et al. compared open surgical technique for FAI to arthroscopic procedures, and their results favored arthroscopic surgery in terms of faster recovery, fewer complications, and similar efficacy [50, 51]. This diversification period is now associated with truly massive numbers of procedures undertaken in some parts of the world, a global expansion of the technique, and multiple manufacturers entering the market. Periarticular surgery is expanding, as is the hip arthroscopic application of orthobiological techniques. Indeed, although hip arthroscopy itself was once regarded as a subspecialist technique, in certain institutions hip arthroscopy is now so routine that some surgeons are beginning to subspecialize even within an already subspecialist area.

Conclusion

Hip arthroscopy has taken a long and arduous journey to its present place in orthopedic surgery. It has now been accepted as a reliable technique with solid indications. It has proved to be a low-risk procedure with potential benefits for treating hip problems by a minimally invasive technique. However, it involves a long learning curve for the surgeon and demands attention to detail. The future for hip arthroscopy is vast but secure and there is hope for further refinement of techniques.

References

1. Montgomery SR, et al. Trends and demographics in hip arthroscopy in the United States. Arthroscopy. 2013;29(4):661–5.
2. Bush RB, et al. Dr. Bozzini's lichtleiter. A translation of his original article (1806). Urology. 1974;3(1):119–23.
3. Jackson RW. Textbook of operative arthroscopy. 3rd ed. Hagerstown: Lippincott Williams & Wilkins; 2003.
4. Kieser CW, Jackson RW. Severin Nordentoft: the first arthroscopist. Arthroscopy. 2001;17(5):532–5.
5. Hatzinger M, et al. [Hans-Christian Jacobaeus (1879-1937): the inventor of human laparoscopy and thoracoscopy]. Urologe A. 2006;45(9):1184–6.

6. Takagi K. The classic. Arthroscope. Kenji Takagi. J. Jap. Orthop. Assoc.,1939. Clin Orthop Relat Res. 1982;167:6–8.
7. Kieser CW, Jackson RW. Eugen Bircher (1882-1956) the first knee surgeon to use diagnostic arthroscopy. Arthroscopy. 2003; 19(7):771–6.
8. Burman MS. Arthroscopy or the direct visualization of joints: an experimental cadaver study. J Bone Joint Surg Am. 1931; 13(4):669–95.
9. Takagi K. The arthroscope: the second report. J Jpn Orthop Assoc. 1939;14:441–66.
10. Watanabe M. Memories of the early days of arthroscopy. Arthroscopy. 1986;2(4):209–14.
11. Jackson RW. A history of arthroscopy. Arthroscopy. 2010; 26(1):91–103.
12. Joyce JJ. History of the Arthroscopy Association of North America. Part I: its origin and growth. Arthroscopy. 1987;3(4):265–8.
13. Aignan M. Arthroscopy of the hip. Rev Int Rheumatol. 1976;33:458.
14. Gross RH. Arthroscopy in hip disorders in children. Orthop Rev. 1977;6:43–9.
15. Holgersson S, et al. Arthroscopy of the hip in juvenile chronic arthritis. J Pediatr Orthop. 1981;1(3):273–8.
16. Shifrin LZ, Reis ND. Arthroscopy of a dislocated hip replacement: a case report. Clin Orthop Relat Res. 1980;146:213–4.
17. Vakili F, Salvati EA, Warren RF. Entrapped foreign body within the acetabular cup in total hip replacement. Clin Orthop Relat Res. 1980;150:159–62.
18. Eriksson E, Sebik A. Arthroscopy and arthroscopic surgery in a gas versus a fluid medium. Orthop Clin North Am. 1982;13(2):293–8.
19. Glick JM, et al. Hip arthroscopy by the lateral approach. Arthroscopy. 1987;3(1):4–12.
20. Eriksson E, Arvidsson I, Arvidsson H. Diagnostic and operative arthroscopy of the hip. Orthopedics. 1986;9(2):169–76.
21. Dvorak M, Duncan CP, Day B. Arthroscopic anatomy of the hip. Arthroscopy. 1990;6(4):264–73.
22. Keene GS, Villar RN. Arthroscopic anatomy of the hip: an in vivo study. Arthroscopy. 1994;10(4):392–9.
23. Byrd JW, Pappas JN, Pedley MJ. Hip arthroscopy: an anatomic study of portal placement and relationship to the extra-articular structures. Arthroscopy. 1995;11(4):418–23.
24. Byrd JW. Hip arthroscopy utilizing the supine position. Arthroscopy. 1994;10(3):275–80.
25. Dorfmann H, Boyer T. Hip arthroscopy utilizing the supine position (letter to editor). Arthroscopy. 1996;12(2):264–6.
26. Dienst M, et al. Hip arthroscopy without traction: in vivo anatomy of the peripheral hip joint cavity. Arthroscopy. 2001;17(9):924–31.
27. Rodeo SA, Forster RA, Weiland AJ. Neurological complications due to arthroscopy. J Bone Joint Surg Am. 1993;75(6):917–26.
28. Lyon T, et al. Pudendal nerve palsy induced by fracture table. Orthop Rev. 1993;22(5):521–5.
29. Funke EL, Munzinger U. Complications in hip arthroscopy. Arthroscopy. 1996;12(2):156–9.
30. Griffin DR, Villar RN. Complications of arthroscopy of the hip. J Bone Joint Surg Br. 1999;81(4):604–6.
31. Clarke MT, Arora A, Villar RN. Hip arthroscopy: complications in 1054 cases. Clin Orthop Relat Res. 2003;406:84–8.
32. Ilizaliturri VM, Acosta-Rodriguez E, Camacho-Galindo J. A minimalist approach to hip arthroscopy: the slotted cannula. Arthroscopy. 2007;23(5):560.e1–3.
33. Ito K, et al. Femoroacetabular impingement and the cam-effect. A MRI-based quantitative anatomical study of the femoral head-neck offset. J Bone Joint Surg Br. 2001;83(2):171–6.
34. Ganz R, et al. Femoroacetabular impingement: a cause for osteoarthritis of the hip. Clin Orthop Relat Res. 2003;417:112–20.
35. Murphy S, et al. Debridement of the adult hip for femoroacetabular impingement: indications and preliminary clinical results. Clin Orthop Relat Res 2004, Dec (429): 178-81 of the hip in athletes. Clin Sports Med. 2006;25(2):327–35.
36. Guanche CA, Bare AA. Arthroscopic treatment of femoroacetabular impingement. Arthroscopy. 2006;22(1):95–106.
37. Sampson TG. Arthroscopic treatment of femoroacetabular impingement: a proposed technique with clinical experience. Instr Course Lect. 2006;55:337–46.
38. National Institute for Health and Care Excellence (NICE). Interventional procedure guidance on femoroacetabular impingement 203. 2007. www.nice.org.uk/guidance/IPG203.
39. Larson CM, Giveans MR. Arthroscopic management of femoroacetabular impingement: early outcomes measures. Arthroscopy. 2008;24(5):540–6.
40. Bardakos NV, Vasconcelos JC, Villar RN. Early outcome of hip arthroscopy for femoroacetabular impingement: the role of femoral osteoplasty in symptomatic improvement. J Bone Joint Surg Br. 2008;90(12):1570–5.
41. Byrd JW, Jones KS. Prospective analysis of hip arthroscopy with 10-year follow-up. Clin Orthop Relat Res. 2010;468(3):741–6.
42. National Institute for Health and Care Excellence (NICE). Interventional procedure guidance on femoroacetabular impingement 408. 2011. www.nice.org.uk/guidance/IPG408.
43. Bajwa AS, Villar RN. Arthroscopy of the hip in patients following joint replacement. J Bone Joint Surg Br. 2011;93(7):890–6.
44. Martin HD, et al. The endoscopic treatment of sciatic nerve entrapment/deep gluteal syndrome. Arthroscopy. 2011;27(2):172–81.
45. Ilizaliturri VM, et al. Soft tissue pathology around the hip. Clin Sports Med. 2011;30(2):391–415.
46. Bardakos NV, Villar RN. The ligamentum teres of the adult hip. J Bone Joint Surg Br. 2009;91(1):8–15.
47. Simpson JM, Field RE, Villar RN. Arthroscopic reconstruction of the ligamentum teres. Arthroscopy. 2011;27(3):436–41.
48. Stafford GH, Bunn JR, Villar RN. Arthroscopic repair of delaminated acetabular articular cartilage using fibrin adhesive. Results at one to three years. Hip Int. 2011;21(6):744–50.
49. Larson CM, Giveans MR, Stone RM. Arthroscopic debridement versus refixation of the acetabular labrum associated with femoroacetabular impingement: mean 3.5-year follow-up. Am J Sports Med. 2012;40(5):1015–21.
50. Botser IB, et al. Open surgical dislocation versus arthroscopy for femoroacetabular impingement: a comparison of clinical outcomes. Arthroscopy. 2011;27(2):270–8.
51. Matsuda DK, et al. Comparative systematic review of the open dislocation, mini-open, and arthroscopic surgeries for femoroacetabular impingement. Arthroscopy. 2011;27(2):252–69.

Indications for Hip Arthroscopy

35

Catherine A. Nosal, Asheesh Bedi, Rebecca M. Stone, and Christopher M. Larson

Introduction

Hip arthroscopy is a rapidly expanding procedure that has been gaining popularity in the medical field since the 1980s [1]. Initially, the indications for hip arthroscopy were much more limited than for other joints because the congruous anatomy of the hip presents additional challenges with respect to access and maneuverability. Instrumentation was also limited to handle the depth of the joint, the thick surrounding soft tissue envelope and joint capsule, and the constrained alignment of the femoral head within the acetabulum [2]. With improved instrumentation, positioning equipment, and capsular management and exposure techniques, the indications for hip arthroscopy have greatly expanded [3]. In experienced hands, this minimally invasive procedure may offer the potential for reduced neurovascular risk, decreased morbidity to periarticular musculature, and an expedited recovery compared to more traditional open exposures of the hip [2].

C.A. Nosal, BS • A. Bedi, MD
University of Michigan Medical School, Department of Orthopaedic Surgery, UMHS, 1500 E Medical Center Dr, Ann Arbor, MI 48109, USA
e-mail: cnosal@med.umich.edu; abedi@med.umich.edu

R.M. Stone, MS, ATC • C.M. Larson, MD (✉)
Minnesota Orthopedic Sports Medicine Institute at Twin Cities Orthopedics, 4010 West 65th Street, Edina, MN 55435, USA
e-mail: chrislarson@tcomn.com

Indications (Table 35.1)

Intra-articular Pathology

FAI

Femoroacetabular impingement (FAI) is a pathomorphology of the hip joint that results in compromised terminal hip range of motion. The resultant abnormal contact between the head-neck junction and acetabulum can lead to chondral and/or labral pathology [4]. Although some individuals with radiographic FAI are asymptomatic, recurrent cyclical impingement, especially in athletic activities requiring excessive hip range of motion gymnastics, or martial arts, often precipitates pain and discomfort and is reported to be one of the predominant causes of arthritis in the non-dysplastic hip [5].

Ganz and colleagues described the open surgical dislocation as an effective and reproducible technique to safely address FAI in symptomatic patients [6]. Recent advances in arthroscopic techniques, however, have allowed for equally effective correction of femoral offset and focal rim impingement lesions with outcomes comparable to open approaches [7]. Arthroscopy also affords the potential advantages of decreased trauma to the periarticular soft tissues without the need for trochanteric osteotomy. Although superoposterior cam deformities can be reached arthroscopically with experience, posteriorly based cam deformities and some global acetabular deformities (i.e., severe acetabular retroversion, protrusion) are better addressed through open approaches to allow for a complete correction of mechanical factors contributing to hip pain [7].

Labral Pathology

The acetabular labrum is a ring of fibrocartilage that acts as a suction seal for lubrication of the hip joint and to distribute contact forces with loading [8]. The seal also contributes to its stability by load sharing [3]. Labral damage can

J.C. McCarthy et al. (eds.), *Hip Joint Restoration*, DOI 10.1007/978-1-4614-0694-5_35

Table 35.1 Current indications of hip arthroscopy

Intra-articular	Periarticular
FAI (cam and pincer type)	Greater trochanteric pain syndrome
Labral pathology	Snapping hip syndromes
Chondral lesions	Proximal hamstring repair
Ligamentum teres injuries	Sciatic nerve entrapment
Loose bodies/synovial chondromatosis	FAI (ischiofemoral and AIIS/ subspine type)
Septic arthritis	
Synovial-based diseases	
Adhesive capsulitis	
Capsular laxity and instability	
Staged interventions	
Adjunct to total hip replacement	

cause pain, mechanical symptoms, and/or a restricted range of motion [9]. Labral pathology can be secondary to FAI, dysplasia, degeneration, or trauma, and the labrum is typically debrided or repaired/refixed based on tear pattern, tissue quality, and vascularity.

While the location of labral pathology has been found to occur most commonly in the anterior and superior margins of the acetabulum, the location typically reflects the areas of mechanical conflict between femoral and acetabular dysmorphology [10]. In the case of dysplasia, anterosuperior, superior, and posterior abnormalities of a hypertrophic labrum have been identified [11]. The objectives for labral repair/preservation are to treat the resultant pain, restore the hip seal/stability, and potentially prevent the premature development of arthritis associated with abnormal contact forces on the articular cartilage. Studies have suggested that labral repair, rather than indiscriminate over-debridement/excision, leads to better outcomes as part of a joint preservation procedure [12–15].

Chondral Lesions

In addition to the labrum, the articular chondral surfaces of the hip confer congruency and provide a smooth, almost frictionless articulation of the femoral head and acetabulum. Derangements of this surface can be traumatic from acute (i.e., subluxation/dislocation/lateral impact) or cyclical trauma (i.e., FAI), or they can be more chronic and degenerative from static overload (i.e., dysplasia). In addition chondral injury can occur from pivoting maneuvers as the hip is extended.

Injury can occur on either the articular surface of the femoral head or on the chondral surface of the acetabulum. Lesions of the femoral head are often the result of hip subluxation/dislocation or traumatic impact injury, which may result in osteochondral defects [1].

Chondral lesions of the acetabulum are frequent findings in patients presenting with intra-articular hip disorders and reflect a morphological incongruity between an aspherical head-neck junction and the acetabular geometry. Loss of femoral offset and sphericity at the head-neck junction can cause a delamination of the chondral surface of the acetabulum. These flaps may result in pain and mechanical symptoms in an otherwise well-preserved joint. Arthroscopic treatment allows for visualization of the entire articular surface of the hip, debridement, and marrow stimulation techniques (i.e., drilling, microfracture) to treat these chondral lesions [10]. Continued evolution of arthroscopic techniques may also allow for whole tissue transplantation of autograft or allograft for more significant osteochondral injuries of the hip.

Ligamentum Teres Injuries

The ligamentum teres is a strong, intra-articular ligament that is important for the stabilization of the hip, particularly in adduction, flexion, and external rotation. Lesions of the ligamentum teres include partial or complete traumatic tears, degenerative tears, and avulsion fractures at the foveal insertion of the femoral head [16]. A complete tear is usually associated with traumatic hip subluxation or a twisting injury. Degenerative tears are caused by chronic inflammation of the joint, which may lead to degeneration of the ligament, or alternatively can be indicative of hip instability [2].

Ligamentum teres injuries may present with mechanical hip pain, and the patient may experience a snapping sensation in the joint. Arthroscopy is an effective technique to resect or debride this ligament. Although reconstruction techniques have been described, there is no current data to support this treatment over conservative debridement. When significant ligamentum tears and or hyperplasia are encountered in the absence of significant degenerative changes, traumatic (subluxation) and atraumatic (dysplasia/multidirectional instability) instability should be suspected. A classification system of ligamentum teres injury as assessed arthroscopically has been recently described [17].

Loose Bodies/Synovial Chondromatosis

Loose bodies are small fragments of cartilage and/or bone that are contained within the central or peripheral compartment of the hip joint. These may develop secondary to a traumatic event or result from degenerative changes and reactive bone formation. Patients with loose bodies often present with mechanical symptoms, such as popping, catching, and locking [9]. Not all loose bodies are visible on radiological imaging, emphasizing the diagnostic and therapeutic value of arthroscopy which can identify and reliably treat these lesions in a minimally invasive fashion [18].

Numerous loose bodies may also be the product of primary or secondary synovial chondromatosis/osteochondromatosis. Primary synovial chondromatosis is a proliferative disease affecting the synovial lining of the joint. This disease causes metaplasia of the synovial membrane which gradually enlarges, calcifies, and breaks off into the joint space which can result in pain and mechanical symptoms [19]. Secondary synovial chondromatosis is more common and typically occurs secondary to trauma. The trauma causes parts of the articular cartilage to break off into the joint space, and calcification of the chondral fragment may or may not be present. Removal of the fragments and treatment of associated chondral pathology can readily be performed arthroscopically [19]. While osseous fragments caused by trauma can often be detected with imaging techniques such as CT or MRI, purely chondral fragments can sometimes only be identified during the arthroscopy [1].

Septic Arthritis

Septic arthritis is an infection of the hip joint proper, caused by a bacteria, fungus, or virus. The infection can cause rapid chondrolysis and irreversible damage to the articular surfaces of the joint, which results in pain, warmth, and/or swelling. Most often, this disorder occurs secondary to a hematogenous infection in infants and young children who are rapidly growing or in immunocompromised patients and older adults.

Arthroscopic drainage for acute septic arthritis has been reported with favorable short-term outcomes, including irrigation, lavage, and debridement of the infected tissue. This approach is often favorable over a conventional open exposure and arthrotomy, which is associated with potentially increased morbidity, greater pain, and an extended hospital stay [18, 20]. However, arthroscopy is not a definitive treatment for sepsis associated with abscess formation, extra-articular involvement, or osteomyelitis.

Synovial-Based Diseases

The synovial membrane is a thin layer of soft tissue that lines the hip joint, functioning not only as a protective barrier for articular cartilage but also as a producer of a lubricant called synovial fluid. The synovial lining of the hip can degenerate over time secondary to trauma, repetitive stress to the joint, and/or inflammatory arthropathies. Pigmented villonodular synovitis (swelling of the synovial lining and an overproduction of the synovial fluid), rheumatoid arthritis (swelling of the synovium due to an autoimmune response), and synovial chondromatosis (previously mentioned) are examples of synovial-based diseases.

Arthroscopy in the setting of synovial-based disease not only allows for treatment but also can confirm the underlying diagnosis. Arthroscopic synovectomy of the joint has proven to be beneficial in slowing the deterioration of the articular cartilage and allow for maintained function of the hip [18]. Focal PVNS located within the lunate fossa and inferomedial femoral neck region may be more effectively treated and eradicated arthroscopically. More diffuse disease, which can extend into the extra-articular soft tissues and posterior hip regions, may be more thoroughly eliminated via surgical dislocation. Arthroscopic techniques also allow for synovial biopsies in a minimally invasive fashion to help confirm the diagnosis of inflammatory arthropathies and guide appropriate treatment with disease-modifying agents.

Adhesive Capsulitis

Adhesive capsulitis is a more recent indication for hip arthroscopy, as it was first clinically recognized in 1999 [21]. It is similar to adhesive capsulitis of the shoulder in that the joint becomes painful and loses range of motion due to inflammation. However, this pathology can be nonspecific in the presence of other hip pathologies that cause pain and a decreased passive range of motion of the joint.

Adhesive capsulitis of the hip is thought to be more prevalent than previously recorded in the literature, but it is likely underreported relative to adhesive capsulitis of the shoulder as decreased range of motion of the hip is perhaps less of a functional limitation for many patients [21]. Arthroscopy can effectively treat these patients in a minimally invasive fashion, allowing for a capsulotomy or capsulectomy of the pathologically thickened capsule and intra-articular synovectomy.

Capsular Laxity and Instability

The cause of capsular laxity and hip instability can be divided into traumatic and atraumatic etiologies. Traumatic injuries can result in capsular incompetence and/or damage to the labrum. Atraumatic hip instability can be the consequence of overuse and may result in anterior subluxation secondary to repetitive external rotation with axial loading. Other individuals may be predisposed to hip instability due to general ligamentous laxity, acetabular dysplasia, or connective tissue disorders such as Ehlers-Danlos syndrome [22, 23].

Capsular laxity, whether traumatic or atraumatic, can be associated with hip pain and subluxation events. Arthroscopic intervention to repair or reconstruct the labrum and capsule may be beneficial for patients with recurrent hip instability, particularly in the setting of prior trauma [23]. Berkes et al. and others have recently described a series of traumatic hip dislocations in which FAI may have predisposed patients to secondary posterior instability and reported favorable outcomes with arthroscopic osteoplasty and labral re-fixation [24, 25]. However, these procedures should be approached with caution in atraumatic cases and primarily employed in patients with capsular or labral insufficiency in the setting of normal bony morphology. When dysplastic features predominate, the hip is best addressed via open procedures to restore the depth, congruity, and kinematics of the joint and correct the underlying mechanical problems which have compromised the secondary soft tissue envelope.

Staged Interventions

Acetabular dysplasia can result in structural instability and static overload of the hip and has been associated with hypertrophy and degeneration of the labrum, chondral surface damage, and hypertrophy/tearing of the ligamentum teres [26]. Correction of the shallow acetabulum can be successfully achieved with a periacetabular osteotomy (PAO), which decreases the force and load on the acetabular surface by mechanically reorienting the acetabulum into a better fit position. PAOs may be performed with an anterior arthrotomy to address any intra-articular pathology, yet arthroscopy in conjunction with PAO may be favorable to allow for a more precise staging of chondral injury, as well as treatment of any associated chondral and labral injury [26].

In severely deformed hips, it may be beneficial to combine a PAO with a proximal femoral osteotomy (PFO) to enhance the stability and restore the function of the hip [27]. With all levels of deformity, arthroscopy can be an effective adjunct tool for the accurate treatment of the intra-articular disease, such as labral re-fixation or debridement [28]. It should not, however, be used in the isolated treatment of dysplasia as correction of the acetabular and femoral morphology may be more definitively addressed with corrective osteotomies. There have been multiple reports of iatrogenic instability with and without bony resection, labral debridement, and capsulotomy in this setting [29–32].

With Total Hip Replacement

Arthroscopy of the hip can be used as a diagnostic tool both before and after traditional total hip replacement surgery. Arthroscopy can aid in establishing whether or not an individual requires a replacement when more advanced degenerative changes are suspected despite fairly well-maintained chondral surfaces on plain radiographs and MRI. Post-arthroplasty arthroscopy is infrequently performed to evaluate the integrity and wear of an acetabular liner several years after surgery, for removal of acetabular screws that have backed out, and potentially perform debridement of soft tissue impingement with an arthroscopic shaver [9].

There have also been reports of psoas pain and impingement after hip arthroplasty with associated component malpositioning (relative cup retroversion, oversized components, and leg length inequalities). While definitive treatment for some may be component revision and reorientation, the morbidity of revision arthroplasty in elderly patients may preclude this intervention. To correct this impingement, psoas lengthening or release, as well as flange trimming, may be performed arthroscopically to reliably improve pain and function. Studies have shown similar results after revision THA and psoas tenotomy in carefully selected individuals [33–35]. In some cases, psoas pain has been documented without any apparent impingement. The psoas has been found to be thicker and under tension, and an arthroscopic transcapsular or lesser trochanteric lengthening can be performed to relieve pain [34]. A release at the level of the lesser trochanter may have the advantage of easier exposure without the risk of iatrogenic infection or instability secondary to capsular damage.

Periarticular Pathology

Greater Trochanteric Pain Syndrome

Greater trochanteric pain syndrome (GTPS) is a term used to describe chronic pain over the lateral aspect of the hip in the region of the greater trochanter [3]. The most common form of GTPS is trochanteric bursitis, which is an inflammatory disorder of the bursa between the trochanteric facets and the gluteus medius, gluteus minimus, and the iliotibial band caused by repetitive trauma. Pain can also be a result of tendonitis or tearing of the abductor musculature [36]. Trochanteric bursitis and focal tears of the gluteus medius and minimus tendon can be effectively treated with arthroscopic bursectomy, iliotibial band release, and/or tendon repair to the greater trochanter [37]. A recent case series of arthroscopic abductor repairs with favorable clinical outcomes has been reported by Voos et al. [38].

Snapping Hip Syndrome

Snapping hip syndrome is characterized by an audible (internal coxa saltans) or visible (external coxa saltans) snapping of the hip when the joint is in motion and may be accompanied by pain. Sources of the snapping include the posterior border of the iliotibial band or the anterior aspect of the gluteus maximus (external coxa saltans) sliding over the greater trochanter when the hip is flexed and extended. The snapping can also be the result of the iliopsoas tendon (internal coxa saltans) being displaced over the iliopectineal eminence, anterior inferior iliac spine (AIIS), acetabular rim, or femoral head. Asymptomatic snapping requires no treatment. Arthroscopic procedures for recalcitrant symptoms include the removal of osseous impingement and/or the release or lengthening of the iliopsoas or iliotibial band to alleviate symptoms [39].

Proximal Hamstring Repair

Avulsion of the hamstring from the ischial tuberosity is a rare injury that occurs during forceful hip flexion and knee extension [40]. This injury is most commonly seen as a result of water-skiing accidents. Reattachment of two or three tendon avulsion injuries with significant retraction is often performed in young and active patients with favorable outcomes and return to sport [41, 42]. With advances in arthroscopy of the deep gluteal space, surgeons are currently exploring the role for endoscopic repair of proximal hamstring tendon avulsion injuries. However, there is no literature to date on the outcomes and complications associated with this procedure. Care must be exercised in the deep gluteal space to visualize and protect the sciatic nerve and gluteal vasculature. Currently, this application may be more predictably used for treatment of recalcitrant proximal hamstring tendinopathy with high-grade tear. The areas of tendinosis can be debrided, followed by creation of a bleeding bony bed at the ischial tuberosity and tendon repair. Chronic ruptures, which may require reconstruction with allograft material, may be best treated via an open surgical approach [43].

Sciatic Nerve Entrapment

The sciatic nerve passes through the sciatic notch inferior to the piriformis muscle. Trauma to this muscle, resulting in spasm or contracture, can cause ensuing compression of the sciatic nerve [44]. Pain can also be secondary to nerve entrapment by the hamstring, quadratus femoris/gemellus inferior, obturator internus/gemellus superior, or scar tissue [45]. Nerve entrapment is aggravated by hip flexion combined with internal or external rotation and can cause pain over the buttock that radiates down the posterior thigh.

Endoscopic treatment has been used to reduce pain associated with the sciatic nerve by releasing the nerve from impinging structures. However, it has been found that the nerve cannot be freed if it is tethered too proximally or distally [45]. Endoscopic decompression of the sciatic nerve involves precision and accurate knowledge of the periarticular space to ensure that all potential impinging structures have been addressed. While this is a relatively new indication for hip endoscopy, it is advisable that this approach be performed by surgeons familiar with the anatomy of the subgluteal space. As an alternative, thorough decompression of the sciatic nerve can be readily accomplished by a mini open posterior approach quite safely.

FAI

Ischiofemoral and AIIS/subspine impingement are extra-articular patterns of hip impingement [46–48]. Impingement occurs between the lesser trochanter and ischium (ischiofemoral) or AIIS and distal femoral neck (AIIS/subspine) regions. Recent reports have shown that decompression of the offending bony anatomy with arthroscopic/endoscopic approaches have led to improved outcomes with appropriate indications [46–48]. Extra-articular greater trochanteric/pelvic impingement, which is classically seen in the setting of Legg-Calve-Perthes, is best treated with open surgical approaches and includes relative neck lengthening/greater trochanteric transfers. Further follow-up and larger numbers, however, are required to better define outcomes and optimal surgical procedures for these extra-articular impingement disorders.

Contraindications (Table 35.2)

A successful outcome for arthroscopy/endoscopy of the hip requires careful patient selection and a keen awareness of factors that may technically preclude the procedure or compromise clinical outcomes.

Relative

Arthroscopy in the setting of obesity is technically more challenging with a greater potential risk for complications and may require longer instruments to access the joint [10]. Obesity and deconditioning may also compromise the ability to participate in rigorous postoperative rehabilitation. Arthroscopic procedures to preserve the integrity of the hip are less effective in the presence of mild to moderate osteoarthritis, dysplasia, and inflammatory arthritis. High failure rates have been reported in the setting of preexisting degenerative changes [49]. It is important to carefully evaluate the osseous morphology and the status of the articular cartilage on preoperative imaging studies. Arthroscopy may be a useful adjunct for diagnostic purposes and treatment of intra-articular pathology in the setting of significant dysplasia but should typically be employed in combination with more definitive open procedures to address the abnormal femoral and acetabular dysmorphology responsible for static overload. Subtle dysplastic features, however, can be seen in the setting of impingement, and arthroscopy may be carefully considered in these cases. Arthroscopic procedures may also be contraindicated for patients with known neurological injury/disorders (i.e., pudendal nerve neuralgia) where traction of the hip may cause a "double crush" phenomenon with greater risk of further neurologic impairment [44, 50]. Chronically retracted proximal hamstring and abductor tendon avulsions can be more technically challenging scenarios and require allograft reconstruction. Open approaches may

Table 35.2 Contraindications for hip arthroscopy/endoscopy

Relative contraindications	Absolute contraindications
Obesity/deconditioning	Advanced osteoarthritis
Moderate osteoarthritis	Septic joint spread
Dysplasia	Ankylosis
Inflammatory arthritis	Dysplasia with femoral head migration
Neurological injury	Greater trochanteric impingement
Chronic proximal hamstring avulsions	Severe acetabular retroversion
Chronic abductor avulsions with severe retraction and fatty atrophy	
Internal snapping hip with severe femoral neck anteversion	

be more predictable in these situations. Finally, internal snapping hip in the setting of severe femoral neck anteversion may be best addressed with a derotational femoral osteotomy in an effort to avoid potentially further destabilizing the hip anteriorly.

Absolute

In cases of severe osteoarthritis, where the articular cartilage has been fully denuded, arthroscopy should not be performed, as universally poor results have been reported [49, 51]. The outcomes after arthroscopic lavage or debridement in severely osteoarthritic joints were found to have results no better than those after a placebo procedure [52]. In the case of a septic joint, arthroscopy should not be performed if the infection has spread beyond the point of the synovial matrix. An open arthrotomy should be implemented if osteomyelitis is suspected [53]. Ankylosis of the joint is an important absolute contraindication. If the hip cannot be distracted or distended properly, then arthroscopic instruments cannot be safely employed [1]. Dysplastic features with femoral head migration (>1 cm lateral, or break in Shenton's line) indicate more severe structural instability and open corrective approaches should be considered. Symptomatic greater trochanteric impingement cannot be reliably managed with an arthroscopic/endoscopic approach at this time, and open procedures might be considered in the presence of significant disability. Finally, rim resection in the presence of severe acetabular retroversion can further destabilize a posteriorly deficient acetabulum and anteversion/reverse PAO should be considered in these situations.

Summary

Until relatively recently, the hip has been largely neglected from an arthroscopic standpoint due to the complexity of the deep joint with thick surrounding tissues and a constrained alignment of the bony anatomy. Arthroscopic and endoscopic hip procedures are now rapidly evolving. These minimally invasive procedures can effectively be performed for various disorders about the hip and pelvis. The use of hip arthroscopy/endoscopy has not only allowed for the precise diagnosis and treatment of hip injuries/disorders but has also allowed for a better understanding of intra- and periarticular hip pathology. Indications and contraindications will likely continue to evolve as new technological advances and longer-term outcomes become available. Adherence to evidence-based indications and contraindications will help to optimize outcomes after arthroscopic and endoscopic hip procedures.

References

1. Byrd JW. Hip arthroscopy. J Am Acad Orthop Surg. 2006;14(7): 433–44.
2. DeLee J, Drez D, Miller MD. DeLee & Drez's orthopaedic sports medicine principles and practice. Philadelphia: Saunders/Elsevier; 2010.
3. Rath E, Tsvieli O, Levy O. Hip arthroscopy: an emerging technique and indications. Isr Med Assoc J. 2012;14(3):170–4.
4. Larson CM, Giveans MR. Arthroscopic management of femoroacetabular impingement: early outcomes measures. Arthroscopy. 2008;24(5):540–6.
5. Byrd JW, Jones KS. Arthroscopic management of femoroacetabular impingement: minimum 2-year follow-up. Arthroscopy. 2011;27(10):1379–88.
6. Leunig M, Beaule PE, Ganz R. The concept of femoroacetabular impingement: current status and future perspectives. Clin Orthop Relat Res. 2009;467(3):616–22.
7. Bedi A, Zalta I, De La Torre K, Keely BT. Radiographic comparison of surgical hip dislocation and hip arthroscopy for treatment of cam deformity in femoroacetabular impingement. Am J Sports Med. 2011;39(Suppl):20S–8.
8. Ferguson SJ, Bryant JT, Ganz R, et al. An in vitro investigation of the acetabular labral seal in hip joint mechanics. J Biomech. 2003;36:171–8.
9. Diulus CA, Krebs VE, Hanna G, Barsoum WK. Hip arthroscopy technique and indications. J Arthroplasty. 2006;21(4 Suppl 1): 68–73.
10. Khanduja V, Villar RN. Arthroscopic surgery of the hip: current concepts and recent advances. J Bone Joint Surg Br. 2006; 88(12):1557–66.
11. Resnick DL, Kang HS, Pretterklieber ML. Internal derangements of joints. Philadelphia: Saunders/Elsevier; 2007.
12. Espinosa N, Rothenfluh DA, Beck M, Ganz R, Leunig M. Treatment of femoro-acetabular impingement: preliminary results of labral refixation. J Bone Joint Surg Am. 2006;88(5):925–35.
13. Larson CM, Giveans MR, Stone RM. Arthroscopic debridement versus refixation of the acetabular labrum associated with femoroacetabular impingement: mean 3.5 year follow-up. Am J Sports Med. 2012;40(5):1015–21.
14. Larson CM, Giveans MR. Arthroscopic debridement versus refixation of the acetabular labrum associated with femoroacetabular impingement. Arthroscopy. 2009;25(4):369–76.
15. Schilders E, Dimitrakopoulou A, Bismil Q, et al. Arthroscopic treatment of labral tears in femoroacetabular impingement: a comparative study of refixation and resection with a minimum two-year follow-up. J Bone Joint Surg Br. 2011;93(8):1027–32.
16. Cerezal L, Kassarjian A, Canga A, Dobado MC, Montero JA, et al. Anatomy, biomechanics, imaging, and management of ligamentum teres injuries. Radiographics. 2010;30(6):1637–51.
17. Botser IB, Martin DE, Stout CE, Domb BG. Tears of the ligamentum teres: prevalence in hip arthroscopy using 2 classification systems. Am J Sports Med. 2011;39(Suppl):117S–25.
18. Fu FH. Sports medicine. Master techniques in orthopaedic surgery. Philadelphia: Wolters Kluwer Health/Lippincott Williams & Wilkins; 2010. p. 640. xxiv.
19. Helms CA, Major NM, Anderson MW, Kaplan P, Dussault R. Musculoskeletal MRI. 2nd ed. Philadelphia: Saunders Elsevier; 2009. p. 442. vii.
20. Rutz E, Brunner R. Septic arthritis of the hip—current concepts. Hip Int. 2009;19 Suppl 6:S9–12.
21. Byrd JW, Jones K. Adhesive capsulitis of the hip. Arthroscopy. 2006;22(1):89–94.
22. Smith MV, Sekiya JK. Hip instability. Sports Med Arthrosc. 2010;18(2):108–12.

23. Tibor LM, Sekiya JK. Differential diagnosis of pain around the hip joint. Arthroscopy. 2008;24(12):1407–21.
24. Berkes MB, Cross MB, Shindle MK, Bedi A, Kelly BT. Traumatic posterior hip instability and femoroacetabular impingement in athletes. Am J Orthop (Belle Mead NJ). 2012;41(4):166–71.
25. Krych AJ, Thompson M, Larson CM, Byrd JW, Kelly BT. Is posterior hip instability associated with cam and pincer deformity? Clin Orthop Relat Res. 2012;470(12):3390–7.
26. Ross JR, Zaltz I, Nepple JJ, Schoenecker PL, Clohisy JC. Arthroscopic disease classification and interventions as an adjunct in the treatment of acetabular dysplasia. Am J Sports Med. 2011;39(Suppl):72S–8.
27. Clohisy JC, St John LC, Nunley RM, Schutz AL, Schoenecker PL. Combined periacetabular and femoral osteotomies for severe hip deformities. Clin Orthop Relat Res. 2009;467(9):2221–7.
28. Kim KI, Cho YJ, Ramteke AA, Yoo MC. Peri-acetabular rotational osteotomy with concomitant hip arthroscopy for treatment of hip dysplasia. J Bone Joint Surg Br. 2011;93(6):732–7.
29. Matsuda DK. Acute iatrogenic dislocation following hip impingement arthroscopic surgery. Arthroscopy. 2009;25(4):400–4.
30. Ranawat AS, McClincy M, Sekiya JK. Anterior dislocation of the hip after arthroscopy in a patient with capsular laxity of the hip. A case report. J Bone Joint Surg Am. 2009;91(1):192–7.
31. Benali Y, Katthagen BD. Hip subluxation as a complication of arthroscopic debridement. Arthroscopy. 2009;25(4):405–7.
32. Mei-Dan O, McConkey MO, Brick M. Catastrophic failure of hip arthroscopy due to iatrogenic instability: can partial division of the ligamentum teres and iliofemoral ligament cause subluxation? Arthroscopy. 2012;28(3):440–5.
33. Van Riet A, De Schepper J, Delport HP. Arthroscopic psoas release for iliopsoas impingement after total hip replacement. Acta Orthop Belg. 2011;77(1):41–6.
34. Jasani V, Richards P, Wynn-Jones C. Pain related to the psoas muscle after total hip replacement. J Bone Joint Surg Br. 2002;84(7):991–3.
35. Dora C, Houweling M, Koch P, Sierra RJ. Iliopsoas impingement after total hip replacement: the results of non-operative management, tenotomy or acetabular revision. J Bone Joint Surg Br. 2007;89(8):1031–5.
36. Benzel EC. Spine surgery: techniques, complication avoidance, and management. 2nd ed. Philadelphia: Churchill Livingstone; 2005.
37. Voos JE, Rudzki JR, Shindel MK, Martin H, Kelly BT. Arthroscopic anatomy and surgical techniques for peritrochanteric space disorders in the hip. Arthroscopy. 2007;23(11):1246.e1–5.
38. Voos JE, Shindle MK, Pruett A, Asnis PD, Kelly BT. Endoscopic repair of gluteus medius tendon tears of the hip. Am J Sports Med. 2009;37(4):743–7.
39. Kelly BT, Williams III RJ, Philippon MJ. Hip arthroscopy: current indications, treatment options, and management issues. Am J Sports Med. 2003;31(6):1020–37.
40. Beltran L, Ghazikhanain V, Padron M, Beltran J. The proximal hamstring muscle-tendon-bone unit: a review of the normal anatomy, biomechanics, and pathophysiology. Eur J Radiol. 2012;81(12): 3772–9.
41. Birmingham P, Muller M, Wickiewicz T, Cavanaugh J, Rodeo S, Warren R. Functional outcome after repair of proximal hamstring avulsions. J Bone Joint Surg Am. 2011;93(19):1819–26.
42. Folsom G, Larson CM. Surgical treatment of acute versus chronic complete proximal hamstring ruptures: results of acute repair and a new allograft technique for chronic reconstructions. Am J Sports Med. 2008;36(1):104–9.
43. Larson CM. Management of chronic proximal hamstring ruptures: surgical treatment. Oper Tech Sports Med. 2009;17(4):210–4.
44. Frontera WR, Micheli LJ, Herring SA, SIlver JK. Clinical sports medicine medical management and rehabilitation. Philadelphia: Saunders/Elsevier; 2007.
45. Martin HD, Shears SA, Johnson JC, Smathers AM, Palmer IJ. The endoscopic treatment of sciatic nerve entrapment/deep gluteal syndrome. Arthroscopy. 2011;27(2):172–81.
46. Stafford GH, Villar RN. Ischiofemoral impingement. J Bone Joint Surg Br. 2011;93(10):1300–2.
47. Larson CM, Kelly BT, Stone RM. Making a case for anterior inferior iliac spine/subspine hip impingement: three representative case reports and proposed concept. Arthroscopy. 2011;27(12):1732–7.
48. Hetsroni I, Larson CM, Dela Torre K, Zbeda RM, Magennis E, Kelly BT. Anterior inferior iliac spine deformity as an extra-articular source for hip impingement: a series of 10 patients treated with arthroscopic decompression. Arthroscopy. 2012;28(11): 1644–53.
49. Larson CM, Giveans MR, Taylor M. Does arthroscopic FAI correction improve function with radiographic arthritis? Clin Orthop Relat Res. 2011;469(6):1667–76.
50. Flierl MA, Stahel PF, Hak DJ, Morgan SJ, Smith WR. Traction table-related complications in orthopaedic surgery. J Am Acad Orthop Surg. 2010;18(11):668–75.
51. Farjo LA, Glick JM, Sampson TG. Hip arthroscopy for acetabular labral tears. Arthroscopy. 1999;15(2):132–7.
52. Haviv B, O'Donnell J. The incidence of total hip arthroplasty after hip arthroscopy in osteoarthritic patients. Sports Med Arthrosc Rehabil Ther Technol. 2010;2:18.
53. Kaminski A, Muhr G, Kutscha-Lissberg F. Modified open arthroscopy in the treatment of septic arthritis of the hip. Ortop Traumatol Rehabil. 2007;9(6):599–603.

Arthroscopic Treatment: Surgical Anatomy

36

Allston J. Stubbs, Todd C. Johnson, and Elizabeth A. Howse

Introduction

A keen understanding of the arthroscopic anatomy of the hip is essential for the identification of pathology, the safety of the patient, and the efficiency of the surgeon. The goal of this chapter is to provide a visual tour of the arthroscopic anatomy of the hip, and this will be accomplished in two parts. First, a discussion on the appropriate operating room setup, patient positioning, and portal placement is essential as success on the arthroscopic scale always begins on the macroscopic scale. Second, detailed descriptions along with arthroscopic pictures from the three compartments of the hip—the central, peripheral, and peritrochanteric/lateral compartments—will be provided as the task of determining the abnormal always begins with defining the normal. Additionally, a knowledge of the associated vascular and ligamentous anatomy will help to avoid intraoperative and postoperative complications.

Operating Room Setup Relative to Arthroscopic Anatomy

The operating room setup, while critical to success in hip arthroscopy, has many individual preferences. The surgeon must find a setup that not only works on an individual level but is also compatible with the capabilities and preferences of the institution. Finding a reproducible, reliable, and cost-efficient system is the goal and is more important than any single preference expressed here.

The patient is placed on a fracture table in the supine position. Both feet are placed in fracture table boots and over-wrapped with 3 in. tape to decrease the chance of intraoperative slippage. The boots are then connected to the fracture table, and a lateralized perineal post from the K.A.F. kit (Bledsoe Philippon K.A.F. positioning kit with perineal post pad kit; Bledsoe, Grand Prairie, TX) is placed in the patient's groin area. The perineal post needs to be firm enough to provide sufficient traction yet soft enough to avoid compression upon the pudendal nerve. The patient's hips and knees are placed in full extension bilaterally. The operative extremity is abducted approximately 25° against the perineal post which produces an oblique traction vector that is roughly in line with the femoral neck [1]. The operative extremity is then internally rotated to orient the femoral neck parallel to the floor, effectively eliminating femoral neck anteversion. This has the additional benefit of increasing the distance to the sciatic nerve posteriorly.

The nonoperative extremity is placed under minimal traction. Under fluoroscopy, the operative extremity is placed under traction until a vacuum sign is noted, indicative of subatmospheric pressure within the hip joint (Fig. 36.1). The time is noted by the circulator to prevent excess traction time. Fluoroscopy is then removed from the room.

Portal Placement Relative to Arthroscopic Anatomy

At our institution, we typically use a two portal technique that includes an anterolateral portal and a modified anterior portal. The combination of these two portals allows for safe and satisfactory access to both the central and peripheral compartments; however, additional portals, at times, become

A.J. Stubbs, MD, MBA (✉)
Division of Sports Medicine, Department of Orthopaedic Surgery, Wake Forest University, 131 Miller St., Winston Salem, NC 27103, USA
e-mail: astubbs@wakehealth.edu

T.C. Johnson, MD
Division of Sports Medicine, Department of Orthopaedics, Wake Forest University, 131 Miller St., Winston Salem, NC 27103, USA
e-mail: todd.johnson@mac.com; tjohnso@wakehealth.edu

E.A. Howse, MD
Department of Emergency Medicine, Hofstra North Shore-LIJ School of Medicine, Long Island Jewish Medical Center, New Hyde Park, NY, USA
e-mail: howseea@gmail.com

J.C. McCarthy et al. (eds.), *Hip Joint Restoration*, DOI 10.1007/978-1-4614-0694-5_36

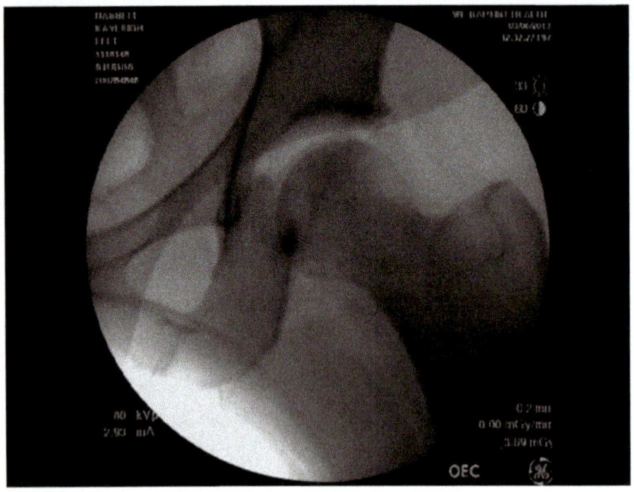

Fig. 36.1 X-ray picture of hip vacuum sign. © Allston J. Stubbs, MD

necessary. A command of the hip anatomy relative to specific portal sites is essential for minimizing risk to the patient and maximizing success for the procedure.

Anterolateral Portal for the Central Compartment

To make the anterolateral portal, the anterior margin of the greater trochanter is defined by palpation. For a left hip, the surgeon's right hand long finger is placed at the tip of the greater trochanter, and a line is drawn on the skin radial to and just beyond the tip of the surgeon's index finger approximately 10 mm superior and 10 mm anterior to the greater trochanter. For a right hip, the surgeon's left hand is used. The skin is incised, and a 6 in., 17-gauge spinal needle is delivered into the joint at an angle measuring approximately 15° cephalad and 15° posterior [2]. The stylet is withdrawn from the spinal needle. A 60 cm^3 syringe is utilized to deliver saline into the joint, and if properly placed into the joint, backflow into the syringe will be noted when pressure is relieved from the plunger. The syringe is removed from the spinal needle and a nitinol wire is delivered into the joint. The spinal needle is then removed over the wire. The wire is tested for placement by a gentle push-pull technique. If it does not slide easily, it may be through the labrum and will need to be adjusted. A cannula is then introduced into the joint. Fluoroscopy may be utilized to facilitate placement.

The anterolateral portal pierces the gluteus medius muscle prior to entering the joint [3]; however, it is possible to deliver the portal between the tensor fascia lata anteriorly and the gluteus medius posteriorly in young active patients who develop a palpable ridge in the region of the anterolateral portal when placed in traction [2]. A nearby structure of importance is the superior gluteal nerve which courses along the deep surface of the gluteus medius from posterior to anterior. It is typically between 44 mm [3] and 64.1 mm [2] away from the portal. The sciatic nerve is 40.2 mm away [2]. Once an anterior portal is placed, this portal is visualized and confirmed to be in a proper position. An arthroscopic blade is then introduced through the cannula, and a portion of the capsule is incised to assist with camera and instrument mobility within the central compartment.

Anterior Portal for the Central Compartment

For the anterior portal, the ASIS is palpated and marked and a straight line is drawn distally along the anterior thigh. A perpendicular line is drawn from the tip of the greater trochanter anteriorly until it intersects with the previous line. The point of intersection is the location for the anterior portal. A spinal needle is then directed approximately 30° toward midline and 45° cephalad into the joint under direct visualization [1]. The path of the portal travels through the sartorius and the rectus femoris. The portal is typically 63 mm distal to the ASIS, and at that point the lateral femoral cutaneous nerve has typically divided into two or three branches and is therefore at risk (within 2–4 mm), while the femoral nerve is 32 mm away [3]. There is variability in the ascending branch of the lateral circumflex femoral artery, but on average it is 36 mm inferior to this portal [1].

Modified Anterior Portal for the Central Compartment

The modified anterior portal is slightly modified from descriptions in the literature as the adjusted position seems to facilitate anchor placement for labral repairs. A line is drawn from the anterior portal to the anterolateral portal. The portal is located approximately 2 cm distal to the midpoint of this line. Robertson and Kelly describe the positioning of the mid-anterior portal as an equilateral triangle with the three points being the anterior portal, the anterolateral portal, and the mid-anterior portal [2]. We prefer a configuration that is best described as an isosceles triangle with the two equal sides being the line from the anterior portal to the modified anterior portal and the line from the anterolateral portal to the modified anterior portal (Fig. 36.2) [4].

The modified anterior portal is made under arthroscopic visualization from the anterolateral portal. Once the spinal needle is visualized in the joint, the skin is incised and a hemostat is utilized to spread the soft tissue in an effort to

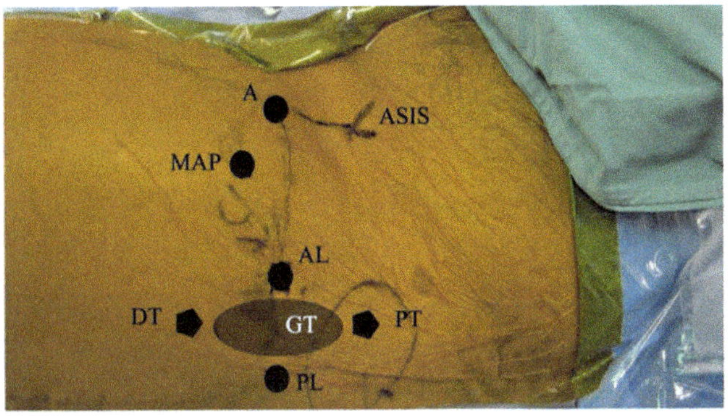

Fig. 36.2 Picture of modified anterior portal showing the isosceles triangle in a left hip. *A* anterior portal, *MAP* modified anterior portal, *AL* anterolateral portal, *PL* posterolateral portal, *GT* greater trochanter, *PT* proximal trochanteric portal, *DT* distal trochanteric. From Stubbs AJ, Mason P. Iliotibial Band Release. In Byrd JWT, editor. Operative Hip Arthroscopy 3rd ed. New York: Springer; 2013. p. 291–8. Reprinted with permission from Springer

avoid the lateral femoral cutaneous nerve branches. The portal pierces the tensor fascia lata and then splits the interval between the gluteus minimus and the rectus femoris [2]. When using the equilateral triangle technique, the lateral femoral cutaneous nerve is 25.2 mm away and has typically already divided into two or more branches at the level of the portal. The ascending branch of the lateral circumflex femoral artery is highly variable, but an average is 19.2 mm from the portal [2].

Posterolateral Portal for the Central Compartment

The posterolateral portal is positioned approximately 1 cm posterior to the tip of the greater trochanter, approximately 20 mm posterior to the anterolateral portal. This portal pierces the gluteus medius and minimus and courses superior and anterior to the piriformis tendon [1]. It is angled 5° cephalad and 5° anterior [2]. The sciatic nerve is anywhere from 21.8 mm [2] to 29 mm away from this portal. The superior gluteal nerve is 44 mm away [1].

Portal Placement for the Peripheral Compartment

At our institution, access to the peripheral compartment is achieved by the anterolateral and modified anterior portals without the use of fluoroscopy or a spinal needle. The patient is taken out of traction, and the peripheral compartment is visualized utilizing various combinations of hip flexion and extension along with internal and external rotation.

Portal Placement for the Peritrochanteric/Lateral Compartment

Access to the peritrochanteric/lateral compartment is accomplished with the leg placed in full extension, 20° of abduction, and 15° of internal rotation. The anterior portal is placed 10 mm lateral to the anterior superior iliac spine and is directed into the interval between the tensor fascia lata and sartorius. Similar to the initial entry into the subacromial space in the shoulder, the cannula is swept back and forth between the iliotibial band and the greater trochanter [5].

The distal trochanteric portal is placed midway between the tip of the greater trochanter and vastus tubercle, along the posterior one-third of the greater trochanteric midline. It can be used for both proximal and distal work and evaluation [5]. The proximal trochanteric portal is placed proximal to the tip of the greater trochanter in line with the distal trochanteric portal. It is predominantly used for proximal work and distal evaluation [5].

The Three Compartments of Arthroscopic Hip Anatomy

Hip arthroscopists typically divide the hip joint into three compartments—the central, peripheral, and peritrochanteric or lateral compartments. The central compartment anatomy is best visualized under traction and includes the femoral head, acetabulum, labrum, ligamentum teres, and psoas tendon. The peripheral compartment is best visualized after releasing traction and contains a portion of the femoral head, the femoral neck, the lateral synovial fold, the ligament of Weitbrecht (medial synovial fold), the zona orbicularis, and the anterior synovial fold. The peritrochanteric or lateral compartment includes the gluteus maximus, medius, and minimus along with the vastus lateralis. The iliotibial band serves as the lateral margin to the space.

Arthroscopic Anatomy of Central Compartment

The central compartment is accessed under traction and is approached initially through the anterolateral portal. With proper placement of the portal and subsequent introduction of the arthroscope, the first visualized structure is typically the superior aspect of the femoral head and the anteromedial acetabulum. A 70° arthroscope allows for visualization of much of the joint with isolated movement of the optics and minimal movement of the arthroscope itself. Adjusting the optics to look anterior displays the anterior triangle, which is bordered by the femoral head, the anterior labrum, and the

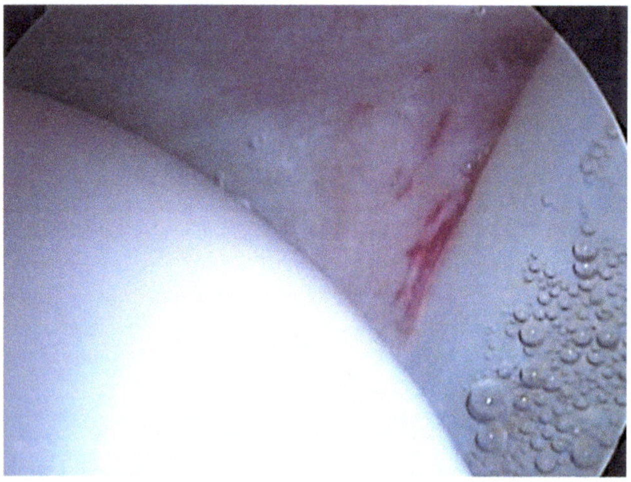

Fig. 36.3 Arthroscopic picture of anterior triangle. © Allston J. Stubbs, MD

edge of the arthroscope superiorly (Fig. 36.3). Under direct visualization, a needle can be introduced into this triangle through the anterior capsule for a second portal.

Femoral Head

The femoral head is two-thirds of a sphere but somewhat flattened in the area where the acetabulum applies its greatest load [6]. Approximately 80% of the femoral head can be visualized arthroscopically [7]. The ligamentum teres inserts at the fovea capitus located on the anteromedial portion of the head [7].

Acetabulum

The acetabulum is a concave structure with a horseshoe-shaped area of hyaline cartilage that extends to the periphery where it is met by the labrum [7]. The inferomedial portion of the acetabulum contains the acetabular fossa. The superior one-third of the fossa has dense fibroconnective tissue without a synovial lining, and the lower two-thirds is filled with pulvinar or fat pad tissue that often appears bulbous [7]. It fills the fossa, is highly vascular, and likely plays a role in joint lubrication [6]. The transverse acetabular ligament traverses the fossa at the inferior margin. A probe can normally be passed between the transverse ligament and the inferior acetabular fossa, entering the inferior recess [7]. The lowest margin of the fossa contains dense synovial tissue that passes beneath the transverse acetabular ligament. The ligamentum teres attaches to the posteroinferior portion of the acetabular fossa (Fig. 36.4) [7]. The physeal scar which is the fused triradiate cartilage in adults typically extends linearly along the medial wall of the acetabulum and can be anterior, posterior, or both anterior and posterior to the acetabular fossa [1]. In adults, the articular cartilage is absent in the fossa and should not be interpreted as a pathologic finding (Fig. 36.5) The stellate crease, located immediately superior to the acetabular fossa, contains a stellate pattern that can be confused for early degenerative changes but is in fact a normally occurring process, even in young adults (Fig. 36.6) [1].

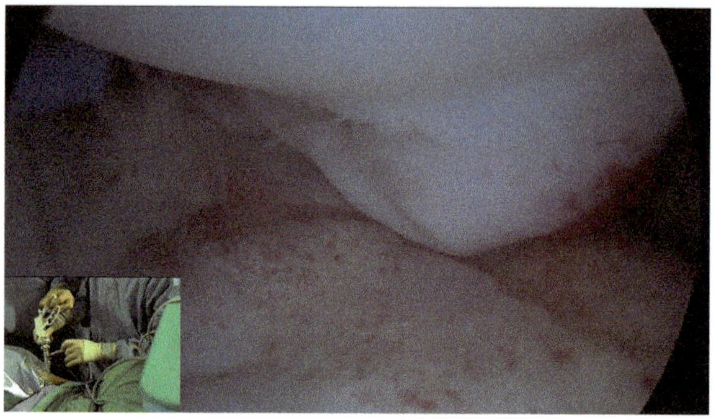

Fig. 36.4 Arthroscopic picture of ligamentum teres attachment to acetabular fossa. © Allston J. Stubbs, MD

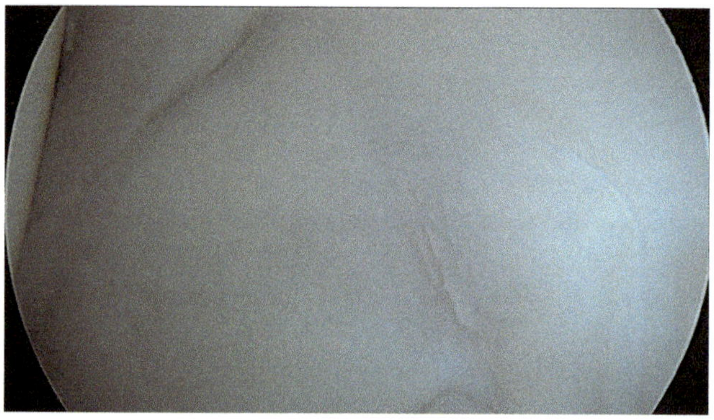

Fig. 36.5 Arthroscopic picture of physeal scar. © Allston J. Stubbs, MD

Fig. 36.6 Arthroscopic picture of stellate crease. © Allston J. Stubbs, MD

Labrum

The labrum is attached circumferentially to the perimeter of the acetabulum with anterior and posterior attachments to the transverse acetabular ligament (Fig. 36.7) [8]. The lateral and anterior portions are the most variable in structure [1].

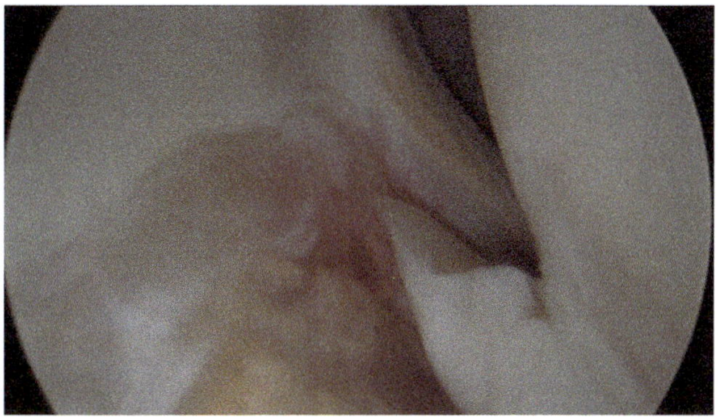

Fig. 36.7 Arthroscopic picture of transverse acetabular ligament and the labral attachments. © Allston J. Stubbs, MD

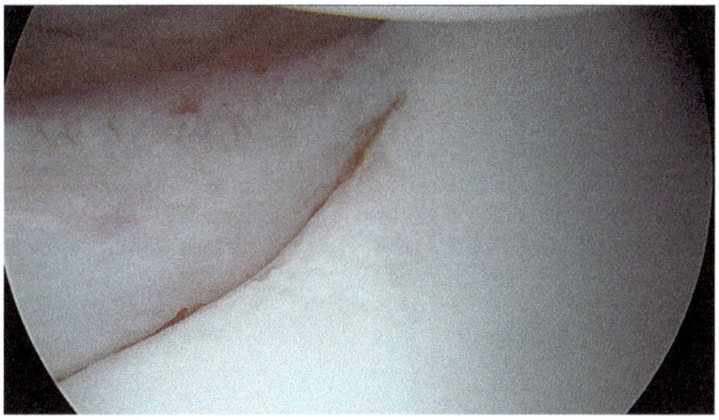

Fig. 36.8 Arthroscopic picture of perilabral sulcus. © Allston J. Stubbs, MD

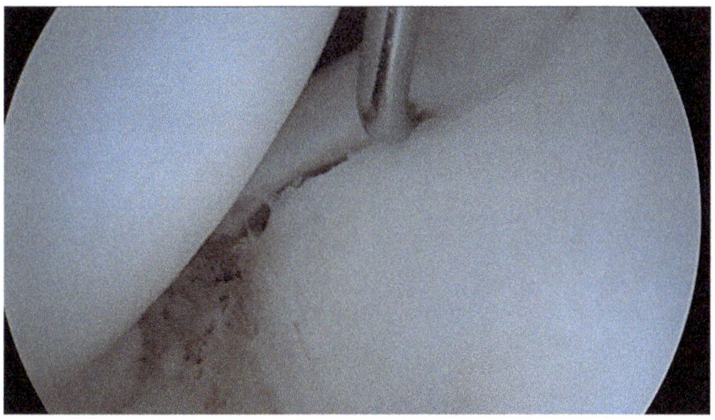

Fig. 36.9 Arthroscopic picture of a labral cleft normal variant. © Allston J. Stubbs, MD

The labrum is more triangular in cross section posterosuperiorly and thinner anteroinferiorly [7]. The vascularity and healing potential are greatest at the peripheral capsulo-labral junction [9]. A perilabral sulcus can be present at the periphery of the labrum (Fig. 36.8). There is a distinct groove at the acetabular fossa that separates labral tissue from hyaline cartilage [7]. The labral cleft separates acetabular articular surface from the labrum and is considered a normal variant as long as the tissue does not appear damaged and there is no healing response (Fig. 36.9) [1].

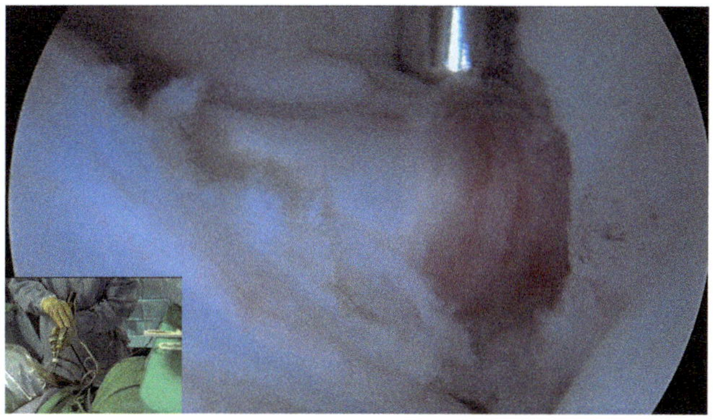

Fig. 36.10 Arthroscopic picture of psoas tendon at the level of the labrum. © Allston J. Stubbs, MD

Ligamentum Teres

The ligamentum teres originates from the posteroinferior acetabular fossa and inserts at the fovea capitus which is a small depressed bare spot on the medial aspect of the femoral head [6]. In a dysplastic hip or in the setting of a deficient labrum, it may function as a secondary stabilizer [10]. Some authors consider it to have an anterior and posterior bundle [6], while others report three bundles including a medial bundle [11]. The average length is between 30 and 35 mm [11]. In external rotation the anterior bundle tightens [6]. Capillaries may be seen, but there is no substantial vasculature visualized [7].

Psoas Tendon

The psoas tendon synovial reflection can be visualized in the central compartment with the arthroscope directed anteromedial. After resection of sufficient capsule in this area, the bursa associated with the tendon is visualized. Gentle debridement of the bursa will reveal the psoas tendon (Fig. 36.10). The tendon is intra-articular in 20 % of people; otherwise, only the bursa communicates with the joint [12]. The tendon typically creates a medial indentation in the anterior labrum referred to as the "psoas U" [5]. At the level of the labrum, the iliopsoas is approximately 40 % tendon and 60 % muscle [13].

Posterior Recess

The posterior recess is a space most often viewed from an anterior portal with the arthroscope facing posterior. Along with the inferior recess, it is a common location for intra-articular loose bodies [6].

Arthroscopic Anatomy of the Peripheral Compartment

Access to the peripheral compartment is best achieved after the release of the traction. The hip is flexed until adequate visualization is achieved. The peripheral compartment is considered extra-articular but intracapsular. At our institution, this compartment is visualized through the anterolateral portal and the modified mid-anterior portal.

Femoral Neck

The femoral head and neck junction is best visualized with the hip in flexion to allow the capsule to relax. The area most commonly associated with a CAM lesion along the anterosuperior neck is easily visualized through the anterolateral portal. The neck gives way to the articular surface of the femoral head more proximally.

Synovial Folds

The synovial folds of the hip can be used as reliable points of reference for peripheral compartment anatomy. The lateral synovial fold is located in a posterosuperior position along the femoral neck. Recognizing the lateral synovial fold is critical to avoiding the primary blood supply to the femoral head as it is slightly anterior to the medial circumflex femoral artery and retinacular vessels (Fig. 36.11) [14]. The medial synovial fold is also known as the ligament of Weitbrecht. It is a capsular reflection located along the inferior femoral neck in the 6 o'clock position (Fig. 36.12) [6]. The anterior synovial fold lies midway between the lateral and medial folds.

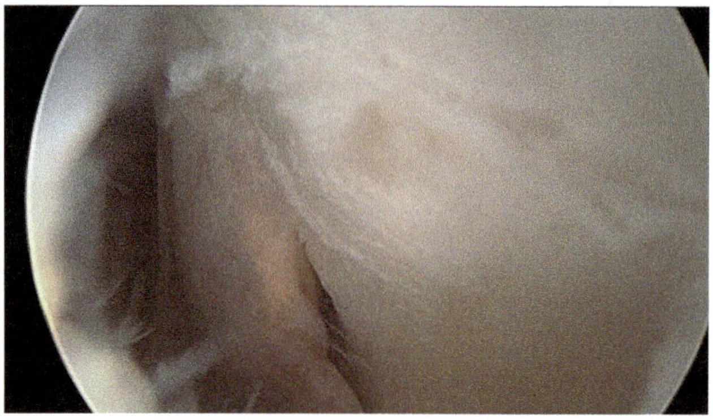

Fig. 36.11 Arthroscopic picture of the lateral synovial fold and retinacular vessels. © Allston J. Stubbs, MD

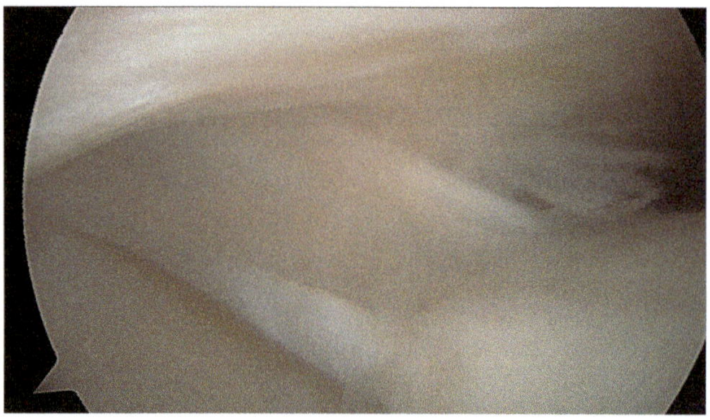

Fig. 36.12 Arthroscopic picture of the ligament of Weitbrecht. © Allston J. Stubbs, MD

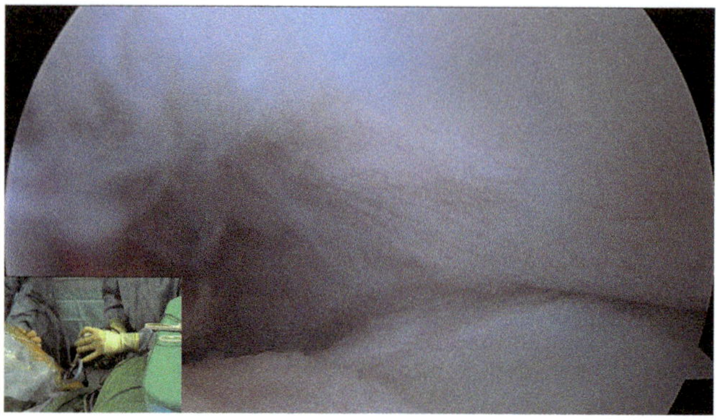

Fig. 36.13 Arthroscopic picture of zona orbicularis. © Allston J. Stubbs, MD

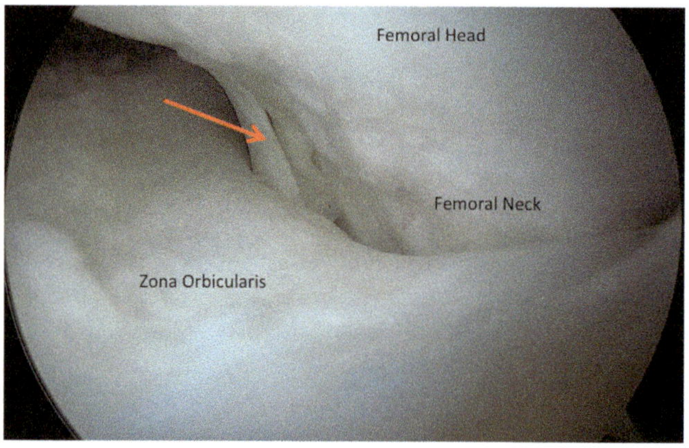

Fig. 36.14 *Red arrow* indicates terminal branches of MFCA. Peripheral compartment view with 70° arthroscope in mid-anterior portal. © Allston J. Stubbs, MD

Zona Orbicularis

The zona orbicularis is a capsular condensation that wraps around approximately three-quarters of the femoral neck [6, 7]. Anteriorly, the capsule blends with the terminal fibers of the iliofemoral ligament to form a leash or a collar around the neck of the femur (Fig. 36.13) [6]. Its function is poorly understood; however, it may contribute to stability in distraction [15]. Its fibers tighten in extension and loosen in flexion and external rotation [16, 17].

Relevant Arthroscopic Anatomy of the Medial Femoral Circumflex Artery

Knowledge of the anatomic location of the medial femoral circumflex artery (MFCA) and its branches is critical to avoiding damage to the vasculature and possible avascular necrosis of the femoral head. The MFCA, along with the lateral femoral circumflex artery, is a branch off of the external iliac system. The MFCA has five main branches, the superficial, ascending, acetabular, descending, and deep branches. The deep branch of the MFCA is the primary blood supply to the femoral head and can be visualized near the lateral synovial fold arthroscopically

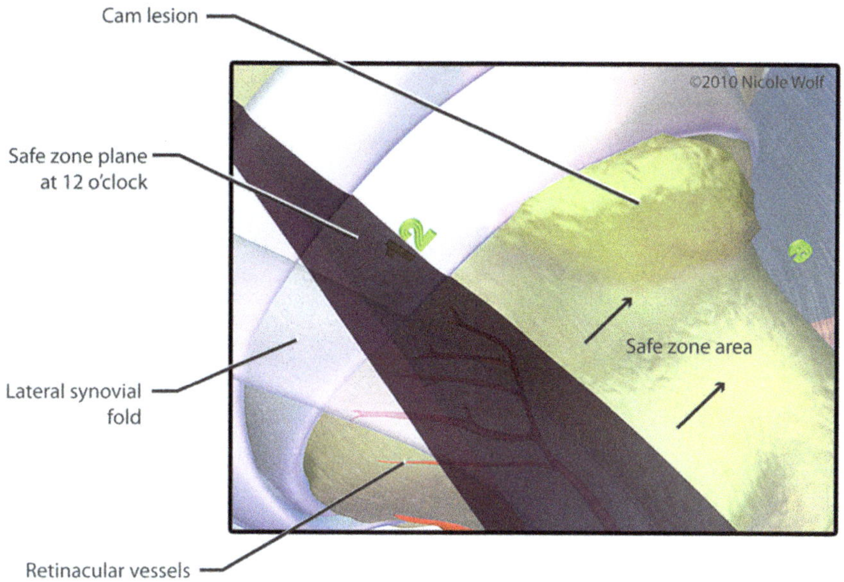

Fig. 36.15 An anterolateral portal perspective on the femoral neck safe zone with labeled anatomic and intracapsular landmarks. The femoral neck safe zone is on the anterior half of the femoral neck. From McCormick F, et al. Vascular safe zones in hip arthroscopy. Am J Sports Med. 2011 Jul;39 Suppl:64S–71S. Reprinted with permission from Sage Publications

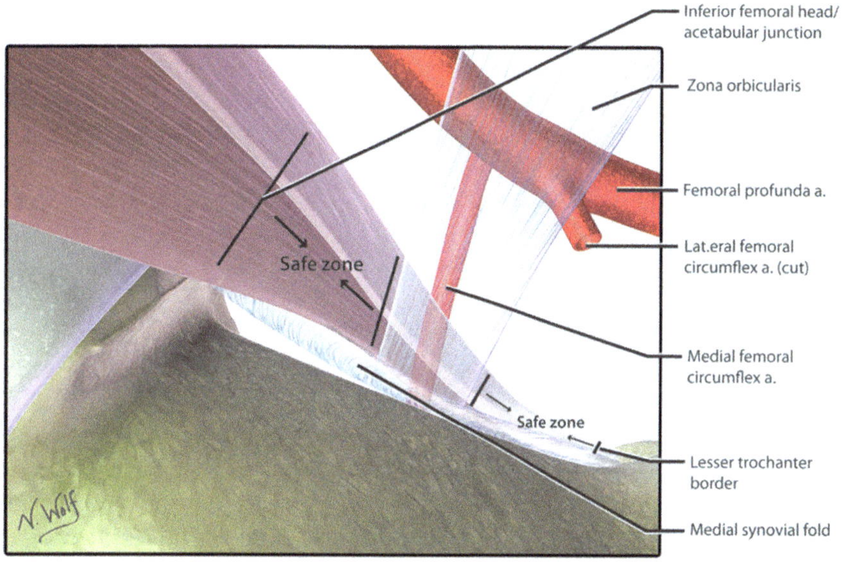

Fig. 36.16 An anterolateral portal perspective of the psoas tendon release safe zone with labeled anatomic and intracapsular landmarks. The psoas tendon release safe zone is astride the middle third of the medial hip capsule (bordered by the lesser trochanter and inferior femoral head/acetabular junction). From McCormick F, et al. Vascular safe zones in hip arthroscopy. Am J Sports Med. 2011 Jul;39 Suppl:64S–71S. Reprinted with permission from SAGE Publications

(Fig. 36.14) [18]. On a right hip, the MFCA inserts on the posterosuperior femoral neck medial to the greater trochanter at the 10:30 to 12 o'clock position with a mean of 11:15, placing it slightly posterior to the lateral synovial fold [14]. Anywhere from two to six retinacular vessels travel medially in the same region of the clock face and then become subchondral at the head-neck junction with 97 % of the vessels being posterior to 12 o'clock (Fig. 36.15) [14]. Therefore, the safe zone is considered to be from 12 to 6 o'clock.

The MFCA anatomy is also relevant when considering a psoas tendon release in the peripheral compartment. The psoas tendon release safe zone is on either side of the middle third of the medial hip capsule. The zone is bordered by the lesser trochanter inferiorly and the inferior femoral head/acetabular junction superiorly. The middle third of this region is the location of the MFCA and should be avoided (Fig. 36.16) [14].

Relative to the inferior femoral head/acetabular junction, the MFCA is 24.3 ± 5 mm distal and lateral. Relative to the medial cortex of the femoral neck, it is 15 mm medial. Relative to the lesser trochanter, it is 22.9 ± 5 mm proximal and medial [14]. In short, a central compartment release accomplishes the task furthest away from the MFCA, while a peripheral compartment release places the MFCA millimeters away.

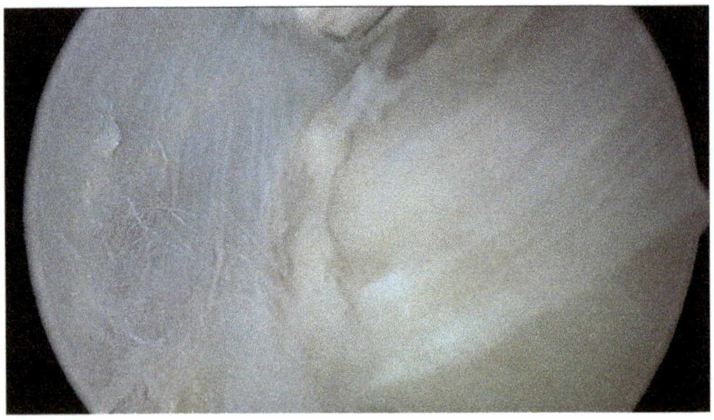

Fig. 36.17 Picture of gluteus maximus inserting along the posterior aspect of the iliotibial band at the linea aspera. © Allston J. Stubbs, MD

Peritrochanteric/Lateral Compartment Endoscopic Anatomy

The peritrochanteric or lateral compartment is visualized without traction and with the operative leg in slight abduction to allow for a potential space. This space is further developed with the introduction of the endoscope as the saline fills the area. Initial anatomic structures are visualized from an anterior portal with the scope directed distally. This view typically includes the gluteus maximus inserting along the posterior aspect of the iliotibial band at the linea aspera (Fig. 36.17) [5]. More proximally, the longitudinal fibers of the vastus lateralis are visible and can be traced to their insertion on the vastus tubercle.

Gluteus Minimus and Medius

The peritrochanteric space also includes the gluteus medius and minimus. Efforts to repair these tendons must be combined with a thorough knowledge of their insertion sites (Fig. 36.18). The gluteus minimus tendon is more anterior and has a single insertion at the inner aspect of the anterosuperior margin of the greater trochanter upon the anterior facet (Fig. 36.19) [19]. The gluteus medius tendon is more posterior and has two separate insertion sites on the greater trochanter [20, 21]. The lateral facet has an insertion site of 428.0 mm^2, and the superoposterior facet has an insertion site of 196.5 mm^2 [20]. The greater trochanteric bursa typically covers the posterior facet and the lateral insertion of the gluteus medius insertion [21].

Iliotibial Band

The iliotibial band may be best visualized from the proximal trochanteric portal, placed a few centimeters proximal to the greater trochanter, and a distal trochanteric portal, placed in line with the proximal trochanteric portal and several centimeters distal to the greater trochanter [22]. The traction is completely relaxed, and the endoscope is placed superficially between the skin and the iliotibial band (Fig. 36.20). Saline from the endoscope helps to develop this potential space. Careful attention is given to the posterior one-third of the iliotibial band as it is implicated in coxa saltans externus [5].

Arthroscopic Anatomy of the Hip Capsular Ligaments

While individual fibers of the hip capsular ligaments cannot be discerned arthroscopically, their anatomic locations remain relevant given their functional importance. An awareness of their locations relative to the hip clock face is helpful for intraoperative decision making (Fig. 36.21). The iliofemoral ligament, also known as the Y-ligament or the ligament of Bigelow, is typically pierced by the anterolateral and anterior portals. On a right hip, the ligament is present from 12:45 to 3 o'clock [23]. The medial and lateral arms limit external rotation, and the lateral arm is particularly effective at limiting external rotation when the hip is flexed and in a neutral position. When the hip is in extension, the lateral arm also limits internal rotation [24]. The pubofemoral ligament is present from the 3:30 to 5:30 position. The lateral border is at the "psoas U," while the medial border is at the junction of the anteroinferior acetabulum and cotyloid fossa [23]. The predominant function of the pubofemoral ligament is to limit external rotation [24]. The ischiofemoral ligament is present from the 7:45 to 10:30 position and limits internal rotation [23, 24].

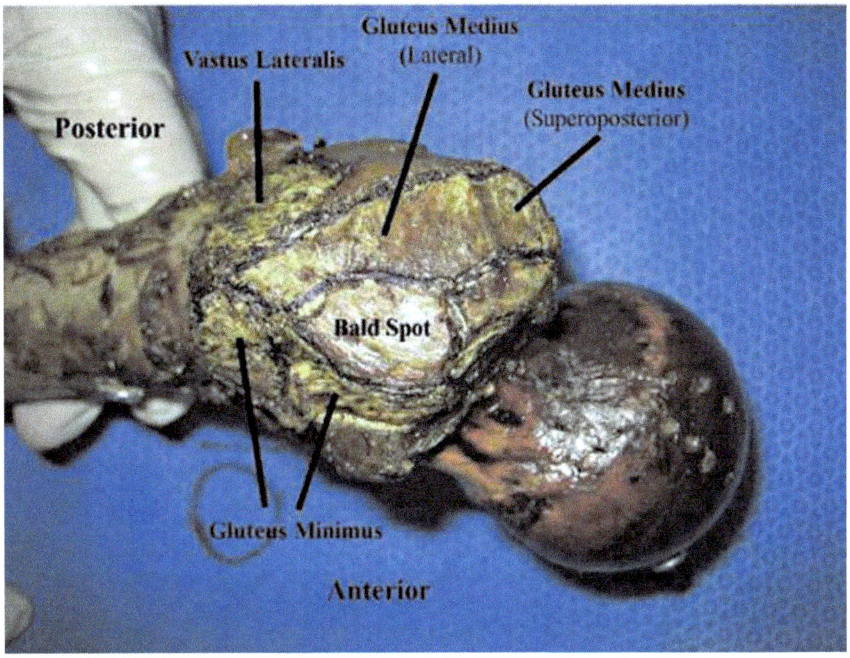

Fig. 36.18 Cadaveric right proximal femur, showing the soft tissue attachments onto the greater trochanter. From Robertson WJ, et al. Anatomy and dimensions of the gluteus medius tendon insertion. Arthrosc. 2008 Feb;24(2):130–136. Reprinted with permission from Elsevier Limited

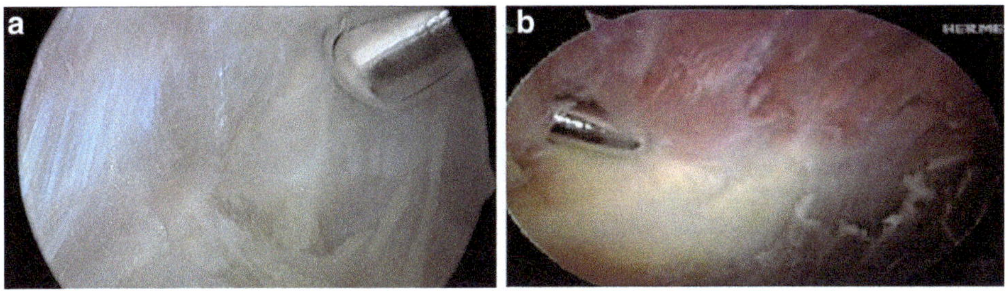

Fig. 36.19 Arthroscopic picture of gluteus minimus and medius pictures: (**a**) right hip and (**b**) left hip. © Allston J. Stubbs, MD

Conclusion

Proper room setup, patient positioning, and portal placement are necessary for reproducible results in the operating room. Attention to those details allows for consistent arthroscopic views that are essential in recognizing the normal and abnormal arthroscopic anatomy of the hip. A command of this anatomy is a powerful tool that will increase the likelihood of success while decreasing the possibility of complications.

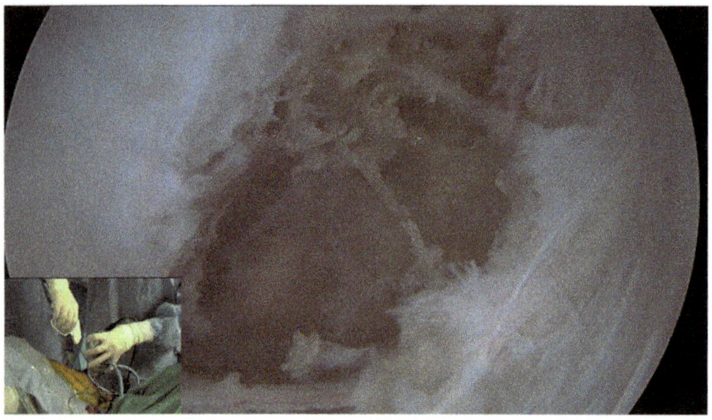

Fig. 36.20 Arthroscopic picture of the iliotibial band. © Allston J. Stubbs, MD

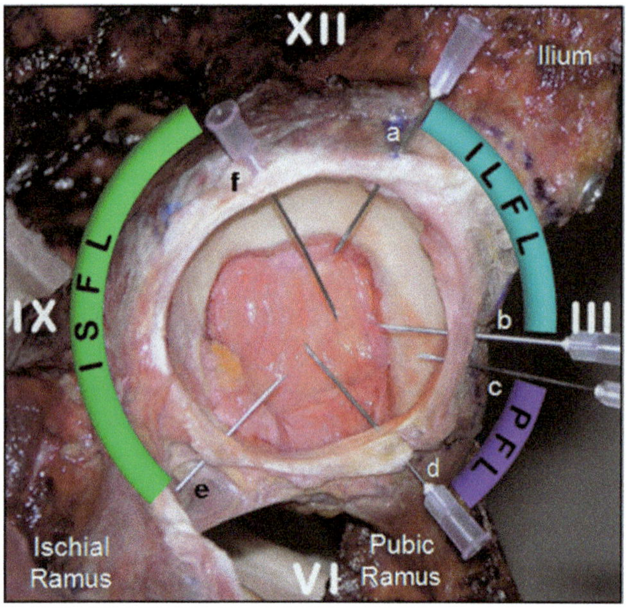

Fig. 36.21 Annotated photograph showing a right acetabulum in situ from one cadaveric specimen. The needles demarcate the borders of the hip capsular ligaments. The roman numerals represent hours on a clock face: 3 o'clock is anterior, 6 o'clock is inferior, 9 o'clock is posterior, and 12 o'clock is lateral. ((*a*) ILFL lateral border, (*b*) ILFL medial border, (*c*) PFL lateral border, (*d*) PFL medial border, (*e*) ISFL inferior/medial border, and (*f*) ISFL superior/lateral border (Courtesy of Marc R. Safran, M.D.)

References

1. Byrd JW. Hip arthroscopy, the supine approach: technique and anatomy of the intraarticular and peripheral compartments. Tech Orthop. 2005;20(1):17–31.
2. Robertson WJ, Kelly BT. The safe zone for hip arthroscopy: a cadaveric assessment of central, peripheral, and lateral compartment portal placement. Arthroscopy. 2008;24(9):1019–26.
3. Byrd JW, Pappas JN, Pedley MJ. Hip arthroscopy: an anatomic study of portal placement and relationship to the extra-articular structures. Arthroscopy. 1995;11(4):418–23.
4. Stubbs AJ, Mason P. Iliotibial band release. In: Byrd JWT, editor. Operative hip arthroscopy. 3rd ed. New York: Springer; 2013. p. 291–8.
5. Voos JE, Rudzki JR, Shindle MK, Martin H, Kelly BT. Arthroscopic anatomy and surgical techniques for peritrochanteric space disorders in the hip. Arthroscopy. 2007;23(11):1246.e1–5.
6. Ranawat AS, Kelly BT. Anatomy of the hip: open and arthroscopic structure and function. Oper Tech Orthop. 2005;15(3):160–74.
7. Keene GS, Villar RN. Arthroscopic anatomy of the hip: an in vivo study. Arthroscopy. 1994;10(4):392–9.
8. Philippon MJ. The role of arthroscopic thermal capsulorrhaphy in the hip. Clin Sports Med. 2001;20(4):817–29.
9. Kelly BT, Shapiro GS, Digiovanni CW, Buly RL, Potter HG, Hannafin JA. Vascularity of the hip labrum: a cadaveric investigation. Arthroscopy. 2005;21(1):3–11.
10. Rao J, Zhou YX, Villar RN. Injury to the ligamentum teres. Mechanism, findings, and results of treatment. Clin Sports Med. 2001;20(4):791–9. vii.
11. Demange MK, Kakuda CMS, Pereira CAM, Sakaki MH, Albuquerque RFM. Influence of the femoral head ligament on hip mechanical function. Acta Orthop Bras. 2007;15(4):187–90.
12. Philippon MJ. Arthroscopy of the hip in the management of the athlete. In: McGinty JB, editor. Operative arthroscopy. 3rd ed. Philadelphia: Lippincott, Williams & Wilkins; 2003. p. 879–83.
13. Blomberg JR, Zellner BS, Keene JS. Cross-sectional analysis of iliopsoas muscle-tendon units at the sites of arthroscopic tenotomies: an anatomic study. Am J Sports Med. 2011;39(Suppl):58S–63.
14. McCormick F, Kleweno CP, Kim YJ, Martin SD. Vascular safe zones in hip arthroscopy. Am J Sports Med. 2011;39(Suppl):64S–71.
15. Ito H, Song Y, Lindsey DP, Safran MR, Giori NJ. The proximal hip joint capsule and the zona orbicularis contribute to hip joint stability in distraction. J Orthop Res. 2009;27(8):989–95.
16. Callaghan J, Rosenburg A, Rubash H, editors. The adult hip. 1st ed. Philadelphia: Lippincott-Raven; 1998.
17. Dvorak M, Duncan CP, Day B. Arthroscopic anatomy of the hip. Arthroscopy. 1990;6(4):264–73.
18. Gautier E, Ganz K, Krugel N, Gill T, Ganz R. Anatomy of the medial femoral circumflex artery and its surgical implications. J Bone Joint Surg Br. 2000;82(5):679–83.
19. Gottschalk F, Kourosh S, Leveau B. The functional anatomy of tensor fasciae latae and gluteus medius and minimus. J Anat. 1989;166:179–89.
20. Robertson WJ, Gardner MJ, Barker JU, Boraiah S, Lorich DG, Kelly BT. Anatomy and dimensions of the gluteus medius tendon insertion. Arthroscopy. 2008;24(2):130–6.
21. Pfirrmann CW, Chung CB, Theumann NH, Trudell DJ, Resnick D. Greater trochanter of the hip: attachment of the abductor mechanism and a complex of three bursae—MR imaging and MR bursography in cadavers and MR imaging in asymptomatic volunteers. Radiology. 2001;221(2):469–77.
22. Ilizaliturri Jr VM, Camacho-Galindo J. Endoscopic treatment of snapping hips, iliotibial band, and iliopsoas tendon. Sports Med Arthrosc. 2010;18(2):120–7.
23. Telleria JJ, Lindsey DP, Giori NJ, Safran MR. An anatomic arthroscopic description of the hip capsular ligaments for the hip arthroscopist. Arthroscopy. 2011;27(5):628–36.
24. Martin HD, Savage A, Braly BA, Palmer IJ, Beall DP, Kelly B. The function of the hip capsular ligaments: a quantitative report. Arthroscopy. 2008;24(2):188–95.

Hip Arthroscopy: Anatomy and Technical Pearls of the Procedure

37

Scott D. Martin and David M. Privitera

Introduction

The hip joint presents challenges not encountered in other joints commonly requiring arthroscopy. The central compartment has strict confines, and many of the instruments used are straight, rigid, and better suited for less constrained joints. The depth of the joint makes triangulation difficult, and the 70° arthroscope has a variable focal length with a small depth of field. Additionally, working in the central compartment requires traction which adds time constraints. These challenges create a steep learning curve for arthroscopist surgeons.

Historically, hip arthroscopy was performed through two portals for diagnostic purposes, as well as to remove loose bodies and debride the labrum and chondral surfaces. With a greater understanding of femoroacetabular impingement and advancements in techniques, complex hip arthroscopic procedures are now performed through additional portals which are safe and reliable and allow additional access to the joint. The indications have expanded to include labral repair and reconstruction, microfracture, femoral and acetabular osteoplasty, and removal of benign tumors.

As the field of hip arthroscopy evolves, the importance of strict adherence to guidelines for surgical indications developed from evidence-based medicine will occur. In addition, residency and sports fellowship training programs will need to provide formal didactic training to better prepare orthopedic surgeons of the future [1]. The purpose of this chapter is to describe current surgical techniques to treat simple, as well as complex, hip joint problems to improve hip joint preservation.

S.D. Martin, MD (✉)
Division of Sports Medicine, Department of Orthopedic Surgery, Brigham and Women's Hospital/Harvard Medical School, 75 Francis Street, Boston, MA 02115, USA
e-mail: sdmartin@partners.org

D.M. Privitera, MD
Division of Sports Medicine, Department of Orthopedic Surgery, Rochester Regional Health System, Rochester, NY, USA
e-mail: dave.privitera@gmail.com

Positioning and Distraction: My Technique

The use of traction for working in the central compartment demands attention to detail, alacrity, and awareness of surgical time. As popularized by Byrd et al. [2], it is our preference to perform hip arthroscopy in the supine position, although the lateral position may also be used. The patient is placed under general anesthesia with complete paralysis to decrease the amount of traction force required during the procedure; regional anesthetics may be used, but it is important to have a good motor block. The patient can also be placed in Trendelenburg position to reduce the amount of traction necessary for hip distraction [3]. We use a specialized table with a hip distraction device. The perineal post is wrapped with a silicone gel pad [4] and is relatively lateralized to the operative side to add a transverse vector to the applied traction. It has been shown that a well-padded, large-diameter (>10 cm) perineal post significantly reduces perineal pressure [5] and minimizes complications to the pudendal nerve [5, 6]. In males, the genitalia are positioned to the opposite side to minimize pressure on the pudendal nerve and reduce the chance of entrapping the genitals. In females, labial trauma has been reported [7], so females must be centered on the post to avoid unnecessary trauma and pressure due to eversion or malpositioning of the labia. In experienced hands, pudendal nerve palsies occur in about 1 % of patients [7], so all measures must be taken to minimize this potential complication. Apply intermittent traction, a technique described later in the chapter; take care to decrease overall traction times from an upper limit of 2 h; and use a padded perineal post. Silicone is ideal, but Webril, bandage pads, and foam are alternative materials that can be substituted to cover the firm rubber post [8, 9].

J.C. McCarthy et al. (eds.), *Hip Joint Restoration*, DOI 10.1007/978-1-4614-0694-5_37

The feet and ankles are well padded with foam boots and secured into traction boots. The nonoperative leg is abducted, so the C-arm fluoroscope has enough room to allow for imaging both AP and lateral views. We place the operative leg in neutral rotation with the patella facing the ceiling and abducted approximately 10°–15°. The arm on the operative side is folded across the chest, so it doesn't interfere with C-arm placement. A gel pad is wrapped around the elbow/forearm like a sugar tong splint, and appropriate padding is used at the wrist/hand to keep the wrist in a neutral position. These precautions are taken so once the arm is taped down, complications to the median nerve at the wrist and ulnar nerve at the elbow can be avoided by preventing unnecessary pressure at these locations. The umbilicus and anterior superior iliac spine (ASIS) are exposed so that they can be incorporated into the sterile field for orientation and anatomic referencing.

Full relaxation with a motor blockade is necessary to reduce the amount of traction needed to distract the hip [10]; it's confirmed with the anesthesiologist at this time. The C-arm is brought in between the legs to view the operative hip, and mild traction is applied to the nonoperative leg to help secure the pelvis against the post. Next, mild traction is applied to the operative leg to achieve 1 cm of distraction. Once sufficient distraction is confirmed with a vacuum sign, the white semilunar signal seen on fluoroscopy created by negative pressure, traction is released and the operative site is prepped and draped.

Portal Placement

The safe portal access zone is defined as a region lateral to a sagittal line from the ASIS to the lateral border of the patella [11, 12]. Traction is reapplied, and the anterolateral (AL) portal is established with fluoroscopic guidance [11]. The portal penetrates the gluteus medius and lies approximately 4–6 cm from the superior gluteal nerve [11, 13]. A 6 in. 17 gauge spinal needle is positioned on top of the skin and viewed via AP fluoroscopic imaging, to get an idea of the entrance angle. This angle, which starts approximately 5–10 mm proximal and anterior to the greater trochanter, is angled 10°–15° cephalad. The needle is inserted in a coronal plane or angled slightly posterior to this plane with the bevel side facing the femoral head. It is positioned just superior to the femoral head, so when the needle is advanced through the capsule, the chance of iatrogenic injury to the labrum is reduced. The stylet is removed from the needle, and a nitinol wire is inserted. As a 5.0 mm cannula is advanced over the nitinol wire, the medial tip of the wire should be free, not lodged against the acetabulum or other firm end point. This avoids coiling and the possibility of wire breakage while advancing the cannula, which has been anecdotally reported. Placement of the nitinol wire should be checked frequently with fluoroscopy while advancing the cannula. While advancing the locked obturator and cannula, a twisting force also prevents scuffing off articular cartilage. Once inside the joint, a 70° arthroscope is placed inside the cannula. The camera is left dry, without inflow, to minimize unnecessary insufflation time and fluid loss. After the AL portal is established, the arthroscope is inserted, and a quick overview of the joint is completed to assess pathology before placing the anterior portal.

Femoral Head Distraction Technique

When appropriate distraction is not achieved with a moderate amount of traction (25–30 lbs), additional distraction is created by injecting the joint with 25–30 mL of saline. This breaks the relative vacuum. If the needle is appropriately placed, pressurized backflow of fluid should follow when the syringe is removed from the needle (Fig. 37.1a). This leads to several additional millimeters of joint distraction with caudal movement of the femoral head (Fig. 37.1b). The needle is reinserted as closely as possible to the femoral head,

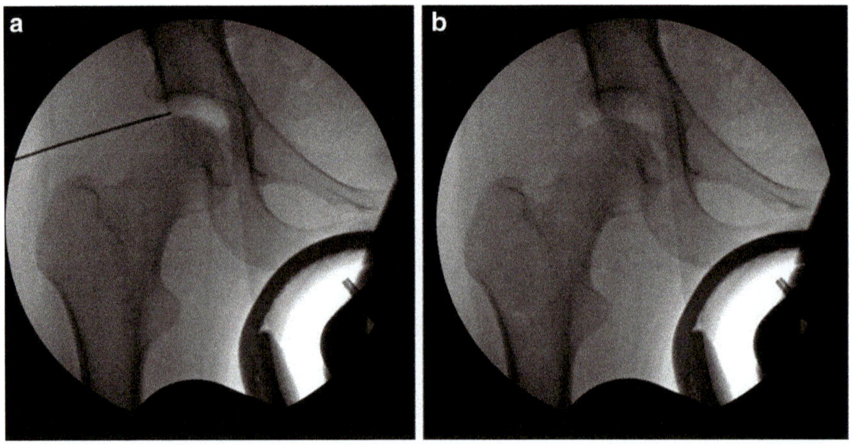

Fig. 37.1 (**a**) AP of the right hip. Vacuum sign with needle penetration of the joint. Needle has cannula inserted. (**b**) AP of the right hip. "Head-drop technique": Injection of 25–30 mL of saline adds several additional millimeters of joint distraction. Published with permission of Scott D. Martin, MD ©2013. All Rights Reserved

and the anterolateral portal is established; backflow of joint fluid verifies needle positioning into the joint. This procedure is helpful in tight hips or in those with a significant pincer overhang and reduces the likelihood of iatrogenic injury to the labrum and/or chondral surfaces during portal placement.

Anterior Portal Placement

The entrance point of the anterior portal is established 1 cm lateral to the safe zone sagittal line and usually 2 cm distal to the transverse line across the tip of the trochanter. The spinal needle is advanced approximately 30° cephalad and 30° toward the midline, which can vary based on the body habitus [5]. Under direct visualization from the anterolateral portal, the needle should penetrate the capsule at the center of an anterior triangle bordered by the femoral head, labrum, and capsular recess. After making a longitudinal skin incision against the needle with a nitinol wire inserted, the subcutaneous soft tissue is freed from the needle with blunt dissection as described below. Be careful not to injure branches of the lateral femoral cutaneous nerve when making the superficial skin incision. The anterior skin of the thigh is quite thin, so only a minimal nick is required followed by dilatation of the portal with a mosquito hemostat.

Cadaveric studies have described the anatomic structures near the anterior portal. Byrd et al. measured, without the use of hip traction, their original anterior portal which is 1 cm medial to our entrance point [11]. They found both the medial branch of the lateral femoral cutaneous nerve and the terminal branch of the ascending branch of the lateral circumflex femoral artery (LCFA) averaged 3 mm from their portal. Anterior portals placed laterally to their location were cautioned as the LFCN has three or more variable, lateral branches at this level which are at high risk for iatrogenic injury [11]. A more recent study using traction and portal placement similar to ours found both the LFCN and terminal branch of the ascending branch of the LCFA an average of 15 mm from the portal, but variant branches were found as close as 1–2 mm [13]. Therefore, the nick-and-spread technique is most important when establishing this portal.

During portal placement, great care is taken to prevent any skin remaining between the portal incision and the nitinol wire. This occurs when the knife penetrates the epidermis but leaves a sliver of dermis around the nitinol wire. As the obturator is advanced in this scenario, a resistance is encountered at the dermis and may lead to wire breakage if aggressively pushed. Usually, a twisting motion with gentle force will free the dermal sliver, but if not, re-incision of the portal may be necessary. After blunt dissection with a mosquito hemostat and removal of the needle, the cannula and obturator are advanced over the nitinol wire.

Joint Inspection

The anterior portal cannula is slightly pulled back to a position just superficial to the capsule. A beaver blade is advanced, and a capsulotomy is made toward the anterolateral portal/camera. The incision only needs to be a few millimeters to loosen the tension around the anterior portal and avoid iatrogenic injury to the chondral surfaces when maneuvering the cannula into the central compartment. The camera should be switched to the anterior portal, and the anterolateral portal is checked for placement. A diagnostic arthroscopic exam of the central compartment is performed. Although we do not routinely use a posterolateral portal for our diagnostic exam, it may be useful for removal of loose bodies and access to the acetabular notch. Please see other reading for additional information [14].

If a labral tear is encountered, a decision must be made as to whether the tear is amenable to repair or needs to be debrided. As long as the tear has sufficient remaining tissue (not too complex), or the labrum is not too degenerated or ossified, we advocate repairing the tear if it is full thickness. If the tear is partial thickness with a high-grade, large surface area and/or associated with a pincer lesion, we also advocate repair. If the tear is repairable, a capsulectomy is performed at the anterior portal by widening with a shaver and thermal device to form a proper viewing portal for labral repair. The use of any thermal device requires high flow through the joint to keep the arthroscopic fluid from warming and damaging the chondrocytes [15]. Consistent with the current literature, we rarely repair labra without concomitantly addressing bony pathology [16].

Additional Portal Placement

If the labral tear is amenable to repair, we establish two additional portals to facilitate the technique; first is a mid-anterolateral (MAL) portal. The MAL portal is utilized for placement of suture anchors and shuttling of sutures. It can also facilitate microfracture of the acetabulum and chondral debridement. This portal is placed approximately 3–5 cm distal to the halfway point between the anterior and anterolateral portal; the points between the anterior, anterolateral, and mid-anterolateral should form approximately an isosceles triangle. The spinal needle is inclined approximately 45° cephalad to enter the joint under direct arthroscopic visualization. The closest structure to this portal is the terminal branch of the ascending LCFA at an average of 10 mm (Robertson, Arthroscopy 2008) [13]. A 5.5 mm cannula is placed to facilitate anchor placement.

Secondly, we establish a proximal mid-anterolateral (PMAL) or “Dienst” portal [12]. The Dienst portal is used to elevate the capsulolabral tissue and recess the acetabular rim

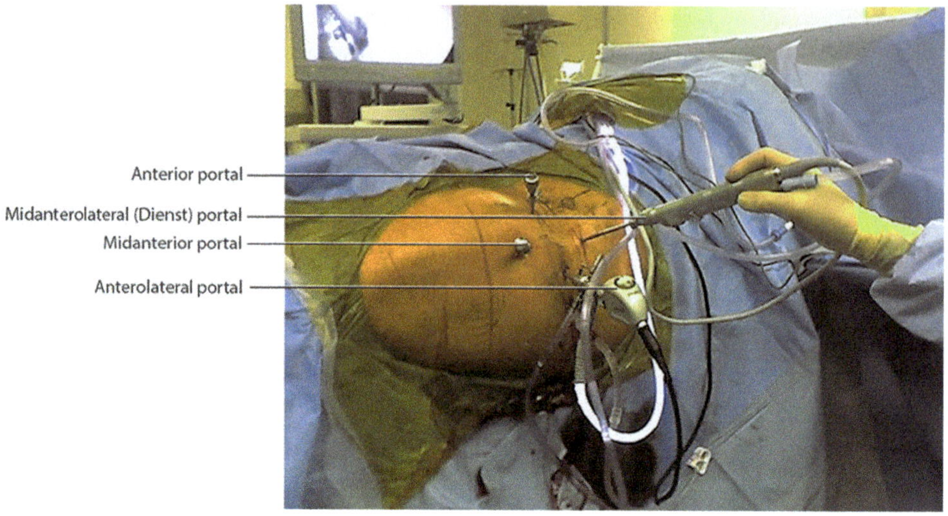

Fig. 37.2 Left hip. Preferred location of our four portals for working in the central compartment. Published with permission of Scott D. Martin, MD ©2013. All Rights Reserved

and for tying sutures. The entrance point is approximately one-third of the distance between the ASIS and the AL portal. The needle is aimed toward the acetabular rim in the location of the labral tear, just lateral to the reflected head of the rectus at the 12 o'clock position on the acetabulum. Alternatively, aim the needle toward the anterior cannula for entry. The closest structure to this portal is the superior gluteal nerve, at an average distance of 50 mm (Robertson, Arthroscopy 2008) [13]. A 5.5 mm cannula is placed to facilitate work in this portal. Figure 37.2 demonstrates our preferred location for all four portals.

Identifying Labral Pathology

Significant advances in magnetic resonance imaging have improved the sensitivity to detect labral tears. Conventional MRI has a sensitivity of 8–30% [17, 18], whereas MR arthrogram (MRA) has improved sensitivity to 90–100% in some series [12, 18, 19]. False-positive MRA findings have misidentified sublabral recesses, defined as stable clefts found between the labrum and articular cartilage, as labral tears [20]. Further study has shown these false-positive sublabral recesses to be read in the inferior half of the acetabulum [20]. Arthroscopy remains the gold standard for diagnosing labral pathology.

Labral tears have been classified in a variety of ways. The Lage arthroscopic method describes tears by etiology and morphology. Morphologic types are described as radial flap, radial fibrillated, longitudinal peripheral, or unstable [21]. Correlation between the Czerny MRA classification and the Lage classification is poor [17, 21, 40]. Rather, Seldes et al. performed a cadaveric study and identified two distinct histological types of labral tears [22]. Type I tears occur through the chondrolabral junction and type II tears occur through the substance of the labrum. Type I tears require repair. Type II tears that are large, longitudinal, and have a stable rim are often repairable. This is particularly important when a type II tear is located in a region of concomitant pincer or cam impingement. Small type II tears may be carefully debrided; however a strong effort is made to repair all labral tears when possible, to maintain the integrity of the hip labral seal.

Factors Predicting Outcomes

Patient selection is a critical factor in optimizing surgical outcomes following labral repair and concomitant osteoplasty surgery. At a minimum of 2-year follow-up, one study found patients younger than 40 and those with less than grade IV Outerbridge articular cartilage changes in the hip had better outcomes [23]. Other studies with similar follow-up have shown better results in patients with higher preoperative hip scores, less than 2 mm radiographic joint space narrowing compared to normal, and those who had a labral repair rather than a debridement [24–26]. Long-term studies of labral debridement without osteoplasty have found better outcomes in patients without significant degenerative changes [27, 28] and in those younger than 40. Ten-year survivorship, measured as a need for a total hip replacement, was 90% for patients with Outerbridge grade II changes or less compared to 12% and 22% for Outerbridge changes greater than grade II on the femoral head or acetabulum, respectively [28]. Other factors associated with better outcomes in hip arthroscopy include patients with mechanical symptoms [29] and nonsmokers [30].

Labral Vascularity

The acetabular labrum consists of fibrocartilage and dense connective tissue. It receives its blood supply peripherally from vessels entering from the joint capsule. Immunostaining studies have confirmed the inner two-thirds of the labrum is relatively avascular [31], and the capsular side of the labrum is two times more vascularized than the articular side [32]. Although about 75% of labral tears occur in the anterior or anterosuperior acetabular quadrant [33, 34], the vascular density of the labrum is similar throughout all quadrants—anterior, posterior, superior, and inferior [34]. Seldes reported that a few small blood vessels travel circumferentially within the labrum at its attachment to the bony acetabulum on the capsular side [33]. Using a sheep model, Philippon et al. evaluated labral repair histologically 12 weeks after surgery [35]. They demonstrated that labral repairs healed via a fibrovascular scar originating from the joint capsule in addition to bony areas near the suture anchor. We believe that preserving this capsular blood supply is integral to optimize healing following labral repairs and is reflected in the senior author's (SDM) labral repair technique [36].

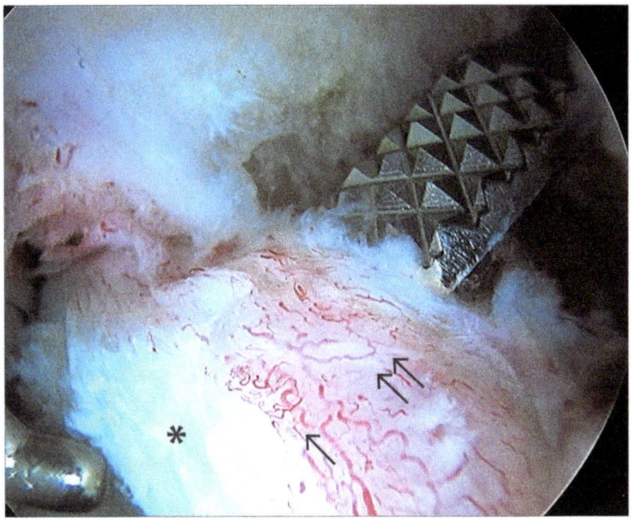

Fig. 37.3 Left hip. Arthroscopic view of 12 o'clock through the AL portal. A knife rasp is used, through the Dienst portal, to elevate 3–5 mm of the capsule (*double arrow*) above the capsulolabral junction (*arrow*). The blood supply to the labrum (*asterisk*) is protected. Published with permission of Scott D. Martin, MD ©2013. All Rights Reserved

Labral Tear Repair and Acetabuloplasty Technique: Acetabular Rim Recession

As previously described, the labral tear is identified and a decision is made to repair the labrum. All four portals are established, and every effort is made to preserve the capsulolabral and chondrolabral junctions via our capsular reflection technique. At the site of the tear, preserve the capsule proximal to the labrum. To avoid injury to the labral blood supply, do not violate the region of the capsulolabral junction [36]. A knife rasp (Smith & Nephew, Andover, MA, USA) is used to elevate the capsule 3–5 mm proximal to the labrum using the Dienst portal. The capsulolabral junction is then elevated subperiosteally to the level of the acetabular rim without violation of the chondrolabral junction. Often at the site of a type II labral tear, an overlying pincer lesion is identified and must be addressed with acetabular recession. The capsulolabral complex is elevated as an entire unit down to the bone along the length of the rim of the pincer lesion, and the chondrolabral junction is preserved. This junction has an elastic quality and can be carefully reflected off the acetabular rim. Tissue ablation should be minimized in clearing soft tissue from the rim to preserve the surrounding blood supply and avoid destabilizing the labrum (Fig. 37.3).

Next, a 4.0 long round abrader is used, through the Dienst portal, to recontour the acetabular rim and recess the pincer lesion while preserving the chondrolabral junction (Fig. 37.4a). The acetabular osteoplasty is performed with most of the traction released, using direct arthroscopic visualization through the AL and MAL portals and fluoroscopic guidance to confirm the level of recession (Fig. 37.4b). It is extremely important to use the burr on reverse at the bony edge of the acetabulum to avoid traumatizing and mutilating the chondrolabral junction. In most cases, 3–5 mm of bone is removed, contingent on the size of the pincer lesion (Fig. 37.4c).

For the labral seal to be reconstituted, the labrum must be anatomically restored to the recessed acetabular rim. Single-loaded 2.3 mm composite suture anchors with number 2 braided suture (Smith & Nephew, Andover MA, USA) are used to repair the labrum, but another anchor type may be substituted. The drill is placed on the acetabular edge at an approximately 45° angle to the rim through the MAL portal. It is aimed away from the articular cartilage of the acetabulum. For tears that extend laterally, the AL portal can be utilized for anchor placement; the arthroscope is switched to the MAL or anterior portal. Appropriate drill position and angle are visualized arthroscopically and confirmed fluoroscopically. Proximal placement of the anchor away from the rim will lead to labral eversion and nonanatomic eccentric placement. This can lead to loss of the labral seal and an "out-of-round" labral reattachment.

If the labral quality is robust, we use a vertical mattress stitch to repair the labrum. However, if the labral tissue lacks sufficient substance, we use a simple loop stitch with capsular augmentation, as described below. Recent evidence in the shoulder demonstrates the mattress stitch is better at restoring the labral height than the simple stitch [37]. To minimize trauma to the labrum when passing the suture through the Dienst portal, a 10 in. 17 gauge spinal needle is used to pierce the labrum about 1–2 mm into the chondrolabral junction, close to the location of the anchor (Fig. 37.5). The stylet of the needle is removed, and a Chia Percpasser (DePuy, Warsaw, IN) is inserted through the needle to shuttle the

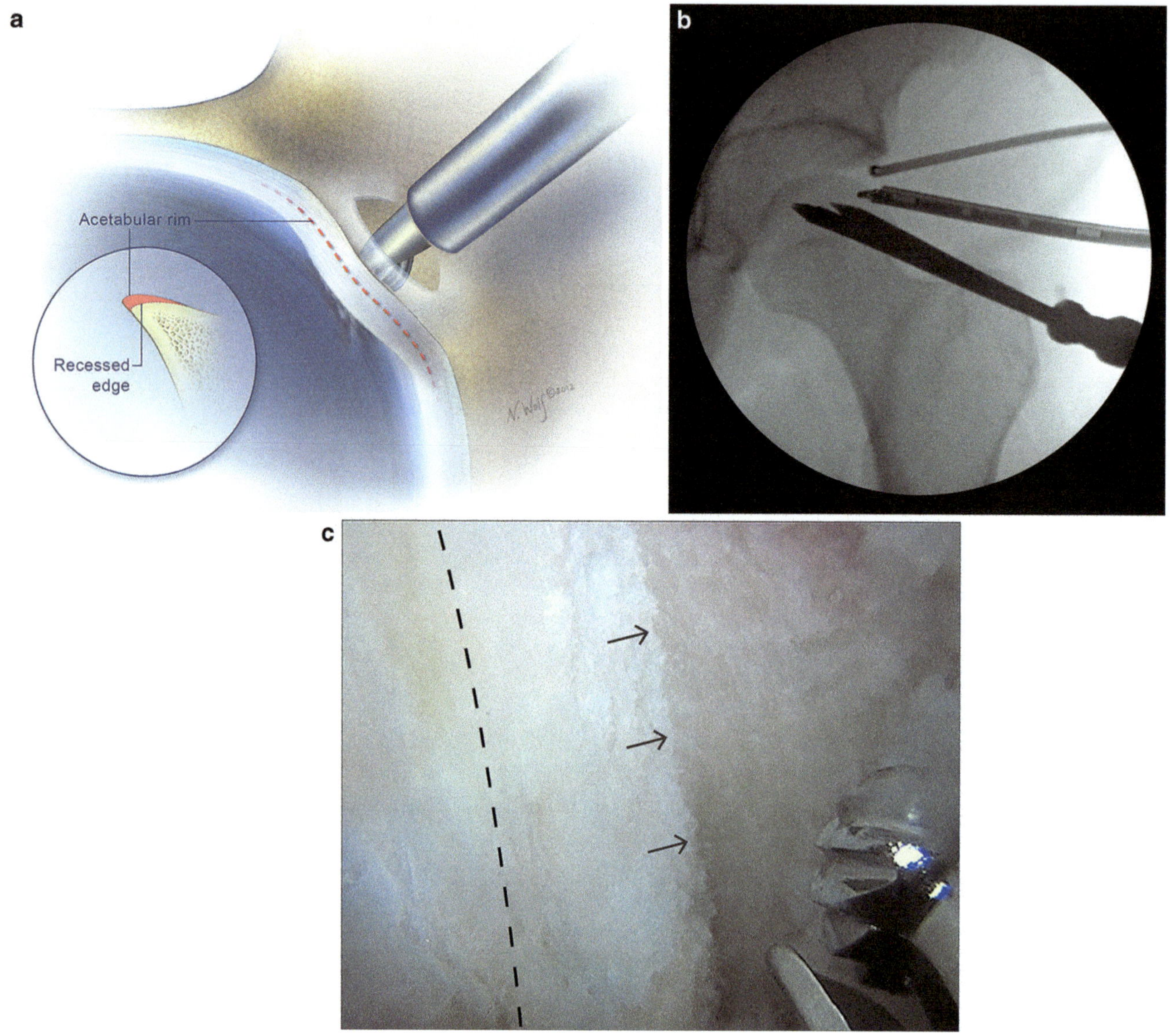

Fig. 37.4 (**a**) Lateral view of acetabular recession of the left hip. A 4.0 round abrader is used, through the Dienst portal, to recontour the acetabular rim and recess the pincer lesion. Published with permission of Nicole Wolf ©2013. All Rights Reserved. (**b**) AP of the left hip. Fluoroscopic guidance of acetabular recession. Published with permission of Scott D. Martin, MD ©2013. All Rights Reserved. (**c**) Left hip. Arthroscopic view of 12 o'clock through the AL portal. Acetabular recession of a pincer lesion (original location at *dashed line*) with a 4.0 round abrader through the Dienst portal. Chondrolabral junction (*arrows*) is preserved. Published with permission of Scott D. Martin, MD ©2013. All Rights Reserved

suture (Fig. 37.6). Any suture relay system that inflicts minimal trauma on the labrum may be used, including the mini-suture lasso.

The vertical stitch (Figs. 37.7, 37.8, and 37.9) or simple stitch is then completed (Fig. 37.10). The post of the suture for the simple stitch is kept on the capsular side; this keeps the knot away from the articular cartilage. We prefer to use the Weston sliding locking knot arthroscopically with additional 3–4 half hitches. Prior to sliding the Weston knot fully down the post (at about halfway), the traction is released. This allows the repaired labrum to conform to the femoral head and restores the anatomic position to the newly contoured acetabular rim. The labral seal is restored naturally and prevents an "out-of-round" repair [38, 39]. The use of intermittent traction also reduces overall traction times and reduces the chance of nerve palsy. Once the traction is fully released, the knot is slid down the post and locked, making sure not to overtighten. Care should be taken to push the knot toward the anchor and avoid pulling up on the suture limbs when tightening. This prevents dislodging the anchor. Thus,

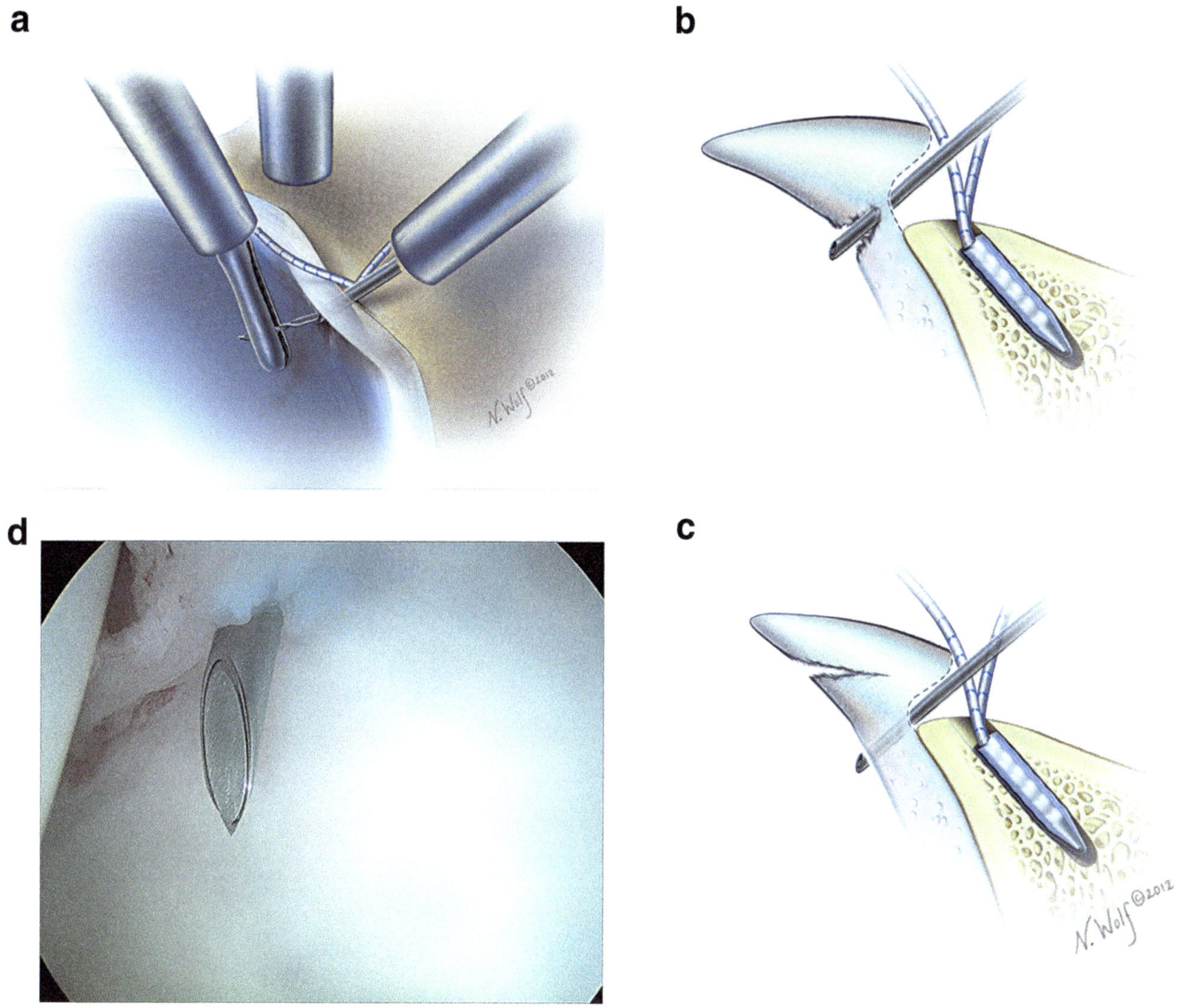

Fig. 37.5 (**a**) Left hip, lateral view. A 10 in. 17 gauge spinal needle, in the Dienst portal, is used to pierce the labrum about 1–2 mm into the chondrolabral junction to improve the strength of repair. (**b**, **c**) Cross-sectional view of the first needle passage. Second passage can be either a loop or vertical mattress, depending on the quality of tissue. (**b**) Pierce at the level of the defect in a type I tear. (**c**) Pierce at the level of the chondrolabral junction in a type 2 tear. Published with permission of Nicole Wolf ©2013. All Rights Reserved. (**d**) Left hip. Arthroscopic view through the AL portal. The needle pierces the labrum through the defect as illustrated in (**a**, **b**). Published with permission of Scott D. Martin, MD ©2013. All Rights Reserved

the repair is finished within the peripheral compartment of the hip. The technique prevents the repaired labrum from everting and losing a tight seal around the femoral head. Three or four half hitches are thrown securely, and the sutures are cut with an arthroscopic suture cutter. Subsequent anchors (as appropriate for the tear size) are placed every 8–10 mm. Traction is reapplied for anchor and suture management and released again for knot tying as described above.

Capsular Augmentation

In cases where the labrum is significantly deficient and will not support suture without pulling through, capsular augmentation may be performed (Fig. 37.11a). The technique utilizes capsular tissue proximal to the labrum to augment the labrum; it supports the suture and maintains the labral seal of the hip.

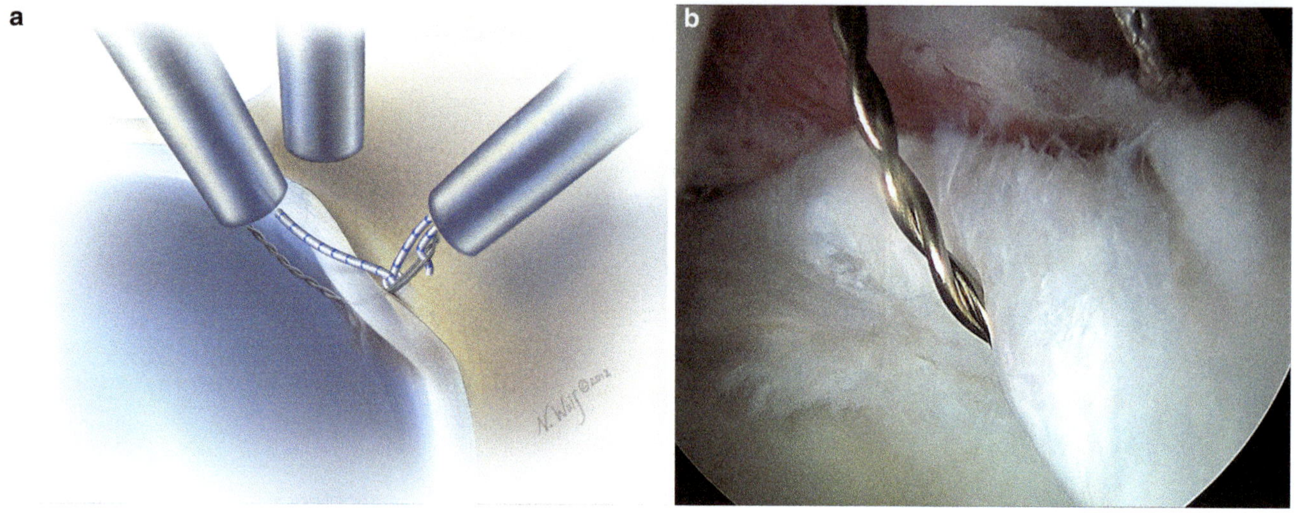

Fig. 37.6 (**a**) Left hip. Lateral view. After the defect is pierced, the suture is passed from the Dienst to MAL portal via a wire suture shuttle relay. Published with permission of Nicole Wolf ©2013. All Rights Reserved. (**b**) Left hip. Arthroscopic view through the AL portal shows the suture shuttle relay between the MAL and Dienst portals as illustrated in (**a**). Published with permission of Scott D. Martin, MD ©2013. All Rights Reserved

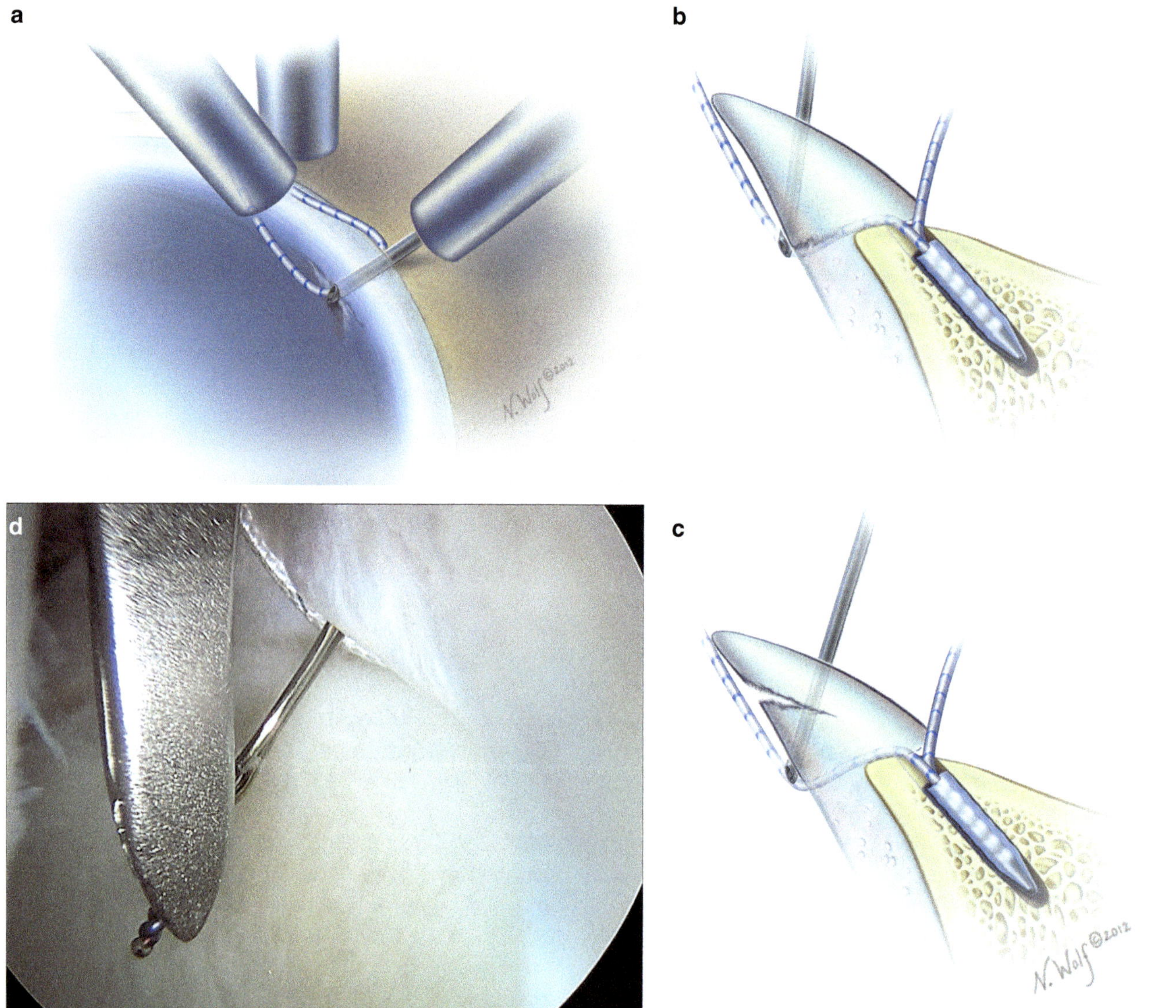

Fig. 37.7 (**a**) Left hip. Lateral view. The second needle passage for the vertical mattress stitch using the Dienst portal. (**b**, **c**) Cross-sectional view of second needle passage to complete the vertical mattress stitch. (**b**) Type I tear. (**c**) Type II tear. Published with permission of Nicole Wolf ©2013. All Rights Reserved. (**d**) Left hip. Arthroscopic view through the AL portal shows the second needle passage as illustrated in (**a**, **b**). Published with permission of Scott D. Martin, MD ©2013. All Rights Reserved

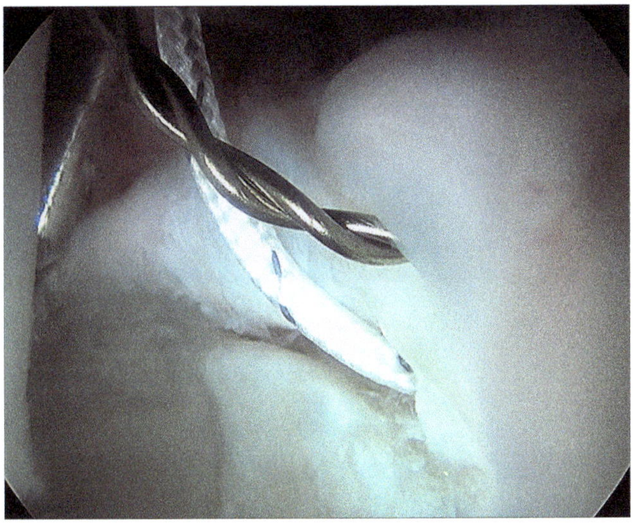

Fig. 37.8 Left hip. Arthroscopic view through the AL portal shows the suture shuttle relay from the MAL to the Dienst portal to complete the vertical mattress stitch. Published with permission of Scott D. Martin, MD ©2013. All Rights Reserved

The procedure requires elevating the labrum approximately 5–8 mm proximal to the capsulolabral junction, down to the acetabular rim (Fig. 37.11b). If a pincer lesion is present, the bone prominence is recessed at this time, taking great care to preserve the chondrolabral junction as described above.

Anchors are placed and simple loop sutures are tied around the labrum and capsule (Fig. 37.11d). The 5–8 mm of capsule augments the labrum and provides structure so the loop sutures do not pull through. Suture limbs are tensioned and the traction is removed prior to tie-down. This technique allows maintenance of a deficient labrum that would otherwise need to be debrided. The labral seal would be lost and reconstruction with graft tissue possibly required.

The labral repair and acetabuloplasty technique offers a few unique advantages. Philippon's histologic study evaluated the repair of surgically created labral tears of the hip in sheep at 12 weeks following arthroscopic repair. The repairs were stable but healing was incomplete. There was a superficial cleft along the articular surface of the repair; the morphology of the labra appeared "bunched" and did not resemble normal labra [35].

It is important to emphasize correct placement of anchors at the acetabular rim. More proximal placement can lead to an "out-of-round" repair with eccentric placement of the labrum and loss of the acetabular vacuum seal. It is possible that by preserving the capsular blood supply to the labrum with this capsular reflection technique, we may improve the healing of labral repairs. Secondly, it has been postulated that restoring the labral seal reestablishes the normal fluid state of the central compartment, may reduce frictional forces in the hip, and offers nutritional benefits to cartilage [39]. We release traction prior to securing knots to help restore this seal; overtightening can inadvertently distort the seal and evert labral tissue.

Integrity of the chondrolabral junction is maintained by this acetabuloplasty rim recession technique. The chondrolabral junction is a region of poor vascularity [32]; surgically incising it to remove the labrum could iatrogenically create healing issues. This could lead to further damage to the chondrolabral junction. In addition, reattachment of a freely detached labrum can lead to out-of-round labral repair and loss of seal (Fig. 37.12).

We feel preservation of the chondrolabral junction is paramount to preserving the joint. If chondral flaps are encountered, microfracture is performed behind the flap to stimulate stem cell release from the bone marrow (Fig. 37.11c). Smaller grade IV chondral defects (<2 cm) at the chondrolabral junction may also be microfractured. However, results are variable; they depend on the size of the lesion and age of the patient. Loss of the chondrolabral junction's integrity can lead to acetabular cartilage delamination and joint deterioration over time.

Peripheral Compartment

After completion of the acetabular osteoplasty and labral repair, the traction is released. The hip is flexed to about 40° to relax the anterior capsule. The peripheral compartment can be entered directly from the central compartment via the anterior portal or indirectly by redirecting the obturator and cannula via the anterolateral portal. For direct entry, the scope is placed in the anterior portal and is maneuvered into the anteromedial region of the hip at the labral junction. As the traction is released and the hip is flexed up to 40°, the scope is passed into the peripheral compartment. Great care must be taken not to lever the scope off of the femoral head to avoid damaging the articular cartilage. In large patients or excessively tight joints, the peripheral compartment is entered using the anterolateral portal.

When entering the peripheral compartment in initial anterolateral portal placement, fluoroscopic guidance is used as necessary. A needle is walked anteriorly along the femoral neck and inserted into the peripheral compartment distal to the head/neck junction. The needle stylet is removed and the backflow of fluid confirms the correct location. Addressing cam lesions and tumors in the peripheral compartment will be discussed elsewhere.

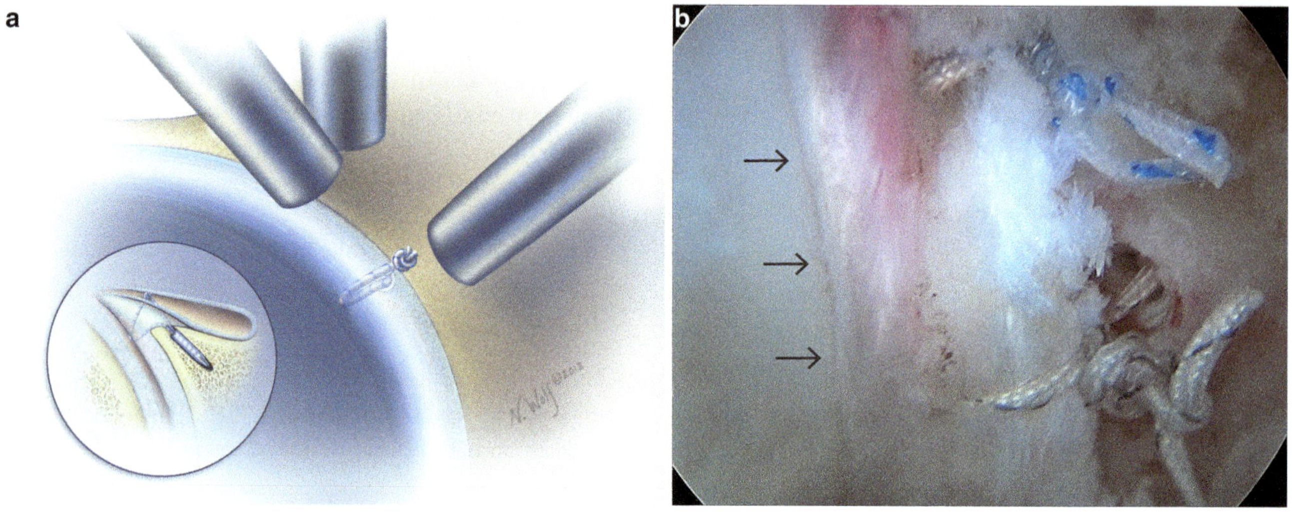

Fig. 37.9 (**a**) Vertical mattress final repair. Published with permission of Nicole Wolf ©2013. All Rights Reserved. (**b**) Left hip. Arthroscopic view through the AL portal in the peripheral compartment. Repair of the labrum with vertical mattress stitches shows restoration of the seal (*arrows*) and no eversion. Traction is released and the head is reduced. Published with permission of Scott D. Martin, MD ©2013. All Rights Reserved

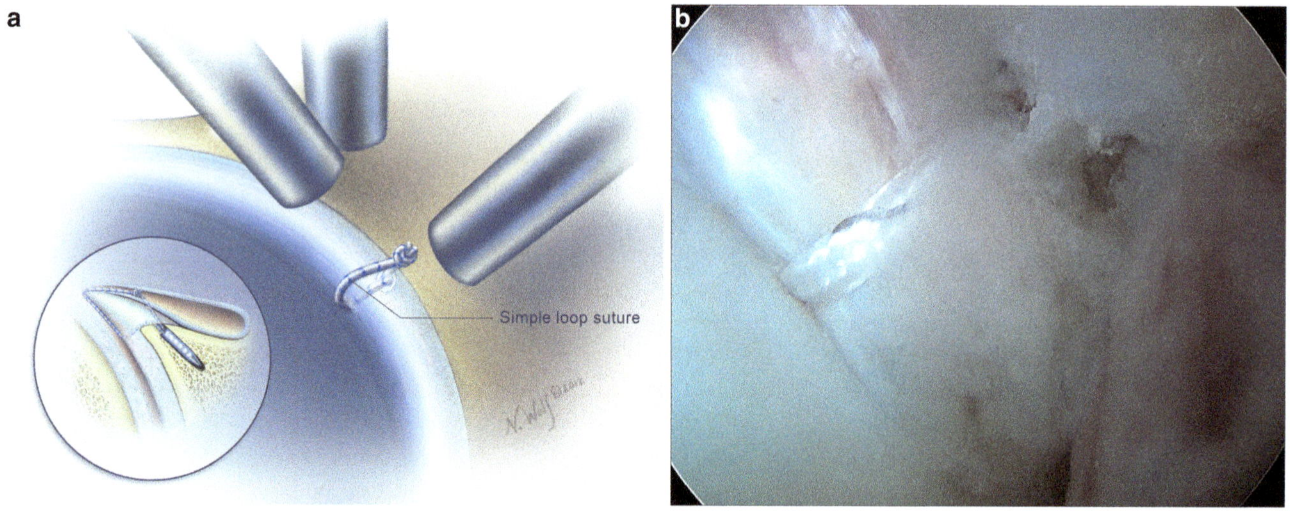

Fig. 37.10 (**a**) Simple loop final repair. Published with permission of Nicole Wolf ©2013. All Rights Reserved. (**b**) Left hip. Arthroscopic view through the AL portal in peripheral compartment. Repair of the labrum with a simple loop stitch shows restoration of the labral seal and no eversion. Traction is released and the head is reduced. Published with permission of Scott D. Martin, MD ©2013. All Rights Reserved

Tumors of the Hip

Hip arthroscopy can be utilized for both definitive diagnosis and treatment of certain lesions about the hip joint: multiple osteochondromatosis, PVNS (Fig. 37.13), and giant cell tumors. Care is taken to meticulously excise all lesions within the central and peripheral compartments. Frequently, PVNS lesions will occur within the gutters of the peripheral compartment and within the femoral neck capsular recess. Surgical technique should include systematic examination of the entire hip joint. Within the central compartment, examine the inferior recess, acetabular fossa, medial joint, and capsular recesses. In the peripheral compartment, examine the medial and lateral gutters, inferior recess, and femoral neck capsular reflection. Flexible instruments, including thermal ablators, can be invaluable in excision of a tumor, especially within the peripheral gutters and acetabular fossa. Multiple accessory utility portals can greatly facilitate access and removal of a tumor. Use meticulous technique to completely

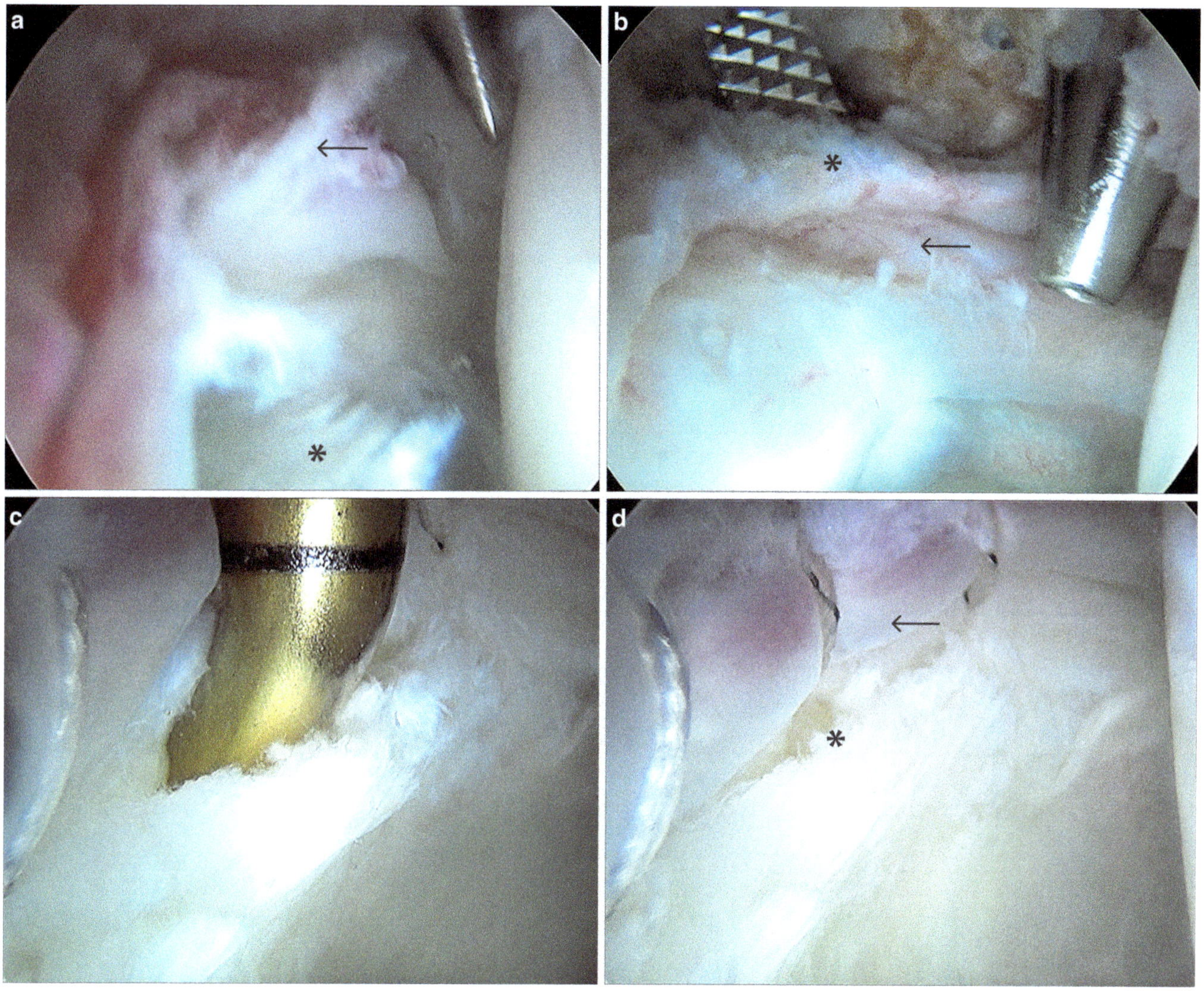

Fig. 37.11 (**a**) Right hip. Arthroscopic view through the AL portal shows a complex tear of a deficient labrum (*black arrow*) and chondrolabral flap (*asterisk*). (**b**) Right hip. Arthroscopic view through the AL portal. A knife rasp elevates both the labrum (*black arrow*) and capsule (*asterisk*). 5–8 mm of capsule is used to augment the deficient labrum. (**c**) Right hip. Arthroscopic view through the AL portal. Microfracture is performed behind the chondral flap into the subchondral plate to stimulate the underlying stem cells. (**d**) Right hip. Arthroscopic view through the AL portal shows the finished repair with an augmented labrum (*black arrow*) and stable chondral flap (*asterisk*). Published with permission of Scott D. Martin, MD ©2013. All Rights Reserved

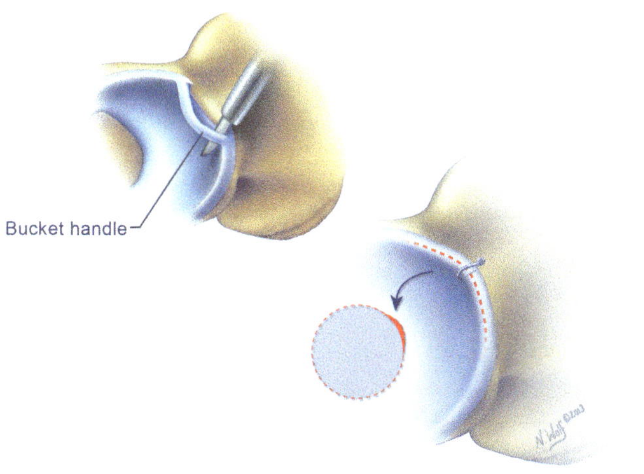

Fig. 37.12 Surgical detachment pitfall: out-of-round repair. Published with permission of Nicole Wolf ©2013. All Rights Reserved

extirpate all evidence of the tumor without residual lesions. Radioablation can provide a few extra millimeters of marginal depth to the excision and excellent homeostasis. Sufficient outflow is needed to prevent thermal chondrolysis of the surrounding cartilage.

Iliopsoas Tendon Recession

Recession of the iliopsoas tendon is performed to relieve impingement on the underlying labrum with partial tearing of the labrum (Fig. 37.14a). In the peripheral compartment, the iliopsoas tendon is viewed at the 12 o'clock position as it passes over the acetabular rim. The capsule of the joint is usually violated and frayed. Frequently, the findings are not well visualized on MRI and are discovered at the time of

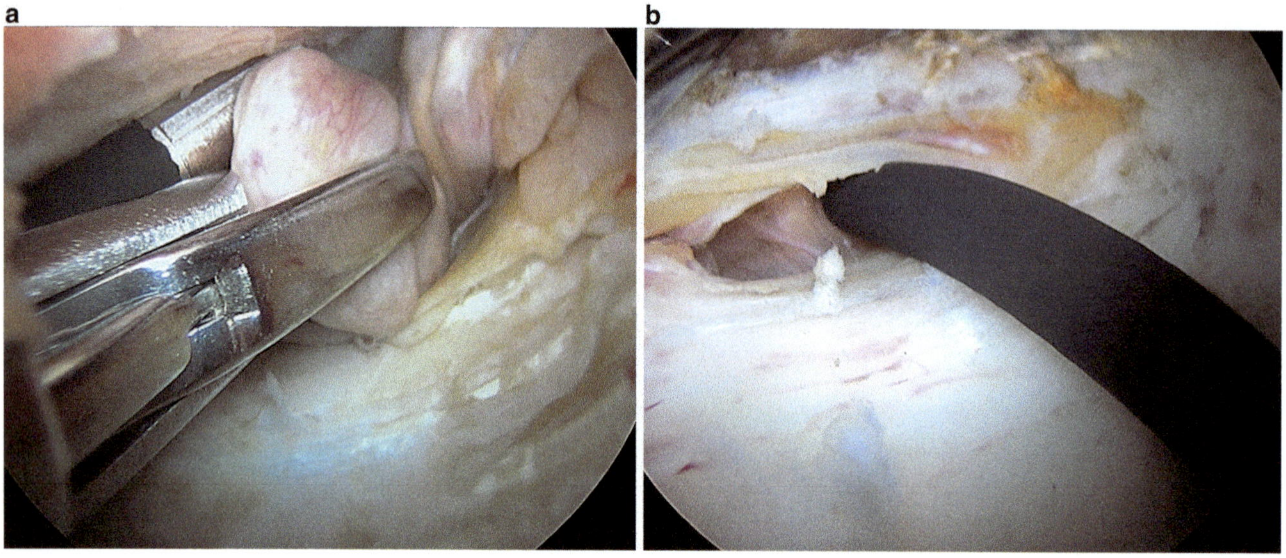

Fig. 37.13 (**a**) PVNS. Left hip. Arthroscopic view through the AL portal shows removal of stalk through the distal anterior portal. (**b**) Left hip. Arthroscopic view through the AL portal shows completed tumor removal. Ablator, through the proximal anterior portal, is used to remove any residual lesions within the medial synovial fold. Published with permission of Scott D. Martin, MD ©2013. All Rights Reserved

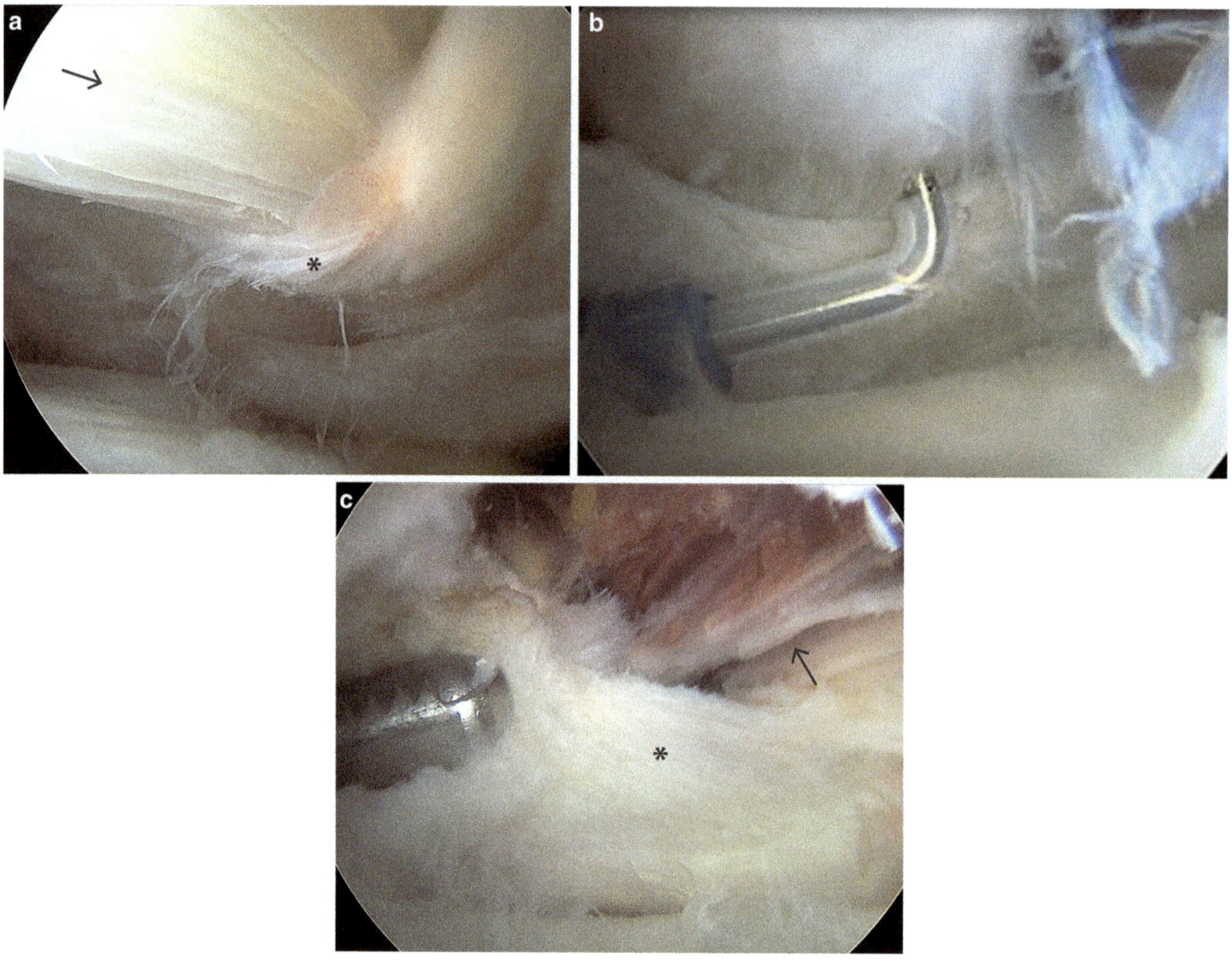

Fig. 37.14 (**a**) Right hip. Arthroscopic view through the AL portal. The iliopsoas tendon (*arrow*) impinges on the underlying labrum (*asterisk*). (**b**) Right hip. Arthroscopic view through the AL portal. The iliopsoas tendon is recessed with electrocautery through the proximal anterior portal. (**c**) Right hip. Arthroscopic view through the AL portal. Recession is complete. The underlying iliacus is exposed (*arrow*) and the labrum (*asterisk*) no longer impinged upon by the iliopsoas. Published with permission of Scott D. Martin, MD ©2013. All Rights Reserved

surgery. With a hooked electrocautery in the anterior portal and the scope in the anterolateral portal, the iliopsoas is recessed in the peripheral compartment just distal to the labrum, leaving the underlying iliacus muscle tendon fibers (Fig. 37.14b). By recessing the tendon at the acetabular rim, the underlying iliacus muscle tendon unit is preserved, and there is less chance of additional hip flexor weakness (Fig. 37.14c).

Postoperative Routine

For most patients, formal physical therapy is not required. Patients are immediately allowed flatfoot ambulation with weight bearing as tolerated. Crutches are used for 6 weeks if labral repair was completed versus 2 weeks if no repair was completed. This allows the pelvis to remain relatively level during ambulation and prevents lurching, which can stress the repair. Weight bearing, with a balanced gait, also allows the femoral head to concentrically load the labrum. This assists in maintaining reduction of the labral repair against the acetabular rim. At 6 weeks postoperative, a low resistance stationary bike is initiated. Swimming with a straight kick may be started at 8 weeks postoperative. If a patient is having difficulty with simple ambulation, therapy is allowed for gait training only. No deep squats are allowed for 4 months. Return to full activities, including impact loading, is often allowed at 4–6 months postoperatively. Complete recovery from surgery may take a year to see the full benefit.

Chapter Pearls

- When entering the hip during anterolateral portal placement, direct the needle in a coronal plane or angled slightly posterior to this plane to facilitate entrance into the joint.
- In tight hips or hips with a significant acetabular overhang, additional distraction can be obtained safely with the "femoral head drop technique." Initially injecting the joint with 30 mL fluid breaks the labral seal and leads to several additional millimeters of joint distraction. The spinal needle can then safely reenter the joint. This technique decreases the incidence of labral penetration and chondral injury when establishing the anterolateral portal.
- Capsulotomy and capsulectomy should not be excessive. This avoids joint instability, need for capsular closure, and formation of heterotopic bone.
- The use of the Dienst portal facilitates labral elevation, repair, and acetabular osteoplasty.
- Acetabular osteoplasty is performed with minimal traction to reduce traction time and with the burr on reverse to prevent damage to the chondrolabral junction.
- Anchors for labral repair should be placed close to the acetabular rim to allow anatomic repair and to avoid everting and/or displacement of the labrum.
- Prior to suture tie-down, the traction should be released to allow the femoral head to concentrically reduce the labrum to the newly recessed acetabular rim. This lessens the possibility for an eccentric reduction and/or eversion on tie-down from over-tensioning of the sutures. The use of intermittent traction for labral repair also lessens traction time.
- In cases where the labrum is excessively attenuated, capsular augmentation can be performed. A 5–8 mm capsular sleeve is elevated with the labrum during labral reconstruction. In this case, simple loop sutures are required to preserve the remaining labrum and maintain the labral seal.

References

1. Crawford JR, Villar RN. Current concepts in the management of femoroacetabular impingement. J Bone Joint Surg Br. 2005;87:1459–62.
2. Byrd JW. Hip arthroscopy utilizing the supine position. Arthroscopy. 1994;10(3):275–80.
3. Mei-Dan O, McConkey MO, Young DA. Hip arthroscopy distraction without the use of a perineal post: prospective study. Orthopedics. 2013;36(1):e1–5. doi:10.3928/01477447-20121217-10.
4. Kong KF, Chien P, Wong JW, Yip DK. Perineal padding: an alternative to a perineal post in hip arthroscopy. Arthroscopy. 2003;19(9): 1027–9.
5. Topliss CJ, Webb JM. Interface pressure produced by the traction post on a standard orthopaedic table. Injury. 2001;32(9):689–91.
6. Flierl MA, Stahel PF, Hak DJ, Morgan SJ, Smith WR. Traction table-related complications in orthopaedic surgery. J Am Acad Orthop Surg. 2010;18(11):668–75.
7. Griffin DR, Villar RN. Complications of arthroscopy of the hip. J Bone Joint Surg Br. 1999;81(4):604–6.
8. Byrd JW, Jones KS. Arthroscopic management of femoroacetabular impingement: minimum 2-year follow-up. Arthroscopy. 2011;27(10):1379–88.
9. Nwachukwu BU, McFeely ED, Nasreddine AY, Krcik JA, Frank J, Kocher MS. Complications of hip arthroscopy in children and adolescents. J Pediatr Orthop. 2011;31(3):227–31.
10. Smart LR, Oetgen M, Noonam B, Medvecky MA. Beginning hip arthroscopy: indications, positioning, portal placement, basic techniques and complications. J Arthrosc Relat Surg. 2007;23(12): 1348–58.
11. Byrd JW, Pappas JN, Pedley MJ. Hip arthroscopy: an anatomic study of portal placement and relationship to the extra-articular structures. Arthroscopy. 1995;11(4):418–23.
12. Dienst M, Seil R, Kohn DM. Safe arthroscopic access to the central compartment of the hip. Arthroscopy. 2005;21(12):1510–4.
13. Robertson WJ, Kelly BT. The safe zone for hip arthroscopy: a cadaveric assessment of central, peripheral, and lateral compartment portal placement. Arthroscopy. 2008;24(9):1019–26.

14. Bond JL, Knutson ZA, Ebert A, Guanche CA. The 23-point arthroscopic examination of the hip: basic setup, portal placement, and surgical technique. Arthroscopy. 2009;25(4):416–29.
15. McCormick F, Alpaugh K, Nwachukwu BU, Xu S, Martin SD. Effect of radiofrequency use on hip arthroscopy irrigation fluid temperature. Arthroscopy. 2013;29(2):336–42.
16. Wenger DE, Kendell KR, Miner MR, Trousdale RT. Acetabular labral tears rarely occur in the absence of bony abnormalities. Clin Orthop Relat Res. 2004;426:145–50.
17. Toomayan GA, Holman WR, Major NM, Kozlowicz SM, Vail TP. Sensitivity of MR arthrography in the evaluation of acetabular labral tears. AJR Am J Roentgenol. 2006;186(2):449–53.
18. Czerny C, Hofmann S, Neuhold A, Tschauner C, Engel A, Techt MP, et al. Lesions of the acetabular labrum: accuracy of MR imaging and MR arthrography in detection and staging. Radiology. 1996;200:225–30.
19. Chan YS, Lien LC, Hsu HL, Wan YL, Lee MS, Hsu KY, Shih CH. Evaluating hip labral tears using magnetic resonance arthrography: a prospective study comparing hip arthroscopy and magnetic resonance arthrography diagnosis. Arthroscopy. 2005; 21(10):1250.
20. Studler U, Kalberer F, Leunig M, Zanetti M, Hodler J, Dora C, Pfirrmann CW. MR arthrography of the hip: differentiation between an anterior sublabral recess as a normal variant and a labral tear. Radiology. 2008;249(3):947–54.
21. Lage LA, Patel JV, Villar RN. The acetabular labral tear: an arthroscopic classification. Arthroscopy. 1996;12(3):269–72.
22. Seldes RM, Tan V, Hunt J, Katz M, Winiarsky R, Fitzgerald Jr RH. Anatomy, histologic features, and vascularity of the adult acetabular labrum. Clin Orthop Relat Res. 2001;382:232–40.
23. McCormick F, Nwachukwu BU, Alpaugh K, Martin SD. Predictors of hip arthroscopy outcomes for labral tears at minimum 2-year follow-up: the influence of age and arthritis. Arthroscopy. 2012; 28(10):1359–64.
24. Philippon MJ, Briggs KK, Yen YM, Kuppersmith DA. Outcomes following hip arthroscopy for femoroacetabular impingement with associated chondrolabral dysfunction: minimum two-year follow-up. J Bone Joint Surg Br. 2009;91(1):16–23.
25. Schilders E, Dimitrakopoulou A, Bismil Q, Marchant P, Cooke C. Arthroscopic treatment of labral tears in femoroacetabular impingement: a comparative study of refixation and resection with a minimum two-year follow-up. J Bone Joint Surg Br. 2011;93(8): 1027–32.
26. Larson CM, Giveans MR, Stone RM. Arthroscopic debridement versus refixation of the acetabular labrum associated with femoroacetabular impingement: mean 3.5-year follow-up. Am J Sports Med. 2012;40(5):1015–21.
27. Byrd JW, Jones KS. Hip arthroscopy for labral pathology: prospective analysis with 10-year follow-up. Arthroscopy. 2009;25(4): 365–8.
28. McCarthy JC, Jarrett BT, Ojeifo O, Lee JA, Bragdon CR. What factors influence long-term survivorship after hip arthroscopy? Clin Orthop Relat Res. 2011;469(2):362–71.
29. Awan N, Murray P. Role of hip arthroscopy in the diagnosis and treatment of hip joint pathology. Arthroscopy. 2006;22:215–8.
30. Kamath AF, Componovo R, Baldwin K, Israelite CL, Nelson CL. Hip arthroscopy for labral tears: review of clinical outcomes with 4.8-year mean follow-up. Am J Sports Med. 2009;37:1721–7.
31. Petersen W, Petersen F, Tillmann B. Structure and vascularization of the acetabular labrum with regard to the pathogenesis and healing of labral lesions. Arch Orthop Trauma Surg. 2003;123(6):283–8.
32. Kelly BT, Shapiro GS, Digiovanni CW, Buly RL, Potter HG, Hannafin JA. Vascularity of the hip labrum: a cadaveric investigation. Arthroscopy. 2005;21(1):3–11.
33. Seldes RM, Tan V, Hunt J, Katz M, Winiarsky R, Fitzgerald Jr RH. Anatomy, histologic features, and vascularity of the adult acetabular labrum. Clin Orthop. 2001;382:232–40.
34. Farjo LA, Glick JM, Sampson TG. Hip arthroscopy for acetabular labral tears. Arthroscopy. 1999;15:132–7.
35. Philippon MJ, Arnoczky SP, Torrie A. Arthroscopic repair of the acetabular labrum: a histologic assessment of healing in an ovine model. Arthroscopy. 2007;23(4):376–80.
36. Syed H, Martin SD. Labral repair with acetabular recession and chondrolabral preservation. J Orthop Surg. 2012.
37. Hagstrom LS, Marzo JM. Simple versus horizontal suture anchor repair of Bankart lesions: which better restores labral anatomy? Arthroscopy. 2013;29(2):325–9.
38. Ferguson SJ, Bryant JT, Ganz R, Ito K. The acetabular labrum seal: a poroelastic finite element model. Clin Biomech (Bristol, Avon). 2000;15(6):463–8.
39. Ferguson SJ, Bryant JT, Ganz R, Ito K. An in vitro investigation of the acetabular labral seal in hip joint mechanics. J Biomech. 2003;36(2):171–8.
40. Blankenbaker DG, De Smet AA, Keene JS, Fine JP. Classification and localization of acetabular labral tears. Skeletal Radiol. 2007;36(5):391–7.

Arthroscopic Treatment: Principles of Hip Distraction

38

Hassan Sadri

Introduction

Hip pain in young adults is often characterized by nonspecific symptoms, normal imaging studies, and vague findings from history and physical examination. As such, identifying the source and mechanism of the pain can be difficult. At the same time, treatment needs to be specific because its effects will be experienced longer in this population. Hip arthroscopy has advanced enormously in the past 10 years and is a very precious tool in treating complex hip pathologies. Hip arthroscopies can be separated into three compartments: the so-called central compartment, peripheral compartment, and extraarticular compartment. Distraction is needed essentially for the central compartment where the most frequent pathologies are found. Very often central compartment surgery is associated with peripheral compartment surgery, such as in femoroacetabular pathology corrections [1–6] and distraction is also needed in these cases. Complex hip arthroscopies of the central compartment include correction of femoroacetabular impingement, labral suturing, labral grafting, ligamentum teres reconstruction, cartilage reconstruction techniques, chondromatosis and osteochondromatosis, acetabular and head (Pipkin type) fractures, etc. A thorough arthroscopic correction of hip pathology must not be hindered by time constraint.

Since these reconstructive procedures are time consuming, have a steep learning curve, and can provoke fearful complications [7–9], surgeons must be aware of the limitations of each distraction technique.

We present the rationale of hip distraction and complications. General tips on how to minimize or avoid these complications are discussed. We also present an innovative distraction method using pin hip distraction (Pin Hip Distractor, Swiss Medical Instruments, Wollerau, Switzerland) in these indications (Figs. 38.1, 38.2, and 38.3). This method entirely avoids the abovementioned complications. The pin hip distractor [6, 10–12] allows the surgeon to perform these time-consuming surgical steps without time pressure with the same degree of precision as in open surgery. The results obtained are, therefore, identical to the open surgical technique. It is also a wonderful teaching tool, since beginners may perform these more complex procedures without worrying about distraction time and the related complications.

H. Sadri, MD (✉)
Department of Orthopaedic Surgery, Clinique Bois-Cerf, Avenue Serran 4, Lausanne 1006, Switzerland
e-mail: sadrih@bluewin.ch

Complications of Hip Distraction

In order to access the central hip compartment, femoroacetabular distraction is necessary. For optimal viewing and safe surgery, at least 12 mm of distraction (Fig. 38.3) of the femoroacetabular joint is ideally required. If less is attained, the insertion of cannulas and instruments put the articular cartilage at risk. Classically and historically, distraction has been obtained on a traction table (Figs. 38.4, 38.5, and 38.6). This implies progressive traction on the foot via some sort of boot (Figs. 38.4 and 38.5) and a perineal post. It has been reported that traction times longer than 90–120 min can provoke severe neurological and perineal skin lesions in up to 15 % of cases [7–9]. It has been suggested that the release of traction after 90–120 min for some time may reduce the neurological complication rate but this has not been clearly demonstrated in the literature. The most frequent neurological lesions reported are pudendal nerve lesions with resultant impotence due to the compression of the nerve on the perineal post. To minimize pudendal compression, the use of a larger diameter post of over 20 cm has been recommended. Although this reduces the incidence of pudendal nerve and perineal skin lesions, it does not completely eliminate it. Additionally, the use of traction creates the risk of sciatic and femoral nerve lesions. These are at risk due to overstretching during longer periods of time (see overstretching of nerves below under

J.C. McCarthy et al. (eds.), *Hip Joint Restoration*, DOI 10.1007/978-1-4614-0694-5_38

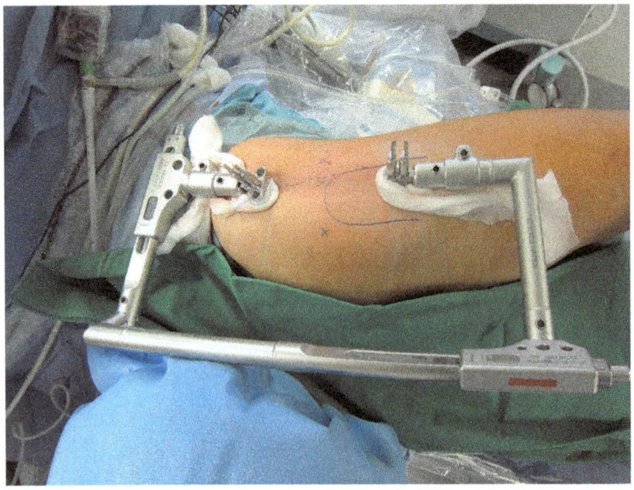

Fig. 38.1 Installation of the pin hip distractor. Posterior view of a right hip in lateral decubitus. The greater trochanter is drawn with a dotted line on the anterior trochanteric margin. The greater trochanter is drawn, as well as the positions of the posterolateral, anterolateral, and anterior portals (drawn as *x* on the skin). The proximal Schanz screws (*left*) are placed in line with the anterior trochanteric margin dotted line drawn on the skin. The proximal acetabular Schanz screws are placed 1 cm above the acetabular sourcil under image intensifier control and the distal (*right*) screws at the level of the lesser trochanter in the middle of the anteroposterior diameter of the proximal femur. Note the anterior to posterior precision screw mechanism (*left*), which allows an increase in the anterior to posterior traction vector, thus opening the anterior joint space. The proximal to distal traction is controlled by the distal (*right*) precision screw mechanism

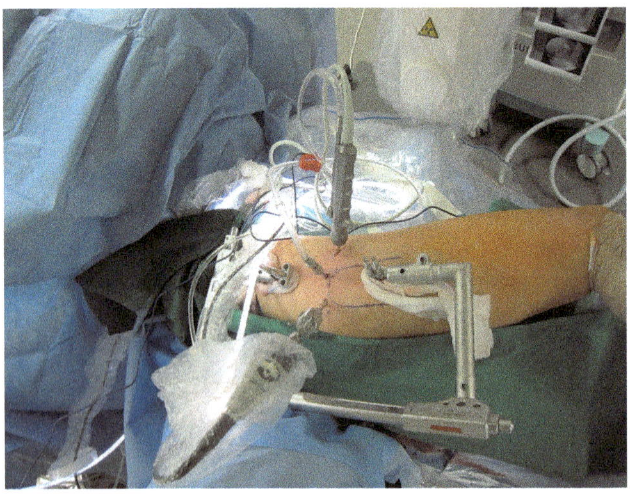

Fig. 38.2 Posterior view of the setup of a right hip with pin hip distractor applied and posterolateral (arthroscope), anterolateral (outflow cannula), and anterior (shaver) portals. The patient is in lateral decubitus with the head on the left and the feet on the right. Note that the leg and foot are draped to be moved freely

basic science). Skin lesions of the foot and arterial spasm, as well as ischemia of the foot, have also been reported. It has also been suggested that pressure [8, 9] plays a role in pudendal nerve and perineal skin compression injuries. Traction

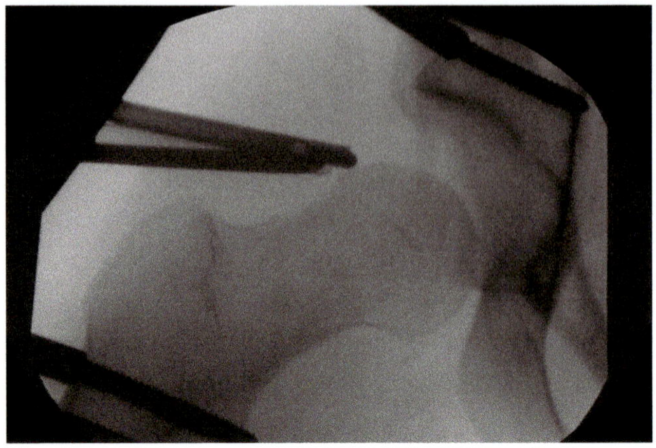

Fig. 38.3 Image intensifier anteroposterior view with pin hip distractor in position and femoroacetabular joint distraction. The proximal acetabular Schanz screw is placed 1 cm above the acetabular sourcil under image intensifier control and the distal screw at the level of the lesser trochanter of the proximal femur. Lower limb in neutral position with traction applied. Note that more than 12 mm of joint space distraction is already visible in this young and muscular patient. The proximal Schanz screws have started to bend, thus signaling sufficient 500 N of distraction force. Femoroacetabular cam (pistol grip head) component correction with a burr

should be viewed in the same way as safe tourniquet time and pressure. A tensiometer has been suggested to monitor the pressure, although this is rarely routinely used.

I and other surgeons have abandoned the use of a traction table in complex arthroscopic hip surgery because of a high neurological complication rate. Although I have followed the standard recommendations to avoid neurological complications of hip arthroscopies in the literature (such as the use of a very large perineal post), in my initial 20 cases, two slowly regressive pudendal nerve lesions, with clinical impotence, were encountered. In one case the symptoms of impotence lasted 1 year. This is probably due to longer than 90 min of traction used in this case to correct the complex acetabular anomalies. It can be very challenging to complete these complex surgeries in under 90 min with large labral tears sometimes needing eight anchors, as well as concomitant reconstruction techniques (matrix autologous cartilage transplantation and matrix-induced chondrogenesis). The major indication for hip arthroscopy worldwide today is the correction of femoroacetabular impingement [1–6]. These cases need complex reconstruction and corrective surgery as mentioned above.

To avoid these numerous distraction complications, the use of the pin hip distractor (Figs. 38.1, 38.2, and 38.3) was initiated. We have currently an experience of over 3000 cases for this indication. We have also noted that our operative time has not changed, nor the traction times. This is due to the fact that increasingly complex cases are operated on arthroscopically and that labral suturing and/or complex reconstruction, such as labral graft reconstruction, is neces-

Fig. 38.4 Patient in supine position on a mobile traction table (Medacta International). The foot is well padded and held in an adequate boot. Traction is applied with the wheel handle seen left. The hip can be flexed, extended, abducted, and adducted. For internal and external rotation, the boot has to be released from the traction mechanism

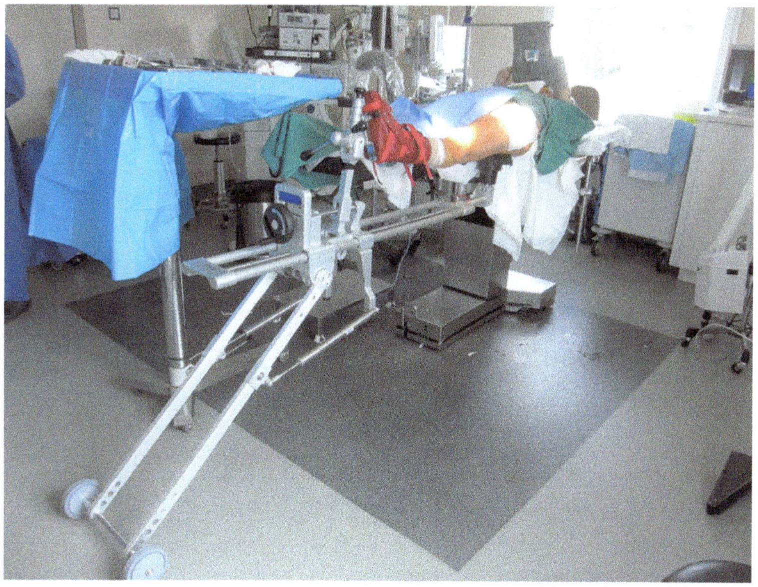

Fig. 38.5 Patient in supine position on a mobile traction table with wheels (Medacta International). Note the progressive traction mechanism and wheel handle

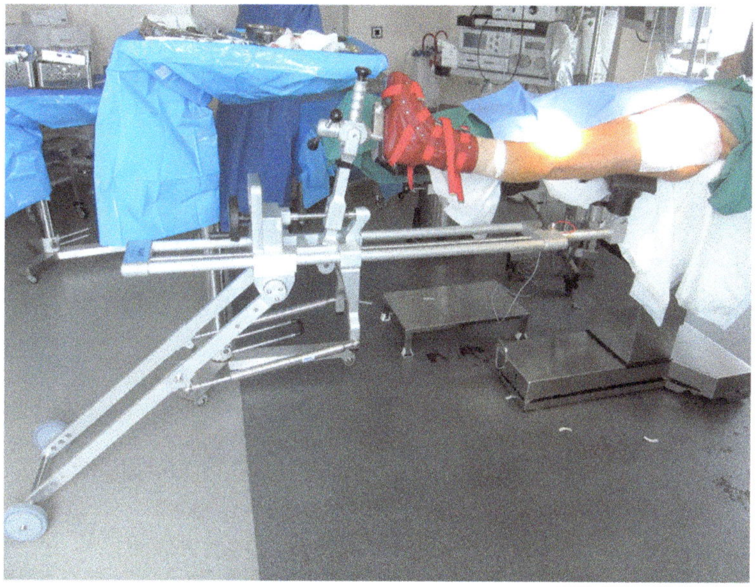

Fig. 38.6 Patient in supine position and traction table draped. Note the pneumatic assistant arm with the blue insert, which helps the surgeon hold the arthroscope

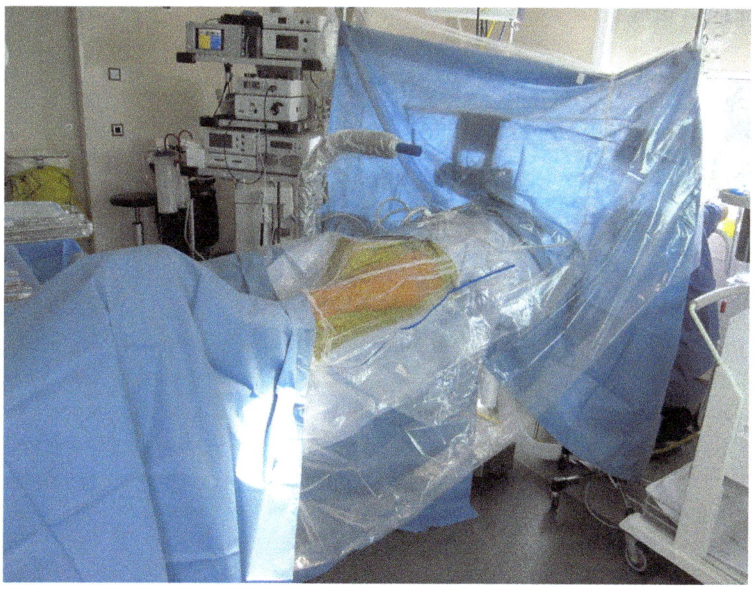

sary in many cases. In the case of labral suturing, on average four anchors are necessary, with some cases requiring eight anchors. This is, of course, time consuming and puts nerves at risk. The pin hip distraction technique [6, 10–12] has been used since the year 2000 and is still in use at our institution. The device not only avoids the perineal post, which is responsible for the pudendal nerve and perineal skin lesions, but also distracts the hip joint without overstretching the femoral and sciatic nerves (see basic science below). In over 3000 cases, we have not documented a single nerve lesion due to traction with this type of hip distraction.

Basic Science and Distraction Technique

Most commonly general anesthesia is used, often with the addition of some type of agent to induce muscle relaxation. The procedure can be performed either in the lateral or supine position. On a traction table (Figs. 38.4, 38.5, and 38.6), the foot is well padded, and the foot holder is applied taking care of the skin. The leg is held in abduction and a large perineal post with a diameter larger than 20 cm is placed. The genitalia are inspected to ensure minimal compression. The foot holder (Figs. 38.4 and 38.5) is connected to the distraction arm. If the table permits a lateralization of the perineal post (elevation in lateral decubitus), this adds a force moment for better distraction. No traction is applied yet. The fluoroscopic C-arm is brought into the field and the hip visualized. A traction test is applied to see if the hip easily distracts (see capsular releases below). The traction is then released and the patient draped. The hip is placed in 15° of flexion, neutral rotation, and 15° of abduction. The hip capsule is maximally relaxed in this position. This is a good starting point, but further adjustments might be necessary during the procedure. Progressive traction is then applied to the foot. Sufficient hip distraction implies traction forces of about 250–500 N (i.e., 25–50 kg). A dedicated spinal needle (e.g., a 14 G) is used under careful fluoroscopic control to break the suction seal. Once the suction seal is broken, the force needed diminishes significantly. However, on a traction table, much of the traction force is lost in uselessly distracting the knee (about 5 mm) and ankle joints (another 5 mm). This extra 10 mm of distraction overstretches the sciatic and femoral nerves putting them in danger of neurapraxia, or even worse axonotmesis. If a traction table is used, distraction time should be carefully recorded. The measurement of pressure by using a tensiometer has been suggested. The lateral decubitus and supine positions have been in use for many years and are equally safe.

The pin hip distractor [6, 10–12], once installed, produces a traction force exclusively on the hip joint, thus avoiding overstretching the sciatic and femoral nerves as mentioned above. No perineal post is needed and this fully avoids pudendal nerve and perineal skin lesions. The initial 500 N of distraction force needed is calculated in the elasticity of the dedicated Schanz screws. Once this traction force is attained, the dedicated Schanz screws will begin to bend on the image intensifier (Fig. 38.3).

Also, on a traction table, the femoral head has a tendency to slide anteriorly and reduce the anterior joint space because of acetabular anteversion. Most often, lesions are in the anterior and superior regions (such as in the often encountered femoroacetabular impingement), and most surgeons prefer to internally rotate the lower extremity to avoid the narrowing of the anterior joint space. Internal rotation moves the sciatic nerve anteriorly and thus puts it at risk if the surgeon creates a posterolateral portal. Pin hip distraction avoids this by allowing a controlled anterior to posterior traction vector in neutral rotation (Fig. 38.1). A posterolateral portal (Fig. 38.2) is thus very safe without putting the sciatic nerve at risk. The posterolateral portal gives a great view of the most frequent lesions that are located in the anterosuperior region of the acetabulum. This is because the camera is farther away from the area visualized and gives a better perspective than an anterolateral or anterior viewing portal.

Complex hip arthroscopy indications where traction times may be greater than 90 min and pin hip distraction may be considered:

1. Complete femoroacetabular impingement correction (head–neck junction correction, labral suturing, labral reconstruction grafting, and cartilage transplantation).
2. Labral suturing.
3. Labral reconstruction grafting (fascia lata, allograft, or semitendinosus graft).
4. Acetabular cartilage transplantation [11] or reconstruction techniques (MACI and AMIC).
5. Osteochondromatosis and chondromatosis.
6. Ligamentum teres reconstruction.
7. Keen hip arthroscopy beginner who wants to progress to more complex surgery.
8. Senior hip arthroscopy surgeons who are teaching procedures to beginners.
9. Other complex hip arthroscopy procedures that were longer than 90 min of hip distraction time are needed.
10. "Nondistractable" hips on traction tables.
11. When traction on the lower limb is not desirable (such as ipsilateral lower limb fracture, recent ligamentous injuries, or knee prosthesis).
12. Obese patients where powerful distraction is needed (invasive hip distraction has been used successfully in patients up to 160 kg of weight).

Surgical Technique of Pin Hip Distractor

We have tried the lateral and supine approaches for this indication. We are largely in favor of the lateral decubitus position and setup is identical to the classical "lateral approach" with some differences. Three standard arthroscopy portals [13] are used: the posterolateral, anterolateral, and anterior portals (Fig. 38.2).

We prefer the lateral approach and pin hip distraction for the following practical reasons:

1. For the beginner it is always possible, if technical difficulties are encountered, to convert to mini open or open surgery without redraping (this would not easily be the case if a standard traction table is used). If necessary, conversion to a mini posterior approach is always possible in the lateral position, but not in the supine. We can compare this to the beach chair position in shoulder arthroscopy. An example would be in the case of instrument breakage. Instruments tend to slide on the posterior rim of the acetabulum in the direction of the ligamentum transversum and extraction can be difficult. In lateral decubitus, these fall into the pulvinar and are stopped from sliding further and extraction is thus easier.
2. Newer arthroscopic techniques for the posterior extraarticular compartments, such as sciatic nerve decompression, are easier to access.
3. Beginners feel no time pressure and more complex hip reconstructions such as labral detachment, graft reconstruction techniques, and suturing are possible.
4. Pin hip distraction can be easily released in order to dynamically test impingement positions of the hip during and after surgery (maximum flexion, 90° flexion and maximum internal rotation, and maximum abduction). These motions can be tested without difficulty to confirm that no impingement is present in the same manner as in open surgery. This can be performed without compromising the sterile field. With a traction table, this would be a more risky task due to the nonsterile traction boot.
5. Finally, in the lateral decubitus, bubbles coming from radiofrequency devices are easily evacuated through the incisions, in contrast with the supine position where they tend to accumulate anteriorly.

The lower extremity is draped so that it can be moved freely (Figs. 38.1 and 38.2). The c-arm fluoroscope is brought under the table and draped, providing a good anterior to posterior view. The pin hip distractor is set up in slight hip flexion. The dedicated Schanz screw is placed 1 cm above the acetabular sourcil under image intensifier control and another at the level of the lesser trochanter (Fig. 38.3). The proximal acetabular Schanz screw is in line with the anterior trochanteric margin (Fig. 38.1). The relative positions of the proximal and distal Schanz screws produce an anterior to posterior traction vector optimizing anterior joint space opening, even if no lower limb internal rotation is applied. The pin hip distractor is installed on the inserted Schanz screws (Fig. 38.1). The device has a precision screw mechanism which can precisely move the tubes so that they fit onto the Schanz screws. Once the distractor is installed, two other Schanz screws, one proximally in the acetabulum and another distally in the femur, are applied through the distractor's guiding tubes (Figs. 38.1 and 38.3). This stabilizes the rotational forces and permits a better anterior to posterior distraction vector. The whole hip distractor is thus an angularly stable construct and improves traction forces. Once the pin hip distractor is installed, distraction is applied on the hip by turning the axial distraction screw. The lower extremity is set in abduction of about 30°–45°. This maneuver, and the abovementioned slight flexion of about 10°–15°, will relax the superior and anterior hip capsule including the iliofemoral ligament and will permit better distraction (Fig. 38.3). With adequate distraction of ideally 12 mm, the hip joint is decompressed with a large spinal needle and the suction seal is broken. However, it is estimated that about 5% of hips are considered insufficiently distractible on traction tables. In these cases, pin hip distraction can be useful by permitting controlled capsular releases (see below). The capsular release technique can also be used on a traction table; however, one must be very prudent with traction times applied. Using a cannulated system, the arthroscope is first introduced in the anterolateral portal. We prefer using the 70° scope which provides a better view initially, especially in tighter joints. The posterolateral and anterior portals are then created under direct visual control, avoiding iatrogenic labral and cartilage lesions.

In the case of insufficiently distractible hips, it is very difficult to visualize the joint without putting the articular cartilage at risk. This is the case with either the traction table or the pin distraction device. If the joint space opening is less than 12 mm, we do not recommend blind and forceful intraarticular penetration. Once the pin distractor is in place, the posterolateral portal is established. The arthroscope is brought onto the hip capsule and the anterolateral and anterior portals are made. While viewing from the posterolateral portal, the superior and anterosuperior capsule are freed from the attachment of the gluteus minimus fibers (extraarticular arthroscopy). An anterosuperior capsulectomy is then performed until the head and neck junction is visible. Progressively, this capsulectomy is made in the direction of the acetabular rim until the labrum is visualized. The joint space will open slowly based on the extent of the superior and anterior capsulectomy. Once this joint space is deemed sufficient, a nitinol guide wire and cannula are inserted between the labrum and the femoral head through the anterolateral portal. The other portals are then established in a similar fashion, as mentioned above, under direct vision.

Postoperative Rehabilitation After Arthroscopies with Pin Hip Distractor

The postoperative program described here is essentially for complex arthroscopic reconstructive surgery, such as femoroacetabular impingement correction. The patients are placed on crutches and partial weight bearing of 5–10 kg is authorized during the first 6 weeks. We have been voluntarily overcautious in weight bearing. Most of the cases have had major head–neck junction osteoplasty. No neck fractures or other proximal femoral fractures around the Schanz screw holes have been observed in over 3000 cases. After 6 weeks, abductor strengthening exercises are allowed. In cases of minor arthroscopic surgery, such as labral resection, weight bearing is as tolerated and strengthening exercises are introduced as soon as pain regresses, often at one postoperative week.

Minor Complications of Pin Hip Distraction

Complications were monitored for the first 1000 cases. Surprisingly, no fractures of the proximal femur or the head–neck junction were observed. We think that this is partially due to the strict partial weight-bearing protocol we apply, thus treating every patient as if they suffered a nondisplaced neck fracture. We have observed three (0.3 %) lateral femoral cutaneous nerve neuropraxias. None were related to traction. Two resolved after 48 h and the other after 6 weeks. This is likely due to the anterior portal, which is very close in proximity to the branches of this nerve. Vigorous instrumentation usually occurs through this portal since most hip pathology is in the anterosuperior region. We usually try to move the anterior portal as laterally as possible, leaving 3 cm between the anterolateral portal and the anterior portal in an attempt to minimize irritation of this cutaneous nerve. No pudendal, sciatic, or femoral nerve lesions and no perineal skin lesions were observed. Five hematomas at the level of the distal Schanz screws were documented and resolved spontaneously. Overall, pin hip distraction for complex reconstructive surgery with longer than 90–120 min traction time is very safe compared to reported complication rates of hip arthroscopy performed on traction tables.

Technical Pearls

1. Lateral decubitus (authors favorite) or supine.
2. Drape the lower limb so that it can be moved freely.
3. If a traction table is used, use a perineal post that has more than a 20 cm diameter.
4. If a traction table is used, limit traction time to 90 min and traction force to 250 N (25 kg).
5. If the pin hip distractor is used:
   - Place the two proximal Schanz screws anteriorly in line with the anterior trochanteric margin, 1 cm above the acetabular sourcil.
   - Place the two distal Schanz screws in the middle of the femur at the level of the lesser trochanter.
   - Apply distraction.
   - Apply 10° of flexion and 30°–45° of abduction.
   - A minimum of 12 mm of distraction should be visible once abduction is applied.
     - If not (5 % cases), use the capsular release technique described.

References

1. Beck M, Leunig M, Parvizi J, et al. Anterior femoroacetabular impingement: part II. Midterm results of surgical treatment. Clin Ortho. 2004;(418):67–73.
2. Espinosa N, Rothenfluh DA, Beck M, et al. Treatment of femoro-acetabular impingement: preliminary results of labral refixation. J Bone Joint Surg Am. 2006;88:925–35.
3. Gautier E, Ganz K, Krugel N, et al. Anatomy of the medial femoral circumflex artery and its surgical implications. J Bone Joint Surg Br. 2000;82:679–83.
4. Ganz R, Parvizi J, Beck M, et al. Femoroacetabular impingement: a cause for osteoarthritis of the hip. Clin Orthop. 2003;417:112–20.
5. Lavigne M, Parvizi J, Beck M, et al. Anterior femoroacetabular impingement: part I. Techniques of joint preserving surgery. Clin Orthop. 2004;418:61–6.
6. Sadri H, Menetrey J, Kraus E, et al. Arthroskopische Behandlung des femoroazetabulären Impingements. Arthroskopie. 2006;19:67–74. German.
7. Funke EL, Munzinger U. Complications in hip arthroscopy. Arthroscopy. 1996;12:156–9.
8. Glick JM. Complications of hip arthroscopy by the lateral approach. In: Sherman OH, Minkoff J, editors. Current management of complications in orthopaedics: arthroscopic surgery. Baltimore: Williams & Wilkins; 1990. p. 193–201.
9. Sampson TG. Complications of hip arthroscopy. Clin Sports Med. 2001;20:831–5.
10. Langlais F, Lambotte JC, Lannou R, et al. Hip pain from impingement and dysplasia in patients aged 20-50 years. Workup and role for reconstruction. Joint Bone Spine. 2006;73:614–23.
11. Sadri H, Dienst M. Eingriffe am hyalinen Knorpel. In: Dienst M, editor. Lehrbuch und Atlas Hüftarthroscopie. München: Elsevier Urban & Fischer; 2010. p. 189–200.
12. http://www.swissmedicalinstruments.ch/.
13. Byrd JW, Pappas JN, Pedley MJ. Hip arthroscopy: an anatomic study of portal placement and relationship to the extra-articular structures. Arthroscopy. 1995;11:418–23.

39 Arthroscopic Treatment: Fundamentals of Hip Joint Instrumentation

Sean Mc Millan, Brian D. Busconi, and Craig M. Roberto

Introduction

Hip arthroscopy has grown exponentially in the past decade. Looking at hip arthroscopy trends occurring from 2004 through 2009, Montgomery et al. in 2012 found a 365 % increase in the rate of hip arthroscopy. The majority of cases were performed in patients aged 20–39 years [1]. A multitude of factors can be identified when examining the growth of hip arthroscopy including heightened awareness of hip pathology, improved radiographic imaging, increased number of hip preservation fellowships available, continued scholarly articles, improved training centers, and advances in arthroscopic instrumentation allowing for easier surgical performance. Within this chapter we will focus on the latter.

Operating Room Tables

Hip arthroscopy has traditionally been performed on standard operating room tables and fracture tables. However, these tables, while usable in skilled hands, were not designed specifically for the needs of hip arthroscopy. As such, problems have been noted during the procedure secondary to table inadequacies. Among these problems have been inability to adequately distract the joint, ankle injury, the inability to maintain distraction, pudendal and/or sciatic nerve injury, and limitations related to fluoroscopy [2–4]. Fracture tables were often ill suited for positioning in the lateral decubitus position, which is the preferred position for a number of surgeons who perform the procedure [5]. Furthermore the limited availability of fracture tables in ambulatory surgery center settings has been cited as a problem as well.

As such, there has been a growth of commercial hip arthroscopy tables and/or table attachments that are designed specifically for the procedure. The first dedicated hip distractors were made by Arthronix and Innomed. The latter, designed by McCarthy, provided significant and effective mechanical distraction in the lateral decubitus position and can be used on a conventional operating table. The Smith and Nephew System allows for surgical performance in the supine or lateral position. Others, such as the Arthrex System, Maquet table, Athello table, and Hanna table, allow for the procedure to be performed in the supine position only (Figs. 39.1 and 39.2). It should be noted that many of these tables, including the Athello, Maquet, and Hanna tables, are also used for other procedures, such as anterior hip replacements.

Improvements in table designs are wide ranging. For one, all newer-generation tables or attachment systems are radiolucent. This facilitates the use of fluoroscopic imaging in either position, lateral or supine. Next the perineal posts have been bulked up to help minimize perineal and pudendal nerve injury. The post comes equipped with a thick cushioned pad that is designed to provide "give" as well as eliminate firm surfaces that may cause injury or bruising to the patient. Additionally the table designs allow for the posts to be lateralized against the inner thigh to further aid against injury [6–8]. Newer modifications have also been made to the foot holder. Fracture tables conventionally utilized a leather boot with friction tensioning to secure the feet into place. However, more current-generation foot holders are in the form of a "ski boot" design. The intent of this modification is to prevent foot slippage during traction, as well as to minimize injury to the foot by distributing the forces across it.

S.M. Millan, DO (✉)
Orthopedic Sports Medicine, Professional Orthopedics at Lourdes Medical Associates, 2103 Burlington-Mount Holly Road, Burlington, NJ 08016, USA
e-mail: mcmillans@lourdesnet.org

B.D. Busconi, MD
Division of Sports Medicine, Department of Orthopaedics, University of Massachusetts Memorial Medical Center, Worcester, MA, USA

C.M. Roberto, DO
Division of Sports Medicine, Department of Orthopaedics, University of Massachusetts, Worcester, MA, USA

J.C. McCarthy et al. (eds.), *Hip Joint Restoration*, DOI 10.1007/978-1-4614-0694-5_39

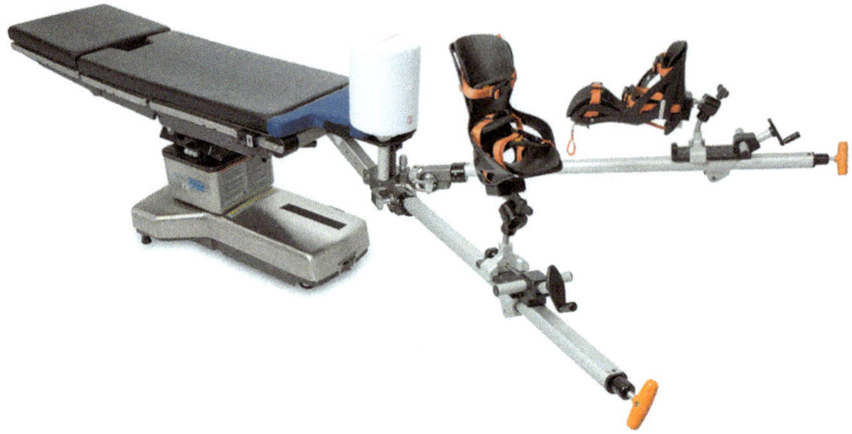

Fig. 39.1 The Smith and Nephew hip distractor allows for nerve protection of both the perineum and the lower leg due to its well-padded post and force distributed foot holder. The table easily converts to positioning in lateral decubitus, making it the only table currently available that can accommodate both positions. Image courtesy of Smith & Nephew, Inc

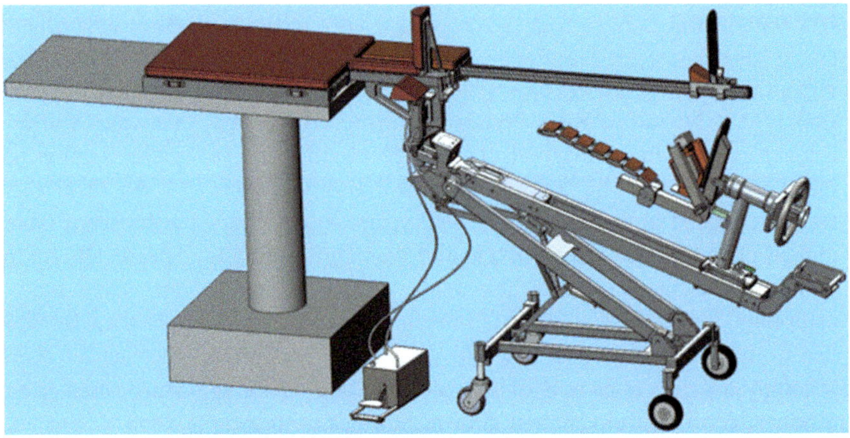

Fig. 39.2 The Athello table is designed to allow anterior hip replacement as well as supine hip arthroscopy. The table is adjustable for height and length for the operative leg and allows for the boot to be detached easily for ranging during femoral osteoplasty. Image courtesy of ATHELLO Inc

Instrumentation

During the early years of hip arthroscopy, specific instrumentation for hip arthroscopy was not available. Instead, instruments from commonly used shoulder trays were utilized for suture passing and manipulation. While crossover is seen in many of the shoulder and hip instruments today, the ability to have instruments designed specifically for hip arthroscopy has facilitated increased procedural indications and has minimized the risk of iatrogenic injury [9].

Standard in numerous hip arthroscopy trays are half skids or cannulas, switching sticks, and metal cannulated obturators. These instruments are available in standard and hip length sizes. Additionally, disposable partially threaded and fully threaded cannulas are available to facilitate delivery of hip length instruments while maintaining portal patency.

Several commercial companies have created hip "length" instruments. These instruments include graspers, suture retrievers, suture passers, and tissue liberators. Hip length instruments are elongated on average 2–8 cm's to facilitate working with the deeply recessed hip joint. The variability of the lengths is company dependent [10–12]. As such, larger patients are now able to undergo the procedure safely. Secondly, many of the hip instruments are designed with a curve at their distal tip to allow work around the spherical femoral head. This advancement has resulted in decreased iatrogenic injury to the cartilage within the tight hip joint. Furthermore, it makes access to the entirety of the hip joint possible through the standard arthroscopic portals.

More recently, articulating instrumentation has arrived to the market. These devices afford the surgeon the ability to safely maneuver about the rounded femoral head and into the acetabulum. These instruments include probes, graspers, suture retrievers, elevation paddles, and radiofrequency devices (Figs. 39.3, 39.4, and 39.5). Designed specifically for hip usage, the shafts to these devices are stiffer than their earlier versions. Additionally, the shafts are of a length suitable for usage in most hips [10].

Options for suture passing around the labrum have grown significantly. These increased options are one of the principal reasons why there has been a shift in philosophy from labral debridement to labral repair. Among these suture passing options are "bird beaks," "Clever hooks", and a variety of

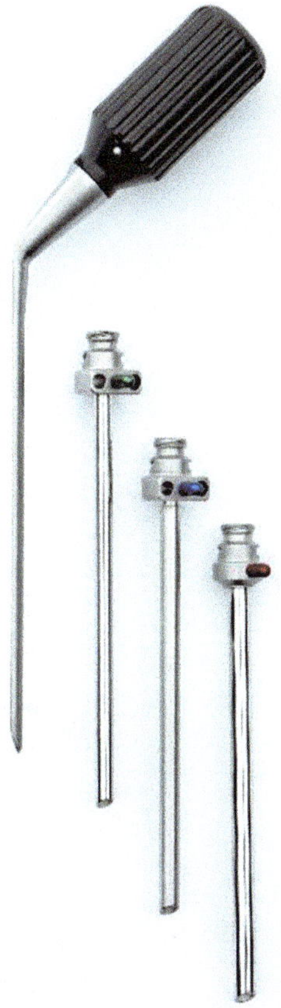

Fig. 39.3 Variable-sized slotted cannulas allow for instrument delivery into the hip joint safely. The metal cannulas for working and viewing are also available in variable sizes with rounded edges to protect the tissues and cartilage. Image courtesy of Smith & Nephew, Inc

boutique instruments that allow for antegrade or retrograde stitch passage [10–12]. Moreover, the diameter of the suture passing devices has been decreased in size to allow for delicate maneuvering around the labrum. The ability to repair the labrum in an atraumatic manner has had a great appeal to hip arthroscopists [13].

For articular cartilage injuries, particularly of the acetabulum, microfracture instrumentation has been designed specifically for hip arthroscopy. Long-handled ring curettes are also available to clear the articular surface to the subchondral bone. Likewise higher caliber shavers have become available, such as the Arthrex torpedo shaver, to allow for cartilage edge stabilization [10]. Finally, long-handled variable angle chondral picks are commercially available for carrying out the micro fracture procedure [10–12].

Capsular closure devices have also gained popularity within the past few years. The need to close the capsule at the completion of the arthroscopic procedure has been debated. The merits of closing the capsule are meant for discussion at a later time; however, the advent of devices that can readily aid the surgeon in repairing the capsule has provided this option for surgeons of all skill levels [10, 13].

Joint Access

Hip access kits have grown in popularity within the past few years. Within these kits are elongated spinal needles ranging from 14 to 18 gauge in thickness [10–13]. Nitinol guide wires are also standard within the access kits, as are a variety of other optional use components, such as syringes for insufflation, rulers, and marking pens. The diameter of the Nitinol wires varies in size from 1.1 to 1.5 mm. These variations are company dependent and it is important to know the diameter of the wire prior to commencement of surgery. The cannulated metal obturators used for joint access are not universal in the size of their cannulation and, as such, may not be able to accommodate the diameter of the guide wire from a different company. Additionally, due to the forces applied across the Nitinol guide wires during access, it is recommended to utilize a new guide wire for each access procedure. As such, the various commercial kits available come standard with 2–3 wires.

Cannulated metal obturators that range from 4.5 to 6.5 mm are available in most hip arthroscopy trays. These cannulas are able to be used in conjunction with the hip arthroscopy access kits to facilitate precise access while minimizing iatrogenic damage. These cannulas are available commercially in variable sizes as well, with diameters that increase incrementally by 0.5 mm. The ability to rapidly change from a 4.5 mm cannula to a larger size cannula has many advantages [12]. Typical hip distraction allows for a working field of 8–10 mm of space between the femoral head and the acetabulum. However, patients with large pincer deformities can sometimes have a field of 6 mm or less. As such, the risk of cartilage damage while accessing the hip joint can be minimized by downsizing the cannula size [14]. A second advantage of the variable diameter sizes relates to fluid management. The metal cannulas' ability to connect easily to a bridge construct allows for manipulation of fluid inflow and outflow. This ability can improve field visualization, as well as limit fluid extravasation. Further technical changes within the newer-generation metal cannulas include rounding of the distal edges of the cannula [10]. This feature limits soft tissue and articular cartilage damage.

The length of the metal cannulas varies dependent upon the commercial system that is employed. Standard hip arthroscopes range from 160 to 180 mm in length. Elongated hip length arthroscopes can range up to 240 mm [10, 12]. As such, the metal cannulas are designed to accommodate their corresponding arthroscope. Marriage of cannulas and camera systems is advisable to avoid intraoperative mismatch.

Once hip access has been achieved, the surgeon has the ability to view with multiple-angle arthroscopes. The use of a 70° arthroscope has allowed increased visualization around the femoral head. This feature has made it easier to avoid missing pathology around the rim and to have a more

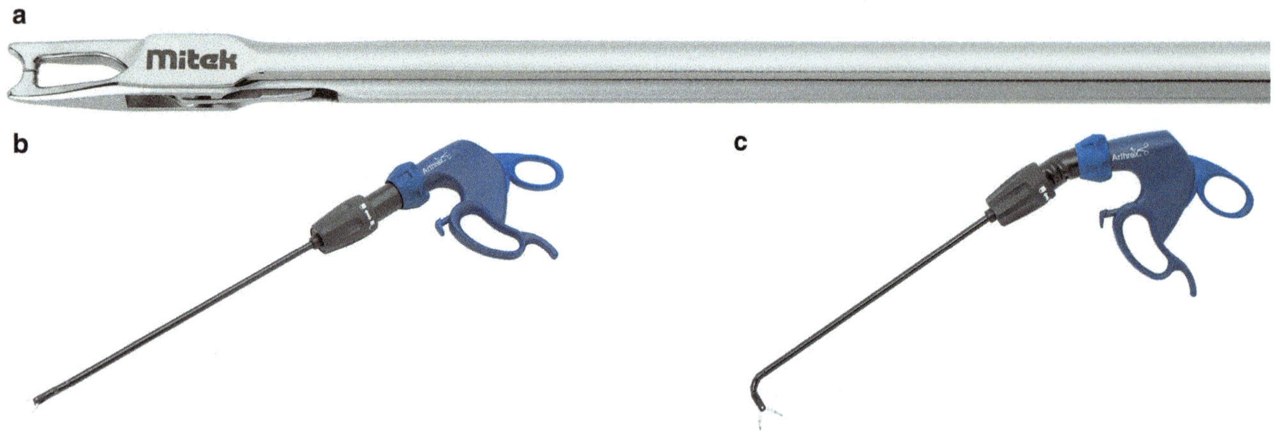

Fig. 39.4 (**a**) Hip length suture graspers with a blunt recessed nose allow the surgeon to safely push or pull within the hip joint. (**b, c**) The articulating instruments are designed with longer, stiffer shafts and contain tips that are able to maneuver 360° within the working field. Images courtesy of Arthrex, Inc

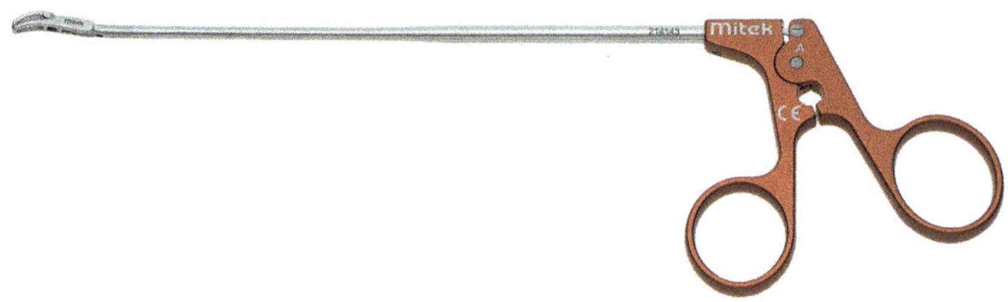

Fig. 39.5 Hip designed instrumentation with left and right angles allow for maneuvering around the femoral head safely. Image courtesy of DePuy Synthes Mitek Sports Medicine

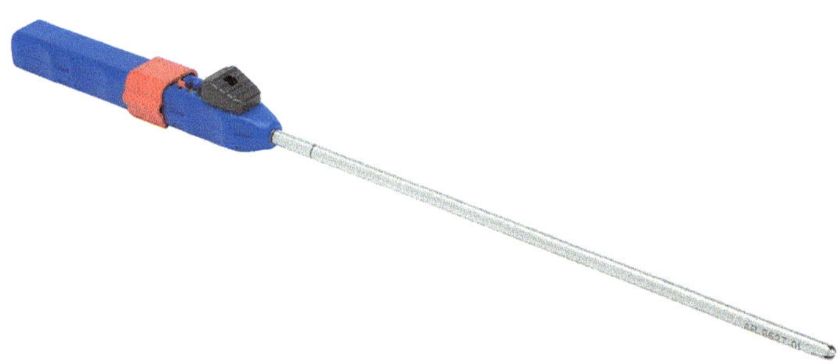

Fig. 39.6 Disposable, retractable blade for arthroscopic capsulotomy and iliopsoas release. The device is cannulated to allow for insertion over a Nitinol guide wire. Image courtesy of Arthrex, Inc

expansive view of the spherical femoral head. The 30° arthroscope also has a role during hip arthroscopy. It is more readily utilized in the peripheral compartment and for visualizing the fovea within the central compartment.

The use of a banana blade to perform the capsulotomy has enabled surgeons to work within the joint more freely. It has also greatly enhanced the ability to perform femoral osteoplasties by creating an increased field of view in the working area. The evolution of these blades has continued to grow, with both reusable and single-use tools available. As the application of these blades has expanded to include usage for other procedures, such as labral takedown and iliopsoas release, the strength and sharpness of the blades has also continued to improve. In addition to the all-metal capsule blades, the grip and contour of the handles have evolved to allow for finer control [10–13]. Additionally, retractable capsule cutting devices are available that work via the guidance of a Nitinol guide wire for targeting and cartilage protection [10] (Fig. 39.6).

Further advancing the ease of hip arthroscopy are targeting guides designed to allow surgeons to triangulate accessory portals by referencing off of the standard anterolateral portal [10, 12] (Fig. 39.7). These targeting guides function by clipping onto the cannula for the arthroscope. The ability to rapidly target and create precise accessory portals can decrease traction and overall surgical time. The increased precision can translate into easier repairs and maneuverability within the working field.

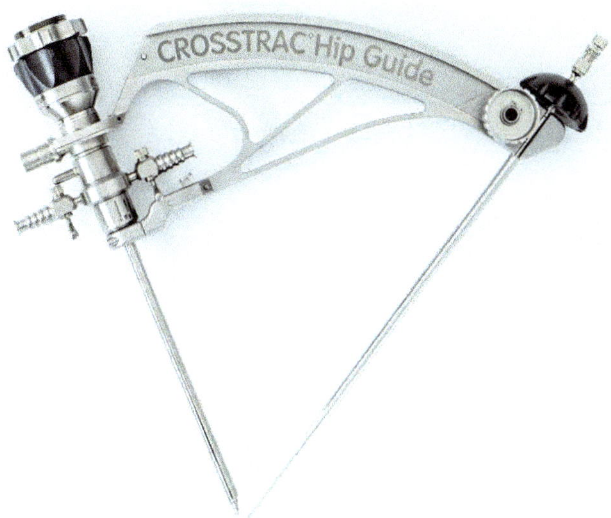

Fig. 39.7 The accessory portal targeting system allows for quick and reproducible placement of portals, referenced off the viewing arthroscope. Image courtesy of Smith & Nephew, Inc

Fluid Management

Fluid extravasation is a known complication of hip arthroscopy. Fluid volumes between 1 and 3 L in the retroperitoneum and abdomen have been reported in symptomatic patients [15, 16]. Several factors have been identified as causes for the extravasation. Among these are wide capsulotomies for osteochondroplasty, normal saline solution usage, arthroscopic equipment, and pump selection [17]. Additionally, certain procedures such as iliopsoas release have also been associated. Sampson recommended the use of an outflow-dependent pump based upon his small case review of fluid extravasation; pressure-sensitive systems have also been recommended [18–20].

The use of cannulas to shuttle instruments into the working field has also been noted to decrease the risk of fluid extravasation. Newer plastic cannulas have come onto the market that allow for telescoping, facilitating a wider working field [13]. Furthermore, improvements made to cannula dams have limited the loss of fluid outside the body, allowing for more precise calculation of fluid input and output.

Shavers, Burrs, and Radiofrequency

Hip length shavers, burrs, and radiofrequency devices have facilitated the expansion of hip arthroscopy indications. Whereas early hip arthroscopy relied upon shoulder designed instruments, these devices are elongated on average 2 cm; and many have been designed specifically for the hip.

Due to the geometry of the femoral head, the use of curved shavers has become preferred by hip arthroscopists. The curve allows for safe passage over the femoral head into the deep foveal region of the hip joint. Likewise, it has made following the curvature of the acetabulum for labral debridement easier to perform.

With the more recent recognition of bony femoroacetabular impingement (FAI), significant advancement in the design of burrs used for acetabular rim resection and femoral neck osteoplasty has occurred. Burrs with an elongated hip length have allowed for increased access while maintaining safety. Additionally, the diameter and shape of the burr tips has allowed the surgeon a variety of options for treatment. The author prefers a round-tip 5.5 mm burr for femoral osteoplasty and a 4.0 mm clear hooded burr for acetabuloplasty. The use of the smaller, clear hooded burr allows for fine boney resection while protecting the labrum.

Similarly, the advent of articulating radiofrequency devices has permitted deep access more readily and safely [10–12]. Articulating wands were initially designed for usage in the supine position; however, a more ergonomic device has been launched that allows for ease of articulation in the lateral positions as well [11]. The articulating wands allow for 360° range of movement within the working field (Fig. 39.8).

Anchors

One of the greatest advances in hip arthroscopy has been the evolving design of anchors and their placement. As labral repair has gained popularity over simple debridement in the last decade, the need for anchors specifically designed to meet the needs of the hip has grown. As noted earlier, the drill guide instrumentation has been modified to accommodate for placement of anchors in the hip. These modifications include elongation of the guides approximately 2–3 cm in length, application of curved guides, and modification to the guide tips (such as dove tails or saw teeth) [10–13].

The unique bony shape of the acetabulum has provided challenges to labral repair. However, with the arthroscopic movement toward labral preservation, the frequency of anchor use has risen in the past 10–15 years. The acetabular rim, where the labrum resides, has a rounded curvature from anterior to posterior. Additionally, the rim is extremely thin and may contain cysts in advanced FAI. As such, the challenge for the surgeon is to place anchors as close to the acetabular rim as possible in order to restore the labral suction seal, without penetrating the articular cartilage.

To help avoid anchor penetration into the joint, as well as to compensate for slight working portal malposition, the use of curved anchor guides has become more prevalent. These guides can be of particular benefit when utilizing the mid-

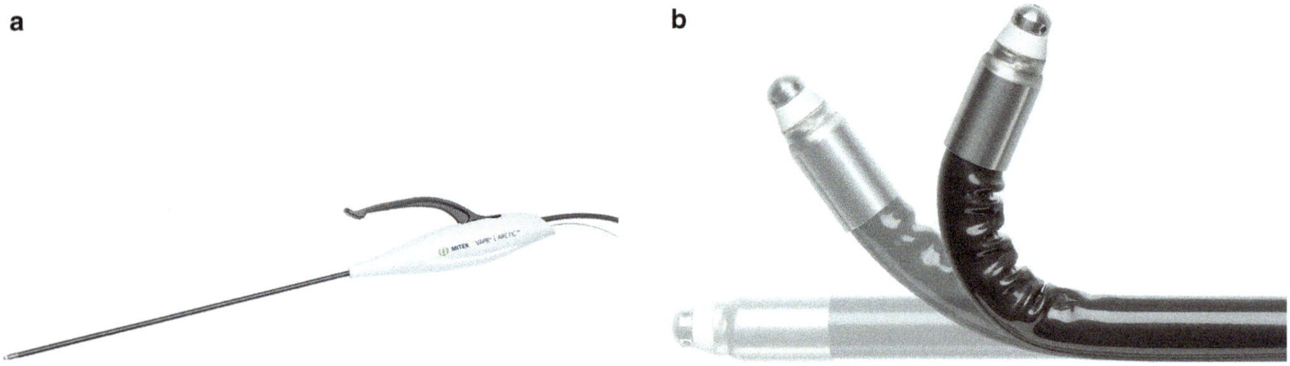

Fig. 39.8 The articulating radiofrequency device allows for 360° of working field. The ergonomic design allows for utilization in either the supine or lateral position. Image courtesy of DePuy Synthes Mitek Sports Medicine

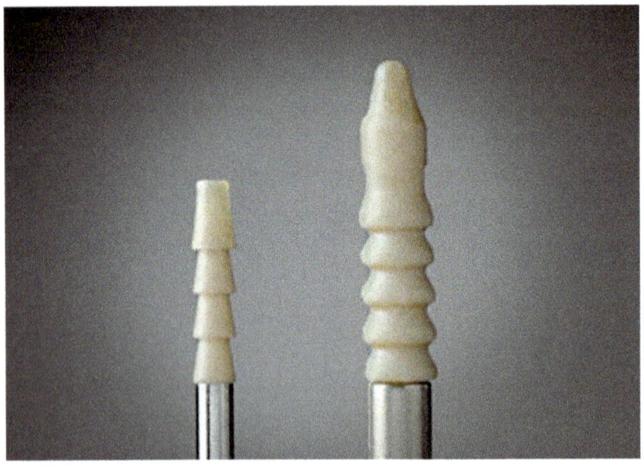

Fig. 39.9 Advances in anchor technology have allowed for reduction in length by roughly half while maintaining acceptable pullout strength. Image courtesy of Pivot Medical, A Stryker Sports Medicine Company

anterior portal for anchor placement, as it can increase anchor divergence from the articular surface. A study by Nho et al. found curved anchor guides to be of greatest benefit when utilized at the 1 o'clock position [21].

The composition and profile of the anchors themselves have also evolved. Currently, anchors for labral repair are available in the form of PEEK (polyetheretherketone), bio-composite, and PLDLA (poly-L/D-lactide) [10–13]. Modifications made to these anchors for the hip include decreasing their diameter, decreasing their length, and decreasing the suture size. Both knotless and knotted anchor systems are available, as well as single- and double-loaded anchor constructs. Currently the smallest anchor with hip labral repair indications is 1.4 mm in diameter [13]. Additional anchor sizes also exist, including 2.3, 2.9, and 3.0 mm. Furthermore, the advent of "short anchors" has gained support due to the decreased drilling depth requirement. These anchors are shortened by approximately 1/3 to 1/2 in length as compared to traditional anchors, with similar pullout strength (Fig. 39.9) [13].

Summary

Hip arthroscopy is an extremely challenging field that has a steep learning curve. Advances in hip arthroscopy instrumentation have facilitated more reproducible outcomes and shorter surgical times. Additionally, these advances have decreased iatrogenic injury. While there is no single commercial system available that is perfect, most of the systems are able to function interchangeably with one another, providing a multitude of options for the surgeon.

References

1. Montgomery SR, Ngo SS, Hobson T. Trends and demographics in hip arthroscopy in the United States. Arthroscopy. 2013;29(4): 661–5.
2. Smart LR, Oetgen M, Noonan B, Medvecky M. Beginning hip arthroscopy: indications, positioning, portals, basic techniques, and complications. Arthroscopy. 2007;23:1348–53.
3. Lo YP, Chan YS, Lien LC, et al. Complications of hip arthroscopy: analysis of seventy three cases. Chang Gung Med J. 2006;29:86–92 [PubMed].
4. Farjo LA, Glick JM, Sampson TG. Hip arthroscopy for acetabular labral tears. Arthroscopy. 1999;15:132–7.
5. Glick JM, Sampson TG, Gordon RB, Behr JT, Schmidt E. Hip arthroscopy by the lateral approach. Arthroscopy. 1987;3:4–12.
6. Byrd JW. Hip arthroscopy: surgical indications. Arthroscopy. 2006;22:1260–2.
7. Sampson TG. Complications of hip arthroscopy. Tech Orthop. 2005;20:63–6.
8. McCarthy JC, Mason JB, Lee JA. Hip arthroscopy in the lateral position. Oper Tech Sports Med. 2002;10:196–9.
9. Ilizaliturri VM Jr, Camacho-Galindo J, Ugalde HG, Evia Ramirez AN. Paper #13: Cartilage injury caused by hip scope. In: Proceedings of the International Society for hip arthroscopy annual scientific meeting, Paris. 2011.
10. http://www.arthrex.com/hip?megamenu=hip.
11. http://www.depuy.com/hiparthroscopy.
12. http://www.smith-nephew.com/professional/products/all-products/hip-arthroscopy-system/.
13. www.pivotmedical.com.

14. Ilizaliturri VM. Complications of arthroscopic femoroacetabular impingement treatment: a review. Clin Orthop Relat Res. 2009;467: 760–8.
15. Haupt U, Völkle D, Waldherr C, Beck M. Intra- and retroperitoneal irrigation liquid after arthroscopy of the hip joint. Arthroscopy. 2008;24:966–8.
16. Stafford GH, Malviya A, Villar RN. Fluid extravasation during hip arthroscopy. Hip Int. 2011;21:740–3.
17. Siegel MG. Irrigation fluid complications. Arthroscopy. 2010; 26:576.
18. Funke EL, Munzinger U. Complications in hip arthroscopy. Arthroscopy. 1996;12:156–9.
19. Byrd JW, Chern KY. Traction versus distension for distraction of the joint during hip arthroscopy. Arthroscopy. 1997;13:346–9.
20. Fabricant PD, Maak TG, Cross MB, Kelly BT. Avoiding complications in hip arthroscopy. Oper Tech Sports Med. 2011;19:108–13.
21. Nho SJ, Freedman RL, Federer AE, Mather III RC, Espinoza Orias AA, Wang VM, Van Thiel GS. Computed tomographic analysis of curved and straight guides for placement of suture anchors for acetabular labral refixation. Arthroscopy. 2013;29(10):1623–7.

Arthroscopic Treatment: Principles and Devices for Hip Joint Access

40

J.W. Thomas Byrd

Introduction

The anatomy of the hip presents unique challenges to arthroscopy. These include its constrained ball and socket architecture, the dense surrounding soft tissue envelope, and the thick capsule with limited compliance. Specialized instrumentation is essential to overcoming each of these barriers (Fig. 40.1). Instruments must be longer and also sturdier to withstand the longer lever arm as well as the bending movements created by maneuvering within the deep soft tissues that encase the joint. Imaginative designs are necessary to navigate through the confines of the hip space and its deeply situated position.

Access

Because of these anatomic factors, access to the hip is more of a challenge and also more critical for effective operative procedures. For example, in the knee or shoulder, access is more of a given, whereas, in the hip, it is more of an essential element bearing close attention in every case. The two principles of access are (1) to be accomplished in an atraumatic fashion, avoiding iatrogenic injury to the joint, and (2) optimal positioning in order to reach the various confines and effectively perform resection, repair, and reconstructive procedures.

Once access to the hip has been achieved, maintaining and working along specifically developed portal tracts is important. The purpose is to be as atraumatic as possible to the surrounding soft tissues. This is important for three reasons. First, minimizing injury to the soft tissues reduces the amount of postsurgical pain, diminishing narcotic needs, and facilitating early recovery and rehabilitation. Second, it reduces the amount of soft tissue extravasation of fluid. Minimizing fluid extravasation aids in accomplishing complex procedures that may take more time and, again, helps reduce the amount of postoperative discomfort. Extravasation and swelling around the joint can start to hinder access, even with longer instruments. Third, complex bony procedures, such as correction of FAI, introduce a small risk of heterotopic ossification (HO). HO is not a consequence of surgical violation of the joint, but surgical violation of the surrounding soft tissues. Thus, lessening violation of the soft tissues lessens the risk of developing HO. Once portal tracts have been developed, it can be easy to maneuver instruments freehand along the soft tissue tracts, but in general, maintenance of the tract with some type of structural device will be preferable.

Technological advances have aided immensely in the technical considerations for effective access to the hip. Cannulated instrumentation allows prepositioning to be performed with needles and the instrumentation then subsequently placed in a reproducible fashion over guide wires (Fig. 40.2). Numerous bridging systems are available to maximize the working length with standard arthroscopes (Fig. 40.3). Various cannula designs emphasize being atraumatic to the joint surfaces and maintaining their position within the joint while moving different instruments and devices in and out (Fig. 40.4). Differing lengths and adjustable designs accommodate the highly variable depth of soft tissues, and large diameter cannulas are available for passage of virtually any instrumentation (Fig. 40.5). Additionally, slotted cannulas provide maximal versatility, accommodating placement of standard-length and long instruments and any curved or large design (Fig. 40.6).

Once the arthroscope has been introduced, placement of supplementary working portals is performed using fundamental triangulation techniques. The use of longer instruments and the constrained joint architecture can create greater challenges for triangulation skills. When necessary, guide systems have been developed that can lessen these hurdles (Fig. 40.7).

J.W.T. Byrd, MD (✉)
Nashville Sports Medicine Foundation,
2011 Church Street, Suite 100, Nashville, TN 37203, USA

Department of Orthopaedic Surgery and Rehabilitation,
Vanderbilt University, Nashville, TN 37232, USA
e-mail: info@nsmoc.com

J.C. McCarthy et al. (eds.), *Hip Joint Restoration*, DOI 10.1007/978-1-4614-0694-5_40

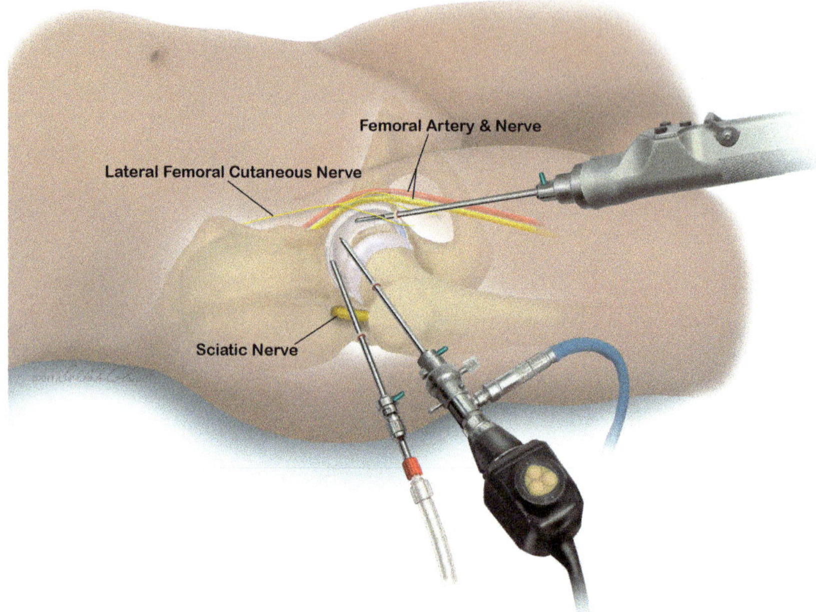

Fig. 40.1 The hip is the diarthrodial joint most deeply situated within the soft tissues. Precise portal placement is essential for navigating around the vital extra-articular structures as well as optimizing access within the joint. Longer instrument designs and special features for maneuvering within the spherical confines facilitate the procedure. Published with kind permission of ©J.W. Thomas Byrd 2015. All Rights Reserved

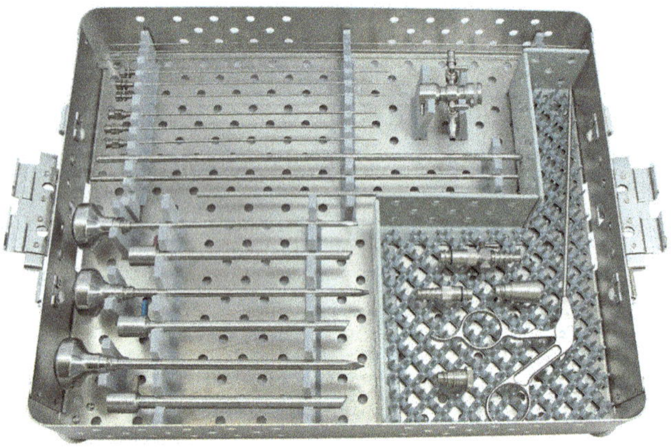

Fig. 40.2 Cannulated instrumentation systems are popular, as illustrated by this Stryker version. Prepositioning is performed with a spinal needle. A guide wire is passed through the needle, and the cannula/obturator assembly then passed over the guide wire. With permission from Stryker®

Fluid Management Systems

The development of reliable fluid management systems significantly influenced the progress of hip arthroscopy. This facilitated the development of more extensive restorative intra-articular procedures and the advancement of extra-articular endoscopic methods. The advantages of a high-flow fluid management system are that it allows prompt flow in response to suction and drainage, thus allowing more optimal visualization through a clear fluid medium without having to necessitate higher pressures that can result in greater unwanted fluid extravasation. Thus, procedures can be performed expanded beyond the confines of the capsule and also complex procedures of greater duration with less extravasation. Gravity flow alone may be less adequate for meeting these needs, although is it known to work well in the hands of some experienced surgeons. Numerous pumps are available that can serve well for hip arthroscopy. Each performs differently and has unique idiosyncrasies. The pumps are not infallible and thus the surgeon must be familiar with the characteristic behavior of whichever pump they choose to use.

Resection

Resection is accomplished in the hip as in other joints with combinations of power shaver blades and hand instruments. The designs are long and sturdy to accommodate maneuvering through the soft tissues and curved features are available to navigate within the constrained spherical anatomy (Fig. 40.8). Other special features with hand instruments are helpful to contend with the thick soft tissues (Fig. 40.9). Sharp dissection is important for both resection and soft tissue preparation for restorative procedures. Specialized arthroscopic knives are available (Fig. 40.10).

Repair

Three current principal areas of repair are the labrum, capsule, and articular surface.

Repair of the acetabular labrum in the hip is more challenging than repair of the glenoid labrum in the shoulder.

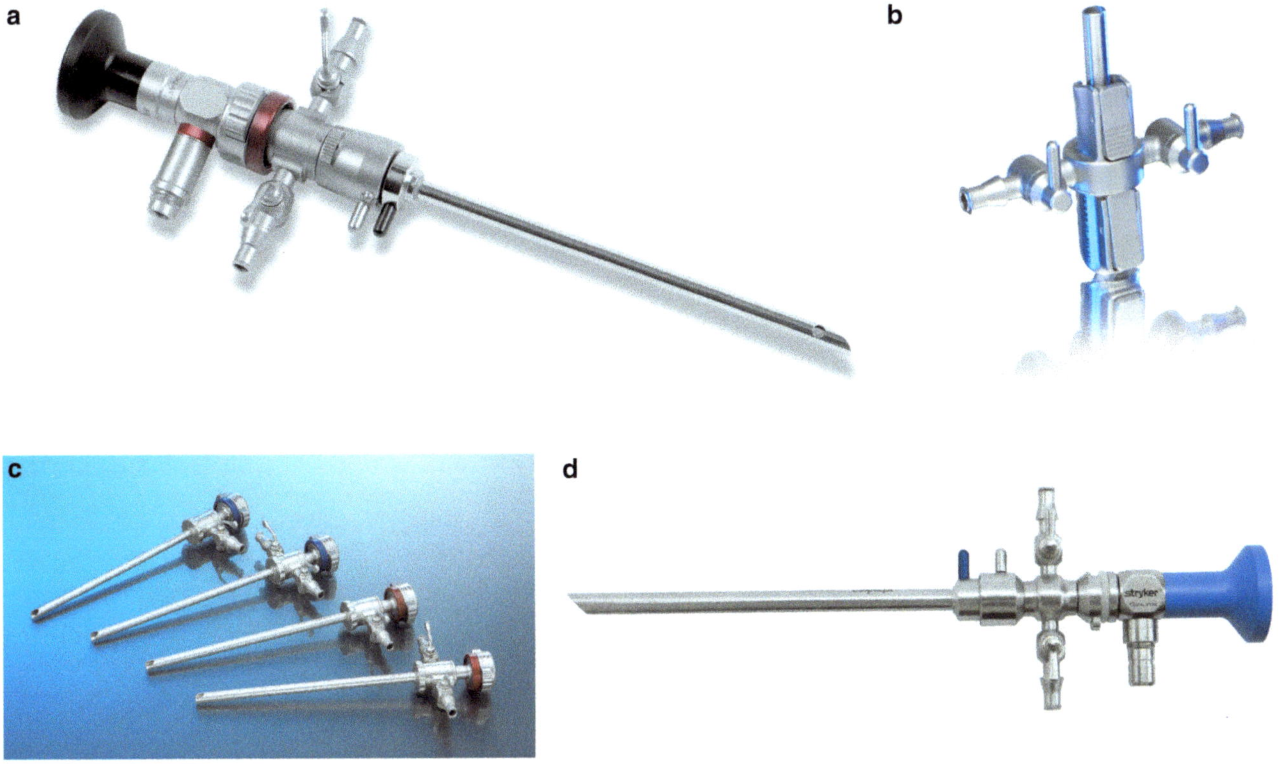

Fig. 40.3 Various bridge systems are available including these illustrated by (**a**) Arthrex (Image provided courtesy of Arthrex, Inc. 2015); (**b**) Conmed-Linvatec (with permission from CONMED Corporation); (**c**) Storz (© 2013 photo courtesy of KARL STORZ Endoscopy-America, Inc.); (**d**) Stryker (with permission from Stryker®)

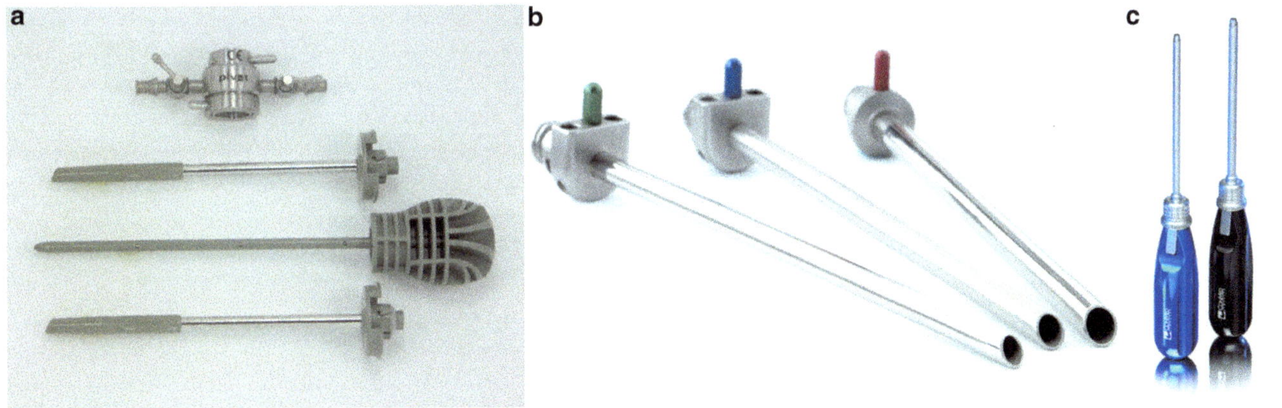

Fig. 40.4 Cannula designs emphasize being atraumatic to the joint surfaces. (**a**) This version by Pivot has soft material on the cannula end within the joint (with permission from Stryker®). (**b**) This Smith & Nephew design features a blunt edge on the cannula end (with permission from Smith & Nephew, Inc.). (**c**) Conmed-Linvatec (with permission from CONMED Corporation)

The anterior face of the acetabulum is more acute than the glenoid, less forgiving, and requiring tighter tolerances in the direction of anchor placement (Fig. 40.11). Also, less maneuvering can be performed through the surrounding soft tissues, and thus anchor placement is critically dependent on the angle from which it enters through the soft tissues. Typically, a more distal entry site is necessary to make sure that the anchor adequately diverges from the articular surface of the acetabulum. Placing portals this far distally may compromise their utility for other routine access to the central compartment. Percutaneous anchor delivery systems obviate the need of routine portals for anchor placement and allow the portals to be positioned for more optimally addressing other joint pathology (Fig. 40.12). Curved delivery designs

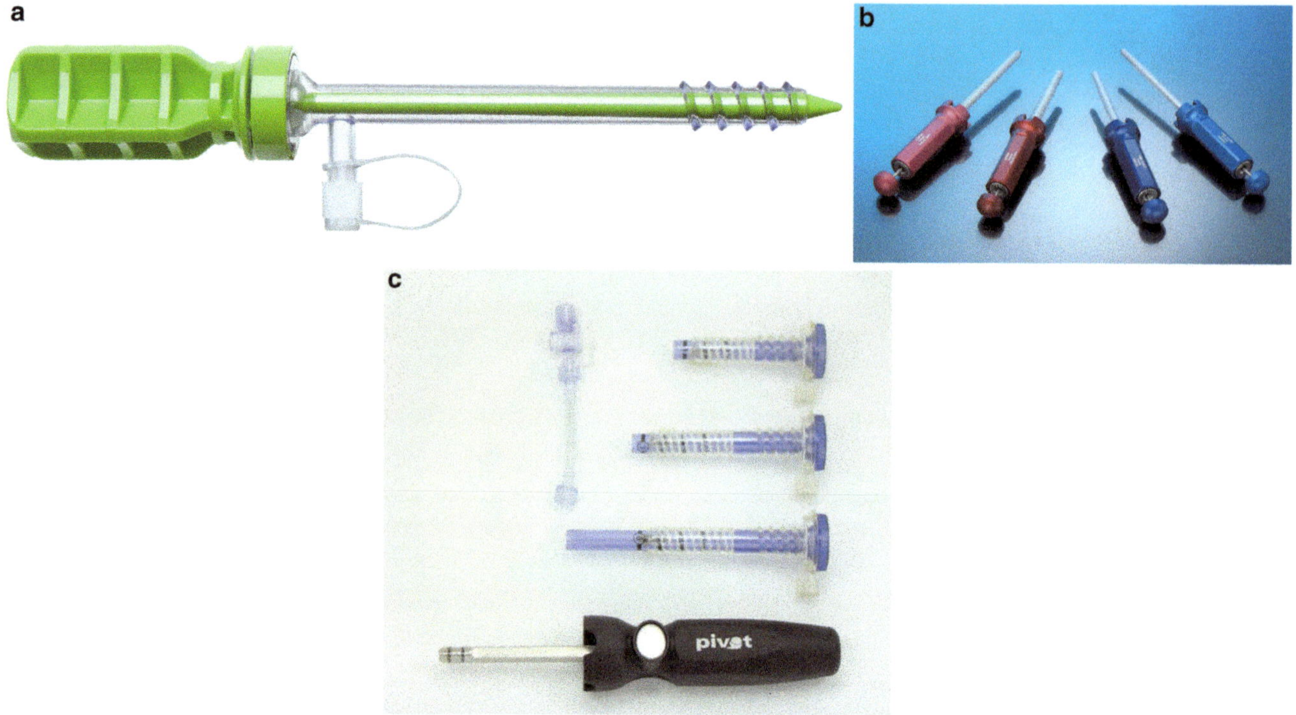

Fig. 40.5 Working cannulas, in various diameters and lengths to accommodate the soft tissues around the hip, such as these examples by (**a**) Mitek (with permission from Mitek Sports Medicine) and (**b**) Storz (© 2013 photo courtesy of KARL STORZ Endoscopy-America, Inc.). (**c**) This Pivot design has an adjustable length (with permission from Stryker®)

are another method for accommodating existing portals for anchor placement while still assuring adequate divergence (Fig. 40.13). In general, smaller anchor designs are more forgiving for placement around the hip (Fig. 40.14). Numerous materials are available including metallic and nonmetallic inert materials and bio-absorbable, osteo-conductive, and all-suture designs. In general nonferrous anchors are preferable to avoid artifact with future MRIs. Pullout strength is sufficient for most anchors and perhaps not as critical in the hip. Repair of the acetabular labrum is simply a matter of reapproximating it to the rim, restoring its anatomy. Unlike the shoulder, there is no capsulolabral complex and no capsular shifts are performed and thus the anchor sees very little resting tension. The necessary pullout strength is essentially needed to make sure that the construct will hold while tying the knots. Knotless designs are also available although they usually require a slightly larger implant for fixation in the bone (Fig. 40.15). Many surgeons adopting the role of hip arthroscopy are experienced hip surgeons and may not be as versed in the use of arthroscopic techniques from other joints, and thus, for them, the knotless features may be more appealing.

There are numerous devices for passing sutures through the labrum to be repaired. Anchor placement in the rim of the acetabulum can be quite standardized, but suture management is highly variable depending on the size, morphology, and pattern of pathology of the damaged labrum (Fig. 40.16). Thus, it is important to have a variety of devices to accommodate various methods of labral repair. Soft tissue-penetrating devices can accommodate antegrade and retrograde suture passage through the labrum in a single step (Fig. 40.17). However, these work better in a robust labrum or in the presence of hardy tissue and are not well suited when the labrum is fragile (Figs. 40.18 and 40.19). A small or tenuous labrum may be better managed with a suture shuttle device which usually provides the smallest instrument to penetrate the tissue (Fig. 40.20). With this, antegrade or retrograde passage of the suture can still be accomplished, although requiring one additional step (Figs. 40.21 and 40.22). Many imaginative technical and technological advancements are underway aimed at improving the ability to restore the labral anatomy. These devices are equally applicable to labral reconstruction where autograft or allograft donor tissue is used to replace the absent native labrum.

Capsular repair is most commonly performed in the presence of a surgically created capsulotomy and where there is a concern of potential iatrogenic instability. Keep in mind that iatrogenic instability is more likely to be caused by excessive or inappropriately selected bone removal, and thus one should not rely on soft tissue closure to solely compensate for bony compromise. Sufficient capsule and reasonably prepared capsular edges are necessary to accommodate

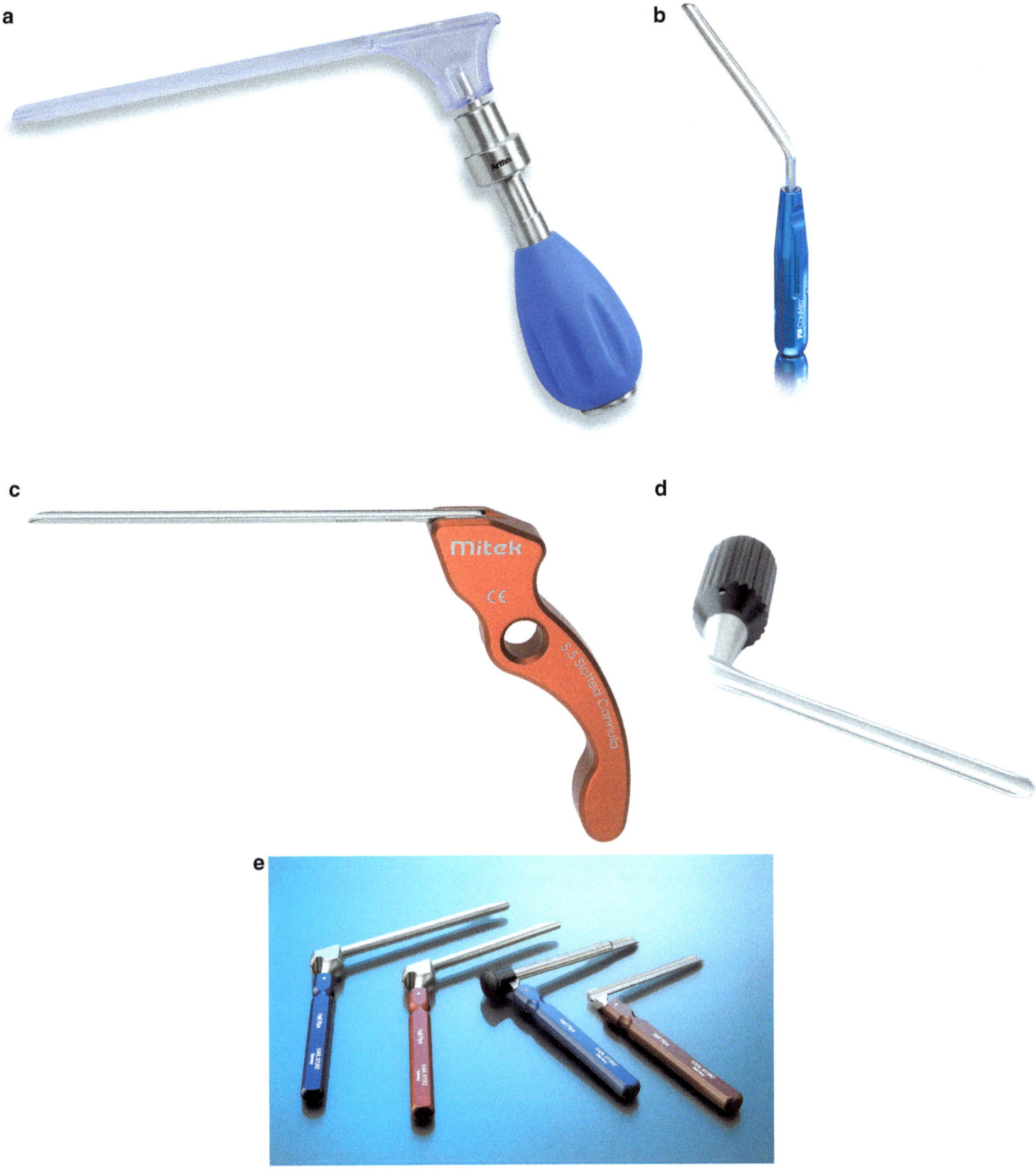

Fig. 40.6 Slotted cannulas provide maximal versatility for introducing instruments while maintaining the portal track. Examples include (**a**) Arthrex (image provided courtesy of Arthrex, Inc. 2015); (**b**) Conmed-Linvatec (with permission from CONMED Corporation); (**c**) Mitek (with permission from Mitek Sports Medicine); (**d**) Smith & Nephew (with permission from Smith & Nephew, Inc.); (**e**) Storz (© 2013 photo courtesy of KARL STORZ Endoscopy-America, Inc.)

capsular repair. The three challenges of capsular repair revolve around suture management. First, the suture must be passed through the superficial surface of the capsule separated from the surrounding soft tissues. Second, it must be retrieved from the deep surface of the capsule, avoiding injury to the labrum or articular surface. Third, tying the sutures is often performed in a blind fashion, or at least with limited visualization as the capsule is approximated.

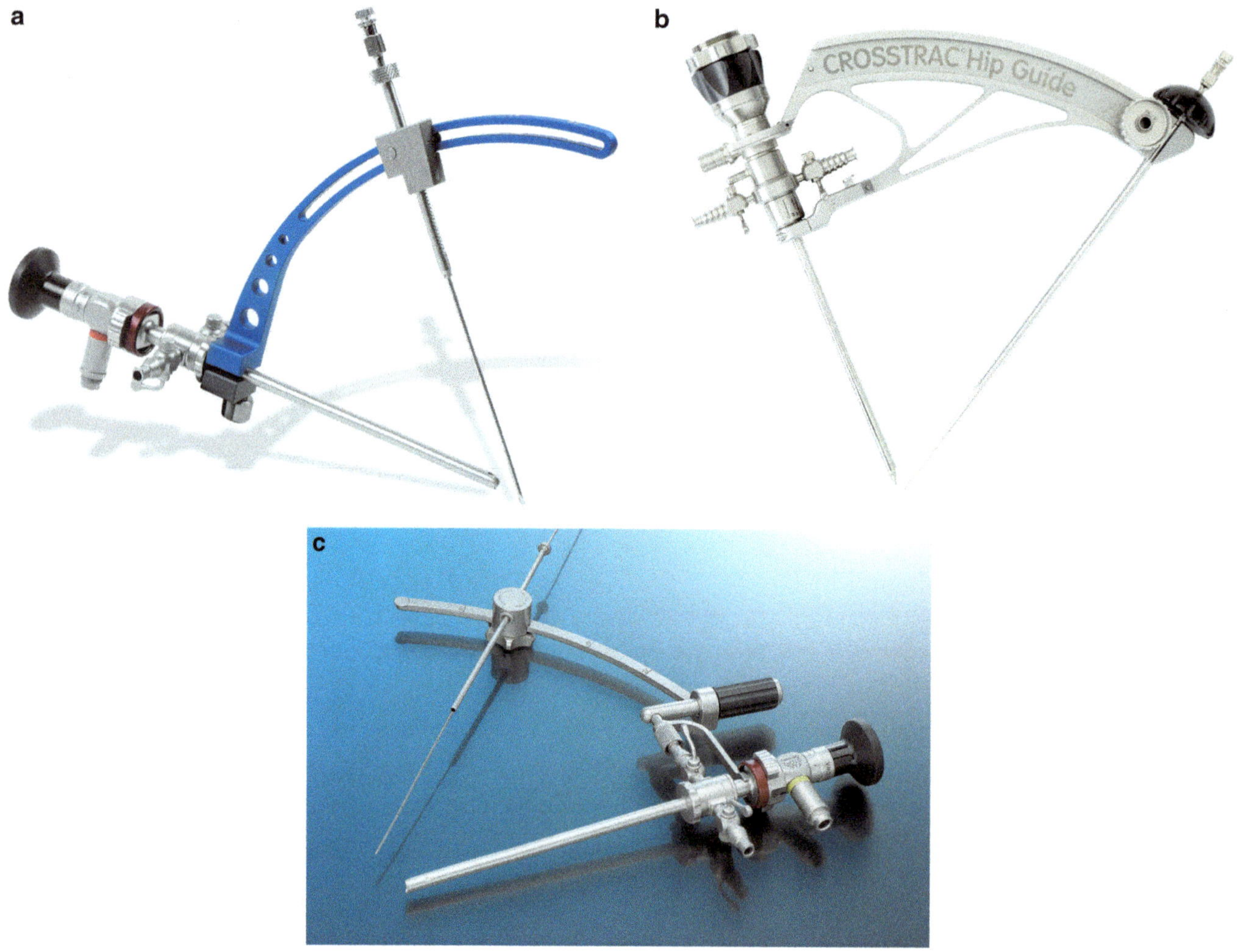

Fig. 40.7 Guide systems can aid in triangulation, facilitating placement of working portals. Examples include (**a**) Arthrex (image provided courtesy of Arthrex, Inc. 2015); (**b**) Smith & Nephew (with permission from Smith & Nephew, Inc.); (**c**) Storz (© 2013 photo courtesy of KARL STORZ Endoscopy-America, Inc.)

Numerous technological advancements have been made to aid in suture passage that complement the technical tips for capsular closure (Fig. 40.23). Less commonly, capsular plication may be performed to eliminate capsular laxity or redundancy even in absence of having performed a surgical capsulotomy.

Articular cartilage repair most frequently consists of simply marrow stimulation techniques with microfracture to potentiate a fibrocartilaginous healing response (Fig. 40.24). Most commonly, this is for a grade IV lesion of the acetabulum, although sometimes the femoral head (Fig. 40.25). Access for properly performing a microfracture can be a challenge, necessitating different positions to address the entirety of the lesion, and is facilitated by a variety of different arthroscopic awls that have been developed specifically for use in the hip (Fig. 40.26). Both transfer of osteochondral autograft plugs and autologous chondrocyte transplantation have each received investigational attention in the hip. Future technological creations will enhance these and other procedures that currently remain restricted because of the joint's anatomy. Fibrin glue and other methods of refixing unstable articular cartilage are also being trialed.

Many refinements are needed in these developed areas of repair and reconstruction. There are also numerous other frontiers that may prove to have merit. Reconstruction of the ligamentum teres has been devised, and there is much that could potentially be accomplished in the management of avascular necrosis both with revascularization and replacement of diseased osseous and osteochondral segments.

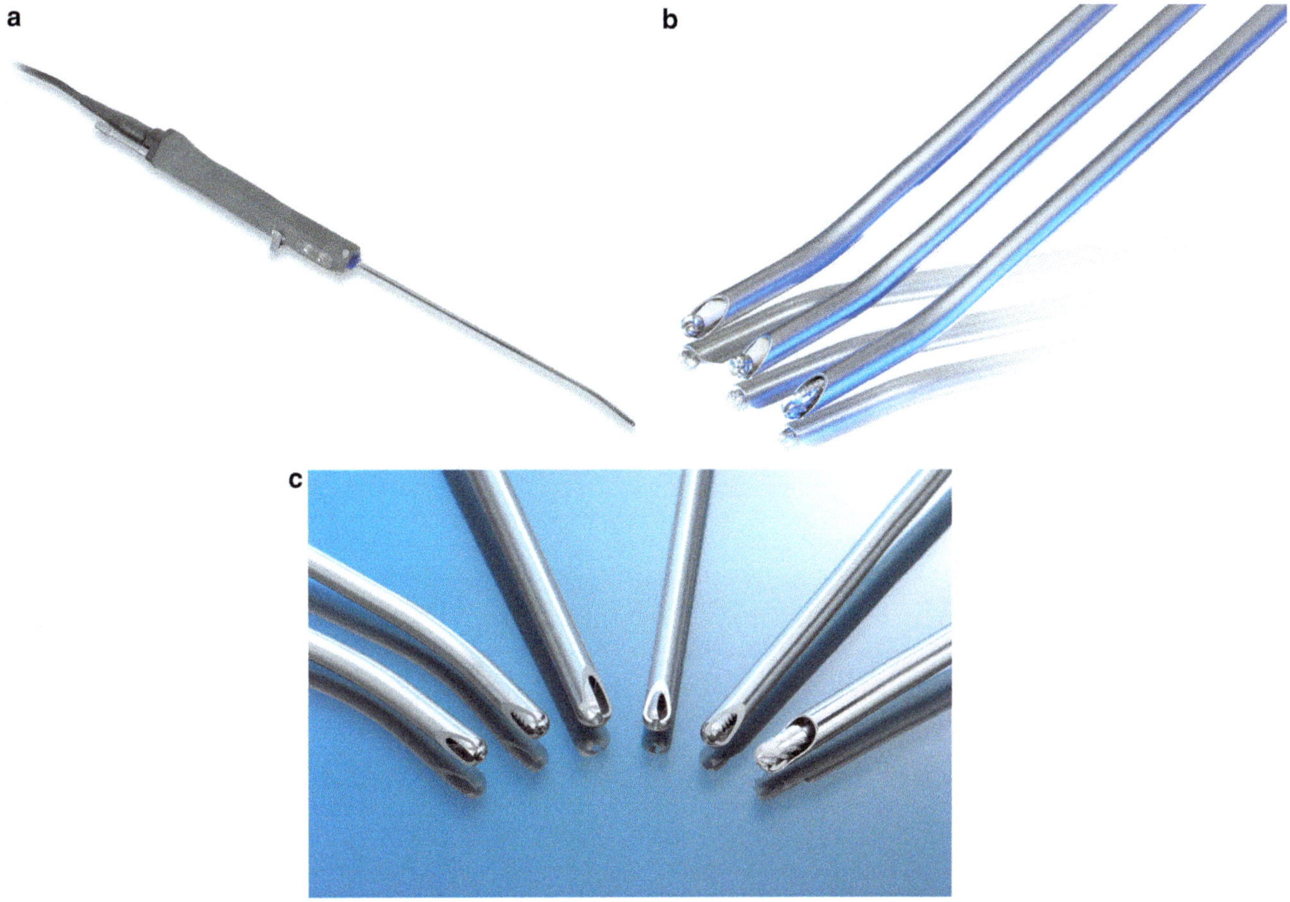

Fig. 40.8 Extra-length and curved blade features facilitate maneuvering within the deeply situated constrained architecture of the hip joint. Examples include (**a**) Arthrex (image provided courtesy of Arthrex, Inc. 2015); (**b**) Conmed-Linvatec (with permission from CONMED Corporation); (**c**) Storz (© 2013 photo courtesy of KARL STORZ Endoscopy-America, Inc.)

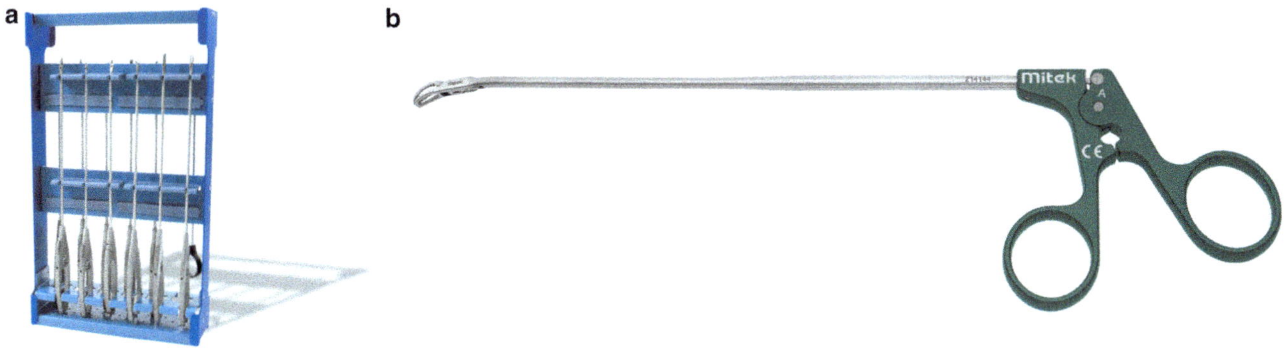

Fig. 40.9 Special features of hand instruments accommodate the dense tissues. (**a**) The grip design on this Arthrex version does not get hindered by the soft tissues (image provided courtesy of Arthrex, Inc. 2015). (**b**) This Mitek version illustrates the advantage of a longer shaft and curved design (with permission from Mitek Sports Medicine)

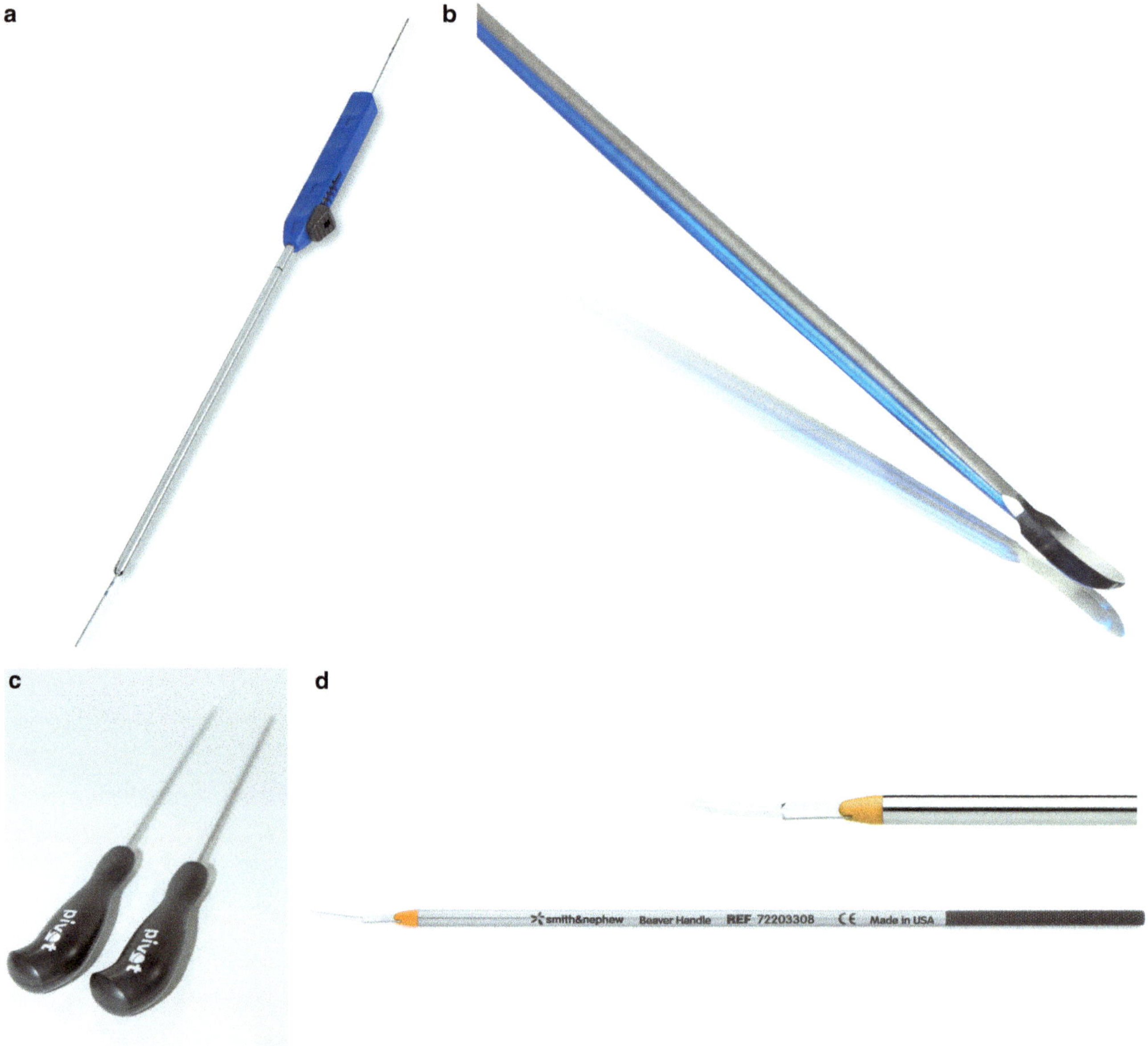

Fig. 40.10 Specialized arthroscopic knives are illustrated including (**a**) Arthrex (image provided courtesy of Arthrex, Inc. 2015); (**b**) Conmed-Linvatec (with permission from CONMED Corporation); (**c**) Pivot (with permission from Stryker®); (**d**) Smith & Nephew (with permission from Smith & Nephew, Inc.)

Radiofrequency Devices

Radiofrequency devices are popular in the hip because they complement the use of mechanical instruments, especially in accessing many of the confines within the joint. Longer and sturdy designs are available. Flexible and steerable features are especially advantageous within the hip (Fig. 40.27). Like any instrument, an RF device must be used properly to avoid iatrogenic injury. It can ablate diseased tissue and cut precisely. At low settings, with thoughtful use, it can complement the use of shavers in the removal of damaged labrum and articular cartilage specifically at the site of creating a stable transition zone (Fig. 40.28a–d). Often due to limited maneuverability of the shavers, resection can result in unnecessary removal of healthy tissue. Tissue responds to thermal treatment by heating water in the cells. Diseased cartilage (labrum and articular surface) has increased water content and selectively responds to thermal treatment. Thus, creation of a stable transition zone can be accomplished by simply watching the brisk response of the diseased portion.

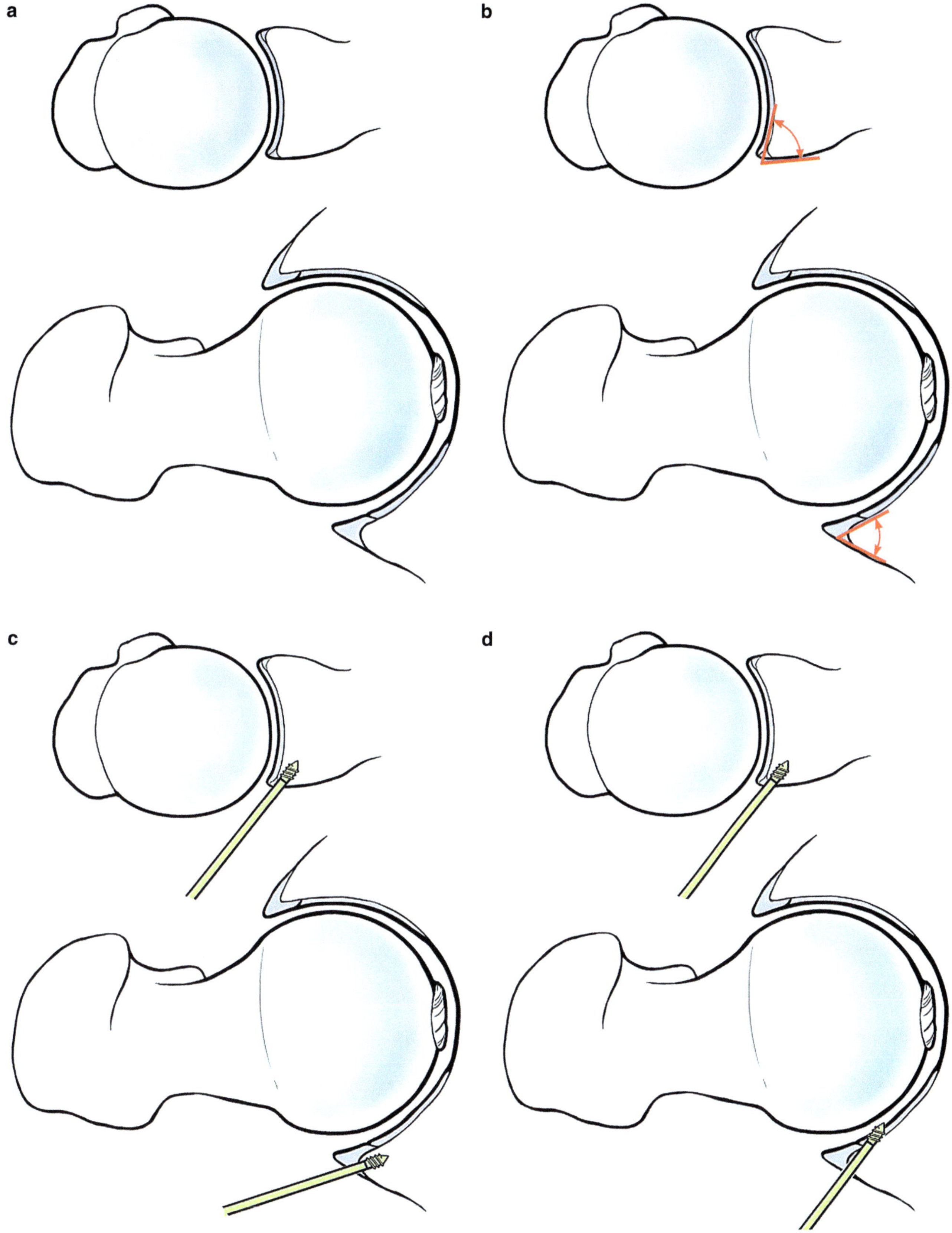

Fig. 40.11 (**a**) Cross-section comparison of the glenoid of the shoulder and the acetabulum of the hip. (**b**) The anterior face of the acetabulum is more acute than then glenoid and, thus, less forgiving to anchor placement. (**c**) The angle of placement of the anchor is dependent on the angle of entry through the deep soft tissues which limit correction of the entry angle. (**d**) The biggest concern is to avoid perforation of the acetabular surface. Typically, this necessitates a distal entry site for adequate anchor divergence. Published with kind permission of ©J.W. Thomas Byrd 2015. All rights reserved

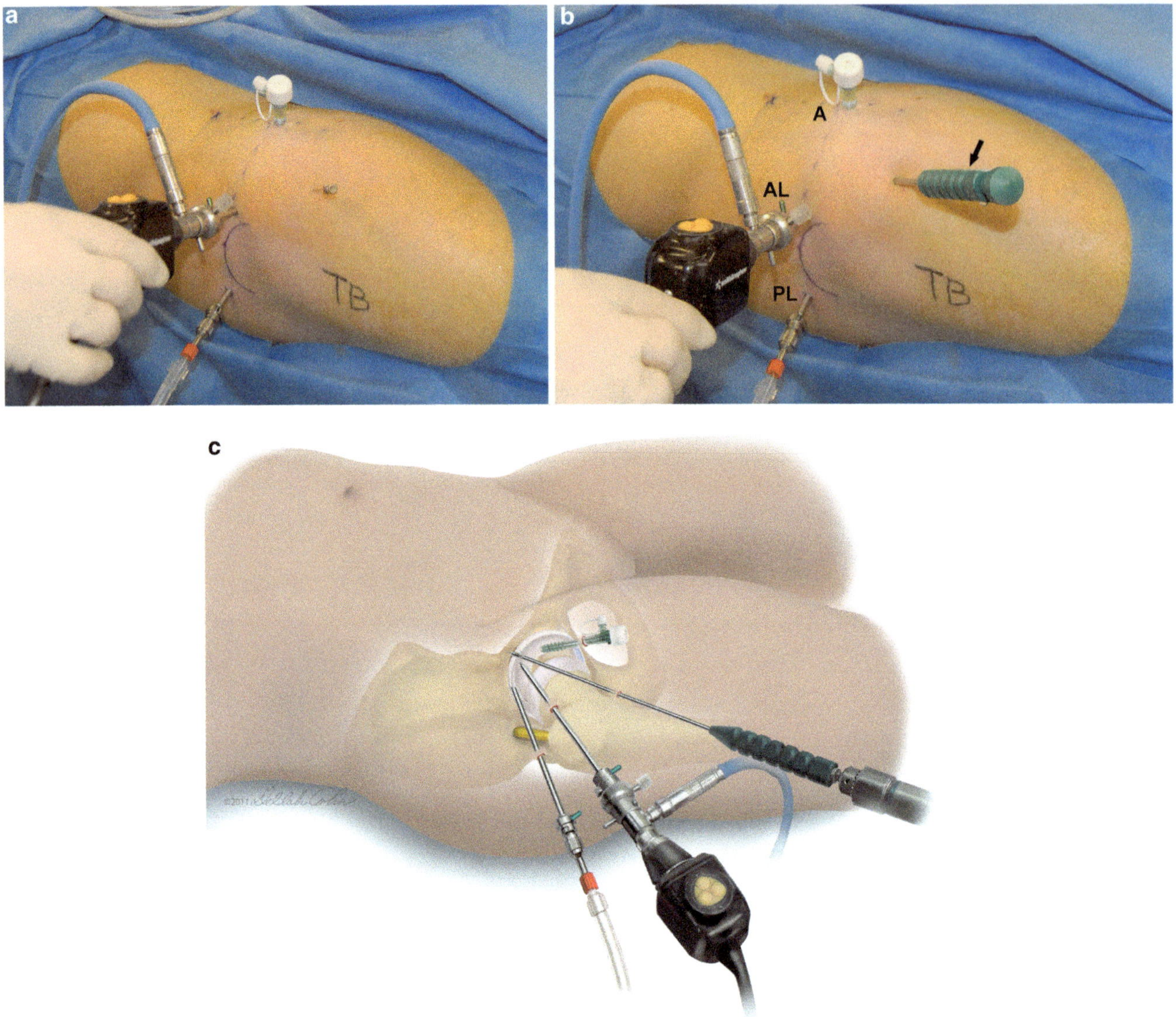

Fig. 40.12 A right hip with three standard portals positioned for optimal access to the central compartment. (**a**) A spinal needle (*arrow*) has been prepositioned distally to assure adequate divergence of the anchor from the acetabular articular surface. (**b**) The cannulated drill sleeve assembly (*arrow*) has replaced the spinal needle, switched over a guide wire. (**c**) Drilling against the rim of the acetabulum is illustrated. Published with kind permission of ©J.W. Thomas Byrd 2015. All rights reserved

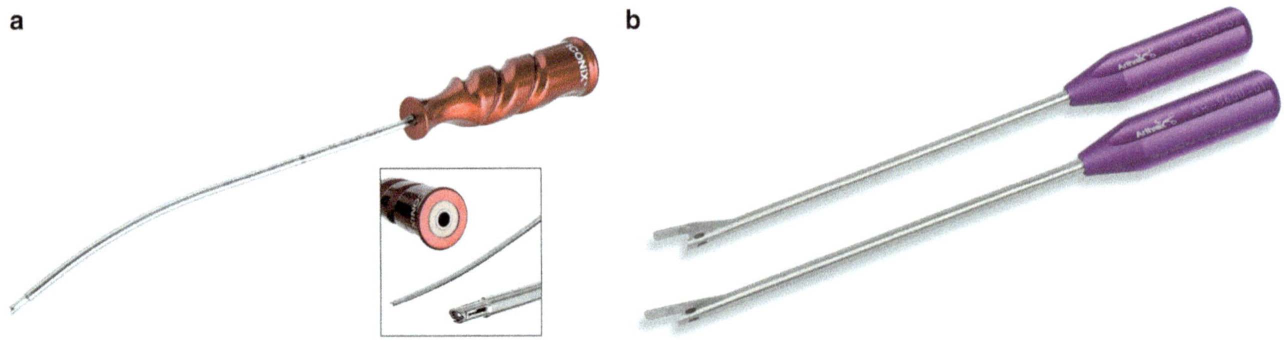

Fig. 40.13 (**a**) This curved Stryker drill guide system provides more divergence from the articular surface of the acetabulum during anchor placement (with permission from Stryker®). (**b**) This Arthrex system includes an outrigger that references the articular surface during anchor placement (image provided courtesy of Arthrex, Inc. 2015)

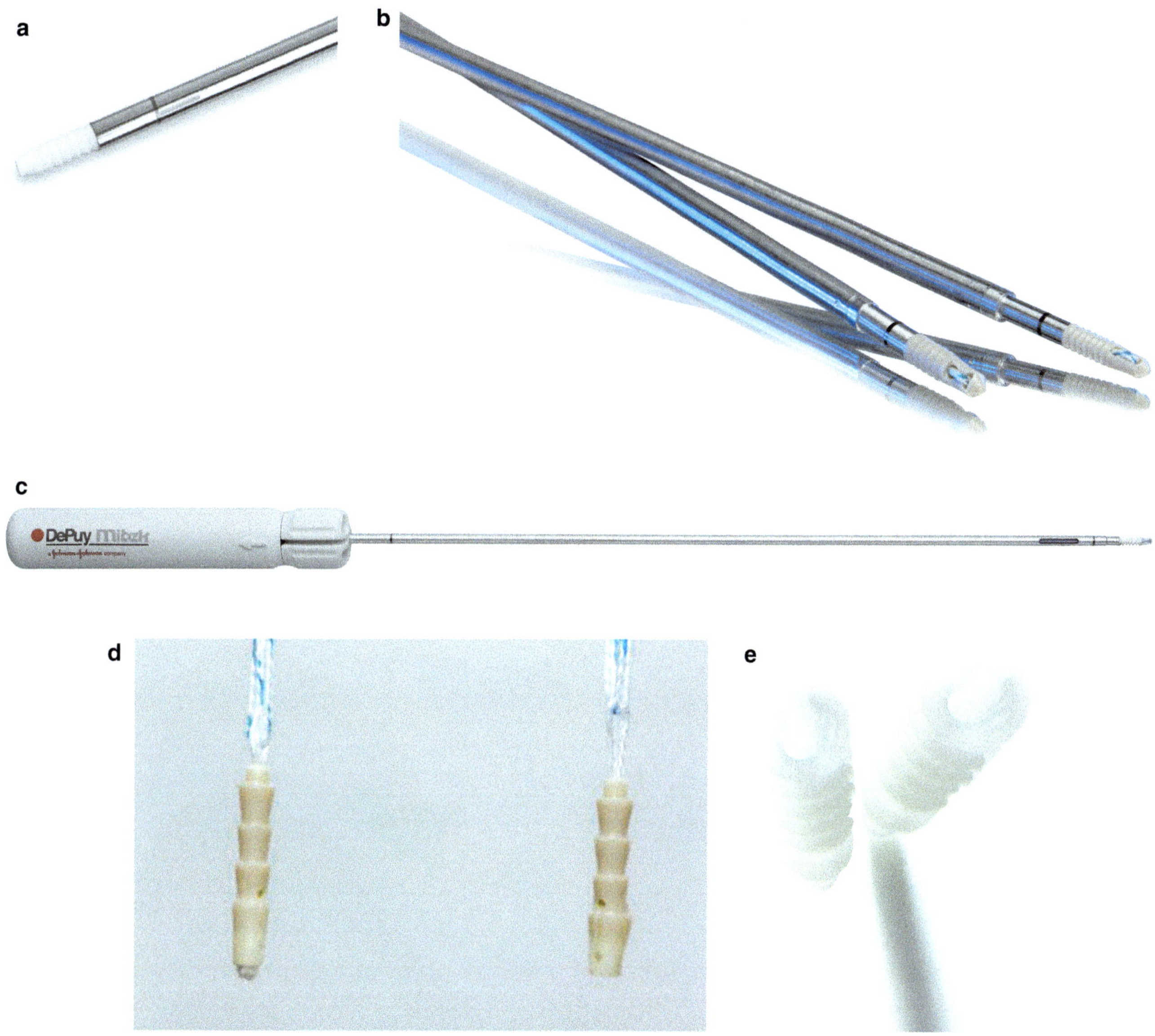

Fig. 40.14 Smaller anchors are preferable around the hip, including these versions from (**a**) Arthrex (image provided courtesy of Arthrex, Inc. 2015); (**b**) Conmed-Linvatec (with permission from CONMED Corporation); (**c**) Mitek (with permission from Mitek Sports Medicine); (**d**) Pivot (with permission from Stryker®); (**e**) Smith & Nephew (with permission from Smith & Nephew, Inc.)

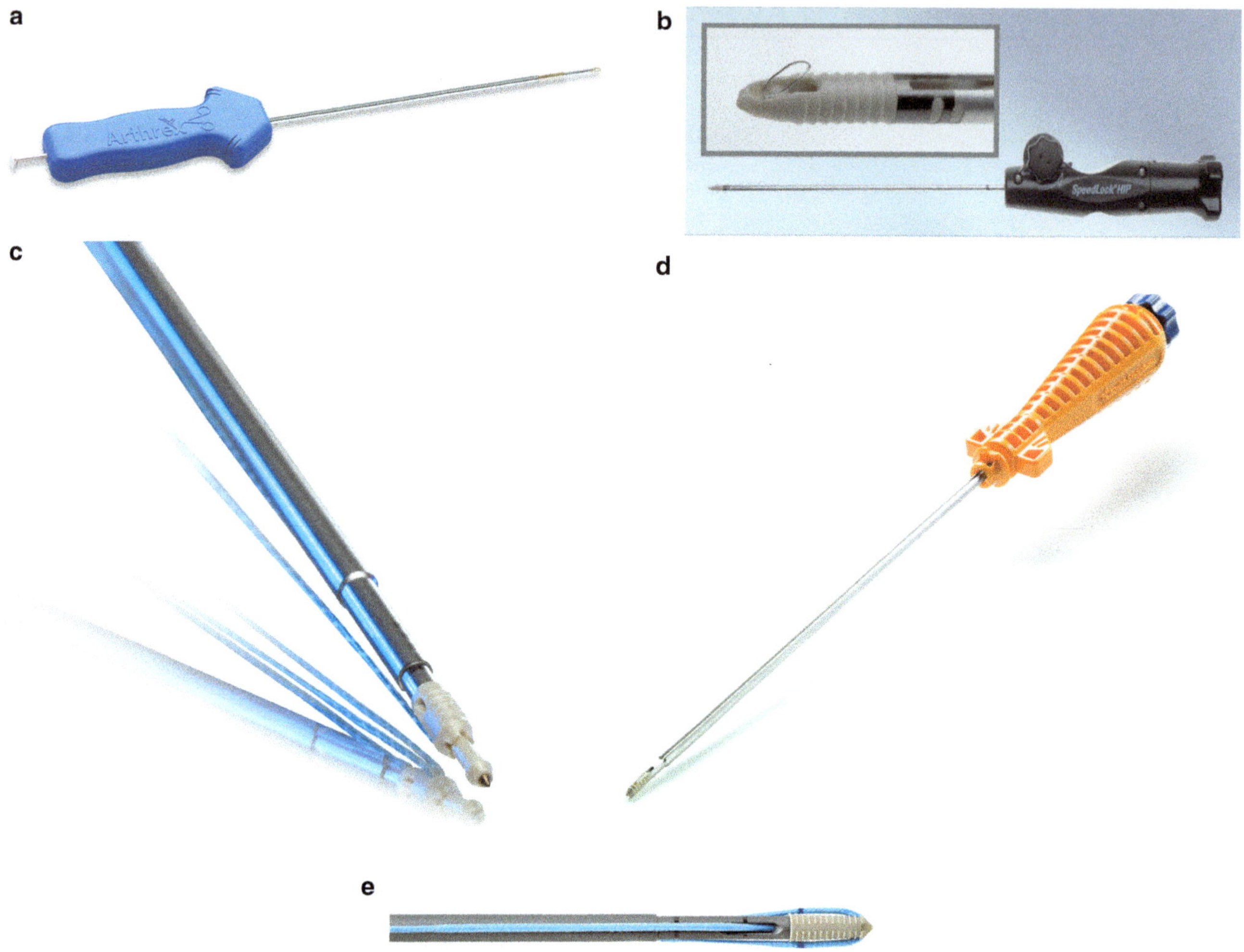

Fig. 40.15 Knotless anchors have application in the hip. Examples include (**a**) Arthrex (image provided courtesy of Arthrex, Inc. 2015); (**b**) ArthroCare (with permission from Smith & Nephew, Inc.); (**c**) Conmed-Linvatec (with permission from CONMED Corporation); (**d**) Smith & Nephew (with permission from Smith & Nephew, Inc.); (**e**) Stryker (with permission from Stryker®)

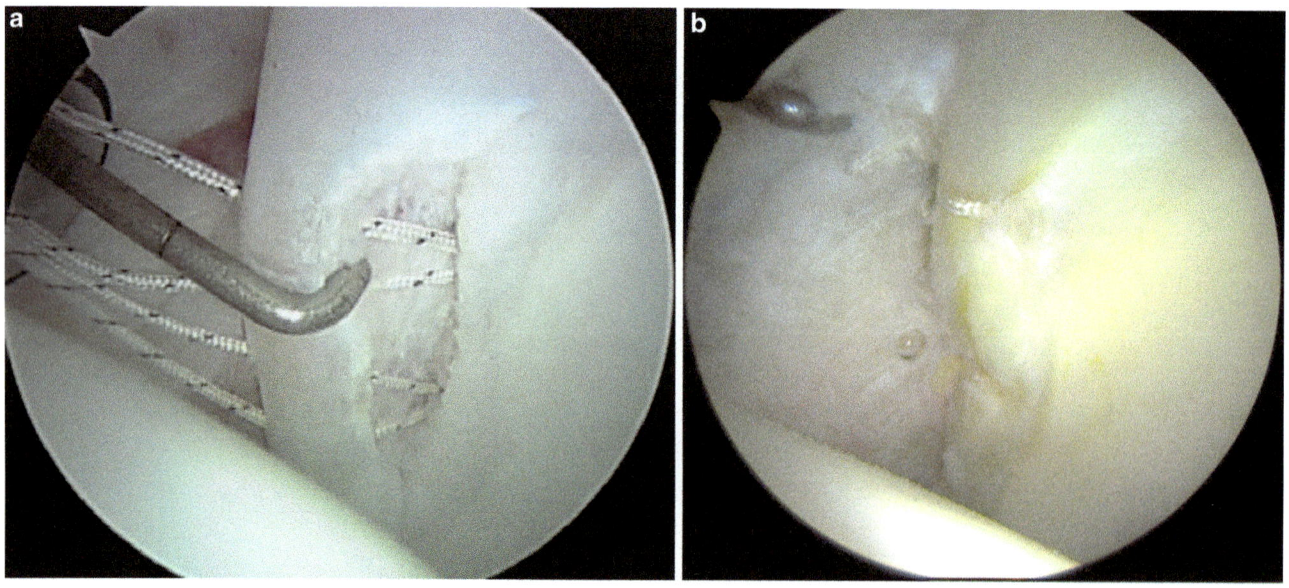

Fig. 40.16 Two different methods of primary labral repair. (**a**) With robust tissue, the sutures are passed in a mattress fashion to securely reapproximate the labrum and avoid suture interposed between the labrum and the articular surface of the femoral head. (**b**) In this example, the labral tissue was tenuous and a simple loop technique was necessary in order to have adequate tissue substance to reapproximate to the rim of the acetabulum. Published with kind permission of

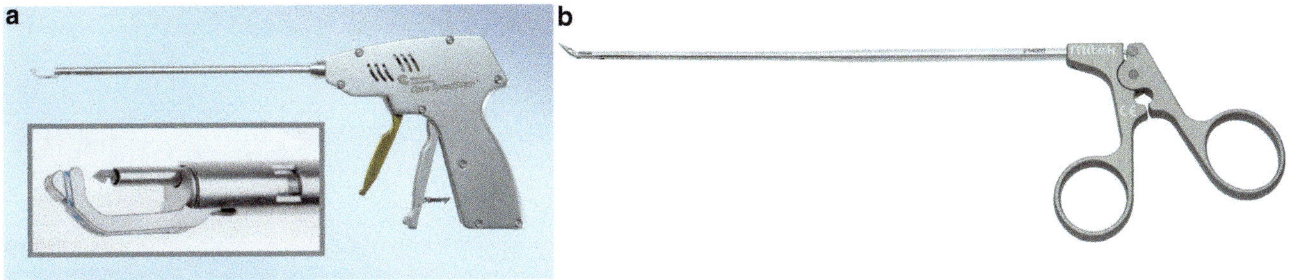

Fig. 40.17 Numerous soft-tissue-penetrating devices are available such as these versions. (**a**) ArthroCare (with permission from Smith & Nephew, Inc.); (**b**) Mitek (with permission from Mitek Sports Medicine)

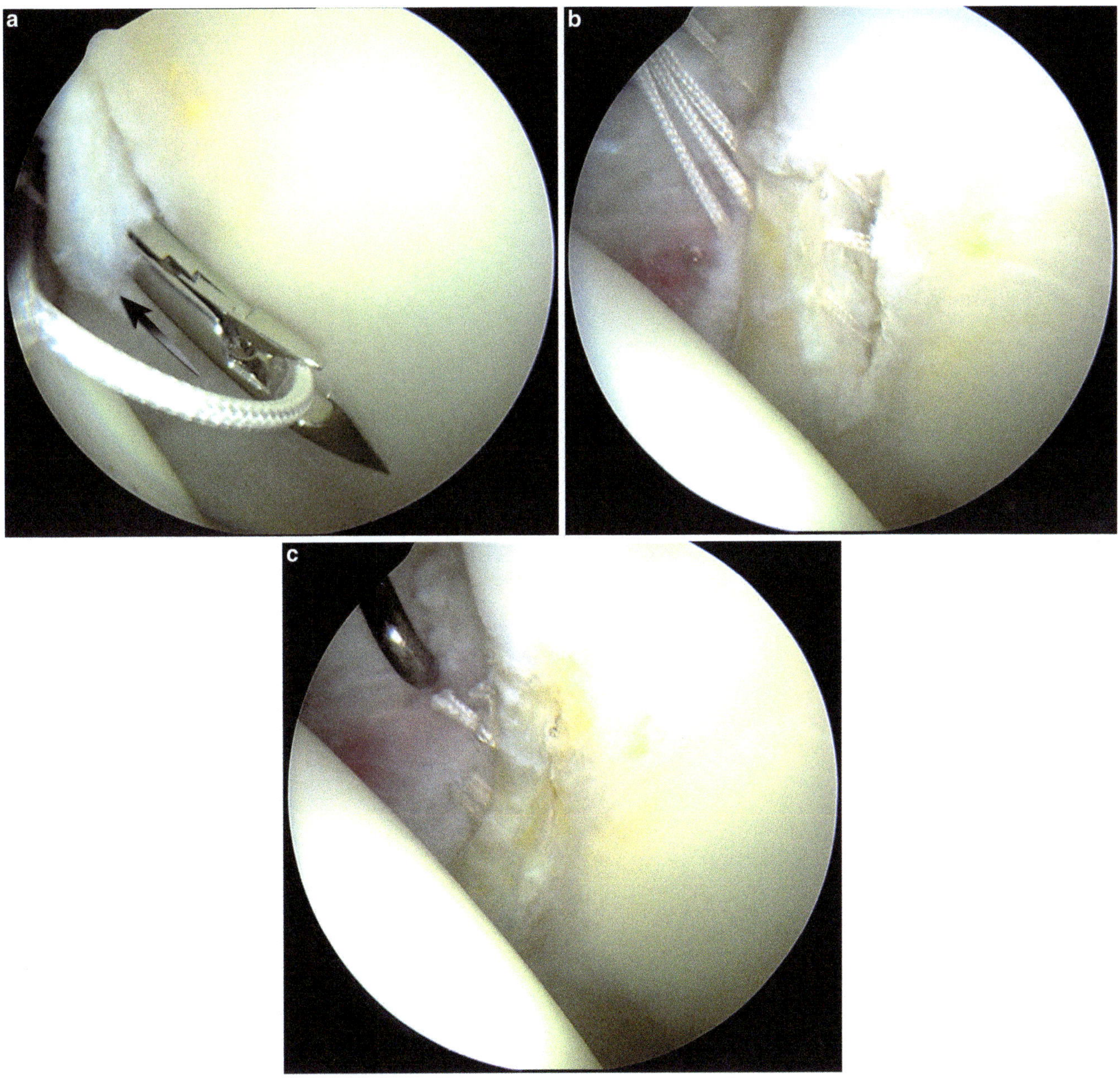

Fig. 40.18 Example of a primary labral repair with mattress sutures. The anchor has been placed against the acetabular rim on the articular side of the labrum. (**a**) The soft tissue-penetrating device pierces the labrum, grasping the suture and then pulling it back through the labrum. (**b**) A mattress configuration has been created with four suture limbs from two anchors. (**c**) The labrum has been reapproximated to the rim of the acetabulum. Published with kind permission of ©J.W. Thomas Byrd 2015. All rights reserved

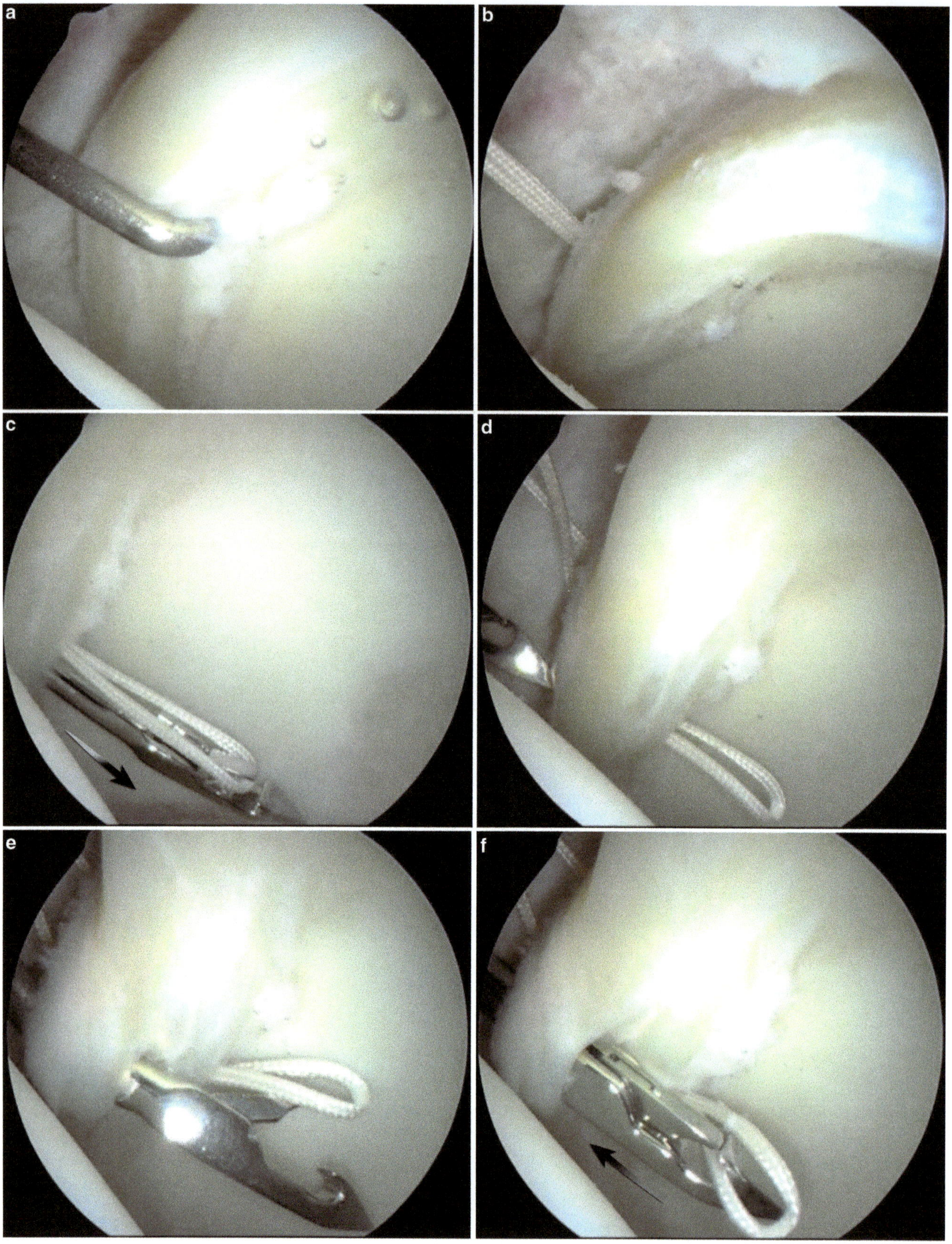

Fig. 40.19 Viewing anteriorly from the anterolateral portal of this left hip. (**a**) The labrum is hypertrophic with tearing at the chondrolabral junction identified with the probe. (**b**) An anchor has been placed with the sutures on the capsular side of the labrum. (**c**) A soft tissue-penetrating device pushes one limb of the suture into the joint at the chondrolabral junction. (**d**) With the suture in the joint, the penetrator is repositioned within the midsubstance of the labral tissue. (**e**) The limb of suture is grasped. (**f**) The suture limb is then retrieved outside the joint creating a single-limb-modified suture pattern. (**g**) Repair has been completed with two suture anchors, securing the labrum, reconstituting the chondrolabral junction without distorting the labral morphology. Published with kind permission of ©J.W. Thomas Byrd 2015. All rights reserved

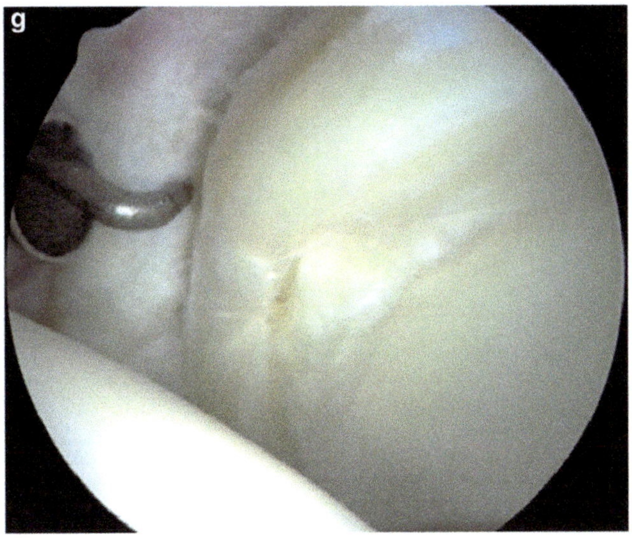

Fig. 40.19 (continued)

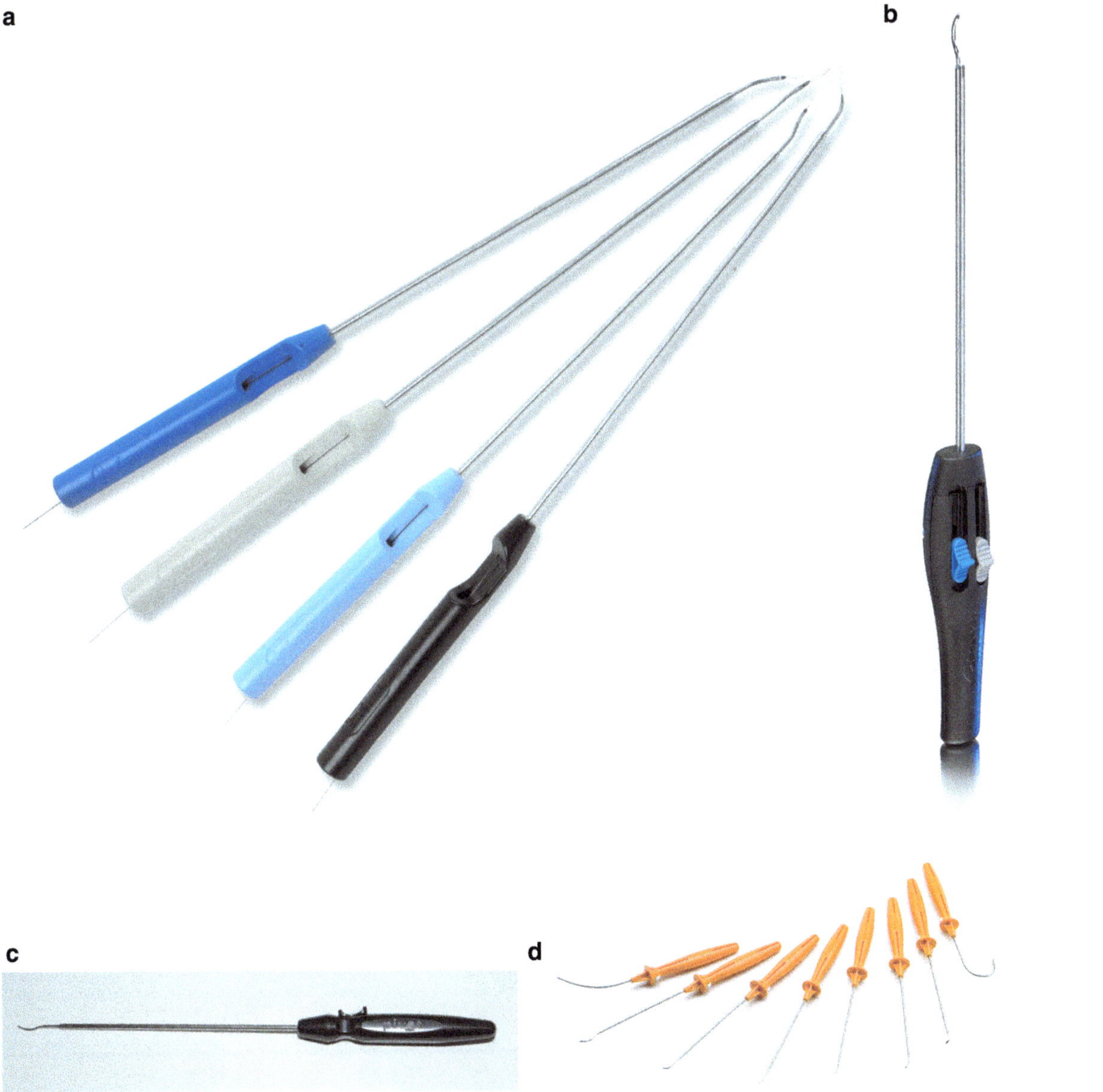

Fig. 40.20 Smaller devices that penetrate the labrum are preferable when the quality of the tissue is tenuous. Examples include (**a**) Arthrex (image provided courtesy of Arthrex, Inc. 2015); (**b**) Conmed-Linvatec (with permission from CONMED Corporation); (**c**) Pivot (with permission from Stryker®); (**d**) Smith & Nephew (with permission from Smith & Nephew, Inc.)

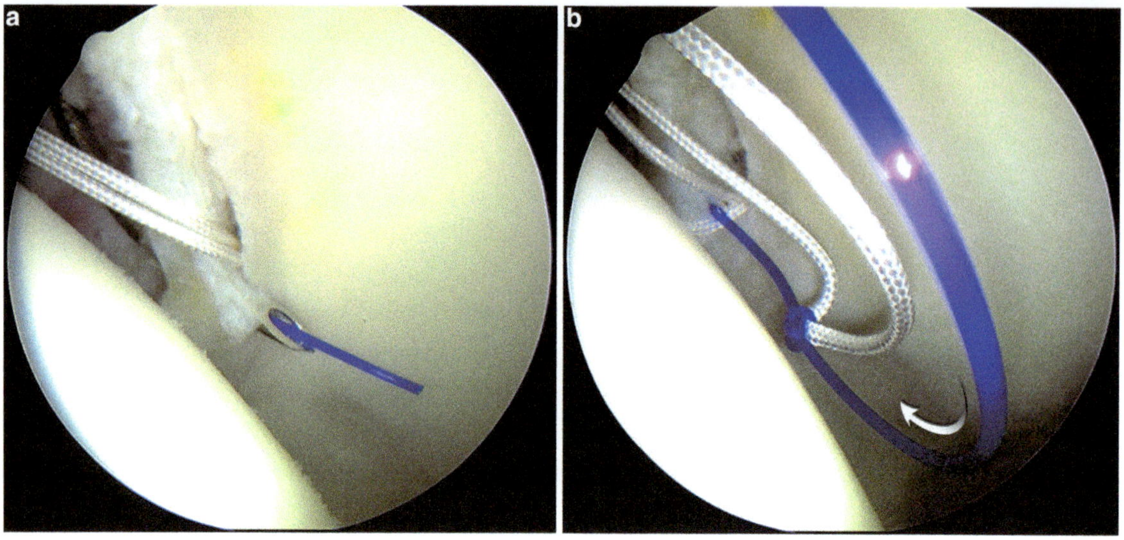

Fig. 40.21 A primary labral repair featuring suture management with a shuttle technique. (**a**) The labrum is pierced by a small diameter instrument sufficient for passing a monofilament suture. (**b**) With a shuttle technique, the monofilament is used to withdraw the braided anchor suture through the labrum. Published with kind permission of ©J.W. Thomas Byrd 2015. All rights reserved

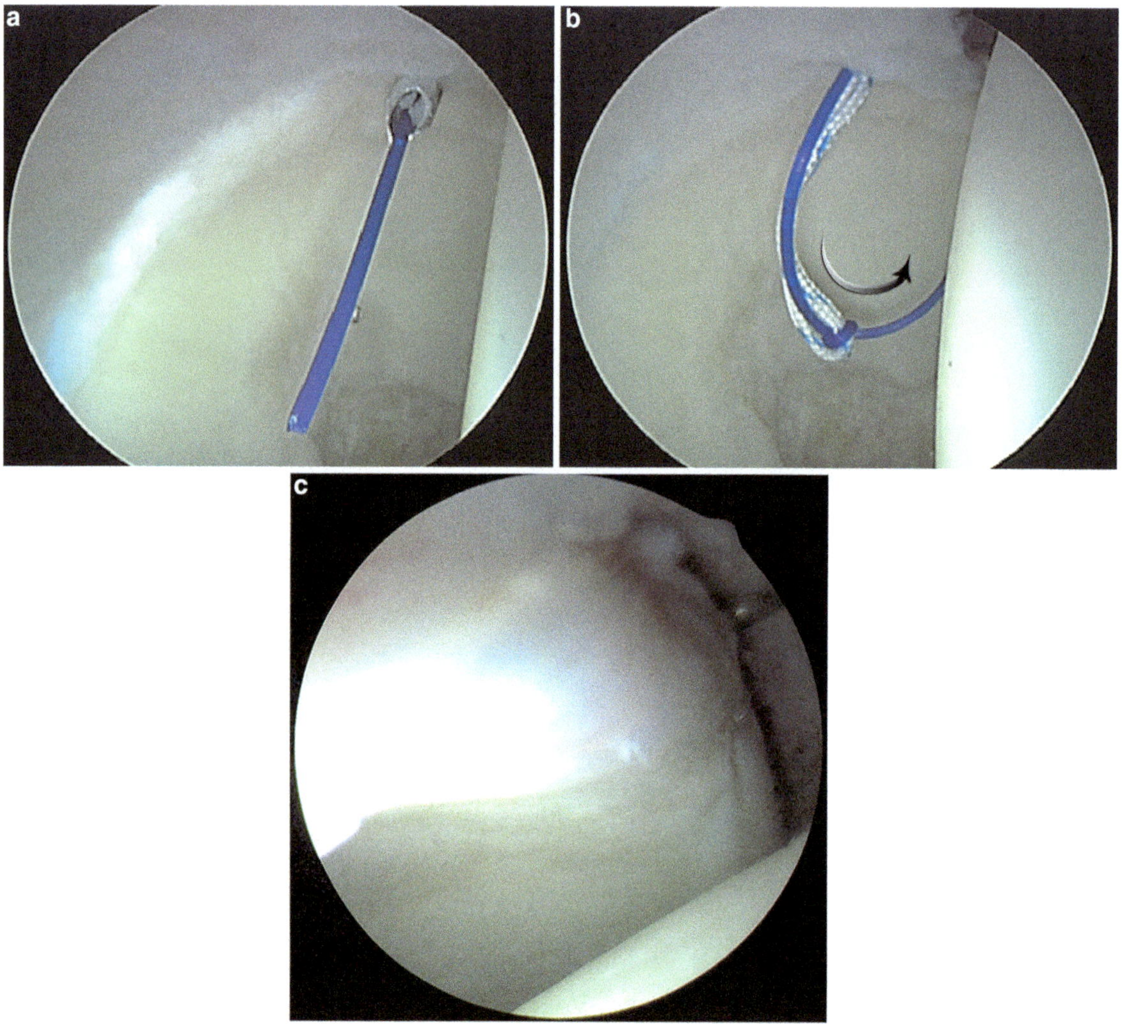

Fig. 40.22 In this case, an acetabular rim trimming has been performed, preserving the chondrolabral junction. Thus, a simple suture through the lateral half of the labrum is used to restore stability to the preserved labrum. (**a**) A monofilament suture is passed through the midsubstance of the labrum. (**b**) This is then used to shuttle the braided suture from the anchor that has been placed on the capsular side of the labrum. (**c**) Multiple sutures have been placed, preserving the labrum against the acetabular rim. Published with kind permission of ©J.W. Thomas Byrd 2015. All rights reserved

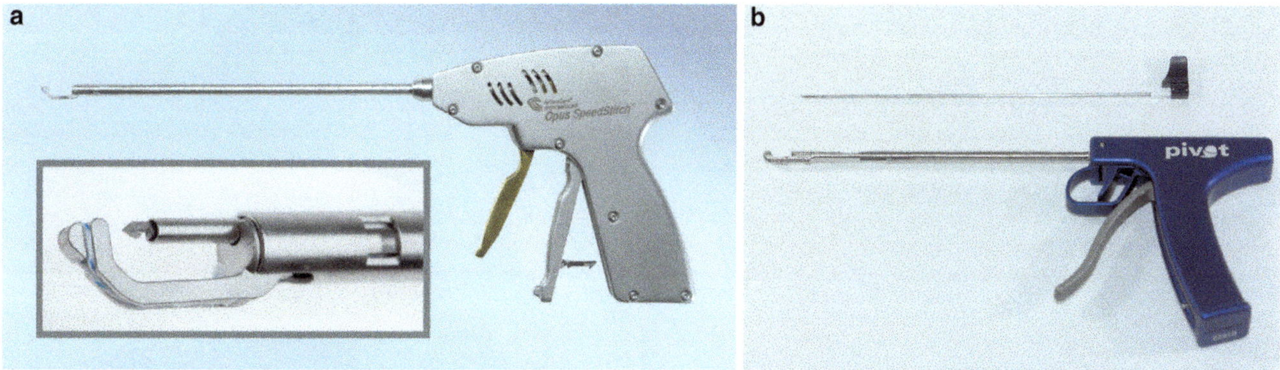

Fig. 40.23 Devices designed for capsular closure. (**a**) ArthroCare (with permission from Smith & Nephew, Inc.); (**b**) Pivot (with permission from Stryker®)

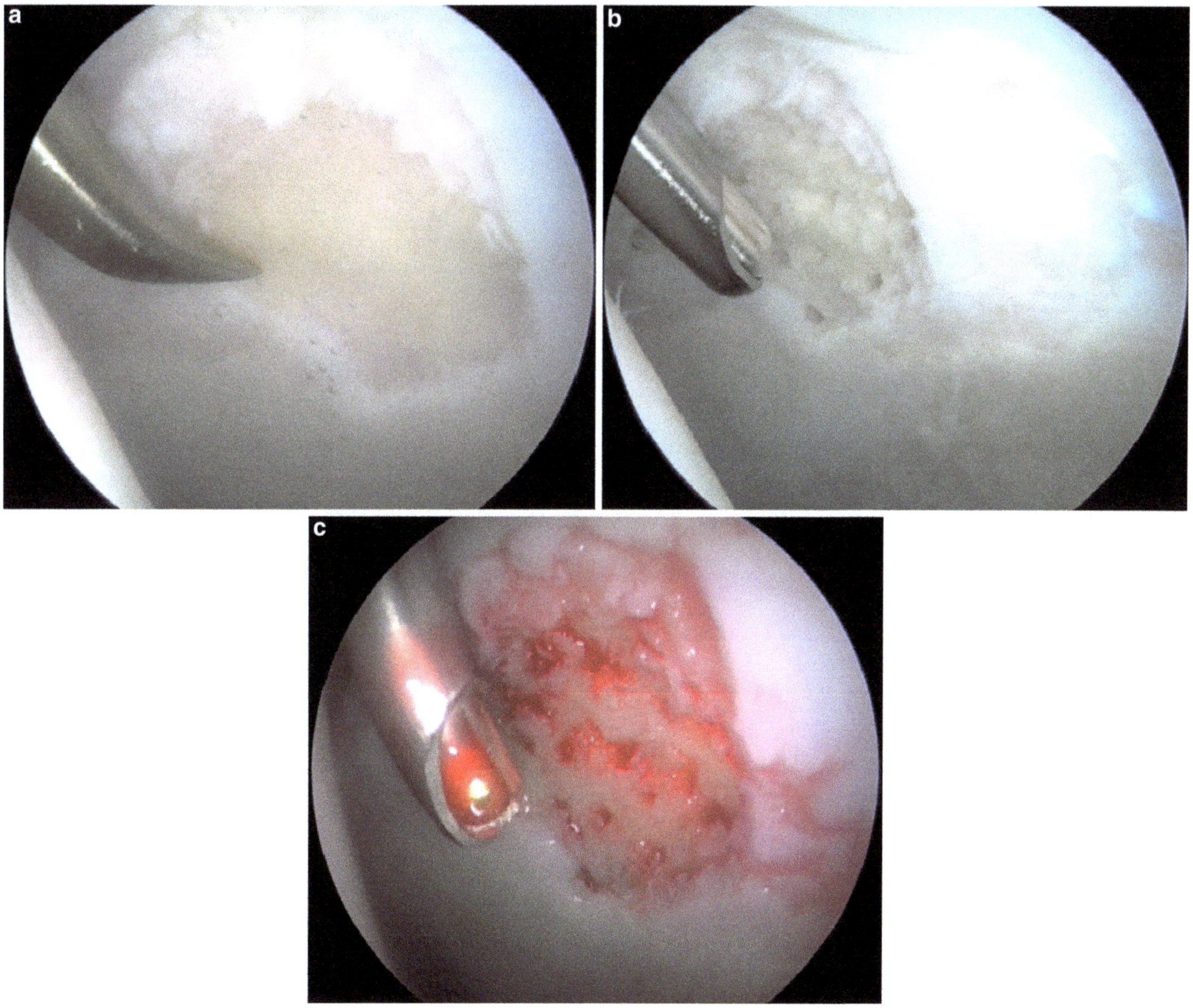

Fig. 40.24 Viewing this left hip from the anterolateral portal, a grade IV chondral lesion of the anterior acetabulum is identified. (**a**) An awl has been introduced to perform a microfracture. (**b**) Microfracture has been completed. (**c**) Vascular return through the perforations is substantiated

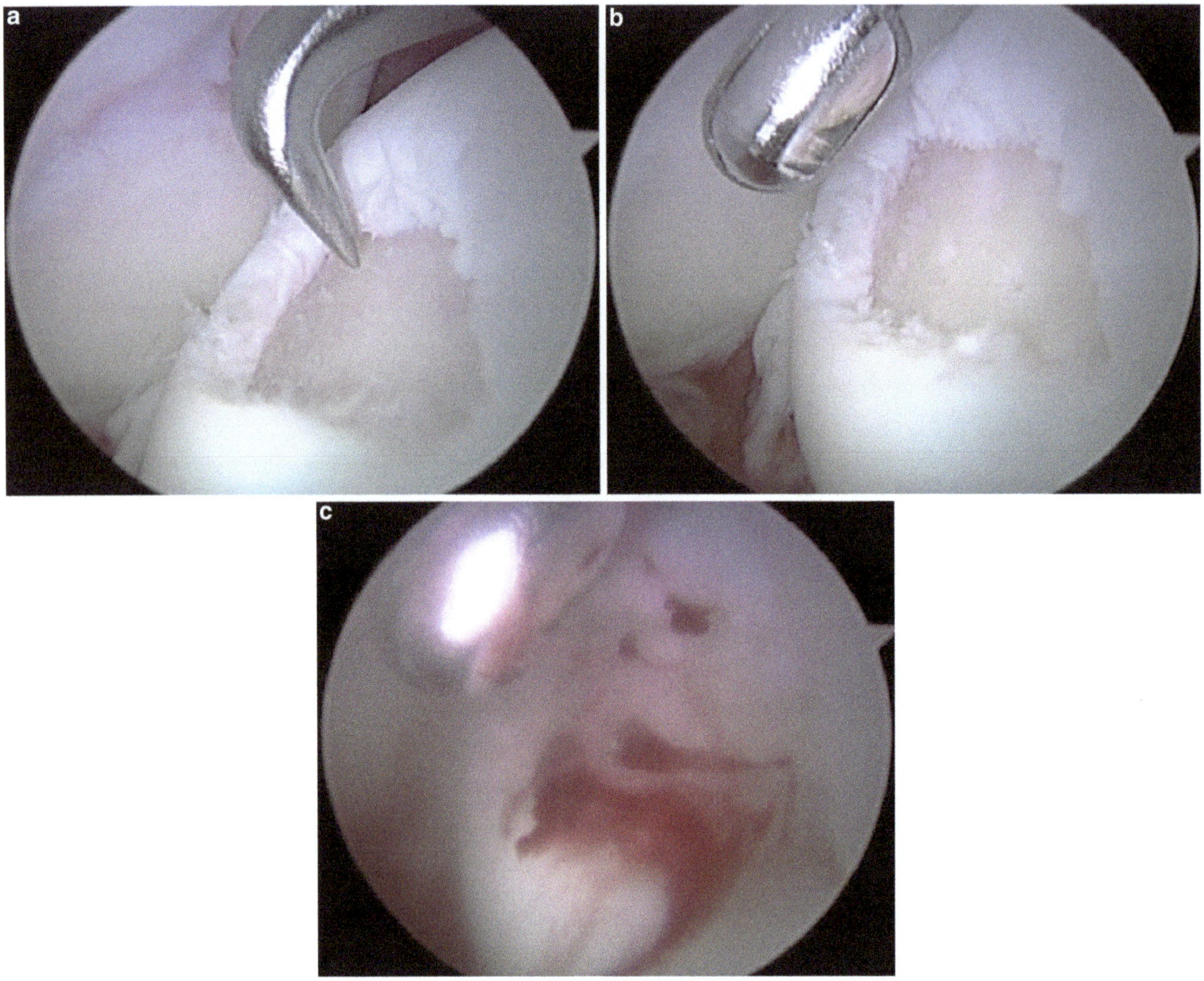

Fig. 40.25 Arthroscopic view of a right hip from the anterolateral portal reveals a grade IV chondral lesion of the femoral head. (**a**) An arthroscopic awl has been introduced to perform a microfracture. (**b**) The microfracture has been completed. (**c**) Occluding the inflow, vascular return is substantiated through the perforations. Published with kind permission of

Conclusions

Collaborations between surgeons and industry have been the cornerstone to all developments in hip arthroscopy. The technical advancements of talented surgeons are complemented by the technological innovations of industry. One could not be successful without the other. This is true in all surgical fields, but is especially highlighted in the technically and technologically advanced discipline of arthroscopy and perhaps most illustrated in the rapidly evolving area of the hip with a focus on joint preserving and restorative procedures.

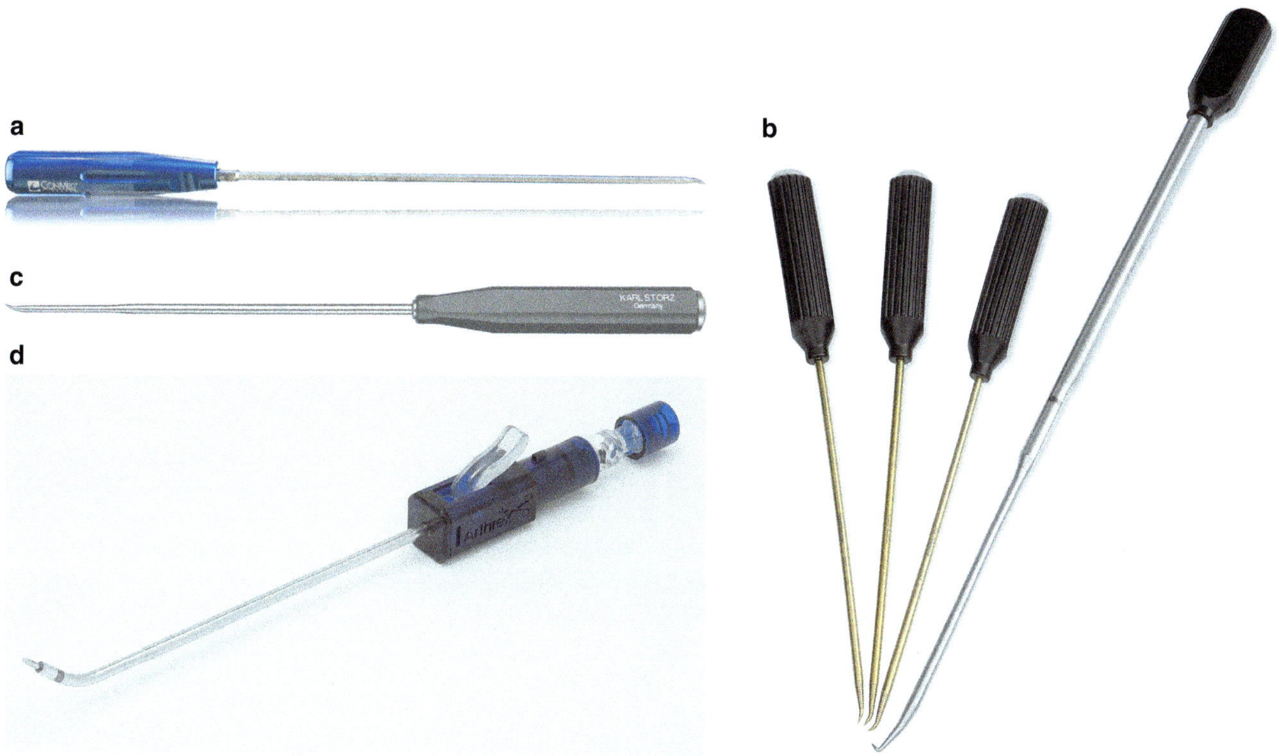

Fig. 40.26 Numerous arthroscopic awls are available including the following examples: (**a**) Conmed-Linvatec (with permission from CONMED Corporation); (**b**) Smith & Nephew (with permission from Smith & Nephew, Inc.); (**c**) Storz (© 2013 photo courtesy of KARL STORZ Endoscopy-America, Inc.); (**d**) Additionally, a power device is available from Arthrex (image provided courtesy of Arthrex, Inc. 2015)

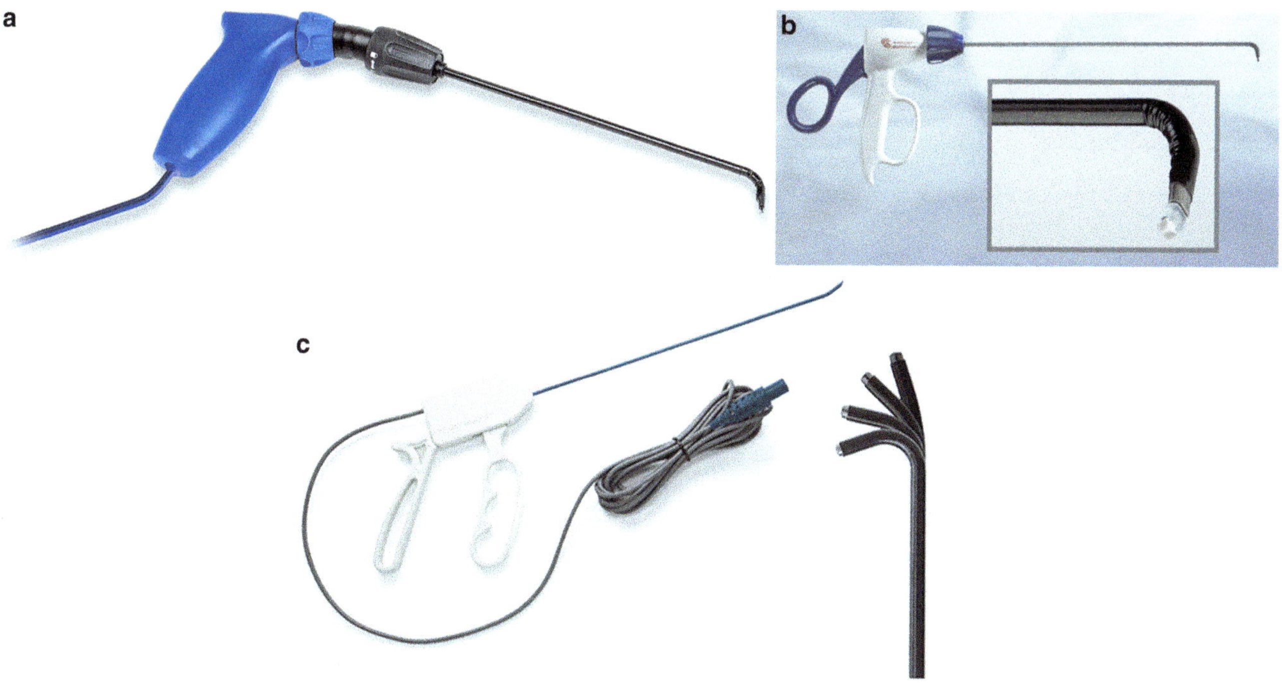

Fig. 40.27 Steerable radiofrequency devices provide better maneuverability within the confines of the hip, including (**a**) Arthrex (image provided courtesy of Arthrex, Inc. 2015); (**b**) ArthroCare (with permission from Smith & Nephew, Inc.); (**c**) Smith & Nephew (with permission from Smith & Nephew, Inc.)

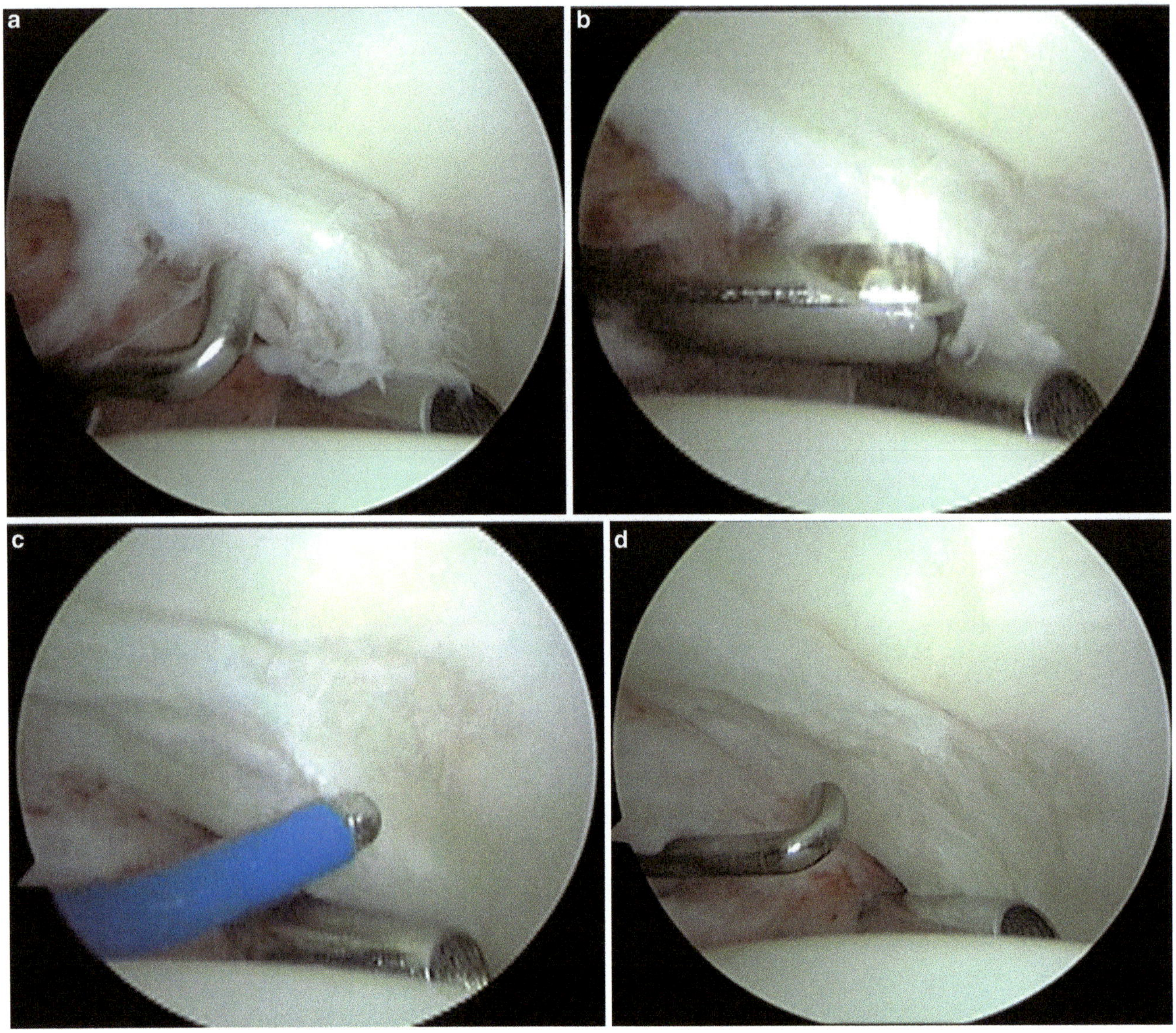

Fig. 40.28 (a) A fragmented labral tear with degeneration within its substance is identified. (b) Debridement is initiated with the power shaver. (c) A portion of the comminuted labral tear is conservatively stabilized with a radiofrequency probe. (d) The damaged portion has been removed, preserving the healthy substance of the labrum. Published with kind permission of ©J.W. Thomas Byrd 2015.

Arthroscopic Treatment: Layout of the Operating Room Surgical Approaches—Lateral

41

Thomas G. Sampson

Introduction and Brief History

Hip arthroscopy was first done in our practice in the early 1980s using the supine approach on a fracture table for distraction. In our early experience, problems of getting into the hip joint and complications such as scuffing of articular cartilage, poor maneuverability, and inability to achieve the anticipated result before extensive fluid extravasation occurred and made the procedure difficult. Specific instruments were not yet developed and distraction parameters were not established. As a result, the procedure was not predictable or reproducible in entering the intra-articular space now known as the central compartment.

History has shown us that Burman [1] in 1931 was the first to arthroscope the hip in a cadaveric study. He was unable to enter the central compartment even with distraction. My associate James M. Glick M.D (JMG) performed 11 cases between 1977 and 1982 and had difficulty getting in on two occasions [2]. Because of my experience with the lateral decubitus positioning in total hip replacements, the idea of approaching hip arthroscopy with a similar approach was developed. We dissected a cadaver hip to determine the most direct access to the intra-articular space and described the anterior peritrochanteric and posterior peritrochanteric portals (Fig. 41.1). Later these have been referred to as the anterolateral and posterolateral portals. Distraction was initially introduced by Eriksson et al. [3] using a fracture table to facilitate entering the central compartment in 1986. We developed a rope and pulley system with weights, similar to what was utilized for shoulder arthroscopy as our first hip distractor (Fig. 41.2). The first patient we arthroscoped with the lateral approach was a massively obese woman with hip pain that JMG had previously arthroscoped without success in the supine position. In the lateral decubitus position, the obese portions of her thigh drooped down to expose a prominent greater trochanter. The neurovascular structures are safely away from the lateral portals, and the surgeon is very familiar with their locations. These portals offer a direct entry into the femoroacetabular joint and do not require imagining the angles of entry as described by Byrd for the supine approach. The few surgeons interested in hip arthroscopy at that time adopted the lateral technique and continue to use it today.

With the interest by industry to develop arthroscopic instruments and distractors, the supine approach was once again used and described by Byrd. There have been editorials, journal articles, and book chapters arguing the advantages of each method over the other, and it is my opinion that the approach used should be based on the surgeon's training and comfort [4–7]. All procedures of hip arthroscopy are done equally well using either technique, and complications are not reported as technique specific. A distractor has been designed to be used on any operating room table for both techniques (Smith and Nephew), and all instruments designed for hip arthroscopy can be used for either position. However, we have found that shorter traditional length instruments work well in the lateral position, as the distance from the skin to the depths of the central compartment seems to be shorter due to the soft tissue dropping away from the portals.

The major advancements in entering the central compartment were from distraction and using cannulated trocars. Later the development of longer arthroscopes, slotted (half pipe) cannulas, and curved and flexible instruments has facilitated advanced techniques, following a similar path as with knee and shoulder arthroscopy (Fig. 41.3).

T.G. Sampson, MD (✉)
Director of Hip Arthroscopy, Post Street Surgery, Post Street Orthopaedics and Sports Medicine, 2299 Post Street Suite 107, San Francisco, CA 94115-3443, USA

Orthopaedic Consultant and Surgeon, Veterans Administration Medical Center at Fort Miley, San Francisco, CA, USA

Associate Clinical Professor Department of Orthopaedics, University of California, San Francisco, CA, USA
e-mail: tgsampsonmd@gmail.com

J.C. McCarthy et al. (eds.), *Hip Joint Restoration*, DOI 10.1007/978-1-4614-0694-5_41

Indications

As Thomas Byrd said: "The key to successful hip arthroscopy lies in selecting appropriate patients." I have stated that: "The patient's expectations should match the surgeon's." Hip arthroscopy in the early 1980s was felt to be a procedure looking for indications. Clearly, over the years, the list of indications has grown with the advancements of the technique. The specific indications and contraindications will be discussed in other chapters in this manuscript.

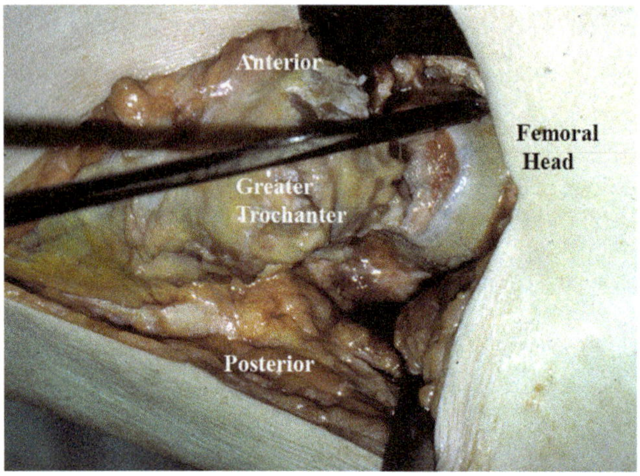

Fig. 41.1 Original cadaver dissection done by James M. Glick and Thomas G. Sampson to develop portals for the lateral approach. With kind permission from Springer Science+Business Media: Nho SJ, Leunig M, Larson CM, Bedi A, Kelly BT. Hip Arthroscopy and Hip Joint Preservation Surgery, Hip Arthroscopy: Lateral Approach to Patient Positioning, Set-Up, and Traction, 2014, p. 304, Thomas G. Sampson, Fig. 1

Femoroacetabular Impingement

The most common reason for arthroscopic surgery of the hip is to treat damage related to femoroacetabular impingement. Femoroacetabular impingement is a mismatch between the shape of the head-neck junction and the acetabulum causing an overload to the labrum and articular cartilage resulting in damage to both. Prior to 2001, this condition was only treated using a surgical dislocation of the hip. The procedure was developed by Reinhold Ganz from an unintended consequence of overcorrection with a pelvic acetabular osteotomy, in which anterior impingement was created. We described an arthroscopic technique to reshape the femoral head-neck junction in 2001 and published in 2005. The arthroscopic technique has evolved from the open technique and today is accepted as a treatment for the condition. Bone reshaping of both the head-neck junction and the acetabular rim along with labral refixation is performed to correct the defects.

Removal of Loose Bodies and Foreign Bodies

Originally, the procedure was done to remove loose bodies and foreign bodies. Today, this has been the clearest indication and has essentially replaced arthrotomy as a much less-invasive alternative. The loose bodies may be from

Fig. 41.2 The first hip distractor (*left*) similar to a shoulder (*right*) design using Buck's traction as a leg holder suspended with ropes and pulleys from the ceiling and the wall with >45 lb of weight. With kind permission from Springer Science+Business Media: Byrd T. Operative Hip Arthroscopy, The Lateral Approach, 2005, p. 132, Thomas G. Sampson, Fig. 9.5

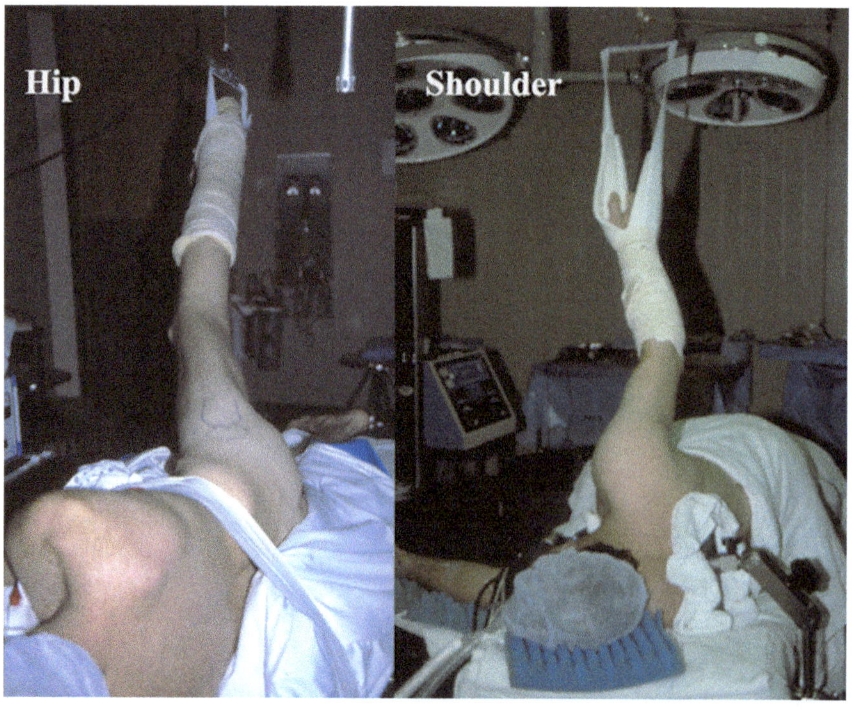

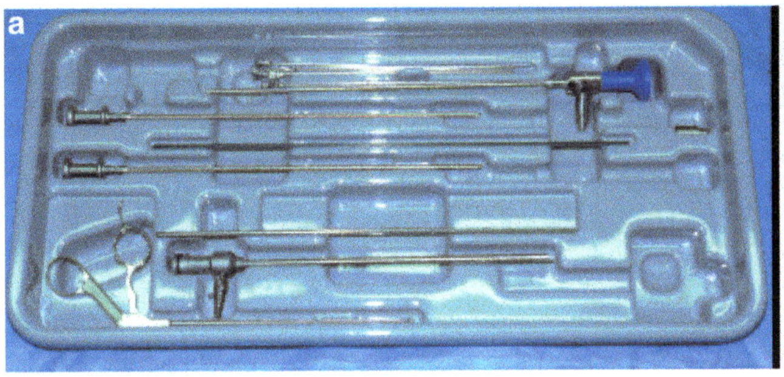

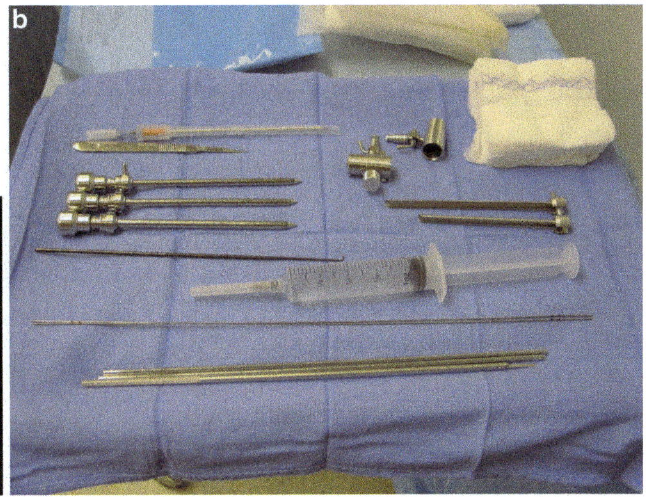

Fig. 41.3 (**a**) The first cannulated long hip scope system developed by Stryker. With kind permission from Springer Science + Business Media: Byrd T. Operative Hip Arthroscopy, The Lateral Approach, 2005, p. 133, Thomas G. Sampson, Fig. 9.9. (**b**) A simplified cannulated system with varying sized sheaths, switching sticks, and slotted cannulas. The arthroscope has a shortened hub and the trocar is cannulated for a Nitinol wire. With kind permission from Springer Science + Business Media: Byrd T. Operative Hip Arthroscopy, The Lateral Approach, 2005, p. 134, Thomas G. Sampson, Fig. 9.11

synovial chondromatosis (rice-like or osteocartilagenous), bullets, or loose cement or wires in total hip replacements.

Removal of Osteochondral Fracture Fragment

Articular cartilage injury from falling directly onto the side of a hip in young people may result in an osteochondral fracture and loose fragment, with the reaction of the head resembling aseptic necrosis. Removal of the fragment and microfracture of the base has been shown to be beneficial.

Labral Lesions

Labral lesions represent the most common indication for hip arthroscopy. In the past, partial or total excision was the treatment of choice. The outcome, however, was not predictable, especially in the presence of articular cartilage damage or arthritis. Primary labral repair was equally controversial and with unpredictable outcomes. Recently, femoroacetabular impingement has helped to explain the etiology of atraumatic labral tears, and its treatment with head-neck osteoplasty, rim trimming, and labral debridement and/or refixation has become more common in treating labral tears.

Developmental Dysplasia

Developmental dysplasia of the hip was in the past a contraindication for hip arthroscopy and osteotomy was recommended. Today, if the dysplasia is borderline (center-edge angle 20°–25°) or in combination with femoroacetabular impingement, the symptomatic patient may benefit from arthroscopic treatment. The intra-articular pathology includes labral tears, articular cartilage damage, and disruption of the ligamentum teres. The peripheral compartment pathology may include a lax capsule and an anterior rim osteophyte. Techniques to treat this condition arthroscopically have had favorable outcomes, obviating arthrotomy. Capsulorrhaphy for laxity can be done and is more successful with less biomechanical instability.

Synovial Diseases

The treatments of synovial diseases with biopsy for rheumatic diseases, or synovectomy for PVNS, synovial chondromatosis, and infection are very effective. The problem has been accessing all of the synovial surfaces within the central and peripheral compartments, which have now been improved with capsulotomy.

Adhesive Capsulitis

Adhesive capsulitis has been recognized as a cause of hip pain similar to that seen in the shoulder. Debridement and synovectomy in primary or revision cases have shown benefit.

Sepsis

Acute sepsis has clearly been successfully treated with hip arthroscopy and treatment for acutely infected total hips with an irrigation and debridement.

Hip Arthritis

The treatment of hip arthritis has had an upsurge in hip arthroscopy as a bridge technique before total hip replacement. With the advent of bone-reshaping techniques done arthroscopically, the results of debridement, microfracture, and resection osteoplasty have improved the outcomes when compared to debridement alone. However, moderate to severe osteoarthritis with loss of joint space and limited range of motion are contraindications.

Staging Aseptic Necrosis

The treatment of end-stage aseptic necrosis is met with poor results; however, staging for open techniques such as vascularized fibular grafts has improved it.

Coxa Saltans

Coxa saltans (snapping hip syndrome) can be treated arthroscopically with releases. The iliopsoas tendon is accessible both at the lesser trochanter or trans-capsular near the inferior synovial fold for an arthroscopically facilitated release. The peritrochanteric region is the latest frontier in hip arthroscopy. Release of the iliotibial band for external snapping and repair of gluteus medius ruptures (rotator cuff of the hip) have been done with success.

Surgical Technique

Anesthesia

Most commonly we use general anesthesia. If regional anesthesia is used, there must be muscle relaxation. Antibiotic prophylaxis is warranted using one of the cephalosporins. DVT prophylaxis is accomplished using compression stockings and a sequential pump on both legs.

Patient Positioning

The patient is placed on a well-padded operating room table in the lateral decubitus position (Fig. 41.4). An axillary roll is placed and hip positioners are used to support the pelvis. By preventing the pelvis from rolling back on the perineal post, the risk of pudendal neuropraxias may be reduced.

The foot is wrapped with padding and the foot holder is applied, taking care to avoid skin pinching by the device. The leg is held in abduction by the assistant for careful placement of the well-padded perineal post. We have determined that the post should have an outer diameter greater than 9 cm for safety. Commercially available hip distractors all exceed this size. The genitalia are inspected to ensure they are free from compression. The foot holder is applied to the distraction arm with enough traction to only support the leg.

The fluoroscopic C-arm is brought in with the apex under the table and centered at the level of the greater trochanter. Preoperative X-rays are done to check for positioning and hip anatomy. A trial of distraction will be of benefit for two reasons: (1) to check for the distractibility of the joint and (2) to ensure the foot is properly secured in the foot holder. If the hip does not distract well, it may be due to a tight or hypertrophic capsule, and a few minutes of traction may allow it to relax. Failure to distract may require greater forces, and necessitate capsulotomy or acetabular rim trimming to avoid femoral head scuffing. If the foot slips out of the holder during the trial, less padding and careful attention to strap placement and tightening may help prevent slippage. Adequate security of the foot in the holder is imperative to prevent an accidental release of distraction while the instruments are in the central compartment, which may result in iatrogenic articular cartilage damage.

Sticky towels or drapes are placed from the iliac crest to six inches below the greater trochanter and a sagittal line lateral to the anterior superior iliac spine anterior and the sciatic notch posterior.

The anesthesiologist is at the head of the table, while the surgeon stands either anterior or posterior with the assistant on the opposite side. The scrub technician stands next to the surgeon with the C-arm in between. A Mayo stand is placed above the patient's shoulder for easy accessibility to the instruments and organization of the arthroscopic cords.

We typically drape with split sheets and use a large plastic pouch to catch fluids.

Distraction

For optimal viewing and safe surgery, at least 1.2 cm of distraction is required to enter the femoroacetabular joint (central compartment). Commercially available distractors for the lateral approach are available and have the ability to move the hip into various positions to optimize surgery in the central, peripheral, and peritrochanteric compartments during surgery (Fig. 41.5).

Not all distractors have a tensiometer to measure the force of distraction. Distraction should be thought of in the same way as a tourniquet. James M. Glick M.D., in a study using evoked potentials, originally concluded that forces less than 75 lb for less than 2 h were safe and did not cause permanent neuropraxias [2, 8]. However, on a later analysis of his original data using modern statistical analysis, the actual force is more pertinent than the time spent in traction [9]. We have done over 1500 cases without a tensiometer, taking care to

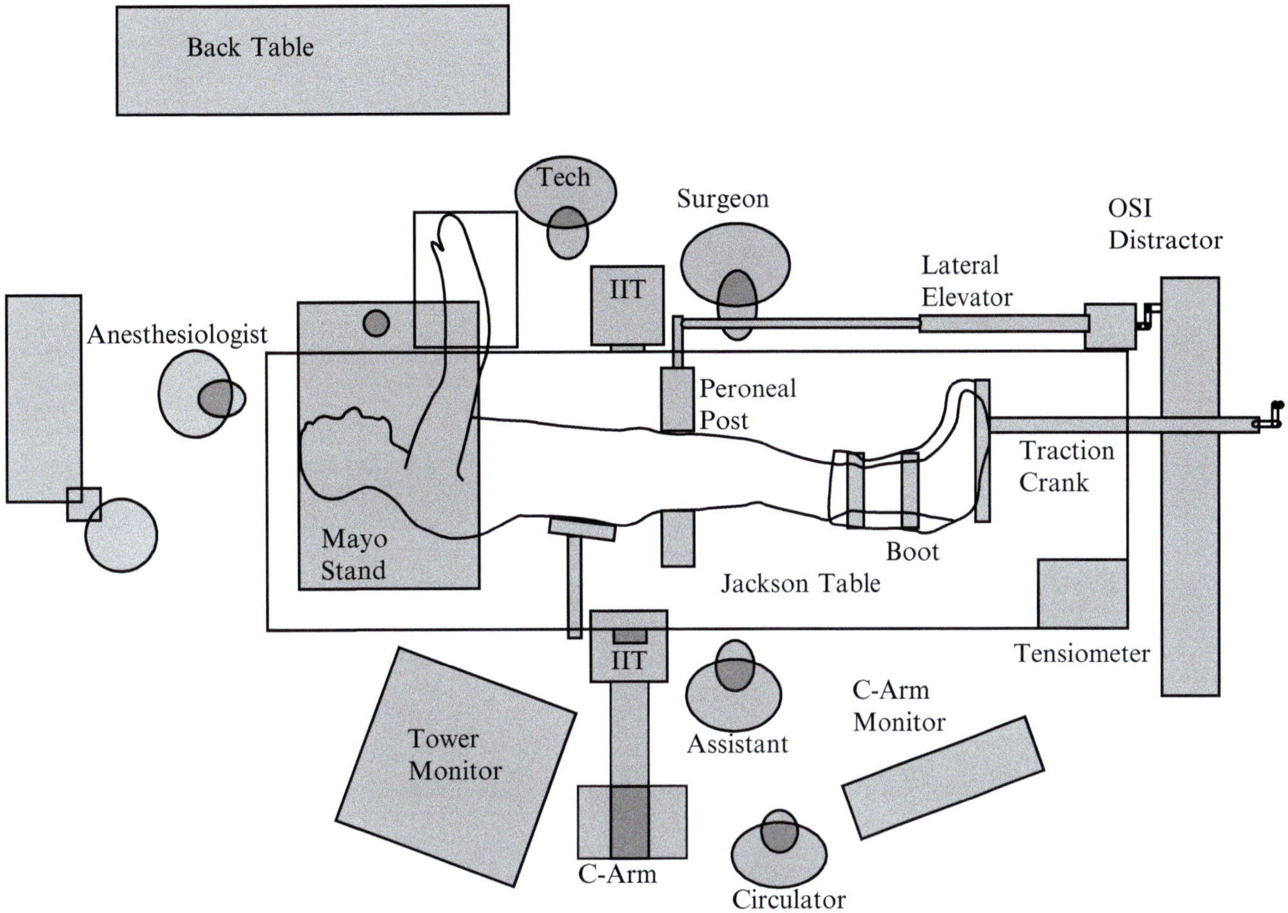

Fig. 41.4 Room setup in the lateral approach. The surgeon stands anterior (some prefer posterior if they do total hips from the posterior approach). The assistant works from the opposite side and the scrub technician to the side of the surgeon. The C-arm lies below the table throughout the case, and a Mayo stand is placed above the shoulder for instruments. With kind permission from Springer Science+Business Media: Byrd T. Operative Hip Arthroscopy, The Lateral Approach, 2005, p. 134, Thomas G. Sampson, Fig. 9.12

keep the distraction time and the forces to a minimum, resulting in no neuropraxias. A well-planned capsulotomy will reduce the forces of distraction necessary to enter the central compartment. The entire team should be aware of when the hip distraction begins and its duration. Realize, however, that complications may occur from too little or too much traction, and to accomplish the procedure, the joint surfaces must be separated to introduce instruments.

The perineal post should have padding of at least 9 cm in diameter and positioned eccentrically over the pubic symphysis with little to no compression to the downside thigh (Fig. 41.6).

We initiate the operative distraction after the case is entirely set up and all the equipment has been turned on and is functioning. We record the traction time, which is entered in the operative record. The assistant or the circulating nurse announces the distraction time at 15 min intervals.

Once the surgery in the central compartment has been completed, all of the distraction forces are released, and the periarticular work in the peripheral compartment can be done without distraction concerns.

Operating Room Setup

Leg Position

In traction, the hip capsule is maximally relaxed in 15 ° of flexion, neutral rotation, and 15 ° of abduction. I use this as a starting position and make positional adjustments during the procedure to facilitate getting into different areas. Additionally, the perineal post may be elevated laterally to add an abduction moment for better viewing.

Instruments

The 30° arthroscope is best for central viewing. It is easier to become oriented with this angle and is the best for getting started using the lateral approach. The 70° arthroscope is best for peripheral viewing, around the femoral head, deep in the fossa, to view the fovea and to create additional portals. On thin patients, standard arthroscopic equipment may be used if the sheath has a short hub. The advantage of commercially available hip kits is that they contain the proper sheath lengths and cannulated systems. The option for longer

a b c d

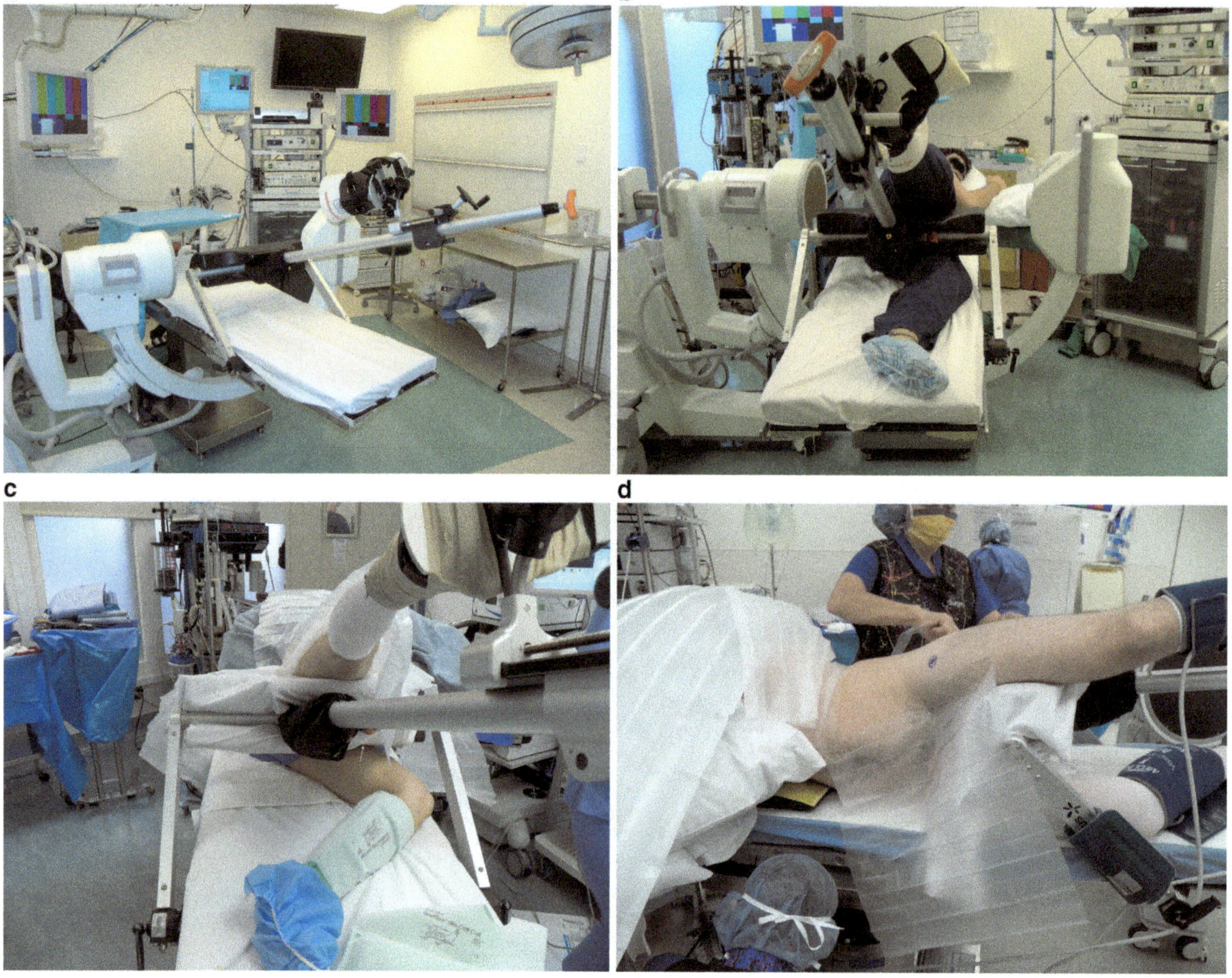

Fig. 41.5 (**a**) The room setup with a commercially available lateral hip distractor made by Smith and Nephew®. The C-arm fluoroscope apexes under the table and monitors are on either side for both the surgeon and assistant to view. (**b**) Patient positioned and in the distractor. (**c**) Note that the large perineal post is off the downside leg and sequential compression devices are used (**d**)

arthroscopes should be available for larger patients and for those cases in which excessive swelling occurs in the thigh during the procedure.

Both straight and curved graspers are necessary, as well as straight and curved shavers. To insert curved instruments, a slotted cannula or a flexible plastic sheath is used.

Radio thermal probes are used for coagulation, cutting, and ablation of tissues such as capsule or labrum. Many are curved or bendable and can reach lesions not accessible to straight shavers. Flexible wands for hips can be manually maneuvered with a trigger handle.

Angled neuro-currettes and angled picks are used to treat arthritic defects and remove attached and loose bodies. These may be located in difficult areas to reach, such as the medial acetabular fossa and anterior medial acetabulum.

The Pump

It is generally accepted to use a pump system since the exact pressure and flow can be controlled and monitored. I recommend using an outflow-dependent pump, which reduces the amount of extravasation into the soft tissues. The pump pressure is set to the same settings as for the shoulder, slightly above diastolic pressure or as low as possible to achieve distention and a clear field without bleeding.

The Tower

The arthroscopic tower with the monitor and instrument boxes should be placed opposite the surgeon and slightly cephalad, adjacent to the C-arm for optimal viewing of all the settings by the surgeon. The cords from the tower are brought onto the Mayo stand and organized for the surgeon

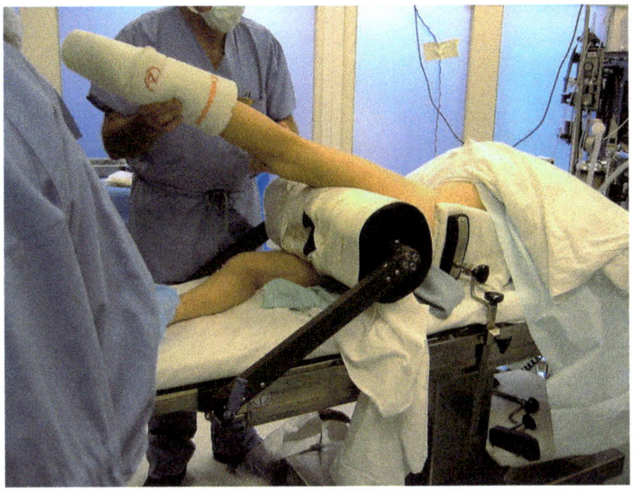

Fig. 41.6 A patient's right leg being placed in the hip distractor. Note the posterior hip positioner, the large perineal pad, and the foot padding. Not seen is the axillary roll

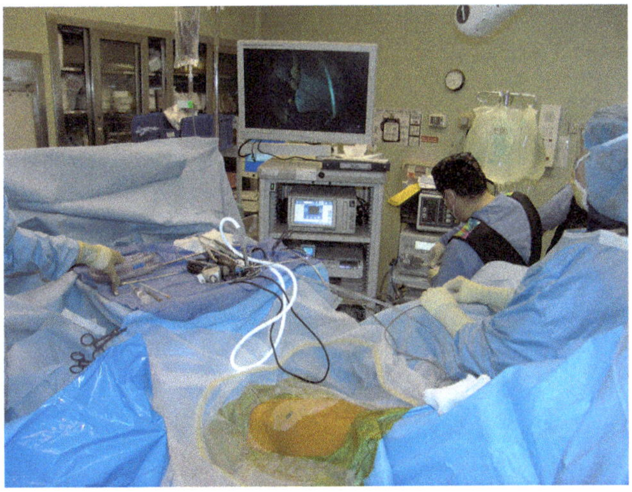

Fig. 41.7 The surgeon's view from the front of the patient. There is a clear view of the tower's instrument boxes, the monitor, and the outflow-dependent pump. The Mayo stand is above the patient's shoulder and is used to organize and make easy access of the instruments. A view of the fluoroscopic monitor is toward the foot of the table

to easily reach the shaver and wands. It is more efficient and safe for the Mayo stand to act as neutral ground, whereby only one person accesses it to avoid accidental glove punctures or lacerations (Fig. 41.7).

The Procedure

The portals for the lateral approach are nearly identical to the supine approach except the anterior portal is located approximately 2 cm. lateral to the ASIS line. As a result, the anterior portal courses in an intermuscular plane between the sartorius and tensor fascia lata (Fig. 41.8).

Distraction should be initiated only after the patient has been prepped and draped, all instruments, camera, and shaver sets have been plugged in, the foot controls are positioned, and everything is functioning correctly. For small and flexible patients, start with 25–50 lb of force and with large stiff patients 50–75 lb if using a tensiometer. Alternatively, attain at least 8–12 mm of separation between the femoral head and the acetabulum on the fluoroscopic view.

Beginning with the anterolateral portal, a long 17-gauge needle is inserted under direct fluoroscopic visualization while observing it pass between the head of the femur and acetabulum (closer to the femur to avoid puncturing the labrum). Listen for a hiss of sound as the joint suction seal is broken and room air is sucked into the joint. Observe for the traction forces to reduce on the tensiometer, or a sudden distal subluxation of the hip. Obtain the desired distraction (usually about 1.2 cm). Insert a Nitinol wire through the needle and incise the skin with a No. 11 blade. Push the cannulated arthroscopic sheath over the wire and into the joint while advancing concentrically over the wire to prevent kinking and wire breakage. Backing the wire out slightly will reduce cartilage trauma.

If it is difficult to advance into the joint, suspect the wire is going through the labrum. In such instances, it is best to start over and reposition the needle to avoid labral avulsions or tears. In some cases with stiff hips, the anterior capsule is very thick and very difficult to penetrate. In that situation it is best to begin with the posterolateral portal or gently cut the capsule with a long Beaver blade through the arthroscopic sheath prior to advancing into the joint. Entry into the joint should always be controlled to avoid damage to the labrum or scuffing of the cartilage. However, pushing a cannula through the anterior hip capsule is difficult and requires a lot of force when compared to any other joint in the body (Fig. 41.9).

Introduce a 30° arthroscope and visually sweep the joint under air or fluid. Next, create the anterior and posterolateral portals using the same technique with the added benefit of viewing entry of the needle, Nitinol wire, and instruments under direct vision to prevent injury to the cartilage and labrum. We feel that it is much safer with this approach in reducing iatrogenic injury. In creating the anterior portal, take care to only incise the skin superficially to avoid laceration of a branch of the lateral femoral cutaneous nerve. Spreading through the subcutaneous tissue with a clamp is also advised for this portal. Slotted or half pipe cannulas may be used to insert larger or curved instruments (Fig. 41.10a).

An alternate way to enter the peripheral and central compartments is through a capsulotomy first approach. We have found that it is easier to teach hip arthroscopy to arthroplasty surgeons using this technique since it is essentially a submuscular arthrotomy of the hip. For most cases, we use the anterolateral and the mid-anterior portals and start with the

Fig. 41.8 Portals for the lateral approach (right hip); anterior superior iliac spine (ASIS), posterolateral (PL), anterolateral (AL), anterior (A), and mid-anterior (MA)

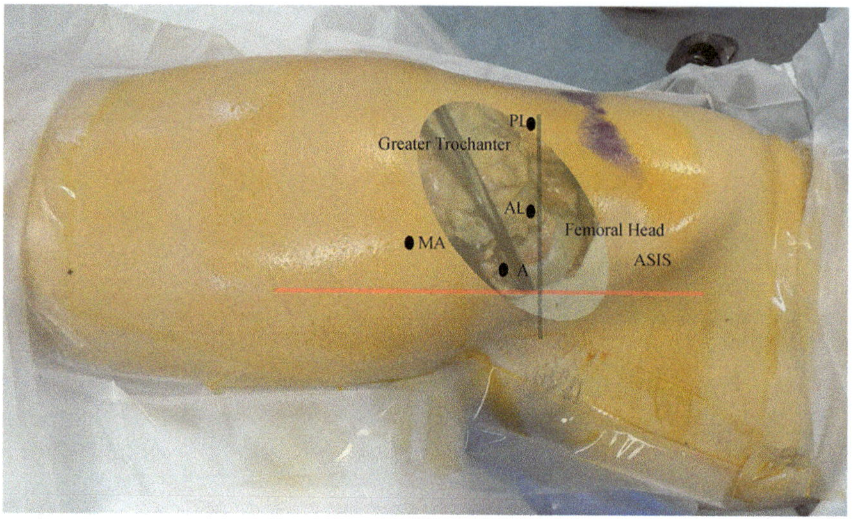

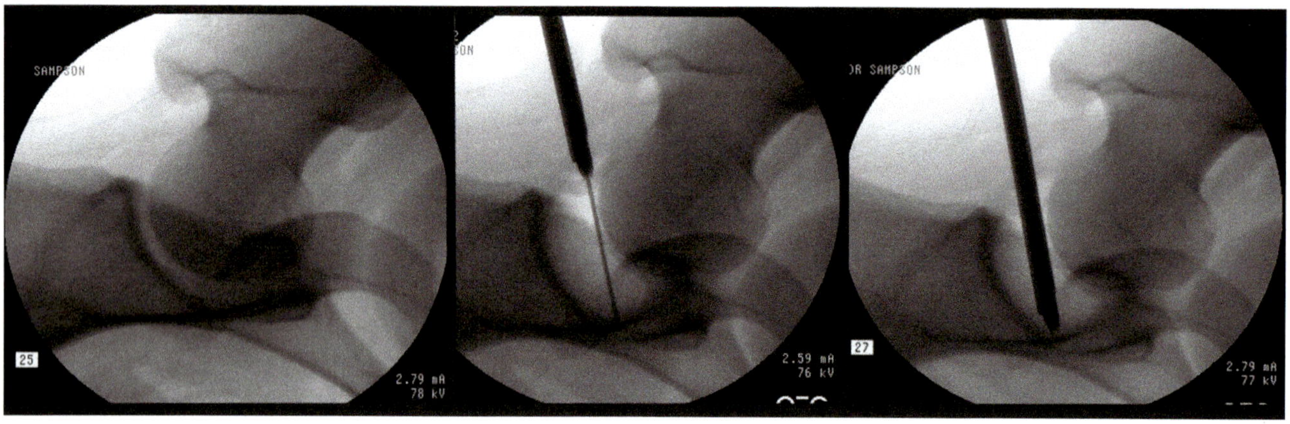

Fig. 41.9 Fluoroscopic view of distracting the hip joint and insertion of the cannulated trocar over the Nitinol wire

hip in a relaxed position without distraction. Using fluoroscopic control, a spinal needle is placed through the anticipated anterolateral portal and aimed at the superior lateral rim of the acetabulum about a half a centimeter toward the head. Using the cannulated system with a Nitinol wire, the 30° arthroscope views the anterior fat pad of the hip distal to the indirect head of the rectus femoris. The mid-anterior portal is created in the same fashion and a 4 mm shaver is used to clear a space anterolaterally. Using a radiofrequency device, the capsule is incised at the base of the neck longitudinally through the zona orbicularis to the acetabular rim while avoiding the labrum so as not to damage it. The capsule is then incised at the labral capsular junction along the rim laterally and anteriorly which gives a global view of the femoral head and neck junction, the labrum, the acetabular rim, the peripheral space, and the subspine space. Distraction is then initiated requiring less force, and the arthroscope is driven into the central compartment under direct view reducing the incidence of chondral or labral damage. We have done over 1500 capsulotomies in this fashion without the complication of subluxation or dislocation. The capsule may be repaired at the end of the case if deemed necessary (Fig. 41.10b).

The central compartment should be inspected in a methodical fashion to plan the necessary treatment. Efficient management of the pathology with careful attention to distraction time while simultaneously monitoring the patient's temperature and presence of abdominal distention will facilitate correction of the problem and reduce the potential for complications.

The Visual Sweep and Anatomy

The acetabulum and its structures are viewed first. Initially the femoral head cannot be entirely viewed with the hip distracted; however, the hidden portions will be observed when looking in the peripheral compartment later in the procedure (Fig. 41.11).

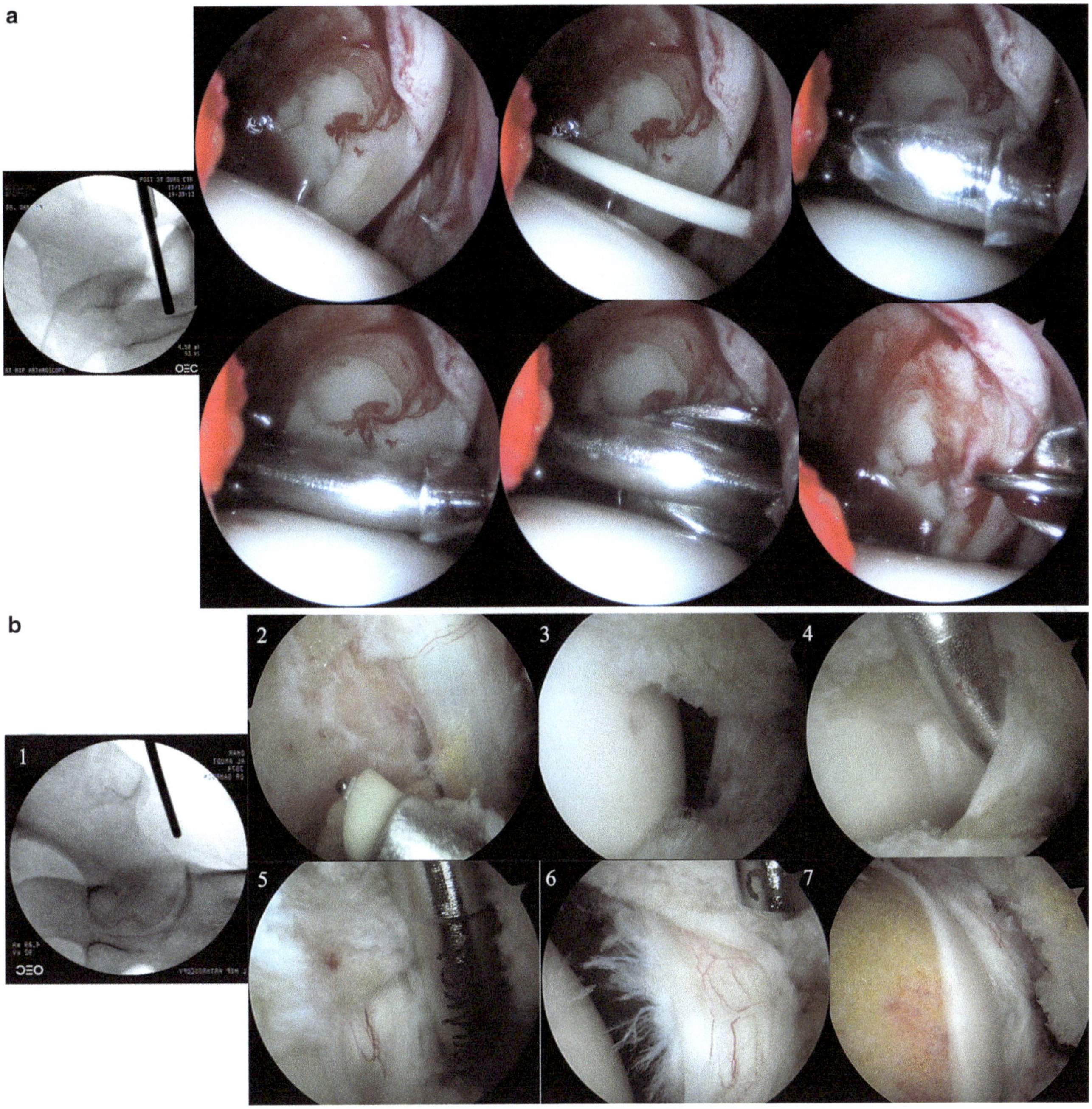

Fig. 41.10 (**a**) Arthroscopic view of a right hip from the anterolateral portal with the progression of steps inserting the needle, the Nitinol wire, the cannulated trocar, the switching stick, the slotted (half pipe) cannula, and finally a probe through the anterior portal. With kind permission from Springer Science+Business Media: Byrd T. Operative Hip Arthroscopy, The Lateral Approach, 2005, p. 139, Thomas G. Sampson, Fig. 9.21b. (**b**) The approach through a capsulotomy viewing from anterolateral. (*1*) Fluoroscopic view of the instrument aiming toward the anterolateral acetabular rim, (*2*) identification of the indirect head of the rectus femoris, (*3*) longitudinal incision of the capsule, (*4*) protecting the labrum while cutting the capsule, (*5*) shaving the capsular labral junction to expose the acetabular rim, (*6*) hip distraction to expose the central compartment, (*7*) at the end of the procedure after rim trimming, labral refixation, and osteoplasty of the head-neck junction

With the 30° scope, start by observing the acetabular fossa and the fat pad. Petechial hemorrhage is normal due to the traction forces pulling negative pressure on the vessels. Atrophy of the fat pad is abnormal. Look for loose bodies and rice bodies and notch osteophytes or masses. Advance the scope deep to view the ligamentum teres. Look for tears or avulsions. The transverse acetabular ligament is very hard to see unless the patient has hyperlaxity.

Rotate the scope posterior and inferior and pick up the posterior labrum at the articular margin noting the posterior third. Look behind the labrum for loose bodies and then follow the labrum lateral and anterior noting a normal cleft in

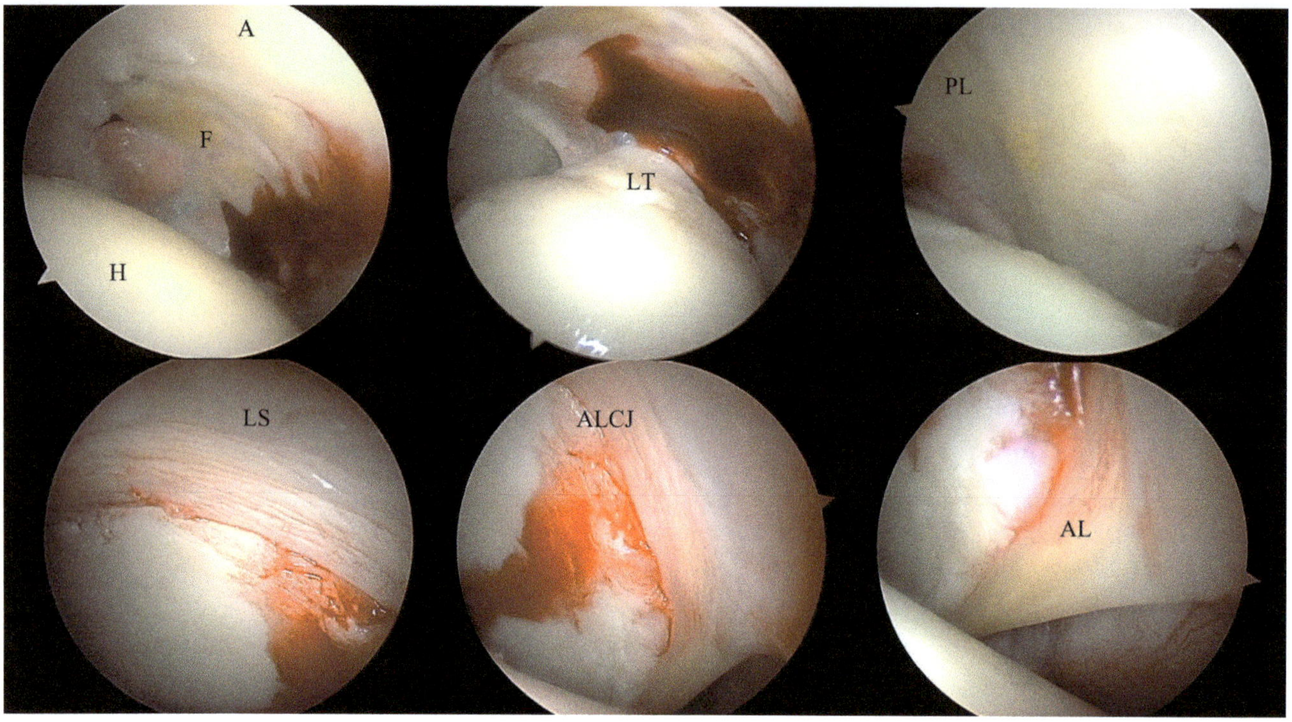

Fig. 41.11 Arthroscopic view of a right hip under room air. Acetabulum (A), head (H), labrum (L), fossa (F), ligamentum teres (LT), posterior labrum (PL), anterior labrum (AL), lateral sulcus (LS), and anterior labrocartilaginous junction (ALCJ). With kind permission from Springer Science+Business Media: Byrd T. Operative Hip Arthroscopy, The Lateral Approach, 2005, p. 140, Thomas G. Sampson, Fig. 9.22

the posterior articular margin with a small labral cartilage sulcus. The sulcus is not an old avulsion fracture, nor from posterior subluxation. Note any labral fraying or tears and articular changes.

Look at the middle third and note any labral cartilage separations or fraying and degenerative changes. The surface may be smooth or have a cobblestone appearance in early degeneration.

As the scope is rotated to the anterior area, look for hypertrophy of the labrum in patients with dysplasia. The acetabular cartilage may be soft or may appear blistered or delaminated in dysplastics with anterior groin pain, instability, or popping. Look anterior beyond the labrum in the sulcus for synovitis and loose bodies. Move the scope to the superior sulcus of the joint to see the nonarticular side of the labrum in the pericapsular space from anterior to posterior. Look for evidence of cysts, spurring, and labral tears. All the while, a probe or switching stick is used to probe.

Next observe as much of the femoral head possible with the same method, and if necessary rotate the leg while in traction. At this point we may switch to a 70° scope to look deeper into the notch and have a better view of the femoral head fovea with its ligamentum teres insertion.

After viewing from the anterolateral portal, the same procedure is carried out from the posterior portal if not satisfied with the initial viewing.

If getting into the central compartment is very difficult, or if the surgical plan is to remove the bone in patients with femoroacetabular impingement, a capsulotomy is accomplished first. The capsule is viewed by sweeping the muscle off with a switching stick and removing the interval bursa with the shaver. The capsule is incised along the neck using an RF cutting probe by positioning the tool near the base of the neck anterior to the lateral neck to avoid damage to the lateral epiphyseal branch of the medial femoral circumflex artery. Care is taken as the labrum is approached so as to not cut it. Many times the zona orbicularis looks like the labrum and is distinguished by its more distal position on the neck as seen on the C-arm X-ray. If the capsule is excessively thick, partial capsulectomy is then performed.

The corrective surgery is then performed depending on the diagnosis, and the distraction is subsequently released to allow the hip to be moved in rotation and flexion.

With the hip in slight flexion and neutral rotation, the 17-gauge needle is inserted through the anterolateral portal aiming along the femoral neck toward the head-neck junction. While observing under fluoroscopy, a small pop is felt as the needle passes through the capsule and the effusion dribbles out of the needle (Fig. 41.12). Pass a Nitinol wire and bounce it off the medial capsule to confirm it is intra-articular. Advance the arthroscopic sheath over the wire and begin viewing the anterior, medial, inferior, and posterior peripheral spaces.

First note the femoral head seated in the labrum, as it transforms into the transverse acetabular ligament. The zona orbicularis crosses the field, and one may see the vincula-like vessel in the lateral synovial fold going into the femoral neck. Push the scope deep and posterior to view the sulcus and look for loose bodies.

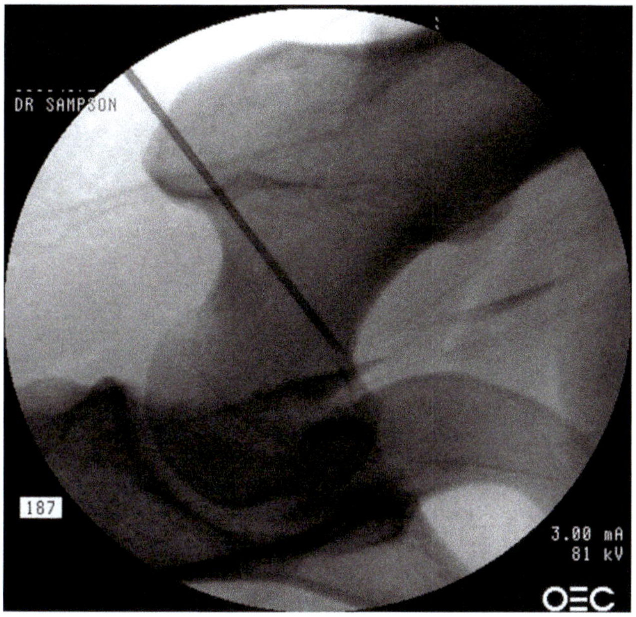

Fig. 41.12 Fluoroscopic view of a left hip with a Nitinol wire in the peripheral compartment touching the medial capsule from the anterior portal

As the scope is withdrawn, rotate it and advance it anterior, medial, and inferior to appreciate the reflection of the iliopsoas tendon on the capsule. The tendinous bulge on the capsule is usually opposite the inferior synovial fold at the head-neck junction and is not to be mistaken for the zona orbicularis. Flexing the hip will relax the capsule for a larger field of view and improves the mobility of the scope and operative instruments (Fig. 41.13). A mid-anterior portal may be created at the level of the femoral neck midway between the head-neck junction and lesser trochanter for both the arthroscope and operative instruments.

A far anteroinferior portal may be used at the level of the lesser trochanter for iliopsoas release.

At the completion of the procedure, close the wounds and apply a standard dressing. An intra-articular injection of a long-acting local anesthetic will make recovery and the trip home from the surgical center more tolerable. Ropivacaine is preferred as it has less chondrotoxic effects.

In the recovery room, have the patient begin both passive and active range of motion of their hip. Crutches are used with the amount of weight bearing dependent on the diagnosis and treatment.

The dressings are removed in 24 h and the patient is allowed to shower. Therapy is started within a week to regain motion and strength.

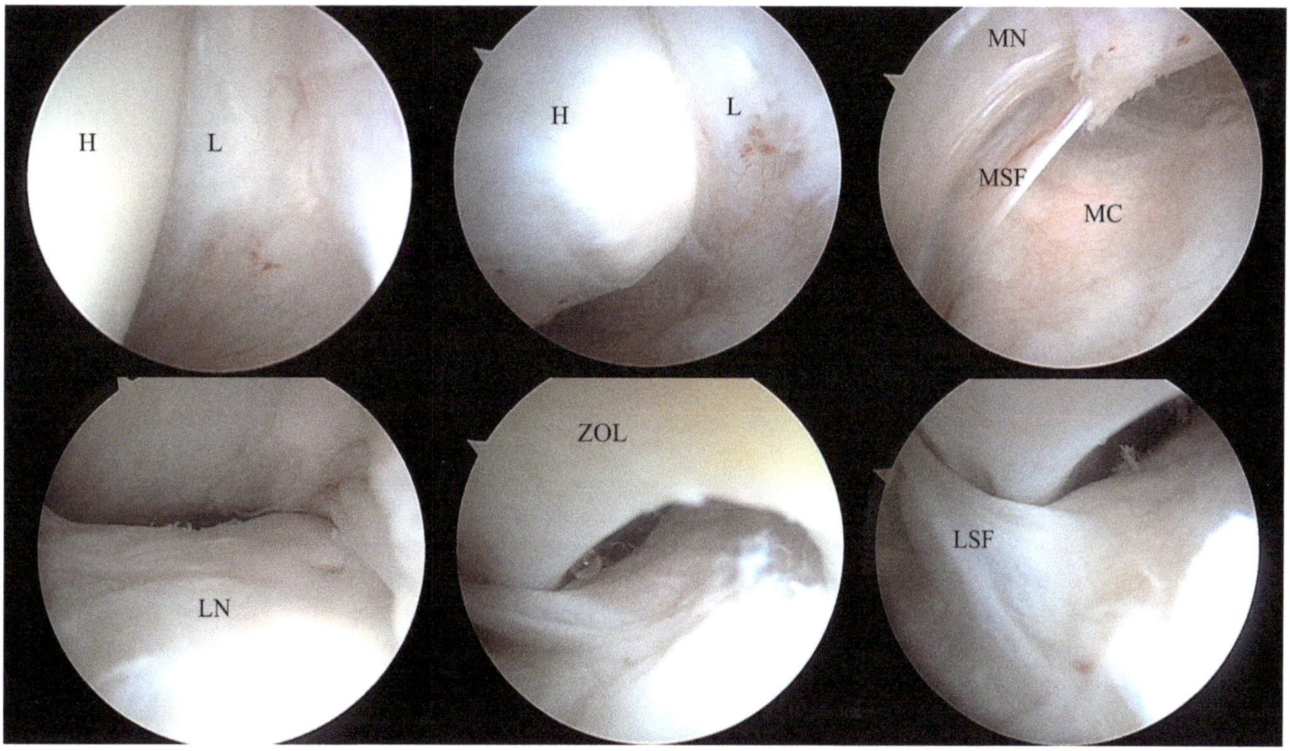

Fig. 41.13 Arthroscopic view of a right hip in the peripheral space. Head (H), labrum (L), zona orbicularis lateral portion (ZOL), medial neck (MN), medial synovial fold (MSF), medial capsule (MC), lateral neck (LN), and lateral synovial fold (LSF)

Postoperative Rehabilitation

Aggressive physical therapy is not necessary after most hip arthroscopic procedures. In some cases, moving too quickly with rehabilitation may cause unnecessary pain, which impedes progress. If a therapist is used, they must have full knowledge of the procedures performed and precautionary restrictions imposed.

We have found that instructions to the patient for self-therapy during the first month have eliminated complications from physical therapy. After a month, prescribed therapy may be used. We initiate the patient on stationary bike and elliptical trainer exercises, followed by swimming and pool exercises. The concept is to allow for early range of motion and weight bearing for better joint mobility and proprioception.

In most cases, repetitive joint percussion such as running is avoided until pain and swelling are gone and the patient has good hip stability (usually 3 months).

Results/Outcomes in Table Format

The success of the lateral approach cannot be measured in a double-blind prospective study; however, it should be judged on the facilitation of entering the central compartment of the hip. In that sense, it was the first, most reproducible, and widely used technique prior to development of specific "hip kits" or hip distractors. Outcomes in treating specific conditions using either the lateral or the supine approaches are the subject of other chapters in the book.

Complications

There are many potential complications; however, with experience and attention to detail, they may be significantly minimized. In the first 60 cases, we had a 15 % complication rate and in the last 1000 cases only 0.4 %. We have never had a deep infection; however, there have been four superficial infections involving the anterior portal. It is not uncommon to have instruments pass in and out of the portals numerous times during a case, which can irritate and injure the skin around the portal.

In the early years of development, there were more extravasations into the thigh. In nine cases extravasation occurred into the retroperitoneal space, requiring an ICU stay with the patient intubated and a pericentesis to drain the fluid in one case. This complication was virtually eliminated with the modern outflow-dependent pumps and attention to operative time.

Neuropraxias of the pudendal nerve were common before the use of more than 9 cm of padding on the peroneal post and its position offset from the pubic symphysis.

Damage to the major nerves has rarely occurred, particularly with modern distractors and attention to minimizing distraction time below 2 h.

Iatrogenic trauma to the articular cartilage occurs even in the most experienced surgeons and is under reported.

Instrument breakage does occur; however, most are successfully retrieved.

Infections are extremely rare. We have never had a patient develop deep sepsis following hip arthroscopy. The treatment is arthroscopic lavage and synovectomy and parenteral antibiotics.

Technical Pearls

- Position the patient on the table closer to the side that the surgeon is working for better ergonomics and less surgeon fatigue.
- Pad down side bony prominences, the peroneal nerve, and the foot.
- Carefully place the axillary roll.
- Check the genitalia against the perineal post.
- Pad the foot going into the distractor and double-check that the foot is well seated and securely strapped in.
- Test the distractor before scrubbing to prevent inadvertent foot slippage.
- Keep the C-arm fluoroscope under the table throughout the case for instrument positioning and checking the surgical progression.
- Always use the C-arm X-ray to confirm needle and cannula placement.
- Choose special instruments ahead of the procedure, such as spinal curettes, heavy graspers for large loose bodies/osteophytectomy, and labral refixation anchors.
- If there is significant resistance on needle placement, it may be hitting the acetabular rim not seen on X-ray or the labrum. Back out and reposition the needle.
- When distracting the hip, if there is poor excursion of the head (<0.5 cm), try to break the suction seal of the labrum with a spinal needle.
- If distraction does not separate the head from the acetabulum despite any amount of distraction in any position, entering the central compartment may be facilitated by extra-articular capsulotomy and rim trimming of the acetabulum.
- Intra-articular capsulotomy facilitates instrument mobility.
- When working in the anterior portion of the central compartment, bringing the leg in more extension will open up the space.
- Any instrument may be placed by using a slotted cannula.
- Use distraction judiciously and only when it is necessary to work in the central compartment. All peripheral compartment work should be done without distraction.

- Flex and externally rotate the hip when accessing the medial and posteromedial peripheral space.
- Do a wide capsulotomy when taking out loose bodies and when treating femoroacetabular impingement.
- Make a new portal if a portal is not working well.

References

1. Burman M. Arthroscopy or the direct visualization of joints: an experimental cadaver study. Clin Orthop Relat Res. 1931;390:5–9.
2. Glick JM, et al. Hip arthroscopy by the lateral approach. Arthroscopy. 1987;3(1):4–12.
3. Eriksson E, Arvidsson I, Arvidsson H. Diagnostic and operative arthroscopy of the hip. Orthopedics. 1986;9(2):169–76.
4. Byrd JW. Hip arthroscopy utilizing the supine position. Arthroscopy. 1994;10(3):275–80.
5. Byrd JW. Hip arthroscopy. The supine position. Clin Sports Med. 2001;20(4):703–31.
6. Byrd JW. Hip arthroscopy: the supine position. Instr Course Lect. 2003;52:721–30.
7. Byrd JW. Hip arthroscopy by the supine approach. Instr Course Lect. 2006;55:325–36.
8. Glick JM. Hip arthroscopy by the lateral approach. Instr Course Lect. 2006;55:317–23.
9. Telleria JJ, et al. Risk of sciatic nerve traction injury during hip arthroscopy—is it the amount or duration? An intraoperative nerve monitoring study. J Bone Joint Surg Am. 2012;94(22):2025–32.

42 Arthroscopic Treatment: Layout of the Operating Room—Surgical Approaches, Supine

Carlos A. Guanche

Introduction

Arthroscopy of the hip can be effectively performed with the patient in either the supine or lateral position. With experience, positioning of the patient is simple and can be accomplished in just a few minutes with either technique. The advantages of the supine position include that it can be performed on virtually any standard fracture table with an orientation to the joint that is familiar to orthopedic surgeons accustomed to managing hip fractures. In addition, the layout of the operating room is user friendly for the entire operating room staff. Most importantly, with many of the newer techniques that are employed around the joint, there is reliable access for all standard portal placements, and the leg can be easily repositioned for arthroscopy of the peripheral compartment, iliopsoas bursa, as well as trochanteric and sciatic pathologies.

With the increasing performance of hip arthroscopy, a direct analysis of the supine and lateral positions was undertaken as it relates to simulated hip arthroscopy [1]. In an analysis of training programs and the efficiency of performing hip arthroscopy, there appears to be some quantifiable advantage as it relates to the establishment of portals in the supine versus the lateral position. The ability to orient oneself during the performance of the procedures was statistically simpler in the supine position in this study. With further analysis of the more complex procedures that are being undertaken in the hip, it may turn out that the supine approach may be more predictable for certain treatments; however, there is no evidence-based data currently available.

One final important advantage of the supine position regards intra-abdominal fluid extravasation. This is a potentially serious complication of hip arthroscopy and has been reported more frequently in the lateral position [2, 3]. With the patient on their side, the abdominal and pelvic cavity lie in a dependent position, creating a reservoir into which gravity flow would theoretically allow fluid to collect, perhaps through a connection of the psoas bursa and the joint. Despite this observation, there is no statistically significant difference in frequency between the two positions for this uncommon complication.

The hip joint has both a central and a peripheral compartment. Although historically, most hip pathology has been documented within the central region, the peripheral compartment has been increasingly recognized as involved in hip pathological conditions. It is important to realize that distraction is necessary to achieve arthroscopic access to the central compartment, but not the peripheral portions of the joint.

Performing hip arthroscopy without traction has not been popular because it does not allow access to the important central compartment. However, this method can be a usefully employed along with the traction technique in select situations [4, 5]. Hip flexion relaxes the anterior capsule and allows access to the peripheral compartment, which is still intracapsular. There are many lesions encountered in this area, and they may be overlooked with traction alone. These include significant synovial disease (such as pigmented villonodular synovitis) and free-floating loose bodies in the medial gutter. Femoral impingement lesions (cam impingement) are also best addressed from the peripheral compartment. Finally, hip flexion also allows a more complete access to the anterior capsule for plication procedures.

Operating Room

Anesthesia

In most cases, the procedure is performed as an outpatient under general anesthesia. Epidural is an appropriate alternative, but requires an adequate motor block to ensure muscle relaxation prior to beginning the procedure. Another approach that can be taken, and used in conjunction with

C.A. Guanche, MD (✉)
Southern California Orthopedic Institute,
6815 Noble Avenue, Van Nuys, CA 91405, USA
e-mail: cguanche@scoi.com

J.C. McCarthy et al. (eds.), *Hip Joint Restoration*, DOI 10.1007/978-1-4614-0694-5_42

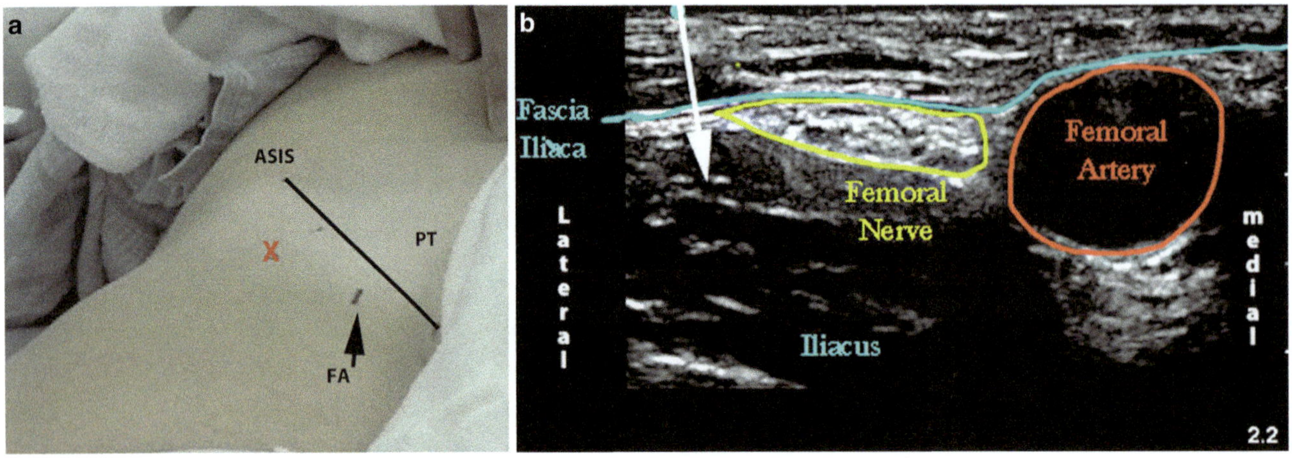

Fig. 42.1 Fascia Iliaca block technique. (**a**) The image is of a right hip being injected. The superficial landmark is a line along the inguinal ligament from the pubic tubercle to the anterior superior iliac spine. The line is trisected and the needle insertion point is 1 cm below the junction of the lateral and middle thirds of the line (2–3 cm lateral to the femoral artery) (*Red X*). The needle is advanced at a 40°–70° angle to the skin until a "loss of resistance" is encountered twice (the fascia lata and fascia iliaca) (*FA* femoral artery; *ASIS* anterior, superior iliac spine; *PT* pubic tubercle). (**b**) Ultrasound sound image depicting the area of entry for the needle (*white arrow*), immediately lateral to the femoral nerve. The image is of a right hip, with the probe in the transverse axis

general anesthesia, is to use a fascia iliaca block for both intraoperative and postoperative pain management [6]. This has been used successfully in several series of hip fracture cases. In the author's experience, most patients obtain significant pain relief for 12–24 h. The procedure is ideally performed following the induction of general anesthesia and in the supine position. The cutaneous projection of the inguinal ligament is drawn from the pubic tubercle to the anterior superior iliac spine and trisected. The needle insertion point for the fascia iliaca compartment approach is 1 cm below the junction of the lateral third and middle third of the cutaneous line, approximately 2–3 cm lateral to the femoral artery, which is palpated and marked. The needle is advanced at a 40°–70° angle to the skin until a "loss of resistance" is encountered twice (first through the fascia lata and then the fascia iliaca), indicating entrance into the fascia iliaca compartment (Fig. 42.1). In our institution, the block is performed under ultrasound guidance. A nerve stimulator technique may also be used. The angle to the skin is then decreased to 30°, and 20 mL of analgesic solution is injected incrementally to expand the compartment of the iliac muscle fascia. A catheter is advanced 15–20 cm cephalad, and an additional 10 mL of analgesic solution is injected incrementally via the catheter [6]. Once the block is placed, the patient is then positioned appropriately for the procedure.

Patient Positioning

For the supine position, a standard fracture table can be used, or several versatile distractors have been developed that can be adapted to a standard operating room table (Hip Positioner; Smith & Nephew, Inc. Andover, MA). The patient is positioned supine and an oversized (12 cm outer diameter) perineal post is used. A large-sized perineal post with generous padding will more safely distribute the pressure on the perineum and facilitate lateralization of the surgical hip. The post is lateral against the medial thigh of the operative leg, with the leg in abduction (Fig. 42.2). Lateralizing the perineal post adds a transverse component to the direction of the traction vector such that the overall moment is lateral as well as distal, yielding concentric displacement of the femoral head from the acetabular fossa (Fig. 42.3). Utilizing the correct vector will decrease the required force to achieve optimal distraction and also distances the post from the area of the pudendal nerve, lessening the risk of compression neuropraxia [2]. In addition,

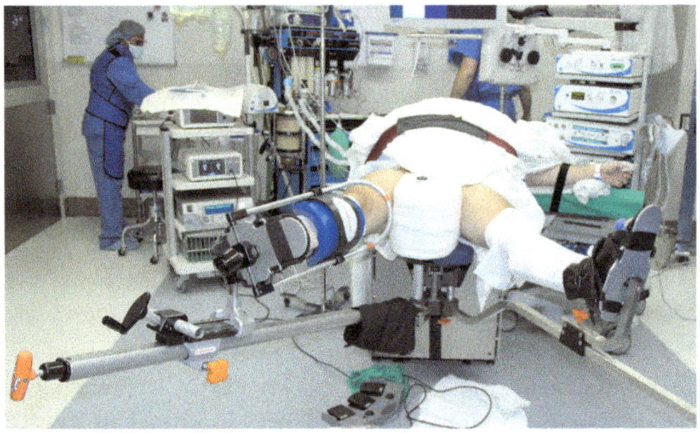

Fig. 42.2 The patient is positioned on the traction table with the perineal post placed as far laterally as possible toward the operative hip (right hip) resting against the medial thigh. The leg is placed in slight abduction, at this point

prolonged traction places the neurovascular structures at risk and one should constantly monitor traction time. The operative hip is then positioned in slight flexion and abduction. While slight flexion may relax the capsule and facilitate distraction, excessive flexion should be avoided because it places tension on the sciatic nerve and may increase the risk of traction neuropraxia. The leg is then maneuvered into

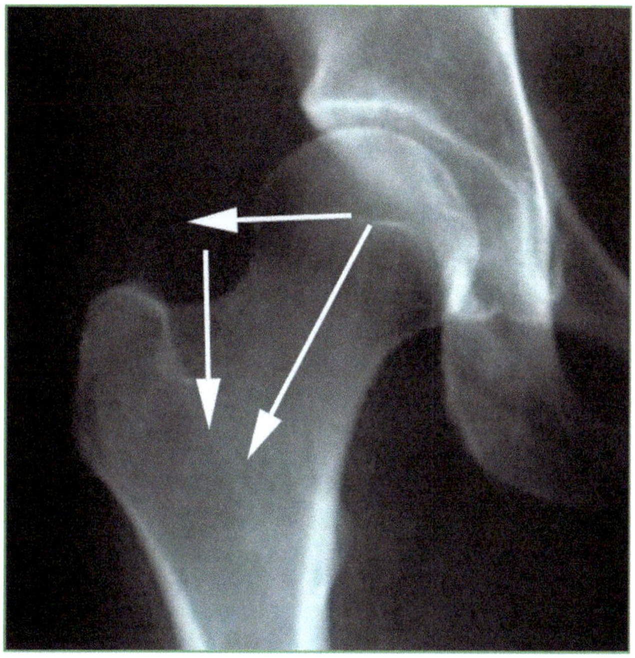

Fig. 42.3 The optimal vector for distraction is oblique relative to the axis of the body and is parallel with the axis of the femoral neck. The resultant vector is created by a combination of abduction of the hip and a transverse component, leading to concentric displacement of the joint

an adducted position in order to effect the desired vector (Fig. 42.4). Neutral to slight internal rotation of the extremity during portal placement is important for proper orientation. However, it is important to have freedom of rotation of the footplate during the procedure, thus facilitating broader visualization of the femoral head intraoperatively.

The contralateral extremity is positioned in about 25° of abduction. Prior to distracting the operative hip, slight traction is applied to the nonoperative leg, in order to stabilize the torso and prevent the pelvis from rotating.

Appropriate sterile preparation of the operative extremity is undertaken. This should include complete access to the buttock, thigh, and anterior groin (Fig. 42.5). An image intensifier is used for all cases to assure precise portal placement and to minimize the risk of iatrogenic injury. Traction is then applied to the operative extremity and distraction of the joint is confirmed by fluoroscopic examination. Approximately 50 lb of traction force is adequate to achieve sufficient distraction. In some cases, more force may be necessary, but application of excessive force should be undertaken with caution (Fig. 42.6).

If adequate distraction is not readily achieved, waiting a few minutes for the capsule to accommodate to the tensile forces often results in capsular relaxation and adequate distraction without excessive force. Also, a vacuum phenomenon will be apparent fluoroscopically (Fig. 42.6). The negative intracapsular pressure caused by distraction creates this phenomenon. This seal will be released when the joint is distended with fluid at the time of surgery and may further facilitate distraction. However, the effect is variable and should not be relied upon to overcome inadequate traction [7]. In situations where no additional distraction is possible,

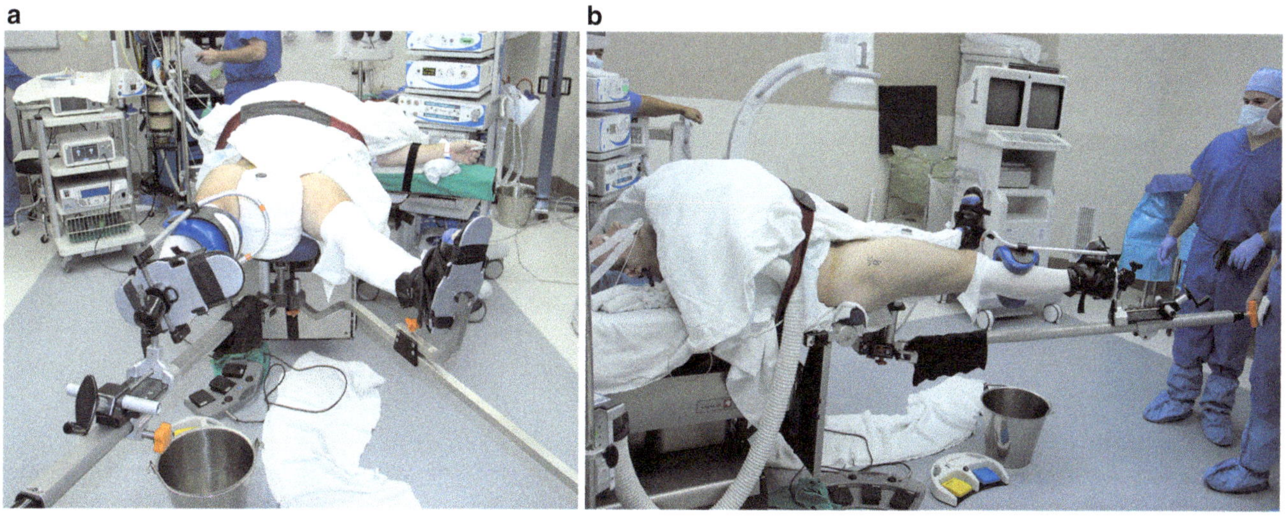

Fig. 42.4 Once the post is in the right position, the leg is then brought into adduction with the foot in slight internal rotation. (**a**) View from the distal aspect. Note the bulge along the medial thigh, indicating that the post is slightly lateral and causing the appropriate moment arm. (**b**) View from the lateral aspect. Note the slight distal position of the post and the internal rotation of the foot

a b

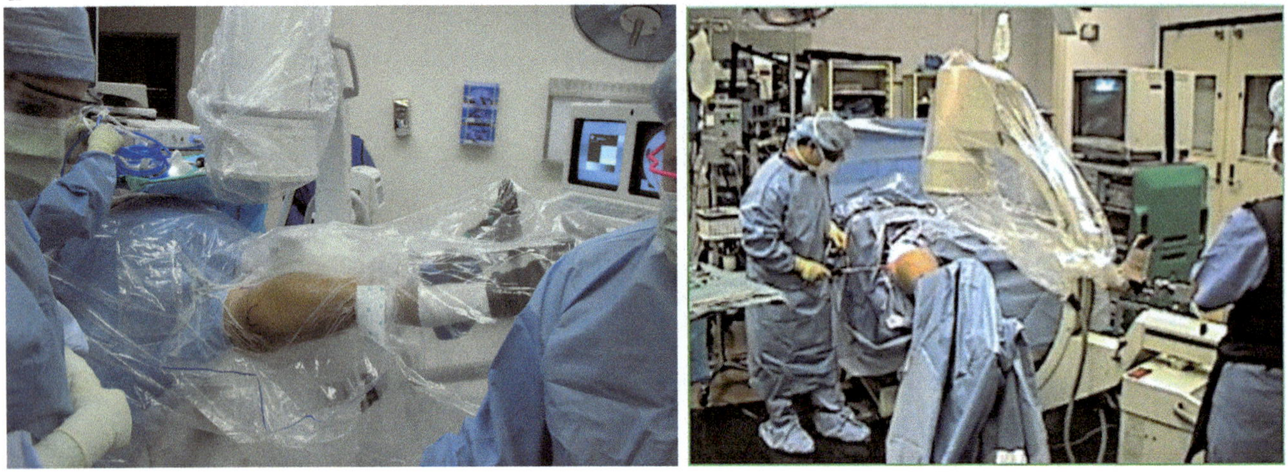

Fig. 42.5 Final positioning of the extremity with draping and equipment in place. (**a**) View with the use of the table attachment hip positioner (Smith & Nephew, Inc.; Andover, MA). Note the Mayo tray on the contralateral side and holding the shaver and arthroscopes in place. The image intensifier is coming in from the contralateral side. (**b**) View with a standard fracture table. The setup is nearly identical, with the exception of the intensifier being brought in between the legs

inserting a needle into the joint to equilibrate the joint and local atmospheric pressure will facilitate further displacement and allow appropriate entry without iatrogenic articular cartilage damage or penetration of the labrum with instrumentation [8–10].

Once the ability to distract the hip joint has been confirmed, the distracted position is marked and then traction is released. The hip is then prepped and draped and traction reapplied when ready to begin arthroscopy. The surgeon, assistant, and scrub nurse are positioned on the operative side of the patient (Fig. 42.7). The monitor and arthroscopy cart with an attached sterile Mayo stand containing the arthroscope and shaver are positioned on the contralateral side (Fig. 42.5).

Both the 30° and 70° arthroscopes are routinely used to optimize visualization. Interchanging the two scopes allows complete joint visualization despite the limited maneuverability due to the bony and soft tissue constraints of the hip. The 30° scope provides the best view of the superior portion of the acetabular fossa and femoral head, while the 70° scope allows for visualizing the periphery of the joint, the labrum, the capsule, and the inferior acetabular fossa.

A fluid pump is employed in all cases and provides optimal visualization. A high flow system can provide adequate flow without excessive pressures. Adequate flow is essential in order to perform the procedure effectively and in a safe and expedient manner. The surgeon must always be cognizant that the pump is functioning properly. Flow cannot be as precisely modulated with a gravity system, creating difficulties both with visualization and extravasation.

A diagnostic algorithm can then be undertaken in the central portion of the joint [11]. This assures a thorough evaluation of the central compartment to elucidate any present pathology. Once the central compartment diagnostics and treatment are completed, the instrumentation is removed from the central compartment and traction is released. The leg is flexed to approximately 45° and entry into the peripheral compartment is established [4, 5]. There are a variety of techniques that are utilized for entry into the periphery. One technique enters the compartment from the anterolateral portal site. A spinal needle penetrates the capsule on the anterior neck of the femur under fluoroscopic control, and subsequent use of dilators and cannulas allows for establishment of multiple portals in this space, if necessary. For instrumentation, an ancillary portal is placed 5 cm distal to the anterolateral portal. Placement is accomplished with a spinal needle, directly observing through the arthroscope where the needle enters the peripheral compartment [12].

The peripheral compartment can contain a variety of pathological entities that are further detailed in this textbook. It is important in all cases of hip arthroscopy to evaluate the peripheral compartment and treat any pathology encountered [4, 5, 11].

Summary

Surgical arthroscopy of the hip can be a challenging procedure. With the improved instrumentation that has been recently developed, including positioning devices, the procedure has become more predictable. The principles are identi-

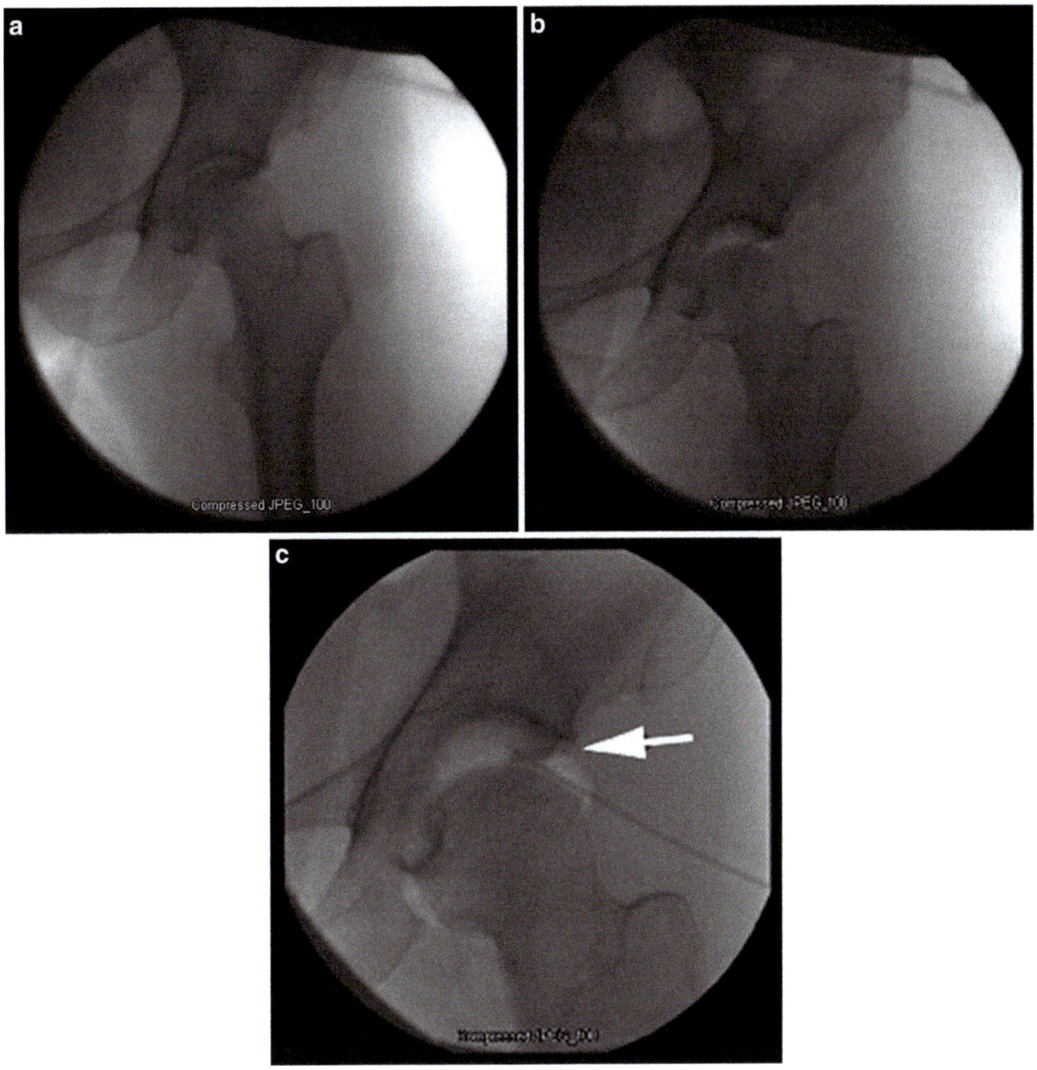

Fig. 42.6 Process for application of traction and assurance of distraction in a left hip. (**a**) AP view prior to the application of any traction. (**b**) Vacuum effect is apparent due to the negative intracapsular pressure created by distraction of the joint. (**c**) A spinal needle is used to position the anterolateral portal. Venting the joint with the needle releases the vacuum effect and creates an air arthrogram that silhouettes the free margin of the lateral labrum (*arrow*)

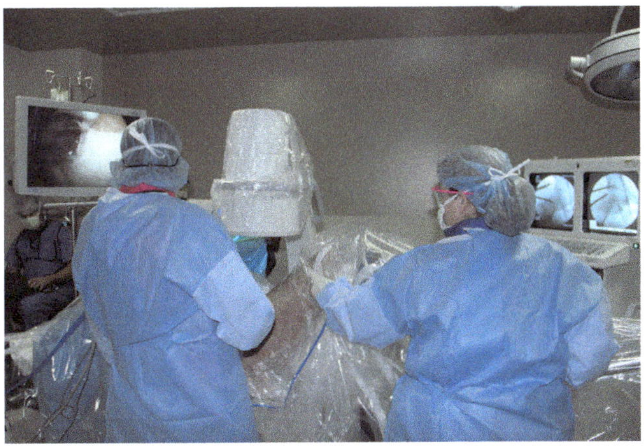

Fig. 42.7 Positioning for entry into the peripheral compartment. The operative area remains covered in sterile drapes while traction is released and the hip flexed to approximately 45°

cal to any other joint arthroscopy and begin with careful positioning. It is paramount to allow access all areas of the joint in both the central and peripheral compartments. The surgical team must be able to easily and reproducibly apply and release traction, as well as reposition the extremity in flexion/extension and internal/external rotation while in the supine position.

References

1. Pollard TC, Khan T, Price AJ, et al. Simulated hip arthroscopy skills: learning curves with the lateral and supine patient positions: a randomized trial. J Bone Joint Surg Am. 2012;94(10):e68.
2. Sampson TG. Complications of hip arthroscopy. Clin Sports Med. 2001;20:831–6.

3. Bartlett CS, DiFelice GS, Buly RL, et al. Cardiac arrest as a result of intraabdominal extravasation of fluid during arthroscopic removal of a loose body from the hip joint of a patient with an acetabular fracture. J Orthop Trauma. 1998;12:294–9.
4. Dienst M, Godde S, Seil R, et al. Hip arthroscopy without traction: in vivo anatomy of the peripheral hip joint cavity. Arthroscopy. 2001;17:924–31.
5. Dienst M. Hip arthroscopy without traction. In: Byrd JWT, editor. Operative hip arthroscopy. 2nd ed. New York: Springer; 2005. p. 170–88.
6. Mouzopoulos G, Vasiliadis G, Lasanianos N, et al. Fascia iliaca block prophylaxis for hip fracture patients at risk for delirium: a randomized placebo-controlled study. J Orthop Traumatol. 2009;10(3):127–33.
7. Byrd JWT, Chern KY. Traction vs distension for distraction of the hip joint during arthroscopy. Arthroscopy. 1997;13:346–9.
8. Byrd JWT. The supine approach. In: Byrd JWT, editor. Operative hip arthroscopy. 2nd ed. New York: Springer; 2005. p. 145–69.
9. Boyle JR, Silva JA, McMillan S. Mechanics of hip arthroscopy. Clin Sports Med. 2011;30(2):285–92.
10. Byrd JWT. Avoiding the labrum in hip arthroscopy. Arthroscopy. 2000;16:770–3.
11. Bond JL, Knutson ZA, Ebert A, et al. The 23-point arthroscopic examination of the hip: basic setup, portal placement, and surgical technique. Arthroscopy. 2009;25:416–29.
12. Byrd JWT. Position and set-up: supine. In: Guanche CA, editor. Hip and pelvic injuries in sports medicine. Philadelphia: Wolters Kluwer; 2009. p. 86–98.

Optimizing Exposure and Accessibility for Arthroscopic Correction of Femoroacetabular Impingement

43

Christopher M. Larson

Introduction

Systematic reviews have supported the role for arthroscopic femoroacetabular impingement (FAI) corrective procedures with outcomes comparable to surgical hip dislocation if performed with appropriate indications [1–4]. Hip arthroscopy's popularity is evolving, and improved techniques and instrumentation have allowed surgeons to access more of the acetabular rim, pelvis, and proximal femur/femoral head–neck junction. Early on, resection of the anterior femoral head–neck junction was demonstrated with resections comparable to open approaches in cadaveric studies [5, 6]. Acetabular rim resection and labral refixation were later described with labral preservation shown to be superior to extensive labral debridement/excision [7–11]. More recently, surgeons have demonstrated the ability to access the majority of the acetabular rim including the posterior rim, as well as AP deformities (posterolateral/posteromedial) at the femoral head–neck junction [12, 13]. In addition, some surgeons have suggested the importance of resection at the distal femoral neck near the intertrochanteric line for patients with mixed impingement/instability patterns, extreme range of motion sports (hockey goalies, dancers), and those with subspine/AIIS impingement [14–17]. The current chapter will discuss technical considerations and PEARLS that can maximize the ability to maximally correct acetabular sided, femoral sided, and subspine/AIIS impingement.

C.M. Larson, MD (✉)
Minnesota Orthopedic Sports Medicine Institute at Twin Cities Orthopedics, 4010 West 65th Street, Edina, MN 55435, USA
e-mail: chrislarson@tcomn.com

The Acetabulum

In the author's experience, the majority of acetabuli require only anterosuperior or no rim resection at all. Acetabular retroversion is a relatively common finding, in particular for males, and does not always result in pincer-type impingement. Peripheral labral bruising and degeneration are findings that may indicate pincer-type impingement. Although global overcoverage (profunda/protrusion) is less common, this entity often requires global rim resection, including a posteriorly based resection, which can be more challenging. Profunda must be managed with experience and typically requires the addition of a posterolateral portal in order to achieve a resection posteroinferiorly. Temporarily increasing the degree of traction and additional posterior capsulotomy helps to access the posteroinferior and anteroinferior rim (Fig. 43.1). In many of these cases, the labrum/rim is ossified and/or severely degenerative and requires labral debridement or resection. Although some authors have recommended a labral reconstruction in this setting, this author reserves labral reconstructions for revision cases with labral deficiency. In some cases overcoverage can be associated with a rim fracture. The current author has previously described management in this setting [18]. If the fragment contributes to impingement but not to stability, the fragment is excised (residual CE angle 20°–25°). If the fragment contributes to both stability and impingement, the fragment is partially excised, fixed with one or two cannulated screws, followed by labral refixation (Fig. 43.2). Often the fragment and native acetabulum have intact articular cartilage at the junction of the two, and the fragment is not formally taken down. A K-wire can be passed across the fibrocartilaginous junction in order to promote ossification. In addition, the labrum is sometimes partially ossified, and the rim is therefore resected without a formal labral takedown in this instance in order to preserve as much labrum as possible for later repair/refixation.

J.C. McCarthy et al. (eds.), *Hip Joint Restoration*, DOI 10.1007/978-1-4614-0694-5_43

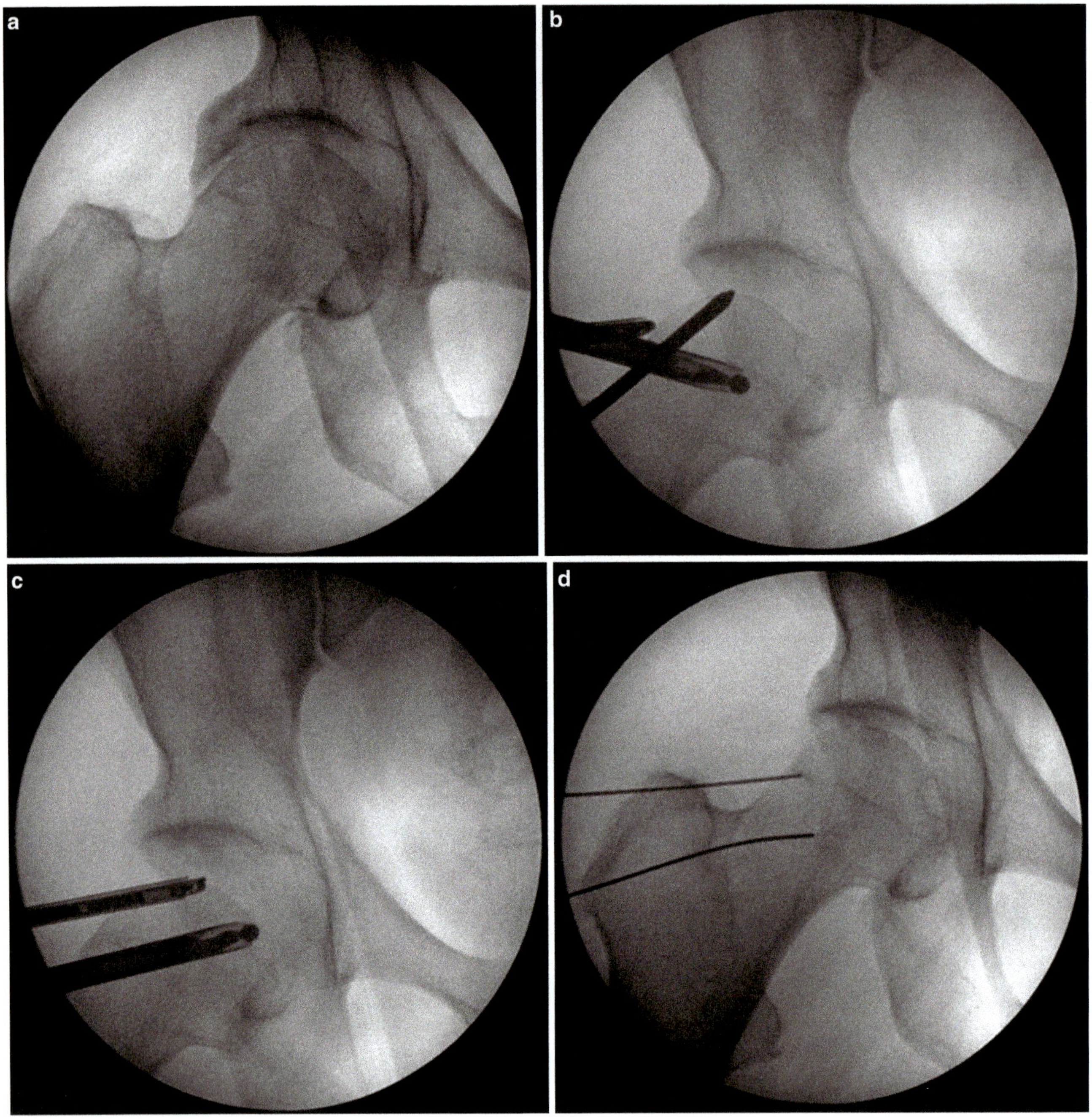

Fig. 43.1 Access to the acetabular rim for global overcoverage. (**a**) Intraoperative fluoroscopic image of the R hip reveals global acetabular overcoverage with labral/rim ossification. (**b**) Additional traction and a posterolateral portal allow access to the posteroinferior acetabular rim. (**c**) Intraoperative fluoroscopic image demonstrating access to the anteroinferior acetabular rim. (**d**) Intraoperative fluoroscopic image after global arthroscopic rim resection

AIIS/Subspine Impingement

The anterior inferior iliac spine (AIIS) can contribute to impingement in some cases and can be the result of a prior apophyseal avulsion, ossification after prior rectus femoris avulsion, overcorrection after periacetabular osteotomy (PAO), or development in etiology and is often seen in the setting of acetabular retroversion [14–17]. In addition, a low AIIS can give the appearance of acetabular retroversion in the setting of an anteverted acetabulum based on a prior study [19]. Straight hip flexion limitations and pain and focal ecchymosis in the region of the AIIS are typically seen in this setting (Fig. 43.3). The AIIS can be located anteriorly between the 1:00 to 1:30 and 2:00 to 2:30 on the clock face for a right hip based on our recent cadaveric

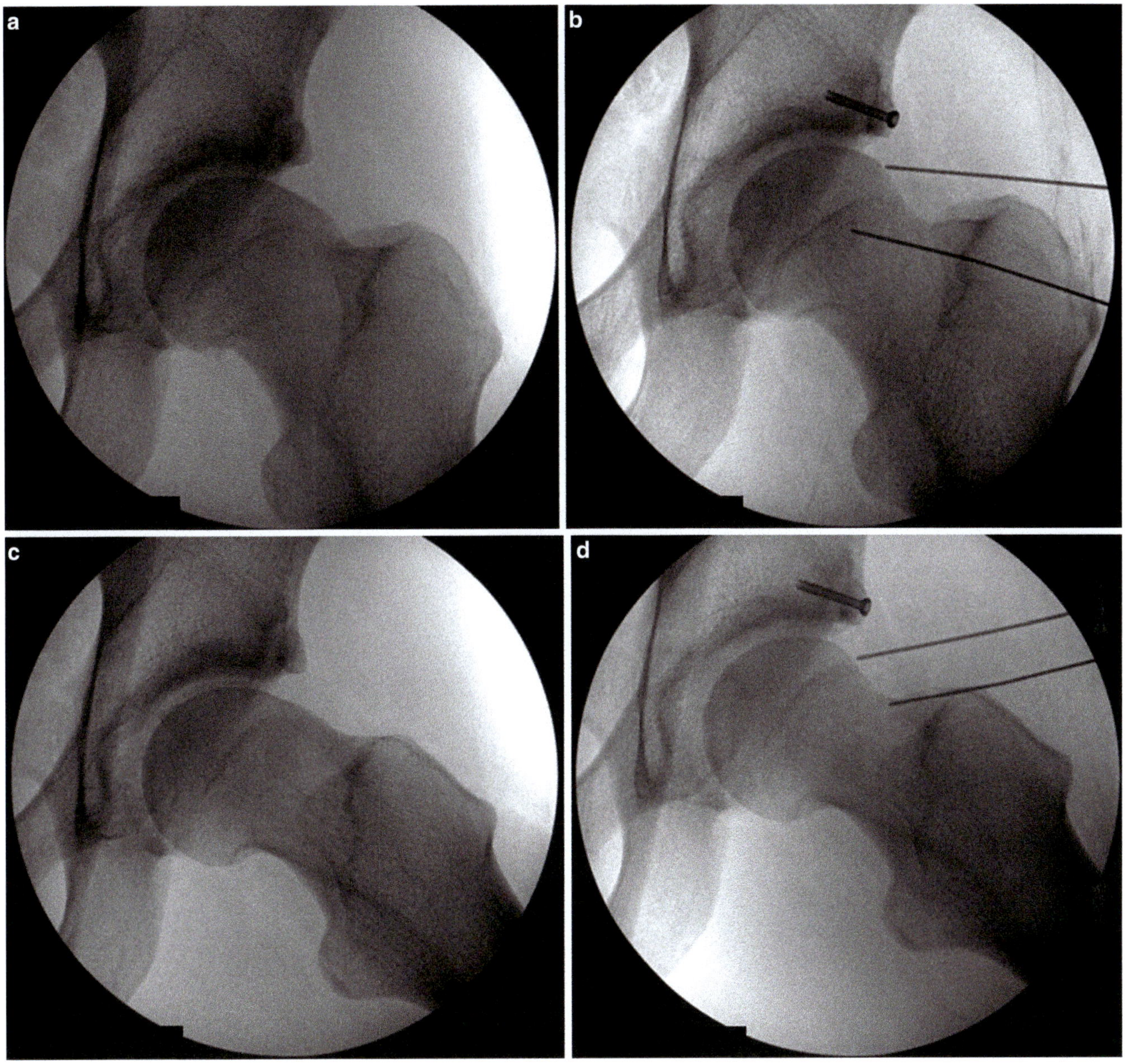

Fig. 43.2 Arthroscopic screw fixation of an acetabular rim fracture. (**a**) Intraoperative anteroposterior fluoroscopic image of the left hip with a rim fracture that contributes to both hip impingement and stability, as well as cam-type morphology (*arrow*). (**b**) Anteroposterior fluoroscopic image after partial rim fracture resection, internal fixation with a cannulated screw, and femoral resection (*arrow*). (**c**) Intraoperative lateral fluoroscopic image reveals cam-type morphology (*arrow*) and a rim fracture. (**d**) Lateral fluoroscopic image after rim fracture fixation and femoral resection (*arrow*)

study [17]. The AIIS can be located by placing the burr on the acetabular rim and localizing it on intraoperative fluoroscopic images. Once located, the capsule can be stripped peripheral to the labrum, and the AIIS resected under direct visualization via the mid-anterior portal. The direct head of the rectus femoris can sometimes limit the proximal extent of resection, and this author occasionally makes a window through the rectus with a beaver blade for further proximal resection, which avoids excessive capsular excision or rectus damage (Fig. 43.3).

The Femur

Management of asphericity of the femoral head–neck junction is one of the most common arthroscopic hip procedures performed. There is significant variability in the morphology of the proximal femur, and therefore different management techniques are required to access these various regions. The current author takes six fluoroscopic images pre- and post-procedure in every case in order to better

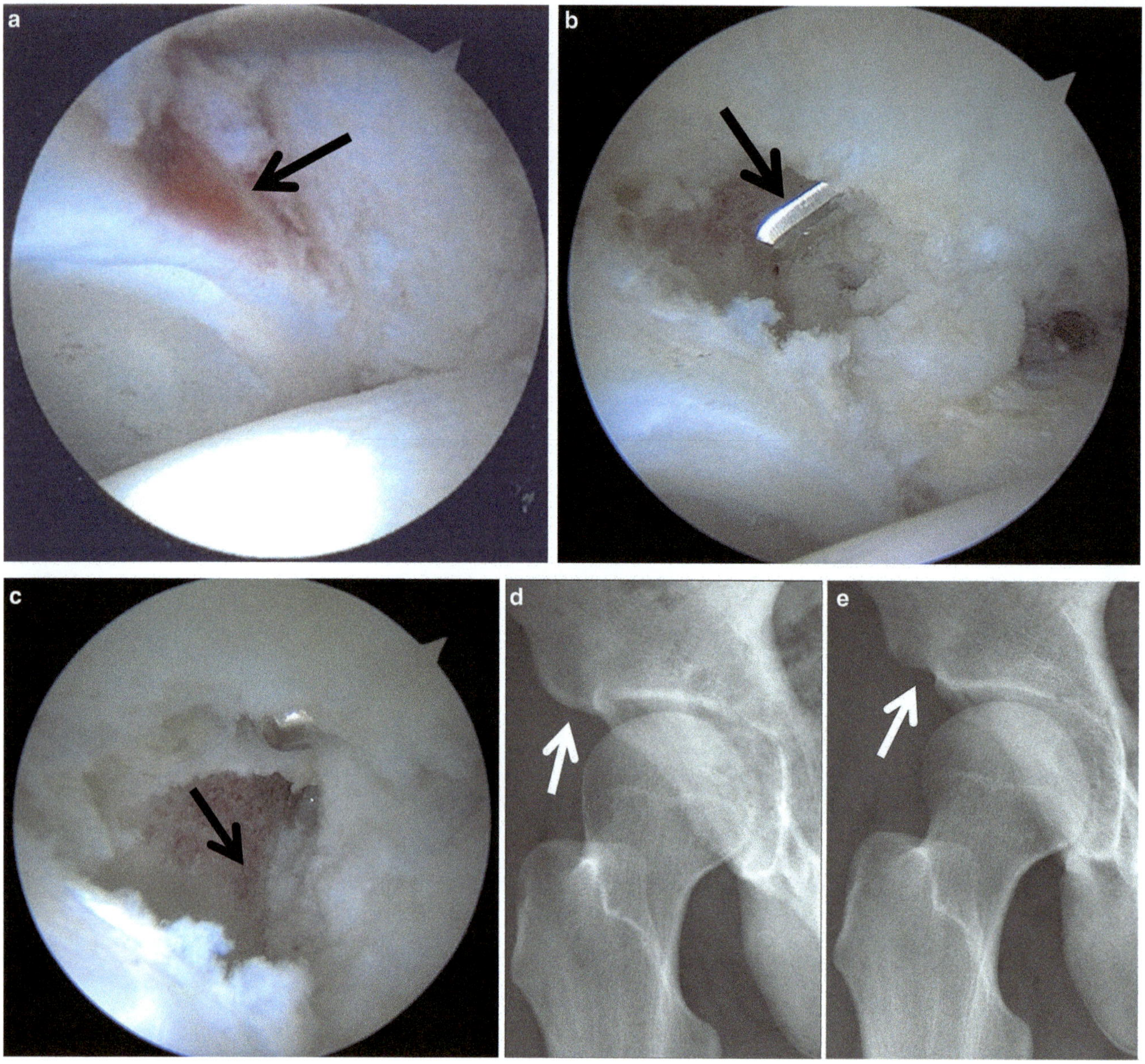

Fig. 43.3 Arthroscopic images of AIIS/subspine impingement/decompression. (**a**) Arthroscopic image of the right hip via the anterolateral portal reveals focal ecchymosis (*arrow*) in the region of the AIIS. (**b**) An arthroscopic knife (*arrow*) is introduced via the mid-anterior portal and used to create a window through the direct head of the rectus and capsule in order to perform more proximal AIIS decompression. (**c**) Arthroscopic image after a burr is used to complete the AIIS/subspine decompression (*arrow*). (**d**) False-profile view of the right hip preoperatively reveals distal and anterior prominence of the AIIS with cortical sclerosis (*arrow*) consistent with AIIS impingement. (**e**) Postoperative false-profile view after AIIS/subspine decompression (*arrow*)

define the head–neck junction and adequacy of resection (Fig. 43.4). Three views are taken in 20–40 degrees of flexion with the hip in neutral, 30° external rotation, and 60° external rotation to better evaluate the anterior and posterior head–neck junction. Three views are taken in full hip extension with the hip in 30° internal rotation, neutral rotation, and 30° external rotation in order to better define the lateral and medial femoral head–neck junction [20, 21]. A recent study performed by the current author comparing these fluoroscopic images with 3D CT scanning showed that the AP (hip extension) external rotation view and lateral (flexion) neutral rotation views best characterized the maximal cam deformity [21]. The anterior head–neck junction can be accessed with a limited capsulotomy, and this region is the most predictably accessed with an arthroscopic approach. Making an interportal capsular cut

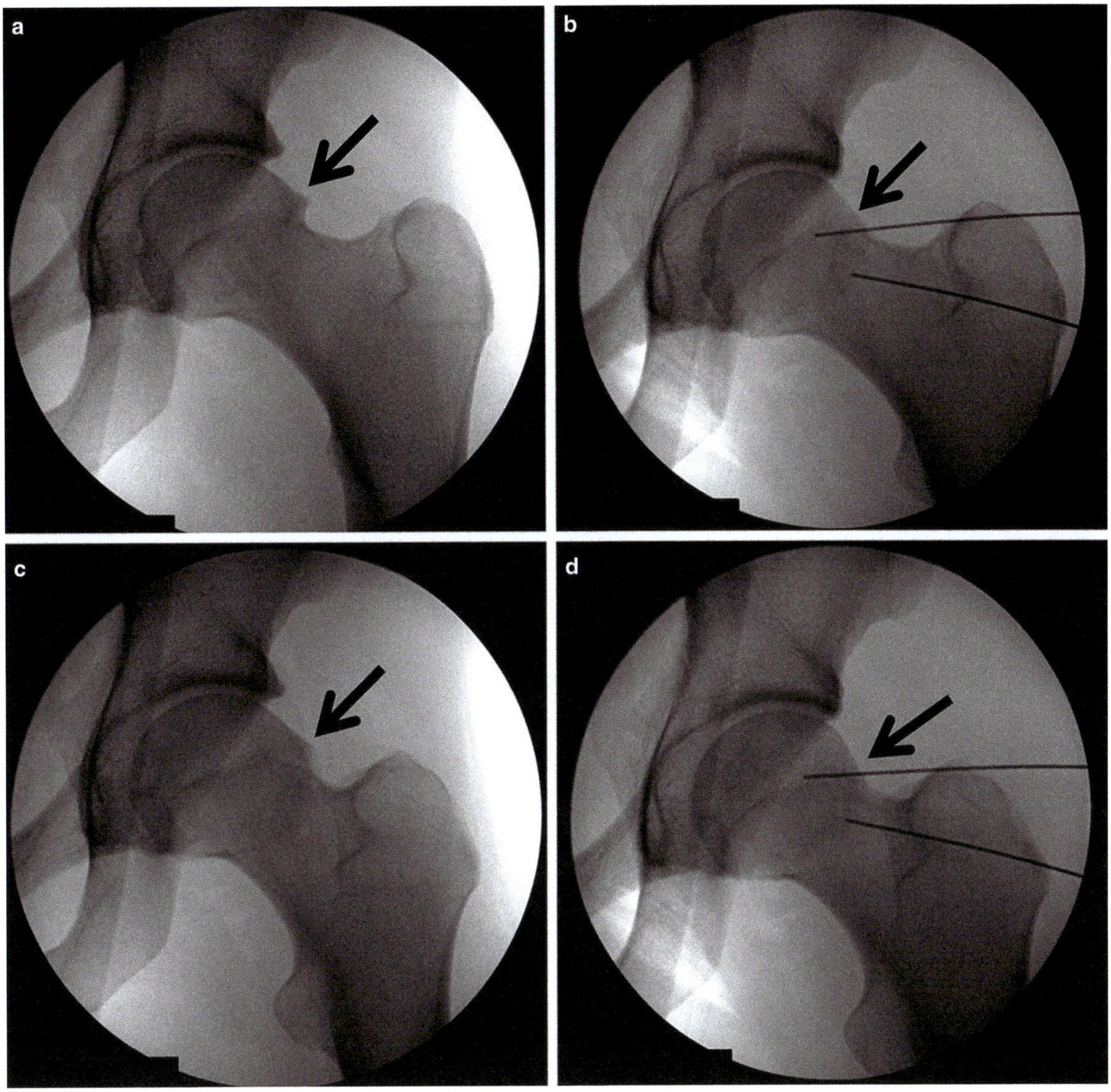

Fig. 43.4 Intraoperative fluoroscopic views used to assess the femoral head–neck junction pre- and post-resection. Anteroposterior (hip extension) views of the femur in 30° internal rotation (**a**, **b**) and neutral rotation (**c**, **d**) evaluate the posterolateral femoral head–neck junction pre-resection (*arrows*) (**a**, **c**) and after femoral resection (*arrows*) and rim resection (**b**, **d**). Lateral (hip flexion) views of the femur in 30° (**e**, **f**) and 60° (**g**, **h**) external rotation evaluate the anterior femoral head–neck junction (*arrows*) pre-resection (**e**, **g**) and after femoral resection and rim resection (**f**, **h**)

from the mid-anterior/anterior portal to the anterolateral/posterolateral portal and placing the hip in 20–40 degrees of flexion gives excellent exposure to the anterior head–neck junction. The current author visualizes the hip with the arthroscope in the mid-anterior portal, while the burr is introduced via the anterolateral portal for the majority of cases. Placing the burr in the anterolateral portal allows for better access to the typical apex of the femoral deformity. The burr can be used to retract the capsule distally to the level of the intertrochanteric line without the addition of a T cut in the current author's experience (Fig. 43.5a–f). The lateral and medial femoral head–neck junctions are best visualized on AP radiographs and are more challenging areas to access (Fig. 43.6). Making an additional cut down the femoral neck (T cut) can help to improve visualization along the posterolateral and posteromedial femoral head–neck junction.

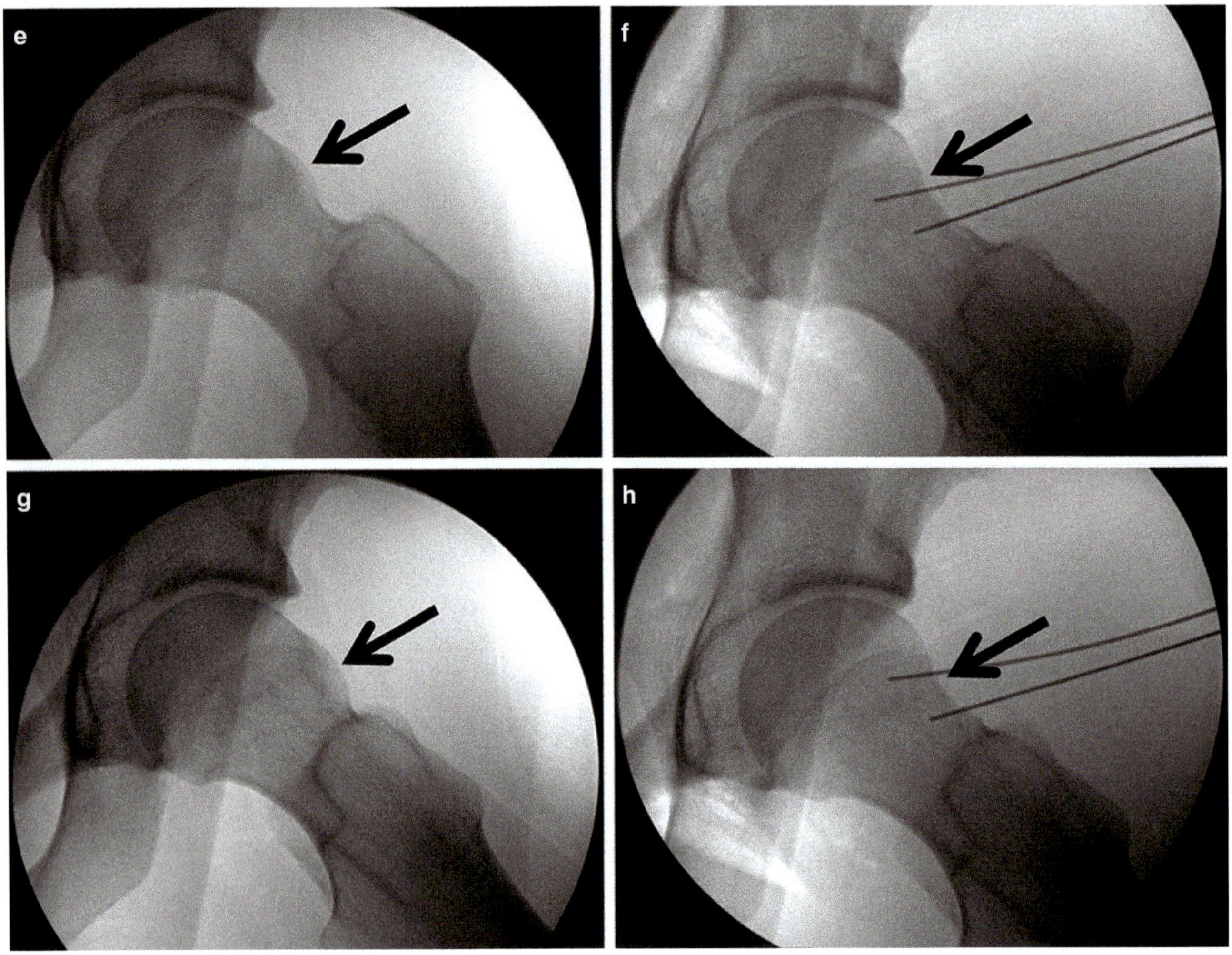

Fig. 43.4 (continued)

The current author, however, does not routinely use this technique and instead relies on varying the position of the leg and sliding the arthroscope under the medial and lateral capsule to access these regions. PEARLS regarding access include greater degrees of flexion/external rotation for accessing the posteromedial femoral head–neck junction and full hip extension/internal rotation with occasional traction applied to access the posterolateral head–neck junction (Fig. 43.5e, f). It is important when working in these regions to only resect/recontour bone proximal to the lateral and medial synovial folds/vessels. Switching the burr to the mid-anterior portal allows for greater access to the medial femoral head–neck junction which may be required when medial deformities are noted on AP radiographs. Although the above techniques allow the surgeon to reach further posteriorly (Fig. 43.5g), posterior femoral head–neck junction deformities seen on the lateral radiograph are not predictably accessed with an arthroscopic approach, and an open surgical approach should be considered in these less common situations. In addition, when large cam deformities are present, it may not be possible to visualize the entire deformity and associated vessels after initially entering the peripheral compartment. These more difficult to access regions, however, can be predictably visualized and accessed after initial femoral resection anteriorly creates more space. Ultimately, a systematic approach for dynamically evaluating the hip should be the primary means of confirming the presence of impingement and verifying appropriate corrections. The current author uses several positions to evaluate the hip arthroscopically, with both direct visualization of impingement and feeling the impingement during range of motion. The anterior head–neck junction and anterior acetabular rim are assessed with 90 degrees of hip flexion and internal rotation. The lateral femur and posterolateral acetabulum are assessed with butterfly testing (abduction of the hip in 20°–40° hip flexion).

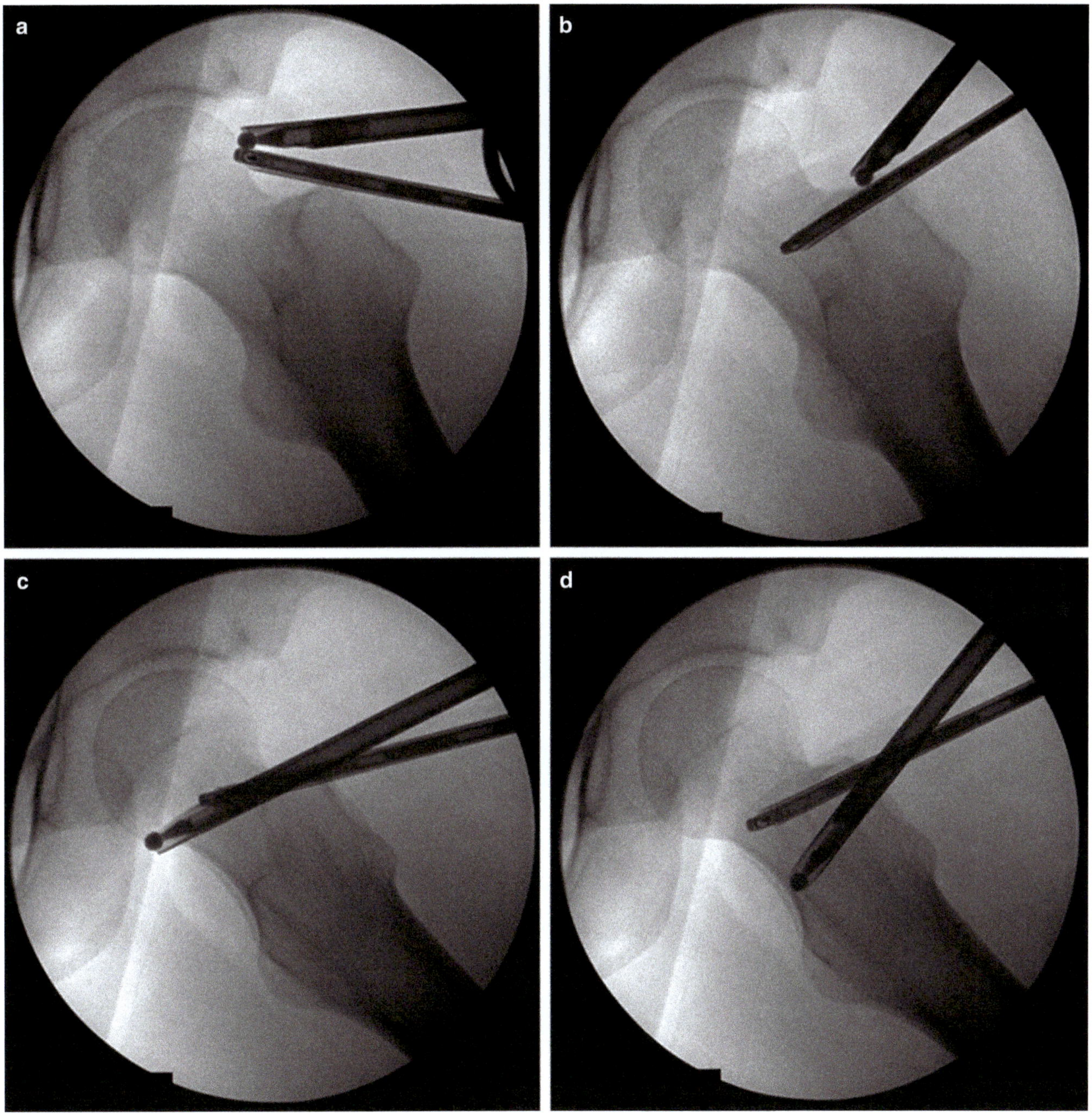

Fig. 43.5 Fluoroscopic images demonstrating access to the femoral head–neck junction. Fluoroscopic images of the left hip after an interportal capsulotomy demonstrate the ability of the burr to access the proximal (**a**) and distal (**b**) anterolateral head–neck junction, the proximal (**c**) and distal (**d**) anteromedial head–neck junction, the proximal (**e**) and distal (**f**) lateral head–neck junction, and the posterolateral (**g**) head–neck junction

The lateral femur and lateral acetabulum are assessed with abduction of the extended hip. In the majority of cases, significant improvements in hip range of motion and radiographic appearance/parameters are appreciated intraoperatively after appropriate resections are completed. The six previously mentioned fluoroscopic views are obtained to evaluate final resections.

Conclusions

There is a significant technical learning curve for arthroscopic FAI corrective surgery. A combination of intraoperative fluoroscopy and dynamic assessment can accurately assess FAI deformities and appropriate corrections. Appropriate use

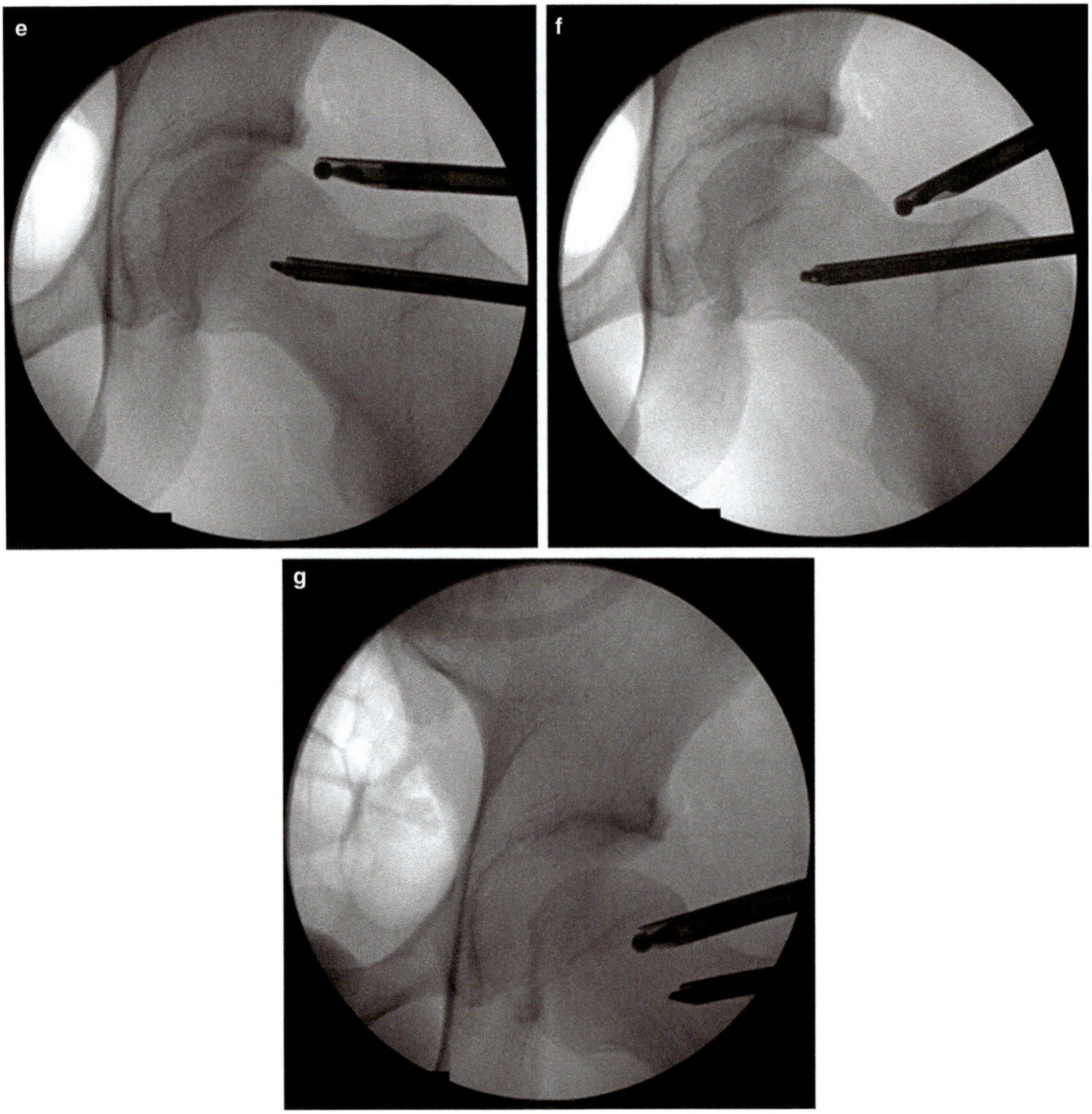

Fig. 43.5 (continued)

of portals, varying the position of the hip, and a systematic approach can allow for correction of the majority of the acetabular rim, as well as the anterior, posterolateral, and posteromedial femoral head–neck junction with experience. Directly posterior femoral deformities are not predictably accessed with an arthroscopic approach, and open surgical approaches should be considered in these situations. Ultimately, the surgical approach chosen to manage these varying patterns of FAI should be based on the surgeon's ability to correct the pathoanatomy present.

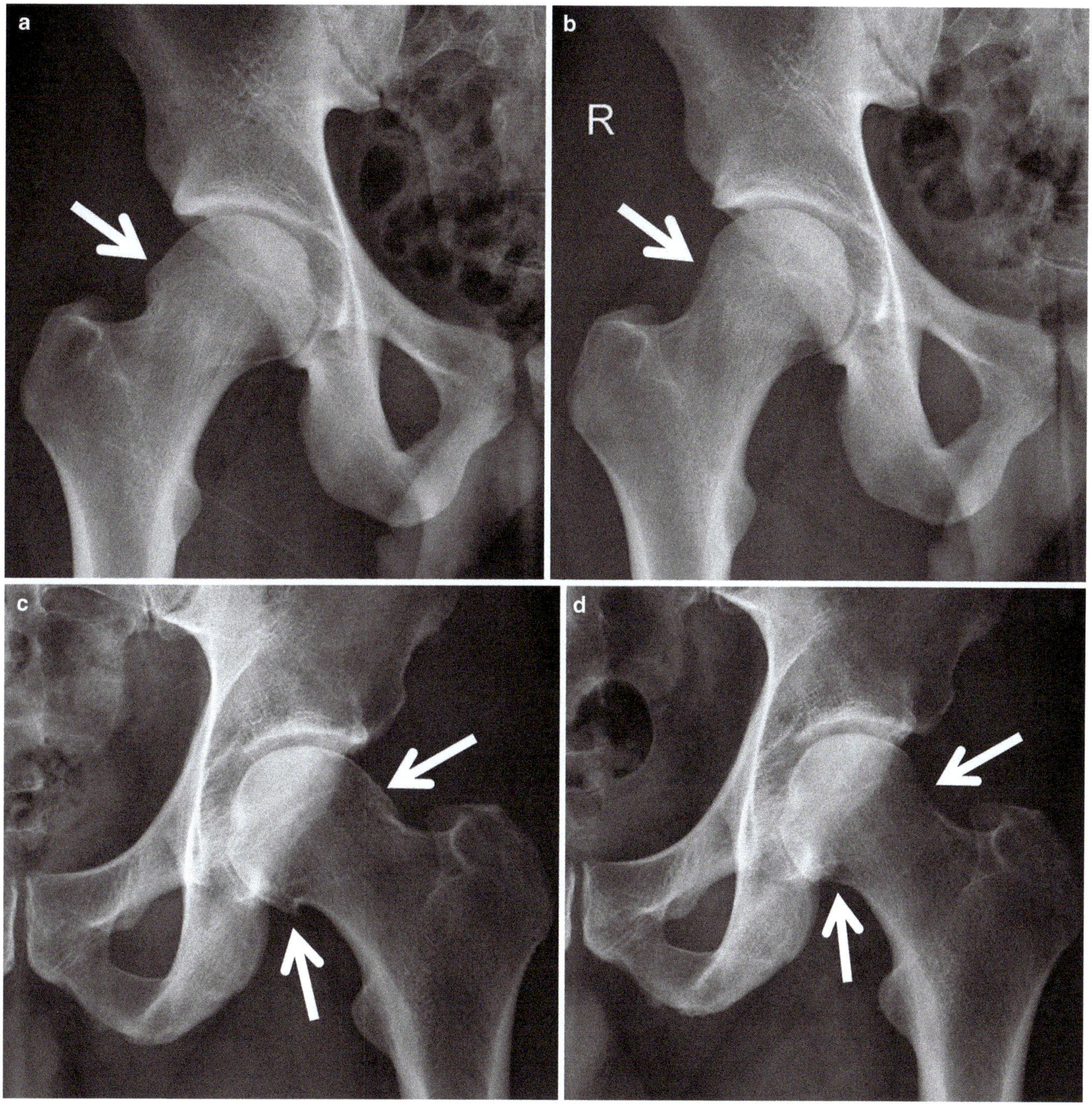

Fig. 43.6 Pre- and postoperative plain radiographs demonstrating the ability to correct the lateral and medial femoral head–neck junction. Anteroposterior plain radiograph of the right hip reveals lateral cam-type deformity (*arrow*) preoperatively (**a**) and improved head–neck offset (**b**) after arthroscopic femoral resection osteoplasty (*arrow*). Anteroposterior plain radiograph of the left hip reveals lateral and medial cam-type deformity (*arrows*) preoperatively (**c**) and improved head–neck offset (**d**) after arthroscopic femoral resection osteoplasty (*arrows*)

References

1. Botser IB, Smith Jr TW, Nasser R, Domb BG. Open surgical dislocation versus arthroscopy for femoroacetabular impingement: a comparison of clinical outcomes. Arthroscopy. 2011;27(2):270–8.
2. Clohisy JC, St John LC, Schutz AL. Surgical treatment of femoroacetabular impingement: a systematic review of the literature. Clin Orthop Relat Res. 2010;468(2):555–64.
3. Matsuda DK, Carlisle JC, Arthurs SC, Wierks CH, Philippon MJ. Comparative systematic review of the open dislocation, mini-open, and arthroscopic surgeries for femoroacetabular impingement. Arthroscopy. 2011;27(2):252–69.
4. Bedi A, Chen N, Robertson W, Kelly BT. The management of labral tears and femoroacetabular impingement of the hip in the young, active patient. Arthroscopy. 2008;24(10):1135–45.
5. Mardones R, Lara J, Donndorf A, et al. Surgical correction of "cam-type" femoroacetabular impingement: a cadaveric compari-

son of open versus arthroscopic debridement. Arthroscopy. 2009;25(2):175–82.
6. Sussman PS, Ranawat AS, Lipman J, Lorich DG, Padgett DE, Kelly BT. Arthroscopic versus open osteoplasty of the head-neck junction: a cadaveric investigation. Arthroscopy. 2007;23: 1257–64.
7. Larson CM, Giveans MR. Arthroscopic debridement versus refixation of the acetabular labrum associated with femoroacetabular impingement. Arthroscopy. 2009;25:369–76.
8. Larson CM, Giveans MR, Stone RM. Arthroscopic debridement versus refixation of the acetabular labrum associated with femoroacetabular impingement: mean 3.5-year follow-up. Am J Sports Med. 2012;40(5):1015–21.
9. Schilders E, Dimitrakopoulou A, Bismil Q, Marchant P, Cooke C. Arthroscopic treatment of labral tears in femoroacetabular impingement: a comparative study of refixation and resection with a minimum two-year follow-up. J Bone Joint Surg Br. 2011;93(8): 1027–32.
10. Philippon MJ, Schenker ML. A new method for acetabular rim trimming and labral repair. Clin Sports Med. 2006;25(2):293–7.
11. Krych AJ, Thompson M, Knutson Z, Scoon J, Coleman SH. Arthroscopic labral repair versus selective labral debridement in female patients with femoroacetabular impingement: a prospective randomized study. Arthroscopy. 2013;29(1):46–53.
12. Matsuda DK. Protrusio acetabuli: contraindication or indication for hip arthroscopy? And the case for arthroscopic treatment of global pincer impingement. Arthroscopy. 2012;28(6):882–8.
13. Matsuda DK, Hanami D. Hip arthroscopy for challenging deformities: posterior cam decompression. Arthrosc Tech. 2013;2(1): e45–9.
14. Hetsroni I, Larson CM, Dela Torre K, et al. Anterior inferior iliac spine deformity as an extra-articular source for hip impingement: a series of 10 patients treated with arthroscopic decompression. Arthroscopy. 2012;28(11):1644–53.
15. Hetsroni I, Poultsides L, Bedi A, Larson CM, Kelly BT. Anterior inferior iliac spine morphology correlates with hip range of motion: a classification system and dynamic model. Clin Orthop Relat Res. 2013;471(8):2497–503.
16. Larson CM, Kelly BT, Stone RM. Making a case for anterior inferior iliac spine/subspine hip impingement: three representative case reports and proposed concept. Arthroscopy. 2011;27(12):1732–7.
17. Hapa O, Bedi A, Gursan O, Akar MS, Guvencer M, Havitcioglu H, Larson CM. Anatomic footprint of the direct head of the rectus femoris origin: cadaveric study and clinical series of hips after arthroscopic AIIS/subspine decompression. Arthroscopy. 2013; 29(12):1932–40.
18. Larson CM, Stone RM. The rarely encountered rim fracture that contributes to both femoroacetabular impingement and hip stability: a report of 2 cases of arthroscopic partial excision and internal fixation. Arthroscopy. 2011;27(7):1018–22.
19. Zaltz I, Kelly BT, Hetsroni I, Bedi A. The crossover sign overestimates acetabular retroversion. Clin Orthop Relat Res. 2013; 471(8):2463–70.
20. Larson CM, Wulf CA. Intraoperative fluoroscopy for evaluation of bony resection during arthroscopic management of femoroacetabular impingement in the supine position. Arthroscopy. 2009;25:1183–92.
21. Ross JR, Bedi A, Stone RM, Sibilsky Enselman E, Leunig M, Kelly BT, Larson CM. Intraoperative fluoroscopic imaging to treat cam deformities: correlation with 3D computed tomography. Am J Sports Med. 2014;42(6):1370–6.

44 Anesthesia and Analgesia for Hip Surgery

Sunit Ghosh, Amo Oduro, and Stephen Webb

Although outcome following orthopedic surgery is determined primarily by the patient's preoperative state and comorbidities rather than by the choice of individual anesthetic agents used, anesthetists can influence outcome by detailed preoperative assessment and attention to optimization of the patient. Intraoperatively, regional or local anesthetic techniques, either as an adjunct to or as an alternative to general anesthesia, may have beneficial effects on recovery. However, the risks and benefits of regional anesthetic techniques for individual patients must always be considered in the context of medical history, medications, and patient choice.

Certain issues have been identified as being critical to improving outcomes; these include minimizing blood loss and consequent transfusion, intraoperative management of fluid balance, maintenance of body temperature, and prevention of deep venous thrombosis (DVT). These issues are discussed further below.

While planning the perioperative management of open procedures, such as arthroplasty, the surgical and anesthetic team should give consideration to techniques that minimize the need for blood transfusion [1–4], for example, by arranging autologous blood collection prior to surgery [5], using cell salvage intra- and postoperatively [5, 6], and utilizing anti-fibrinolytics in complex cases [7]. In patients who do not have a history of significant cardiovascular or cerebrovascular disease, judicious use of a hypotensive anesthetic technique improves visualization of the surgical field and reduces blood loss [8].

Intraoperatively, there is evidence to suggest that prevention of hypothermia [9, 10] and control of fluid balance using a goal-directed fluid therapy protocol may reduce the incidence of complications and enhance recovery. In the United Kingdom, the National Institute for Health and Care Excellence (NICE) has recommended considering the use of noninvasive cardiac output monitoring devices, for example, the esophageal Doppler monitor, to optimize fluid therapy during all major surgery [11].

In the perioperative period, prevention of DVT is a critical issue, and a variety of pharmacological measures are employed. No single technique has yet to be established as clearly superior. The key to successful reduction in the incidence of DVT is having clear guidelines in place for the choice of agent, timing, and duration of administration, coupled with a program for early mobilization [12, 13].

Postoperatively, it is helpful to have guidelines in place for pain management and the treatment of postoperative nausea and vomiting. In general "multimodal analgesia," the combination of analgesics from different pharmacological groups, tends to provide the most consistent method of pain relief [14]. Commonly, a rapid progression from intravenous boluses of narcotic delivered using a patient-controlled analgesia infusion pump (PCA) to oral opioids, nonsteroidal anti-inflammatory drugs (NSAIDs), and simple analgesics such as paracetamol provides a route to mobilization without the adverse consequences of prolonged narcotic analgesia or the encumbrance of infusion pumps. In some centers, the use of epidural analgesia by infusion of local anesthetic solutions or mixtures of local anesthetic and opiates is routine practice for major hip surgery. Best practice requires a higher level of nursing observation and monitoring for patients with epidural infusions than for those without epidurals, and this increases the burden on healthcare systems without necessarily improving outcome. Undoubtedly, certain subgroups of patients, such as those with debilitating respiratory disease, benefit from the use of epidural analgesia extended into the postoperative period. Perhaps the use of such techniques is best reserved for those whose recovery would be compromised by the use of systemic opiates [15].

Current recommendations [16] for the management of postoperative nausea and vomiting include prophylactic administration of antiemetics such as ondansetron. Repeat

S. Ghosh, BSc, MBBS, FRCA, FFICM (✉) • A. Oduro, MBBS, FRCA, FRCP • S. Webb, MBBCh, FRCA, FFICM
Anaesthesia and Intensive Care, Papworth Hospital, Papworth, Cambridge CB23 3RE, UK
e-mail: ghoshs@btinternet.com; stephen.webb@papworth.nhs.uk

J.C. McCarthy et al. (eds.), *Hip Joint Restoration*, DOI 10.1007/978-1-4614-0694-5_44

doses may be given as required during recovery in conjunction with an alternative agent such as cyclizine if necessary. The routine use of steroids, such as dexamethasone, to counteract nausea remains of unproven benefit but may be of value in those patients with a known history of postoperative nausea.

In relation to the diagnosis and treatment of hip disorders, the four commonest procedures encountered in anesthetic practice are (1) manipulation under anesthesia (MUA), sometimes combined with intra-articular injection of local anesthetic and steroids; (2) arthroscopy, (3) total hip replacement (THR); and (4) fixation of femoral neck fractures.

Manipulation Under Anesthetic/Intra-articular Injection

MUA of the hip, often in combination with intra-articular injection of steroids and/or local anesthetic, is sometimes performed under general anesthesia to facilitate mobilization of the joint and for patient comfort. As the procedure is of relatively short duration (usually about 10–20 min depending on whether radiographic imaging is required) and with minimal post-procedural discomfort, either no narcotic or a minimal dose of narcotic is required. Induction of anesthesia with propofol, maintenance with an inhalational agent, and airway control with a laryngeal mask (LMA) are usually satisfactory. Anesthesia should be targeted at having the patient in a safely ambulatory state for discharge from the hospital soon after the procedure. In some centers, sedation with a benzodiazepine or low-dose propofol infusion is routinely used as an alternative to general anesthesia.

Hip Arthroscopy

Since the 1990s hip arthroscopy has evolved from being primarily a diagnostic procedure to being a therapeutic entity in its own right. This is a result of increasing expertise in accessing the joint cavity, development of endoscopic equipment, and wider acceptance of the surgical indications. Debridement of articular surfaces, repair of cartilage, and excision of soft tissue and bone to treat femoro-acetabular impingement are now all routinely performed arthroscopically.

There is little published material relating to anesthesia for hip arthroscopy; our own experience with the procedure extends over 20 years and includes over 4000 cases. The operation is best performed under general anesthesia, as considerable traction is applied to ensure ease of access to the joint cavity. This places mechanical stress not only on the lower limb but also the spine. General anesthesia, with the use of muscle relaxant agents, reduces the force required to distract the joint and thus reduces the stresses applied to the limb and spine. Our practice is to induce anesthesia with propofol (2 mg/kg) and fentanyl (1–2 μg/kg), secure the airway with an LMA, and maintain anesthesia with sevoflurane or desflurane. As bradycardia sometimes accompanies application of traction, use of a low dose of anticholinergic agent, either atropine 0.3 mg or glycopyrrolate 0.2 mg with additional doses given if required, is advisable. Morphine (2–2.5 mg/kg) or Diamorphine (0.5–1 mg/kg) is administered in divided increments intravenously during the procedure, and intravenous paracetamol (15 mg/kg) and an NSAID, e.g., parecoxib (40 mg) or diclofenac (50 mg), are routinely given for analgesia. The antiemetic ondansetron (4 mg) is administered prophylactically.

It is essential to ensure that the airway is satisfactorily secured with respiration clearly maintainable and that well-functioning venous access has been established before the procedure commences. Once surgical preparation and draping is completed, and with traction applied, there is limited facility for the anesthetist to manipulate the airway or gain venous access.

The procedure is conducted with the patient either supine or in the lateral position and with the operative limb placed securely in a traction boot linked to a traction frame. A fluoroscopic "C arm" is positioned around the hip with images acquired prior to and following distraction of the joint. Once the operative field has been prepared, the entire patient is covered in surgical drapes, and we have found that using a transparent, impermeable plastic drape permits visualization of the patient during the procedure.

Maintenance of body temperature using an active warming mattress or blanket is recommended, as several liters of intra-articular irrigation fluid are used during the arthroscopy.

We have found that reduction of intra-articular hemorrhage, particularly in those procedures requiring synovial tissue resection, with consequent improvement of the visual field, can be achieved by adding Adrenaline to the irrigation fluid. Our practice is to add 1 mg Adrenaline per 4 L bag of irrigant.

It should be emphasized that constant awareness of the vital signs is requisite especially for those bony resection procedures requiring a large capsulotomy. Egress of irrigating fluid from the joint can produce a large retroperitoneal collection, resulting in hypotension and patient morbidity.

The most physiologically stimulating points of the procedure, which usually takes in the region of 60–90 min including time for positioning and imaging, are not only the insertion of the arthroscope at the start of the procedure but also debridement of the peripheral compartment during the later part of the operation. Our practice has been to administer a bolus of narcotic to deepen anesthesia if, and when, the peripheral compartment is accessed.

At the end of the surgical procedure, the surgeon injects chirocaine or bupivacaine (10–20 mL of 0.5 %) periarticularly and subcutaneously at the arthroscopic portal sites to reduce postoperative pain. Until relatively recently, local anesthetic was instilled within the joint cavity, but this has been discon-

Summary of a Consensus Document Produced by Expert Members of a Working Party on the Management of Proximal Femoral Fractures Established by the Association of Anesthetists of Great Britain and Ireland (AAGBI) [1].

- There should be protocol-driven, fast-track admission of patients with hip fractures through the emergency department.
- Patients with hip fractures require multidisciplinary care, led by orthogeriatricians.
- Surgery is the best analgesic for hip fractures.
- Surgical repair of hip fractures should occur within 48 h of hospital admission.
- Surgery and anesthesia must be undertaken by appropriately experienced surgeons and anesthetists.
- There must be high-quality communication between clinicians and allied health professionals.
- Early mobilization is a key part of the management of patients with hip fractures.
- Preoperative management should include consideration of planning for discharge from hospital.
- Measures should be taken to prevent secondary falls.
- Continuous audit and targeted research is required in order to inform and improve the management of patients with hip fracture.

tinued in the light of evidence of potential articular chondrolysis caused by this practice.

In some centers anesthetists combine general anesthesia with a regional anesthetic technique for hip arthroscopy. Regional techniques suitable for the procedure include intrathecal, epidural, or lumbar plexus block. Use of such techniques may, however, prevent same-day discharge from the hospital because of residual motor deficit. Local anesthetic blockade of the lateral cutaneous nerve of the thigh to reduce postoperative discomfort is currently being investigated.

Postoperatively, Toradol and/or incremental doses of morphine (1 mg) may be given intravenously as required, but the majority of patients find a combination of oral analgesics such as paracetamol, NSAIDs, and tramadol satisfactory.

Hip Fracture Surgery

Patients with hip fractures present significant challenges for anesthetists, as they tend to be elderly and frail, often with limited mobility, cognitive impairment, and multiple comorbidities. Urgent surgery allows early rehabilitation and is a key factor in improving outcome together with multidisciplinary collaboration from the time of admission until discharge. A number of organizations have recently produced guidelines for the management of the hip fracture patient [17–20]. A priority for this patient group is the organization of services to create a comprehensive hip fracture program incorporating fast-track hospital admission, urgent access to the operating room, adequate analgesia, surgery and anesthesia delivered by experienced personnel, preoperative and postoperative orthogeriatric management, and early rehabilitation.

Prior to fracture surgery, acute pain should be adequately controlled. Pain scoring systems are recommended to clearly assess pain at rest and on movement and to guide the provision of analgesia [21]. Preoperative peripheral nerve blocks (femoral nerve block and fascia iliaca block) provide effective pain relief after hip fracture [22, 23] and should be considered if pain is not well controlled with paracetamol, NSAIDs, and opioids.

Preoperative assessment involves multidisciplinary input from orthogeriatricians, anesthetists, surgeons, nurses, and physiotherapists. Early orthogeriatric input into the management of patients with hip fracture is advisable to rapidly optimize fitness for surgery. Surgery should be performed within 48 h of admission [18]. Postponing surgery to permit extensive preoperative investigations and protracted preoperative physiological stabilization does not appear to improve outcome. Treatment for acute medical disorders should be initiated rapidly and without delaying surgery. Preoperative assessment by the anesthetist allows recognition of comorbidities, planning of anesthetic technique, and estimation of perioperative risk. The Nottingham Hip Fracture Score has recently been developed to predict postoperative mortality according to age, male gender, anemia, cognitive impairment, malignancy, number of comorbidities, and place of residence [24].

Fat embolism syndrome, causing respiratory and cognitive dysfunction, is not uncommon and may manifest acutely or progressively at any point in the perioperative period.

Either general anesthesia or regional anesthesia is acceptable for hip fracture surgery. There is no strong evidence that one method is better than the other in terms of outcome, and hence the decision should be based on patient preference and anesthetist's expertise [25, 26]. Central neuraxial (spinal or epidural) anesthesia is necessary for hip surgery if a regional anesthetic technique alone is used.

Spinal (subarachnoid/intrathecal) anesthesia is commonly employed for hip fracture surgery. The use of lower doses of bupivacaine (e.g., 2–3 mL 0.5%) and the use of hyperbaric bupivacaine may reduce the hypotension associated with spi-

PROSPECT Summary Recommendations 2011 for Pain Management for Total Hip Arthroplasty [15]

Recommended preoperative interventions:

- COX-2-selective inhibitors in time to provide sufficient analgesia when the patient wakes

Recommended postoperative interventions:

- COX-2-selective inhibitors or conventional NSAIDs in combination with paracetamol and/or strong opioids for high-intensity pain or with paracetamol and/or weak opioids for moderate or low-intensity pain
- Strong opioids in combination with non-opioid analgesia to manage high-intensity pain, in time to provide analgesia in the early postoperative recovery period, administered by IV patient-controlled analgesia or IV titrated for pain intensity
- Weak opioids for moderate or low-intensity pain if conventional NSAIDs or COX-2-selective inhibitors are insufficient or are contraindicated
- Paracetamol in combination with conventional NSAIDs or COX-2-selective inhibitors, with or without rescue opioids
- Epidural infusion with local anesthetic plus opioid for cardiopulmonary risk patients, in time to provide analgesia in the early postoperative recovery period
- Posterior lumbar plexus block or femoral nerve block or single-bolus spinal morphine as a part of spinal anesthesia, depending on the balance of efficacy and risks for the individual patient
- Intraoperative high-volume, low-concentration wound infiltration (local infiltration analgesia)

nal anesthesia. The use of spinal opioids as an adjunct to spinal local anesthetics prolongs postoperative analgesia. Epidural anesthesia (including combined spinal-epidural anesthesia) may hinder postoperative mobilization and is less commonly used. Sedation may be used along with regional anesthesia to enhance patient comfort during the procedure, particularly as this procedure is performed on a traction table with the operative limb in traction. Intraoperative peripheral nerve blocks, which provide prolonged analgesia postoperatively, should be considered as an adjunct to general or spinal anesthesia. Posterior lumbar plexus block (psoas compartment block) provides blockade of the femoral nerve, obturator nerve, and lateral cutaneous nerve of the thigh, but is associated with the risks of deep hematoma and inadvertent neuraxial block. Femoral nerve block and fascia iliaca block do not reliably block all three nerves, but require less expertise than posterior lumbar plexus block. Local infiltration analgesia using high-volume, low-concentration injection of local anesthetic may be of value for hip fracture surgery, but has not been well evaluated in this context.

Hip Arthroplasty

Hip arthroplasty is associated with significant postoperative pain, and the choice of anesthetic and analgesic techniques may influence postoperative mobilization and hospital length of stay. The recent focus on enhancing recovery and reducing length of stay after surgery has led to increasing interest in optimizing perioperative analgesia [27]. Enabling fast-track hip arthroplasty recovery involves early mobilization, attention to fluid management, nutritional support, and prevention of nausea and constipation. The use of multimodal opioid-sparing techniques combining systemic analgesia and regional anesthesia is recommended to allow rapid postoperative recovery [28, 29]. PROSPECT (procedure-specific postoperative pain management) has recently updated its evidence-based guidelines for hip arthroplasty [30].

Patients undergoing hip arthroplasty are often elderly and may have significant comorbidities. In contrast to hip fracture surgery, hip arthroplasty is performed as an elective procedure, and time is available to fully optimize the patient's general medical condition before surgery. Information about postoperative pain relief and the importance of active participation in early mobilization and physiotherapy should be given preoperatively.

One notable aspect of hip arthroplasty is the adverse physiological effect of bone cement used to secure certain types of prostheses. Release of methyl methacrylate from the cement into the bloodstream may lead to varying degrees of cardiovascular and respiratory compromise. If a cemented prosthesis is used, the anesthetist needs to be particularly vigilant to note and treat changes in blood pressure, heart rate, and oxygen saturation immediately following bone cement implantation [31].

No specific intraoperative anesthetic technique can be recommended as being superior, and the choice should be based on the patient's and anesthetist's choice. While either general anesthesia or central neuraxial anesthesia (with or without sedation) is satisfactory, general anesthesia alone is not recommended and should be supplemented by some form of regional analgesia initiated intraoperatively to enhance postoperative pain relief.

Spinal anesthesia with local anesthetic and opioid is a commonly used technique for hip arthroplasty. Spinal long-acting opioids (e.g., morphine) are preferred to short-acting opioids (e.g., fentanyl) to provide prolonged postoperative analgesia, but may be associated with late respiratory depression, nausea, vomiting, and urinary retention. Spinal clonidine and continuous spinal anesthesia are not recommended because of their cardiovascular side effects.

Continuous epidural analgesia with local anesthetic and opioid may be considered for patients at high risk of postoperative cardiac and respiratory complications. Epidural clonidine, magnesium, and extended-release morphine are not recommended because of cardiovascular and respiratory side effects [32].

Posterior lumbar plexus block or femoral nerve block may be used to supplement general anesthesia or spinal anesthesia for hip arthroplasty. Posterior lumbar plexus block provides more effective analgesia than femoral nerve block, but may be associated with major complications involving epidural or intrathecal spread or deep hematoma formation in a small number of cases. Alternatively, a femoral nerve block with high volume of a local anesthetic solution, termed the "3 in 1" block, may be used to block the obturator nerve and the lateral cutaneous nerve of the thigh in addition to the femoral nerve. Continuous regional analgesia may be established using local anesthetic infusion via an indwelling catheter placed in, or close to, the neural sheath. Peripheral nerve blocks can cause prolonged motor block which may delay mobilization.

Local infiltration analgesia using high-volume, low-concentration local anesthetic is emerging as a potentially beneficial technique in hip arthroplasty. Intraoperative periarticular local infiltration analgesia may improve postoperative pain relief, but more convincing evidence is required. Continuous wound local infiltration analgesia does not appear to be beneficial [33].

Conclusion

Anesthesia techniques for current hip procedures continue to evolve. Over the past decade the use of preemptive multimodal analgesic medications has dramatically improved perioperative patient comfort, reduced complications, and facilitated more rapid recovery. For hip surgery the combination of a comprehensive preoperative medical evaluation and intraoperative close communication between the anesthetist and surgeon remarkably improves patient safety and outcome.

References

1. Moonen AF, Neal TD, Pilot P. Peri-operative blood management in elective orthopaedic surgery. A critical review of the literature. Injury. 2006;37 Suppl 5:S11–6.
2. Tenholder M, Cushner FD. Intraoperative blood management in joint replacement surgery. Orthopedics. 2004;27(6 Suppl):s663–8.
3. Sculco TP. Minimally invasive total hip arthroplasty: in the affirmative. J Arthroplasty. 2004;19(4 Suppl 1):78–80.
4. Muñoz M, García-Erce JA, Villar I, Thomas D. Blood conservation strategies in major orthopaedic surgery: efficacy, safety and European regulations. Vox Sang. 2009;96(1):1–13.
5. Keating EM, Meding JB. Perioperative blood management practices in elective orthopaedic surgery. J Am Acad Orthop Surg. 2002;10(6):393–400.
6. Ashworth A, Klein AA. Cell salvage as part of a blood conservation strategy in anesthesia. Br J Anaesth. 2010;105(4):401–16.
7. Ker K, Edwards P, Perel P, Shakur H, Roberts I. Effect of tranexamic acid on surgical bleeding: systematic review and cumulative meta-analysis. BMJ. 2012;344:e3054.
8. Sharrock NE, Salvati EA. Hypotensive epidural anesthesia for total hip arthroplasty: a review. Acta Orthop Scand. 1996;67(1):91–107.
9. Moola S, Lockwood C. Effectiveness of strategies for the management and/or prevention of hypothermia within the adult perioperative environment. Int J Evid Based Healthc. 2011;9(4):337–45.
10. Scott EM, Buckland R. A systematic review of intraoperative warming to prevent postoperative complications. AORN J. 2006;83(5):1090–104. 1107–13.
11. Ghosh S, Arthur B, Klein AA. NICE guidance on CardioQ(TM) oesophageal Doppler monitoring. Anesthesia. 2011;66(12):1081–3.
12. Falck-Ytter Y, Francis CW, Johanson NA, Curley C, Dahl OE, Schulman S, Ortel TL, Pauker SG, Colwell Jr CW. Prevention of VTE in orthopedic surgery patients: antithrombotic therapy and prevention of thrombosis, 9th ed: American College of Chest Physicians Evidence-Based Clinical Practice Guidelines. Chest. 2012;141(2 Suppl):e278S–325.
13. Kakkos SK, Warwick D, Nicolaides AN, Stansby GP, Tsolakis IA. Combined (mechanical and pharmacological) modalities for the prevention of venous thromboembolism in joint replacement surgery. J Bone Joint Surg Br. 2012;94(6):729–34.
14. Savoia G, Alampi D, Amantea B, et al. Postoperative pain treatment SIAARTI Recommendations 2010. Minerva Anestesiol. 2010;76(8):657–67.
15. Rawal N. Epidural technique for postoperative pain: gold standard no more? Reg Anesth Pain Med. 2012;37(3):310–7.
16. Fero KE, Jalota L, Hornuss C, Apfel CC. Pharmacologic management of postoperative nausea and vomiting. Expert Opin Pharmacother. 2011;12(15):2283–96.
17. Membership of the Working Party, Griffiths R, Alper J, Beckingsale A, Goldhill D, Heyburn G, Holloway J, Leaper E, Parker M, Ridgway S, White S, Wiese M, Wilson I. Management of proximal femoral fractures 2011. Anesthesia. 2012;67:85–98.
18. Scottish Intercollegiate Guidelines Network. Management of hip fracture in older people. National Clinical Guideline 111. 2009.
19. British Orthopaedic Association and British Geriatrics Society. The care of patients with fragility fracture. 2007.
20. The National Institute for Health and Clinical Excellence. Clinical Guideline 124. The management of hip fracture in adults. 2011.
21. Royal College of Physicians, British Geriatrics Society, The British Pain Society. The assessment of pain in older people. 2007.
22. Cuvillon P, Ripart J, Debureaux S, et al. Analgesia after hip fracture repair in elderly patients: the effect of a continuous femoral nerve block: a prospective and randomised study. Ann Fr Anesth Reanim. 2007;26:2–9.
23. Parker MJ, Griffiths R, Appadu BN. Nerve blocks (subcostal, lateral cutaneous, femoral, triple, psoas) for hip fractures. Cochrane Database Syst Rev. 2002;1:CD001159.
24. Maxwell MJ, Moran CG, Moppett IK. Development and validation of a preoperative scoring system to predict 30 day mortality in patients undergoing hip fracture surgery. Br J Anaesth. 2008;101:511–7.
25. Parker MJ, Handoll HHG, Griffiths R. Anesthesia for hip fracture surgery in adults. Cochrane Database Syst Rev. 2004;18:CD000521.

26. Luger TJ, Kammerlander C, Gosch M, et al. Neuraxial versus general anesthesia in geriatric patients for hip fracture surgery: does it matter. Osteoporos Int. 2010;21:S555–72.
27. Kehlet H, Wilmore DW. Evidence-based surgical care and the evolution of fast-track surgery. Ann Surg. 2008;248:189–98.
28. Hebl JR, Dilger JA, Byer DE, et al. A pre-emptive multimodal pathway featuring peripheral nerve block improves perioperative outcomes after major orthopedic surgery. Reg Anesth Pain Med. 2008;33:510–7.
29. Raphael M, Jaeger M, van Vlymen J. Easily adoptable total joint arthroplasty program allows discharge home in two days. Can J Anaesth. 2011;58:902–10.
30. Kehlet H, Wilkinson RC, Fischer HB, et al. PROSPECT: evidence-based, procedure-specific postoperative pain management. Best Pract Res Clin Anaesthesiol. 2007;21:149–59.
31. Donaldson AJ, Thomson HE, Harper NJ, Kenny NW. Bone cement implantation syndrome. Br J Anaesth. 2009;102(1):12–22.
32. Choi PT, Bhandari M, Scott J, et al. Epidural analgesia for pain relief following hip or knee replacement. Cochrane Database Syst Rev. 2003;3:CD003071.
33. Kehlet H, Anderson L. Local infiltration analgesia in joint replacement: the evidence and recommendations for clinical practice. Acta Anaesthesiol Scand. 2011;55:778–84.

Part VII

Surgical Treatment of Specific Hip Conditions

Rodrigo Mardones

Biologic Labrum

45

Joseph C. McCarthy, Leah Elson, and JoAnn Lee

Healthy Labrum

The labrum is a fibrocartilaginous structure consisting of Type I collagen and hyaline cartilage [1]. The labrum extends the rim and is derived from the iliac, pubic, and ischium bones. The structural labral fibers run in a circumferential direction around the acetabulum, continuing across the acetabular notch (located inferiorly) to the region in which the labrum joins with the transverse ligament to completely encapsulate the femoral head [2]. In the anterior aspect (near the pubis) of the acetabulum, labral fibers are parallel to the acetabulum, whereas posterior labral fibers grow perpendicularly. It has been suggested by several authors that this difference in growth pattern between the two types of fibers, located in the anterior aspect of the labrum, could be a contributing factor to the higher prevalence of tearing in that area [2–4]. The labrum is thickest in the superior aspect of the acetabulum and widest anteriorly [3]. Microscopically, the articulating surface of the labrum (between acetabulum and femoral head) attaches indirectly to the hip, located on top of and merging with articular hyaline cartilage [3]. However, at the nonarticular surface, the labrum is in direct contact with the bone, where the neurovascular bundle transverses in order to supply the labrum [5] (Fig. 45.1).

The acetabular labrum receives blood and nourishment primarily from the highly vascularized synovium on the outer surface of the acetabulum [3]. Macroscopically, the blood supply originates from the obturator and both the superior and inferior gluteal arteries [1, 6]. A cadaveric study of 54 hips showed no evidence of penetration of vessels from underlying bone into the labrum [5]. This fact was supported by the lack of laminin in immunohistochemical staining of the inner labrum observed by several authors, demonstrating that the inner two-thirds of the labrum is, indeed, avascular [1, 5, 7]. The lack of vascularization within the inner labrum becomes critical when considering the likelihood of a labral tear healing without surgical intervention (see Surgery/Treatment section).

While Kim et al. showed the presence of numerous nerve endings throughout the entirety of the labrum, these nerves were more densely located in the anterior and superior aspects of the labrum [8]. In the same study Kim et al. also found sensory nerve organs including Vater-Pacini corpuscles, Krause corpuscles, Golgi-Mazzoni corpuscles, and Ruffini corpuscles. The presence of these structures within the acetabular labrum suggests that the labrum is involved in nociception and proprioception of the body.

The exact function of the labrum has been a matter of debate for some time; however, it is suspected that the labrum increases the stability of the hip and aids in distributing forces at the articular surface of the acetabulum [9–12]. The labrum also increases the stability of the hip by creating a seal that opposes the flow of synovial fluid from the central to the peripheral compartment and vice versa. This sealing property creates a negative pressure that resists femoral head distraction from the socket by counteracting the increased joint force that may occur when the hip is articulating in extreme ranges of motion.

The labrum further increases the stability of the hip joint by deepening the acetabular socket, increasing the surface area of the articulating surface, and expanding the volume of

J.C. McCarthy, MD (✉)
Kaplan Joint Center, Newton-Wellesley Hospital, Green Bldg, Suite 361, 2000 Washington St., Newton, MA 02462, USA

Department of Orthopedic Surgery, Massachusetts General Hospital, Boston, MA, USA
e-mail: JCMCCARTHY1@PARTNERS.ORG; JCMCCARTHY1@mgh.harvard.edu

L. Elson, BSc
Harris Laboratory, Department of Orthopedics, Massachusetts General Hospital, Boston, MA, USA
e-mail: leelson@gmail.com

J. Lee, MS
Department of Orthopedics, Newton Wellesley Hospital, Newton, MA, USA
e-mail: jlee76@partners.org

J.C. McCarthy et al. (eds.), *Hip Joint Restoration*, DOI 10.1007/978-1-4614-0694-5_45

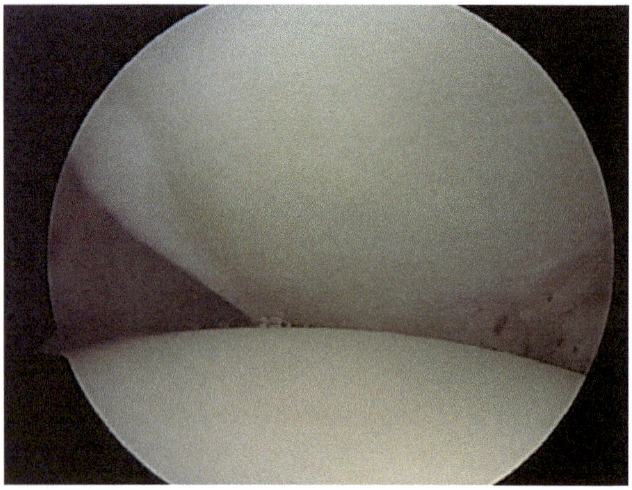

Fig. 45.1 An intraoperative photo of the femoral head articulating with the labro-chondral surface in the anterior quadrant

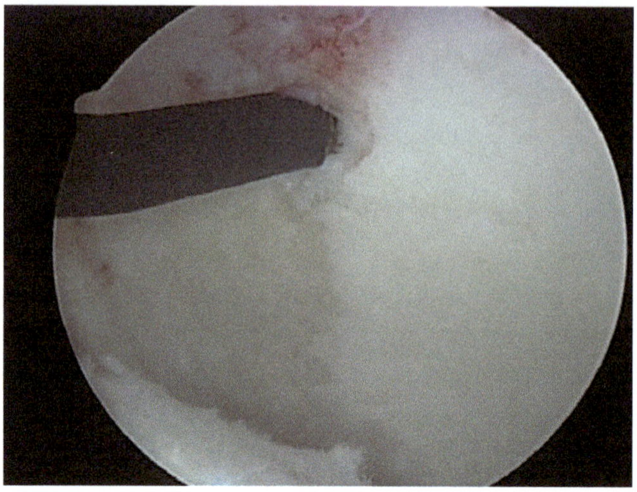

Fig. 45.2 An intraoperative photo showing a degenerated labrum with extensive degenerative joint disease of the adjacent acetabular cartilage

the acetabulum itself by approximately 21 %, 22 %, and 33 %, respectively [3, 13]. This combination of increased structural support and surface area reduces the risk of damage to the articular surface that may occur as a result of contact stress between the acetabulum and femoral head [12, 13].

Furthermore, Ferguson et al. demonstrated that the removal of the labrum from the acetabular rim increased the contact stress by a factor of 92 %. Additionally, this study showed that the removal of the labrum also increased the rate at which the acetabulum and femoral head approached one another (creep consolidation rate) by 40 % [14]. In another study, Ferguson et al. showed in six cadaveric hips the consolidation rate was increased 22 %, and final displacement was increased 21 % in hips that had their labrum removed [15]. Smith et al. showed in 22 cadaveric hips that circumferential labral tears greatly reduce hip stability and radial labral tears can reduce stability but only after the tear is greater than 2 cm [16]. Crawford et al. showed in six cadaveric hips that labral tears decreased hip stability especially when the hip was put into extreme range of motions [17]. They showed that 60 % less force was needed in order to distract the femur by 3 mm suggesting that an intact labrum is important in keeping the femoral head in the acetabulum at extreme positions. In all, as one can see from these studies, the acetabular labrum plays a crucial role in maintaining hip stability and preventing articular surface degeneration.

Diseased Labrum

The precise biomechanical role of the acetabular labrum is still being evaluated. However, research studies have begun to reveal that this peripheral cartilaginous structure may be integral to the overall kinematic function of the hip joint [16–22].

As an extension of the acetabulum itself, the labrum deepens the socket making it more difficult for the femoral head to undergo subluxation [16, 17, 20]. Additionally, the labrum contributes to the intra-articular pressure seal that exists within the joint. This sealing action may ultimately aid in the dispersion of compressive forces on the articulating surface of the acetabulum as well as contribute to the reduction of the joint during extreme ranges of motion [17]. These crucial contributions to the overall functioning of the hip joint make the labrum an aspect of anatomy that is well worth consideration. Thus, it is critical to understand how the integrity of this structure may dictate patient clinical outcomes.

A damaged labrum can cause localized pain, usually in the groin, or it may be associated with indirect pain radiating from the spine, inguinal region, musculature surrounding the hip joint, or the adjacent pelvic structures. If left untreated, these painful lesions, and the etiology thereof, may ultimately lead to disability [16].

Labral damage does not often occur as an isolated problem but manifests itself in concert with one or more various other pathological afflictions. Etiologically, lesions of the labrum have shown to be concurrent with degenerative disease, dysplasia, femoroacetabular impingement (FAI), and traumatic injury [21–25] (Fig. 45.2). Typically, most labral lesions have been shown to occur in the anterior or anterior-superior regions of the acetabulum [25–28]. However, the location, extent, and classification of damage can be variable based on the aforementioned associations. Three common categories of labral lesions, classified by morphology, are the separation of the labrum from the rim of the acetabulum, radial tears or fraying of the labral body, and idiopathic damage [20, 24, 25, 27–31].

The separation of the labrum at the labral-chondral junction typically leaves the bulk of the labrum unscathed.

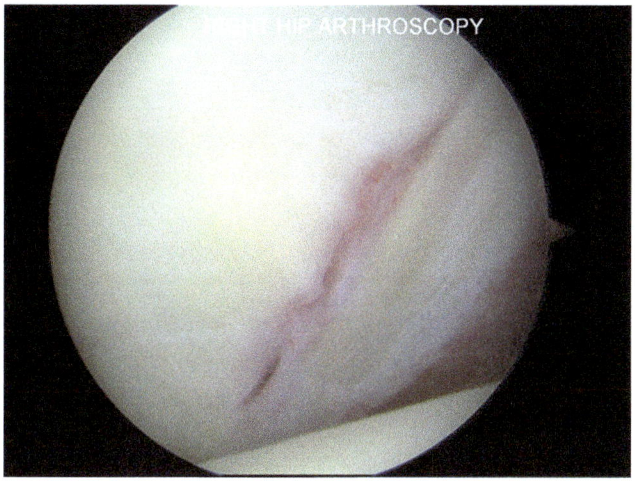

Fig. 45.3 This intraoperative photo shows an anteromedial labral tear at the labro-chondral junction

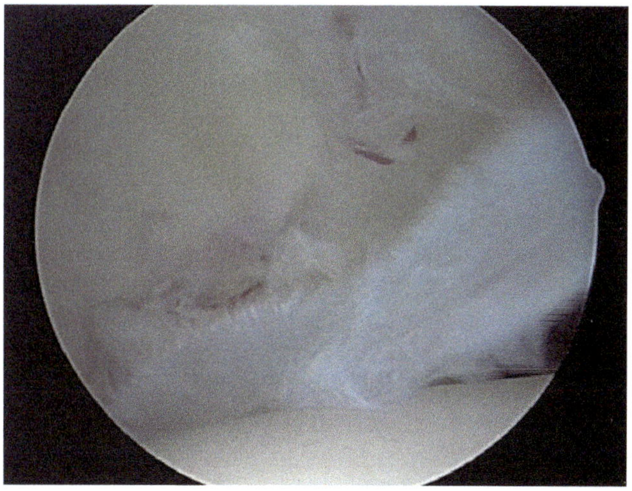

Fig. 45.4 This is an intraoperative photo of an enlarged and torn labrum in a patient with acetabular dysplasia

This particular pattern of damage has been associated with traumatic injury and FAI. For low-grade trauma without dislocation (i.e., repetitive loading due to certain pivoting motions occurring in athletes), the circumferential tearing typically occurs at the anterior region of the acetabulum (Fig. 45.3). However, the location and extent of this lesion is specific to the cause of trauma itself. Nonconcentric loading in the hip joint caused by structural abnormalities—such as the cam and pincer bony anomalies inherent in FAI—can also cause a separation of the labrum at the acetabular rim. As the nonspherical structure of the femoral head and acetabulum articulate against one another, they crush the labral tissue, thereby damaging and separating it from the rim [20]. Findings from cadaveric studies demonstrate that circumferential tears do not disrupt the stability of the hip joint until the tear reaches 3 cm in length and beyond [16, 17].

Radial tears and fraying cause damage to the body of the labrum itself, disrupting the integrity of the circular fibers (Fig. 45.4). These lesions are often associated with dysplasia. Dysplastic abnormalities—including a decrease in acetabular or femoral anteversion, acetabular retroversion, shallow acetabula, or a decreased head offset—force the femoral head to load in nonconcentric patterns [20, 32–40]. This adverse loading can reduce joint stability by increasing stress on the intra-articular surface, and at the labrum, which may eventually lead to damage at the labral and chondral surfaces [20, 23, 24, 32, 41–43] (Fig. 45.5).

Idiopathic damage can be variable in its extent, type, and location, and its causes are either obscure, such as from genetic predisposition, or completely unknown. While this type of lesion varies from patient to patient, it nonetheless causes mechanical symptoms [20, 25, 44].

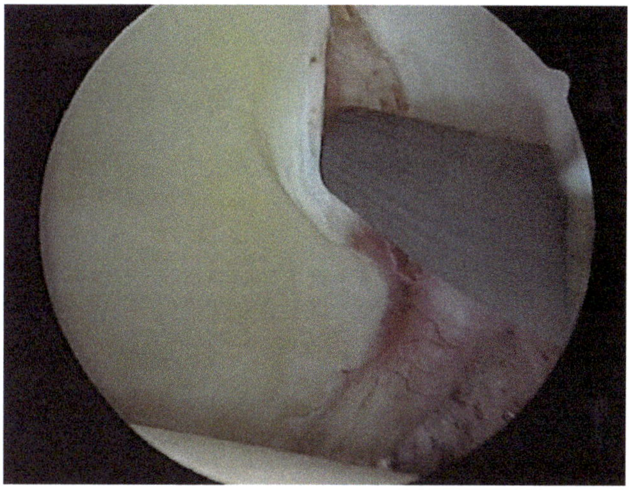

Fig. 45.5 This is an intraoperative photo of an anterior labral tear with adjacent acetabular chondral damage

Clinical Presentation

Typically, symptoms associated with labral lesions occur in a younger, more active population. These symptoms include mechanical abnormalities such as locking, clicking, or weakness; partial joint space preservation; and a suboptimal rotational range of motion [20].

The progression of symptoms is often gradual. Patients may report an onset of variable pain, aggravated while engaging in impact activities such as jumping, running, or walking. However, some patients may also experience discomfort while sitting or in the supine position for extended periods of time [20, 45].

These patients may have also had prior failure of nonoperative treatment, including rehabilitation and/or a regiment of anti-inflammatory medications. As with any operative treatment, the proper selection of patients is integral to ensuring clinical success. With this in mind, ideal candidates for arthroscopic intervention would present the aforementioned symptoms for longer than a period of 6 months and have reasonable expectations for their postoperative outcomes [18–20].

The incidence of labral lesions has been reported to be in as many as 55 % of patients exhibiting pain from the hip or groin [12, 26, 32, 46]. Due to the inconsistency in diagnostic methods, as well as to the need for diagnostic tools crafted specifically for the discovery of labral tears, it is not uncommon for these types of injuries to go undiagnosed [20].

There are several reliable physical examination abnormalities that can be tested in patients with suspected labral lesions. The first is a positive anterior hip impingement test [45, 47, 48]. With the patient in the supine position—hip and knee flexed at 90°—the hip is internally rotated, and an adductive force is applied. A positive indication of labral damage results in pain originating from the anterolateral hip or groin area. A second test that can be performed to identify labral tearing is the posterior hip impingement test. In this examination, the patient is prone with hip and knee extended. The affected hip is then extended, adducted, and externally rotated. A positive indication of labral damage produces posterior pelvic and/or anterior hip pain and discomfort [20, 45]. There is also a positive McCarthy sign. The patient is supine with both hips fully flexed; the patient's pain is reproduced by extending the affected hip, first in external rotation, then in internal rotation. Hip terminal extension will produce a painful click, a catching sensation or in rare cases locking of the joint. Physical examination may not yield a clear enough indication that labral damage is present, thus it is necessary to use imaging for further confirmation.

Radiographic Imaging

Initially, diagnostic imaging begins with plain radiographs. These films are taken to evaluate other potential causes for pain and mechanical symptoms, including degenerative disease, avascular necrosis, slipped capital femoral epiphysis (SCFE), and dysplasia. The three standard film views used for bony diagnosis are anteroposterior pelvis, cross-table lateral, and frog lateral views. Specialized views such as a false-profile Lequesne view may be helpful in identifying bony morphologic abnormalities, especially of the anterior acetabular rim. When appropriate a Dunn view, with the hip in 45 or 90 degrees of flexion, can also define femoral bony abnormalities [49]. Once any bony abnormalities have been identified, soft tissue imaging must be performed. Noncontrast magnetic resonance imaging (MRI) and computed tomography (CT) scans have been shown to be unreliable for

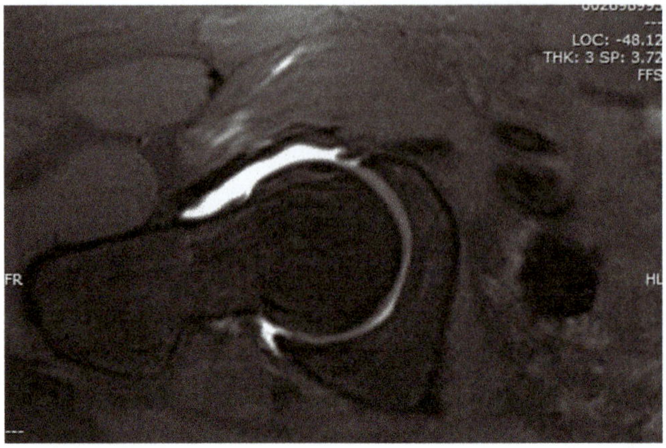

Fig. 45.6 This is an oblique sagittal image on an MR arthrogram demonstrating a labral tear

diagnosis of chondral or labral lesions. Thus magnetic resonance arthrography (MRA) is the preferred diagnostic imaging method [20, 24, 32, 45, 50–52] (Fig. 45.6).

Once a diagnosis has been confirmed, a course of treatment must be decided upon between the patient and physician. Nonoperative treatment is typically offered first. This may include rest of the affected joint (or a complete non-weight-bearing protocol), with a combined nonsteroid anti-inflammatory medication. Physical therapy may also be offered for a 10–12-week period. Depending entirely upon the patient-specific symptoms, pain, and mechanical limitations, the physical therapy protocol may focus on gait correction or strengthening of weakened musculature. Often, patients will report a decrease in pain; however, it is not uncommon for it to return once the patient is allowed to resume normal activities [32, 45].

When conservative options of treatment for the patient have failed, and a patient remains dissatisfied with their functional limitations, a surgical consult becomes necessary. Current arthroscopic treatment focuses on the repair of damaged tissue surrounding labral tears and correcting any structural abnormalities thereof [5, 28, 41, 45, 47, 53–55]. This reparative procedure can encourage the healing of peripheral labral tears, reduce pain, and restore proper joint function [56–59].

Conclusion

Despite the disagreement surrounding the precise kinematic role of the acetabular labrum, it is becoming clear that this small structure contributes to a fully functioning and healthy hip joint. With its variable pathologies—causing a diverse array of pain and dissatisfaction—it is critical to fully understand the best methods with which to treat labral lesions. In most cases, arthroscopy is proving to be the best method with which to treat pain and instability of the hip joint. Validated outcome scoring tests, such as the NAHS and the IHOT, have demonstrated not only short-term symptom resolution but also long-term, now out beyond 15 years, maintenance of comfort and function, if performed prior to advanced joint cartilage damage.

References

1. Petersen W, Petersen F, Tillmann B. Structure and vascularization of the acetabular labrum with regard to pathogenesis and healing of labral lesions. Arch Orthop Trauma Surg. 2003;123(6):283–8.
2. Cashin M, Uhthoff H, O'Neill M, Beaule PE. Embryology of the acetabular labral-chondral complex. J Bone Joint Surg Br. 2008;90:1019–24.
3. Seldes RM, Tan V, Hunt J, Katz M, Winjarsky R, Fitzgerald RH. Anatomy, histologic features, and vascularity of the adult acetabular labrum. Clin Orthop Relat Res. 2001;382:232–40.
4. Safran MR. The acetabular labrum: anatomic and functional characteristics and rationale for surgical intervention. J Am Acad Orthop Surg. 2010;18:338–45.
5. McCarthy JM, Noble P, Aluisio FV, Schuck M, Wright J, Lee JA. Anatomy, pathologic features, and treatment of acetabular labral tears. Clin Orthop Relat Res. 2003;406(1):33–47.
6. Kalhor M, Horowitz K, Beck M, Bashir B, Ganz R. Vascular supply to the acetabular labrum. J Bone Joint Surg Am. 2010;93(15): 2570–5.
7. Haviv B, O'Donnell J. Arthroscopic treatment for acetabular labral tears of the hip without bony dysmorphism. Am J Sports Med. 2001;39:79S.
8. Kim YT, Azuma H. The nerve endings of the acetabular labrum. Clin Orthop Relat Res. 1995;320:176–81.
9. Henak CR, Ellis BJ, Harris MD, Anderson AE, Peters CL, Weiss JA. Role of acetabular labrum in load support across the hip joint. J Biomech. 2011;44(12):2201–6.
10. Takechi H, Nagashima H, Ito S. Intra-articular pressure of the hip joint outside and inside the limbus. Nippon Seikeigeka Gakkai Zasshi. 1982;56:529–36.
11. Ueo T, Suzuki S, Iwasaki R, Yosikawa J. Rupture of the labra acetabularis as a cause of hip pain detected arthroscopically, and partial limbectomy for successful pain relief. Arthroscopy. 1990;6:48–51.
12. McCarthy JC, Noble PC, Schuck MR, et al. The Otto E. Aufranc Award: the role of labral lesions to development of early degenerative hip disease. Clin Orthop. 2001;393:25–37.
13. Tan V, Seldes RM, Katz MA, et al. Contribution of acetabular labrum to articulating surface area and femoral head coverage in adult hip joints: an anatomic study in cadavera. Am J Orthop. 2001;30:809–12.
14. Ferguson SJ, Bryant JT, Ganz R, Ito K. The influence of the acetabular labrum on hip joint cartilage consolidation: a poroelastic finite element model. J Biomech. 2000;33:953–60.
15. Ferguson SJ, Bryant JT, Ganz R, Ito J. An in vitro investigation of the acetabular labral seal in hip joint mechanics. J Jpn Orthop Assoc. 1982;56(6):529–36.
16. Smith MV, Panchal HB, Ruberte RA, Sekiya JK. The effect of acetabular labrum tears on hip stability and labral strain in a joint compression model. Am J Sports Med. 2011;39:103S.
17. Crawford JC, Dy CJ. The biomechanics of the hip labrum and the stability of the hip. Clin Orthop Relat Res. 2007;465:16–22.
18. Shetty V. Hip arthroscopy: current concepts and review of literature. J Sports Med. 2007;41:64–8.
19. Byrd JWT. Hip arthroscopy: its role in osteoarthritis. J Bone Joint Surg Br. 2004;86:207.
20. Groh MM. A comprehensive review of labral tears. Curr Rev Musculoskelet Med. 2009;2(2):105–17.
21. Harris WH, Bourne RB. Intra-articular acetabular labrum: a possible etiological factor in certain cases of osteoarthritis of the hip. J Bone Joint Surg Am. 1979;61:510–4.
22. Ueo T, Hamabuchi M. Hip pain caused by cystic deformation of the labrum acetabulare. Arthritis Rheum. 1984;27:947–50.
23. Dorrell JH, Catterall A. The torn acetabular labrum. J Bone Joint Surg Br. 1986;68:400–3.
24. Klaue K, Durnin CW. The acetabular rim syndrome, a clinical presentation of dysplasia of the hip. J Bone Joint Surg Br. 1991;73:423–9.
25. Lage LA, Patel JV. The acetabular labral tear: an arthroscopic classification. Arthroscopy. 1996;12:269–72.
26. McCarthy JC, Busconi B. The role of hip arthroscopy in the diagnosis and treatment of hip disease. Orthopedics. 1995;18:753–6.
27. Byrd JW. Labral lesions: an elusive source of hip pain case reports and literature review. Arthroscopy. 1996;12:603–12.
28. Fitzgerald RH Jr. Acetabular labrum tears. Diagnosis and treatment. Clin Orthop. 1995;(311):60–8.
29. Ikeda T, Awaya G, Suzuki S. Torn acetabular labrum in young patients. Arthroscopic diagnosis and management. J Bone Joint Surg Br. 1988;70:13–6.
30. Hase Y, Ueo T. Acetabular labral tear: arthroscopic diagnosis and treatment. Arthroscopy. 1999;15:138–41.
31. Keene GS, Villar RN. Arthroscopic anatomy of the hip: an in vivo study. Arthroscopy. 1994;10:392–9.
32. Lewis CL, Sahrmann SA. Acetabular labral tears. Phys Ther. 2006;86:110–21.
33. Ganz R, Parvizi J, Beck M. FAI: a cause for osteoarthritis of the hip. Clin Orthop Relat Res. 2003;417:112–20.
34. Ito K, Minka II MA. Femoroacetabular impingement and the cam-effect: an MRI-based quantitative anatomical study of the femoral head-neck offset. J Bone Joint Surg Br. 2011;83:171–6.
35. Siebenrock KA, Schoeniger R, Ganz R. Anterior femoro-acetabular impingement due to acetabular retroversion: treatment with periacetabular osteotomy. J Bone Joint Surg Am. 2003;85:278–86.
36. Coleman SS. Congenital dysplasia and dislocation of the hip. St. Louis: Mosby; 1978.
37. Li PL, Ganz R. Morphologic features of congenital acetabular dysplasia: one in six retroverted. Clin Orthop Relat Res. 2003;416:245–53.
38. Robertson DD, Essinger JR, Imura S. Femoral deformity in adults with developmental hip dysplasia. Clin Orthop Relat Res. 1996;327:196–206.
39. Siebenrock KA, Wahab KH, Werlen S. Abnormal extension of the femoral head epiphysis as a cause of cam impingement. Clin Orthop Relat Res. 2004;418:54–60.
40. Lavigne M, Parvisi J, Beck M. Anterior femoroacetabular impingement, part I: techniques of preserving surgery. Clin Orthop Relat Res. 2004;418:61–6.
41. Mason JB. Acetabular labral tears in the athlete. Clin Sports Med. 2001;20:779–90.
42. Lane NE, Lin P, Christiansen L, Gore LR. Association of mild acetabular dysplasia with an increased risk of incident hip osteoarthritis in elderly white women: the study of osteoporotic fractures. Arthritis Rheum. 2000;43:400–4.
43. Hickman JM, Peters CL. Hip pain in the young adult: diagnosis and treatment of disorders of the acetabular labrum and acetabular dysplasia. Am J Orthop. 2001;30:459–67.
44. Schmerl M, Pollard H, Hoskins W. Labral injuries of the hip: a review of diagnosis and management. J Manipulative Physiol Ther. 2005;28(8):632.

45. Hunt D, Clohisy J, Prather H. Acetabular tears of the hip in women. Phys Med Rehabil Clin N Am. 2007;18(3):497–520.
46. Narvani AA, Tsiridis E, Kendall S, Chaudhuri R, Thomas P. A preliminary report on prevalence of acetabular labrum tears in sports patients with groin pain. Knee Surg Sports Traumatol Arthrosc. 2003;11:403–8.
47. Burnett S, Della Rocca G, Prather H. Clinical presentation of patients with tears of the acetabular labrum. J Bone Joint Surg Am. 2006;88(7):1448–57.
48. Saw T, Villar R. Footballer's hip: a report of six cases. J Bone Joint Surg Br. 2004;86(5):655–8.
49. Lequesne MG. Femorocoxometry: angles and segments characteristic of dysplastic and dysmorphic hip conditions in adult: measurement using a femorocoxometer for standard or reduced (digitized) films. Rev Rhum Engl Ed. 1999;66:136–42.
50. Altenburg AR. Acetabular labrum tears: a cause of hip pain and degenerative arthritis. South Med J. 1977;70:174–5.
51. Bonnomet F, et al. Arthroscopic treatment of acetabular labrum lesions: a series of 12 patients with a 4-year follow-up. Rev Chir Orthop Reparatrice Appar Mot. 2000;86:787–93.
52. Santori N, Villar RN. Acetabular labral tears: results of arthroscopic partial limbectomy. Arthroscopy. 2000;16(1):11–5.
53. O'Leary JA, Berend K, Vail TP. The relationship between diagnosis and outcome in arthroscopy of the hip. Arthroscopy. 2001;17(2):181–8.
54. Clohisy JC, Keeney JA, Schoenecker PL. Preliminary assessment and treatment guidelines for hip disorders in young adults. Clin Orthop Relat Res. 2005;441:168–79.
55. Clohisy JC, McClure JT. Treatment of anterior FAI with combined hip arthroscopy and limited open osteoplasty. Iowa Orthop J. 2005;25:164–71.
56. Kelly BT, Shapiro GS, Digiovanni CW, Buly RL, Potter HG, Hannafin JA. Vascularity of the hip labrum: a cadaveric investigation. Arthroscopy. 2005;21(1):3–11.
57. Kelly BT, Weiland DE, Schenker ML, Philippon MJ. Arthroscopic labral repair in the hip: surgical technique review of literature. Arthroscopy. 2005;21:1496–504.
58. Philippon MJ. New frontiers in hip arthroscopy: the role of arthroscopic hip labral repair and capsulorrhaphy in the treatment of hip disorders. Instr Course Lect. 2006;55:309–16.
59. Peterson W, Peterson F, Tillmann B. Structure and vascularization of the acetabular labrum with regard to pathogenesis and healing of labral lesions. Arch Orthop Trauma Surg. 2003;11:403–8.

Specific Tissues and Conditions: Chondral Lesions

46

Daniel L. Skinner, Edward D.R. Bray, Giles H. Stafford, and Richard N. Villar

Cartilage Histology

In healthy synovial joints, the articulating surfaces are covered in avascular, translucent hyaline cartilage [1, 2]. The most abundant constituent of hyaline cartilage is the extracellular matrix (ECM). Water constitutes 60–85 % [3] along with other substances such as glycoprotein and salts. Approximately 15–22 % of hyaline articular cartilage is composed of type II collagen fibres, whilst the principal cell, the chondrocyte, only makes up 10 % of the structure. The final constituent is proteoglycans (4–7 %) [1, 3]. Proteoglycans are proteins with covalently bonded glycosaminoglycans (GAG), such as chondroitin sulphate, attached.

The articular cartilage is arranged into four zones overlying the subchondral bone. The most superficial zone is the "superficial tangential zone" (STZ) [1, 3, 4]. It forms 10–20 % of the cartilage thickness and is composed of collagen fibres closely packed and orientated in parallel alignment to the articulating surface [1, 3, 4]. Directly under this layer is the "middle (transitional) zone" (40–60 % of the thickness) [1, 3, 4] which has loosely packed and disorganised collagen fibres. Inferiorly, the "deep (radial) zone" (30–40 % of the thickness) [1, 3, 4] has compact, large diameter collagen fibres that are organised in a perpendicular, radial configuration. At the deep surface of the "radial zone", the fibres penetrate into the underlying "calcified zone" at the Tidemark, adhering the cartilage to the subchondral bone beneath (Fig. 46.1).

The structural proteoglycan, aggrecan, creates an oncotic affect, drawing water into the cartilage whilst simultaneously contributing to a stiff architectural framework through its bonds with collagen fibres [2, 5]. In addition, the glycoprotein chondronectin binds collagen fibres to the proteoglycans, entrapping the chondrocytes within the ECM [6]. Chondrocytes are responsible for the maintenance of the ECM and production of collagen. Subsequently, their orientation mirrors that of the collagen fibres as they progress through the differentiation zones [3, 6–8].

Microscopic Cartilage Degeneration Pathophysiology

Hyaline articular cartilage provides a low-friction, resistant, load-bearing surface that distributes compression and sheer stresses placed upon it [2, 6]. The outermost layers of the STZ are collectively known as the lamina splendens. In addition to being formed from densely packed parallel collagen fibres, the lamina splendens is also infiltrated by the proteoglycan lubricin, a component of synovial fluid [3, 9] to aid with these functions.

Articular cartilage is described as having biphasic viscoelastic properties [7]. The "solid phase" represents the increased stiffness created by the aggrecan/collagen interface [2, 7], whilst the "fluid phase" occurs due to the high osmotic draw and water content within the ECM. This allows articular cartilage to be resistant to sudden loading forces, whilst simultaneously being able to dissipate low continuous loads [2]. Consequently, the STZ is able to distort up to 25 times more than the underlying *transitional* zone [7].

Degenerative changes and cyclical stress loading have been shown to promote transformation within chondrocytes that are not typically observed in preserved hyaline cartilage [9]. Chondrocyte-induced up-regulation of matrix metalloproteases (MMPs) results in the degradation of proteoglycans,

D.L. Skinner, MBChB, BSc (Hons) (✉) • E.D.R. Bray, MBBS, BSc (Hons) • G.H. Stafford, MBBS, BSc (Hons), FRCS
Orthopaedic Department, Research Division, The South West London Elective Orthopaedic Centre, Epsom General Hospital, Dorking Road, Epsom KT18 7EG, Surrey, UK
e-mail: danielskinner@doctors.org.uk; edbray86@gmail.com; giles.stafford@eoc.nhs.uk

R.N. Villar, MS, FRCS
The Richard Villar Practice, Spire Cambridge Lea Hospital, 30 New Road, Impington, Cambridge CB24 9EL, UK
e-mail: rnv1000@aol.com

J.C. McCarthy et al. (eds.), *Hip Joint Restoration*, DOI 10.1007/978-1-4614-0694-5_46

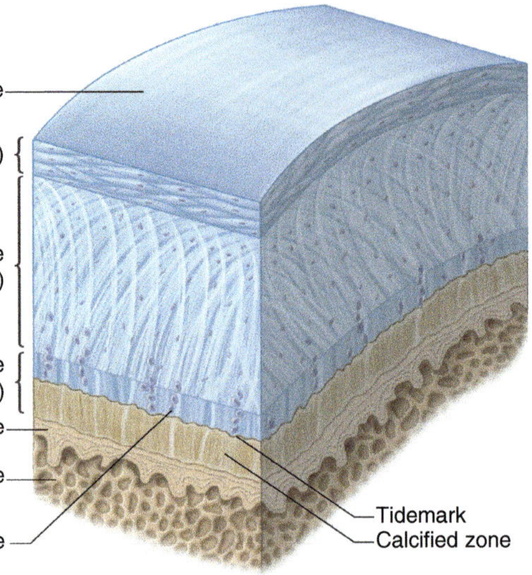

Fig. 46.1 Cross section of articular cartilage showing chondrocyte and collagen fibre orientation

Table 46.1 Outerbridge classification [16]

Grade	Description
0	Normal
1	Cartilage softening and swelling
2	Fragmentation and fissuring in an area half an inch or less in diameter
3	Fragmentation and fissuring in an area more than half an inch in diameter
4	Erosion of cartilage down to bone

collagen and ECM [5, 7]. Furthermore, the up-regulation of pro-inflammatory cytokines TNF-α, IL-1β and IL-6 is responsible for assisting MMPs in cartilage degeneration and promoting synovitis [5, 7, 10]. The net consequence of collagen and matrix degradation is an increased permeability and water loss from the tissues causing a failure of the articular cartilage biphasic properties. As a result, there is a reduced resistance to stress, leading to fatigue and, ultimately, chondromalacia [7].

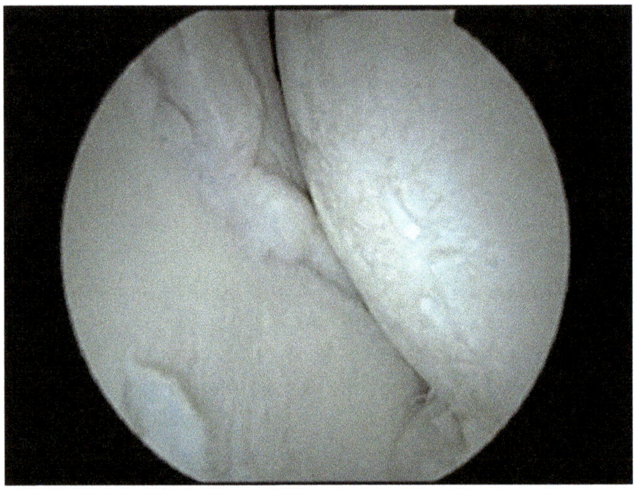

Fig. 46.2 Outerbridge grade 3 defect (with permission of Mr G Stafford)

Macroscopic Cartilage Degeneration and Patterns of Wear in the Hip Joint

There are a number of pathologies which result in chondral defects; these include hip dysplasia, femoroacetabular impingement (FAI), trauma, degenerative disease and slipped upper femoral epiphysis (SUFE) [11–13]. Classification systems have been devised to assist with localising and grading chondral defects [14, 15].

The Outerbridge classification (Table 46.1), developed in 1961, is a descriptive system originally designed for grading patellar chondral defects [16]. The grading scale describes the macroscopic changes associated with the aforementioned microscopic histopathological process (Fig. 46.2). However, despite its popular and frequent use, it has been labelled as ambiguous due to the difficulty differentiating between grades 2 and 3 [15, 16].

As the causative relationship between FAI and early osteoarthritis was identified, a more specific system than the Outerbridge classification was needed to grade acetabular cartilage defects. In 2004, the Beck classification (Table 46.2) was developed for patients who underwent surgical dislocation and offset modification for FAI [14]. This classification, however, has not escaped criticism as it only provided a descriptive analysis and failed to chart the progression of the injury [15].

An alternative grading system (Table 46.3) showing good inter-observer and intra-observer reliability was developed to provide a more advanced interpretation of chondral defect progression [15] (Fig. 46.3). Each chondral lesion (except grade 2—cleavage defects) is provided with an alphabetical subclass (A–C) dependent on the distance the defect spanned.

Table 46.2 Beck classification of acetabular chondral defects [14]

Stage	Description	Criteria
0	Normal	Macroscopically sound cartilage
1	Malacia	Roughening of surface, fibrillation
2	Pitting malacia	Roughening, partially thinning and full-thickness defects or deep fissuring to the bone
2	Debonding	Loss of fixation to the bone, macroscopically sound; carpet phenomenon
3	Cleavage	Loss of fixation to the subchondral bone, frayed edges, thinning of the cartilage
5	Defect	Full-thickness defect

Table 46.3 The University College London (UCL) chondral classification and defect sub-classification [15]

Grade	Description
0	Normal
1	Loss of fixation to the subchondral bone with a positive wave sign
2	Cleavage tear
3	Delamination of articular cartilage
4	Exposed bone in the acetabulum
Defect progression sub-classification	
A	<1/3 from the acetabulum rim to the cotyloid fossa
B	1/3–2/3 of this distance
C	> than 2/3's distance

Grade 2 lesions do not receive a sub-classification as cleavage tears do not result in delamination [15].

In order to accurately record acetabular chondral defects, a clock-face approach was historically used, but with the advancement of arthroscopy techniques, this method has now been superseded by dividing the acetabulum into six regional anatomical zones [15, 17] (Fig. 46.4).

Acetabular Chondral Defects

During hip arthroscopy for FAI, lesions affecting the acetabular cartilage at the chondrolabral junction are the dominant finding [15, 18]. CAM deformities are irregular osteocartilaginous protuberances [11, 19, 20] at the femoral head/neck junction leading to a nonspherical femoral head [19–21]. When the hip is moved into flexion, abduction or internal rotation, the protuberance abuts the superior acetabular rim and labrum causing compressive shear forces that lead to an "outside-in" defect at chondrolabral junction [18, 22]. This can be seen clinically with the presence of a "wave sign" during hip arthroscopy [15], indicating fatigue of the collagen fibres within the *radial zone*.

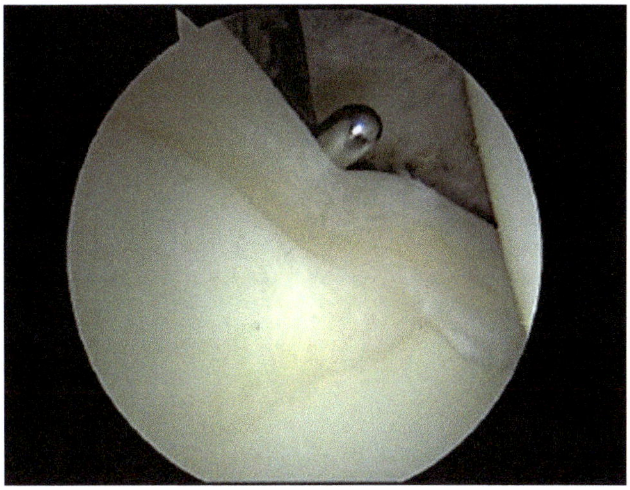

Fig. 46.3 Grade 1 defect with positive wave sign (with permission of Mr G Stafford)

Once there is failure of the anchoring radial collagen fibres, delamination of the articular cartilage occurs through avulsion of the cartilage from the underlying subchondral bone, causing a cleavage tear [15, 22]. Chondrolabral defects increase stress through the hip joint by up to 92 % [13, 23], promoting intra-articular extension of the cleavage tear and enhancing chondral degeneration [24]. Observed patterns of chondral defects in CAM lesions have shown to be classically Beck grade 3 or 4 (cleavage flap) lesions [18], occurring predominantly in the anterior-superior acetabular zones 2, 3 and 4 [20, 21].

In contrast, pincer deformities occur due to overcoverage of the acetabular rim, acetabular retroversion or coxa profunda [20–22, 25]. Biomechanically, this deepens the acetabulum causing the rim to compress the femoral neck and lever the femoral head inside the acetabulum leading to radial cartilaginous tears [18, 22, 26]. Along with defects in zone 2 and 3, chronic pincer impaction and resultant femoral head leverage have been observed to cause a "contrecoup" posterior inferior defect in the acetabulum at zones 4 and 5 [22].

Femoral Head Chondral Lesions

Chondral lesions of the femoral head have historically been demonstrated following hip dysplasia, SUFE, osteonecrosis, osteochondritis dissecans and Perthes and traumatic dislocation [19, 27, 28]. Hip arthroscopy has moved away from a diagnostic procedure and towards a joint-preserving intervention. This has led to greater identification of femoral head chondral defects associated with FAI [27]. Along with the contrecoup lesion, the altered biomechanics associated with CAM lesions have been demonstrated to cause a transient subluxation or non-concentric motion between the femoral

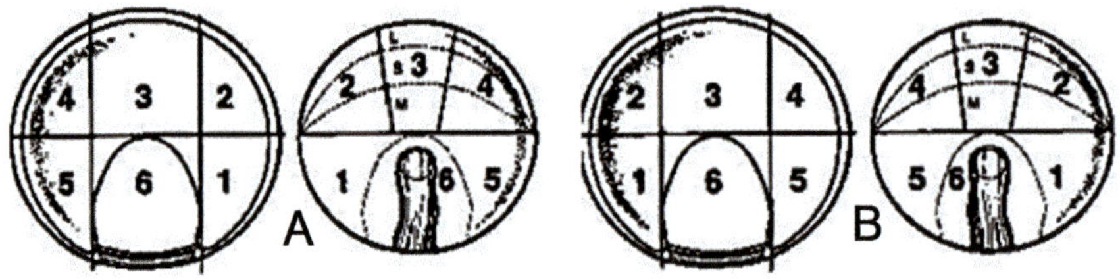

Fig. 46.4 Ilizaliturri regional acetabular zones. (a) Left hip joint. (b) Right hip joint. From Ilizaliturri VJ et al. A geographic zone method to describe intra-articular pathology in hip arthroscopy: cadaveric study and preliminary report. Arthroscopy. 2008;24(5):534–9. Reprinted with permission from Elsevier Limited

head and acetabulum [19, 29–31]. This causes characteristic posterior-superior defects, often lateral to the fovea [19] to develop. Interestingly, when intraoperative findings have been correlated with preoperative diagnostic radiographs, it was observed that these defects often mimicked osteonecrosis or end-stage arthritis [19, 29].

Clinical Presentation

As chondral defects are often secondary consequences of an underlying hip pathology, symptoms typically relate to the primary cause. Over time, as the chondral defect progresses in size and location, patients describe anterior groin pain, with or without anterior thigh, buttock or lateral hip pain. Associated symptoms such as clicking, a feeling of instability, stiffness and reduction in the range of motion are often described.

On clinical examination, patients often express deep anterior groin pain which can refer, to a lesser extent, into the lateral thigh or buttock [32]. This pattern of distribution results in a positive C-sign [32, 33], which refers to the shape formed between the patients' index finger and thumb when holding the lateral thigh. Limitation in active hip range of motion is dependent on the magnitude of chondral defects, but when associated with FAI, pain is reproduced with the combined movements of hip flexion, internal rotation and adduction.

Imaging

Multiple modalities are used in the diagnosis of hip chondral lesions [32]. Anterior posterior pelvis and lateral hip radiographs are the most frequently used method [32]; however, there are multiple reports of poor correlation between radiographic findings and cartilage status [34–36].

Higher-resolution imaging techniques including computed tomography (CT) arthrography, bone scintigraphy and magnetic resonance imaging (MRI) [34] are more sensitive to morphological changes in the articular surface however; they fail to identify early cartilage degeneration [34].

The MRI techniques, 3 T MRI with T2 cartilage mapping and delayed gadolinium-enhanced MRI of cartilage (dGEMRIC), are sensitive to early biophysical changes in cartilage degeneration. These are therefore useful with relation to joint preservation surgery. dGEMRIC scanning requires negatively charged gadolinium to be injected prior to the imaging. Both gadolinium and glycosaminoglycans in cartilage are negatively charged. Therefore, the gadolinium penetrates the cartilage inversely proportional to the GAG content and provides information with regard to the health of cartilage [37, 38].

MRI with T2 cartilage mapping assesses the transverse relaxation time and water mobility within cartilage [39, 40]. The degradation of collagen increases tissue permeability resulting in water loss, and this is reflected by a lower T2 value. Clinically, the T2 value is represented on an image using a colour spectrum. Green indicates healthy cartilage, whilst blue (decreasing value) and red (increasing value) are both pathological (Figs. 46.5 and 46.6). A T2 hip cartilage mapping study showed mean T2 values for Outerbridge grade 0 chondral defects as 25.2 ms; grade 1, 18.1 ms, grade 2, 16.3 ms; and grade 3, 13.8 ms [41].

Management

Management for cartilage delamination and flaps is wide ranging and includes resection, subchondral microfracture, autologous chondrocyte implantation (ACI) and fibrin glue repair [28]. Recent histological studies have shown that between 40 and 90 % of chondrocytes in chondral flaps are still viable, and there is continued deposition of hyaline and fibrocartilage indicating attempted repair [18, 26]. These findings, along with positive follow-up results after refixation of chondral defects, are encouraging when considering repair over debridement [18, 42].

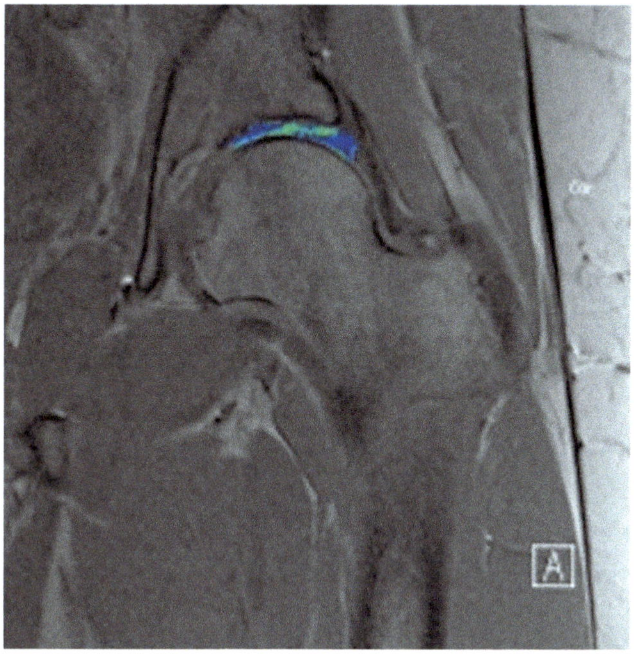

Fig. 46.5 MRI with T2 cartilage mapping showing T2 cartilage mapping (with permission of Mr G Stafford)

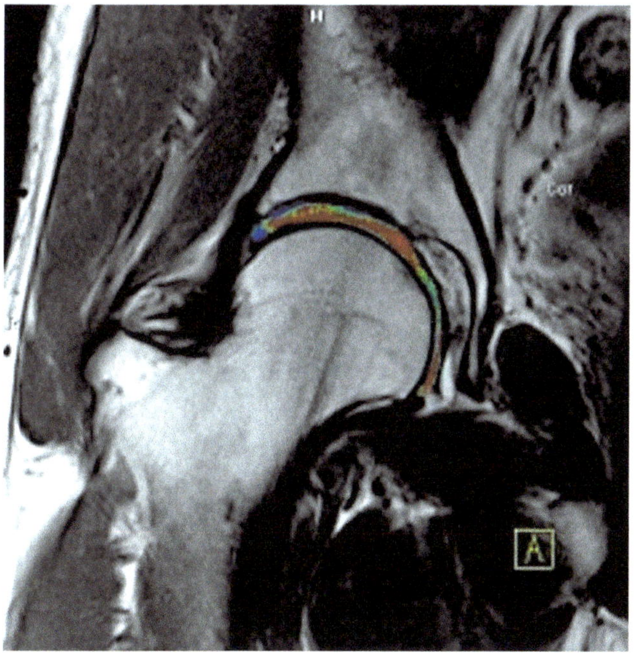

Fig. 46.6 MRI with T2 cartilage mapping. *Blue* and *red* zones indicate severe cartilage defects (with permission of Mr G Stafford)

Summary

In summary, chondral defects are the collective result of abnormal stress placed upon a joint coupled with a predisposing factor, such as morphological irregularity or injury. Advancements in joint preservation surgery have resulted in a greater understanding of the evolution of lesions from subtle cartilage fibrillation to full-thickness defects along with their encroachment into the joint. Consequently, new techniques identifying early changes are at the forefront of joint preservation surgery allowing management to take place whilst viable chondrocytes are still present in the damaged tissue.

References

1. Mow VC, Hung C. Chapter 3: Biomechanics of articular cartilage. In: Nordin M, Frankel VH, editors. Basic biomechanics of the musculoskeletal system. 3rd ed. Pennsylvania: Lippincott Williams & Wilkins; 2001. p. 60–100.
2. Kiani C, Chen L, Wu YJ, Yee AJ, Yang BB. Structure and function of aggrecan. Cell Res. 2002;12(1):19–32.
3. Fox AJS, Bedi A, Rodeo SA. The basic science of articular cartilage structure, composition, and function. Sports Health. 2009;1(6): 461–8.
4. Buckwalter JA, Mow VC, Ratcliffe A. Restoration of injured or degenerated articular cartilage. J Am Acad Orthop Surg. 1994;2(4):192–201.
5. Findlay DM, Atkins GJ. Osteoblast-chondrocyte interactions in osteoarthritis. Curr Osteoporos Rep. 2014;12(1):127–34.
6. Junqueira LC, Carneiro J. Chapter 7: Cartilage. In: Jason Malley, Harriet Lebowitz, Peter J. Boyle, editors. Basic histology text & atlas. 11th ed. New York: McGraw-Hill Companies; 2005. p. 128–33.
7. Pearle A, Warren RF, Rodeo SA. Basic science of articular cartilage and osteoarthritis. Clin Sports Med. 2005;24(1):1–12.
8. Jazrawi L, Alaia MJ, Chang G, Fitzgerald EF, Recht MP. Advances in magnetic resonance imaging of articular cartilage. J Am Acad Orthop Surg. 2011;19(7):420–9.
9. Jay G, Torre JR, Warman ML, Laderer MC, Breuer KS. The role of lubricin in the mechanical behavior of synovial fluid. Proc Natl Acad Sci U S A. 2007;104(15):6194–9.
10. van de Loo F, Joosten LA, van Lent PL, Arntz OJ, van den Berg WB. Role of interleukin-1, tumour necrosis factor alpha, and interleukin-6 in cartilage proteoglycan metabolism and destruction. Effect of in situ blocking in murine antigen-andzymosan-induced arthritis. Arthritis Rheum. 1995;38(2):164–72.
11. Zebala L, Schoenecker PL, Clohisy JC. Anterior femoroacetabular impingement: a diverse disease with evolving treatment options. Iowa Orthop J. 2007;27:71–81.
12. Harris W. Etiology of osteoarthritis of the hip. Clin Orthop. 1986;213(2):20–33.
13. Jordan M, Van Thiel GS, Chahal J, Nho SJ. Operative treatment of chondral defects in the hip joint: a systematic review. Curr Rev Musculoskelet Med. 2012;5(3):244–53.
14. Beck M, Leunig M, Parvizi J, Boutier V, Wyss D, Ganz R. Anterior femoroacetabular impingement. Part II: midterm results of surgical treatment. Clin Orthop. 2004;418:67–73.
15. Konan S, Rayan F, Meermans G, Witt J, Haddad FS. Validation of the classification system for acetabular chondral lesions identified at arthroscopy in patients with femoroacetabular impingement. J Bone Joint Surg Br. 2011;93-B(3):332–6.
16. Outerbridge RE. The etiology of chondromalacia patellae. J Bone Joint Surg Br. 1961;43-B:752–7.
17. Ilizaliturri VJ, Byrd JW, Sampson TG, Guanche CA, Philippon MJ, Kelly BT, Dienst M, Mardones R, Shonnard P, Larson CM. A geographic zone method to describe intra-articular pathology in hip arthroscopy: cadaveric study and preliminary report. Arthroscopy. 2008;24(5):534–9.

18. Meulenkamp B, Gravel D, Beaulé PE. Viability assessment of chondral flap in patients with cam-type femoroacetabular impingement: a preliminary report. Can J Surg. 2014;57(1):44–8.
19. Zaltz I, Leunig M. Parafoveal chondral defects associated with femoroacetabular impingement. Clin Orthop Relat Res. 2012; 470(12):3383–9.
20. Tannast M, Goricki D, Beck M, Murphy SB, Siebenrock KA. Hip damage occurs at the zone of femoroacetabular impingement. Clin Orthop Relat Res. 2008;466(2):273–80.
21. Sampson T. Arthroscopic treatment for chondral lesions of the hip. Clin Sports Med. 2011;30(2):331–48.
22. Ganz R, Parvizi J, Beck M, Leunig M, Nötzil H, Siebenrock KA. Femoroacetabular impingement. A cause for osteoarthritis of the hip. Clin Orthop Relat Res. 2003;417:112–20.
23. Ellis H, Briggs KK, Philippon MJ. Innovation in hip arthroscopy. Is hip arthritis preventable in the athlete? Br J Sports Med. 2011;45(4):253–8.
24. Ganz R, Leunig M, Leunig-Ganz K, Harris WH. The etiology of osteoarthritis of the hip: an integrated mechanical concept. Clin Orthop. 2008;466(2):264–72.
25. Beck M, Kalhor M, Leunig M, Ganz R. Hip morphology influences the pattern of damage to the acetabular cartilage. Femoroacetabular impingement as a cause of early osteoarthritis of the hip. J Bone Joint Surg Br. 2005;87-B(7):1012–8.
26. Kohl S, Hosalkar HS, Manil-Varlet P, Krueger A, Buechler L, Siebenrock K. Histology of damaged acetabular cartilage in symptomatic femoroacetabular impingement: an observational analysis. Hip Int. 2011;21(2):154–62.
27. Yen Y, Kocher M. Chondral lesions of the hip microfracture and chondroplasty. Sports Med Arthrosc Rev. 2010;18(2):83–9.
28. Philippon MJ, Briggs KK, Yen YM, Kuppersmith DA. Outcomes following hip arthroscopy for femoroacetabular impingement with associated chondrolabral dysfunction: minimum two-year follow-up. J Bone Joint Surg Br. 2009;91(1):16–23.
29. Weaver CJ, Major NM, Garrett WE, Urbaniak JE. Femoral head osteochondral lesions in painful hips of athletes: MR imaging findings. AJR Am J Roentgenol. 2002;178(4):973–7.
30. Charbonnier C, Kolo FC, Duthon VB, Magnenat-Thalmann N, Becker CD, Hoffmeyer P, Menetrey J. Assessment of congruence and impingement of the hip joint in professional ballet dancers: a motion capture study. Am J Sports Med. 2011;39(3):557–66.
31. Charbonnier C, Magnenat-Thalmann N, Becker CD, Hoffmeyer P, Menetrey J. An integrated platform for hip arthritis analysis: design, implementation and results. Int J Comput Assist Radiol Surg. 2010;5(4):351–8.
32. Larson CM, Swaringen J, Morrison G. A review of hip arthroscopy and its role in the management of adult hip pain. Iowa Orthop J. 2005;25:172–9.
33. Byrd JW. Hip arthroscopy: patient assessment and indications. Instr Course Lect. 2003;52:711–9.
34. Nishii T, Tanaka H, Sugano N, Sakai T, Hananouchi T, Yoshikawa H. Evaluation of cartilage matrix disorders by T2 relation time in patients with hip dysplasia. Osteoarthritis Cartilage. 2008;16(2):227–33.
35. Fife RS, Brandt KD, Braunstein EM, Katz BP, Shelbourne KD, Kalasinski LA, Ryan S. Relationship between arthroscopy evidence of cartilage damage and radiographic evidence of joint space narrowing in early osteoarthritis of the knee. Arthritis Rheum. 1991;34(4):377–82.
36. Felson DR. The course of osteoarthritis and factors that affect it. Rheum Dis Clin North Am. 1993;19(3):607–15.
37. Li X, Cheng J, Lin K, Saadat E, Bolbos RI, Jobke B, Ries MD, Horvai A, Link TM, Majumdar S. Quantitative MRI using T1ρ and T2 in human osteoarthritic cartilage specimens: correlation with biochemical measurements and histology. Magn Reson Imaging. 2011;29(3):324–34.
38. Hesper T, Hosalkar HS, Bittersohl D, Welsch GH, Krauspe R, Zilkens C, Bittersohl B. T2 mapping for articular cartilage assessment: principles, current applications, and future prospects. Skeletal Radiol. 2014;43(10):1429–45. doi:10.1007/s00256-014-1852-3.
39. Mosher TJ, Dardzinski BJ. Cartilage MRI T2 relaxation time mapping: overview and applications. Semin Musculoskelet Radiol. 2004;8(4):355–68.
40. Harrison R, Bronskill MJ, Henkelman RM. Magnetization transfer and T2 relation components in tissue. Magn Reson Med. 1995; 33(4):490–6.
41. Bittersohl B, Miese FR, Hosalkar HS, Mamisch TC, Antoch G, Krauspe R, Zilkens C. T2* mapping of acetabular and femoral hip joint cartilage at 3 T: a prospective controlled study. Invest Radiol. 2012;47(7):392–7.
42. Stafford GH, Bunn JR, Villar RN. Arthroscopic repair of delaminated acetabular articular cartilage using fibrin glue adhesive. Results at one to three years. Hip Int. 2011;21(6):744–50.

Special Patients and Conditions: Femoroacetabular Impingement

47

Óliver Marín-Peña and Lissette Horna-Castiñeiras

Introduction

During the last century, some authors proposed that the early onset of hip osteoarthritis was related to a nonspherical femoral head [1]. Smith-Petersen described an anterior approach to the hip to reach the "deformity" of the anterior acetabular wall and femoral head–neck junction [2]. The concept of femoroacetabular impingement (FAI) has been popularized as a mechanical cause of hip pain and development of osteoarthritis in the hip [3–6]. Since that time, more than 500 papers on this subject have been published in peer-review journals. However, studies with high-quality evidence have been scarce [7].

FAI has been proposed as one of the major causes of osteoarthritis of the hip [3, 4, 8]. It has been defined as a dynamic impingement between the anterior femoral head–neck junction and anterior acetabular rim, causing chondrolabral damage as a consequence of repetitive hip motion. Impingement can result from structural abnormalities including reduced anterolateral femoral head–neck offset and overcoverage of the antero-superior acetabular rim. During flexion, internal rotation and adduction of the hip, the femoral head–neck junction may contact the acetabular rim, thus leading to the development of lesions at the labrum and acetabular cartilage [3, 9, 10] (Fig. 47.1). With time, this repetitive trauma leads to progressive cartilage damage [11–15] and eventually to early osteoarthritis [4, 16–18], but this aspect is not completely clear in current literature [19, 20]. The incidence of FAI has been estimated to be around 15–20 % in an asymptomatic Caucasian population [21, 22]. Athletes have been considered a high-risk group, with an estimated prevalence, including asymptomatic cases, greater than 65 % in men and 50 % in women [23, 24]. If we consider patients under 55 years who underwent total hip arthroplasty, from 36 to 60 % of the Caucasian patients had radiological signs of FAI [22, 25–27] as a significant cause of its osteoarthritis, in contrast to 0.6 % in Japanese population [28] or 11.7 % in Indian population [29]. Based on the osseous deformities present, two distinct types of FAI have been identified, cam and pincer [6, 8, 13, 30, 31], but these morphological variations are not mutually exclusive.

Cam impingement appears frequently in men where a nonspherical femoral head with a "bump" along the anterior lateral head–neck junction contacts and elevates the labrum during flexion and internal rotation. This "out-in" mechanism results in tearing of the labrum or its avulsion from the rim. At the same time, antero-superior acetabular cartilage may be delaminated and separated from the subchondral bone [4, 12, 14, 17] (Fig. 47.1). This nonspherical femoral head has been related to an abnormal closure of the proximal femoral physis during skeletal growth and development [32] and frequently is bilateral [33].

Pincer impingements are more common in middle-aged women in which there is overcoverage of the femoral head because of a prominent anterior acetabular rim. The prominent acetabulum contacts the femoral neck in extreme flexion and internal rotation. Conditions such as coxa profunda, coxa vara or acetabular retroversion are frequently associated with pincer impingement [34, 35]. The labrum is injured in a localized area at the antero-superior margin [18], but a repetitive pincer mechanism can result in a chondral injury at the antero-superior acetabular cartilage as well as in the postero-inferior acetabulum (contrecoup effect) (Fig. 47.2). Commonly, patients have a combination of cam and pincer, and it is estimated that more than 70 % of patients present with this mixed type.

When we evaluate painful hips in young adults, FAI is frequently present. FAI is often confused with adductor

Ó. Marín-Peña, MD (✉) • L. Horna-Castiñeiras, MD
Hip and Knee Unit at Orthopedic Surgery and Traumatology Department University Hospital Infanta Leonor, Madrid, Spain
e-mail: olivermarin@yahoo.es; olivermar@gmail.com

J.C. McCarthy et al. (eds.), *Hip Joint Restoration*, DOI 10.1007/978-1-4614-0694-5_47

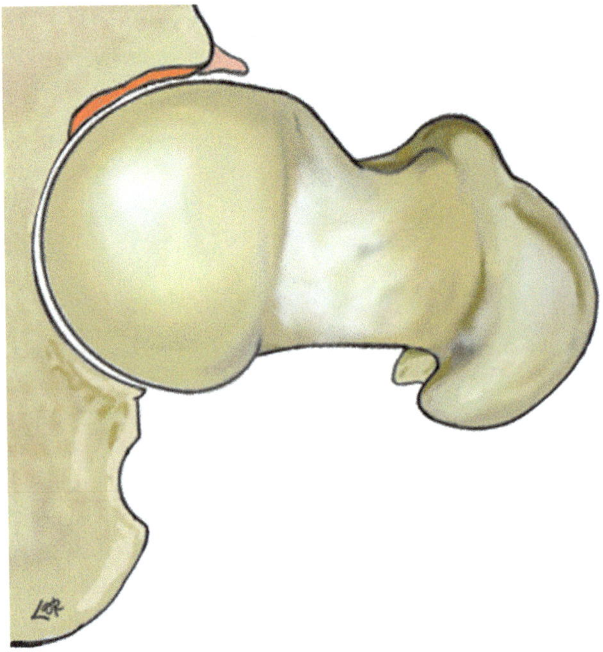

Fig. 47.1 FAI cam deformity at the femoral head–neck junction that induce acetabular chondro-labral damage (*red coloured*). From Marín-Peña, Ó. Open Surgical Treatment of FAI: Safe Surgical Dislocation of the Femoral Head. In: Femoroacetabular Impingement. Leunig M et al., eds. Springer Berlin Heidelberg. 2012:77–86. Reprinted with permission from Springer

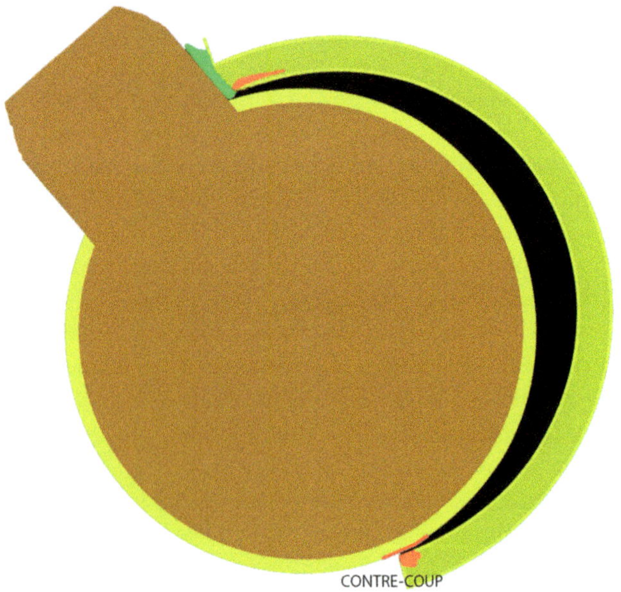

Fig. 47.2 FAI pincer deformity. Acetabular chondro-labral damage (*red coloured* superiorly) and contrecoup effect (*red coloured* inferiorly)

tendonitis, inguinal hernia or pubic osteopathy. Among the articular causes, imaging tests can help to differentiate such diseases as avascular necrosis of the femoral head, Legg–Calvé–Perthes disease or hip dysplasia.

Medical History and Physical Exam

It is very important to perform a comprehensive physical examination that must include evaluating the range of motion. The limitation of motion in FAI usually restricts flexion, adduction and internal rotation, being more pronounced when the hip was flexed 90° [4, 36–38]. The conventional FAI patient is an active 20–50-year-old person that complains about progressive pain without traumatic injury. The location of the pain is usually in the groin, greater trochanter and buttocks and may even radiate to the knee. Frequently, patients describe the pain using their thumb and index finger around the hip ("pain in C"). Initially, the pain was intermittent and increased with activities such as taking long walks and hyperflexion activities (sitting down and crossing their legs, hitting a ball, jumping fences, practicing martial arts and driving). Sometimes pain appeared after being in a prolonged sitting position or after a minor trauma [18, 38]. It has been stated that FAI is the most frequent cause of hip pain in athletes [39]. There are several specific physical tests to identify symptomatic FAI. During the impingement test [4], the patient complains of groin pain in 90° of flexion, internal rotation and adduction of the hip (Fig. 47.3). This manoeuvre is sensitive but not specific to FAI. When the impingement test is positive, we often repeat the test after an intra-articular injection of local anaesthetic to determine the extent of intra-articular pain. The apprehension test should be performed with the patient in the supine position and the affected leg in extension. If positive, moderate pain should appear when gentle external rotation was applied. Although not specific, a positive apprehension test can be related to an injury in the acetabular labrum in cases of mild acetabular dysplasia. During the flexion–abduction–external rotation (FABER) test, the patient's leg is placed in a position of "four". We apply a slight pressure on the knee and measure the vertical distance from the knee to the edge of the stretcher. The result is con-

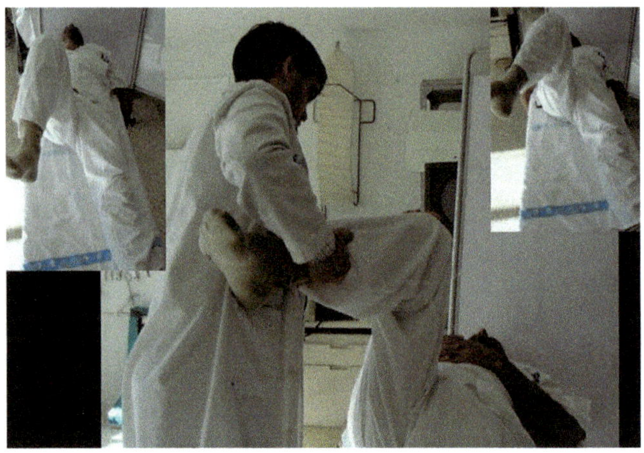

Fig. 47.3 Impingement test. Detail of the painful position (*upper right* and *left*)

sidered positive if this distance was higher in the affected limb compared with the contralateral [38]. Other physical tests such as rolling test or dial test have been describe for the diagnoses of hip pathology, but a recent systematic literature review concluded that no physical tests are available that can reliably confirm the diagnoses of FAI or labral pathology of the hip in clinical practice [40].

Radiological Evaluation

Standard X-Ray

Plain X-ray is helpful in the diagnosis of FAI. We routinely take more than one standard view to evaluate FAI. An AP pelvis and especially Lequesne false-profile view is useful to establish the extent of joint degeneration [41]. The remaining joint space greater than 2 mm is critical in selecting the best treatment option [42–44]. The best views for diagnosing a cam FAI are the antero-posterior pelvic orthostatic projection, Dunn view at 45° and "frog-leg" view (Fig. 47.4). We also take a "cross-table" lateral view to assess the more antero-superior femoral head–neck bumps [45–48] (Fig. 47.5). The bone bump in cam-type FAI is known as a "pistol grip sign" [37]. Measurement of the bump is made by the determination of the alpha angle. That is the angle between the femoral neck axis and a line connecting the head centre with the point where the asphericity of the head–neck contour begins (Fig. 47.6) [14]. It is increased in cam-type FAI and can be measured on standard X-ray, CT slices or MRI. A 60° alpha-angle threshold value gave a sensitivity of 72–80 % and specificity of 73–76 % [49–51]. There are some attempts in the literature to design a simple template tool for measuring the preoperative alpha angle and planning the amount of bone to resect until normalization of the alpha angle [52]. Another measurement in cam-type FAI is anterior offset, which is the difference in radius between the anterior femoral head and the anterior femoral neck on a cross-table axial view. We can also determine the offset ratio that can be calculated as the ratio between the anterior offset and the diameter of the head [53].

For the assessment of pincer FAI, an antero-posterior (AP) pelvic view should be taken, centred at the coccyx. The distance between the coccyx and pubic symphysis should be around 1–2 cm [18]. These technical aspects influence the assessment of acetabular inclination and the overcoverage of femoral head. It has been recommended to take an orthostatic AP pelvis to obtain a more physiological pelvic tilt and control the lumbar lordosis [45] (Fig. 47.7). In pincer type, the AP pelvic view showed the overlay of the anterior and posterior wall of the acetabulum. This radiographic finding is called crossover sign (COS) (Fig. 47.8). To rule out a dysplastic acetabulum in an AP pelvis X-ray, we measure the lateral centre-edge angle (normal value should be between 25° and 39°) and the acetabular index (normal value between 0° and 10°) [54]. We also evaluate the coverage of the femoral head with the extrusion index, which represents the percentage of the femoral head that is uncovered when a horizontal line is drawn parallel to the inter-teardrop line. An extrusion index higher than 25 % is associated with dysplasia [55]. Other radiological signs in pincer FAI are the ischial spine sign (positive when the ischial spine is visible in standard AP pelvis) [30] and the posterior wall sign (defined as positive when the posterior wall extends medially to the centre point of the femoral head). When we evaluate a cross-table view in pincer FAI, at the head–neck junction, a linear indentation may be observed [6, 31, 56–58].

Computerized Tomography (CT)

A more detailed diagnosis of acetabular retroversion can be established with CT scan. Coronal, sagittal and transverse slices will help to identify degenerative stage and acetabular anteversion, although different authors mentioned some

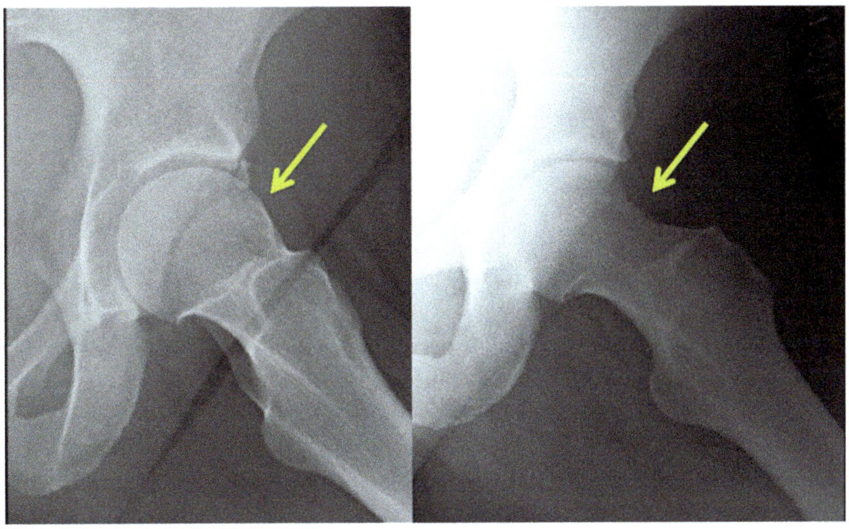

Fig. 47.4 Dunn view of showing the correction of cam FAI; preoperative (*left*) and postoperative (*right*)

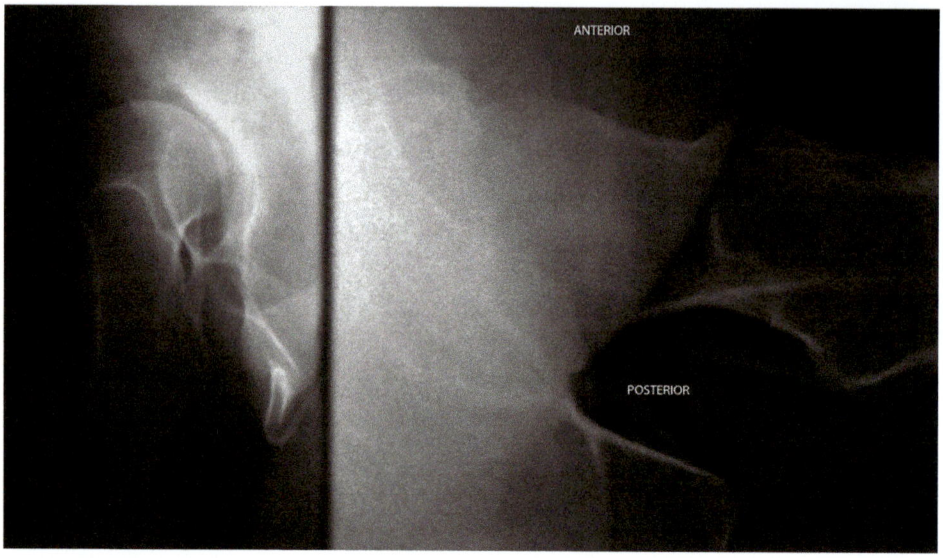

Fig. 47.5 False-profile hip view (*left*) and "cross-table" projection (*right*) to evaluate FAI

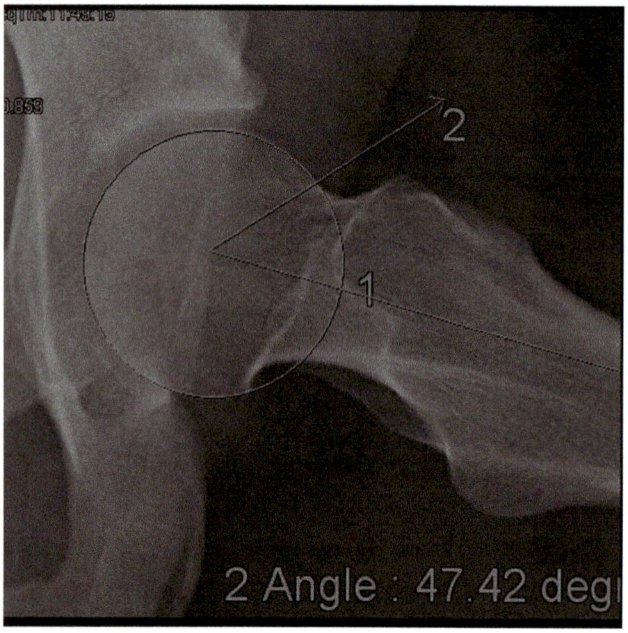

Fig. 47.6 Normal alpha angle

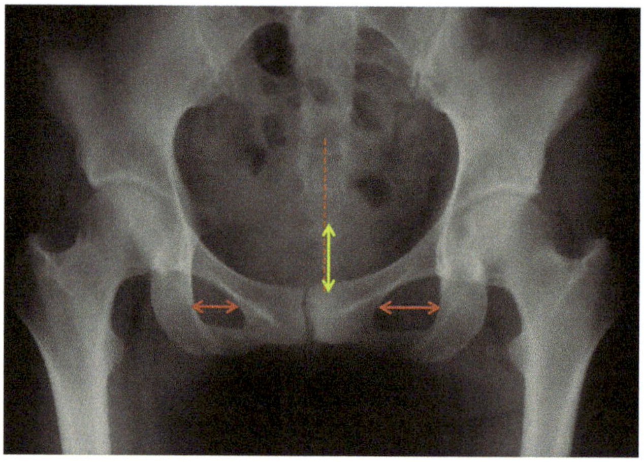

Fig. 47.7 AP pelvic X-ray. *Discontinued red line* shows that pelvis is not centre in coccyx-pubic axis and asymmetry in obturator foramens is detected (*red arrows*). *Yellow arrow* measures the coccyx-pubic distance (pelvic tilt)

concerns about this measurement [31, 57, 59]. The three-dimensional (3D) representation is useful in preoperative planning of the osteoplasty [60, 61] (Fig. 47.9).

Magnetic Resonance Imaging (MRI)

Conventional (non-arthrographic) MRI of the hip should include T1-weighted imaging (WI) without fat suppression, fluid-sensitive sequences as T2 or proton density (PD) and short tau inversion recovery (STIR) [62]. Achieving oblique-axial slices along the neck axis can display degenerative labrum tears, labral cysts and the presence of bone bumps in the head–neck junction [36]. MR T2 mapping technique can indirectly assess cartilage and may be a significant prognostic indicator [63].

Direct magnetic resonance arthrography (MRA) is the combination of MRI with the intra-articular injection of gadolinium-based contrast agents. It is often used to facilitate evaluation of the labrum, hyaline cartilage and loose bodies [12, 36], but there are certain limitations in detecting chondral delamination [10]. Cam-type impingement has a characteristic sequence of pathological findings: increased alpha angle, antero-superior labrum injury and antero-superior acetabular cartilage injury [64] (Fig. 47.10).

Indirect MRA involves intravenous injection of gadolinium contrast, followed by a variable delay or physical

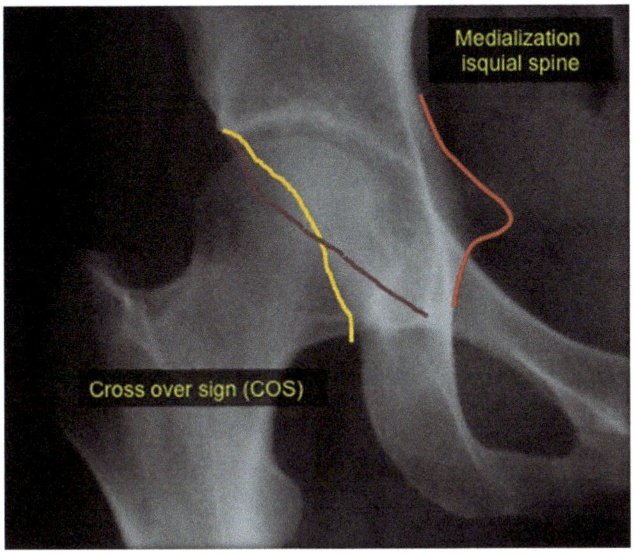

Fig. 47.8 Pincer type. Crossover sign delimitated the anterior acetabular wall (brown line) and posterior wall (*yellow line*). Ischial spine sign is drawn in *red*

activity [65]. Delayed gadolinium-enhanced MR imaging of cartilage (dGEMRIC) uses the properties of intravenously injected gadolinium to indirectly assess the biochemical composition of cartilage [66]. The main advantage of dGEMRIC is that it may demonstrate abnormal biochemical properties of grossly morphologically normal cartilage of the hip [67].

Treatment

Surgical treatment of FAI is becoming a worldwide current practice, with different surgical approaches proposed. A recent systematic literature review concluded that open dislocation, mini-open and arthroscopic methods for treating symptomatic FAI are effective in improving pain and function in short-term to midterm studies and are relatively safe procedures [68, 69]. Nevertheless, open dislocation surgery has a comparatively high major complication rate, and mini-open method shows a significant incidence of iatrogenic injury to the lateral femoral cutaneous nerve. The arthroscopic approach has a lower rate of major complications but only when performed by experienced surgeons [70]. Accurate preoperative clinical evaluation and radiological imaging are the key factors to establish a correct surgical indication. Surgical indications include groin pain, symptom reproducing impingement exam findings, impingement osseous abnormalities on imaging and prearthritic hip disease (Tönnis scale <2) [41]. The ultimate goal of treatment in carefully selected patients is relief of hip pain and preservation of the hip joint.

When pincer FAI is detected, labral repair has historically been performed more frequently with open surgical dislocation and combined approach procedures than in arthroscopic surgeries [69]. There are two ways to correct pincer deformity. First, the labrum can be detached off and rim trimming is performed with a burr. Afterwards, the labrum is reattached to the acetabulum using anchors. A second technique starts with rim trimming, while the labrum is still attached to acetabular margin. The paralabral sulcus is cleaned with a radiofrequency probe, and then the acetabular margin is resected using a burr. Routinely, an image intensifier is used to verify a good acetabular correction. If labral tears are irreparable, then the labrum could be debrided, although labral refixation compared with focal labral debridement resulted in better outcomes and a greater percentage of good to excellent results [68, 71]. When an insufficient labrum is presented (usually less than 5 mm width), due to congenital hypoplasia or secondary to previous surgical labral treatment, labral grafting with iliotibial band [72], capsule or even labral transplantation [73] is also recommended. Excessive acetabular rim trimming in a dysplastic joint may lead to an unstable hip. There is a correlation between the amount of resection and the correction of the centre-edge angle (CE). One millimetre acetabular resection will decrease the CE angle by approximately 2.4°, while 5 mm trimming will decrease the CE angle by approximately 5°. The resection should never reduce the CE angle to less than 25° [74]. Cartilage injury ranges from stable delaminated lesions to full width and depth chondral damage. Multiple repair options have been proposed for the treatment of hip chondral lesions, such as resection of unstable chondral fragments, use of fibrin glue [75], sutured stable flaps, autologous osteochondral graft [76], autologous chondrocyte transplantation [77] or microfractures in full-thickness chondral lesions [78]. Delaminated cartilage should not be debrided; only unstable cartilage should be removed.

When cam FAI deformity is assessed, the specific location of the sphericity must be clearly delineated preoperatively using appropriate tools. Typically, bone deformity is at the antero-superior head–neck junction. Abnormal cartilage has a moderate pink appearance due to hypervascularity [79]. Femoral head deformity usually extends from the medial synovial fold to the anterolateral insertion of the retinacular vessels. These vessels can be seen clearly in most cases and must be preserved. Intraoperative radiographic evaluation of the accurate bump resection can diminish the risk of femoral neck fracture and maintain the labral seal effect with the femoral head [80]. Also, surgical navigation might increase the safety of osteochondroplasty procedures [81]. The presence of a cyst at the antero-superior head–neck junction may correlate with the impinging zone. Femoral bump resection should be done cautiously to avoid overresection that could weaken the femoral head–neck junction. Restoration of the normal head–neck junction offset and clearance of the femoral head within the acetabulum should

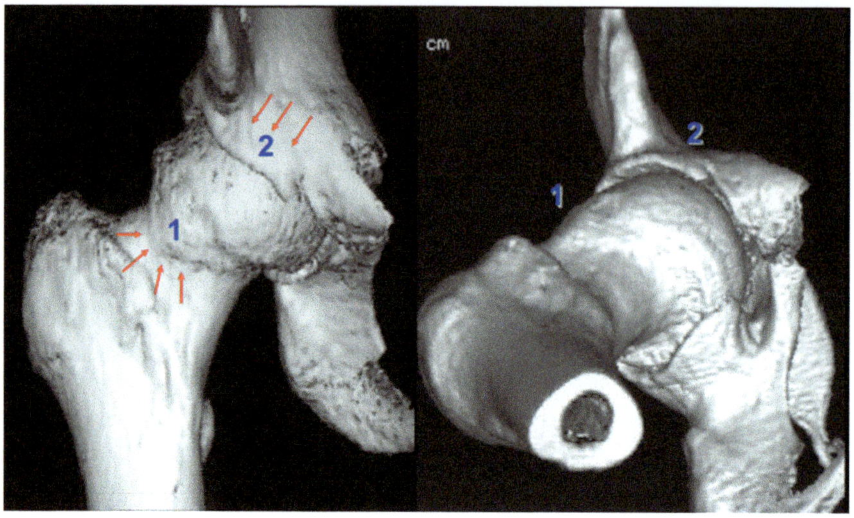

Fig. 47.9 The three-dimensional CT representation in combined FAI

be the aim of the femoral side correction. Despite an excellent femoral head correction, postoperative clinical results generally depend on the extent of articular damage [16, 82–84].

Nonoperative Treatment

Nonoperative treatment should be tailored to the patient. In most cases, conservative treatment is attempted initially. Conservative management consists of activity restriction or modification and non-steroidal anti-inflammatory medications. Physical therapy should focus on abdominal, lower back and hip flexor and abductor strengthening.

Because of the possibility of progressive chondral damage, conservative treatment often results in high rates of failure, especially in the setting of mechanical symptoms. Attempts by physical therapists to improve passive range of motion are not often beneficial and may be counterproductive since limitation of internal rotation in FAI is due to abnormal osseous morphology. Conservative treatment has been proposed recently as an initial option for FAI patients with an alpha angle less than 60° [85].

Safe Surgical Dislocation Approach

Safe surgical dislocation of the hip was described by Ganz [11], offering a full access to the complete femoral head and acetabulum while allowing identification of chondral lesions. Although this approach demonstrated excellent results in conventional FAI cases [86, 87], it also allows treatment of large deformities not amenable to other approaches or failed arthroscopic treatment [11, 35, 48]. The patient is placed in the lateral decubitus positions, and a straight lateral incision is done. From a posterolateral conventional approach, the trochanteric flip osteotomy can now be performed (Fig. 47.11). Ideally, the osteotomy fragment should provide continuity between the gluteus medius and minimus proximally and the vastus lateralis distally [88]. The medial femoral circumflex artery (MFCA) remained protected even during controlled surgical dislocation [89]. The osteotomy is then mobilized, and hip capsule is exposed between the interval of gluteus minimus and the piriformis. A z-shaped capsulotomy is performed, and the femoral head is then dislocated anteriorly (Fig. 47.11). Damage to the acetabular cartilage and labrum is documented and then repaired. Postoperatively, the patient should be on crutches with partial weight bearing for 6–8 weeks, and hip flexion is limited to 70°. Full activities are allowed usually at 3 months.

Mini-Anterior Approach Arthroscopically Assisted

Combined techniques using an anterior approach and arthroscopic support have been used by several noted surgeons to avoid trochanteric osteotomy and to diminish complications of hip arthroscopy during the learning curve [18, 90–101]. Arthroscopic support provides the ability to precisely assess intra-articular lesions, while the limited open exposure provides direct access to anterior acetabular rim and head–neck junction. The main advantages of this technique are avoidance of trochanteric osteotomy and hip dislocation, the ability to directly visualize and correct cam and pincer deformities and less technically demanding than arthroscopic osteochondroplasty. Nevertheless, there is limited ability to work on posterior acetabular rim lesions and moderate risk of injury to the lateral femoral cutaneous nerve. The patient is placed supine on a traction table, and a

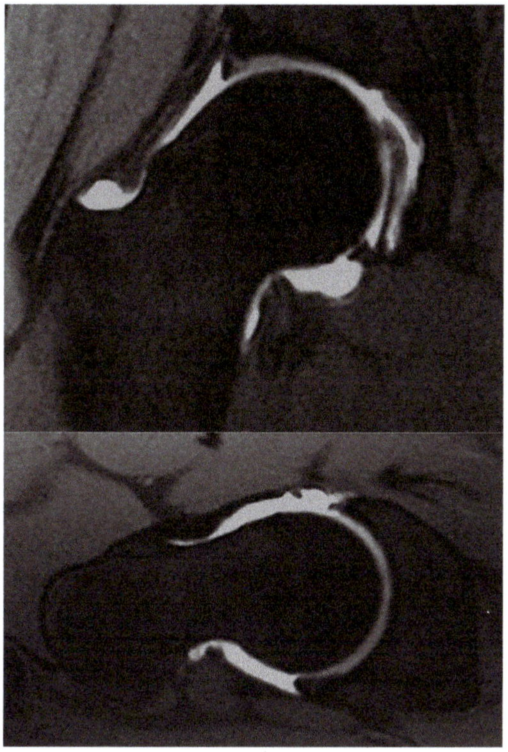

Fig. 47.10 Direct MRA. Coronal slice (superior image) and oblique-axial slice along the neck axis (inferior image)

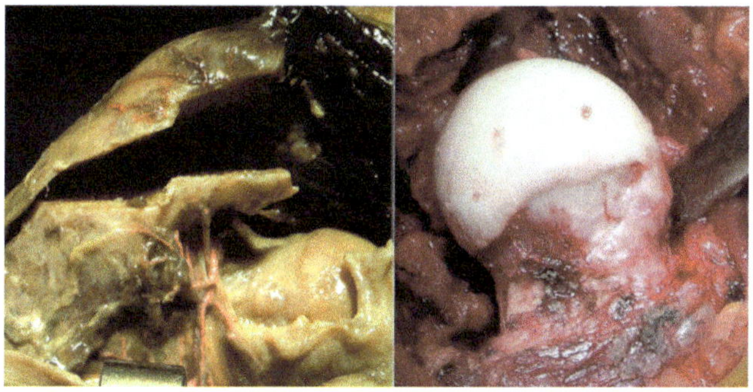

Fig. 47.11 Femoral head dislocation approach. Lateral view of trochanteric osteotomy. A step is performed at the middle osteotomy site to enhance stability (*left image*). Femoral head dislocation (*right image*). Cam deformity is detected at the femoral head–neck junction (*right image*)

modified Hueter mini-anterior approach is performed. The skin incision begins 1 cm distal and lateral to the anterosuperior iliac spine (ASIS) and is extended 6–8 cm distally oriented towards the fibular head (Fig. 47.12). The intermuscular space between sartorius and tensor fascia latae muscles is obtained. A gentle 30° hip flexion is applied and detachment of the reflected portion of rectus femoris muscle is performed to allow a wide exposure of the hip capsule that is opened through a "capital-I"- or "capital-H"-shaped interligamentous capsulotomy. The cam deformity is then

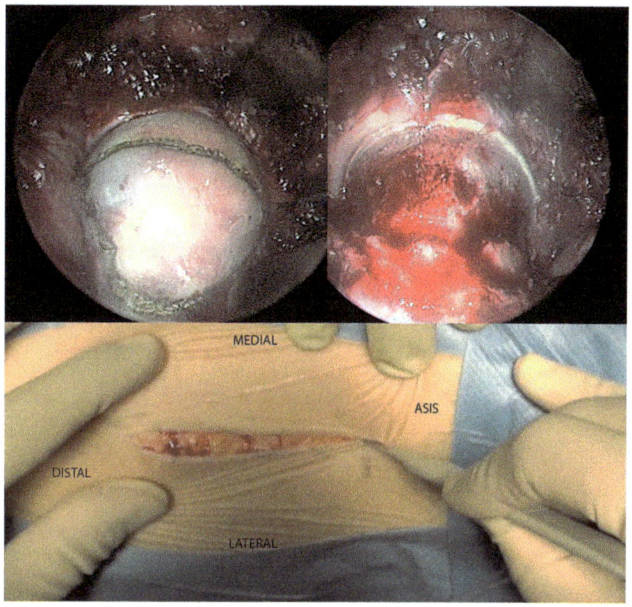

Fig. 47.12 Mini-anterior approach arthroscopically assisted. Skin incision (*bottom image*). Delimitation of cam deformity to be resected (*upper left image*). Final aspect after bone bump resection at femoral head–neck junction (*upper right image*)

visualized, and gentle traction is applied to get enough access to central compartment. A 70° arthroscope is then introduced into the hip joint without fluid. Dry arthroscopic visualization gives information about the extent of chondro-labral damage. Labral and acetabular cartilage repair and osteochondroplasty are done with less traction time than in the pure arthroscopy technique (Fig. 47.12). Capsule closure should be initiated with slight hip extension followed by the superficial fascia, subcutaneous and skin layers. The patient remains on crutches with a partial weight bearing for 3 weeks. Patients were encouraged to start biking as soon as they can, but in cases of labral reattachment, hip flexion restriction to 80°–90° is recommended at the initial rehabilitation phase. Patients are allowed to resume low-impact sports after 12 weeks [79]. Several studies show promising midterm results with this procedure, improving pain and allowing return to activity in young patients with FAI [94]. Even in an athletic population, it has been demonstrated to be an effective surgical procedure that allows patients a successful return to high activity levels and may be comparable with open and arthroscopic treatment of FAI in high expectation patients [96].

Arthroscopic Treatment

Hip arthroscopy has become the most published surgical method to treat FAI [69]. Advances in hip arthroscopy have allowed surgeons to examine the hip joint and treat FAI deformities [102–104]. Although arthroscopic treatment of FAI has increased in popularity in the orthopaedic surgeon community, a lack of consensus on clinical and radiographic indications for the arthroscopic management of FAI has been reported [105]. A recent study demonstrated that hip arthroscopy in patients with FAI without arthritis (joint space greater than 2 mm) is considered a cost-effective intervention [106]. Surgeon experience is the greatest variable when treating FAI through the arthroscopic technique [107, 108]. During the learning curve, it is recommended to avoid complex FAI cases [109]. Arthroscopy can be performed in either the supine or the lateral position based upon the surgeon preference [110, 111]. The surgical technique in FAI requires dynamic intraoperative evaluation, and the surgeon must release traction and mobilize the hip joint intraoperative. Most surgeons start the procedure by entering the central compartment with traction, but other authors access the peripheral compartment first without traction, followed by moving to central compartment under direct arthroscopic visualization and traction [112]. Portal placement should be started by marking the greater trochanter and the anterior superior iliac spine (ASIS) as skin landmarks [113]. The anterolateral portal is situated at the antero-superior corner of the greater trochanter, the posterolateral portal is situated at the postero-superior corner of the greater trochanter, and the anterior portal is situated at the intersection of a horizontal line running anteriorly from the tip of the greater trochanter with a vertical line running down from the ASIS (Fig. 47.13). The central compartment is the space between femoral head and the acetabulum. It is bounded by the acetabular labrum, and at least 10 mm of joint space via traction is required to access it easily. Within this compartment, pincer-type deformities and intra-articular pathology are treated. The anterolateral portal is always the first portal to be established with fluoroscopic assistance. A 70° arthroscope is introduced through this portal into the central compartment. The posterolateral and anterior portals can then be established under direct visualization to avoid iatrogenic injury to the labrum or the cartilage surfaces. A systematic inspection is then performed, by identifying the labrum, acetabular cartilage, cotyloid fossa, ligamentum teres, stellate creases, transverse ligament and weight-bearing portion of femoral head (Fig. 47.13).

The peripheral compartment is the space surrounding the femoral neck, lateral to the labrum. We can easily move from central to peripheral space with traction release and

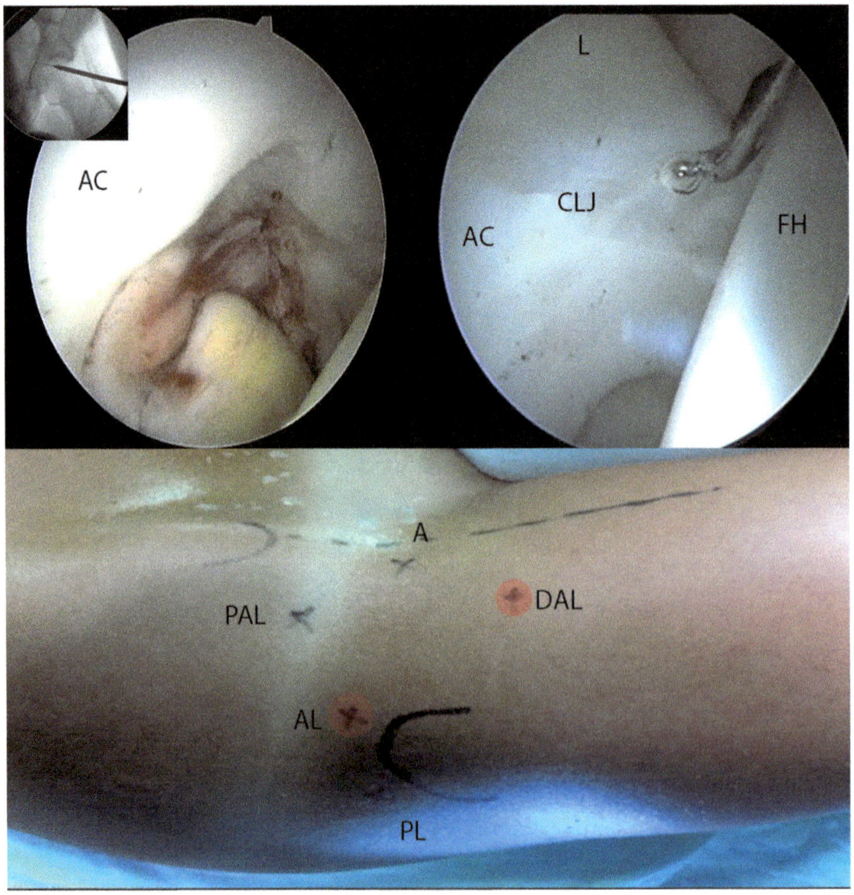

Fig. 47.13 Arthroscopic approach. Arthroscopic hip portals (*bottom image*): anterior (A), anterolateral (AL), posterolateral (PL), distal anterolateral (DAL), proximal anterolateral (PAL). Central compartment arthroscopic view through anterolateral portal (*upper left image*). Acetabular cartilage (AC) and femoral head (FH) are inspected. Chondro-labral injuries are detected and repair at the chondro-labral junction (CLJ) by introducing instruments through distal anterolateral portal (*upper right image*)

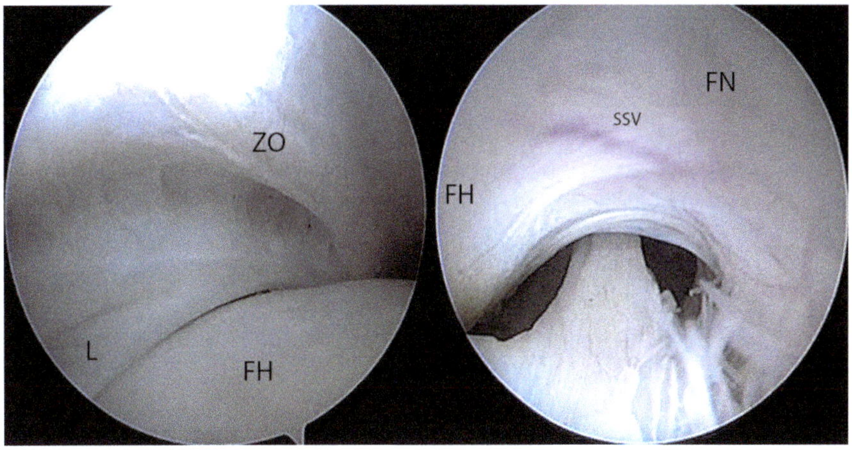

Fig. 47.14 Arthroscopic peripheral compartment. Non-weight-bearing femoral head area (FH), extra-articular labrum zone (L) and zona orbicularis (ZO) can be detected (*left image*). Subsynovial vessels (SSV) can be observed entering to the femoral head (FH) at the femoral neck junction (FN) (*right image*)

flexion of the hip. The key factor to obtain a wide view of the peripheral compartment is a wide anterior capsulotomy [114, 115]. In this compartment, we can detect cam deformity that should be delineated by performing an intraoperative impingement test. Once the size and the location of the cam lesion are verified, the bump is resected with an arthroscopic burr that is introduced through a second portal. Dynamic arthroscopy and fluoroscopy are performed to confirm the absence of any residual impingement (Fig. 47.14).

Although current evidence indicates that hip arthroscopy can significantly reduce pain and improve function in patients with intra-articular hip pathology [116], we should diminish the complication rate that is associated with the learning curve by increasing in the number of programmes offering training in hip arthroscopy [117]. The most common intra-articular structure damaged during hip arthroscopy is the articular cartilage [118] and iatrogenic lesions of the labrum [119, 120]. Neurological complications (sciatic nerve, pudendal nerve, femorocutaneous nerve and femoral nerve injuries) can be related to portal placement, excessive articular distraction and direct compression. Arthroscopic osteochondroplasty has been shown to be equivalent to open procedures [121, 122]. Multiple articles have shown promising early- to midterm results with arthroscopic treatment of FAI reaching up to 80 % of good or excellent clinical results at more than 3 years [123]. Even in patients older than 50 years who underwent hip arthroscopy for FAI, improvement in hip pain and function initially occurs, but 43 % of patients finally require total hip replacement (THR) when less than 2 mm of joint space is present preoperatively [42]. The articular joint space width is the main risk factor regardless of age [124]. When the benefit of hip arthroscopy to treat FAI was analysed in terms of quality of life (QoL) at one year, scores improved in 76.6 % of patients, remained unchanged in 14.4 % and deteriorated in 9.0 % [125].

In conclusion, FAI is a frequent condition in the general population that can cause important limitations in young patients. When left untreated, it could cause degenerative disease of the hip joint. Determining proper surgical indications in a symptomatic patient is an important prerequisite to obtain a successful long-term outcome. When surgical treatment is performed, several surgical techniques are available. Safe surgical dislocation of the femoral head provides excellent visualization of FAI lesions, but it has some disadvantages related to trochanteric osteotomy. Mini-anterior approach arthroscopically assisted is a valuable option with excellent results, but a pure arthroscopic approach of FAI is actually the most popular option despite its large learning curve.

References

1. Harrison MH, Schajowicz F, Trueta J. Osteoarthritis of the hip: a study of the nature and evolution of the disease. J Bone Joint Surg Br. 1953;35-B(4):598–626. Epub 1953/11/01.
2. Smith-Petersen MN. The classic: treatment of malum coxae senilis, old slipped upper femoral epiphysis, intrapelvic protrusion of the acetabulum, and coxa plana by means of acetabuloplasty. 1936. Clin Orthop Relat Res. 2009;467(3):608–15. Epub 2008/12/18.
3. Beck M, Kalhor M, Leunig M, Ganz R. Hip morphology influences the pattern of damage to the acetabular cartilage: femoroacetabular impingement as a cause of early osteoarthritis of the hip. J Bone Joint Surg Br. 2005;87(7):1012–8. Epub 2005/06/24.
4. Ganz R, Parvizi J, Beck M, Leunig M, Notzli H, Siebenrock KA. Femoroacetabular impingement: a cause for osteoarthritis of the hip. Clin Orthop Relat Res. 2003;417:112–20. Epub 2003/12/04.
5. Myers SR, Eijer H, Ganz R. Anterior femoroacetabular impingement after periacetabular osteotomy. Clin Orthop Relat Res. 1999;363:93–9. Epub 1999/06/24.
6. Siebenrock KA, Schoeniger R, Ganz R. Anterior femoroacetabular impingement due to acetabular retroversion. Treatment with periacetabular osteotomy. J Bone Joint Surg Am. 2003;85-A(2):278–86. Epub 2003/02/07.
7. Haviv B, Burg A, Velkes S, Salai M, Dudkiewicz I. Trends in femoroacetabular impingement research over 11 years. Orthopedics. 2011;34(5):353. Epub 2011/05/24.

8. Ganz R, Leunig M, Leunig-Ganz K, Harris WH. The etiology of osteoarthritis of the hip: an integrated mechanical concept. Clin Orthop Relat Res. 2008;466(2):264–72. Epub 2008/01/16.
9. Ito K, Leunig M, Ganz R. Histopathologic features of the acetabular labrum in femoroacetabular impingement. Clin Orthop Relat Res. 2004;429:262–71. Epub 2004/12/04.
10. Leunig M, Podeszwa D, Beck M, Werlen S, Ganz R. Magnetic resonance arthrography of labral disorders in hips with dysplasia and impingement. Clin Orthop Relat Res. 2004;418:74–80. Epub 2004/03/27.
11. Ganz R, Gill TJ, Gautier E, Ganz K, Krugel N, Berlemann U. Surgical dislocation of the adult hip a technique with full access to the femoral head and acetabulum without the risk of avascular necrosis. J Bone Joint Surg Br. 2001;83(8):1119–24. Epub 2002/01/05.
12. Ito K, Minka 2nd MA, Leunig M, Werlen S, Ganz R. Femoroacetabular impingement and the cam-effect. A MRI-based quantitative anatomical study of the femoral head-neck offset. J Bone Joint Surg Br. 2001;83(2):171–6. Epub 2001/04/04.
13. Lavigne M, Parvizi J, Beck M, Siebenrock KA, Ganz R, Leunig M. Anterior femoroacetabular impingement: part I. Techniques of joint preserving surgery. Clin Orthop Relat Res. 2004;418:61–6. Epub 2004/03/27.
14. Notzli HP, Wyss TF, Stoecklin CH, Schmid MR, Treiber K, Hodler J. The contour of the femoral head-neck junction as a predictor for the risk of anterior impingement. J Bone Joint Surg Br. 2002;84(4):556–60. Epub 2002/06/05.
15. Clohisy JC, Dobson MA, Robison JF, Warth LC, Zheng J, Liu SS, et al. Radiographic structural abnormalities associated with premature, natural hip-joint failure. J Bone Joint Surg Am. 2011;93 Suppl 2:3–9. Epub 2011/05/13.
16. Beck M, Leunig M, Parvizi J, Boutier V, Wyss D, Ganz R. Anterior femoroacetabular impingement: part II. Midterm results of surgical treatment. Clin Orthop Relat Res. 2004;418:67–73. Epub 2004/03/27.
17. McCarthy JC, Noble PC, Schuck MR, Wright J, Lee J. The Otto E. Aufranc Award: the role of labral lesions to development of early degenerative hip disease. Clin Orthop Relat Res. 2001;393:25–37. Epub 2002/01/05.
18. Parvizi J, Leunig M, Ganz R. Femoroacetabular impingement. J Am Acad Orthop Surg. 2007;15(9):561–70. Epub 2007/09/01.
19. Audenaert EA, Peeters I, Van Onsem S, Pattyn C. Can we predict the natural course of femoroacetabular impingement? Acta Orthop Belg. 2011;77(2):188–96. Epub 2011/06/15.
20. Bardakos NV, Villar RN. Predictors of progression of osteoarthritis in femoroacetabular impingement: a radiological study with a minimum of ten years follow-up. J Bone Joint Surg. 2009;91(2):162–9. Epub 2009/02/05.
21. Laborie LB, Lehmann TG, Engesaeter IO, Eastwood DM, Engesaeter LB, Rosendahl K. Prevalence of radiographic findings thought to be associated with femoroacetabular impingement in a population-based cohort of 2081 healthy young adults. Radiology. 2011;260(2):494–502. Epub 2011/05/27.
22. Gosvig KK, Jacobsen S, Palm H, Sonne-Holm S, Magnusson E. A new radiological index for assessing asphericity of the femoral head in cam impingement. J Bone Joint Surg Br. 2007;89(10):1309–16. Epub 2007/10/25.
23. Gerhardt MB, Romero AA, Silvers HJ, Harris DJ, Watanabe D, Mandelbaum BR. The prevalence of radiographic hip abnormalities in elite soccer players. Am J Sports Med. 2012;40(3):584–8. Epub 2012/02/22.
24. Nepple JJ, Brophy RH, Matava MJ, Wright RW, Clohisy JC. Radiographic findings of femoroacetabular impingement in National Football League Combine athletes undergoing radiographs for previous hip or groin pain. Arthroscopy. 2012; 28(10):1396–403. Epub 2012/06/16.
25. Marin-Peña O, Gebhard C, Velev K, Ribas-Fernandez M, Plasencia-Arriba M, Marin-Peña O, Gebhard C, Velev K, Ribas-Fernandez M, Plasencia-Arriba M. Femoroacetabular impingement: first step on the way to hip arthroplasty in young patients. J Bone Joint Surg Br. 2006;88-B Suppl 2:329.
26. Ipach I, Mittag F, Syha R, Kunze B, Wolf P, Kluba T. Indications for total hip arthroplasty in young adults—idiopathic osteoarthritis seems to be overestimated. Rofo. 2012;184(3):239–47. Epub 2012/01/26.
27. Lung R, O'Brien J, Grebenyuk J, Forster BB, De Vera M, Kopec J, et al. The prevalence of radiographic femoroacetabular impingement in younger individuals undergoing total hip replacement for osteoarthritis. Clin Rheumatol. 2012;31(8):1239–42. Epub 2012/05/04.
28. Takeyama A, Naito M, Shiramizu K, Kiyama T. Prevalence of femoroacetabular impingement in Asian patients with osteoarthritis of the hip. Int Orthop. 2009;33(5):1229–32. Epub 2009/03/12.
29. Malhotra R, Kannan A, Kancherla R, Khatri D, Kumar V. Femoral head-neck offset in the Indian population: a CT based study. Indian J Orthop. 2012;46(2):212–5. Epub 2012/03/27.
30. Kalberer F, Sierra RJ, Madan SS, Ganz R, Leunig M. Ischial spine projection into the pelvis: a new sign for acetabular retroversion. Clin Orthop Relat Res. 2008;466(3):677–83. Epub 2008/02/12.
31. Siebenrock KA, Kalbermatten DF, Ganz R. Effect of pelvic tilt on acetabular retroversion: a study of pelves from cadavers. Clin Orthop Relat Res. 2003;407:241–8. Epub 2003/02/05.
32. Johnson AC, Shaman MA, Ryan TG. Femoroacetabular impingement in former high-level youth soccer players. Am J Sports Med. 2012;40(6):1342–6. Epub 2012/03/24.
33. Allen D, Beaule PE, Ramadan O, Doucette S. Prevalence of associated deformities and hip pain in patients with cam-type femoroacetabular impingement. J Bone Joint Surg Br. 2009;91(5):589–94. Epub 2009/05/02.
34. Ganz R, Klaue K, Vinh TS, Mast JW. A new periacetabular osteotomy for the treatment of hip dysplasias. Technique and preliminary results. Clin Orthop Relat Res. 1988;232:26–36. Epub 1988/07/01.
35. Reynolds D, Lucas J, Klaue K. Retroversion of the acetabulum. A cause of hip pain. J Bone Joint Surg Br. 1999;81(2):281–8. Epub 1999/04/16.
36. Beall DP, Sweet CF, Martin HD, Lastine CL, Grayson DE, Ly JQ, et al. Imaging findings of femoroacetabular impingement syndrome. Skeletal Radiol. 2005;34(11):691–701. Epub 2005/09/21.
37. Jager M, Wild A, Westhoff B, Krauspe R. Femoroacetabular impingement caused by a femoral osseous head-neck bump deformity: clinical, radiological, and experimental results. J Orthop Sci. 2004;9(3):256–63. Epub 2004/05/29.
38. Philippon MJ, Maxwell RB, Johnston TL, Schenker M, Briggs KK. Clinical presentation of femoroacetabular impingement. Knee Surg Sports Traumatol Arthrosc. 2007;15(8):1041–7. Epub 2007/05/15.
39. Philippon MJ, Schenker ML. Arthroscopy for the treatment of femoroacetabular impingement in the athlete. Clin Sports Med. 2006;25(2):299–308. ix. Epub 2006/04/28.
40. Tijssen M, van Cingel R, Willemsen L, de Visser E. Diagnostics of femoroacetabular impingement and labral pathology of the hip: a systematic review of the accuracy and validity of physical tests. Arthroscopy. 2012;28(6):860–71. Epub 2012/03/01.
41. Tonnis D. Normal values of the hip joint for the evaluation of X-rays in children and adults. Clin Orthop Relat Res. 1976;119:39–47. Epub 1976/09/01.
42. Philippon MJ, Schroder ESBG, Briggs KK. Hip arthroscopy for femoroacetabular impingement in patients aged 50 years or older. Arthroscopy. 2012;28(1):59–65. Epub 2011/10/11.

43. Larson CM, Giveans MR, Taylor M. Does arthroscopic FAI correction improve function with radiographic arthritis? Clin Orthop Relat Res. 2011;469(6):1667–76. Epub 2010/12/25.
44. Philippon MJ, Briggs KK, Yen YM, Kuppersmith DA. Outcomes following hip arthroscopy for femoroacetabular impingement with associated chondrolabral dysfunction: minimum two-year follow-up. J Bone Joint Surg Br. 2009;91(1):16–23. Epub 2008/12/19.
45. Miguel OF, Cabrita HB, Rodrigues MB, Croci AT. A comparative radiographic investigation of femoroacetabular impingement in young patients with and without hip pain. Clinics (Sao Paulo). 2012;67(5):463–7. Epub 2012/06/06.
46. Cavaignac E, Chiron P, Espie A, Reina N, Lepage B, Laffosse JM. Experimental study of an original radiographic view for diagnosis of cam-type anterior femoroacetabular impingement. Int Orthop. 2012;36(9):1783–8. Epub 2012/05/04.
47. Domayer SE, Ziebarth K, Chan J, Bixby S, Mamisch TC, Kim YJ. Femoroacetabular cam-type impingement: diagnostic sensitivity and specificity of radiographic views compared to radial MRI. Eur J Radiol. 2011;80(3):805–10. Epub 2010/11/16.
48. Meyer DC, Beck M, Ellis T, Ganz R, Leunig M. Comparison of six radiographic projections to assess femoral head/neck asphericity. Clin Orthop Relat Res. 2006;445:181–5. Epub 2006/02/04.
49. Sutter R, Dietrich TJ, Zingg PO, Pfirrmann CW. How useful is the alpha angle for discriminating between symptomatic patients with cam-type femoroacetabular impingement and asymptomatic volunteers? Radiology. 2012;264(2):514–21. Epub 2012/06/02.
50. Kumar R, Aggarwal A. Femoroacetabular impingement and risk factors: a study of 50 cases. Orthop Surg. 2011;3(4):236–41. Epub 2011/10/25.
51. Pollard TC, Villar RN, Norton MR, Fern ED, Williams MR, Simpson DJ, et al. Femoroacetabular impingement and classification of the cam deformity: the reference interval in normal hips. Acta Orthop. 2010;81(1):134–41. Epub 2010/02/24.
52. Marin-Pena O, Ribas-Fernandez M, Valles-Purroy A, Pareja JA, Benito E, Plasencia-Arriba MA, et al. Preoperative planning in femoroacetabular impingement: a novel template tool. Hip Int. 2008;18(2):173–89.
53. Eijer H, Leunig M, Mahomed MN, Ganz R. Crosstable lateral radiograph for screening of anterior femoral head–neck offset in patients with femoro-acetabular impingement. Hip Int. 2001;11:37–41.
54. Murphy SB, Ganz R, Muller ME. The prognosis in untreated dysplasia of the hip. A study of radiographic factors that predict the outcome. J Bone Joint Surg Am. 1995;77(7):985–9. Epub 1995/07/01.
55. Li PL, Ganz R. Morphologic features of congenital acetabular dysplasia: one in six is retroverted. Clin Orthop Relat Res. 2003;416:245–53. Epub 2003/12/04.
56. Kappe T, Kocak T, Neuerburg C, Lippacher S, Bieger R, Reichel H. Reliability of radiographic signs for acetabular retroversion. Int Orthop. 2011;35(6):817–21. Epub 2010/05/11.
57. Wassilew GI, Heller MO, Diederichs G, Janz V, Wenzl M, Perka C. Standardized AP radiographs do not provide reliable diagnostic measures for the assessment of acetabular retroversion. J Orthop Res. 2012;30(9):1369–76. Epub 2012/03/14.
58. Werner CM, Copeland CE, Ruckstuhl T, Stromberg J, Turen CH, Kalberer F, et al. Radiographic markers of acetabular retroversion: correlation of the cross-over sign, ischial spine sign and posterior wall sign. Acta Orthop Belg. 2010;76(2):166–73. Epub 2010/05/28.
59. Dandachli W, Ul Islam S, Tippett R, Hall-Craggs MA, Witt JD. Analysis of acetabular version in the native hip: comparison between 2D axial CT and 3D CT measurements. Skeletal Radiol. 2011;40(7):877–83. Epub 2010/12/25.
60. Heyworth BE, Dolan MM, Nguyen JT, Chen NC, Kelly BT. Preoperative three-dimensional CT predicts intraoperative findings in hip arthroscopy. Clin Orthop Relat Res. 2012;470(7):1950–7. Epub 2012/04/25.
61. Beaule PE, Zaragoza E, Motamedi K, Copelan N, Dorey FJ. Three-dimensional computed tomography of the hip in the assessment of femoroacetabular impingement. J Orthop Res. 2005;23(6):1286–92. Epub 2005/06/01.
62. Kassarjian A, Brisson M, Palmer WE. Femoroacetabular impingement. Eur J Radiol. 2007;63(1):29–35. Epub 2007/05/09.
63. Mosher TJ, Smith H, Dardzinski BJ, Schmithorst VJ, Smith MB. MR imaging and T2 mapping of femoral cartilage: in vivo determination of the magic angle effect. AJR Am J Roentgenol. 2001;177(3):665–9. Epub 2001/08/23.
64. Kassarjian A, Yoon LS, Belzile E, Connolly SA, Millis MB, Palmer WE. Triad of MR arthrographic findings in patients with cam-type femoroacetabular impingement. Radiology. 2005;236(2):588–92. Epub 2005/06/24.
65. Steinbach LS, Palmer WE, Schweitzer ME. Special focus session. MR arthrography. Radiographics. 2002;22(5):1223–46. Epub 2002/09/18.
66. Bashir A, Gray ML, Boutin RD, Burstein D. Glycosaminoglycan in articular cartilage: in vivo assessment with delayed Gd(DTPA)(2-)-enhanced MR imaging. Radiology. 1997;205(2):551–8. Epub 1997/11/14.
67. Bittersohl B, Hosalkar HS, Haamberg T, Kim YJ, Werlen S, Siebenrock KA, et al. Reproducibility of dGEMRIC in assessment of hip joint cartilage: a prospective study. J Magn Reson Imaging. 2009;30(1):224–8. Epub 2009/06/27.
68. Papalia R, Del Buono A, Franceschi F, Marinozzi A, Maffulli N, Denaro V. Femoroacetabular impingement syndrome management: arthroscopy or open surgery? Int Orthop. 2012;36(5):903–14. Epub 2011/12/23.
69. Botser IB, Smith Jr TW, Nasser R, Domb BG. Open surgical dislocation versus arthroscopy for femoroacetabular impingement: a comparison of clinical outcomes. Arthroscopy. 2011;27(2):270–8. Epub 2011/01/27.
70. Matsuda DK, Carlisle JC, Arthurs SC, Wierks CH, Philippon MJ. Comparative systematic review of the open dislocation, mini-open, and arthroscopic surgeries for femoroacetabular impingement. Arthroscopy. 2011;27(2):252–69. Epub 2011/01/27.
71. Larson CM, Giveans MR, Stone RM. Arthroscopic debridement versus refixation of the acetabular labrum associated with femoroacetabular impingement: mean 3.5-year follow-up. Am J Sports Med. 2012;40(5):1015–21. Epub 2012/02/07.
72. Philippon MJ, Briggs KK, Hay CJ, Kuppersmith DA, Dewing CB, Huang MJ. Arthroscopic labral reconstruction in the hip using iliotibial band autograft: technique and early outcomes. Arthroscopy. 2010;26(6):750–6. Epub 2010/06/01.
73. Tey M, Erquicia JI, Pelfort X, Miquel J, Gelber PE, Ribas M. Allogenic labral transplantation in hip instability following arthroscopic labrectomy. Hip Int. 2011;21(2):260–2. Epub 2011/04/13.
74. Philippon MJ, Wolff AB, Briggs KK, Zehms CT, Kuppersmith DA. Acetabular rim reduction for the treatment of femoroacetabular impingement correlates with preoperative and postoperative center-edge angle. Arthroscopy. 2010;26(6):757–61. Epub 2010/06/01.
75. Stafford GH, Bunn JR, Villar RN. Arthroscopic repair of delaminated acetabular articular cartilage using fibrin adhesive. Results at one to three years. Hip Int. 2011;21(6):744–50. Epub 2011/11/26.
76. Leunig M, Tibor LM, Naal FD, Ganz R, Steinwachs MR. Surgical technique: second-generation bone marrow stimulation via surgical dislocation to treat hip cartilage lesions. Clin Orthop Relat Res. 2012;470(12):3421–31. Epub 2012/07/10.

77. Fontana A, Bistolfi A, Crova M, Rosso F, Massazza G. Arthroscopic treatment of hip chondral defects: autologous chondrocyte transplantation versus simple debridement—a pilot study. Arthroscopy. 2012;28(3):322–9. Epub 2011/12/07.
78. Philippon MJ, Schenker ML, Briggs KK, Maxwell RB. Can microfracture produce repair tissue in acetabular chondral defects? Arthroscopy. 2008;24(1):46–50. Epub 2008/01/10.
79. Marín-Peña Ó. Femoroacetabular impingement. New York: Springer; 2012.
80. Mardones RM, Gonzalez C, Chen Q, Zobitz M, Kaufman KR, Trousdale RT. Surgical treatment of femoroacetabular impingement: evaluation of the effect of the size of the resection. J Bone Joint Surg Am. 2005;87(2):273–9. Epub 2005/02/03.
81. Ecker TM, Puls M, Steppacher SD, Bastian JD, Keel MJ, Siebenrock KA, et al. Computer-assisted femoral head-neck osteochondroplasty using a surgical milling device an in vitro accuracy study. J Arthroplasty. 2012;27(2):310–6. Epub 2011/05/31.
82. Beaule PE, Le Duff MJ, Zaragoza E. Quality of life following femoral head-neck osteochondroplasty for femoroacetabular impingement. J Bone Joint Surg Am. 2007;89(4):773–9. Epub 2007/04/04.
83. Espinosa N, Rothenfluh DA, Beck M, Ganz R, Leunig M. Treatment of femoro-acetabular impingement: preliminary results of labral refixation. J Bone Joint Surg Am. 2006;88(5):925–35. Epub 2006/05/03.
84. Murphy S, Tannast M, Kim YJ, Buly R, Millis MB. Debridement of the adult hip for femoroacetabular impingement: indications and preliminary clinical results. Clin Orthop Relat Res. 2004;429:178–81. Epub 2004/12/04.
85. Emara K, Samir W, el Motasem H, Ghafar KA. Conservative treatment for mild femoroacetabular impingement. J Orthop Surg (Hong Kong). 2011;19(1):41–5. Epub 2011/04/27.
86. Peters CL, Stronach BM, Pelt CE, Erickson JA. Open surgical dislocation for the treatment of femoroacetabular impingement: past, present, and future. Instr Course Lect. 2012;61:273–86. Epub 2012/02/04.
87. Naal FD, Miozzari HH, Schar M, Hesper T, Notzli HP. Midterm results of surgical hip dislocation for the treatment of femoroacetabular impingement. Am J Sports Med. 2012;40(7):1501–10. Epub 2012/05/05.
88. Mercati E, Guary A, Myquel C, Bourgeon A. [A postero-external approach to the hip joint. Value of the formation of a digastric muscle]. J Chir. 1972;103(5):499–504. Epub 1972/05/01. Une voie d'abord postero-externe de la hanche. Interet de la realisation d'un muscle digastrique.
89. Locher S, Werlen S, Leunig M, Ganz R. [MR-Arthrography with radial sequences for visualization of early hip pathology not visible on plain radiographs]. Z Orthop Ihre Grenzgeb. 2002;140(1):52–7. Epub 2002/03/19. Arthro-MRI mit radiarer Schnittsequenz zur Darstellung der praradiologischen Huftpathologie.
90. Ribas M, Vilarrubias JM, Ginebreda I, Silberberg J, Leal J. [Atrapamiento o choque femoroacetabular]. Rev Ortop Traumatol. 2005;49:390–403.
91. Ribas M, Marin-Pena OR, Regenbrecht B, De La Torre B, Vilarrubias JM. Hip osteoplasty by an anterior minimally invasive approach for active patients with femoroacetabular impingement. Hip Int. 2007;17(2):91–8. Epub 2007/04/01.
92. Clohisy JC, McClure JT. Treatment of anterior femoroacetabular impingement with combined hip arthroscopy and limited anterior decompression. Iowa Orthop J. 2005;25:164–71. Epub 2005/08/11.
93. Laude F, Sariali E, Nogier A. Femoroacetabular impingement treatment using arthroscopy and anterior approach. Clin Orthop Relat Res. 2009;467(3):747–52. Epub 2008/12/18.
94. Parvizi J, Huang R, Diaz-Ledezma C, Og B. Mini-open femoroacetabular osteoplasty: how do these patients do? J Arthroplasty. 2012;27(8 Suppl):122–5.e1. Epub 2012/06/12.
95. Barton C, Banga K, Beaule PE. Anterior Hueter approach in the treatment of femoro-acetabular impingement: rationale and technique. Orthop Clin North Am. 2009;40(3):389–95. Epub 2009/07/07.
96. Cohen SB, Huang R, Ciccotti MG, Dodson CC, Parvizi J. Treatment of femoroacetabular impingement in athletes using a mini-direct anterior approach. Am J Sports Med. 2012;40(7):1620–7. Epub 2012/05/09.
97. Malik AK, Chou DT, Witt JD. Anterior approaches to the hip for the treatment of femoro-acetabular impingement: a cadaveric study. Hip Int. 2010;20(4):482–8. Epub 2010/12/16.
98. Trevino-Garza O, Rivas-Fernandez M, Marin-Pena O, Esteban-Ledezma R, Vilarubias-Guillament JM. [Treatment of femoroacetabular impingement by a minimally invasive approach. Results at 2 years follow-up]. Acta Ortop Mex. 2009;23(2):57–69. Epub 2009/05/13. Tratamiento del pinzamiento femoro-acetabular mediante abordaje minimo invasivo. Resultados con 2 anos de seguimiento.
99. Lincoln M, Johnston K, Muldoon M, Santore R. Combined arthroscopic and modified open approach for cam femoroacetabular impingement: a preliminary experience. Arthroscopy. 2009;25(4):392–9. Epub 2009/04/04.
100. Hartmann A, Gunther KP. Arthroscopically assisted anterior decompression for femoroacetabular impingement: technique and early clinical results. Arch Orthop Trauma Surg. 2009;129(8):1001–9. Epub 2009/01/07.
101. Chiron P, Espie A, Reina N, Cavaignac E, Molinier F, Laffosse JM. Surgery for femoroacetabular impingement using a minimally invasive anterolateral approach: analysis of 118 cases at 2.2-year follow-up. Orthop Traumatol Surg Res. 2012;98(1):30–8. Epub 2012/01/20.
102. Byrd JW. Hip arthroscopy by the supine approach. Instr Course Lect. 2006;55:325–36. Epub 2006/09/09.
103. Philippon MJ, Stubbs AJ, Schenker ML, Maxwell RB, Ganz R, Leunig M. Arthroscopic management of femoroacetabular impingement: osteoplasty technique and literature review. Am J Sports Med. 2007;35(9):1571–80. Epub 2007/04/11.
104. Bardakos NV, Vasconcelos JC, Villar RN. Early outcome of hip arthroscopy for femoroacetabular impingement: the role of femoral osteoplasty in symptomatic improvement. J Bone Joint Surg Br. 2008;90(12):1570–5. Epub 2008/12/02.
105. Ayeni OR, Wong I, Chien T, Musahl V, Kelly BT, Bhandari M. Surgical indications for arthroscopic management of femoroacetabular impingement. Arthroscopy. 2012;28(8):1170–9. Epub 2012/04/27.
106. Shearer DW, Kramer J, Bozic KJ, Feeley BT. Is hip arthroscopy cost-effective for femoroacetabular impingement? Clin Orthop Relat Res. 2012;470(4):1079–89. Epub 2011/08/16.
107. Sampson TG. Arthroscopic treatment of femoroacetabular impingement: a proposed technique with clinical experience. Instr Course Lect. 2006;55:337–46. Epub 2006/09/09.
108. Byrd JW. Hip arthroscopy: surgical indications. Arthroscopy. 2006;22(12):1260–2. Epub 2006/12/15.
109. Kelly BT, Williams III RJ, Philippon MJ. Hip arthroscopy: current indications, treatment options, and management issues. Am J Sports Med. 2003;31(6):1020–37. Epub 2003/11/19.
110. Mason JB, McCarthy JC, O'Donnell J, Barsoum W, Mayor MB, Busconi BD, et al. Hip arthroscopy: surgical approach, positioning, and distraction. Clin Orthop Relat Res. 2003;406:29–37. Epub 2003/02/13.
111. Byrd JW. Hip arthroscopy. The supine position. Clin Sports Med. 2001;20(4):703–31. Epub 2001/10/26.

112. Dienst M, Seil R, Kohn DM. Safe arthroscopic access to the central compartment of the hip. Arthroscopy. 2005;21(12):1510–4. Epub 2005/12/27.
113. Byrd JW, Pappas JN, Pedley MJ. Hip arthroscopy: an anatomic study of portal placement and relationship to the extra-articular structures. Arthroscopy. 1995;11(4):418–23. Epub 1995/08/01.
114. Ilizaliturri Jr VM. Complications of arthroscopic femoroacetabular impingement treatment: a review. Clin Orthop Relat Res. 2009;467(3):760–8. Epub 2008/11/20.
115. Dienst M, Godde S, Seil R, Hammer D, Kohn D. Hip arthroscopy without traction: in vivo anatomy of the peripheral hip joint cavity. Arthroscopy. 2001;17(9):924–31. Epub 2001/11/06.
116. Kemp JL, Collins NJ, Makdissi M, Schache AG, Machotka Z, Crossley K. Hip arthroscopy for intra-articular pathology: a systematic review of outcomes with and without femoral osteoplasty. Br J Sports Med. 2012;46(9):632–43. Epub 2011/12/24.
117. Colvin AC, Harrast J, Harner C. Trends in hip arthroscopy. J Bone Joint Surg Am. 2012;94(4):e23. Epub 2012/02/18.
118. Dorfmann H, Boyer T. Arthroscopy of the hip: 12 years of experience. Arthroscopy. 1999;15(1):67–72. Epub 1999/02/19.
119. McCarthy JC, Lee JA. Hip arthroscopy: indications, outcomes, and complications. Instr Course Lect. 2006;55:301–8. Epub 2006/09/09.
120. Domb B, Hanypsiak B, Botser I. Labral penetration rate in a consecutive series of 300 hip arthroscopies. Am J Sports Med. 2012;40(4):864–9. Epub 2012/03/01.
121. Sussmann PS, Ranawat AS, Lipman J, Lorich DG, Padgett DE, Kelly BT. Arthroscopic versus open osteoplasty of the head-neck junction: a cadaveric investigation. Arthroscopy. 2007;23(12):1257–64. Epub 2007/12/08.
122. Mardones R, Lara J, Donndorff A, Barnes S, Stuart MJ, Glick J, et al. Surgical correction of "cam-type" femoroacetabular impingement: a cadaveric comparison of open versus arthroscopic debridement. Arthroscopy. 2009;25(2):175–82. Epub 2009/01/28.
123. Byrd JW, Jones KS. Arthroscopic management of femoroacetabular impingement: minimum 2-year follow-up. Arthroscopy. 2011;27(10):1379–88. Epub 2011/08/25.
124. Cooper AP, Basheer SZ, Maheshwari R, Regan L, Madan SS. Outcomes of hip arthroscopy. A prospective analysis and comparison between patients under 25 and over 25 years of age. Br J Sports Med. 2013;47(4):234–8. Epub 2012/07/17.
125. Malviya A, Stafford GH, Villar RN. Impact of arthroscopy of the hip for femoroacetabular impingement on quality of life at a mean follow-up of 3.2 years. J Bone Joint Surg Br. 2012;94(4):466–70. Epub 2012/03/22.

Arthroscopic Treatment of Combined Cam- and Pincer-Type Femoroacetabular Impingement

48

Christopher M. Larson, Rebecca M. Stone, and Patrick M. Birmingham

Introduction

Femoroacetabular impingement (FAI) is a disorder associated with labrochondral injury and the potential development of osteoarthritis [1–6]. The two most common types of FAI are cam and pincer [1–6]. Cam-type impingement is the result of asphericity and decreased head-neck offset of the femoral head-neck junction, whereas pincer-type impingement results from acetabular overcoverage [1–3, 5, 6]. FAI can also be secondary to extra-articular sources such as anterior inferior iliac spine (AIIS) impingement/subspine impingement [7, 8] and ischiofemoral impingement [9–11]. Pathomechanics, common subtypes of FAI, clinical presentation, imaging, surgical indications, surgical techniques, and outcomes will be described.

Anatomy and Pathomechanics

Pincer-type FAI results in crushing of the acetabular rim and labrum against the femoral neck or femoral head-neck junction. Isolated pincer-type impingement leads to edge loading of the acetabular rim and labrum (Fig. 48.1a) without separation of the labrochondral junction [1–6]. Pincer-type pathology can also lead to posterior subluxation of the femoral head with resultant "contrecoup" posterior acetabular chondromalacia [1–6]. There are three primary types of pincer-type impingement: focal anterior overcoverage, relative anterior overcoverage as seen in acetabular retroversion, and global acetabular overcoverage.

The pathogenesis of cam-type FAI is unclear. It has been suggested that excessive loading secondary to athletic activities during adolescence may result in adaptive physeal remodeling and bony apposition at the head-neck junction leading to this asphericity [12]. Excessive coxa vara and relative femoral neck retroversion can also contribute to proximal femoral impingement. Isolated cam-type FAI generally produces shear forces, resulting in eventual disruption of the acetabular articular cartilage from the labrum (Fig. 48.1b) [1, 12–15].

Extra-articular sources of impingement have been recently described. AIIS impingement is a less common type of acetabular-based impingement. The AIIS serves as the origin of the direct head of the rectus femoris, and impingement can be secondary to prior avulsion injury, pelvic osteotomy, or developmental as seen in the setting of acetabular retroversion [7, 8]. Ischiofemoral impingement is a rare type of proximal femoral-based impingement that occurs between the lesser trochanter and the ischial tuberosity. The quadratus femoris occupies this space and may be compressed when this space is reduced. The normal distance between the lesser trochanter and the ischial tuberosity is said to be 20 mm [9]. This space is said to be reduced to around 13 mm in patients with ischiofemoral impingement. Also, women because of the wider positioning of their ischial tuberosities appear to be more at risk [10].

Clinical Presentation

Patients complain primarily of intermittent activity-related anterior groin pain during activities which can progress to limiting pain during and after activity. Patients may complain of pain with torsional activities, getting in and out of a car, difficulty with prolonged sitting, difficulty putting on socks and shoes, and a history of the inability to sit in a figure of

C.M. Larson, MD (✉) • R.M. Stone, MS, ATC
Minnesota Orthopedic Sports Medicine Institute at Twin Cities Orthopedics, 4010 West 65th Street, Edina, MN 55435, USA
e-mail: chrislarson@tcomn.com; beckystone@tcomn.com

P.M. Birmingham, MD
Division of Sports Medicine, Department of Orthopaedic Surgery, Northshore University Health System Chicago, Chicago, IL, USA
e-mail: patrickbirmingham@gmail.com

J.C. McCarthy et al. (eds.), *Hip Joint Restoration*, DOI 10.1007/978-1-4614-0694-5_48

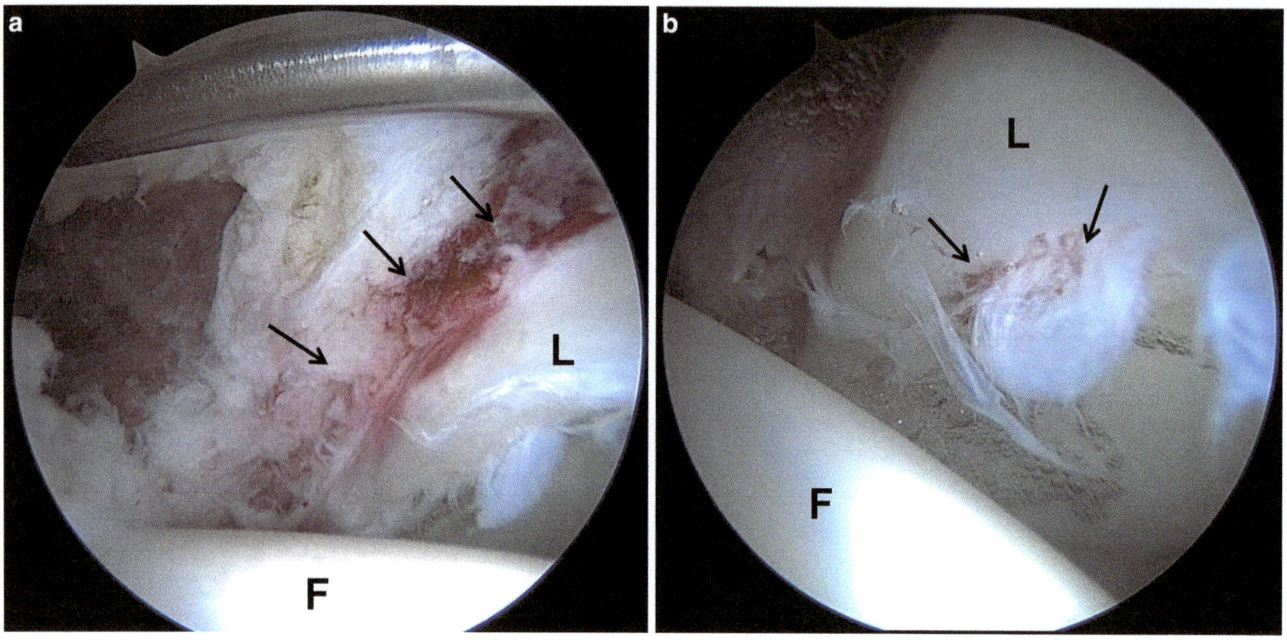

Fig. 48.1 (**a**) An arthroscopic image of the left hip reveals peripheral labral bruising (*arrows*) consistent with pincer-type impingement. (**b**) Arthroscopic image reveals a labral chondral disruption (*arrows*) consistent with cam-type impingement. *F* femoral head, *L* labrum

four position, or with their legs crossed. Cam impingement, combined cam- and pincer-type pathology, and, to a lesser degree, isolated pincer-type pathology can lead to significant motion limitations. Subspine (AIIS) impingement typically presents with groin pain with hip flexion-based activities and limitations in hip flexion [7]. Patients with ischiofemoral impingement present with chronic pain in the groin or buttock in the absence of any history of injury. The pain may radiate distally and may present in association with chronic psoas and/or proximal hamstring tendonitis [11].

Physical Examination

In the presence of FAI, range of motion (ROM) assessment may reveal limitations in forward flexion (FF), internal rotation (IR), abduction, as well as an increased distance from the lateral knee to the examination table with FABER's testing. Relatively decreased internal rotation and increased external rotation may be indicative of femoral neck retroversion. Obligate abduction and external rotation (ER) of the hip during FF ROM testing can also be indicative of anterolateral hip impingement. Groin pain elicited with the anterior impingement test (forward flexion, internal rotation, and adduction of the hip) may indicate anterolateral rim pathology, whereas posterolateral pain with posterior impingement testing (extension, abduction, external rotation of the hip) can be indicative of posterolateral rim pathology [16–19]. Apprehension and anterior pain with hip extension and external rotation may be indicative of structural instability. A low volume intra-articular anesthetic injection (<5 cm^3) followed by physical examination or performing the inciting activities can be invaluable to confirm the hip joint as a source of pain.

In the presence of AIIS impingement, hip flexion ROM is limited, and palpation over the AIIS reproduces the typical pain. An intra-articular injection will give partial relief if intra-articular pathology coexists, but the restricted ROM persists. A subspine injection may be diagnostic. For ischiofemoral impingement, the symptoms can be reproduced by a combination of extension, adduction, and external rotation [9]. Temporary relief of the symptoms can be provided by CT-guided injection around the quadratus femoris [20].

Imaging

We routinely obtain an anteroposterior (AP) pelvis of both hips, a modified 45° flexion Dunn view, cross-table lateral, and false-profile view of the affected hip. It is imperative that the AP pelvis has the coccyx centered over the pubic symphysis with 0–3 cm between these two structures in order to accurately evaluate acetabular version [21]. The three previously mentioned types of pincer impingement are best evaluated by plain radiographs as follows. Focal anterior overcoverage (cranial retroversion) is indicated by a positive

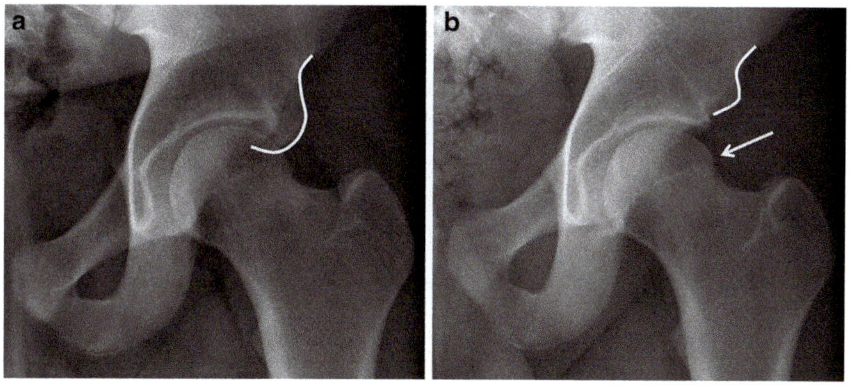

Fig. 48.2 (**a**) Preoperative plain AP radiograph of the left hip reveals a distal anterior inferior iliac spine deformity (*curved line*) and mild superior cam morphology (*arrow*). (**b**) Postoperative AP plain radiograph after arthroscopic anterior inferior iliac spine decompression and minimal cam decompression

crossover sign, negative posterior wall sign, and lateral center-edge angle (LCE) of greater than 25°. True acetabular retroversion is indicated by a crossover sign, a positive posterior wall sign, and positive ischial spine sign. Global acetabular overcoverage is typically secondary to coxa profunda or protrusio acetabuli. Coxa profunda is diagnosed by plain radiographs when the teardrop lies medial to the ilioischial line with a LCE of greater than 35°. Protrusio acetabuli is diagnosed by plain radiographs when the medial aspect of the femoral head lies medial to the ilioischial line. Findings consistent with cam-type FAI include an elevated alpha angle of greater than 55° and or decreased head-neck offset of <8–10 mm [13, 21–24]. Superior and inferior cam morphology can be visualized on the AP radiograph, whereas anterior and posterior cam morphology is seen on the lateral radiographs.

Subspine impingement is evaluated on the standard AP pelvis and false-profile views. Evidence of prior AIIS avulsion and calcification within the rectus origin can be seen in this setting. Extension of the AIIS below the sourcil on an AP radiograph (Fig. 48.2) may be indicative of AIIS impingement, and excessive anterior and distal extension of the AIIS can be further defined on the false-profile view.

Advanced Imaging

MRI has been shown to be accurate for evaluation of labral greater than chondral abnormalities [25, 26]. Axial and radial imaging of the femoral head-neck junction also allows for an evaluation of the proximal femoral head-neck junction morphology [13, 27]. For ischiofemoral impingement, radiographs are not typically diagnostic, and MRI and CT appear to be the best diagnostic tools. MRI axial and coronal T2-weighted images typically show edema in the muscle belly of the quadratus femoris without disruption of its fibers [28].

Although MRI can be used to evaluate bony pathology, we find that three-dimensional computerized tomography (3-D CT) is invaluable. Rim hyperostosis, rim fractures/os acetabuli, and AIIS deformity are well visualized, and axial images allow for evaluation of acetabular version and anterior and posterior coverage. The extent of the cam deformity and its proximity to the retinacular vessels can be evaluated, and sections through the knee can be obtained in order to assess femoral neck version in an effort to better globally assess the hip joint. Although the radiation dose can be minimized with specific CT protocols, there remains some concern regarding radiation exposure.

Arthroscopic Surgical Indications

Anteriorly based cam-type morphology can be addressed with an arthroscopic approach. Cam-type morphology that is visible on AP radiographs, indicating extension beyond the lateral retinacular vessels (superoposterior) and medial synovial fold (inferoposterior), is much more technically challenging to address arthroscopically but can be managed with experience. Two cadaveric studies comparing open versus arthroscopic femoral resection osteochondroplasty showed no clear advantage for either approach with respect to depth or arc of resection [29, 30]. A clinical study evaluated pre- and postoperative radiographs of patients that underwent open versus arthroscopic femoral resection osteochondroplasty and found no differences between approaches for anteriorly based cam morphology; however, better resections were noted superiorly on anteroposterior radiographs with an open approach [31]. Focal anterior overcoverage (cranial retroversion), moderate degrees of acetabular retroversion, coxa profunda, and, in some instances, protrusio can be managed with an arthroscopic approach. The majority of the acetabular rim can be addressed with experience.

Contraindications

Symptomatic posterior femoral head-neck deformities are not predictably accessed arthroscopically, and a surgical dislocation should be considered in these situations. Moderate to severe deformities (i.e., moderate to severe slipped capital femoral epiphysis [SCFE], complex Perthes) may require open corrective procedures. Additionally, cam deformities are not infrequent findings in the setting of hip dysplasia. When dysplastic features predominate, corrective osteotomies should be considered when contemplating surgical treatment. The senior author will consider referral for corrective osteotomies when the LCE is less than 20°, anterior center-edge angle (ACE) is less than 15°, and Tonnis angle is greater than 15° and when there is lateralization of the femur greater than 1 cm and/or a break in Shenton's line.

Protrusio can be very challenging to manage arthroscopically as arthroscopic dynamic assessment is limited in comparison to a surgical dislocation. In addition, there is some evidence supporting increased stress in protrusio hips at the medial aspect of the hip rather than the rim, and some authors have proposed an anteversion pelvic osteotomy (PAO), posterior rim resection, and possible proximal femoral osteotomy in these instances [32]. In addition, severe acetabular retroversion may be better addressed with an anteversion PAO.

Surgical Technique

The current authors perform arthroscopy in the supine position with a two to three portal technique and typically use the anterolateral portal and mid-anterior portal and occasionally formally establish the posterolateral portal for posterior rim resection in the setting of profunda [33, 34]. Labral preservation is preferred to indiscriminate debridement/excision whenever possible [2, 33, 35]. If the labrum has significant intrasubstance/cytic/calcific deposits or is ossified, a debridement is appropriate. Labral preservation in the setting of pincer impingement and rim resection can be performed with one of two primary techniques: takedown and no takedown [36]. For the "no takedown" technique, a 5.5 mm burr is introduced via the mid-anterior portal, and the rim is resected peripheral to the labrum from anterior to superior (Fig. 48.3a, b). The burr is then introduced via the anterior portal to resect the superior to posterior rim when indicated and to verify resection immediately adjacent to the labrum (Fig. 48.3c). For resections further posteriorly, it can be helpful to temporarily increase traction and/or place the burr in the posterolateral portal. Suture anchors (typically 3–4) are then placed close (1–2 mm) to the articular margin while avoiding penetration of the acetabular articular cartilage and approximately 1 cm apart. Further distal portals are helpful to achieve a safe and effective angle for anchor placement. One limb of the suture is then placed under the labrum, and one limb is passed through the labrum creating a mattress suture, which may better recreate the labral seal, followed by standard knot tying (Fig. 48.4). Alternatively, the labrum can be sharply detached from the acetabular rim with an arthroscopic knife, followed by rim resection, suture anchor placement, and knot tying as previously described. We prefer a takedown when greater degrees of rim resection are performed in order to remove the transition zone articular cartilage between the labrum and rim. If AIIS impingement is present, the resection is carried further proximal at the anterior rim to identify and decompress the prominent AIIS (Fig. 48.5). A thermal device can be used to better define the AIIS proximally, and occasionally, a longitudinal window can be made in the rectus for more proximal resection. We supplement our arthroscopic evaluation of pincer-type impingement with an intraoperative fluoroscopic assessment [37].

After completion of labral refixation, traction is released, the hip is flexed 20°–40°, and the cam deformity is inspected (Fig. 48.6a, b). We then perform dynamic assessment (Fig. 48.6c) in positions of hip flexion, abduction, and internal and external rotation (superoposterior impingement) and maximal hip flexion (typically 100° with a fracture table), adduction, and internal rotation (anterior impingement). If the femoral neck and or head-neck junction impinges against the labrum or results in levering of the femoral neck, cam decompression is indicated. The magnitude of femoral resection should be estimated by preoperative radiographs and confirmed with intraoperative findings. An additional "T" incision can be made down the anterior femoral neck in order to improve visualization although the senior author rarely performs this. The anteroinferior head-neck junction is best accessed with the hip in flexion external rotation (Fig. 48.6d), and the superoposterior head-neck junction is best accessed with the hip in extension, internal rotation. Typically the resection is performed from the medial synovial fold (Fig. 48.6e) to the lateral retinacular vessels (Fig. 48.6f), but this is quite variable. With the arthroscope in the mid-anterior portal and the burr in the anterolateral portal, the proximal extent of the resection is performed, and underlying sclerotic bone indicates the regions of impingement (Fig. 48.7a). The resection is then performed with an attempt to recreate the normal sphericity and offset of the head-neck junction from the medial synovial fold to the retinacular vessels (Fig. 48.7b–d). The burr can be placed in the mid-anterior portal

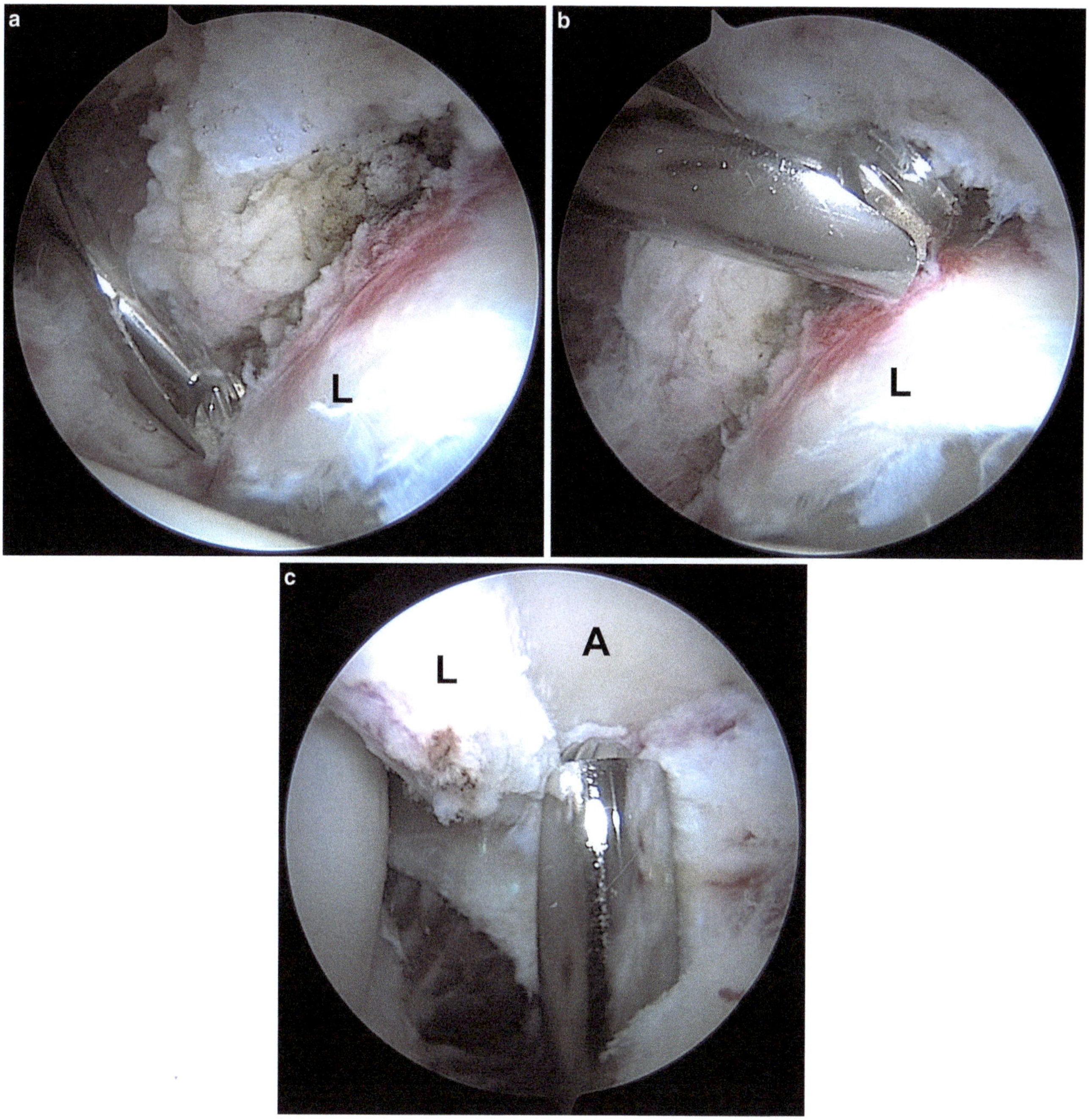

Fig. 48.3 Arthroscopic image of the left hip showing the area for rim resection with a burr anterior (**a**) and superior (**b**). (**c**) The burr is then introduced via the anterolateral portal to complete the resection adjacent to the labrum without formal labral takedown in this case. *L* labrum, *A* acetabulum

with the hip in flexion to reach beyond the medial synovial fold. Introducing the burr via the anterolateral portal with the hip in extension and the occasional use of traction allows the surgeon to extend the resection beyond the vessels. When working beyond the lateral synovial fold, it is important to stay proximal to the retinacular vessels. The osteoplasty is complete when there are impingement-free ROM arthroscopically and normal sphericity and offset with intraoperative fluoroscopy on AP and lateral imaging (Fig. 48.8). The capsule can then be repaired (Fig. 48.9a) by placing a looped monofilament suture through the distal limb of the capsulotomy (Fig. 48.9b) and retrieving it through the proximal limb

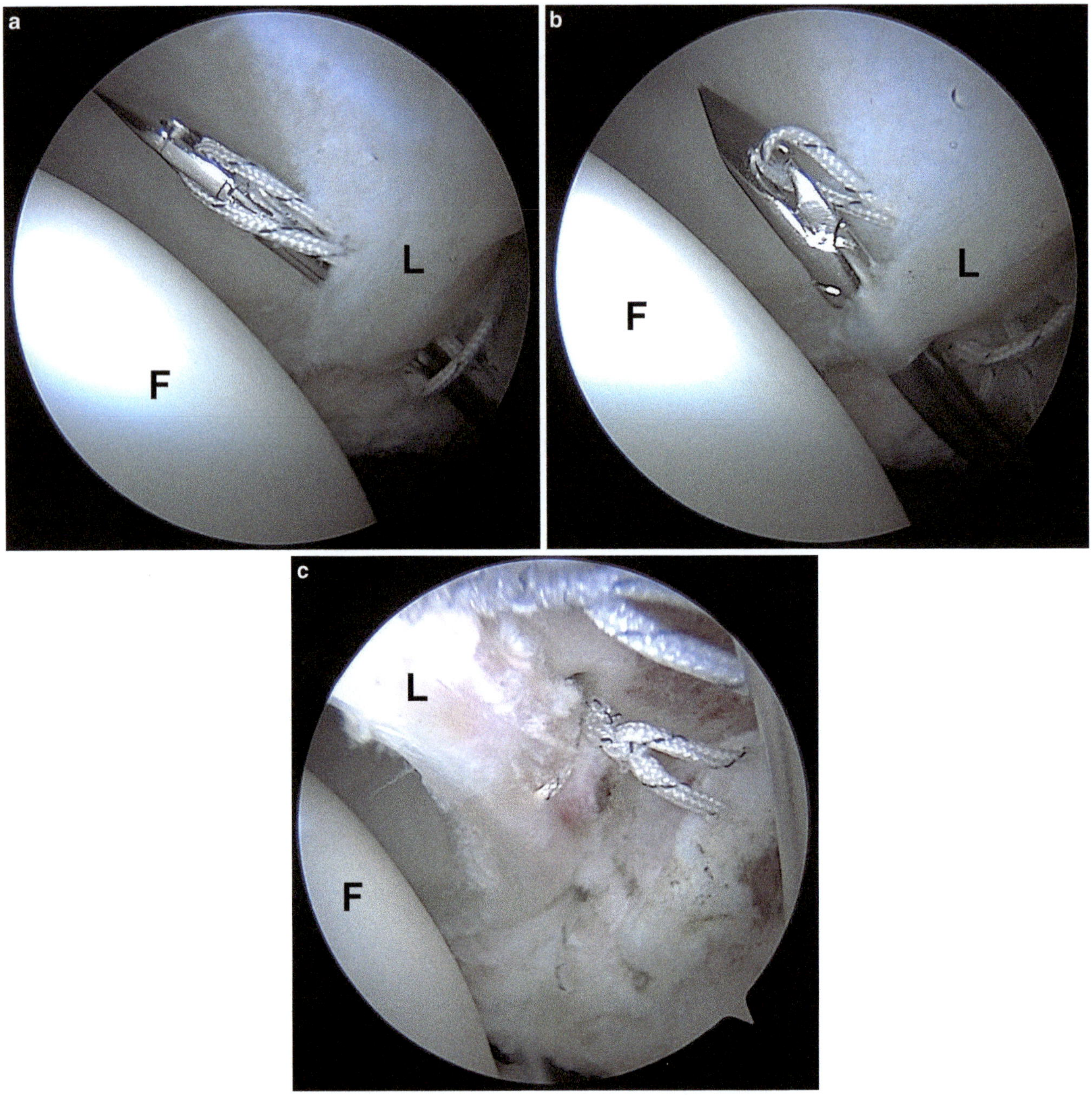

Fig. 48.4 Labral repair/refixation is typically performed with a mattress suture technique. One limb of the suture is placed through the labrochondral junction (**a**) and then retrieved through the midsubtance of the labrum (**b**). (**c**) Final arthroscopic image after labral repair/refixation. *F* femur, *L* labrum

of the capsulotomy (Fig. 48.9c). A #2 vicryl suture is then shuttled across the capsulotomy, and standard knot tying is performed (Fig. 48.9d). The senior author typically places 2–4 sutures which closes approximately 50–90% of the capsulotomy.

If ischiofemoral impingement is present, access to the lesser trochanter can be established, and two methods have been described for this. Ilizaliturri describes the use of two anterior portals, a superior accessory portal 2 cm distal and 2 cm anterior to the tip of the greater trochanter with a sec-

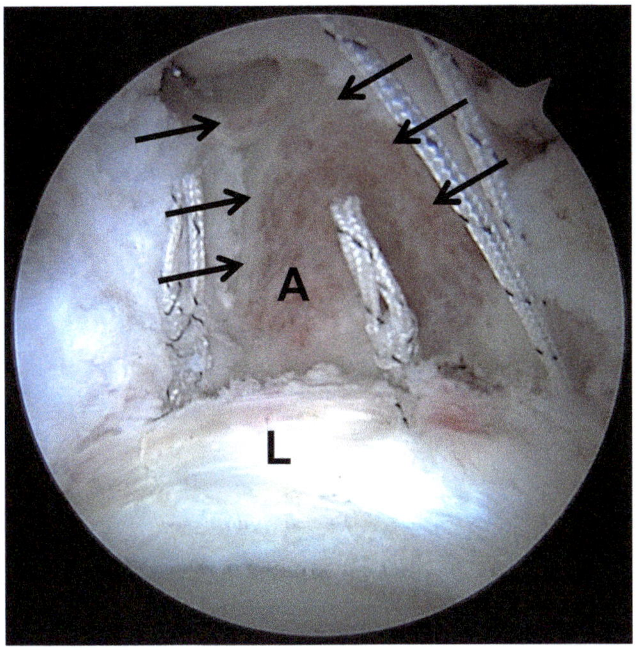

Fig. 48.5 Arthroscopic image of the left hip after labral repair and decompression of the anterior inferior iliac spine (*arrows*). *L* labrum, *A* acetabulum

ond 3–4 cm distal to the first [38]. Martin describes the use of two posterolateral portals in the supine position with the leg internally rotated. The posterolateral portal is made 3 cm posterior to the tip of the greater trochanter, and the auxiliary posterolateral portal is made 3 cm superior to the posterolateral portal [39]. Once this space is accessible, the lesser trochanter can be resected with a motorized burr to decompress the ischiofemoral space [9, 11]. Alternatively, a mini-open procedure, as an outpatient, can be performed to address the quadratus impingement under direct vision and avoid the risk of circumflex vessel bleeding.

Outcomes and Complications

Outcomes after arthroscopic management of FAI are increasingly reported in the literature [2, 33, 34, 40–46]. The available studies have shown improved outcomes comparable to that seen after an open surgical dislocation. Studies comparing labral resection versus labral preservation/refixation have shown significantly better outcomes and less degenerative changes on radiographs in the refixation group at early up to 3.5-year follow-up [2, 34, 35, 40].

Systematic reviews have been performed looking at the efficacy of treating FAI and included arthroscopic management [47–50]. In one study, the evidence supporting arthroscopic treatment of FAI was fair [48]. Two other studies combined open and arthroscopic approaches and found that the majority of patients improved, with pain relief in 68–96% of patients as a result of surgical management [47, 50]. Another study compared outcomes after arthroscopic, open, and combined approaches for treating FAI and found no significant differences for eventual outcome based on the surgical approach [49].

Complications related to hip arthroscopy include iatrogenic labral [51, 52] and chondral injury; traction-related neuropraxias to the femoral, pudendal, sciatic, and peroneal nerves [53]; lateral femoral cutaneous nerve neuropraxia related to its proximity to the anterior and mid-anterior portals; intra-abdominal fluid extravasation; skin breakdown in the perineal region secondary to traction [53];and deep venous thrombosis [53, 54]. Potential complications related to arthroscopic femoral osteochondroplasty include femoral neck fractures, avascular necrosis, and residual impingement. Femoral neck fractures have been reported after arthroscopic femoral resection osteochondroplasty, and a cadaveric study reported that resection of greater than 30% of the width of the anterolateral femoral neck significantly decreased the load to failure in a cadaveric model [53, 55–57]. Although disruption of the lateral retinacular vessels poses the potential risk of avascular necrosis, this has yet to be reported in the literature after femoral resection osteochondroplasty. Osteonecrosis has been reported after rim resection in one report; however, this was felt to be secondary to traction [58]. There have been multiple reports of iatrogenic instability with and without rim resections, and care must be taken to avoid over-resection of the rim for any patient and indiscriminate labral excision and unrepaired capsulotomies in patients with subtle dysplastic features [59–62].

Conclusions

The growing arthroscopic literature reveals excellent outcomes in the majority of patients and improvements comparable to that seen after open surgical dislocation for carefully selected individuals with FAI. A thorough understanding of hip mechanics and pathology is required to properly select individuals that may benefit from an arthroscopic approach. With careful patient selection and appropriate indications, arthroscopic treatment will lead to improved outcomes in the majority of patients.

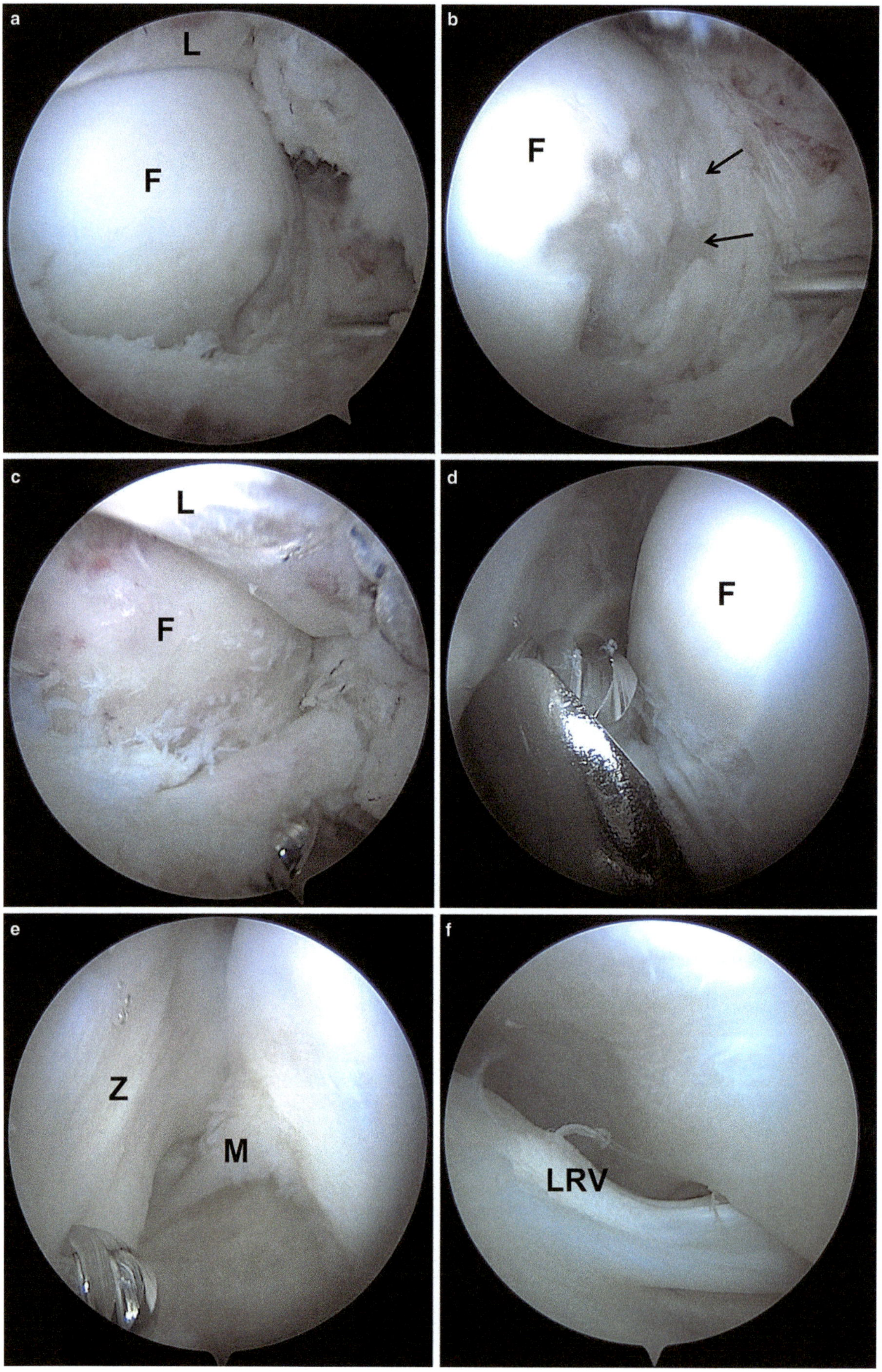

Fig. 48.6 (continued)

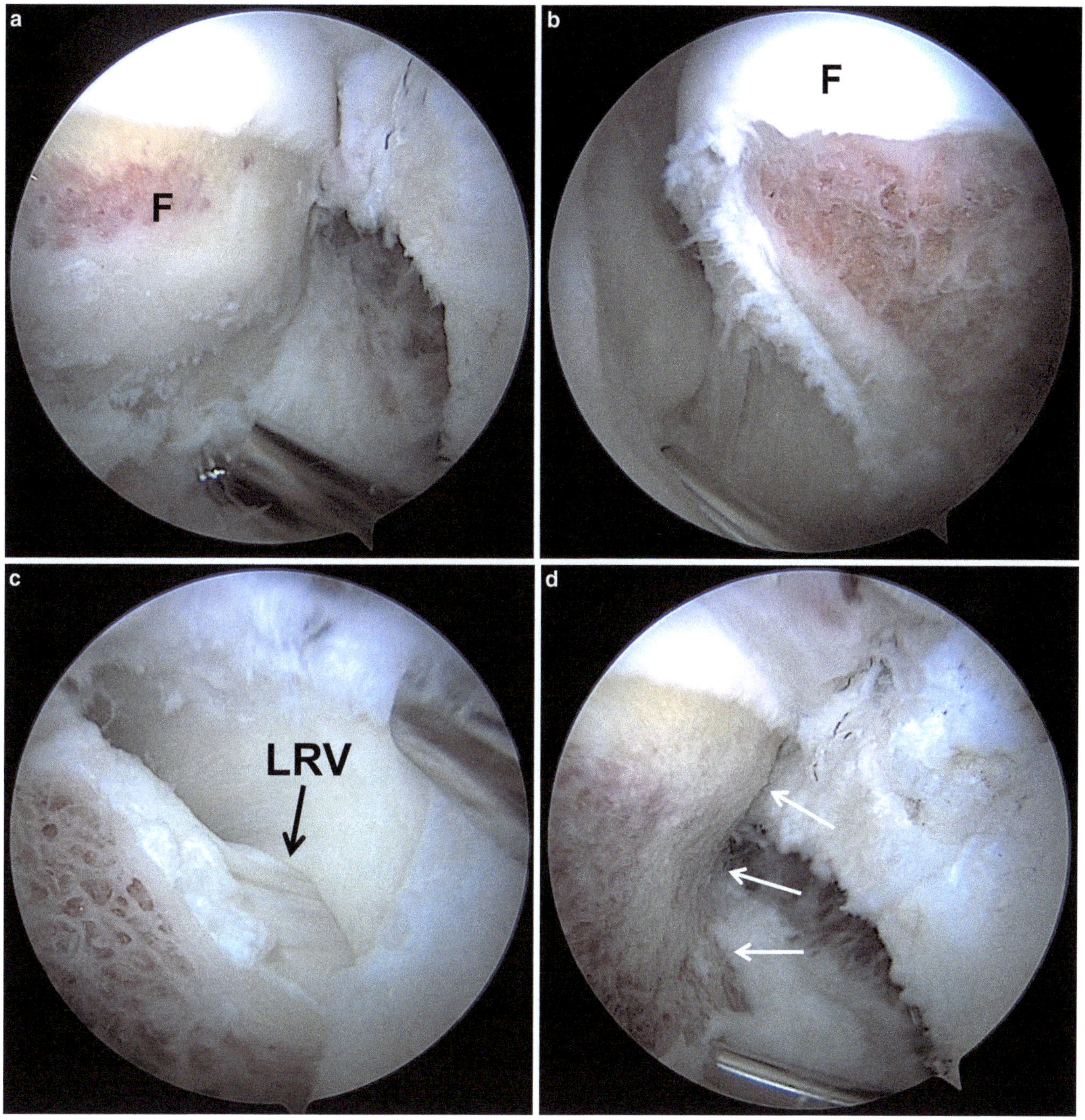

Fig. 48.7 (**a**) Arthroscopic view of the left hip reveals sclerotic bone in the region of femoral-sided impingement. The extent of the femoral resection runs extends from the medial synovial fold (**b**) to the lateral retinacular vessels (**c**). (**d**) The final cam decompression reveals improved sphericity and head-neck offset (*arrows*). *F* femoral head, *LRV* lateral retinacular vessels

Fig. 48.6 (**a**) Arthroscopic image of the left hip after release of traction reveals maintenance of the labral seal, cam-type morphology anteriorly (**a**) and damage at the femoral head-neck junction (**b**, *arrows*) consistent with cam-type impingement. Dynamic assessment (**c**) reveals limited range of motion and impingement between the femoral head-neck junction and labrum/acetabulum. (**d**) The inferior extent of the resection is identified with a burr. (**e**) The inferior extent of the resection is typically near the medial synovial fold (M), and the superior extent is typically the lateral retinacular vessels (**f**, LRV). *F* femoral head, *L* labrum, *Z* zona orbicularis, *M* medial synovial fold, *LRV* lateral retinacular vessels

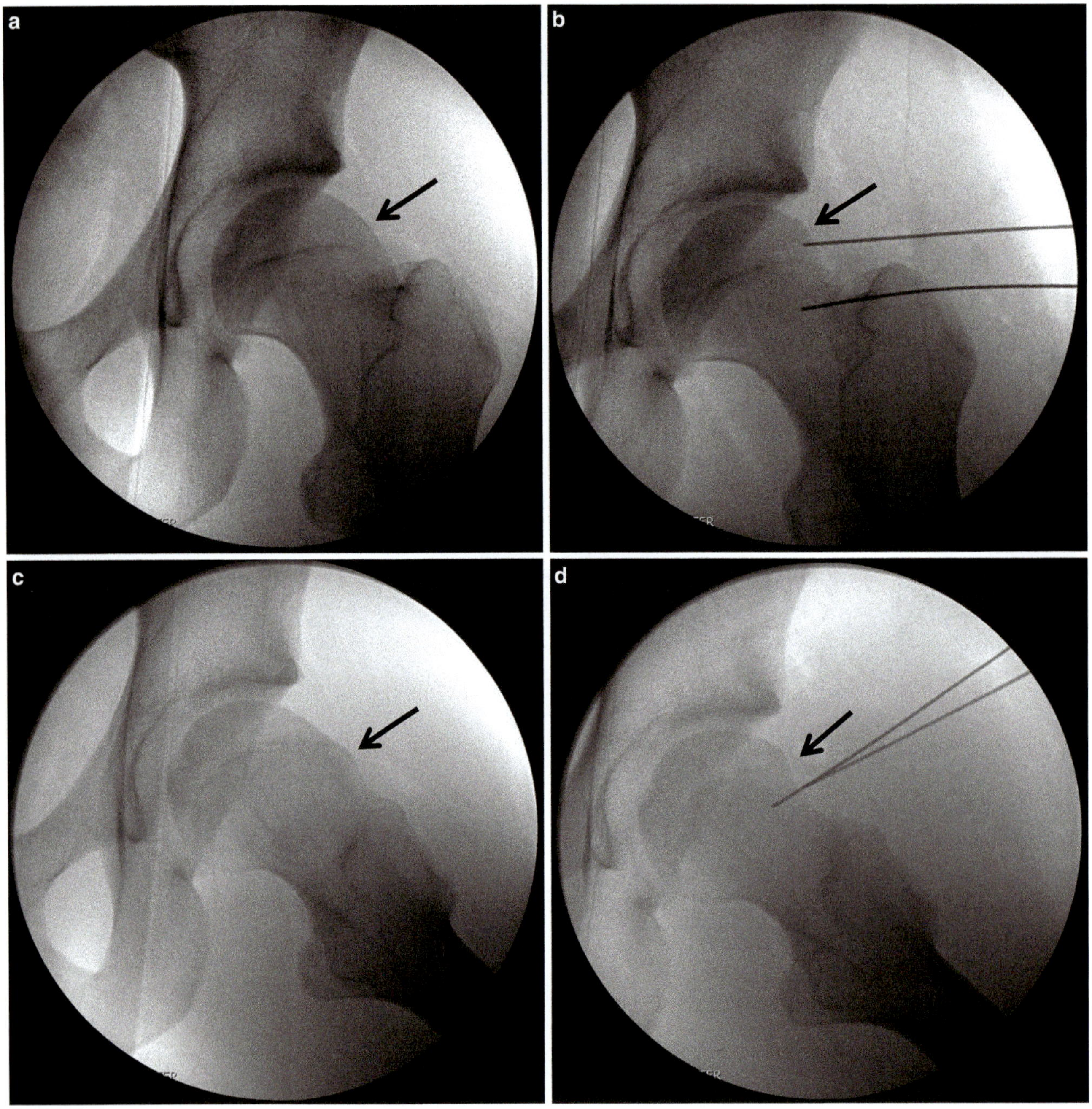

Fig. 48.8 (**a**) Preoperative AP fluoroscopic image demonstrates cam-type morphology (*arrow*). (**b**) Postoperative fluoroscopic AP image demonstrates improved sphericity and improved head-neck offset (*arrow*). (**c**) Preoperative lateral fluoroscopic image demonstrates a large cam-type deformity (*arrow*). (**d**) Postoperative lateral fluoroscopic image shows improved sphericity and improved head-neck offset (*arrow*). The two wires on the postoperative images are nitinol guide wires used to maintain the portal sites if further resection is deemed necessary after fluoroscopic evaluation

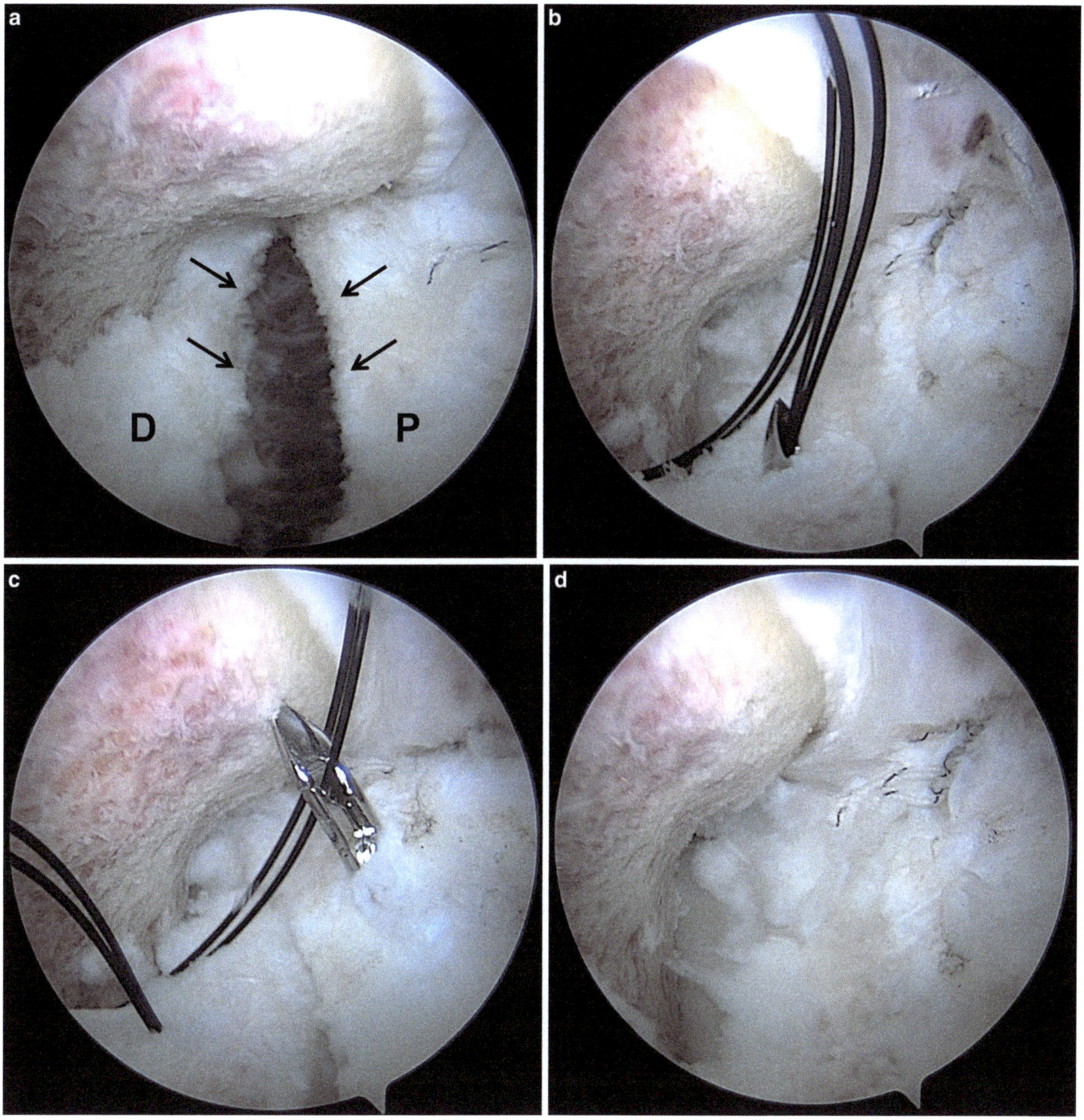

Fig. 48.9 (**a**) Arthroscopic image of the left hip demonstrates the femoral resection and capsulotomy margins (*arrows*). (**b**) A suture passer is used to pass a looped monofilament suture through the distal limb of the capsulotomy toward the acetabulum. (**c**) A penetrating device is then passed through the proximal limb of the capsulotomy and the suture is retrieved. (**d**) The looped suture is then used to shuttle a #2 vicryl suture across the capsulotomy and secured with standard knot tying in order to close the capsular incision

References

1. Beck M, Leunig M, Parvizi J, Boutier V, Wyss D, Ganz R. Anterior femoroacetabular impingement: part II. Midterm results of surgical treatment. Clin Orthop Relat Res. 2004;418:67–73.
2. Espinosa N, Rothenfluh DA, Beck M, Ganz R, Leunig M. Treatment of femoro-acetabular impingement: preliminary results of labral refixation. J Bone Joint Surg Am. 2006;88(5):925–35.
3. Ganz R, Parvizi J, Beck M, Leunig M, Nötzli H, Siebenrock KA. Femoroacetabular impingement: a cause for osteoarthritis of the hip. Clin Orthop Relat Res. 2003;417:112–20.
4. Leunig M, Beck M, Dora C, Ganz R. Femoroacetabular impingement: etiology and surgical concept. Oper Tech Orthop. 2005; 15(3):247–55.
5. Philippon MJ, Stubbs AJ, Schenker ML, Maxwell RB, Ganz R, Leunig M. Arthroscopic management of femoroacetabular impingement: osteoplasty technique and literature review. Am J Sports Med. 2007;35(9):1571–80.
6. Larson CM, Guanche CA, Kelly BT, Clohisy JC, Ranawat AS. Advanced techniques in hip arthroscopy. Instr Course Lect. 2009;58:423–36.
7. Larson CM, Kelly BT, Stone RM. Making a case for anterior inferior iliac spine/subspine hip impingement: three representative case reports and proposed concept. Arthroscopy. 2011;27(12):1732–7.
8. Pan H, Kawanabe K, Akiyama H, Goto K, Onishi E, Nakamura T. Operative treatment of hip impingement caused by hypertrophy of the anterior inferior iliac spine. J Bone Joint Surg Br. 2008; 90(5):677–9.
9. Johnson KA. Impingement of the lesser trochanter on the ischial ramus after total hip arthroplasty. Report of three cases. J Bone Joint Surg Am. 1977;59(2):268–9.
10. Torriani M, Souto SC, Thomas BJ, Ouellette H, Bredella MA. Ischiofemoral impingement syndrome: an entity with hip pain and abnormalities of the quadrates femoris muscle. AJR Am J Roentgenol. 2009;193(1):186–90.
11. Stafford HG, Villar RN. Ischiofemoral impingement. J Bone Joint Surg Br. 2011;93(10):1300–2.
12. Ng VY, Ellis TJ. More than just a bump: cam-type femoroacetabular impingement and the evolution of the femoral neck. Hip Int. 2011;21(1):1–8.
13. Notzli HP, Wyss TF, Stoecklin CH, Schmid MR, Treiber K, Hodler J. The contour of the femoral head-neck junction as a predictor for the risk of anterior impingement. J Bone Joint Surg Br. 2002;84(4): 556–60.
14. Ganz R, Leunig M, Leunig-Ganz K, Harris WH. The etiology of osteoarthritis of the hip: an integrated mechanical concept. Clin Orthop Relat Res. 2008;466(2):264–72.
15. Siebenrock KA, Wahab KH, Werlen S, Kalhor M, Leunig M, Ganz R. Abnormal extension of the femoral head epiphysis as a cause of cam impingement. Clin Orthop Relat Res. 2004;418:54–60.
16. Martin RL, Enseki KR, Draovitch P, Trapuzzano T, Philippon MJ. Acetabular labral tears of the hip: examination and diagnostic challenges. J Orthop Sports Phys Ther. 2006;36(7):503–15.
17. Reider B, Martel J. Pelvis, hip and thigh. In: Reider B, Martel J, editors. The orthopedic physical examination. Philadelphia: WB Saunders; 1999. p. 159–99.
18. McCarthy JC, Busconi BD, Owens BD. Assessment of the painful hip. In: McCarthy JC, editor. Early hip disorders. New York: Springer; 2003. p. 3–6.
19. Meyers WC, McKechnie A, Philippon MJ, Horner MA, Zoga AC, Devon ON. Experience with "sports hernia" spanning two decades. Ann Surg. 2008;248(4):656–65.
20. Ali AM, Whitwell D, Ostlere SJ. Case report: imaging and surgical treatment of a snapping hip due to ischiofemoral impingement. Skeletal Radiol. 2011;40(5):653–6.
21. Clohisy JC, Carlisle JC, Beaule PE, Kim YJ, Trousdale RT, Sierra RJ, et al. A systematic approach to the plain radiographic evaluation of the young adult hip. J Bone Joint Surg Am. 2008;90 Suppl 4:47–66.
22. Eijer H, Leunig M, Mahomed MN, Ganz R. Crosstable lateral radiograph for screening of anterior femoral head–neck offset in patients with femoro-acetabular impingement. Hip Int. 2001;11: 37–41.
23. Wenger DE, Kendell KR, Miner MR, Trousdale RT. Acetabular labral tears rarely occur in the absence of bony abnormalities. Clin Orthop Relat Res. 2004;426:145–50.
24. Peele MW, Della Rocca GJ, Maloney WJ, Curry MC, Clohisy JC. Acetabular and femoral radiographic abnormalities associated with labral tears. Clin Orthop Relat Res. 2005;441:327–33.
25. Czerny C, Hofmann S, Neuhold A, Tschauner C, Engel A, Recht MP, et al. Lesions of the acetabular labrum: accuracy of MR imaging and MR arthrography in detection and staging. Radiology. 1996;200(1):225–30.
26. Kenney JA, Peelle MW, Jackson J, Rubin D, Maloney WJ, Clohisy JC. Magnetic resonance arthrography versus arthroscopy in the evaluation of articular hip pathology. Clin Orthop Relat Res. 2004;429:163–9.
27. Hack K, Di Primio G, Rakhra K, Beaule PE. Prevalence of cam-type femoroacetabular impingement morphology in asymptomatic volunteers. J Bone Joint Surg Am. 2010;92(14):2436–44.
28. Kassarjian A. Signal abnormalities in the quadratus femoris muscle: tear or impingement? AJR Am J Roentgenol. 2008;190(6):W379. Author reply W380–1.
29. Mardones R, Lara J, Donndorf A, Barnes S, Stuart MJ, Glick J, et al. Surgical correction of "cam-type" femoroacetabular impingement: a cadaveric comparison of open versus arthroscopic debridement. Arthroscopy. 2009;25(2):175–82.
30. Sussman PS, Ranawat AS, Lipman J, Lorich DG, Padgett DE, Kelly BT. Arthroscopic versus open osteoplasty of the head-neck junction: a cadaveric investigation. Arthroscopy. 2007;23(12): 1257–64.
31. Bedi A, Zaltz I, De La Torre K, Kelly BT. Radiographic comparison of surgical hip dislocation and hip arthroscopy for treatment of cam deformity in femoroacetabular impingement. Am J Sports Med. 2011;39(Suppl):20S–8.
32. Larson CM. Letter to the editor. Protrusio acetabuli: some questions. Arthroscopy. 2012;28(9):1193.
33. Larson CM, Giveans MR. Arthroscopic management of femoroacetabular impingement: early outcomes measures. Arthroscopy. 2008;24(5):540–6.
34. Larson CM, Giveans MR. Arthroscopic debridement versus refixation of the acetabular labrum associated with femoroacetabular impingement. Arthroscopy. 2009;25(4):369–76.
35. Larson CM, Giveans MR, Stone RM. Arthrosopic debridement versus refixation of the acetabular labrum associated with femoroacetabular impingement: mean 3.5 year follow-up. Am J Sports Med. 2012;40(5):1015–21.
36. Philippon MJ, Schenker ML. A new method for acetabular rim trimming and labral repair. Clin Sports Med. 2006;25(2):293–7.
37. Larson CM, Wulf CA. Intra-operative fluoroscopy for evaluation of bony resection during arthroscopic management of femoroacetabular impingement in the supine position. Arthroscopy. 2009; 25(10):1183–92.
38. Ilizaliturri Jr VM, Camacho-Galindo J. Endoscopic treatment of snapping hips, iliotibial band, and iliopsoas tendon. Sports Med Arthrosc. 2010;18(2):120–7.
39. Martin HD, Shears SA, Johnson JC, Smathers AM, Palmer IJ. The endoscopic treatment of sciatic nerve entrapment/deep gluteal syndrome. Arthroscopy. 2011;27(2):172–81.
40. Philippon MJ, Briggs KK, Yen YM, Kuppersmith DA. Outcomes following hip arthroscopy for femoroacetabular impingement

with associated chondrolabral dysfunction: minimum two-year follow-up. J Bone Joint Surg Br. 2009;91(1):16–23.
41. Byrd JW, Jones KS. Arthroscopic femoroplasty in the management of cam-type femoroacetabular impingement. Clin Orthop Relat Res. 2009;467(3):739–46.
42. Bedi A, Chen N, Robertson W, Kelly BT. The management of labral tears and femoroacetabular impingement of the hip in the young, active hip. Arthroscopy. 2008;24(10):1135–45.
43. Ilizaliturri Jr VW, Orozco-Rodriguez L, Acosta-Rodriguez E, Camacho-Galindo J. Arthroscopic treatment of cam-type femoroacetabular impingement: preliminary report at 2 years minimum follow-up. J Arthroplasty. 2008;23(2):226–34.
44. Philippon MJ, Schenker ML. Arthroscopy for the treatment of femoroacetabular impingement in the athlete. Clin Sports Med. 2006;25(2):299–308.
45. Guanche CA, Bare AA. Arthroscopic treatment of femoroacetabular impingement. Arthroscopy. 2006;22(1):95–106.
46. Philippon MJ, Schenker M, Briggs K, Kuppersmith D. Femoroacetabular impingement in 45 professional athletes: associated pathologies and return to sport following arthroscopic decompression. Knee Surg Sports Traumatol Arthrosc. 2007;15(7):908–14.
47. Ng VY, Arora N, Best TM, Pan X, Ellis TJ. Efficacy of surgery for femoroacetabular impingement: a systematic review. Am J Sports Med. 2010;38(11):2337–45.
48. Stevens MS, Legay DA, Glazebrook MA, Amirault D. The evidence for hip arthroscopy: grading the current indications. Arthroscopy. 2010;26(10):1370–83.
49. Botser IB, Smith Jr TW, Nasser R, Domb BG. Open surgical dislocation versus arthroscopy for femoroacetabular impingement: a comparison of clinical outcomes. Arthroscopy. 2011;27(2):270–8.
50. Clohisy JC, St John LC, Schutz AL. Surgical treatment of femoroacetabular impingement: a systematic review of the literature. Clin Orthop Relat Res. 2010;468(2):555–64.
51. Domb B, Hanypsiak B, Botser I. Labral penetration rate in a consecutive series of 300 hip arthroscopies. Am J Sports Med. 2012;40(4):864–9.
52. Badylak JS, Keene JS. Do iatrogenic punctures of the labrum affect the clinical results of hip arthroscopy? Arthroscopy. 2011;27(6):761–7.
53. Ilizaliturri Jr VM. Complications of arthroscopic femoroacetabular impingement treatment: a review. Clin Orthop Relat Res. 2009;467(3):760–8.
54. Verma M, Sekiya JK. Intrathoracic fluid extravasation after hip arthroscopy. Arthroscopy. 2010;26(9 Suppl):S90–4.
55. Mardones RM, Gonzalez C, Chen Q, Zobitz M, Kaufman KR, Trousdale RT. Surgical treatment of femoroacetabular impingement: evaluation of the effect of the size of the resection. Surgical technique. J Bone Joint Surg Am. 2006;88 Suppl 1:84–91.
56. Sampson TG. Arthroscopic treatment of femoroacetabular impingement: a proposed technique with clinical experience. Instr Course Lect. 2006;55:337–46.
57. Ayeni OR, Bedi A, Lorich DG, Kelly BT. Femoral neck fracture after arthroscopic management of femoroacetabular impingement: a case report. J. Bone Joint Surg Am. 2011;93(9):e47.1–8.
58. Scher DL, Belmont Jr PJ, Owens BD. Case report: osteonecrosis of the femoral head after hip arthroscopy. Clin Orthop Relat Res. 2010;468(11):3121–5.
59. Matsuda DK. Acute iatrogenic dislocation following hip impingement arthroscopic surgery. Arthroscopy. 2009;25(4):400–4.
60. Ranawat AS, McClincy M, Sekiya JK. Anterior dislocation of the hip after arthroscopy in a patient with capsular laxity of the hip. A case report. J Bone Joint Surg Am. 2009;91(1):192–7.
61. Benali Y, Katthagen BD. Hip subluxation as a complication of arthroscopic debridement. Arthroscopy. 2009;25(4):405–7.
62. Mei-Dan O, McConkey MO, Brick M. Catastrophic failure of hip arthroscopy due to iatrogenic instability: can partial division of the ligamentum teres and iliofemoral ligament cause subluxation? Arthroscopy. 2012;28(3):440–5.

49 Special Patients and Conditions: Other Forms of Impingement (Ischiofemoral, Pectineofoveal)

J.W. Thomas Byrd

Overview

The concept of femoroacetabular impingement as a cause of secondary joint damage in the native hip was first published by Ganz and colleagues in 2003. In a brief period of time, it has been recognized as a common cause of hip pathology. FAI is not the source of all hip problems, and its rapid acceptance reflects that we must remain open minded of other forms of pathology that have only recently been proposed or have yet to be elucidated. This chapter focuses on two alternate forms of impingement, ischiofemoral and pectineofoveal [1–4].

Ischiofemoral Impingement

With regard to snapping hip syndromes, we coined the adage "if you can hear it from across the room, it's the iliopsoas tendon and if you can see it from across the room, it's the iliotibial band." With this understanding, you can diagnose 90 % of snapping hip syndromes before placing a hand on the patient. It is the other 10 % that will challenge the clinician's acumen. We described a 4.5 % failure rate in our cases of endoscopic release of the iliopsoas tendon performed to eliminate its snapping [5]. In some of these, even revision surgery failed to eliminate the snapping. Eventually, it became evident to us that it was not a technical failure of the procedure but simply having performed the wrong operation because the snapping was likely due to something other than the iliopsoas tendon. It is likely that, in this subgroup, ischiofemoral impingement may be a common culprit.

Impingement between the ischium and the lesser trochanter as a cause of hip pain was first described as an iatrogenic phenomenon in a case series of three patients who underwent total hip arthroplasty (THA) in conjunction with severe proximal femoral deformities [6]. The diagnosis was based on radiographic evidence of ischiofemoral narrowing. Symptoms were relieved in these three patients who underwent resection of the lesser trochanter.

More recently, Torriani and coauthors described a case of ischiofemoral impingement as a cause of pain in a native hip and then followed this with a case series [1, 7]. This condition was an MRI diagnosis characterized by edema and fatty infiltration of the quadratus femoris and narrowing of the bony and soft tissue ischiofemoral space in which it is contained. Limited information was available on the clinical presentation, treatment, and outcomes. In a retrospective review of a large institutional database, Tosun et al. identified 50 cases with MRI evidence of ischiofemoral impingement [8]. However, a nexus with this being the source of the patient's symptoms was not established.

Diagnosis

A precise clinical presentation for ischiofemoral impingement has not been clearly defined. Groin and/or buttock pain that may radiate distally has variously been noted [2]. To date, clinically documented cases of ischiofemoral impingement have only been reported in women. In our experience, it is a painful popping or grating sensation that precipitates the patient to seek treatment. Examination findings are variable as far as slight hip irritability or tenderness to palpation. Particular attention is given to palpating posteriorly over

J.W.T. Byrd, MD (✉)
Nashville Sports Medicine Foundation, 2011 Church Street, Suite 100, Nashville, TN 37203, USA

Department of Orthopaedic Surgery and Rehabilitation, Vanderbilt University, Nashville, 37232, TN, USA
e-mail: info@nsmoc.com

J.C. McCarthy et al. (eds.), *Hip Joint Restoration*, DOI 10.1007/978-1-4614-0694-5_49

the area of the quadratus femoris insertion. The most remarkable finding is the popping or grating sensation that occurs with ambulation. Specifically, it tends to occur at the end of the stance phase of gait as the hip is extending. Patients will tend to describe the origin of the pain as being more posterior but sometimes anterior and rarely is conclusive. Snapping due to ischiofemoral impingement is most easily confused with snapping of the iliopsoas tendon which much be ruled out.

Routine radiographs of the pelvis and affected hip should be obtained but are likely to be unremarkable. Attention should be given to assess for coxa valga and excessive femoral anteversion, especially if unilateral, which may be associated with narrowing of the ischiofemoral space.

MRI should reveal abnormality of the quadratus femoris muscle, characterized by intramuscular edema and sometimes focal fatty infiltration or partial tearing (Fig. 49.1). Torriani et al. described two measurements [1]. The ischiofemoral space was defined as the smallest distance between the lateral cortex of the ischial tuberosity and the medial cortex of the lesser trochanter. The quadratus femoris space was defined as the smallest space for passage of the quadratus femoris muscle, being limited by the superolateral surface of the hamstring tendons and the posteromedial surface of the iliopsoas tendon. They found the ischiofemoral space to be narrowed in patients with ischiofemoral impingement (13±5 mm) compared to control subjects (23±8 mm). The quadratus femoris space was also narrowed (7±3 mm) compared to controls (12±4 mm). Ali et al. described deterioration of the quadratus femoris [9]. Tosun et al. also described greater cross-sectional area of the proximal hamstring tendon and a larger neck shaft angle (coxa valga) as being more prevalent in their cases with MRI findings of quadratus femoris pathology [8]. O'Brien and Bui-Mansfield described quadratus femoris tears in four women in whom no narrowing of the ischiofemoral space was documented [10]. In our experience of eight women with pathology of the quadratus femoris and painful snapping, the ischiofemoral and quadratus femoris spaces were normal.

Treatment

A trial of conservative treatment is appropriate although no specific strategy has been described. The mainstay includes anti-inflammatory medication and efforts to avoid offending activities. This is difficult because often the painful popping simply occurs with normal ambulation. CT-guided injection of the quadratus femoris within the ischiofemoral space has been described, and we have had some experience with this as well [9]. The results are often equivocal, both in terms of diagnostic and therapeutic value. Ultrasound guidance has been reported and may prove to be equally effective at reaching the region [11].

Although the entity of ischiofemoral impingement has been described, the precise clinical presentation and pathomechanics have been only partly elucidated, and thus surgical intervention should be considered only with cau-

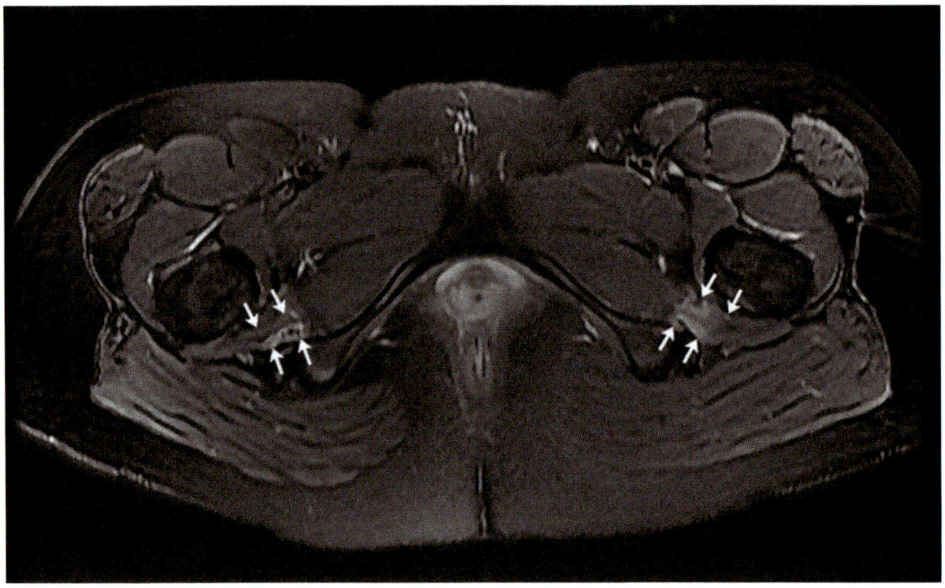

Fig. 49.1 A 20-year-old female with bilateral painful snapping symptoms of ischiofemoral impingement. A T2-weighted axial MR image of the pelvis illustrates edema and cystic changes within the muscle belly of the quadratus femoris bilaterally (*arrows*). Published with kind permission of ©J.W. Thomas Byrd 2015. All Rights Reserved

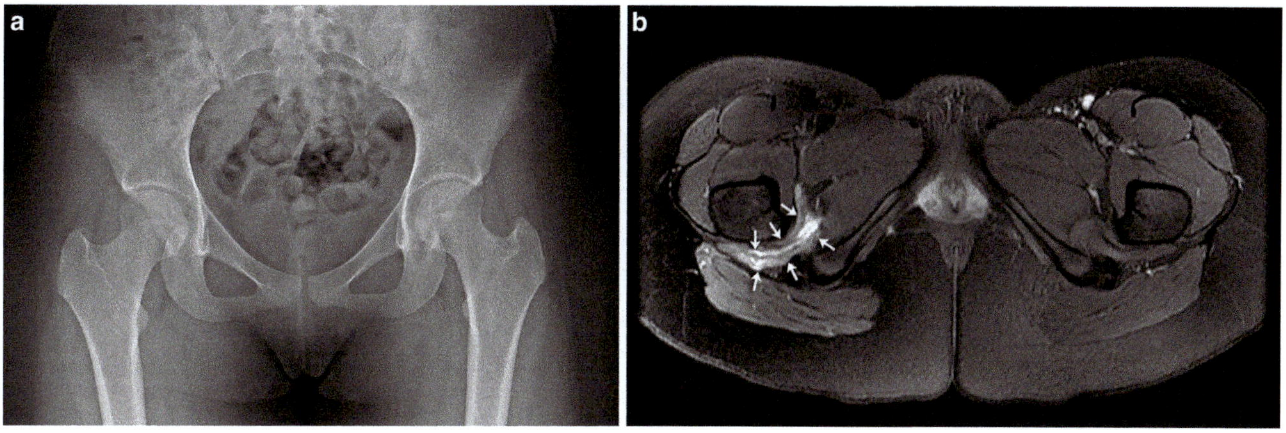

Fig. 49.2 A 17-year-old female with recalcitrant right-sided findings of ischiofemoral impingement characterized by painful grating/popping with ambulation. (**a**) AP pelvis radiograph is unremarkable. (**b**) Axial T2-weighted MR image demonstrates severe edema within the quadratus femoris muscle (*arrows*). Published with kind permission of ©J.W. Thomas Byrd 2015. All Rights Reserved

tion. Johnson, in his first report of impingement of the lesser trochanter against the ischium following THA, noted successful treatment with resection of the lesser trochanter [6]. Ali et al. reported a successful outcome with open resection of the lesser trochanter exposed by releasing the origin of the quadratus femoris and the insertion of the iliopsoas, both of which were reattached at the completion of the procedure [9]. However, follow-up was only 10 weeks. We are aware of another case, treated by arthroscopic resection of the lesser trochanter resulting in a protracted recovery process but eventually a successful outcome. In six cases of painful snapping due to ischiofemoral impingement with quadratus femoris pathology, but a normal space, we performed an endoscopic resection of the quadratus from the subgluteal region (Figs. 49.2 and 49.3). We selected this approach, choosing not to resect the lesser trochanter because the space was normal and we did not want to compromise the uninvolved iliopsoas tendon. The results have been mixed and the data not yet conclusive enough to advocate this as a reliable surgical technique to correct the problem. The two concerns of resecting the quadratus femoris are (1) that the sciatic nerve must be carefully protected during the resection and (2) there is an uncertain risk of whether the medial circumflex femoral artery could be injured where it emerges posteriorly underneath the obturator externus at the superior margin of the quadratus femoris. Our most complete success was a case in which we did resect a substantial portion of the lesser trochanter via iliopsoas bursoscopy in a patient with both ischiofemoral and iliopsoas symptoms (Figs. 49.4 and 49.5).

Conclusions

Ischiofemoral impingement can be a cause of painful snapping around the hip area. The imaging criteria have been well described. Interpretation of the clinical presentation is being better formulated, but a reliable treatment strategy, including predictable surgical correction and an understanding of its consequences, remains to be defined.

Pectineofoveal Impingement

Pectineofoveal impingement has been described as a cause of hip pain due to pathology of the medial synovial fold and, when symptoms are recalcitrant, treated by excision [3, 4]. We have encountered one such case in an elite female sprinter. She demonstrated evidence of joint pain as well as recalcitrant hip flexor irritability that failed to resolve despite training modifications and concerted physical therapy. Arthroscopy revealed an isolated area of synovial thickening and hypertrophy contiguous with the medial synovial fold (Fig. 49.6a). The lesion was excised (Fig. 49.6a–c) with prompt resolution of her pain. The pectineofoveal (medial synovial) fold is a normal anatomic structure that may exhibit some natural morphological variation. It is likely that aberrations and disease may exist in conjunction with other joint pathology and may rarely be an isolated source of symptoms. Further research will provide a more comprehensive understanding of this condition.

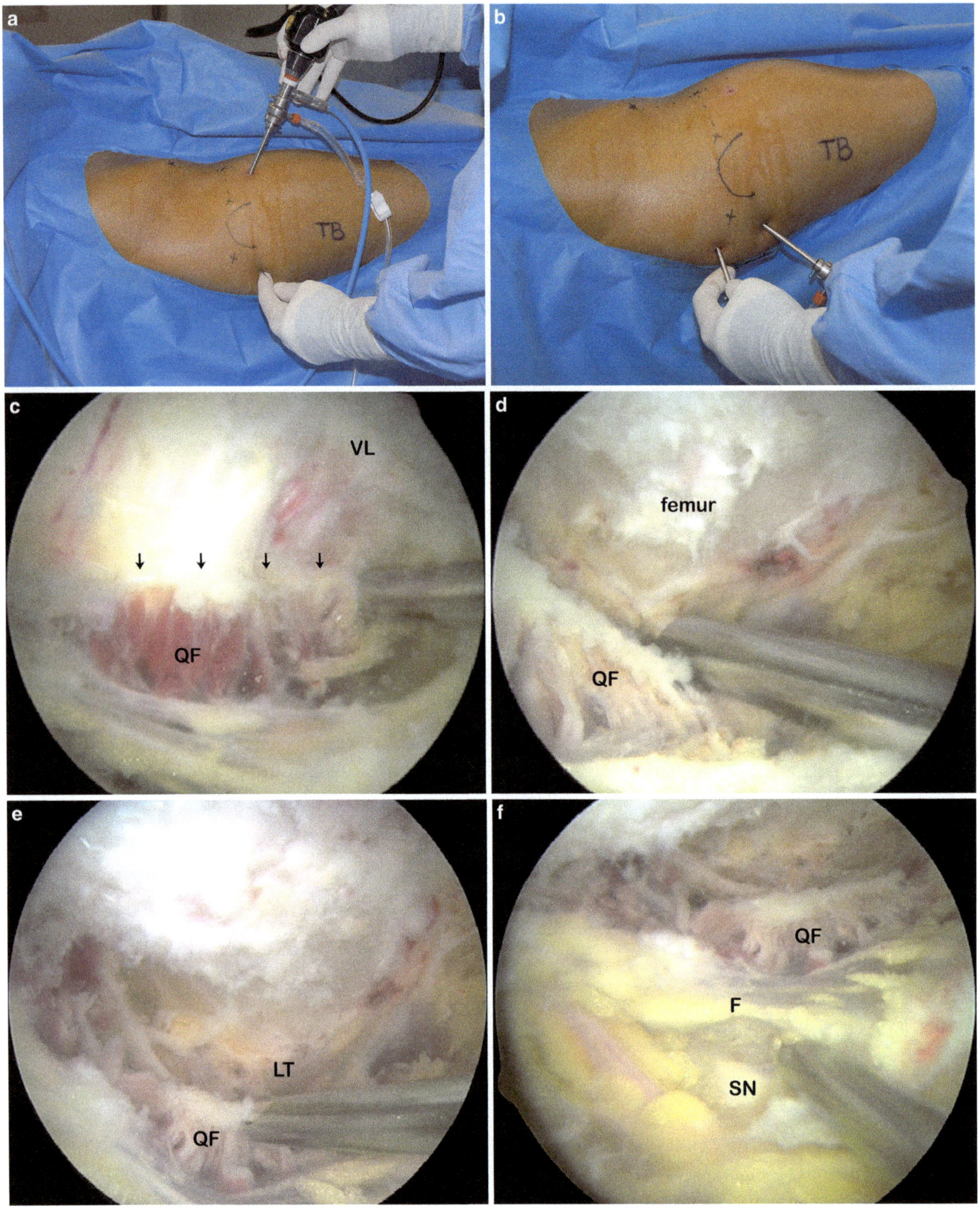

Fig. 49.3 (**a**) Viewing with the arthroscope in the peritrochanteric space, positioning of a spinal needle is being performed for access to the subgluteal region. (**b**) The arthroscope and instrumentation are positioned in the subgluteal space. (**c**) Viewing from the subgluteal space, the quadratus femoris muscle (QF) is inserting along the posterolateral aspect of the proximal femur (*arrows*) posterior to the vastus lateralis (VL). (**d**) Excision of the quadratus femoris (QF) from its insertion skeletonizes the posterior aspect of the proximal femur (femur). (**e**) Release of the quadratus femoris (QF) is complete when the lesser trochanter (LT) has been exposed medially. (**f**) Viewing posteriorly, the sciatic nerve (SN) is surrounded by a thin veil of fat (F) posterior to the remnant of the quadratus femoris (QF). Published with kind permission of ©J.W. Thomas Byrd 2015. All Rights Reserved

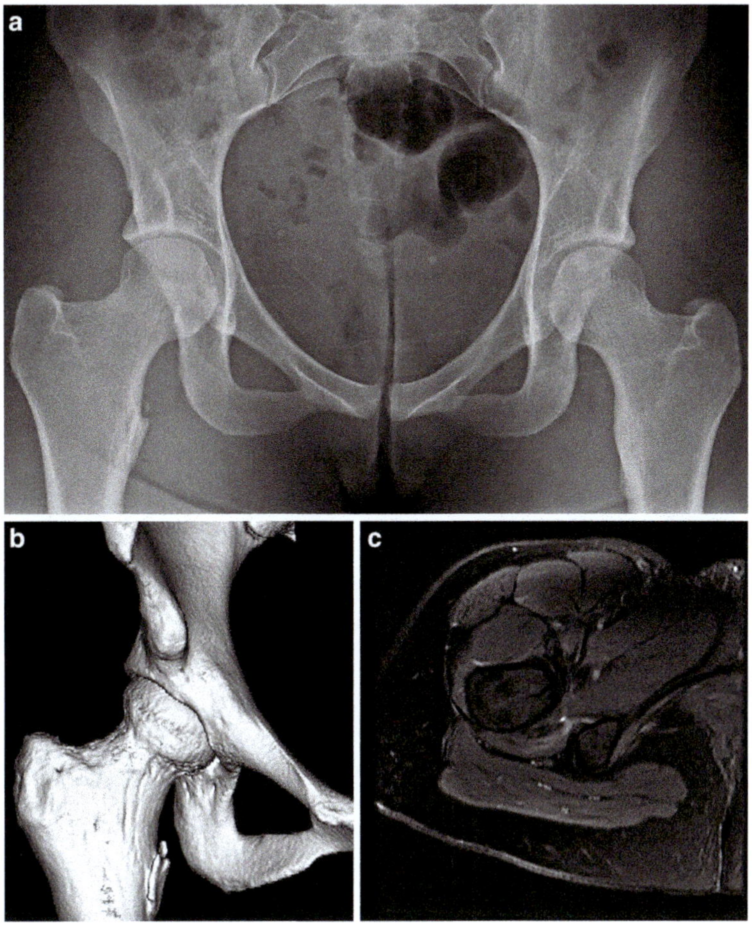

Fig. 49.4 A 25-year-old female presents with recurrent painful right hip snapping 8 years following previous successful correction with endoscopic release of the iliopsoas from the lesser trochanter. Examination findings are more consistent with ischiofemoral impingement and painful popping with every step. (**a**) AP pelvis radiograph reveals slight bone density adjacent to iliopsoas insertion on the lesser trochanter. (**b**) Computed tomography demonstrated a normal ischiofemoral space, and 3-D reconstruction revealed slight spurring around the lesser trochanter (*arrows*). (**c**) Axial T2-weighted MR image reveals slight edema within the quadratus femoris (*arrows*). Published with kind permission of ©J.W. Thomas Byrd 2015. All Rights Reserved

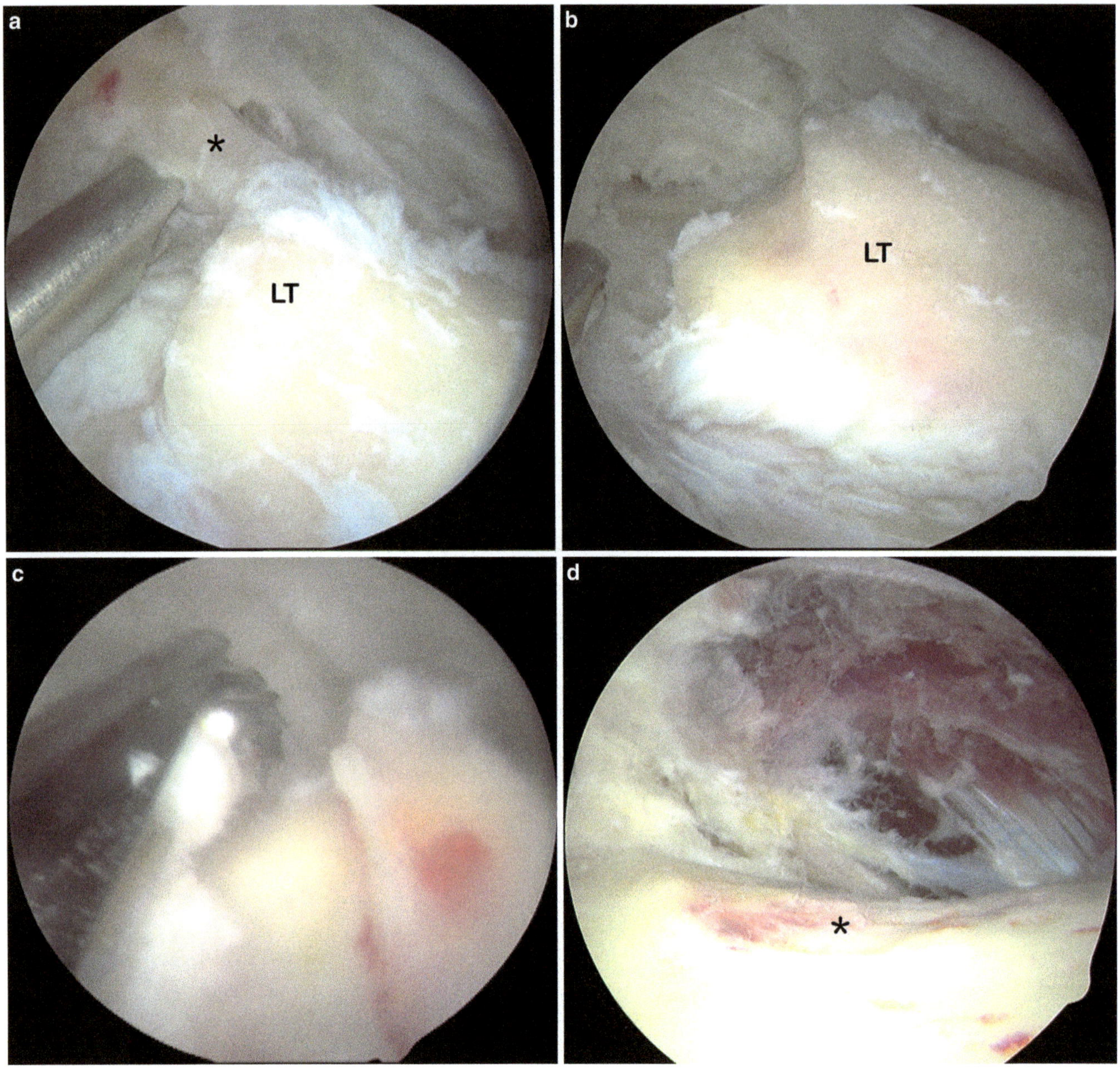

Fig. 49.5 Resection of the lesser trochanter was selected to address the iliopsoas tendon as well as decompress the ischiofemoral space. (**a**) Viewing from the iliopsoas bursa, the iliopsoas tendon (*asterisk*) is identified at its insertion to the lesser trochanter (LT). (**b**) The tendon has been released, skeletonizing the lesser trochanter (LT). (**c**) Resection of the lesser trochanter is being performed with a burr. (**d**) Resection has been completed removing approximately 2/3 of the lesser trochanter (*asterisk*). Published with kind permission of ©J.W. Thomas Byrd 2015. All Rights Reserved

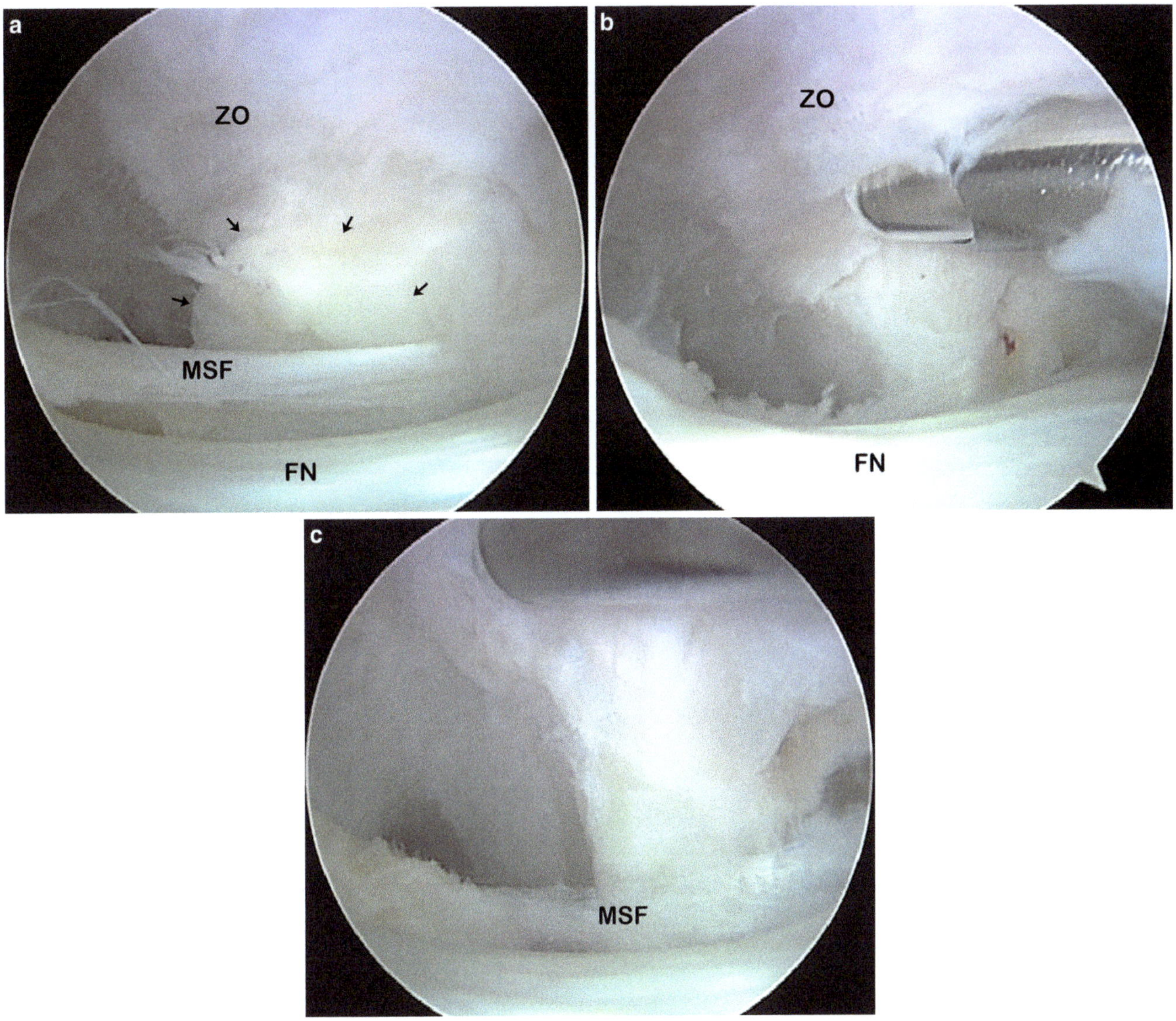

Fig. 49.6 A 17-year-old elite level female sprinter had findings of recalcitrant right hip irritability and hip flexor symptoms. (**a**) Arthroscopy of the peripheral compartment reveals pathological synovial thickening (*arrows*) embedded between the medial synovial fold (MSF) and zona orbicularis (ZO) anterior to the femoral neck (FN). (**b**) A shaver has been introduced excising the lesion between the zona orbicularis (ZO) and the femoral neck (FN). (**c**) Excision has been completed preserving the normal portion of the medial synovial fold (MSF). Published with kind permission of ©J.W. Thomas Byrd 2015. All Rights Reserved

References

1. Torriani M, Souto S, Thomas B, Ouellette H, et al. Ischiofemoral impingement syndrome: an entity with hip pain and abnormalities of the quadratus femoris muscle. Am J Roentgenol. 2009; 193(1):186–90.
2. Stafford G, Villar R. Ischiofemoral impingement. J Bone Joint Surg Br. 2011;93(10):1300–2.
3. May O, Boyer T. Dorfmann: pathologie du repli pectineofoveal et treatment arthroscopie. Rev Chir Orthop. 2004;90:182.
4. Boyer T, May O. Pektineofoveales impingement. Arthroskopie. 2009;22:290–2.
5. Byrd JWT, Polkowski G, Jones KS. Endoscopic management of the snapping iliopsoas tendon (SS-33). Arthroscopy. 2009;25 (6 Suppl):e18.
6. Johnson KA. Impingement of the lesser trochanter on the ischial ramus after total hip arthroplasty. J Bone Joint Surg Am. 1977;59(2):268–9.
7. Patti JW, Ouellette H, Bredella MA, Torriani M. Impingement of lesser trochanter on ischium as a potential cause for hip pain. Skeletal Radiol. 2008;37(10):939–41.
8. Tosun O, Algin O, Yalcin N, Cay N, et al. Ischiofemoral impingement: evaluation with new MRI parameters and assessment of their reliability. Skeletal Radiol. 2012;41:575–87.
9. Ali AM, Whitwell D, Ostlere SJ. Case report: imaging and surgical treatment of a snapping hip due to ischiofemoral impingement. Skeletal Radiol. 2011;40:653–6.
10. O'Brien SD, Bui-Mansfield LT. MRI of quadratus femoris muscle tear: another cause of hip pain. Am J Roentgenol. 2007;189:1185–9.
11. Klinkert Jr P, Porte RJ, de Rooij TPW, deVries AC. Quadratus femoris tendinitis as a cause of groin pain. Br J Sports Med. 1997;31:348–50.

Synovial Disease

50

J.W. Thomas Byrd

Introduction

There is little published literature specifically on the role of arthroscopic synovectomy in the hip. There are two review articles but no original scientific studies [1, 2]. Generally, the indications for arthroscopic synovectomy in the hip are comparable to those reported for other joints. Perhaps, a truly complete synovectomy cannot be performed arthroscopically, but with thorough techniques addressing the central and peripheral compartments, a sufficiently complete synovectomy can be performed to justify its less-invasive nature compared to an open procedure. Synovial disease of the hip may also extend into the iliopsoas bursa, sometimes requiring concomitant iliopsoas bursoscopy.

Hajdu developed a classification system for soft tissue tumors based on the tissue of origin [3]. Tumors of tenosynovial tissue seem to have the greatest predilection for the hip and include synovial).chondromatosis and pigmented villonodular synovitis (PVNS).

This is consistent with our observations as the two most common disorders that we have treated are synovial chondromatosis ($n=38$) and PVNS ($n=13$). Additionally, we have treated a number of PVNS-like cases ($n=4$) characterized by patients with all of the clinical, imaging, and arthroscopic findings of PVNS, yet lacked histologic confirmation because of absence of giant cells on histology. Rarely has arthroscopy been performed for inflammatory arthritides, the most common of which would be rheumatoid disease. As with other joints, improved pharmacological management has eliminated the need for most surgical synovectomies.

J.W.T. Byrd, MD (✉)
Nashville Sports Medicine Foundation, 2011 Church Street, Suite 100, Nashville, TN 37203, USA

Department of Orthopaedic Surgery and Rehabilitation, Vanderbilt University, Nashville, 37232, TN, USA
e-mail: info@nsmoc.com

Nonspecific synovial metaplasia is often observed within the acetabular fossa in conjunction with other damage to the joint. The pulvinar tissue (fat pad lined by synovium) within the fossa is the "canary in the coal mine" among various hip disorders. This tissue demonstrates some type of reaction in conjunction with most any other hip pathology.

Chondrocalcinosis is a metabolic problem, not a synovial-based disorder. However, it is included in this chapter because of its common inflammatory component.

Synovial Chondromatosis (Figs. 50.1, 50.2, and 50.3)

The correct term is synovial chondromatosis. Synovial osteochondromatosis implies ossification of the loose bodies, which does not always occur and is partly responsible for why such an obvious disease is not always so evident on preliminary evaluation. McCarthy reported that half of the cases were unrecognized prior to arthroscopy [4]. While this number may be high with the current quality of imaging, the diagnosis may still not be obvious. An MRI will reveal synovial disease, but it may appear nonspecific. The synovial disorder may not be evident at all when intra-articular contrast has been used and close attention must be given to look for the loose bodies, which sometimes measure only a few millimeters.

We have seen a number of cases of classic femoroacetabular impingement compounded by the presence of synovial chondromatosis. With the obvious impingement as an explanation for problems, closer scrutiny for the synovial disorder may be lacking. The clinical assessment will provide obvious clues. Patients with protracted synovial chondromatosis tend to be very painful even with inactivity and painful with range of motion of the hip in all planes. This is in contrast to the more specific findings typically associated with simple impingement.

J.C. McCarthy et al. (eds.), *Hip Joint Restoration*, DOI 10.1007/978-1-4614-0694-5_50

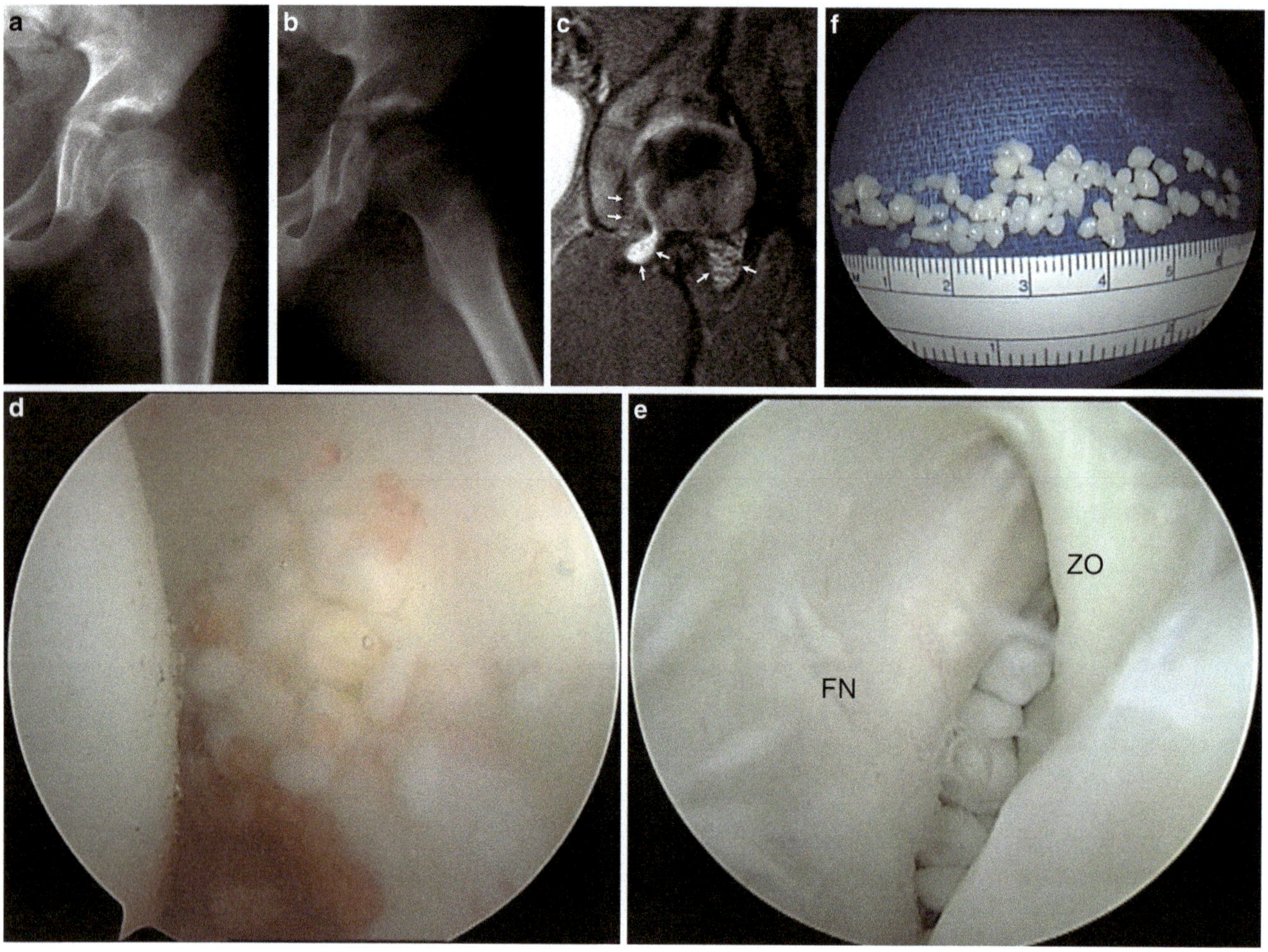

Fig. 50.1 A 10-year-old male with a 2-year history of left hip pain. (**a**, **b**) AP and lateral radiographs reveal numerous densities consistent with synovial chondromatosis. (**c**) Coronal MRI reveals more numerous filling defects (*arrows*) indicative of ossified and non-ossified loose bodies. (**d**) Arthroscopic view of the central compartment reveals clusters of loose bodies. (**e**) Viewing the periphery, more loose bodies are embedded posterior to the femoral neck (FN) underneath the zona orbicularis (ZO). (**f**) Most were debrided with a shaver, but loose bodies expressed through the cannula are illustrated. Published with kind permission of ©J.W. Thomas Byrd 2015. All Rights Reserved

The hip is surpassed only by the knee and elbow as the site of involvement of synovial chondromatosis [5, 6]. Milgram described three phases of synovial chondromatosis based on a temporal sequence [7]. During phase I, the synovial disease is active, but no loose bodies are yet present. The second phase is transition, in which there is active synovial proliferation and loose bodies are present. In the third phase, the synovium becomes quiescent with no demonstrable disease, but the loose bodies remain. Because of the insidious nature of the disease, by the time symptoms become significant enough to incite diagnosis and surgical intervention, the synovial process has long since receded, leaving behind only the loose bodies to create symptoms. Thus, the histologic diagnosis is often in limbo unless synovium can be identified actively producing loose bodies. Recurrence of disease is possible, but recurrence of symptoms following arthroscopy is usually more accurately the result of residual disease, because it can be difficult to ensure that an absolutely thorough debridement has been performed.

Boyer and Dorfmann have reported the largest series of synovial chondromatosis treated by arthroscopy with 120 cases [8]. Twenty-three patients required repeat arthroscopy, while 42 went on to open surgery and another 22 had gone on to total hip replacement. Many of these patients were treated with arthroscopy only of the peripheral compartment without traction. Current techniques would routinely incorporate traction to address the central (intra-articular) compartment as well as the periphery for more thorough management.

In our experience, we have had a 20 % reoperation rate, but repeat arthroscopy can still result in successful outcomes. More than one-third of our patients had concomitant findings of FAI.

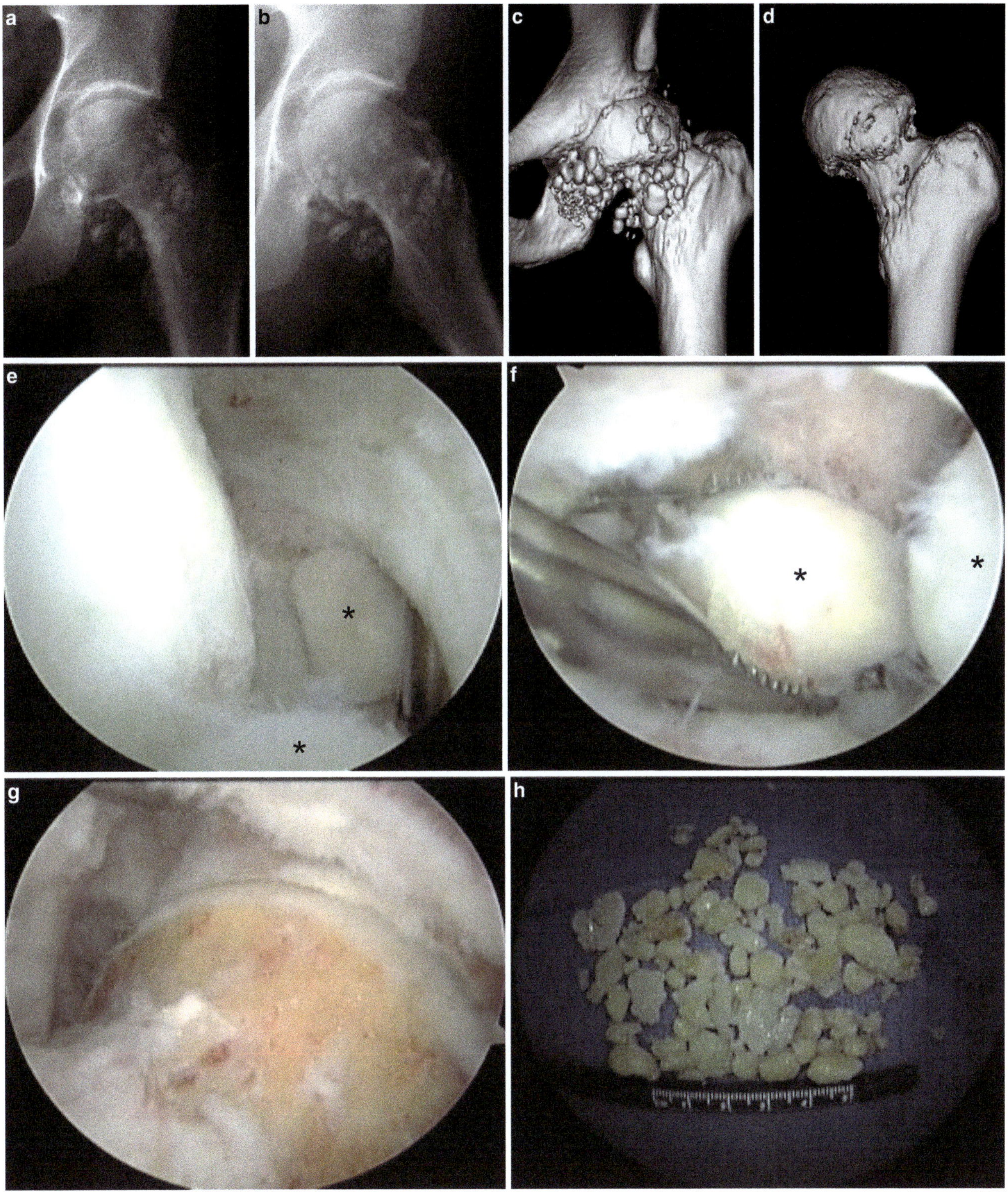

Fig. 50.2 A 48-year-old male presented for evaluation of chronic left knee pain. Examination revealed his knee symptoms to be referred from his hip. (**a**, **b**) AP and lateral radiograph reveal evidence of synovial chondromatosis. (**c**) Loose bodies are further evident on CT scan with 3D reconstruction. (**d**) A digital subtraction image reveals significant cam morphology. (**e**) Viewing from the central compartment, loose bodies are identified (*asterisks*). (**f**) Viewing peripherally, the loose bodies were large (*asterisk*) and required removal with hand instruments. (**g**) Femoroplasty has been completed. (**h**) Some of the removed fragments are shown. Published with kind permission of ©J.W. Thomas Byrd 2015. All Rights Reserved

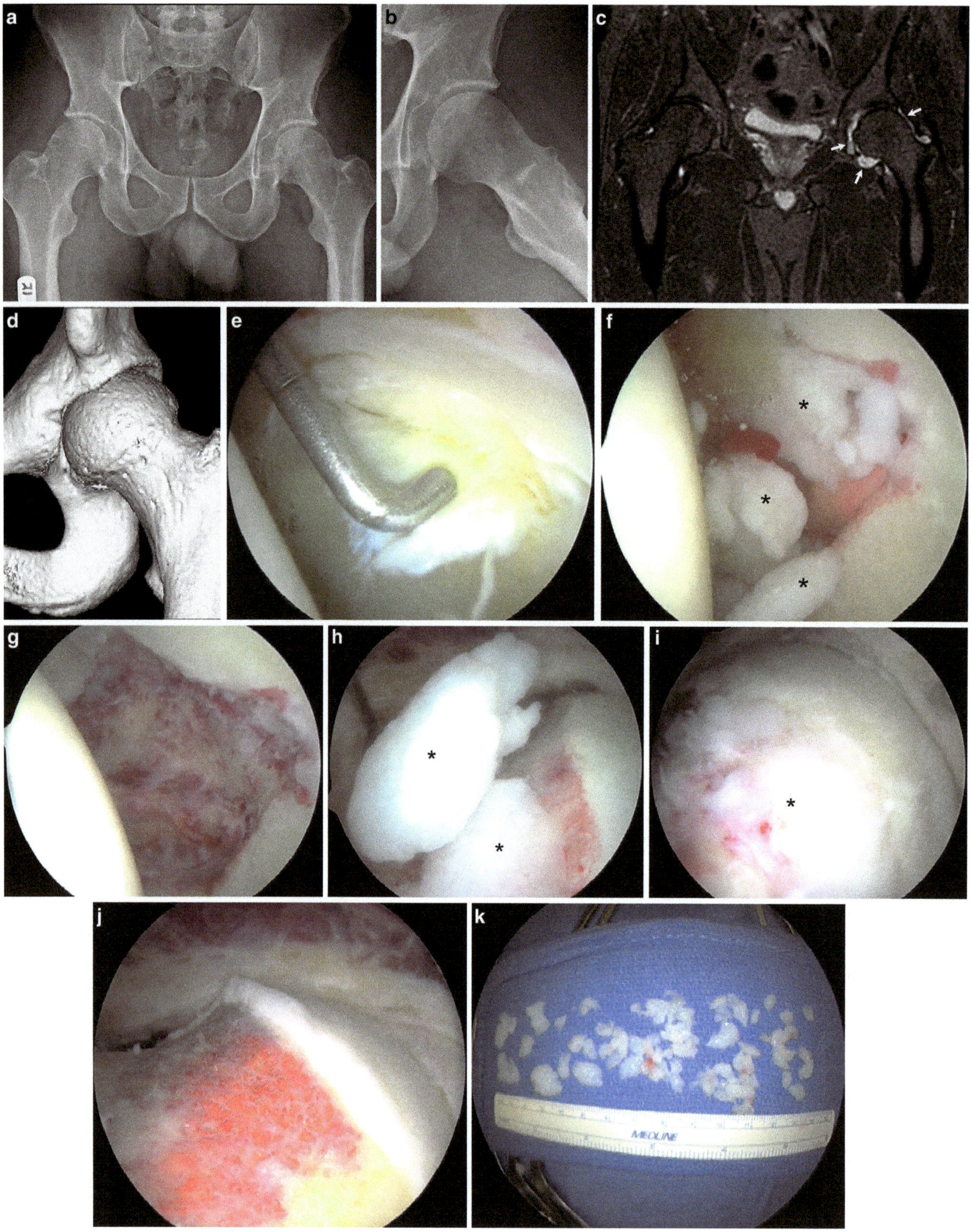

Fig. 50.3 A 36-year-old male miner with a 10-month history of left hip pain following a squatting injury. (**a**) AP pelvis reveals cam morphology with a herniation pit bilaterally and dysplasia with a CE angle of 19 on the left. (**b**) Lateral radiograph reveals loss of normal anterior femoral offset. (**c**) Coronal T2-weighted large field of view MRI reveals a left hip effusion. (**d**) 3D CT scan reveals findings consistent with cam impingement and borderline dysplasia. (**e**) Arthroscopy reveals articular delamination of the anterior acetabulum being probed consistent with pathological cam impingement. (**f**) Loose bodies (*asterisks*) are identified within the acetabular fossa. (**g**) The fossa has been cleared. (**h**) Loose bodies (*asterisks*) are identified in the periphery. (**i**) After loose body removal, the cam lesion is identified (*asterisk*). (**j**) The cam lesion has been corrected. (**k**) Some of the removed debris is illustrated. Published with kind permission of

Pigmented Villonodular Synovitis (Figs. 50.4 and 50.5)

PVNS has been described as having a nodular and a diffuse pattern [9]. The hip is the second most frequent site of involvement with both patterns having been encountered [6, 10].

Synovectomy is the recommended treatment. Many of these patients have significant secondary joint destruction due to the disease by the time the diagnosis is made. Thus, the less-invasive nature of the arthroscopic approach can be especially appealing in this group. In our experience, the diagnosis was established preoperatively in less than half of these patients. Arthroscopic synovectomy can result in good to excellent outcomes and allows treatment of the secondary damage to the joint as well. .Almost one-third had accompanying FAI. In these cases, the primary synovial disease may be overlooked on imaging studies and misinterpreted as simply a secondary synovitis.

Treatment may be as simple as removing a single or multiple nodules, or may require more extensive synovectomy of the central and peripheral compartments and possibly iliopsoas bursa in diffuse patterns. Our results have been comparable with both nodular and diffuse types, with none requiring

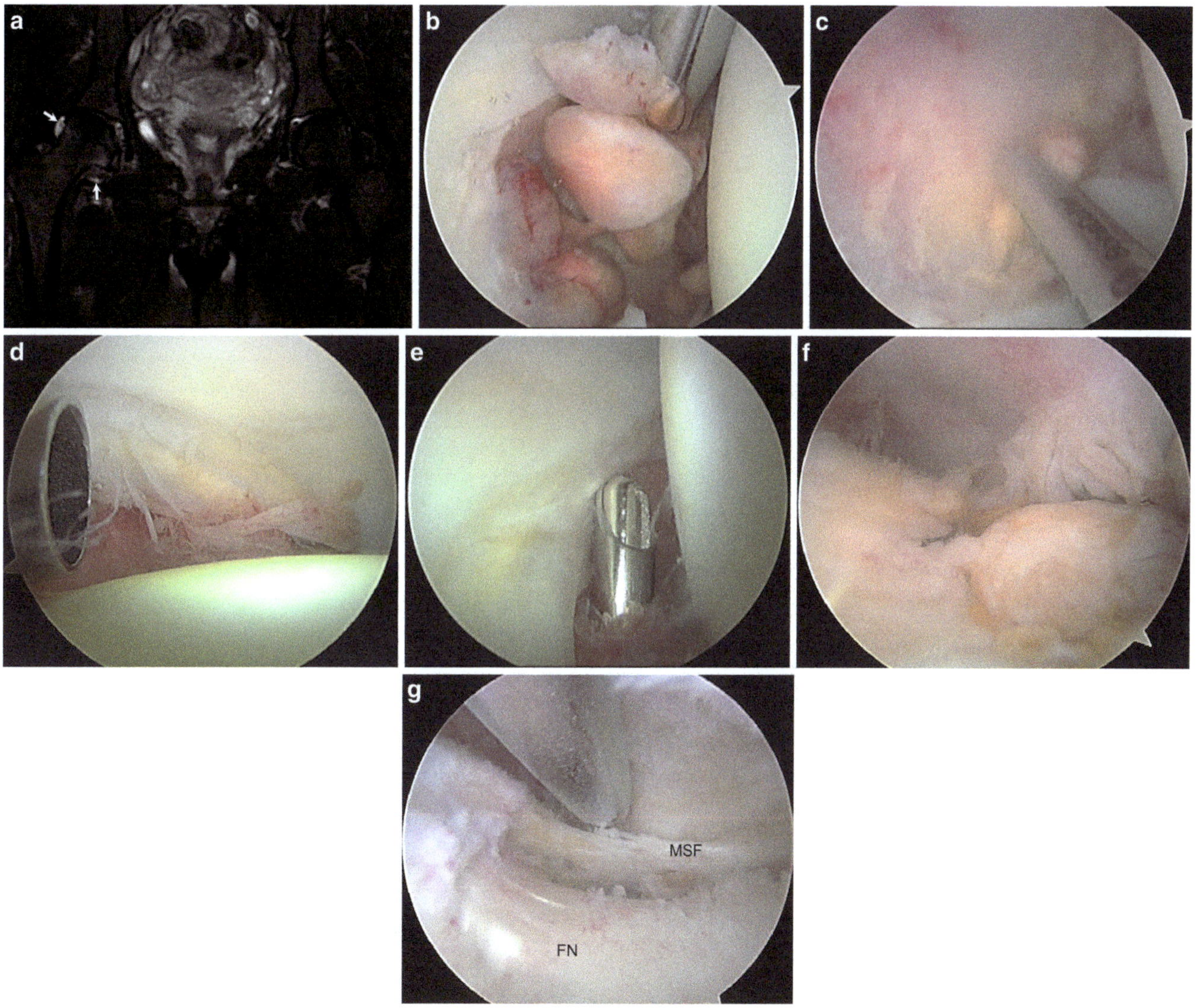

Fig. 50.4 A 23-year-old female with a 2-year history of right hip pain. Radiographs were unrevealing. (**a**) Large field of view T2-weighted coronal image demonstrates a right hip effusion (*arrows*). (**b**) Looking medially, synovial disease consistent with a diffuse pattern of pigmented villonodular synovitis is identified within the acetabular fossa. Debridement begun with the shaver from the anterior portal. (**c**) Synovectomy of the fossa is completed with the shaver from the posterolateral portal. (**d**) Looking posteriorly, further synovial disease is evident behind the labrum. (**e**) Synovectomy of the posterior capsule is accomplished from the posterolateral portal. (**f**) Now viewing in the periphery, the normal anatomy is obscured by synovial disease. (**g**) The save view after synovectomy reveals the anterior neck of the femur (FN) and medial synovial fold (MSF). Published with kind permission of ©J.W. Thomas Byrd 2015. All Rights Reserved

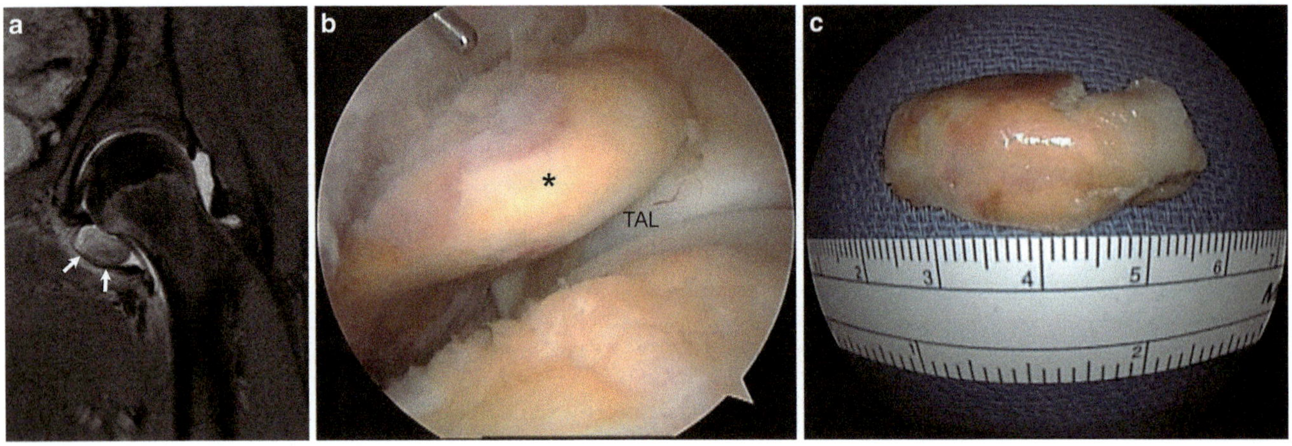

Fig. 50.5 A 14-year-old female dancer with a 3-month history of worsening left hip pain. Radiographs are unremarkable. (**a**) Coronal MRI reveals a nodular lesion (*arrows*) adjacent to the medial base of the femoral neck. (**b**) Arthroscopy reveals a nodular lesion (*asterisk*) underneath the transverse acetabular ligament (TAL). C. The nodular PVNS lesion has been excised. Published with kind permission of ©J.W. Thomas Byrd 2015. All Rights Reserved

further surgery for recurrent synovial disease. The future outlook is often dictated by the severity of secondary damage present at the time of the index arthroscopic procedure. Thus, it is possible that some may still be facing the prospect of a future arthroplasty even with successful management of the synovial disease.

Intra-articular radioisotope injection has been described as an ionizing method of synovectomy [11, 12]. However, there is little information on its application in the hip and the success is limited. Perhaps it might be considered as adjuvant therapy with arthroscopic synovectomy, but its role is not yet defined, and, thus far, we have found satisfactory results with arthroscopy alone.

Nonspecific Inflammatory Disorders of the Pulvinar

The pulvinar tissue has been reported as an important trigger of joint pain with a substantial pattern of nociceptive innervation [13]. It undergoes significant upregulation of these neurons in painful conditions such as osteoarthritis. We have observed that lesions in this area can be quite painful and may represent the neural equivalent of the fat pad in the knee as described by Scott Dye's neural mapping.

Metaplasia of this synovial tissue can occasionally be a primary pain generator in the hip and frequently occurs in association with numerous types of joint pathology [14]. These metaplastic changes are variable and may be characterized as typical villous synovitis, fibrous hyperplasia, or dense contracted fibrosis. As stated in the opening comments, the pulvinar tissue is the canary in the coal mine for the hip and reacts with almost any joint problem.

Primary synovial lesions in this area can be quite painful and respond very well to debridement. Thus, our tendency is to remove the abnormal tissue when present in conjunction with other disorders. It is important to preserve the ligamentum teres, if it is intact, and avoid unnecessarily violating this structure. Also, for some hips, if access to the fossa is difficult, then the surgeon should not risk damaging the joint surfaces in an effort to remove the diseased tissue. For aggressive synovial disorders such as PVNS, thermal ablation can be performed with a flexible radiofrequency device. Additional access to the most medial and inferior portions of the fovea can usually be obtained by temporarily increasing the distraction, creating an additional portal, and using curved or flexible extended length instruments.

Chondrocalcinosis (Fig. 50.6)

Chondrocalcinosis is most commonly caused by calcium pyrophosphate deposition (CPPD; or pseudogout) [15]. Gout typically attacks peripheral joints, such as the foot or knee, with lower temperature that promotes precipitation of calcium urate crystals and would be very uncommon in the hip [16]. In fact there is only one reported case of monarticular gouty arthritis of the hip [17].

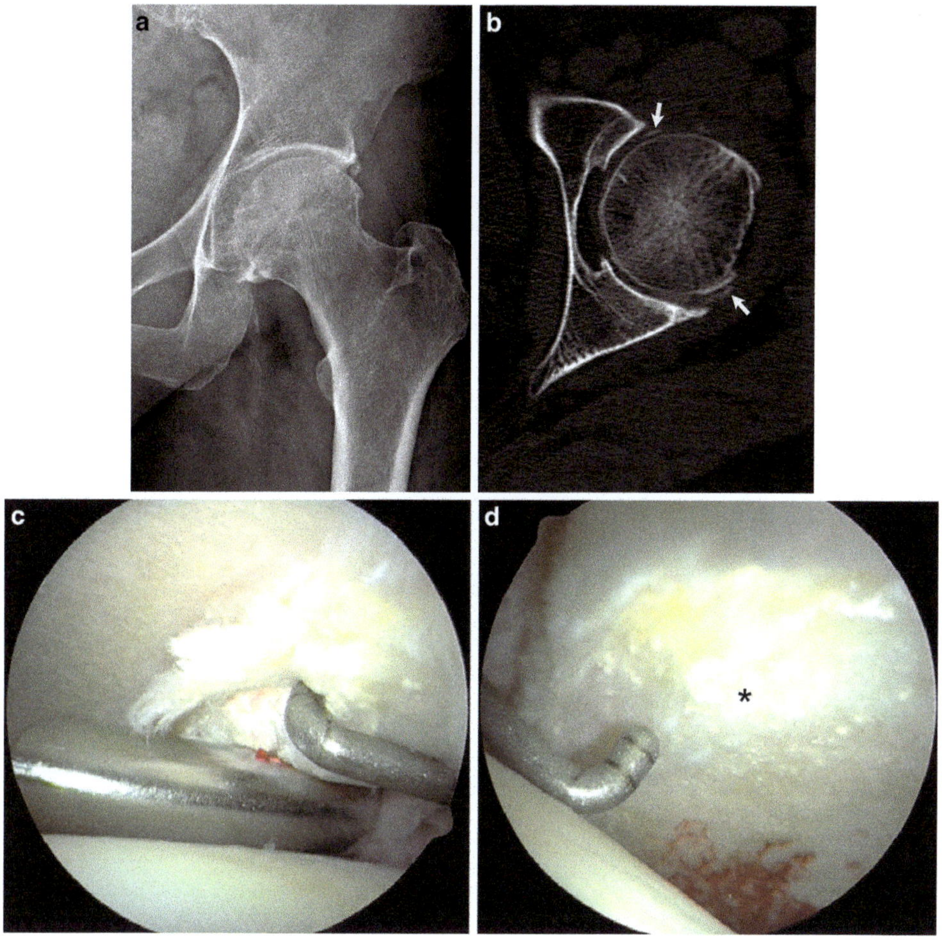

Fig. 50.6 A 59-year-old female with- long-standing left hip pain. (**a**) AP radiograph left hip reveals some densities around the acetabulum. (**b**) Axial CT scan reveals evidence of calcification embedded within the articular surface. (**c**) Arthroscopy reveals calcific deposition is embedded within the substance of the degenerated labrum which is being probed. (**d**) A stippled pattern of calcific deposition within the articular surface of the acetabulum is revealed (*asterisk*). Published with kind permission of ©J.W. Thomas Byrd 2015. All Rights Reserved

Chondrocalcinosis is characterized by the crystallite material embedded within the hyaline cartilage and sometimes the labrum. This is different than amorphous globular calcific deposits that may develop within diseased labrum (Fig. 50.7). This occurs because the diseased labrum loses its inhibitory properties to prevent these deposits. This type of calcific deposition is more comparable to the pathophysiology of calcific deposits within a diseased rotator cuff.

Chondrocalcinosis in the hip is not as radiographically evident as it is in the knee, where the meniscus is often silhouetted by the depositions. The deposits alter the structural properties of the articular surface and labrum, making them more susceptible to breakdown. Treatment typically consists of treating the damaged cartilage. Sometimes superficial deposits can be swept off, generally using a blunt-tipped probe, but aggressive efforts to excise the embedded material are not necessary. In the knee, arthroscopic surgery in the presence of chondrocalcinosis is often followed by a stormy early postoperative course due to recurrent painful effusions. Fortunately, in the hip, only occasionally is this observation made. It is worthy to be aware of this scenario and warn patients so that they will be prepared in case the initial few days of recovery are difficult.

Summary

Arthroscopic synovectomy is appropriately indicated in the hip for a variety of conditions. Often, the secondary damage to the joint is significant and further emphasizes the advantage of a less-invasive arthroscopic approach for these patients who are often still facing a future arthroplasty.

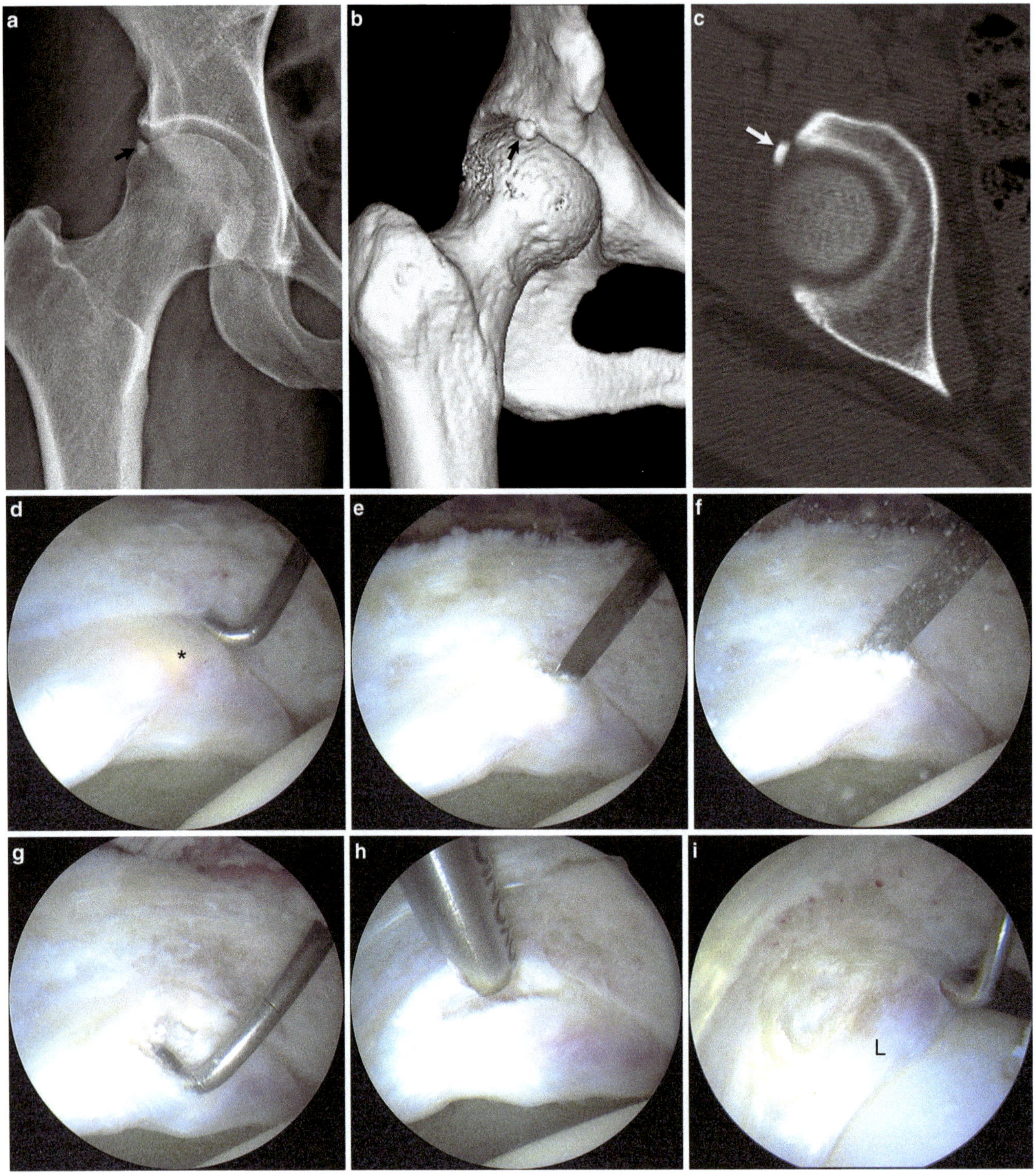

Fig. 50.7 A 41-year-old female with calcific deposition within the substance of the anterolateral labrum of her right hip. (**a**) AP radiograph reveals a small density (*arrow*). (**b**) 3D CT scan demonstrates the density geographically within the area of the anterolateral labrum (*arrow*). (**c**) Axial CT image reveals increased homogeneous density compared to bone, suggesting calcification instead of ossification (*arrow*). (**d**) Arthroscopic view from the anterolateral portal reveals the area of calcific deposition within the anterolateral labrum (*asterisk*). (**e**) An arthroscopic knife is being used to open the area of calcific deposit. (**f**) A slurry of calcific debris is expressed creating the snow field appearance. (**g**) The pocket has been opened. (**h**) Debridement is completed with a shaver. (**i**) Viewing with the traction released, excision has been completed, preserving the structural integrity of the labrum (L). Published with kind permission of

References

1. Godde S, Kusma M, Dienst M. Synovial disorders and loose bodies in the hip joint. Arthroscopic diagnostics and treatment. Orthopade. 2006;35(1):67–76.
2. Krebs VE. The role of hip arthroscopy in the treatment of synovial disorders and loose bodies. Clin Orthop Relat Res. 2003;406:48–59.
3. Hajdu SI. Tumors of tendosynovial tissue. In: Hajdu SI, editor. Pathology of soft tissue tumors. Philadelphia: Lea & Febiger; 1979. p. 165–226.
4. McCarthy JC, Bono JV, Wardell S. Is there a treatment for synovial chondromatosis of the hip joint? Arthroscopy. 1997;13(3):409–10.
5. Villacin AB, Brigham LN, Bullough PG. Primary and secondary synovial chondrometaplasia. Hum Pathol. 1979;10(4):439–51.
6. Spjut JH, Dorfmann HD, Fechner RD, Ackerman LV, Firminger HI, editors. Tumors of bone and cartilage, Atlas of tumor pathology, second series. Washington: Armed Forces Institute of Pathology; 1983. p. 391–410.
7. Milgram JW. Synovial osteochondromatosis. J Bone Joint Surg Br. 1977;59:792–801.
8. Boyer T, Dorfmann H. Arthroscopy in primary synovial chondromatosis of the hip: description and outcome of treatment. J Bone Joint Surg Br. 2008;90(3):314–8.
9. Enneking WF. Musculoskeletal tumor surgery. New York: Churchill Livingstone; 1983. p. 1167–74.
10. Danzig LA, Gershuni DH, Resnick D. Diagnosis and treatment of diffuse pigmented villonodular synovitis of the hip. Clin Orthop. 1982;168:42–77.
11. Shabat S, Kollender Y, Merimsky O. The use of surgery and yttrium 90 in the management of extensive and diffuse pigmented villonodular synovitis of large joints. Rheumatology. 2002;41:1113–8.
12. Zook JE, Wurtz DL, Cummings JE, et al. Intra-articular chromic phosphate (^{32}P) in the treatment of diffuse pigmented villonodular synovitis. Brachytherapy. 2011;10(3):190–4.
13. Saxler G, Loer F, Skumavc M, et al. Localization of SP- and CGRP-immunopositive nerve fibers in the hip joint of patients with painful osteoarthritis and of patients with painless failed total hip arthroplasties. Eur J Pain. 2007;11(1):67–74.
14. Byrd JWT. Indications and contraindications. In: Byrd JWT, editor. Operative hip arthroscopy. 2nd ed. New York: Springer; 2005. p. 6–35.
15. Rosenthal AK. Update in calcium deposition diseases. Curr Opin Rheumatol. 2007;19:158–62.
16. Fitzgerald BT, Setty A, Mudgal CS. Gout affecting the hand and wrist. J Am Acad Orthop Surg. 2007;15:625–35.
17. Parhami N, Feng H. Gout in the hip joint. Arthritis Rheum. 1993;36(7):1026.

Surgical Treatment of Specific Hip Conditions: Ligamentum Teres Injuries

51

Alexandra Dimitrakopoulou and Richard N. Villar

Introduction

The awareness of ligamentum teres pathology has increased in recent years, alongside improvements in surgical techniques and imaging modalities. Injury to the ligamentum teres has been identified as a significant source of hip pain and has also been demostrated that contributes to mechanical instability of the hip joint.

Ligamentum Teres Injuries

Epidemiology

In the literature the prevalence of ligamentum teres tears during hip arthroscopy is reported to be between 4 % and 17.5 % [1–3]. Byrd et al. [2] reported 24 cases, in which 40 % were isolated tears of the ligamentum and 60 % had other associated intra-articular lesions. A more recent study [4], demonstrated that 51 % (284 cases) had a ligamentum tear in a cohort of 558 hip arthroscopies. The most common type (43 %) was a partial tear, followed by 4.5 % for a degenerate tear and 3.7 % for a complete rupture. In an athletic population, rupture of the ligamentum teres has been reported as the third most common problem affecting the hip joint [5].

Aetiology

Isolated ligamentum teres ruptures are rare [6, 7] although have been reported in the literature, as well as tears in conjunction with other intra-articular pathologies of the hip. Aetiologies include trauma, repetitive stress or micro-instability and degeneration [4]. In a cohort study [8] of 48 patients with dysplasia, 13 patients (27 %) were identified with a rupture of the ligamentum teres, suggesting that the ligamentum may be vulnerable in the presence of dysplasia.

A. Dimitrakopoulou, MD
The London Hip Arthroscopy Center, Orthopaedics, The Wellington Hospital and Leeds Metropolitan University, London, UK
e-mail: alexdimitr@yahoo.gr

R.N. Villar, MS, FRCS (✉)
The Richard Villar Practice, Spire Cambridge Lea Hospital, 30 New Road, Impington, Cambridge CB24 9EL, UK
e-mail: rnv1000@aol.com

Mechanism of Injury

Usually, ruptures of the ligamentum are associated with major trauma such as a road traffic accident [2, 9], falling from a height or sporting activities [10]. Philippon et al. [10] published a series of athletes (14 hockey players) with a traumatic dislocation of the hip joint during athletic activities and found that 12 patients (85.7 %) had a torn ligamentum. Ilizaliturri et al. [9] reported on 17 patients with hypertrophic tissue (scar tissue) around the ligamentum teres after a traumatic posterior dislocation of the hip. Meanwhile avulsion fractures of the ligamentum teres, normally from its femoral attachment, may also occur [7, 11].

Several case reports [6, 7, 12] have been published on ligamentum rupture after minor injury; they occurred after a hyperabduction injury [6, 12]. A twisting injury has also been described as a mechanism for rupture of the ligamentum teres [2, 13].

In DDH, entrapment of the ligamentum teres can be a source of pain with mechanical symptoms, because of its special structure or degeneration [8]. Of interest is a study [14] of 19 hips in the early stage of Perthes' disease. The authors measured the sphericity and subluxation of the hip after an arthrography. They reported no correlation between sphericity and subluxation and it seems that subluxation precedes deformation. Re-examining all the arthrograms they identified that swelling of the ligamentum teres caused a lateral subluxation of the femoral head.

Meanwhile, ossification of the ligamentum teres has been reported in certain enthesopathies (Ankylosing Spondylitis and Diffuse Idiopathic Skeletal Hyperostosis) [15, 16]. This has been reported as a possible mechanism of lateral subluxation of the femoral head, resulting in superolateral narrowing of the joint space [15].

J.C. McCarthy et al. (eds.), *Hip Joint Restoration*, DOI 10.1007/978-1-4614-0694-5_51

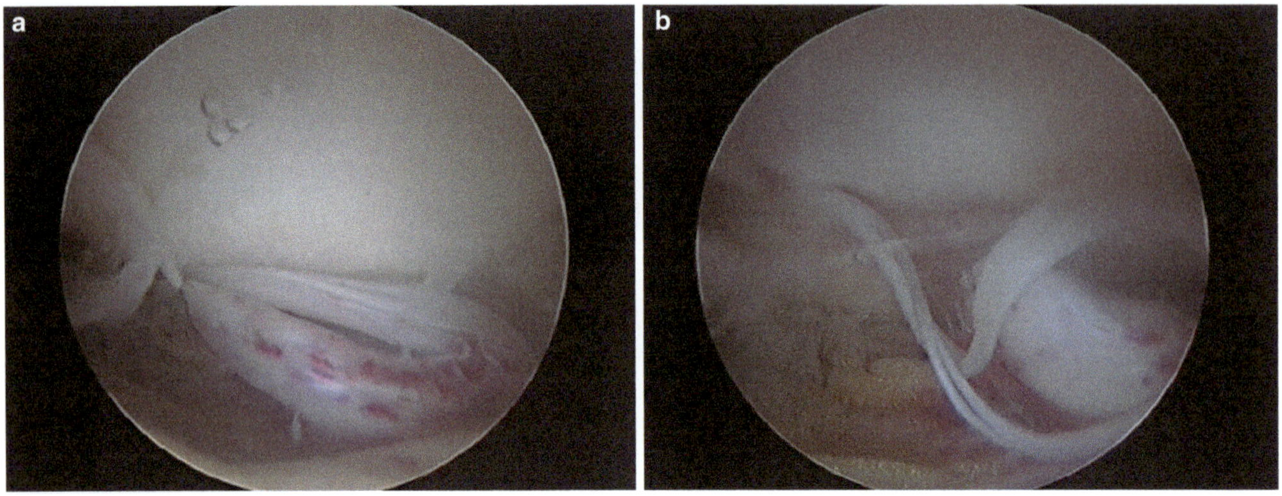

Fig. 51.1 Arthroscopic images revealing a possible rupture of the ligamentum teres during internal rotation (**a**), which is completely revealed in external rotation (**b**)

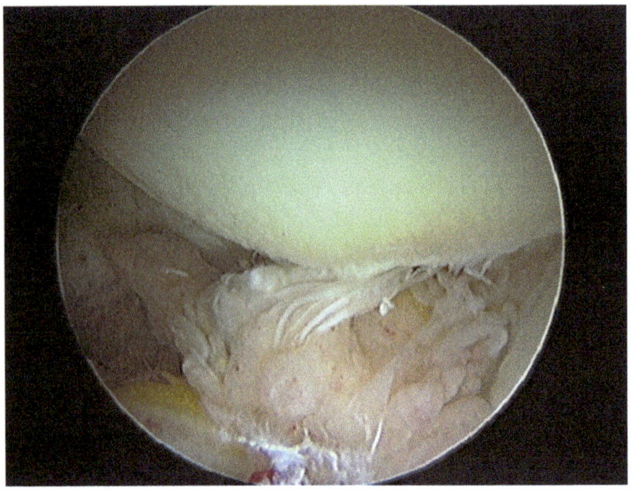

Fig. 51.2 Arthroscopic image of a partially ruptured ligamentum teres

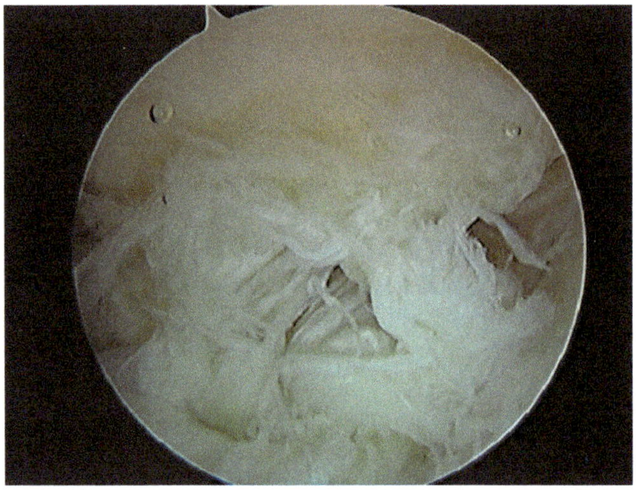

Fig. 51.3 Arthroscopic image showing a degenerate, frayed ligamentum combined with generalised degenerative changes of the femoral head

A potential mechanism of injury to the ligamentum may occur in femoroacetabular impingement. During flexion-abduction, additional strain is placed on the ligamentum as it provides a sling-like support to prevent inferior subluxation of the femoral head [17].

Classification of Injury

Gray and Villar [18] were the first to categorise pathology of the ligamentum teres. According to their classification there are three types of injury: Group 1 is a complete rupture of the ligamentum caused by injury (Fig. 51.1), Group 2 is a partial rupture with no specific injuries but long-standing hip problems (Fig. 51.2). Group 3 refers to a degenerate, frayed ligament combined with generalised degenerative changes of the joint (Fig. 51.3). A new descriptive classification based on the intra-operative findings and the tear percentage of the ligamentum has been proposed [4]. Grade 0 is normal, grade 1 is a low-grade partial tear <50 %, grade 2 is a high-grade partial tear >50 % and grade 3 is a full-thickness tear.

Diagnosis of Ligamentum Teres Injury

Clinical Presentation

The onset of pain can be acute after a traumatic event [4]. Patients can present with persistent, deep anterior groin pain or thigh pain during activities with loss of movement and stiffness. Mechanical symptoms such as catching, popping, locking, and giving way can be present but are non-specific for ligamentum pathology [2]. Limping can also be apparent. A detailed clinical history with careful analysis of the mechanism of injury may help in diagnosing ligamentum injuries.

Physical Examination

Physical examination of the hip is challenging. There is no specific examination that can reveal a ligamentum teres injury. A test has been proposed with the patient supine and the knee flexed to 90^0 while moving the leg through a full range of internal and external rotation. The test is positive when pain is elicited during rotational movements [19]. The sensitivity of the test is 83 % and the specificity 90 %, with a positive predictive value of 93 % and a negative predictive value of 77 % [19].

Log-rolling can be a useful test for distinguishing intra-articular from extra-articular pathology of the hip. The external rotation dial test can show hip laxity and more specifically assesses anterior capsular laxity [20]. Manual external rotation is applied to the leg and the test becomes positive when the leg lies externally rotated or there is no end point reached with external rotation. The impingement test can cause some discomfort and straight leg raise can be painful. Meanwhile the axial traction apprehension test assesses global instability of the hip [20]. For this, manual axial traction is applied to the leg, thereby applying distraction, the test being positive when the patient demonstrates apprehension. Combined flexion, adduction and external rotation of the affected leg may reproduce painful symptoms by stressing a partially torn ligamentum teres.

The range of movement can be reduced, while there may be painful internal rotation and extension [1, 2]. Botser et al. [4] reported an increased range of movement especially in flexion and internal rotation after injury to the ligamentum teres. Audible or palpable clicking of the hip may be manifest during clinical examination.

Differential Diagnosis

The differential diagnosis should include a hip flexor strain, internal snapping of the hip and other intra-articular pathologies such as a labral tear, osteochondral defect, or loose bodies.

Radiographic Assessment

Detection of ligamentum pathology is difficult as the hip is a deeply seated and tight joint, its intra-articular structures are very closely opposed, so it can be difficult to assess accurately.

Under fluoroscopy, laxity of the hip can be assessed using axial traction. It is positive when a "vacuum sign" is evident [20]. Computed tomography (CT) and magnetic resonance imaging (MRI) can reveal ligamentous pathology (Fig. 51.4). Rao et al. [3] identified only 4 % of patients with Group 1 tears and 4 % with Group 2 and 3 tears. However, a

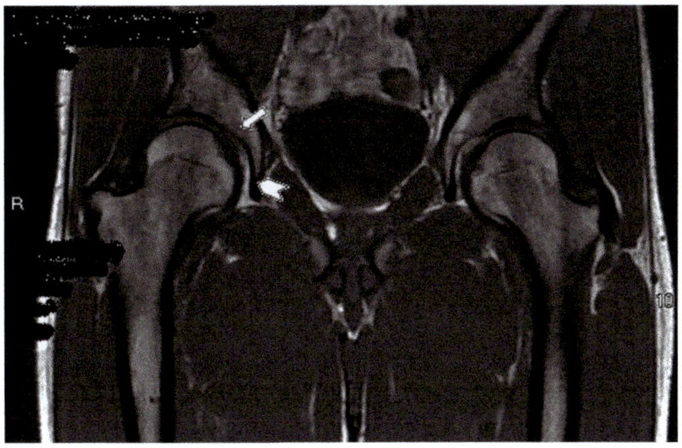

Fig. 51.4 A coronal T1-weighted fat-suppressed MRI shows a complete rupture of the ligamentum (*arrow*) with widened joint space (*arrowhead*)

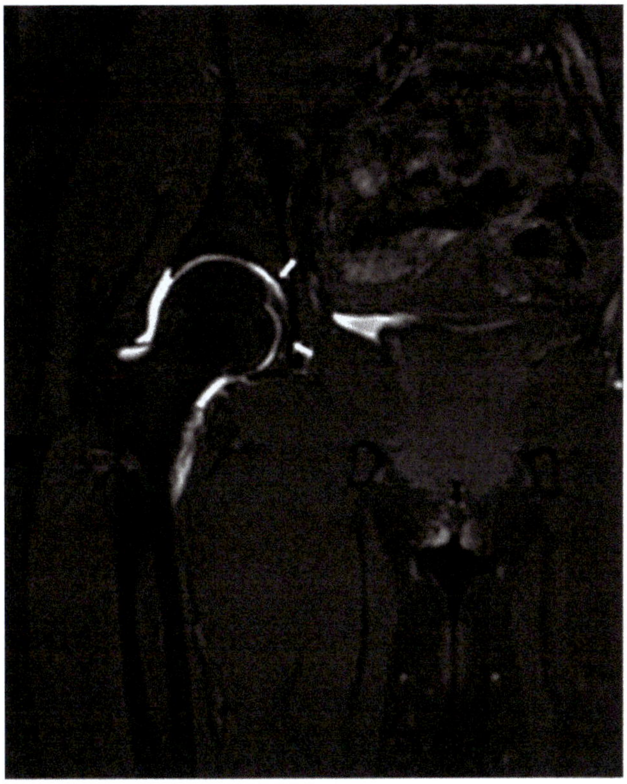

Fig. 51.5 A coronal T1-weighted fat-suppressed MR arthrogram can reveal the continuity and entire length of the ligamentum teres (the *double arrow* shows the origin at the acetabular transverse ligament and the *single arrow* shows its insertion at the fovea capitis femoris)

3-T MRI scan without contrast can reveal the ligamentous pathology [20].

Magnetic resonance arthrography (MRA) with gadolinium-enhancement and CT arthrography are the preferred imaging modalities for detection of ligamentum tears (Fig. 51.5). The best images for identifying the ligamentum are coronal, axial and axial oblique. Discontinuity, waviness

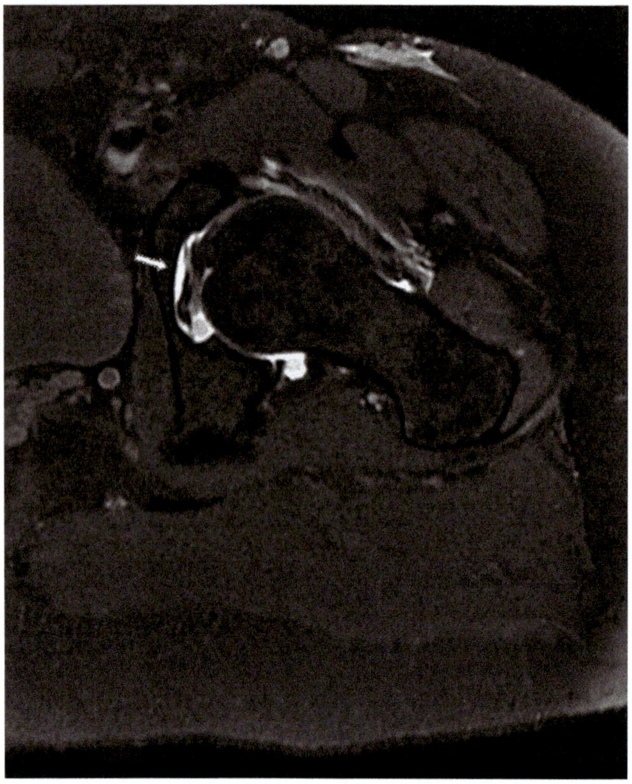

Fig. 51.6 Axial oblique fat-suppressed MR arthrogram shows a partial tear of the ligamentum teres (the *arrow* shows the discontinuity of the ligamentum)

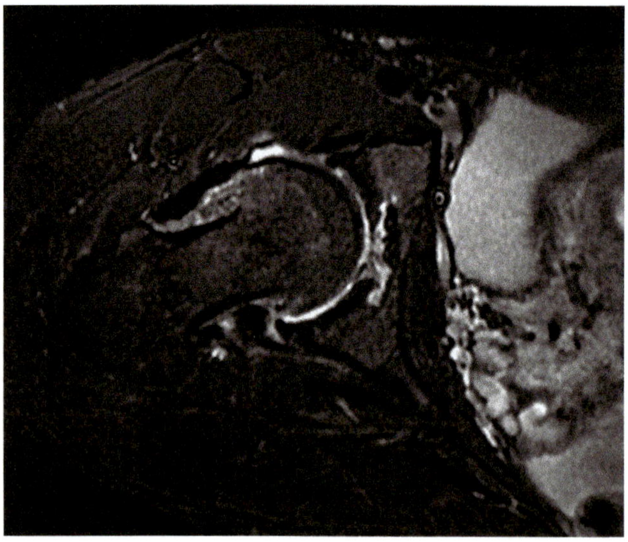

Fig. 51.7 Axial oblique fat-suppressed MR arthrogram shows a complete tear of the ligamentum teres

or a lax contour are signs of an acute tear (Fig. 51.6 and Fig. 51.7). Meanwhile, focal loss of continuity, elongation or attenuation with an irregular or lax contour are signs of a chronic tear. Mucinous or mucoid degeneration represent a degenerate (Fig. 51.8) or chronic tear. Avulsion fractures of

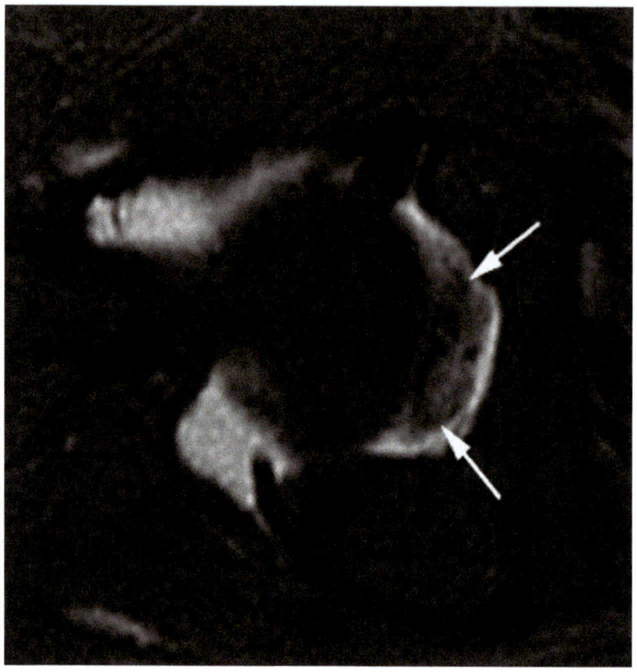

Fig. 51.8 Axial MR arthrogram shows diffuse degenerative thickening of the ligamentum teres (*arrows*)

the foveal attachment of the ligamentum teres may be non-displaced, partially or completely displaced [21]. Abnormalities of the ligament include hypertrophy, fraying, elongation or absence.

For tears of the ligamentum teres, Botser et al. [4] reported a very low sensitivity, (<2 %), a low accuracy, with positive and negative predictive values of 56 % and 49 %, respectively, on MRA.

Treatment

When lesions of the ligamentum teres are diagnosed, the treatment may involve arthroscopic surgery. Although isolated tears can occur, most tears are associated with other intra-articular pathologies, which should also be addressed.

Debridement of frayed, torn fibres relieves pain and mechanical symptoms [1, 2]. It should be performed with the hip in slight external rotation as this improves the visualisation and access to the area. A more posteriorly situated portal is sometimes better for access to structures within the cotyloid fossa. However, careful attention should be paid to surgery in this area as a complete resection of the ligamentum may result in iatrogenic instability of the hip. In case of partial tears, shrinkage of the ligament with a radiofrequency device, while the hip is in a neutral position, can be performed (Fig. 51.9). Radiofrequency instruments also permit haemostasis within the vascular pulvinar.

After this procedure a fibroblastic response may improve the biomechanical strength of the remaining fibres of the ligament. Over-shrinkage may lead to limitation of external

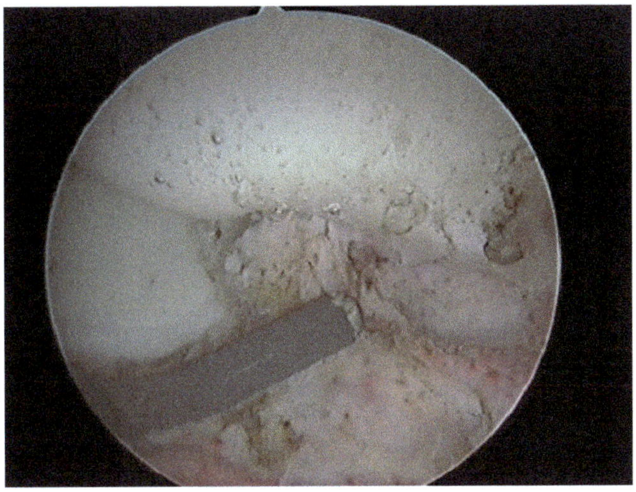

Fig. 51.9 Shrinkage of the ligament with a radiofrequency device in progress

rotation of the hip postoperatively. In addition, a complete tear and avulsion fracture of the ligamentum can be treated with arthroscopic debridement [12, 22]. Arthroscopic debridement for degenerative rupture of the ligamentum teres has proved successful with immediate relief of symptoms [23].

Short-term outcomes with arthroscopic debridement in small series and case report studies showed favourable-to-excellent results [2, 12, 18, 22, 23]. Haviv and O'Donnell [24] evaluated 29 patients with isolated ligamentum injuries. At 12 months' follow-up the mean mHHS (modified Harris Hip Score) improved from 70 to 86 and the mean NAHS (non-Arthritic Hip Score) improved from 64 to 86. Continued improvement was observed in 82.7 % of cases but 17.3 % (5 cases) developed recurrent symptoms and subsequently underwent a second arthroscopy. All the cases had recurrent partial tears and were treated by re-debridement and capsular tightening, resulting in reduction of external rotation (10°–15°) both in flexion and extension of the hip.

Regeneration of the ligamentum teres has been reported in two cases after a traumatic hip dislocation [25]. A soft-tissue connection between the cotyloid fossa and the femoral head was evident during hip arthroscopy.

Arthroscopic reconstruction of the ligamentum teres has been undertaken. Simpson et al. [26] were the first to publish an arthroscopic reconstruction in one patient, a dancer, using an artificial graft (Ligament Augmentation & Reconstruction System-LARS, LARS (France)). At 10 weeks' follow-up the patient was asymptomatic although external rotation was restricted to 50 % compared with the contralateral hip. At 8 months the patient showed continued improvement and by 1 year had returned to dance. Arthroscopic reconstruction using a double-stranded semitendinosus tendon as a graft has been reported in one female patient by Amenabar and O'Donnell [27]. At 12 months after surgery the mHHS improved from 53 to 100 and NAHS increased from 73 to 95. At a repeat arthroscopy 15 months postoperatively, the graft had resorbed but the two stitches remained firmly attached and were acting as a synthetic ligament. More recently, Philippon et al. [20] reported an arthroscopic reconstruction of the ligamentum teres using an iliotibial band autograft in four female athletes. At a mean of 31 months after surgery all patients reported resolution of symptoms and had returned to their desired level of sport. At 3 years' follow-up one patient underwent a hip replacement. Future studies with larger series and longer follow-up are required to assess the efficacy of this procedure. Postoperative rehabilitation involves immediate weight-bearing as tolerated, with early movement of the hip.

References

1. Bardakos NV, Villar RN. The ligamentum teres of the adult hip. J Bone Joint Surg (Br). 2009;91-B:8–15.
2. Byrd JWT, Jones KS. Traumatic rupture of the ligamentum teres as a source of hip pain. Arthroscopy. 2004;20:385–91.
3. Rao J, Zhou YX, Villar RN. Injury to the ligamentum teres. Mechanism, findings, and results of treatment. Clin Sports Med. 2001;20:791–9.
4. Botser IB, Martin DE, Stout CE, Domb BG. Tears of the ligamentum teres. Prevalence in hip arthroscopy using 2 classification systems. Am J Sports Med. 2011;39(Suppl):17–25.
5. Byrd JWT, Jones KS. Hip arthroscopy in athletes. Clin Sports Med. 2001;20:749–62.
6. Delcamp DD, Klaaren HE, Pompe van Meerdervoort HF. Traumatic avulsion of the ligamentum teres without dislocation of the hip. J Bone Joint Surg Am. 1988;70(6):933–35.
7. Barrett IR, Goldberg JA. Avulsion fracture of the ligamentum teres in a child. J Bone Joint Surg Am. 1989;1-A:438–9.
8. Byrd JWT, Jones KS. Hip arthroscopy in the presence of dysplasia. Arthroscopy. 2003;19:1055–60.
9. Ilizaliturri VM, Gonzalez-Gutierrez B, Gonzalez-Ugalde H, Camacho-Galindo J. Hip arthroscopy after traumatic hip dislocation. Arthroscopy. 2011;39S:50–7.
10. Philippon MJ, Kuppersmith DA, Wolff AB, Briggs KK. Arthroscopic findings following traumatic hip dislocation in 14 professional athletes. Arthroscopy. 2009;25:169–74.
11. Krych AJ, Thompson M, Larson CM, Byrd JWT, Kelly BT. Is posterior hip instability associated with cam and pincer deformity? Clin Orthop Relat Res. 2012;470:3390–7.
12. Kusma M, Jung J, Dienst M, et al. Arthroscopic treatment of an avulsion fracture of the ligamentum teres of the hip in an 18-year-old horse rider. Arthroscopy. 2004;20(Suppl):64–6.
13. Yamamoto Y, Villar RN, Papavasileiou A. Supermarket hip: an unusual cause of injury to the hip joint. Arthroscopy. 2008;24: 490–3.
14. Kamegaya M, Moriya H, Tsuchiya K, Akita T, Ogata S, Someya M. Arthrography of early Perthes' disease. J Bone Joint Surg Br. 1989;71(3):413–17.
15. Innoue K, Schichikawa K, Takenaka Y, et al. Ossification of the ligamentum teres as a possible mechanism of lateral subluxation in coxopathy associated with ankylosing spinal hyperostosis. Ann Rheum Dis. 1993;52:306–7.

16. Gillet P, Pere P, Jouzeau JY, Floquet J, Gaucher A. Enthesitis of the ligamentum teres during ankylosing spondylitis: histopathological report. Ann Rheum Dis. 1994;53:82–3.
17. Kivlan BR, Clemente FR, Martin RL, Martin HD. Function of the ligamentum teres during multi-planar movement of the hip joint. Knee Surg Sports Traumatol Arthrosc. 2013;21(7):1664–8.
18. Gray AJ, Villar RN. The ligamentum teres of the hip: an arthroscopic classification of its pathology. Arthroscopy. 1997;13:575–8.
19. Bates D, Pritchard M, O'Donnell J, Singh P. Ligamentum teres test. 2013. http://www.lakesidesmc.com.au. Accessed 21 Jun 2013.
20. Philippon MJ, Pennock A, Gaskill TR. Arthroscopic reconstruction of the ligamentum teres. J Bone Joint Surg Br. 2012;94(11): 1494–98.
21. Cerezal L, Kassarjian A, Canga A, et al. Anatomy, biomechanics, imaging, and management of ligamentum teres injuries. Radiographics. 2010;30:1637–51.
22. Kashiwagi N, Suzuki S, Seto Y. Arthroscopic treatment for traumatic hip dislocation with avulsion fracture of the ligamentum teres. Arthroscopy. 2001;17:67–9.
23. Yamamoto Y, Usui I. Arthroscopic surgery for degenerative rupture of the ligamentum teres femoris. Arthroscopy. 2006;22:689e1–e3.
24. Haviv B, O'Donnell J. Arthroscopic debridement of the isolated ligamentum teres rupture. Knee Surg Sports Traumatol Arthrosc. 2011;19:1510–3.
25. Schaumkel JV, Villar RN. Healing of the ruptured ligamentum teres after hip dislocation-an arthroscopic finding. Hip Int. 2009;19: 64–6.
26. Simpson JM, Field RE, Villar RN. Arthroscopic reconstruction of the ligamentum teres. Arthroscopy. 2011;27:436–41.
27. Amenabar T, O'Donnell J. Arthroscopic ligamentum teres reconstruction using semitendinosus tendon: surgical technique and an unusual outcome. Arthrosc Tech. 2012;2:e169–74.

Treatment of Specific Conditions: Loose Bodies

52

Matías Salineros and Rodrigo Mardones

With the development of arthroscopic surgery, one of its most remarkable advantages is the ability to remove loose bodies from synovial lined joints without an arthrotomy. It's been reported as successful and effective in almost every joint accessed such as the shoulder, wrist, elbow, knee, and now the hip [1–3].

The early reports on loose bodies extraction from the hip occurred during the 1980s [4, 5]. Since then a number of paper/case reports have been recorded including resection of bullets, osteochondral fragments, and metal debris [6].

During the last 10 years the use of hip arthroscopy has been widely applied to treat a vast number of problems around the joint.

Reports on hip arthroscopy were limited until the early 1980s as seen when the editors of *Arthroscopy* reviewed their rate of hip arthroscopy-related publications. There was approximately one article each year from 1984 to 1994. A more recent literature review demonstrated that there have been ten or more articles published yearly from 2003 onward. The number of reports regarding loose bodies management has been also increasing [7].

Open arthrotomy used to be the gold standard technique due to direct visualization and full access of the hip joint, but now hip arthroscopy is preferred mostly because of the morbidity associated with the open procedure. During arthrotomy, in order to have a full view of the hip joint, the femoral head has to be dislocated and the ligamentum teres sacrificed. Using the arthroscopic technique an excellent visualization of the joint can be obtained with distraction, not dislocation, and thus can be performed on an outpatient basis with a low reported complication rate [8–11]. The postoperative recovery period and rehabilitation process is significantly lower in comparison with the open procedure [12, 13]. The most important issue is that attempting arthroscopic removal of loose bodies does not preclude, complicate, or "burn bridges" for future procedures if ever they should be necessary.

M. Salineros, MD (✉)
Orthopaedic Department, Joint Reconstruction, Clinica Las Condes, Berna 4751, Santiago, Chile
e-mail: msalineros@clc.cl

R. Mardones, MD
Tissue Engineering Lab, Orthopaedic Department, Clinica Las Condes, Berna 4751, Santiago, Chile
e-mail: rmardones@clc.cl

Clinical Presentation

Loose bodies in the hip are the direct result of either previous trauma or hip disease. A careful history may reveal a minor injury, trauma, or a persistent increasing pain. In the case of traumatic injury or dislocation of the hip joint, the diagnosis and source of the loose fragments within the joint should be apparent, or at least highly suspected.

Loose bodies will present with a wide number and severity of symptoms. Groin pain will be the capital and most frequent complaint. Hip locking and clicking are also very common, usually during flexion and internal rotation motions. Buttock pain could be also present and is related with loose bodies in the posterior and inferior aspect of the acetabulum. McCarthy et al. demonstrated that the most common symptoms associated with loose bodies inside the hip joint were locking episodes associated with anterior inguinal pain [14, 15].

Plain X-rays should be taken in every patient with the clinical history suspicious of a loose body. The recommended views are an AP pelvis, AP of the affected hip, and a cross-table view. Ossified and osteocartilaginous loose bodies will be identified or suspected with X-rays. In order to complete the study, a CT scan with a 2 mm slice acquisition sequence will confirm the diagnosis. With these two exams the majority of loose bodies will be seen because the most common are ossified, but there are some that will not be addressed using these methods because they are non-ossified, fibrous, and

J.C. McCarthy et al. (eds.), *Hip Joint Restoration*, DOI 10.1007/978-1-4614-0694-5_52

cartilaginous. That is why, in symptomatic patients, MRI scanning has become the gold standard in visualizing both the loose bodies and the joint synovitis [16–19].

Types of Loose Bodies

As was previously alluded to, there are two principal groups of loose bodies in the hip joint, the ossified and non-ossified ones. They could be also divided into cartilaginous, osteocartilaginous, fibrous, and foreign bodies.

- Ossified
  - Calcified single or multiple
- Non-ossified
  - Cartilaginous
  - Osteocartilaginous
  - Fibrous
  - Foreign

Osteocartilaginous loose bodies may originate from several sources in the hip. Osteophytes, osteochondritis dissecans, synovial osteochondromatosis, and osteochondral fractures are the most common causes. Foreign loose bodies have occurred as a result of broken materials during hip arthroscopy, such as metal debris from the shaver. Additionally, broken wires from prior surgery as well as bullets in the hip joint have been reported, and arthroscopically removed.

Post-traumatic Loose Bodies

Hip dislocation with or without acetabular fractures can be associated with osteochondral fractures. These are usually the result of a high-energy injury of the hip, such as traumatic dislocation. This type of injuries occurs mostly in young adults as a result of a motor vehicle accident or sports, such as skiing. Substantial force is required to dislocate a native hip [20]. The combination of young age and damaging force applied to the joint may lead to prolonged disability and dysfunction due to subsequent complications such OA and osteonecrosis. The rate of coxarthrosis after hip dislocations is between 24 and 88 % depending on the extent of acetabular damage and fracture [20, 21]. To rule out the presence of loose bodies after closed reduction, plain X-rays and a thin slice CT scan cuts must be performed (2 mm). Studies from Mullis et al. have shown that there is a high prevalence of intra-articular loose bodies despite negative radiographs and CT scan [22]. Thus, patients may potentially have debris within the joint that goes unrecognized and untreated. MRI may be useful to evaluate this debris, and also soft tissue interposition. A nonconcentric reduction should alert the clinician to the presence of cartilage or osteochondral fragments. Some fragments may be located within the pulvinar area. If that is the case a congruent reduction may be obtained. Evans et al. provided basic science evidence in rabbits that cartilage debris causes a joint effusion, synovitis, and degradation to the intact articular cartilage. Dahners et al. performed 39 hip arthroscopies following reduction of posterior dislocations and found loose bodies in 92 % of the cases. Foulk et al. found loose bodies in 78 % of 9 cases that were predicted to be free of intra-articular pathology by radiograph and CT. Although there is basic science that supports the beneficial use of arthroscopy after hip dislocation to remove loose bodies, there is no prospective evidence-based study so far. The indication at this point for hip arthroscopy after hip dislocation reduction is if there are any signs on the CT or MRI that demonstrate a nonconcentric reduction or loose bodies in a weight bearing area of the joint or patient functional impairment (Fig. 52.1) [20].

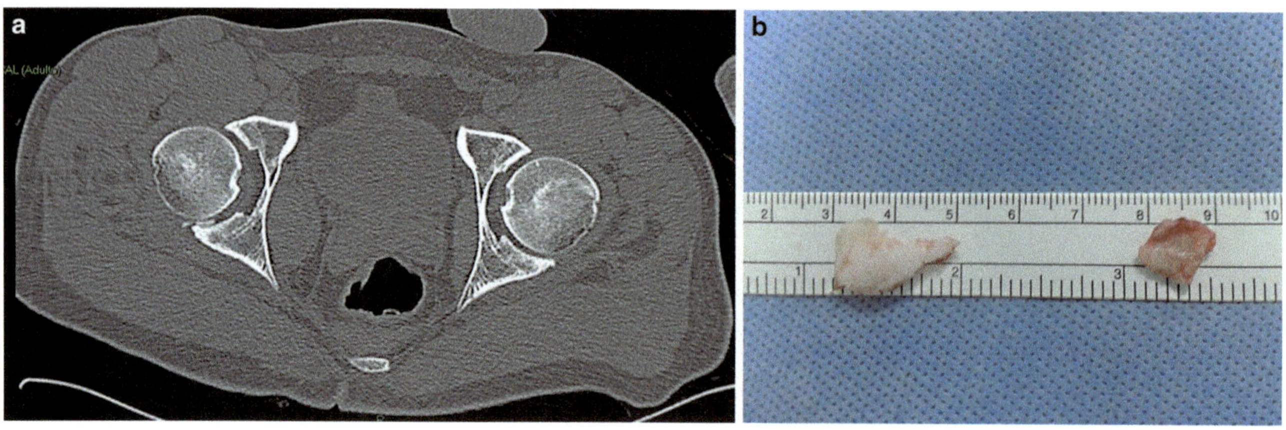

Fig. 52.1 (**a**) Intra-articular loose body after reduction of a posterior hip dislocation. The reduction in comparison with the other side is not concentric due to the interposed fragments. (**b**) Using hip arthroscopy with anterior and anterolateral portals, two major osteochondral fragments were removed from the joint

Secondary Loose Bodies

Osteochondritis dissecans (OCD) is a common pathology in adolescents and young adults that can affect any diarthrodial joint. In the hip joint only a few cases have been reported as isolated lesions from the acetabular or femoral side. The process begins with repeated low energy trauma to the joint that leads to avascular necrosis with involvement of the underlying cartilage. When the lesion becomes unstable, presenting as a cartilage flap or complete detachment, the patient may benefit from arthroscopic intervention, usually involving fixation or debridement. Bowen et al. described the removal of loose bodies due to OCD associated with Legg-Calvé-Perthes disease. The rate of occurrence of these lesions is around 3% of the cases of Legg-Calvé-Perthes disease in children [23, 24]. In symptomatic patients, an arthroscopy procedure was employed to remove the loose osteocartilaginous fragment, with good and excellent results. Filipe et al. concluded that loose fragments in patients with previous Legg-Calvé-Perthes should be removed surgically when it's bulging into the joint space, or when there are signs of early arthrosis [25].

Cartilaginous loose bodies are difficult to diagnosis, because regular MRI usually fails to identify them [26]. A high index of suspicion associated with physical exam will direct the approach. These lesions are less common in the hip than in other joints because of the constrained mechanism of the hip joint. Usually a traumatic event or direct fall on the lateral aspect of the hip or extreme axial compression may lead to chondral injury [27]. Avascular necrosis of the femoral head may also result in deterioration of the articular cartilage; the cartilage starts as a flap lesion that becomes loose and initiates mechanical symptoms of the hip.

Osteochondromatosis is a rare benign disease of unknown cause. It is characterized by formation of cartilage nodules that detach from the synovial membrane resulting in intra-articular fragments that become ossified or undergo endochondral ossification. The hip is the second most commonly involved joint after the knee. The chondral damage that this disease produces is due to mechanical friction. Surgical removal is the treatment of choice and it can performed both open and arthroscopically. Open surgery has shown good results but is an invasive procedure, with significant potential risk. Hip arthroscopy allows adequate debridement, synovectomy, and removal of loose bodies with a less invasive approach. Crnobaric et al. published a case series of hips treated arthroscopically [28]. Patients were satisfied with the operative advantages of the arthroscopic procedure when compared to an open procedure, the lesser operative morbidity and faster postoperative recovery. We recommend the procedure done arthroscopically if the surgeon has adequate surgical skills to perform it. We also advise patients that the procedure may not be definitive to treat the disease but the authors' results and the low morbidity associated will support the arthroscopic treatment as first choice.

Foreign Loose Bodies

Foreign bodies of the hip have been reported. Needles, bullets, shrapnel, drain tubes, broken arthroscopic instruments, and even fragments of total joint replacement parts have been removed using the arthroscope [29–31].

Surgical Pearls

Before hip arthroscopy was widely developed, "creative solutions" to remove loose bodies were published. During the last 10 years, specialized instruments, long grasper tools, and the 70° arthroscope allow removal of the majority of bodies in almost every location of the hip joint. Preoperative planning is crucial in order to remove the loose bodies, minimizing complications from the procedure. Preoperative studies, including MRI and CT scan, will tell the surgeon which one of the arthroscopic portals may be necessary for the procedure. If the loose bodies are located close to the transverse ligament for example, the posterolateral portal will be very useful.

Preferably the surgeon should start with simple cases and, when necessary, extend the capsulotomy to minimize damage to the femoral head and to allow the instruments to explore the joint without excessive difficulties. Adequate distraction is mandatory in order to obtain good visualization. Do not exceed the 2 h limit for traction to avoid neurological complications. Mechanical morcellation of the fragments must be performed with appropriate instruments, to avoid breakage of inadequate instruments. Start with the smaller fragments first. If you start with the larger ones the portals will probably need to be extended and significant irrigation leakage will occur. The slotted cannula that is in almost all hip arthroscopy trays is extremely helpful, especially when curved instruments are required. This half pipe instrument will prevent the loose bodies from staying in the soft tissues during extraction.

Conclusion

Loose bodies inside the hip joint will often lead to chondral damage when untreated. If the mechanical damage is sustained it will ultimately end in premature arthritic degeneration. The significance of the wear damage should not be understated, and the surgical treatment should not be delayed. Epstein demonstrated a very poor prognosis associated with intra-articular loose bodies in a long-term follow-up study of patients who suffered posterior fracture dislocation of the hip. Santora showed good to excellent results in loose body removal in adolescents even in cases of late diagnosis [32]. Only in cases of traumatic intra-articular pathology does the literature show prevention of future articular damage. In cases of pathological conditions that produce loose bodies, the treatment improves symptoms, but the effect on the future of the joint depends on the natural history of the underlying condition (AVN, Synovial chondromatosis).

The low morbidity and early recovery associated with hip arthroscopy make this procedure an excellent choice of treatment when surgery is indicated. Short- and mid-term studies comparing open and arthroscopic technique demonstrate equivalent outcomes but with marked reduction in complications and cost with the arthroscopic procedure.

References

1. Beaule PE, et al. Hip arthroscopy: an emerging gold standard. Arthroscopy. 2007;23(6):682.
2. McCarthy JC. The role of hip arthroscopy in the diagnosis and treatment of hip disease. Can J Surg. 1995;38 Suppl 1:S13–7.
3. Jackson RW. A history of arthroscopy. Arthroscopy. 2010;26(1):91–103.
4. Glick JM. Hip arthroscopy using the lateral approach. Instr Course Lect. 1988;37:223–31.
5. Glick JM, et al. Hip arthroscopy by the lateral approach. Arthroscopy. 1987;3(1):4–12.
6. Singleton SB, et al. Arthroscopic bullet removal from the acetabulum. Arthroscopy. 2005;21(3):360–4.
7. Lubowitz JH, Poehling GG. Hip arthroscopy: an emerging gold standard. Arthroscopy. 2006;22(12):1257–9.
8. Martin RL, Philippon MJ. Evidence of reliability and responsiveness for the hip outcome score. Arthroscopy. 2008;24(6):676–82.
9. Philippon MJ. New frontiers in hip arthroscopy: the role of arthroscopic hip labral repair and capsulorrhaphy in the treatment of hip disorders. Instr Course Lect. 2006;55:309–16.
10. Philippon MJ, et al. Arthroscopic findings following traumatic hip dislocation in 14 professional athletes. Arthroscopy. 2009;25(2):169–74.
11. Sampson TG. Complications of hip arthroscopy. Clin Sports Med. 2001;20(4):831–5.
12. Bozic KJ, et al. Trends in hip arthroscopy utilization in the United States. J Arthroplasty. 2013;28(8 Suppl):140–3.
13. Cooper AP, et al. Outcomes of hip arthroscopy. A prospective analysis and comparison between patients under 25 and over 25 years of age. Br J Sports Med. 2013;47(4):234–8.
14. McCarthy JC, Busconi B. The role of hip arthroscopy in the diagnosis and treatment of hip disease. Orthopedics. 1995;18(8):753–6.
15. McCarthy JC, Busconi B. The role of hip arthroscopy in the diagnosis and treatment of hip disease. Can J Surg. 1995;38 Suppl 1:S13–7.
16. Sheikh A, et al. MR imaging of osseous lesions of the hip. Magn Reson Imaging Clin N Am. 2013;21(1):111–25.
17. Chang CY, Huang AJ. MR imaging of normal hip anatomy. Magn Reson Imaging Clin N Am. 2013;21(1):1–19.
18. Guanche CA. Clinical update: MR imaging of the hip. Sports Med Arthrosc. 2009;17(1):49–55.
19. Conway WF, Totty WG, McEnery KW. CT and MR imaging of the hip. Radiology. 1996;198(2):297–307.
20. Foulk DM, Mullis BH. Hip dislocation: evaluation and management. J Am Acad Orthop Surg. 2010;18(4):199–209.
21. Matta JM and Evarts CM. Dislocations of the Hip and Fractures of the acetabulum, in Surgery of the Musculoskeletal System. 1990
22. Mullis BH, Dahners LE. Hip arthroscopy to remove loose bodies after traumatic dislocation. J Orthop Trauma. 2006;20(1):22–6.
23. Bowen JR, et al. Osteochondritis dissecans following Perthes' disease. Arthroscopic-operative treatment. Clin Orthop Relat Res. 1986;209:49–56.
24. Lecuire F. The long-term outcome of primary osteochondritis of the hip (Legg-Calve-Perthes' disease). J Bone Joint Surg (Br). 2002;84(5):636–40.
25. Filipe G, et al. Osteochondritis dissecans of the hip in Legg-Perthes-Calve disease. Rev Chir Orthop Reparatrice Appar Mot. 1985;71(1):55–61.
26. Edwards DJ, Lomas D, Villar RN. Diagnosis of the painful hip by magnetic resonance imaging and arthroscopy. J Bone Joint Surg (Br). 1995;77(3):374–6.
27. Keene GS, Villar RN. Arthroscopic loose body retrieval following traumatic hip dislocation. Injury. 1994;25(8):507–10.
28. Crnobaric A, Blagojevic Z, Stevanovic V. Arthroscopy of the hip--surgical treatment of synovial osteochondromatosis. Acta Chir Iugosl. 2006;53(4):121–3.
29. Cory JW, Ruch DS. Arthroscopic removal of a .44 caliber bullet from the hip. Arthroscopy. 1998;14(6):624–6.
30. Luchetti WT, et al. Drain entrapment and titanium to ceramic head deposition: two unique complications following closed reduction of a dislocated total hip arthroplasty. J Arthroplasty. 1998;13(6):713–7.
31. Papavasiliou AV, Bardakos NV. Complications of arthroscopic surgery of the hip. Bone Joint Res. 2012;1(7):131–44.
32. Santora SD, Stevens PM, Coleman SS. Intraarticular loose bodies in the adolescent hip: results of treatment of those recognized late. J Pediatr Orthop. 1990;10(2):261–4.

Specific Tissues and Conditions: Trauma

53

Christopher Betz, Michael A. Flaherty, Craig M. Roberto, Scott King, Joshua A. Tuck, and Brian D. Busconi

Injuries of the hip most frequently involve the muscles or soft tissues and typically resolve with rest, anti-inflammatory medication, and physical therapy exercises. This chapter will focus on recognition and treatment of traumatic injuries about the Hip.

Apophyseal Avulsion Injuries

The apophysis is a secondary ossification center that appears during the adolescent stage of growth; between the ages of 13–15. While the epiphysis provides mainly longitudinal growth, the apophysis provides the shape and contour of bone. In children and adolescents, the ligaments, tendons, and muscles are much stronger than the secondary ossification centers, therefore injury mechanisms that would typically lead to muscle strains in adults may lead to avulsion injuries in the developing adolescent [1].

On one end of the spectrum, constant, repetitive pull of a musculotendinous unit can produce inflammation of the apophysis leading to apophysitis. This presents with the insidious onset of localized pain, generally made worse with activity and dissipating with rest. For complete recovery, the recommended treatment consists of a short period of rest from previous activities, followed by a physical therapy program focusing on stretching and conditioning the surrounding muscles, with a controlled return to sports [1].

Apophyseal avulsion fractures of the pelvis have increased in prevalence over the last few decades, likely due to the increased participation of adolescents in competitive sports. These injuries usually occur from a sudden forceful concentric or eccentric muscle contraction, in an attempt to rapidly accelerate/decelerate, or change direction. This leads to a forceful pull against the apophysis and its separation from the rest of the pelvis [1–4]. Sports that require rapid acceleration/deceleration or a sudden change in direction include football, soccer, track, baseball, tennis, and gymnastics [1]. Avulsion injuries may also arise from activities causing sudden excessive passive lengthening of muscles, as seen when a cheerleader or dancer performs a split, which may lead to avulsion injuries of the ischial tuberosity [3]. Avulsion injuries are more common in males, although the incidence in females is increasing [1, 3]. In a case series, reported in 1985, of 27 avulsion fractures of the pelvis reported by Metzmaker and Pappas, 22 (88 %) were male [3]. Rossie and Dragoni published in 2001 (information collected over 22 years, from 1976 to 1998) one of the largest collection of acute avulsion fractures involving the pelvis, with 203 cases, the distribution of injuries involved 139 males (68.5 %) vs 64 females (31.5 %) [4].

The adolescent athlete may describe hearing a "pop" or feeling a snapping sensation, with a sudden onset of pain at the time of injury. The pain can be acutely debilitating, with athletes unable to ambulate comfortably [1]. On physical exam, the patient will typically guard the affected region, and will maintain a position that relieves the tension in the involved muscle group, leading to a reduced range of motion on exam. There may be swelling or crepitation over the involved region, with localized tenderness to palpation.

Avulsion fractures of the pelvic apophyses most commonly involve the ischial tuberosity, followed by the anterior inferior iliac spine (AIIS), the anterior superior iliac spine (ASIS), and lastly the lesser trochanter [1]. In Rossi

C. Betz, DO • C.M. Roberto, DO • S. King, DO
Orthopaedics, Sports Medicine, University of Massachusetts, Worcester, MA, USA
e-mail: cbetz09@gmail.com

M.A. Flaherty, MD
Orthopaedic Surgery, Albany Medical College, Albany, NY, USA
e-mail: mflaherty@caportho.com

J.A. Tuck, DO, MS
Department of Orthopaedic Surgery, Sports Medicine, University of Massachusetts Medical School, University of Massachusetts Memorial Medical Center, Worcester, MA, USA

B.D. Busconi, MD (✉)
Orthopaedics, Sports Medicine, University of Massachusetts Memorial Medical Center, Worcester, MA, USA
e-mail: Brian.Busconi@umassmemorial.org

J.C. McCarthy et al. (eds.), *Hip Joint Restoration*, DOI 10.1007/978-1-4614-0694-5_53

and Dragoni's study, 53.7 % of the apophyseal avulsion fractures involved the ischial tuberosity, with 22.2 % involving the AIIS, and 19.2 % ASIS [4].

The majority of these cases are treated nonoperatively with an initial period of non-weight bearing with crutches to help minimize discomfort. The patient can progress to weight-bearing as tolerated, which can take 2–4 weeks [1]. Per Moeller et al., once the patient is able to tolerate full weight-bearing and activities of daily living, then gentle range of motion and flexibility training can be initiated, with gradual strengthening added-on as tolerated. Proprioception and balance are also addressed. Once the patient is able to do the stretching and strengthening exercises without pain, which can take 3–12 weeks depending on the injury site, then jogging and sports-specific activities are initiated; followed by a gradual increase in intensity and eventual return to full activity [1].

Avulsion Fractures of the Ischial Tuberosity

The ischial tuberosity is the origin of the semitendinosus and semimembranosus muscles, as well as the long head of the biceps femoris (Fig. 53.1). Avulsion fractures usually occur after the appearance of the secondary ossification center. Altered growth rates during adolescence correlate to decreased flexibility and increased stress in the apophysis [5]. As the ischial apophysis of the adolescent pelvis is relatively weak compared to the hamstring muscles, ischial tuberosity avulsion fractures (ITAF) occur most commonly in the young (12–18 years) active population, typically in sports that involve sprinting such as football, soccer, and tennis [6–8]. Traumatic avulsion injuries can also occur in the skeletally mature pelvis; however, in the adult, the presence of a pelvic avulsion fracture in the absence of trauma should be considered a pathological lesion until proven otherwise.

Ischial tuberosity avulsion fractures (Fig. 53.2) occur acutely and are characterized by a sudden onset of pain within the posterior thigh and buttock that immediately disables the athlete from participation in activities involving hamstring contraction. On occasion, sciatica symptoms may be present due to the close proximity of the site of avulsion to the sciatic nerve [9–11].

ITAFs should be distinguished from a more chronic and slowly progressing apophysitis. Like hamstring strains, patients with ITAFs present with bruising of the posterior thigh; however, the presence of point tenderness at the ischial tuberosity should lead the clinician to order radiographs of the pelvis to provide a definitive diagnosis. Views should include an AP of the pelvis, and AP and lateral views of the

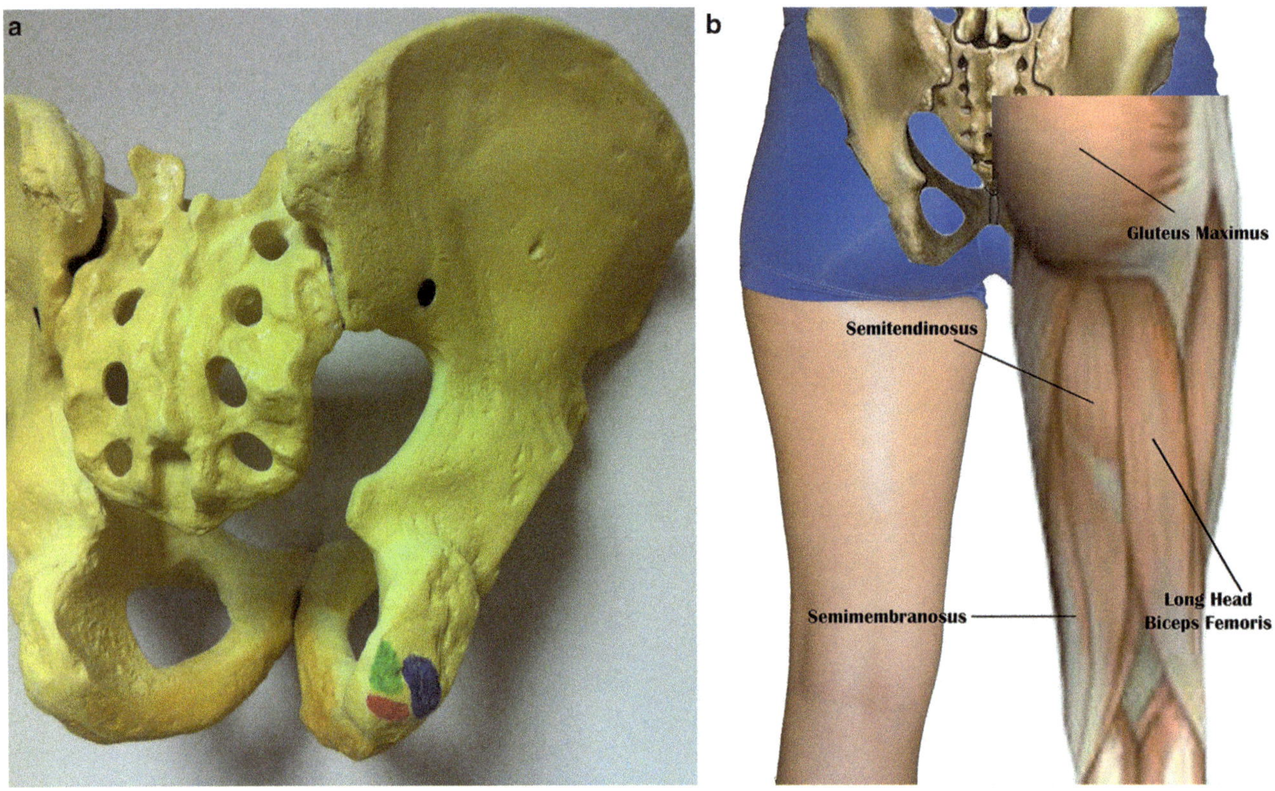

Fig. 53.1 (a) Origin in the ischial tuberosity of the semitendinosus, semimembranosus, and long head of biceps femoris. (b) Surface and deep anatomy of the hamstrings

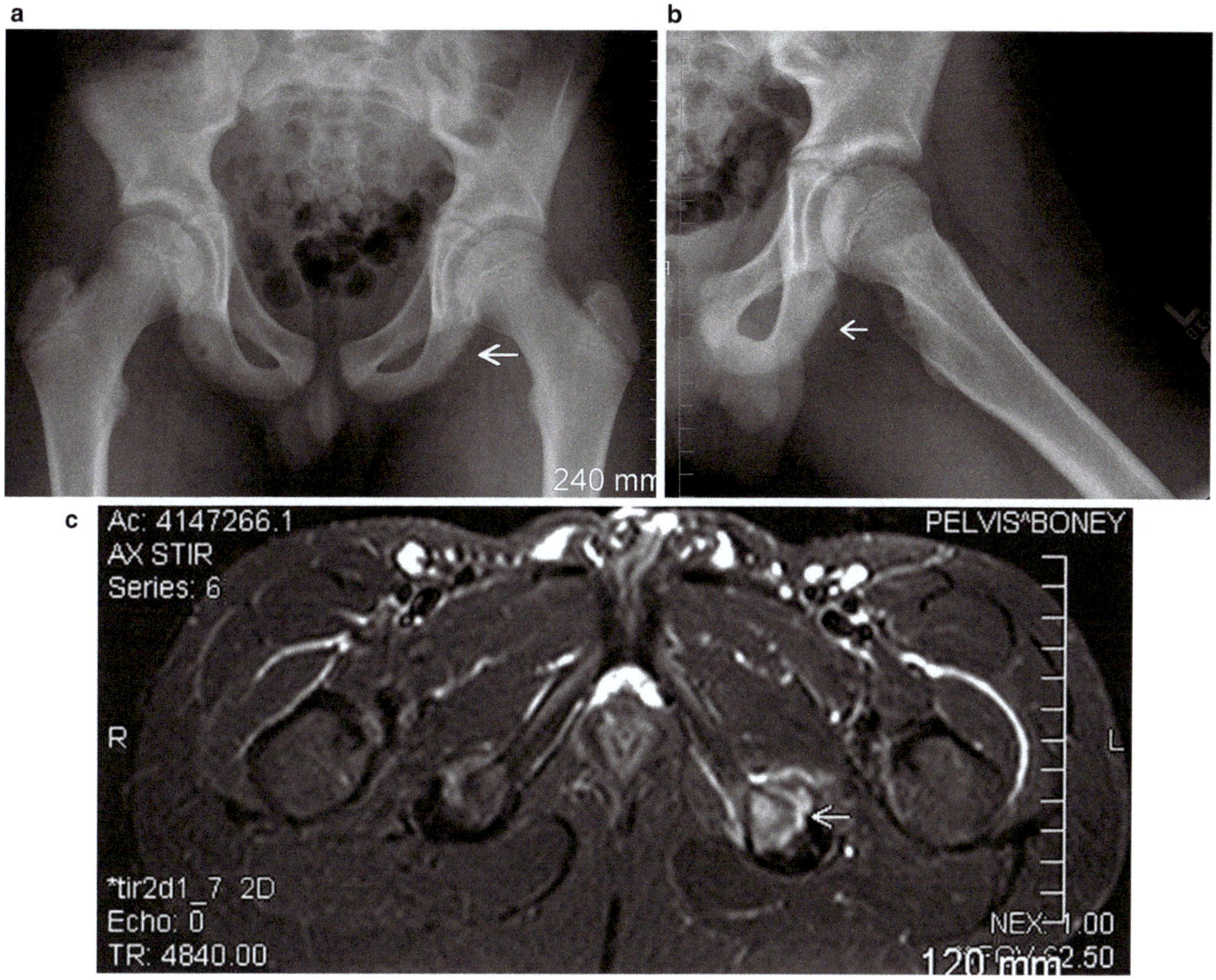

Fig. 53.2 Ischial tuberosity apophyseal avulsion fracture. (**a**) and (**b**). *Arrows* are suggestive of avulsion which was (**c**). confirmed with MRI

affected hip. In the acute setting, cortical irregularities can be seen as well as inferior displacement of the apophysis. In the chronic setting, exuberant callus may be present, causing misinterpretation as a neoplasm [12]. CT scans can help to better delineate fragments and assess for callus formation. MRI is the most sensitive and specific imaging modality.

Treatment for ITAF is based on the amount of displacement of the apophyseal fragment. For nondisplaced or minimally displaced fractures, treatment consists of rest, activity limitation followed by rehabilitation and then sport-specific training once the patient is pain-free. Although no strong evidence is available, many authors advocate open reduction and internal fixation for avulsions with 2 cm or more of retraction [13, 14]. Operative treatment is based on the belief that widely separated fragments are likely to heal with a fibrous nonunion that often gives rise to buttock pain, an ischial mass, or significant weakness of knee flexion, leading to a reduced level of athletic performance. In those cases in which satisfactory reduction cannot be achieved, excision of the avulsed fragment may be necessary [7, 13]. Outcomes of surgical management for fractures displaced more than 2 cm are limited to several case reports or small case series, but have been reported as favorable.

ASIS/AIIS Avulsion Fractures

As with the other apophyseal ossification centers of the pelvis, the anterior superior iliac spine (ASIS) and anterior inferior iliac spine (AIIS) ossification centers appear between the ages of 13–15 in most adolescents. The ASIS is the origin for the musculotendinous units of the sartorius and tensor fascia lata muscles, whereas, the direct head of the rectus femoris muscle originates off the AIIS. An injury to both of these apophyseal centers occurs from similar mechanisms, most commonly involving either sprinting or kicking. With sprinting, the greatest amount of eccentric load on the ASIS and AIIS occurs at push-off at the start of the activity, with the hip extended and the knee flexed [1]. With kicking, an initial concentric force occurs with a forceful flexion of the hip and extension of the knee, which is then suddenly converted to an eccentric load as the foot meets the resistive force of the ground [1].

Rotational loading of the hip may also cause apophyseal injuries to the AIIS with generation of a significantly larger avulsion fragment through eccentric contraction of the tensor fascia lata [15]. White et al. described two similar cases of baseball injuries in which a sudden onset of pain was felt during the initial swing phase of batting [15]. During this phase of batting, the back leg is fixed, and eccentric contraction of the tensor fascia lata of the fixed leg occurs with the twisting motion of the swing. The larger avulsed fragment is displaced laterally, in contrast to the inferior displacement typically seen with avulsion injuries created by the sartorius muscle.

The athletes with ASIS or AIIS avulsions will experience a sudden onset of pain in the anterior pelvic area, with either an audible "pop" or sensation of a "pop." The athlete will have trouble bearing weight on the injured side and will typically hold the involved side in some degree of hip flexion to reduce tension on the involved musculotendinous unit. The involved area can be swollen, and will be tender to palpation. Pain will be exacerbated by active hip flexion. Passive hip extension will also produce discomfort, especially if coupled with passive knee flexion [1].

Plain films should be obtained of the pelvis, including AP and oblique views. The oblique view will allow a better evaluation of the AIIS avulsion injury, since, in contrast to ASIS avulsions, there may be minimal displacement of the bony fragment due to the greater amount of soft-tissue attachments surrounding the site of injury [1]. Again, the fragments will typically displace in a caudal direction due to the pull of either the sartorius or the rectus femoris muscle, but can be displaced laterally if the avulsion involves the action of the tensor fascia lata. MRI is required for further soft tissue evaluation (see Figs. 53.3 and 53.4).

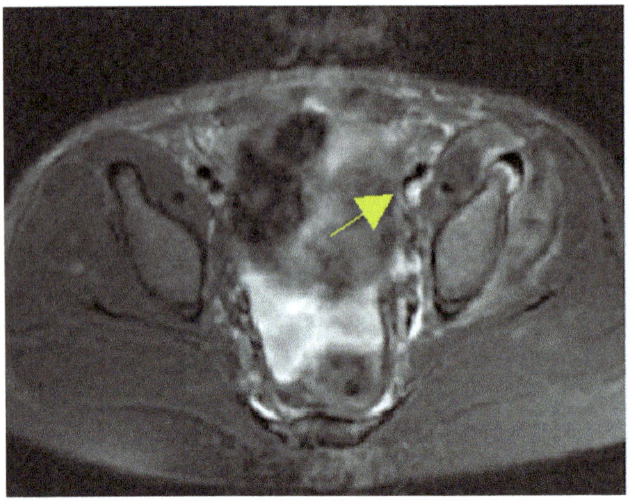

Fig. 53.3 T2-weighted, axial MRI image demonstrating an avulsion fracture involving the left anterior inferior iliac spine in a 13-year-old adolescent male. There is edema interposed within the displacement site

Treatment is similar to the other apophyseal avulsion injuries, including symptomatic rest, with an initial period of crutch use until the pain level improves, with progressive weight bearing as tolerated. Typically, athletes will have a full recovery, with no issues of weakness or lingering pain, and without limitations of athletic activities at 2–4 months from the time of the injury [16, 17].

Although the majority of athletes have done well with conservative treatment, there is debate regarding surgical indications for apophyseal avulsion fractures of the ASIS and the AIIS. Rosenberg et al. [18] reported that the follow-up radiographs of patients following conservative treatment showed that the avulsed fragment reattached more distally than the original site, without a significant clinical deficit in the majority of patients. Patients can develop abundant callus formation, exostosis, malunions, and symptomatic nonunions. There are those that feel that surgical open reduction and internal fixation, even in the acute setting, can lead to a quicker return to full activity, a lesser chance of malunion/nonunion, with good results [19]. Veselko and Smrkolj presented two cases of ASIS avulsion fractures that were treated with open reduction and internal fixation 2 days after the injury [19]. Both athletes returned to training 3–4 weeks after the injury with no significant decrease in strength or residual symptoms and ultimately played at the same level of performance as before the injury. This has led to the conclusion that

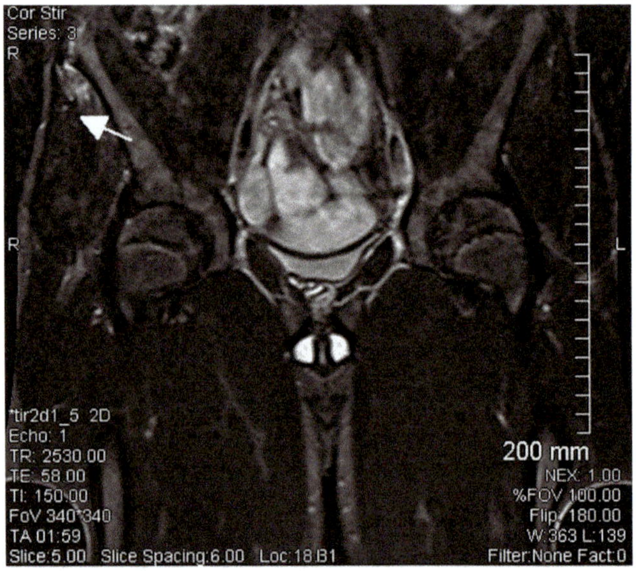

Fig. 53.4 T2-weighted, coronal MRI demonstrating an apophyseal avulsion fracture involving the right anterior superior iliac spine in an adolescent male. From Hsu JC. Proximal Rectus Femoris Avulsions in National Football League Kickers A Report of 2 Cases. Am J Sports Med. 2005. 33; 1085–1087. Reprinted with permission from Sage Publications

surgery may be an option in the treatment of competitive athletes seeking a quick return to activity, regardless of the extent of displacement of the avulsed fragment.

Kameyama and Ogawa [20] reported on 30 avulsion fractures involving the iliac spines (20 ASIS, 10 AIIS), with 11 athletes treated by open reduction and internal fixation (ORIF), and 19 treated nonoperatively. The ORIF group was treated with either a screw or Kirschner wires. The results showed that all of the 19 patients treated conservatively showed good fracture union, with all the patients reporting satisfactory function with activities of daily living, and with the majority able to participate with sporting activities at the same level as they did before surgery; except for two patients who reported occasional fatigue with certain sporting activities. Both patients had ASIS fractures with a large deformity, with one of the two patients having returned to sports activity sooner than recommended and had developed a largely displaced fragment with a bony bar. The authors postulate that the marked displacement of the muscle and its attachment to the fragment that had healed distal to its original site may have lead to the fatigue in the patients.

The main debate is in regards to significantly displaced fragments and whether surgery should be indicated in these cases; to prevent large deformities with large bony bars, and to possibly prevent fatigue of the musculotendinous unit and malunions that cause shortening of the unit [19, 20]. Although the results, for the most part, are similar between those treated conservatively and those treated with surgical ORIF, according to Moeller's and Veselko's articles, surgery should be recommended in the acute setting if the avulsed fragment is displaced more than 2 cm for the above-stated concerns. These fractures are relatively uncommon; we would need further studies to investigate these concerns.

Proximal Hamstring Injuries

The hamstring muscles originating from the ischial tuberosity are the long head of the biceps femoris, semitendinosus, and semimembranosus (Fig. 53.1). All three of these muscles cross both the hip and the knee joints. Feely et al. [21] studied the epidemiology of injuries in the training camps of one team from the National Football League and found that between 1998 and 2007 there were 2.2 hamstring strains per 1000 athletic exposures. While injuries to the hamstring muscles are relatively common, a complete avulsion from the ischial tuberosity is rare. The true incidence of these complete avulsions is difficult to assess because this condition is often misdiagnosed. Patients are usually in their thirties and forties. A review of 18 studies [22] reported an average age of 39.7 years.

Proximal hamstring avulsion injuries typically present with a sudden excruciating pain along the posterior thigh causing cessation of athletic activity. The most common mechanism is a sudden eccentric load resisted by the powerful hamstring muscles [23]. It has been described in multiple sports that involve that eccentric mechanism, especially during sprinting, including rugby, tennis, baseball, and in activities such as water skiing [24]. Patients typically report that, at the time of injury, the affected hip was in a position of near maximal flexion with the knee in extension, similar to the stretch position of hurdling, creating a sudden eccentric load. They often report a "pop" or "tearing" sensation in their proximal posterior thigh. Upon examination, an extensive ecchymosis and swelling of the posterior thigh is noticed [25–27]. Patients will typically avoid hip or knee flexion. Knee flexion weakness is easily tested in the prone position. On occasion, a palpable gap can be felt, although this is often disguised by edema. Some cases of transient sciatica have also been reported due to the close proximity of this nerve to the area of injury. Proximal hamstring avulsion injuries are often misdiagnosed as hamstring strains causing a delay in the initiation of treatment. In their series of 25 proximal hamstring repairs, Folsom and Larson [24] reported that five patients had chronic tears and were operated between 4 and 116 months after the injury. Evaluation for signs of compartment syndrome is advised as the occurrence of this sequela has been previously reported [28].

Both ultrasound and MRI are very sensitive for the diagnosis of proximal hamstring avulsion injuries, although MRI is generally considered more useful for evaluating the anatomy [29–31] (Fig. 53.5). Even with a confident diagnosis from the history and physical exam, MRI is very helpful for identifying the exact anatomy of the tear, including the tendons involved and the magnitude of the retraction. Axial views help identify which tendons are torn. Sagittal and coronal views can help determine the extent of the injury and the magnitude of the retraction.

Several classification schemes of hamstring avulsion injuries have been developed. It is convenient and simple to describe these tears as acute or chronic, to separate them according to the number of tendons involved, and to describe other factors such as sciatic nerve involvement. The original classification was described by Wood et al. [32] and then modified by Sallay [33]. Acute injuries are those less than 4 weeks of evolution, early chronic are between 4 and 12 weeks, and chronic injuries have more than 12 weeks. Incomplete tears are those of one or two tendons, while complete tears involve all three tendons. Both complete and incomplete tears can be further subdivided according to the size of the displacement (more or less than 2 cm).

No formal controlled studies have been reported examining treatment options for proximal hamstring avulsion injuries and guidelines are formed from expert recommendation. Nonsurgical management is reserved for older, less-active patients with less-severe injuries, including all incomplete

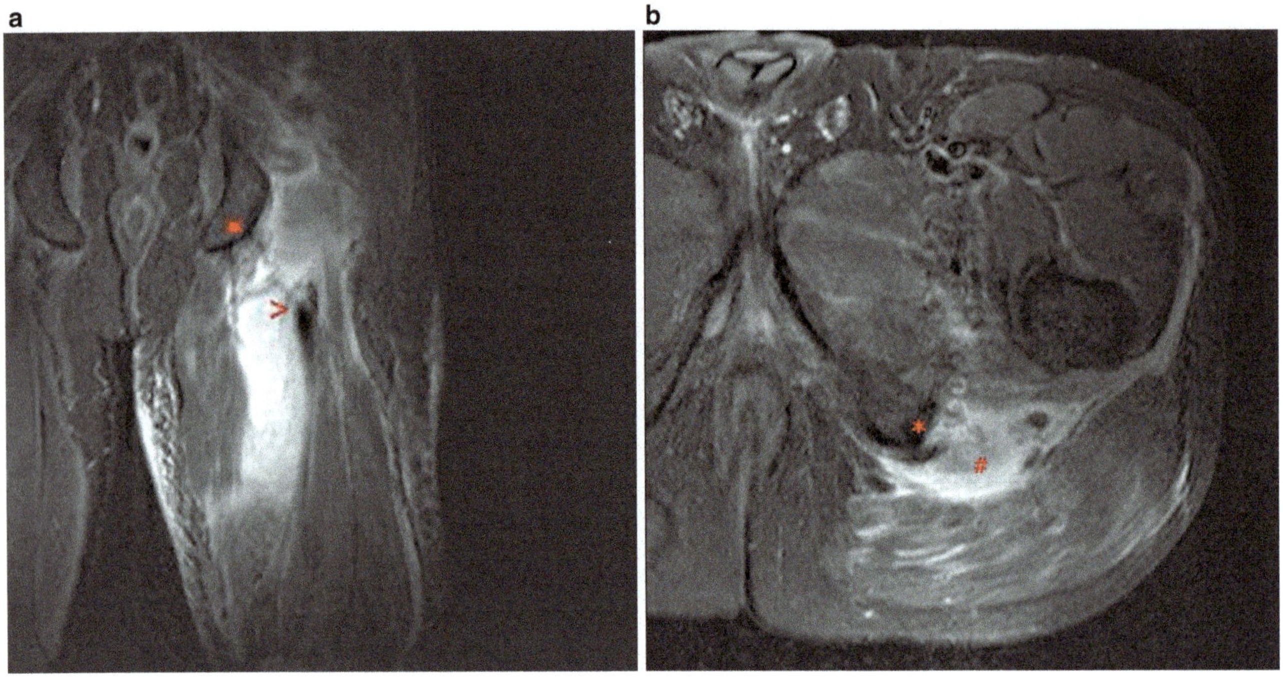

Fig. 53.5 (**a**) *Coronal view* showing the ischial tuberosity (*) and the stump of the proximal hamstring (>). (**b**) *Axial view* showing the ischial tuberosity (*) and abundant inflammation (#) without hamstring muscles attached

tears, and a complete tear (all three tendons) with less than 2 cm of retraction [34]. If these patients continue to be symptomatic, delayed surgical management is usually feasible due to minimal retraction and myostatic contracture [35]. Nonsurgical management consists of protective ambulation, cryotherapy, and analgesics. Early mobilization is recommended in an attempt to avoid venous thrombosis and pharmaceutical agents can be considered in at risk patients. Gentle therapy is then started with pain modalities (i.e. ultrasound and electrical stimulation), and normal joint motion is regained as tolerated. Therapeutic stretches, and range of motion exercises are utilized and patients gradually return into athletic activities once pain-free and strength has been regained.

Surgical management is recommended for active individuals with three tendon tears with more than 2 cm retraction. In counseling the patient prior to surgical repair, it is important to disclose the risk of surgery and explain the postoperative rehab phase to ensure compliance. Surgery is performed in the prone position and careful dissection is performed to expose the ischial tuberosity and the proximal hamstring stump while protecting the sciatic nerve and the posterior cutaneous nerve of the thigh. Superior retraction of the gluteus maximus should be performed with caution as the inferior gluteal nerve can also be injured. If there is adequate residual stump at the proximal tendon, a direct repair is performed. If there is no proximal stump available for adequate direct repair, the bony surface of the ischium is prepared with a periosteal elevator and a curette, and suture anchors are then placed to repair the proximal tendon in its anatomic position.

Postoperatively, patients are placed on a harness or brace that keeps the knee in flexion. This protects the repair by preventing weight-bearing on the affected extremity during the first month after surgery, while still allowing ambulation with crutches (phase 1) [35]. Depending on surgeon preferences, the harness is only worn when the patient is ambulating. Weaning from the harness or brace is performed at the fourth week and then from the crutches as tolerated (phase 2). The goal of this second phase is restoration of normal gait and return to pain-free activities of daily living. Phase 3 of rehabilitation (2–4 months) involves hamstring strengthening and pain-free aerobic activities. Phase 4 (4–6 months) proceeds with advanced proprioceptive training and return to the patient's specific athletic activities. Most patients are able to return to jogging and other sporting activities by 6 months and to full sports participation once the strength of the affected hip is similar to that of the contralateral side.

Birmingham et al. [36] reported a series of 9 acute and 14 chronic repairs of complete tears followed for an average of 43.3 months. Almost all patients (95 %) returned to their pre-injury activity level by 9.8 months, and 78 % of patients reported excellent results at follow-up, with restoration of more than 90 % of hamstring strength compared to the contralateral side. In a recent systematic review of 18 studies involving a total of 298 patients (300 tears), surgical treatment (286 injuries) was compared to nonsurgical management (14 injuries) [22]. Surgical repair resulted in significantly ($p<0.05$) better subjective outcomes, greater rate of return to pre-injury level of sport, and greater strength/

endurance than nonsurgical management, though the number of patients managed nonsurgically was very small. In the surgical group, acute repairs performed better than chronic repairs and had less complications and risk of re-rupture.

Complications after surgical management are those associated to other lower extremity surgeries such as infection, wound dehiscence, seromas, and DVT [26, 36, 37]. Re-tears can also occur. As stated earlier, neurologic structures at risk are the sciatic nerve, the posterior cutaneous femoral nerve (PCFN) and the inferior gluteal nerve from excessive superior retraction of the gluteus maximus. PCFN injury can give symptoms of neuralgia, hyperesthesia, or sensory loss in the posterior thigh. These symptoms usually resolve with time.

Iliac Crest Contusion ("Hip Pointer")

Muscle contusions are commonly seen in sports medicine, especially in contact sports such as football, ice hockey, and rugby. "Hip pointers," as they are described in layman's terms, are contusions involving the iliac crest and the overlying soft tissues. The injury is caused by a direct blow to the iliac crest, typically in patients participating in contact sports wearing inadequate or ill-fitting hip pads.

The iliac crest contusion can be quite painful and debilitating. Surrounding structures can also be injured including the gluteal muscles, the tensor fascia lata, and the adjacent abdominal muscles. Hematomas are also common and can dissect the interval between the iliac crest and the surrounding soft-tissues, contributing to the debilitating pain [38]. The athlete will typically present with pain, with related tenderness to palpation of tissues overlying the iliac crest and the adjacent surrounding soft-tissues, often in the presence of ecchymosis and swelling. The patient may also have an antalgic gait, depending on the severity of the injury. Although the diagnosis is primarily made through the history and physical examination, plain radiographs are important to obtain to rule out possible iliac wing fractures, or apophyseal fractures in the adolescent athlete [38].

Treatment consists of rest, ice, and anti-inflammatory medication. Once tolerable, physical therapy focusing on stretching and strengthening can be initiated to increase range of motion of the ipsilateral hip. Complete recovery typically takes 2 to 4 weeks, depending on the severity of the contusion. Complications can include myositis ossificans and muscle fibrosis [38].

Muscle Strains

Muscle strains are the most common muscle injury suffered in sports, and commonly result from a forcible stretching of the muscle, either actively or passively, but more often through eccentric contraction during activity [39]. Muscles at risk of strains control the range of joint motion, with those spanning both the hip and knee being at greatest risk. These muscles are typically involved in controlling high-speed activities, and contain a relatively high percentage of fast-twitch (type II) muscle fibers [39]. Sporting activities most commonly associated with this form of injury involve rapid acceleration/deceleration, and cutting/pivoting.

Histologic studies show that the muscle fibers are disrupted near the myotendinous junction [39]. At the time of injury, hemorrhage is seen within the muscle. Surrounding edema settles in from an inflammatory process that typically occurs a day or 2 after the injury. After about a week, the inflammatory phase is replaced by fibrous tissue; which persists [39].

Muscle strains involving the adductors are among the most common injuries seen in ice hockey, with an incidence of 43 % of all muscle strains reported in one study of Finnish ice hockey players [40, 41]. The adductor strains in ice hockey can be caused by the rapid and forceful external rotation of the hip during the "push off" movement to initiate the glide stroke [42]. Breaststroke swimmers are also likely to suffer adductor strains during training and competition when the hips are forcefully adduced with the knees flexed, right before the powerful kick that characterizes the breaststroke [43, 44].

The athlete will typically experience an acute episode of pain during an intense activity. This may prevent further participation in the sport depending on the severity of the strain. The athlete will experience further pain after the initial injury if the involved muscle is activated; being more pronounced with eccentric activation [39]. Upon exam, the athlete will have localized tenderness, with possible swelling and ecchymosis being present. There may be guarding, limited range of motion, along with weakness secondary to the pain.

Imaging is for the most part not necessary, as the diagnosis can be made from the history and physical examination. The MRI is the modality that will typically show the localized edema, hemorrhage, and muscle fiber disruption near the musculotendinous unit, but again, is not necessary to make the diagnosis.

In general, the acute treatment includes rest, ice, anti-inflammatory medication, compression to reduce swelling and relieve pain. Once the pain and swelling subside, physical therapy can be initiated to increase range of motion, and restore muscle strength. Athletes typically return to competitive activity once full range of motion and strengthening has been achieved. Studies show that in those athletes who are prone to the muscular strains, a weakness of the involved muscles was present at the start of the season [40, 45]. Orchard et al. reported the association of relative hamstring weakness with the incidence of hamstring strains in Australian rules football [40, 45]. Preseason hamstring strength was 16 % lower on the side that sustained a muscular strain during the season. Hamstring flexibility was not a significant risk factor. Tyler et al. emphasize strengthening exercises to minimize the risk of muscular strains and reoccurrences [40]. A program that focuses on active strengthening, with a progressive increase in resistive exercises, should be used to reduce the rate of injuries and the rate of recurrences. A physical therapy program should also include balance training and core strengthening to increase the overall strength of the surrounding muscles.

Besides strengthening, an adequate pre-exercise warm-up, specifically involving the 'at risk' muscles, may be the most important preventative step [46]. A study by Ekstrand et al. showed that the incidence of hip adductor strains decreased by 75 % in a group of soccer players that used a warm-up and stretching regimen [47].

Athletic Pubalgia

(Please refer to the chapter dealing specifically with athletic pubalgia for full details.) Although athletic pubalgia is a syndrome that typically develops with repetitive stress to the anterior pelvis over time, the injury can occur acutely. The likely injury pattern involves an insertional tear at the origin of the rectus abdominis muscle on the anterior pelvis, with eventual weakening and possible bulging of the posterior wall of the inguinal canal. As mentioned by Meyers et al. [48], the proposed mechanism of injury seems to involve a hyper-extension of the abdomen with hyper-abduction of the hip, leading to the increased stress on the anterior pelvic stabilizers. Acute injuries of this type are seen in bull riders, who experience an exaggeration of the injury pattern, with cases of complete avulsions of the rectus abdominis or adductor muscles on the anterior pelvis [48]. These acute cases are treated surgically, with good outcomes reported [48].

Conclusion

Traumatic injuries are frequent around the hip, especially in adolescents and athletes. These pelvic and peri articular lesions should not be confused with intra-articular joint pathology. On occasion, however, labral, chondral injury may be coexistent with pelvic abnormalities, such as pubic symphysitis or sports hernias. A thorough history, physical exam, and appropriate radiographic imaging will facilitate correct diagnosis.

References

1. Moeller JL. Pelvic and hip apophyseal avulsion injuries in young athletes. Curr Sports Med Rep. 2003;2:110–5.
2. Fernbach SK, Wilkinson RH. Avulsion injuries of the pelvis and proximal femur. Am J Rad. 1981;137:581–4.
3. Metzmaker JN, Pappas AM. Avulsion fractures of the pelvis. Am J Sports Med. 1985;13(5):349–58.
4. Rossi F, Dragoni S. Acute avulsion fractures of the pelvis in adolescent competitive athletes: prevalence, location and sports distribution of 203 cases collected. Skeletal Radiol. 2001;30:127–31.
5. Micheli LJ, Slater JA, Woods E, et al. Patella alta and the adolescent growth spurt. Clin Orthop Relat Res. 1986;213:159–62.
6. Kocis J, Visna P, Vesely R. Traumatic avulsion of the tuberosity of the ischium. Acta Chir Orthop Traumatol Cech. 2003;70(5):311–3.
7. Kujala UM, Orava S, Karpakka J, et al. Ischial tuberosity apophysitis and avulsion among athletes. Int J Sports Med. 1997;18(2):149–55.
8. Sulko J, Olipra W, Oberc A. Ischial tuberosity fractures in children. Chir Narzadow Ruchu Ortop Pol. 2011;76(3):134–7.
9. Dosani A, Giannoudis PV, Waseem M, et al. Unusual presentation of sciatica in a 14-year-old girl. Injury. 2004;35(10):1071–2.
10. Miller A, Stedman GH, Beisaw NE, et al. Sciatica caused by an avulsion fracture of the ischial tuberosity. A case report. J Bone Joint Surg Am. 1987;69(1):143–5.
11. Spinner RJ, Atkinson JL, Wenger DE, et al. Tardy sciatic nerve palsy following apophyseal avulsion fracture of the ischial tuberosity. Case report. J Neurosurg. 1998;89(5):819–21.
12. Bahk WJ, Brien EW, Luck Jr JV. Avulsion of the ischial tuberosity simulating neoplasm--a report of 2 cases. Acta Orthop Scand. 2000;71(2):211–4.
13. Wootton JR, Cross MJ, Holt KW. Avulsion of the ischial apophysis. The case for open reduction and internal fixation. J Bone Joint Surg (Br). 1990;72(4):625–7.
14. Servant CT, Jones CB. Displaced avulsion of the ischial apophysis. A hamstring injury requiring internal fixation. Br J Sports Med. 1998;32(3):255–7.
15. White KK, Williams SK, Mubarak SJ. Definition of two types of anterior superior iliac spine avulsion fractures. J Pediatr Orthop. 2002;22:578–82.
16. Sundar M, Carty H. Avulsion fractures of the pelvis in children: a report of 32 fractures and their outcome. Skeletal Radiol. 1994;23:85–90.
17. Oldenburg FP, Smith MV, Thompson GH. Simultaneous ipsilateral avulsion of the anterior superior and anterior inferior iliac spines in an adolescent. J Pediatr Orthop. 2009;29(1):29–30.
18. Rosenberg N, Noiman M, Edelson G. Avulsion fractures of the anterior superior iliac spine in adolescents. J Orthop Trauma. 1996;10(6):440–3.
19. Veselko M, Smrkolj V. Avulsion of the anterior superior iliac spine in athletes: case reports. J Trauma. 1994;36(3):444–6.
20. Kameyama O, Ogawa R. Avulsion fracture of the iliac spine during sporting activity: report of 30 fractures and their outcome. J Orthop Sci. 1996;1:356–62.
21. Feely BT, Kennelly S, Barnes RP, et al. Epidemiology of National Football League training camp injuries from 1998 to 2007. Am J Sports Med. 2008;36:1597–603.
22. Harris JD, Griesser MJ, Best TM. Treatment of proximal hamstring ruptures - a systematic review. Int J Sports Med. 2011;32(7):490–5.
23. Garrett Jr WE. Muscle strain injuries: clinical and basic aspects. Med Sci Sports Exerc. 1990;22(4):436–43.
24. Folsom GJ, Larson CM. Surgical treatment of acute versus chronic complete proximal hamstring ruptures: results of a new allograft technique for chronic reconstructions. Am J Sports Med. 2008;36(1):104–9.
25. Carlson C. The natural history and management of hamstring inures. Curr Rev Musculoskelet Med. 2008;1(2):120–3.
26. Klingele KE, Sallay PI. Surgical repair of complete proximal hamstring tendon rupture. Am J Sports Med. 2002;30(5):742–7.
27. Johnson AE, Granville RR, DeBerardino TM. Avulsion of the common hamstring tendon origin in an active duty airman. Mil Med. 2003;168(1):40–2.
28. Kwong Y, Patel J, Ramanathan EB. Spontaneous complete hamstring avulsion causing posterior thigh compartment syndrome. Br J Sports Med. 2006;40:723–4.

29. De Smet AA, Best TM. MR imaging of the distribution and location of acute hamstring injuries in athletes. AJR Am J Roentgenol. 2000;174:393–9.
30. Brandser EA, El-Khoury GY, Kathol MH, et al. Hamstring injuries: radiographic, conventional tomographic, CT and MR imaging characteristics. Radiology. 1995;197:257–62.
31. Schneider-Kolsky ME, Hoving JL, Warren P. A comparison between clinical assessment and magnetic resonance imaging of acute hamstring injuries. Am J Sports Med. 2006;34(6):1008–15.
32. Wood DG, Packham I, Trikha SP, et al. Avulsion of the proximal hamstring origin. J Bone Joint Surg Am. 2008;90(11):2365–74.
33. Sallay PI. Diagnosis, classification, and management of acute proximal hamstring avulsion injuries. Oper Tech Sports Med. 2009;17:196–204.
34. Cohen S, Bradley J. Acute proximal hamstring rupture. J Am Acad Orthop Surg. 2007;15(6):350–5.
35. Hamersly SF, Schrader M. Post operative rehabilitation of proximal hamstring tendon tears. Oper Tech Sports Med. 2009;17:219–24.
36. Birmingham P, Muller M, Wickiewicz T, et al. Functional outcome after repair of proximal hamstring avulsions. J Bone Joint Surg Am. 2011;93(19):1819–26.
37. Sarimo J, Lempainen L, Mattila K, et al. Complete proximal hamstring avulsions: a series of 41 patients with operative treatment. Am J Sports Med. 2008;36(6):1110–5.
38. Mora SA, Mandelbaum BR, Byrd JW. Hip and groin injuries. Orthopaedic knowledge update sports medicine 3. Am Acad Ortho Surg. 2004;3:141.
39. Noonan TJ, Garrett WE. Muscle strain injury: diagnosis and treatment. J Am Acad Orthop Surg. 1999;7:262–9.
40. Tyler TF, Nicholas SJ, Campbell RJ. The association of hip strength and flexibility with the incidence of adductor muscle strains in professional ice hockey players. Am J Sports Med. 2001;29(2):124–8.
41. Molsa J, Airaksinen O, Nasman O, et al. Ice hockey injuries in Finland: a prospective epidemiologic study. Am J Sports Med. 1997;25:495–9.
42. Merrifield HH, Cowans RF. Groin strain injuries in ice hockey. J Sports Med. 1973;1:41–2.
43. Grote K, Lincoln TL, Gamble JG. Hip adductor injury in competitive swimmers. Am J Sports Med. 2004;32(1):104–8.
44. Rodeo S. Knee pain in competitive swimming. Clin Sports Med. 1999;18:379–87.
45. Orchard J, Marsden J, Lord S, et al. Preseason hamstring muscle weakness associated with hamstring muscle injury in Australian footballers. Am J Sports Med. 1997;25:81–5.
46. Safran MR, Garrett WE, Seaber AV, et al. The role of warm-up in muscular injury prevention. Am J Sports Med. 1988;16:123–9.
47. Ekstrand J, Gillquist J, Liljedahl SO. Prevention of soccer injuries. Am J Sports Med. 1983;11:116–20.
48. Meyers WC, Yoo E, Devon ON, et al. Understanding "Sports Hernia" (Athletic Publagia): the anatomic and pathophysiologic basis for abdominal and groin pain in athletes. Oper Tech in Sports Med. 2007;15:165–77.

Arthroscopic Treatment: Bony Lesions

54

Thomas G. Sampson

Introduction

The treatment of bony lesions around the hip has advanced exponentially in the last few years because of the recognition of joint pathology associated with femoroacetabular impingement [1–8]. The evolution of arthroscopic excision of the CAM and pincer lesions began initially with working only on the femoral side for nearly 4 years and subsequently treating the rim impingement syndrome and the associated pathology on the acetabular side [9, 10].

Consequently in the earlier years, very few acetabular rims were trimmed and few labrums were repaired [11, 12]. Currently, rim trimming with labral cartilage refixation along with femoroplasty is performed on each of those cases where bony collision can be demonstrated dynamically.

In this chapter we will discuss osseous abnormalities of the hip that cause a pathologic process. It is difficult to discuss bony lesions without regarding the labrum and cartilage lesions and their destructive forces leading to injury or arthritis [7, 13]. Most of this chapter was based on observations at hip arthroscopy over the last 30 years and opinions derived from the literature, experience and outcomes derived from over 1500 cases of bony lesions treated with hip arthroscopic techniques. The discussion will be derived from those conditions related to femoral acetabular impingement. Although most FAI is felt to be of two types, CAM and pincer [3, 7, 14], our observation is that there is a large gray area in which the femoral head junction reacts to the rim overgrowth and vice versa which cannot be classified into the above (Fig. 54.1). The final surgical decision as to the amount of bone removed from the head neck junction of the femur and the acetabular rim, therefore, is predicated on the relationship of the acetabular rim overgrowth, the labral and cartilage damage, the observation using dynamic motion during surgery showing conflict, and the deformity of the head neck junction (Fig. 54.2).

Femoroacetabular impingement was brought to our attention by Prof. Reinhold Ganz et al. nearly 15 years ago, and initially described CAM type and pincer type [1]. His studies showed that the abnormal morphology did not damage the hip statically, but required increased loading with movement. The major destructive changes from CAM type were to the inner 1–2 cm of the articular cartilage of the acetabulum, and with pincer type, the destruction was mostly at the rim and to the labrum. Most literature describes the two distinct types; however in our experience we rarely see one without the other [4–7, 14–18].

When planning correction of the bony lesions, the surgeon should take into account the increased alpha angle if it is greater than 55° [19, 20]. In addition he should also be aware of the reaction of the head neck junction to impaction and its effect on the anterior rim of the acetabulum which may cause nonossified bony deformities *not* measured on x-rays, CT scans, or MRIs. Additionally, when planning removal of rim overgrowth or osteophytes, it is best to not over-resect bone by leaving at least 20–25° for both the lateral center edge angle and the anterior center edge angle (Fig. 54.3).

The articular cartilage and labral damage will further define the effects of the abnormal bony morphology from which the correction should be a balance between labral cartilage preservation and osseous excision [8, 21–23]. Surgical outcomes and ultimate results are directly affected by the degree of articular cartilage and labral damage identified at the time of surgery (Fig. 54.4) [8, 21–31]. Additionally, age, gender, activity level, and desired goals will have a major impact on the individual's satisfaction.

T.G. Sampson, MD (✉)
Director of Hip Arthroscopy, Post Street Surgery, Post Street Orthopaedics and Sports Medicine, 2299 Post Street Suite 107, San Francisco, CA 94115-3443, USA

Orthopaedic Consultant and Surgeon, Veterans Administration Medical Center at Fort Miley, San Francisco, CA, USA

Associate Clinical Professor Department of Orthopaedics, University of California, San Francisco, CA, USA
e-mail: tgsampsonmd@gmail.com

J.C. McCarthy et al. (eds.), *Hip Joint Restoration*, DOI 10.1007/978-1-4614-0694-5_54

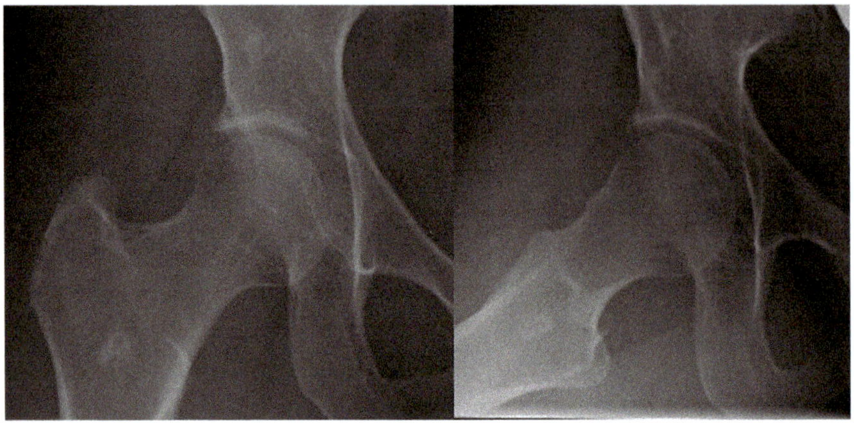

Fig. 54.1 AP and frog leg lateral right hip showing a small femoral neck dent and bump from anterior acetabular rim impingement

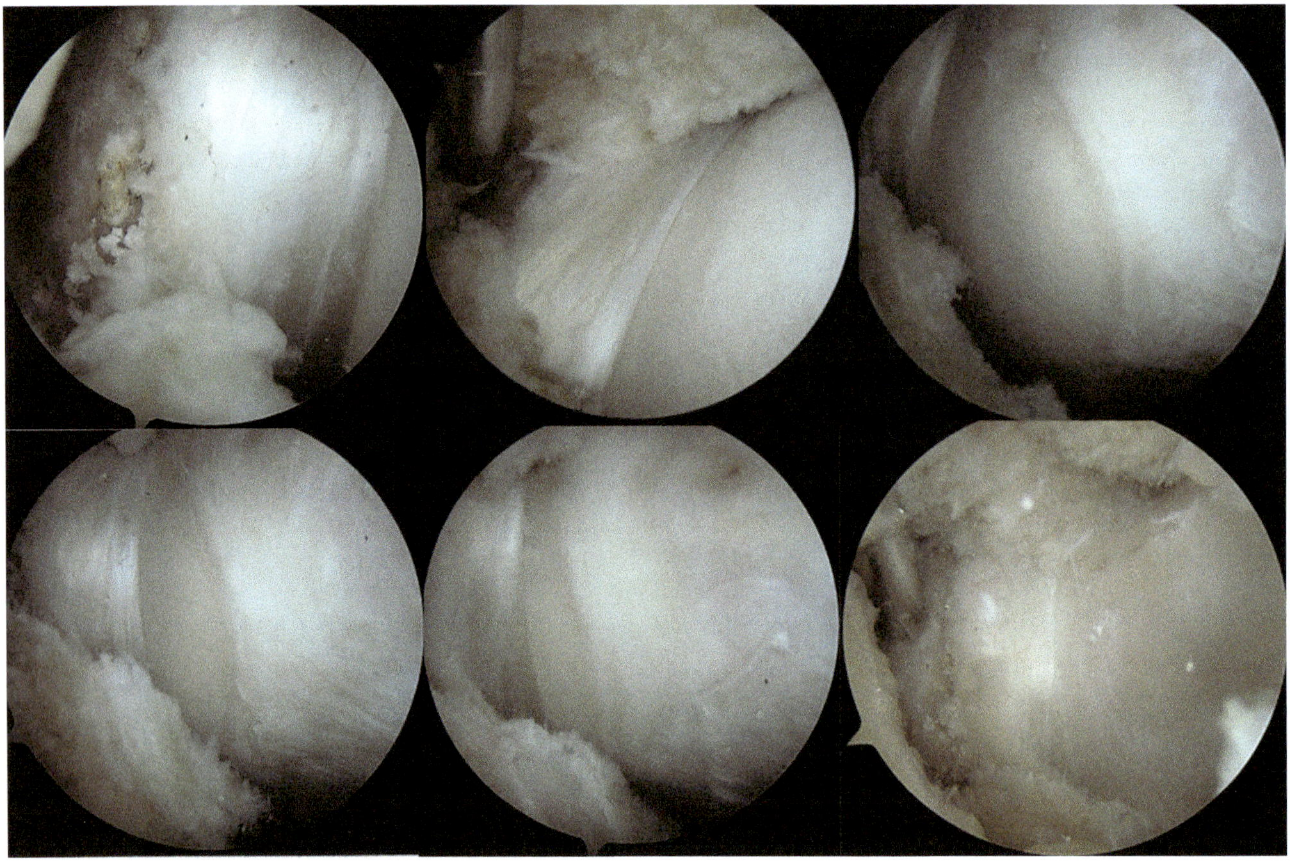

Fig. 54.2 Motion study to determine head neck (H) conflict with the acetabular rim (AR). Note the demarcation zone (DZ), the cut capsule (C), and labrum (L)

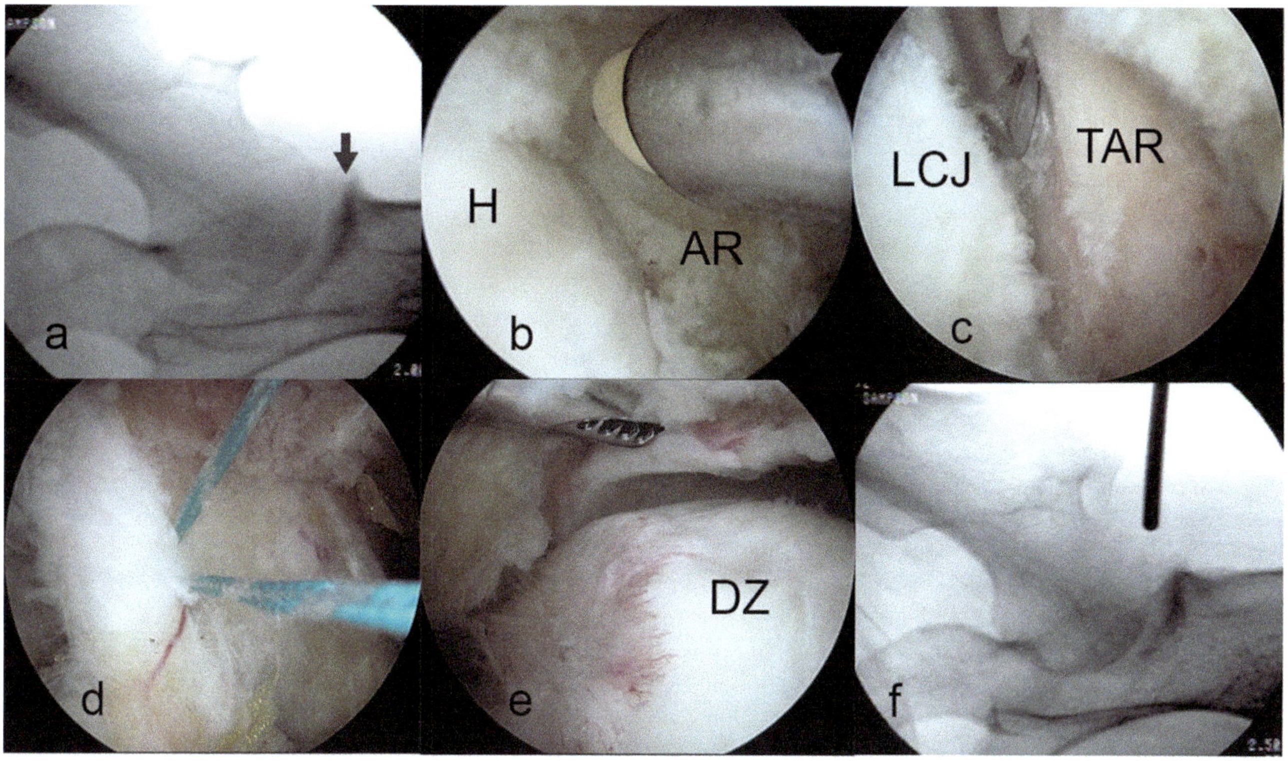

Fig. 54.3 (**a**) Preoperative fluoroscopic view right hip with DDH and excess anterior rim (*arrow*), (**b**) anterior rim (AR) exposed, (**c**) after trimmed anterior rim (TAR) preparing for repair, note labro-cartilage junction (LCJ), (**d**) labrum reattached to the acetabular rim, (**e**) the head is distracted showing a dent at the demarcation zone (DZ) from impaction by the rim, (**f**) postoperative fluoroscopic view after rim trimmed anteriorly, note the LCEA is unchanged from preoperative fluoroscopic view

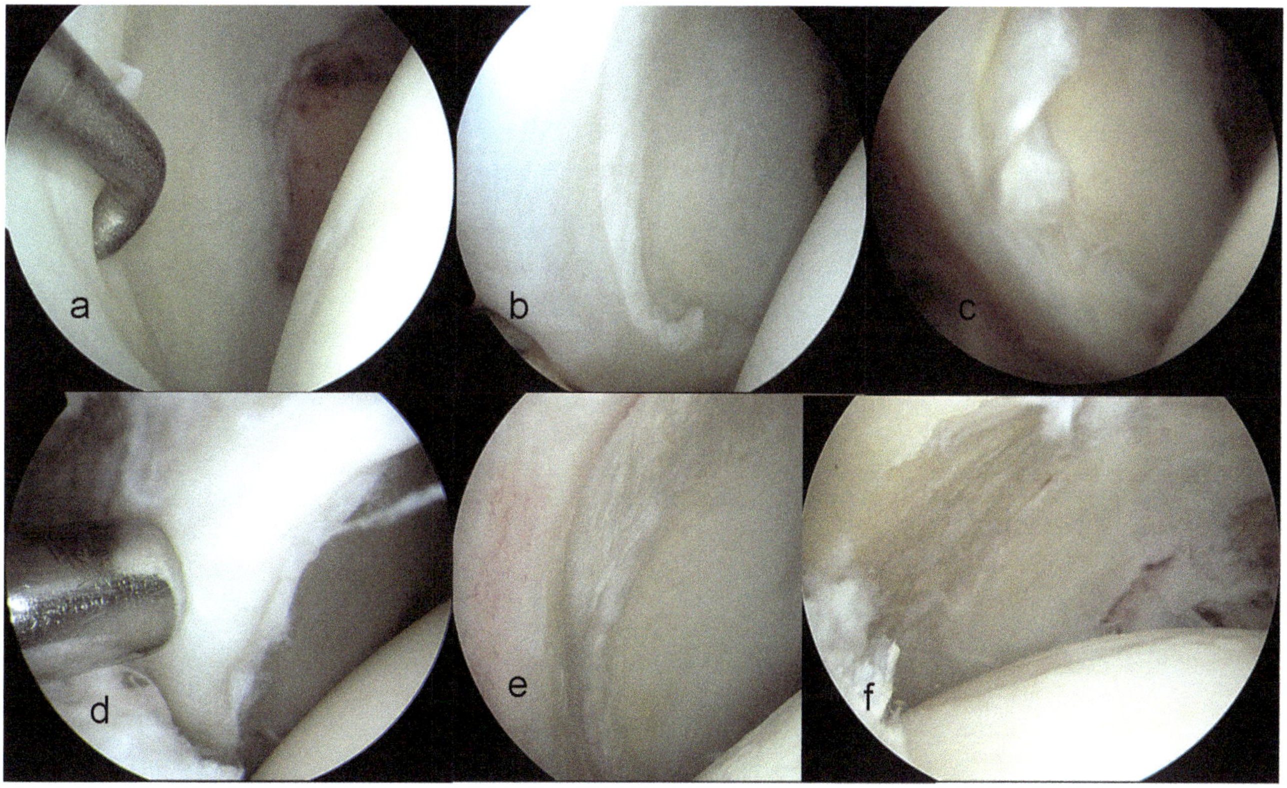

Fig. 54.4 Left hips viewed through the mid-anterior portal showing progression of damage from more pincer effect than CAM (**a**, **b**), mixed effect (**c**, **d**) and more severe damage from more CAM effect (**e**, **f**)

Approach to the Diagnosis

Most patients with FAI complain of hip pain perceived in the groin, but it may also be perceived laterally around the trochanter or beneath the tensor fascia lata or gluteal muscles, and posteriorly beneath the gluteus maximus. John Hilton's law describes why pain is perceived from a joint through the muscles across the joint [32]. The hip joint is a good example of this law, as pain may be perceived as far proximal as the middle of the spine through the iliopsoas, to distal to the insertion of the tensor fascia lata at the knee.

A pop or click may be observed, and only when it occurs 100% with flexion and extension of the hip, will it involve iliopsoas pathology. Random pops or clicks may occur from labral cartilage junctional pathology as well as abnormal bony shapes impacting the soft tissues.

Many individuals lack range of motion, or may have different ranges of motion in the contralateral hip. Lack of internal rotation is common with CAM type impingement; however we have found it associated with anterior rim pincer lesions or soft tissue impingement as well. Most labral and cartilage pathology associated with bony lesions occurs in zones 1 through 3 on the acetabular face, with large cam deformities and large anterior rim lesions can cause the femoral head to partially sublux creating posterior acetabular damage.

The Bony Impingement Mapping Test

With the patient lying in a supine position, the affected leg is held by the examiner with the knee flexed at 90° and the hip also flexed at 90°. The hip is externally rotated to a comfortable position, and then rotated internally adding a bit more flexion until the patient begins to complain of a groin pain or pinch. Next the leg is extended, internally rotated maximally and then slowly flexed, stopping when the patient reports a similar pain or pinch. The position of the leg is noted in both positions that cause symptoms and correlated to the acetabular zones. Those zones are then carefully checked for correlation with bony pathology and changes on the MRA or MRI. It is our observation that there is a strong correlation between this test and the pathology observed that surgery. There is a strong correlation with a full thickness acetabular articular cartilage delamination (FAACD) (Fig. 54.5).

Imaging

Radiographic imaging of bony defects is helpful when the lesions are obvious, and many use a three-dimensional CT scan for their delineation. We are concerned about the levels of radiation exposure with CT, as there is no current safety standard regarding the lower levels of radiation exposure to patients. For that reason we rely on plain radiographs, MRI or MRA, and intraoperative rotational fluoroscopic views to help map out the bony pathology. We look for subtle abnormalities such as "femoral head neck dents or bumps," minor bony excrescences on the anterior acetabular rim, and abnormal shapes on the head neck junction of the femur that would not be described by an abnormal alpha angle. It is often that in young individuals, the MRI or MRA is entirely normal, yet they may have a full thickness acetabular articular cartilage delamination associated with anterior rim bone overgrowth.

Planning the Procedure

When treating bony lesions with an open surgical dislocation, the surgeon has a planned sequence of steps to resolve the pathology. It is our opinion that hip arthroscopic surgery should abide by the same sequence of events to achieve optimum results.

The sequence includes:

- Exposure
- Identification of the abnormal anatomy, morphology, and pathology with dynamic testing
- Correction of the abnormal morphology
- Repair the pathology
- Close

Most hip arthroscopic surgeons approach the central compartment first using distraction, then visualize the peripheral compartment, and finally do a capsulotomy to treat the bony lesions. We have adopted the technique of a planned capsulotomy going from out-to-in in all cases. The advantages are that exposure is reproducible on nearly all hips, and whether the capsule is left open, excised, or repaired (plicated) may be determined prior to surgery based on their acetabular index, center edge angle, and hip laxity index. Additionally, during initial exposure to the peripheral compartment, no . distraction is needed, thus reducing the potential for traction complications (Fig. 54.6).

Fig. 54.6 Left hip capsulotomy approaching from outside the capsule to inward similar to an open capsulotomy. (**a**) fluoroscopic A-P view left hip, (**b**) exposure of capsule (**c**), and reflected head of rectus femoris (rh), (**d**) exposure of the head neck junction, (hnj) and cut-capsular edge (cc), femoral neck (n) and CAM bump (*arrows*), (**e**) cut capsule (*arrows*), (**f**) labral exposure (l), (**g**) removal of soft tissue on CAM bump and cut zona orbicularis (czo), (**h**) exposure of the medial neck noting synovitis and osteophytes

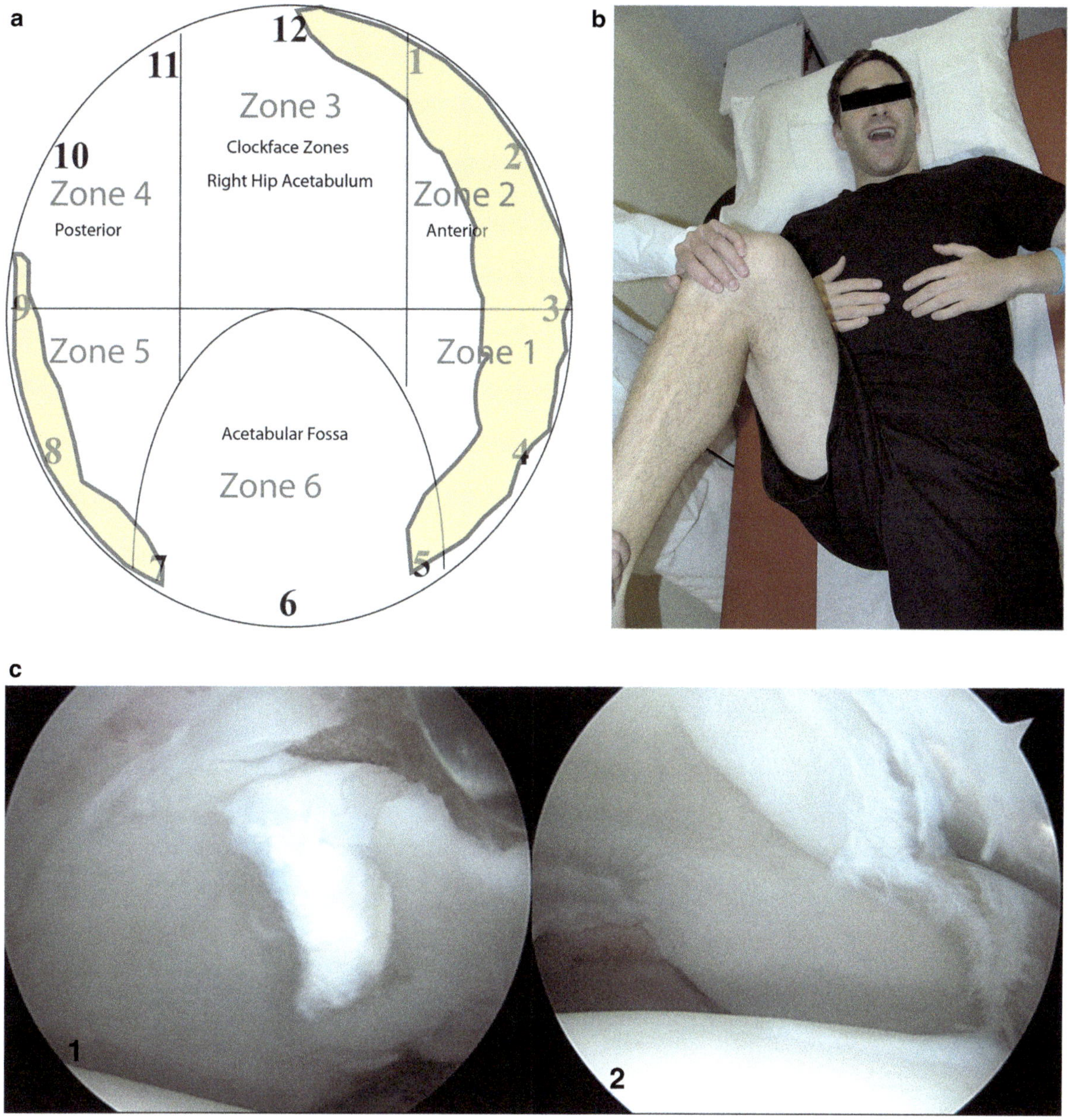

Fig. 54.5 Mapping the lesion on the acetabulum. (**a**) Clock face with zones of a right acetabulum, (**b**) patient showing pain with flexion and internal rotation, (**c**) the arthroscopic correlation (*a*) view right hip zones 3–5, (*b*) view zones 1–3; note the anterior delamination and posterior excoriation of the articular cartilage

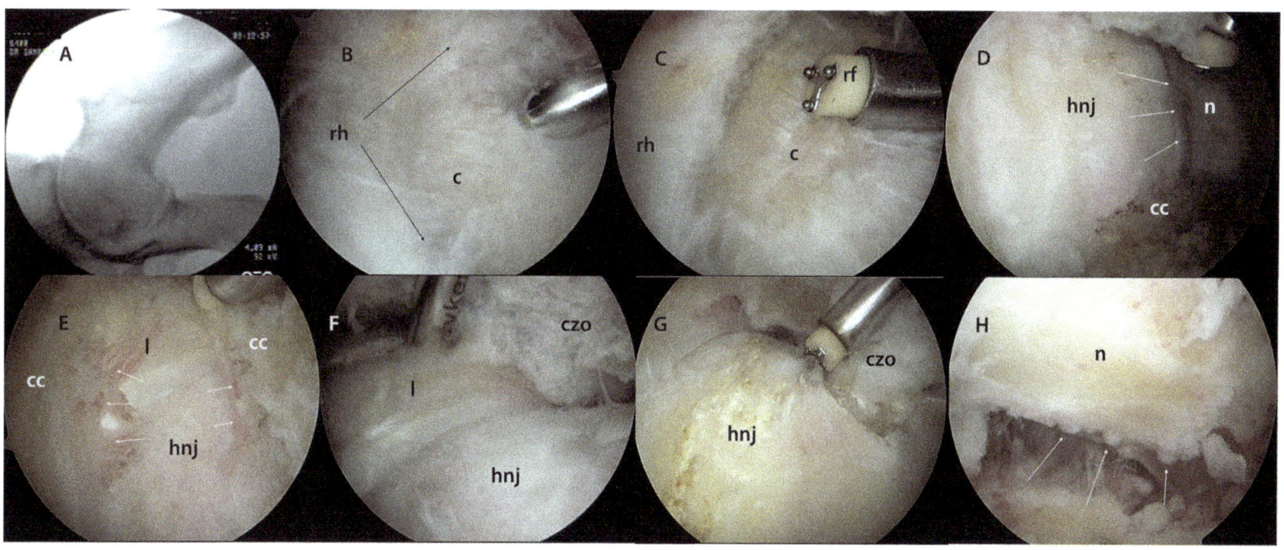

Surgical Technique

We favor the lateral approach to hip arthroscopy; however the procedure may be done in a supine position (Fig. 54.7).

Preoperative Fluoroscopy

Prior to prepping and draping the patient, multiple fluoroscopic views are taken A-P, looking for both obvious and subtle bony deformities of the femoral head neck junction and the relationship to the acetabular rim. They include slight abduction with neutral, external rotation, internal rotation, flexion to 45° with extra rotation 45° (Dunn view), abduction maximally with extra rotation maximally, and internal rotation. These views will alert the surgeon to where most of the conflict occurs on the head neck junction. Most commonly the maximal amount of bone to be removed is anterolateral between the lateral and medial synovial folds (Fig. 54.8).

Portals

Nearly all surgery is performed through a two portal technique; anterolateral and mid-anterior. Additional portals may be necessary, such as a posterior lateral to reach the more posterior aspects of the acetabulum and femoral neck junc-

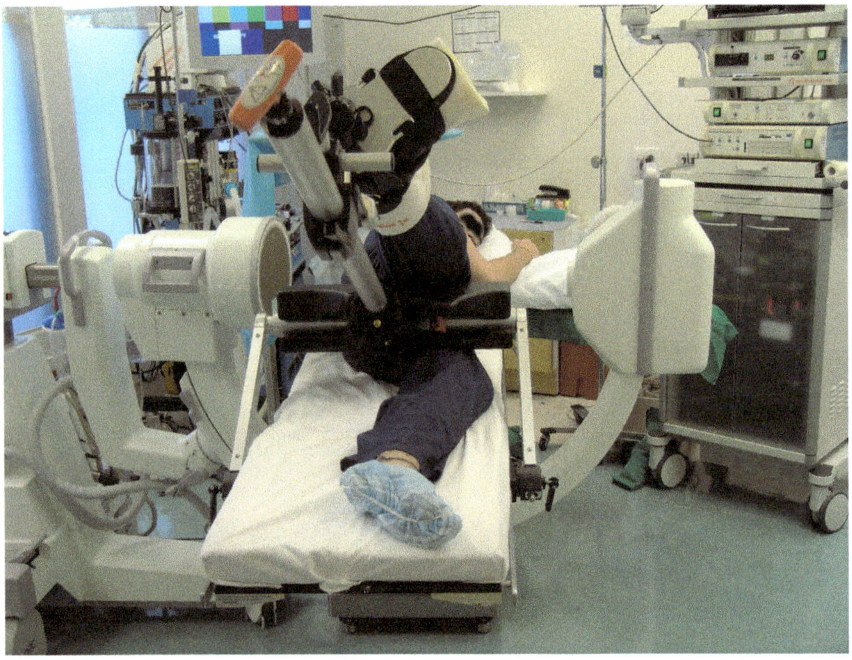

Fig. 54.7 Position of patient for lateral approach. The right leg is in a distractor and the C-Arm fluoroscope lies beneath the patient

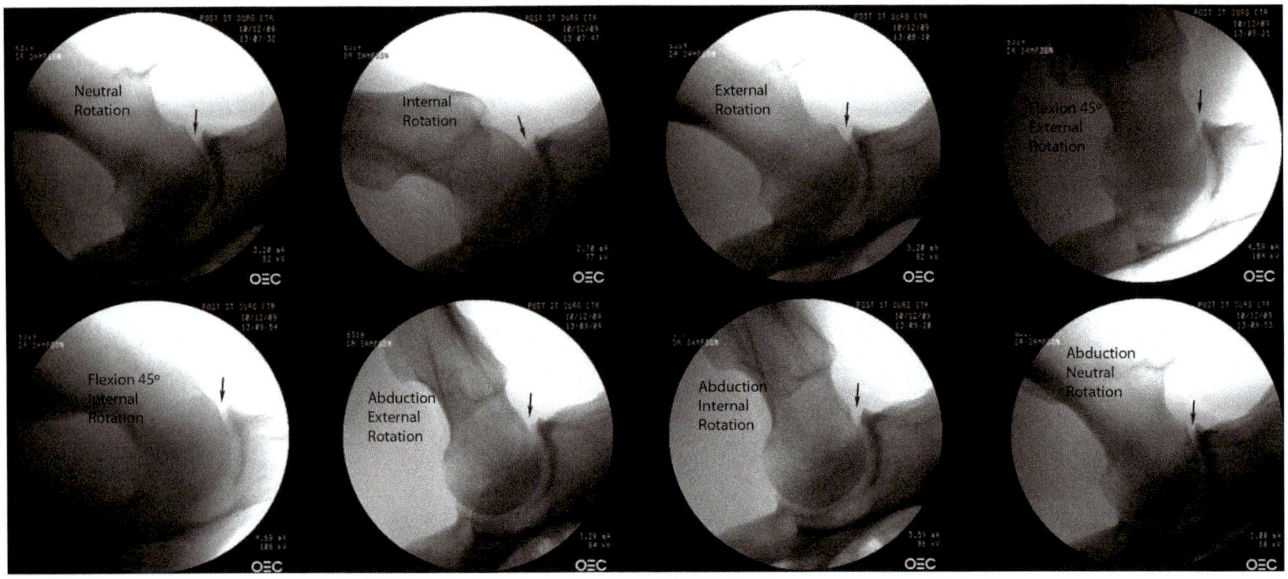

Fig. 54.8 Preoperative fluoroscopic views in lateral decubitus position in multiple rotation and abduction

tion, or accessory portals for suture management during labral repair. Using the standard techniques, the scope and instruments are placed through the portals to the level of the capsule (Fig. 54.9).

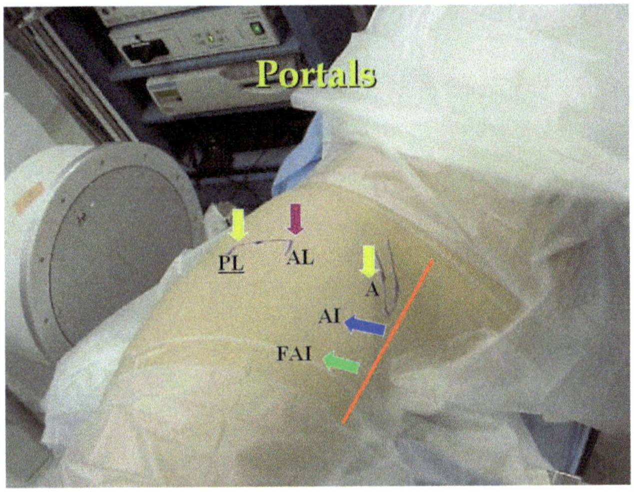

Fig. 54.9 Lateral view right hip of the portals, postero-lateral (PL), antero-lateral (AL), anterior (A), mid-anterior (AI), far anterior inferior (FAI)

Capsulotomy

With the 30° arthroscope looking through the anterolateral portal, and the operative instruments, the anterior fat pad and the reflected head of the rectus femoris are identified. Using a 4 mm shaver, a portion of the anterior fat pad is excised, exposing the anterior lateral capsule. Next, using an RF probe, the capsule is incised from the base of the neck of femur to a position proximal to the labrum on the acetabular rim taking care not to damage the acetabular labrum. The dissection is then carried lateral through zone 3 and anterior through zone 1. A portion of the superior edges of the cut capsule is then removed with the motorized shaver. The bony deformities of the head neck junction and the rim are then visualized. A motion study may then be accomplished to determine conflict between the head neck junction and acetabular rim while observing the effect on the labrum. The function and quality of the labrum may then be assessed as well as it sealing effect on the head. In some cases, there is no seal because of degeneration of the labrum or retraction from the rim overgrowth (Fig. 54.10).

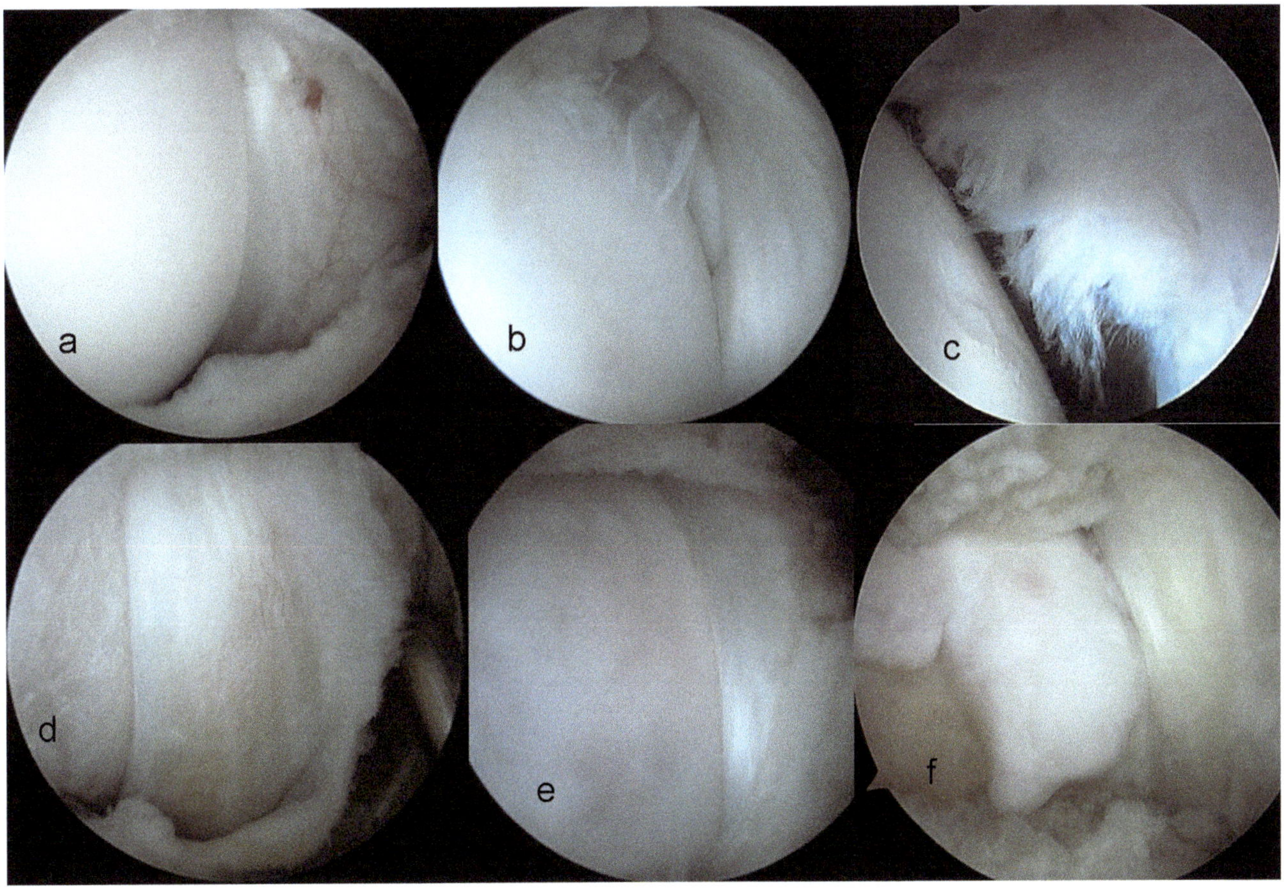

Fig. 54.10 Labral seal evaluated (**a**) excellent seal, (**b**) retracted seal, (**c**) no seal, (**d**) good seal with degeneration (*yellow discoloration*), (**e**) good seal with reaction on head neck (erythema), (**f**) poor seal because of head neck osteophyte

Distraction

Once the capsulotomy has been completed, the hip is distracted to allow entry into the central compartment. This separation allows for direct visualization on entry and therefore reducing the potential damage to the labrum and the articular cartilage of the head and the acetabulum. If there is excessive rim anteriorly or global overcoverage, the rim will need to be trimmed with a burr prior to entry. The central compartment is then inspected for damage and the planned repair of the labral cartilage junction, treatment of cartilage defects, and bony resection of the rim and/or head neck junction may be planned (Fig. 54.11).

The Acetabular Rim

Typically the acetabular rim is exposed external to zones 1 through 3 as that is the most common areas of damage of the acetabular articular cartilage and labrum. Viewing from the anterolateral portal a 4 mm hip burr is used to trim the excess anterior acetabular bone. The labrum is left attached during this process and the amount of bone to be removed is determined to change a convex osteophyte to a shallow concave contour to accommodate the new shape of the head neck junction. The labral cartilage junction is intentionally left intact so as not to disturb its contiguous relationship and sealing effect. The arthroscope is then transferred to the mid-anterior portal with the operative instruments through the anterior lateral portal, and the rim trimming is completed laterally beneath the insertion of the reflected head of the rectus femoris (Fig. 54.12). With global pincer, resection is carried further posteriorly into zone 5. The amount of bone taken off laterally may be determined preoperatively by technique described by Matsuda in which the fluoroscopic image is marked with a sharpie, and intermittent fluoroscopic images are taken until the bone beneath the markings are erased from the image [33].

Femoroplasty

It is our opinion that a methodically planned technique for the excision of the cam bump or any pathologic shape of the head neck junction will facilitate adequacy of the resection. The technique involves first removing the soft tissue over the areas of resection, and then using the 5 mm burr, an outline of the area to be resected is created (Fig. 54.13). We typically will start at a demarcation zone at the head neck junction, if it is present, then work anteriorly to anterolateral, and finally complete the resection posterior lateral.

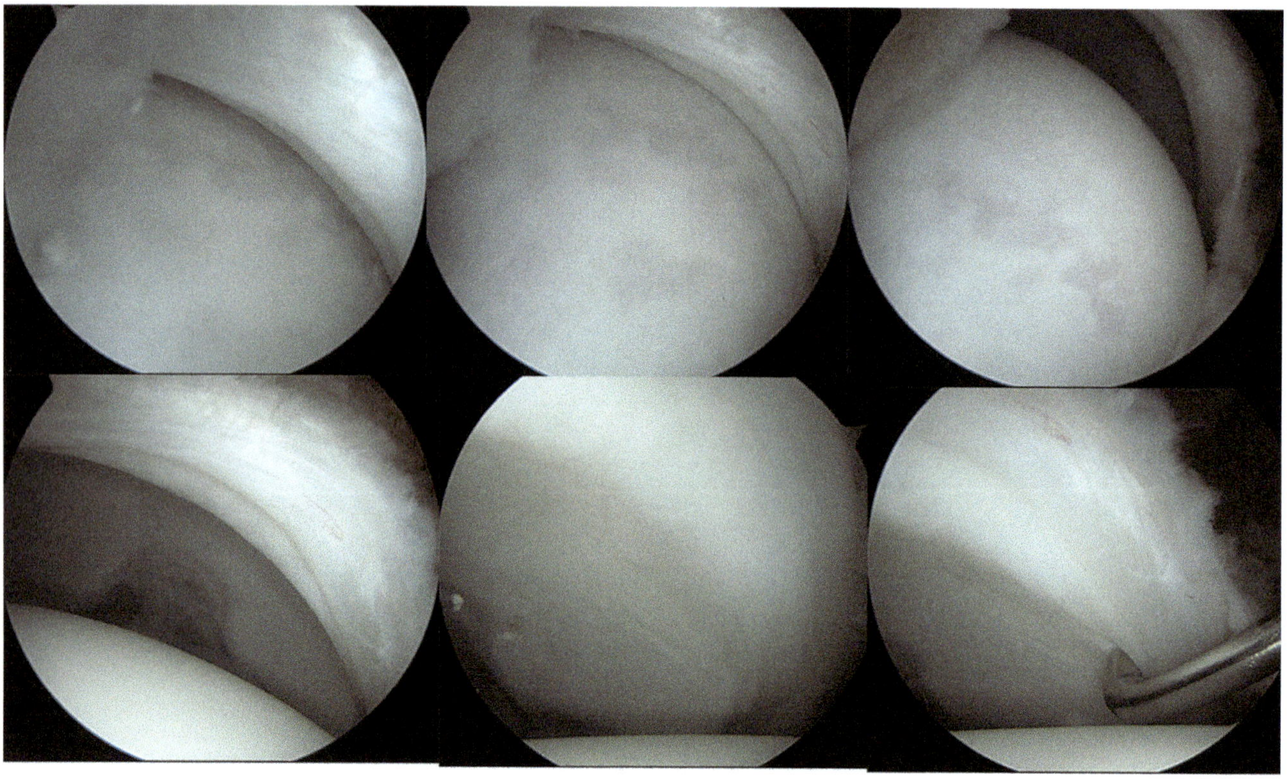

Fig. 54.11 Distraction after a capsulotomy of a right hip viewed through the anterolateral portal

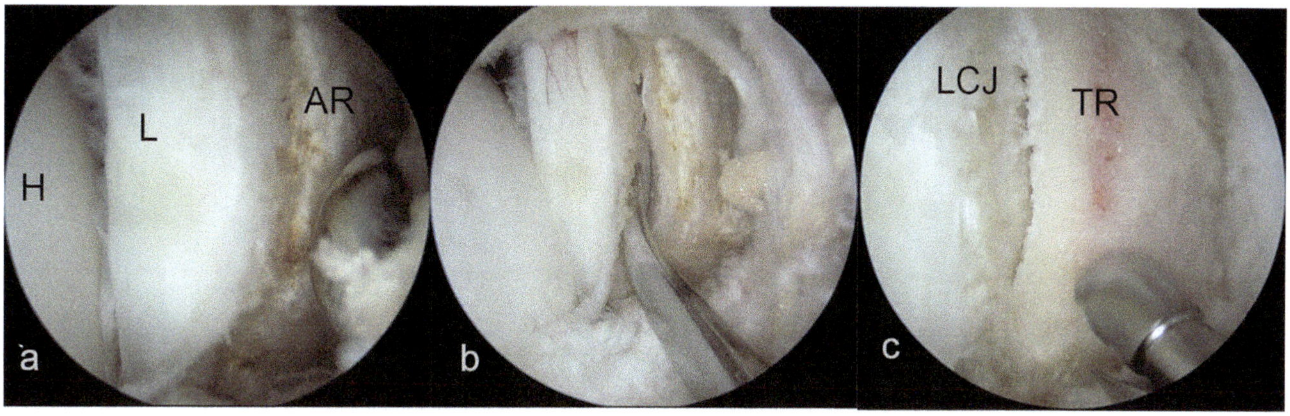

Fig. 54.12 Rim trimming of a right hip viewing from anterolateral portal. (**a**) Exposure through a capsulotomy, head (H), labrum (L), acetabular rim (AR), (**b**) Reflecting the labrum (L), (**c**) trimming with a 4.0 mm burr adjacent to the labro-cartilage junction (LCJ)

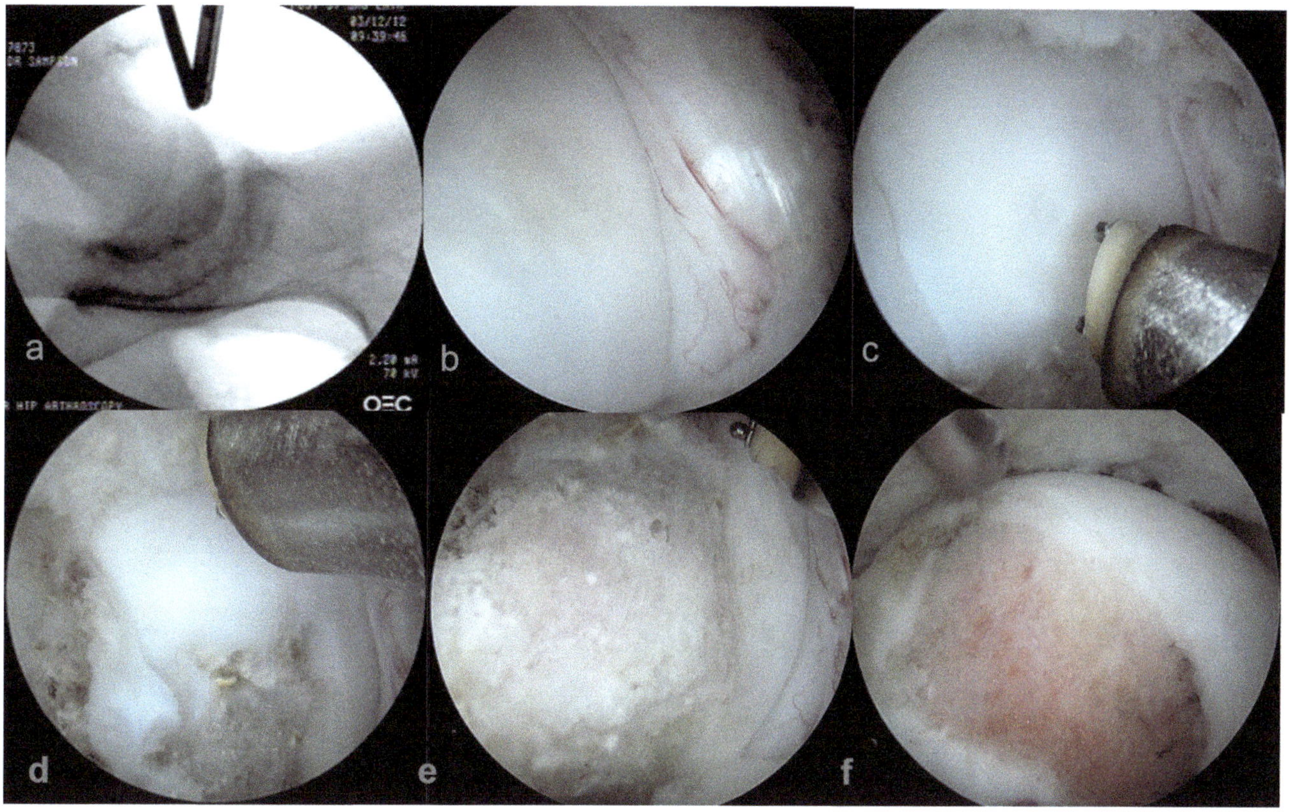

Fig. 54.13 Soft tissue excised from head neck junction prior to femoroplasty. (**a**) Fluoroscopic view A-P right hip lateral position (note scope and instrument position in the following images), (**b**) exposure of a right hip viewing through anterolateral portal, (**c**) RF probe positioned to excise soft tissue over head neck junction at demarcation zone, (**d**) partial soft tissue excised, (**e**) cartilage and periosteum excised, (**f**) partial femoroplasty completed

During the resection, no distraction is necessary until the final bony resection is done posterior lateral as it is needed to expose that area and bring it far enough away from the rim to prevent damage to the labrum (Fig. 54.14). Flexion to 45° with external rotation gives excellent exposure to the anterior aspect of the neck junction (Fig. 54.15).

Labral Refixation and Cartilage Repair

With the bony resection of the acetabular rim and the head neck junction of the femur, labral cartilage delamination, labral tears, or labral separations from the acetabular rim may then be fixed under direct visualization. The planned

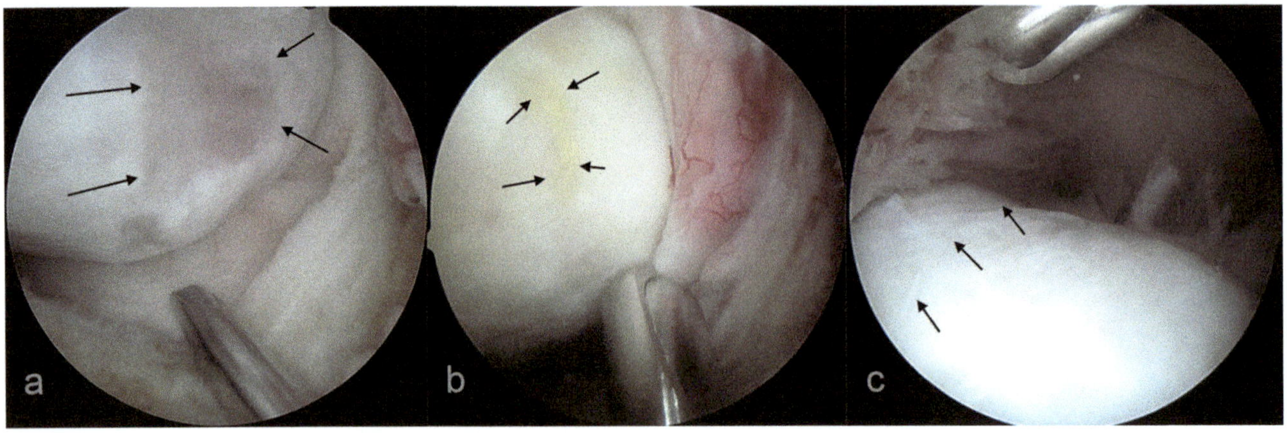

Fig. 54.14 Demarcation zone head neck junction (*arrows*). (**a**) Right hip seen through anterolateral portal, note the area of erosion and clear delineation between healthy cartilage and erythema on the junction from impaction, (**b**) *yellowish staining* of the cartilage at the junction, and (**c**) change in shape of the head at the junction

Fig. 54.15 View improved with flexion to 45° and external rotation using a 30° scope through an anterolateral portal into the anterior peripheral space with the instrument coming through the mid-anterior portal

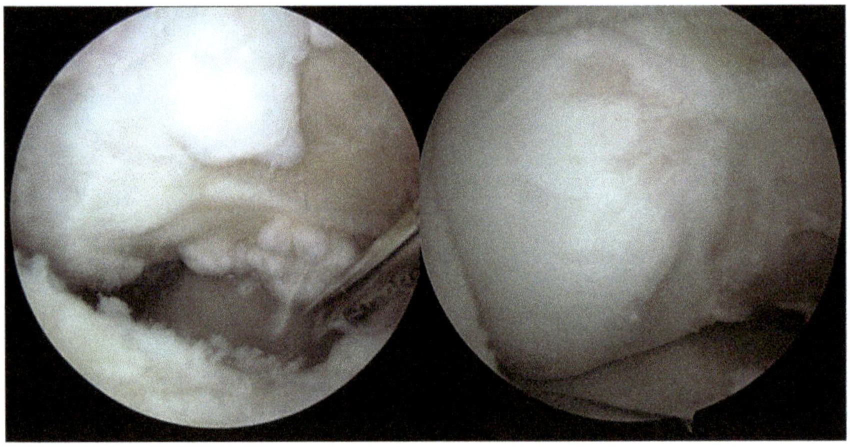

Fig. 54.16 A view of a right acetabular rim through the anterolateral portal with the drill coming through the mid-anterior portal. The acetabular rim is predrilled before suturing the labrum

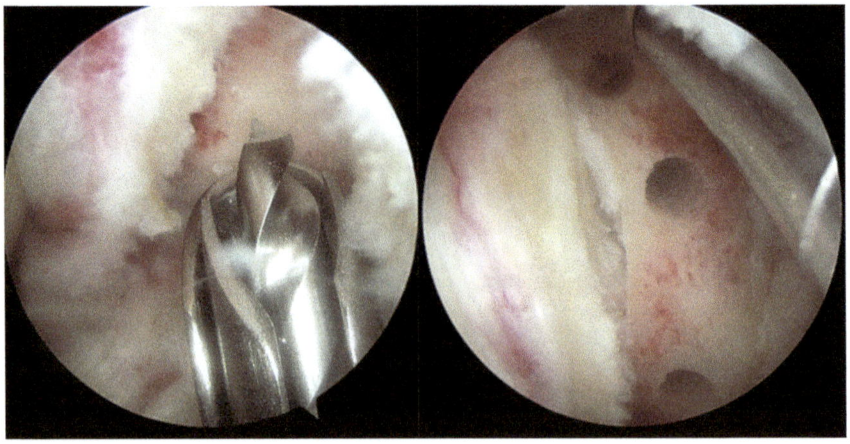

area of repair is identified and all anchor holes are drilled (Fig. 54.16). With the hip in distraction, sequential sutures are placed using a base repair technique, using high-strength suture through the labrum and then secured with a bone anchor (Fig. 54.17). The labrum can be tensioned appropriately to its new position on the acetabular rim to ensure an excellent gasket seal. If there is a cartilage delamination (full thickness acetabular articular cartilage delamination), we favor preparing the bone with curettage of the acetabulum followed by microfracture to promote a fracture healing response prior to refixation of the labrum (Fig. 54.18).

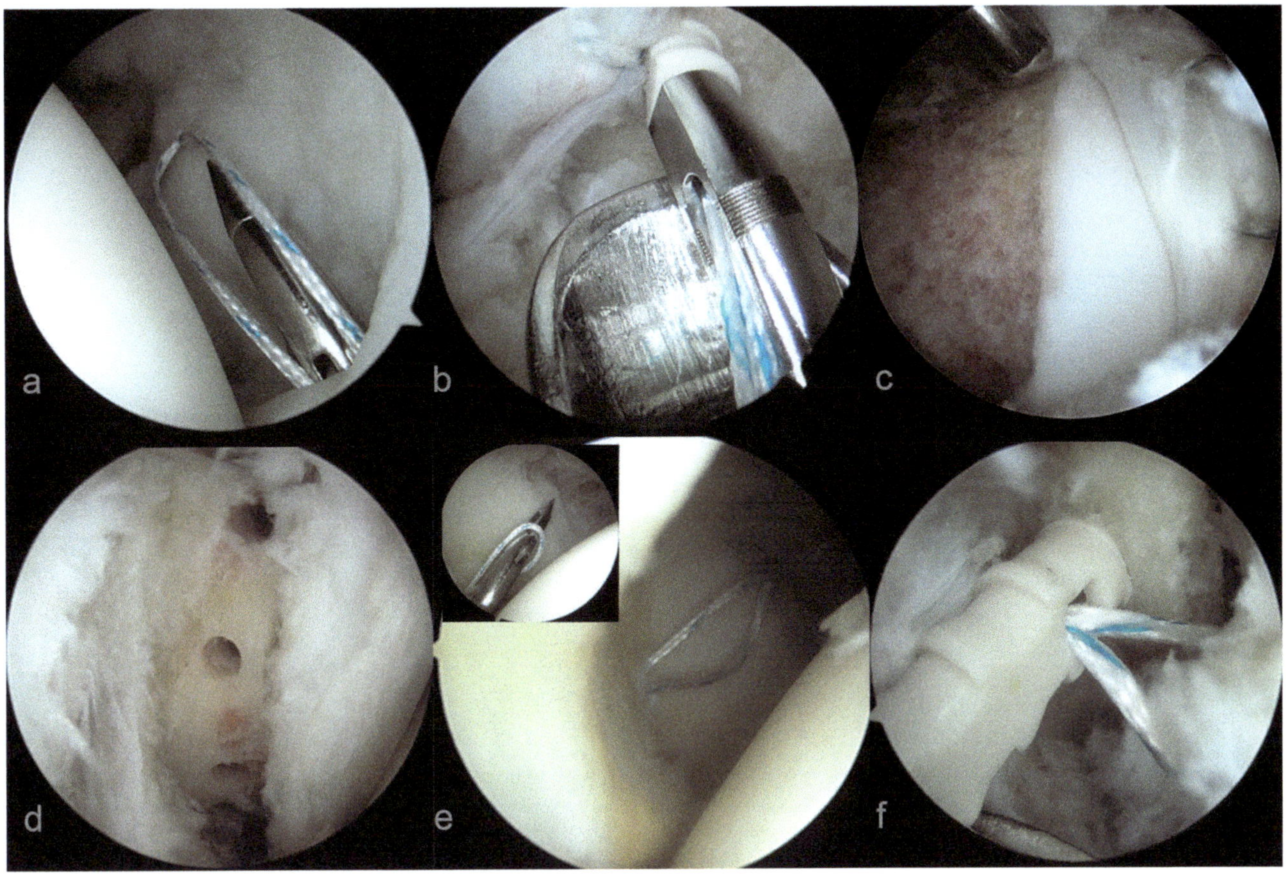

Fig. 54.17 Labral base repair. (**a**) View of right hip through the anterolateral portal showing penetrator and suture though the labro-cartilage junction, (**b**) after the second pass through the labrum, the anchor is impacted into the drill hole, (**c**) the head is sealed by the labrum (note the base sutures), (**d**) left hip showing predrilled holes, (**e**) suture through the base of the labrum (*inset* shows second pass of the penetrator to retrieve the suture, (**f**) impaction of the anchor into the drill hole (note the suture is located at the base of the labrum)

Evaluation of the Bony Resection and Labral Repair

A fluoroscopic motion study is then performed to evaluate for any conflicts between the head and neck junction and the acetabular labrum, which, if not optimal, may result in further resection of the head neck defect. Finally, a repeat of the fluoroscopic images showing no remaining conflict is completed before the procedure is done (Fig. 54.19).

Capsular Management

For the majority of our cases, the capsule is left open. If there is a concern of potential instability due to developmental dysplasia of the hip (DDH), or the laxity index is greater than 3, the capsule is closed partially at the Zona Orbicularis.

Postoperative

A long-acting local anesthetic is administered into the area of surgery, and standard dressings are applied. The patient is then instructed on the use of crutches and encouraged to fully weight bear when tolerated. Sutures are removed in 1 week.

Rehabilitation

Patients are encouraged to start working on a stationary bicycle to regain motion followed by an elliptical trainer and then a treadmill. They are checked at 4 weeks, and if their range of motion is limited they are started with a physical therapist to obtain better movement. If there is a concern about the patient's ability to self-rehabilitate, a physical therapist is utilized at the outset.

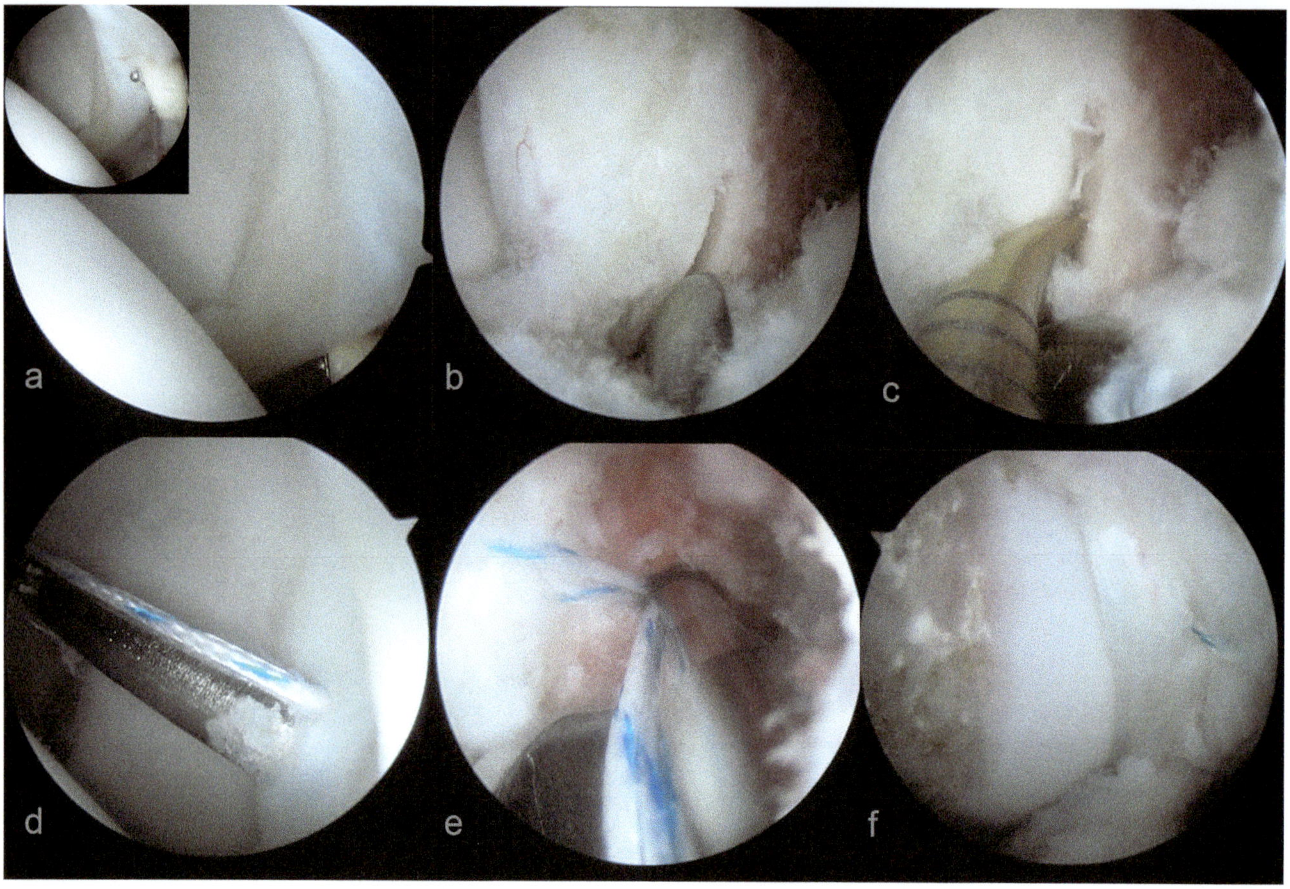

Fig. 54.18 Repair of a full-thickness acetabular articular cartilage defect (FAACD). (**a**) View of a right hip through the anterolateral portal noting the demarcation of the delamination of the articular cartilage (*inset* probing defect), (**b**) elevation of the loose cartilage from the face of the acetabulum, (**c**) microfracture of the acetabular face, (**d**) base repair of the labro-cartilage, (**e**) anchor delivery and tensioning the labrum to the rim, (**f**) head reduced noting excellent seal

Fig. 54.19 Final resection of the head neck junction after a motion study. (**a**) Preoperative fluoroscopy noting the CAM bump, (**b**) initial resection with the burr (*inset* shows some residual bump), (**c**) fine tuning the resection, (**d**) postoperative fluoroscopy showing the desired resection

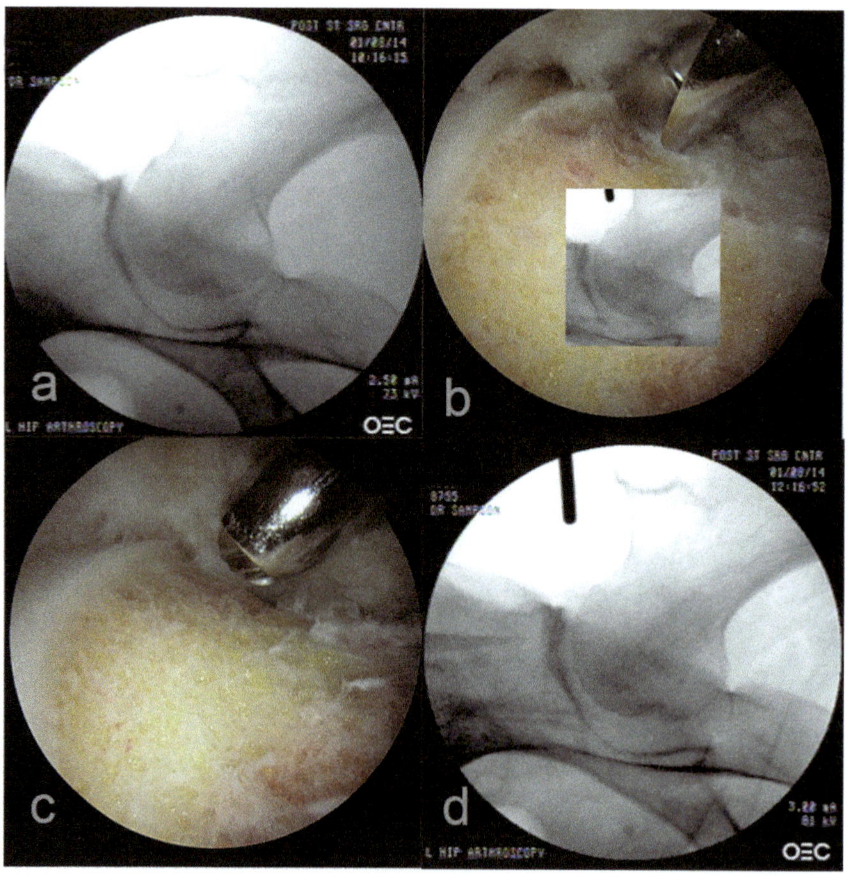

Results

From January 2002 through December 2012, 1532 hips in 1302 patients were treated for FAI. Revisions comprised 154 hips. Females predominated with 794 hips versus males 738 with average age 39.7 years (12–73 years). The Average follow-up was 97 months (range 6–119 months) with an average preop MHHS of 68.9 and average postop mHHS of 91.7. The complication rate was 0.5 % for transient neuropraxias of the lateral femoral cutaneous nerve. The most serious complications were one retroperitoneal abdominal fluid extravasation which resolved with an overnight observation and analgesics, three femoral neck fractures, and one anterior dislocation.

Conclusions

The arthroscopic treatment of bony lesions around the hip has advanced exponentially in the last few years and has become accepted as the treatment of choice when compared to open surgical dislocation. We advise a methodical approach similar to open surgery to gain optimum visualization and access to obtain reproducible results. Recognition of and comprehensive treatment of all bony abnormalities and the labral and cartilage injuries and pathology will give optimum outcomes. We believe the amount of bony excision on the femoral head neck area and the acetabular rim should be based on preoperative signs and symptoms with a correlative physical exam as well as X-rays and MRI, operative fluoroscopy with the final decision based on surgical findings, and intraoperative motion studies. Careful attention to the type of damage to the labrum and articular cartilage will dictate the location and amount of bony resection on the acetabular rim and femoral head neck junction.

Our results have shown the procedure is beneficial in providing pain relief in mid-term follow-up, with few complications.

References

1. Myers SR, Eijer H, Ganz R. Anterior femoroacetabular impingement after periacetabular osteotomy. Clin Orthop Relat Res. 1999;363:93–9.
2. Eijer H, Myers SR, Ganz R. Anterior femoroacetabular impingement after femoral neck fractures. J Orthop Trauma. 2001;15(7):475–81.
3. Ito K, et al. Femoroacetabular impingement and the cam-effect. A MRI-based quantitative anatomical study of the femoral head-neck offset. J Bone Joint Surg Br. 2001;83(2):171–6.
4. Beck M, et al. Anterior femoroacetabular impingement: part II. Midterm results of surgical treatment. Clin Orthop Relat Res. 2004;418:67–73.
5. Lavigne M, et al. Anterior femoroacetabular impingement: part I. Techniques of joint preserving surgery. Clin Orthop Relat Res. 2004;418:61–6.
6. Beall DP, et al. Imaging findings of femoroacetabular impingement syndrome. Skeletal Radiol. 2005;34(11):691–701.
7. Beck M, et al. Hip morphology influences the pattern of damage to the acetabular cartilage: femoroacetabular impingement as a cause of early osteoarthritis of the hip. J Bone Joint Surg Br. 2005;87(7):1012–8.
8. Sampson T. Hip morphology and its relationship to pathology: dysplasia to impingement. Oper Tech Sports Med. 2005;13(1):37–45.
9. Sampson T. Arthroscopic treatment of femoroacetabular impingement. Tech Orthop. 2005;20:56–62.
10. Carlos AG, Aaron AB. Arthroscopic treatment of femoroacetabular impingement. Arthroscopy. 2006;22(1):95–106.
11. Kelly BT, et al. Arthroscopic labral repair in the hip: surgical technique and review of the literature. Arthroscopy. 2005;21(12):1496–504.
12. Philippon MJ, Schenker ML. A new method for acetabular rim trimming and labral repair. Clin Sports Med. 2006;25(2):293–7. ix.
13. Ganz R, et al. Femoroacetabular impingement: a cause for osteoarthritis of the hip. Clin Orthop Relat Res. 2003;417:112–20.
14. Bredella MA, Stoller DW. MR imaging of femoroacetabular impingement. Magn Reson Imaging Clin N Am. 2005;13(4):653–64.
15. Ito K, Leunig M, Ganz R. Histopathologic features of the acetabular labrum in femoroacetabular impingement. Clin Orthop Relat Res. 2004;429:262–71.
16. Murphy S, et al. Debridement of the adult hip for femoroacetabular impingement: indications and preliminary clinical results. Clin Orthop Relat Res. 2004;429:178–81.
17. Siebenrock KA, et al. Abnormal extension of the femoral head epiphysis as a cause of cam impingement. Clin Orthop Relat Res. 2004;418:54–60.
18. Tanzer M, Noiseux N. Osseous abnormalities and early osteoarthritis: the role of hip impingement. Clin Orthop Relat Res. 2004;429:170–7.
19. Naal FD, et al. Surgical hip dislocation for the treatment of femoroacetabular impingement in high-level athletes. Am J Sports Med. 2011;39(3):544–50.
20. Naal FD, et al. Midterm results of surgical hip dislocation for the treatment of femoroacetabular impingement. Am J Sports Med. 2012;40(7):1501–10.
21. Sampson TG. Arthroscopic treatment for chondral lesions of the hip. Clin Sports Med. 2011;30(2):331–48.
22. Martin HD, et al. The pattern and technique in the clinical evaluation of the adult hip: the common physical examination tests of hip specialists. Arthroscopy. 2010;26(2):161–72.
23. Sampson TG. Arthroscopic treatment of femoroacetabular impingement. Am J Orthop (Belle Mead NJ). 2008;37(12):608–12.
24. Browne JA. The mature athlete with hip arthritis. Clin Sports Med. 2011;30(2):453–62.
25. Byrd JW, Jones KS. Arthroscopic management of femoroacetabular impingement in athletes. Am J Sports Med. 2011;39(Suppl):7S–13.
26. McCarthy JC, et al. What factors influence long-term survivorship after hip arthroscopy? Clin Orthop Relat Res. 2011;469(2):362–71.
27. Philippon MJ, et al. Early outcomes after hip arthroscopy for femoroacetabular impingement in the athletic adolescent patient: a preliminary report. J Pediatr Orthop. 2008;28(7):705–10.
28. Sink EL, et al. Acetabular cartilage and labral damage observed during surgical hip dislocation for stable slipped capital femoral epiphysis. J Pediatr Orthop. 2010;30(1):26–30.
29. Stevens MS, et al. The evidence for hip arthroscopy: grading the current indications. Arthroscopy. 2010;26(10):1370–83.
30. Vaughn ZD, Safran MR. Arthroscopic femoral osteoplasty/cheilectomy for cam-type femoroacetabular impingement in the athlete. Sports Med Arthrosc. 2010;18(2):90–9.
31. Walton NP, Jahromi I, Lewis PL. Chondral degeneration and therapeutic hip arthroscopy. Int Orthop. 2004;28(6):354–6.
32. Brand RA. John Hilton, 1805–1878. Clin Orthop Relat Res. 2009;467(9):2208–9. doi:10.1007/s11999-009-0927-2.
33. Matsuda DK. Fluoroscopic templating technique for precision arthroscopic rim trimming. Arthroscopy. 2009;25(10):1175–82.

Specific Tissues and Conditions: Osteonecrosis, Avascular Necrosis

55

Athanasios V. Papavasiliou and Ioannis Gliatis

Abbreviations

AVN Avascular necrosis
BMP Bone morphogenic proteins
CT Computerized tomography
FAI Femoroacetabular impingement
MRI Magnetic resonance imaging
ON Osteonecrosis
PRP Platelet rich plasma

Osteonecrosis (ON), or avascular necrosis (AVN), of the femoral head commonly affects relatively young, active patients in the third or fourth decade of their life (mean age mid-30s) and frequently follows a course that can result in considerable disability [1, 2]. The accurate prevalence of the disease is unknown, but 10,000–20,000 new cases are diagnosed in the United States per year [3]. The 2013 National Joint Registries of England and Wales and of Australia suggest that hip joint replacement surgery performed with a primary diagnosis of osteonecrosis accounts for 2 and 3.5 % of the total number of these operations, respectively [4]. In the United States, the corresponding rate was estimated to be about 10 % [5].

Magnetic resonance imaging (MRI) is the most sensitive imaging method for diagnosing ON. It is 99 % sensitive and 98 % specific for the disease and can detect early marrow necrosis and ingrowth of vascularized mesenchymal tissue, before changes become detectable on plain radiographs [1, 2, 6]. The multiplanar imaging capability of MRI also allows the accurate sizing and location of the ON lesion and with application of appropriate high resolution images it can even image subchondral fractures equally or better than a CT [7, 8]. Using these imaging capabilities, MRI even appears to have a good prognostic value for femoral head collapse [9]. Despite these advances and its ability to evaluate the presence of intra-articular lesions (labral tears, loose bodies etc.), MRI or MR-arthrography still fails to fully evaluate the articular cartilage of the hip joint [4, 8, 10, 11]. A recent meta-analysis comparing MRI, MRa, MDCT (multidetector arrays in computer tomography-CT), and CT-arthrography, for the assessment of articular cartilage in comparison to surgical findings (arthroscopic or open) as reference, confirmed that arthroscopy remains the most accurate method assessing the cartilage in the hip joint [12].

The development of a successful strategy to treat ON of the femoral head is not easy, all the more so because neither the etiology nor the natural history of osteonecrosis of the hip is clearly defined. Published treatment algorithms have been based on staging the lesion and on patient-specific factors, with numerous radiographic classification systems having been proposed [1, 13–18]. The imaging findings that would influence a treatment plan are: (1) the lesion being pre- or post-collapse, (2) the size of the necrotic segment, (3) the extent of femoral head depression, and (4) the presence of acetabular involvement [1, 2]. Patient-specific factors that should be taken into account include (1) coexisting comorbidities (2) the etiology of osteonecrosis—if identified, (3) patient compliance with postoperative instructions, (4) patients age, (5) expectations, and (6) presence of mechanical symptoms. The weak link in this decision-making process is the inability of the current imaging techniques to fully evaluate the integrity of the articular cartilage which should also be taken into account in selecting the best possible treatment.

A.V. Papavasiliou, BSc, MD, PhD (✉)
Blue Cross Euromedica, Orthopaedic Department, Vizyis - Vyzantos 1, Thessaloniki, 54636, Greece
e-mail: apapavasiliou@aol.com

I. Gliatis, MD, PhD
Department of Orthopaedics, University Hospital of Patras, Patras, Greece

J.C. McCarthy et al. (eds.), *Hip Joint Restoration*, DOI 10.1007/978-1-4614-0694-5_55

Treatment

Nonoperative Treatment

Nonoperative treatment consisting of observation or prolonged weight bearing with a crutch or cane has a limited role in the treatment of ON of the femoral head since even asymptomatic small lesions will often demonstrate collapse [6].

Pharmacologic Agents

Several pharmacological agents that try to address the proposed pathophysiology of ON have been assessed as potential treatment agents. The use of bisphosphonates (alendronate) which inhibit osteoclast activity and influence bone turnover and remodeling is associated with a reduction in the prevalence of femoral head collapse [3, 6]. However larger patient cohorts with longer follow-up randomized control trials are necessary to fully evaluate the efficacy of this therapy.

Operative Treatment

Operative treatment of hip osteonecrosis can be divided broadly into femoral head-sparing or arthroplasty procedures. Candidates for joint-preserving procedures are usually at the pre- or early post-collapse stage [1]. Historically, such procedures have included core decompression with or without bony augmentation, free vascularized and nonvascularized bone grafting and osteotomies. In large pre- and post-collapse lesions, however, attempts at joint preservation do not yield predictable results; these patients are best treated with joint arthroplasty procedures.

The Role of Hip Arthroscopy

Diagnostic

As a diagnostic tool, hip arthroscopy is useful in enhancing the ability of the surgeon to accurately stage the disease by directly evaluating the state of the articular cartilage in the weight-bearing area of the femoral head and acetabulum.

Addressing Intra-articular Pathology

Experience shows that hip arthroscopy may also have a therapeutic role in patients with ON of the femoral head by addressing mechanical pathology commonly found in those hips. It is often that these patients complain of mechanical symptoms such as clicking, catching, and buckling secondary to chondral flap lesions, labral tears, or even loose bodies which are amenable to arthroscopic treatment which can improve the clinical outcome, by eliminating mechanical symptoms [19–21].

The intra-articular pathology is thought to be secondary to the periodic and momentary loss of the sphericity of the femoral head which is unable to withstand the weight-bearing forces over the softened necrotic cancellous bone causing mechanical disruption of the cartilage or labrum [4, 22]. Arthroscopic evaluation will reveal localized chondromalacia of the femoral head and a positive ballottement test. This test, described by Sekiya, assesses the stability of the articular cartilage over the infarcted segment [22]. In a positive test, gentle pressure with a probe will cause the articular cartilage to buckle over the infarcted segment (Fig. 55.1a) and to spring back to its original state upon release of pressure. In the presence of a positive ballottement test, labral pathology is frequently encountered (Fig. 55.1b). The identification of this area can also help to guide the core drill during arthroscopic assisted core decompression (Fig. 55.1c). Joint effusion and synovitis are often associated with ON [7]. It is the authors opinion that arthroscopic joint washout and synovectomy in selected cases can be of clinical benefit since it can reduce pain, effusion, improve range of motion and possibly by reducing the capsular stress from the joint collection it can improve the blood supply [4].

Femoroacetabular Impingement (FAI)

The incidence of coexistence of FAI and ON is unknown. They both present at similar age with no good clinical way to differentiate which pathology is responsible for the clinical symptoms. This clinical problem can be addressed with a diagnostic hip injection which will reduce pain from the intra-articular symptoms but not the osseous pain from ON. The accuracy of this "test" is considered to be high [23, 24]. Some authors advocate the correction of cam and pincer at the index operation [25]. It is the author's opinion that in these patients one should be cautious, with ON being the priority and if any FAI surgery is needed it can be addressed at a later date.

Surgical Techniques

Core decompression is commonly performed in ON for small- or medium-sized lesions, especially at the pre-collapse stage [1, 26, 27]. It is a technically demanding procedure, requiring biplanar imaging for proper placement of the core drill [28, 29]. Hip arthroscopy can assist the antegrade drilling of the femoral head, allowing accurate placement of the

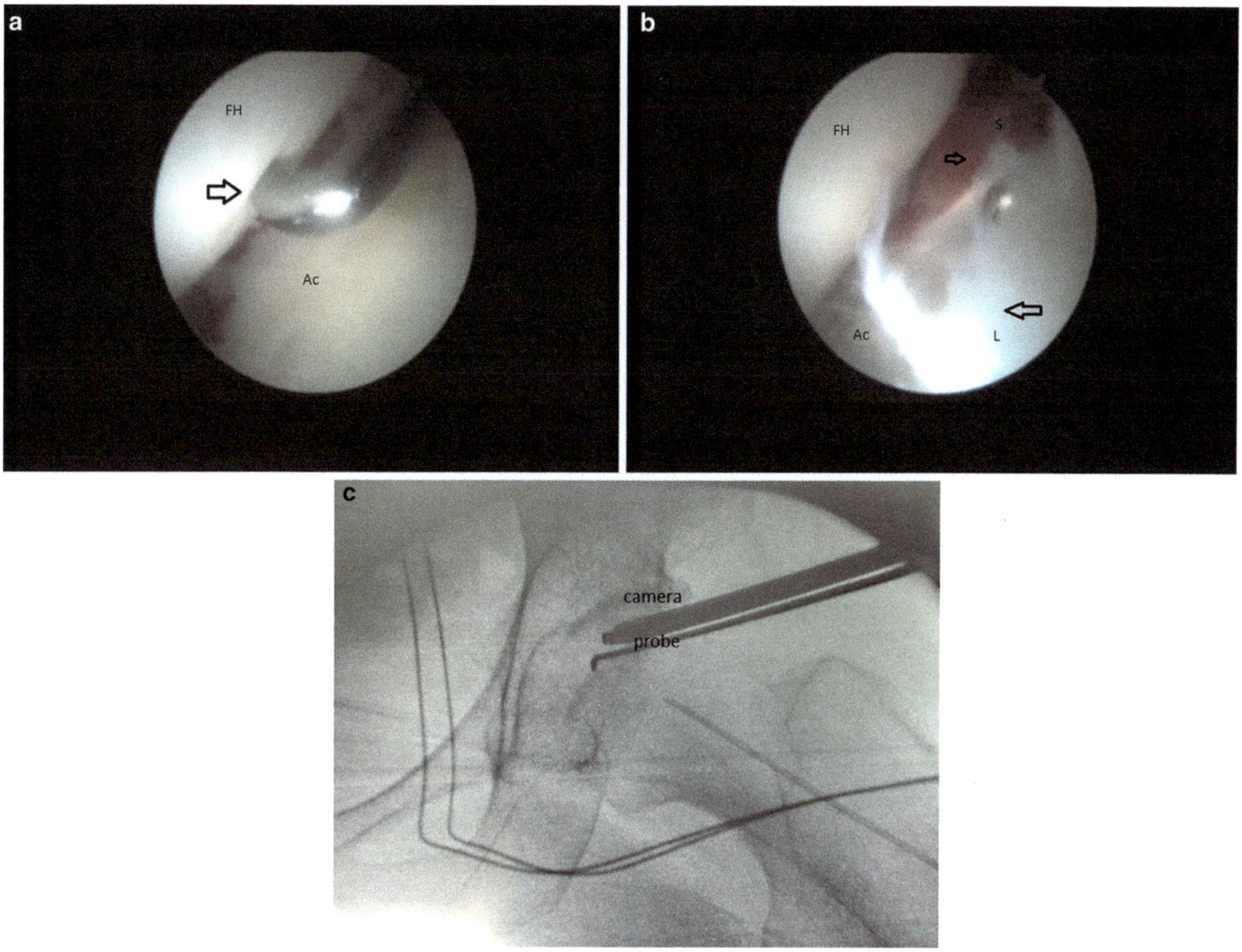

Fig. 55.1 (**a**) Arthroscopic appearance of a positive ballottement test where the articular cartilage buckles (*arrow*) with ease under the pressure of the probe to assume its original state upon release. (**b**) In the same hip associated synovitis (S-*small arrow*) and a degenerative labral tear (L-*large arrow*) are seen. (*FH* femoral head, *Ac* acetabulum). (**c**) The guide wire is aimed at the tip of the probe which is seating at the area where the ballottement test was positive ensuring at the same time that the articular cartilage is not violated

tip of the drill at the level of the area overlying the necrotic segment of the femoral head where chondromalacia and fibrillation of the articular cartilage are seen (Fig. 55.1c). This reduces the possibility of missing the lesion and minimizes the chances for overdrilling and penetration of the articular cartilage which in author's opinion should be avoided.

Meduloscopy (bone endoscopy) can also verify the correct placement of the bone channel during core decompression since the appearance of "white," necrotic bone confirms its correct placement (Fig. 55.2) [30]. Core decompression can also be supplemented with injection of biological factors such as PRP, BMP, or stem cells [1, 6, 31].

Drilling can also be guided arthroscopically by direct visualization of the wire by inserting it through one of the arthroscopic portals, opening under direct vision a cortical window for grafting (light bulb approach) [31]. Graft can also be introduced through the core track to the necrotic lesion. Recently reports have described arthroscopically assisted core decompression curettage of the necrotic lesion and retrograde impaction of autologous bone cylinders or synthetic grafts with promising results [32–34]. The authors have used this technique and agree that the initial results are indeed encouraging (Fig. 55.3).

In summary, there is enough published clinical evidence to support hip arthroscopy as a safe and reliable adjunct in the management of osteonecrosis of the femoral head for improving the accuracy of staging alone or in conjunction with core decompression. Current literature agrees that hip arthroscopy is best indicated in patients with mechanical symptoms and intra-articular pathology in the absence of osteoarthritic changes and at the pre-collapse stage. The presence of advanced OA at the index procedure is a bad indicator with uniformly poor results [4, 19, 35–37].

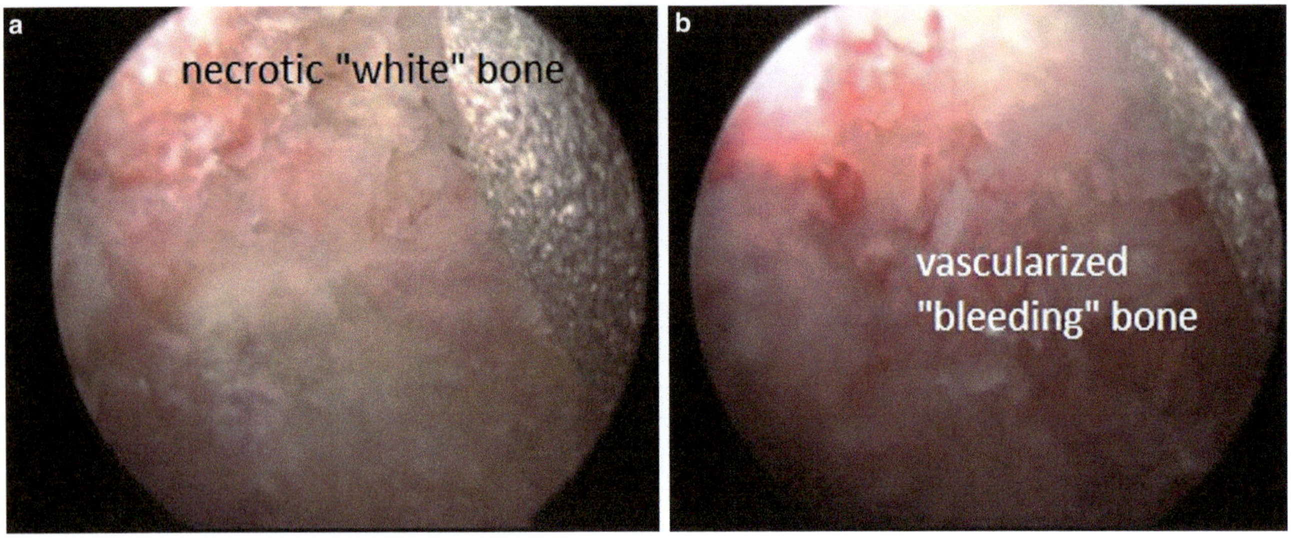

Fig. 55.2 (**a**) During bone endoscopy the necrotic area of the bone is seen as *white*, sclerotic. (**b**) During bone endoscopy when the camera is withdrawn away of the ON area, it reveals *red*, bleeding bone

a b

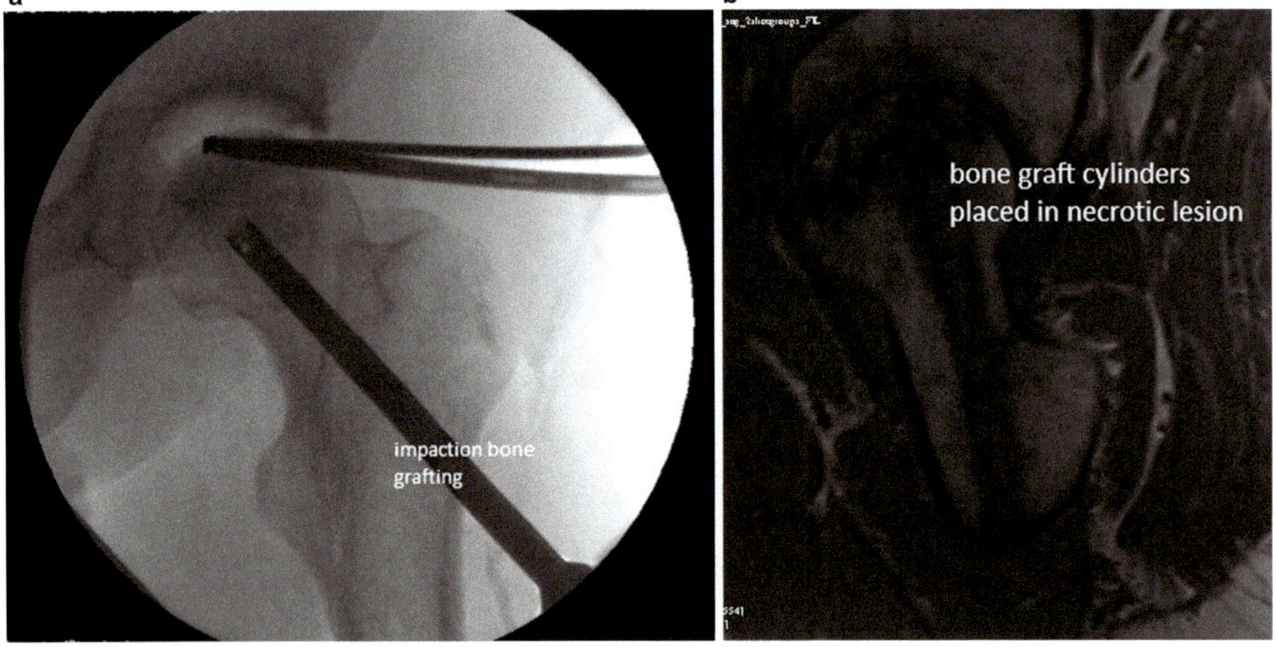

Fig. 55.3 (**a**) Arthroscopic assisted bone graft impaction of bone cylinders harvested from the iliac crest using the knee osteochondral autograft transfer system (OATS). (**b**) Early (4 months postop) magnetic resonance image showing the position of the graft within the necrotic lesion, filing of the femoral tunnel and the maintained congruity of the joint

Symptomatic improvement, at best, is brief and rarely justifies the procedure [35]. As the surgical instrumentation and skills evolve, hip arthroscopy could become an integral part of treatment of osteonecrosis. Comparative clinical studies of high levels of evidence are also needed to better assess outcomes using hip arthroscopy against other ways of management.

References

1. Mont MA, Jones LC, Hungerford DS. Nontraumatic osteonecrosis of the femoral head: ten years later. J Bone Joint Surg Am. 2006;88:1117–32.
2. Lieberman JR, Berry DJ, Mont MA, Aaron RK, Callaghan JJ, Rajadhyaksha AD, Urbaniak JR. Osteonecrosis of the hip: management in the 21st century. Instr Course Lect. 2003;52:337–55.

3. Babis GC, Sakellariou V, Parvizi J, Soucacos P. Osteonecrosis of the femoral head. Orthopedics. 2011;34(1):39–48.
4. Papavasiliou A, Yercan HS, Koukoulias N. The role of hip arthroscopy in the management of osteonecrosis. J Hip Preserv Surg. 2014;1(2):56–61.
5. Mont MA, Hungerford DS. Non-traumatic avascular necrosis of the femoral head. J Bone Joint Surg Am. 1995;77:459–74.
6. Petrigliano FA, Lieberman JR. Osteonecrosis of the hip: novel approaches to evaluation and treatment. Clin Orthop Relat Res. 2007;465:53–62.
7. Karantanas AH. Accuracy and limitations of diagnostic methods for avascular necrosis of the hip. Expert Opin Med Diagn. 2013;7:179–87.
8. Potter HG, Schachar J. High resolution noncontrast MRI of the hip. J Magn Reson Imaging. 2010;31:268–78.
9. Ha YC, Jung WH, Kim JR, Seong NH, Kim SY, Koo KH. Prediction of collapse in femoral head osteonecrosis: a modified Kerboul method with use of magnetic resonance images. J Bone Joint Surg Am. 2006;88 Suppl 3:35–40.
10. Keeney JA, Peelle MW, Jackson J, Rubin D, Maloney WJ, Clohisy JC. Magnetic resonance arthrography versus arthroscopy in the evaluation of articular hip pathology. Clin Orthop Relat Res. 2004;429:163–9.
11. Zlatkin MB, Pevsner D, Sanders TG, et al. Acetabular labral tears and cartilage lesions of the hip: indirect MR arthrographic correlation with arthroscopy–a preliminary study. Am J Roentgenol. 2010;194:709–14.
12. Smith TO, Simpson M, Ejindu V, et al. The diagnostic test accuracy of magnetic resonance imaging, magnetic resonance arthrography and computer tomography in the detection of chondral lesions of the hip. Eur J Orthop Surg Traumatol. 2013;23:335–44.
13. Marcus ND, Enneking WF, Massam RA. The silent hip in idiopathic aseptic necrosis. Treatment by bone grafting. J Bone Joint Surg Am. 1973;55:1351–66.
14. Ficat RP. Idiopathic bone necrosis of the femoral head. Early diagnosis and treatment. J Bone Joint Surg Br. 1985;67:3–9.
15. Gardeniers JWM. A new international classification of osteonecrosis of the ARCO committee on terminology and classification. ARCO Newsletter. 1992;4:41–6.
16. Steinberg ME, Hayken GD, Steinberg DR. A quantitative system for staging avascular necrosis. J Bone Joint Surg Br. 1995;77:34–41.
17. Plakseychuk AY, Shah M, Varitimidis SE, Rubash HE, Sotereanos D. Classification of osteonecrosis of the femoral head. Reliability, reproducibility, and prognostic value. Clin Orthop Relat Res. 2001;386:34–41.
18. Jawad MU, Haleem AA, Scully SP. In brief: Ficat classification: avascular necrosis of the femoral head. Clin Orthop Relat Res. 2012;470:2636–9.
19. O'leary JA, Berend K, Vail TP. The relationship between diagnosis and outcome in arthroscopy of the hip. Arthroscopy. 2001;17(2): 181–8.
20. McCarthy J, Puri L, Barsoum W, Lee JA, Laker M, Cooke P. Articular cartilage changes in avascular necrosis: an arthroscopic evaluation. Clin Orthop Relat Res. 2003;406:64–70.
21. Khanduja V, Villar RN. Arthroscopic surgery of the hip: current concepts and recent advances. J Bone Joint Surg Br. 2006;88(12): 1557–66.
22. Sekiya JK, Ruch DS, Hunter DM, Pope Jr TL, Koman LA, Poehling GG, Russell GB. Hip arthroscopy in staging avascular necrosis of the femoral head. J South Orthop Assoc. 2000;9:254–61.
23. Byrd JW, Jones KS. Diagnostic accuracy of clinical assessment, magnetic resonance imaging, magnetic resonance arthrography, and intra-articular injection in hip arthroscopy patients. Am J Sports Med. 2004;32:1668–74.
24. Kivlan BR, Martin RL, Sekiya JK. Response to diagnostic injection in patients with femoroacetabular impingement, labral tears, chondral lesions, and extra-articular pathology. Arthroscopy. 2011;27: 619–27.
25. Beck DM, Park BK, Youm T, et al. Arthroscopic treatment of labral tears and concurrent avascular necrosis of the femoral head in young adults. Arthrosc Tech. 2013;2:e367–71.
26. Marker DR, Seyler TM, Ulrich SD, Srivastava S, Mont MA. Do modern techniques improve core decompression outcomes for hip osteonecrosis? Clin Orthop Relat Res. 2008;466(5): 1093–103.
27. Scully SP, Aaron RK, Urbaniak JR. Survival analysis of hips treated with core decompression or vascularized fibular grafting because of avascular necrosis. J Bone Joint Surg Am. 1998;80: 1270–5.
28. Ruch DS, Satterfield W. The use of arthroscopy to document accurate position of core decompression of the hip. Arthroscopy. 1998;14(6):617–9.
29. Mont MA, Ragland PS, Etienne G. Core decompression of the femoral head for osteonecrosis using percutaneous multiple small-diameter drilling. Clin Orthop Relat Res. 2004;429:131–8.
30. Govaers K, Meermans G, Bortier H, Londers J. Endoscopically assisted core decompression in avascular necrosis of the femoral head. Acta Orthop Belg. 2009;75(5):631–6.
31. Guadilla J, Fiz N, Andia I, Sánchez M. Arthroscopic management and platelet-rich plasma therapy for avascular necrosis of the hip. Knee Surg Sports Traumatol Arthrosc. 2012;20:393–8.
32. Ellenrieder M, Tischer T, Kreuz PC, et al. [Arthroscopically assisted therapy of avascular necrosis of the femoral head] (in German). Oper Orthop Traumatol. 2013;25:85–94.
33. Cetinkaya S, Toker B, Taser O. Arthroscopic retrograde osteochondral autologous transplantation to chondral lesion in femoral head. Orthopedics. 2014;37(6):e600–4.
34. Gupta AK, Frank RM, Harris JD, McCormick F, Mather RC, Nho SJ. Arthroscopic-assisted core decompression for osteonecrosis of the femoral head. Arthrosc Tech. 2013;3(1):e7–11.
35. McCarthy JC, Lee JA. Arthroscopic intervention in early hip disease. Clin Orthop Relat Res. 2004;429:157–62.
36. Larson CM, Swaringen J, Morrison G. A review of hip arthroscopy and its role in the management of adult hip pain. Iowa Orthop J. 2005;25:172–9.
37. Ruch DS, Sekiya J, Dickson Schaefer W, Koman LA, Pope TL, Poehling GG. The role of hip arthroscopy in the evaluation of avascular necrosis. Orthopedics. 2001;24:339–43.

Specific Tissues and Conditions: Pediatric Conditions

56

Giancarlo C. Polesello, Miguel Akkari, and Marcelo C. Queiroz

Introduction

Minimally invasive procedures are growing in all areas of medicine. Orthopedics has had special importance in this development with the creation and improvement of arthroscopic surgeries. The use of this technique in the hip joint, however, had a long lag period since its initial description had been made in 1931, by Michael Samuel Burman. For many decades, there were few publications. After the 1980s, with the improvement distraction and positioning techniques, this method of approach received a boost. We believe that the diseases that affect the hips of children and adolescents are very peculiar. While in adults traumatic injuries and degenerative diseases predominate, children have different conditions.

There are few references related to hip arthroscopy in children and adolescents [1, 2], mostly case series. They also do not address in depth the technical details and difficulties involved in adolescent surgical procedures.

Our goal in this chapter is to present the indications, surgical technique, and complications of hip arthroscopy in the pediatric population.

G.C. Polesello, PhD (✉)
Department of Orthopedic Surgery and Traumatology, Hip Group, Faculdade de Ciências Médicas, Santa Casa de São Paulo, São Paulo, Brazil

Rua Dr. Cesário Motta Júnior, 112, Prédio Ortopedia, 2° andar, Sala Quadril, 01221-020 São Paulo, SP, Brazil
e-mail: giancarlopolesello@hotmail.com

M. Akkari, MD, PhD
Department of Orthopedic Surgery and Traumatology, Pediatric Orthopaedics, Faculdade de Ciências Médicas, Santa Casa de São Paulo, São Paulo, Brazil

M.C. Queiroz, MD
Department of Orthopedic Surgery and Traumatology, Hip Group, Faculdade de Ciências Médicas, Santa Casa de São Paulo, São Paulo, Brazil

Indications

Hip arthroscopy, as well as any other surgical procedure, must be indicated with great care. We do not know the limits of its application in pediatric hip. Studies in cadavers of newborns performed by Oliveira et al. [3] describe the minimum weight for its realization as being 1700 g. We find references to its successful application in children as the minimum age of 2 years and 4 months by Chung et al. [4]. In our experience, our youngest patient was 11 months (8 kg) with femoral neck osteomyelitis and pyoarthritis of the hip (Fig. 56.1).

We do not recommend arthroscopy as explorative or random. The doubtful cases should undergo a detailed investigation including a thorough medical history, complete physical examination, and radiological exams sufficient to a precise diagnosis, or at least that allow us an adequate strategic planning.

Contraindications

Skin infection, cellulitis, extra-articular abscesses, and cutaneous lesions that may predispose to infection are contraindications to this procedure.

Ankylosis or arthrofibrosis are considered contraindications by many authors, by hindering the achievement of a efficient joint space, preventing intra-articular access, but we believe that arthroscopy, in specific clinical situations, has its usefulness by potentially promoting the release of the lock, resection of fibrosis, and peri- and intra-articular ossifications, aiming to gain mobility.

Acetabular fractures are also relative contraindications, as they may predispose excessive leakage of fluid into the abdominal cavity.

Avascular necrosis is cited as a relative contraindication in adults; however in children it may be used in patients with Legg-Calvé-Perthes (LCP) disease in the active phase of the disease, without progression of necrosis.

J.C. McCarthy et al. (eds.), *Hip Joint Restoration*, DOI 10.1007/978-1-4614-0694-5_56

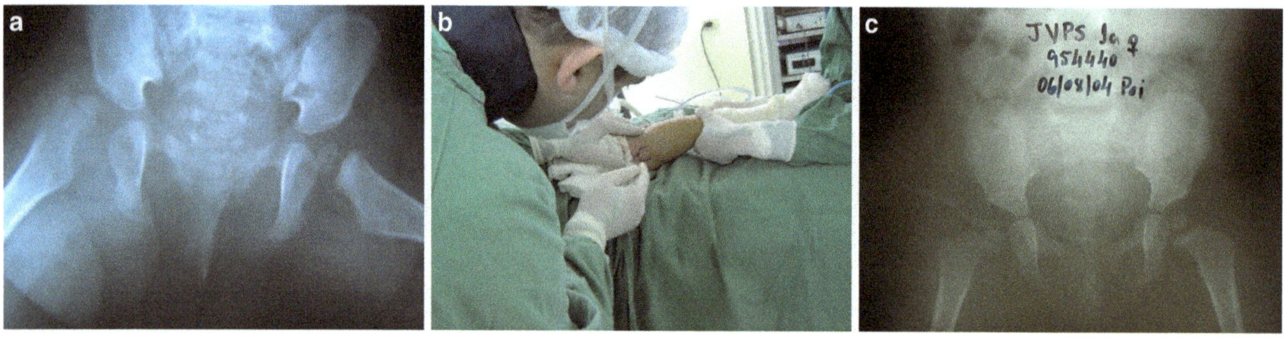

Fig. 56.1 11-month-old child with right hip osteomyelitis and pyoarthritis treated arthroscopically. (**a**) Pre-op X-ray with subluxation of the hip. (**b**) Image of lateral portal being made. (**c**) Post-op X-ray with reduced hip and drain

In our experience, special care should be taken with patients with chondrolysis; despite the apparent improvement in mobility at the time of anesthesia and after resection of bone blocks, there is a great tendency for loss of mobility postoperatively.

Surgical Technique

Positioning

There are two options for positioning: lateral or supine. The lateral decubitus position has the advantage of facilitating traction while allowing the fatty tissue of obese patients to fall away by gravitational action, thus facilitating joint access via lateral portals. The supine position has the advantage of using a conventional orthopedic table, available on most services. This is also our choice of positioning.

Use of Traction

Basically, the surgery may be performed with or without traction. Sometimes it is necessary to use the two techniques.

Traction is obtained with the patient positioned on orthopedic table, feet and ankles carefully protected and secured to the table. The pin properly padded when placed eccentrically allows the facilitation of lateral force vector. If the table does not have the option of the lateralized pin, an alternative is to adapt a large foam around it functioning as lateralization vector and protecting the perineal region. The contralateral limb is held in abduction, thus facilitating the use of fluoroscopy.

Our choice in performing arthroscopy in children is the use of table with a central pin. The common orthopedic table can easily be used in adolescents and children over 5 years, provided that the lower limbs fit the table leg extension. In younger children, we developed a specific traction table, allowing better positioning. We also adapted the foam around the central pin of the table, varying its diameter according to the size of the child. Traction is done manually. In children, the joint space is achieved with ease. Remember that the protection of traction areas, especially the perineum, must be done carefully (Fig. 56.2).

Manual traction may be done in young children. We carried out this method in two patients, achieving a relative gain in joint space, but we do not recommend this form of traction due to the risk of provoking a joint injury when positioning the portals.

In the technique without traction, the patient is positioned on a conventional radiolucent table, lower limbs loose, allowing them to move freely. This is our choice when needed to address only the peripheral and lateral compartments, or when the hip is dislocated.

Equipment

Adequate table and fluoroscopy are essential. 4.5, 5.0, and 5.5 mm cannulas are usually used. Exceptionally, 2.7 mm cannulas can be used in very small children, but they are not cannulated, thus hindering access to the joint. The most often used arthroscope was the 70° scope, and less frequently the 30°.

Portals

The portals usually used are the anterior, lateral, and posterior [5]. In young children, because of the greater proximity between the portals there is an increased difficulty in handling the instruments; also they are located closest to important neurovascular structures, and, therefore, care must be constant (Fig. 56.3).

Some anatomic conditions as coxa vara, pelvic osteotomies, and high-riding trochanter can make the execution of these portals difficult.

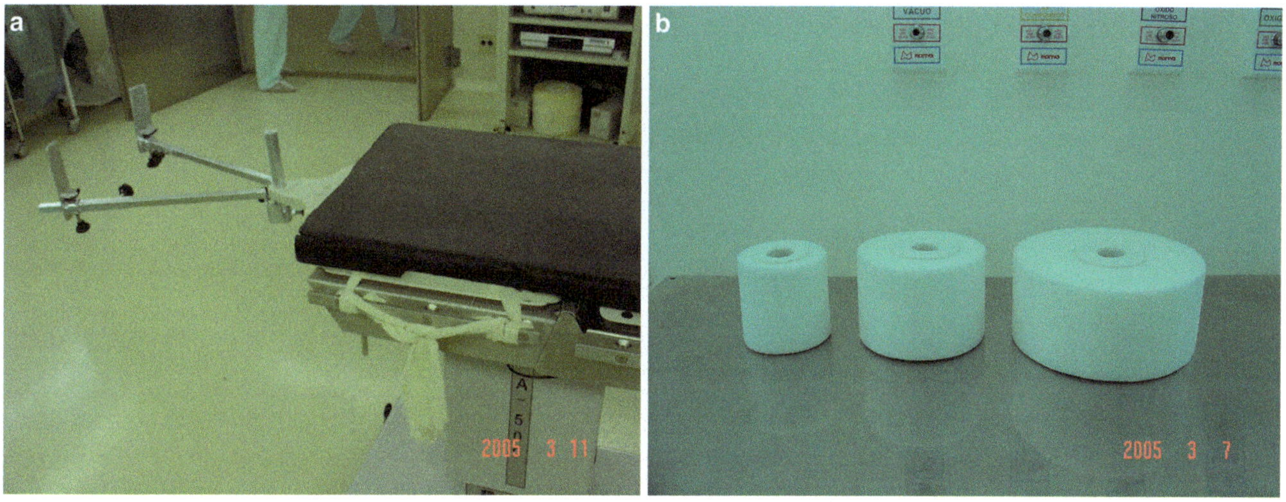

Fig. 56.2 (**a**) Adapter for an orthopedic fracture table and (**b**) foam posts of different diameters to promote a lateral vector of traction

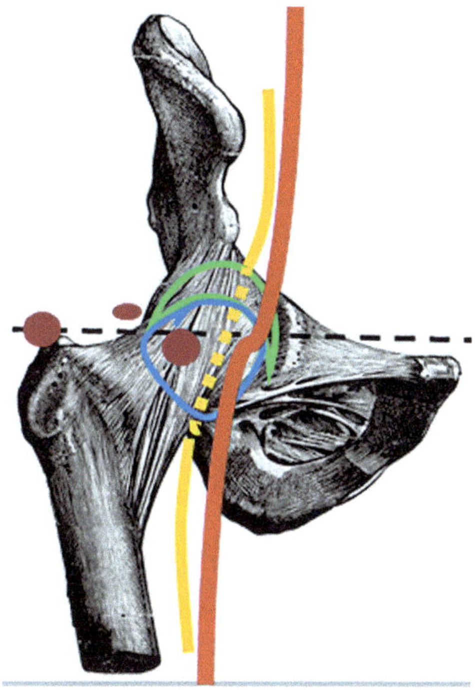

Fig. 56.3 Always consider that in a child the arteries and nerves are closer to the anterior portal than in the adult. *Red line*: Femoral artery, *yellow line*: femoral nerve. *Red dots*: Anterior, anterolateral and posterolateral portals, *blue circle*: peripheral compartment, *green circle*: central compartment

Knowledge of the cartilaginous thickness is very important, because it cannot be identified by fluoroscopy. To avoid unwanted injuries, air may be injected during portal placement, identifying the cartilaginous limits. The greater trochanter also has a cartilaginous part that may hinder the lateral portal [6].

Pediatric Conditions

Etiological Investigation, Biopsies, and Joint Cleaning

Arthroscopy may be useful in the etiological investigation of the child's painful hip, allowing a direct view of the joint and also obtaining tissue for pathological and microbiological studies.

Chronic inflammation may promote articular cavity filling with inflammatory and fibrous tissue, causing a subluxation of the hip and thus perpetuating the pain. In situations like this, hip arthroscopy may be useful to perform a cleanup of the joint cavity and reduction of subluxation. One advantage of the arthroscopic approach compared with open access is not causing instability of the hip joint, eliminating the use of braces, casts, or traction postoperatively.

Septic Arthritis

Septic arthritis of the hip is a serious and relatively common condition and can lead to crippling deformities. Surgical drainage of the infected joint is indicated in most patients. Several open approaches have historically been used, but more recently arthroscopy has many advantages: it allows efficient articular cleaning with copious irrigation, a detailed investigation of the cavity, adds no joint instability, allows the installation of irrigation with negative aspiration, rapid rehabilitation, shorter hospital stay, and better aesthetics [7–9] (Fig. 56.4).

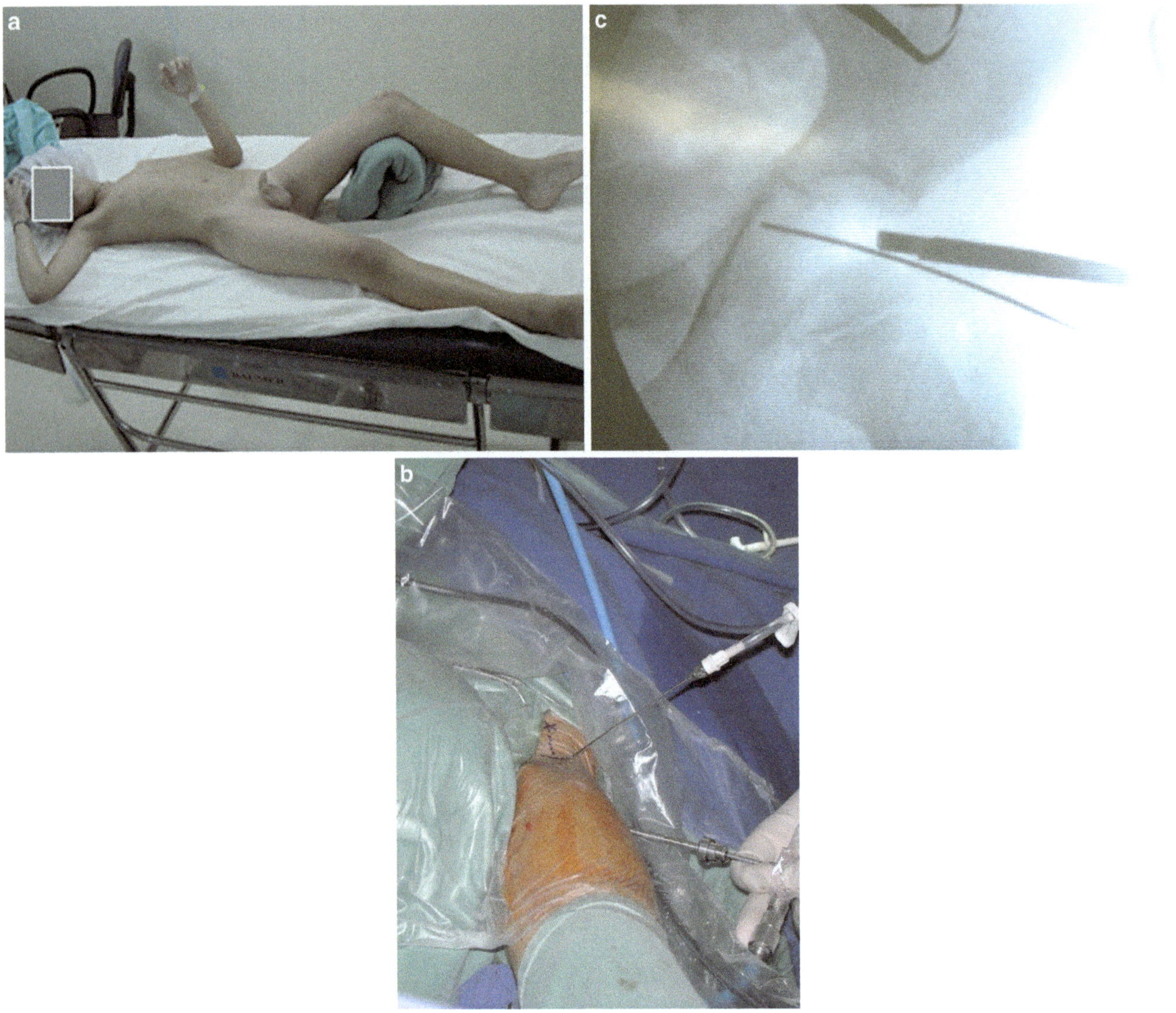

Fig. 56.4 Seven-year-old boy with septic arthritis of the left hip treated arthroscopically. (**a**) Patient with hip flexion due to septic arthritis. (**b**) Anterior and anterolateral used to drain. (**c**) Good joint space

Developmental Dislocation of the Hip

Arthroscopy may have its indication at different times during the treatment of developmental dislocation of the hip (DDH) [10, 11], these being the following:

Acetabular Cleaning to Facilitate Reduction

In attempting closed reduction of DDH, we may have some unwanted situations such as inability to obtain a reduction or an unstable reduction. In these situations, an alternative is open reduction, with the risk of necrosis or cicatricial retraction. Arthroscopy may be applied in lieu of open reduction, with exploration of the joint cavity, articular cleaning, and consequent increase in the security zone of the reduction (Fig. 56.5).

As Adjunctive Procedure to Pelvic Osteotomies

Arthroscopy can be helpful in exploring and articular cleaning or repair as an adjunct to pelvic osteotomies.

Postoperative Exploration for Persistence of Joint Incongruity

The persistence of hip subluxation postoperatively may have several causes: inadequate capsuloplasty, insufficient acetabular cleaning, femoral or acetabular deformities, or a persistent mechanical obstacle among others. We had the opportunity to explore one of these situations and we observed that the cause of subluxation resulted from the interposition of the suture used in capsuloplasty.

Labrum and Cartilage Debridement

Hip arthroscopy may be used to repair or debride labral or cartilage lesions.

Release of Postoperative Arthrofibrosis

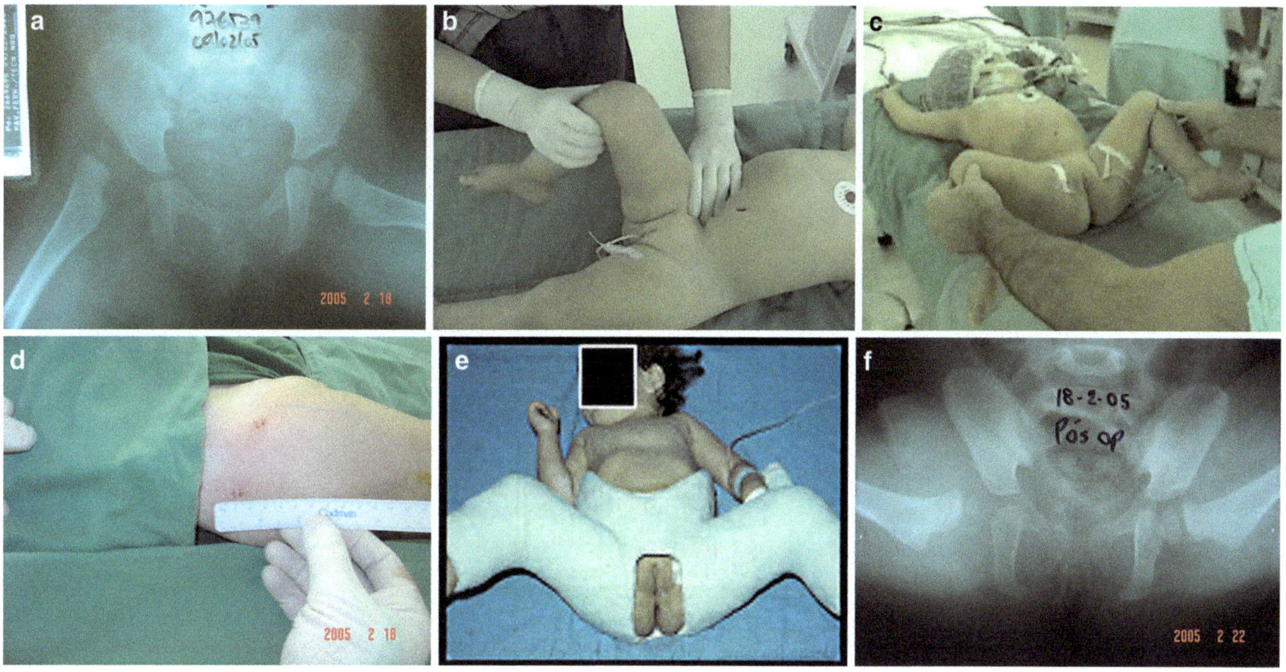

Fig. 56.5 16-month-old girl with right hip DDH and unstable reduction, arthroscopically acetabular cleaning was done to facilitate reduction. (**a**) Right hip subluxed. (**b**) Unstable reduction. (**c**) Reduction after arthroscopy. (**d**) Anterior and anterolateral portal. (**e**) Spica cast. (**f**) Post-op X-ray with reduced right hip

One of the most feared complications in surgical treatment of DDH is postoperative stiffness. Despite the articular fibrosis being described as one of the contraindications of hip arthroscopy, we have had the opportunity to perform the arthroscopic release in a patient with postoperative stiffness, achieving a significant mobility improvement.

Legg-Calvè-Perthes Disease

Pain in adolescents and young adults with previous LCP can have several causes: acetabular and femoral deformities, lesions of the articular cartilage or labrum, lesions of the teres ligament, osteochondritis, loose bodies, hyperpressure on the psoas tendon, or muscle fatigue due to biomechanical changes among others.

Hip arthroscopy may be useful to treat several of these different clinical situations.

Loose Body Removal: Sometimes during the regeneration process of the femoral epiphysis loose bodies may be formed. Arthroscopic removal is very advantageous when compared to open surgery.

Articular Cleaning in Synovitis: Articular cleaning may be effective in improving mobility and decreasing pain in these patients.

Teres Ligament Treatment: Changes of the teres ligament may cause pain in patients previously affected by LCP disease, among the most common injuries found: hypertrophy, rupture, anomalous insertions, or degenerative lesions. Arthroscopic surgery is very useful in addressing the round ligament and may have both diagnostic and therapeutic purposes.

Femoroacetabular impingement (FAI) treatment and *labrum and cartilage debridement.*

Myo-Tendinous Structures Treatment

The psoas tendon may be the cause of anterior hip pain. This diagnosis is often difficult and can be aided by therapeutic tests.

It is possible to approach endoscopically the tendon of the psoas muscle in both its intrapelvic portion (trans-articular), but also in its femoral insertion (extra-articular), as described by Ilizaliturri, 2005 [12].

Slipped Capital Femoral Epiphysis (SCFE)

Arthroscopy has been very helpful in dealing with these patients, among the indications we quote [13].

Osteochondroplasty for FAI Treatment

In order to correct the femoral bump impingement and gain mobility in the hip, femoral osteoplasty can be accomplished. Arthroscopy has proven to be a good option in this procedure [14, 15] (Fig. 56.6).

Trapezoidal Femoral Neck Bone Correction Through Arthroscopy

The trapezoidal femoral neck osteotomy is used to correct severe deformities in open physis patients, reducing the incidence of necrosis. We have done this fully arthroscopic surgery associated with percutaneous fixation of the femoral epiphysis. This procedure is indicated in very specific situations, mainly severe slips with very limited range of motion.

We have published a mean 2-year follow-up of five patients with severe SCFE that underwent trapezoidal femoral neck correction through arthroscopy [16]. The mean age at the time of surgery was 13.2 years. Mean modified Harris hip score was 17.2 points preoperatively and 86.6 points at the last assessment. The mean epiphyseal deviation ranged from 82° at the initial presentation to 14° postoperatively. There were no intraoperative complications, and there was one case of avascular necrosis [13] (Fig. 56.7).

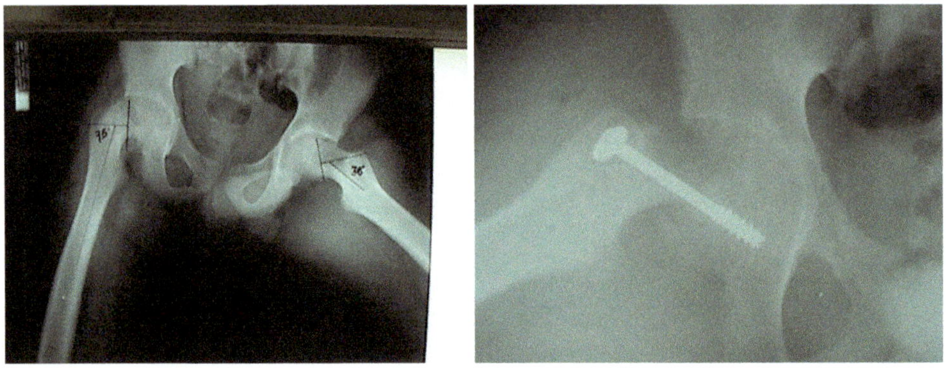

Fig. 56.6 14-year-old boy with SCFE treated with in situ fixation and femoral neck arthroscopic osteochondroplasty. (**a**) Pre-op X-ray. (**b**) Pos-op X-ray

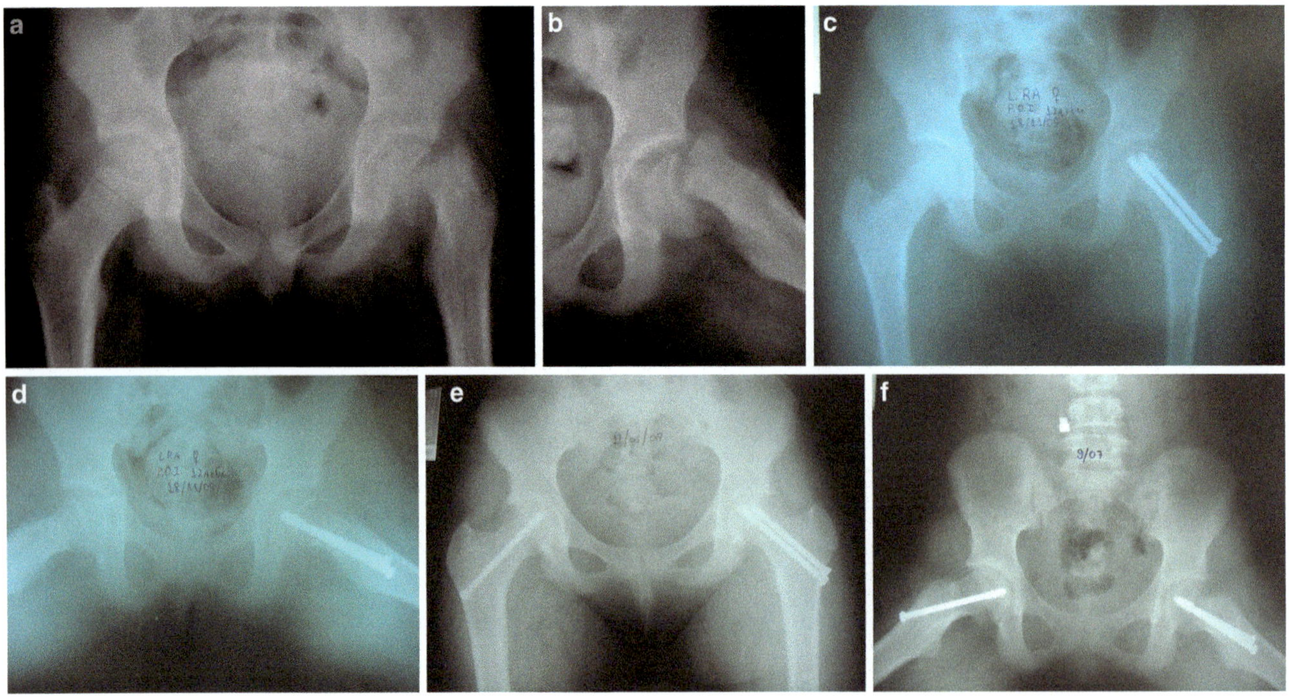

Fig. 56.7 12-year-old male with severe left hip SCFE treated with arthroscopic trapezoidal femoral neck bone correction, and right hip prophylactic fixation. (**a**) Left hip SCFE. (**b**) Left profile with severe SCFE. (**c**) Immediate post-op arthroscopic trapezoidal femoral neck bone correction fixed with two screws. (**d**) Profile immediate post-op. (**e/f**) 2-year follow-up

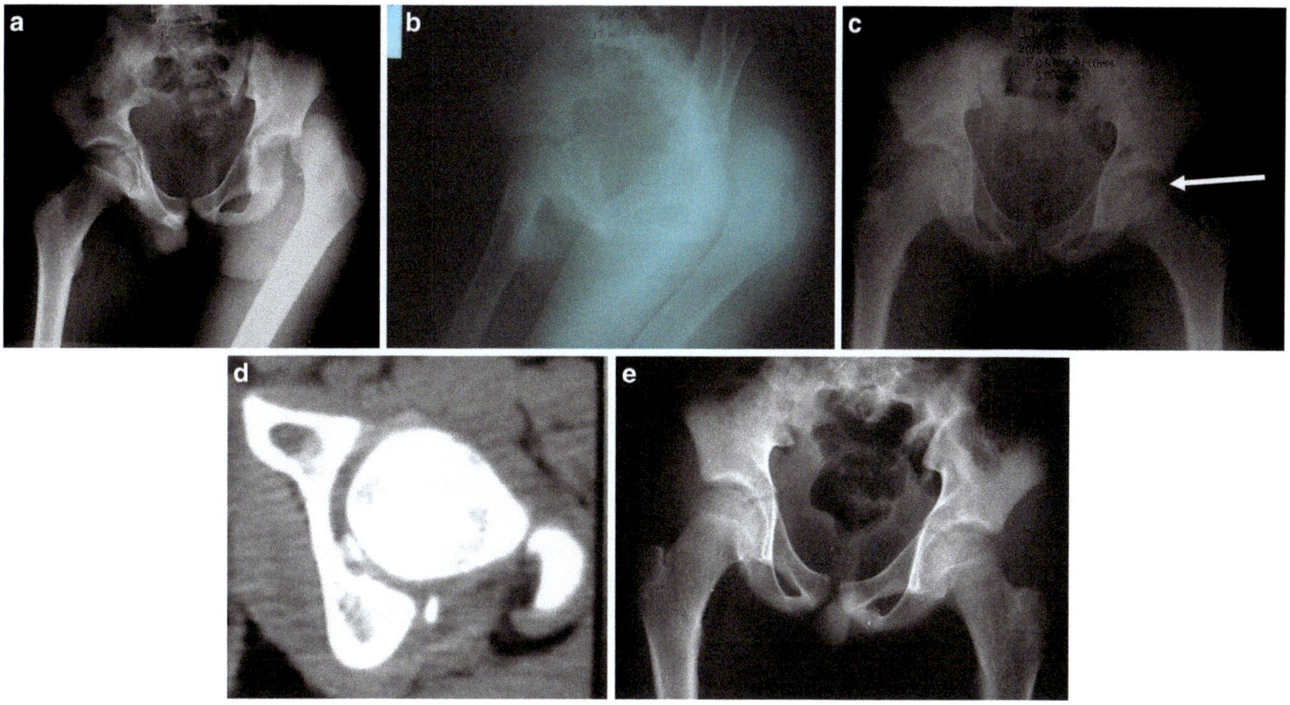

Fig. 56.8 12-year-old male with left hip fracture dislocation of left hip with subluxation after reduction due to osteochondral articular loose body that was removed arthroscopically, achieving adequate reduction. (**a/b**) Fracture-dislocation. (**c**) Persistent subluxation after closed reduction. (**d**) CT with subluxation and loose bodies. (**e**) Post-op arthroscopic removal with good reduction

Pediatric Traumatology

Fracture-dislocations of the hip: May help in loose body removal and chondrolabral junction repair (Fig. 56.8).

Sequelae resulting from epiphyseal necrosis of the femoral neck: Bone resection and osteoplasties of the femoral epiphysis.

Inveterate traumatic dislocation of the hip: Articular cleaning, reduction, and congruence analyses (Fig. 56.9).

Resection of bone tumors: Arthroscopy may be used to resect osteoid osteoma, osteoblastoma, bone cyst, synovial chondromatosis among others.

Complications

Nwachukwu et al. have described a 1.8% complication rate in his series, the most common complications being transient pudendal nerve palsy, instrument breakage, and suture abcess [17]. We found few other papers mentioning complications of hip arthroscopy in children [18–20]. In our series so far we had a case in which damage to the cartilage of the femoral head caused the introduction of cannulae; this was due to inefficient traction. In another patient removal of articular loose bodies was incomplete, requiring a second arthroscopic surgery.

Conclusion

Arthroscopy should be seen as an adjunct in the treatment of hip disorders of children and adolescents. This minimally invasive procedure should not change the basics of treatment. The successful results are independent of the route of approach but the correct management of each patient.

The option of performing an arthroscopic surgery seeks to bring comfort to the patient, minimizing tissue damage with a low incidence of complications, allowing for a faster recovery and better aesthetics.

We believe that surgery makes sense only when its benefits outweigh the morbidity of the procedure. For this we recommend a great familiarity with pediatric hip diseases, a good surgical experience by conventional methods, and also a theoretical and practical study of hip arthroscopy.

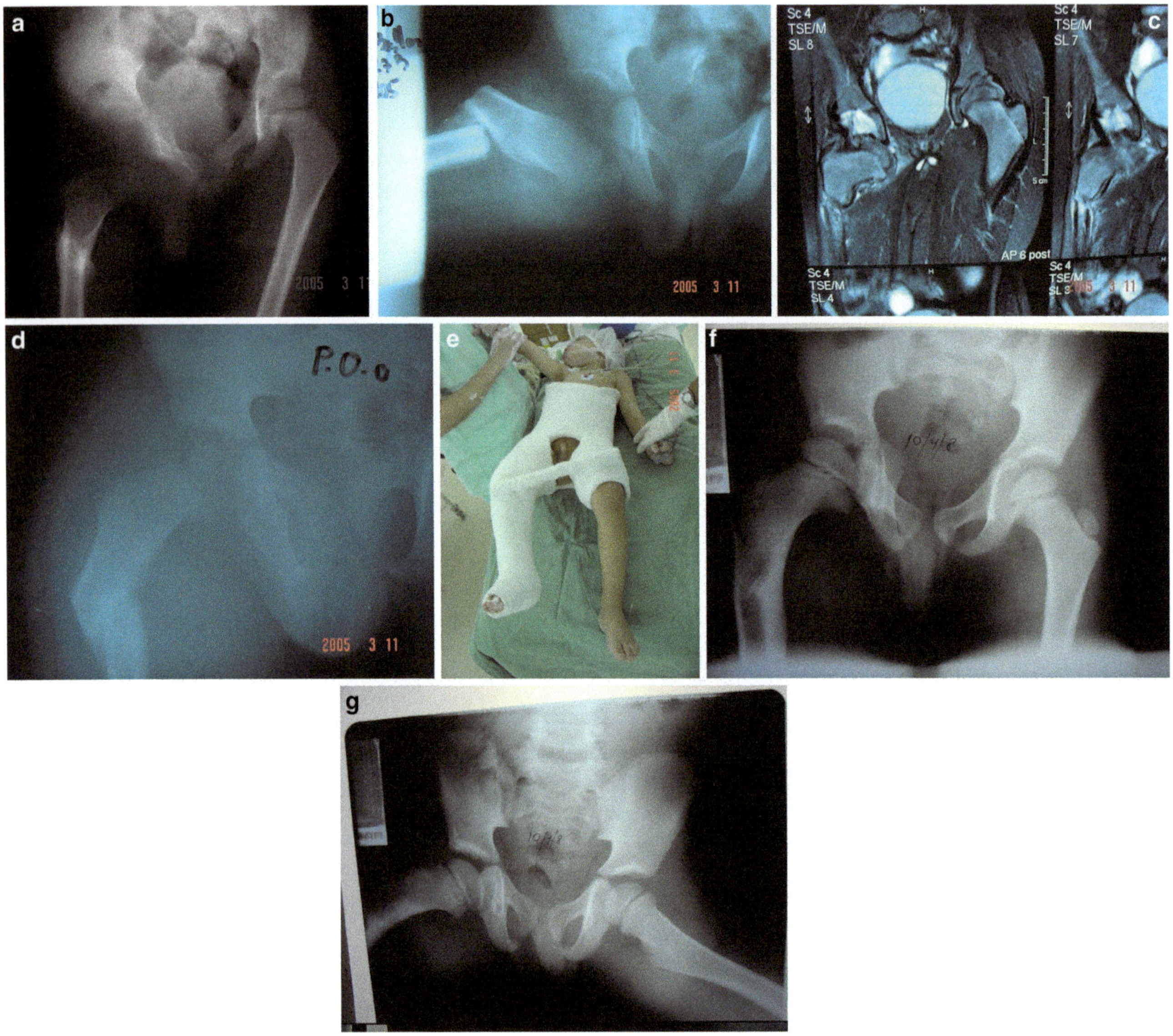

Fig. 56.9 3-year-old boy with inveterate traumatic dislocation of right hip that closed reduction was not possible was treated with arthroscopic removal of interposed tissue, reduction, and spica cast. (**a/b**) Inveterate traumatic hip dislocation. (**c**) MRI with interposed tissue. (**d**) Post-op arthroscopic removal of interposed tissue and reduction. (**e**) Post-op arthroscopic removal of interposed tissue, reduction, and spica cast. (**f/g**) 3-year post-op

References

1. Berend KR, Vail TP. Hip arthroscopy in adolescence and childhood. In: Byrd JWT, editor. Operative hip arthroscopy. 2nd ed. New York: Springer; 2005. p. 204–19.
2. Byrd JWT. Operative hip arthroscopy. 2nd ed. New York: Springer; 2005.
3. Oliveira RS, Leite JAD, Patrocínio RMSV, et al. Modelo experimental de artroscopia do quadril em cadáveres de recém-nascidos. Acta Ortop Bras. 2005;13(2):86–90.
4. Chung WK, Slater GL, Bates EH. Treatment of septic arthritis of the hip by arthroscopic lavage. J Pediatr Orthop. 1993;13: 444–6.
5. DeAngelis NA, Busconi BD. Hip arthroscopy in the pediatric population. Clin Orthop Relat Res. 2003;406:60–3.
6. Dvorak M, Duncan CP, Day B. Arthroscopic anatomy of the hip. Arthroscopy. 1990;6(4):264–73.
7. Fontana A, Battistella F, Randelli P. Hip arthroscopy for treatment of septic arthritis in children. J Bone Joint Surg [Br]. 1999;81-B(Suppl II):169.
8. Fernandez FF, Langendörfer M, Wirth T, Eberhardt O. Treatment of septic arthritis of the hip in children and adolescents. Z Orthop Unfall. 2013;151(6):596–602.
9. Nusem I, McAlister A. Arthroscopic lavage for the treatment of septic arthritis of the hip in children. Acta Orthop Belg. 2012;78(6):730–4.
10. Oztürk H, Oztemür Z, Bulut O, Tezeren G, Bulut S. Arthroscopic-assisted surgical treatment for developmental dislocation of the hip before the age of 18 months. Arch Orthop Trauma Surg. 2013;133(9):1289–94.
11. Eberhardt O, Fernandez FF, Wirth T. Arthroscopic reduction of the dislocated hip in infants. J Bone Joint Surg Br. 2012;94(6):842–7.

12. Ilizaliturri Jr VM, Villalobos Jr FE, Chaidez PA, Valero FS, Aguilera JM. Internal snapping hip syndrome: treatment by endoscopic release of the iliopsoas tendon. Arthroscopy. 2005;21(11):1375–80.
13. Futami T, Kasahara Y, et al. Arthroscopy for slipped capital femoral epiphysis. J Pediatr Orthop. 1992;12:592–7.
14. Philippon MJ, Patterson DC, Briggs KK. Hip arthroscopy and femoroacetabular impingement in the pediatric patient. J Pediatr Orthop. 2013;33 Suppl 1:S126–30.
15. Philippon MJ, Ejnisman L, Ellis HB, Briggs KK. Outcomes 2 to 5 years following hip arthroscopy for femoroacetabular impingement in the patient aged 11 to 16 years. Arthroscopy. 2012;28(9):1255–61.
16. Akkari M, Santili C, Braga SR, Polesello GC. Trapezoidal bony correction of the femoral neck in the treatment of severe acute-on-chronic slipped capital femoral epiphysis. Arthroscopy. 2010;26(11):1489–95.
17. Nwachukwu BU, McFeely ED, Nasreddine AY, Krcik JA, Frank J, Kocher MS. Complications of hip arthroscopy in children and adolescents. J Pediatr Orthop. 2011;31(3):227–31.
18. Schindler A, Lechevallier JJC, Rao NS, Bowen R. Diagnostic and therapeutic arthroscopy of the hip in children and adolescents: evaluation of results. J Pediatr Orthop. 1995;15:317–21.
19. Jayakumar P, Ramachandran M, Youm T, Achan P. Arthroscopy of the hip for paediatric and adolescent disorders: current concepts. J Bone Joint Surg Br. 2012;94(3):290–6.
20. Griffin DR, Villar RN. Complications of arthroscopy of the hip. J Bone Joint Surg [Br]. 1999;81-B:604–6.

57 Specific Tissues and Conditions: Extra-articular Pathologic Conditions

Shane J. Nho, Richard C. Mather III, Andrew E. Federer, Ryan Freedman, Frank McCormick, and Michael J. Salata

Introduction

Hip arthroscopy has expanded greatly over the past decade and remains one of the orthopedic field's fastest developing areas of treatment. Current techniques of diagnoses and treatment have facilitated evolving interventions for these conditions. With the growth of intra-articular surgical interventions, orthopedic surgeons are now venturing extracapsularly to treat soft tissue ailments. The use of the endoscope provides improved visualization of extra-articular pathology that previously required large open incisions for diagnosis and treatment.

Arthroscopic or endoscopic approaches are now effective in treating: transarticular or extra-articular lengthening of the iliopsoas in internal coxa saltans; extra-articular access to the iliotibial band for external coxa saltans; and endoscopic repair of gluteus medius tears (Table 57.1). The purpose of the present chapter is to characterize the extra-articular pathology around the hip joint and provide nonoperative and operative treatment of these disorders.

S.J. Nho, MD, MS (✉) • A.E. Federer, BS • R. Freedman, BS, MS
F. McCormick, MD
Department of Orthopedic Surgery, Hip Preservation Center, Section of Sports Medicine, Rush Medical College of Rush University, 1611 W. Harrison St., Suite 300, Chicago, IL 60612, USA
e-mail: shane.nho@rushortho.com

R.C. Mather III , MD
Department of Orthopaedic Surgery, Duke University Medical Center, Durham, NC, USA

M.J. Salata, MD
Department of Orthopaedic Surgery, Center for Joint Preservation and Cartilage Restoration, University Hospitals Case Medical Center, Case Western Reserve University, Cleveland, OH, USA

Disorders of the Peritrochanteric Space

Abductor Muscle Tendinopathy and Tears

Greater trochanteric pain syndrome (GTPS) is characterized by lateral-sided hip pain and includes trochanteric bursitis, gluteus medius or minimus tears, and external coxa saltans [16, 17]. Gluteus medius or minimus tears, also known as "rotator cuff tear of the hip" [18], is the most common presentation and is often found in patients with ostensible recalcitrant trochanteric bursitis [18, 19]. The natural progression of hip abductor tendinopathy is similar to the pathogenesis of tendon degeneration elsewhere in the body and generally begins sequentially with bursitis, tendonitis, tendinopathy, partial thickness tears, full thickness tears, and massive tears.

Patients may present with a constellation of buttock, lateral hip, and groin pain which is due, in part, to the varying nerve supply to the peritrochanteric compartment. Inflammation in this area may cause radiating pain and paresthesia often leading to wide differential diagnoses. Patients may complain of activities that engage the hip abductors such as getting up from a seated position or difficulty climbing stairs. In most cases, the onset of symptoms is insidious, but there are some patients that report an acute exacerbation of symptoms after a recent fall [1]. Patients suffering specifically from a gluteus medius avulsion often present with an obvious limp, necessitating the use of a walker [20, 21]. Due to the stress placed on the greater trochanter, patients complain of pain in a lateral decubitus position that may awaken them at night. Certain anatomic abnormalities such as a high valgus knee angles and a leg length discrepancy have been known to cause mechanical abrasion and subsequent abductor tears due to the increased ITB tension [22].

Physical exam of the hip begins with observation of the patient for Trendelenburg gait followed by performing the Trendelenburg fatigue test. A distinct drop of the non-support pelvis indicates weakness or loss of function of the abductors. With the patient in a lateral decubitus position, the examiner

J.C. McCarthy et al. (eds.), *Hip Joint Restoration*, DOI 10.1007/978-1-4614-0694-5_57

Table 57.1 The diagnostic and treatment courses of the conditions comprising GTPS

Pathology	Clinical presentation	Pathology	Treatment	Outcomes
Abductor tendinopathy	– Lateral hip, buttock, and groin pain. Difficulty climbing stairs, pain with lateral decubitus position, night pain, "grinding sensation," weak ABD – Palpable pain at the gluteus medius insertion or directly over greater trochanter (GT). (+) Trendelenburg fatigue test – MRI T2 shows hyperintensity at superior GT	– Degenerative tears at anterior third due to frictional trauma from tight ITB, osteophytes at anterior intertrochanteric line or ischemia with resulting degenerative tears – 3 types: intrasubstance, partial, and complete tears	– NSAID – Physical therapy – Cortisone injections – Open or endoscopic repair	– Surgical repair may provide pain relief and improvement in functional outcome – Endoscopic gluteus medius repairs of 10 patients with metal suture anchors, all had complete pain relief and regained abductor strength at 25 months [1]
External coxa saltans	– Observable/palpable catching or impingement of ITB over GT during flexion/extension – Increased snapping with hip adduction and knee extension. (+) Ober test	– Increased adduction angle secondary to pelvic morphology, greater femoral neck angle and gait kinetics causing increased thickness to the posterior 1/3 of the ITB	– NSAIDs – Physical therapy to stretch the ITB – Cortisone injections – Surgery: ITB release at posterolateral portion of GT. From vastus tubercle to GT, Z-type release, longitudinal incisions distally to proximally in ITB, or diamond defect technique	– Most cases improve with PT, NSAIDs, corticosteroid injections for resultant bursitis – Endoscopic bursectomy and longitudinal ITB release of 11 hips saw absence of pain and return to previous activity level at 2 years in all except one patient [2, 3]
Internal coxa saltans	– Audible snapping in the anterior aspect of hip is common – Diagnosis is confirmed when the physician uses finger pressure over the area of the snapping sensation and successfully blocks the symptom [4, 5] – Physical exam can reproduce the clicking sensation by extending a flexed, abducted, and externally rotated hip with the patient in a supine position [5–7]	– Audible and *painful* displacement of the iliopsoas tendon over pectineal eminence or prominent pincer or cam deformity	– Physical therapy is successful in the majority of cases – Cortisone injections into the iliopsoas bursa – Open and arthroscopic iliopsoas release has proven to be extremely effective at relieving pain and symptomatic snapping	– Arthroscopic or endoscopic techniques are relatively new but have been shown to be equal to or better than open techniques – Open iliopsoas lengthening involves complications that include recurrence, hip flexor weakness, cosmetic disturbances, and loss of sensation [6]
Ischiofemoral femoral impingement	– No classical examination finding – Case reports show pain with hip flexion/extension, internal/external rotation, and abduction/adduction – Tosun et al. showed findings of pain with internal rotation, flexion, and abduction, with pain being localized to the posterior of the hip in most patients [8–13]	– Entrapment of the quadratus femoris muscle between the ischial tuberosity and the lesser trochanter of the femur – In older patients, IFI may be acquired through fractures of lesser trochanter, valgus-producing intertrochanteric osteotomy and osteoarthritis that can lead to superior and medial migration of the femur	– Surgical approaches can entail partial resection of the hip external rotators at the site of impingement, or bony recession at the lesser trochanter and ischium at the site of impingement	– Addressing the impingement endoscopically is currently investigational
Subspine (AIIS) hip impingement	– Anterior hip and groin pain exacerbated by straight hip flexion as well as prolonged hip flexion, noticed when sitting – This pain and limited range of motion can also be elicited with hip adduction, internal rotation. A "grinding" sensation is noted on hip flexion and lateral movements – Palpation of the tender AIIS can recreate the typical pain	– Impingement of the direct head of the rectus femoris tendon with the distal femoral neck – Can be developmental but is often secondary to prior AIIS avulsion or pelvic osteotomy [14]	– Arthroscopic or open decompression of the AIIS deformity	– In a 3 case study of arthroscopic decompression, both modified Harris Hip Score (HSS) and visual analog scale (VAS) improved. On average, the HHS increased from 75.6 preoperatively to 93.3 postoperatively and VAS improved from 6.18 to 1.13 [15]

should palpate the anterior, lateral, and posterior aspect of the greater trochanter for tenderness. Abductor strength testing can be performed with knee flexed and extended, enabling gravity strength testing. Provocative maneuvers can be performed including the "trochanteric pain sign" which is performed with the patient in a supine position with the hip flexed to 90°, abducted, and externally rotated. If there is pain with external rotation, then the test is considered to be positive. In addition, flexion, abduction, and external rotation (FABER) test may also elicit pain in patients with GTPS. A resisted external rotation should be performed while the patient is in the supine position with the hip flexed at 90° [23, 24].

Plain radiographs can be helpful to rule out osteoarthritis and may demonstrate evidence of calcific tendonitis. MRI and ultrasonography are the primary imaging modalities used to diagnose tendon pathology. Often concomitant with this tendinopathy are subminimus and submedius bursitis, enthesopathic changes along trochanteric insertion, and fatty atrophy [22]. On T2 MRI, hyperintensity is often seen due to thickened hip abductor tendons, tendinopathy, or tendon tears. Though the overall specificity of MRI is debated [25], Kingzett-Taylor et al. found T2-weighted MRI of the superior greater trochanter to be diagnostic of a partial abductor tendon tear with the highest sensitivity (73%) and specificity (95%) [17].

Surgical Technique

Endoscopic treatment of GTPS can be performed in either the lateral position on a standard table or in the supine position on the fracture table. The authors' preference is to perform the procedure in the supine position. After general endotracheal anesthesia, the patient is positioned in a hip traction table until the hip joint has been distracted approximately 1 cm. The patient is prepped and draped ensuring the anterior superior iliac spine (ASIS) and greater trochanter are readily accessible. Once the tip of the greater trochanter is identified, an anterolateral portal (ALP) is established approximately 1 cm anterior and 1 cm proximal to the anterior aspect of the greater trochanter (Fig. 57.1a). A diagnostic arthroscopy is performed in the central compartment to determine whether or not any intra-articular pathology is identified. After addressing any intra-articular pathologies the traction is then released and the leg is abducted 15–20°.

The peritrochanteric space is entered using a 5.0 mm metal cannula through the mid-anterior portal (MAP) over the vastus ridge. The cannula is directed between the iliotibial band (ITB) and the lateral aspect of the proximal greater trochanter. Once the cannula is in the appropriate interval, then the cannula is swiped from proximal to distal to open the potential space. The arthroscope and light source are both directed proximally so that the distal aspect of the peritrochanteric space is visualized. Using spinal needle localization, the 4.5 mm shaver is introduced over a Wissinger rod and 5.0 mm metal cannula. The arthroscopic shaver is then used to perform a thorough bursectomy until the tendon of the gluteus maximus is identified distally, the ITB is identified laterally, the undersurface of the gluteus maximus is identified proximally, and the abductor tendons and vastus lateralis are identified medially.

The arthroscope is then placed in the ALP and the arthroscopic shaver is placed in the MAP to continue to debride any excessive bursal tissue. The gluteus medius and minimus are readily identified and the tear pattern can be recognized at this point. An attempt is then made to characterize the mobility of the torn tendons, the quality of the tissue, and the size of the tear. A grasper is then used to ensure the tendon can be approximated to the gluteus medius footprint without tension. Using a 5.0 mm cylindrical burr the footprint is debrided to punctate cortical bleeding (Fig. 57.1b). For small and medium tears, a single row with one to two suture anchors is preferred. For large and massive tears, a double-row suture bridge is the preferred fixation construct. Anchors are inserted percutaneously via a posterolateral portal (PLP), which is 1 cm posterior and 1 cm proximal to the tip of the posterolateral aspect of the greater trochanter. Next, two 5.5 mm biocomposite anchors double-loaded with #2 high strength sutures (Biocorkscrew, Arthrex, Naples, Fl) are placed at the medial border of the gluteus medius footprint (Fig. 57.1c). Next, sutures are passed through the tendon with tissue penetrating device (InJector, Pivot Medical, Sunnyvale, CA) or suture shuttling device (Crescent SutureLasso, Arthrex, Naples, FL) and grasped through the MAP for suture management. In general, two sets of horizontal mattress stitches are passed per anchor and subsequently tied using reverse half hitches and alternating posts (RHAP). An 8.5 mm clear plastic cannula is placed in the PLP. One limb from each stitch is retrieved for the first lateral row anchor (Swivelock, Arthrex, Naples, FL), and the remaining limb is retrieved for the second lateral row anchor (Swivelock, Arthrex, Naples, FL) (Fig. 57.1d). The ends of the sutures are cut, and the hip is rotated to ensure anatomic reduction and fixation of the torn gluteus medius tendon.

Our postoperative protocol consists of bracing with partial weight bearing for the first 6 weeks after surgery. Gentle passive range of motion is performed for the first 6 weeks to prevent adhesions. From 6 to 8 weeks, the patient will progress to full weight bearing but continues to use assistive devices. The patient may continue to use a walker or cane until 3 months from surgery.

Repair of chronic tears may have limits. In a study using MRI to evaluate progress in a late abductor avulsion repair following a THA, it was found that fatty degeneration of the anterior gluteus medius did not reverse or improve at a 1-year follow-up. This illuminates the limitation of late stage abductor avulsion repairs and the possibility that fatty degeneration cannot be reversed [26].

In a study by Lequesne et al. [27], eight MRI diagnosed gluteus medius tears were repaired. Complete remission of spontaneous and provoked pain was seen in seven patients

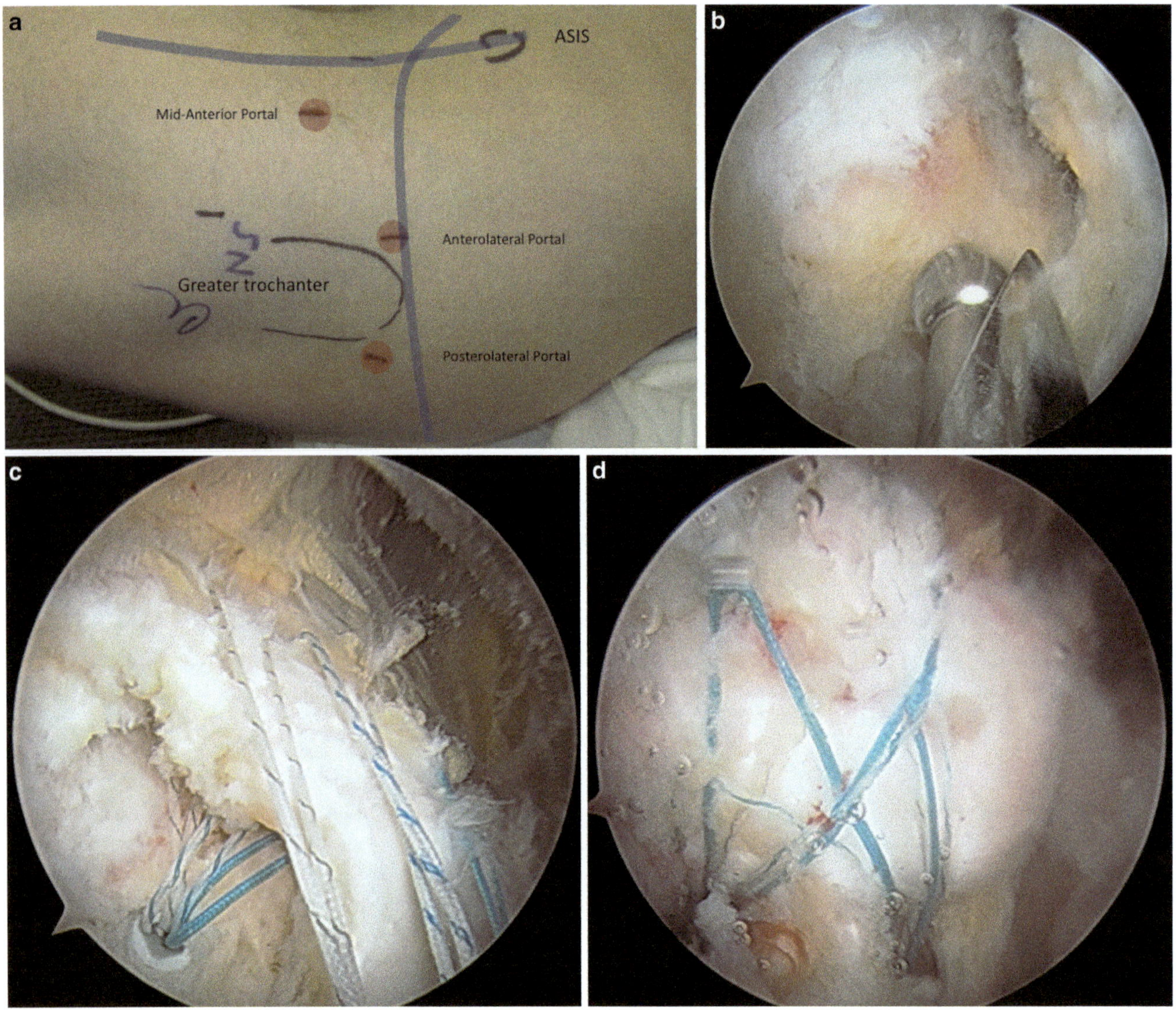

Fig. 57.1 (**a**) Landmarks for portals for peritrochanteric space. (**b**) Large gluteus medius tear. (**c**) Medial row suture anchor in the greater tuberosity. (**d**) Double-row suture bridge construct for repair of gluteus tendon

with partial submission in one patient. Six MRIs performed at 20.5 months showed good reinsertion of tendon. In a study by Voos et al. [1], ten patients with MRI diagnosed and endoscopically confirmed hip abductor tears with endoscopic repair had HHS of 94 and hip outcome scores of 95 at average 1-year follow-up. Seven of ten patients said their hip felt "normal" while three of ten reported "nearly normal" at 25-month follow-up.

Coxa Saltans Externa (External Snapping Hip Syndrome)

Snapping hip, or coxa saltans, has two variant etiologies. External snapping hip syndrome is often secondary to the thickening of the posterior third of the ITB that lies posterior to the greater trochanter in neutral position [22]. Repeated flexion and extension of the overly taut ITB will show signs of "catching" or "impingement" on the trochanter. Further tightening of the ITB and its resultant "snapping" is emphasized by hip adduction and extension at the knee [28]. Women with a large pelvis or more prominent greater trochanters have a predilection for external snapping hip. This is most commonly seen in women who adduct beyond their midline in their stride [28].

The actual snapping of the ITB itself is usually nonpainful [22]; however, the pathology of external coxa saltans lies in resultant complications. As commonly reported, inflammation of the trochanteric bursae may result from the abrasive wear characteristic of external coxa saltans [29]. Additionally, Kingzett-Taylor et al. [17] supported the notion that both abductor tendinopathy and trochanteric bursitis could be secondary to the frictional trauma caused by high tension of the ITB, backing the idea that one cause of GTPS begets other conditions and symptoms, making the disorder largely multifactorial.

The physical exam for external snapping hip syndrome includes a palpable or observable snapping of the ITB over the greater trochanter upon flexion and subsequent extension. The patient can be placed in a lateral decubitus position and a single leg bicycle maneuver can be performed which may reproduce ITB snapping. A significant tightening of the ITB can be observed, characterized by a positive Ober test, qualifying the patient for ITB release with concomitant removal of the symptomatic bursa [30].

Surgical Technique

Prior to surgery, the area of tenderness and snapping on the skin is marked in the preop area to guide the location of our release. The access to the peritrochanteric space is the same as previously described in the surgical technique for gluteus medius repairs. Once the trochanteric bursectomy is completed, the ITB lengthening can be performed (Fig. 57.2a, b). The endoscope is placed in the MAP portal and light source is directed medially to visualize the ITB. The spinal needle is used to localize the posterior third of the ITB at the level of the PLP. Next, an 11 blade on a scalpel is used to create a portal then passed deeper to incise the ITB. The blade is then passed in line with the ITB fibers approximately 2–3 cm. At the midpoint of the incised ITB, the perpendicular incision is then created anteriorly and posteriorly approximately 1.5 cm in each direction (Fig. 57.2c). Next, the 4.5 mm arthroscopic shaver is passed through the PLP and used to debride the flaps of the ITB so that a diamond configuration is visible at the conclusion of the ITB lengthening (Fig. 57.2d).

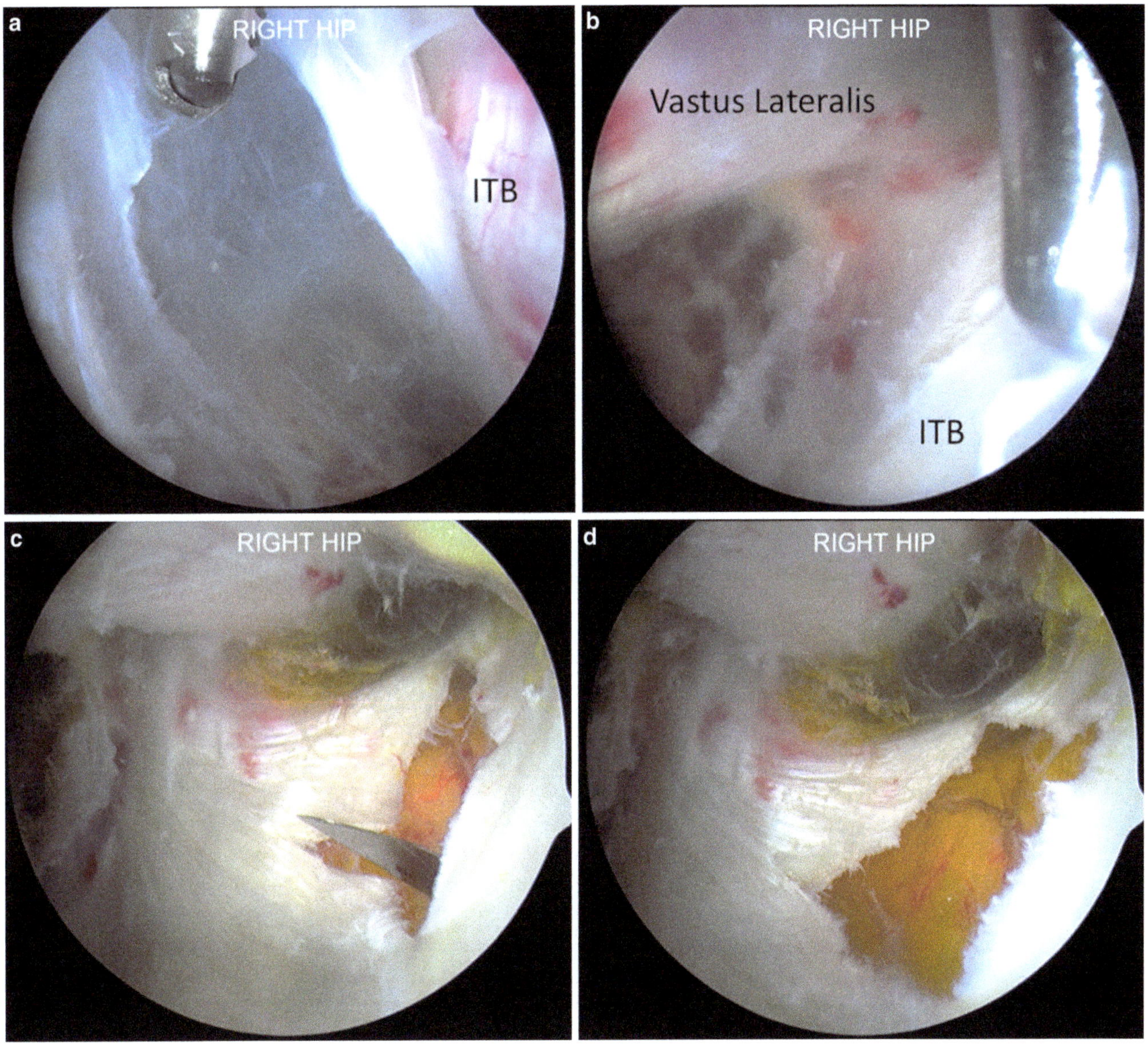

Fig. 57.2 Iliotibial Band Lengthening. (**a**) Endoscopic trochanteric bursectomy in the peritrochanteric space. ITB, Iliotibial band. (**b**) Complete exposure of the ITB and the insertion of the gluteus maximus tendon under the vastus lateralis. (**c**) Scalpel used to percutaneously incise parallel with the ITB then perpendicular to the ITB. (**d**) Final appearance of ITB lengthening with diamond configuration

Table 57.2 Result of endoscopic and open ITB release for external snapping hip

Author, year	Approach	Patient #/age	Mean follow-up/results
Provencher et al. [31], 2004	Open ITB Z-plasty	8 consecutive hips, 1 bilateral; mean age 25.6 years old	22.9 months f/u. 8/9 (89 %) complete resolution of snapping hip, all but one returned to unrestricted activities due to persistent groin pain, but no snapping
White et al. [32], 2004	Open ITB release consisting of single longitudinal cut with 6 stepwise transverse cuts	16 patients (13 female, 3 male); mean age 33 years old	32.5 months f/u. 14/16 (88 %) had ultimate resolution of snapping including 2 revisions due to recurrence. 12/12 patients contacted via phone were satisfied with procedure
Ilizaliturri et al. [3], 2005	Endoscopic ITB release	11 hips (9 f one bilateral, 1 m); mean age 26 years old	24 months f/u. 10/11 (91 %) complete resolution of hip pain, 1/11 (9 %) had nonpainful snapping
Zini et al. [33], 2013	Endoscopic ITB release	15 hips (12 f, 3 m); mean age 25 years old	33 months f/u. Resolution of snapping in all patients, but only 9/15 (60 %) pain free. VAS score improved from 5.5 to 0.53 postop ($p<0.0001$). HHS 97.5 postop
Polesello et al. [34], 2013	Endoscopic release of gluteus maximus tendon on ITB	9 hips (7 f one bilateral, 1 m); mean age 35 years old	32 months f/u. 7/9 (78 %) complete resolution of pain. 1/9 (11 %) needing reoperation for no symptom relief. HHS preop 61–78 postop. All returned to previous level of activity including one revision

The clinical studies on the endoscopic treatment of external coxa saltans have been reported to be promising (Table 57.2). Ilizaliturri et al. reported on 11 patients with ITB release—10/11 had complete resolution of painful snapping [22]. In 15 patients who underwent endoscopic ITB release, Zini et al. saw average visual analog scale (VAS) improvement from 5.5 to 0.53 with 9/15 patients having complete resolution of pain [cite ZINI].

Coxa Saltans Interna (Internal Snapping Hip)

Internal snapping hip, another etiology of snapping hip syndrome, was first described by Nunziata and Blumenfeld in 1954 as a slippage of the iliopsoas tendon over the iliopectineal line [35]. It has since been described as snapping of the iliopsoas tendon as it crosses the femoral head and anterior capsule during hip flexion to extension [6]. Internal snapping hip can be thought of as an audible and painful displacement of the iliopsoas tendon over bony pelvic or femoral prominences [4, 36]. The typical patient with internal snapping hip syndrome will present with a snapping sensation during walking, long distance running, and other physical activities [6].

Physical exam can reproduce the snapping sensation by extending a flexed, abducted, and externally rotated hip with the patient in a supine position [5–7]. Diagnosis is confirmed when the physician uses finger pressure over the area of the snapping sensation and successfully blocks or palpates the snapping [4, 5].

Iliopsoas bursography, once a popular modality, has been supplanted by more dynamic imaging tools to visualize the snapping of the iliopsoas [5–7, 37]. Recently, the inexpensive combination of radiographs and ultrasound has shown to be effective in diagnosis [5–7, 37, 38]. Nonetheless, MRI also continues to be the most effective diagnostic tool.

Internal snapping hip syndrome can be treated conservatively with a period of rest and activity modification. Physical therapy is the mainstay for the treatment of internal coxa saltans with an emphasis on deep tissue massage or active release therapy and stretching [4, 5]. For patients with persistent painful internal snapping, an image-controlled cortisone injection in the iliopsoas bursa can be effective. In rare cases, iliopsoas lengthening can be performed when refractory to nonsurgical treatment. Compared to open techniques, arthroscopic or endoscopic techniques have been shown to be equal to or better than open techniques. Given the comparable outcomes, endoscopic techniques tend to avoid the complications of open treatment including recurrence, hip flexor weakness, cosmetic disturbances, and loss of sensation [6]. In addition, arthroscopic techniques allow for visualization of the intra-articular space, allowing for a comprehensive diagnostic examination [39]. There is no endoscopic technique proven to be more effective than another [40].

There are currently three described locations for iliopsoas lengthening, and the more distal the lengthening the greater the proportion of tendon to muscle (Table 57.3). The iliopsoas tendon can be released through the central compartment at the reflection of the rectus femora's head and acetabular rim while the leg is in traction through the anterior portal with anterolateral visualization [45]. An arthroscopic psoas tendon release is also possible from the peripheral compartment at the femoral head neck junction, proximal to the zona orbicularis and anterior to the medial synovial fold insertion. This is best done with traction removed, the leg

Table 57.3 Results of open and endoscopic treatment for internal snapping hip

Author, year	Technique	Patient #/age	Results/complications
Dobbs et al. [41], 2002	Open modified iliofemoral approach, fractional lengthening at musculotendinous junction	9 adolescent patients (11 hips), means age 15 years old	1/9 (11 %) had recurrence of nonpainful snapping. 9/9 returned to preop level of activities with no detectable loss of hip flexion strength. 2/9 (22 %) had transient anterolateral numbness
Gruen et al. [42], 2002	Open ilioinguinal intrapelvic approach, fractional tendon lengthening	11 patients, 12 hips; mean age 31.5 years old	11/11 resolution of snapping without recurrence, 9/11 (82 %) satisfactory pain relief, 7/11 (64 %) total resolution of pain, 3/11 (27 %) could not return to previous level of activity, 3/11 (27 %) returned but to a lesser level of activity, 5/11 (45 %) reported subjective hip flexion weakness
Hoskins et al. [4], 2004	Open iliofemoral approach, iliopsoas lengthening	92 consecutive hips (80 patients); mean age 27.3 years old	40/92 (43 %) hips had complications: 6/92 (7 %) had recurrent pain, 20 (22 %) failures/recurrences of snapping, 8 (9 %) anterior thigh sensory deficits, 11/92 (12 %) wound problems. Still, overall satisfaction rate was 89 %
Flanum et al. [43], 2007	Endoscopic release of iliopsoas tendon	6 hips/patients; mean age 38.8 years old	Preop HHS avg 58, postop 6 weeks scores 62, 12 weeks 85, 6 months 90, 12 months HHS 96. 2/5 (40 %) had occasional slight pain at 1 year but 6/6 reported no painful snapping
Ilizaliturri et al. [40], 2009	Endoscopic: iliopsoas release at lesser trochanter (LT) vs. transcapsular (TC) release from peripheral compartment	– LT:10 hips (5 male, 5 female); mean age 29.5 years old – TC: 9 hips (8 f, 1 m); mean age 32.6 years old	LT: preop WOMAC improved 70.1 ± 10.7 to 83.7 ± 7.1 (p=0.0001). TC: preop WOMAC 67 ± 11.4 to 83.5 ± 5.9 (p=0.001). No statistical difference in preop Western Ontario MacMaster (WOMAC) scores, every patient in all groups had statistically significant improvement in WOMAC scores, no complications in either group
Ilizaliturri et al. [44], 2014	Endoscopic: peripheral/lesser trochanter (LT) release vs. central compartment/ transcapsular (CC)	– LT: 6 hips (4 m, 2 f); mean age 35.7 years old – CC: 14 hips (5 m, 9 f); mean age 30.9 years old	LT: preop WOMAC 46.33 ± 21.83 improved to 89.33 ± 1.36. CC: preop WOMAC 56 ± 13.21 improved to 89.57 ± 3. One patient in CC group had recurrence of snapping that required surgical intervention. All have improvement of WOMAC scores

flexed 30°, with the anterolateral portal used for visualization [46]. Finally, an endoscopic iliopsoas tendon release is done at the lesser trochanter insertion, with the leg externally rotated and flexed 30° [47]. The surgeon should be aware of the proximity of the MFCA during this procedure [48].

Surgical Technique

Once the patient is placed in appropriate distraction, a standard ALP is established as previously described. An anterior portal is established at the intersection of the vertical line from the ASIS and the horizontal line from the tip of the greater trochanter. A guide wire is passed through the spinal needle and a 5.0 mm metal cannula is passed. In most cases labral contusion is visualized at the 3 o'clock position and most pronounced at the capsular side of the labrum (Fig. 57.3a). At this location, the capsulotomy is widened to about 1 cm and the tendinous portion of the iliopsoas is visualized. Next, a bipolar radiofrequency device is used to lengthen the tendinous portion without releasing the muscular portion of the iliopsoas (Fig. 57.3b, c). The tendinous portion can extend more distal but adjacent to the anterior hip capsule and needs to be recognized. There are case reports of bifid tendons of the iliopsoas and the entire tendinous portion needs to be addressed to prevent recurrent snapping [49]. Meticulous hemostasis must be performed and the area of the middle third between the proximal head neck junction and the lesser trochanter much be avoided to prevent injury to a branch of the medial femoral circumflex artery [48].

Ischiofemoral Impingement

Ischiofemoral impingement (IFI) is described as the entrapment of the quadratus femoris muscle between the ischial tuberosity and the lesser trochanter of the femur. Johnson [8] first described this pathology in a study that found profound symptomatic relief in patients with prior hip surgery after removal of the lesser trochanter. More recently, it has been discovered that IFI can be found in a native hip as a result of trauma, diseases that alter bone architecture such as hereditary multiple exostoses, or congenital abnormalities [8–11]. In older patients, IFI may be acquired through fractures involving the lesser trochanter, valgus-producing intertrochanteric osteotomy, and osteoarthritis that can lead to superior and medial migration of the femur [10, 50].

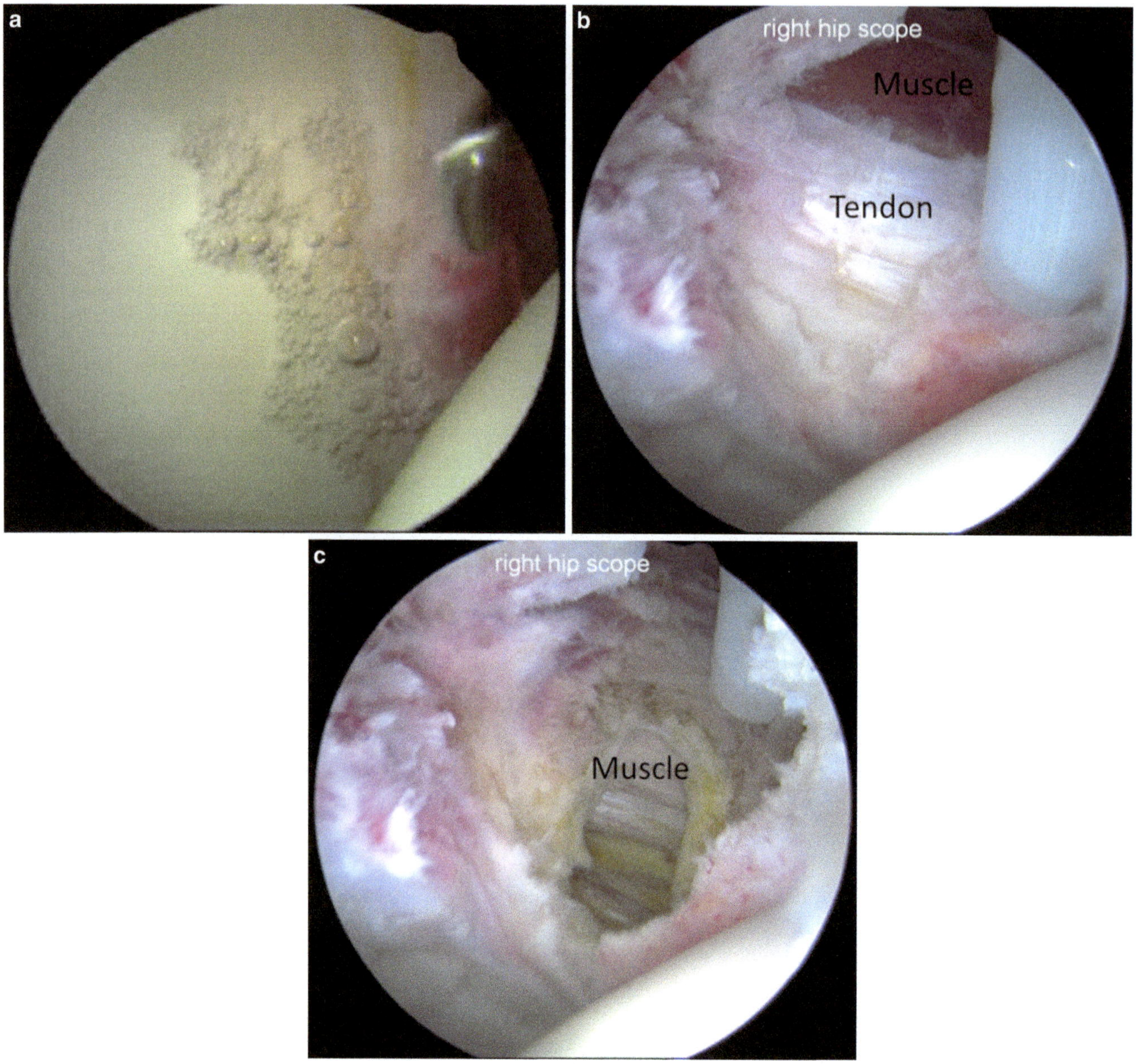

Fig. 57.3 Iliopsoas Impingement. (**a**) Labral contusion at the 3 o'clock position that suggests external compression from snapping iliopsoas tendon. (**b**) Iliopsoas tendon and muscle unit at the central compartment. (**c**) Iliopsoas lengthening of the tendon at the central compartment

Ischiofemoral impingement is more commonly found in females. This has been thought to be due to ischiofemoral space narrowing secondary to wider and shallower pelvises [10] typical of females, as well as larger lesser trochanter prominences [51].

There is no classical examination finding with IFI. Case reports have shown that pain can be elicited with hip flexion/extension, internal/external rotation, and abduction/adduction [8–12]. The most recent retrospective study by Tosun et al. [13] showed findings of pain with internal rotation, flexion, and abduction, with pain being localized to the posterior aspect of the hip in most patients. Diagnosis of this process is more helpful by examining the clinical picture and diagnostic imaging.

Magnetic resonance imaging (MRI), in a study by Torriani et al. [12], showed abnormal MR signal intensity of the quadratus femoris muscle and a narrowing of the space between the ischial tuberosity and lesser trochanter. This space narrowing is thought to be due to congenital ischiofemoral narrowing with bilateral involvement of 25 % of patients.

The diagnosis of IFI can be complicated, as there is minimal literature and discussion on to develop the proper diagnostic tools. To date, there is no gold standard diagnostic tool or exam to diagnose IFI. It is important to correlate physical exam findings with MR imaging when IFI is suspected as the cause of hip pain. Once a diagnosis is established, physicians can apply conservative management or surgical techniques for correcting IFI.

Addressing the impingement endoscopically is currently investigational. Surgical approaches can entail partial resection of the hip external rotators at the site of impingement, or bony recession at the lesser trochanter and ischium at the site of impingement.

Subspine (Anterior Inferior Iliac Spine) Hip Impingement

Cam and pincer femoroacetabular impingement (FAI) have been well researched in recent years [52–54]; however extra-articular impingement conditions have been increasingly recognized as a source of hip and groin pain and restriction [14, 55]. Rectus bony impingement or anterior inferior iliac spine (AIIS)/subspine hip impingement, as described by Larson and Kelly, is the impingement of the direct head of the rectus femoris tendon with the distal femoral neck [15]. While AIIS impingement can be developmental, it is often secondary to prior AIIS avulsion or pelvic osteotomy [14]. Developmental AIIS impingement is commonly seen in the setting of acetabular retroversion and can be mistaken for acetabular retroversion in certain radiographs. In a study using an osteology collection of 3954 hemipelvi, there was found to be a prevalence of 6.4 % with a higher prevalence in males and African Americans, and three subtypes were described: columnar, bulbous, and hooked (Fig. 57.4) [56]. In a study by Hetsroni et al. three-dimensional CT reconstructions were used to classify AIIS morphology into three morphological types that correlated to hip range of motion [57]. In type I AIIS variant, there is smooth ilium between the caudad level of the AIIS and the labrum. Type II variant has either bony prominence between the caudad area and the acetabular rim, or the caudad area is at the level of the acetabular rim. In the type III variant, the caudad level extends distally to the anterosuperior acetabular rim. Type II and III variants result in decreased hip flexion and internal rotation supporting AIIS decompression in certain cases of subspine impingement [57].

The patient generally presents with anterior hip and groin pain exacerbated by straight hip flexion as well as prolonged hip flexion, noticed when sitting. This pain and limited range of motion can also be elicited with hip adduction and internal rotation. A "grinding" sensation is noted on hip flexion and lateral movements. Palpation of the tender AIIS can recreate the typical pain.

Radiographic findings consistent with AIIS impingement include AIIS avulsion, acetabular retroversion with anterior rim sclerosis calcific deposits at the rectus femoris origin as well as impingement cysts at the distal femoral neck [15]. The distal location of these impingement cysts can help differentiate cam and pincer FAI from AIIS impingement. AP pelvis radiograph can show extension of the AIIS below the acetabular sourcil while anterior and distal extension can be seen on false-profile radiograph. Similarly, three-dimensional computed tomography can show AIIS avulsion deformities, excessive anterior and distal extension of the AIIS below the acetabular rim. Larson and Kelly cited the three-dimensional imaging as an invaluable diagnostic tool in evaluating cases of developmental AIIS impingement [15].

Treatment is arthroscopic or open decompression of the AIIS. This is achieved with extension of the acetabuloplasty superiorly with the use of the shaver, radiofrequency device and burr, above the capsule to the insertion of the rectus femoris. In a recent case series, the authors report both modified Harris Hip Score (HSS) and visual analog scale (VAS) improved. On average, the HHS increased from 75.6 preoperatively to 93.3 postoperatively and VAS improved from 6.18 to 1.13 [15]. Further work is warranted to identify risk factors, radiographic findings, and surgical techniques.

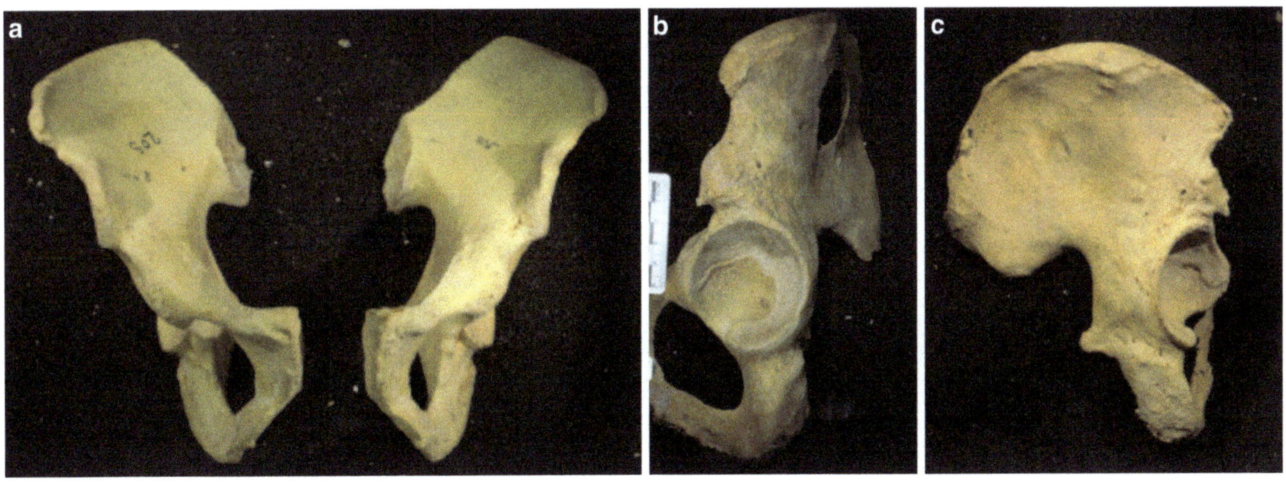

Fig. 57.4 Subspine (AIIS) Impingement. (**a**) Columnar Type. (**b**) Bulbous Type. (**c**) Hooked Type

Limitations and Potential Complications of the Technique

Endoscopy of the extra-articular hip conditions is a relatively new frontier. Techniques and instruments should continue to evolve to allow broader adoption and greater efficiency. Possibly the greatest limitation is understanding of the disease processes and patient selection. Further clinical and scientific research will be critical to advancing the treatment of extra-articular hip conditions.

Complications after endoscopy of extra-articular hip conditions have not been well described but thought to be less frequent and less severe than complications after intra-articular hip arthroscopy. The peritrochanteric space is outside the pelvis, and therefore, potentially severe complications such as fluid extravasation have not been reported. Other major complications such as avascular necrosis, femoral neck fracture, postoperative instability, or adhesions have also not been reported. Iatrogenic injury to the gluteal vessels or sciatic nerve is a possibility if entry into the space is either too proximal or too posterior. Walsh et al. [58] reported a study of 89 patients receiving endoscopic repair for abductor tendon tears from 2000 to 2008, in which the most frequent complication (6 %) was deep vein thrombosis, which is low relative to other lower extremity orthopedic procedures.

Summary

Extra-articular hip disorders are a rapidly evolving field in terms of diagnosis and treatment. There is a considerable amount of excitement as indications for surgery begin to expand and our understanding of conditions that are effectively treated with minimally invasive surgery [59]. Although the treatment of extra-articular hip diseases is becoming more widely performed, the procedures are considered to be relatively safe with few reported complications. Additional clinical and scientific research will be paramount to determining which patients will benefit from the treatment of extra-articular hip conditions and for the advancement of the field.

References

1. Voos JE, Shindle MK, Pruett A, et al. Endoscopic repair of gluteus medius tendon tears of the hip. Am J Sports Med. 2009;37:743–7.
2. Farr D, Selesnick H, Janecki C, et al. Arthroscopic bursectomy with concomitant iliotibial band release for the treatment of recalcitrant trochanteric bursitis. Arthroscopy. 2007;23:905.e1–e5.
3. Ilizaliturri Jr VM, Martinez-Escalante FA, Chaidez PA, et al. Endoscopic iliotibial band release for external snapping hip syndrome. Arthroscopy. 2006;22:505–10.
4. Hoskins JS, Burd TA, Allen WC. Surgical correction of internal coxa saltans: a 20-year consecutive study. Am J Sports Med. 2004;32:998–1001.
5. Allen WC, Cope R. Coxa saltans: the snapping hip revisited. J Am Acad Orthop Surg. 1995;3:303–8.
6. Jacobson T, Allen WC. Surgical correction of the snapping iliopsoas tendon. Am J Sports Med. 1990;18:470–4.
7. Schaberg JE, Harper MC, Allen WC. The snapping hip syndrome. Am J Sports Med. 1984;12:361–5.
8. Johnson KA. Impingement of the lesser trochanter on the ischial ramus after total hip arthroplasty. Report of three cases. J Bone Joint Surg Am. 1977;59:268–9.
9. Ali AM, Whitwell D, Ostlere SJ. Case report: imaging and surgical treatment of a snapping hip due to ischiofemoral impingement. Skeletal Radiol. 2011;40:653–6.
10. Tosun O, Cay N, Bozkurt M, et al. Ischiofemoral impingement in an 11-year-old girl. Diagn Interv Radiol. 2012;18(6):571–3.
11. Viala P, Vanel D, Larbi A, et al. Bilateral ischiofemoral impingement in a patient with hereditary multiple exostoses. Skeletal Radiol. 2012;41:1637–40.
12. Patti JW, Ouellette H, Bredella MA, et al. Impingement of lesser trochanter on ischium as a potential cause for hip pain. Skeletal Radiol. 2008;37:939–41.
13. Tosun O, Algin O, Yalcin N, et al. Ischiofemoral impingement: evaluation with new MRI parameters and assessment of their reliability. Skeletal Radiol. 2012;41:575–87.
14. Pan H, Kawanabe K, Akiyama H, et al. Operative treatment of hip impingement caused by hypertrophy of the anterior inferior iliac spine. J Bone Joint Surg Br. 2008;90:677–9.
15. Larson CM, Kelly BT, Stone RM. Making a case for anterior inferior iliac spine/subspine hip impingement: three representative case reports and proposed concept. Arthroscopy. 2011;27:1732–7.
16. Bard H. Tendinopathy of the gluteus medius tendon. Rev Prat. 2009;59:463–8.
17. Kingzett-Taylor A, Tirman PF, Feller J, et al. Tendinosis and tears of gluteus medius and minimus muscles as a cause of hip pain: MR imaging findings. AJR Am J Roentgenol. 1999;173:1123–6.
18. Kagan II A. Rotator cuff tears of the hip. Clin Orthop Relat Res. 1999;368:135–40.
19. Lachiewicz PF. Abductor tendon tears of the hip: evaluation and management. J Am Acad Orthop Surg. 2011;19:385–91.
20. Svensson O, Skold S, Blomgren G. Integrity of the gluteus medius after the transgluteal approach in total hip arthroplasty. J Arthroplasty. 1990;5:57–60.
21. Weber M, Berry DJ. Abductor avulsion after primary total hip arthroplasty. Results of repair. J Arthroplasty. 1997;12:202–6.
22. Ilizaliturri Jr VM, Camacho-Galindo J, Evia Ramirez AN, et al. Soft tissue pathology around the hip. Clin Sports Med. 2011;30:391–415.
23. Bird PA, Oakley SP, Shnier R, et al. Prospective evaluation of magnetic resonance imaging and physical examination findings in patients with greater trochanteric pain syndrome. Arthritis Rheum. 2001;44:2138–45.
24. Domb BG, Nasser RM, Botser IB. Partial-thickness tears of the gluteus medius: rationale and technique for trans-tendinous endoscopic repair. Arthroscopy. 2010;26:1697–705.
25. Blankenbaker DG, Ullrick SR, Davis KW, et al. Correlation of MRI findings with clinical findings of trochanteric pain syndrome. Skeletal Radiol. 2008;37:903–9.
26. Miozzari HH, Dora C, Clark JM, et al. Late repair of abductor avulsion after the transgluteal approach for hip arthroplasty. J Arthroplasty. 2010;25:450–457.e1.
27. Lequesne M, Djian P, Vuillemin V, et al. Prospective study of refractory greater trochanter pain syndrome. MRI findings of gluteal tendon tears seen at surgery. Clinical and MRI results of tendon repair. Joint Bone Spine. 2008;75:458–64.
28. Anderson K, Strickland SM, Warren R. Hip and groin injuries in athletes. Am J Sports Med. 2001;29:521–33.

29. Voos JE, Rudzki JR, Shindle MK, et al. Arthroscopic anatomy and surgical techniques for peritrochanteric space disorders in the hip. Arthroscopy. 2007;23:1246.e1–e5.
30. Strauss EJ, Nho SJ, Kelly BT. Greater trochanteric pain syndrome. Sports Med Arthrosc. 2010;18:113–9.
31. Provencher MT, Hofmeister EP, Muldoon MP. The surgical treatment of external coxa saltans (the snapping hip) by Z-plasty of the iliotibial band. Am J Sports Med. 2004;32:470–6.
32. White RA, Hughes MS, Burd T, et al. A new operative approach in the correction of external coxa saltans: the snapping hip. Am J Sports Med. 2004;32:1504–8.
33. Zini R, Munegato D, De Benedetto M, et al. Endoscopic iliotibial band release in snapping hip. Hip Int. 2013;23:225–32.
34. Polesello GC, Queiroz MC, Domb BG, et al. Surgical technique: endoscopic gluteus maximus tendon release for external snapping hip syndrome. Clin Orthop Relat Res. 2013;471:2471–6.
35. Nunziata A, Blumenfeld I. Snapping hip; note on a variety. Prensa Med Argent. 1951;38:1997–2001.
36. Beals RK. Painful snapping hip in young adults. West J Med. 1993;159:481–2.
37. Harper MC, Schaberg JE, Allen WC. Primary iliopsoas bursography in the diagnosis of disorders of the hip. Clin Orthop Relat Res. 1987;221:238–41.
38. Wunderbaldinger P, Bremer C, Matuszewski L, et al. Efficient radiological assessment of the internal snapping hip syndrome. Eur Radiol. 2001;11:1743–7.
39. Byrd JW. Evaluation and management of the snapping iliopsoas tendon. Instr Course Lect. 2006;55:347–55.
40. Ilizaliturri Jr VM, Chaidez C, Villegas P, et al. Prospective randomized study of 2 different techniques for endoscopic iliopsoas tendon release in the treatment of internal snapping hip syndrome. Arthroscopy. 2009;25:159–63.
41. Dobbs MB, Gordon JE, Luhmann SJ, et al. Surgical correction of the snapping iliopsoas tendon in adolescents. J Bone Joint Surg Am. 2002;84-A:420–4.
42. Gruen GS, Scioscia TN, Lowenstein JE. The surgical treatment of internal snapping hip. Am J Sports Med. 2002;30:607–13.
43. Flanum ME, Keene JS, Blankenbaker DG, et al. Arthroscopic treatment of the painful “internal” snapping hip: results of a new endoscopic technique and imaging protocol. Am J Sports Med. 2007;35:770–9.
44. Ilizaliturri Jr VM, Buganza-Tepole M, Olivos-Meza A, et al. Central compartment release versus lesser trochanter release of the iliopsoas tendon for the treatment of internal snapping hip: a comparative study. Arthroscopy. 2014;30:790–5.
45. Contreras ME, Dani WS, Endges WK, et al. Arthroscopic treatment of the snapping iliopsoas tendon through the central compartment of the hip: a pilot study. J Bone Joint Surg Br. 2010;92:777–80.
46. Wettstein M, Jung J, Dienst M. Arthroscopic psoas tenotomy. Arthroscopy. 2006;22:907.e1–e4.
47. Ilizaliturri Jr VM, Villalobos Jr FE, Chaidez PA, et al. Internal snapping hip syndrome: treatment by endoscopic release of the iliopsoas tendon. Arthroscopy. 2005;21:1375–80.
48. McCormick F, Kleweno CP, Kim YJ, et al. Vascular safe zones in hip arthroscopy. Am J Sports Med. 2011;39(Suppl):64S–71.
49. Shu B, Safran MR. Case report: bifid iliopsoas tendon causing refractory internal snapping hip. Clin Orthop Relat Res. 2011;469:289–93.
50. Anderson SE, Siebenrock KA, Tannast M. Femoroacetabular impingement: evidence of an established hip abnormality. Radiology. 2010;257:8–13.
51. Torriani M, Souto SC, Thomas BJ, et al. Ischiofemoral impingement syndrome: an entity with hip pain and abnormalities of the quadratus femoris muscle. AJR Am J Roentgenol. 2009;193:186–90.
52. Beck M, Leunig M, Parvizi J, et al. Anterior femoroacetabular impingement: part II. Midterm results of surgical treatment. Clin Orthop Relat Res. 2004;418:67–73.
53. Ganz R, Parvizi J, Beck M, et al. Femoroacetabular impingement: a cause for osteoarthritis of the hip. Clin Orthop Relat Res. 2003;417:112–20.
54. Larson CM. Arthroscopic management of pincer-type impingement. Sports Med Arthrosc. 2010;18:100–7.
55. Macnicol MF, Makris D. Distal transfer of the greater trochanter. J Bone Joint Surg Br. 1991;73:838–41.
56. Fortun C, Schilf C, Nho S, et al. Anterior Inferior Iliac Spine Morphology And Implications For Subspine Impingement: An Anatomic Study Of 3594 Cadaveric Specimens. ISHA Annual Meeting. 2012
57. Hetsroni I, Poultsides L, Bedi A, et al. Anterior inferior iliac spine morphology correlates with hip range of motion: a classification system and dynamic model. Clin Orthop Relat Res. 2013;471: 2497–503.
58. Walsh N, Walsh M, Walton J, et al. Surgical repair of the abductor mechanism of the Hip. Orthop Proc. 2011;93-B, 25–25.
59. Griffiths EJ, Khanduja V. Hip arthroscopy: evolution, current practice and future developments. Int Orthop. 2012;36:1115–21.

Part VIII

Special Patients and Conditions

John M. O'Donnell

Special Patients and Conditions: Elite Athletes

58

John M. O'Donnell, Michael George Pritchard, Mohamed S. Gobba, George Chukwuka Ozoude, Philip C. Noble, and Parminder J. Singh

Introduction

Treating elite athletes can be challenging on many fronts. The extreme joint loads generated by sporting activities make athletes more susceptible to musculoskeletal injuries at an earlier age compared to the general population, whether the cause is direct trauma or repetitive loading. Because of the demand for elite athletes to perform at their peak, treatment may be sought for relatively minor injuries that more sedentary individuals may ignore or never notice. Because most elite athletes are highly motivated and strive to maintain their position at the highest levels of their sport, they will generally do everything possible to return to their level of performance prior to the onset of hip pathology. However this level of motivation is double-edged as elite athletes have so much personally invested in the success or failure of a course of orthopedic treatment. This brings into focus issues that are normally not significant in the treatment of patients whose livelihood is not determined by peak physical performance.

Major challenges facing physicians in treating athletes arise from secondary factors not directly related to the physiologic processes of injury, diagnosis, treatment and healing. In the context of elite sporting activity, these processes do not play out in a vacuum isolated from sport, but are often affected by the conflicting interests of the athlete, the sports medicine physician, and external parties with an interest in the outcome of treatment [1–6]. This 'Conflict of Interest' is particularly understandable in professional sports and colours many facets of the doctor-patient relationship, potentially undermining the normal tension between the aspirations of the athlete and the professional obligations of the physician. The independent judgement of the physician is often tested by the overarching desire for the player to return to play as early as possible, but at the pre-injury level of performance. This is understandable, as the health of elite athletes is often tied to the success of a team, and the competing interests of multiple stakeholders, including health care providers, athletes, management, agents, family members and fans [7]. After injury, the financial and competitive incentives for the physician to allow the elite athlete to return to sport are magnified. As the team physician, it becomes critically important to recognise this fact while still managing to deliver the accepted standard of care.

Issues of maintaining patient confidentiality and privacy are also cited among the top challenges of team physicians [8]. Other challenges include pressure to use the latest in emerging technology in diagnosis and treatment modalities despite lack of high quality evidence [9]. Still, other obstacles include legal and malpractice implications of the medical decisions that are made [10]. These conflicts lead to

J.M. O'Donnell, MBBS, FRACS, FAOrthA (✉)
Hip Arthroscopy Australia, St. Vincents Private Hospital, East Melbourne, Richmond, Victoria, Australia
e-mail: john@johnodonnell.com.au

M.G. Pritchard, BMedSci, MBBS(Hons), FRACS(Orth)
Wellington Orthopaedics, University of Tasmania, Calvary Hospital Hobart, St. Johns Campus CA, Hobart, Tasmania, Australia
e-mail: michael@wellingtonorthopaedics.com.au

M.S. Gobba, MD
Department of Orthopedics and Traumatology, Cairo University, Cairo, Egypt
e-mail: dr_mgobba@yahoo.com

G.C. Ozoude, MD
Orthopaedic Surgery, Sports Medicine, University of Texas Health Science Center at Houston, Houston, TX, USA
e-mail: george.ozoude@gmail.com

P.C. Noble, PhD
Director of Research, Institute of Orthopedic Research and Education, 6550 Fannin Street, Suite 2501, Houston, TX 77030, USA
e-mail: pnoble@bcm.edu

P.J. Singh, MBBS, MRCS, FRCS(Tr&Orth), MS, FRACS
Division of Orthopaedic Surgery, University of Ottawa, Ottawa, Ontario, Canada

Orthopaedic Surgery, The Ottawa Hospital, Ottawa, Ontario, Canada
e-mail: drparm@gmail.com

J.C. McCarthy et al. (eds.), *Hip Joint Restoration*, DOI 10.1007/978-1-4614-0694-5_58

an array of ethical dilemmas including patient confidentiality, the patient's right to informed consent, drug use and the use of emerging technology [6]. Many of these studies also highlight the absence of clear guidelines on the appropriate ethical behaviour of a sports team physician.

Clinical challenges also exist in managing hip conditions in elite athletes. Often, guidelines have not been clearly established for defining 'normal' recovery and return-to-play which makes it difficult to validate post-operative rehabilitation protocols. We don't always have clear-cut objective measures of recovery from musculoskeletal injury and must often depend upon the patient's evaluation of their own symptoms. This often places the team physician in the dilemma of deciding whether an athletic patient has healed faster than other patients in the general population, or whether an athlete with be exposed to an unacceptable risk of re-injury due to premature return to elite-level competition.

Nonetheless, hip arthroscopy has played a valuable role in the diagnosis and treatment of injuries involving the hip and limiting athletic performance. In the elite athlete, this has been shown to improve performance post-injury and accelerate return to sport. In this chapter we identify those factors which differentiate the treatment of elite athletes from other patients with hip complaints. General principles and procedures common to all patients will not be presented in any detail in this chapter and can be found elsewhere in this book.

Mechanisms for Loss of Performance with Hip Injury

Hip pathology and underlying bony morphology can dramatically affect the function of the hip during sporting activities. In a study looking at hip joint range of motion in elite female soccer players from the high school to the professional level, a decrease in internal rotation, external rotation and hip flexion was seen for professional athletes compared to all other groups (IR: 28° vs. 34°; ER: 40° vs. 56°; HF: 105° vs. 115°) [11]. The average values of hip range of motion for the professional athletes were also found to be decreased compared to a cohort of young adult non-athletes in a similar study from the same authors [12].

The first and most obvious factor impacting athletic performance is the presence of pain caused by intra-articular pathology of the hip joint, or surrounding structures. Thus, for example, a labral tear or chondral injury, a ligamentum teres tear, a psoas bursitis or tendon irritation or a gluteal strain or tear can cause enough pain to limit the function of the hip and reduce performance.

The second mechanism of reducing performance is a limitation of range of motion, as may occur with femoroacetabular impingement (FAI). Specific considerations regarding baseline hip morphology need to be considered when examining the elite athlete. Every athlete has an innate range of motion of their hip determined by bony structures, capsular structures and ligamentous structures. For every sport there will be a variation in the required range of motion required to compete the tasks of that particular sport at a high level. Patients with a decreased range of motion due to CAM deformity, pincer type impingement or acetabular overhang, femoral retroversion or acetabular retroversion, or other abnormalities relating to hip dysplasia will find that their best possible performance may be compromised, and they can attempt to compensate through other mechanisms.

Diminished range of movement of the hips may cause the stride length and speed of an athlete to be reduced. It may alter the biomechanics of cyclists so that their knees are no longer able to maintain a biomechanically strong position next to the top bar of the bike. An elite rower may find that their stroke is altered due to lack of flexion, resulting in overuse of the lumbar and thoracic spine, leading to rib stress fractures. There are many variations and permutations of this type of alteration in range of motion, which can affect sports.

In addition to this, athletes have different degrees of ligamentous laxity. There are athletes who have greater flexibility of the soft tissues in the form of ligamentous laxity which allow a greater freedom of movement of the joint before the check-rein effect of those soft tissues is applied to the joint. This check-rein effect will prevent the labral and articular structures of the hip colliding during range of motion. Those with increased laxity of their ligaments and capsule will have greater range of motion and may not have a check-rein effect which prevents them impinging on the acetabulum to the femur resulting in damage also.

The third major way an athlete's performance is diminished is more subtle, and is due to changes in muscle strength and balance. There is reduction in muscle strength of certain agonist and antagonist muscle groups within directions of movement. These alterations in muscle strength are affected through pain. Pain can be mediated through the labral structures, the chondral structures and sub-chondral bone and also the ligamentous structures around the hip including the ligamentum teres.

In our experience, the muscle groups first affected by pathological conditions involving the hip include psoas, the hip flexors, the adductors, tensor fasciae latae, and the gluteus medius. Certainly from a clinical point of view, these muscle groups are the first to become sore and have been shown to have decreased strength [13]. The external rotator muscles, particularly quadratus femoris, have also been shown to lose strength early which compromises their ability to stabilise the hip during movement of the prime muscle mover groups of the hip joint leading to abnormal kinematics [13]. An athlete will usually feel an increase in discomfort or tightness within the adductor, tensor fasciae latae, psoas and gluteus medius muscle groups. This perceived change in laxity may be related to fatigue rather than true loss of strength. It has been demonstrated previously that measured weakness in a hip joint, particularly through the adductors and external rotators, can be reversed with a local anaesthetic injection within the hip joint itself [13]. This then provides a pain pathway for these muscles' inhibition and perceived weakness.

Considerations Relating to Individual Sports

Several sports have been shown to be associated with a high incidence of symptomatic femoro-acetabular impingement (FAI), including ice hockey, Australian Rules football, other kicking sports such as soccer/football, and martial arts. Research studies performed in young, active adult men support the conclusion that the cam deformity of the femur develops during adolescence after long periods of repetitive loading during sporting activities during skeletal growth and maturation [14]. It has been suggested that large shear stresses developed at the head/neck junction during high-impact sports, such as basketball, ice hockey, and soccer, predispose the hip to development of the cam-type deformity [15]. However, definitive proof of this connection is still awaited. Other sports which involve extreme movement, such as ballet, dancing and gymnastics, tend to select athletes with more generalised ligamentous laxity, and sometimes acetabular dysplasia, as they tend to start off with an increased range of hip movements. With additional stretching they seem to be particularly prone to instability, ligamentum teres tears and labral tears.

Ice Hockey

Ice Hockey is a high contact sport in which players have a greatly increased risk of time loss injuries, especially of the hip [15]. Hip and groin injuries are a major cause of morbidity, with a cumulative incidence rate of 19.87 injuries per 100 players per year reported amongst players competing in the National Hockey League in the United States (NHL) [16]. In a similar study, Molsa et al. calculated the overall risk of injury amongst members of elite ice hockey teams in Finland to be 66 injuries per 1000 player-game hours [14].

Approximately 1 of 5 elite ice hockey players present with a painful hip during each season, compared to only 1.5 % of Swiss army recruits of a similar age, suggesting a 15-fold increase in relative risk of hip symptoms in those participating in ice hockey [17, 18]. Ice hockey athletes sought treatment at a mean age of only 15.5 years, which is younger than in any other sports, including basketball (17.6 years) [18]. The most common injuries presented by elite skaters are muscle strains and labral injuries. Adductor strains are particularly common and typically occur in athletes with an imbalance in the relative strength of the hip abductors and adductors [19].

The high risk of hip injury associated with the sport may be attributed to several factors, principally the prevalence of physical contact and high-energy collisions in professional competition, and the mechanical demands of skating as a repetitive physical activity. As a sporting activity, ice skating often imposes large forces on the hip in positions of internal and external rotation. During the sprint start, players push-off with the hip placed in external rotation and abduction, to be followed by internal rotation and increasing hip flexion during the recovery phase, placing the player in an 'at-risk' hip position [20]. Goaltenders, in particular, have been reported to be at an increased risk due to the unique style of joint position known as the butterfly technique in which the goaltender attempts to cover the goal net by 'laying out' their lower-leg pads. This is performed by kneeling on the ice with both femurs maximally internally rotated. Owing to the combined motions of hip flexion and internal rotation, the butterfly technique has been associated with the development of overuse hip injuries (FAI), especially in elite players [21].

As ice hockey places such extreme loads on the hip, and as so many athletes participate in the sport from childhood through adolescence to adulthood, there has been significant study of the interaction of sports participation and normal skeletal development [17, 18, 22]. In a descriptive study of 77 elite-level players from the recruitment programme of the first national ice hockey league of Switzerland, Siebenrock et al. reported the results of data obtained from a questionnaire, clinical examination, and magnetic resonance imaging [17]. These athletes showed an increased prevalence for a cam-type deformity of the proximal femur with 56 % of the cases having α angle in excess of 55° at some point around the circumference of the head-neck axis. Larger values of the α angle were observed in athletes with closed versus open physes (58° vs. 49°, respectively; $P<.001$), and in symptomatic versus asymptomatic athletes (62° vs. 52°; 1-o'clock position; $p<0.001$).

In ice skaters playing competitively, abnormalities of the femoral head-neck junction are seen at an early age. In a study of adolescent athletes (ages 10–18), Philippon et al. found a higher prevalence of cam-type FAI in ice hockey players compared to age-matched skiers leading them to suspect that unique properties of the sport lead to FAI pathology [23]. Overall, 75 % of the ice hockey players had an alpha angle >55°, compared to 42 % of the youth skiers. The α-angles were also found to increase with age in keeping with observations of players participating in several other sports.

With the growing popularity of ice hockey both at the youth and professional level, the prevalence of intra-articular hip injuries is expected to rise, not only impacting performance and longevity of players within the sport, but also increasing the risk of degenerative joint disease in the years after competing at the elite level. This suggests that radiographic screening of players prior to reaching elite competition may play a useful role in counselling players with increased risk of intra-articular damage.

American Football

In impact sports, as typified by American football, loading of the hip has been estimated to be up to 12 times body weight during competition, leading to a substantial incidence of hip injuries [24]. The 'sports hip triad' of soft tissue injuries is (labral tear, rectus strain, and adductor strain) commonly observed due to repetitive loading in flexion, abduction, and external rotation in combination with the presence of any abnormality of the femoral head-neck junction [24, 25]. When this occurs in combination with morphological alterations of the femur or acetabulum femoro-acetabular impingement may occur with restriction of joint motion and damage to the labrum and the acetabular rim [25].

Deformities of the femur and acetabulum are ubiquitous amongst elite footballers at both the collegiate and professional levels. Among college athletes being evaluated for recruitment into the National Football League (NFL) 94 % of those reporting hip pain also have radiographic indicators of FAI [26]. Similarly Larson et al. [25] noted that radiographic signs of FAI were seen frequently in collegiate-level NFL prospects, with 90 % having radiographic evidence of cam or pincer impingement. There was also a correlation between increased alpha angle and mixed cam/pincer impingement and the incidence of groin and hip pain. In a similar report, Kapron et al. presented the results of physical and radiographic examination of the hips of 67 Division 1A collegiate football players [27]. Using an alpha angle of 50° as the cut-off, 78 % of femora had at least one sign of a cam deformity (alpha angle >50° or anterior head offset <8 mm), and 95 % had at least one sign of a cam or pincer deformity.

Basketball

Hip pathology is frequently seen in elite basketball athletes, with a 15 % incidence reported for a positive anterior hip impingement test in combination with a history of hip pain [28]. The general hypothesis based on research on young, active adult men is that the cam deformity develops during adolescence after a long period of excessive sports practice during growth [28]. Recently, Siebenrock et al. showed that young basketball players are at higher risk for having a cam-type deformity, which developed especially around the time of physeal closure with a prevalence of 89 % in elite (national league) basketball players [28]. A comparison of basketball players of 8–28 years of age with age-matched non-sporting controls revealed no difference in the alpha angles of the youngest players when compared to controls. However, during puberty and young adulthood there was a progressive increase in the mean alpha angle of the athletic group with a concomitant loss of hip internal rotation in flexion.

Overhead Athletes

The high functional requirements of overhead athletes make them more prone to hip injury more than the usual spectrum of FAI [29]. One study has shown sports imposing high axial and torsional loads on the hips may predispose elite athletes to increased laxity leading to intra-articular pathology [31]. Most commonly, the joint is exposed to excessive external or internal rotational torque causing permanent stretching of the ilio-femoral or ischio-femoral ligaments respectively [30]. Forces leading to instability are often associated with manoeuvres involving hip rotation with rapid acceleration and deceleration [30, 32, 33]. In the presence of acquired capsular laxity this may cause excessive loading of the anterior-superior labrum leading to chondrolabral injury [32, 34].

Assessment—History, Examination and Investigations

In assessing the elite athlete, a careful history is required with a detailed review of the demands associated with each patient's sport, including the physical requirements of the position played in terms of range of motion, loading and strength.

In the early phases of hip dysfunction, patients often report a loss of strength around the joint, particularly in sprinting, jumping or kicking. There will be a reduction in performance, noticeable with sustained activity, and perhaps more evident when returning to the field after a short break in play. This is probably the first sign of pain inhibition of muscle contraction. The athlete may not voice specific complaints of groin pain, lateral hip pain, or discomfort. At this stage, temporary relief is often obtained using physical therapy and massage.

Patients may be unable to run due to discomfort felt through the anterior groin or anterolateral groin at the anterior boarder of the tensor fasciae latae, inferior to the anterior iliac spine. This may be the most common site of discomfort, radiating from the hip. Pain may also be felt through the adductor origin more medially, and laterally running posterior into the gluteals at the back. Patients will sometimes grasp their hip in a C sign. They may describe locking or jamming of the hip which could indicate loose bodies, articular flaps, labral instability or ligamentum teres tear. They may complain of an inability to flex the leg and straight leg raise which may indicate them having some psoas pathology. Their pain is not always present without activity thus careful description of their onset of pain, or discomfort or cause of decreased performance the history may need to be taken.

The examination of an elite athlete with hip pain should include appropriate functional assessment, such as an assessment of gait, hopping test or single leg squat. It may be helpful to stress the athlete (e.g. send them for a run) to provoke pain and then repeat these tests. Evaluation of the hip during the motions required for the patient's sporting activities is also critical. In some cases this necessitates examining the patient while they actually perform their sport. For example, in the case of a rower it may be necessary to see them in a boat to evaluate the range of hip flexion required to perform a full stroke. Pain may be elicited repeatedly during a part of the recurring movement cycle that the athlete performs. This will help in determining what part of the range of motion needs to be changed.

Physical examination should include palpation over the hip joint itself and the associated muscles. It should also include the inguinal canal to check for hernia and if the history suggests, an assessment of the testicular structures. An assessment should be made of the lumbar spine and particularly of the sacroiliac joints which can often be tender and inflamed in association with hip pathology. It is important to perform an accurate assessment of the range of motion of the hip with special tests for impingement and instability, including the FADIR (Impingement) test, the FABER test, and a ligamentum teres test.

Capsular injuries may be revealed by assessment of the leg in the resting position looking for signs of asymmetry particularly increased external rotation. The absence of a positive recoil sign (or Dial Test) may indicate capsular laxity or a tear. A positive apprehension test will provide further evidence to support such a diagnosis.

Radiographic Assessment

As for most patients, the first imaging study that should be requested is plain radiographs of the hips. These should comprise an AP standing view of both hips, a standard lateral of the affected hip and a Dunn view (90° flexion, 20° abduction) [30]. When a cam deformity is suspected, the shape of the femoral head neck junction may be evaluated using CT 3D surface reconstructions which allow bony lesions to be visualised and surgical resections planned (Fig. 58.1) [28]. In addition, if excessive anteversion or retroversion is suspected then a CT scan can be helpful to assess the version of the femoral neck [32, 33].

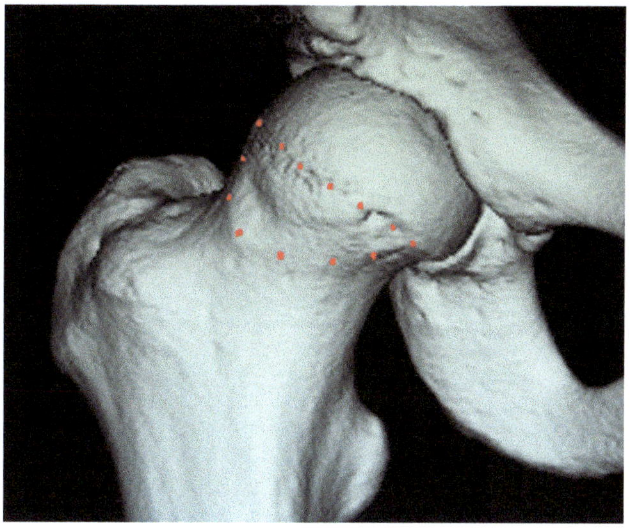

Fig. 58.1 A pre-operative plan showing the area of bone delineated for surgical resection

The CT protocol can be varied to allow the hip to be placed in positions eliciting symptoms. For example, a tennis player may describe pain provocation with extreme abduction, and this position can be reproduced in the scanner. Similarly, a football player may be scanned in a supine position with the hip flexed, adducted and internally rotated simulating a kicking type activity. This latter projection is termed the 'Position of Discomfort' (POD) view and is particularly useful for demonstrating FAI lesions and areas of impingement (Fig. 58.2) [34, 35].

MRI and MRA scans are also extremely useful to examine intra-articular structures in all patients [36–40]. In athletes, magnetic resonance imaging is also valuable for investigating extra-articular symptoms, particularly athletic pubalgia.

Ultrasound imaging may also be useful in the identification of muscle and ligament injuries, particularly when the individual performing the examination has extensive experience in the interpretation of ultrasound images of structures around the hip. When doubt remains about the origin of an athlete's pain, guided local anaesthetic injections may be extremely helpful and have been shown to be approximately 90 % accurate.

Surgical Treatment

Apart from normal operative planning, there are several additional factors to consider when treating elite athletes. It is important to remember that time off training and competition is of paramount importance. Athletes require early

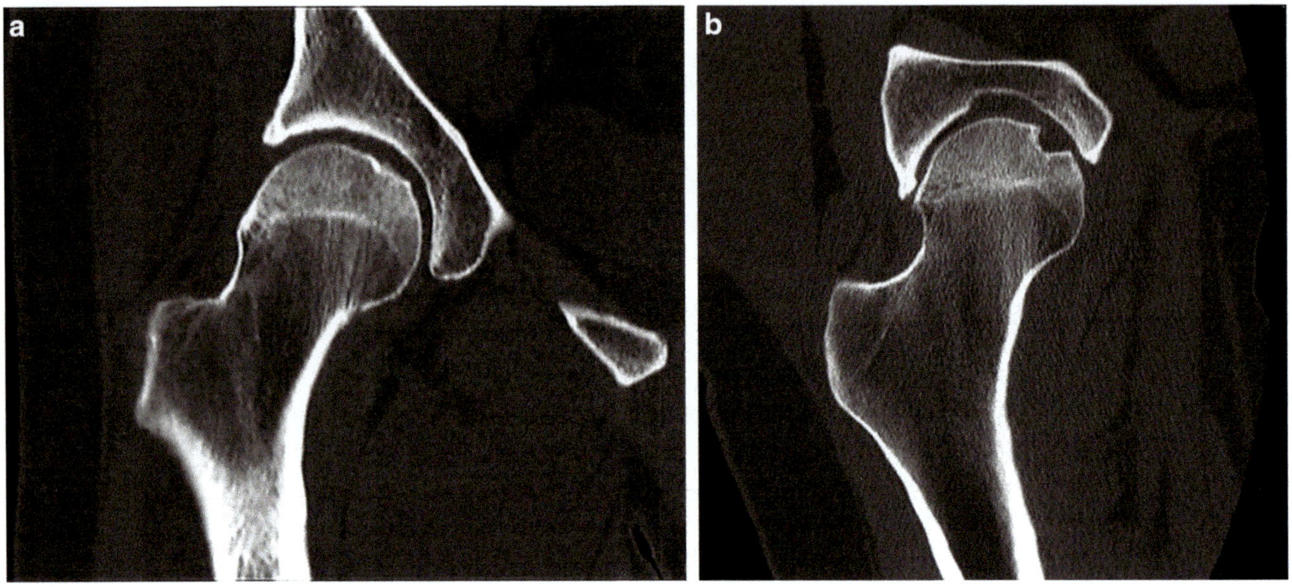

Fig. 58.2 (**a**) An axial CT slice taken through the hip of a patient with a typical cam deformity. A fibrocystic impingement lesion of the anterior head neck junction is seen but no evidence of joint space compromise (with thanks to Dr. James Linklater). (**b**) The same hip as in (**a**) scanned in the 'Position of Discomfort' (POD) position simulating a kicking activity. The scan reveals the impingement lesions and also confirms articular cartilage loss at the point of impingement

mobilisation, early return to function and early ability to continue with their usual fitness and strength regime. Also the timing of surgery is extremely important to minimise time away from sport. Sometimes it will be possible to continue competition until the end of season when surgery can be planned. This will largely depend on the level of impairment and pain that the athlete is experiencing, as well as the importance of the player to the team. At other times, the athlete will be so severely impaired that immediate surgery is required.

Under most circumstances, elite athletes will not accept extended periods away from competition. So, athletic patients will often refuse to undergo peri-acetabular osteotomies and femoral osteotomies for correction of version abnormalities because of the length of recovery and the uncertainty of whether the athlete will regain their previous level of performance. Sometimes a temporising procedure may be indicated to allow an athlete to finish a career before undertaking a more definitive treatment.

In any case, the athlete has already reached an elite level in their sport despite the presence of an underlying 'imperfection' in musculoskeletal anatomy or function. Thus it is possible to consider arthroscopic correction of an abnormality which is clearly impeding normal function without undertaking an extensive reconstruction of a joint to render the athlete theoretically perfect. The more minimalist approach will often be sufficient to enable the athlete to return to previous levels of activity with increased range of motion and decreased inhibition and loss of function, while still minimising the time away from their sport.

In keeping surgical procedures simple and minimal, pathological changes are repaired and optimised for healing. Intra-articular pathology is often secondary to a range of motion deficit which must be corrected to enable the athlete to avoid continuing problems. Thus, we do not routinely take down the labrum and resect rim unless significant labral damage is present. It is far more common for us to see a reduction in head neck offset or CAM lesions and for this to be resected with a debridement of the chondrolabral junction. Often in those athletes with CAM impingement, the acetabulum is more shallow than deep and thus a rim resection is not required in addition to substantial femoral bony resections.

To enable an adequate access to the femoral head neck junction, various techniques can be utilised. Our preference is to perform a limited capsulotomy, extending it where appropriate and repairing it if large. The capsule acts a substantial check rein to prevent further impingement event. A capsulectomy will require longer rehabilitation times to allow healing and maturation of the resulting scar tissue, and more risk for the athlete to return early.

Rehabilitation

Rehabilitation guidelines for both the elite athlete and the general population after FAI surgery are also not very prevalent in the literature at this time. Most of what is currently available is not firmly based in high level evidence and addresses the general population. Few studies specifically investigate rehabilitation in elite athletes. Philippon et al. [41] report the success of 4-phase programme in a case study of a professional football player. Cheathem et al. [42] describe the results of a case study involving an 18-year-old high school football player who underwent labral repair along with osteoplasty of acetabulum and femoral neck. Spencer-Gardner et al. [43] describe a 5-phase programme that was successful in a cohort of 52 patients; however it is unclear if these were elite-level athletes. Several other studies provide anecdotal literature about rehabilitation protocols after hip arthroscopy [44–46]. While these efforts can provide some platform in this emerging field, validation with well-controlled studies in elite athlete populations is needed.

The variations of hip morphology and function with respect to age, gender and sport must be taken into account when guiding rehabilitation protocols in elite athletes. Pierce et al. described a functional programme for ice hockey goaltenders, which can also be adapted to other on-ice positions, to assist in rehabilitation post-arthroscopic hip surgery with an expected on-ice return of 4 months [47]. The programme is divided into a four-phase rehabilitation protocol with six phases dedicated to an on-ice programme. The phases are athlete dependent, meaning that the individual athlete's rehabilitation abilities should be taken into consideration. The completion of the programme will be decided when the injured player obtains successful pass of a score higher than 17/20 or 20/20 (for professional athletes) in the Vail Hip Sports test without pain or swelling during drills.

As with any joint, physical therapy is an integral part of facilitating and optimising recovery after arthroscopic surgery of the hip. Several centres have developed specific rehabilitation protocols to use following arthroscopic hip surgery. There has been little work done yet to determine the relative merits of these different methods. Our method has been described elsewhere [47, 48].

Outcomes

Surgical treatment of the non-arthritic hip in athletes has become increasingly common over the past decade, with many players returning to their previous level of competitive athletic activity [47, 50]. Singh and O'Donnell reported the outcomes of treatment in 26 elite-level Australian Rules Football (AFL) players, with a minimum follow-up of 2 years (range: 2–8 years) [49]. All but 1 returned to play at, or above, their pre-injury level of performance. The mean modified Harris Hip Scores improved from 83.6 to 98, and Non-arthritic Hip Scores from 85 to 97, and these improvements were maintained for up to 8 years after surgery [51].

Many of the reports of outcomes in elite athletes have come from studies of arthroscopic treatment of FAI and labral lesions in professional ice hockey players. In this patient group, successful short-term outcomes have been reported with early return to practice and a prompt return to sport, with the time to participating in skating/hockey drills averaging 3–4 months following surgery. This recovery of performance has been associated with a substantial improvement in the Modified Harris Hip Score from a pre-operative value averaging 70 points to 95 points at an average of 24 months post-surgery. A large proportion of athletes treated with hip arthroscopy regain their original level of sporting competition after treatment. In one clinical study, 93 % of 45 professional ice hockey players returned to professional competition after arthroscopic treatment of FAI, with 78 % still paying professionally at 1.6 years after surgery [47]. In this study, the longer the delay in surgical treatment the greater the extent of chondral damage present at surgery and the more prolonged the period of recovery before players returned to play. On average, players who underwent hip arthroscopy more than 1 year after injury took an additional 1.1 months to return to sport than those having surgery less than 1 year after injury, which highlights the benefit of early intervention in management of professional hockey players.

Several studies have also focused on differences in the outcomes of elite versus recreational athletes after arthroscopic osteochondroplasty [52–55]. Malviya et al. found that professional athletes returned to their previous level of play at similar rates when compared to recreational athletes after arthroscopy for FAI, 88 % and 73 % respectively at 1 year ($P=0.09$), but did so significantly sooner as the average time to return was 4.2 versus 6.8 months, respectively ($P=0.03$) [53]. Similarly, in a systematic review involving studies on open and arthroscopic intervention, Alradwan et al. found rate of return-to-sport and return-to-previous level tended to be higher in professional athletes compared to recreational athletes, RTS: 95 % versus 87 %; RTPL: 92 % versus 84 %, respectively [54]. Although it is understood that socioeconomic motivations may drive professional athletes to return sooner to play, it is nonetheless important for a team physician to understand these trends and manage recovery expectations in elite athletes. In a similar vein, team physicians should be aware that professional athletes are less likely to report complications or poor outcomes while still active.

Conclusions

The findings reported in this chapter support future research to identify risk factors for developing intra-articular hip injuries to allow timely and effective efforts in both prevention and treatment. Additionally, the information contained in this article should allow physicians and athletic trainers to better counsel athletes and coaches regarding the nature and incidence of these injuries.

In this chapter we have endeavoured to identify deficits in hip function that are known to impact sports performance at the elite level. Our goal, as sports medicine physicians, is to correct these deficits when necessary whilst also trying to minimise time away from sport. This requires care in selecting the surgery to be undertaken so as to allow early, or accelerated, rehabilitation, without prolonged joint protection, but also to provide a durable, long-term solution.

References

1. Boyd JL. Understanding the politics of being a team physician. Clin Sports Med. 2007;26(2):161–72.
2. Goforth M, Almquist J, Matney M, et al. Understanding organization structures of the college, university, high school, clinical and professional settings. Clin Sports Med. 2007;26(2):201–26.
3. Johnson R. The unique ethics of sports medicine. Clin Sports Med. 2004;23(2):175–82.
4. Mathias MB. The competing demands of sport and health: an essay on history of ethics in sports medicine. Clin Sports Med. 2004;23(2):195–214.
5. Tucker AM. Ethics and the professional team physician. Clin Sports Med. 2004;23(2):227–41.
6. Dunn WR, George MS, Churchill L, et al. Ethics in sports medicine. Am J Sports Med. 2007;35(5):840–4.
7. Greenfield BH, West CR, et al. Ethical issues in sports medicine: a review and justification for ethical decision making and reasoning. Sports Health. 2012;4(6):475–9.
8. Anderson LC, Gerrard DF. Ethical issues concerning New Zealand sports doctors. J Med Ethics. 2005;31(2):88–92.
9. Bernstein J, Perlis C, Bartolozzi AR. Ethics in sports medicine. Clin Orthop Relat Res. 2000;378:50–60.
10. Gould MT, Hansted KT. The "fix" is in: legal and malpractice standards regarding the treatment of athletic injuries. Clin Sports Med. 2003;22(3):631–8.
11. Agel J, Dompier TP, Dick R, Marshall SW. Descriptive epidemiology of collegiate men's ice hockey injuries: National Collegiate Athletic Association Injury Surveillance System, 1988–1989 through 2003–2004. J Athl Train. 2007;42(2):241–8.
12. Tegner Y, Lorentzon R. Ice hockey injuries: incidence, nature and causes. Br J Sports Med. 1991;25(2):87–9.
13. Kemp JL, Schache AG, Makdissi M, Sims KJ, Crossley KM. Greater understanding of normal hip physical function may guide clinicians in providing targeted rehabilitation programmes. J Sci Med Sport. 2013;16(4):292–6.
14. Molsa J, Airaksinen O, Nasman O, Torstila I. Ice hockey injuries in Finland: a prospective epidemiologic study. Am J Sports Med. 1997;25:495–9.
15. Byrd JW. Femoroacetabular impingement in athletes: current concepts. Am J Sports Med. 2014;42(3):737–51.
16. Emery CA, Meeuwisse WH, Powell JW. Groin and abdominal strain injuries in the National Hockey League. Clin J Sport Med. 1999;9(3):151–6.
17. Siebenrock KA, Kaschka I, Frauchiger L, Werlen S, Schwab JM. Prevalence of cam-type deformity and hip pain in elite ice hockey players before and after the end of growth. Am J Sports Med. 2013;41:2308.
18. Reichenbach S, Jüni P, Werlen S, et al. Prevalence of cam-type deformity on hip magnetic resonance imaging in young males: a cross-sectional study. Arthritis Care Res (Hoboken). 2010;62(9):1319–27.
19. Tyler TF, Nicholas SJ, Campbell RJ, McHugh MP. The association of hip strength and flexibility with the incidence of adductor muscle strains in professional ice hockey players. Am J Sports Med. 2001;29(2):124–8.
20. Stull JD, Philippon MJ, LaPrade RF. "At-risk" positioning and hip biomechanics of the Peewee ice hockey sprint start. Am J Sports Med. 2011;39(1 suppl):29S–35.
21. Torry MR, Schenker ML, Martin HD, Hogoboom D, Philippon M. Neuromuscular hip biomechanics and pathology in the athlete. Clin Sports Med. 2006;25:179–97.
22. Murray RO, Duncan C. Athletic activity in adolescence as an etiological factor in degenerative hip disease. J Bone Joint Surg (Br). 1971;53(3):406–19.
23. Philippon MJ, Ho CP, Briggs KK, Stull J, LaPrade RF. Prevalence of increased alpha angles as a measure of cam-type femoroacetabular impingement in youth ice hockey players. Am J Sports Med. 2013;41(6):1357–62.
24. Feeley BT, Powell JW, Muller MS, et al. Hip injuries and labral tears in the National Football League. Am J Sports Med. 2008;36:2187–95.
25. Larson CM, Sikka RS, Sardelli MC, Byrd JW, Kelly BT, Jain RK, et al. Increasing alpha angle is predictive of athletic-related "hip" and "groin" pain in collegiate national football league prospects. Arthroscopy. 2013;29(3):405–10.
26. Nepple JJ, Brophy RH, Matava MJ, Wright RW, Clohisy JC. Radiographic findings of femoroacetabular impingement in National Football League Combine athletes undergoing radiographs for previous hip or groin pain. Arthroscopy. 2012;28(10):1396–403.
27. Kapron AL, Anderson AE, Aoki SK, Phillips LG, Petron DJ, Toth R, et al. Radiographic prevalence of femoroacetabular impingement in collegiate football players AAOS Exhibit Selection. J Bone Joint Surg. 2011;93(19):e111 1–10.
28. Siebenrock KA, Ferner F, Noble PC, Santore RF, Werlen S, Mamisch TC. The cam-type deformity of the proximal femur arises in childhood in response to vigorous sporting activity. Clin Orthop Relat Res. 2011;469(11):3229–40.
29. McCarthy J, Barsoum W, Puri L, Lee JA, Murphy S, Cooke P. The role of hip arthroscopy in the elite athlete. Clin Orthop Relat Res. 2003;406:71–4.
30. Meyer DC, Beck M, Ellis T, Ganz R, Leunig M. Comparison of six radiographic projections to assess femoral head/neck asphericity. Clin Orthop Relat Res. 2006;445:181–5.
31. Dolan MM, Heyworth BE, Bedi A, Duke G, Kelly BT. CT reveals a high incidence of osseous abnormalities in hips with labral tears. Clin Orthop Relat Res. 2011;469(3):831–8.
32. Dandachli W, Islam SU, Liu M, Richards R, Hall-Craggs M, Witt J. Three-dimensional CT analysis to determine acetabular retroversion and the implications for the management of femoroacetabular impingement. J Bone Joint Surg Br. 2009;91(8):1031–6.
33. Dandachli W, Islam SU, Tippett R, Hall-Craggs MA, Witt JD. Analysis of acetabular version in the native hip: comparison between 2D axial CT and 3D CT measurements. Skelet Radiol. 2011;40(7):877–83.
34. Haviv B, Singh PJ, Takla A, O'Donnell J. Arthroscopic femoral osteochondroplasty for cam lesions with isolated acetabular chondral damage. J Bone Joint Surg Br. 2010;92(5):629–33.
35. Grabinski R, Ou D, Saunder K, Rotstein A, Singh P, Pritchard M, et al. Protocol for CT in the position of discomfort: preoperative assessment of femoroacetabular impingement - how we do it and what the surgeon wants to know. J Med Imaging Radiat Oncol. 2014;58:649–56. doi:10.1111/1754-9485.12201.
36. Schmid MR, Notzli HP, Zanetti M, Wyss TF, Hodler J. Cartilage lesions in the hip: diagnostic effectiveness of MR arthrography. Radiology. 2003;226:382–6.
37. Kramer J, Recht MP. MR arthrography of the lower extremity. Radiol Clin North Am. 2002;40:1121–32.
38. Kassarjian A, Yoon LS, Belzile E, Connolly SA, Millis MB, Palmer WE. Triad of MR arthrographic findings in patients with

cam-type femoro-acetabular impingement. Radiology. 2005;236: 588–92.

39. Mintz DN, Hooper T, Connell D, Buly R, Padgett DE, Potter HG. Magnetic resonance imaging of the hip: detection of labral and chondral abnormalities using non-contrast imaging. Arthroscopy. 2005;21:385–93.
40. Byrd JW, Jones KS. Diagnostic accuracy of clinical assessment, magnetic resonance imaging, magnetic resonance arthrography, and intra-articular injection in hip arthroscopy patients. Am J Sports Med. 2004;32:1668–74.
41. Philippon MJ, Christensen JC, Wahoff MS. Rehabilitation after arthroscopic repair of intra-articular hip disorders of a professional football athlete. J Sports Rehabil. 2009;18(1):118–34.
42. Cheathem SW, Kolber MJ. Rehabilitation after hip arthroscopy and labral repair in a high school football athlete. Int J Sports Phys Ther. 2012;7(2):173–84.
43. Spencer-Gardner L, Eischen JJ, Levy BA, et al. A comprehensive five-phase rehabilitation programme after hip arthroscopy for femoroacetabular impingement. Knee Surg Sports Traumatol Arthrosc. 2013;22(4):849–59.
44. Wahoff M, Ryan M. Rehabilitation after hip femoroacetabular impingement arthroscopy. Clin Sports Med. 2011;30(2):463–82.
45. Enseki KR, Martin R, Kelly BT. Rehabilitation after arthroscopic decompression for femoroacetabular impingement. Clin Sports Med. 2010;29(2):247–55.
46. Edlestein J, Ranawat A, Enseki KR, et al. Post-operative guidelines following hip arthroscopy. Curr Rev Musculoskelet Med. 2012; 5(1):15–23.
47. Pierce CM, LaPrade RF, Wahoff M, O'Brien L, Philippon MJ. Ice hockey goaltender rehabilitation, including on-ice progression, after arthroscopic hip surgery for femoroacetabular impingement. J Orthop Sports Phys Ther. 2013;43(3):129–41.
48. Bennell KL, O'Donnell JM, Takla A, Spiers LN, Hunter DJ, Staples M, et al. Efficacy of a physiotherapy rehabilitation program for individuals undergoing arthroscopic management of femoroacetabular impingement - the FAIR trial: a randomised controlled trial protocol. BMC Musculoskelet Disord. 2014;15:58. doi:10.1186/1471-2474-15-58.
49. Larson CM, Pierce BR, Giveans MR. Treatment of athletes with symptomatic intra-articular hip pathology and athletic pubalgia/sports hernia: a case series. Arthroscopy. 2011;27(6):768–75.
50. Singh PJ, O'Donnell J. The outcome of hip arthroscopy in Australian Football League players. A review of 27 hips. Arthroscopy. 2010;26(6):743–9.
51. Amenabar T, O'Donnell J. Return to sport in Australian Football League Footballers after hip arthroscopy and midterm outcome. Arthroscopy. 2013;29(7):1188–94.
52. Philippon MJ, Zehms CT, Briggs KK, Manchester DJ, Kuppersmith DA. Hip instability in the athlete. Operat Tech Sports Med. 2007;15(4):189–94.
53. Byrd JW, Jones KS. Arthroscopic management of femoroacetabular impingement in athletes. Am J Sports Med. 2011; 39(Suppl):7S–13.
54. Malviya A, Paliobeis CP, Villar RN. Do professional athletes perform better than recreational athletes after arthroscopy for femoroacetabular impingement. Clin Orthop Relat Res. 2013;471(8): 2477–83.
55. Alradwan H, Philippon MJ, Farrokhyar F, et al. Return to preinjury activity levels after surgical management in femoroacetabular impingement in athletes. Arthroscopy. 2012;28(10):1567–76.

Special Patients and Conditions: Capsular Laxity Including Ehlers-Danlos

59

Lourenço P. Peixoto, Peter Goljan, Brian M. Devitt, and Marc J. Philippon

Introduction

As a ball and socket joint, the hip consists of the femoral head snugly fitting into the semi-hemispheric acetabular fossa. Surrounding the acetabulum is a fibrocartilaginous rim known as the acetabular labrum, which effectively increases the surface area and volume of the acetabular socket by up to 28.3 and 30 %, respectively [1, 2]. Within and surrounding the hip joint are the iliofemoral, pubofemoral, and ischiofemoral ligaments, as well as the zona orbicularis and ligamentum teres, all of which play a critical role as static stabilizers. The iliofemoral ligament is a band of great strength which lies across the anterior of the joint, and serves to strengthen the area between 12:45 and 3 o'clock [3]. Originating at the lower aspect of the anterior inferior iliac spine, the ligament commonly divides into two bands as it crosses the joint, one of which continues downward before attaching to the lower portion of the intertrochanteric line, while the other moves laterally as well as downward before attaching on the same line just proximal to the other band. A thin region of capsule commonly runs in the space between the two bands. In some anatomic variants no division occurs, and instead the ligament fans out into a flat triangular band which then attaches along the entire length of the intertrochanteric line. Due to its unique anatomic shape, this ligament is frequently referred to as the Y ligament of Bigelow, and it is the primary restraint to external rotation in all degrees of hip flexion and extension, accounting for more than 50 % contribution [4]. The lateral arm of the ligament also plays a small role as a secondary restrictor to internal rotation. The pubofemoral ligament arises from the obturator crest and superior ramus of the pubis, and inserts onto the intertrochanteric line, blending with the capsule as well as with the deep surface of the vertical band of the iliofemoral ligament. This ligament acts to limit the degree of external rotation in both flexion and extension of the hip, but it provides its greatest contribution (34 %) when the hip is fully extended. The ischiofemoral ligament consists of a triangular band of strong fibers which originate from the posterior ischium just inferiorly to the acetabulum, and inserts superiorly onto the femoral neck, blending with the circular fibers of the capsule. The main function of this ligament is restricting internal rotation in all degrees of hip flexion and extension. The ligamentum teres femoris is a triangular, somewhat flattened band originating at the anterosuperior aspect of the fovea capitis femoris, and divides into an anterior and posterior bundle before inserting directly adjacent to the transverse acetabular ligament on either side of the acetabular notch. The ligament tightens with flexion, adduction, and external rotation of the hip. The zona orbicularis is a circular structure formed by the terminal fibers of the iliofemoral ligament, and wrapping around the femoral neck just distally to the femoral head, it constitutes the narrowest area of the hip capsule. It is the most important structure for hip stability in distraction [5], effectively acting as a locking ring during the swing phase of gait.

Concerning the dynamic stabilizers of the hip joint, the two most important structures for stability are the iliocapsularis muscle and iliopsoas tendon. Originating from the inferior border of the anterior inferior iliac spine, the iliocapsularis muscle overlies the anteromedial hip capsule, and inserts onto the femur just distal to the lesser trochanter. When contracted, this muscle acts to tighten the hip capsule which in turn stabilizes the femoral head. The location of the iliopsoas tendon varies depending on hip position; it is intimately

L.P. Peixoto, MD • P. Goljan, MD • B.M. Devitt, MD, FRCSI
Center for Outcomes-Based Orthopaedic Research,
The Steadman Philippon Research Institute, Vail, CO, USA

M.J. Philippon, MD (✉)
The Steadman Clinic, Vail, CO, USA

Department of Surgery, McMaster University,
Hamilton, Ontario, Canada

Department of Orthopaedic Surgery, Unviersity of Pittsburgh
School of Medicine, Pittsburgh, PA, USA
e-mail: mjp@sprivail.org

J.C. McCarthy et al. (eds.), *Hip Joint Restoration*, DOI 10.1007/978-1-4614-0694-5_59

related to the anteromedial joint capsule when the hip is fully extended, but during hip flexion the tendon is displaced laterally across the iliopectineal eminence.

All of the aforementioned structures play an integral role in maintaining normal joint biomechanics, and the ability to accurately diagnose and treat any dysfunction among them is vital for the restoration of normal hip functionality. This is especially important in the case of recurrent hip instability secondary to the loss of static hip stabilizers such as the labrum and capsular ligaments, as contraction of the dynamic stabilizers is then the only remaining method available to maintain proper joint stability.

Atraumatic Instability

Atraumatic causes of hip instability include repetitive external rotation with axial loading, generalized ligamentous laxity, and collagen disorders such as Ehlers-Danlos. Due to the lack of a definable event, atraumatic hip instability symptoms often have an insidious onset.

Professional athletes who participate in sports requiring repetitive hip rotation with axial loading (e.g., golf, football, and ballet) can develop labral or ligamentous injuries within the hip that result in capsular redundancy and relative instability. When injuries to these static stabilizers of the hip occur, contraction of secondary stabilizers such as the psoas tendon and iliotibial band becomes necessary in order to attempt to maintain stability. Over time, this may lead to secondary problems such as psoas tendinitis, snapping of the iliopsoas or iliotibial band over bony prominences, or lateral hip pain from iliotibial band contracture. This highlights the challenge associated with diagnosing atraumatic hip instability, as patients can present with a wide array of hip symptoms while demonstrating only subtle findings suggestive of capsular laxity. Thus, a high degree of clinical suspicion must be combined with a detailed history, thorough physical examination, and appropriate imaging modalities [6].

Hyperlaxity states should be suspected in active patients presenting with symptoms of hip instability who lack a definable traumatic event or who do not participate in a sport which involves repetitive hip movement. The Beighton modification of the Carter and Wilkinson [7] scoring system is a helpful screening guide that can be utilized to diagnose a generalized hyperlaxity state. Within those patients with increased joint laxity, however, it is still essential to differentiate between idiopathic hyperlaxity and pathological forms such as Ehlers-Danlos syndrome. Patients suffering from this syndrome will often present with the characteristic triad of joint hypermobility, skin hyperelasticity, and fragility of the skin and blood vessels. The spectrum of clinical symptoms is very wide, however, with the mildest cases showing only a slight deviation from normal and the most severe presenting with life-threatening collagen tissue dysfunction and major disabilities secondary to widespread tissue deformity. The classic form of Ehlers-Danlos syndrome is an inheritable autosomal dominant disease, and the major diagnostic findings include skin hyperextensibility, widened atrophic scars (manifestation of tissue fragility), and multiple joint hypermobility. Minor diagnostic findings include positive family history, smooth velvety skin, molluscoid pseudotumors, subcutaneous spheroids, repetitive joint dislocations or subluxations, muscle hypotonia, delayed gross motor development, and manifestations of tissue fragility, such as easy bruising, hiatal hernia, anal prolapse in childhood, cervical insufficiency, and postoperative hernias. The classic Ehlers-Danlos syndrome will often display abnormal electrophoretic mobility of the proα1(V) or proα2(V) chains of collagen type V, but as of now, a highly sensitive screening method has not yet been developed, so the absence of detectible abnormalities by biochemical or molecular analysis does not necessarily rule out a defect in collagen type V.

When considering treatment options for hip instability, patients with a confirmed treatment utilizing either open or arthroscopic capsular plication should be seriously considered once patients have become symptomatic.

Traumatic Instability

Hip dislocations and subluxation are historically associated with high-energy mechanisms involving an external force exerted on the hip joint, such as with motor vehicle accidents, falls, and contact sports [8, 9]. These injuries are initially treated with urgent reduction, preferably closed, in an attempt to prevent osteonecrosis. Patients infrequently go on to develop recurrent anterior or posterior hip dislocation that necessitates surgical intervention. Anterior hip dislocations are relatively rare injuries, comprising approximately 9 % of all hip dislocations, and as initially described by Epstein, can be further classified as superior (inguinal) or inferior (obturator) [8]. Amongst cases of anterior dislocations, the inferior subset is more common and accounts for 92 %. Posterior dislocations of the hip are much more common, and usually occur secondary to direct or indirect trauma against a flexed and adducted hip joint.

Traumatic joint dislocation can also damage many of the surrounding structures of the hip. Philippon et al. showed that the most common intra-articular hip pathologies found at arthroscopy following a posterior dislocation were labral tears, chondral defects, and loose bodies [10]. In that study, the mean time from the initial traumatic event to when the patient underwent surgery was 125 days, and 14 % (2/14) of patients had capsular lesions that required repair at the time of surgery. Moorman et al. observed that in a cohort of seven patients who underwent an MRI of their hips acutely following joint subluxation, all seven had disruption of the iliofemoral ligament, posterior rim fracture, and evidence of hemarthrosis [11]. These results indicate that the iliofemoral ligament can be damaged acutely as a result of hip dislocation. Once damaged, symptoms of instability could potentially develop if the ligament is not allowed to heal properly, especially in highly active patients.

Following a hip dislocation, there must be a high degree of clinical suspicion regarding hip instability for any patient who fails the standard conservative protocol and in which osteonecrosis has already been excluded as the source of continued hip pain. It is also important to keep in mind the possibility of a labral or chondral lesion, intra-articular loose fragment, or ligamentum teres tear, as those are the most common intra-articular hip joint pathologies associated with dislocation, and could contribute to the symptoms of instability.

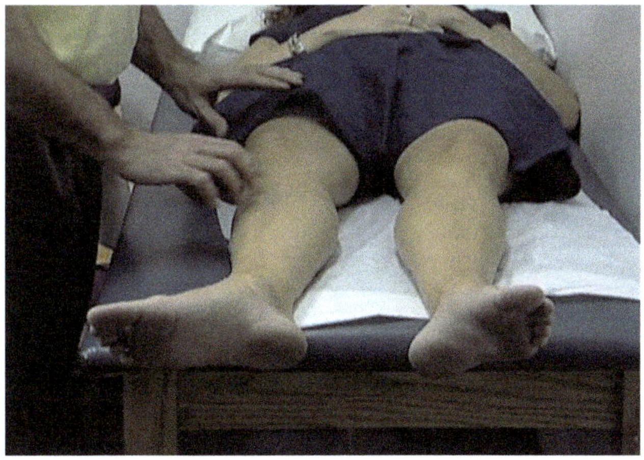

Fig. 59.1 Evidence of increased external rotation on hip dial test

Physical Exam

It is always important to rule out generalized hyperlaxity in any patient presenting with hip instability. Again, the Beighton modification of the Carter and Wilkinson [7] scoring system is a useful screening guide for diagnosing generalized hyperlaxity. Based on clinical experience, laxity can be classified into four categories (Table 59.1). Patients who present acutely following a traumatic episode of hip dislocation or subluxation will usually demonstrate both a painful and limited range of motion on physical exam. In comparison, patients with chronic hip instability may be able to voluntarily reproduce their instability mechanism in the examination room. During the physical exam, the pain associated with hip instability may be reproduced by stretching the capsular structures with passive extension and external rotation while the patient is in the prone position [12]. Range of motion (ROM) testing is critical in order to determine the functionality of both osseous and ligamentous structures. Internal and external rotation is commonly assessed in a supine or seated position, with the hip flexed to 90°. It can also be helpful to compare these values with those obtained while the hip is extended, which is performed in the prone position. In the flexed position, the medial and lateral bundles of the iliofemoral ligament, which controls external rotation, are relaxed. However, the dominant control for internal rotation, the ischiofemoral ligament, remains tight in both extension and flexion. ROM is dictated either by a firm endpoint or by patient pain [13]. The hip dial test should also be performed, as it is usually positive in the setting of an unstable hip (Fig. 59.1). In that test, the patient lies supine on the examination table and the examiner internally rotates the affected leg. The limb is then released and allowed to passively rotate externally. The test is considered positive if the leg externally rotates >45° from vertical in the axial plane and lacks a definitive end point. A positive axial distraction test may also be present, which can be confirmed by the presence of a vacuum sign on dynamic fluoroscopic examination.

Table 59.1 Classification system for hip laxity

Classification of hip laxity[a]		
Grade	Vacuum sign and/or laxity on axial distraction	Clinical feel
1 (mild)	No (negative pain on axial distraction test)	Soft end point
2 (moderate)	Yes (positive pain)	Laxity at 45°
3 (severe)	Yes (pistoning and pain)	Patient can demonstrate subluxation/dislocation (history of previous dislocation) No end point at 45°
4 (collagen disease)	Ehlers-Danlos syndrome, Down syndrome, Marfan syndrome	Upper extremities and lower extremity joint laxity

[a]Acetabular and femoral neck version must be taken into account

Radiographic and MRI Evaluation

Radiographs and magnetic resonance imaging (MRI) are required in order to effectively evaluate for intra-articular pathology of the hip. Our radiographic series includes supine anteroposterior pelvic, lateral cross-table, and false profile radiographs of the hip [13]. Radiographs are used to assess for acetabular retroversion, hip dysplasia, femoroacetabular impingement, as well as degenerative changes. The radiographic measurements obtained include the acetabular version, center-edge angle of Wiberg, joint space along the weight-bearing surface, Sharp's angle, and alpha angle [13]. Magnetic resonance imaging can be used to further characterize the presence of any avascular necrosis as well as impingement or labral pathology. When MRI is performed in the acute setting following traumatic dislocation it is possible to detect iliofemoral ligament rupture, labral tears,

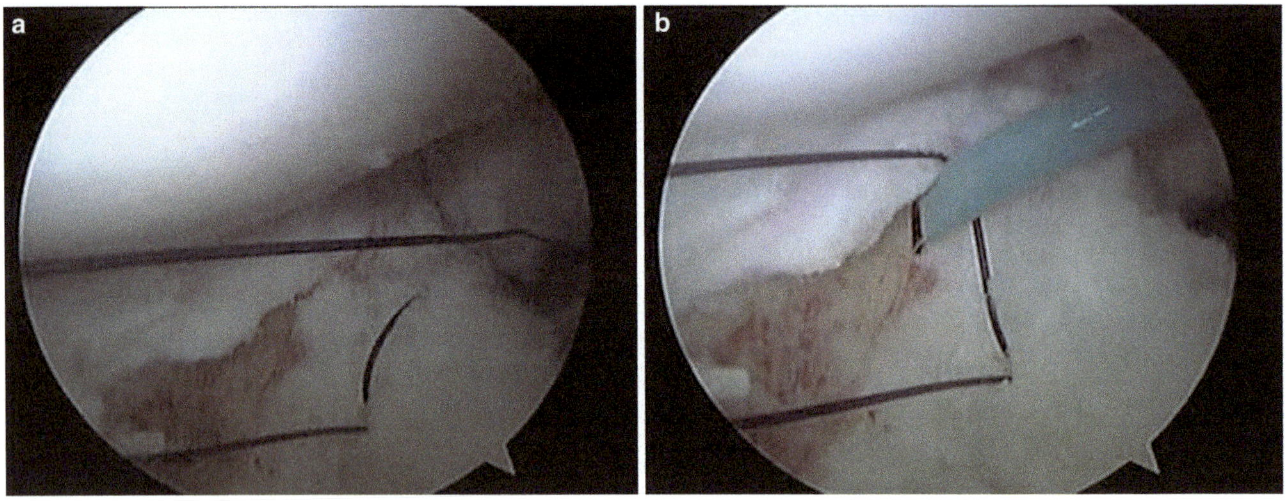

Fig. 59.2 Capsular plication. (**a**) Capsular suture placement, (**b**) Precise suture placement using ligament chisel

and hemarthrosis [11]. In patients with chronic atraumatic instability, it is possible to detect secondary capsular thickening anteriorly, which presents as increased signal intensity. In cases where the origin of pain is unclear, the use of injected anesthetic into the hip joint at the time of MRI can help confirm the source of pain as intra-articular.

Treatment

Patients who are evaluated acutely following a traumatic hip dislocation or subluxation are submitted to our standardized radiographic protocol. Clinical indications for acute surgical intervention consist of the radiographic presence of an intra-articular fragment or a posterior rim fracture of 30% or more. If no surgical indications are detected immediately, the patient is instructed to use crutches with only toe-touch weight-bearing allowed for 6 weeks. A physical therapy program is recommended to decrease the inflammation process as well as to strengthen the secondary hip restrictors. Magnetic resonance imaging is repeated 6 weeks after the initial episode of trauma, and if no avascular osteonecrosis is detected, the patient is allowed to gradually increase their activity level and return to play as tolerated.

If a patient fails to improve following a conservative management protocol, there should be an increased degree of suspicion regarding secondary hip pathologies such as labral tears or intra-articular loose bodies, as well as ligamentum teres, chondral, or capsular lesions, all of which must be addressed surgically [10].

Patients with suspected atraumatic hip instability should also undergo a trial of conservative management, consisting of modification of daily activities, nonsteroidal anti-inflammatories, and physical therapy. If the hip pain continues to persist despite conservative treatment, surgical intervention may be indicated in order to address any possible capsular laxity or labral tears. To treat capsular laxity we recommend capsular plication, in which the goal is to place sutures within the incised capsule to remove any redundancy and decrease the overall volume (Fig. 59.2). A curved suture-passing device is utilized to penetrate one of the capsular flaps, and the suture loop is then grasped by a penetrator through the opposite side. The stitches are then tied in standard arthroscopic fashion. Plication sutures are placed between the lateral arm of the iliofemoral ligament and the ischiofemoral ligament. Care must be taken not to overtighten the capsule, as that may lead to limitations in external rotation postoperatively.

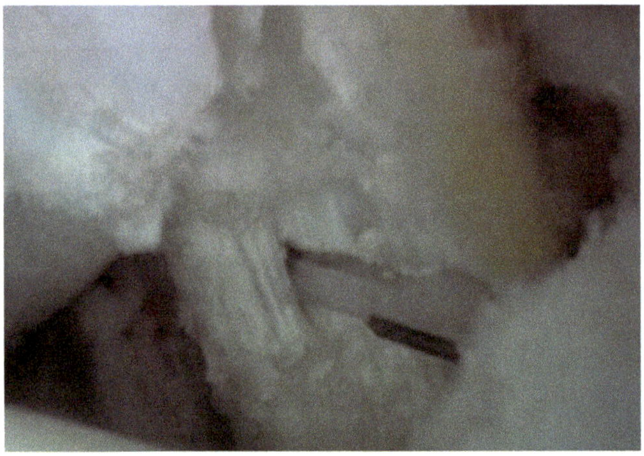

Fig. 59.3 Release of the iliopsoas tendon

At that time, either the psoas tendon or the iliotibial band may require surgical release, depending on the anatomic findings intraoperatively [14] (Fig. 59.3). Philippon et al. have already published good results utilizing thermal capsulorrhaphy in conjunction with partial labral resection in 12 patients treated for redundant or attenuated capsular tissue secondary to atraumatic hip instability [15]. Similarly, Epstein et al. have published a case report regarding recurrent anterior instability which was treated successfully by means of arthroscopic capsular plication and labral repair [16].

We emphasize the importance of diagnosing severely dysplastic hips preoperatively because in our experience these patients will usually benefit from surgical procedures to address their bony deformity, especially acetabular undercoverage. It is also critical to differentiate between idiopathic hyperlaxity and inherited collagen diseases, as those patients in the latter group require continued multidisciplinary medical treatment as well as careful consideration for capsular tightening when surgery is deemed necessary. In addition, there is a subset of instability patients who as a result of long-term alteration of the hip mechanics can develop concomitant femoroacetabular impingement, which then may be addressed along with the primary instability during surgery [17].

Conclusion

Considering the increasing number of patients diagnosed with hip instability each year, and the percentage of those patients who desire a therapeutic intervention in order to remain active, the treatment of hip instability has rapidly become a new frontier for arthroscopic surgeons. In our experience, the results obtained following arthroscopic treatment for hip instability indicate that the repair of the static hip stabilizers along with capsular plication is the correct and appropriate way to treat this pathologic occurrence. Further evidence-based research will help to clarify the most optimal long-term treatment for these conditions.

References

1. Tan V, Seldes RM, Katz MA, Freedhand AM, Klimkiewicz JJ, Fitzgerald Jr RH. Contribution of acetabular labrum to articulating surface area and femoral head coverage in adult hip joints: an anatomic study in cadavera. Am J Orthop. 2001;30:809–12.
2. Seldes RM, Tan V, Hunt J, Katz M, Winiarsky R, Fitzgerald RH. Anatomy, histologic features, and vascularity of the adult acetabular labrum. Clin Orthop Relat Res. 2001;382:232–40.
3. Telleria JJM, Lindsey DP, Giori NJ, Safran MR. An anatomic arthroscopic description of the hip capsular ligaments for the hip arthroscopist. Arthroscopy. 2011;27:628–36.
4. Martin HD, Savage A, Braly BA, Palmer IJ, Beall DP, Kelly B. The function of the hip capsular ligaments: a quantitative report. Arthroscopy. 2008;24:188–95.
5. Ito H, Song Y, Lindsey DP, Safran MR, Giori NJ. The proximal hip joint capsule and the zona orbicularis contribute to hip joint stability in distraction. J Orthop Res. 2009;27:989–95.
6. Smith MV, Sekiya JK. Hip instability. Sports Med Arthrosc. 2010;18:108–12.
7. Carter C, Wilkinson J. Persistent joint laxity and congenital dislocation of the hip. J Bone Joint Surg (Br). 1964;46:40–5.
8. Epstein HC. Traumatic dislocations of the hip. Clin Orthop Relat Res. 1973;92:116–42.
9. Tornetta P. Hip dislocations and fractures of the femoral head. In: Bucholz RW, Heckman JD, Court-Brown C, Tornetta P, Koval KJ, Wirth MA, editors. Rockwood and Green`s fractures in adults. 5th ed. Philadelphia, Pennsylvania: Lippincott Williams & Wilkins; 2002. p. 1547–78.
10. Philippon MJ, Kuppersmith DA, Wolff AB, Briggs KK. Arthroscopic findings following traumatic hip dislocation in 14 professional athletes. Arthroscopy. 2009;25:169–74.
11. Moorman CT, Warren RF, Hershman EB, Crowe JF, Potter HG, Barnes R, et al. Traumatic posterior hip subluxation in American football. J Bone Joint Surg Am. 2003;85:1190–6.
12. Tibor LM, Sekiya JK. Differential diagnosis of pain around the hip joint. Arthroscopy. 2008;24:1407–21.
13. Philippon MJ, Maxwell RB, Johnston TL, Schenker ML, Briggs KK. Clinical presentation of femoroacetabular impingement. Knee Surg Sports Traumatol Arthrosc. 2007;15:1041–7.
14. Shindle MK, Ranawat AS, Kelly BT. Diagnosis and management of traumatic and atraumatic instability in the athletic patient. Clin Sports Med. 2006;25:309–26.
15. Philippon MJ. The role of arthroscopic thermal capsulorrhaphy in the hip. Clin Sports Med. 2001;20:817–29.
16. Epstein DM, Rose DJ, Philippon MJ. Arthroscopic management of recurrent low energy anterior hip dislocation in a dancer. A case report and review of literature. Am J Sports Med. 2010;38: 1250–4.
17. Ranawat AS, McClincy M, Sekiya JK. Anterior hip dislocation after hip arthroscopy in a patient with capsular laxity of the hip. A case report. J Bone Joint Surg Am. 2009;91:192–7.

Current Procedures and Techniques for the Treatment of Osteonecrosis of the Hip

60

Samik Banerjee, Bhaveen H. Kapadia, Jeffrey J. Cherian, and Michael A. Mont

Introduction

Osteonecrosis of the hip is a devastating condition, which typically affects the young and active population in their third to fifth decades of life. To diagnose patients who present early in the natural history of the disease, an understanding of the various associated risk factors for osteonecrosis is essential. These risk factors and the etiopathogenesis in the development of osteonecrosis have been elaborated in detail in a previous chapter. Formulating an optimal treatment plan for osteonecrosis requires a thorough history, physical examination, and radiographic evaluation. Once a diagnosis is made it is imperative to classify the disease-based size of the lesion, amount of depression, extent of depression, presence of acetabular involvement, and existence of arthritis [1]. The primary goal of treatment for early stage osteonecrosis is joint preservation; thus, it is imperative to diagnose the condition as soon as possible and prevent progression to articular surface collapse. Development of articular surface collapse is a critical step in the pathophysiology of the disease and has been associated with pain, progression to secondary degenerative arthritis, and the need for total hip arthroplasty. Although a multitude of nonsurgical and surgical treatment options are currently available, there are no gold standards for treating this condition, and management of these patients often constitutes a therapeutic challenge. This chapter aims to provide an algorithm to aid in the diagnosis and optimize surgical management of patients who are diagnosed with osteonecrosis of the hip.

S. Banerjee, MD • J.J. Cherian, DO • M.A. Mont, MD (✉)
Rubin Institute for Advanced Orthopedics, Center for Joint Preservation and Replacement, Sinai Hospital of Baltimore, 2041 West Belvedere Avenue, Baltimore, MD 21215, USA
e-mail: mmont@lifebridgehealth.org; Rhondamont@aol.com

B.H. Kapadia, MD
Rubin Institute for Advanced Orthopedics, Center for Joint Preservation and Replacement, Sinai Hospital of Baltimore, 2041 West Belvedere Avenue, Baltimore, MD 21215, USA

Department of Orthopaedic Surgery and Rehabilitation Medicine, State University of New York (SUNY) Downstate Medical Center, Brooklyn, NY, USA
e-mail: bhaveen.k@gmail.com

Patient Evaluation

History

Elaborate history taking is crucial, as with any other diagnosis. Various associated factors that have been postulated to have a cause-and-effect relationship in the development of osteonecrosis of the hip need to be considered when eliciting the history. These have been elaborated in a previous chapter.

Clinical Features

Patients typically present with groin pain, which increases on weight bearing, although the disease can be clinically silent in the early stages of the disease. A small percentage of patients can present with nonspecific symptoms of trochanteric or buttock pain or referred pain to the knee. The groin pain is typically described as deep, throbbing, intermittent pain that is usually insidious, although sometimes it can be sudden. Usually these symptoms precede any radiographic changes and a high index of suspicion, especially in a susceptible patient, is crucial for early diagnosis.

Physical Examination

Physical examination in the early stages of the disease may be unremarkable or reveal anterior hip joint tenderness or subtle loss of motion, particularly internal rotation. Muscle wasting in the thigh and buttock may be present and occasionally clicking of the joint may be elicited when collapse is present.

J.C. McCarthy et al. (eds.), *Hip Joint Restoration*, DOI 10.1007/978-1-4614-0694-5_60

However, fixed deformities and leg length discrepancy may occur as the disease advances. A thorough and systematic examination of the opposite hip joint is essential as the disease can be bilateral in 40–80 % of cases. Moreover, about 10 % of patients may present with other joint involvement, especially in the presence of systemic risk factors (for e.g., corticosteroid use) and examination of other joints is essential to avoid missing early stage disease in the remaining joints [2].

Diagnosis

Definitive diagnosis requires radiographic imaging. The two commonly performed investigations for diagnosis of osteonecrosis of the hip are plain radiographs and magnetic resonance imaging [3].

Plain Radiographs

Plain radiographs are the first investigation performed after history and physical examination (Fig. 60.1). Two orthogonal radiographic views (antero-posterior and frog-leg lateral) should be commonly obtained. It is also essential to obtain images of the opposite hip due to bilaterality of involvement in a high percentage of cases. However, as early radiographic changes in the form of cysts, sclerosis, or a "crescent sign" usually take many months to appear after disease onset, it is not a sensitive test for early stage disease. Once radiographic diagnosis is made, it is essential to estimate the size, determine the location of the lesions, and calculate the Kerboul's combined necrotic angle. Kerboul's angle is defined as the combined arc of surface involvement of osteonecrosis in antero-posterior and lateral radiographs and is graded as small (<150°), medium (150–200°), and large (>200°) [4]. It is also critical to evaluate the presence of subchondral fracture, acetabular involvement, and degenerative arthritis [5]. These factors are important for classifying the disease and formulating a plan of management [1].

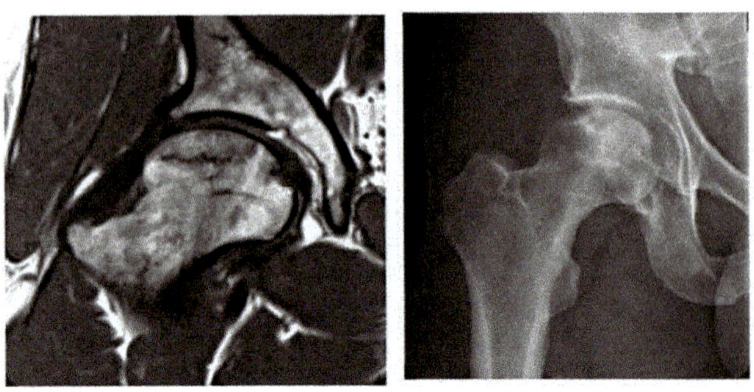

Fig. 60.1 Magnetic resonance imaging (*left*) and antero-posterior radiograph (*right*) of a 39-year-old female with Ficat and Arlet Grade III osteonecrosis of the right femoral and acetabulum. Used with permission from Sinai Hospital of Baltimore, Inc

Magnetic Resonance Imaging

It is one of the most sensitive and specific imaging modalities used for the diagnosis of osteonecrosis of the hip and is considered the next line of investigation in the presence of strong clinical suspicion and lack of radiographic findings (Fig. 60.1) [6]. Magnetic resonance scans have reported sensitivities in the range of 80–100 %, which is considered to be higher than other contemporary imaging tests such as plain radiographs, computed tomography scans, and nuclear scintigraphy. Moreover, its specificity in differentiating other hip pathologies from osteonecrosis is also reported to be very high, which makes it the modality of choice. A double line signal on T2-weighted images is virtually diagnostic of osteonecrosis, while a single density line surrounding the osteonecrotic lesion in T1-weighted image is considered highly specific for the diagnosis. In addition to the diagnosis, MRI scans can be used to assess the extent of involvement (MRI estimation of the Kerboul's angle), condition of the acetabular and femoral head cartilage, the presence of a labral lesion, and revascularization of the lesions following treatment which may predict the prognosis and guide further treatment. Ancillary tests such as bone marrow pressure measurements, bone biopsy, or venography are rarely performed due to their invasive nature and the high accuracy of MRI scans. Similarly, bone scans are no longer recommended and have limited value due to their lack of accuracy and high false negative rates between 25 and 45 %.

In conclusion, when clinical suspicion remains high after a thorough history and physical examination, a low threshold for ordering an MRI is needed to diagnose this condition early. Staging of the disease based on radiographs and MRI scans is essential to counsel patients about the prognosis and guide appropriate treatment.

Differential Diagnosis

Transient osteoporosis of the hip, a self-limiting condition, is one of the most important conditions to consider in the differential diagnosis that closely resembles osteonecrosis. Patients with transient osteoporosis are usually men in their fifth or sixth decades of life or it is found to occur in women in their third trimester of pregnancy. These patients often present with an antalgic hip and complain of severe pain in their groin. Magnetic resonance imaging often shows presence of bone marrow edema in the femoral neck and the metaphyseal region of the proximal femur, which rarely occurs with osteonecrosis. However, these patients need to be carefully followed up until resolution of their symptoms, as 2–5 % of patients who initially had transient osteoporosis may go on to develop osteonecrosis of the hip.

Staging of Osteonecrosis

A number of classification systems are currently available to stratify patients according to radiographic stage. This is essential to guide further management and also to compare outcomes of various modalities of treatment. Of these, the Ficat and Arlet, Japanese Investigation Committee on osteonecrosis, Steinberg, University of Pennsylvania, and the ARCO classification systems have been more commonly used [7]. The common theme in all the classification systems is the recognition of subchondral fracture and development of collapse as a crucial point in the radiographic staging of the disease, beyond which rapid and relentless disease progression occurs, leading to the development of degenerative arthritis. However, it is also essential to identify the size of the lesions (for e.g., <15, 15–30, and >30 % head involvement), location of the lesion (medial, central, and lateral), and extent of depression (<2, 2–5, and >5 mm) as the overall prognosis may vary based on lesion characteristics.

The Ficat and Arlet classification system is based on radiographic findings and describes the four stages of the natural history and progression of the disease (Table 60.1). This classification describes the four stages of the natural history of the disease and its progression. In the preradiographic stage, the patient often has clinical symptoms suggestive of osteonecrosis; however, no radiographic signs are present. Radiographic stage II disease is diagnosed in the presence of multiple cysts and sclerotic regions in the femoral head. A crescent sign, when present, marks the transition between stage II and stage III disease and represents the occurrence of subchondral fracture. Collapse and flattening of the head is found in stage III disease, while presence of degenerative changes with loss of joint space signifies stage IV disease. The Steinberg classification is a more exhaustive classification that takes into account the extent of collapse and the presence of acetabular involvement, and is based on both plain radiographic and magnetic resonance imaging (MRI). The Japanese Orthopaedic Association classification included the location of the lesion, while the ARCO classification included both extent of involvement and location of the lesions as a guide to treatment (Table 60.2). Even though we classify these lesions, we typically utilize the presence or absence of a few radiographic features to plan for treatment (please see patient considerations section).

Table 60.1 Ficat and Arlet staging

Ficat and Arlet staging	Radiographic findings
1	None (only evident on magnetic resonance images)
2	Diffuse sclerosis, cysts (visualized on radiographs)
3	Subchondral fracture (crescent sign)
4	Femoral head collapse, acetabular involvement, and joint destruction (osteoarthritis)

Table 60.2 ARCO staging of osteonecrosis

Stage	Findings	Techniques	Subclassification	Quantification
0	None	Radiography, computed tomography, scintigraphy, magnetic resonance imaging	NO	NO
1	Radiography and computed tomography normal. At least ONE of the other techniques is positive	Scintigraphy, magnetic resonance imaging	Location of lesion Medial Central Lateral	Area of involvement (percentage) A: Minimal (<15 %) B: Moderate (15 % to 30 %) C: Extensive
2	Sclerosis, osteolysis, focal porosis	Radiography, computed tomography, scintigraphy, and magnetic resonance imaging	Location of lesion Medial Central Lateral	Area of involvement (percentage) A: Minimal (<15 %) B: Moderate (15 % to 30 %) C: Extensive
3	CRESCENT SIGN and/or flattening of articular surface	Radiography and computed tomography	Location of lesion Medial Central Lateral	Length of crescent A: <15 % B: 15 % to 30 % C: >30 % Surface collapse and dome depression A: <15 % and <2 mm B: 15 % to 30 % and 2 mm to 4 mm C: >30 % and >4 mm
4	Osteoarthritis, acetabular changes, joint destruction	Radiography only	NO	NO

Staging System of Steinberg

IA:	Mild (<15 % of femoral head affected)
IB:	Moderate (15–30 % of femoral head affected)
IC:	Severe (>30 % of femoral head affected)
II	Cystic and sclerotic changes in the femoral head
IIA:	Mild (<15 % of femoral head affected)
IIB:	Moderate (15–30 % of femoral head affected)
IIC:	Severe (>30 % of femoral head affected)
III	Subchondral collapse (crescent sign) without flattening
IIIA:	Mild (<15 % of femoral head affected)
IIIB:	Moderate (15–30 % of femoral head affected)
IIIC:	Severe (>30 % of femoral head affected)
IV	Flattening of femoral head
IVA:	Mild (<15 % of surface and <2-mm depression)
IVB:	Moderate (15–30 % of surface or 2- to 4-mm depression)
IVC:	Severe (30 % of surface)
V	Joint narrowing and/or acetabular changes (this stage can be graded according to severity)
VI	Advanced degenerative changes

Surgical Management

Patient Considerations

An assessment of the age, activity levels, disease etiology, type of prior treatment, bilaterality of involvement, and health status is essential to individualize treatment for this condition. In young and active patients, all efforts should be directed towards head salvage, and if that is not possible, consideration should be given towards choosing the appropriate bearing surface and fixation interface to improve implant longevity when performing a total joint arthroplasty. Disease etiology also needs to be taken into consideration when planning treatment as some of these may predispose patients to further complications. For example patients with human immunodeficiency virus infections may have risks for wound infection and delayed wound healing.

Many of the affected patients are young and may often undergo multiple head preserving procedures in their lifetime and these may need to be considered when planning further treatment. Although prior core decompression or multiple drilling rarely affects the outcome of future arthroplasty procedures, distortion of the morphology of the proximal femur after proximal femoral osteotomy or vascularized fibular grafting may increase the complexity of primary total hip arthroplasty in these patients. As the disease is often bilateral and patients may need bilateral total hip arthroplasty, it may be beneficial to consider deferring further treatment on the opposite hip until rehabilitation of the operated hip is complete. However, if the opposite hip is in early stage and may need a less extensive procedure, such as multiple drilling, both the procedures can be performed simultaneously in one sitting. Commonly, the more severely affected hip is treated first, unless the opposite hip is in early stage and necessitates prompt treatment to prevent collapse. The presence of a severe systemic disease or limited life expectancy may preclude a head salvaging procedure and the tip the balance in favor of a definitive procedure (for e.g., a total hip arthroplasty). Thus, treatment may need to be tailored according to patient demands, demographics, lifestyle needs, and activity.

Our selection, most often, is based on a number of radiographic features over any other patient demographic factors. The four radiographic features we typically use are (1) pre- or post-collapse; (2) size of the lesion; (3) size of the head depression (>2 mm vs. <2 mm); and (4) acetabular involvement (or evidence of arthritis). A joint-preserving procedure is classically indicated for pre-collapse, small- to medium-sized lesions. However, in the presence of marked cartilage delamination, large lesions, substantial head depression (>2 mm), acetabular involvement, or degenerative arthritis, total joint arthroplasty remains the only reliable treatment option. In the sections below, a broad overview is provided regarding the surgical treatment options for atraumatic osteonecrosis of the hip. The various techniques described are as follows: (1) core decompression and multiple drilling; (2) bone grafting procedures; (3) proximal femoral osteotomies; (4) resurfacing arthroplasty; and (5) total hip arthroplasty.

Head Preserving Procedures

Core Decompression

Initially described by Ficat and Arlet in 1964 as a diagnostic procedure, core decompression alone or in combination with bone grafting is commonly performed today as a therapeutic procedure for osteonecrosis of the femoral head. It is based on the principle that it leads to a reduction in intraosseous hypertension, which is often present during the early stages of the disease process. This decrease in intraosseous pressure leads to an improvement in the blood flow to the ischemic zone which aids the reparative process of new bone formation in the necrotic region. In addition to the increase in blood flow, it is believed that removal of a core of tissue relieves pain and stimulates vascular ingrowth that aids in healing of these lesions.

Despite its universal acceptance as a surgical option for early stage lesions, its efficacy in the presence of potential adverse risk factors, such as head involvement of >50 %,

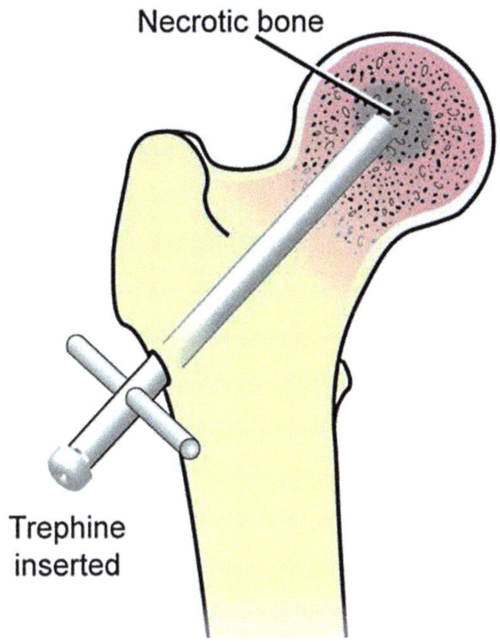

Fig. 60.2 Core decompression technique. Used with permission from Sinai Hospital of Baltimore, Inc

affection of the weight-bearing dome, presence of collapse ≤2 mm, and sickle cell disease, is debatable. However, when the indications are restricted to small size (<50 % head involvement) Ficat Arlet Stage I and II lesions and Kerboul's combined necrotic angles <200°, favorable outcomes may be achieved with core decompression [8–10]. The standard technique of core decompression as described by Ficat and Arlet involves drilling the femoral head with a large diameter (8–10 mm) reamer or trephine under fluoroscopic guidance to remove a core of tissue from the center of the necrotic region in order to relieve the intraosseous pressure within the femoral head (Fig. 60.2). However, drilling such a large diameter bore within the femoral head can substantially weaken the femoral head and increase the risks of head penetration and subtrochanteric fractures.

Various modifications to the classical technique, such as the Steinberg technique and the multiple drilling technique as popularized by Kim et al. [11] and Mont et al. [12], have been described to decrease these risks. The Steinberg technique involves drilling two additional 6 mm holes in the head to remove core tissues from the periphery of the lesion, although there remains a single external entry point in the lateral cortex. The viable bone harvested from the trochanteric region during this process is loosely packed into the central core. In the multiple drilling technique described by Song et al. [13], a 3.2 mm drill bit is used to make 1–8 drill holes in the osteonecrotic region of the femoral head, while Mont et al. [12] used 1–3 drill holes into the osteonecrotic region.

Historically, core decompression has been one of the most common procedures performed for early stage osteonecrosis, with success rates varying between 40 and 80 % (Table 60.3) [14, 15]. In a systematic review of 2605 hips, Marker et al. compared the outcomes of core decompression in osteonecrotic hips operated prior to 1992 ($n = 1337$ hips) to those who had undergone surgery after this period ($n = 1268$ hips) [16]. The authors reported that the mean rates of additional surgery were significantly lower in patients operated with modern techniques after 1992 compared to comparison controls (30 % versus 41 %; $p < 0.05$). In addition, the authors found that higher rates of clinical failure and radiographic progression in patients with stage III lesions compared to early stage disease.

In another systematic review, Rajagopal et al. found that the risk of progression to THA varied according to radiographic stage. Ficat stage I lesions had a 0–17 % risk, stage II lesions had a 17–44 % risk, and stage III lesions had a 66 % risk of conversion to total hip arthroplasty [8]. Israelite et al. evaluated the outcomes of simultaneous bilateral core decompressions in 152 osteonecrotic hips in University of Pennsylvania staging I to IV, at a mean follow-up of 56 months (range, 24–136 months) [17, 18]. The authors found that the 32 % of hips with bilateral disease required conversion to total hip arthroplasty at final follow-up.

In a report of 45 hips with Ficat stage I to II osteonecrosis, Mont et al. found an overall success rate of 71 % (32 out of 45 hips) following multiple drilling at a mean follow-up of 2 years (range, 1.7–3.3 years) [19]. The authors found that stage I hips with small- to medium-sized lesions (<50 % lesion size) were more likely to have better outcomes than those with stage II disease with large sized lesions (80 % versus 57 %). Similarly, Song et al. [13] also reported success rates of 88 % (52 out of 59 hips) in small- to medium-sized lesions with multiple drilling at a mean follow-up of approximately 7 years (range, 5–11.2 years).

In summary, core decompression appears to be beneficial in relieving pain and preventing radiographic progression in patients who have early stage, small sized, pre-collapse lesions. It is believed that the outcomes of core decompression may be improved with the addition of bone graft substitutes and growth factors that aid in healing of the osteonecrotic lesions through their osteoinductive and angiogenic properties. Moreover, due to the high incidence of bilaterality (up to 60 %) in this condition, it may be advisable to simultaneously treat both sides to prevent progression of the disease. Recently, the technique of multiple drilling has gained in popularity as a simpler, less invasive alternative to the traditional technique of core decompression. However, further research is needed to explore these options.

Bone marrow instillation and mesenchymal stem cell therapy have been used to fill defects following core decompression procedures with the aim of augmenting the repair

Table 60.3 Outcomes of core decompression

Author (year)	Level of evidence	Hips				Mean age (years)	Follow-up (years)	Survivorship (%)			Survivorship
		Stage 1	Stage 2a	Stage 2b	Stage 3			Stage 1	Stage 2a	Stage 2b	Stage 3
Al Omran et al. [96] (2013)	III	13	25	23	–	26	6.1	100	80	52	–
Lieberman et al. [97] (2004)	IV	–	15	1	1	47	4.4	–	93	0	0
Aigner et al. [98] (2002)	IV	30	9	-	6	41	5.7	97	44	–	33
Lavernia et al. [99] (2000)	IV	15	30*	–	22	40.2	3.4	100	83*	–	44
Maniwa et al. [100] (2000)	IV	10	16*	–	–	46	7.8	100	56.4*	–	–
Bozic et al. [101] (1999)	IV	12	12	2	0	38	10	92	52	20	0
Iorio et al. [102] (1998)	IV	7	20	6	–	41	5	71	45	33	–
Powell et al. [103] (1997)	IV	18	8*	–	–	35	4	80	37*	–	–
Markel et al. [104] (1996)	IV	10	32	7	4	38	4	45	38	14	25
Fairbank et al. [15] (1995)	IV	25	51	–	52	40	11	88	72	–	26
Saito et al. [32] (1988)	III	17	–	–	–	33	4	100	–	–	–

and remodeling process in the osteonecrotic lesions [20–22]. The bone marrow stromal cells are known to secrete angiogenic growth factors that stimulate the development of blood vessels which ultimately leads to osteogenesis.

Liu et al. [23], in a retrospective study of 53 osteonecrotic hips, compared the outcomes of bone marrow instillation and core decompression with core decompression only. At a mean follow-up of 2 years (range, 1–3.3 years), the authors found that the bone marrow group had significantly higher radiographic and clinical success, and lower rates of radiographic progression (21.4 %; vs. 59.3 %) compared to the core decompression only group. In a prospective randomized trial, Gangji et al. compared the outcomes of autologous bone marrow instillation with core decompression-only in 24 hips at ARCO stages I and III [24]. At a final follow-up of 5 years, the authors found lower rates of radiographic progression in the bone marrow cohort compared to the core decompression group (23 % vs. 73 %). However, no significant differences were found in the functional outcomes or the eventual need for a total hip arthroplasty between the two groups.

Initial reports on bone marrow instillation suggest that this procedure appears to be efficacious in the treatment of early stage osteonecrotic lesions to delay disease progression. This appears to be related to the availability of pluripotent mesenchymal cells with angiogenic and osteogenic properties. However, further larger randomized trials are necessary to better evaluate the outcomes of bone marrow use in osteonecrosis of the hip.

Vascularized and Nonvascularized Bone Grafting

Nonvascularized Bone Grafting

Phemister first described the use of nonvascularized bone in the treatment of osteonecrosis [25]. Later, Bonfiglio and Bardenstein in 1958 reported on the use of nonvascularized fibular grafting in this condition [26]. The aim of any bone grafting procedure is to stimulate healing and enhance repair of osteonecrotic lesions following removal of dead bone. Bone grafts provide a scaffold for new bone formation and, depending on the type of graft used, may also provide structural stability to prevent collapse of the overlying cartilage.

Typically the indication for nonvascularized bone grafting is limited to the treatment of small- to medium-sized (<50 %) early stage lesions (Ficat stage 1 and 2; ARCO stage 1 to 3A). Less optimal outcomes have been reported in hips that present with cartilage delamination, acetabular involvement, or collapse of more than 2 mm.

A variety of techniques have been used historically, such as the Phemister technique, trapdoor procedure, and the light bulb procedure. The Phemister technique involves insertion of a nonvascularized tibial strut graft through a bored channel in the femoral neck. A formal core decompression and curettage of the necrotic bone is performed prior to insertion of the strut grafts. Two other techniques of nonvascularized bone

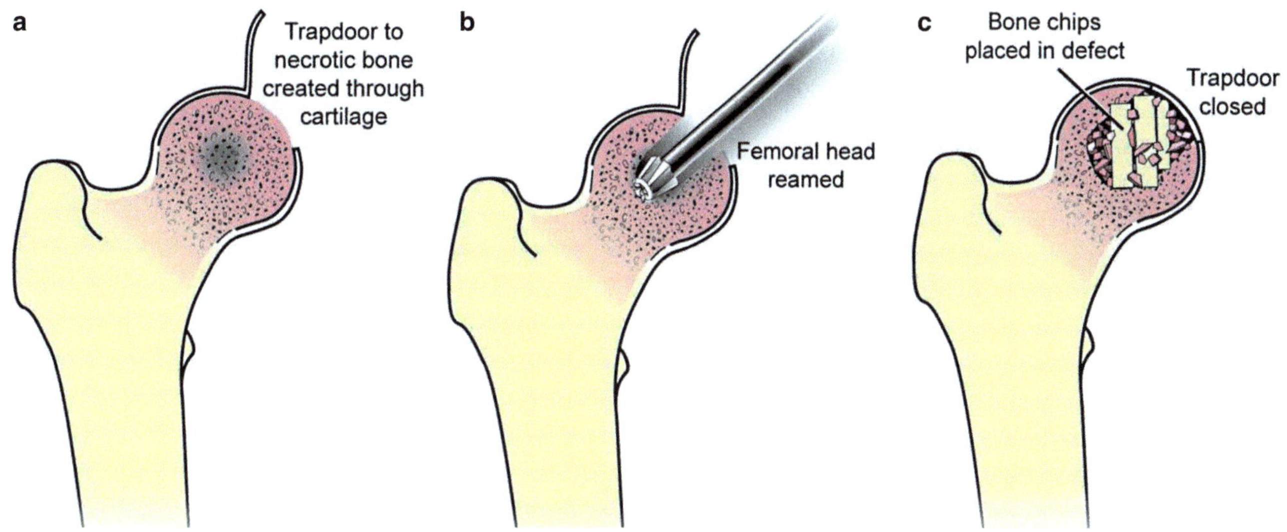

Fig. 60.3 (**a–c**) Trapdoor procedure for removal of necrotic bone and bone grafting. Used with permission from Sinai Hospital of Baltimore, Inc

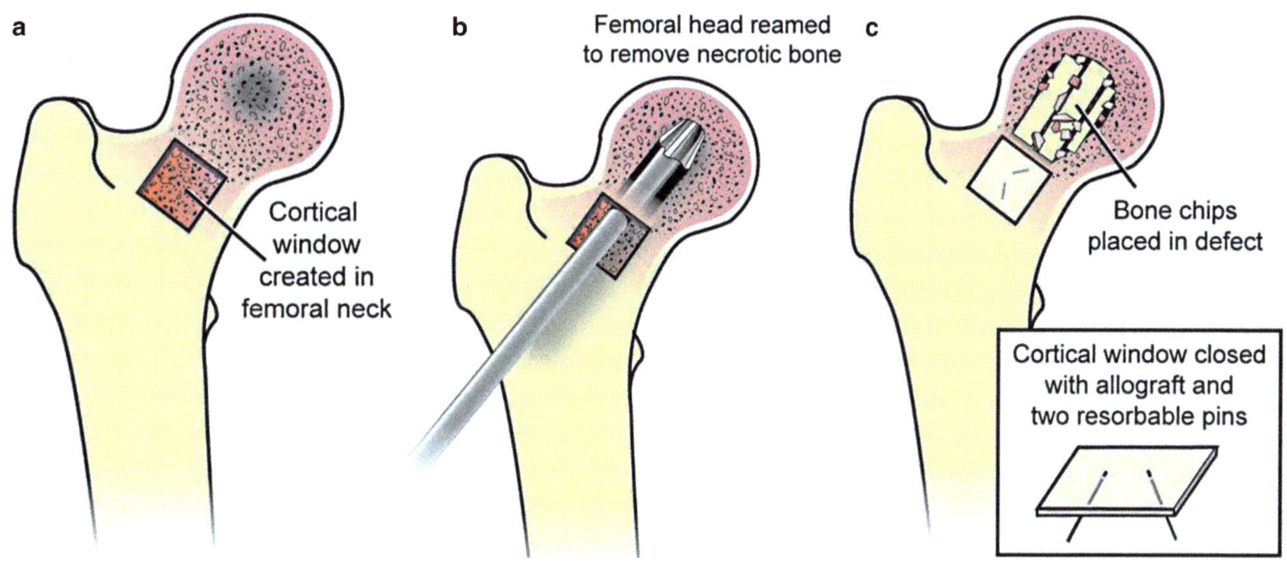

Fig. 60.4 (**a–c**) Light bulb procedure for removal of necrotic bone and bone grafting. Used with permission from Sinai Hospital of Baltimore, Inc

grafting involve creating either a trapdoor in the articular cartilage (trapdoor technique) or a window in the femoral neck (light bulb procedure) for insertion of bone grafts or bone graft substitutes (Figs. 60.3 and 60.4). The trapdoor procedure requires the hip to be surgically dislocated for access to the diseased portion of the head. The key step in the procedure involves removal of an intact cortico-cancellous plug from the head-neck junction followed by thorough debridement and curettage of the lesions followed by packing of autogenous cancellous bone grafts. The cortico-cancellous plug is replaced following insertion of the grafts. Similarly, in the light bulb technique, following completion of the cortical window, debridement of the necrotic bone and packing of the defect with cancellous bone grafts are performed.

Multiple studies on nonvascularized bone grafts have reported varying success rates of 70 to 90 % based on the stage of the disease (Tables 60.4 and 60.5) [27]. The Phemister technique has reported success rates varying between 17 and 90 % at approximately 2–7 year follow-up [18, 28, 29]. Keizer et al. in a report of 78 osteonecrotic hips in Ficat stages I–IV reported a survivorship of 59 % following the Phemister technique at an approximate mean follow-up of 5 years. With the light bulb technique the reported radiographic success varies between 60 and 80 % [30, 31]. In a study of 39 osteonecrotic hips in Ficat stage I and II, Seyler et al. reported survivorship of 78 % with the light bulb procedure, at 2–4 year follow-up [30]. Rosenwasser et al. also evaluated the outcomes of the light bulb procedure in a study of 13 hips at a mean follow-up

Table 60.4 Nonvascularized bone grafting

Author/year	Level of evidence	Stage	Number of hips	Mean age	Mean follow-up	Survivorship
Zhang et al. (2012)	IV	Steinberg II to IV	85	31.4	2.3	85.4
Wei et al. (2011) [105]	IV	ARCO II to III	223	33.5	2	81
Wang et al. (2010) [106]	IV	ARCO IIA to IIIA	138	32.3	2	68
Yuhan et al. (2009) [107]	IV	ARCO IIC to III A	11	37	5	73
Seyler et al. (2008) [30]	IV	Ficat 2 and 3	39	35	3	67
Mont et al. (2003) [108]	IV	Ficat 2 and 3	19	31	4	86
Mont et al. (1998) [109]	IV	Ficat 3 and 4	30	26	56	80

Table 60.5 Vascularized bone grafting

Author/year	Level of evidence	Stage	Number of hips	Mean age	Mean follow-up	Survivorship
Eward et al. (2012) [37]	IV	Ficat 1 and 2	65	32.1	14.4	75
Yin et al. (2011)	IV	Steinberg II to IV	14	34	3.3	100
Chen et al. (2009) [110]	IV	ARCO IIIA and IIIB	33	37	6.2	24
Sun et al. (2009)	IV	Steinberg II to V	80	31	4.3	100
Babhulkar et al. (2009)	IV	ARCO IIB and IIIC	31	32	8	96.7
Bakshi et al. (2009) [39]	IV	Ficat stage 1 to 3	187	35.5	16.5	71
Kawate et al. (2007) [111]	IV	Steinberg IB to V	71	39	7	83
Marciniak et al. (2005)	IV	Marcus Enneking stage 2 to 4	101	37	8	42
Hasegawa et al. (1997) [112]	IV	Inoue and Ono I and II	31	38.3	8	70

of 12 years (range, 10–15 years) [31]. The authors reported that 87 % patients were symptom free and had minimal radiographic progression to osteoarthritis at final follow-up. Saito et al. in a report of 18 patients with stage II and III osteonecrosis reported an overall clinical success of 72 % at an approximate mean follow-up of 48 months (range, 2–14 years) [32]. However, the radiographic success was only 60 % in their report. In a study of 21 patients, Seyler et al. [30] evaluated the outcomes of bone morphogenetic protein enriched allografting using the light bulb procedure, in 21 osteonecrotic hips at a mean follow-up of 4 years (range, 36–55 months). The authors found that 86 % of the hips were clinically successful at final follow-up.

In conclusion, nonvascularized bone grafting procedures are simple, reproducible techniques for early stage osteonecrosis. Strict patient selection, removal of the necrotic lesions, and packing of the defects with donor grafts are essential to optimize outcomes. The availability of the stem cells bestowed with osteogenic properties in the autografts may be potentially related to the success of these techniques, since a decrease in the mesenchymal stem cell pool in the proximal femur may not be adequate during healing.

Vascularized Bone Grafting

To improve blood flow and healing, Meyers et al. [33] in 1978 introduced muscle pedicle bone grafting, and later, Judet et al. [34] in 1980 described free fibular vascularized grafting for the treatment of osteonecrosis and this was further popularized by Urbaniak et al. in the 1990s [35]. The principles of vascularized grafting include decompression and removal of the necrotic bone followed by replacement with grafts that provide an osteoconductive, viable strong mechanical support to the overlying cartilage and subchondral bone during the process of repair and remodeling of the osteonecrotic lesions. This is believed to expedite revascularization and prevent collapse.

Vascularized bone grafts are predominantly indicated for Ficat stages I to II osteonecrosis. Although proponents of this technique have reported successful outcomes in patients with post-collapse disease (<2 mm), it is controversial whether these patients may benefit from this procedure. Adverse risk factors that can potentially affect the rate of healing of osteonecrotic lesions include patients who are current smokers or had a history of heavy smoking, and those who abuse alcohol. These patients need to be carefully screened before the procedure.

The common techniques of vascularized bone grafting that have been described in literature include the vascularized free fibular grafting, iliac crest, sartorius, gluteus medius, and quadratus femoris muscle pedicle bone grafting. The vascularized free fibula graft is often harvested from the ipsilateral side along with the peroneal vascular pedicle for microsurgical anastomosis with the ascending branches of the lateral circumflex femoral vessels. A core tract of 16–19 mm is drilled in the head of the femur from just distal to the vastus lateralis ridge. The necrotic bone is then removed from the head and the area is packed with autologous cancellous bone from the trochanteric region. The vascularized fibula is then inserted through the core decompression tract to within 3–5 mm from the subchondral bone and is stabilized with a 0.62 mm Kirschner wire. Microvascular anastomosis is performed between the peroneal vessels and the ascending cervical branches of the lateral circumflex vessels. Patency of the anastomosis is checked when back bleeding is present from the exposed endosteum of the fibula.

The type of muscle pedicle grafting used is based on the location of the lesion. The iliac crest graft or the sartorius muscle pedicle graft is often preferable for anteriorly located lesions, while the quadratus femoris grafts are used for posterior lesions.

Although varying reports have shown between 60 and 90 % success rates with the use of vascularized grafts in osteonecrosis, less optimal outcomes are noted to occur in hips with more than 2 mm of collapse on presentation. In a study of 103 osteonecrotic hips with Ficat stage II and III, Urbaniak et al. reported on the outcomes of vascularized fibular grafting at a mean follow-up of approximately 5 years. The authors found that the overall survivorship for stage II lesions was 91 %, while stage III lesions had success rates of 77 % at final follow-up [35]. Similarly, Yoo et al. reported a survivorship of 89 % in hips with Ficat stage II and III at a follow-up of approximately 10 years (mean, 13.9; range, 10–23.7 years) [36]. Edward et al. also reported that 75 % of the hips in pre-collapse stage (49 out of 65 hips) survived following vascularized fibular grafting without needing a conversion to total hip arthroplasty at a minimum follow-up of 10 years [37]. However, despite these improved results, the potential risks of donor site morbidity as high as 25 % and risks of subtrochanteric of 2.5 % must be taken into consideration when selecting this treatment.

Although some authors have reported successful outcomes with muscle pedicle bone grafting in the treatment of osteonecrosis of the hip, this procedure is currently less popular in the United States [38–41]. Baksi et al. evaluated the outcomes of tensor fascia lata or sartorius muscle grafting in a study of 187 osteonecrotic hips in 152 patients who were in Ficat stages I to III [39]. At a mean follow-up of approximately 17 years (range, 10–21.5 years), radiological improvement was found in 81 % of patients in stage II and 70 % of patients in stage III disease. Similarly, Stein et al. evaluated the outcomes of tensor fascia lata muscle pedicle bone grafting in 37 patients with symptomatic osteonecrosis of the hip in ARCO stage 2 and 3. The authors found that 89 % of patients had a successful outcome and did not require conversion to total hip arthroplasty at 12 year during a 12-year study period [40].

In summary, vascularized bone grafts offer the advantage of restoring circulation and providing structural support to the overlying cartilage and are considered as a biological head preserving technique that may potentially maintain coxofemoral joint congruity and prevent development of arthritis. Although long-term head preservation has been reported from a few centers using free vascularized fibular grafting, universal acceptance of this procedure has been limited by its technically complexity, complications with fibular harvesting, and the need for microsurgical anastomosis.

Bone Morphogenetic Proteins (BMP)

Bone morphogenic proteins have been used as an osteoconductive agent in the treatment of osteonecrosis to stimulate the process of repair and remodeling [42, 43]. In a study of 17 osteonecrotic hips, Lieberman et al. reported successful outcomes in 82 % of patients treated with nonvascularized bone grafting and bone morphogenetic proteins at a mean follow-up of 4.4 years (range, 2.2–7.8 years) [43].

Although limited data is currently available on the outcomes of bone morphogenetic proteins in the treatment of osteonecrosis, early results appear promising. Further research will indicate whether outcomes are superior to conventional bone grafting procedures.

Proximal Femoral Osteotomies

A variety of osteotomies have been described for the treatment of osteonecrosis of the femoral head. The two main types of osteotomies that have been described in literature are the intertrochanteric varus and valgus and the transtrochanteric rotational osteotomies.

Intertrochanteric Osteotomies

Merle D'Aubigne in 1965 [44], and later Pauwels in 1968, described angular osteotomies for osteonecrosis of the hip [45]. The aim of all proximal femoral osteotomies in osteonecrosis of the hip is to rotate the osteonecrotic segment of the femoral head away from the load bearing area to prevent progression to collapse and replace it with healthy intact bone. Some authors have postulated that the beneficial effects of these osteotomies occur through reduction in venous hypertension and subsequent decrease in intraosseous pressures.

Typically, favorable outcomes with proximal femoral osteotomies are reported in hips with Ficat stage II and III disease, with combined necrotic angles less than 200°, and intact ratios of more than 35–40 % (ratio of intact segment of the head articulating with the weight-bearing segment of the acetabulum), compared to those that have larger necrotic angles and smaller intact ratios.

The technique of angular osteotomy involves the removal of a wedge of bone from the per-trochanteric region and is dependent on the location and size of the lesion in the femoral head. A varus osteotomy is often chosen when the lesion involves the medial part of the head, thereby changing the location of the weight-bearing portion of the head to the uninvolved antero-superior part. Conversely, a valgus osteotomy is chosen when the antero-superior part of the femoral head is involved, to transfer the medial unaffected region of the head in line with the weight-bearing axis. However, due to concerns of abductor weakness, limb-length discrepancy, and elevation of the greater trochanter, a number of modifications to the classical technique of varus wedge osteotomy have been described, such as the curved intertrochanteric and the varus half wedge osteotomy. Curved osteotomies are biomechanically more stable due to the wide surface area of bone contact. However, these are technically more demanding to perform compared to conventional wedge osteotomies. Although these modifications have the advantage of less reduction in limb length and abductor power, it is unsuitable for varus corrections of more than 25° [46].

Multiple reports on intertrochanteric osteotomies have described success rates up to 90 % at mid- to long-term follow-up. However, a majority of these have been single-surgeon series with Level IV evidence [46, 47]. Few prospective randomized studies comparing the outcomes of trochanteric osteotomies with other head preserving surgical treatment options are currently reported in literature [17, 47–52]. In a study of 73 osteonecrotic hips in 62 patients, Zhao et al. reported on the outcomes of curved intertrochanteric osteotomies at a mean follow-up of approximately 13 years. The authors found that only 6 out of 73 hips (8 %) required conversion to total hip arthroplasty at final follow-up [52].

In summary, intertrochanteric proximal femoral osteotomies for the treatment of osteonecrosis have diminished in popularity in the United States due to a lack of reproducible results, in addition to concerns about the perceived difficulties encountered if a conversion to a total hip arthroplasty is needed in future. Moreover, due to the complex nature of the osteotomies, they should preferably be performed only by experienced surgeons.

Transtrochanteric Rotational Osteotomy

Transtrochanteric rotational osteotomies were originally described by Wagner and Zeiler [53] in the 1960s and later popularized by Sugoika [48] in the 1970s. These osteotomies involve either anterior or posterior rotation of the head through the longitudinal axis of the femoral neck to transfer the weight-bearing forces through the intact healthy part of the head with the aim of increasing joint congruity. Following trochanteric rotational osteotomy, healing is believed to occur through ingrowth of vascular connective tissue and appositional new bone formation occurs over the dead trabeculae. However, radiographically 70 % of patients continue to demonstrate an osteosclerotic zone, while 30 % of patients have a normal radiographic appearance at long-term follow-up.

Although Sugoika [48] initially recommended these osteotomies could be performed even in patients with articular collapse, other groups of researchers have found the outcomes to be inconsistent when performed for post-collapse lesions. This may be due to instability associated with large post-collapse lesions [54]. Most researchers believe that these rotational osteotomies are indicated in localized Ficat stage II and in stage III lesions when less than 2 mm of collapse is present with intact ratios more than 35–40 %.

Various reports, mostly from Japan and other Asian countries, have demonstrated varying success rates ranging from 17 to 94 % with transtrochanteric rotational osteotomy. However, reports from Europe and America have found high failure rates with rotational osteotomies [55, 56]. In a study of 27 osteonecrotic hips in 22 patients who had a mean age of 16 years, Ikemura et al. reported on the outcomes of transtrochanteric osteotomy. The authors found that at a mean follow-up of approximately 15 years (range, 2–32 years), only 7.4 % of the hips needed conversion to total hip arthroplasty [57]. Similarly, in a study of 51 hips in Ficat stage III and IV, Zhao et al. reported on the outcomes of posterior rotational osteotomy at a mean follow-up of approximately 11 years follow-up [52]. Of these 51 hips, 31 had collapse less than 3 mm, 18 had collapse more than 3 mm, and 2 had radiographic evidence of osteoarthritis. The authors found that patients with minimal collapse (<3 mm) and intact ratios more than 37 % had better outcomes and were less likely to progress to collapse and osteoarthritis compared to those who had more substantial collapse and less intact ratios. Hasegawa et al. [17] compared the outcomes of rotational osteotomy with vascularized bone grafting in a study of 86 hips. At approximately mean 5-year follow-up, the authors reported similar survivorship of 67 and 85 % between the two cohorts and these outcomes were also maintained at 10-year follow-up (61 and 71 %). However, the authors reported better outcomes with rotational osteotomy in patients with Ficat stage II disease compared to those who had stage III disease on presentation. However, other authors have reported less optimal outcomes with transtrochanteric osteotomies. At a mean follow-up of approximately 9 years, Rijnen et al. [58] reported on the outcomes of rotational osteotomy in 26 hips. The authors reported unsatisfactory outcomes in 56 % of their patients who needed conversion to total hip arthroplasty at 7-year follow-up. The majority of the current literature in favor of proximal femoral osteotomy is based on single-surgeon series with low level evidence. Transtrochanteric rotational osteotomies require considerable planning, substantial surgical skill, high level of training, and can be extremely demanding for the less experienced surgeon. Limiting the indications to a select group of patients is crucial in order to obtain successful outcomes with proximal femoral osteotomies. Moreover, concerns related to abnormal femoral version, greater trochanter overhang, presence of previous hardware, location of previous incisions, and the potential for increased blood loss need to be considered, if these procedures fail and conversion to a total hip arthroplasty is needed.

Head Sacrificing Procedures: Arthroplasty Options

Resurfacing Arthroplasty

Historically, less optimal outcomes were reported with total hip arthroplasty in patients with osteonecrosis due to their relative youth and various other implant-related factors including the use of earlier generation of ceramic and polyethylene bearings. This led to interest in more bone conserving options such as hemi- and total hip resurfacing. With similar reported improvements in quality of life, activity levels, pain relief, and function compared to a conventional total hip arthroplasty, proponents of resurfacing arthroplasty believe that it remains a viable treatment option for Ficat stage III and stage IV osteonecrosis of the hip [59–63]. In addition, it is argued that resurfacing procedures provide a more normal gait, maintain physiological stresses in the proximal femur, reduce risk of dislocations, and require a less technically demanding revision should a conversion to total hip arthroplasty become necessary [59, 61, 64–68]. Despite these advantages, the use of resurfacing in osteonecrosis of the hip has been debated upon as it involves cementing the prosthesis in a bed of dead bone, in addition to recent concerns of metal hypersensitivity, metallosis, and adverse local tissue reactions with metal-on-metal bearings [69, 70].

Hemiresurfacing Arthroplasty

In a hemiresurfacing procedure, the native femoral head is replaced with a hemispherical prosthesis that roughly matches the diameter of the acetabulum. The acetabular cartilage itself is not resurfaced. Hemiresurfacing was proposed as a time buying procedure and a reasonable option in the treatment of Ficat stage II, III osteonecrosis in young patients [71]. However, the efficacy of the procedure, in terms of pain relief, is reported to be lower in the presence of marked acetabular cartilage degeneration and in the presence of short duration of the disease [62, 63]. Most authors have reported acetabular erosion or groin pain as the two common causes for revision surgery following hemiresurfacing procedures.

In a report of 54 osteonecrotic hips in stage II–IV, Amstutz et al. [72] evaluated the outcomes of hemiresurfacing arthroplasty. The authors found that the cumulative implant survivorship was 63.3 % (95 % CI; 45.0–77.0 %) at 10 years, and 36.4 % (95 % CI; 17.3–55.9 %) at 15 years. However, Cuckler et al. found inferior outcomes in their report of 59 patients who had undergone a hemiresurfacing procedure for stage III osteonecrosis [71]. The authors found a cumulative failure of 32 % at a mean follow-up of approximately 5 years.

It is controversial whether hemiresurfacing results in delaying the need for a total hip arthroplasty. Current evidence suggests that restricting the indications to hips with intact acetabular cartilage may optimize the results. Since most patients who present with stage III or stage IV disease have some evidence of cartilage degeneration, the role for hemiresurfacing in osteonecrosis of the hip appears limited at best.

Total Resurfacing Arthroplasty

Patient selection is crucial to improve outcomes and reduce complications after resurfacing arthroplasty in osteonecrosis. To improve longevity, it has been suggested by some authors that the friable, yellowish necrotic bone needs to be adequately debrided down to normal reactive bone. This is believed to be necessary to avoid placing implants over dead bone that may provide less mechanical support. However, others recommend placing implants after minimal reaming of the necrotic region, enough to debride away the loose fibrous tissue [73]. Multiple perforations of the dead bone in the femoral head with a 3 mm drill bit are recommended by most authors to improve cement fixation. However, care should be taken to avoid excessive cement penetration in the head to reduce thermal damage in the remaining viable bone. It has been reported that more favorable outcomes are achieved in young males (<55 years) who have head sizes >50 mm and in the presence of head defects more than 1 cm [74–77]. A more exacting surgical technique is necessary in resurfacing procedures to avoid edge-loading from cup inclination angles of more than 55°, which have been reported to adversely affect the outcomes [74–77]. Some of the reported contraindications of the procedure include documented cobalt or chromium allergy, presence of multiple cysts, and marked osteopenia in the head and proximal femur.

Nevertheless, multiple authors have reported durable aseptic implant survivorship at short-to-mid-term follow-up (Fig. 60.5) [63, 70, 78, 79]. Sayeed et al. evaluated the outcomes of resurfacing arthroplasty in 16 patients (20 osteonecrotic hips) who were less than 25 years of age [78]. At approximately 7.5-year follow-up, the authors reported that the cumulative aseptic implant survivorship was 100 %. Mont et al., in a matched pair analysis, compared the outcomes of

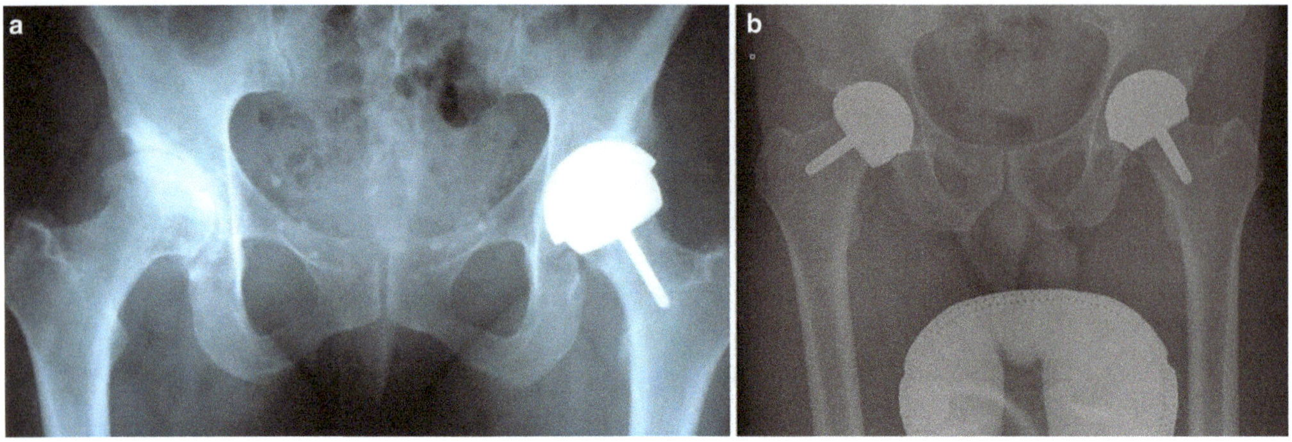

Fig. 60.5 (**a** and **b**) Resurfacing arthroplasty for end-stage osteonecrosis. Used with permission from Sinai Hospital of Baltimore, Inc

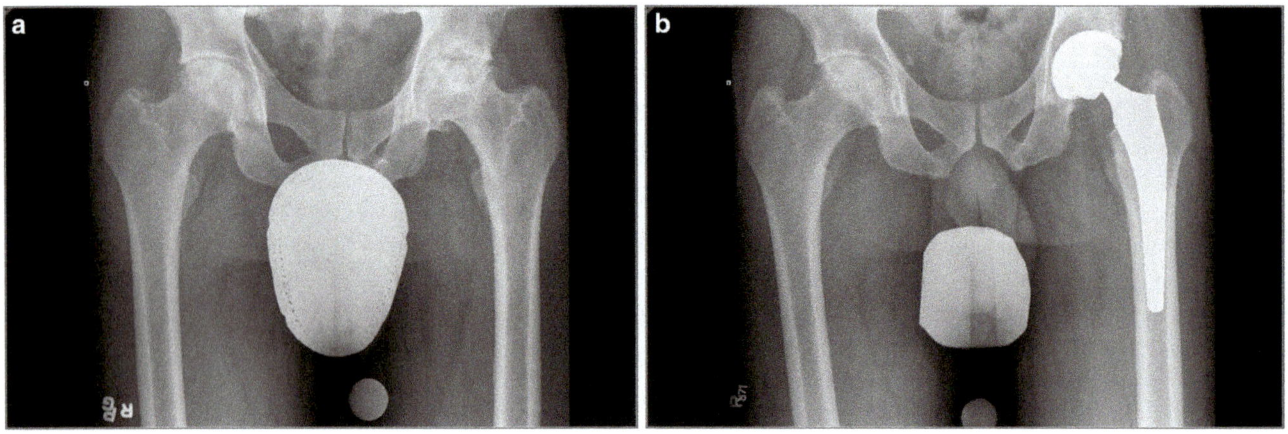

Fig. 60.6 Antero-posterior radiographs of a 43-year-old male with bilateral hip osteonecrosis, which demonstrates (**a**) the Ficat and Arlet stage IV lesion in the left femoral head treated with a (**b**) total hip arthroplasty. Used with permission from Sinai Hospital of Baltimore, Inc

resurfacing arthroplasty in osteonecrosis ($n=42$) and in patients with osteoarthritis ($n=42$). The authors reported excellent results in both groups, with 93 % survival in the osteonecrotic cohort, and 98 % in the osteoarthritis group at a minimum follow-up of 2 years (range, 2–6 years) [59]. In a study of hip 94 osteonecrotic hips, Bose et al. [80] reported on the outcomes of hip resurfacing arthroplasties at a mean follow-up of 5.4 years (range, 4–8.1 years). At final follow-up the authors reported significant improvements in the UCLA scores from a mean of approximately 3 points preoperatively, to a mean of 7 points postoperatively, and a cumulative implant survivorship of 95.4 %.

Hip resurfacing arthroplasty has excellent functional outcomes and survivorship in patients with osteonecrosis at mid-term follow-up. However, most of these reports are from surgeons with extensive experience. With strict patient selection and exacting surgical technique, more predictable outcomes can be expected with resurfacing arthroplasty for end-stage osteonecrosis. Long-term outcome studies are currently awaited to better evaluate the clinical and radiological outcomes in this patient population.

Total Hip Arthroplasty

Of all the treatment options available for end-stage osteonecrosis, total hip arthroplasty has the highest likelihood of providing the most predictable clinical and functional improvement and relief of pain. The general consensus is that total hip arthroplasty is indicated when osteonecrosis of the hip is associated with advanced degenerative arthritis (Ficat stage IV; ARCO stage IV) in the presence of severe damage to the femoral head and acetabular cartilage and in a severely symptomatic low-demand patient with radiographic evidence of extensive collapse of the femoral head (Ficat stage III; ARCO stage III C) (Fig. 60.6) [11].

Most early reports found high rate of failures due to bearing wear as well as aseptic loosening in this patient group compared to patients with osteoarthritis, potentially related to the increased activity levels in the younger population [81–87]. Other factors that may have been causally related to the poor survivorship include poor bone quality and presence of dense sclerotic bone in the proximal femur and acetabulum that impedes both cement interdigitation and osseointegration with cementless implants. Recent evidence suggests more durable aseptic implant survivorship in patients with osteonecrosis. Johansson et al., in a systematic review on 3277 hips, found that the overall revision rate reported in studies on osteonecrotic patients prior to 1990 was 17 % (range, 0–50 %) at a mean approximate follow-up of 9 years, compared to 3 % (range, 0–7 %) in studies after 1990 at a mean follow-up of 6 years [88].

Advances in bearing technology have led to the development of third generation ceramic bearings and highly cross-linked polyethylene. The modern generations of ceramic-on-ceramic bearings developed after 1994 have better scratch resistance, higher wettability, increased burst strength, and greater lubrication [81, 82]. These improved properties have been postulated to provide an advantage over the predicate designs when used in younger populations with osteonecrosis. Highly cross-linked polyethylene, which is produced by gamma irradiation of cross-linked polyethylene, is also believed to substantially reduce adhesive and abrasive wear [89, 90]. Some of the initial success reported with these bearings is potentially related to the lower rates of osteolysis as a result of decreased number of wear particles generated with the use of these bearings.

In a study of 162 osteonecrotic hips (140 patients), Min et al. evaluated the outcomes of highly cross-linked bearings in total hip arthroplasty. At mean follow-up of 7.2 years (range, 5–10.6 years), the authors found the cumulative implant survivorship for component revision from any cause was 100 % at 10 years follow-up. The authors reported a very low rate of linear polyethylene wear of 0.037 mm/year (range, 0–0.099 mm/year), which was found to be well below the osteolysis threshold of 0.1 mm/year [81, 82]. Similarly, Byun et al. [91] reported on the outcomes of third generation ceramic-on-ceramic bearings in 41 patients with osteonecrosis. The authors reported 100 % implant survivorship at a mean follow-up of 7.7 years (range, 6.0–8.5 years). Most importantly, the authors did not find any case of radiographic loosening, liner fracture, or osteolysis. At present, mid-term data suggests excellent survivorship, clinical, and functional outcomes with these newer bearing options. However, long-term data concerning these bearings are necessary to better evaluate these outcome metrics.

Furthermore, with the development of ultra-porous biomaterials for cementless acetabular fixation, modern generation of cementless implants, and improved cementing techniques, better overall outcomes have been reported recently in osteonecrotic patients undergoing total hip arthroplasty. In a study of 148 osteonecrotic hips, Kim et al. compared the outcomes of hybrid and cementless fixation [11]. The authors found that at a mean follow-up of approximately 17 years, (range, 16–18 years), the implant survivorship was 98 % in both cemented and cementless stems. They also reported that the cementless acetabular component survivorship was 85 % in comparison to 83 % in the hybrid cohort. It was found that periacetabular osteolysis and wear were the main causes of failure at final follow-up. In a study reporting on the long-term outcomes of cementless total hip arthroplasty, at a mean follow-up of 12 years (range, 10–16 years), Bedard et al. [92] reported cumulative aseptic survivorship of 100 %. Despite these improved outcomes, the authors found a 21 % incidence of proximal femoral osteolysis and 7.5 % incidence of pelvic osteolysis at follow-up. The authors found that hips with moderately cross-linked polyethylene demonstrated significantly lower wear linear and volumetric wear (0.06 mm/year and 20.76 mm^3/year) compared to hips with conventional polyethylene (0.22 mm/year and 70.85 mm^3/year; $p<0.0001$).

A number of previous studies have reported lower implant survivorship in certain select patient groups with osteonecrosis of the hip. Johansson et al. reported in a systematic review that patients with sickle cell disease, Gaucher's disease, and renal failure had less optimal outcomes following total hip arthroplasty compared to heart transplant recipients and patients who had systemic lupus erythematosus or idiopathic disease [88]. Similarly, in a study of 41 patients (55 osteonecrotic hips) who had undergone total hip arthroplasty, Radl et al. [93] reported on the outcomes at a mean follow-up of 6.4 years (range, 2–12.8 years). The authors found significantly lower 10-year cumulative implant survivorship in osteonecrotic patients with systemic risk factors (57 %) compared to patients who had idiopathic or post-traumatic osteonecrosis (100 %).

High risks of infections secondary to immunosuppression and osteopenia and higher perioperative medical and surgical complication in patients with sickle cell disease were causally related to these poor outcomes. More recently, a number of authors have refuted these results. In a comparison study, Issa et al. [94] found similar outcomes in sickle ($n=42$ hips) and non-sickle cell patients ($n=102$ hips) undergoing total hip arthroplasty. The authors found comparable aseptic implant survivorship (95 % versus 97 %; $p=0.85$), SF-36 scores ($p=0.84$), and Harris hip scores (87 and 88 points; $p=0.75$) between the two cohorts. Similarly, Chang et al. [95] evaluated the outcomes of cementless total hip arthroplasty in a study of 74 osteonecrotic hips in 52 patients who were renal transplant recipients. The authors reported 100 % aseptic stem survivorship at a mean follow-up of approximately 10 years. Although encouraging outcomes are reported in recent literature describing the outcomes of total hip arthroplasty in patients with osteonecrosis, further long-term data is necessary to evaluate the efficacy of these modern bearings and fixation interfaces.

Summary

The treatment of osteonecrosis of the hip is challenging. Having a low threshold for imaging with radiographs and magnetic resonance scans in young patients who present with groin pain or have risk factors for developing osteonecrosis is the key to early diagnosis. It is important to classify the disease in order to select the appropriate treatment option based on staging to halt the progression of disease. The goal of early stage disease is hip preservation while end-stage disease usually requires a total hip arthroplasty. Although initial reports on the use of stem cells as an adjuvant therapy with core decompression have shown encouraging results, long-term data is currently not available. Recent studies on total hip arthroplasty with modern generation bearings and fixation interfaces in patients with osteonecrosis have shown to have substantial improvements in implant longevity at mid-term follow-up. Moreover, better outcomes have been reported in recent reports on high-risk patients groups such as sickle cell patients and renal transplant recipients undergoing total hip arthroplasty. Despite these improved outcomes, it is imperative that the operating surgeon counsel patients about the possibility of a revision surgery and the need to avoid high impact and strenuous activities in an effort to increase the longevity of their prostheses.

References

1. Mont MA, Jones LC, Hungerford DS. Nontraumatic osteonecrosis of the femoral head: ten years later. J Bone Joint Surg Am. 2006;88:1117–32.
2. Zalavras CG, Lieberman JR. Osteonecrosis of the femoral head: evaluation and treatment. J Am Acad Orthop Surg. 2014;22: 455–64.
3. Stulberg BN. Osteonecrosis: what to do, what to do! J Arthroplast. 2003;18:74–9.
4. Ha YC, Jung WH, Kim JR, Seong NH, Kim SY, Koo KH. Prediction of collapse in femoral head osteonecrosis: a modified Kerboul method with use of magnetic resonance images. J Bone Joint Surg Am. 2006;88 Suppl 3:35–40.
5. Ikemura S, Yamamoto T, Motomura G, Nakashima Y, Mawatari T, Iwamoto Y. MRI evaluation of collapsed femoral heads in patients 60 years old or older: differentiation of subchondral insufficiency fracture from osteonecrosis of the femoral head. AJR Am J Roentgenol. 2010;195:W63–8.
6. Lee GC, Khoury V, Steinberg D, Kim W, Dalinka M, Steinberg M. How do radiologists evaluate osteonecrosis? Skelet Radiol. 2014;43:607–14.
7. Mont MA, Marulanda GA, Jones LC, Saleh KJ, Gordon N, Hungerford DS, et al. Systematic analysis of classification systems for osteonecrosis of the femoral head. J Bone Joint Surg Am. 2006;88 Suppl 3:16–26.
8. Rajagopal M, Balch Samora J, Ellis TJ. Efficacy of core decompression as treatment for osteonecrosis of the hip: a systematic review. Hip Int. 2012;22:489–93.
9. Yoon TR, Song EK, Rowe SM, Park CH. Failure after core decompression in osteonecrosis of the femoral head. Int Orthop. 2001;24:316–8.
10. Mont MA, Carbone JJ, Fairbank AC. Core decompression versus nonoperative management for osteonecrosis of the hip. Clin Orthop Relat Res 1996:169–78.
11. Kim YH, Kim JS, Park JW, Joo JH. Contemporary total hip arthroplasty with and without cement in patients with osteonecrosis of the femoral head: a concise follow-up, at an average of seventeen years, of a previous report. J Bone Joint Surg Am. 2011;93:1806–10.
12. Mont MA, Ragland PS, Etienne G. Core decompression of the femoral head for osteonecrosis using percutaneous multiple small-diameter drilling. Clinical orthopaedics and related research. 2004:131–138.
13. Song WS, Yoo JJ, Kim YM, Kim HJ. Results of multiple drilling compared with those of conventional methods of core decompression. Clin Orthop Relat Res. 2007;454:139–46.
14. Ficat RP. Idiopathic bone necrosis of the femoral head. Early diagnosis and treatment. J Bone Joint Surg Br. 1985;67:3–9.
15. Fairbank AC, Bhatia D, Jinnah RH, Hungerford DS. Long-term results of core decompression for ischaemic necrosis of the femoral head. J Bone Joint Surg Br. 1995;77:42–9.
16. Marker DR, Seyler TM, Ulrich SD, Srivastava S, Mont MA. Do modern techniques improve core decompression outcomes for hip osteonecrosis? Clin Orthop Relat Res. 2008;466:1093–103.
17. Hasegawa Y, Sakano S, Iwase T, Iwasada S, Torii S, Iwata H. Pedicle bone grafting versus transtrochanteric rotational osteotomy for avascular necrosis of the femoral head. J Bone Joint Surg Br. 2003;85:191–8.
18. Israelite C, Nelson CL, Ziarani CF, Abboud JA, Landa J, Steinberg ME. Bilateral core decompression for osteonecrosis of the femoral head. Clin Orthop Relat Res. 2005;441:285–90.
19. Mont MA, Ragland PS, Etienne G. Core decompression of the femoral head for osteonecrosis using percutaneous multiple small-diameter drilling. Clin Orthop Relat Res 2004;131–8.
20. Hernigou P, Poignard A, Zilber S, Rouard H. Cell therapy of hip osteonecrosis with autologous bone marrow grafting. Indian J Orthop. 2009;43:40–5.
21. Hernigou P, Daltro G, Filippini P, Mukasa MM, Manicom O. Percutaneous implantation of autologous bone marrow osteoprogenitor cells as treatment of bone avascular necrosis related to sickle cell disease. Open Orthop J. 2008;2:62–5.
22. Hernigou P, Poignard A, Manicom O, Mathieu G, Rouard H. The use of percutaneous autologous bone marrow transplantation in nonunion and avascular necrosis of bone. J Bone Joint Surg (Br). 2005;87:896–902.
23. Liu Y, Liu S, Su X. Core decompression and implantation of bone marrow mononuclear cells with porous hydroxylapatite composite filler for the treatment of osteonecrosis of the femoral head. Arch Orthop Trauma Surg. 2013;133:125–33.
24. Gangji V, De Maertelaer V, Hauzeur JP. Autologous bone marrow cell implantation in the treatment of non-traumatic osteonecrosis of the femoral head: Five year follow-up of a prospective controlled study. Bone. 2011;49:1005–9.
25. Phemister DB. Treatment of the necrotic head of the femur in adults. J Bone Joint Surg Am. 1949;31A:55–66.

26. Bonfiglio M, Bardenstein MB. Treatment by bone-grafting of aseptic necrosis of the femoral head and non-union of the femoral neck (Phemister technique). J Bone Joint Surg Am. 1958;40-A: 1329–46.
27. Gaskill TR, Urbaniak JR, Aldridge 3rd JM. Free vascularized fibular transfer for femoral head osteonecrosis: donor and graft site morbidity. J Bone Joint Surg Am. 2009;91:1861–7.
28. Buckley PD, Gearen PF, Petty RW. Structural bone-grafting for early atraumatic avascular necrosis of the femoral head. J Bone Joint Surg Am. 1991;73:1357–64.
29. Plakseychuk AY, Kim SY, Park BC, Varitimidis SE, Rubash HE, Sotereanos DG. Vascularized compared with nonvascularized fibular grafting for the treatment of osteonecrosis of the femoral head. J Bone Joint Surg Am. 2003;85-A:589–96.
30. Seyler TM, Marker DR, Ulrich SD, Fatscher T, Mont MA. Nonvascularized bone grafting defers joint arthroplasty in hip osteonecrosis. Clin Orthop Relat Res. 2008;466:1125–32.
31. Rosenwasser MP, Garino JP, Kiernan HA, Michelsen CB. Long term followup of thorough debridement and cancellous bone grafting of the femoral head for avascular necrosis. Clin Orthop Relat Res 1994:17–27.
32. Saito S, Ohzono K, Ono K. Joint-preserving operations for idiopathic avascular necrosis of the femoral head. Results of core decompression, grafting and osteotomy. J Bone Joint Surg (Br). 1988;70:78–84.
33. Meyers MH. The treatment of osteonecrosis of the hip with fresh osteochondral allografts and with the muscle pedicle graft technique. Clin Orthop Relat Res 1978:202–9.
34. Judet J, Judet H, Gilbert A. Trial revascularization of the femur head with a pediculed fibular transplant. Rev Chir Orthop Reparatrice Appar Mot. 1980;66 Suppl 2:65.
35. Urbaniak JR, Coogan PG, Gunneson EB, Nunley JA. Treatment of osteonecrosis of the femoral head with free vascularized fibular grafting. A long-term follow-up study of one hundred and three hips. J Bone Joint Surg Am. 1995;77:681–94.
36. Yoo MC, Kim KI, Hahn CS, Parvizi J. Long-term followup of vascularized fibular grafting for femoral head necrosis. Clin Orthop Relat Res. 2008;466:1133–40.
37. Eward WC, Rineer CA, Urbaniak JR, Richard MJ, Ruch DS. The vascularized fibular graft in precollapse osteonecrosis: is long-term hip preservation possible? Clin Orthop Relat Res. 2012;470:2819–26.
38. Baksi DP. Treatment of osteonecrosis of the femoral head by drilling and muscle-pedicle bone grafting. J Bone Joint Surg (Br). 1991;73:241–5.
39. Baksi DP, Pal AK, Baksi DD. Long-term results of decompression and muscle-pedicle bone grafting for osteonecrosis of the femoral head. Int Orthop. 2009;33:41–7.
40. Stein H, Volpin G, Horer D. Vascularized muscle pedicle flap for osteonecrosis of the femoral head. Orthopedics. 2002;25:485–8.
41. Meyers MH. Osteonecrosis of the femoral head treated with the muscle pedicle graft. Orthop Clin N Am. 1985;16:741–5.
42. Shi SH, Li ZR, Wang BL, et al. Study on the relationship between sclerosis rim and bone morphogenetic proteins of osteonecrosis of the femoral head. Zhonghua Wai Ke Za Zhi. 2010;48: 1305–8.
43. Lieberman JR, Conduah A, Urist MR. Treatment of osteonecrosis of the femoral head with core decompression and human bone morphogenetic protein. Clin Orthop Relat Res. 2004;139–45.
44. d' Aubigne RM. Treatment of juxta-articular nonunion associated with joint stiffness. Clinical orthopaedics and related research. 1965; 43: 149–159.
45. Merle D'Aubigne R, Postel M, Mazabraud A, Massias P, Gueguen J, France P. Idiopathic necrosis of the femoral head in adults. J Bone Joint Surg (Br). 1965;47:612–33.
46. Ito H, Tanino H, Yamanaka Y, et al. Long-term results of conventional varus half-wedge proximal femoral osteotomy for the treatment of osteonecrosis of the femoral head. J Bone Joint Surg (Br). 2012;94:308–14.
47. Zhao G, Yamamoto T, Ikemura S, et al. Radiological outcome analysis of transtrochanteric curved varus osteotomy for osteonecrosis of the femoral head at a mean follow-up of 12.4 years. J Bone Joint Surg (Br). 2010;92:781–6.
48. Sugioka Y. Transtrochanteric anterior rotational osteotomy of the femoral head in the treatment of osteonecrosis affecting the hip: a new osteotomy operation. Clin Orthop Relat Res. 1978;191–201.
49. Sugioka Y, Katsuki I, Hotokebuchi T. Transtrochanteric rotational osteotomy of the femoral head for the treatment of osteonecrosis. Follow-up statistics. Clin Orthop Relat Res. 1982;115–26.
50. Sugioka Y, Hotokebuchi T, Tsutsui H. Transtrochanteric anterior rotational osteotomy for idiopathic and steroid-induced necrosis of the femoral head. Indications and long-term results. Clin Orthop Relat Res. 1992;111–20.
51. Zhao G, Yamamoto T, Ikemura S, et al. Clinico-radiological factors affecting the joint space narrowing after transtrochanteric anterior rotational osteotomy for osteonecrosis of the femoral head. J Orthop Sci. 2012;17:390–6.
52. Zhao G, Yamamoto T, Motomura G, et al. Radiological outcome analyses of transtrochanteric posterior rotational osteotomy for osteonecrosis of the femoral head at a mean follow-up of 11 years. J Orthop Sci. 2013;18(2):277–83.
53. Wagner H, Zeiler G. Idiopathic avascular necrosis of the femoral head. Results of intertrochanteric osteotomy and resurfacing (author's transl). Orthopade. 1980;9:290–310.
54. Lee YK, Ha YC, Kim KC, Yoo JJ, Koo KH. Total hip arthroplasty after previous transtrochanteric anterior rotational osteotomy for femoral head osteonecrosis. J Arthroplasty. 2009;24:1205–9.
55. Belal MA, Reichelt A. Clinical results of rotational osteotomy for treatment of avascular necrosis of the femoral head. Arch Orthop Trauma Surg. 1996;115:80–4.
56. Eyb R, Kotz R. The transtrochanteric anterior rotational osteotomy of Sugioka. Early and late results in idiopathic aseptic femoral head necrosis. Arch Orthop Trauma Surg. 1987;106:161–7.
57. Ikemura S, Yamamoto T, Nakashima Y, Mawatari T, Motomura G, Iwamoto Y. Transtrochanteric anterior rotational osteotomy for osteonecrosis of the femoral head in patients 20 years or younger. J Pediatr Orthop. 2009;29:219–23.
58. Rijnen WH, Gardeniers JW, Westrek BL, Buma P, Schreurs BW. Sugioka's osteotomy for femoral-head necrosis in young Caucasians. Int Orthop. 2005;29:140–4.
59. Mont MA, Seyler TM, Marker DR, Marulanda GA, Delanois RE. Use of metal-on-metal total hip resurfacing for the treatment of osteonecrosis of the femoral head. J Bone Joint Surg Am. 2006;88 Suppl 3:90–7.
60. Schmalzried TP. Total resurfacing for osteonecrosis of the hip. Clin Orthop Relat Res. 2004;151–6.
61. McGrath MS, Marker DR, Seyler TM, Ulrich SD, Mont MA. Surface replacement is comparable to primary total hip arthroplasty. Clin Orthop Relat Res. 2009;467:94–100.
62. Rahman WA, Greidanus NV, Siegmeth A, Masri BA, Duncan CP, Garbuz DS. Patients report improvement in quality of life and satisfaction after hip resurfacing arthroplasty. Clin Orthop Relat Res. 2013;471:444–53.
63. Aulakh TS, Rao C, Kuiper JH, Richardson JB. Hip resurfacing and osteonecrosis: results from an independent hip resurfacing register. Arch Orthop Trauma Surg. 2010;130:841–5.
64. Burroughs BR, Hallstrom B, Golladay GJ, Hoeffel D, Harris WH. Range of motion and stability in total hip arthroplasty with 28-, 32-, 38-, and 44-mm femoral head sizes. J Arthroplasty. 2005;20:11–9.

65. Aqil A, Drabu R, Bergmann JH, et al. The gait of patients with one resurfacing and one replacement hip: a single blinded controlled study. Int Orthop. 2013;37(5):795–801.
66. Shrader MW, Bhowmik-Stoker M, Jacofsky MC, Jacofsky DJ. Gait and stair function in total and resurfacing hip arthroplasty: a pilot study. Clin Orthop Relat Res. 2009;467:1476–84.
67. Wera GD, Gillespie RJ, Petty C, Petersilge WJ, Kraay MJ, Goldberg VM. Revision of hip resurfacing arthroplasty. Am J Orthop (Belle Mead NJ). 2010;39:E78–83.
68. Ball ST, Le Duff MJ, Amstutz HC. Early results of conversion of a failed femoral component in hip resurfacing arthroplasty. J Bone Joint Surg Am. 2007;89:735–41.
69. Gross TP, Liu F. Comparative study between patients with osteonecrosis and osteoarthritis after hip resurfacing arthroplasty. Acta Orthop Belg. 2012;78:735–44.
70. Kabata T, Maeda T, Tanaka K, et al. Hemi-resurfacing versus total resurfacing for osteonecrosis of the femoral head. J Orthop Surg (Hong Kong). 2011;19:177–80.
71. Cuckler JM, Moore KD, Estrada L. Outcome of hemiresurfacing in osteonecrosis of the femoral head. Clin Orthop Relat Res. 2004;146–50.
72. Amstutz HC, Esposito C, Campbell P. Long term preservation of femoral bone following hemiresurfacing. Hip Int. 2010;20:236–41.
73. Mont MA. CORR Insights: Does the extent of osteonecrosis affect the survival of hip resurfacing? Clin Orthop Relat Res. 2013;471(6):1935–6.
74. Hart AJ, Muirhead-Allwood S, Porter M, et al. Which factors determine the wear rate of large-diameter metal-on-metal hip replacements? Multivariate analysis of two hundred and seventy-six components. J Bone Joint Surg Am. 2013;95:678–85.
75. Johnson AJ, Zywiel MG, Hooper H, Mont MA. Narrowed indications improve outcomes for hip resurfacing arthroplasty. Bull NYU Hosp Jt Dis. 2011;69 Suppl 1:S27–9.
76. Schmalzried TP. Why total hip resurfacing. J Arthroplasty. 2007;22:57–60.
77. Liu F, Gross TP. A safe zone for acetabular component position in metal-on-metal hip resurfacing arthroplasty: winner of the 2012 HAP PAUL award. J Arthroplasty. 2013;28(7):1224–30.
78. Sayeed SA, Johnson AJ, Stroh DA, Gross TP, Mont MA. Hip resurfacing in patients who have osteonecrosis and are 25 years or under. Clin Orthop Relat Res. 2011;469:1582–8.
79. Stulberg BN, Fitts SM, Zadzilka JD, Trier K. Resurfacing arthroplasty for patients with osteonecrosis. Bull NYU Hosp Jt Dis. 2009;67:138–41.
80. Bose VC, Baruah BD. Resurfacing arthroplasty of the hip for avascular necrosis of the femoral head: a minimum follow-up of four years. J Bone Joint Surg Br. 2010;92:922–8.
81. Ortiguera CJ, Pulliam IT, Cabanela ME. Total hip arthroplasty for osteonecrosis: matched-pair analysis of 188 hips with long-term follow-up. J Arthroplasty. 1999;14:21–8.
82. Issa K, Naziri Q, Maheshwari AV, Rasquinha VJ, Delanois RE, Mont MA. Excellent results and minimal complications of total hip arthroplasty in sickle cell hemoglobinopathy at mid-term follow-up using cementless prosthetic components. J Arthroplasty. 2013;28(9):1693–8.
83. Ritter MA, Meding JB. A comparison of osteonecrosis and osteoarthritis patients following total hip arthroplasty. A long-term follow-up study. Clin Orthop Relat Res. 1986;139–46.
84. Saito S, Saito M, Nishina T, Ohzono K, Ono K. Long-term results of total hip arthroplasty for osteonecrosis of the femoral head. A comparison with osteoarthritis. Clin Orthop Relat Res. 1989;198–207.
85. Issa K, Johnson AJ, Naziri Q, Khanuja HS, Delanois RE, Mont MA. Hip osteonecrosis: does prior hip surgery alter outcomes compared to an initial primary total hip arthroplasty? J Arthroplasty. 2014;29(1):162–6.
86. Fyda TM, Callaghan JJ, Olejniczak J, Johnston RC. Minimum ten-year follow-up of cemented total hip replacement in patients with osteonecrosis of the femoral head. Iowa Orthop J. 2002;22:8–19.
87. Issa K, Naziri Q, Rasquinha VJ, Tatevossian T, Kapadia BH, Mont MA. Outcomes of primary total hip arthroplasty in systemic lupus erythematosus with a proximally-coated cementless stem. J Arthroplasty. 2013;28(9):1663–6.
88. Johannson HR, Zywiel MG, Marker DR, Jones LC, McGrath MS, Mont MA. Osteonecrosis is not a predictor of poor outcomes in primary total hip arthroplasty: a systematic literature review. Int Orthop. 2011;35:465–73.
89. McKellop H, Shen FW, Lu B, Campbell P, Salovey R. Development of an extremely wear-resistant ultra high molecular weight polyethylene for total hip replacements. J Orthop Res. 1999;17:157–67.
90. Muratoglu OK, Bragdon CR, O'Connor DO, Jasty M, Harris WH. A novel method of cross-linking ultra-high-molecular-weight polyethylene to improve wear, reduce oxidation, and retain mechanical properties. Recipient of the 1999 HAP Paul Award. J Arthroplasty. 2001;16:149–60.
91. Byun JW, Yoon TR, Park KS, Seon JK. Third-generation ceramic-on-ceramic total hip arthroplasty in patients younger than 30 years with osteonecrosis of femoral head. J Arthroplast. 2012;27: 1337–43.
92. Bedard NA, Callaghan JJ, Liu SS, Greiner JJ, Klaassen AL, Johnston RC. Cementless THA for the treatment of osteonecrosis at 10-year follow-up: have we improved compared to cemented THA? J Arthroplast. 2013;28:1192–9.
93. Radl R, Egner S, Hungerford M, Rehak P, Windhager R. Survival of cementless femoral components after osteonecrosis of the femoral head with different etiologies. J Arthroplast. 2005;20:509–15.
94. Issa K, Johnson AJ, Naziri Q, Khanuja HS, Delanois RE, Mont MA. Hip osteonecrosis: does prior hip surgery alter outcomes compared to an initial primary total hip arthroplasty? J Arthroplast. 2014;29:162–6.
95. Chang JS, Han DJ, Park SK, Sung JH, Ha YC. Cementless total hip arthroplasty in patients with osteonecrosis after kidney transplantation. J Arthroplast. 2013;28:824–7.
96. Al OA. Multiple drilling compared with standard core decompression for avascular necrosis of the femoral head in sickle cell disease patients. Arch Orthop Trauma Surg. 2013;133:609–13.
97. Lieberman JR, Conduah A, Urist MR. Treatment of osteonecrosis of the femoral head with core decompression and human bone morphogenetic protein. Clin Orthop Relat Res. 2004;139–145.
98. Aigner N, Schneider W, Eberl V, Knahr K. Core decompression in early stages of femoral head osteonecrosis--an MRI-controlled study. Int Orthop. 2002;26:31–5.
99. Lavernia CJ, Sierra RJ. Core decompression in atraumatic osteonecrosis of the hip. J Arthroplasty. 2000;15:171–8.
100. Maniwa S, Nishikori T, Furukawa S, Kajitani K, Iwata A, Nishikawa U, et al. Evaluation of core decompression for early osteonecrosis of the femoral head. Arch Orthop Trauma Surg. 2000;120:241–4.
101. Bozic KJ, Zurakowski D, Thornhill TS. Survivorship analysis of hips treated with core decompression for nontraumatic osteonecrosis of the femoral head. J Bone Joint Surg Am. 1999;81: 200–9.
102. Iorio R, Healy WL, Abramowitz AJ, Pfeifer BA. Clinical outcome and survivorship analysis of core decompression for early osteonecrosis of the femoral head. J Arthroplast. 1998;13:34–41.
103. Powell ET, Lanzer WL, Mankey MG. Core decompression for early osteonecrosis of the hip in high risk patients. Clin Orthop Relat Res. 1997;181–189.

104. Markel DC, Miskovsky C, Sculco TP, Pellicci PM, Salvati EA. Core decompression for osteonecrosis of the femoral head. Clin Orthop Relat Res. 1996:226–233.
105. Wei BF, Ge XH. Treatment of osteonecrosis of the femoral head with core decompression and bone grafting. Hip Int. 2011;21: 206–10.
106. Wang BL, Sun W, Shi ZC, Zhang NF, Yue DB, Guo WS, et al. Treatment of nontraumatic osteonecrosis of the femoral head using bone impaction grafting through a femoral neck window. Int Orthop. 2010;34:635–9.
107. Yuhan C, Hu CC, Chen DW, Ueng SW, Shih CH, Lee MS. Local cancellous bone grafting for osteonecrosis of the femoral head. Surg Innov. 2009;16:63–7.
108. Mont MA, Etienne G, Ragland PS. Outcome of nonvascularized bone grafting for osteonecrosis of the femoral head. Clin Orthop Relat Res. 2003;84–92.
109. Mont MA, Einhorn TA, Sponseller PD, Hungerford DS. The trapdoor procedure using autogenous cortical and cancellous bone grafts for osteonecrosis of the femoral head. J Bone Joint Surg (Br). 1998;80:56–62.
110. Chen CC, Lin CL, Chen WC, Shih HN, Ueng SW, Lee MS. Vascularized iliac bone-grafting for osteonecrosis with segmental collapse of the femoral head. J Bone Joint Surg Am. 2009;91:2390–4.
111. Kawate K, Yajima H, Sugimoto K, Ono H, Ohmura T, Kobata Y, et al. Indications for free vascularized fibular grafting for the treatment of osteonecrosis of the femoral head. BMC Musculoskelet Disord. 2007;8:78.
112. Hasegawa Y, Iwata H, Torii S, Iwase T, Kawamoto K, Iwasada S. Vascularized pedicle bone-grafting for nontraumatic avascular necrosis of the femoral head. A 5- to 11-year follow-up. Arch Orthop Trauma Surg. 1997;116:251–8.

Special Patients and Conditions: Sports Hernia

61

Michael A. Flaherty, Joshua A. Tuck, Jeffrey F. Murray, and Brian D. Busconi

Introduction

Injuries to the lower abdomen and groin region are frequent in certain sports, such as soccer, football, rugby, tennis, ice hockey, and field hockey [1]. These sports require repetitive twisting and turning at an elevated speed, leading to an overall rate of about 6% of all athletic injuries involving the lower abdomen and groin region [2]. The majority of these injuries are muscular strains that are self-limiting, and typically resolve within a few weeks. However, there are several causes of chronic pain involving the lower abdomen and groin region that can be debilitating and even career ending for an athlete. The differential diagnosis is broad and spans many medical subspecialities, from orthopedics and sports medicine to urology and general surgery. Besides a vast differential diagnosis, the lower abdomen and pelvic region have a complex overlapping anatomy, making a clear, objective diagnosis difficult as the athlete may present with multiple coexisting injuries in the same region.

M.A. Flaherty, M.D.
Orthopaedic Surgery, Albany Medical College, Albany, NY, USA

J.A. Tuck, D.O., M.S.
Department of Orthopaedic Surgery, Sports Medicine, University of Massachusetts Medical School, University of Massachusetts Memorial Medical Center, Worcester, MA, USA

J.F. Murray, D.O. • B.D. Busconi, M.D. (✉)
Orthopedics, Sports Medicine, University of Massachusetts Memorial Medical Center, Worcester, MA, USA
e-mail: Brian.Busconi@umassmemorial.org

Athletic Pubalgia or "Sports Hernia" is a syndrome of the lower abdomen and groin region that can present a challenge to the treating physician and lead to frustration amongst competitive athletes. It is a syndrome first defined as "pubalgia" by Taylor et al. [3], with the term reinforced by Meyers et al. [4] who support the idea that the "pubalgia" can affect a variety of anatomical structures around the hip joint, including the abdomen and anterior pelvis. Injuries can involve the lower abdominal muscles as well as the muscles that attach to the anterior pelvis, specifically the hip adductors and flexors. Meyers et al. [4] believe that as evaluating physicians, we should view injuries to this area as caused by an imbalance between the many overlapping muscles, leading to muscular strains, tears, and further soft tissue injuries. As we review the local anatomy and appreciate the mechanism of injury later in the chapter, the typical injury pattern involves a tear of the rectus abdominis insertion on the superior pubic ramus, with associated findings of a weakened posterior wall, and strains involving the surrounding musculature, specifically the hip adductors [4–6]. So, the term "pubalgia" appropriately fits the diagnosis, as the injury can involve a variety of the surrounding abdominal and anterior pelvic muscles.

It is easy to go through the past literature about such injuries and come out being confused. Historically two schools of thought have developed over the decades in viewing athletic pubalgia [5]. There have also been many different terms used to describe the presenting signs, symptoms, and pathology related to what we now describe as athletic pubalgia. Terms such as sports hernia, sportsman's hernia, Gilmore's groin, hockey groin, osteitis pubis, and pectineus syndrome have all been used to describe the different entities that cause chronic lower abdomen and groin pain. In fact, athletic pubalgia does not involve a hernia at all, as once believed, leading to a number of unwarranted hernia repairs with poor results. The misnomer of sports hernia should not be used interchangeably when talking about athletic pubalgia since it leads one to think of a hernia as the main offending problem, as well as leading the treating physician to think of one

J.C. McCarthy et al. (eds.), *Hip Joint Restoration*, DOI 10.1007/978-1-4614-0694-5_61

specific pathologic entity [7]. Athletic pubalgia involves a complex of a close and overlapping group of muscles around the lower abdomen and anterior pelvis, and can present with a variable presentation. The goal of this chapter is to provide a clear understanding of what athletic pubalgia represents, how it manifests, and the current workup and treatment options.

History

Issues with chronic lower abdominal and groin pain have plagued many athletes in past decades, and have even ended the career of many professionals. In 1980, O.J. Gilmore was one of the first to recognize the problem of chronic lower abdominal and groin pain in soccer players, and took the initiative to surgically repair the groin disruption, which was described as an attenuation of the external oblique, with separation of the conjoint tendon from the inguinal ligament, and laxity of the transversalis fascia [5, 8, 9]. He described these findings in a 1992 paper, where he reported his surgical experience involving 313 athlete cases, most of whom were soccer players in Europe, from which the term "Gilmore's Groin" was coined to describe the symptomatic condition [5]. In the mid-1980s, before the experience of dealing with this injury was widely published, Meyers had come across Duke University athletes who presented with chronic lower abdominal and groin injuries. At the time, Meyers admitted that he did not have much experience in dealing with these vague injury patterns, as many others were still coming across and learning of this debilitating condition [4]. After listening to a Yugoslavian physician named Nesovic, Meyers through his experience at Duke developed, with Drs. Basset and Garrett, the concept of viewing the anterior pelvis centered around a "pubic joint," and that injuries to the lower abdomen and groin region emanated from an imbalance at this joint [4]. We will review this concept of the "pubic joint" later in the chapter.

When Gilmore first started treating groin disruptions with the thought that the injury was primarily a muscle injury, others in Europe at the time felt that the chronic injury was the result of a developing posterior inguinal wall hernia. This was first described by Gullmo in 1980 [4, 10]. Others in the early 1990s described similar findings at the time of operative repair of these developing, weakened posterior walls of the inguinal canal. Polglase et al. [11] reported a weakened posterior wall in 85% of 64 Australian Rules football players, treated surgically for chronic lower abdominal and groin pain. In 1991, Taylor et al. also reported their results of athletes with chronic pain and found both palpable and nonpalpable hernias at the time of surgery, as well as microscopic tears involving the lower abdominal muscles [12]. Taylor termed the amalgam of various muscular injuries and abdominal wall weaknesses in this lower abdominal and groin area as "pubalgia" to reflect the vagueness of the clinical presentation for this injury.

As physicians searched and theorized the etiology of athletic pubalgia in the 1980s and early 1990s, two schools of thought developed regarding the underlying cause: (1) that the injury was due to a muscular disruption or was (2) due to an early developing inguinal hernia [4]. In order to appreciate how these two underlying theories developed, we must first review the pertinent anatomy and function of the muscles of the lower abdomen and anterior pelvis, and discuss the pathophysiologic processes that are theorized to cause the athletic pubalgia syndrome.

Anatomy

The pelvic bony complex is composed of the sacrum and the two innominate bones joined anteriorly at the pubic symphysis and posteriorly at the paired sacroiliac joints. The innominate bones are formed from the fusion of the triradiate cartilage at the acetabulum, composed of the ilium, ischium, and pubic ossification centers. The stability to the bony pelvic ring is mainly provided by the pubic symphysis, the paired sacroiliac joints, and the pelvic floor [13]. The anterior pubic symphysis and pubic rami provide 40% of the stiffness to the bony pelvic ring, while the posterior sacroiliac complex contributes 60% of the stability [13]. Further stability to the pelvis is imparted by the surrounding soft tissue complex, including the complexity of overlapping and joint crossing muscles, as well as the surrounding ligaments. The main function of the pelvis is to provide a center of balance for the body, transfer weight from the upper body to the axial skeleton and lower extremities, to protect the organs within the pelvic "bowl," and to withstand and dissipate compression forces imparted from one's body weight and activity [2, 7, 13]. The surrounding anatomy is complex, with Meyers stating that "there are more muscles, ligaments, bones and other soft tissues in the pelvis than anywhere else" [14].

The injuries pertinent to athletic pubalgia involve the anterior pelvis. The pubic symphysis is viewed as the centerpoint upon which the majority of forces are imparted during movement [7]. The pubic symphysis is an amphiarthrodial joint with a fibrocartilaginous disc interposed between the two pubic bones joined anteriorly [6]. There are four ligaments that surround the pubic symphysis, providing stability. The superior and inferior ligaments provide most of the resistance to shear forces [6]. Extending laterally from the pubic symphysis are the superior and inferior pubic rami. These structures, just as the pubic symphysis, provide insertional sites for surrounding muscles and also help dissipate the compressive forces from the pubic symphysis, transmitting them to the rest of the pelvis [6].

The pubic symphysis is the main fulcrum which serves as the attachment site for numerous musculotendinous units that help provide dynamic stability to the anterior pelvis [6]. The primary stabilizing muscle complex to this fulcrum, and the main musculotendinous unit injured in athletic pubalgia, is composed of the rectus abdominis musculature and the opposing adductor longi [2–4, 6, 7]. The rectus abdomini are paired, midline muscles which originate at the pubic symphysis and insert onto the inferior margin of the xiphoid process, and the fifth-seventh costal cartilages. The paired strap muscles are broader at their proximal attachment on the lower rib cage and taper towards the attachment on the pubic symphysis [6]. According to Omar et al., the tapered origin of these paired recti muscles on the pubic region may play a factor in generating concentrated forces here during strenuous and/or repetitive activities, potentially leading to injury [6]. The main function of the rectus abdomini muscles is to help flex the trunk, provide muscle tone to the anterior abdominal wall, and form an anchor for hip movement [6, 7].

The adductor longus takes off as a narrow tendinous origin off the anterior margin of the pubic symphysis, below the pubic crest, and travels distally to insert on the linea aspera of the femur. This muscle broadens as it inserts on the linea aspera, assisting in adduction at the hip, as well as flexion and internal rotation [6]. The adductor longus provides an anteroinferior force vector that is opposite that provided by the rectus abdominis muscle, with the fulcrum being the pubic symphysis. An anterior tilt of the pelvis is created with the composite force vectors [7]. As we review the pathophysiology, we will see how these opposing muscles provide stability to the anterior pelvis, and that imbalance between muscle groups may be a cause of pubalgia.

Although the midline rectus abdominis muscles and the adductor longus muscles are the main dynamic stabilizers to the anterior pelvis, it is important to discuss and understand the other surrounding abdominal wall muscles as well, as injuries to these dynamic stabilizers will also manifest in the syndrome of athletic pubalgia. The muscles around the rectus abdominis muscles that make up the abdominal wall are the external oblique, internal oblique, and transversus abdominis muscles and fascia, as well as the transversalis fascia [15]. The internal oblique and transverses abdominis aponeuroses blend as they travel midline to form a "conjoined tendon," which inserts onto the pubic tubercle [15]. They may frequently be found to have tearing at its insertion along with the rectus abdominis with an athletic pubalgia injury.

Distal to the pubic symphysis, the other adductor tendons can also be involved in athletic pubalgia injuries. The adductors brevis and magnus, just like the longus, originate from the inferior pubic ramus and insert onto the linea aspera of the femur. The function of the adductors is to adduct the thigh, assist with hip flexion, along with the iliopsoas and sartorius muscles, and with external rotation, along with the obturator externus. The adductors also help stabilize the anterior pelvis during the swing phase of gait [6]. The gracilis muscle, originating from the pubic arch and inserting at the pes anserine on the proximal medial tibia, is also contained within the medial compartment of the thigh, along with the adductors. The gracilis also helps with hip adduction and internal rotation, and helps flex the knee. The last muscle in the medial compartment of the thigh is the obturator externus, which originates off the obturator foramen of the pelvis and inserts on the trochanteric fossa of the femur [6]. The main function of the obturator externus is to externally rotate at the hip.

The muscles of the anterior thigh are also involved with athletic pubalgia injuries but are usually uncommon variants [7]. These anterior thigh muscles include the pectineus, sartorius, psoas, iliacus, rectus femoris, vastus lateralis, vastus medialis, and the vastus intermedius. The psoas tendon arises from the T12-L5 vertebrae and discs, as well as the transverse processes of the lumbar vertebrae, and inserts onto the lesser trochanter. The iliacus muscle arises from inner table of the iliac fossa of the pelvis, and travels distally to blend in with the psoas muscle as they insert onto the lesser trochanter as the iliopsoas tendon. These iliopsoas muscle functions as the "chief" flexor of the hip. This tendon has been implicated as a cause of internal snapping hip syndrome, which can be a painful snapping as the tendon slips from lateral to medial over the femoral head, or the iliopectineal ridge, as the hip is brought from flexion into extension. The pectineus muscle originates from the superior pubic ramus and inserts onto the femoral pectineal line. The pectineus muscle helps with adduction and flexion of the hip, and also assists with internal rotation. The sartorius muscle originates off the anterior superior iliac spine, and inserts onto the proximal medial tibia at the pes anserinus along with the gracilis. The sartorius flexes, adducts, and externally rotates the hip. The rectus femoris originates from the anterior inferior iliac spine, crosses both the hip and knee joint, and inserts onto the patella and tibial tubercle along with the other quadriceps muscles. The vastus lateralis, intermedius, and medialis originate off the greater trochanter, proximal femoral shaft, and intertrochanteric line, respectively. The rectus femoris, because it crosses the hip and knee joint, helps flex the hip and extend the knee, whereas the other quadriceps muscles help extend the knee.

The muscles of the posterior thigh are the least important in terms of involvement with the stability of the anterior pelvis [7]. The posterior thigh muscles include the hamstring muscles, made up of the long and short heads of the biceps femoris, the semitendinosus, and the semimembranosus.

Pathophysiology

Understanding the anatomy of the region and the forces of the individual musculotendinous units on the stability of the anterior pelvis helps demonstrate the imbalance that is created with an injury to the area, leading to the various manifestations of athletic pubalgia syndrome.

Meyers et al. describe the anterior pelvis as a "pubic joint," similar to the knee joint, composed of "both pubic symphyseal bones and the entire anterior pelvic musculoskeleton around these bones" [4]. The main stabilizers of this "pubic joint" are the central rectus abdominis musculotendinous unit on the abdominal side of the joint, and the adductor longus musculotendinous unit on the opposite, inferior side of the anterior pelvis. This opposing muscle complex is seen as being analogous to the location of the cruciate ligaments of the knee [4, 14]. The more lateral, surrounding ligaments and muscles such as the psoas, sartorius, and rectus muscles around the anterior pelvis are viewed as being analogous to the collateral ligaments of the knee [14]. As per Meyers [14], these lateral structures "provide important support, but are not as important for stability, and heal quickly without surgery."

It is believed that sports that require repetitive twisting and rapid changes in direction can lead to injuries involving the anterior pelvis. According to Meyers et al. [4], the most common mechanism of injury is believed to be a combination of "hyperextension of the abdomen and/or hyperabduction of the thigh." These forces are most dramatically seen with bull riders, who exhibit the extremes of the proposed mechanism of injury, with cases of complete avulsion of the rectus abdominis muscles or adductor muscles being reported [4]. The tremendous torque placed on the anterior pelvic muscles usually causes injury to the weaker abdominal muscles first either acutely or with repetitive force. This affects the midline rectus abdominis with insertional tears at the pubic symphysis. An imbalance of opposing forces is created, which leads to a greater force vector within the adductors. It is then postulated that this imbalance of unopposed forces leads to a propagation of the tear across the aponeurosis on the pubic symphysis to involve the adductor longus tendon first followed by increased stress on the other adductors with further propagation of injury [4, 6]. The injury pattern can then disrupt lateral balance and involve the contralateral side.

Prior to this hypothesis, there were two schools of thought, as mentioned earlier, regarding the basis of athletic pubalgia injury. On one side, the etiology behind the vague presentation of pubalgia was thought to originate from an incipient inguinal hernia [5]. That repetitive twisting motion produced a weakness involving the posterior wall of the inguinal canal. At the time of surgery for many of these chronic lower abdominal and groin injuries, a bulge was appreciated involving the posterior wall, which was then repaired with traditional hernia repair techniques. Some patients came out doing well from the surgery, but the majority still suffered from anterior pelvic pain and could not return to the same level of performance in their respective sport. The other stance was that the initial injury was muscular in origin, either a chronic strain or tear involving the lower abdominal or anterior pelvic muscles.

It is now appreciated that likely a muscular injury takes place first with disruption and attenuation of the lower abdominal muscles, with an eventual failure of the transversalis fascia in the posterior wall of the inguinal canal, leading to the bulge appreciated at the time of surgery [5]. Although Meyers postulates that the injury is muscular in origin, his group did find that at the time of surgery involving 157 athletes, that 57 % of them had a "loose feeling" involving the inguinal floor [16]. Polglase et al., who believed that the injury was primarily a developing inguinal hernia, found "an apparent splitting of the conjoined tendon" in 26 % of their patients at the time of the hernia repair [5, 11]. Athletic pubalgia is likely muscular in origin but subsequently has an associated weakening of the posterior inguinal wall.

The injury can involve any of the lower abdominal or anterior pelvic muscles, and may present with a variable set of vague complaints; however, with the above understanding of the mechanism of injury and the muscles involved, the athletic pubalgia injury usually involves the rectus abdominis and the adductor unit (Fig. 61.1).

Epidemiology

As the diagnosis of athletic pubalgia is becoming better recognized amongst physicians, athletic trainers, physical therapists, and radiologists, we have a better understanding of the patient most likely to develop the associated injury patterns.

According to Meyers et al., "forces in the pelvis increase as the muscle strength increases," and in their experience, it explains why the majority of the athletic pubalgia cases occurs in the most physically conditioned patients [7]. Most of the patients tend to be male, and although the age range is widening, the typical patient is under the age of 40 [6]. Two or three decades ago, it was thought that the male predominance with athletic pubalgia was due to a disparity between the sexes in athletic participation. According to Meyers et al., in the mid-80s, there were no females reflected in the literature with athletic pubalgia, but in a recent profile, women represented 8.2 % of those with this condition [17]. However, despite the increased participation of females in sports that require rapid changes in direction, with cutting and pivoting, the gender disparity continues to exist.

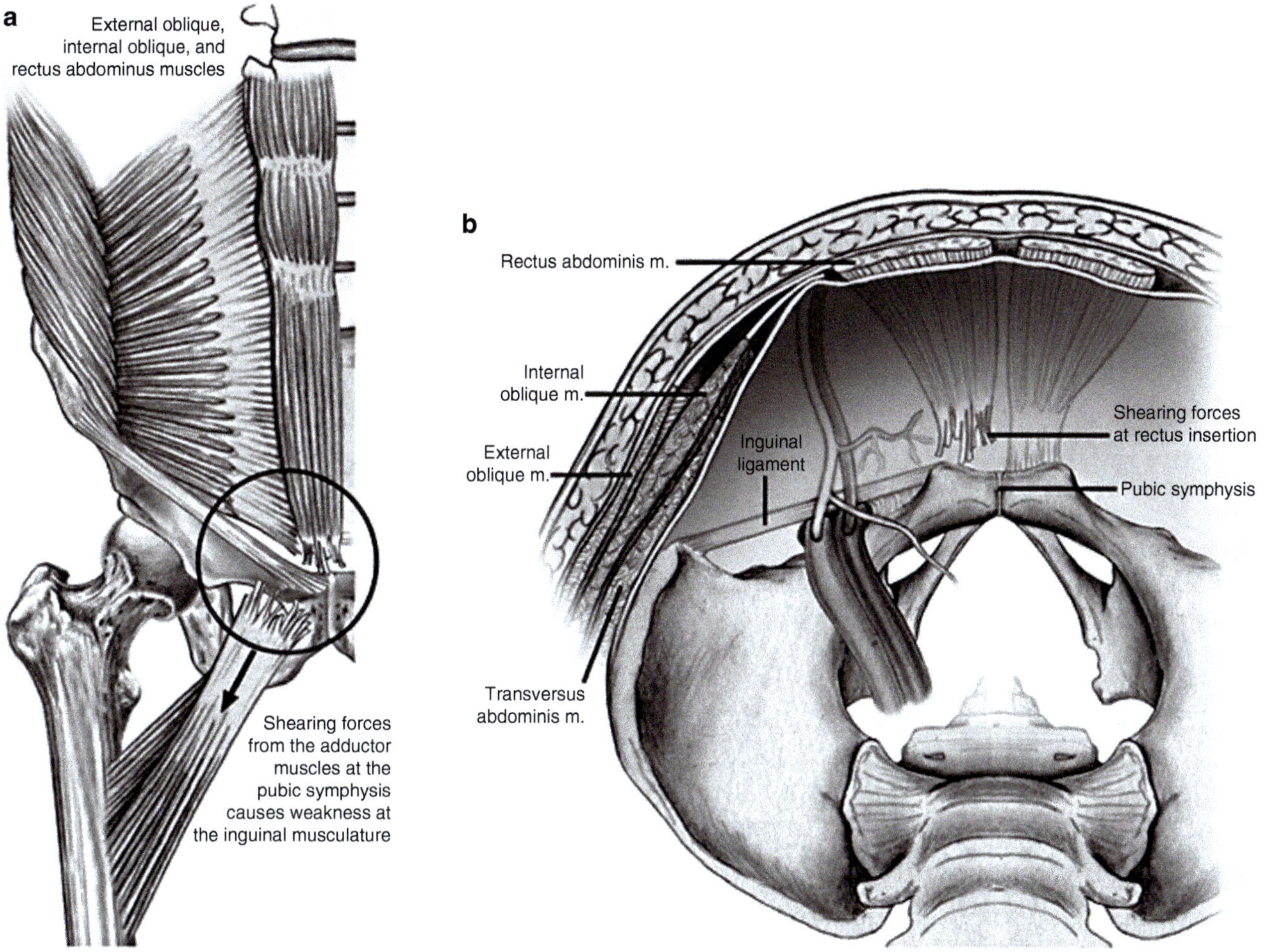

Fig. 61.1 Anatomy and proposed shearing pathophysiology of athletic pubalgia. (**a**) Extra-abdominal view (**b**) Intra-abdominal view. (Courtesy Barre AA, Guanche CA [35])

It has been theorized that the anatomical differences between the male and female pelvis, as well as differences in the musculotendinous attachments on the anterior pelvis, have led to the greater incidence of pubalgia-type injuries in males. Firstly, the female pelvis is wider, with a larger subpubic angle than the male pelvis, which may help dissipate the forces away from the anterior pelvis to the more narrow stance of the female knees [4, 6]. This may partially help explain why females are more likely to suffer injuries to the knees during landing than males. The male pelvis is also thicker and heavier than the female pelvis, which causes greater shifts in the forces during activity, and further stress to the anterior pelvis [7]. Also the musculotendinous origin of the rectus abdominis muscles is broader in females than in males, which dissipates the contractile forces of the muscles over a broader area. Females are also more likely to suffer musculotendinous injuries involving the more lateral muscles, such as the sartorius, rectus femoris, or psoas muscles due to the wider female pelvis and its mechanical dependence on the lateral supporting structures [7].

Table 61.1 Distribution of athletic pubalgia by sport [7]

Top six sports (total 8490 athletes)	
Sport	%
Soccer	44.6
Football	22.3
Hockey	8.1
Baseball	6.3
Basketball	6.2
Distance running	1.2

The distribution of sports played that had the highest incidence of athletic pubalgia is listed in Table 61.1.

Differential Diagnosis

The differential diagnosis for lower abdominal and groin pain is vast.

Differential diagnosis of lower abdomen/groin pain in athletes
Musculoskeletal causes
Hip-related pathology
• Acetabular labral tear
• Femoroacetabular impingement
• Femoral neck stress fracture
• Internal/external snapping hip syndrome
• Slipped capital femoral epiphysis
• Legg-Calve-Perthes disease
– Avascular necrosis of the femoral head
– Osteoarthritis
– Rheumatoid arthritis
– Trochanteric bursitis
Pelvic-related pathology
• Osteitis pubis
• Apophysitis
• Apophyseal avulsion fracture
• Sacroiliitis
• Piriformis syndrome
• Proximal hamstring strain/rupture
• Hip flexor/adductor strain
• Iliac crest contusion (hip pointer)
Other
• Lumbosacral pain/herniated disc
Infectious causes
• Osteomyelitis
• Septic arthritis
• Orchitis
• Epididymitis
• Urinary tract infection
• Diverticulitis
• Prostatitis
Inflammatory causes
• Endometriosis
• Pelvic inflammatory disease
• Inflammatory bowel disease
Neoplastic causes
• Testicular cancer
• Metastatic lesions of the hip/pelvic/lumbosacral spine
• Ovarian cancer
• Primary bone tumor
Other causes
• Testicular torsion
• Ovarian cyst
• Hydrocele
• Nerve entrapment (Obturator nerve)

Varying clinical problems may present with similar signs and symptoms, as well as similar and overlapping clinical exam findings. Patients may have other orthopedic, neurological, gastrointestinal, genitourinary, gynecological, oncological, and/or abdominal pathology present that may require attention. Meyers analyzed 100 consecutive pelvic MRIs of patients with athletic pubalgia, and found that just over 15 % of the patients also had concomitant hip pathology present [17]. It is up to the treating physician to consider all the different clinical entities that may potentially exist, or co-exist, and evaluate them based on the history, physical exam, and imaging studies.

In the past, as we were still learning of the pathophysiology and presentation of athletic pubalgia, it often took months to years before athletes were diagnosed for chronic lower abdominal and groin pain due to pubalgia. However, with a better understanding of this syndrome, there are clear historical findings, characteristic physical exam findings, and better MRI imaging protocols that have allowed us to hone in on the diagnosis.

Presentation

The pain associated with athletic pubalgia is most commonly insidious in onset, unilateral, deep seated, sharp to burning in character, and may radiate down to the scrotum, perineum, the inner thigh, the low back, or even the contralateral side, depending on the patterns of compensation [4–6, 14, 15]. Although the injury is usually insidious in onset, some athletes do recall a traumatic event that may have initiated the injury [5]. The pain is typically aggravated by activity and relieved by rest. Patients may have trouble getting up in the mornings due to stiffness [5]. The pain may also be brought on by Valsalva pressure such as coughing or sneezing. The pain becomes lingering as a dull ache at rest that takes longer to resolve after stopping the aggravating activity. An athlete may try to participate in their sport through the pain, but will either not perform at the same level or may not tolerate the pain to continue participating [5].

Kachingwe et al. provide a cluster of signs and symptoms that they feel summarize the characteristic presentation: (1) the athlete complaining of deep groin pain, (2) pain that is aggravated by activities, such as sports involving twisting, turning, kicking, etc., and relieved by rest, (3) tenderness upon exam over the pubic ramus, where the rectus abdominis muscle inserts, (4) pain with resisted hip adduction, (5) and lastly, pain with a resisted sit-up [5, 18].

In contrast to the muscular pain associated with athletic pubalgia, that is exacerbated by activity, hip-related pain is typically present with minimal activity, such as sitting or standing for a prolonged period of time, walking, or going up and down stairs [14]. According to Meyers, hip pain is typically "more sporadic and less predictable" [14].

Pain related to other lower abdominal pathology will typically present with either continuous or sporadic pain, typically unrelated to activity [14]. Meyers et al. evaluated the cause of lower abdominal or inguinal pain in high-performance athletes, and found that in 16 out of 20 women in their study, the cause of the pain was not related to athletic pubalgia [16]. The women in that study were discovered to have either endometriosis, ovarian cysts, pelvic inflammatory disease, Crohn's disease, or pain related to the menstrual cycle [16]. In that same study, during the preoperative workup, it was found that the most common cause of lower abdominal or inguinal pain was due to inflammatory bowel disease [16]. Along with the history, the physical exam and different imaging modalities will help make the diagnosis.

Physical Examination

Patients presenting with athletic pubalgia will have localized tenderness at the origin of the rectus abdominis muscle on the pubic tubercle/crest, proximally over the musculotendinous unit, and involving the conjoined tendon [5, 15]. Although a true inguinal hernia is not present with athletic pubalgia, a dilated and tender superficial inguinal ring may be palpated [5]. It is also important to check the contralateral side to evaluate for bilateral involvement. Pain can also be elicited in the region of the rectus abdominis origin with a resisted sit-up, which is a characteristic provocative test for athletic pubalgia. Patients frequently have tenderness over the adductor origin, and along the proximal musculotendinous unit of the adductors. Pain involving the adductors can also be elicited with active adduction of the thigh, which may also exacerbate the rectus abdominis symptoms [5].

It is also important to evaluate for intra-articular hip pathology, since hip pathology can be present in the face of athletic pubalgia. Range of motion of the hip in flexion, extension, internal and external rotation, as well as abduction and adduction must be evaluated. Patients with femoral acetabular impingement (FAI) have been found to have limitations with internal rotation. The log roll test of the lower extremity can produce pain with intra-articular hip pathology. Rotational tests such as the FABER (flexion, abduction, external rotation) and the FADIR (flexion, adduction, internal rotation) tests can produce pain related to FAI during the maneuvers. The FABER test can also produce pain at the sacroiliac joint if there is inflammation present in the posterior pelvis.

Palpation over the anterior hip region, overlying the psoas tendon, may identify psoas-related pathology as a source of anterior hip pain, which may co-exist with athletic pubalgia. Resistive hip flexion may also produce pain involving the psoas musculotendinous unit. Positioning the patient in the lateral decubitus position with the unaffected side down allows evaluation of the lateral and posterior aspects of the hip region. Palpation over the greater trochanteric region and distal to the greater trochanter over the iliotibial band will isolate any irritation of the trochanteric bursa. Ober's test (extending the thigh and then allowing the thigh to adduct) is sensitive in evaluating for iliotibial band contracture. If the thigh does not adduct towards the opposite side in this position, then a positive Ober's test is present. Palpation of the piriformis region can also be performed to evaluate for piriformis syndrome in the lateral decubitus position. It is imperative to check for an inguinal hernia in the standing position, evaluate the thoracolumbar spine for any etiological factors that may generate radicular symptoms into the lower extremities, and examine the gait for a Trendelenburg sign.

Imaging

The diagnosis of athletic pubalgia is made primarily from the history and physical examination. Imaging studies are used to exclude other potential causes of lower abdominal or groin pain. MR imaging has come a long way in helping reinforce the diagnosis, or helping to confer the presence or absence of other potential pathology.

Plain radiographs of the lumbar spine, pelvis, and hips should be obtained in the evaluation of athletic pubalgia, mainly to rule out any other pathology that may be present. Irregularity, bone resorption, sclerosis, and symphyseal widening may be present with osteitis pubis [15]. The hip joint should be evaluated for developmental dysplasia, avascular necrosis, and femoroacetabular impingement or arthritic changes. Evaluating the lumbar spine for arthritic changes, spondylolisthesis, spondylosis or any other process that has the potential of encroaching on a nerve, and causing referred pain in the groin region is imperative in the radiographic examination. Evaluate the sacroiliac joints for signs of arthritic changes, or the pelvis for signs of an apophyseal avulsion injury that are typically seen in the adolescent athletic population.

Bone scans may be used to exclude other potential causes for lower abdominal or groin pain. Increased uptake can be appreciated with osteitis pubis, osteoarthritis, the presence of certain tumors, and osteomyelitis. The bone scan is not the best test for the evaluation or diagnosis of athletic pubalgia; it can be used however to evaluate a larger area of bony structures. Although increased uptake may be appreciated at the origin of the rectus abdominis or adductor muscles, bone scans, overall, have a lack of specificity [19].

Dynamic ultrasound has been used by some clinicians in making the diagnosis of athletic pubalgia. The ultrasound is used to detect for any protrusion that might be present in the posterior wall of the inguinal canal during a Valsalva maneuver [15]. Although a weakness of the posterior wall may be seen secondary to a tear involving the rectus abdominis or conjoint tendon attachments, the use of an ultrasound does not provide much appreciation for the inciting pathology. The ultrasound can be used to appreciate primary hernias of the abdomen or inguinal region that may be present, or for other pathologic processes, such as ovarian cysts, endometriosis, as well as other soft tissue masses or tumors. Dynamic ultrasound is a noninvasive modality, and readily available; however it is highly operator-dependent in evaluating for athletic pubalgia [19].

Herniography, popularized in Europe, provides similar information as an ultrasound, providing a detailed outline of the peritoneal cavity and the presence of any hernias within the lower abdomen or groin region. It is an invasive diagnostic technique that involves the injection of a contrast dye into the peritoneal space, with fluoroscopic views taken as the patient performs Valsalva maneuvers [15, 19]. The test is considered positive if a herniation is appreciated within the normal contour of the peritoneal cavity [15]. However, the primary etiology of athletic pubalgia seems to involve a tear of the rectus abdominis or adductor muscle complex, and therefore, does not make the use of herniography beneficial to confirm the diagnosis. The invasive procedure also carries the risk of potential complications such as infection, hollow viscus perforation, hematomas, vasovagal reactions, and dye reactions [19]. The complication rates range anywhere from 3 to 6 % [19–22]. Herniography should not play a role in the diagnosis of athletic pubalgia [5].

Compared to the other imaging modalities, MRI has been most reliable in providing imaging of the complex soft tissue anatomy of the lower abdomen and groin region. In the early 1990s, MRI identified specific musculoskeletal pathology only 10–15 % of the time, mostly providing evidence of other soft tissue diagnoses [4]. At the time, clinicians could occasionally correlate "soft" findings in patients with a working diagnosis of athletic pubalgia, including tiny avulsion fractures and edema patterns on the side of injury [4, 17]. The constellation of "soft" findings on the side of injury helped bring attention to the area, and allowed radiologists to study the various attachments to the anterior pelvic region, and refine the MRI imaging techniques [4, 17].

Omar et al. have developed a specific MRI protocol to enhance the diagnostic findings of athletic pubalgia [6]. Initially a large field, scout view is taken of the pelvis to reveal any suspected lesions that may be present in association with the typical athletic pubalgia findings. If a lesion is found within the pelvic region, further high-resolution small field-of-view images can be focused on that particular area [6]. The MRI is centered on the pubic symphysis to obtain dedicated images that better define the region of suspected pathology in athletic pubalgia [6]. Images are taken in the axial, sagittal, and coronal planes, with both non-fat-suppressed T1 images and fat-suppressed fluid-sensitive T2 images [6]. Fluid-sensitive sequences are beneficial in finding areas where tears may be present, with fluid undermining the torn region; seen as increased signal intensity on the T2 images [6]. According to Omar et al., the tenoperiosteal disruption that occurs at the rectus abdominis-adductor aponeurosis on the anterior aspect of the pubic body is best visualized on the axial and sagittal T2 images approximately 1–2 cm lateral to the pubic symphysis [6]. The area of the rectus abdominis tendinous insertion on the pubic symphysis may appear edematous or atrophic on the sequences [6]. Also described is a "secondary cleft sign" on the ipsilateral side of suspected injury [6, 23, 24]. The "secondary cleft sign" is thought to be a microtear in the origin of the adductors, and appears as a "curvilinear region of high signal intensity adjoining the pubic symphysis" [6, 23, 24]. The adductor tendons, with the adductor longus being most commonly involved, can also appear edematous, thickened, disrupted, or frankly torn from their pubic body attachments [6].

Meyers et al. analyzed 100 consecutive MRIs of patients with athletic pubalgia, and the most common finding (93 %) was a soft tissue disruption involving both the rectus abdominis and adductor attachment sites on the ipsilateral side of the pubic body [17]. The adductor longus was most frequently involved, followed by the pectineus, and the adductor brevis [17]. The most frequently involved muscles outside of the adductors and rectus abdominis muscles were the iliopsoas, rectus femoris, and sartorius [17].

Meyers et al. also found that 15 % of patients with MRI findings related to athletic pubalgia also had associated hip pathology [17]. It is important to make the distinction between these two pathologic entities that can produce groin pain, along with other pathologies that can produce referred pain in and around the pelvis. If there is high suspicion of hip-related pathology, obtaining an MR arthrogram with gadolinium contrast can be used to provide evidence of any suspected hip pathology; labral tears, or acetabular chondral injury. A local anesthetic can also be injected into the hip at the time of the arthrogram, both for diagnostic and therapeutic purposes.

MRI can provide diagnostic findings that are confirmed at surgery in 91 % of cases [17, 25]. Despite continued improvement in MRI evaluation the diagnosis of athletic pubalgia is still made with history and clinical exam [26]. With the evolving MRI technology, and with better understanding of the complex and overlapping anatomy of the anterior pelvis, the pathophysiology of athletic pubalgia can be more accurately studied.

Nonoperative Treatment

The majority of injuries involving the lower abdomen and groin region respond well to nonoperative treatment, including rest, modification of activity, anti-inflammatory medication, ice and physical therapy. Meyers et al. describe many different patterns of musculotendinous involvement as athletic pubalgia, with some patterns responding better to conservative measures than others. Surgical intervention is usually required for the most common pattern of athletic pubalgia, involving the "central" region of the rectus abdominis-adductor complex on the pubic body [14]. The "non-central" patterns that typically respond well to nonoperative treatment can also become chronic in nature and may require surgical intervention [5].

There is no formal algorithm for the management of athletic pubalgia. According to Litwin et al., a trial of nonoperative treatment for at least 3 months, from the onset of symptoms, should be conducted [5]. For in-season athletes, Litwin et al. allowed a 4-week period of rest for the athlete, and the option of a corticosteroid injection at the insertion of the rectus abdominis or the adductors on the pubic body to provide therapeutic relief, versus a short course of oral steroids [5]. The treatment should also include the above stated treatment modalities for typical groin strains, as well as closed-chain lower extremity workouts, and core strengthening, focusing on the abdominal muscles, the lumbar spine, hips, and thigh muscles. The goal of therapy is to balance the hip and pelvic stabilizers [14, 15]. After the 4-week period of rest is completed, the athlete may participate in functional activities related to his or her sport to assess if the athlete is comfortable and can perform their respective activity at a desired performance level [5]. If the pain continues to linger, the decision is left to the athlete whether to continue participating or undergo surgical treatment. Insertional tears of the rectus or adductor tendons are not made worse with athletic activity [5].

Surgical Treatment

Surgical intervention is only undertaken after the failure of nonoperative management for 3 months or more and usually after the completion of the patient's athletic season. Surgery should only be considered when careful elicitation of the history and physical has excluded other potential causes of chronic lower abdominal and groin pain.

At the present time, there is no consensus on the preferred surgical technique, as practitioners are still learning the complexities of the anterior pelvis and still debating the underlying pathophysiology. There are three main categories of surgical intervention under which several different operative techniques fall for the treatment of athletic pubalgia [5, 15]. The categories are: open repair with sutures (no mesh), open repair with mesh, and laparoscopic repair with mesh. There are also combinations of the three categories, such as combining the suture repair of the anterior pelvis with mesh on-lay, or operations which add a nerve release, or a muscle release [5]. All the techniques are variations of the traditional, established surgical techniques for conventional inguinal hernia repairs [5].

Under the laparoscopic category, there are two variations of the technique that both introduce a mesh over the inguinal region, where a defect may be present, but differ in how they approach the preperitoneal space laparoscopically [5, 27, 28]. With the transabdominal preperitoneal (TAPP) approach, the peritoneal cavity is entered, a flap is created in the peritoneum over the inguinal region where a defect is present, and a mesh is then placed over the space created from the flap [5]. Per Litwin et al. the mesh covers "the entire myopectineal orifice and thereby occludes any defect that may be present in the direct, indirect, or femoral space" [5]. In the totally extraperitoneal (TEP) approach, the peritoneal space is not entered, and the dissection is carried out in the preperitoneal space, until a plane is developed that allows visualization of the inguinal region where a weakness is suspected, and a mesh is then similarly placed over this area [5].

The open suture repair technique and the open mesh on-lay technique are selected based on the primary pathophysiology, which is still under debate. The suture technique is used to primarily repair the rectus insertion to the pubis, while the mesh technique is used to prevent bulging and defects (classical hernia repair). In contrast to the laparoscopic technique, the open approach allows better visualization of the anterior pelvic structures, and allows the surgeon to combine suture repair with the mesh on-lay technique if needed. The primary goal of the suture repair is to bring down the inferolateral border of the rectus abdominis muscle with its fascial attachment to the pubic tubercle, establishing a broader attachment of its insertion to help balance the anterior pelvis with the adductor insertion on the inferior aspect of the pubic body [15, 16]. Tightening and broadening the musculotendinous insertion of the rectus abdominis muscle may also help reinforce the posterior inguinal wall, making the use of mesh unnecessary.

The open suture repair technique that broadens the insertion of the rectus abdominis muscle was initially described by Meyers [16]. Meyers believes that the pathology related to athletic pubalgia is due to an imbalance between the soft tissue structures of the anterior pelvis, and that surgery should involve either "tightening" or "loosening" of the "involved" structures [14]. He feels that the use of mesh in athletic pubalgia cases is unnecessary and should be avoided, and that if the surgery is unsuccessful, it can become challenging determining whether the failure occurred due to the mesh or missed pathology [14].

Muschaweck and Berger also describe an open suture repair technique that is described as a "minimal repair" technique with good results [29]. However, in contrast to Meyers, Muschaweck and Berger believe that the diagnosis of athletic pubalgia is made by the presence of a localized bulge in the posterior wall of the inguinal canal during a Valsalva maneuver [29]. This localized bulge leads the rectus abdominis muscle to retract cranially and medially, exerting tension on the anterior pelvis, producing the pain related to athletic pubalgia [29]. Per Muschaweck and Berger, this localized bulge in the posterior wall of the inguinal canal can also compress the genital branch of the genitofemoral nerve and produce related pain in the groin region [29].

The open suture "minimal repair" technique described by Muschaweck and Berger involves opening only the defect of the posterior wall without enlarging the area into the surrounding soft tissues [29]. The posterior wall is then stabilized by a "nearly tension-free suture" with "doubling of the fascia transversalis [enclosing] only the area of fascial weakness" [29]. The suture repair also incorporates lateralizing the rectus abdominis insertion, which helps counteract the increased tension created on the pubic body from the cranially and medially retracted rectus muscle [29]. If it was determined that the genital branch of the genitofemoral nerve was compressed by the bulge of the posterior wall, this branch was then sacrificed [29].

Unpublished data from JB Hanks, 2009, reports the results of a series of patients with athletic pubalgia treated with either the Meyer's technique or the Muschaweck and Berger technique [15]. In one group, 17 athletes underwent a primary repair of the rectus abdominis muscle, similar to the technique described by Meyers, with an adductor release included in 16 of the athletes [15]. In the other group, 10 athletes were treated with the "minimal repair" technique described by Muschaweck and Berger. The patients in both groups had similar results with respect to patient satisfaction and return to the same level of performance, but the patients in the "minimal repair" technique returned to their respective sport sooner (averaging 4.5 weeks) compared to the group treated with Meyer's technique (averaging 16.5 weeks return to sporting activity) [15].

A literature review on the surgical treatment of athletic pubalgia showed that 35 % of open and 100 % of laparoscopic procedures used mesh [27]. Meyers, Muschaweck, and Berger all feel that mesh should not be included in the treatment of athletic pubalgia [14, 29, 30]. Per Muschaweck and Berger, "the inserted mesh results in localized stiffening of the abdominal muscles and, therefore, restricted movement…in athletes who require full elasticity and movement in their abdominal muscles" [29]. Mesh can also lead to complications of infection, fistula formation, migration, and foreign body reactions [29]. For those surgeons who do use mesh, whether for conventional inguinal hernia repair or for athletic pubalgia, there is controversy regarding the weight and porosity of the mesh, as this affects the extent of scarring [5].

The results overall seem comparable with suitable outcomes regardless of the varying approaches or thoughts on pathophysiology [5]. Success rates for both laparoscopic and open techniques range from 63 to 97 % for improvement of symptoms and returning to a pre-injury level of athletic participation [27]. Based on a systematic literature review by Caudill et al., there is a comparable success rate between open and laparoscopic athletic pubalgia repair, with 92.8 % (SD 9.9 %) of open cases and 96.0 % (SD 4.5 %) of laparoscopic cases successfully returning to sporting activity [27]. In a similar review article published by Nam and Brody, there were 12 studies of open repair compared to 7 studies of laparoscopic repair [5, 31]. The results showed that the open repair studies reported a success rate from 77 to 100 %, which was comparable to the laparoscopic studies showing a range of 87 to 100 % [5, 31].

Litwin et al. believe there may be "unifying principles of treatment that are satisfied to some extent by all of these operations." Most of the reported successful open and laparoscopic operations contain (1) reinforcement of the posterior wall of the inguinal canal and (2) fixation of the rectus abdominis or rectus/conjoined tendon complex [5]. The use of mesh to reinforce the posterior wall may also inadvertently tighten and broaden the fixation of the rectus abdominis muscle through fibrosis between the mesh and rectus muscle, which fixates the muscle [5].

An adductor release can also be added in the surgical treatment of athletic pubalgia. According to Meyers et al., if the rectus abdominis muscle complex is disrupted, this can lead to an unopposed pull from the adductor muscles which may create a compartment syndrome phenomenon within the adductor compartment, and the related adductor pain [16]. The adductor component may be a "secondary phenomenon," with associated edema seen on MRI, reflective of tendinopathy at the origin of the adductors [16]. At the time of surgery, an epimysial adductor release can provide relief of this increased pressure within the adductor compartment. Meyers describes the adductor release as a "complete division of all the anterior epimysial fibers of the adductor longus muscle about 2–3 cm from the pubic insertion, leaving the muscle belly intact. Multiple longitudinal incisions are also made into the tendinous insertion site on the pubis, similar to the incisions into the tendinous insertion site in treatment for lateral epicondylitis [16].

Muschaweck and Berger feel that a significant cause of groin pain associated with athletic pubalgia is due to the compression of the genital branch of the genitofemoral nerve from the bulge of the posterior wall [29]. As there are so many variations of procedures for the treatment of athletic pubalgia, there is increasing speculation that nerve release may play an important step [5].

Further studies are needed to explore the etiology of athletic pubalgia. There is a need for prospective randomized controlled studies that compare the open suture repair techniques with the on-lay mesh techniques, as well as studies that gauge the successful outcome of surgery solely not only based on whether the athlete returned to sports activity but also based on patient-directed outcome measures.

Postoperative Rehabilitation

After the open procedure, the postoperative rehabilitation involves a 4-week period of relative rest, which does not preclude activities of daily living but does not allow activities such as heavy lifting or any strenuous exercise. The use of a stationary bike, gentle stretching, or pool walking is allowed during this time period. After 4 weeks, core strengthening, closed-chain exercises, as well as exercises that work on improving endurance and coordination are added [5, 32]. At the 6–8-week mark progressive running is started, and by the 3-month mark, sprinting, cutting, pivoting, as well as other sports-specific activities can begin [24, 32]. Most protocols allow return to full competitive sports by 3 months if no pain is experienced. In general, after a laparoscopic repair, most athletes are able to return to full competition at around 6–8 weeks [27].

The open "minimal repair" technique described by Muschaweck and Berger allows a more aggressive rehabilitation protocol, with lifting up to 44 pounds immediately after surgery, running and cycling on postoperative day 2, and starting sport-specific training by postoperative day 4 [29]. This protocol allows an athlete to return to play much sooner than the traditional 3 months described by other open techniques, as well as much earlier than the laparoscopic techniques.

Most preventative programs focus on reducing the risk of muscular strains in the lower abdomen and groin region, by working on trying to balance the abdominal and pelvic musculature, stretching and core exercises [15]. Orchard et al. report using ultrasound as a screening tool for asymptomatic soccer players in the preseason for evaluation of the posterior wall [33]. Hogan et al. have created an adductor squeeze test using a blood pressure cuff to evaluate reduced adductor power and identify early microtear pathology [34]. The squeeze test is performed weekly and those with noted weakness have reduced training load and increased core stability training. Future research exploring the effectiveness of these preventative exercise programs is needed.

Summary

Athletic pubalgia is a syndrome of the lower abdomen and groin region, predominantly affecting athletes involved with repetitive twisting and turning in their respective sports. This repetitive load leads to increased torque and tension on the dynamic stabilizers of the anterior pelvis. The injury is most likely muscular in origin, most frequently involving the rectus abdominis-adductor complex, with eventual failure of the transversalis fascia, and the resultant formation of a bulge in the posterior wall of the inguinal canal. The athlete can sustain an acute injury, but typically the syndrome develops insidiously, with pain developing and increasing in the lower abdomen and groin region with increased activity negatively affecting the level of athletic performance. With increased awareness of the syndrome, physicians and trainers are becoming better educated on diagnosing the injury sooner, treating the athlete sooner and returning the athlete to sports. Nonsurgical treatment for athletic pubalgia has typically been found not to provide long-term relief, with surgical intervention often being necessary. A variety of surgical treatment options are used today, as surgeons are still debating the underlying etiology of athletic pubalgia. However, the underlying principles of surgery do involve reinforcement of the posterior wall of the inguinal canal and fixation of the rectus abdominis tear, whether through suturing techniques or inadvertent scarring from mesh placement. Future research is needed to explore and compare the different surgical treatment modalities, and evaluate the etiology of a syndrome that has been described vaguely in the past, and is only now becoming better defined through experience and an appreciation of the complex anatomy of the anterior pelvis.

References

1. Meyers WC, McKechnie A, Philippon MJ, Horner MA, Zoga AC, Devon ON. Experience with "sports hernia" spanning two decades. Ann Surg. 2008;248(4):656–65.
2. Swan Jr KG, Wolcott M. The athletic hernia: a systematic review. Clin Orthop Relat Res. 2007;455:78–87.
3. Taylor DC, Meyers WC, Moylan JA, Lohnes J, Bassett FH, Garrett Jr WE. Abdominal musculature abnormalities as a cause of groin pain in athletes. Inguinal hernias and pubalgia. Am J Sports Med. 1991;19(3):239–42.
4. Meyers WC, Foley DP, Garrett WE, Lohnes JH, Mandlebaum BR. Management of severe lower abdominal or inguinal pain in high-performance athletes. PAIN (Performing Athletes with Abdominal or Inguinal Neuromuscular Pain Study Group). Am J Sports Med. 2000;28(1):2–8.
5. Gilmore J. Groin pain in the soccer athlete: fact, fiction, and treatment. Clin Sports Med. 1998;17(4):787–93. vii.
6. Omar IM, Zoga AC, Kavanaugh EC, Koulouris G, Bergin D, Gopez AG, et al. Athletic pubalgia and "sports hernia"; optimal MR imaging technique and findings. Radiographics. 2008;28(5):1415–38.
7. Shortt CP, Zoga AC, Kavanaugh EC, Meyers WC. Anatomy, pathology and MRI findings in sports hernia. Semin Musculoskelet Radiol. 2008;12(1):54–61.
8. Brannigan AE, Kerin MJ, McEntee GP. Gilmore's groin repair in athletes. J Orthop Sports Phys Ther. 2000;30(6):329–32.
9. Williams P, Foster ME. 'Gilmore's groin'-or is it. Br J Sports Med. 1995;29(3):206–8.
10. Gullmo A. Herniography. The diagnosis of hernia in the groin and the incompetence of the pouch of Douglas and pelvic floor. Acta Radiol Suppl. 1980;361:1–76.
11. Polglase AL, McMurrick PJ. Laparoscopic or open repair of inguinal hernias? Med J Aust. 1994;16(4):238–9.
12. Taylor DC. Abdominal musculature abnormalities as a cause of groin pain in athletes. Am J Sports Med. 1991;19(4):421.
13. Garvey JF, Read JW, Turner A. Sportsman hernia: what can we do? Hernia. 2010;14(1):17–25.

14. Meyers WC, Lanfranco A, Castellanos A. Surgical management of chronic lower abdominal and groin pain in high performance athletes. Curr Sports Med Rep. 2002;1(5):301–5.
15. Ekstrand J, Hilding J. The incidence and differential diagnosis of acute groin injuries in male soccer players. Scand J Med Sci Sports. 1999;9(2):98–103.
16. Meyers WC, Kahan DM, Joseph T, Butrymowicz A, Poor AE, Schoch S, et al. Current analysis of women athletes with pelvic pain. Med Sci Sports Exerc. 2011;43(8):1387–93.
17. Albers SL, Spritzer CE, Garrett Jr WE, Meyers WC. MR findings in athletes with pubalgia. Skeletal Radiol. 2001;30(5):270–7.
18. Kachingwe AF, Grech S. Proposed algorithm for the management of athletes with athletic pubalgia (sports hernia): a case series. J Orthop Sports Phys Ther. 2008;38(12):768–81.
19. Davies AG, Clarke AW, Gilmore J, Wotherspoon M, Connell DA. Review: imaging of groin pain in the athlete. Skeletal Radiol. 2010;39(7):629–44.
20. Butsch JL, Kuhn JP. Intramural hematoma of the small bowel: a possible lethal complication of herniography. Surgery. 1978;83(1): 121–2.
21. Ekberg O, Lasson A, Kesek P, Olsson R, Gustafson T. Post-herniographic abdominal pain syndrome. Acta Radiol. 2004; 45(1):3–6.
22. Brierly RD, Hale PC, Bishop NL. Is herniography an effective and safe investigation? J R Coll Surg Edinb. 1999;44(6):374–7.
23. Cunningham PM, Brennan D, O'Connell M, Macmahon P, O'Neill P, Eustace S. Patterns of bone and soft-tissue injury at the symphysis pubis in soccer players: observations at MRI. AJR Am J Roentgenol. 2007;188(3):W291–6.
24. Khan W, Zoga AC, Meyers WC. Magnetic resonance imaging of athletic pubalgia and the sports hernia: current understanding and practice. Magn Reson Imaging Clin N Am. 2013;21(1):97–110.
25. Mullens FE, Zoga AC, Morrison WB, Meyers WC. Review of MRI technique and imaging findings in athletic pubalgia and the "sports hernia". Eur J Radiol. 2012;81(12):3780–92.
26. Farber AJ, Wilckens JH. Sports hernia: diagnosis and therapeutic approach. J Am Acad Orthop Surg. 2007;15:507–14.
27. Caudill P, Nyland J, Smith C, Yerasimides J, Lach J. Sports hernias: a systematic literature review. Br J Sports Med. 2008;42(12): 954–64.
28. Novitsky YW, Czerniach DR, Kercher KW, Kaban GK, Gallagher KA, Kelly JJ, et al. Advantages of laparoscopic transabdominal preperitoneal herniorrhaphy in the evaluation and management of inguinal hernias. Am J Surg. 2007;193(4):466–70.
29. Muschaweck U, Berger L. Minimal Repair technique of sportsmen's groin: an innovative open-suture repair to treat chronic inguinal pain. Hernia. 2010;14(1):27–33.
30. Muschaweck U, Berger LM. Sportsmen's groin-diagnostic approach and treatment with the minimal repair technique: a single-center uncontrolled clinical review. Sports Health. 2010;2(3): 216–21.
31. Nam A, Brody F. Management and therapy for sports hernia. J Am Coll Surg. 2008;206(1):154–64.
32. Litwin DE, Sneider EB, McEnaney PM, Busconi BD. Athletic pubalgia (sports hernia). Clin Sports Med. 2011;30(2):417–34.
33. Orchard JW, Read JW, Neophyton J, Garlick D. Groin pain associated with ultrasound finding of inguinal canal posterior wall deficiency in Australian Rules footballers. Br J Sports Med. 1998;32(2): 134–9.
34. Malliaras P, Hogan A, Nawrocki A, Crossley K, Schache A. Hip flexibility and strength measures: reliability and association with athletic groin pain. Br J Sports Med. 2009;43(10):739–44.
35. Johnson DH, Pedowitz RA. Practical orthopaedic sports medicine and arthroscopy. Williams and Wilkins: Lippincott; 2006.

Acetabular Dysplasia: Aetiological Classification

62

Jason Brockwell, John N. O'Hara, and David A. Young

Introduction

Acetabular dysplasia is a cause of hip pain and osteoarthritis. Various radiological measurements have been described to quantify acetabular dysplasia. With increasing interest in hip preservation surgery, there is a need for a classification of different types of acetabular dysplasia to guide surgical management. Our proposed aetiological classification encompasses abnormalities of direction, deficient total available bony cover for the head and ultimately subluxation and dislocation.

Aetiological Classification of Acetabular Dysplasia

TYPE I—Primary or 'Classical' Dysplasia

1. The salient feature is a sloping acetabular roof, i.e. Tönnis sourcil angle greater than 10°.
2. Shallow socket with reduced lateral centre-edge angle of Wiberg, thus giving a 'short roof'.
3. The joint is relatively incongruent.
4. Acetabular version may be increased, normal or decreased.
5. Often there is 'caput cor'—a deformed heart-shaped femoral head and/or other abnormalities of the femoral head shape.
6. Often increased femoral version.
7. Increased neck-shaft angle with a high fovea, which does not line up with the acetabular notch.
8. Often associated with ligamentous laxity.

TYPE II—Impingement or 'Flat Roof' Dysplasia

1. The salient feature is a 'flat acetabular roof', i.e. Tönnis sourcil angle less than 10°.
2. Shallow socket with a reduced lateral centre-edge angle of Wiberg, thus giving a 'short roof'.
3. The joint is congruent.
4. Acetabular version is usually normal.
5. Impingement type proximal femoral morphology, e.g. pistol grip deformity of femoral head-neck junction from slipped upper femoral epiphysis or from playing sport in adolescence.
6. Normal or decreased femoral version.
7. Normal neck-shaft angle.
8. No particular association with ligamentous laxity.
9. Intraosseous femoral neck impingement cysts.

TYPE III—'Abnormal Acetabular Version'

1. The salient feature is abnormal acetabular version in the presence of a normal depth socket.
2. Normal lateral centre-edge angle of Wiberg.
3. Normal or increased Tönnis sourcil angle.
4. Femur may be normal or abnormal.

TYPE IV—Vascular

1. Hyperaemia: (usually secondary to inflammation) causes coxa magna and subluxation because the head enlarges faster than the acetabulum. Usually there is a shallow

J. Brockwell, FRCSEdOrth, FHKAMOrth (✉) • J.N. O'Hara, FRCS, FRCSI, MCh • D.A. Young, FRACS
Asia Medical Specialists, 8/F China Bldg., 29 Queen's Rd Central, Hong Kong, People's Republic of China

The Birmingham Hip Clinic, Birmingham, UK

Melbourne Orthopaedic Group, Melbourne, Australia
e-mail: jason.brockwell@asiamedical.hk

J.C. McCarthy et al. (eds.), *Hip Joint Restoration*, DOI 10.1007/978-1-4614-0694-5_62

socket with a sloping roof, subluxation and coxa magna, with slight loss of sphericity.
2. Necrosis: e.g. fracture; sickle cell disease; Gaucher's & Perthes': Usually features are the same as in pure hyperaemia, but there is often more severe femoral head asphericity.

TYPE V—Infection

Infection: Typically destroys the longitudinal growth plate of the femur, causing coxa brevia, or damages the triradiate cartilage, resulting in a small diameter socket.

TYPE VI—Trauma

Trauma: Damage to the triradiate cartilage will produce a small diameter socket. Damage to the secondary ossification centres will produce a shallow socket. The effects of damage to the femoral head are mainly dependent on whether there is damage to the longitudinal growth plate, and/or avascular necrosis of the femoral head.

TYPE VII—Iatrogenic

The features vary depending on the nature of the damage. Common findings include:

1. Failure of deepening of the acetabulum following excision of the secondary ossification centres as part of an open reduction of DDH.
2. Early fusion of the triradiate cartilage following damage during osteotomy.
3. Excessive acetabular anteversion or retroversion, typically after a pelvic osteotomy.
4. Reduced anterior and superior acetabular coverage, typically after arthroscopic acetabular rim recession.

Development of the Hip Joint

An overall understanding of the development of the hip joint allows the surgeon to appreciate the development of different patterns of acetabular dysplasia in response to the nature and timing of joint injuries. Siffert has written an excellent article on this subject, which we commend to interested readers [1].

The cartilage models of the acetabulum and femoral head evolve from a single mesenchymal mass early in foetal life. As the hip moves after birth it develops by the principle of 'companion coaptation'—in other words the femoral head and acetabulum mould each other. If the pressure between them is too high, cartilage growth will be inhibited, if it is too low, the unopposed cartilage will overgrow.

There are three areas of growth in the proximal femur: the longitudinal growth plate, which is mainly responsible for growth in the length of the femur; and the trochanteric growth plate and the femoral neck isthmus (on the lateral aspect of the femoral neck), which are physically continuous and are responsible for broadening of the femoral neck. The resultant vector of the longitudinal and trochanteric growth plates is along the axis of the femur. Disturbances to this balance will produce valgus or varus angulation of the neck.

Prior to adolescence, the acetabulum grows via the triradiate cartilage (Figs. 62.1, 62.2, and 62.3), which is primarily responsible for increasing its diameter. After fusion of the triradiate cartilage, three secondary ossification centres appear (Figs. 62.4, 62.5, and 62.6), each associated with one of the innominate bones, which mainly increase its depth while the femoral head continues to grow.

There is some disagreement about relevant terminology [2] (Table 62.1). Ponseti [3] uses the terms 'os acetabulare' for the pubic epiphysis, which mainly forms the anterior wall, 'lateral acetabular epiphysis' for the iliac epiphysis, which forms the superior wall, and 'ischial epiphysis' for the epiphysis forming the posterior wall. Zander [4] noted the use of

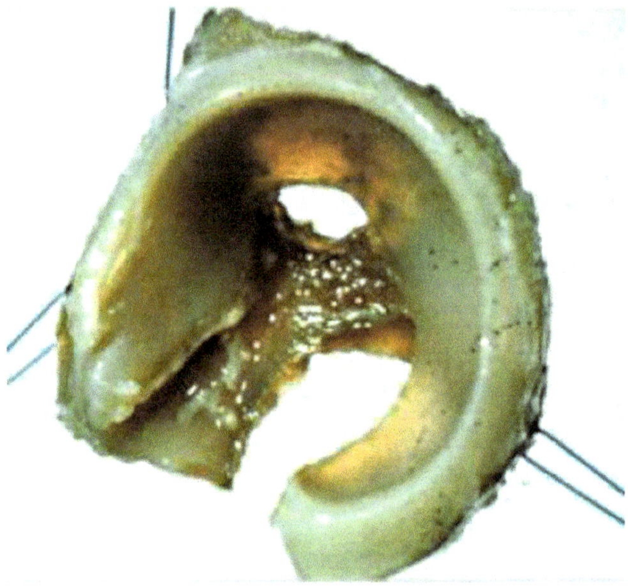

Fig. 62.1 The normal left acetabular cartilage complex of a one-day infant. The adjacent bone has been removed. The translucent iliac area is uppermost and is separated from the ischial area, below and to the right by the posterior limb of the triradiate cartilage [TRC]. The area of the pubic bone lies behind the thick cartilage to the left and is continuous with the anterior and vertical limbs of the TRC, which separate it from the ilium and ischium respectively. This *lateral view* also shows the concavity of the socket and the continuity of the acetabular cartilage and the labrum. Reprinted from J Bone Joint Surg Am, 1978 60(5):575–85 with permission

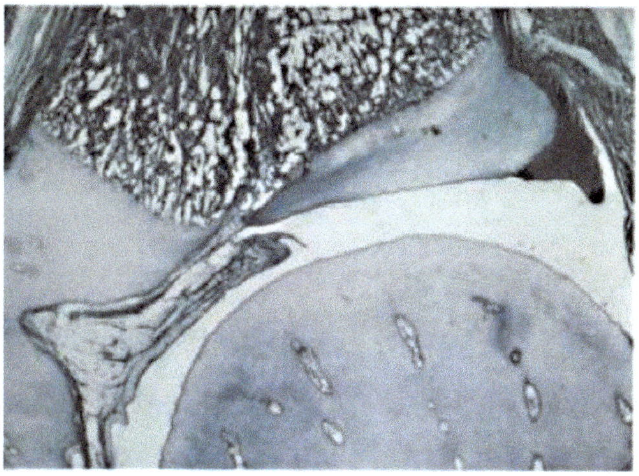

Fig. 62.2 A section through the hip of a newborn child (trichrome ×30). The acetabulum is composed of hyaline articular cartilage, which is in naked-eye continuity with the labrum distinguished by staining. The hyaline cartilage has three layers, the superficial articular layer, with flattened cells; the metaphyseal growth cartilage next to the ilium; and the vacuolated pre-osseous cartilage between these two. Medially, the vertical limb of the TRC can be seen. Reprinted from J Bone Joint Surg Am, 1978 60(5):575–85 with permission

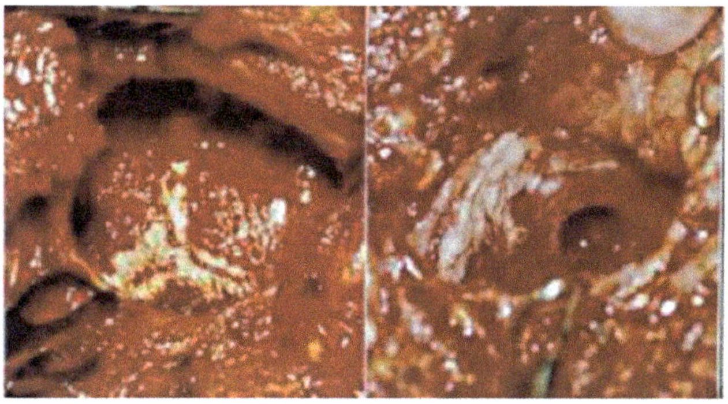

Fig. 62.3 *Left*, the reamed acetabulum of an 8-year-old exposed during hip disarticulation for a malignant tumour. Two fronts of ossification can be seen in all three limbs of the TRC. *Right*, a similar exposure in a 13-year-old girl. The TRC has fused and the iliac acetabular epiphysis lies within the unossified peripheral cartilage mass

the terms 'radiological os acetabulare' for the ischial epiphysis, and 'anatomical os acetabulare' for the pubic epiphysis. Other authors have used other terms. We propose the terms 'pubic, iliac and ischial acetabular epiphyses' and suggest that the term 'os acetabulare' be abandoned entirely, as it is, incorrectly in our opinion, being used to describe any ossification in the lateral acetabulum, including an ununited iliac epiphysis and osseous metaplasia in the base of the labrum.

According to Scheueur [2] the pubic acetabular epiphysis appears around 9–10 years of age; the ischial around 10–11 years; and the iliac around 12–14 years. All unite by about 18 years.

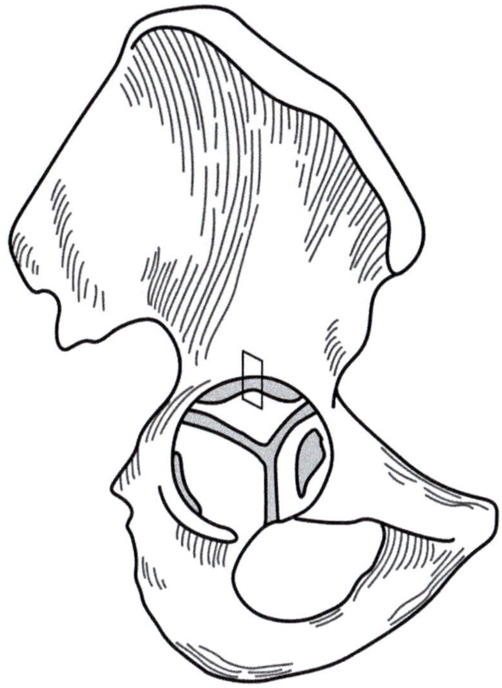

Fig. 62.4 Diagram of the right pelvis in an adolescent (after Dr. I. Ponseti). The epiphyses, including the triradiate cartilage, are *grey*. The pubic acetabular epiphysis lies within the cartilage adjoining the pubis. The iliac acetabular epiphysis lies within the cartilage adjoining the ilium and is shown in cross-section in subsequent illustrations (indicated by the parallelogram). The ischial acetabular epiphysis lies within the cartilage adjoining the ischium

Several studies have described the effects of iatrogenic damage to the secondary ossification centres in early childhood [5, 6]. O'Hara [5] described more severe dysplasia in children in whom limbectomy (excision of the inverted labrum and associated articular cartilage) was performed as part of the open reduction of DDH; in these cases, the iliac epiphysis failed to appear by age 13 years, leading to loss of coverage of the femoral head in patients followed up until the third decade. The lateral acetabular epiphysis appeared in all remaining patients in whom reduction was achieved without limbectomy. Bohler used the term 'anti-Chiari effect', to describe loss of coverage from damage to the iliac acetabular epiphysis during Chiari osteotomy. If the osteotomy damaged the iliac acetabular epiphysis, an 'anti-Chiari' effect would be seen, and if the osteotomy was cephalad to the iliac acetabular epiphysis, it would not occur [6].

The trochanteric growth plate is a traction epiphysis, which is stimulated by the normal force of contraction of the abductor muscles and inhibited by a reduction of their pull, as in cases of muscle weakness. The femoral neck isthmus tends to follow the trochanteric growth plate, as it is stimulated or retarded by the action of the same forces.

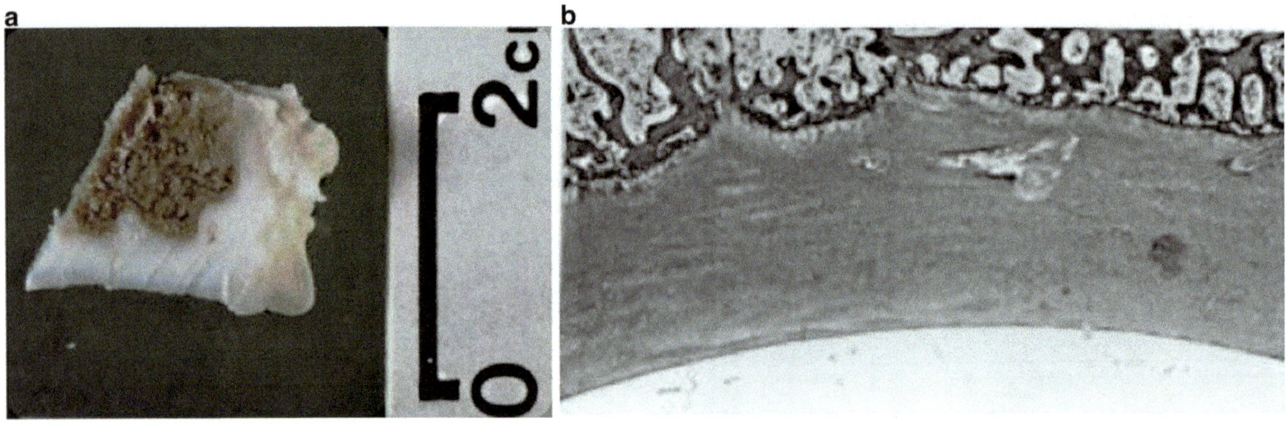

Fig. 62.5 (**a**) A coronal section (as indicated by the parallelogram in Fig. 62.4) from a 9-year-old's hip, disarticulated for osteosarcoma, shows the corresponding unossified part of the acetabulum. (**b**) Histological section (trichrome ×100). Note the area of destruction, vascular invasion, and partial calcification in the pre-osseous cartilage

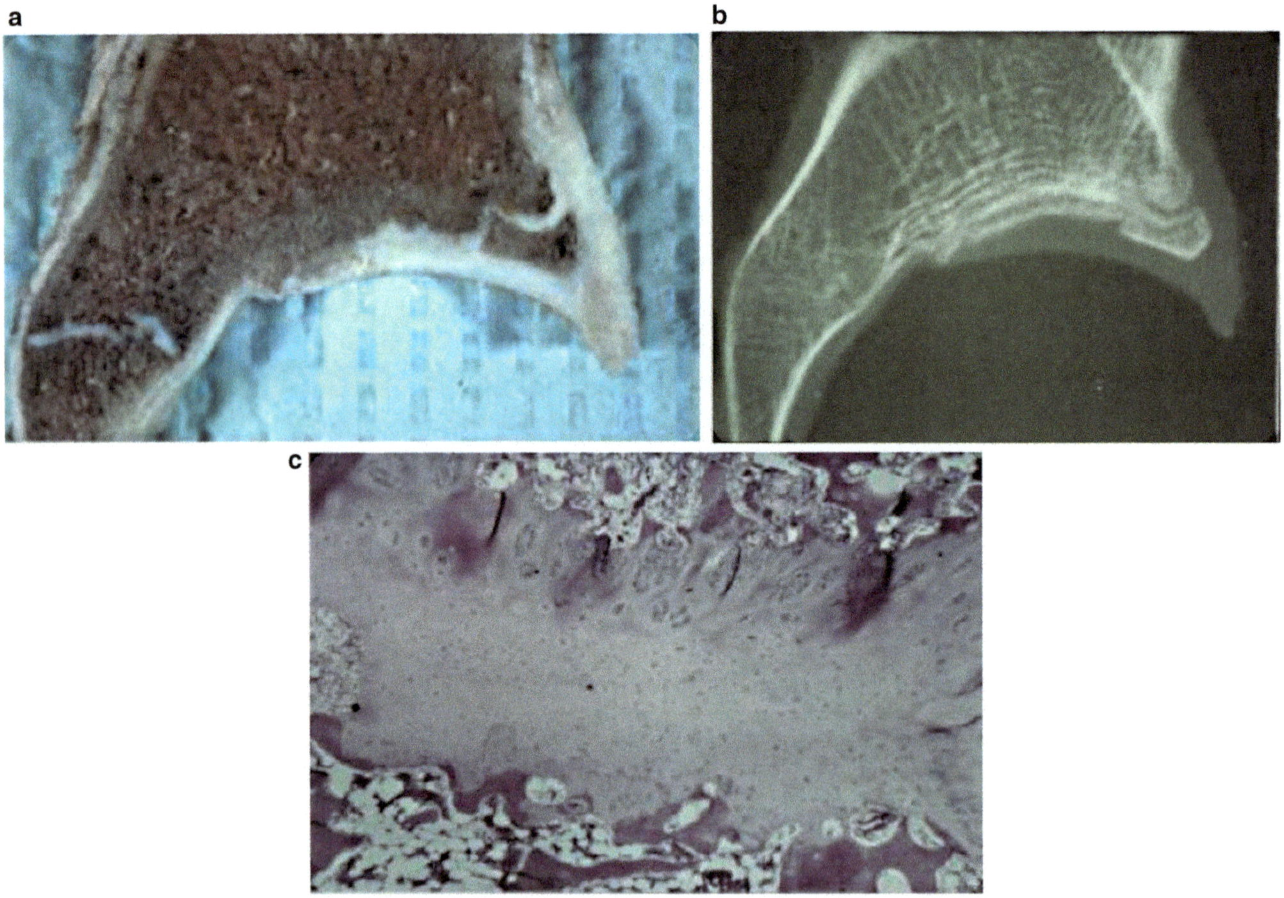

Fig. 62.6 (**a**) Slab section through the hip of a 14-year-old boy who died of multiple injuries shows the iliac acetabular epiphysis. Note that the triradiate cartilage is almost fully closed. Reprinted from J Bone Joint Surg Am, 1978 60(5):575–85 with permission. (**b**) Radiograph of the same. Reprinted from J Bone Joint Surg Am, 1978 60(5):575–85 with permission. (**c**) Coronal section through the same specimen (haematoxylin & eosin ×100). At this stage the iliac acetabular epiphysis has separated from the ilium (above) by hyaline cartilage and a growth plate (Courtesy Dr. I. Ponseti)

Table 62.1 Nomenclature of secondary ossification centres and ossicles

Location	Proposed term	Other terms
Base of superior labrum	Osseous metaplasia	Os acetabulare
Anterior acetabular wall	Pubic acetabular epiphysis	Os acetabulare; anatomical os acetabulare
Superior acetabular wall	Iliac acetabular epiphysis	Os acetabulare; lateral acetabular epiphysis
Posterior acetabular wall	Ischial acetabular epiphysis	Radiological os acetabulare; os marginalis superior acetabuli; nucleus osseous superior marginalis acetabuli

The Spectrum of Dysplasia

TYPE I Primary or 'Classical' Dysplasia

In Type I ('classical') hip dysplasia, the acetabular roof is sloping (i.e. is not horizontal), and the shallow acetabular socket fails to adequately cover the femoral head. Thus, the centre-edge angle of Wiberg [7] is reduced and the Tönnis sourcil angle [8] is increased. Symptoms are usually experienced first during weight-bearing exercises. A history of gradual withdrawal from sporting activities, long walks and shopping at the larger stores and supermarkets is the most usual presentation.

Aetiology

Classical dysplasia is probably caused by a mixture of genetic and mechanical factors [9]. Intrauterine mechanical factors may be the commonest cause. It is more common if babies are swaddled with their hips extended as demonstrated by the Japanese [9, 10] and Navajo [9, 11] experience. Until recently, Japanese babies were swaddled with their hips extended, and Japan had a very high rate of dysplastic disease of the hip and acetabular dysplasia. Following a public health campaign in the mid-1970s, the rate dropped to equal that of the rest of the world [9, 10]. The likely cause is the failure of distribution of companion coaptation forces because of lack of motion, leading to deformity.

Muscle imbalance: Cerebral palsy; Myelodysplasia; Poliomyelitis; Charcot-Marie-Tooth disease [12]. Lack of muscular pull on the trochanteric growth plate, because of abductor weakness, reduces its growth, so, in order to produce a resultant vector along the axis of the femur, the longitudinal growth plate remains more horizontal, producing a valgus femoral neck [1].

Ligamentous laxity: This form of dysplasia is often associated with ligamentous laxity, and is 4–5 times more common in females than males. A normal hip at birth which partially subluxes because of ligamentous laxity may go on to develop dysplasia because of failure of companion coaptation [1].

When seen in combination, the high femoral head fovea does not line up with the acetabular notch, giving the impression that there is incongruous weight-bearing (Figs. 62.7 and 62.8).

A sloping acetabular roof and shallow acetabulum occur because of unopposed thickening of the deeper growth cartilage of the triradiate cartilage once it loses the inhibitory effect of the femoral head. As the hip subluxes, the femoral head will apply excessive force to the lateral edge of the acetabulum, inhibiting its development [1].

Secondary developmental anomalies are often present, including abnormalities of femoral version, which is most often increased [13], although the causes are not clear.

An increased femoral neck-shaft angle may be present, probably as a consequence of muscle inhibition because of pain and alteration of the centre of rotation, leading to a reduction in the force on the trochanteric growth plate. This allows the longitudinal growth plate to remain relatively horizontal, giving a valgus neck, but maintaining a straight femur, with the resultant vector of the trochanteric and longitudinal growth plates in line with the shaft of the femur [1].

Very often, patients with 'classical' hip dysplasia have a deformed 'heart-shaped' femoral head [9]—possibly because the high neck-shaft angle and/or valgus femoral head places the fovea and the ligamentum teres in contact with the articular cartilage instead of the notch (Fig. 62.7 and 62.8). Therefore there is no space for the ligamentum teres; thus it compresses a dimple into the femoral head—leading to the appearance of *'caput cor'*—a heart-shaped deformity.

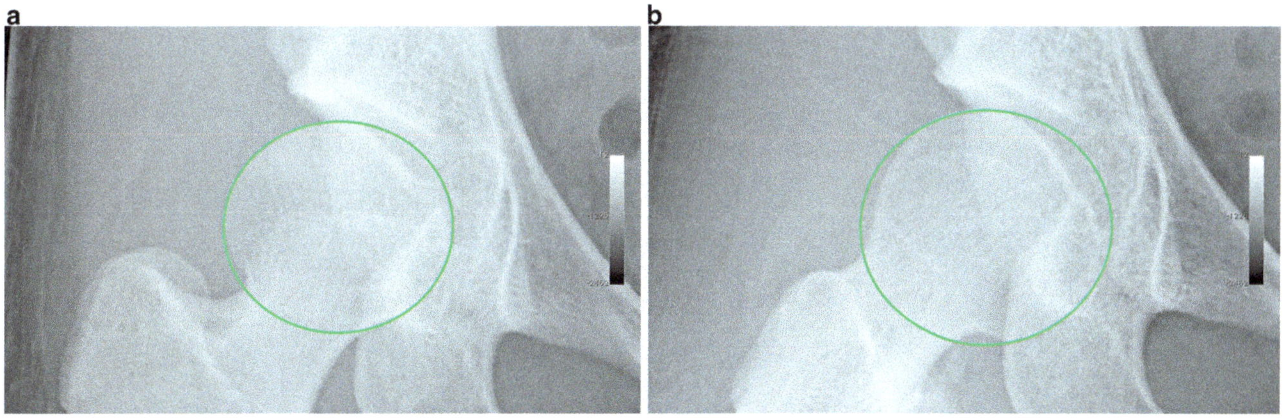

Fig. 62.7 (**a**) Classical dysplasia AP X-ray with 'endospherical' femoral head with perifoveal flattening. The fovea is high and adjacent the horseshoe instead of the notch. Note that there can often be lateral flattening of the head, of no consequence, provided the whole head above its centre fits within a sphere allowing easy abduction into a corrected socket. (**b**) Classical dysplasia with 'caput cor'—heart-shaped head—in *45 degree Dunn projection*

The 'heart-shaped' femoral head may easily be mistaken for the pistol grip deformity of cam impingement, tempting the arthroscopist to perform a femoroplasty. The distinguishing features are the symmetry of the proximal femur in a profile view, e.g. modified frog lateral radiograph (Fig. 62.9) or Dunn view, with a heart-shaped appearance instead of a pistol grip appearance, and the dimple at the fovea (Table 62.2).

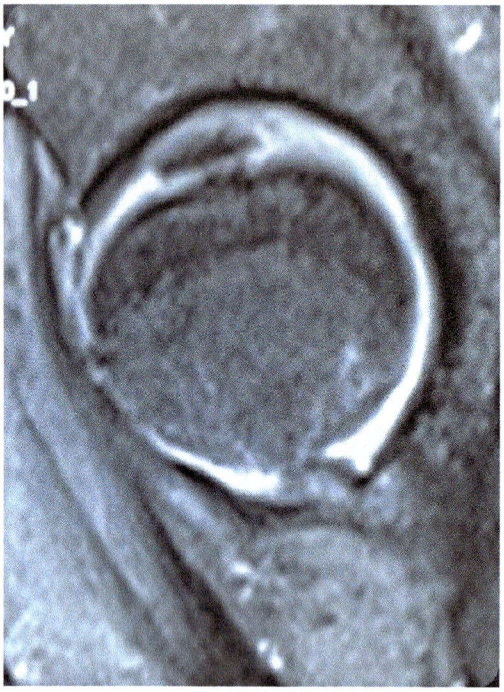

Fig. 62.8 Sagittal MRI shows flattening of femoral head around fovea where ligamentum teres abuts horseshoe instead of notch, causing heart-shaped or 'caput cor' appearance

TYPE II Impingement or 'Flat Roof' Dysplasia

The salient feature of this form of hip dysplasia is a flat acetabular roof, i.e. a Tönnis sourcil angle of less than 10°, as well as a shallow socket with a reduced lateral centre-edge angle of Wiberg (Fig. 62.10). Symptoms are usually first experienced when sitting for long periods, sometimes in a car on the long journey to a hospital appointment. The later onset of symptoms in association with weight-bearing is suggestive of articular cartilage damage.

Aetiology

The abnormality of the acetabular roof is caused by chronic impingement after fusion of the triradiate cartilage up to skeletal maturity, with damage to the iliac acetabular epiphysis. Cam-type femoro-acetabular impingement (FAI) causes attrition injury to the iliac acetabular cartilage and the unfused iliac acetabular epiphysis, at a critical period of growth.

The pattern of deformity depends on the time of occurrence of the impingement. If the deformity causing impingement occurs before fusion of the triradiate cartilage, for example in Perthes' disease, growth of the central acetabular cartilage is unopposed, causing a shallow acetabulum with a sloping roof-giving the appearance of 'classical' dysplasia. In addition, subluxation of the head overloads the edge of the acetabulum, and the iliac acetabular epiphysis fails to unite or disappears, causing a deficient lateral acetabulum as well.

If the deformity occurs after fusion of the triradiate cartilage, but before fusion of the iliac acetabular epiphysis, the central acetabulum has normal depth and a normal flat roof,

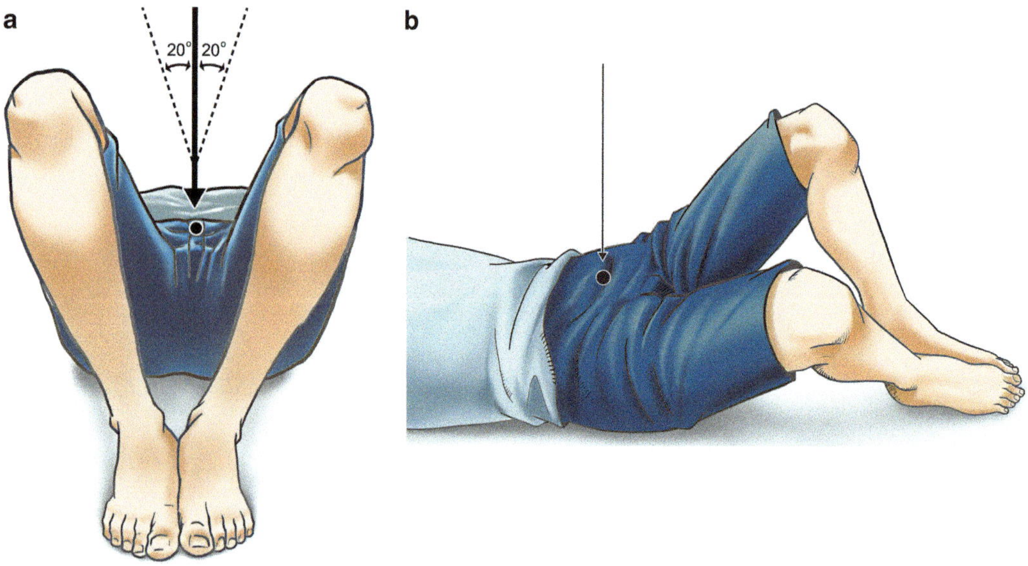

Fig. 62.9 Positioning for modified frog lateral X-ray. Each hip is flexed 70° and abducted 20°, and the soles of the feet are on the table, rather than facing each other, as in conventional frog lateral projection. This is similar to a Dunn projection. The modified frog lateral demonstrates the head-neck junction clearly, whereas this area is usually obscured by the greater trochanter in a conventional frog lateral radiograph

Table 62.2 Distinguishing between femoral deformities in type I 'classical' and type II 'impingement' dysplasia

Appearance	Normal	Type I 'classical'	Type II 'impingement'
Profile of proximal femur	Symmetrical light bulb	Symmetrical heart shaped	Asymmetrical pistol grip deformity
Fovea	Normal-aligns with notch	Enlarged-abuts horseshoe	Normal-aligns with notch
Cam deformity	Absent	Present	Present

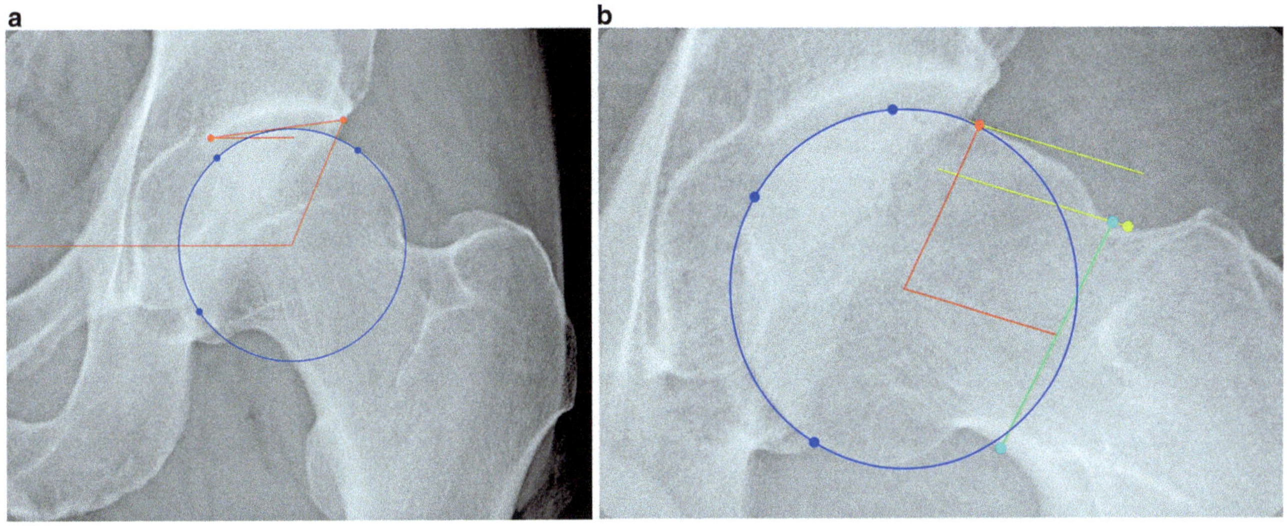

Fig. 62.10 (**a**) Flat roof dysplasia with impingement—AP view. This is a subtle case, with a Wiberg CE angle of 23°, which most surgeons would classify as pure impingement. We have deliberately chosen this case to demonstrate the spectrum of impingement-associated dysplasia. (**b**) Flat roof dysplasia with impingement-modified frog lateral view. The Notzli alpha angle [29] is increased at 80° (*red*) and the Murray Head-Neck Offset Ratio [30] (*yellow lines*) decreased at 0.15. It would be appropriate to treat this combination of severe cam impingement with mild acetabular dysplasia with an isolated femoroplasty. Acetabular rim trimming would be counter-productive

but the iliac acetabular epiphysis is affected. Resorption of the iliac acetabular epiphysis secondary to impingement damage leads to a deficient lateral acetabulum with the typical appearance of 'short' or 'flat roof' dysplasia, with a normal Tönnis sourcil angle, but a reduced Wiberg CE angle. If the iliac acetabular epiphysis is not destroyed, but is prevented from fusing, a large unfused iliac acetabular epiphysis is present, which, recently, and in our opinion, incorrectly, has been called 'os acetabulare'. We believe this should logically be called an 'unfused iliac acetabular epiphysis'.

The commonest causes of cam-type FAI are late-onset Perthes'; Slipped Capital Femoral Epiphysis (SCFE) (Fig. 62.11); and 'idiopathic' pistol grip deformity of the proximal femur, which we believe is associated with sport in adolescence [14, 15]. Alternatively, it may begin as a very mild SCFE, causing pressure inhibition of the postero-inferior aspect of the longitudinal growth plate, causing increased retroversion and relative varus without further slip. Impingement can also be caused by relative acetabular or femoral retroversion (Fig. 62.12) in the absence of a pistol grip deformity.

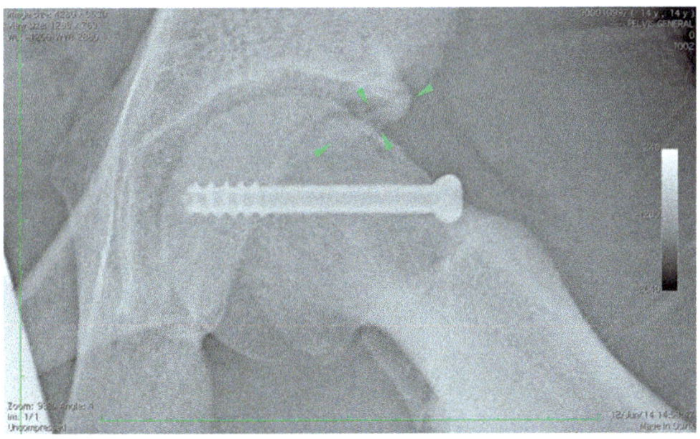

Fig. 62.11 A 14-year-old boy with SCFE and an unfused iliac acetabular epiphysis (*arrows*). The iliac acetabular epiphysis may fail to fuse because of impingement from the bone or from the screw, and remain unfused beyond skeletal maturity, or may be resorbed, causing type II 'impingement dysplasia'

If the iliac acetabular epiphysis is not destroyed, it may not fuse, which is a *forme fruste* of 'flat roof' or impingement dysplasia.

It is unusual to see a large iliac acetabular epiphysis in the absence of a pistol grip deformity or some other cause of cam-type FAI. Being secondary to Perthes' disease; SUFE; or adolescent sport; this is more common in men.

Klaue, Durnin and Ganz divided dysplasia into the same type I and type II forms, and coined the term 'short roof dysplasia' [16]; however the salient feature of the roof which distinguishes type I from type II dysplasia is not the length of the roof (it is short in both cases), but its slope: it is excessively sloping in type I and normal in type II-hence our use of the term 'flat roof'. There is debate over whether ossicles at the anterosuperior acetabular rim represent stress fractures of the rim, or unfused epiphyses. If the plane of separation is vertical it is more likely that this is a stress fracture, and if the plane follows the physis it is more likely to be an unfused epiphysis [17].

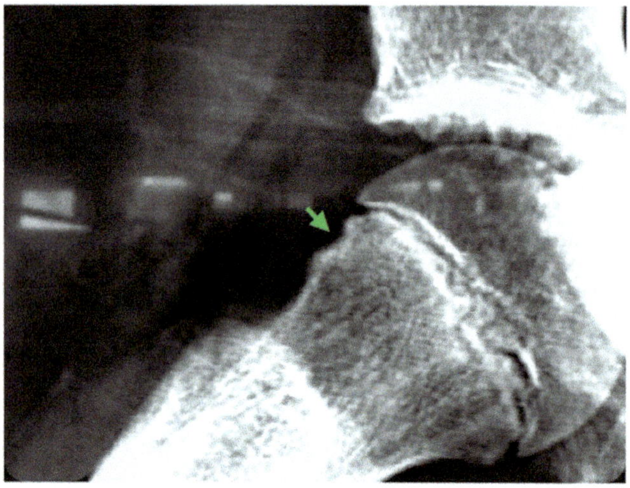

Fig. 62.12 The earliest example (a boy of 10 years) we have seen of an impingement divot on the front of the femoral neck (*arrow*) caused by femoral retroversion. Some blunting of the acetabular edge is already evident. In this case there was 10° of retroversion, which was treated successfully with a 30° internal rotation osteotomy

TYPE III 'Abnormal Acetabular Version'

The salient feature of this form of hip dysplasia is abnormal acetabular version in the presence of a normal depth socket, as reflected by a normal lateral centre-edge angle of Wiberg. The Tönnis sourcil angle may be normal or slightly increased. Femoral morphology may be normal or abnormal.

Aetiology

It is not clear how most pure version abnormalities develop. We have seen a handful of pre-adolescent patients with painful hip flexion and normal femoral version in whom we have suspected slight acetabular retroversion. We are unable to accurately measure the acetabular version at this age because of the unossified cartilage and are unable to predict its adolescent ossification.

In Perthes' disease, the acetabulum has normal anteversion initially but progressively develops retroversion [18], probably by relative overgrowth of the anterior (pubic) portion of the lateral acetabular cartilage. It has been proposed that this occurs as a consequence of loss of inhibition from the femoral head due to anterosuperior necrosis [1].

We believe the mechanism of pure version abnormalities is likely to be either abnormal orientation of the foetal mesenchymal cleft or abnormal companion coaptation, with relative overgrowth or inhibition of the pubic acetabular epiphysis and/or the ischial acetabular epiphysis.

TYPE IV Vascular

The features of hip dysplasia secondary to vascular injury vary as a function of the timing and nature of the damage. Avascular necrosis due to fracture, sickle disease, Gaucher's and Perthes' (Fig. 62.13) initially causes loss of head bulk due to necrosis, reducing pressure on the acetabular cartilage and allowing it to overgrow; as the head revascularises there is hyperaemia and overgrowth resulting in coxa magna,

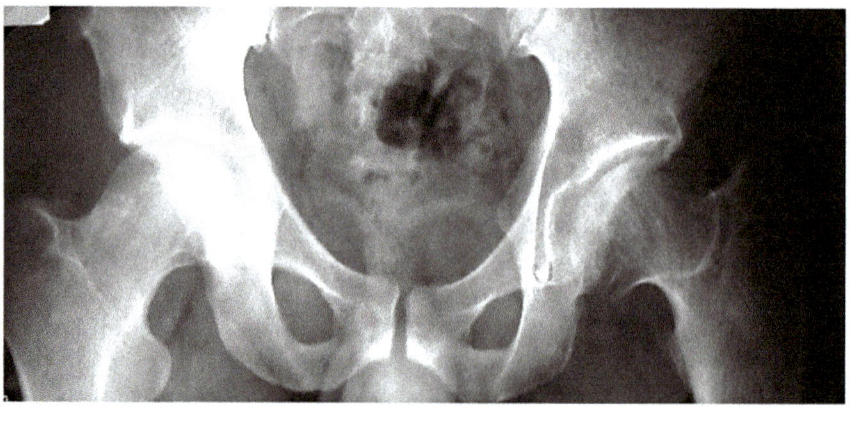

Fig. 62.13 A 28-year-old man with an enlarged femoral head and secondary acetabular dysplasia on the left, following childhood Perthes' disease. There is no incongruity, but function is compromised by acetabular dysplasia, a short leg, and potential extra-articular impingement. This was treated by contemporaneous Birmingham Interlocking Peri-Acetabular Osteotomy [31] and valgus femoral osteotomy

which, combined with the overgrowth of the acetabular cartilage, causes subluxation, with further reduced pressure on the femoral head and further femoral head overgrowth. The femoral head will be aspherical if subluxation occurs before or during revascularisation, but will be more spherical if the head remains in the acetabulum. In pure hyperaemia without necrosis the features are similar, with head and acetabular overgrowth giving a shallow socket and large head, and therefore subluxation, but without the additional insult of femoral head necrosis and revascularisation, so there is usually less severe femoral head asphericity.

TYPE V Infection

The effects of infection depend on the location of the infection and the damage caused. It most commonly damages the longitudinal growth plate of the femur, causing coxa brevia. The effects of damage to the femoral head are mainly dependent on whether there is damage to the longitudinal growth plate, and/or avascular necrosis of the femoral head.

TYPE VI Trauma

The effects of trauma depend on the location and timing of the infection: Damage to the triradiate cartilage will cause a small diameter socket. Damage to secondary acetabular ossification centres will cause a low volume socket. Damage to the longitudinal growth plate of the femur will cause coxa brevia.

TYPE VII Iatrogenic

The features vary depending on the nature of the damage. Common findings include:

1. Failure of deepening of the acetabulum following excision of the secondary ossification centres as part of an open reduction of the hip in treatment of DDH [5].
2. Early fusion of the triradiate cartilage following damage during acetabular osteotomies [19].
3. Excessive acetabular anteversion or retroversion, typically after a pelvic osteotomy. The Salter osteotomy, because it hinges on the symphysis pubis, retroverts as it closes. Any pelvic osteotomy producing a completely free central acetabular fragment may lead to a variety of unintended positions.
4. Reduced anterior and superior acetabular coverage, typically after arthroscopic acetabular rim recession [20–22].

Management Considerations

In this era of increased awareness of femoro-acetabular impingement, we fear that dysplasia is becoming an overlooked diagnosis. We have found that the anterior impingement (flexion/adduction/internal rotation-FADDIR) test is just as valid in dysplasia as it is in FAI. This is because the internal rotation of the femoral neck against the tender labrum is as painful in dysplasia as in FAI, though a positive result is usually elicited in greater internal rotation in the cases of hip dysplasia.

The femoral head may look a little 'heart-shaped' (caput cor) (Fig. 62.7b) and *may* be a little eccentric in type I classical dysplasia. However a large majority are 'endospherical'—i.e. they will fit inside a sphere—above the centre of the head (Fig. 62.7a), so allowing unimpaired adjustment of the socket.

The classification system guides management by alerting clinicians to the presence of dysplasia in combination with impingement and to impingement after treatment of dysplasia if the cam deformity has not been corrected.

In classical dysplasia it is usually sufficient to perform an isolated pelvic osteotomy even in the presence of mild femoral head deformity, as significant post-operative impingement is unlikely. Conversely, in impingement dysplasia, it is usually necessary to perform a femoroplasty together with the pelvic osteotomy to avoid significant post-operative impingement.

Radiographic Assessment

We believe the basic screening examination should be a plain AP pelvis radiograph and a 'modified frog lateral' radiograph—taken with each hip flexed 70° and abducted 20° (Fig. 62.9). The modified frog lateral demonstrates the head-neck junction clearly, whereas this area is usually obscured by the greater trochanter in a conventional frog lateral radiograph.

The two most useful radiological parameters are the centre-edge angle of Wiberg and the Tönnis sourcil angle.

On the plain radiograph one can also assess acetabular version by noting the distance between the anterior and posterior edges of the acetabulum, as described by Tönnis [8]. Tönnis describes a distance of 1.5 cm as normal, a greater distance represents increased anteversion and a lesser distance relative retroversion, though one can calculate the distance as a percentage of the femoral head diameter, to compensate for patient size and magnification. We use <25 % to define relative retroversion and >33 % to define increased anteversion. This technique is only accurate for normal volume acetabulae. If the acetabulum is low volume, i.e. deficient both anteriorly and posteriorly, with the lateral walls medial to the centre of the femoral head, this method is not accurate.

On CT or MRI, we feel the most important assessment of acetabular version is the version of the weight-bearing surface, as defined by the roof edge angle [23]. In addition, we agree with Tönnis that it is appropriate to measure 'deep socket' acetabular version at about the centre of the head [8], though this measurement can be confounded by marginal osteophytes.

It is difficult to accurately assess femoral version by X-ray, and we believe all patients should have CT or MR assessment of femoral version. Various methods exist for making measurements from CT or MRI, but we feel the most consistent is Murphy's method [24], which defines the proximal femur with reference to the centroids of the head and the shaft at the level of the lesser trochanter. No further investigations are necessary for planning treatment: CT or MRI will demonstrate the joint space.

Modern software, such as that from Clinical Graphics, allows animation of a virtual 3D hip joint created from the patient's CT or MRI data. It is intended to demonstrate and plan treatment of femoro-acetabular impingement. In principle, this software will allow the surgeon to perform a virtual pelvic and/or femoral osteotomy, and predict any post-operative FAI, and, if so, treat this by modifying the index procedure by additional open or arthroscopic Heyman-type femoroplasty [25].

In some cases we perform examination under anaesthesia, sometimes using local anaesthetic injected into the hip joint freehand in the office, a technique which we find to be accurate [26, 27]. Imaging under anaesthesia allows checking if there is incongruity on abduction of the hip—for example hinge abduction in Perthes' or where there is a large pistol grip deformity.

Treatment of Acetabular Dysplasia

Type I Primary or 'Classical' Dysplasia

- Core stability exercises
- Hip capsule tightening
- Heyman-type femoroplasty to correct minor cam-type impingement—this may be open or arthroscopic. It is important to recognise that the underlying condition is dysplasia, not impingement, and to do nothing to destabilise the hip.
- Rotational femoral osteotomy
- Pelvic osteotomy

Note: Do not confuse this with impingement—the heart-shaped femoral head may cause a minor cam effect, but this is not primarily an impingement problem.

Type II Impingement Dysplasia

- Avoid impingement positions and activities
- Surgical repair of any large unfused iliac epiphysis
- Heyman-type femoroplasty
- Pelvic osteotomy

Note: The primary problem is impingement, but it is important to recognise the severity of acetabular dysplasia, and treat if appropriate. If a pelvic osteotomy is performed, there will be increased impingement unless a femoroplasty is also performed.

Type III Abnormal Acetabular Version

- Rotational periacetabular osteotomy or femoral osteotomy.

Assess femoral version as well as acetabular version-if femoral version is abnormal it may be possible to correct the McKibbin [28] *index with an isolated femoral osteotomy. We tend to treat the most abnormal bone.*

Type IV Vascular

- The principle is to correct the anatomy as far as possible. In general we accept a large femoral head, and aim to correct the acetabulum and femoral version as far as possible. A large, aspherical head may function remarkably well in a deeper socket with a horizontal sourcil despite residual incongruity. Valgising femoral osteotomy and/or trochanteric advancement may help abductor leverage.

Type V Infection

- The principle is to correct the anatomy as far as possible—we use the same approach as in vascular dysplasia.

Type VI Trauma

- The principle is to correct the anatomy as far as possible—we use the same approach as in vascular dysplasia.

Type VII Iatrogenic

- The principle is to correct the anatomy as far as possible—we use the same approach as in vascular dysplasia.

Note: Common iatrogenic problems are failure to recognise acetabular dysplasia and treat dysplasia as impingement via *arthroscopic acetabular rim trimming +/– femoroplasty. Often abnormal femoral version will be unrecognised and untreated.*

Pelvic osteotomies can be malpositioned to produce retroversion and anterior impingement or anteversion and posterior impingement.

Treatment of Acetabular Dysplasia

Type I: Primary or 'Classical' Dysplasia

Conservative treatment, such as core stability exercises and operations to tighten the hip capsule, do not, in our experience, produce predictable or durable benefits. The bedrock of effective treatment of this condition is the accurate surgical correction of all the underlying bony misalignments by pelvic osteotomy, femoral osteotomy, or both, with intra-articular procedures, as required.

Where there is measurable deformity on both sides of the joint, and where one is more marked than the other; we may have to choose whether to perform one versus two procedures. In these circumstances we tend to opt for correction of the most severe deformity. An example is femoral anteversion; the normal (95 %) range is taken to be 11–29°. As it is difficult to accurately and predictably adjust femoral anteversion by less than 15°, due to imperfect techniques, we do not usually try to adjust anteversion presenting in the range 5–35°. Similarly, adjustment of lateral acetabular cover of less than 15° may be difficult to achieve accurately and should not be attempted by the inexperienced. However, we have not experienced the same difficulty in accurately adjusting acetabular anteversion by as little as 10°.

Type II: Impingement Dysplasia

In understanding the pathology, it is important to remember that SCFE virtually never occurs in the absence of relative femoral retroversion, itself an important cause of impingement pathology. Lifestyle modifications such as avoiding impingement positions and activities may help control symptoms.

Evaluation with MRI scans and CT scans with femoral version views is recommended. Treatment can include intra-articular procedures such as femoroplasty and labral repair, combined with pelvic osteotomy +/– femoral osteotomy as required by the bony configuration. Surgical repair of large unfused iliac acetabular epiphysis may be required.

Type III Abnormal Acetabular Version

Assess femoral version as well as acetabular version—if femoral version is abnormal it may be possible to correct the McKibbin index [28] with an isolated femoral osteotomy (Fig. 62.12). If the acetabulum is high volume, it may be possible to perform a rim trimming; if the volume is small, it will be necessary to perform a rotational acetabular osteotomy.

Type IV Vascular

The principle is to correct the anatomy as far as possible. In general we accept a large femoral head, and aim to correct the acetabular and femoral version as far as possible. A large, aspherical head may function remarkably well in a deeper socket with a horizontal sourcil despite residual incongruity. Valgising femoral osteotomy and/or trochanteric advancement may help abductor leverage.

Type V Infection

The principle is to correct the anatomy as far as possible—we use the same approach as in vascular dysplasia.

Type VI Trauma

The principle is to correct the anatomy as far as possible—we use the same approach as in vascular dysplasia.

Type VII Iatrogenic

The principle is to correct the anatomy as far as possible—we use the same approach as in vascular dysplasia.

Common iatrogenic problems are failure to recognise acetabular dysplasia and treatment as impingement via arthroscopic acetabular rim trimming +/– femoroplasty. Often abnormal femoral version will be unrecognised and untreated.

Pelvic osteotomies can be malpositioned in almost any direction, most commonly in retroversion, causing anterior impingement, or in anteversion, producing posterior impingement. The condition should be evaluated as described in section III and treated as required. Patient's expectations after a revision procedure should be tempered.

Proximal Femoral Morphology in Hip Dysplasia

In classical dysplasia there is often perifoveal flattening—i.e. a divot in the femoral head from the ligamentum teres (Fig. 62.8). Because of the valgus neck-shaft angle, the fovea does not line up with the acetabular notch, and the ligamentum is compressed by the articular cartilage of the horseshoe (Fig. 62.7 and 62.8). We call the distinctive deformity 'caput cor' (*heart-shaped head*). The proximal femur may also have an increased Notzli alpha angle [29] and a reduced Murray head-neck offset ratio [30] giving a cam deformity.

References

1. Siffert RS. Patterns of deformity of the developing hip. Clin Orthop Relat Res. 1981;160:14–29.
2. Scheuer L, Black SM. The juvenile skeleton. Cambridge, MA: Elsevier Academic; 2004.
3. Ponseti IV. Growth and development of the acetabulum in the normal child. Anatomical, histological, and roentgenographic studies. J Bone Joint Surg Am. 1978;60(5):575–85.
4. Zander G. Os acetabuli and other bony periarticular calcifications at the hip joint. Acta Radial Diagn. 1943;24:317.
5. O'Hara JN. Congenital dislocation of the hip: acetabular deficiency in adolescence (absence of the lateral acetabular epiphysis) after limbectomy in infancy. J Pediatr Orthop. 1989;9(6):640–8.
6. Osebold WR, Lester EL, Watson P. Observations on the development of the acetabulum following Chiari osteotomy. Iowa Orthop J. 2002;22:66–74.
7. Wiberg G. The anatomy and roentgenographic appearance of a normal hip joint. Acta Chir Scand. 1939;83 Suppl 58:7–38.
8. Tonnis D, Heinecke A. Acetabular and femoral anteversion: relationship with osteoarthritis of the hip. J Bone Joint Surg Am. 1999;81(12):1747–70.
9. Loder RT, Skopelja EN. The epidemiology and demographics of hip dysplasia. ISRN Orthop. 2011;2011:238607.
10. Ishida K. Prevention of the development of the typical dislocation of the hip. Clin Orthop Relat Res. 1977;126:167–9.
11. Rabin DL et al. Untreated congenital hip disease. A study of the epidemiology, natural history, and social aspects of the disease in a Navajo population. Am J Public Health Nations Health. 1965;55(SUPPL):1–44.
12. Stover MD et al. Early results of the Bernese periacetabular osteotomy for symptomatic dysplasia in Charcot-Marie-Tooth disease. Hip Int. 2013;23 Suppl 9:S2–7.
13. Sugano N et al. The morphology of the femur in developmental dysplasia of the hip. J Bone Joint Surg (Br). 1998; 80(4):711–9.
14. Agricola R et al. A cam deformity is gradually acquired during skeletal maturation in adolescent and young male soccer players: a prospective study with minimum 2-year follow-up. Am J Sports Med. 2014;42(4):798–806.
15. Murray RO, Duncan C. Athletic activity in adolescence as an etiological factor in degenerative hip disease. J Bone Joint Surg (Br). 1971;53(3):406–19.
16. Klaue K, Durnin CW, Ganz R. The acetabular rim syndrome. A clinical presentation of dysplasia of the hip. J Bone Joint Surg (Br). 1991;73(3):423–9.
17. Martinez AE et al. Os acetabuli in femoro-acetabular impingement: stress fracture or unfused secondary ossification centre of the acetabular rim? Hip Int. 2006;16(4):281–6.
18. Sankar WN, Flynn JM. The development of acetabular retroversion in children with Legg-Calve-Perthes disease. J Pediatr Orthop. 2008;28(4):440–3.
19. Leet AI et al. Injury to the growth plate after Pemberton osteotomy. J Bone Joint Surg Am. 1999;81(2):169–76.
20. Matsuda DK. Acute iatrogenic dislocation following hip impingement arthroscopic surgery. Arthroscopy. 2009;25(4):400–4.
21. Ranawat AS, McClincy M, Sekiya JK. Anterior dislocation of the hip after arthroscopy in a patient with capsular laxity of the hip. A case report. J Bone Joint Surg Am. 2009;91(1):192–7.
22. Rosenbaum A et al. Posterior dislocation of the hip following arthroscopy - a case report and discussion. Bull Hosp Jt Dis. 2013;72(2):181–4.
23. Reynolds D, Lucas J, Klaue K. Retroversion of the acetabulum: a cause of hip pain. J Bone Joint Surg Br. 1999;81-B(2):281–8.
24. Murphy SB et al. Femoral anteversion. J Bone Joint Surg Am. 1987;69(8):1169–76.
25. Heyman CH, Herndon CH, Strong JM. Slipped femoral epiphysis with severe displacement; a conservative operative treatment. J Bone Joint Surg Am. 1957;39-A(2):293–303. passim.
26. Masoud MA, Said HG. Intra-articular hip injection using anatomic surface landmarks. Arthrosc Tech. 2013;2(2):e147–9.
27. Mei-Dan O et al. The anterior approach for a non-image-guided intra-articular hip injection. Arthroscopy. 2013; 29(6):1025–33.
28. McKibbin B. Anatomical factors in the stability of the hip joint in the newborn. J Bone Joint Surg (Br). 1970;52(1):148–59.
29. Notzli HP et al. The contour of the femoral head-neck junction as a predictor for the risk of anterior impingement. J Bone Joint Surg (Br). 2002;84(4):556–60.
30. Murray RO. The aetiology of primary osteoarthritis of the hip. Br J Radiol. 1965;38(455):810–24.
31. Kumar D, Bache CE, O'Hara JN. Interlocking triple pelvic osteotomy in severe Legg-Calve-Perthes disease. J Pediatr Orthop. 2002;22(4):464–70.

Quality-of-Life After Hip Arthroscopic Surgery

63

Nicholas G.H. Mohtadi

Introduction

In order to appreciate "Quality-of-Life" after the treatment of hip disorders it is necessary to have a clear understanding of what the term means.

Every person has an intuitive understanding of what is meant by quality-of-life and therefore the term is used in many different ways. It may represent health and wellness, satisfaction, happiness, or even income level. The World Health Organization (WHO) defines Quality-of-Life as individuals' perception of their position in life in the context of the culture and value systems in which they live and in relation to their goals, expectations, standards, and concerns. It is a broad-ranging concept affected in a complex way by the person's physical health, psychological state, level of independence, social relationships, personal beliefs, and their relationship to salient features of their environment [1]. This definition is clearly matched to the constitution of the WHO, which states that health is a state of complete physical, mental, and social well-being not merely the absence of disease. To a greater or lesser extent this definition is reflective of the socioeconomic impact on health and disease; crucial in the global context.

However, in the context of the treatment of hip disorders one must consider a more focused definition that can be used to evaluate patients across regions, countries, and continents. Health-related quality-of-life (HRQL or HRQOL) is the term that is more appropriate for this chapter [2]. HRQOL has been defined in many ways but the one that is generally accepted is the following: HRQOL is thus subjective and multidimensional, encompassing physical and occupational function, psychological state, social interaction, and somatic sensation [3].

Therefore, if we are interested in measuring quality-of-life after Hip arthroscopic surgery we must have a means of addressing what is inherently subjective and multidimensional.

Measuring Health-Related Quality-of-Life

In simplest form quality-of-life can be measured by asking a patient "How is your quality-of-life?" [4] This approach assumes that the answer is both subjective which it is, but that it is reflective of many dimensions. It is not possible to identify what specific dimensions are being measured or which one(s) the patient may be emphasizing. The idea of using a single question such as the assessment of pain on a visual analogue scale or using the Single Assessment Numeric Evaluation is inherently reasonable. In reality these simple measures correlate with more complex outcome quality-of-life measure [5]. However, there is a great deal of information that is unknown or lost with this approach.

It is also very important to distinguish health-related quality-of-life assessment from other similar evaluative patient outcomes. Clinicians sometimes confuse or use interchangeably the terms "functional assessment" or even "patient satisfaction" with HRQOL. Patient satisfaction is indeed a multifaceted concept but includes the interpretation of external services such as access to care, interaction with staff and healthcare providers, costs, as well as, the outcome of treatment [6]. A functional assessment may involve objective measures such as gait, strength, or range of motion [7].

All areas of outcome assessment have their own specific merits and limitations. Therefore it is paramount that the clinician understands several specific concepts of what exactly is being measured. Quality-of-life outcome measures can be called instruments, tools, scales, scores, indices, measures, outcomes, or questionnaires. These terms are used interchangeably for the purpose of this chapter. The purpose of outcome measures can be classified as either disease specific,

N.G.H. Mohtadi, MD, MSc, FRCSC (✉)
Section of Orthopaedics, Department of Surgery, Peter Lougheed Centre, University of Calgary Sport Medicine Centre, 2500 University Dr. NW, Calgary, AB T2T 3Y4, Canada
e-mail: mohtadi@ucalgary.ca

J.C. McCarthy et al. (eds.), *Hip Joint Restoration*, DOI 10.1007/978-1-4614-0694-5_63

such as those tools created to assess osteoarthritis, or joint specific, such as those created to assess the outcome of any pathology of the hip. These measures can also be classified according to the person who completes the assessment. Traditionally, combined scoring systems have been used by clinicians which included physical examination findings and objective measures such as radiographic assessments. The clinician also asked the patient about pain and other subjective measures. These "clinician-based" or "clinician-administered" tools may introduce bias due to the way they are administered but more importantly may not capture the patient's perceived outcomes [8]. More recently, patient-based and administered tools have been created [5, 9–18]. These patient-reported outcomes (PROs) are typically self-administered and can be completed in a non-threatening environment to the patient. Patient-Reported Outcomes are considered to be the reference standard for reporting clinical trials. It is necessary to distinguish between self-administered (i.e., by the patient) outcomes from those, which are not only self-administered but are also **patient-derived** outcomes. There is some debate regarding what constitutes a Patient-Reported Outcome [19–23]. The commonly accepted definition is: "any report coming directly from patients, without interpretation by physicians or others, about how they function or feel in relation to a health condition and its therapy" [21]. This definition works very well for simple outcomes such as measuring pain intensity over-time using a visual analogue scale. The PRO takes on a different context when one is attempting to measure more complicated concepts such as HRQOL. A more complete definition of a PRO is that it is collected from a patient but more importantly the "information gained is necessarily of direct concern to the patient" [19]. It is well recognized that the patient perspective is different from that of the clinician and most importantly the surgeon [8]. Therefore, if we accept the first and simple definition of a Patient-Reported Outcome, i.e., the patient is the source of the information it becomes critical to define and or label the content, construct or concept of the specific PRO [24]. Typically, this content has included measures "that includes direct subjective assessment by the patient of elements of their health including: symptoms, function, well-being, health-related quality-of-life (HRQoL), perceptions about treatment, satisfaction with care received, and satisfaction with professional communication. The patient is asked to summarize his or her evaluation of the disease, treatment, or health-care system interactions through various modes, providing perceptions related to the condition, its impact, and its functional implications" [22]. It is evident from the literature that there is discussion and debate regarding the definition of a PRO, what context it is measuring, the importance of patient input, not to mention how it is analyzed and reported [19–25].

The objective of the tool must also be considered. If the goal is to follow patients over time and to assess changes, an evaluative index is necessary, because it can measure the magnitude of longitudinal change in an individual or a group of individuals [26]. If the objective is to differentiate among patients to determine treatment, a discriminative index should be used, because it distinguishes between individuals or groups [26]. It is important to recognize that the properties of each outcome measure are different, depending on the objective of the tool. Discriminative instruments need to be highly reliable and the questions included in these instruments must enhance the ability to measure variability. In essence this type of questionnaire should have unique items that are different from each other that all patients would be able to respond to. Redundant questions would add nothing to the ability to discriminate and therefore would add nothing to a discriminative questionnaire. One of the key properties of an evaluative index is the demonstration of responsiveness [26]. Responsiveness refers to the ability of the outcome measure or instrument **to detect within patient change over time** [2]. A discriminative index needs to **differentiate**, **between patients**, **at a particular point in time**. In other words, being able to distinguish patients with more- or less-severe "disease" states. Guyatt has explained the differences between these two types of instruments by using the statistical concept of quantifying the signal-to-noise ratio [2]. The better the signal-to-noise ratio the better the instrument. "If the variability between patients (the signal) is much greater than the variability within patients (the noise), an instrument will be deemed reliable" [2]. Evaluative instruments are subtly different in that they need to detect change over time and responsiveness is a reflection of that change. Responsiveness is "directly related to the magnitude of the difference in score in patients who have improved or deteriorated (the signal) and the extent to which patients who have not changed provide more or less the same scores (the noise)" [2]. If the change over time is clinically meaningful, then a responsive instrument will be able to measure whether or not specific treatment (i.e., surgery) has improved a patient's outcome. Finally, it is essential to understand how each item in a PRO is determined. It is the initial item pool through the process of item generation that is critical [2, 27]. Once a comprehensive item pool is identified then the final set of items is reduced and formulated into the questionnaire [27]. "The procedure for achieving comprehensiveness is different when selecting an item pool for an evaluative instrument than for either a discriminative or predictive tool" [26]. In a discriminative index it would be important to have the majority of the respondents to answer the questions. Whereas in an evaluative index all relevant and important aspects should be included in order to measure clinically important outcomes [26].

When it comes to HRQOL this can be determined by using **generic** instruments that are designed to be applicable to multiple diseases or conditions and to be administered to a variety of patients [28]. Then there are instruments, which are **condition (disease) or joint specific**.

Generic Health Related Quality-of-life Instruments

Generic instruments include examples such as the Medical Outcomes Study 36-item Short Form (SF-36) health survey, the Sickness Impact Profile (SIP) and the EuroQol Instrument (EQ-5D) [3, 4, 28–32]. The literature includes comparisons of these and other generic outcomes [28, 31]. The SF-36 health survey is the most commonly used measure. It measures eight separate health concepts, which are analyzed into Physical and Mental Component Scales (PCS and MCS). It can be patient self-administered in a short period of time. The SIP is a behaviorally based measure that includes 136 items in 12 separate categories [30]. The SIP was developed as an outcome to be used in the evaluation of healthcare, program planning and policy development [28]. The EuroQOL or EQ-5D, is considered a preference-based measure that was intended to be used in conjunction with a condition-specific outcome. It is self-administered and includes two parts. The patient identifies his or her current state based on five dimensions of health including: mobility, self-care, usual activity, pain/discomfort and anxiety/depression and then rates his or her own health on a 20 cm Visual Analogue Scale (VAS) from 0 indicating his or her worst imaginable health state to 100 which represents his or her best imaginable health state. Separate comparisons of these and other similar generic instruments have shown that they are all well developed [28, 31]. They all demonstrate good psychometric properties and there is no specific recommendation of which one to use [28, 31]. Generic health status measures are helpful when comparing different populations of patients with different disease states. They typically do not provide clinicians, researchers, or more importantly patients with information that is as specific or valid, compared to condition or joint-specific outcome measures [13, 33].

Condition (Disease) of Joint-Specific Quality-of-Life Outcomes

With respect to quality-of-life after hip arthroscopy there are two ways to approach this aspect of outcome assessment. One would be to consider the condition or disease and utilize a HRQOL instrument developed and validated for the specific disorder. The second approach is to consider using a joint-specific outcome that is germane to the hip joint or region.

Arthroscopic treatment of the hip addresses several disparate diseases or conditions. It is reasonable that we could classify "hip" conditions as those that are related to the soft tissues in the hip and groin region, pre-arthritic conditions, and those that are arthritic in nature. It is important from the perspective of measuring outcomes that although the focus is on arthroscopic treatment, one must consider using outcome measures that can be used to compare non-surgical to surgical treatment, and open to arthroscopic techniques. The other important concept is that it is necessary to distinguish whether we are using the outcome to categorize the conditions, determine the severity of disease or determine whether a patient is needing surgery or not. These characteristics would require a discriminative HRQOL instrument [27, 34]. Whereas, if the goal is to follow patients over time and compare treatments to one another, then an evaluative instrument is necessary [27, 34]. The clinician is ideally looking for an outcome that serves both purposes equally well and from the perspective of the healthcare system an outcome that is reflective of the quality-of-care [35].

There are three outcome measures that could be considered in the category of condition- or joint-specific HRQOL outcomes. The first would be the Western Ontario and McMaster Universities Osteoarthritis Index (WOMAC) [36, 37]. Strictly speaking the WOMAC was designed to measure pain (5-items), stiffness (2-items), and physical function (17-items); in patients with hip and/or knee osteoarthritis. It has been characterized as a HRQOL measure and compared to the SF-36 [33]. However, there are no questions related to occupational function, psychological state, or social interaction and therefore it is limited in its capacity to measure all the characteristic dimensions of quality-of-life [3, 27]. The WOMAC is otherwise a highly recognized disease-specific PRO that has been validated in every respect, has been translated into 65 alternate language forms, has two question response formats (Likert and VAS), can be administered on paper, computer, telephone, and mobile devices; and it has been utilized for almost 30 years.

The second outcome measure that can be considered for the assessment of quality-of-life is the Copenhagen Hip and Groin Outcome Score (HAGOS) [38]. The goal of this "joint-specific" outcome is to evaluate hip and/or groin disability related to impairment (body structure and function), activity (activity limitations), and participation (participation restrictions) according to the International Classification of Functioning, disability, and health (ICF), in young to middle-aged physically active patients with hip and/or groin pain [38]. The final version of the HAGOS includes 37 items in six separate subscales: Pain (10 items), Symptoms (7 items), ADL (5 items), Sport/Rec (8 items), PA (2 items), and QOL (5 items). The HAGOS was initially derived from pre-existing published questionnaires (WOMAC and Hip disability and osteoarthritis outcome score (HOOS)), of which the quality-of-life component can be traced back to the ACL-QOL questionnaire [16, 36, 39]. Additional items were added to the quality-of-life subscale and based on the validation this subscale demonstrated the best responsiveness characteristics [38]. The HAGOS has been demonstrated to be valid reliable and responsive with a quality-of-life subscale and therefore fits some of the criteria for a HRQOL outcome measure.

Finally, the only outcome that was specifically designed to address quality-of-life is the International Hip Outcome Tool (iHOT-33 and iHOT-12) [11, 18]. The iHOT was developed to evaluate the young active patient with a hip disorder, utilized the input from more than 400 patients and was developed de novo to ensure that all questions were patient generated and therefore important to patients with hip problems [11, 18]. The iHOT-33 includes 33 questions and four domains (Symptoms and Functional Limitations 16-items; Sports and Recreational Activities 6-items; Job Related Concerns 4-items; and Social, Emotional and Lifestyle Concerns 7-items) [18]. The iHOT-12 includes 12 questions covering the same domains. The iHOT questionnaires are designed for self-administration, utilize 100-point VAS scale response formats for ease of analysis and have demonstrated reliability, validity, and responsiveness [18]. The iHOT-33 is recommended for use in clinical trials as a responsive evaluative outcome tool, whereas the iHOT-12 is recommended for easy use in clinical practice. The iHOT-12 may also prove to be a simple discriminative outcome since it has less redundancy, high reliability, and all questions are relevant to patients [11].

Summary

Understanding quality-of-life after hip arthroscopic surgery depends on defining health-related quality-of-life (HRQOL), how it is measured, and through an appreciation of the measurement tools. Health-related quality-of-life is a multidimensional construct that includes symptoms, function, psychological, and social domains. There are commonly used generic tools, which are not as responsive as the condition or joint-specific measures. The iHOT-33 is the only outcome specifically designed to measure HRQOL in patients with hip disorders and with arthroscopic treatment.

References

1. Kuyken W, Orley J. Development of the Whoqol - rationale and current status. Int J Ment Health. 1994;23(3):24–56.
2. Guyatt GH, Feeny DH, Patrick DL. Measuring health-related quality of life. Ann Intern Med. 1993;118(8):622–9.
3. Schipper H, Clinch J, Olweny C. Quality of life Studies: definitions and conceptual issues. In: Spilker B, editor. Quality of life and pharmacoeconomics in clinical trials. Philadelphia: Lippincott-Raven; 1996. p. 11–23.
4. Torrance G. Measurement of health state utilities for economic appraisal. J Health Econ. 1986;5:1–30.
5. Williams GN, Gangel TJ, Arciero RA, Uhorchak JM, Taylor DC. Comparison of the Single Assessment Numeric Evaluation method and two shoulder rating scales. Outcomes measures after shoulder surgery. Am J Sports Med. 1999;27(2):214–21. Epub 1999/04/02.
6. Krywulak SA, Mohtadi NG, Russell ML, Sasyniuk TM. Patient satisfaction with inpatient versus outpatient reconstruction of the anterior cruciate ligament: a randomized clinical trial. Can J Surg. 2005;48(3):201–6. Epub 2005/07/15.
7. Bizzini M, Notzli HP, Maffiuletti NA. Femoroacetabular impingement in professional ice hockey players: a case series of 5 athletes after open surgical decompression of the hip. Am J Sports Med. 2007;35(11):1955–9. Epub 2007/07/05.
8. Martin RL, Mohtadi NG, Safran MR, Leunig M, Martin HD, McCarthy J, et al. Differences in physician and patient ratings of items used to assess hip disorders. Am J Sports Med. 2009;37(8):1508–12. Epub 2009/05/07.
9. Dawson J, Fitzpatrick R, Carr A. A self-administered questionnaire for assessment of symptoms and function of the shoulder. J Bone Joint Surg Am. 1998;80(5):766–7. Epub 1998/06/04.
10. Dawson J, Fitzpatrick R, Carr A. The assessment of shoulder instability. The development and validation of a questionnaire. J Bone Joint Surg Br. 1999;81(3):420–6. Epub 2000/06/29.
11. Griffin DR, Parsons N, Mohtadi NG, Safran MR. A short version of the International Hip Outcome Tool (iHOT-12) for use in routine clinical practice. Arthroscopy. 2012;28(5):611–6. quiz 6–8. Epub 2012/05/01.
12. Hatta T, Shinozaki N, Omi R, Sano H, Yamamoto N, Ando A, et al. Reliability and validity of the Western Ontario Shoulder Instability Index (WOSI) in the Japanese population. J Orthop Sci. 2011;16(6):732–6. Epub 2011/08/26.
13. Hollinshead RM, Mohtadi NG, Vande Guchte RA, Wadey VM. Two 6-year follow-up studies of large and massive rotator cuff tears: comparison of outcome measures. J Shoulder Elb Surg. 2000;9(5):373–81. Epub 2000/11/15.
14. Kirkley A, Alvarez C, Griffin S. The development and evaluation of a disease-specific quality-of-life questionnaire for disorders of the rotator cuff: the Western Ontario Rotator Cuff Index. Clin J Sport Med. 2003;13(2):84–92. Epub 2003/03/12.
15. Lo IK, Griffin S, Kirkley A. The development of a disease-specific quality of life measurement tool for osteoarthritis of the shoulder: the Western Ontario Osteoarthritis of the Shoulder (WOOS) index. Osteoarthritis Cartilage. 2001;9(8):771–8. Epub 2002/02/14.
16. Mohtadi N. Development and validation of the quality of life outcome measure (questionnaire) for chronic anterior cruciate ligament deficiency. Am J Sports Med. 1998;26(3):350–9.
17. Salomonsson B, Ahlstrom S, Dalen N, Lillkrona U. The Western Ontario Shoulder Instability Index (WOSI): validity, reliability, and responsiveness retested with a Swedish translation. Acta Orthop. 2009;80(2):233–8. Epub 2009/05/01.
18. Mohtadi NG, Griffin DR, Pedersen ME, Chan D, Safran MR, Parsons N, et al. The Development and validation of a self-administered quality-of-life outcome measure for young, active patients with symptomatic hip disease: the International Hip Outcome Tool (iHOT-33). Arthroscopy. 2012;28(5):595–605. quiz 6–10 e1. Epub 2012/05/01.
19. Doward LC, McKenna SP. Defining patient-reported outcomes. Value Health. 2004;7 Suppl 1:S4–8. Epub 2004/09/16.
20. Fairclough DL. Patient reported outcomes as endpoints in medical research. Stat Methods Med Res. 2004;13(2):115–38. Epub 2004/04/08.

21. Patrick DL, Burke LB, Powers JH, Scott JA, Rock EP, Dawisha S, et al. Patient-reported outcomes to support medical product labeling claims: FDA perspective. Value Health. 2007;10 Suppl 2:S125–37. Epub 2007/11/13.
22. Rothman ML, Beltran P, Cappelleri JC, Lipscomb J, Teschendorf B. Patient-reported outcomes: conceptual issues. Value Health. 2007;10 Suppl 2:S66–75. Epub 2007/11/13.
23. Scoggins JF, Patrick DL. The use of patient-reported outcomes instruments in registered clinical trials: evidence from ClinicalTrials.gov. Contemp Clin Trials. 2009;30(4):289–92. Epub 2009/03/12.
24. Patrick DL. Patient-reported outcomes (PROs): an organizing tool for concepts, measures and applications. Qual Life Newsl. 2003; 31(Fall Issue):1–5.
25. Wright JG, Rudicel S, Feinstein AR. Ask patients what they want. Evaluation of individual complaints before total hip replacement. J Bone Joint Surg (Br). 1994;76(2):229–34.
26. Kirshner B, Guyatt G. A methodological framework for assessing health indices. J Chronic Dis. 1985;38(1):27–36.
27. Guyatt GH, Bombardier C, Tugwell PX. Measuring disease-specific quality of life in clinical trials. CMAJ. 1986;134(8):889–95. Epub 1986/04/15.
28. Coons SJ, Rao S, Keininger DL, Hays RD. A comparative review of generic quality-of-life instruments. PharmacoEconomics. 2000; 17(1):13–35. Epub 2000/04/05.
29. The EuroQol Group. EuroQol--a new facility for the measurement of health-related quality of life. Health Policy. 1990;16(3): 199–208. Epub 1990/11/05.
30. Bergner M, Bobbitt RA, Carter WB, Gilson BS. The Sickness Impact Profile: development and final revision of a health status measure. Med Care. 1981;19(8):787–805. Epub 1981/08/01.
31. Essink-Bot ML, Krabbe PF, Bonsel GJ, Aaronson NK. An empirical comparison of four generic health status measures. The Nottingham Health Profile, the Medical Outcomes Study 36-item Short-Form Health Survey, the COOP/WONCA charts, and the EuroQol instrument. Med Care. 1997;35(5):522–37. Epub 1997/05/01.
32. Ware Jr JE, Gandek B. Overview of the SF-36 Health Survey and the International Quality of Life Assessment (IQOLA) Project. J Clin Epidemiol. 1998;51(11):903–12. Epub 1998/11/17.
33. Hawker G, Melfi C, Paul J, Green R, Bombardier C. Comparison of a generic (SF-36) and a disease specific (WOMAC) (Western Ontario and McMaster Universities Osteoarthritis Index) instrument in the measurement of outcomes after knee replacement surgery. J Rheumatol. 1995;22(6):1193–6. Epub 1995/06/01.
34. Guyatt GH. A taxonomy of health status instruments. J Rheumatol. 1995;22(6):1188–90. Epub 1995/06/01.
35. Treurniet HF, Essink-Bot ML, Mackenbach JP, van der Maas PJ. Health-related quality of life: an indicator of quality of care? Qual Life Res. 1997;6(4):363–9. Epub 1997/05/01.
36. Bellamy N. Pain assessment in osteoarthritis: experience with the WOMAC osteoarthritis index. Semin Arthritis Rheum. 1989;18(4 Suppl 2):14–7. Epub 1989/05/01.
37. Bellamy N, Buchanan WW, Goldsmith CH, Campbell J, Stitt LW. Validation study of WOMAC: a health status instrument for measuring clinically important patient relevant outcomes to antirheumatic drug therapy in patients with osteoarthritis of the hip or knee. J Rheumatol. 1988;15(12):1833–40. Epub 1988/12/01.
38. Thorborg K, Holmich P, Christensen R, Petersen J, Roos EM. The Copenhagen Hip and Groin Outcome Score (HAGOS): development and validation according to the COSMIN checklist. Br J Sports Med. 2011;45(6):478–91. Epub 2011/04/12.
39. Klassbo M, Larsson E, Mannevik E. Hip disability and osteoarthritis outcome score. An extension of the Western Ontario and McMaster Universities Osteoarthritis Index. Scand J Rheumatol. 2003;32(1):46–51.

Evaluating the Outcome of Hip Preserving Procedures: Patient Function, Satisfaction, and Impairment

64

Maureen K. Dwyer and Philip C. Noble

The advancement of hip arthroscopic procedures has contributed to improvements in the identification and treatment of hip disorders. While originally used for diagnosis and debridement of acetabular labral pathology, arthroscopy is now frequently used to perform complex procedures such as osteochondroplasty for treatment of abnormal bony morphology. As the complexity of arthroscopic procedures continues to increase, assessing the success of these procedures is of utmost importance to determine appropriate treatment plans for patients. Given that hip arthroscopy is a relatively new procedure for the management of hip disorders, evaluation of long-term patient function and satisfaction following surgery is limited. In addition, few measurement tools have been validated to specifically assess outcomes of patients undergoing these procedures. Many hip arthroscopy patients are younger and more active, and have different goals and expectations than patients undergoing more traditional open hip procedures. As such, the evaluation of outcomes for hip arthroscopy patients is restricted by the limitations of the measurement tools available. Nonetheless, the available evidence derived from outcome instruments derived from older patients demonstrates that many hip preservation procedures performed via arthroscopy lead to marked improvement in pain and function for many patients. This chapter will review patient function, satisfaction, and impairment following hip arthroscopy, including potential confounding variables which may improve or limit the success of these procedures. Understanding what factors contribute to good and poor outcomes is essential for surgeons to plan appropriate surgical options for future patients.

M.K. Dwyer, PhD, ATC
Orthopedics, Kaplan Joint Center, Newton Wellesley Hospital, Newton, MA, USA

Orthopedics, Massachusetts General Hospital, Boston, MA, USA

P.C. Noble, PhD (✉)
Director of Research, Institute of Orthopedic Research and Education, 6550 Fannin Street, Suite 2501, Houston, TX 77030, USA
e-mail: pnoble@bcm.edu

Patient Function and Impairment Following Hip Arthroscopy: Reported Results Based on Common Outcome Instruments

The Modified Harris Hip Score

As patients elect to undergo hip arthroscopy primarily to return to full, pain-free function, quantification of patient function pre- and post-surgery is central to the evaluation of the success of arthroscopic surgery. Though multiple outcome instruments have been employed to assess patient-reported function following hip arthroscopy, most studies have utilized the Modified Harris Hip Score (MHHS), which is an adaptation of the original Harris Hip Score designed for patients undergoing hip arthroplasty [1–14]. The modified score includes items assessing pain, impairments during gait (limp, assistive devices), walking distance, and the ability to climb stairs, put on socks and shoes, sit, and use public transportation. Items on the original Harris Score relating to deformity and range of motion have been omitted [15]. In calculating the MHHS, the total of all items is multiplied by a factor of 1.5 to yield a total possible score of 100 points. The MHHS has been used to assess outcomes following hip arthroscopy for patients of all ages and ranges of physical abilities. As many of these patients are young and active without chronic disabling hip disease, a ceiling effect has been commonly reported for the MHHS. Despite this, a plethora of information regarding patient function following hip arthroscopy is available in the form of MHHS scores, allowing direct comparison between studies as well as the opportunity to combine data from different studies to examine comprehensive trends.

Patient outcomes have been reported using the MHHS for up to 10 years after arthroscopic treatment of labral derangement in hips without bony abnormalities [2–14, 16]. In these studies the MHHS has increased from an average of 59 points pre-surgery to 82 points post-surgery, a 39 % improvement. When examining short term (1–3 years) [2, 4, 7, 8, 10, 13, 15], midterm (3–5 years) [9, 11, 14, 16], and

J.C. McCarthy et al. (eds.), *Hip Joint Restoration*, DOI 10.1007/978-1-4614-0694-5_64

long term (5–10 years) [3, 5, 6, 12] outcomes individually, similar patterns of improvement have been reported. Studies examining short term functional outcomes reported improvements of 38 %. MHHS scores increased from an average of 60 points to 82 points, with 80 % of outcomes rated as good to excellent. Midterm outcomes were slightly inferior, with scores increasing from 55 points to 75 points; however, only 56 % were rated as good to excellent. Superior outcomes were observed for the three studies reporting long term outcomes. MHHS scores increased from 62 points to 90 points, a 45 % improvement. Sixty-two percent of outcome scores were rated as good to excellent in this cohort. In a single study assessing outcomes following arthroscopic labral reconstruction using an iliotibial band graft, MHHS scores were shown to improve from 62 points to 85 points, suggesting this technique may be a viable alternative to arthroscopic debridement of labral tears. Based on these findings, patient-reported pain and function is improved following hip arthroscopy for labral pathology without bony abnormalities.

For patients undergoing hip arthroscopy for femoroacetabular impingement (FAI), MHHS scores have been reported up to 4 ½ years following surgery [1, 17–36]. Overall, the total score was shown to increase from 64 points to 87 points, a 37 % improvement. Improvements reported for short term (1–3 years) outcomes (64–88 points; 38 % increase) [1, 18, 21–24, 26, 27, 29, 30, 32–34, 36–39] were identical to those reported for midterm (3–5 years) outcomes (63–86 points; 37 % increase) [17, 19, 20, 25, 28, 31, 35, 40]. Additionally, 77 % of patients reported good to excellent outcomes. Age at time of surgery may play a role in postoperative outcomes scores for patients undergoing osteochondroplasty. For the three studies examining an adolescent population [29, 31, 32], postoperative MHHS scores averaged 87 points at 1–3 years following surgery, compared to an average of 78 points at 2–3 years following surgery for the two studies examining patients greater than 50 years of age. In addition to age, whether a labral repair or resection was performed in concert with osteochondroplasty was shown to affect postoperative MHHS scores. For patients with concomitant labral repair, MHHS scores improved from 60 points to 94 points, while those with labral resection improved from 63 points to 88 points. Additionally, only 68 % of patients with labral resection reported good to excellent outcomes, compared to 92 % with repair. In general, clinical outcomes support the use of hip arthroscopy for patients with symptomatic FAI.

There is limited data documenting the outcome of arthroscopic procedures for treatment of conditions other than FAI and labral repair (e.g. synovial chondromatosis, ligamentum teres ruptures). In a cohort of patients presenting with synovial chondromatosis, only half (48 %) reported good to excellent outcomes at an average of 5 years following surgery [41]. This sub-group was shown to have only grade I or II cartilage lesions of the hip at the time of surgery, suggesting arthroscopy for synovial chondromatosis may be an effective in the setting of limited joint degeneration, but not in those with more advanced joint disease. More favorable outcomes were reported following arthroscopic treatment of traumatic ruptures of the ligamentum teres. At an average of 29 months following surgery, MHHS scores were shown to improve from 43 points to 90 points. In addition, 96 % of patients reported a greater than 20 point improvement in pain and function. While these two examples provide preliminary information which may be useful in designing treatment plans for patients, more research is needed to assess the efficacy of arthroscopic procedures for the treatment of hip pathologies other than labral derangement and FAI.

As stated previously, a ceiling effect has been observed for the MHHS; therefore, scores for higher functioning patients may be inflated compared to lower functioning patients. In fact, studies which examined hip arthroscopy for labral debridement without bony abnormality in an athletic population ($n=3$) reported higher postoperative scores (94 points) compared to all other studies (80 points) ($n=13$), regardless of time from surgery. Specifically comparing 10-year outcomes after arthroscopy performed by the same surgeon, MHHS scores reported for athletes (96 points) were higher than non-athletes (81 points). In contrast, there was no difference in overall postoperative MHHS scores for an athletic population (88 points; $n=9$) compared to others (86 points; $n=13$) for studies which examined hip arthroscopy for femoroacetabular impingement. Therefore, activity level of patients should to be taken into account when examining outcomes following hip arthroscopy for labral debridement without bony abnormality.

Other confounding factors have been shown to significantly affect postoperative MHHS scores following hip arthroscopy with or without bony abnormality. The presence of concomitant chondral pathology has been identified as an independent predictor of poor outcome following hip arthroscopy [3, 15, 17]. Patients with arthritis were 2.5 times more likely to have a poor outcome compared to patients without arthritis at an average of 4 years post-surgery [17]. For patients 8 years following hip arthroscopy, the presence of arthritis at the time of surgery was the strongest predictor of poor outcome, with only 19 % reporting good to excellent results using the MHHS [3]. Secondary gain issues (disability, potential litigation, worker's compensation) were also shown to be negative predictors of outcome following hip arthroscopy [4, 17]. Patients with issues involving secondary gain were found to have poorer outcomes and were less likely to return to their prior activity level following surgery. In fact, no patient with secondary gain issues in either study reported a good to excellent outcome. Younger age was shown to be an independent predictor of good to excellent outcome. Patients less than 39 years of age were 7 times more likely to report good to excellent outcomes compared to their elder counterparts [17]. As a result, chondral pathology, disability status, and patient age should to be taken into account when interpreting outcomes for patients following hip arthroscopy for labral pathology.

The Nonarthritic Hip Score

The Nonarthritic Hip Score (NAHS) was developed to assess patients performing at a higher level of functioning. The NAHS assesses pain during daily activities; symptoms of joint catching, instability, and stiffness; function during daily activities; and function during recreation and sporting activities [42]. One study employed the NAHS for patients undergoing hip arthroscopy for labral tear without bony abnormality. At 3 years following surgery, total NAHS scores improved from 61 points to 78 points for all types of labral derangement. In this group of patients, the presence of chondral lesions at the time of surgery was shown to negatively affect outcome. For patients undergoing hip arthroscopy for femoroacetabular impingement, NAHS scores improved 38 %, from an average of 61 points to 83 points [1, 22, 25, 35–40]. Postoperative NAHS scores reported for short-term (1–3 years; 84 points) were similar to those reported for midterm outcomes (3–5 years; 81 points).

Less information exists regarding potential confounding factors for patient outcomes using the NAHS compared to the MHHS. A single study examined the use of a computer navigation system for improving surgical performance during osteochondroplasty [39]. At an average of 27 months following surgery, NAHS scores for patients who underwent surgery with navigation (90 points) were slightly higher than without navigation (82 points). These results suggest improved surgical technique during osteochondroplasty may positively affect patient outcome as assessed with the NAHS. In contrast, the presence of chondral pathology at the time of surgery appears to have a negative effect on the postoperative NAHS score. Scores for studies examining outcomes for patients with chondral pathology ($n=3$; 77 points) were less than those for patients without chondral pathology ($n=8$; 85 points). Interestingly, while a slight difference in NAHS score was observed between athletes (87 points) and others (81 points) following osteochondroplasty, athletes received virtually the same average outcome score whether assessed with the NAHS (87 points) or the MHHS (88 points). Given that the NAHS was created to address some of the ceiling effects seen by scores like the MHHS, use of the total score on NAHS for reporting outcomes may not offer any additional information from the total score of the MHHS. More detailed understanding of outcomes for athletic populations may be best accomplished by reporting average scores for each domain of each measurement tool.

Instruments for Pain Measurement: The Visual Analog Scale

Pain is one of the main reasons patients elect to undergo arthroscopic procedures for hip pathology. Although scores such as the MHHS and the NAHS both have questions which specifically address a patient's level of pain, most studies only report the total outcome score, which also includes functional questions. Thus, the extent to which joint pain is specifically relieved by arthroscopic surgery must be assessed through additional investigation. A handful of studies of patients undergoing hip arthroscopy for FAI have used the Visual Analog Scale (VAS) to assess pain levels independent of hip function [20, 37, 39, 40]. Patients were asked to rate their pain on a scale of 1–10, with 10 being the worst pain. Pain was shown to improve from an average of 5.7 presurgery to 1.6 at 1–3 years following surgery. The use of computer navigation during surgery may result in greater improvements in pain [39]. At an average of 27 months following surgery, patients who underwent surgery with navigation reported pain scores of 1 compared to scores of 2 for those without navigation. In addition, those patients for whom a labral repair was performed reported slightly lower pain scores (0.7) compared to those for whom labral debridement was performed (1.7) [20]. Overall, these results suggest osteochondroplasty performed via hip arthroscopy results in pain relief for patients.

Patient Satisfaction

Patients who elect to undergo arthroscopic surgery for treatment of hip disorders do so for a variety of reasons—pain relief, restoration of joint mobility and function, and/or return to recreational and sporting activities. As such, available measurement tools may not accurately address all constructs which are important in determining a good or poor outcome for each patient. To compensate for this, assessing patient satisfaction in addition to patient function can provide valuable information regarding overall surgical outcomes. For patients undergoing hip arthroscopy for labral derangement without bony abnormalities, few studies have reported patient satisfaction rates [3–5, 9]. Overall, 75 % of patients reported being satisfied with their outcomes following surgery. Studies describing short-term (1–3 years) patient satisfaction rates report similar rates (75 %) [4, 43] as those reporting midterm (3–5 years) satisfaction rates (67 %) [9] and long term (5–10 years) satisfaction rates (82 %) [3, 5].

For patients undergoing hip arthroscopy for FAI, numerous authors have reported patient satisfaction rates [17, 22–25, 27, 31, 35, 36]. Short term satisfaction rates (1–3 years; 80 %) were slightly lower than midterm satisfaction rates (3–5 years; 89 %) as a whole. In general, the majority of patients appear satisfied with their outcome following arthroscopy.

Certain factors were found to affect patient satisfaction after hip arthroscopy. The presence of articular cartilage degeneration at the time of surgery was shown to negatively affect patient satisfaction [3, 5]. Similarly, for patients involved in disability proceedings, reduced satisfaction rates (50 %) were reported when compared to patients not involved in such proceedings (84 %) [4]. Therefore, while the evidence is limited, these variables should be taken into account when interpreting patient satisfaction after hip arthroscopy.

Conclusion

As arthroscopic procedures for hip pathologies are still in their infancy compared to other joints, assessing the success of these procedures is paramount to advancing treatment techniques. For patients with labral derangement with or without concomitant bony abnormalities, the evidence suggests patient function is improved and pain is reduced following surgery. In addition, the majority of patients report being satisfied with their outcomes. However, there is a subset of patients for whom arthroscopic treatment of their hip disorder is not successful. For these patients, the presence of chondral defects at the time of surgery is the most common cofounding factor. Patient age and level of functioning may also affect postoperative pain and function. Understanding the goals of each patient prior to surgery and creating a treatment plan which best addresses those goals and expectations is paramount to successful outcomes.

References

1. Haviv B, Singh PJ, Takla A, O'Donnell J. Arthroscopic femoral osteochondroplasty for cam lesions with isolated acetabular chondral damage. J Bone Joint Surg Br. 2010;92(5):629–33.
2. Byrd JT, Jones K. Hip arthroscopy in athletes. Clin Sports Med. 2001;20(4):749–62.
3. Meftah M, Rodriguez JA, Panagopoulos G, Alexiades MM. Long-term results of arthroscopic labral debridement: predictors of outcomes. Orthopedics. 2011;34(10):e588–92.
4. Potter BK, Freedman BA, Andersen RC, Bojescul JA, Kuklo TR, Murphy KP. Correlation of Short From-36 and disability status with outcomes of arthroscopic acetabular labral debridement. Am J Sports Med. 2005;33(6):864–70.
5. Londers J, Van Melkebeek J. Hip arthroscopy: outcome and patient satisfaction after 5 to 10 years. Acta Orthop Belg. 2007; 73(4):478–83.
6. Byrd JWT, Jones KS. Prospective analysis of hip arthroscopy with 10-year followup. Clin Orthop Relat Res. 2010;468(3):741–6.
7. Farjo LA, Glick JM, Sampson TG. Hip arthroscopy for acetabular labral tears. Arthroscopy. 1999;15(2):132–7.
8. McCarthy JC, Barsoum W, Puri L, Lee J-A, Murphy S, Cooke P. The role of hip arthroscopy in the elite athlete. Clin Orthop Relat Res. 2003;206:71–4.
9. Santori N, Villar RN. Acetabular labral tears: result of arthroscopic partial limbectomy. Arthroscopy. 2000;16(1):11–5.
10. Burnett SJ, Della Rocca GJ, Prather H, Curry M, Maloney WJ, Clohisy JC. Clinical presentation of patients with tears of acetabular labrum. J Bone Joint Surg. 2006;88:1448–57.
11. Kamath AF, Componovo R, Baldwin K, Israelite CL, Nelson CL. Hip arthroscopy for labral tears: review of clinical outcomes with 4.8-year mean follow-up. Am J Sports Med. 2009;37(9): 1721–7.
12. Byrd JWT, Jones KS. Hip arthroscopy in athletes: 10-year follow-up. Am J Sports Med. 2009;37(11):2140–3.
13. Freedman BA, Potter BK, Dinauer PA, Giuliani JR, Kuklo TR, Murphy KP. Prognostic value of magnetic resonance arthrography for Czerny stage II and III acetabular labral tears. Arthroscopy. 2006;22(7):742–7.
14. Streich NA, Gotterbarm T, Barié A, Schmitt H. Prognostic value of chondral defects on the outcome after arthroscopic treatment of acetabular labral tears. Knee Surg Sports Traumatol Arthrosc. 2009;17(10):1257–63.
15. Byrd JT, Jones KS. Prospective analysis of hip arthroscopy with 2-year follow-up. Arthroscopy. 2000;16(6):578–87.
16. Haviv B, O'Donnell J. Arthroscopic treatment for acetabular labral tears of the hip without bony dysmorphism. Am J Sports Med. 2011;39:79S–84.
17. McCormick F, Nwachukwu B, Alpaugh K, Martin S. Predictors of hip arthroscopy outcomes for labral tears at minimum 2-year follow-up: the influence of age and arthritis. Arthroscopy. 2012;28: 1359–64.
18. Kang C, Hwang D-S, Cha S-M. Acetabular labral tears in patients with sports injury. Clin Orthop Surg. 2009;1(4):230–5.
19. Cooper A, Basheer S, Maheshwari R, Regan L, Madan S. Outcomes of hip arthroscopy. A prospective analysis and comparison between patients under 25 and over 25 years of age. Br J Sports Med. 2012;47(4):234–8.
20. Larson CM, Giveans MR, Stone RM. Arthroscopic debridement versus refixation of the acetabular labrum associated with femoroacetabular impingement: mean 3.5-year follow-up. Am J Sports Med. 2012;40(5):1015–21.
21. Byrd JWT, Jones KS. Arthroscopic management of femoroacetabular impingement in athletes. Am J Sports Med. 2011;39(Suppl): 7S–13.
22. Javed A, O'Donnell JM. Arthroscopic femoral osteochondroplasty for cam femoroacetabular impingement in patients over 60 years of age. J Bone Joint Surg Br. 2011;93(3):326–31.
23. Gedouin JE, May O, Bonin N, et al. Assessment of arthroscopic management of femoroacetabular impingement. A prospective multicenter study. Orthop Traumatol Surg Res. 2010;96(8 Suppl): S59–67.
24. Gédouin JE, Duperron D, Langlais F, Thomazeau H. Update to femoroacetabular impingement arthroscopic management. Orthop Traumatol Surg Res. 2010;96(3):222–7.
25. Malviya A, Stafford GH, Villar RN. Impact of arthroscopy of the hip for femoroacetabular impingement on quality of life at a mean follow-up of 3.2 years. J Bone Joint Surg Br. 2012;94(4):466–70.
26. Nho SJ, Magennis EM, Singh CK, Kelly BT. Outcomes after the arthroscopic treatment of femoroacetabular impingement in a mixed group of high-level athletes. Am J Sports Med. 2011; 39(Suppl):14S–9.

27. Philippon MJ, Briggs KK, Yen YM, Kuppersmith DA. Outcomes following hip arthroscopy for femoroacetabular impingement with associated chondrolabral dysfunction: minimum two-year follow-up. J Bone Joint Surg Br. 2009;91(1):16–23.
28. Philippon MJ, Schroder E, Souza BG, Briggs KK. Hip arthroscopy for femoroacetabular impingement in patients aged 50 years or older. Arthroscopy. 2012;28(1):59–65.
29. Fabricant PD, Heyworth BE, Kelly BT. Hip arthroscopy improves symptoms associated with FAI in selected adolescent athletes. Clin Orthop Relat Res. 2012;470(1):261–9.
30. Philippon MJ, Weiss DR, Kuppersmith DA, Briggs KK, Hayy CJ. Arthroscopic labral repair and treatment of femoroacetabular impingement in professional hockey players. Am J Sports Med. 2010;38(1):99–104.
31. Philippon MJ, Ejnisman L, Ellis HB, Briggs KK. Outcomes 2 to 5 years following hip arthroscopy for femoroacetabular impingement in the patient aged 11 to 16 years. Arthroscopy. 2012;28(9):1255–61.
32. Philippon MJ, Yen Y-M, Briggs KK, Kuppersmith DA, Maxwell RB. Early outcomes after hip arthroscopy for femoroacetabular impingement in the athletic adolescent patient: a preliminary report. J Pediatr Orthop. 2008;28(7):705–10.
33. Schilders E, Dimitrakopoulou A, Bismil Q, Marchant P, Cooke C. Arthroscopic treatment of labral tears in femoroacetabular impingement: a comparative study of refixation and resection with a minimum two-year follow-up. J Bone Joint Surg Br. 2011;93(8):1027–32.
34. Larson CM, Giveans MR. Arthroscopic management of femoroacetabular impingement: early outcomes measures. Arthroscopy. 2008;24(5):540–6.
35. Singh PJ, O'Donnell JM. The outcome of hip arthroscopy in Australian football league players: a review of 27 hips. Arthroscopy. 2010;26(6):743–9.
36. Malviya A, Stafford GH, Villar R. Is hip arthroscopy for femoroacetabular impingement only for athletes. Br J Sports Med. 2012;46(14):1016–8.
37. Horisberger M, Brunner A, Herzog RF. Arthroscopic treatment of femoroacetabular impingement of the hip: a new technique to access the joint. Clin Orthop Relat Res. 2010;468(1):182–90.
38. Brunner A, Horisberger M, Herzog RF. Sports and recreation activity of patients with femoroacetabular impingement before and after arthroscopic osteoplasty. Am J Sports Med. 2009;37(5):917–22.
39. Brunner A, Horisberger M, Herzog RF. Evaluation of a computed tomography-based navigation system prototype for hip arthroscopy in the treatment of femoroacetabular cam impingement. Arthroscopy. 2009;25(4):382–91.
40. Horisberger M, Brunner A, Herzog RF. Arthroscopic treatment of femoral acetabular impingement in patients with preoperative generalized degenerative changes. Arthroscopy. 2010;26(5):623–9.
41. Marchie A, Panuncialman I, McCarthy JC. Efficacy of hip arthroscopy in the management of synovial chondromatosis. Am J Sports Med. 2011;39(Suppl):126S–31.
42. Christensen C, Althausen P, Mittleman M, Lee JL, McCarthy JC. The Nonarthritic Hip Score: reliable and validated. Clin Orthop Relat Res. 2003;406:75–83.
43. Philippon MJ, Briggs KK, Hayy CJ, Kuppersmith DA, Dewing C, Huang M. Arthroscopic labral reconstruction in the hip using iliotibial band autograft: technique and early outcomes. Arthroscopy. 2010;26(6):750–6.

Part IX

Articular Lesions: Prevention and Treatment

Marc R. Safran

Biology of Cartilage Regeneration

65

Cecilia Pascual-Garrido and Scott A. Rodeo

Articular Cartilage Structure and Composition

The function of the articular cartilage is to provide for smooth, pain-free gliding of the joints during skeletal motion. Articular cartilage is composed of a large extracellular matrix, synthesized by the chondrocytes, including type II collagen and proteoglycan aggregates. Collagen fibers give cartilage its form and tensile strength, and water constitutes 75–80 % of cartilage weight, functioning largely in compression. Chondrocytes are responsible for maintaining the matrix, which involves degradation by proteinases, aggrecanase, and oxygen free radicals, which may be generated by the chondrocyte [1]. The structure of articular cartilage can be divided into zones—superficial, middle, and deep—each of which imparts mechanical properties contributing to the articular surface [1] (Fig. 65.1). In the superficial zone, the chondrocytes are flattened and collagen fibrils are aligned parallel to the surface. The primary function of this layer is to resist shear forces. Cells in this zone synthesize a molecule called "superficial zone protein" providing the almost frictionless articulation by the articular cartilage. The middle zone is composed of obliquely oriented collagen fibers and primarily resists compression forces. In the deep zone, fibers are oriented perpendicular to the subchondral plate, resisting both compression and shear forces. Calcified cartilage in the deep layer provides a buffer with intermediate mechanical properties between the more superficial uncalcified cartilage and the underlying subchondral bone. The avascular nature of articular cartilage makes it dependent on diffusion through the matrix for nutrition. Diffusion of nutrients from subchondral bone vessels and synovial tissue play a critical role in maintaining normal adult cartilage homeostasis and function [2].

Healing Capacity of the Cartilage

Both partial and full-thickness lesions have limited capacity for repair. In animal models, after the creation of osteochondral defects, generally good reconstitution of the articular cartilage is observed as early as four weeks. However, early traces of degeneration are seen after 12 weeks and continue to progress with time [3]. Not only is the immediate area of the defect affected but the articular cartilage adjacent to defect also degenerates, suggesting a "zone of influence" which may explain the progression of a focal chondral defect to more diffuse degeneration [4]. Differences in the potential for cartilage repair separate acute injuries of articular cartilage into three general types: (1) loss of matrix macromolecules or disruption of the macromolecular framework without visible tissue disruption, (2) mechanical disruption of articular cartilage alone, and (3) mechanical disruption of articular cartilage and subchondral bone:

1. *Loss of matrix macromolecules*: This may alter chondrocyte function or even damage the chondrocytes. Chondrocytes can sense changes in matrix composition and synthesize new molecules, which allow the cells to repair damage to the macromolecular framework. Available evidence indicates that repair of the matrix in response to loss of proteoglycans may require many weeks and possibly months. If the cells fail to repair significant matrix macromolecular abnormalities, or if the loss of matrix molecules progresses, the tissue will deteriorate with time. The threshold for irreversible injury and progressive loss of articular cartilage is unknown [5, 6].

C. Pascual-Garrido, MD
Hip Preservation, Sports Medicine, University of Colorado, Boulder, CO, USA

S.A. Rodeo, MD (✉)
Orthopedics Department, Sports Medicine and Shoulder Service, The Hospital for Special Surgery, 535 East 70th Street, New York, NY 10021, USA
e-mail: rodeos@hss.edu

J.C. McCarthy et al. (eds.), *Hip Joint Restoration*, DOI 10.1007/978-1-4614-0694-5_65

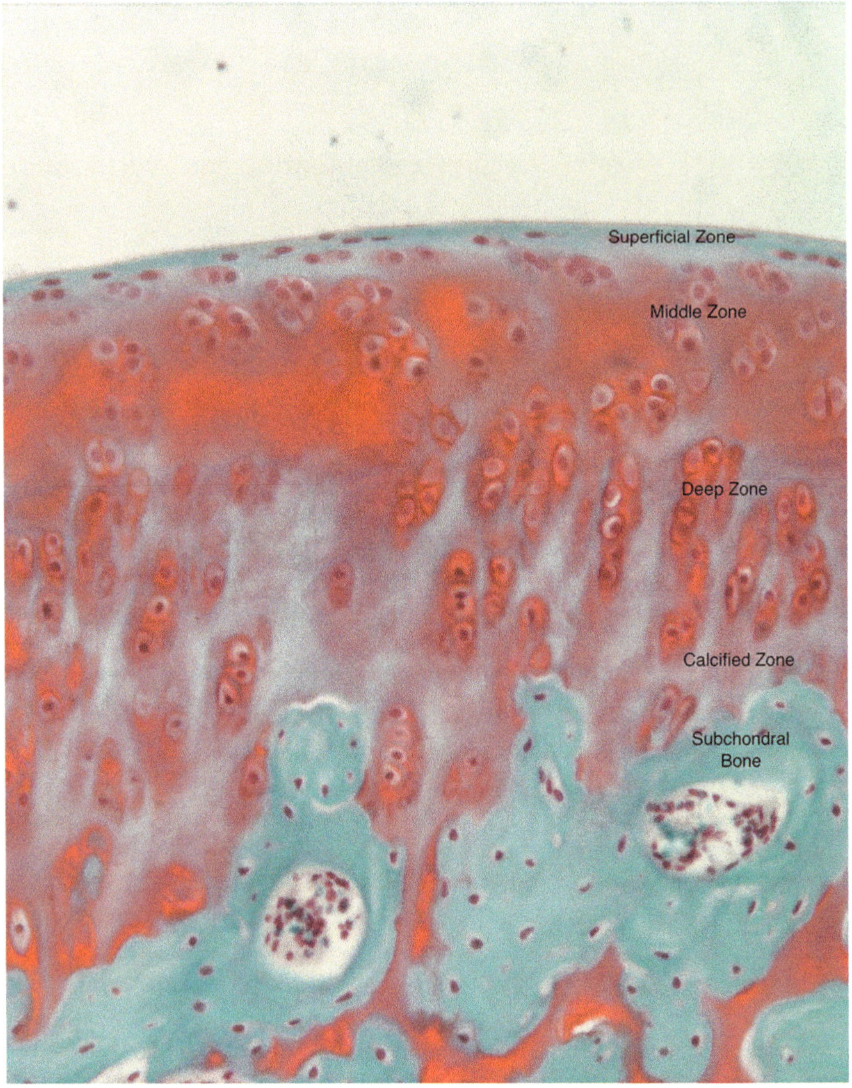

Fig. 65.1 Microscopic anatomy of articular cartilage. Safranin O staining. Note the superficial, middle, and deep zone with the decreased content of aggrecan

2. *Mechanical disruption of articular cartilage alone*: When injury is limited to the cartilage tissue, the local response depends entirely on the chondrocytes. Undifferentiated mesenchymal cells cannot migrate from blood vessels to the site of injury. The chondrocytes near the injury site respond to tissue injury by proliferating and increasing synthesis of matrix macromolecules, however, the newly synthesized matrix and proliferating chondrocytes are unable to fill the tissue defect, and soon after injury, the increased proliferation and synthetic activity ceases [7].
3. *Injuries affecting Cartilage and Subchondral Bone*: When a joint injury extends into the subchondral bone, hemorrhage occurs with fibrin clot formation and activation of an inflammatory response. In animal experiments, repair tissue fills about two-thirds of the total volume of the chondral portion but most of the filling is performed in the bone portion of the osteochondral defect [8]. The tissue in the chondral and bone portions of the defect differs significantly in composition. The chondral repair tissue does not contain bone or blood vessels and has a significantly higher proportion of hyaline-like cartilage or fibrocartilage. Whereas, the repair tissue within the subchondral bone is highly vascular and endochondral bone formation is normally evident [3]. With time the cartilage repair tissue occasionally persists unchanged or progressively remodels. Most of the time, the chondral repair tissue begins to show depletion of matrix proteoglycans, with progressive degeneration through fibrillation and fragmentation.

Many factors that prevent cartilage from healing have been suggested, including joint environment, age, changes in epigenetics, apoptosis, and biochemical constitution of the repair tissue [9–11].

Several factors are felt to contribute to the failure of attempts to perform surgical repair of cartilage lesions, including abnormalities in the biochemical constitution of the repaired tissue, the quality of its physicochemical binding to the adjacent cartilage, and the altered stiffness of the repaired subchondral bone [12]. The reparative tissue is weaker, with higher water and lower proteoglycan content compared to normal-appearing cartilage [13].

The potential for cartilage healing is also strongly influenced by the age of the patient, with repair usually occurring in the growing child but not in the adult [12, 14]. Cartilage matrix turnover and remodeling is much more rapid in a child as part of the growth process. In adults, although synthesis increases in damaged cartilage, these newly synthesized molecules are degraded [15, 16]. Stimulation of matrix synthesis alone is not sufficient to ensure the success of a reparative process, as the newly synthesized molecules must be protected from proteolysis to ensure their incorporation and retention in the newly repaired matrix [17].

Changes in the joint environment after cartilage injury have also been implicated in cartilage degeneration. After cartilage trauma, there is an increased expression of metalloproteinases (MMP), (ADAMTS-5), and caspases (3–9), which promote chondrocyte apoptosis [11, 18–21]. There are also inflammatory mediators, such as interleukin-1 beta, which have degradative effects on cartilage matrix.

Ongoing research to identify the factors that prevent cartilage from healing will allow development of interventions that may enhance cartilage repair or even prevent cartilage from degeneration.

Current Techniques for Cartilage Regeneration in the Hip

The options for surgical treatment of articular cartilage lesions can be divided into palliative, reparative, and restorative procedures. Palliative procedures, including debridement and lavage, are done primarily for symptomatic relief and have little potential for cartilage regeneration. Reparative techniques attempt to restore the integrity of the native subchondral interface and preserve the overlying articular cartilage [22]. These include drilling and ORIF, normally used for OCD lesions in the talus and knee [23]. Finally, restorative procedures attempt to replace damaged cartilage with hyaline or hyaline-like tissue [24]. When performing the treatment of cartilage lesions, the surgeon must consider the "next step" option if initial surgical management fails. The treatment algorithm proceeds from the least destructive and invasive methodologies, to preserve the ability to use additional options should initial treatment fail. Although there has not been any published data yet on how to proceed with cartilage lesions in the hip, one should assume that the treatment algorithm should be similar to other joints [25]. Thus the algorithm for treatment of hip lesions is likely to include consideration of the anatomic location of the lesion (acetabulum versus femoral head), and its size (small vs big), and depth (superficial versus deep). Concomitant pathology such as FAI (femoro-acetabular impingement) (Cam-Pincer lesion), labrum tears, or hip dysplasia should always be considered and treated simultaneously.

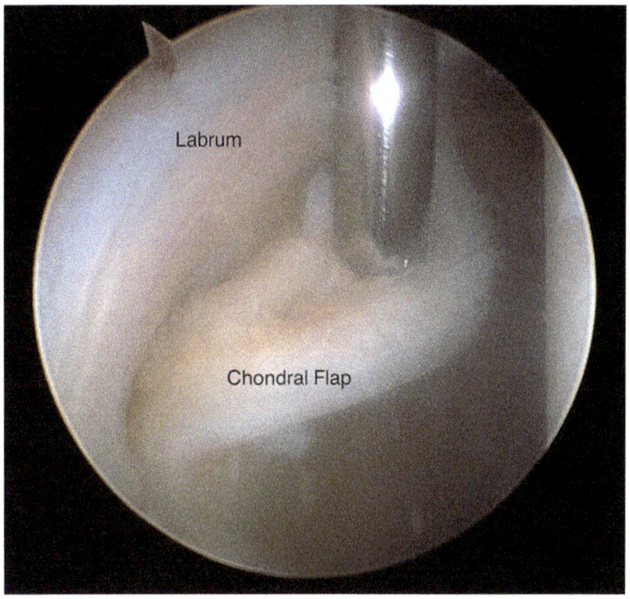

Fig. 65.2 Note typical flap chondral lesion that is observed in patients with a CAM lesion. Location is normally in the acetabulum and in the anterosuperior area

Table 65.1 Classification of cartilage damage

Description	Criteria
Normal	Macroscopically sound cartilage
Malacia	Roughening of surface, fibrillation
Debonding	Loss of fixation to the subchondral bone, macroscopically sound cartilage; carpet phenomenon
Cleavage	Loss of fixation to the subchondral bone; frayed edges, thinning of cartilage, flap
Defect	Full-thickness defect

Intraoperative classification for chondral lesions in the hip as proposed by Beck et al. [30]

Cartilage lesions have a typical pattern in patients with CAM lesions [26, 27] and are most commonly located in the anterosuperior area of the acetabulum [28]. The commonly accepted mechanism of injury is exposure of the labrochondral junction to repetitive compression and shear that occurs when the CAM lesion slides into the anterosuperior acetabulum during flexion and internal rotation. This causes the labrum to be stretched and displaced peripherally while the cartilage is compressed and pushed centrally resulting in separation between the labrum and cartilage, and, in many cases, a typical flap chondral lesion (Fig. 65.2). These chondral defects may cause pain, and, if left untreated, will likely progress to more generalized degeneration [27, 29]. Classification of cartilage damage in the acetabulum has been proposed by Beck et al. [30] (Table 65.1).

Cartilage restorative procedures such as marrow stimulation or microfracture, fresh osteochondral allografts, osteochondral autografts (OATS), and autologous chondrocyte implantation (ACI) have been extensively described in different joints including knees, shoulders, and ankles [25] (Figs. 65.3 and 65.4). However, there is currently very little published data on the outcome of cartilage repair in the hip.

Microfracture is one of most widely cartilage therapy used to treat cartilage lesions in the hip. This technique is normally indicated for small chondral lesions, no bigger than 10 mm in any dimension. These lesions are normally seen in patients with CAM lesions in the anterosuperior area of the acetabulum (Figs. 65.5 and 65.6).

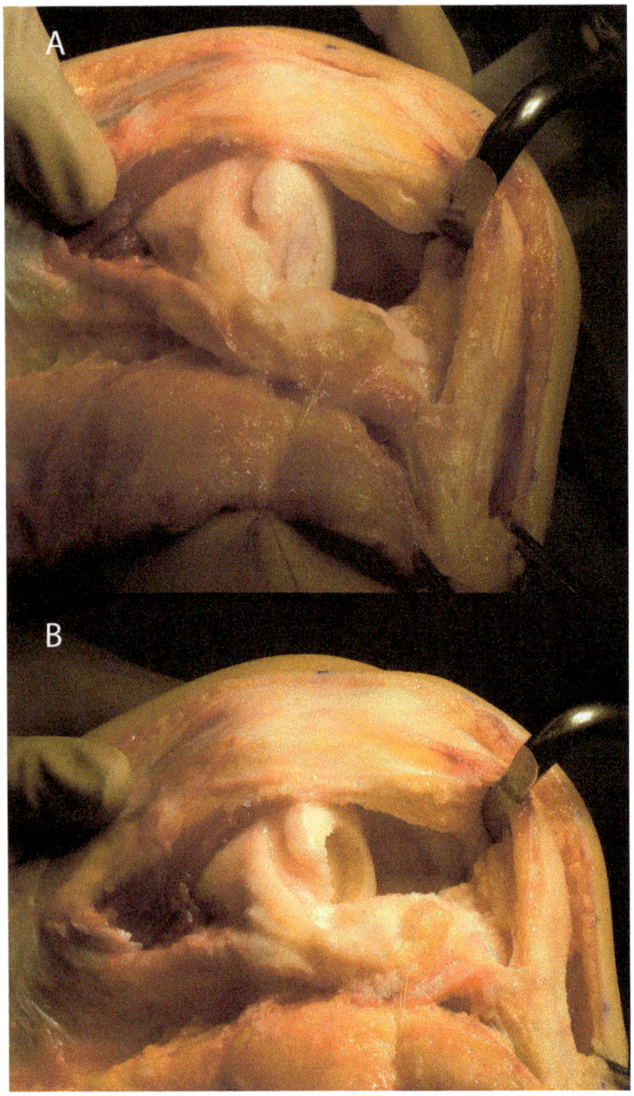

Fig. 65.3 (**a**) A chondral defect is evident in the lateral femoral condyle. This patient underwent a combined distal femoral osteotomy, osteochondral allograft, and meniscus allograft transplantation. An arthrotomy with a proximal extension for exposure of the distal femur was performed. (**b**) The defect was prepared using the recipient harvester instrument

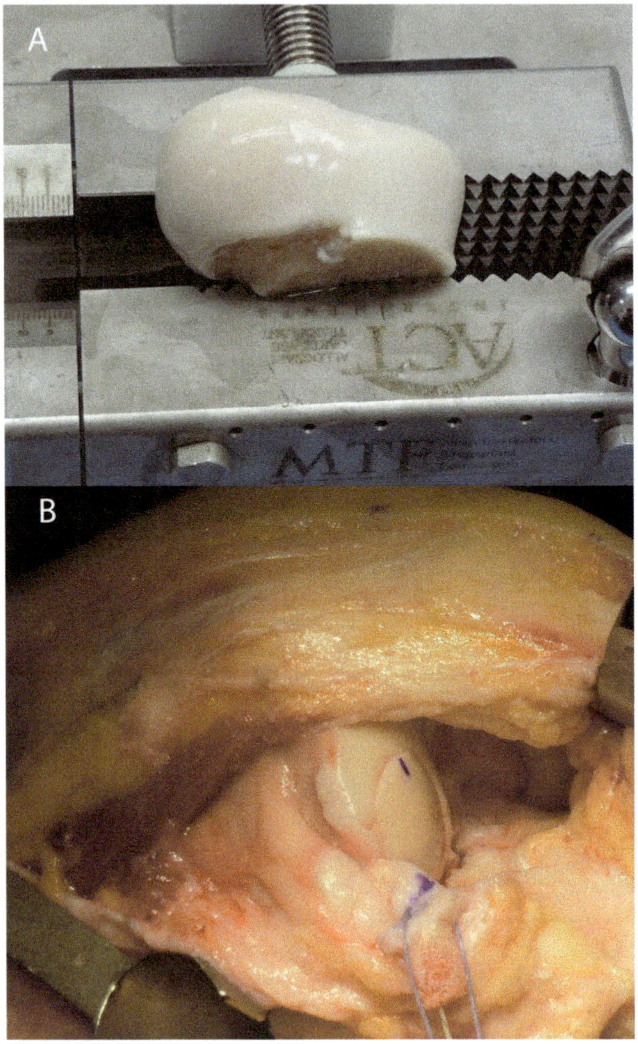

Fig. 65.4 (**a**) Donor condyle secured on a device that holds the graft while the donor segment is harvested. (**b**) The osteochondral plug was placed into the recipient defect. The 12 o clock position was marked on the allograft, representing the most superior point of the defect

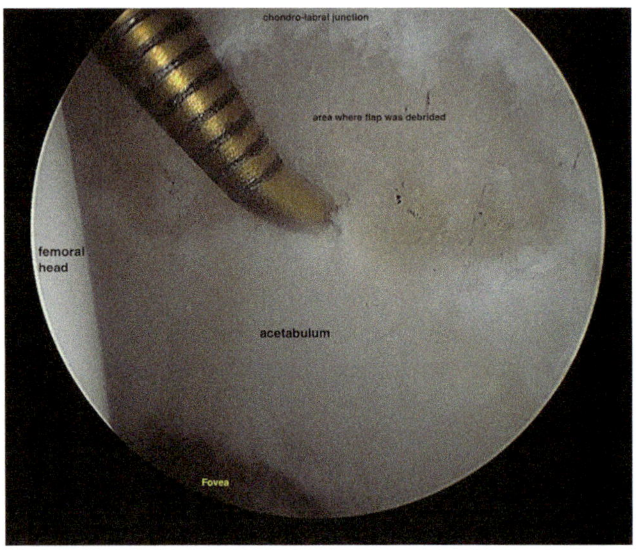

Fig. 65.5 Note the chondral lesion, already debrided and prepared for microfracture. Using an awl, microfracture was performed

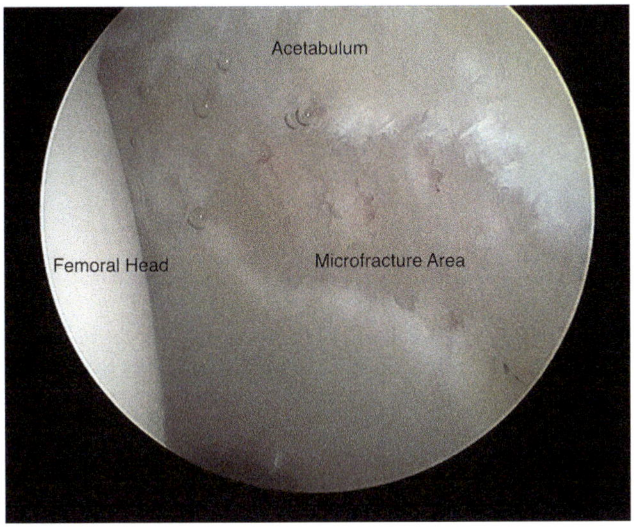

Fig. 65.6 Microfracture was performed. The microfracture holes are evident in the chondral lesion

Clinical results have been encouraging [31–33]. Karthikeyan et al. recently published the results observed with microfracture for acetabular chondral defects in patients with FAI [33]. All patients had a second look arthroscopy at an average 17 months post microfracture. Repair tissue was assessed as described by Blevins et al. [34]. Fill rate of the chondral lesions were reported in 93 % of the patients. Clinically, the NHS (nonarthritic hip score) improved from 55 to 78 after microfracture. Histologically, the tissue appeared to be fibrocartilage. Collagen type I and II was present in most samples. Philippon et al. [32] reported 95–100 % fill in eight of the nine patients who had second-look hip arthroscopic surgery after microfracture for acetabular cartilage lesions. They demonstrated an average fill of 91 % at an average follow-up of 20 months. No clinical evaluation was performed in this study.

Mosaicplasty or OATS should be considered for larger cartilage lesions or those with involvement of the subchondral bone. These lesions normally occur over the femoral surfaces of patients who sustain traumatic hip dislocations or patients with AVN (avascular necrosis). Mosaicplasty has shown excellent results in the knee [35, 36]. However, in the hip, literature is lacking with only isolated case reports. In all of these reports, short-term outcomes are encouraging, suggesting patients may return to normal activity with no progression of cartilage degeneration. Gagala et al. recently published clinical and radiological results for the treatment of AVN (avascular necrosis) of the femoral head using OATS in 20 patients [37]. At 18 months post operative, they reported clinical improvement (HHS from 42 to 87) with only one patient requiring a THR. At the moment, this technique can only be performed with an open dislocation of the hip, which adds morbidity. Future studies of a larger series of patients will further evaluate the effectiveness of this technique for traumatic osteochondral injury of the femoral head.

Autologous chondrocyte implantation (ACI) has been widely used in the last 15 years for the repair of cartilage defects [38]. It has been shown to be successful in the treatment of full-thickness defects in the knee and ankle, especially in young and active patients. There is only on case report of ACI for AVN of the hip [25, 39, 40]. Similar to OATS, this procedure was performed with an open dislocation.

More advanced techniques such as use of juvenile allograft cartilage (De Novo NT ®), CAIS (cartilage autograft implantation system), MACI (matrix autologous chondrocyte implantation), second- and third-generation ACI and characterized chondrocyte implantation (CCI) are becoming popular in the treatment for chondral lesions in the knee and may play a future role in cartilage restoration in the hip [34–36, 41]. Clinical results of MACI technique in the hip have been reported. The technique proposed is performed arthroscopically. At 5 years post-operative, patients improved clinically with no reported failures or adverse events [42, 43]. Continued development of an arthroscopic surgical technique for the treatment of chondral lesions in the hip with cell therapies will improve future applicability [44].

Future Directions

Future directions in cartilage regeneration are focusing on growth factors, stem cells, and new biomaterials, together with improvement in early diagnosis using MRI imaging and novel biomarkers [45]. Various growth factors continue to be investigated as a treatment for early joint pain or osteoarthritis and for cartilage regeneration, and they were recently reviewed [46]. Combinations of anabolic growth factors such as OP-1 and IGF-1 appear to be the most promising growth factor approach due to a synergistic effect [47]. The use of stem cells to regenerate articular cartilage remains a topic of active investigation. Novel biomaterials that are able to recruit endogenous stem cells to the site of injury rather than implanting exogenous cells is also a promising area of investigation. Ongoing studies are aimed at understanding why and how stem cells "home" to sites of injury. Progenitor stem cells have been identified in normal human articular cartilage. These studies have suggested that cartilage progenitor cells may be a superior cell source to mesenchymal stem cells. Additional studies are required to understand how to recruit these resident cartilage progenitor cells to the site of damage [48–50].

The therapeutic use of autologous platelet-rich plasma (PRP) constitutes a relatively new biotechnology that may play a role in the stimulation and acceleration of cartilage healing [51–53]. Chondrocytes and MSCs (mesenchymal stem cells) exposed to PRP both have increased cell proliferation and cartilage extracellular matrix synthesis of proteoglycans and collagen type II compared with controls [54].

There is very little data on clinical results of the treatment of early OA of the hip with PRP. The optimal PRP formulation, timing, and number of injections are still controversial. Different PRP preparations are available, which makes it even more difficult to compare results. Battaglia et al. recently reported the outcomes of injection of PRP for OA of the hip. All patients had significantly improved clinical symptoms at short-term follow-up. No major complications or adverse events occurred at the time of injection or in the follow-up period [55].

Magnetic resonance imaging (MRI) of cartilage continues to be the optimal modality for detailed cartilage imaging. In addition to the traditional morphologic assessment, more advanced quantitative cartilage imaging techniques, such as T1ρ, T2 mapping, and dGEMRIC are increasingly being used to noninvasively assess the biochemistry of the cartilage repair and to diagnose preclinical disease. The concept is that if signatures of cartilage damage could be detected early, prior to development of morphologic abnormalities, then early interventional therapies could be applied to prevent rather than to slow or diminish the degenerative process.

References

1. Schuurman W, Gawlitta D, Klein TJ, ten Hoope W, van Rijen MH, Dhert WJ, et al. Zonal chondrocyte subpopulations reacquire zone-specific characteristics during in vitro redifferentiation. Am J Sports Med. 2009;37 Suppl 1:97S–104.
2. Wang Y, Wei L, Zeng L, He D, Wei X. Nutrition and degeneration of articular cartilage. Knee Surg Sports Traumatol Arthrosc. 2013;21(8):1751–62.
3. Jackson DW, Lalor PA, Aberman HM, Simon TM. Spontaneous repair of full-thickness defects of articular cartilage in a goat model. A preliminary study. J Bone Joint Surg Am. 2001;83-A(1):53–64.
4. Messner K, Maletius W. The long-term prognosis for severe damage to weight-bearing cartilage in the knee: a 14-year clinical and radiographic follow-up in 28 young athletes. Acta Orthop Scand. 1996;67(2):165–8.
5. Guilak F, Fermor B, Keefe FJ, Kraus VB, Olson SA, Pisetsky DS, et al. The role of biomechanics and inflammation in cartilage injury and repair. Clin Orthop Relat Res. 2004;(423):17–26.
6. Beris AE, Lykissas MG, Papageorgiou CD, Georgoulis AD. Advances in articular cartilage repair. Injury. 2005;36 Suppl 4:S14–23.
7. Ouzzine M, Venkatesan N, Fournel-Gigleux S. Proteoglycans and cartilage repair. Methods Mol Biol. 2012;836:339–55.
8. Frisbie DD, Morisset S, Ho CP, Rodkey WG, Steadman JR, McIlwraith CW. Effects of calcified cartilage on healing of chondral defects treated with microfracture in horses. Am J Sports Med. 2006;34(11):1824–31.
9. Lee CM, Kisiday JD, McIlwraith CW, Grodzinsky AJ, Frisbie DD. Synoviocytes protect cartilage from the effects of injury in vitro. BMC Musculoskelet Disord. 2013;14:54.
10. Kamm JL, Frisbie DD, McIlwraith CW, Orr KE. Gene biomarkers in peripheral white blood cells of horses with experimentally induced osteoarthritis. Am J Vet Res. 2013;74(1):115–21.
11. Bajaj S, Shoemaker T, Hakimiyan AA, Rappoport L, Pascual-Garrido C, Oegema TR, et al. Protective effect of P188 in the model of acute trauma to human ankle cartilage: the mechanism of action. J Orthop Trauma. 2010;24(9):571–6.
12. Strauss EJ, Goodrich LR, Chen CT, Hidaka C, Nixon AJ. Biochemical and biomechanical properties of lesion and adjacent articular cartilage after chondral defect repair in an equine model. Am J Sports Med. 2005;33(11):1647–53.
13. Wei X, Gao J, Messner K. Maturation-dependent repair of untreated osteochondral defects in the rabbit knee joint. J Biomed Mater Res. 1997;34(1):63–72.
14. Bernstein B, Forrester D, Singsen B, King KK, Kornreich H, Hanson V. Hip joint restoration in juvenile rheumatoid arthritis. Arthritis Rheum. 1977;20(5):1099–104.
15. Antoniou J, Steffen T, Nelson F, Winterbottom N, Hollander AP, Poole RA, et al. The human lumbar intervertebral disc: evidence for changes in the biosynthesis and denaturation of the extracellular matrix with growth, maturation, ageing, and degeneration. J Clin Invest. 1996;98(4):996–1003.
16. Nelson F, Dahlberg L, Laverty S, Reiner A, Pidoux I, Ionescu M, et al. Evidence for altered synthesis of type II collagen in patients with osteoarthritis. J Clin Invest. 1998;102(12):2115–25.
17. Poole AR. What type of cartilage repair are we attempting to attain? J Bone Joint Surg Am. 2003;85-A Suppl 2:40–4.
18. Pascual Garrido C, Hakimiyan AA, Rappoport L, Oegema TR, Wimmer MA, Chubinskaya S. Anti-apoptotic treatments prevent cartilage degradation after acute trauma to human ankle cartilage. Osteoarthritis Cartilage. 2009;17(9):1244–51.
19. Green DM, Noble PC, Ahuero JS, Birdsall HH. Cellular events leading to chondrocyte death after cartilage impact injury. Arthritis Rheum. 2006;54(5):1509–17.
20. D'Lima DD, Hashimoto S, Chen PC, Colwell Jr CW, Lotz MK. Human chondrocyte apoptosis in response to mechanical injury. Osteoarthritis Cartilage. 2001;9(8):712–9.
21. D'Lima DD, Hashimoto S, Chen PC, Colwell CW Jr, Lotz MK. Impact of mechanical trauma on matrix and cells. Clin Orthop Relat Res. 2001; (391 Suppl):S90–9.
22. Mithoefer K, Scopp JM, Mandelbaum BR. Articular cartilage repair in athletes. Instr Course Lect. 2007;56:457–68.
23. Pascual-Garrido C, Friel NA, Kirk SS, McNickle AG, Bach Jr BR, Bush-Joseph CA, et al. Midterm results of surgical treatment for adult osteochondritis dissecans of the knee. Am J Sports Med. 2009;37 Suppl 1:125S–30.
24. Lewis PB, McCarty III LP, Kang RW, Cole BJ. Basic science and treatment options for articular cartilage injuries. J Orthop Sports Phys Ther. 2006;36(10):717–27.
25. Cole BJ, Pascual-Garrido C, Grumet RC. Surgical management of articular cartilage defects in the knee. Instr Course Lect. 2010;59:181–204.
26. Kaya M, Suzuki T, Emori M, Yamashita T. Hip morphology influences the pattern of articular cartilage damage. Knee Surg Sports Traumatol Arthrosc. 2014. DOI 10.1007/s00167-014-3297-6.
27. Beck M, Kalhor M, Leunig M, Ganz R. Hip morphology influences the pattern of damage to the acetabular cartilage: femoroacetabular impingement as a cause of early osteoarthritis of the hip. J Bone Joint Surg (Br). 2005;87(7):1012–8.
28. Bedi A, Kelly BT. Femoroacetabular impingement. J Bone Joint Surg Am. 2013;95(1):82–92.
29. McCarthy JC, Lee JA. Arthroscopic intervention in early hip disease. Clin Orthop Relat Res. 2004;(429):157–62.
30. Beck M, Leunig M, Parvizi J, Boutier V, Wyss D, Ganz R. Anterior femoroacetabular impingement: part II. Midterm results of surgical treatment. Clin Orthop Relat Res. 2004;(418):67–73.
31. Haviv B, Singh PJ, Takla A, O'Donnell J. Arthroscopic femoral osteochondroplasty for cam lesions with isolated acetabular chondral damage. J Bone Joint Surg (Br). 2010;92(5):629–33.

32. Philippon MJ, Schenker ML, Briggs KK, Maxwell RB. Can microfracture produce repair tissue in acetabular chondral defects? Arthroscopy. 2008;24(1):46–50.
33. Karthikeyan S, Roberts S, Griffin D. Microfracture for acetabular chondral defects in patients with femoroacetabular impingement: results at second-look arthroscopic surgery. Am J Sports Med. 2012;40(12):2725–30.
34. Blevins FT, Steadman JR, Rodrigo JJ, Silliman J. Treatment of articular cartilage defects in athletes: an analysis of functional outcome and lesion appearance. Orthopedics. 1998;21(7):761–7. discussion 767–8.
35. Gudas R, Kalesinskas RJ, Kimtys V, Stankevicius E, Toliusis V, Bernotavicius G, et al. A prospective randomized clinical study of mosaic osteochondral autologous transplantation versus microfracture for the treatment of osteochondral defects in the knee joint in young athletes. Arthroscopy. 2005;21(9):1066–75.
36. Horas U, Pelinkovic D, Herr G, Aigner T, Schnettler R. Autologous chondrocyte implantation and osteochondral cylinder transplantation in cartilage repair of the knee joint. A prospective, comparative trial. J Bone Joint Surg Am. 2003;85-A(2):185–92.
37. Gagala J, Tarczynska M, Gaweda K. Clinical and radiological outcomes of treatment of avascular necrosis of the femoral head using autologous osteochondral transfer (mosaicplasty): preliminary report. Int Orthop. 2013;37(7):1239–44.
38. Brittberg M, Lindahl A, Nilsson A, Ohlsson C, Isaksson O, Peterson L. Treatment of deep cartilage defects in the knee with autologous chondrocyte transplantation. N Engl J Med. 1994;331(14):889–95.
39. Bentley G, Biant LC, Carrington RW, Akmal M, Goldberg A, Williams AM, et al. A prospective, randomised comparison of autologous chondrocyte implantation versus mosaicplasty for osteochondral defects in the knee. J Bone Joint Surg (Br). 2003;85(2):223–30.
40. Akimau P, Bhosale A, Harrison PE, Roberts S, McCall IW, Richardson JB, et al. Autologous chondrocyte implantation with bone grafting for osteochondral defect due to posttraumatic osteonecrosis of the hip--a case report. Acta Orthop. 2006;77(2):333–6.
41. Nam D, Shindle MK, Buly RL, Kelly BT, Lorich DG. Traumatic osteochondral injury of the femoral head treated by mosaicplasty: a report of two cases. HSS J. 2010;6(2):228–34.
42. Korsmeier K, Classen T, Kamminga M, Rekowski J, Jager M, Landgraeber S. Arthroscopic threedimensional autologous chondrocyte transplantation using spheroids for the treatment of full-thickness cartilage defects of the hip joint. Knee Surg Sports Traumatol Arthrosc. 2014 DOI 10.1007/s00167-014-3293-x.
43. Mancini D, Fontana A. Five-year results of arthroscopic techniques for the treatment of acetabular chondral lesions in femoroacetabular impingement. Int Orthop. 2014;38(10):2057–64.
44. Kruse DL, Ng A, Paden M, Stone PA. Arthroscopic De Novo NT((R)) juvenile allograft cartilage implantation in the talus: a case presentation. J Foot Ankle Surg. 2012;51(2):218–21.
45. Gulotta LV, Wiznia D, Cunningham M, Fortier L, Maher S, Rodeo SA. What's new in orthopaedic research. J Bone Joint Surg Am. 2011;93(22):2136–41.
46. Fortier LA, Barker JU, Strauss EJ, McCarrel TM, Cole BJ. The role of growth factors in cartilage repair. Clin Orthop Relat Res. 2011;469(10):2706–15.
47. Anderson DD, Chubinskaya S, Guilak F, Martin JA, Oegema TR, Olson SA, et al. Post-traumatic osteoarthritis: improved understanding and opportunities for early intervention. J Orthop Res. 2011;29(6):802–9.
48. Toh WS, Spector M, Lee EH, Cao T. Biomaterial-mediated delivery of microenvironmental cues for repair and regeneration of articular cartilage. Mol Pharm. 2011;8(4):994–1001.
49. Williams R, Khan IM, Richardson K, Nelson L, McCarthy HE, Analbelsi T, et al. Identification and clonal characterisation of a progenitor cell sub-population in normal human articular cartilage. PLoS One. 2010;5(10):e13246.
50. Pretzel D, Linss S, Rochler S, Endres M, Kaps C, Alsalameh S, et al. Relative percentage and zonal distribution of mesenchymal progenitor cells in human osteoarthritic and normal cartilage. Arthritis Res Ther. 2011;13(2):R64.
51. Moran CJ, Barry FP, Maher SA, Shannon FJ, Rodeo SA. Advancing regenerative surgery in orthopaedic sports medicine: the critical role of the surgeon. Am J Sports Med. 2012;40(4): 934–44.
52. Rodeo SA, Ma R, Moran C, Fortier L, Frawley RJ, Cunningham M, et al. What's new in orthopaedic research. J Bone Joint Surg Am. 2012;94(24):2289–95.
53. Mei-Dan O, Lippi G, Sanchez M, Andia I, Maffulli N. Autologous platelet-rich plasma: a revolution in soft tissue sports injury management? Phys Sportsmed. 2010;38(4):127–35.
54. Akeda K, An HS, Okuma M, Attawia M, Miyamoto K, Thonar EJ, et al. Platelet-rich plasma stimulates porcine articular chondrocyte proliferation and matrix biosynthesis. Osteoarthritis Cartilage. 2006;14(12):1272–80.
55. Battaglia M, Guaraldi F, Vannini F, Buscio T, Buda R, Galletti S, et al. Platelet-rich plasma (PRP) intra-articular ultrasound-guided injections as a possible treatment for hip osteoarthritis: a pilot study. Clin Exp Rheumatol. 2011;29(4):754.

Microfracture in the Hip

66

Fernando Portilho Ferro, Peter Goljan, and Marc J. Philippon

Introduction

Articular cartilage defects have been shown to rarely heal spontaneously, regardless of whether they are acute, chronic, or degenerative in nature [1]. As an avascular lining of joint surfaces, cartilage has little innate ability to heal on its own once damaged [2]. Therefore, in order to prevent subsequent and continued degradation of the joint space, surgical intervention is usually required. Prior to the development of cartilage repair techniques, treatment options were very limited, leaving joint replacement as the only effective treatment to restore function in patients inhibited by severe osteoarthritic pain. Currently there is a multitude of different procedures utilized by surgeons for cartilage repair, including abrasion chondroplasty, osteochondral drilling, osteoarticular autograft or allograft plugs, bulk allograft, chondrocyte implantation, and microfracture [3–6].

First introduced in the early 1980s, the microfracture technique was developed as a means to utilize the healing potential of the body's own pluripotential stem cells as a means to stimulate cartilage repair [6–8]. This approach was proposed as a "marrow-based strategy" to stimulate cartilage repair by creating a suitable environment within the joint space to allow autogenous stem cells to migrate to the site of cartilage lesions and form new articular tissue [9].

F.P. Ferro, MD
Hospital de Acidentados, Goiânia, Goiás, Brazil

P. Goljan, MD
Center for Outcomes-Based Orthopaedic Research, The Steadman Philippon Research Institute, Vail, CO, USA

M.J. Philippon, MD (✉)
The Steadman Clinic, Vail, CO, USA

Department of Surgery, Faculty of Health Sciences, McMaster University, Hamilton, ON, Canada

Department of Orthopaedic Surgery, Unviersity of Pittsburgh School of Medicine, Pittsburgh, PA, USA
e-mail: drphilippon@sprivail.org

The goal of microfracture is to stimulate a patient's own bone marrow cells to fill the defect with repair tissue. In the procedure, the subchondral plate just beneath the damaged area is punctured, which allows pluripotential stem cells to migrate upwards to the desired region and form a marrow-rich clot. Once the clot is in place, these stem cells may then differentiate into repair tissue and fill up the damaged area. The technique has the advantage of being a technically simple, cost-effective procedure with low associated morbidity, while also leaving other options open in case further treatment is required. Since its development, microfracture has become one of the most frequently used techniques to treat small symptomatic lesions in the knee [10], and this treatment now has been applied to other joints, including the hip.

Hip Cartilage Damage

Cartilage damage in the hip can be secondary to a multitude of etiologies, ranging in severity from acute traumatic high-energy damage as seen in acetabular or femoral fracture dislocations [11] to the more insidious onset secondary to capsular laxity, labral tears, loose bodies, hip dysplasia, or femoro-acetabular impingement (FAI), among others [12, 13]. Among patients with FAI, chondral defects may be present on articular surfaces of both the acetabulum and the femoral head, and even then the exact location can vary depending on which impingement subset is more predominant. Acetabular lesions are common in cam-type impingement [14, 15], particularly in the anterior acetabulum [16, 17] as a result of the shear forces that occur when the irregularly shaped femoral head is levered into the joint space. Injuries at the chondrolabral junction (the "watershed area") are often described as acetabular "peel-off" lesions, as the true severity of the cartilage delamination is only revealed by thorough examination of the cartilage flap, producing the "carpet" or "wave phenomenon" due to delamination of the articular tissue from subchondral bone [18]. Although pincer-type impingement typically leads to more labral than

J.C. McCarthy et al. (eds.), *Hip Joint Restoration*, DOI 10.1007/978-1-4614-0694-5_66

cartilaginous damage, a rim of superior acetabular chondral damage can exist circumferentially at the chondro-labral junction [16], and "contre-coup" lesions of the postero-inferior acetabulum may also occur secondary to subtle posterior subluxation of the femoral head [15].

Although less common, articular lesions of the femoral head are also observed in patients with FAI. Damage may occur when the femoral head impacts against the acetabulum, as is seen in the pathomechanics of "contre-coup" lesions, or potentially from increased translational movement between the femoral head and acetabulum within the hip joint itself. Zaltz et al. reported a series of patients with parafoveal femoral head cartilage defects; proposing that in some patients with FAI the continued impingement alters the normal joint biomechanics, resulting in instability and ultimately translation between the femoral head and acetabulum. This increased intraarticular shifting may in turn create a cartilage defect at the point of contact between the two articular surfaces [19].

Preoperative Planning

Preoperative identification of suitable candidates for hip microfracture remains a challenge, and often the decision to perform microfracture is made intraoperatively. There is currently no physical exam maneuver specific enough to diagnose the type of full-thickness cartilage lesions which merit treatment by microfracture [20]. Surgeons are therefore more dependent on imaging studies, and in particular advanced imaging modalities such as Magnetic Resonance Imaging (MRI) and MRI arthrogram (MRA). The most important element of diagnosis, however, remains direct observation of the defects by intraoperative examination. Plain radiographs remain a useful component of preoperative planning despite their inability to identify chondral lesions. Radiographs enable the surgeon to ascertain the degree of degenerative disease present, determine the severity of the impingement, and identify any bony lesions, dysplastic changes, or loose bodies [21].

MRI and MRA provide improved visualization of the soft tissues surrounding the hip joint as well as the cartilaginous articular surfaces. Although in the past MRI has been thought to be less effective than MRA in identifying soft tissue pathology—including chondral defects–within the hip [22, 23], advancements in hip imaging protocols as well as hip specific MRI coils [24] have led to a reevaluation of the value of this modality. Just as our knowledge of hip arthroscopy has improved over the past decade, so too has our understanding of and experience with hip imaging modalities, so much so that leading international centers feel confident using standard MRI for intraarticular hip pathology, and rely on MRA only for complex cases or when noncontrast MRI is inconclusive [24].

Regardless of the imaging modality employed preoperatively, a thorough and complete intraoperative inspection of the joint space remains of paramount importance, in order to provide a complete diagnosis of hip pathology, including the presence or absence of cartilage damage.

Microfracture: Indications, Contraindications, and Operative Technique

Indications for microfracture include focally contained cartilage lesions, typically less than 4 cm in size. Acceptable chondral damage for the procedure can range from unstable partial thickness lesions to full-thickness lesions, including the previously mentioned acetabular "peel-off" lesions. Patients with degenerative joint disease may still be candidates for this procedure, as long as the changes are focal, the surrounding rim of cartilage is adequate to hold the clot, and diffuse grade IV changes are not seen throughout the joint, an observation that would warrant total joint replacement.

Contraindications to microfracture are stable partial thickness defects and chondral lesions with associated bony defects. Patients with <2 mm of joint space are not recommended to undergo microfracture, as it has been demonstrated that those patients have poorer outcomes following hip arthroscopy and are more likely to ultimately require conversion to total hip replacement [25, 26]. The postoperative protocol, if followed correctly, is also extensive, and therefore patients who are unwilling to follow it exactly should not have this procedure done. Patients with systemic immune-mediated disease and polyarthritis are also not good candidates [13].

At the time of arthroscopy, the patient is positioned on a standard fracture table in the modified supine position, with the hip in 10° of flexion, 15° of internal rotation, 10° of lateral tilt, and neutral abduction. A well-padded perineal post is employed in order to prevent pudendal nerve injury. Traction is required in order to adequately separate the femoral head from the acetabulum and view the articular surfaces, and is applied to the affected limb, with gentle counter-traction on the contralateral limb. Between 25 and 50 lbs of force is normally required to create the necessary 8–10 mm of distraction in order to adequately view structures. Two portals, an antero-lateral and mid-anterior, are establish and are normally sufficient to provide access to all desired areas within the joint. A 70° arthroscope is utilized at all times. Once access to the intraarticular compartment is obtained, but prior to addressing any suspected chondral lesions, a complete intraoperative diagnostic examination

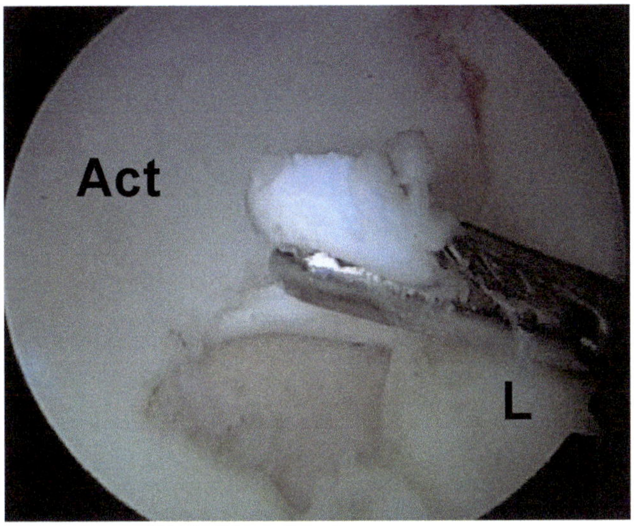

Fig. 66.1 Unstable cartilage is removed and bone is exposed from a lesion at the chondrolabral junction (*Act* acetabulum; *L* labrum)

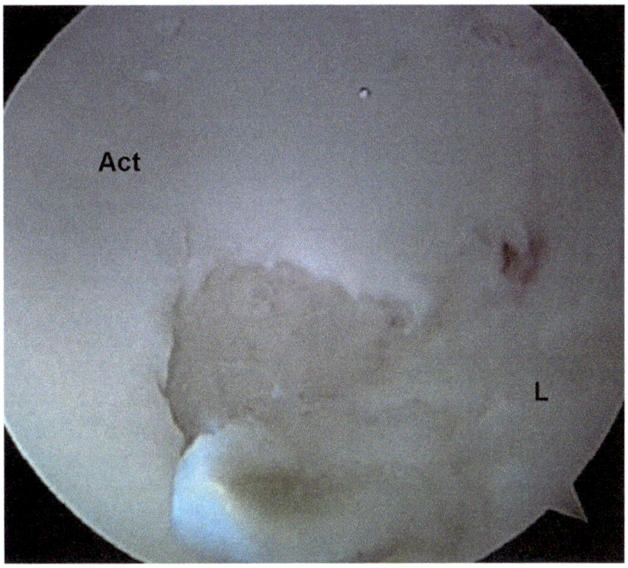

Fig. 66.2 Unstable cartilage is removed until a stable rim of cartilage surrounds the defect to hold the clot (*Act* acetabulum; *L* labrum)

of the hip joint is performed to ensure that all damaged areas are identified.

When a cartilage defect is found, any unstable cartilage present surrounding the exposed bone should be debrided using a resector and curette (Fig. 66.1), until only a buffer of healthy cartilage is present around the damaged area. It is critical to ensure that all unstable cartilage has been identified and removed, and this process should be done carefully and meticulously in order to preserve the integrity of what will be the encompassing healthy cartilage buffer. The debridement must be deep enough to sufficiently remove the layer of calcified cartilage present, however, not so deep as to disrupt the integrity of the subchondral plate (Fig. 66.2). Removal of the calcified cartilage layer is critical to the success of the procedure, as it allows for proper clot adhesion to the site [27].

After preparing the bed, arthroscopic awls are used to penetrate the subchondral plate. Awls of a variety of angles should be employed so that the tip will always remain perpendicular to the subchondral surface. Multiples holes (microfractures) are then made in the exposed bone (Fig. 66.3). The depth of each microfracture should be 2–4 mm, which is typically enough to allow migration of marrow elements, with 3–4 mm spacing between microfractures. Once all of the microfractures have been created, the emergence of blood and fat droplets from each site may be observed after reducing the irrigation pressure within the joint (Fig. 66.4). Ultimately a marrow clot cap will form over the microfractured area, providing an environment rich in mesenchymal stem cells to then differentiate into repair tissue (Fig. 66.5). Once the fat droplets have been visualized, the instruments are withdrawn, the portals closed in a standard fashion, and a sterile dressing is placed over the wound.

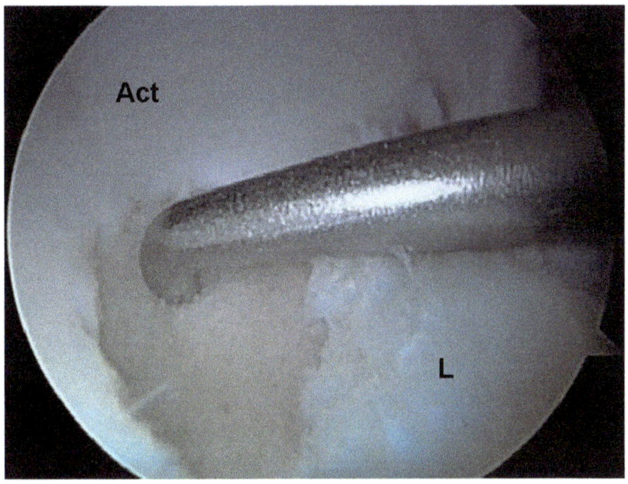

Fig. 66.3 Microfracture awl is used to penetrate the subchondral plate. The tip of the awl is perpendicular to the subchondral bone

Postoperative Care and Rehabilitation

Postoperative management of microfracture patients is similar to the standard hip arthroscopy postoperative regimen, with the exception of the duration of restricted weight-bearing. Following microfracture, crutch-assisted touch-down weight-bearing is allowed for 6–8 weeks, tapering to full weight bearing, in contrast to the 4–6 week duration for nonmicrofracture hip arthroscopy patients [28]. The longer period of restricted weight-bearing is prescribed to allow time for the newly recruited mesenchymal stem cells and growth factors to form a satisfactory repair surface [6, 9, 30]. This process is slow, and the blood clot cap can be quite fragile, requiring protection from disruptive forces [27, 29, 30, 31].

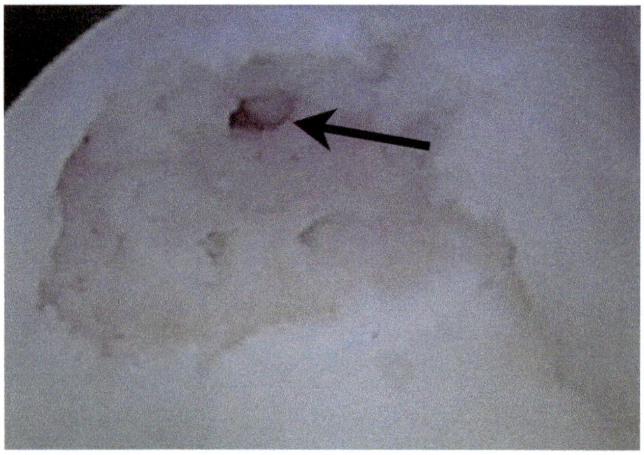

Fig. 66.4 Depth of each microfracture should be 2–4 mm, which will allow migration of marrow elements from the hole (*arrow*). Distance between each microfracture is 3–4 mm

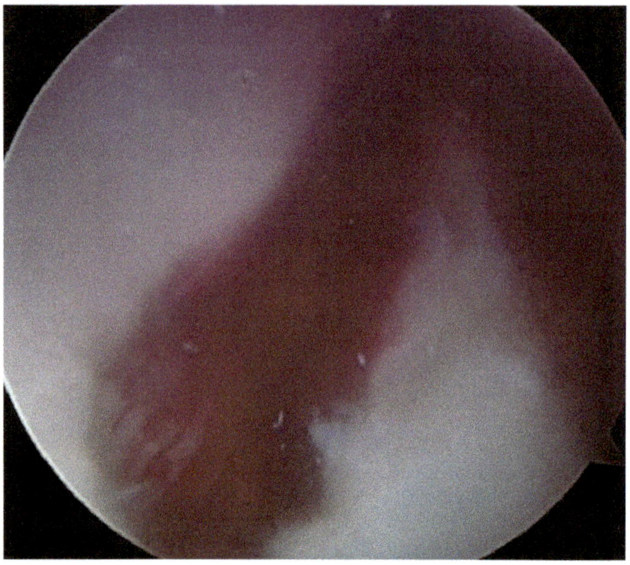

Fig. 66.5 When the irrigation pressure is reduced, blood covers the microfracture site

Although early range of motion is advocated immediately following surgery, patients are still advised to avoid excessive hip flexion, abduction, or external rotation, in order to minimize stress on the capsule-ligamentous structures. Circumduction of the hip remains critical in the early phases of rehabilitation to prevent adhesion formation.

The cooperation of the patient with the demands of the rehabilitation program is crucial to optimize final results. The types of exercises, including range of motion and strengthening programs, might vary depending on what other procedures were executed during the same surgery. However, respecting the period of limited weight bearing is essential to ensure formation of the fibrocartilaginous repair tissue on the articular surface.

Early Published Results

While the results of microfracture in the knee have been widely reported [9, 10, 30], there is a relative paucity of data regarding microfracture within the hip. Early results by Byrd et al. were generally favorable, with one study reporting 86 % success rate at 2-year follow-up among 21 patients [32, 33]. Philippon et al. investigated the ability of microfracture to fill chondral defects in a series of nine patients who underwent second look hip arthroscopy. In that study, they determined that at an average of 20 months, eight of nine patients had 95–100 % coverage of previously diagnosed lesions [18]. Similar results were also found in a separate study by Karthikean et al., in which an average of 96 % fill of prior lesions was documented in 19 of 20 patients at second-look arthroscopy, performed at an average of 17 months' follow-up [34]. Biopsies of the repaired tissue obtained in that study consisted primarily of fibrocartilage, with some aspects of type II collagen at the region closest to the bone.

Microfracture has also been shown to be a successful treatment in high-level athletes in terms of their ability to return to play. A recent study by McDonald et al. compared the return to play statistics for two groups of athletes who underwent arthroscopic treatment of FAI with and without addition of microfracture treatment [35]. No significant difference between the two groups was found at short-term follow-up (3 years), and both groups returning to a high level of competition [35]. These findings are similar to those of Singh et al. [36], in which five of six professional soccer players treated with microfracture successfully returned to their preoperative level of professional sport.

Microfracture in the hip still remains a relatively new procedure, however, and as a result, the majority of published studies involve short-term data. Long-term follow-up studies are required before the efficacy of hip microfracture in preventing the onset of osteoarthritis can truly be determined.

Conclusions

Microfracture has been proven to successfully repair isolated cartilage defects in the hip over the short-term. In order to achieve optimal results, meticulous surgical technique is required, and strong emphasis on strict adherence to the postoperative rehabilitation regimen must be relayed to the patient. With appropriate patient selection and proper surgical technique, microfracture has become an excellent option for full-thickness cartilage lesions within the hip.

Potential Conflict of Interest Smith & Nephew[a,b], Arthrosurface[a], HIPCO[a], MIS[a], Bledsoe[a], DonJoy[a], Slack[a], Ossur[b], Arthrex[b], Siemens[b]

[a]Consulting/Royalty payments (MJP), [b]Research support of the Steadman Philippon Research Institute

References

1. Buckwalter JA. Articular cartilage: injuries and potential for healing. J Orthop Sports Phys Ther. 1998;28:192–202.
2. Cohen NP, Foster RJ, Mow VC. Composition and dynamics of articular cartilage: structure, function, and maintaining a healthy state. J Orthop Sports Phys Ther. 1998;28:203–15.
3. Gross AE. Repair of cartilage defects in the knee. J Knee Surg. 2002;15:167–9.
4. Breinan HA, Minas T, Hsu HP, Nehrer S, Sledge CB, Spector M. Effect of cultured autologous chondrocytes on repair of chondral defects in a canine model. J Bone Joint Surg Am. 1997;79:1439–51.
5. Brittberg M, Lindahl A, Nilsson A, Ohlsson C, Isaksson O, Peterson L. Treatment of deep cartilage defects in the knee with autologous chondrocyte transplantation. N Engl J Med. 1994;331:889–95.
6. Steadman JR, Rodkey WG, Rodrigo JJ. Microfracture: surgical technique and rehabilitation to treat chondral defects. Clin Orthop Relat Res. 2001;391:S362–9.
7. Steadman JR, Rodkey WG, Briggs KK. Microfracture chondroplasty. Sports Med Arthrosc Rev. 2003;11(4):236–44.
8. Steadman JR, Rodkey WG, Briggs KK. Microfracture: its history and experience of the developing surgeon. Cartilage. 2010;1(2):78–86.
9. Steadman JR, Briggs KK, Rodrigo JJ, Kocher MS, Gill TJ, Rodkey WG. Outcomes of microfracture for traumatic chondral defects of the knee: average 11-year follow-up. Arthroscopy. 2003;19(5):477–84.
10. Bedi A, Feeley BT, Williams III RJ. Management of articular cartilage defects of the knee. J Bone Joint Surg Am. 2010;92:994–1009.
11. Kelly BT, Philippon MJ. Arthroscopic techniques of the hip: a visual guide. Thorofare: Slack; 2009. p. 143–51.
12. Jordan MA, Van Thiel GS, Chahal J, Nho SJ. Operative treatment of chondral defects in the hip joint: a systematic review. Curr Rev Musculoskelet Med. 2012;5:244–53.
13. Crawford K, Philippon MJ, Sekiya JK, Rodkey WG, Steadman JR. Microfracture of the hip in athletes. Clin Sports Med. 2006;25(2):327–35. x.
14. Philippon MJ, Schenker ML. Arthroscopy for the treatment of femoroacetabular impingement in the athlete. Clin Sports Med. 2006;25:299–308.
15. Beck M, Kalhor M, Leunig M, Ganz R. Hip morphology influences the pattern of damage to the acetabular cartilage: femoroacetabular impingement as a cause of early osteoarthritis of the hip. J Bone Joint Surg (Br). 2005;87:1012–8.
16. Yen Y, Kocher M. Chondral lesions of the hip: microfracture and chondroplasty. Sports Med Arthrosc Rev. 2010;18(2):83–9.
17. Ganz R, Parvizi J, Beck M, Leunig M, Nötzli H, Siebenrock KA. Femoroacetabular impingement: a cause for osteoarthritis of the hip. Clin Orthop Relat Res. 2003;417:112–20.
18. Philippon MJ, Schenker ML, Briggs KK, Maxwell RB. Can microfracture produce repair tissue in acetabular chondral defects? Arthroscopy. 2008;24:46–50.
19. Zaltz I, Leunig M. Parafoveal chondral defects associated with femoroacetabular impingement. Clin Orthop Relat Res. 2012;470(12):3383–9.
20. Lienert JJ, Rodkey WG, Steadman JR, Philippon MJ, Sekiya JK. Microfracture techniques in hip arthroscopy. Oper Tech Orthop. 2005;15:267–72.
21. Tannast M, Siebenrock KA, Anderson SE. Femoroacetabular impingement: radiographic diagnosis—what the radiologist should know. AJR Am J Roentgenol. 2007;188:1540–52.
22. Smith TO, Hilton G, Toms AP, Donell ST, Hing CB. The diagnostic accuracy of acetabular labral tears using magnetic resonance imaging and magnetic resonance arthrography: a meta-analysis. Eur Radiol. 2011;21:863–74.
23. Keeney JA, Peelle MW, Jackson J, Rubin D, Maloney WJ, Clohisy JC. Magnetic resonance arthrography versus arthroscopy in the evaluation of articular hip pathology. Clin Orthop Relat Res. 2004;429:163–9.
24. Mintz DN, Hooper T, Connell D, Buly R, Padgett DE, Potter HG. Magnetic resonance imaging of the hip: detection of labral and chondral abnormalities using noncontrast imaging. Arthroscopy. 2005;21:385–93.
25. Philippon MJ, Briggs KK, Yen YM, Kuppersmith DA. Outcomes following hip arthroscopy for femoroacetabular impingement with associated chondrolabral dysfunction: minimum two-year follow-up. J Bone Joint Surg (Br). 2009;91:16–23.
26. Philippon MJ, Briggs KK, Carlisle JC, Patterson DC. Joint space predicts THA after hip arthroscopy in patients 50 years and older. Clin Orthop Relat Res. 2013;471(8):2492–6.
27. Frisbie DD, Morisset S, Ho CP, Rodkey WG, Steadman JR, McIlwraith CW. Effects of calcified cartilage on healing of chondral defects treated with microfracture in horses. Am J Sports Med. 2006;34(11):1824–31.
28. Wahoff M, Ryan M. Rehabilitation after hip femoroacetabular impingement arthroscopy. Clin Sports Med. 2011;30:463–82.
29. Steadman JR, Rodkey WG, Briggs KK. Microfracture to treat full-thickness chondral defects: surgical technique, rehabilitation, and outcomes. J Knee Surg. 2002;15(3):170–6.
30. Frisbie DD, Trotter GW, Powers BE, Rodkey WG, Steadman JR, Howard RD, et al. Arthroscopic subchondral bone plate microfracture technique augments healing of large chondral defects in the radial carpal bone and medial femoral condyle of horses. Vet Surg. 1999;28(4):242–55.
31. Hurst JM, Steadman JR, O'Brien L, Rodkey WG, Briggs KK. Rehabilitation following microfracture for chondral injury in the knee. Clin Sports Med. 2010;29(2):257–65. viii.
32. Byrd JWT, Jones KS. Osteoarthritis caused by an inverted acetabular labrum: radiographic diagnosis and arthroscopic treatment. Arthroscopy. 2002;18:741–7.
33. Byrd JW, Jones KS. Microfracture of grade IV chondral lesions of the hip. Arthroscopy. 2004;20 Suppl 1:e41.
34. Karthikean S, Roberts S, Griffin D. Microfracture for acetabular chondral defects in patients with femoroacetabular impingement: results at second-look arthroscopic surgery. Am J Sports Med. 2012;40:2725–30.
35. McDonald JE, Herzog MM, Philippon MJ. Return to play after hip arthroscopy with microfracture in elite athletes. Arthroscopy. 2013;29:330–5.
36. Singh PJ, O'Donnell JM. The outcome of hip arthroscopy in Australian football league players: a review of 27 hips. Arthroscopy. 2010;26:743–9.

Cartilage Grafting

67

Andrea Fontana

Introduction

Hip pain can be a debilitating condition that can be caused by a variety of conditions, from injury to dysplasia and degenerative disease. Femoro-acetabular impingement (FAI) is a common cause of hip pain, most frequently present in athletes or active young individuals [1, 2].

Acetabular cartilage damage is estimated to be present in 73 % of patients in association with a frayed or torn labrum. In almost all patients (94 %) the labral and articular lesions are located in the same zone of the acetabulum [3].

Apart from decreased range of motion, causing discomfort and pain resulting in cartilage damage and labrum tears, impingement may lead to degenerative changes in the hip, such as osteoarthritis [4, 5].

Arthroscopy has been established as diagnostic standard in patients with hip pain and has been shown to provide more accurate diagnosis than radiological examination, arthrography, computed tomography (CT) or magnetic resonance imaging (MRI) [6].

Current treatment options for cartilage defects in the hip include arthroscopic debridement, microfracture and mosaicplasty, performed as an open procedure. Small, partial-thickness defects are often just debrided [1]. Full-thickness defects smaller than 2–4 cm^2 are generally treated with microfracture with good results [1, 7–9]. Most patients treated with microfracture showed improved function and no complications, and the majority were able to return to sport [3, 10–13]. In patients with concomitant chondromalacia (femoral or acetabular) or arthritic changes, microfracture has been found to be less effective [9, 14].

In the knee, larger chondral defects have been treated with autologous chondrocyte implantation (ACI) or matrix-associated autologous chondrocyte implantation (MACI). In ACI/MACI, chondrocytes are harvested from a healthy cartilage site and expanded in vitro. In a second procedure the expanded chondrocytes are injected under a periosteal flap or an artificial membrane or matrix. In MACI, the harvested chondrocytes are seeded onto a matrix and the resulting graft is then implanted. Both ACI and MACI have been used extensively in the knee [15, 16]; however; there are only a few reports on the use of ACI in the hip [17–19].

AMIC is an alternative technique for cartilage defect repair. It is a single-step procedure involving microfracture followed by implantation of a collagen I/III matrix (Chondro-Gide®, Geistlich Pharma AG, Wolhusen, Switzerland), which serves as a scaffold for bone marrow cells released by microfracture. In previous reports this technique has been used to repair chondral and osteochondral defects of the knee [20–24] and the talus [25] but not the hip.

Treating hip pathologies arthroscopically is challenging and often reserved for specialists. Increasing use has been fuelled by greater understanding of hip pathology, advances in techniques and instruments and appropriate physician training.

Methods

Study Population

This retrospective, non-randomised study included 142 patients, 82 female and 60 male, with FAI (Table 67.1). A majority of patients presented with isolated cam pathology (80, 56 %) compared to pincer (37, 26 %) and combined lesions (24, 18 %). Patients enrolled early in the study were treated with ACI either a polymeric (46 cases) or hyaluronic acid (HA) scaffold (34 cases), while those enrolled later were treated with AMIC (62 cases). The age of patients ranged from 18 to 51 years, and was similar for all three treatment groups (ACI/polymer scaffold: 39 years, ACI/HA scaffold: 40 years and AMIC: 38 years).

A. Fontana, MD (✉)
Ortopedia, COF Lanzo Hospital, Località Caslè, 5, 22020 Ramponio Verna (Lanzo D'Intelvi), Como, Italy
e-mail: dr.andreafontana@libero.it

J.C. McCarthy et al. (eds.), *Hip Joint Restoration*, DOI 10.1007/978-1-4614-0694-5_67

Table 67.1 Patient baseline characteristics

	ACI hyaluronic acid scaffold (n=34)	ACI polymer scaffold (n=46)	AMIC (n=62)
Sex (M/F)	12/22	20/26	28/34
Age in years, mean (SD) Range in years	40.26 (8.19) 19–51	38.91 (8.80) 19–50	38.48 (9.94) 18–50
Type of FAI			
cam (n)	17	26	36
pincer (n)	12	13	13
cam+pincer (n)	5	7	13
Average lesion size	3.7±1.8	3.4±1.7	3.6±1.8
Baseline MHHS, mean (SD) Range	44.65 (5.71) 34–56	45.30 (6.68) 34–62	44.58 (6.34) 34–60

ACI autologous chondrocyte implantation, *AMIC* arthroscopic autologous matrix-induced chondroplasty, *FAI* femoro-acetabular impingement, *MHHS* modified Harris hip score

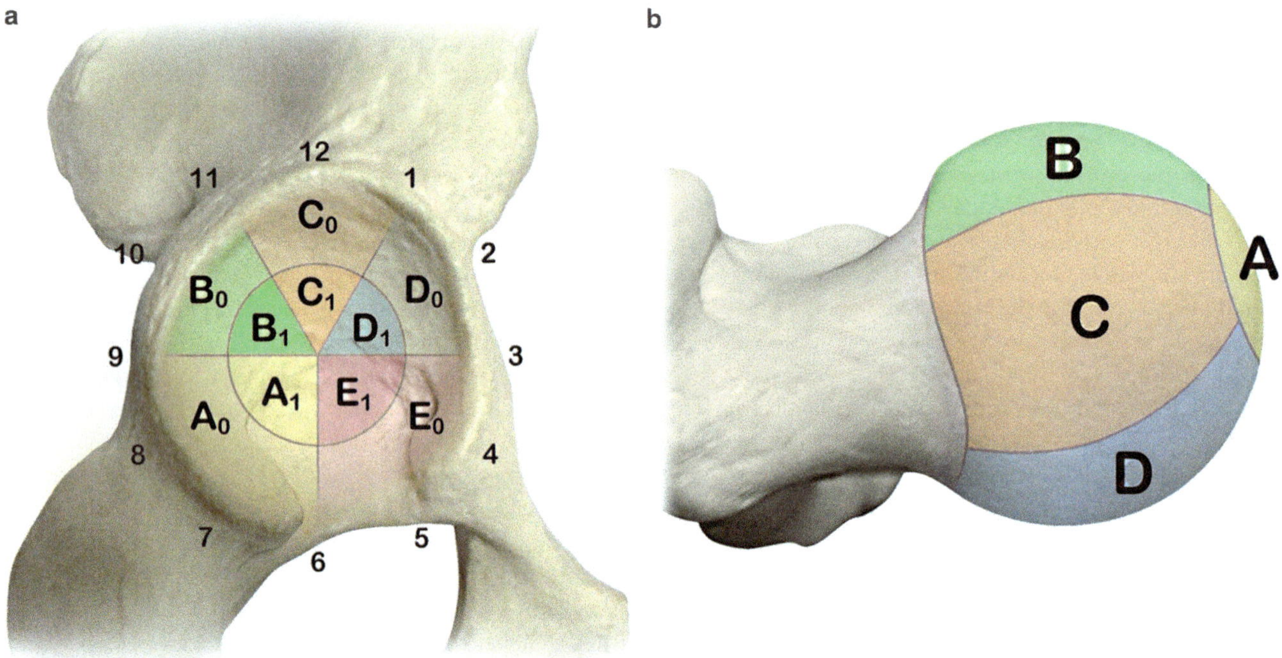

Fig. 67.1 Mapping system for cartilage lesions of the hip joint. (**a**) Mapping of the acetabulum. (**b**) Mapping of the femoral head

Cartilage Lesions Treated

Arthroscopic evaluation of the cartilage defect was performed according to the Outerbridge classification [26], while the localisation of the defect was determined and recorded using the mapping system shown in Fig. 67.1. All lesions were larger than 2 cm^2 in area and were assessed as grade III or IV on the Outerbridge scale [26]. The average lesion size across all groups was 3.6±1.8 cm^2 (range 2–12 cm^2; 3.5±1.7 for ACI and 3.6±1.8 for AMIC). Twenty-seven patients in both the ACI and AMIC groups had concomitant femoral lesions of grades II, III or IV on the Outerbridge scale and average size 2.4±0.5 cm^2 (range 2–3 cm^2) for the ACI group and 3.0±1.7 cm^2 (range 2–10 cm^2) for the AMIC group. The second cartilage defect was treated with microfracture only.

Two patients in the ACI treatment group (with polymer scaffold) had other hip pathologies in addition to FAI (one detached labrum and one bucket handle labrum lesion) and seven patients in the AMIC treatment group had additional pathologies (one bucket handle labrum lesion, one previous femoral head fracture, one flap labrum lesion, one previous femoral neck fracture, one lateral snapping hip, one Perthes disease and one epiphysiolysis).

Surgical Techniques

ACI/MACI

Matrix-assisted ACI was carried out as previously described [27]. Briefly, diagnostic arthroscopy was first performed to evaluate the chondral damage and to take a cartilage biopsy from the area surrounding the pulvinar. Chondrocytes were harvested from the joint and expanded within the laboratory. The expanded cells were seeded on either a polymer scaffold (a resorbable composite material of polyglactin 910 and poly-*p*-dioxanone) [Bioseed®-C, BioTissue AG, Freiburg, Germany] or on a hyaluronic acid scaffold [Hyalograft C®, Fidia Farmaceutici S.p.A., Abano Terme, Italy]. Graft implantation of the expanded and embedded chondrocytes was performed arthroscopically [27].

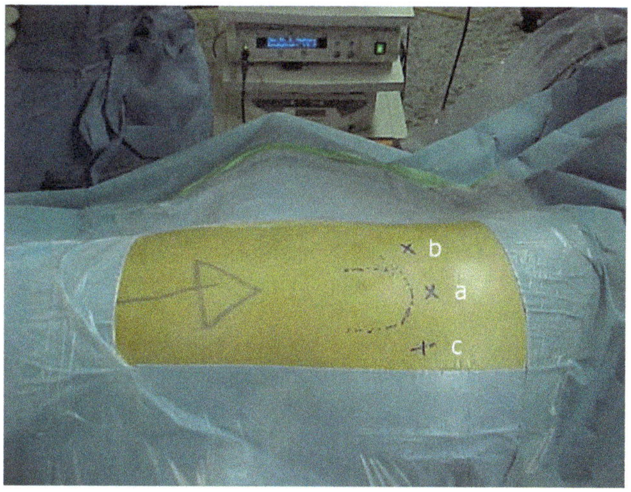

Fig. 67.2 Arthroscopic accession portals for the hip. *GT* greater trochanter, *a* sovra-trochanter portal, *b* anterior-paratrochanter portal, *c* posterior-paratrochanter portal

AMIC

AMIC was performed in a single-step procedure using a fully arthroscopic approach developed at our centre.

For this procedure, the patient was placed in a lateral decubitus position. The hip was accessed via the sovra-trochanter, anterior-paratrochanter and posterior-paratrochanter portals (Fig. 67.2). The cartilage defect was evaluated while combined longitudinal and inguinal traction was being applied (Fig. 67.3). If the evaluated cartilage lesion (Fig. 67.4a) was indicated for an arthroscopic AMIC treatment, the defect was accurately debrided. Chondrectomy was performed using angled curettes or motorised shavers to expose the subchondral bone in order to create clear margins between the healthy cartilage and the cartilage lesion (Fig. 67.4b). The size of the exposed chondral defect was measured with an arthroscopic probe. Accurate chondrectomy is important, leaving very sharp edges to impart sufficient stability to the matrix implant once traction is released. Microfracture was performed using well-established previously reported techniques (REFS), and involved perforation of the subchondral bone plate to release bone marrow blood, containing a cell and growth factor mix, to initiate new tissue formation. The subchondral bone was penetrated approximately 2–4 mm deep with an arthroscopic awl (30 and 45° angles are preferable because of the sphericity of the hip) to create V-shaped holes of 1.5–2 mm diameter (Fig. 67.4c). Microfracturing was started at the periphery proceeding toward the centre at a distance of 5 mm. The subchondral bone was penetrated perpendicularly. Bone marrow bleeding from the holes was verified after reducing the irrigation pressure within the joint (Fig. 67.4d).

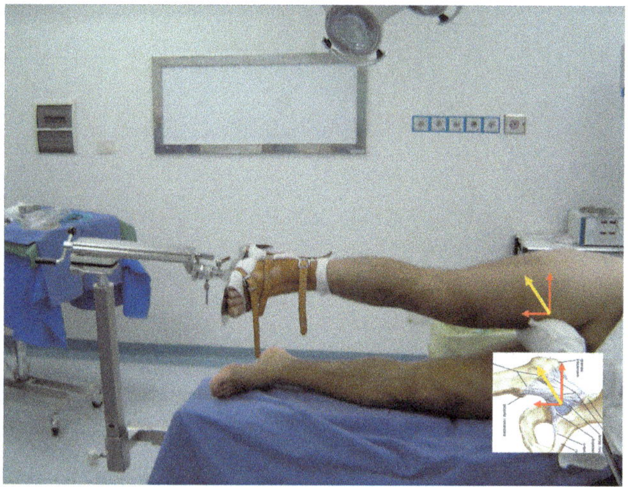

Fig. 67.3 Patient positioning for hip arthroscopy. With the patient in lateral decubitus position, traction to the groin is applied following two forces: L, longitudinal and G, lateral. The resulting force "R" is a force along the femoral neck that allows an appropriate distraction of the femoral head from the acetabulum (1.5–2.0 cm). The created space is just enough to safely insert the arthroscopic instruments without damaging the hip

The dry collagen matrix was trimmed to be slightly smaller than the measured size of the defect, to compensate for the increase in size after moistening. Before introduction of the matrix into the joint, lines were drawn on the smooth layer of the implant with a surgical marker pen to distinguish the layers and aid insertion. The matrix was then inserted directly into the articular space with its porous layer facing the bony surface. This was performed via an arthroscopic cannula to prevent loss of the implant in the surrounding tissues. The implant matrix was modified as necessary to completely fill the chondral defect (Fig. 67.4e).

After having positioned the matrix on the cartilage defect, the traction was released and a series of 4–6 extension and rotation movements were performed. Traction was then reapplied, and the position of the transplant was arthroscopically verified. Fibrin glue was used to fix the matrix if it did not show acceptable stability.

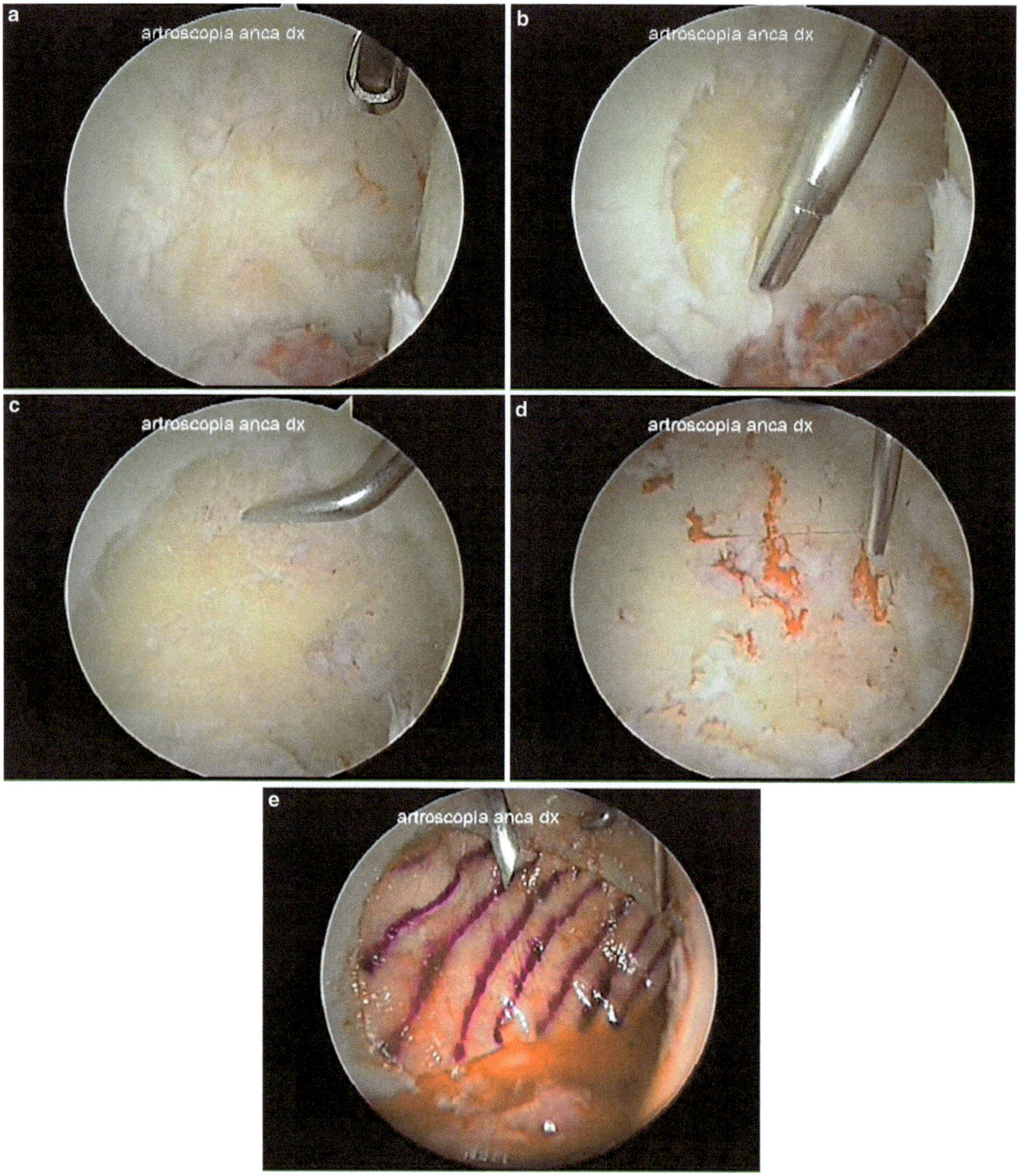

Fig. 67.4 Autologous matrix-induced chondrogenesis (AMIC) for the treatment of a chondral defect in the hip. (**a**) A third/fourth degree chondral defect is located on the anterior area of the acetabulum. (**b**) Debridement and chondrectomy of the area are performed to expose the subchondral bone. (**c**) Once the subchondral bone is fully exposed, microfracturing is performed. (**d**) Bleeding of the area is checked after microfracturing. (**e**) The Chondro-Gide® matrix is inserted and applied to cover the defect. The smooth surface of the matrix is marked with lines to ensure that the rough surface faces the subchondral bone

Post-operative Rehabilitation Programme

Post-operatively, all the patients underwent physiokinesiotherapy. Exercises began from the first post-operative day with isotonic and isometric quadriceps exercises. Continuous passive motion at 60° of hip flexion was also applied. Patients were discharged on the second day and were subject to both active and passive physiotherapy to regain complete range of motion. Partial loading of the joint was permitted for the first 4 weeks after the procedure, including exercising with a stationary bicycle and swimming. After 4 weeks, crutches were no longer required and the patients were allowed to return to normal work activity. Jogging was allowed after 3 months, while a complete return to sports activities was recommended 6 months after the surgical procedure.

Assessment of Clinical Outcomes

All patients were assessed before and after the procedure with the modified Harris hip score (MHHS). The score is reported as 90–100 for excellent results, 80–89 for good, 70–79 for fair, 60–69 for poor and below 60 for a failed result [28]. Pre-operative MHHS scores were similar for all groups, with mean scores of 44.7 ± 5.7 (range: 34–56) for patients treated with ACI/hyaluronic acid scaffold, 45.3 ± 6.7 (34–62) for the ACI/polymer scaffold and 44.6 ± 6.3 (34–60) for AMIC.

Results

The mean follow-up time was 74 ± 10 months (range 48–84 months) for patients undergoing ACI and 51 ± 9 months (range 36–60 months) for AMIC. Over the course of the study the MHHS improved in all patients (Fig. 67.5). Patients in all three groups had similar values of the MHHS at the end of the study (EOS) (ACI/hyaluronic acid scaffold: 81.1 ± 6.7 points (range: 70–100), ACI/polymer scaffold: 80.1 ± 6.1 points (70–98) and AMIC: 84.0 ± 6.4 points (72–100)). The greatest improvement was observed in the first 6 months and up to 1 year after surgery. After 1 year, the MHHS remained fairly constant, with no notable decrease over time.

Good or excellent outcome scores (MHHS ≥80) were achieved at EOS by 68 % (23 of 34) of patients who were treated with ACI with a hyaluronic acid scaffold, and 61 % (28 of 46) treated with ACI with a polymer scaffold. Good or excellent improvement was noted in 49 out of 62 patients (79 %) treated with AMIC. Patients who did not improve their MHHS to >80 tended to have presented also with a lower baseline MHHS score, but the level of improvement (change from baseline) was similar to those who had EOS score >80 points. It is important to note that no patient received a failing (<60) or poor (<70) MHHS. In both groups, unsatisfactory results were recorded mostly in those patients suffering from a cartilage defect on the femoral head or where standard X-rays showed a reduced or compromised joint space.

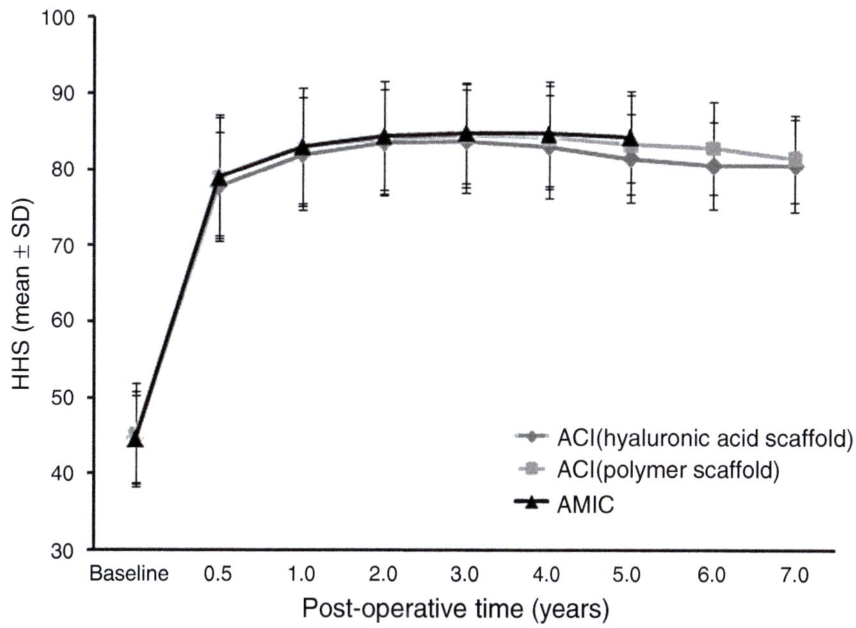

Fig. 67.5 MHHS at baseline and up to 7 years after ACI and AMIC. MHHS was recorded before the procedure (baseline) and up to the end of the study (5 years for AMIC and 7 years for ACI). *ACI* autologous chondrocyte implantation, *AMIC* arthroscopic autologous matrix-induced chondroplasty, *MHHS* modified Harris hip score

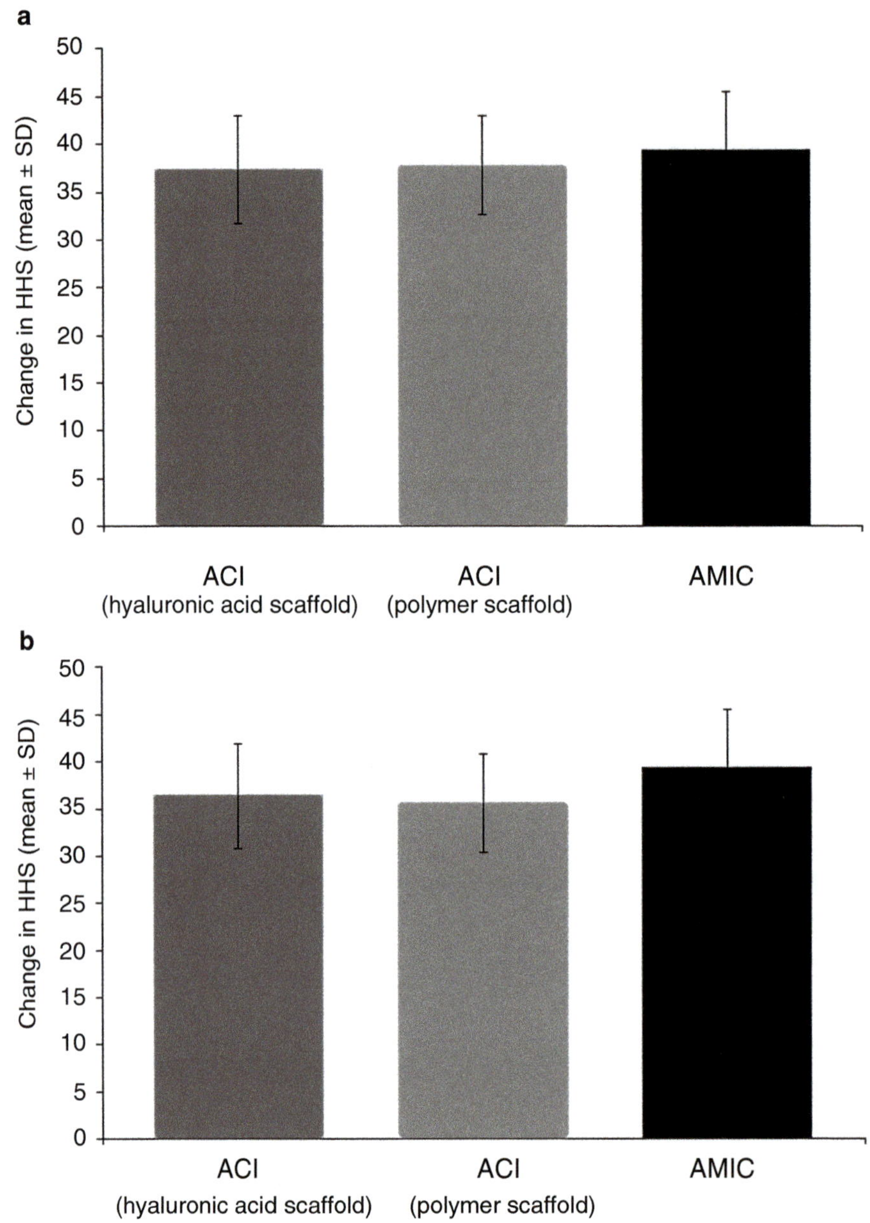

Fig. 67.6 Improvement in MHSS after ACI and AMIC. Improvement in MHHS is shown at 5 years (maximum follow-up time for AMIC) after the study (**a**) and EOS (5 years for AMIC and 7 years for ACI) (**b**). *ACI* autologous chondrocyte implantation, *AMIC* arthroscopic autologous matrix-induced chondroplasty, *EOS* end of study, *MHHS* modified Harris hip score

Mean MHHS improvement from baseline to EOS was calculated for all patients. For patients who underwent ACI with a hyaluronic acid scaffold, the mean MHHS change from baseline to EOS was 36.4 ± 5.6 points (26–48), compared to 35.7 ± 5.2 points (24–46) in ACI/polymer scaffold group, and 39.4 ± 6.2 points (26–50) in the AMIC group (Fig. 67.6). Analysis of subgroups by age (≤35 years vs. >35 years or ≤40 years vs. >40 years), gender or type of FAI (pincer vs. cam) showed no appreciable difference in the change in the MHHS.

No patient in both groups underwent a secondary procedure, including total hip replacement, during the period of follow-up.

Discussion

This study evaluated clinical outcomes for up to 7 years in patients with medium-to-large chondral defects due to FAI who were treated with AMIC or ACI.

In the knee, arthroscopy is common and allows diagnosis of knee pathologies, cartilage damage included. The use of arthroscopy in the hip is considerably less common, as the hip is surrounded by large muscular masses and deep articulation that make surgical access difficult. Historically, arthrotomy has been the gold standard therapeutic approach in the hip because it allows for open dislocation and a nearly

360° access to the joint. However, open dislocation of the hip exposes the articulation to the serious risk of aseptic necrosis of the femoral head [29]. The development of arthroscopic approaches to treat hip chondropathies seeks to address the arthrotomy-associated side effects. A recent review evaluating clinical results of open dislocation, arthroscopy and a combined approach for the treatment of FAI in 1462 hips noted that patients treated with arthroscopic methods had highest improvement in the MHHS after surgery, a higher rate of return to sport and lowest incidence of complications (1.7 % for arthroscopy, 9.2 % for open dislocation and 16 % for the combined approach) [30]. Similarly, another review found that mini-open and arthroscopic methods had similar clinical efficacy for repair of FAI as open dislocation surgery, but that the arthroscopic procedure had lower rates of major complications (0–20 % with open dislocation, 0–17 % in mini-open studies and 0–5 % in the arthroscopic studies) [31].

Several arthroscopic techniques are used for the treatment of full-thickness hip chondropathies. Microfracture is currently the treatment of choice for smaller chondral defects in the hip (≤2 cm^2). It is minimally invasive and no major postoperative complications have been reported. A number of published studies examined clinical outcomes after microfracture and have shown satisfactory results in the majority of patient with small defects [7, 8].

Published literature on the use of open dislocation ACI for the treatment of medium-to-large chondral defects in the hip is scarce. The first published case report utilising ACI in the hip reported a patient who underwent bone grafting and ACI using a collagen I/III matrix for treatment of extensive loss of cartilage and osteonecrosis [17]. Sixteen months after the procedure, the patient's condition had improved and he was able to return to daily activities. Another case report documented a patient with a previous autologous osteochondral mosaicplasty with full-thickness loss around the osteochondral plugs [18]. ACI was performed by implanting chondrocytes harvested from the knee under a collagen I/III matrix. At 2-year follow-up, the patient remained pain free and contrast-enhanced MRI showed good tissue repair and normal joint space.

We performed ACI using either a polymer scaffold or hyaluronic acid scaffold to cover the defect. Scaffolds are preferred to periosteal flaps in part because they eliminate the need for harvesting periosteum and its associated problems. It is also not clear whether cells injected in suspension under the flap have the proper infrastructure to grow into structures that resemble normal cartilage. Hyaluronic acid- and polymer-based scaffolds are non-toxic, fully resorbable and mechanically stable, providing a temporary support for cultured chondrocytes that will be replaced by the extracellular matrix synthesised by the cells themselves [32]. Human chondrocytes seeded on hyaluronic acid-based scaffolds have been shown to express and produce collagen type II and aggrecan and down-regulate the production of collagen type I, and polymer scaffolds are similarly able to support regeneration of cartilage. In the AMIC procedure, we used a collagen type I/III matrix (Chondro-Gide®), as support for the cells released by microfracture. Collagen matrices are becoming the scaffold of choice for repair of cartilage damage. Cultured chondrocytes seeded onto the matrix have been shown to differentiate into chondrocyte-like cells [33] and expressed markers of hyaline chondrocytes [34].

The most desirable techniques for chondral defect repair are those that are easily performed, reduce surgical morbidity, do not require harvesting of other tissues, allow enhanced cell proliferation and maturation and phenotype maintenance and allow for efficient and complete integration of new tissue with surrounding articular cartilage [32]. While ACI has yielded good results in the knee and hip, it has several drawbacks, and AMIC may offer potential advantages over ACI, especially to patients with medium-to-large chondral defects. ACI requires two surgical procedures: an arthroscopy to harvest chondrocytes and a cell implantation step, which is often performed as open surgery, exposing the patient to a risk of infection and requiring a long recovery period. Obtaining a sufficient number of cells for implantation requires external laboratory support for in vitro culturing of chondrocytes, making this a cost-intensive procedure. With AMIC, no cells have to be harvested, cultured and reimplanted and therefore no harvest-site morbidity occurs. The operation can be performed as a single-step procedure with potential time and cost savings. Furthermore, AMIC does not require complex and costly cell expansion techniques, therefore eliminating the need for specialised centres and laboratory support and potentially reducing costs.

Encouraging outcomes for the treatment of cartilage defects in the knee with AMIC have been reported [20–24]. For example, in a recent clinical study of 27 patients [22], all patients experienced significant improvement in five different outcome scores at 12 months and up to 24 months after the procedure. These findings are in line with our results of treating chondral lesions of the hip with AMIC.

AMIC has been previously performed as an open procedure [22], raising issues associated with all arthrotomies, such as the risk of infection and prolonged recovery time. The development of a fully arthroscopic procedure for the use of AMIC in the hip represents a major advance with potential associated advantages.

One of the limitations of this study is that it is retrospective analysis of the data collected over years of treatment. Patients were not randomised, but rather those who enrolled earlier underwent ACI and those who enrolled later underwent AMIC when this treatment option became available. Despite this, the patient baseline characteristics for the two groups were comparable. Another limitation is that clinical improvement was judged only based on the patients' MHHS. Although this test has high validity and reliability [35], it is most suitable for assessment of functionality in elderly arthritic patients and might not be sensitive enough to assess subtle changes in function in young, otherwise healthy patients. Nevertheless, the improvement in these scores suggests that both ACI and AMIC provide clinical benefits to patients with FAI.

Conclusions

Long-term follow-up of 142 patients undergoing AMIC or ACI for the treatment of chondral defects due to FAI showed marked clinical improvement in all patients. Clinical improvement, as measured by MHHS, was similar in the two groups. This study suggests that arthroscopic AMIC may be a viable and cost-effective alternative to ACI in patients with medium-to-large chondral defects of the hip.

Acknowledgements Medical writing was supported by nspm ltd, Meggen, Switzerland and by Geistlich Pharma AG.

Disclosure: The author declares that he has no conflict of interest.

References

1. Yen YM, Kocher MS. Chondral lesions of the hip: microfracture and chondroplasty. Sports Med Arthrosc. 2010;18(2):83–9.
2. Lavigne M, Parvizi J, Beck M, Siebenrock KA, Ganz R, Leunig M. Anterior femoroacetabular impingement: part I. Techniques of joint preserving surgery. Clin Orthop Relat Res. 2004;418:61–6.
3. McCarthy J, Noble P, Aluisio FV, Schuck M, Wright J, Lee JA. Anatomy, pathologic features, and treatment of acetabular labral tears. Clin Orthop Relat Res. 2003;406:38–47.
4. Ganz R, Parvizi J, Beck M, Leunig M, Notzli H, Siebenrock KA. Femoroacetabular impingement: a cause for osteoarthritis of the hip. Clin Orthop Relat Res. 2003;417:112–20.
5. Tanzer M, Noiseux N. Osseous abnormalities and early osteoarthritis: the role of hip impingement. Clin Orthop Relat Res. 2004;429: 170–7.
6. Baber YF, Robinson AH, Villar RN. Is diagnostic arthroscopy of the hip worthwhile? A prospective review of 328 adults investigated for hip pain. J Bone Joint Surg (Br). 1999;81(4):600–3.
7. McGill KC, Bush-Joseph CA, Nho SJ. Hip microfracture: indications, technique, and outcomes. Cartilage. 2011;1(2):127–36.
8. Crawford K, Philippon MJ, Sekiya JK, Rodkey WG, Steadman JR. Microfracture of the hip in athletes. Clin Sports Med. 2006; 25(2):327–35. x.
9. Philippon MJ, Schenker ML, Briggs KK, Maxwell RB. Can microfracture produce repair tissue in acetabular chondral defects? Arthroscopy. 2008;24(1):46–50.
10. Byrd JW, Jones KS. Osteoarthritis caused by an inverted acetabular labrum: radiographic diagnosis and arthroscopic treatment. Arthroscopy. 2002;18(7):741–7.
11. Byrd JW, Jones KS. Microfracture for Grade IV chondral lesion of the hip (SS-89). Arthroscopy. 2004;20:e41.
12. Bharam S. Labral tears, extra-articular injuries, and hip arthroscopy in the athlete. Clin Sports Med. 2006;25(2):279–92. ix.
13. Philippon M, Schenker M, Briggs K, Kuppersmith D. Femoroacetabular impingement in 45 professional athletes: associated pathologies and return to sport following arthroscopic decompression. Knee Surg Sports Traumatol Arthrosc. 2007;15(7):908–14.
14. Farjo LA, Glick JM, Sampson TG. Hip arthroscopy for acetabular labral tears. Arthroscopy. 1999;15(2):132–7.
15. Vasiliadis HS, Wasiak J, Salanti G. Autologous chondrocyte implantation for the treatment of cartilage lesions of the knee: a systematic review of randomized studies. Knee Surg Sports Traumatol Arthrosc. 2010;18(12):1645–55.
16. Gikas PD, Bayliss L, Bentley G, Briggs TW. An overview of autologous chondrocyte implantation. J Bone Joint Surg (Br). 2009;91(8):997–1006.
17. Akimau P, Bhosale A, Harrison PE, et al. Autologous chondrocyte implantation with bone grafting for osteochondral defect due to posttraumatic osteonecrosis of the hip--a case report. Acta Orthop. 2006;77(2):333–6.
18. Ellender P, Minas T. Autologous chondrocyte implantation in the hip: case report and technique. Oper Tech Sports Med. 2008;16: 201–6.
19. Murakibhavi V, Ahmed N, Raj V, Richardson J. Early results of autologous chondrocyte implantation in the hip. J Bone Joint Surg (Br). 2010;92B(Suppl IV):526.
20. Benthien JP, Behrens P. Autologous matrix-induced chondrogenesis (AMIC) A one step procedure for retropatellar articular resurfacing. Acta Orthop Belg. 2010;76(2):260–3.
21. Benthien JP, Behrens P. Autologous matrix-induced chondrogenesis (AMIC): combining microfracturing and a collagen I/III matrix for articular cartilage resurfacing. Cartilage. 2010;1(1):65–8.
22. Gille J, Schuseil E, Wimmer J, Gellissen J, Schulz AP, Behrens P. Mid-term results of autologous matrix-induced chondrogenesis for treatment of focal cartilage defects in the knee. Knee Surg Sports Traumatol Arthrosc. 2010;18(11):1456–64.
23. Benthien JP, Behrens P. The treatment of chondral and osteochondral defects of the knee with autologous matrix-induced chondrogenesis (AMIC): method description and recent developments. Knee Surg Sports Traumatol Arthrosc. 2011;19(8):1316–9.
24. Dhollander AA, De NF, Almqvist KF, et al. Autologous matrix-induced chondrogenesis combined with platelet-rich plasma gel: technical description and a five pilot patients report. Knee Surg Sports Traumatol Arthrosc. 2011;19(4):536–42.
25. Wiewiorski M, Leumann A, Buettner O, Pagenstert G, Horisberger M, Valderrabano V. Autologous matrix-induced chondrogenesis aided reconstruction of a large focal osteochondral lesion of the talus. Arch Orthop Trauma Surg. 2010;131(3):293–6.
26. Outerbridge RE. The etiology of chondromalacia patellae. J Bone Joint Surg (Br). 1961;43-B:752–7.
27. Fontana A, Zanasi S, Brittberg M, Marcacci M. Arthroscopic approach in hip defects. In: Basic science, clinical repair and reconstruction of articular cartilage defects: current status and prospects. Bologna, Italy: Timeo Editore; 2006. p. 419–22.
28. Harris WH. Traumatic arthritis of the hip after dislocation and acetabular fractures: treatment by mold arthroplasty. An end-result study using a new method of result evaluation. J Bone Joint Surg. 1969;51(4):737–55.

29. Sanders S, Tejwani N, Egol KA. Traumatic hip dislocation--a review. Bull NYU Hosp Jt Dis. 2010;68(2):91–6.
30. Botser IB, Smith Jr TW, Nasser R, Domb BG. Open surgical dislocation versus arthroscopy for femoroacetabular impingement: a comparison of clinical outcomes. Arthroscopy. 2011;27(2): 270–8.
31. Matsuda DK, Carlisle JC, Arthurs SC, Wierks CH, Philippon MJ. Comparative systematic review of the open dislocation, mini-open, and arthroscopic surgeries for femoroacetabular impingement. Arthroscopy. 2011;27(2):252–69.
32. Safran MR, Kim H, Zaffagnini S. The use of scaffolds in the management of articular cartilage injury. J Am Acad Orthop Surg. 2008;16(6):306–11.
33. Fuss M, Ehlers EM, Russlies M, Rohwedel J, Behrens P. Characteristics of human chondrocytes, osteoblasts and fibroblasts seeded onto a type I/III collagen sponge under different culture conditions. A light, scanning and transmission electron microscopy study. Ann Anat. 2000;182(4):303–10.
34. Gigante A, Moschini A, Verdenelli A, Del TM, Ulisse S, de Palma L. Open versus percutaneous repair in the treatment of acute Achilles tendon rupture: a randomized prospective study. Knee Surg Sports Traumatol Arthrosc. 2008;16(2):204–9.
35. Soderman P, Malchau H. Is the Harris hip score system useful to study the outcome of total hip replacement? Clin Orthop Relat Res. 2001;384:189–97.

The Use of Fibrin Adhesive for Cartilage Repair in Hip Arthroscopy

68

Samuel J. Barke, and Richard N. Villar

Introduction

Femoroacetabular impingement is a well-recognised cause of articular cartilage damage leading to osteoarthritis of the hip. Articular cartilage flaps are a common finding both at arthroscopic and open surgery [1] with one of the earliest signs of flap formation being the delamination of the articular cartilage form the underlying subchondral bone [2]. At arthroscopy of the hip, this delamination produces bulging of the affected articular cartilage when pressure is applied to the adjacent labrum resulting in the 'wave' or 'carpet' sign (see Fig. 68.1).

There is still debate about how best to treat this delaminated acetabular cartilage. Various techniques have been described to deal with chondral injury in the knee [3–5]. The options currently available to the hip surgeon tend to have evolved from these techniques. In general, the surgeon may choose to leave the chondral defect alone but deal with the cause – generally a cam and/or pincer deformity at the femoral head/neck junction. However, perhaps the most commonly used method employed by arthroscopic surgeons is to excise the articular flap and to perform microfracture on the underlying bone with the aim of encouraging the formation of a fibrocartilage layer which is more stable and halt the progression of the hyaline cartilage delamination. This technique was first described by Steadman [6] for the knee and later extended to the hip by Philippon [7]. Early results are encouraging and have been widely adopted because of the ease of the technique.

S.J. Barke, MBBS
South West London Elective Orthopaedic Centre,
Dorking Road, Epsom, Surrey KT18 7EG, UK
e-mail: giles.stafford@eoc.nhs.uk

R.N. Villar, MS, FRCS
Villar Bajwa Practice, Spire Cambridge Lea Hospital,
30 New Road, Impington, Cambridge CB24 9EL, UK
e-mail: rnv1000@aol.com

Histological studies, however, have shown that delaminated articular cartilage contains viable chondrocytes, although at a reduced level to undamaged cartilage [8, 9]. This would suggest that removing the area of chondral damage is unnecessary and attempts at anatomical repair are therefore reasonable.

As a result, a cartilage repair technique has been introduced by the senior author [1, 10] with the aim of rebonding the native hyaline cartilage to subchondral bone with fibrin adhesive, rather than excising it. The technique is suggested for use in cases where there is delamination in the presence of a macroscopically sound articular surface (no thinning, roughening or fibrillation). The theory is that mesenchymal stem cells may cross the fibrin clot to repopulate the now stable hyaline cartilage differentiating into chondrocytes. The rationale for this is described below.

Fibrin Glue

The first documented use of fibrin as a haemostat was in 1909 by Bergel et al. [11] and the first evidence of its use as an adhesive was in 1940 when Young and Medawar utilised fibrinogen to achieve peripheral nerve attachment [12]. Four years later, in 1944, the use of fibrinogen and thrombin as a biological glue was described as a method to secure skin grafts [13]. Further significant advances were not made until the late 1970s/early 1980s when methods for producing concentrated fibrinogen were developed creating a far more effective fibrin adhesive [14, 15].

Fibrin glue is formed through the conversion of fibrinogen to fibrin in a reaction catalysed by thrombin (see Fig. 68.2). There are various methods of delivery available, but perhaps the most commonly used holds the components in two separate chambers. The first contains the fibrinogen and Factor XIII (a fibrin stabiliser) and usually an agent to inhibit fibrinolysis (aprotinin or tranexamic acid). The second contains thrombin, reconstituted in an aqueous solution of

J.C. McCarthy et al. (eds.), *Hip Joint Restoration*, DOI 10.1007/978-1-4614-0694-5_68

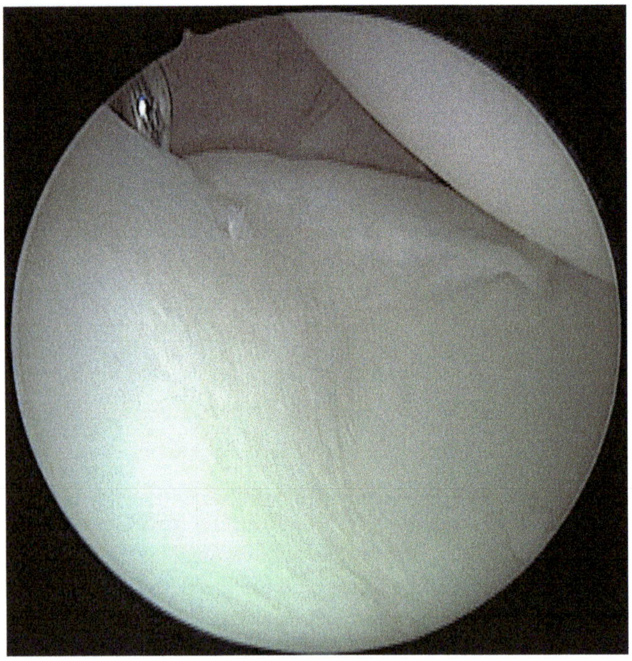

Fig. 68.1 The 'wave' sign – bulging of the delaminated articular cartilage

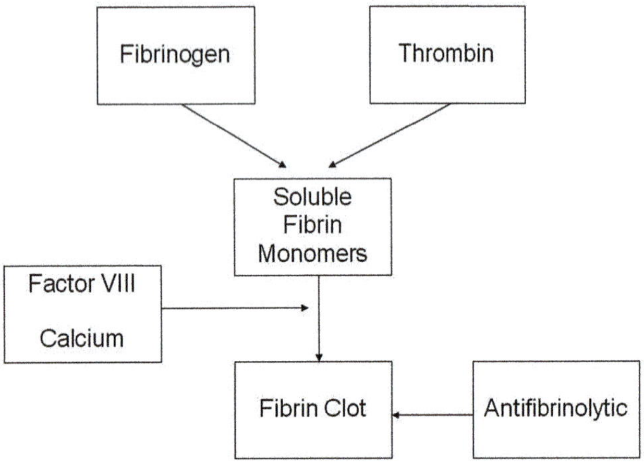

Fig. 68.2 Pathway of formation of fibrin clot

calcium chloride. The contents of the two chambers are mixed in a common lumen on application.

Fibrinogen is a high molecular weight protein (340,000 Da), which is composed of two polypeptide chains. Thrombin acts by cleaving the fibrinopeptides to leave soluble fibrin molecules that form into a three-dimensional network of fibres and fibrils [16]. In the presence of Factor VIII and calcium there is cross-linking of this lattice of fibres, which results in the final, insoluble fibrin clot. Antifibrinolytics such as aprotinin or tranexamic acid can be added to the mixture at varying concentrations to control the rate of fibrinolysis and thus the survival of the fibrin sealant.

As well as playing an integral role as a sealant and haemostatic agent, fibrin adhesive has been shown to promote a variety of cellular responses, mainly through the action of thrombin. These responses include increased cell migration [17, 18], proliferation [19] and survival [20, 21] and are mediated through thrombin's specific interactions with various cell surface receptors.

Surgical Uses of Fibrin Glue

Developments in the manufacturing of fibrin adhesive allowed it to become a commercially viable product and its possible benefits to be realised by various surgical specialties.

Fibrin glue has been shown to be of particular use in cardiac surgery [22] where the risk of bleeding is increased because of fibrinolysis and platelet destruction caused by cardiopulmonary bypass. In both cardiac and peripheral vascular surgery it is common to utilise a fibrin sealant on vascular anastomoses prior to pressurising; its use has been shown to be superior to other available techniques [23]. It has also been used to attach endothelial cells to artificial grafts with the aim of creating a new endothelial lining [24] and also as an external support to vein grafts that will be subjected to arterial pressures [25].

In thoracic surgery fibrin adhesive has been advocated for sealing air leaks from both the parenchyma and the bronchial tree following lung resection [26] and has also been described as a method to stop persistent parenchymal air leaks thoracoscopically [27].

The haemostatic properties of fibrin adhesive make it of particular use in resection of the liver, spleen and pancreas where there are often large areas of bleeding that are difficult to control with conventional methods. It has been shown to considerably reduce blood loss and the need for transfusion [28, 29]. It has also been shown to be of use in traumatic abdominal injury where its application to damaged liver and spleen parenchyma has allowed organ salvage [30]. In addition, fibrin adhesive has been used by general surgeons to seal intestinal anastomoses, restoring the continuity of the intestinal tract and reducing the rates of dehiscence [31], and in the conservative treatment of peri-anal fistulae [32].

In oncological surgery fibrin glue has been suggested as a method of eliminating fluid collection post resection of tumour, mainly in the breast or axilla [33]. Applied between the skin and underlying muscle, the fibrin adhesive seals the layers together reducing the residual space. It is put to a similar use in plastic surgery when there is significant soft tissue dissection in forming muscle flaps, as a haemostatic agent following burn debridement, and for attachment of skin grafts [16].

The structure of fibrin makes it useful as a drug delivery tool as well as a scaffold for tissue engineering applications [16]. The glue allows diffusion of molecules which are able to diffuse through fibrin glue encapsulating layers, thus making it an effective vehicle for drug delivery. Fibrin glue constructs have performed successfully in delivery of antibiotics in the treatment of ocular infections [34], osteomyelitis [35] and localised peritoneal infections [36]. It is also capable of delivering chemotherapeutic agents in treating solid and bony tumours [37, 38].

Specific Uses in Orthopedic Surgery

Currently, the most common clinical uses for fibrin glue in orthopedic surgery utilise its adhesive properties and its ability to support cell growth. It has been employed as a method of haemostasis in total knee replacement (TKR) but, although being effective at reducing blood loss, did not offer any improvement over the use of intravenous tranexamic acid [39] which is easier to administer.

Fibrin adhesive has played a significant role in the repair of injured articular cartilage. In its early use, it was hypothesised to be a suitable method of reattaching post-traumatic chondral and osteo-chondral fragments with promising results being demonstrated by Kaplonyi et al. [40]. However, internal fixation remains the preferred method as it appears to give more reliable results [41].

Both autologous chondrocyte implantation (ACI) and matrix-induced autologous chondrocyte implantation (MACI) utilise fibrin adhesive to secure implanted chondrocytes within articular defects. In ACI, chondrocytes, having been harvested and grown in vitro, are held in the cartilage defect by a periosteal or collagenous membrane, which is sealed with the fibrin adhesive. MACI involves implanting chondrocytes that are held on a matrix that allows fixation exclusively with fibrin adhesive [42]. Although its primary use in these procedures is as a sealant, there is evidence to suggest that fibrin adhesive also promotes migration and proliferation of chondrocytes. These properties have led to it being used to suspend cultured chondrocytes before being applied directly to chondral defects. This method is reported to be technically simpler and less invasive as well as allowing access to sites not usually amenable to traditional ACI [43].

The use of fibrin glue in both meniscal and ligament repair has been explored. However, failure rate of meniscal repair using glue is comparable to that of modern direct surgical repair techniques which, given their relative ease, remains the preferred option. Similarly, the success of hamstring grafts in anterior cruciate ligament (ACL) repair has meant the techniques developed to utilise fibrin adhesive [44] are now largely out of favour.

Rationale for Use in Hip Arthroscopy

As already discussed, it is known that viable chondrocytes are present, at a reduced level, in damaged cartilage [8, 9]. Equally it is known that fibrin glue is effective in securing chondral defects [40, 45] to subchondral bone. This alone is perhaps enough to make securing chondral flaps with fibrin glue during hip arthroscopy a reasonable method.

However, on top of this, fibrin glue has also been shown to promote cell proliferation and migration. Kirilak et al. [46] showed, in vitro, that the thrombin in fibrin glue promoted significant proliferative activity of chondrocytes as well as promoting migration. This might suggest that, even if the area of damaged cartilage has a reduced number of viable chondrocytes, the application of fibrin glue would promote proliferation to more normal levels and migration of chondrocytes from areas of undamaged cartilage.

In the senior author's technique, described below, microfracture of the subchondral bone is performed before fibrin adhesive is applied and the area of delaminated cartilage secured. Microfracture allows the release of marrow elements, including mesenchymal stem cells (MSCs) and growth factors, into the chondral defect [47]. Given that fibrin glue allows the migration of cells, we hypothesis that it is possible for these MSCs to reach the area of delaminated cartilage, differentiate, and repopulate it with chondrocytes. The microfracture holes are also hypothesised to allow a more stable fixation of the fibrin clot.

Surgical Technique

Access is gained to the area behind the delaminated cartilage by developing the perilabral sulcus with a radiofrequency ablation probe and then making a small incision, extending from the outer aspect of the labrum into the area of delamination (see Fig. 68.3). Once access is gained, a microfracture awl is passed into the 'pocket' behind the area of chondral delamination allowing microfracture of the underlying subchondral bone (see Fig. 68.4). Care must be taken to ensure no further damage is done to the overlying cartilage. Before the fibrin adhesive can be applied, the joint must be drained of irrigation fluid. This is achieved through two arthroscopy needles inserted through the anterolateral portal, one into the base of the central compartment (cotyloid fossa), and one into the pocket behind the delaminated cartilage (see Fig. 68.5). The joint is then aspirated dry, the needle in the central compartment is withdrawn, but the needle

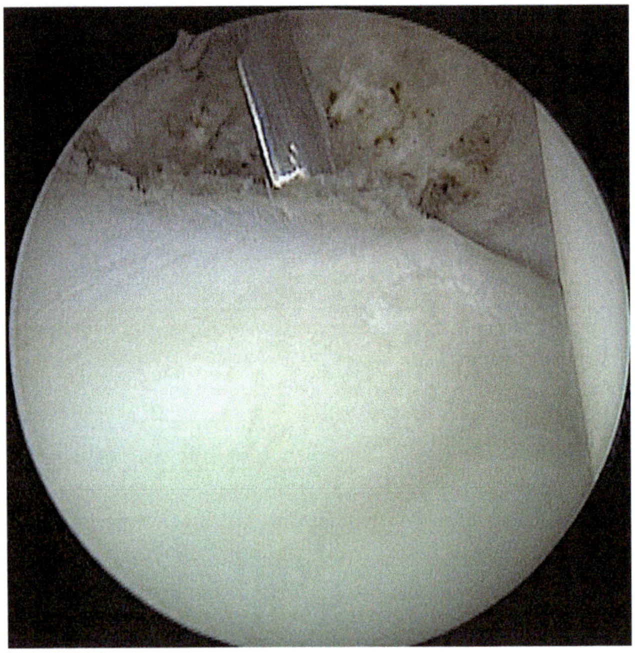

Fig. 68.3 Gaining access to the area of delamination with an arthroscopic knife

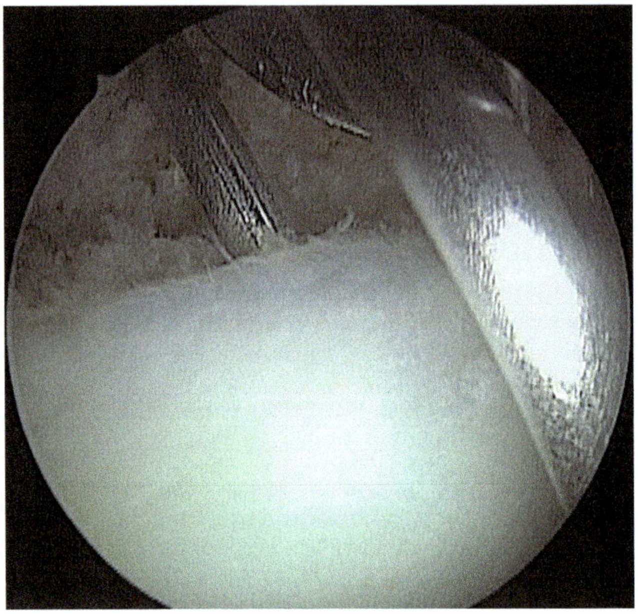

Fig. 68.5 Arthroscopy needle inserted into the 'pocket' and fibrin adhesive applied

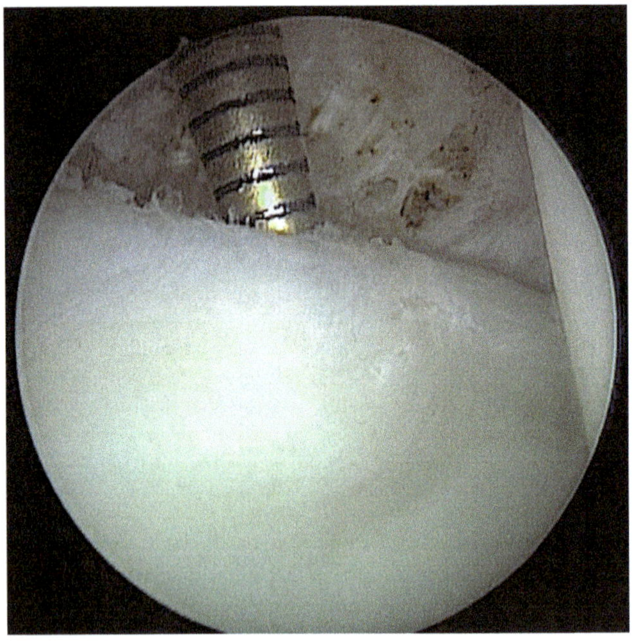

Fig. 68.4 Microfracture of the underlying subchondral bone

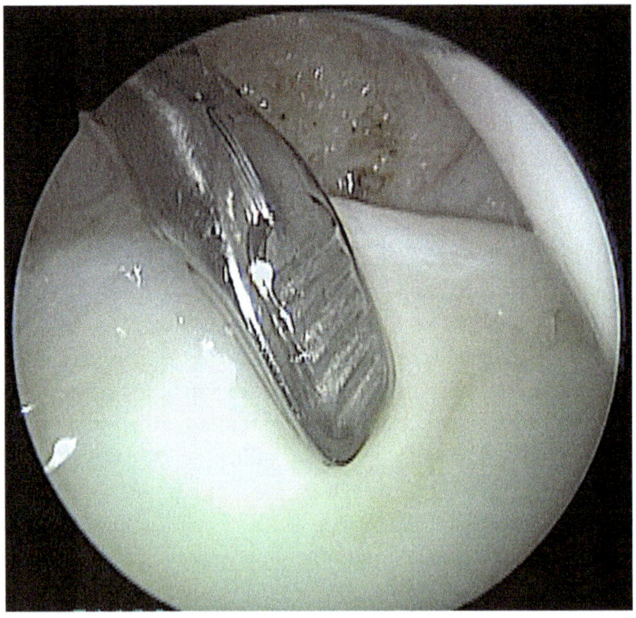

Fig. 68.6 Arthroscopic punch used to ensure contact between delaminated cartilage and subchondral bone

between the subchondral bone and delaminated cartilage is retained. Fibrin adhesive is then injected into the subchondral pocket through the remaining needle. The delaminated chondral surface is firmly pressed against bone with an angled arthroscopic punch while the fibrin adhesive sets (see Fig. 68.6). The fibrin adhesive cures within 2 min, rebonding the delaminated chondral surface. Excess fibrin adhesive often spills into the central compartment and can be removed with arthroscopic graspers. Further compression of the previously delaminated cartilage surface occurs when the femoral head is reduced into the acetabulum on release of limb traction. Post-operatively, the patients are given simple analgesia, reviewed by a physiotherapist and discharged with a standardised rehabilitation programme.

Results

Evidence of the efficacy of this technique is limited to the results of a case series at 1 and 3 years [1, 10]. The clinical results of 43 patients with feremoacetabular impingement were reviewed, with completion of Modified Harris Hip Scores (MHHS) pre- and post-operatively. Average MHHS pain scores (on a scale where 0 indicated totally disabling pain, and 44 indicated completely pain free) improved from 21.8 pre-operatively to 35.8 at a mean of 28 months post-operatively ($p<0.0001$). MHHS functional score (on a scale where 0 indicated a severe disturbance in function, and 47 indicated no functional impairment at all) also improved post-operatively from 40.0 to 43.6 ($p=0.0006$). There was not found to be a statistically significant change in scores between 1 and 3 years post-procedure.

During the follow-up period, three patients underwent repeat hip arthroscopy because of persistent symptoms, all arising from iliopsoas irritation. At the time of repeat arthroscopy, the area of previous chondral delamination was inspected and appeared to be macroscopically intact and well fixed to subchondral bone. Samples were not taken for histological analysis.

The Future

There are some developments that may add to the effectiveness of this technique in the future. Fibrin glue can offer a scaffold to substances that promote tissue healing. A number of studies have looked at using fibrin glue as a transport medium in the repair of meniscal injuries in animal models. Ishimura et al. [48] found that there was earlier mature healing in those treated with standard fibrin glue compared to a control with this effect being enhanced when marrow cells were incorporated into the fibrin glue. Izuta et al. [49] had similarly positive results using fibrin glue as a scaffold for MSCs. No extracellular matrix invasion was seen in the control group, there was invasion in 25 % of samples with fibrin glue alone which increased to 75 % of samples when fibrin glue was embedded with MSCs. The addition of MSCs to fibrin glue has also shown improved healing in various other settings [50–54].

The described technique appears to offer an option in the treatment of early chondral damage of the hip with the aim of preventing progression to osteoarthritis. However, although the results described above are from largest case series to date, published series are all small. In order to properly evaluate the technique, a double-blinded randomised controlled trial is needed. There have also been no histological studies yet undertaken to ascertain the quality and constituency of the repaired delaminated cartilage to confirm whether the technique does indeed allow regeneration of normal articular cartilage in an anatomical repair. Nonetheless, the results of fibrin-assisted cartilage repair appear to be, at least, comparable to that of excision and microfracture.

References

1. Tzaveas AP, Villar RN. Arthroscopic repair of acetabular chondral delamination with fibrin adhesive. Hip Int. 2010;20(1):115–9.
2. Beck M, Leunig M, Parvizi J, Boutier V, Wyss D, Ganz R. Anterior femoroacetabular impingement: part II. Midterm results of surgical treatment. Clin Orthop Relat Res. 2004;418:67–73.
3. Hubbard MJ. Arthroscopic surgery for chondral flaps in the knee. J Bone Joint Surg. 1987;69:794–6.
4. Miller BS, Steadman JR, Briggs KK, Rodrigo JJ, Rodkey WG. Patient satisfaction and outcome after microfracture of the degenerative knee. J Knee Surg. 2004;17(1):13–7.
5. Brittberg M, Lindahl A, Nilsson A, Ohlsson C, Isaksson O, Peterson L. Treatment of deep cartilage defects in the knee with autologous chondrocyte transplantation. N Engl J Med. 1994;331:889–95.
6. Steadman JR, Rodkey WG, Simgleton SB, Briggs KK. Microfracture technique for full-thickness chondral defects: technique and clinical results. Oper Tech Orthop. 1997;7(4):300–4.
7. Philippon MJ, Schenker ML, Briggs KK, Maxwell RB. Can microfracture produce repair tissue in acetabular chondral defects? Arthroscopy. 2008;24(1):46–50.
8. Hembree WC, Ward BD, Furman BD, et al. Viability and apoptosis of human chondrocytes in osteochondral fragments following joint trauma. J Bone Joint Surg (Br). 2007;89:1388–95.
9. Ball ST, Jadin K, Allen RT, Schwartz AK, Sah RL, Brage ME. Chondrocyte viability after intra-articular calcaneal fractures in humans. Foot Ankle Int. 2007;28:665–8.
10. Stafford GH, Bunn JR, Villar RN. Arthroscopic repair of delaminated acetabular articular cartilage using fibrin adhesive. Results at one to three years. Hip Int. 2011;21(6):744–50.
11. Bergel S. Uber Wirkungen des Fibrins. Dtsch Med Wochenschr. 1909;35:633.
12. Young JZ, Medawar PB. Fibrin suture of peripheral nerves. Lancet. 1940;275:126–32.
13. Cronkite EP, Lozner EL, Deaver J. Use of thrombin and fibrinogen in skin grafting. JAMA. 1944;124:976–8.
14. Siedentop KH, Harris DM, Sanchez B. Autologous fibrin tissue adhesive. Laryngoscope. 1985;95:1074–6.
15. Spotnitz WD, Mintz PD, Avery N, et al. Fibrin glue from stored human plasma: an inexpensive and efficient method for local blood bank preparation. Am Surg. 1987;53:460–4.
16. Spotnitz WD, Burks SG, Prabhu R. Fibrin-based adhesives and hemostatic agents. In: Quinn JV, editor. Tissue adhesives in clinical medicine. Hamilton, Ontario: BC Decker; 2005. p. 77–112.
17. Karp JM, Tanaka TS, Zohar R, Sodek J, Shoichet MS, Davies JE, Stanford WL. Thrombin mediated migration of osteogenic cells. Bone. 2005;37:337–48.
18. Brown LF, Lanir N, McDonagh J, Tognazzi K, Dvorak AM, Dvorak HF. Fibroblast migration in fibrin gel matrices. Am J Pathol. 1993;142:273–83.
19. Tani K, Yasuoka S, Ogushi F, Asada K, Fujisawa K, Ozaki T, Sano N, Ogura T. Thrombin enhances lung fibroblast proliferation in bleomycin-induced pulmonary fibrosis. Am J Respir Cell Mol Biol. 1991;5:34–40.
20. Chinni C, De Niese MR, Tew DJ, Jenkins AL, Bottomley SP, Mackie EJ. Thrombin, a survival factor for cultured myoblasts. J Biol Chem. 1999;274:9169–74.

21. Pagel CN, De Niese MR, Abraham LA, Chinni C, Song SJ, Pike RN, Mackie EJ. Inhibition of osteoblast apoptosis by thrombin. Bone. 2003;33:733–43.
22. Rousou J, Gonzalez-Lavin L, Cosgrove D, et al. Randomized clinical trial of fibrin sealant in patients undergoing resternotomy or reoperation after cardiac operations. J Thorac Cardiovasc Surg. 1989;97:194–203.
23. Schenk W, Burks S, Gagne P, et al. Fibrin sealant improves hemostasis in peripheral vascular surgery: a randomized prospective trial. Ann Surg. 2003;237:871–6.
24. Geissler HP, Gosselin C, Ren D, et al. Biointeractive polymers and tissue engineered blood vessels. Biomaterials. 1996;17:329–36.
25. Stoker W, Nissen HW, Waldeau WR, et al. Perivenous application of fibrin glue reduces early injury of the human saphenous vein graft wall in an ex vivo model. Eur J Cardiothorac Surg. 2002;21:212–7.
26. Fabian T, Federico JA, Ponn RB. Fibrin glue in pulmonary resection: a prospective, randomized, blinded study. Ann Thorac Surg. 2003;75:1587–92.
27. Thistlethwaite PA, Luketich JD, Ferson PF, et al. Ablation of persistent air leaks after thoracic procedures with fibrin sealant. Ann Thorac Surg. 1999;67:575–7.
28. Noun R. Fibrin glue effectiveness and tolerance after elective liver resection: a randomized trial. Hepatogastroenterology. 1996;43: 221–4.
29. Uranues S, Mischinger HJ, Pfeifer J, et al. Hemostatic methods for the management of spleen and liver injuries. World J Surg. 1996; 20:1107–12.
30. Ochsner MG. Fibrin solutions to control hemorrhage in the trauma patient. J Long Term Eff Med Implants. 1998;8:161–73.
31. Fernandez L, Tejero E, Tieso A. Randomized trial of fibrin glue to seal mechanical oesophagojejunal anastomosis. Br J Surg. 1995; 83:40–1.
32. Patrlj L, Kocman B, Martinac M, et al. Fibrin glue–antibiotic mixture in the treatment of anal fistulae: experience with 69 cases. Digest Surg. 2000;17:77–80.
33. Langer S, Guenther JM, DiFronzo LA. Does fibrin sealant reduce drain output and allow earlier removal of drainage catheters in women undergoing operation for breast cancer? Am Surg. 2003;69:77–81.
34. Marone P, Monzillo V, Segu C, Antoniazzi E. Antibiotic-impregnated fibrin glue in ocular surgery: in vitro antibacterial activity. Ophthalmologica. 1999;213:12–5.
35. Mader JT, Stevens CM, Stevens JH, et al. Treatment of experimental osteomyelitis with a fibrin sealant antibiotic implant. Clin Orthop. 2002;403:58–72.
36. Woolverton CJ, Fulton JA, Salstrom SJ, et al. Tetracycline delivery from fibrin controls peritoneal infection without measurable systemic antibiotic. J Antimicrob Chemother. 2001;48:861–7.
37. Kitazawa H, Sata H, Adachi I, et al. Microdialysis assessment of fibrin glue containing sodium alginate for local delivery of doxorubicin in tumor-bearing rats. Biol Pharm Bull. 1997;20:278–81.
38. Miura S, Mii Y, Miyauchi Y, et al. Efficacy of slow-releasing anticancer drug delivery systems on transplantable osteosarcomas in rats. Jpn J Clin Oncol. 1995;25:61–71.
39. Molloy DO, Archbold HA, Ogondo L, et al. Comparison of topical fibrin spray and tranexamic acid on blood loss after total knee replacement: a prospective, randomised controlled trial. J Bone Joint Surg (Br). 2007;89-B:306–9.
40. Kaplonyi G, Zimmerman I, Frenyo AD, Farkas T, Nemes G. The use of fibrin adhesive in the repair of chondral and osteochondral injuries. Injury. 1988;19:267–72.
41. Plaga BR, Royster RM, Donigian AM, Wright GB, Caskey PM. Fixation of osteochondral fractures in rabbit knees: a comparison of Kirschner wires, fibrin sealant, and polydioxanone pins. J Bone Joint Surg (Br). 1992;74-B:292–6.
42. Patel S, Rodrigues-Merchan EC, Haddad FS. The use of fibrin glue in surgery of the knee. J Bone Joint Surg (Br). 2010;92-B: 1325–31.
43. Kim MK, Choi SW, Kim SR, Oh IS, Won MH. Autologous chondrocyte implantation in the knee using fibrin. Knee Surg Sports Traumatol Arthrosc. 2010;18:528–34.
44. Aubart F, Roger B, Zeine G. Repair by glueing under arthroscopic control of ruptures of the anterior cruciate ligament: preliminary study of 10 cases controlled by magnetic resonance imaging. Rev Chir Orthop Reparatrice Appar Mot. 1991;77:267–72 (in French).
45. Schlag G, Redil H. Fibrin sealant in orthopaedic surgery. Orthop Relat Res. 1988;227:269–85.
46. Kirilak Y, et al. Fibrin sealant promotes migration and proliferation of human articular chondrocytes: Possible involvement of thrombin and protease-activated receptors. Intl J Molecular Med. 2006;17: 551–8.
47. Steadman JR, Rodkey WG, Rodrigo JJ. Microfracture: surgical technique and rehabilitation to treat chondral defects. Clin Orthop Relat Res. 2001;(391 Suppl):S362–9.
48. Ishimura M, Ohgushi H, Habata T, Tamai S, Fujisawa Y. Arthroscopic meniscal repair using fibrin glue. Part I: experimental study. Arthroscopy. 1997;13:551–7.
49. Izuta Y, Ochi M, Adachi N, et al. Meniscal repair using bone marrow-derived mesenchymal stem cells: experimental study using green fluorescent protein transgenic rats. Knee. 2005;12:217–23.
50. Wing K, et al. Fibrin glue with autogenic bone marrow mesenchymal stem cells for urethral injury repair in rabbit model. Tissue Eng Part A. 2012;18(23–24):2507–17.
51. Yamada Y, et al. Bone regeneration following injection of mesenchymal stem cells and fibrin glue with a biodegradable scaffold. J Craniomaxillofac Surg. 2003;31(1):27–33.
52. Lim JK, Hui J, Li L, et al. Enhancement of tendon graft osteointegration using mesenchymal stem cells in a rabbit model of anterior cruciate ligament reconstruction. Arthroscopy. 2004;20:899–910.
53. Falanga V, et al. Autologous bone marrow-derived cultured mesenchymal stem cells delivered in a fibrin spray accelerate healing in murine and human cutaneous wounds. Tissue Eng. 2007;13(6): 1299–312.
54. Haleem AL, et al. The clinical use of human culture-expanded autologous bone marrow mesenchymal stem cells transplanted on platelet-rich fibrin glue in the treatment of articular cartilage defects: a pilot study and preliminary results. Cartilage. 2010;1(4): 253–61.

Novel Techniques in the Treatment of Chondral Lesions of the Hip

69

Rodrigo Mardones and Catalina Larrain Birrell

Introduction

Chondral lesions of the hip represent a diagnostic challenge and can be an elusive source of pain. Treatment may present difficulties due to access and spherical form of the joint, having few options for the management of chondral lesions of the femoral head, and is most commonly limited to excision, debridement, thermal chondroplasty, and microfracture [1]. This chapter focuses on new technologies to enhance the standard techniques for treating chondral lesions within the hip joint using two approaches: (1) the use of mesenchymal stem cells and platelet-rich plasma, and (2) the implantation of autologous chondrocytes and other differentiated stem cell lines. This review discusses the basis, techniques, and preliminary results obtained with the use of mesenchymal stem cells and platelet-rich plasma (PRP).

Chondral Lesions

Femoroacetabular impingement is frequently associated with chondral damage to the articulating surfaces of the femoral head and the acetabulum [2]. Most commonly, abnormal contact between the femoral neck and the acetabular rim leads to labral detachment and acetabular chondral damage [3]. The incidence of chondral lesions in patients with femoroacetabular impingement has been reported to be 67.3% at arthroscopy, as described by Nepple et al. [4]. Risk factors include the presence of radiographic signs of mild or moderate OA (Tonnis grades 1 or 2) and an alpha angle over 50° [4].

R. Mardones, MD (✉)
Tissue Engineering Lab, Orthopedics Department, Clinica Las Condes, Lo Fontecilla 441, Las Condes, RM, Santiago, Chile
e-mail: rmardones@clc.cl

C.L. Birrell, MD
Department of Orthopedic Surgery, Clinica Las Condes, Santiago, Región Metropolitana, Chile

A characteristic feature observation of chondral lesions of the hip is delamination of cartilage from the subchondral bone (the “wave sign”), leading to a “bag lesion” and chondral flaps. Though the Outerbridge classification system has been adopted from the knee literature to grade the severity of chondral lesions in the hip, it does not include delamination as a criterion for defining joint degeneration (although cases with a “wave sign” would be classified as Grade III on the Outerbridge [5]). Konan et al. recently described a new classification system for chondral lesions in the hip which includes the wave sign, and the extent and location of chondral delamination and chondrolabral lesions [6].

Standard Treatment for Chondral Lesions

Arthroscopic treatment of chondral lesions of the hip consists of excision of the presumed cause of the lesion (rim trimming and femoral neck osteoplasty), debridement, chondroplasty, and microfracture. Rim trimming and femoral neck osteoplasty could lead to the complete excision of the chondral lesion when it is located within the area of over-coverage of the femoral head. However, when the area of chondral damage extends beyond the region of over-coverage, treatment is chosen according to the severity of chondral damage, was expressed by the Outerbridge or Konan classifications.

Type I or II

The treatment of choice in this type of lesions is thermal chondroplasty. It has shown to be a safe technique for closed chondral lesions leading to morphologic changes with better structural characteristics than mechanical debridement [7–10].

Delamination

Delamination represents a treatment challenge among chondral lesions. Excising such an area of chondral instability seems counterproductive, particularly if the articular cartilage itself contains a significant number of viable chondrocytes [11]. The main objective is the reattachment of the cartilage

J.C. McCarthy et al. (eds.), *Hip Joint Restoration*, DOI 10.1007/978-1-4614-0694-5_69

Table 69.1 Commercial presentations of platelet-rich plasma

	Blood volume (ml)	Number of spins	Time (min)	Final PRP volume (ml)	Final platelet concentration	Leukocytes	Activator
Cascade® (PRFM)	9–18	2	21	4–9	1–1.5×	No	$CaCl_2$
GPS®	27–110	1	15	3–12	3–8×	Yes	Autologous thrombin + $CaCl_2$
Magellan®	30–60	2	4–6	6	3–7×	Yes	$CaCl_2$
BioPlat®	40	2	14	4	7–11×	No	Autologous thrombin

Cascade®: MTF, New Jersey, US
GPS®: Biomet, Warsaw, Indiana, US
Magellan®: Medtronic, Minneapolis, US
BioPlat®: Bioteccel, Santiago, Chile

to the underlying subchondral bone, which may be achieved with transchondral microfracture to generate an adherent retrolabral clot or with the use of an adhesive such as fibrin glue. Tzaveas and Villar have reported a series of 19 patients treated with fibrin adhesive showing improvement in pain and function at 6 months and 1 year after surgery [12].

Type III or IVChondral lesions: (Full Thickness Chondral Lesion)

Microfracture is the treatment of choice for full thickness lesions, with indications in the hip being similar to those in the knee and including focal and contained lesions, typically less than 2–4 cm^2 in size, including delamination. Microfracture is a marrow-stimulating procedure that brings undifferentiated stem cells from a subchondral perforation into the chondral defect [13]. A clot formed in the microfractured area provides an environment for both pluripotent marrow cells and mesenchymal stem cells to differentiate into a stable fibrocartilaginous tissue [14, 15]. Several studies had shown good midterm results with this technique; however, we know that this fibrocartilaginous tissue does not have the required mechanical properties and eventually will fail, leading to Chondral lesions:advanced chondral damage and osteoarthritis [15, 16].

Novel Treatments for Chondral Lesions

As mentioned above, the fibrocartilage newly formed at the microfractured area is unsuitable for weight-bearing function in the long term. Therefore, we will describe some techniques that may lead to the formation of hyaline-like cartilage with greater potential for articular function in the long term. The use of these novel technologies, including PRP and mesenchymal stem cells, has demonstrated promising results to date, both in animal and clinical studies.

Platelet-rich plasma (PRP)

PRP is an autologous natural concentrate of growth factors that can be obtained with a minimal, simple, and low-cost procedure from peripheral blood. The sample is centrifuged, one to three times depending on the commercial kit, generating a platelet concentrate, of 4–10 times the normal platelet count. This concentrate can be activated with the addition of calcium chloride or thrombin, autologous or heterologous, the latter with potential disadvantages including a slight increase in the risk of infection and adverse reactions. The absence of leukocytes in some commercial kits could play a role reducing the inflammation at the site of application, enhancing the effect of PRP [17, 18]. Commercial systems marketed for intraoperative ("point-of-care") operation are summarized in Table 69.1.

The mode of action of PRP is based on platelet function and the activation of alpha granules [19]. During the clotting phase, degranulation occurs with the subsequent activation of these granules. This process leads to the release of mitogenic, chemotactic, and morphogenic growth factors, which play an important role in the healing and repair process [20, 21].

PRP use began in the 1990s as a co-adjuvant therapy in maxillofacial surgery [22]. Ten years later, its use was popularized in orthopedic surgery [23]. The indications for this therapy have increased exponentially, not always based on good evidence to support its use. Published studies in orthopedics describe the use of PRP in treating overuse pathologies (epicondylitis [24], patellar [25], and Achilles [26] tendinopathies), sports medicine (anterior cruciate ligament reconstruction [27–31] and rotator cuff repair [32–35]), chondral pathology (osteoarthritis and focal chondral lesions [36–40]), spine [41, 42], trauma (fractures and pseudoarthrosis [43, 44]), and management of skin lesions (acute and chronic [45, 46]). However, the results of the clinical studies are dissimilar, with proven usefulness in some pathologies such as epicondylitis, patellar tendinopathy, pseudoarthrosis, and chronic wound management. It is likely that inter-patient variability and diversity of commercial kits, preparation, implementation, and applied concentrations may play an important role in product efficacy, thus influencing the results [47, 48]. Despite this, the studies agree on the anti-inflammatory and pro-coagulant effect of the PRP.

Hip chondral lesions traditionally have been handled equal to other joints, with similar results of that obtained at the knee for small lesions, but the spherical form of the hip, the composition and anatomy of the cartilage, and the unique types of chondral lesions (delamination) make the techniques and the results obtained at other joints not replicable at the hip for larger lesions. Hip chondral lesion clinical studies are limited to treatment with microfracture and fibrin clot (fibrin glue®) for delamination [12, 16]. These, though they are small clinical series, show some promising results in localized chondral lesions. Milano et al., in a study conducted in sheep, demonstrated that the use of a PRP clot associated with microfracture achieved a complete filling of the chondral lesion with macroscopic, biomechanic, and microscopic characteristics similar to normal hyaline cartilage [49].

Currently, the PRP clot is used as a carrier or membrane carrier of mesenchymal stem cells, a technique which will be explained later.

In summary, the use of a PRP clot in hip chondral lesions has little published evidence; however, the minimal cost and risks of the procedure associated with promising results obtained in both animal and preliminary clinical studies support its use in the clinical practice of arthroscopic hip surgery.

Mesenchymal Stem Cells (MSCs)

For any discussion of stem cells it is crucial to understand what specifically one is referring to, regarding the cellular origin, differentiation potential, and possible adverse effects, which may vary according to each of the subtypes.

Stem cells (SC) have the ability to divide indefinitely in culture and the potential to give rise to mature tissues. SC can be classified according to their origin and potentiality. Thus there are, by origin, *embryonic stem cells* that can be divided by its potentiality in **totipotent** (originating from the zygote and early blastomeres of an embryo) and **pluripotent** (derived from the blastocyst inner cell mass); and *somatic or adult stem cells*, which can be found in a fully developed organism. These may be *mesenchymal* or *hematopoietic* according to the tissue that may give rise and are referred as **multipotent** [50].

Embryonic stem cells have greater potential for differentiation, response, and growth than somatic stem cells and, in the past years have been widely studied in animals [51]. However this vast potential could generate an excessive response to local stimuli at the implantation site, giving rise to teratomas [52, 53].

Hematopoietic stem cells are found mainly in the bone marrow of adult specimens, in a proportion of 1 in 10,000 nucleated cells. Their clinical application has been extensively studied in the management of hematologic diseases.

Mesenchymal stem cells (***MSCs***) are also found in the bone marrow of adult specimens, in a proportion of 1 in 100,000 nucleated cells, decreasing with age [54]. These cells have differentiation potential into bone, fat, chondral, tendinous, ligamentous, neural and muscular tissue, according to the growth factors released by the injury site. MSCs from adult specimens can be obtained from fat tissue, bone marrow, and other tissues; however, bone marrow has several advantages as a donor site compared to other locations because of its ease of procurement, greater purity of the sample, and greater cell growth potential.

The cells are extracted from a bone marrow sample harvested from the iliac crest with a trocar. The marrow sample is first filtered and then centrifuged to separate its cellular components by density. The mononuclear cell layer is then identified and aspirated, obtaining a mononuclear cell concentrate (MCC) containing the MSCs. This concentrate can be applied directly to the implantation site or can undergo expansion and differentiation of the mesenchymal stem cells in a specialized laboratory (Fig. 69.1).

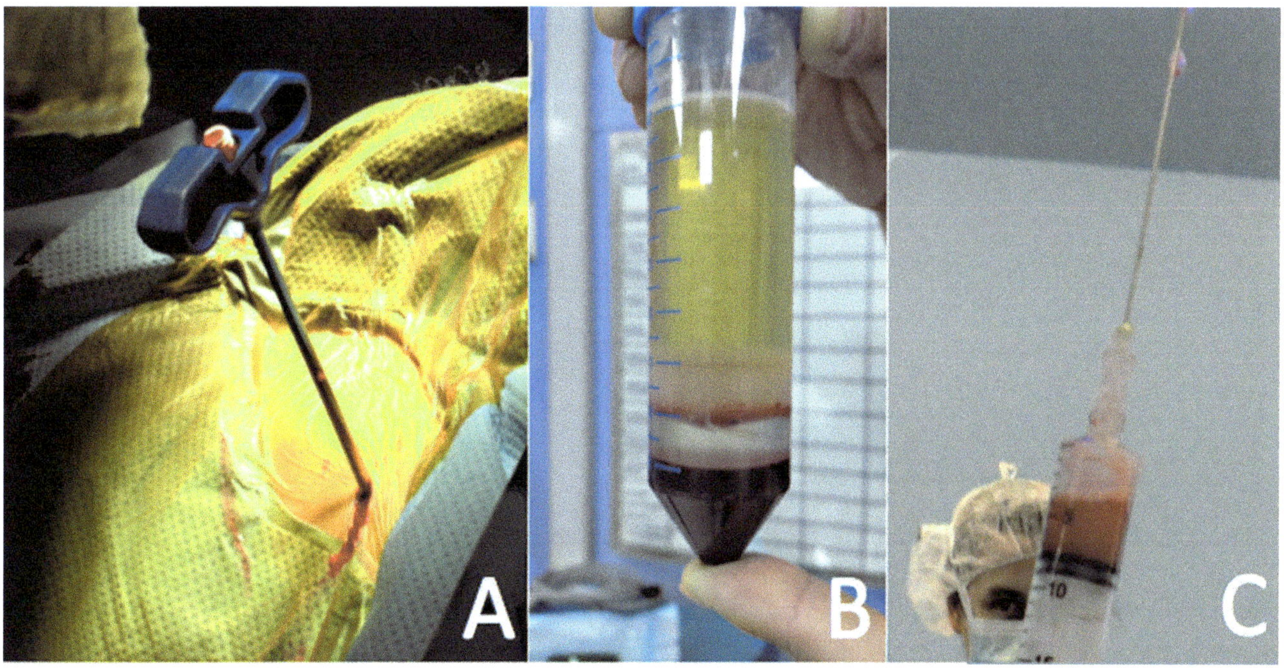

Fig. 69.1 Autologous mesenchymal stem cells concentrate. (**a**) Autologous bone marrow autograft. (**b**) Layer separation by a density filter and identification of mononuclear cells layer after centrifugation process. (**c**) Autologous mononuclear cells concentrate—final view

Clinical use of MCC has been described for avascular necrosis of the femoral head [55–57] and lately in the management of knee chondral lesions showing arthroscopic and histologic hyaline-like cartilage neoformation [58–61].

In summary, the use of MCC in hip pathology has proven benefits for avascular necrosis treatment and its use may be justified for other hip pathologies, such as chondral lesions, based on its potential benefits and favorable preliminary reports. The procedure is simple to perform and has minimal risks and is a promising alternative to established approaches, given the catastrophic consequences of failed treatment of chondral lesions in young patients.

Our Treatment of Choice

In our clinical practice, the treatment of choice for hip chondral lesions is the use of a platelet-rich plasma clot and MCC over the microfractured area (Fig. 69.2). The surgical technique, described below, has led to excellent results, with restoration of the glycosaminoglycan concentration of the regenerated tissue as demonstrated by MRI imaging with dGEMRIC (Delayed Enhanced Magnetic Resonance Imaging Gadolium of Cartilage) sequences (Fig. 69.2f, g).

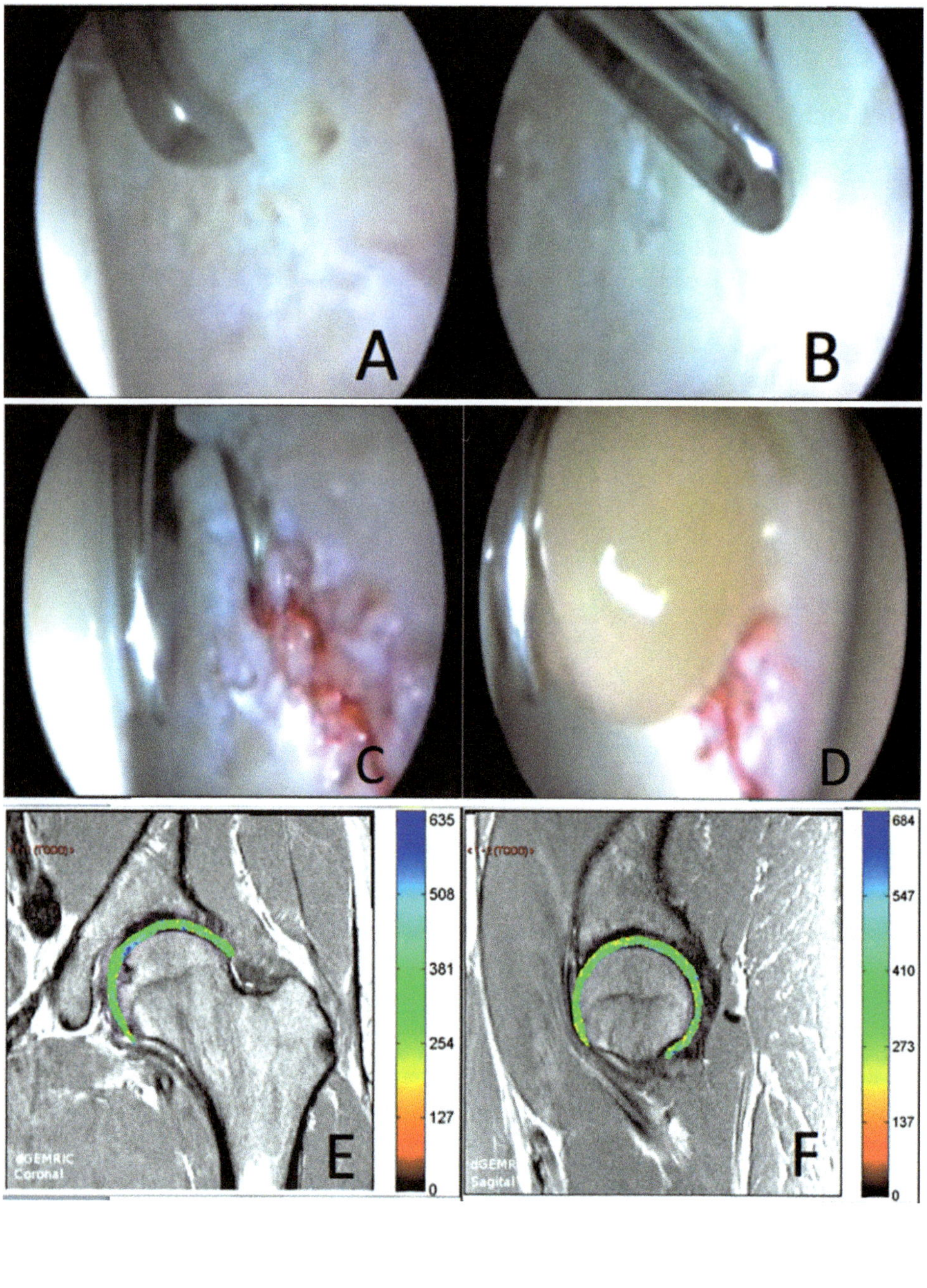

Fig. 69.2 Hip chondral lesions: Surgical alternatives and novel technique with platelet-rich plasma and mononuclear cells concentrate. (**a**) and (**b**): Standard alternatives for hip chondral lesions. (**a**) Microfracture. (**b**) Chondral flap resection. (**c**): Novel Surgical Technique. Insertion of the slotted cannula and position of the needle facing the chondral lesion. (**d**) The PRP clot is positioned over the microfractured area and a mononuclear cells concentrate is instilled under it. (**e**) and (**f**): dGEMRIC images at 6 months postop of the same patient, in which an homogeneous captation of gadolinium is observed meaning the restoration of glycosaminoglycan content

Surgical Technique (Fig. 69.2)

After rim trimming and labrum refixation, the status of the remaining cartilage is assessed. If a chondral lesion exists (>2 cm^2), we prepare a mesenchymal stem cell concentrate (average 14 millions of nucleated cells/cc^3) by harvesting 2–4 cc of bone marrow and processing it with centrifugation. At the same time, 4 cc of PRP (6–9×)) is prepared by centrifuging 50 cc of peripheral blood twice, in readiness for activation with autologous thrombin. Treatment of the chondral lesion is made as described by Steadman in the knee, with debridement of all remaining unstable cartilage, followed for the removal of the calcified plate. After preparation of the bed, multiple holes in the exposed subchondral bone plate are made, leaving about 3–4 mm between each (Fig. 69.2a). Once the microfracture is complete, traction is released and a femoral osteoplasty is performed, obtaining free range of motion with no abnormal contact between acetabular rim and femoral neck–head junction. At the end of the procedure, traction is reapplied and we proceed to the final part of the procedure. After activation of platelet-rich plasma and clot formation, a slotted cannula is inserted via the anterior portal. Platelet-rich plasma clot is inserted through the cannula and positioned over the microfractured area (Fig. 69.2d, e). A 21-gauge trocar is then inserted through the previously located clot and autologous bone marrow. The mesenchymal stem cells concentrate is introduced into the hip beneath the PRP clot. Traction is then released and the procedure is finished.

Rehabilitation protocol: Passive motion device is maintained for 8 h a day. Two crutches with partial weight bearing are indicated for 6–8 weeks. Progressive physical activities are allowed.

Conclusions

Large hip chondral lesions represent a treatment challenge using arthroscopy due to localization and the spherical form of the joint, limiting the use of other methods that require direct visualization. Approaches to this problem are most commonly limited to excision, debridement, thermal chondroplasty, and microfracture.

A novel treatment for chondral lesions of the hip is under investigation by the authors. This involves the administration of a mesenchymal stem cell concentrate harvested from autologous bone marrow, in combination with a platelet-rich plasma clot derived from the patient's own peripheral blood. This may be an effective approach to promote the repair of articular cartilage defects of the hip. Further study is currently underway to identify medium and long-term effects in terms of patient outcomes and cartilage regeneration.

References

1. Yen YM, Kocher MS. Chondral lesions of the hip: microfracture and chondroplasty. Sports Med Arthrosc. 2010;18(2):83–9.
2. Ganz R, Parvizi J, Beck M, et al. Femoroacetabular impingement: a cause for osteoarthritis of the hip. Clin Orthop Relat Res. 2003;417:112–20.
3. Johnston TL, Schenker ML, Briggs KK, Philippon MJ. Relationship between offset angle alpha and hip chondral injury in femoroacetabular impingement. Arthroscopy. 2008;24(6):669–75.
4. Nepple JJ, Carlisle JC, Nunley RM, et al. Clinical and radiographic predictors of intra-articular hip disease in arthroscopy. Am J Sports Med. 2011;39(2):296–303.
5. Outerbridge RE. The etiology of chondromalacia patellae. J Bone Joint Surg (Br). 1961;43:752–7.
6. Konan S, Rayan F, Meermans G, et al. Validation of the classification system for acetabular chondral lesions identified at arthroscopy in patients with femoroacetabular impingement. J Bone Joint Surg (Br). 2011;93(3):332–6.
7. Kaplan LD, Chu CR, Bradley JP, Fu FH, Studer RK. Recovery of chondrocyte metabolic activity after thermal exposure. Am J Sports Med. 2003;31(3):392–8.
8. Lotto ML, Wright EJ, Appleby D, Zelicof SB, Lemos MJ, Lubowitz JH. Ex vivo comparison of mechanical versus thermal chondroplasty: assessment of tissue effect at the surgical endpoint. Arthroscopy. 2008;24(4):410–5.
9. Edwards RB, Lu Y, Cole BJ, Muir P, Markel MD. Comparison of radiofrequency treatment and mechanical debridement of fibrillated cartilage in an equine model. Vet Comp Orthop Traumatol. 2008;21(1):41–8.
10. Voss JR, Lu Y, Edwards RB, Bogdanske JJ, Markel MD. Effects of thermal energy on chondrocyte viability. Am J Vet Res. 2006;67(10):1708–12.
11. Safran MR, Hariri, S, Smith, L, Truntzer, J. Are acetabular chondral flaps worth repairing? A biochemical assessment. 8th Annual meeting ISAKOS, Rio de Janeiro, 15–19 May 2011.
12. Tzaveas AP, Villar RN. Arthroscopic repair of acetabular chondral delamination with fibrin adhesive. Hip Int. 2010;20(1):115–9.
13. Frisbie DD, Oxford JT, Southwood L, Trotter GW, Rodkey WG, Steadman JR, Goodnight JL, McIlwraith CW. Early events in cartilage repair after subchondral bone microfracture. Clin Orthop Relat Res. 2003;407:215–27.
14. Steadman JR, Rodkey WG, Rodrigo JJ. Microfracture: surgical technique and rehabilitation to treat chondral defects. Clin Orthop Relat Res. 2001;(391 Suppl):S362–9.
15. Steadman JR, Rodkey WG, Briggs KK. Microfracture to treat full-thickness chondral defects: surgical technique, rehabilitation, and outcomes. J Knee Surg. 2002;15(3):170–6.
16. Philippon MJ, Schenker ML, Briggs KK, Maxwell RB. Can microfracture produce repair tissue in acetabular chondral defects? Arthroscopy. 2008;24(1):46–50.
17. Davis VL, Abukabda AB, Radio NM, Witt-Enderby PA, Clafshenkel WP, Cairone JV, Rutkowski JL. Platelet-rich preparations to improve healing. Part II: platelet activation and enrichment, leukocyte inclusion, and other selection criteria. J Oral Implantol. 2014;40(4):511–21.
18. Davis VL, Abukabda AB, Radio NM, Witt-Enderby PA, Clafshenkel WP, Cairone JV, Rutkowski JL. Platelet-rich preparations to improve healing. Part I: workable options for every size practice. J Oral Implantol. 2014;40(4):500–10.
19. Mascarenhas R, Saltzman BM, Fortier LA, Cole BJ. Role of platelet-rich plasma in articular cartilage injury and disease. J Knee Surg. 2015;28(1):3–10.
20. Anitua E, Andia I, Ardanza B, Nurden P, Nurden AT. Autologous platelets as a source of proteins for healing and tissue regeneration. Thromb Haemost. 2004;91:4–15.

21. Lopez-Vidriero E, Goulding KA, Simon DA, Sanchez M, Johnson DH. The use of platelet-rich plasma in arthroscopy and sports medicine: optimizing the healing environment. Arthroscopy. 2010;26(2):269–78.
22. Anitua E. Plasma rich in growth factors: preliminary results of use in the preparation of future sites for implants. Int J Oral Maxillofac Implants. 1999;14:529–35.
23. Sanchez M, Anitua E, Orive G, Mujika I, Andia I. Platelet-rich therapies in the treatment of orthopaedic sports injuries. Sports Med. 2009;35:1–10.
24. Gosens T, Peerbooms JC, van Laar W, den Oudsten BL. Ongoing positive effect of platelet-rich plasma versus corticosteroid injection in lateral epicondylitis: a double-blind randomized controlled trial with 2-year follow-up. Am J Sports Med. 2011;39(6):1200–8.
25. Filardo G, Kon E, Della Villa S, Vincentelli F, Fornasari PM, Marcacci M. Use of platelet-rich plasma for the treatment of refractory jumper's knee. Int Orthop. 2010;34(6):909–15.
26. Sanchez M, Anitua E, Azofra J, Andia I, Padilla S, Mujika I. Comparison of surgically repaired Achilles tendon tears using platelet-rich fibrin matrices. Am J Sports Med. 2007;35:245–51.
27. Murray MM, Spindler KP, Ballard P, Welch TP, Zurakowski D, Nanney LB. Enhanced histologic repair in a central wound in the anterior cruciate ligament with a collagen-platelet-rich plasma scaffold. J Orthop Res. 2007;25:1007–17.
28. Radice F, Gutierrez V, Ibarra A, Verdugo A. Arthroscopic, histologic and MRI correlation in the maturation process of the graft in ACL reconstruction in humans. Arthroscopy. 1998;14 Suppl 1:S20.
29. Ekdahl M, Wang JH, Ronga M, Fu FH. Graft healing in anterior cruciate ligament reconstruction. Knee Surg Sports Traumatol Arthrosc. 2008;16:935–47.
30. Orrego M, Orrego M, Larrain C, Rosales J, Valenzuela L, Matas J, Durruty J, Sudy H, Mardones R. Effects of platelet concentrate and a bone plug on the healing of hamstring tendons in a bone tunnel. Arthroscopy. 2008;24(12):1373–80.
31. Figueroa D, Melean P, Calvo R, Vaisman A, Zilleruelo N, Figueroa F, Villalón I. Magnetic resonance imaging evaluation of the integration and maturation of semitendinosus-gracilis graft in anterior cruciate ligament reconstruction using autologous platelet concentrate. Arthroscopy. 2010;26(10):1318–25.
32. Barber FA, Hrnack SA, Snyder SJ, Hapa O. Rotator cuff repair healing influenced by platelet-rich plasma construct augmentation. Arthroscopy. 2011;27(8):1029–35.
33. Gamradt SC. Short-term positive effects of platelet-rich plasma in arthroscopic rotator cuff repair. J Bone Joint Surg Am. 2011;93(13):1–3.
34. Rodeo SA, Delos D, Williams RJ, Adler RS, Pearle A, Warren RF. The effect of platelet-rich fibrin matrix on rotator cuff tendon healing: a prospective, randomized clinical study. Am J Sports Med. 2012;40(6):1234–41.
35. Jo CH, Kim JE, Yoon KS, Shin S. Platelet-rich plasma stimulates cell proliferation and enhances matrix gene expression and synthesis in tenocytes from human rotator cuff tendons with degenerative tears. Am J Sports Med. 2012;40(5):1035–45.
36. Kon E, Mandelbaum B, Buda R, Filardo G, Delcogliano M, Timoncini A, Fornasari PM, Giannini S, Marcacci M. Platelet-rich plasma intra-articular injection versus hyaluronic acid viscosupplementation as treatments for cartilage pathology: from early degeneration to osteoarthritis. Arthroscopy. 2011;27(11):1490–501.
37. Sanchez M, Anitua E, Azofra J, Aguirre JJ, Andia I. Intra-articular injection of an autologous preparation rich in growth factors for the treatment of knee OA: a retrospective cohort study. Clin Exp Rheumatol. 2008;26:910–3.
38. Klatt BA, Lopez HH, Segal NA, Chimes GP. Treatment options in knee osteoarthritis: total knee arthroplasty versus platelet-rich plasma. PM R. 2011;3(4):377–86.
39. Sampson S, Reed M, Silvers H, Meng M, Mandelbaum B. Injection of platelet-rich plasma in patients with primary and secondary knee osteoarthritis: a pilot study. Am J Phys Med Rehabil. 2010;89(12):961–9.
40. Dhillon M, Patel S, Bali K. Platelet-rich plasma intra-articular knee injections for the treatment of degenerative cartilage lesions and osteoarthritis. Knee Surg Sports Traumatol Arthrosc. 2011;19(5):863–4.
41. Hartmann EK, Heintel T, Morrison RH, Weckbach A. Influence of platelet-rich plasma on the anterior fusion in spinal injuries: a qualitative and quantitative analysis using computer tomography. Arch Orthop Trauma Surg. 2010;130(7):909–14.
42. Landi A, Tarantino R, Marotta N, Ruggeri AG, Domenicucci M, Giudice L, Martini S, Rastelli M, Ferrazza G, De Luca N, Tomei G, Delfini R. The use of platelet gel in postero-lateral fusion: preliminary results in a series of 14 cases. Eur Spine J. 2011;20 Suppl 1:S61–7.
43. Galasso O, Mariconda M, Romano G, Capuano N, Romano L, Iannò B, Milano C. Expandable intramedullary nailing and platelet rich plasma to treat long bone non-unions. J Orthop Traumatol. 2008;9(3):129–34.
44. Mariconda M, Cozzolino F, Cozzolino A, D'Agostino E, Bove A, Milano C. Platelet gel supplementation in long bone non-unions treated by external fixation. J Orthop Trauma. 2008;22(5):342–5.
45. De Leon JM, Driver VR, Fylling CP, Carter MJ, Anderson C, Wilson J, Dougherty RM, Fuston D, Trigilia D, Valenski V, Rappl LM. The clinical relevance of treating chronic wounds with an enhanced near-physiological concentration of platelet-rich plasma gel. Adv Skin Wound Care. 2011;24(8):357–68.
46. Dougherty EJ. An evidence-based model comparing the cost-effectiveness of platelet-rich plasma gel to alternative therapies for patients with nonhealing diabetic foot ulcers. Adv Skin Wound Care. 2008;21(12):568–75.
47. Mazzocca AD, McCarthy MB, Chowaniec DM, Cote MP, Romeo AA, Bradley JP, Arciero RA, Beitzel K. Platelet-rich plasma differs according to preparation method and human variability. J Bone Joint Surg Am. 2012;94(4):308–16.
48. Tschon M, Fini M, Giardino R, Filardo G, Dallari D, Torricelli P, Martini L, Giavaresi G, Kon E, Maltarello MC, Nicolini A, Carpi A. Lights and shadows concerning platelet products for musculoskeletal regeneration. Front Biosci. 2011;3:96–107.
49. Milano G, Sanna Passino E, Deriu L, Careddu G, Manunta L, Manunta A, Saccomanno MF, Fabbriciani C. The effect of platelet rich plasma combined with microfractures on the treatment of chondral defects: an experimental study in a sheep model. Osteoarthritis Cartilage. 2010;18(7):971–80.
50. Broxmeyer HE. Insights into the biology of cord blood stem/progenitor cells. Cell Prolif. 2011;44 Suppl 1:55–9.
51. Leeb C, Jurga M, McGuckin C, Forraz N, Thallinger C, Moriggl R, Kenner L. New perspectives in stem cell research: beyond embryonic stem cells. Cell Prolif. 2011;44 Suppl 1:9–14.
52. Kimura T, Nakano T. Induction of pluripotency in primordial germ cells. Histol Histopathol. 2011;26(5):643–50.
53. Fong CY, Gauthaman K, Bongso A. Teratomas from pluripotent stem cells: a clinical hurdle. J Cell Biochem. 2010;111(4):769–81.
54. Caplan AI. Adult mesenchymal stem cells for tissue engineering versus regenerative medicine. J Cell Physiol. 2007;213(2):341–7.
55. Feng Y, Yang SH, Xiao BJ, Xu WH, Ye SN, Xia T, Zheng D, Liu XZ, Liao YF. Decreased in the number and function of circulation endothelial progenitor cells in patients with avascular necrosis of the femoral head. Bone. 2010;46(1):32–40.

56. Gangji V, Toungouz M, Hauzeur JP. Stem cell therapy for osteonecrosis of the femoral head. Expert Opin Biol Ther. 2005;5(4): 437–42.
57. Hernigou P, Beaujean F. Treatment of osteonecrosis with autologous bone marrow grafting. Clin Orthop Relat Res. 2002;405: 14–23.
58. Gobbi A, Karnatzikos G, Scotti C, Mahajan V, Mazzucco L, Grigolo B. One-step cartilage repair with bone marrow aspirate concentrated cells and collagen matrix in full-thickness knee cartilage lesions: results at 2-year follow-up. Cartilage. 2011;2: 286–99.
59. de Girolamo L, Bertolini G, Cervellin M, Sozzi G, Volpi P. Treatment of chondral defects of the knee with one step matrix-assisted technique enhanced by autologous concentrated bone marrow: in vitro characterisation of mesenchymal stem cells from iliac crest and subchondral bone. Injury. 2010;41(11):1172–7.
60. Haleem AH, El Singergy AA, Sabry D, Atta HM, Rashed LA, Chu CR, El Shewy MT, Azzam A, Abdel Aziz MT. The clinical use of human culture–expanded autologous bone marrow mesenchymal stem cells transplanted on platelet-rich fibrin glue in the treatment of articular cartilage defects: a pilot study and preliminary results. Cartilage. 2010;4:253–61.
61. McIlwraith CW, Frisbie DD, Rodkey WG, Kisiday JD, Werpy NM, Kawcak CE, Steadman JR. Evaluation of intra-articular mesenchymal stem cells to augment healing of microfractured chondral defects. Arthroscopy. 2011;27(11):1552–61.

Osteochondral Allografting of the Hip

70

Simon Görtz and William D. Bugbee

Introduction

Recent advances in hip arthroscopy and cartilage imaging have led to increased understanding and acceptance of the concept of femoroacetabular impingement [1, 2], which in turn has fueled an emerging trend toward biological restoration and hip preservation as an alternative to prosthetic joint replacement. Although total hip arthroplasty remains the gold standard treatment for end-stage osteoarthritis and failure endpoint in most clinical studies, longevity concerns make it a reluctant choice in an exceedingly active and actively aging patient population. The focus of treatment has thus been shifted to correcting morphological conflicts and addressing focal chondral or osteochondral lesions to prevent disease progression to end-stage joint degeneration.

Over the last four decades, the use of osteochondral transplants has established itself as a viable option for biological reconstruction in diarthrodial joints, addressing a wide spectrum of osteochondral conditions [3–11]. Fresh osteochondral allografts are composite grafts consisting of a viable mature hyaline cartilage portion anchored to a nonviable subchondral bone portion. This forms a structural and functional osteoarticular unit that may replace a corresponding segment of a recipient joint in the face of disease or injury. Although multiple studies have reported encouraging results for osteochondral allografting in the knee [12–16], studies involving the hip are not yet sufficiently robust to allow absolute conclusions to be drawn regarding best practices. While indications for the use of this approach in the hip continue to evolve, many of the technique points in this chapter have been extrapolated from the literature relating to allografting in the knee [17].

S. Görtz, MD
Washington University Orthopedics, Sports Medicine Campus, Box 8233/OC, 14532 S. Outer Forty Drive, MO 63017, USA

Orthopaedic Surgery, Sports Medicine, Washington University in St. Louis, Chesterfield, MO, USA

W.D. Bugbee, MD (✉)
Division of Orthopaedics, Scripps Clinic, University of California, San Diego, 10666 North Torrey Pines Rd, La Jolla, CA 92037, USA
e-mail: bugbee.william@scrippshealth.org

Graft Acquisition and Storage

Recovery, processing, and testing of donor tissue follow guidelines established by the American Association of Tissue Banks (AATB) and are under supreme authority of the Food and Drug Administration (FDA) [18, 19]. Most tissue banks have a 24-h time limit for retrieval of tissue from refrigerated cadaveric donors. Of those, donors between the ages of 15 and 35 years are generally considered for inclusion in the donor pool if their articular surfaces pass a visual and tactile inspection for cartilage quality. Donor tissue is generally recovered using aseptic technique and cleansed with saline pulse lavage. This may not prevent or remove all contamination and thus the graft tissue should not be considered sterile. Strict and consistent adherence to tissue-banking standards and transplantation protocols is important, and these criteria ensure, but do not guarantee, the availability of tissues of acceptable quality for implantation.

Common to all allografting procedures is matching the donor with the recipient on the basis of size. In the hip, an AP radiograph with a standardized magnification marker is generally used in combination with advanced imaging such as CT or MR to measure the diameter of the femoral head. This measurement is accurately adjusted for magnification, and the tissue bank makes a direct caliper measurement on the donor femoral head. A match is considered acceptable at ±1 mm; however, it should be noted that there is a possible variability in morphology, which is not necessarily reflected in simple measurements that assume sphericity of the head. The surgeon is responsible for inspecting the tissue intended for transplantation, optimally before beginning the actual procedure. This should include affirming graft size, ascertaining

J.C. McCarthy et al. (eds.), *Hip Joint Restoration*, DOI 10.1007/978-1-4614-0694-5_70

integrity of the tissue as well as its packaging, and adequacy of storage and refrigeration.

Federal law requires donor screening for infectious diseases, a process that regularly includes detailed medical histories and physical examinations of donor bodies as well as serological and bacteriological testing. Osteochondral allograft tissue is aseptically procured, but not sterilized, which reduces but does not eliminate the risk of graft contamination during recovery, via postmortem invasion by the gastrointestinal flora or occult infection in the donor. With any transplantation of allogeneic organs or tissue, there is a residual risk of transmission of infectious disease, despite donor screening and testing, and rare allograft-associated bacterial infections have been reported. Advances in serological testing for HIV, hepatitis, etc. have improved the safety of allograft tissue, but a minute risk does remain. As both the surgeon and the patient should be well aware of the risk for the transmission of serious disease when using allograft tissue, the risk of bacterial or viral disease transmission should be discussed as an essential part of the informed consent process. Unfortunately, there are no available published data quantifying the risk of disease transmission from allogeneic tissues. In the 40-year experience at our institution, utilizing almost 1000 fresh allografts, there have been no documented cases of transmission of disease from donor to recipient.

Indications

While several restorative options for biomimetic replacement in acquired articular cartilage defects do exist, allografts currently remain the only treatment option that restores mature orthotopic hyaline cartilage in acquired articular cartilage defects. Due to their osteoarticular nature, fresh allografts are uniquely suited to treat a wide variety of articular and osteoarticular pathology, including large compound osteochondral lesions.

Current indications for osteochondral allografting in the hip include symptomatic lesions with limited head involvement that have not responded to other treatments. These include:

- Osteochondritis dissecans of the hip.
- Highly selected cases of focal osteonecrosis (stage II or III with a small necrotic segment) (Fig. 70.1).
- Osteochondral fractures with or without traumatic hip dislocation.
- Cystic lesions in early hip osteoarthritis.

Concomitant pathology, such as femoroacetabular impingement, must be addressed at the time of cartilage repair surgery. Patients should be of an age and activity level that are not optimally suited for total hip arthroplasty, and present with focal lesions lacking irreversible global osteoarthritic changes. The presence of inflammatory arthritis is a contraindication to osteochondral allografting in the hip.

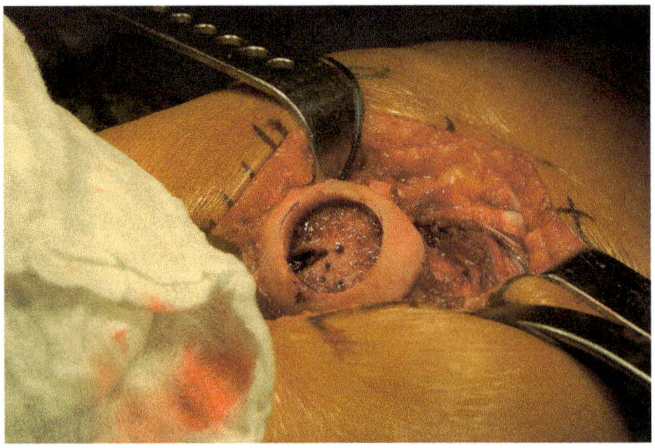

Fig. 70.1 Prepared graft recipient site. Note the minimal depth of resection, with drilled perforation of sclerotic subchondral areas and a curetted segmental defect

Surgical Technique

Osteochondral allografting of the hip relies on a surgical dislocation of the hip joint with a stepped “flip” trochanteric osteotomy, as has been discussed in detail elsewhere [20]. After the femoral head has thus been exposed, the symptomatic lesion is identified. There are several similar proprietary instrumentation systems that are currently available for the preparation and press fit implantation of circular dowel allografts of up to 35 mm in diameter. A size determination of the treated lesion is made after a guide wire has been driven into the center of the lesion, perpendicular to the curvature of the articular surface. The size of the proposed graft then is determined utilizing sizing dowels, remembering that overlapping dowels (in a “snowman” configuration) can possibly deliver the best area fit. The remaining articular cartilage is scored to the calcified layer to prevent fraying of adjacent cartilage, and a core reamer is used to remove the remaining articular cartilage and at least 3–4 mm of subchondral bone (Fig. 70.2). If multiple overlapping grafts are used, varying the thickness of the individual plugs can add rotational stability to the final graft construct. In deeper lesions, fibrous tissue and sclerotic bone are removed until a healthy, bleeding osseous base is exposed, usually at a depth of less than 10 mm (Fig. 70.1). More extensive osseous lesions should be manually curetted and later packed with morselized autologous bone graft salvaged from the reamings. Sclerotic subchondral bone can be perforated using a drill to invite bleeding. The guide pin then is removed, and circumferential depth measurements are made of the prepared recipient site (Fig. 70.3).

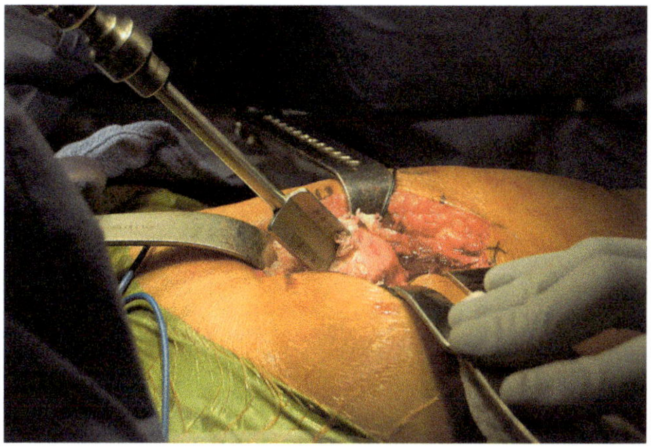

Fig. 70.2 Intraoperative view of a right hip after successful surgical dislocation, exposing the femoral head. After the appropriate graft diameter has been determined, the lesion is reamed with a corresponding core reamer

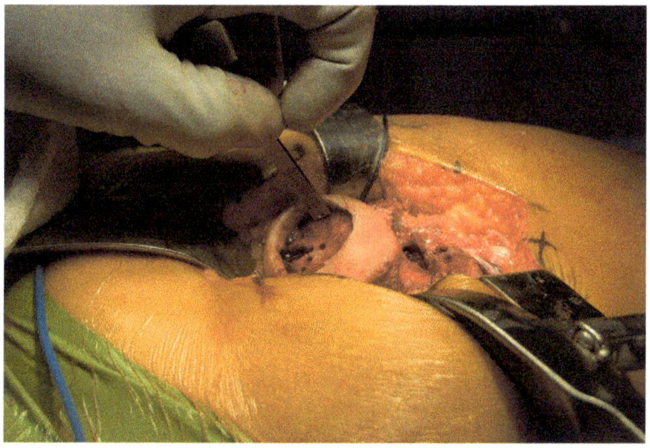

Fig. 70.3 Depth of the prepared graft bed is measured in four quadrants. Measurements are recorded and templated onto the allograft core

The corresponding orthotopic location of the recipient site then is identified on the femoral head allograft. The graft is placed into a graft holder (or alternately, held securely with bone-holding forceps). A saw guide then is placed in the corresponding position and alignment, again perpendicular to the articular surface; and an appropriate sized tube saw is used to core out the graft under continuous irrigation (Fig. 70.4). Prior to removing the graft dowel from the donor femoral head, an identifying mark is made with a surgical pen as a reference for rotational orientation. Once the graft cylinder is amputated using an oscillating saw (Fig. 70.5) and removed, depth measurements, which were taken from the recipient, are transferred to the bony portion of the graft. This graft then is cut with an oscillating saw (Fig. 70.6) and trimmed with a rasp to the appropriate thickness in all four quadrants. Often, this must be repeated multiple times, to ensure precise thickness, preferably refashioning the graft rather than the recipient site and

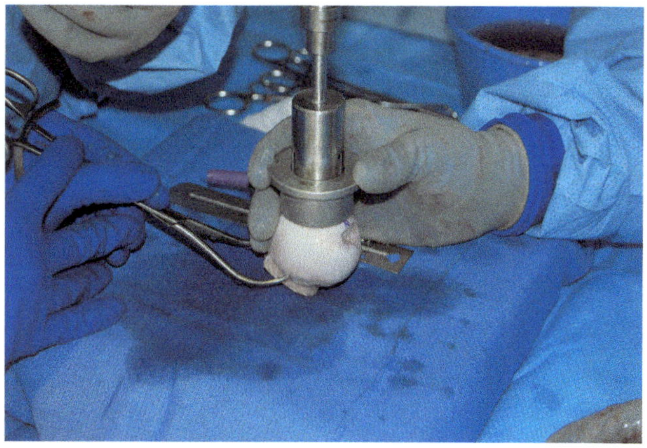

Fig. 70.4 The saw guide is positioned on the corresponding, orthotopic area of the allograft femoral head, and a cylindrical osteochondral core is generated under irrigation

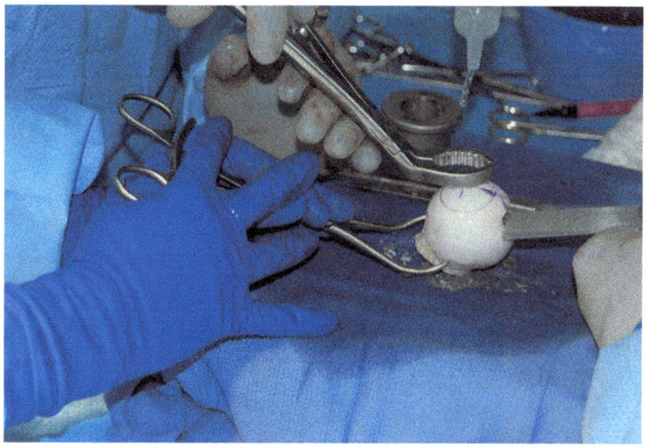

Fig. 70.5 The osteochondral allograft dowel is removed using the oscillating saw

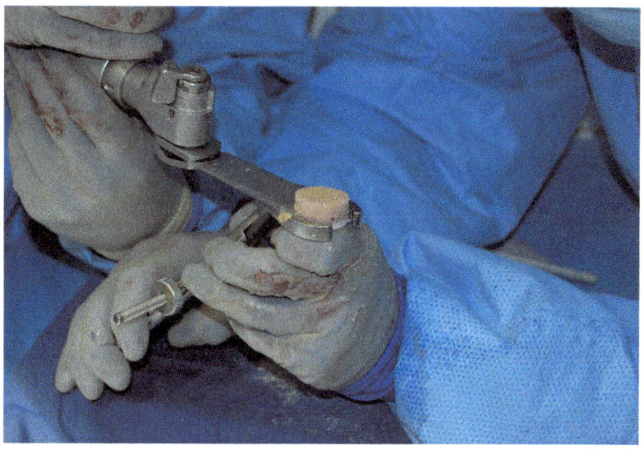

Fig. 70.6 The allograft dowel is trimmed to the templated thickness

optimally keeping the allograft and host cartilage moist throughout the procedure. The deep edges of the bone plug are then beveled with a rongeur or bone rasp to ease insertion (Fig. 70.7).

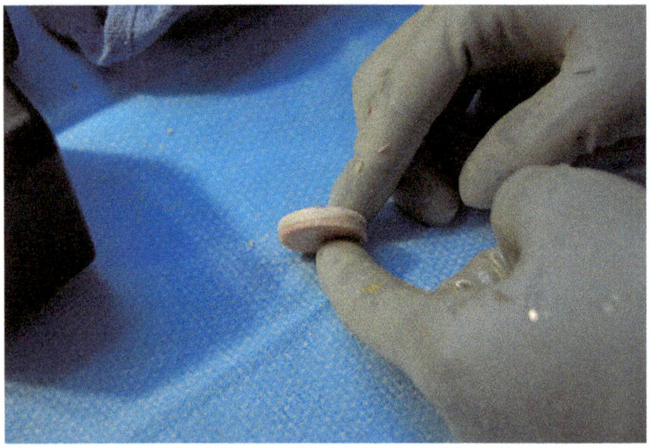

Fig. 70.7 The prepared osteochondral allograft dowel. Note the minimal bone thickness in relationship to the overlying cartilage

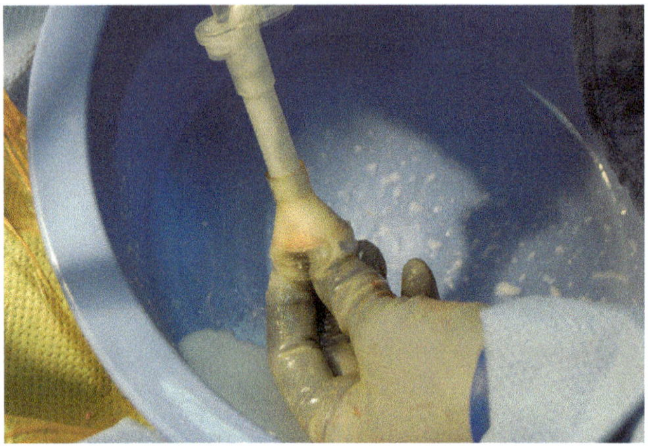

Fig. 70.8 Copious pulsatile lavage is employed to remove marrow elements and debris from the allograft dowel

The graft is then irrigated copiously with a high-pressure pulsatile lavage system to remove marrow elements and debris (Fig. 70.8). The recipient site can be dilated using a slightly oversized tamp in order to ease the insertion of the graft to prevent excessive impact loading of the articular surface when the graft is inserted (Fig. 70.9). At this point, any remaining osseous defects are bone grafted, as described above (Fig. 70.10). The allograft is then inserted by hand in the appropriate rotation. In case of a line-to-line fit, it is often possible to seat the graft with gentle manual pressure only. Alternatively, a cupped mallet can be used to gently tamp the graft into place until it is flush, again minimizing mechanical insult to the articular surface of both the native and graft tissues.

Once the graft is seated, a determination is made whether additional fixation is required. Typically, bioabsorbable pins are utilized, particularly if the graft is large or multiple dowels have been employed. Once it is confirmed that the graft is stable and congruent (Fig. 70.11), the wound is irrigated copiously, and, if no further adjunct procedures are planned, routine closure is performed.

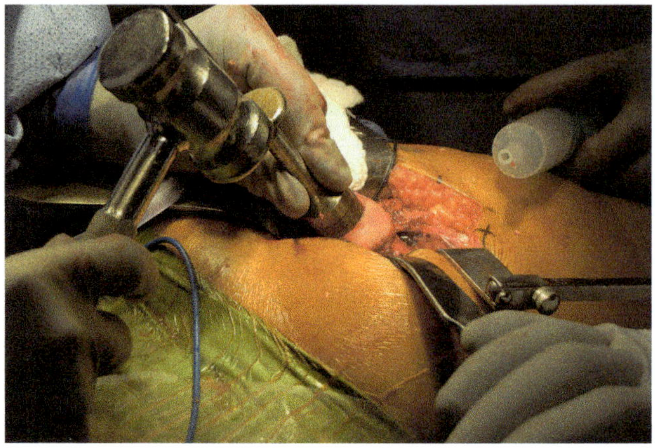

Fig. 70.9 The recipient site is slowly expanded using a dilator to ease insertion of the graft and facilitate press fit

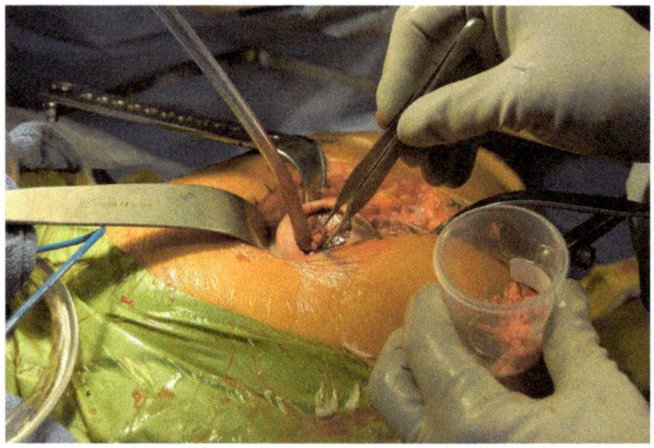

Fig. 70.10 Residual osseous defects of the graft bed are bone grafted with autologous bone reamings prior to implantation of the graft

Postoperatively, patients generally are maintained in a toe-touch-only weight-bearing status for 8–12 weeks or until radiographic evidence of graft incorporation and healing of the trochanteric osteotomy. Full range of motion is usually allowed, unless there are other additional reconstructive procedures, such as a labral repair, that would alter the rehabilitation plan. Closed-chain exercises are introduced at 4 weeks and return to unrestricted activities of daily living by 3–4 months. Appropriate sports and recreation can be reintroduced 6 months postoperatively once functional rehabilitation is complete, usually with impact loading restrictions.

Clinical Outcomes

The published literature on osteochondral allografting of the hip is sparse, comprising a total of only five published papers. The concept of osteochondral allografting of the hip was initially introduced by Meyers et al. in 1983, when they published

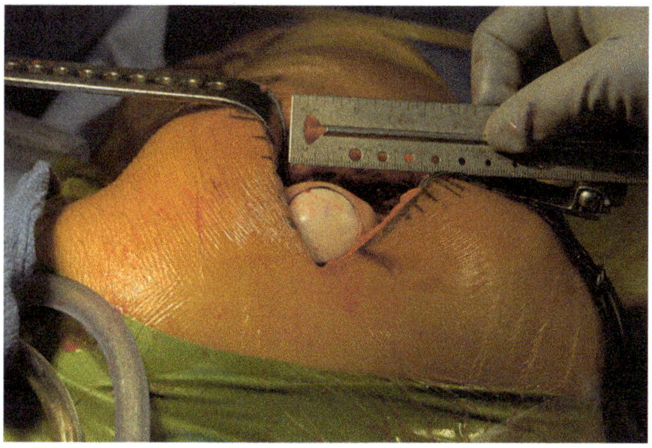

Fig. 70.11 The implanted graft in situ. Please note the surface congruency to the surrounding cartilage, and press fit without additional fixation

their results of allografting for osteonecrosis of the femoral head with segmental collapse [21]. Their technique involved implanting 5 mm thick osteoarticular allografts with morselized bone graft through a posterior approach. Failure in this study was defined as symptomatic collapse of the allograft and/or conversion to total hip arthroplasty. They reported successful outcomes in 15 of the 21 studied hips (71 %) after a follow-up of 18 months. The success rate in patients with steroid-associated osteonecrosis, however, was only 50 %. They concluded that osteochondral allografting is a viable treatment option for nonsteroid induced osteonecrosis of the femoral head.

Evans and Providence published a case report describing the use of an osteochondral allograft in a single case of a traumatic osteochondral lesion in the weight-bearing area of the femoral head of a 32-year-old man [22]. They used a 12-mm thick allograft dowel via a trochanteric osteotomy. At 1-year follow-up, the Harris Hip Score had improved from 69 preoperatively to 94 points, and the patient had full, painless hip range of motion.

Kosashvili et al. reported results of fresh stored osteochondral allografts for symptomatic osteochondral lesions in eight consecutive patients [23]. Their cohort included four cases of osteochondritis dissecans, three cases of osteonecrosis, and one osteochondral fracture without dislocation. All operations involved dowel grafts that were performed via modified trochanteric osteotomy and surgical dislocation. The average age of their patients was 24 years, with an average follow-up of 41 months. The average Harris hip scores improved from 58 points preoperatively to 84 points at latest follow-up. One patient was converted to a total hip arthroplasty due to disease progression and worsening symptoms. One case of graft subsidence was addressed with a successful repeat transplantation. One patient required hardware removal of her trochanteric fixation due to persistent irritation. Overall, seven of eight symptomatic patients did not require conversion to THA after an average follow-up of 3.5 years.

These eight patients were part of a follow-up study published by Khanna et al., who reported on long-term results of fresh osteochondral allografting of the femoral head in 17 patients followed prospectively [24]. Eight of these patients were treated for osteochondritis dissecans, six had osteonecrosis of the femoral head, two had Legg-Calve-Perthes, and one a traumatic femoral head fracture. All patients underwent surgical hip dislocation with a trochanteric slide osteotomy for placement of a dowel allograft. The mean age at surgery was 25.9 years and the mean follow-up was 41.6 months. They noted significant improvement in the mean Harris hip score postoperatively ($p<0.01$), and 13 of 17 patients had fair to good outcomes. One patient required a repeat allograft, and a total of three patients underwent or were awaiting hip replacement. Of note, these three cases included both Perthes patients and a patient with steroid-associated osteonecrosis who remained on high-dose corticosteroid therapy after her osteochondral transplantation. The authors of both studies concluded that osteochondral allograft transplantation is a viable treatment option for femoral head defects in young patients.

Krych et al. reported on management of osteochondral defects of the acetabulum in two patients [25]. They used an open dislocation and dowel grafts procured from a donor acetabulum in one case, and from a medial tibial plateau allograft in the other. They noted that the medial tibial plateau provided improved congruence. Both grafts were press fit without supplemental fixation. MRIs performed 12 months (patient 1) and 18 months (patient 2) postoperatively demonstrated incorporation of the osteochondral allograft to the host bone with maintenance of joint congruity in both cases. At 24 months in patient 1 and 42 months in patient 2, radiographs showed absence of progressive joint space narrowing compared to preoperative radiographs. Modified Harris Hip Scores improved in both patients, from 75 preoperatively to 97 at 2-year follow-up in patient 1, and from 79 preoperatively to 100 at the time of 3-year follow-up in patient 2, while Hip Outcome Score subsets for activities of daily living and sports score were 100 points each. Their observations in these cases suggest osteochondral allograft transplantation may be an appropriate alternative to consider when treating osteochondral defects of the acetabulum in young and active patients.

Summary and Future Outlook

While fresh osteochondral allografts have application in the treatment of a wide spectrum of articular pathology, the indications with respect to their use as a primary treatment of focal femoral head and acetabular lesions are still evolving, and should be limited to carefully selected patients with thorough consideration of mechanical and biological contraindication. The operative procedure for most osteochondral lesions is straightforward but demands precision to achieve reproducible results and to minimize early graft failures related to surgical technique. Many clinical and basic scientific studies support the theoretical foundation and efficacy of small fragment allografting, although more scientific validation of empirical clinical practice is still needed to verify the long-term durability of osteochondral allograft transplantation in the hip joint.

References

1. Apprich S, et al. Evaluation of articular cartilage in patients with femoroacetabular impingement (FAI) using T2* mapping at different time points at 3.0 Tesla MRI: a feasibility study. Skeletal Radiol. 2012;41(8):987–95.
2. Philippon MJ, et al. Outcomes following hip arthroscopy for femoroacetabular impingement with associated chondrolabral dysfunction: minimum two-year follow-up. J Bone Joint Surg (Br). 2009;91(1):16–23.
3. Shasha N, et al. Long-term follow-up of fresh tibial osteochondral allografts for failed tibial plateau fractures. J Bone Joint Surg Am. 2003;85-A Suppl 2:33–9.
4. Emmerson BC, et al. Fresh osteochondral allografting in the treatment of osteochondritis dissecans of the femoral condyle. Am J Sports Med. 2007;35(6):907–14.
5. Gross AE, et al. Fresh osteochondral allografts for posttraumatic knee defects: long-term followup. Clin Orthop Relat Res. 2008;466(8):1863–70.
6. Provencher MT, et al. Anatomic osteochondral glenoid reconstruction for recurrent glenohumeral instability with glenoid deficiency using a distal tibia allograft. Arthroscopy. 2009;25(4):446–52.
7. Görtz S, De Young AJ, Bugbee WD. Fresh osteochondral allografting for osteochondral lesions of the talus. Foot Ankle Int. 2010;31(4):283–90.
8. Görtz S, De Young AJ, Bugbee WD. Fresh osteochondral allografting for steroid-associated osteonecrosis of the femoral condyles. Clin Orthop Relat Res. 2010;468(5):1269–78.
9. Bugbee WD, et al. Bipolar fresh osteochondral allografting of the tibiotalar joint. J Bone Joint Surg Am. 2013;95(5):426–32.
10. Gracitelli GC, et al. Fresh osteochondral allograft transplantation for isolated patellar cartilage injury. Am J Sports Med. 2015;43(4):879–84.
11. Meric G, et al. Fresh osteochondral allograft transplantation for bipolar reciprocal osteochondral lesions of the knee. Am J Sports Med. 2015;43(3):709–14.
12. Levy YD, et al. Do fresh osteochondral allografts successfully treat femoral condyle lesions? Clin Orthop Relat Res. 2013;471(1):231–7.
13. Bugbee WD. Fresh osteochondral allografts. J Knee Surg. 2002;15(3):191–5.
14. McCulloch PC, et al. Prospective evaluation of prolonged fresh osteochondral allograft transplantation of the femoral condyle: minimum 2-year follow-up. Am J Sports Med. 2007;35(3):411–20.
15. LaPrade RF, et al. Refrigerated osteoarticular allografts to treat articular cartilage defects of the femoral condyles. A prospective outcomes study. J Bone Joint Surg Am. 2009;91(4):805–11.
16. Raz G, et al. Distal femoral fresh osteochondral allografts: follow-up at a mean of twenty-two years. J Bone Joint Surg Am. 2014;96(13):1101–7.
17. Görtz S, Bugbee WD. Allografts in articular cartilage repair. J Bone Joint Surg Am. 2006;88(6):1374–84.
18. Food and Drug Administration. Guidance for industry: screening and testing of donors of human tissues intended for transplantation. http://www.fda.gov/. Accessed 1 Mar 2006
19. Görtz S, Bugbee WD. Fresh osteochondral allografts: graft processing and clinical applications. J Knee Surg. 2006;19(3):231–40.
20. Ganz R, et al. Surgical dislocation of the adult hip a technique with full access to the femoral head and acetabulum without the risk of avascular necrosis. J Bone Joint Surg (Br). 2001;83(8):1119–24.
21. Meyers MH, et al. Fresh autogenous grafts and osteochondral allografts for the treatment of segmental collapse in osteonecrosis of the hip. Clin Orthop Relat Res. 1983;174:107–12.
22. Evans KN, Providence BC. Case report: fresh-stored osteochondral allograft for treatment of osteochondritis dissecans the femoral head. Clin Orthop Relat Res. 2010;468(2):613–8.
23. Kosashvili Y, et al. Fresh-stored osteochondral allografts for the treatment of femoral head defects: surgical technique and preliminary results. Int Orthop. 2013;37(6):1001–6.
24. Khanna V, et al. Cartilage restoration of the hip using fresh osteochondral allograft: resurfacing the potholes. Bone Joint J. 2014;96-B(11 Supple A):11–6.
25. Krych AJ, Lorich DG, Kelly BT. Treatment of focal osteochondral defects of the acetabulum with osteochondral allograft transplantation. Orthopedics. 2011;34(7):e307–11.

Part X

Hip Osteotomies

Richard F. Santore

Special Patients and Conditions: Acetabular Dysplasia

71

Cara Beth Lee and Young-Jo Kim

Background

Acetabular dysplasia (AD) is a hip condition in which the weight-bearing surface of the acetabulum is shallow and steeply oriented. The femoral head is insufficiently supported, which results in shear forces to the acetabular rim and labrum [1] that can lead to premature osteoarthritis (OA). AD affects females 4–5 times more frequently than males [2, 3] and has a familial predisposition. Acetabular dysplasia may be a sequela of childhood developmental dysplasia of the hip (DDH) [4] or it may present in adolescence or early adulthood in patients with no history of infantile hip disease [5].

An association between acetabular dysplasia and OA has been recognized for decades. In 1939, Wiberg described the center-edge (CE) angle as a method to quantify acetabular deformity [6]. He noted that low femoral head coverage and subluxation had a linear correlation with earlier development of OA. Subsequent authors similarly observed acetabular dysplasia in 25–50 % of patients with idiopathic osteoarthritis [2–4]. Recently, a retrospective evaluation determined that acetabular dysplasia was the predisposing factor for OA in 48 % of patients who had total hip arthroplasty (THA) under age 50 [7]. Although dysplasia is linked to OA, it remains unclear which hips are at risk for early failure. In a series that followed the contralateral hip in 286 patients after THA, no patient with a CE angle less than 16° and acetabular roof index greater than 15° reached age 65 with a well-functioning hip [8]. In contrast, a radiographic review of patients with CE angles less than 20° in the absence of subluxation found no parameters that were predictive for rapid progression of OA [9].

Several pelvic osteotomies have been developed to reorient the acetabulum in patients with symptomatic acetabular dysplasia. Although they are technically complex, these procedures can dramatically improve the quality of life in well-selected patients. They aim to reposition the acetabular weight-bearing zone, increase femoral head coverage, and improve stability without introducing femoroacetabular impingement (FAI). The primary goal is to normalize hip mechanics in an effort to resolve symptoms and potentially prolong the longevity of the native hip.

Good results have been reported at mid- to long-term follow-up in patients with minimal arthrosis at the time of surgery [10–12], even in those previously considered to be at risk for failure, such as older patients [13–15] and those with severe preoperative pain [11].

Patient Evaluation

History and Physical Examination

The majority of patients with acetabular dysplasia present with insidious onset of groin or lateral hip pain that is exacerbated with activities [16]. Lateral pain and "giving way" episodes are due to abductor muscle weakness and fatigue; groin pain may be associated with labral pathology. Patients often report clicking or popping in the hip that is typically from extra-articular sources, such as the iliopsoas tendon as it moves over the iliopectineal eminence or the iliotibial band at the greater trochanter.

In addition to a baseline examination of stance, gait, and hip motion, there are several tests to screen for impingement, instability, and abductor function. The anterior impingement test is performed by flexing the hip to 90°, combined with adduction and internal rotation. In this test, the femoral head-neck junction compresses structures at the anterior rim and is considered positive if the patient experiences groin pain with

C.B. Lee, MD (✉)
Department of Orthopaedics, Center for Hip Preservation, Virginia Mason Medical Center, 925 Seneca Street, Lindeman Pavilion, Level 6, Seattle, WA 98111, USA
e-mail: carabeth.lee@vmmc.org

Y.-J. Kim, MD, PhD
Child and Young Adult Hip Preservation Program, Department of Orthopaedics, Boston Children's Hospital, Harvard School of Medicine, Boston, MA, USA

J.C. McCarthy et al. (eds.), *Hip Joint Restoration*, DOI 10.1007/978-1-4614-0694-5_71

the maneuver. The test is nonspecific, but is often positive if there is damage to the acetabular rim or labrum [1, 17]. It should be noted however than any anterior structure will be compressed by this maneuver, and, if irritated (such as iliopsoas bursitis), will also provoke a positive test. In a report of clinical findings in patients with acetabular dysplasia, 97 % had a positive impingement sign, nearly 50 % had a limp, and 40 % had a positive Trendelenburg sign [16]. Steppacher et al. found that a preoperative limp and positive anterior impingement test were associated with worse outcome after periacetabular osteotomy (PAO), likely due to more advanced articular damage [11].

The apprehension test assesses anterior stability and rim damage in the hip [18]. The contralateral hip is hyperflexed to the chest, while the affected hip being tested is passively extended beyond neutral, combined with extension, abduction, and external rotation. In this position, the anteriorly directed femoral head stresses the anterior rim structures. The test is positive if the patient experiences apprehension or anterior hip pain. Discomfort in the posterior hip or buttock may be indicative of posterior impingement.

The bicycle test can detect subtle abductor weakness or insufficiency [18]. Lying on his or her side with the upper leg in slight abduction, the patient simulates a bicycle-riding motion as the examiner applies downward resistance at the mid-thigh. The test is positive test if the patient experiences discomfort in the groin, lateral hip, or focal tenderness at the posterior greater trochanter. The side-lying position is the most valid and reliable to perform manual assessment of hip abductor strength [19].

It can often be challenging to distinguish intra- and periarticular sources of hip pain. In-office ultrasound [20] with differential injections can be a valuable extension of the physical examination to determine the site of discomfort.

Imaging

Plane film imaging is a mainstay for diagnosis and preliminary surgical planning for patients with acetabular dysplasia. The recommended initial views include an anterior-posterior (AP) pelvis, lateral (frog-leg, cross-table or 45° Dunn), and false profile. If pelvic osteotomy is being considered, a functional image taken in abduction/internal rotation [21, 22] and standing AP pelvis views [23] are useful.

The AP pelvis view should be well centered with the sacrum and coccyx in line with the pubic symphysis, and the sacrococcygeal joint to pubic symphysis distance between 2 and 5 cm [24, 25]. If the sacrococcygeal joint is obscured, a distance of 0–2 cm from the tip of the coccyx to the pubic symphysis is acceptable [26]. Three measures are commonly used to screen for dysplasia on the AP view: the lateral center-edge angle (CE angle) of Wiberg [6], the acetabular roof, or Tönnis, angle [27], and the Shenton line [28]. The lateral CE angle is formed by the intersection of a line from the center of the femoral head to the lateral rim of the acetabulum and a second line through the femoral head center that is perpendicular to the transverse pelvic axis (Fig. 71.1). The original description used a line perpendicular to the vertical axis of the sacrum to represent the transverse pelvic axis, but it can also

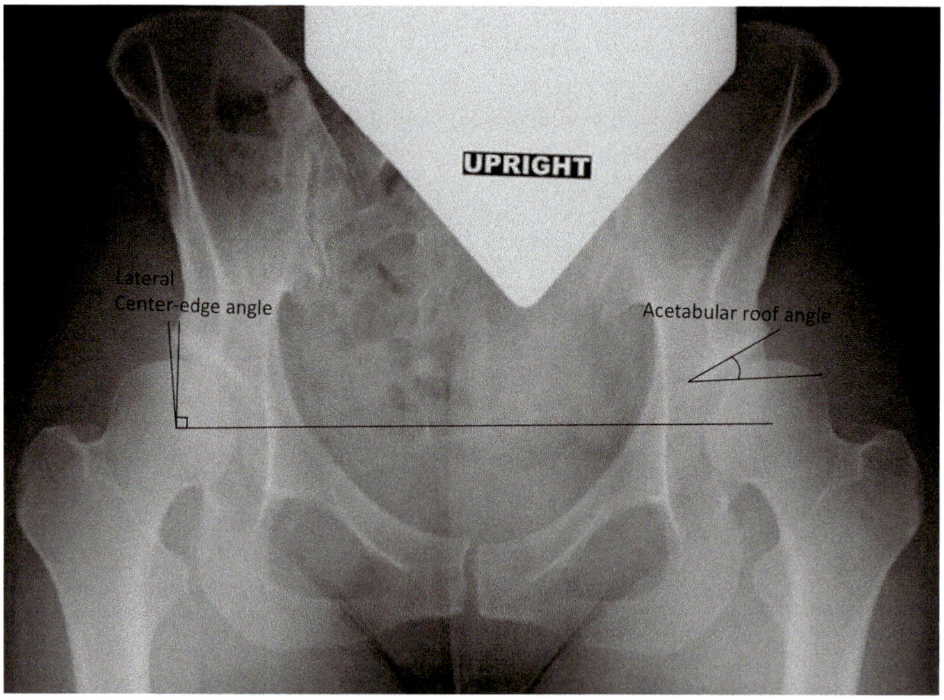

Fig. 71.1 Methods to measure lateral center-edge (CE) angle and acetabular roof, or Tönnis, angle on AP pelvis X-ray. This patient has a low CE angle and a steep roof angle, consistent with acetabular dysplasia

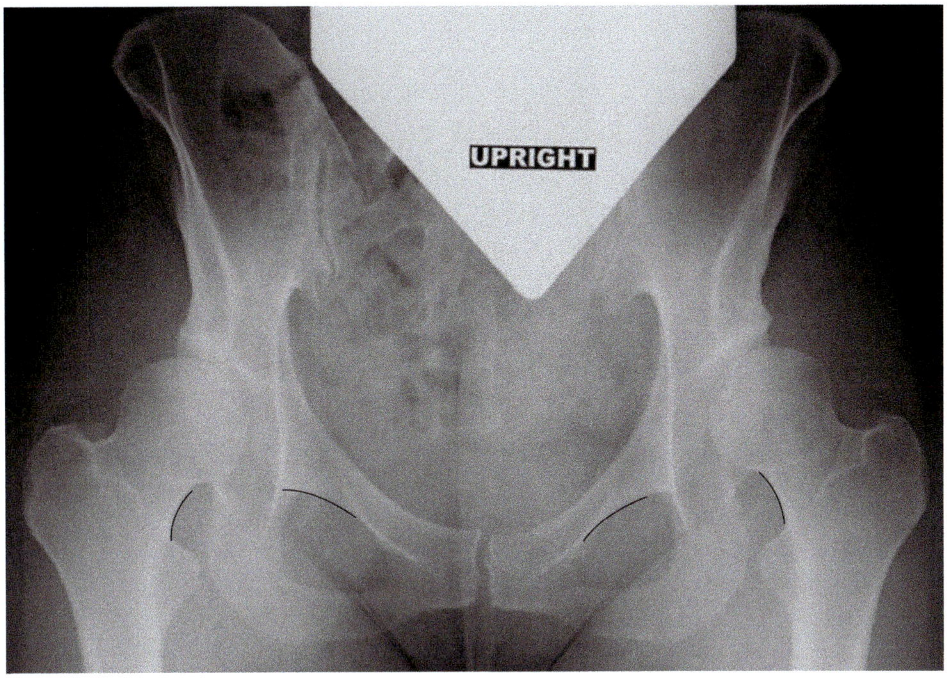

Fig. 71.2 Shenton line. In a normal hip, the arc along the superior obturator ring should continue as a smooth contour with the inferior surface of the femoral neck. This patient (same as Fig. 71.1) with acetabular dysplasia has mild disruption on the right and more pronounced disruption on the left hip

be denoted by a line connecting the centers of the femoral heads. The normal lateral CE angle is 25°–35°; less than 20° is dysplastic [6]. The acetabular roof angle is formed by a line parallel to the transverse pelvic axis and a second line that connects the most medial and lateral margins of the acetabular weight-bearing zone, represented by the sclerotic sourcil (Fig. 71.1). The normal acetabular roof angle ranges between 0 and 10° with greater than 10° considered dysplastic [27]. The Shenton line is a curved arc along the inferior surface of the superior pubic ramus that continues as smooth contour along the medial, inferior femoral neck in a normal hip (Fig. 71.2) [28]. Disruption of this line greater than 5 mm indicates dysplasia with femoral head subluxation [9]. Three additional measures on the AP view, the crossover sign [29], the ischial spine sign [30], and the posterior wall sign [29], are useful to screen for acetabular retroversion and global dysplasia. The superior pubic ramus extends laterally to form the horizontally oriented anterior acetabular wall, and the lateral ischium projects to form the vertically oriented posterior acetabular wall. On an AP pelvis image of a normal hip, the anterior and posterior acetabular walls converge at the lateral rim. The crossover sign is positive if the anterior wall is lateral to the posterior wall at the lateral rim, and is indicative of acetabular retroversion or focal anterior overcoverage (Fig. 71.3) [29]. Pelvic position affects the crossover sign with increased inclination being a potential risk for a false-positive finding. The ischial spine sign is positive if the spine projects medial to the iliopectineal line on an AP pelvis image (Fig. 71.3) [30]. It is also indicative of acetabular retroversion but is less affected by pelvic tilt than the crossover sign [31]. On an AP pelvis image of a normal hip, the posterior wall of the acetabulum aligns with the center of the femoral head. If the posterior wall sign is medial to the center of the head, this sign is positive (Fig. 71.3). This finding denotes insufficient posterior coverage and confirms acetabular retroversion if it is observed in association with a crossover sign, or it suggests global acetabular dysplasia if the crossover sign is negative [29].

The false-profile image is a tangential view of the anterior acetabular rim [32] that can detect mild dysplasia or decreased joint space not evident on the AP view [33]. The anterior (or vertical) center-edge angle quantifies anterior coverage of the femoral head. It is formed by a line from the center of the femoral head to the anterior, sclerotic rim of the weight-bearing zone of the acetabulum and a vertical line that passes through the center of the femoral head (Fig. 71.4). Similar to the lateral CE angle, anterior CE angles between 25 and 35° are considered normal and less than 20° is dysplastic [32].

The lateral radiograph is primarily used to screen for proximal femoral abnormalities and examine femoral head-neck morphology. Coxa valga and increased femoral anteversion are commonly associated with acetabular dysplasia. With improved understanding of FAI, it has been noted that over 70 % of patients with acetabular dysplasia have femoral head-neck deformities [34], and correction of anterior coverage with pelvic osteotomy can result in impingement [35]. Although the frog-leg lateral and cross-table lateral views are most commonly used, there is no consensus on which lateral view is preferable [36, 37]. The 45° Dunn lateral view is increasingly used and was found to have over 96 % sensitivity to detect a cam lesion in a study using radial MRI views as the control [38]. The alpha angle (α angle) is a measure of the contour of the femoral head-neck junction [39]

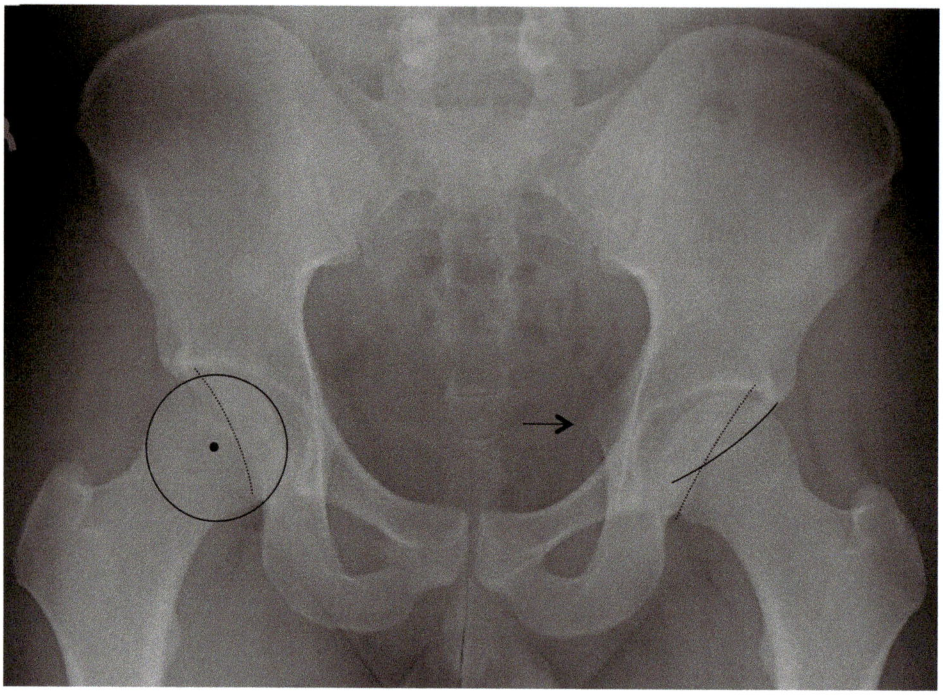

Fig. 71.3 Crossover, ischial spine and posterior wall signs. In a normal hip, the posterior (*dashed line*) and anterior (*solid line*) acetabular walls should meet at the lateral border of the acetabulum on an AP pelvis X-ray. The crossover sign is positive if the anterior wall is lateral to the posterior wall. The ischial spine sign is positive if the spine projects medial to the iliopectineal line (*arrow*). The posterior wall sign is positive if the center of the femoral head (*black dot*) is lateral to the lateral border of the posterior wall. All three signs are positive on both hips in this patient

that was originally determined from oblique axial MR images but is now widely applied to lateral radiographs. After superimposing a spherical template on the femoral head, the α angle is formed by a line drawn along (or parallel to) the central axis of the femoral neck that passes through the center of the femoral head and a second line from the center of the femoral head to the point where the femoral head-neck becomes aspherical (Fig. 71.5). The normal α angle is 55° or less [40].

The abduction/internal rotation, or von Rosen, view [41] is a functional radiograph that simulates the lateral coverage and congruence that can be obtained after acetabular reorientation (see Fig. 71.7b). Incongruence or joint space narrowing seen on an AP pelvis view that persists or worsens on the functional view is predictive of a poor result after PAO [22].

Computed tomography (CT) is a powerful tool to depict two- and three-dimensional pelvic anatomy, and it correlates well with radiographic measures in dysplasia [42]. CT has been used to simulate femoral head coverage and individualize surgical planning prior to pelvic and femoral osteotomy [43–46]. The drawbacks of CT are that it can be subject to positional error [47], similar to plane radiographs, and it introduces the possible risk of radiation-associated cancers [48]. Due to this concern in the dysplastic population, which

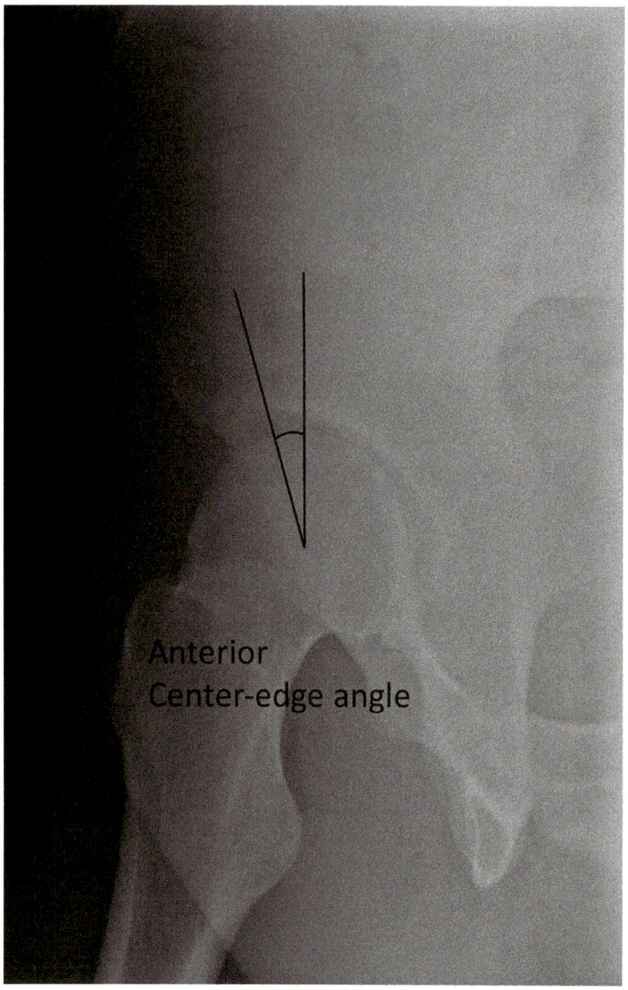

Fig. 71.4 The anterior center-edge angle measured on the false profile view. This angle is formed by a line from the center of the femoral head to the anterior, sclerotic rim of the weight-bearing zone of the acetabulum and a vertical line that passes through the center of the femoral head

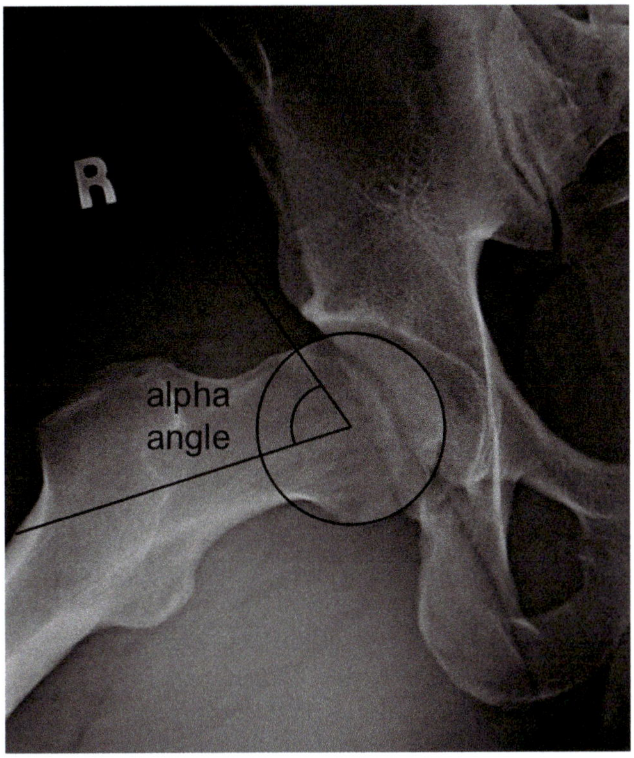

Fig. 71.5 The alpha (α) angle measured on the 45° Dunn lateral view. The α angle is formed by a line parallel to the axis of the femoral neck that passes through the center of the femoral head and a second line from the center of the femoral head to the point where the femoral head-neck becomes aspherical. The normal α angle is 55° or less

is primarily comprised of young, female patients for whom the radiation risks are highest [49], our institutions no longer use CT in the routine preoperative evaluation.

Similar to CT, magnetic resonance imaging (MRI) provides excellent detail of bony, soft-tissue, and intra-articular anatomy [50]. Radial views allow circumferential evaluation of femoral head-neck morphology and may identify subtle deformities and labral damage [51, 52] not detected on radiographs [53, 54]. Acetabular version can be assessed with axial views through the roof of the acetabulum, and femoral version can be measured by the angle between axial cuts through the center of the femoral neck and at the level of the femoral condyles [55].

The results of pelvic osteotomy are influenced by the degree of osteoarthritis at the time of surgery [11, 56, 57]. Biochemical MRI techniques depict the layered structure and molecular composition of cartilage [58] and can identify cartilage deterioration before it is evident on standard MRI or plane radiographs. Although there are several biochemical MRI modalities in clinical use, such as T2 mapping, T1rho, and delayed-gadolinium-enhanced MRI of cartilage (dGEMRIC), the latter has been most widely studied for hip disorders. The dGEMRIC index demonstrates good correlation with pain and the severity of acetabular dysplasia and is a better indicator of early OA than plane radiographs in this population [59]. The dGEMRIC index has also been shown to predict short- to mid-term outcome after PAO compared to standard MRI, radiographs, and clinical measures [60].

Surgical Options

In 1957, Dr. Robert Salter first performed an innominate osteotomy to *reorient* the position of the native acetabulum in patients with dysplasia [61]. Previous techniques sought to *augment* the deficient femoral head coverage. Multiple modifications of Salter's osteotomy have led to improved versatility in addressing the dysplastic hip, particularly in adults. The most commonly used in current practice are the triple pelvic osteotomy; the rotational, or spherical, acetabular osteotomy (RAO); and the PAO.

Triple Pelvic Osteotomy

Salter's technique osteotomizes the pelvis from just proximal to the anterior inferior iliac spine transversely to the sciatic notch. The pubic symphysis acts as a hinge, and the acetabular fragment is rotated anteriorly and laterally [61]. Mobility of the fragment can be limited by stiffness at the pubic symphysis, particularly in adolescents and adults. Multiple modifications have been reported, which include double [62] and triple osteotomies [63–66] through several incisions to improve mobility and correction. The current technique for the triple pelvic osteotomy [67, 68] places the cuts closer to the acetabulum. In particular, osteotomizing the ischium proximal to the ischial spine eliminates tethering from the sacrospinous and sacrotuberous ligaments that limited correction in earlier methods. Tönnis employs a two-stage procedure beginning with the patient prone for the ischial cut and then turned supine for the iliac and pubic ramus osteotomies. Further modifications include a medial approach for the ischial cut to avoid the need for patient repositioning [69], and a single incision, abductor-sparing technique [70, 71].

At an average follow-up of 15 years in a series of 48 hips that had undergone triple pelvic osteotomy, Van Hellemondt et al. reported that 88 % were preserved and 64 % had good-to-excellent functional ratings [10]. Of the hips with no OA at surgery, 80 % showed no radiographic progression at the 15-year evaluation. In another series of 50 patients (60 hips) at an average of 9 years after surgery, 98 % were satisfied, though 27 % of the hips were failures as defined intractable pain or conversion to total hip arthroplasty [72].

Compared to previous techniques of double and triple innominate osteotomies, the triple pelvic osteotomy as modified by Tönnis can achieve much larger corrections and medialize the joint. It is effective in severe dysplasia, even in patients with persistent subluxation or dislocation [67]. In addition, it can be used in patients with an open triradiate cartilage with extraperiosteal dissection of the superior public ramus [70, 73]. Because this technique disrupts both columns of the pelvis, the true pelvis is altered, which can impact childbirth. In addition, there is the potential for instability and a higher nonunion rate, particularly in cases that require a major correction that introduces large gaps at the osteotomy sites [74–76].

Rotational Acetabular Osteotomy

Osteotomy adjacent to the acetabulum was initially described by Blavier and Blavier in 1962 [77]; similar techniques were subsequently reported by Wagner [78] in Germany (Fig. 71.6), Eppright [79] in the USA, and Ninomiya and Tagawa [80] in Japan where it is most widely used. In each method, the osteotomy is carried out 1.5 cm proximal to the joint with curved osteotomes that follow the acetabular contour. Wagner's approach utilizes an extensive anterior iliofemoral dissection [78]; Ninomiya and Tagawa employ both anterior iliofemoral and posterior approaches in the lateral position [80]; subsequent modifications employ a transtrochanteric approach [81] with bioabsorbable fixation [82, 83].

The RAO has demonstrated good success in well-selected patients. At 20-year follow-up of spherical osteotomies performed according to Wagner's technique, Kaplan-Meier survivorship was 86 % at 20 years with conversion to total hip arthroplasty as the end point [84]. Postoperative joint congruence was a key factor in preservation of the native hip. At an average follow-up of 13 years, Nakamura et al. similarly reported 80 % good-to-excellent long-term results in patients with minimal arthrosis at the time of surgery [12]. Several reports have shown RAO to be effective in decreasing pain at 8- to 12-year follow-up in patients with established osteoarthritis [85–89]. Factors associated with improved results are a minimum of 2.5 mm joint space [89], and joint congruence on preoperative imaging [90]. In the absence of severe OA, RAO can yield good outcomes in patients with severe dysplasia [91–94] and advanced age [13, 14]. Undercorrection and persistent lateralization of the femoral head are technical factors that can result in progressive osteoarthritis [95, 96].

A primary advantage of the RAO is that major correction can be achieved while preserving the shape of the true pelvis, and thus maintaining the diameter of the birth canal [97]. One drawback of the procedure is that the small bone surrounding the acetabular fragment can be difficult to stabilize adequately to allow early weight bearing. In addition, due to the close proximity of the osteotomy to the joint, there are risks of acetabular osteonecrosis [18, 98, 99] and fracture [85, 100]. The procedure is contraindicated in patients with joint incongruity or an open triradiate cartilage and should be used with caution in those with abductor muscle weakness, because prolonged limp can be a sequela of the surgery [80].

Periacetabular Osteotomy

The PAO was first performed in 1984 with a description and preliminary report published by Ganz and colleagues in 1988 [57]. It combines the advantages of both the RAO and triple pelvic osteotomy. The PAO is performed through a single surgical approach with osteotomy sites close enough to the acetabulum to allow for a large, multi-planar correction, yet adequate bony bridge to avoid osteonecrosis of the acetabular fragment (Fig. 71.7). The PAO preserves the integrity of the posterior column and the true pelvis. Recent modifications offer the additional advantages of an abductor-sparing [71] and limited-incision approach [101]. Similar to the RAO and triple pelvic osteotomy, the PAO is effective in severe cases of dysplasia with femoral head subluxation [102]. The primary drawback of the technique is that it disrupts the triradiate cartilage, and thus is not recommended in skeletally immature patients.

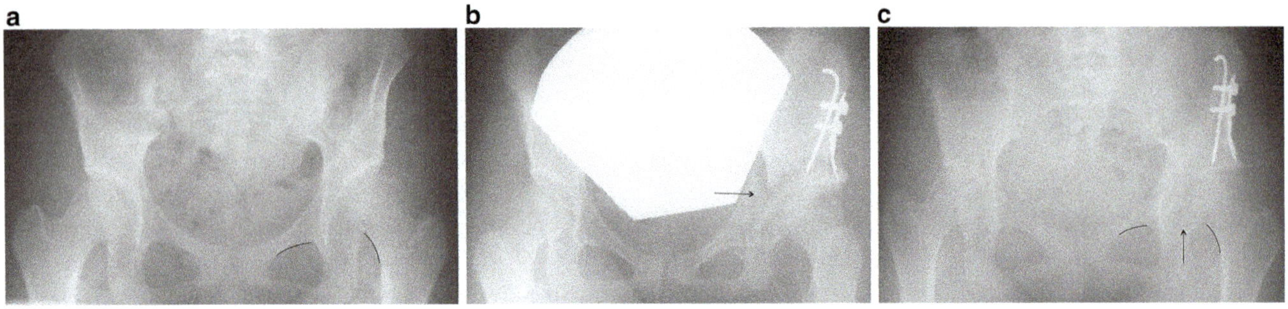

Fig. 71.6 (**a**) Preoperative AP pelvis image of a patient with bilateral acetabular dysplasia. (**b**) Postoperative image after Wagner type III rotational acetabular osteotomy. The type III technique combines osteotomy adjacent to the rim of the acetabulum with a complete osteotomy of the ilium (*arrow*). (**c**) The same patient 2 years after surgery. The superior subluxation is improved, though the femoral head is still lateralized. The *arrow* points to the increased medial joint space

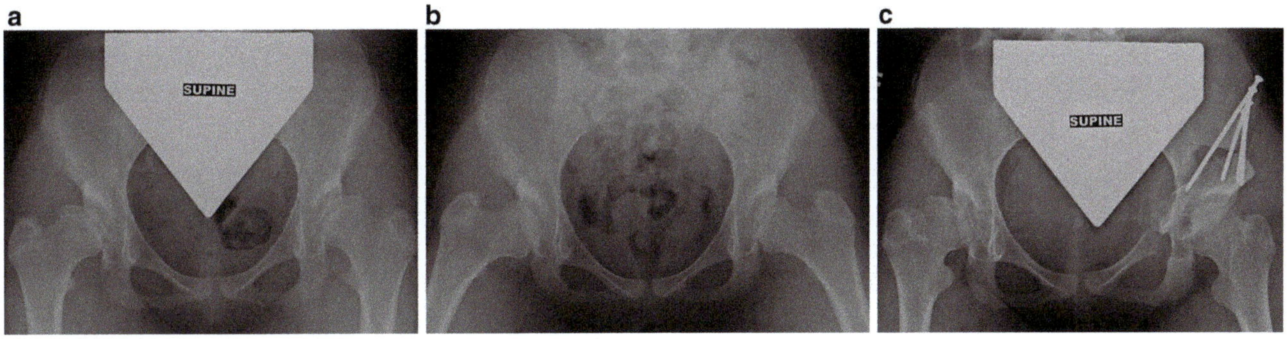

Fig. 71.7 (**a**) AP image of a patient with multiple epiphyseal dysplasia and acetabular dysplasia. (**b**) Functional image in maximal abduction and internal rotation demonstrates good congruence of the femoral head and acetabulum and improvement in superior subluxation as seen by the continuity of the Shenton line. (**c**) The same patient after left PAO

The PAO has demonstrated results similar to the RAO and triple pelvic osteotomy. At an average of 9 years after surgery, Matheney et al. reported that 76 % of 135 native hips (109 patients) were maintained [56]. However, 24 % (33 hips) were considered failures due to pain or need for conversion to hip arthroplasty. Age over 35 years and poor-to-fair preoperative joint congruency were independent factors predictive of failure. In patients who were both over age 35 and had less than "good" congruency, the probability of failure was 95 %, whereas it was 36 % with one, and only 14 % with neither factor. At an average of 11.3-year follow-up of 71 of Ganz's original cohort of 75 dysplastic hips (63 patients), the native hip was preserved in 82 % with good-to-excellent functional results in 73 % [103] as measured by the Merle d'Aubigné rating system [104]. At 20 years, 60 % of hips in this patient group were preserved, although functional scores had decreased from the previous report to match preoperative levels [11]. Factors associated with poor results in the initial report were age > 30 years, labral damage, and higher grades of OA. At the subsequent follow-up, three additional preoperative variables correlated with worse outcomes: limp, positive anterior impingement sign, and lower functional scores.

Borderline Cases: Advanced Age and Arthrosis

Although multiple reports of reorienting pelvic osteotomies correlate worse outcomes with older patients, age may simply be a surrogate for joint damage. In the absence of advanced OA, osteotomy can be successful in this population. Millis et al. reported improved pain and function at 5-year follow-up of patients with a mean age of 43.6 years at surgery with 12 % conversion to THA in patients with Tönnis grades 0–1 OA [27] compared to 27 % in those with grade 2 changes at the time of surgery [15]. In another study comparing the results of RAO between patients over 45 years and those 45 and younger, both groups had statistically significant improvement in radiographic and clinical measures at a mean 8.2 years after surgery [13]. The predicted 10-year survivorship of the native hip was 70.0 % in the older group and 93.7 % in the younger group. In a similar comparison of patients older than 50 years to those 50 and younger, there were equivalent improvements in function but lower 15-year survivorship, 71 % vs. 81 %, respectively [14].

Patients with dysplasia commonly have early OA and labral pathology, because symptoms are often silent until damage occurs. Several approaches, such as evaluation of congruence on preoperative AP and functional radiographs [22], cartilage grading with biochemical MRI [60], and, in some cases, hip arthroscopy [105], can guide prognosis and help select good candidates for pelvic osteotomy.

Okano et al. correlated joint congruity in abduction with OA progression at a mean 12-year follow-up of 90 hips with early OA at the time of RAO [106]. Of 82 hips with good or excellent congruence preoperatively, only six had progression of OA, five of which had femoral head deformities. The eight hips that were rated as having fair congruence all had progression of OA postoperatively. Murphy and Deshmukh reported similar findings in looking at radiographic factors that were associated with failure at a minimum of 2 years after PAO [22]. In hips with Tönnis grades 0–2, only 1 of 40 hips that were congruent on AP and functional views failed. Further, there was only one failure in eight hips with grade 3 OA preoperatively; the failed hip demonstrated decreased joint space on the preoperative functional view.

In patients with degenerative changes on plane films, biochemical MRI can quantify the degree of OA. At present, only dGEMRIC has been correlated with the results after pelvic osteotomy. In a prospective cohort study that compared a group with satisfactory outcome to one with early failure after PAO, lower preoperative dGEMRIC scores and break in the Shenton line were predictive of failure [60]. There were no differences in pre- or postoperative anterior or lateral center-edge angles or Tönnis angle. The dGEMRIC index was the most important predictor of failure of the osteotomy by multivariate analysis.

Hip arthroscopy is increasingly performed in conjunction with pelvic osteotomy [105] and may become a useful adjunct to determine whether joint damage is too advanced to warrant preservation. In follow-up of patients after RAO, Fujii et al. found that severe intra-articular lesions, particularly exposure of femoral head subchondral bone, were associated with progression of OA, even in hips with only mild radiographic OA at the time of surgery [107].

Conclusion

Acetabular dysplasia is a hip condition that can cause pain, functional limitation, and premature osteoarthritis. Radiographic imaging to evaluate these patients should include supine and standing AP pelvis images, false profile, 45° Dunn lateral, and functional views. The best mid- and long-term outcomes are associated with patients younger than 35 years who have good range of motion, no limp, no anterior impingement, and only mild-to-moderate pain. Favorable findings on imaging are a congruent joint with minimal arthrosis, reduction of subluxation, if present, on functional views, and no labral or chondral pathology on MRI. In indeterminate cases with early radiographic osteoarthritis, biochemical MRI and arthroscopy provide further information about the health of the articular cartilage. Reorienting pelvic osteotomy is a technically complex procedure that can correct deformity and improve symptoms in properly selected patients.

References

1. Klaue K, Durnin CW, Ganz R. The acetabular rim syndrome. A clinical presentation of dysplasia of the hip. J Bone Joint Surg (Br). 1991;73(3):423–9.
2. Murray RO. The aetiology of primary osteoarthritis of the hip. Br J Radiol. 1965;38(455):810–24.
3. Stulberg SC, Cordell LD, Harris WH, Ramsey PL, MacEwen GD. Unrecognized childhood hip disease: a major cause of idiopathic osteoarthtis of the hip. The hip, proceedings of the third open scientific meeting of the Hip Society. St. Louis: C.V. Mosby; 1975, pp. 212–28.
4. Aronson J. Osteoarthritis of the young adult hip: etiology and treatment. Instr Course Lect. 1986;35:119–28.
5. Tonnis D, Remus W. Development of hip dysplasia in puberty due to delayed ossification of femoral nucleus, growth plate and triradiate cartilage. J Pediatr Orthop B. 2004;13(5):287–92.
6. Wiberg G. Studies on dysplastic acetabula and congenital sublixation of the hip joint. Acta Chir Scand. 1939;83 Suppl 58:5–135.
7. Clohisy JC, Dobson MA, Robison JF, Warth LC, Zheng J, Liu SS, et al. Radiographic structural abnormalities associated with premature, natural hip-joint failure. J Bone Joint Surg Am. 2011;93 Suppl 2:3–9.
8. Murphy SB, Ganz R, Muller ME. The prognosis in untreated dysplasia of the hip. A study of radiographic factors that predict the outcome. J Bone Joint Surg Am. 1995;77(7):985–9.
9. Cooperman DR, Wallensten R, Stulberg SD. Acetabular dysplasia in the adult. Clin Orthop Relat Res. 1983;175:79–85.
10. van Hellemondt GG, Sonneveld H, Schreuder MH, Kooijman MA, de Kleuver M. Triple osteotomy of the pelvis for acetabular dysplasia: results at a mean follow-up of 15 years. J Bone Joint Surg (Br). 2005;87(7):911–5.
11. Steppacher SD, Tannast M, Ganz R, Siebenrock KA. Mean 20-year followup of Bernese periacetabular osteotomy. Clin Orthop Relat Res. 2008;466(7):1633–44.
12. Nakamura S, Ninomiya S, Takatori Y, Morimoto S, Umeyama T. Long-term outcome of rotational acetabular osteotomy: 145 hips followed for 10-23 years. Acta Orthop Scand. 1998;69(3): 259–65.
13. Yasunaga Y, Takahashi K, Ochi M, Ikuta Y, Hisatome T, Nakashiro J, et al. Rotational acetabular osteotomy in patients forty-six years of age or older: comparison with younger patients. J Bone Joint Surg Am. 2003;85-A(2):266–72.
14. Yamaguchi J, Hasegawa Y, Kanoh T, Seki T, Kawabe K. Similar survival of eccentric rotational acetabular osteotomy in patients younger and older than 50 years. Clin Orthop Relat Res. 2009;467(10):2630–7.
15. Millis MB, Kain M, Sierra R, Trousdale R, Taunton MJ, Kim YJ, et al. Periacetabular osteotomy for acetabular dysplasia in patients older than 40 years: a preliminary study. Clin Orthop Relat Res. 2009;467(9):2228–34.
16. Nunley RM, Prather H, Hunt D, Schoenecker PL, Clohisy JC. Clinical presentation of symptomatic acetabular dysplasia in skeletally mature patients. J Bone Joint Surg Am. 2011;93 Suppl 2:17–21.
17. Macdonald SJ, Garbuz D, Ganz R. Clinical evaluation of the symptomatic young adult hip. Seminars in Arthroplsaty. 1997;8:3–9.
18. Leunig M, Siebenrock KA, Ganz R. Rationale of periacetabular osteotomy and background work. Instr Course Lect. 2001;50:229–38.
19. Widler KS, Glatthorn JF, Bizzini M, Impellizzeri FM, Munzinger U, Leunig M, et al. Assessment of hip abductor muscle strength. A validity and reliability study. J Bone Joint Surg Am. 2009;91(11):2666–72.
20. Smith J, Hurdle MF. Office-based ultrasound-guided intra-articular hip injection: technique for physiatric practice. Arch Phys Med Rehabil. 2006;87(2):296–8.
21. Vonrosen S. Treatment of congenital dislocation of the hip in the newborn. Diagnosis and treatment. Proc R Soc Med. 1963;56:801–3.
22. Murphy S, Deshmukh R. Periacetabular osteotomy: preoperative radiographic predictors of outcome. Clin Orthop Relat Res. 2002;405:168–74.
23. Troelsen A, Jacobsen S, Romer L, Soballe K. Weightbearing anteroposterior pelvic radiographs are recommended in DDH assessment. Clin Orthop Relat Res. 2008;466:813–9.
24. Tannast M, Zheng G, Anderegg C, Burckhardt K, Langlotz F, Ganz R, et al. Tilt and rotation correction of acetabular version on pelvic radiographs. Clin Orthop Relat Res. 2005;438:182–90.
25. Siebenrock KA, Kalbermatten DF, Ganz R. Effect of pelvic tilt on acetabular retroversion: a study of pelvis from cadavers. Clin Orthop Relat Res. 2003;407:241–8.
26. Mast JW, Brunner RL, Zebrack J. Recognizing acetabular version in the radiographic presentation of hip dysplasia. Clin Orthop Relat Res. 2004;418:48–53.
27. Tonnis D. Congenital dysplasia and dislocation of the hip in children and adults. New York, NY: Springer; 1987.
28. Shenton E. Disease in bone and its detection by X-rays. London: Macmillan; 1911.

29. Reynolds D, Lucas J, Klaue K. Retroversion of the acetabulum. A cause of hip pain. J Bone Joint Surg (Br). 1999;81(2):281–8.
30. Kalberer F, Sierra RJ, Madan SS, Ganz R, Leunig M. Ischial spine projection into the pelvis: a new sign for acetabular retroversion. Clin Orthop Relat Res. 2008;466(3):677–83.
31. Kakaty DK, Fischer AF, Hosalkar HS, Siebenrock KA, Tannast M. The ischial spine sign: does pelvic tilt and rotation matter? Clin Orthop Relat Res. 2010;468(3):769–74.
32. Lequesne M, de Seze S. False profile of the pelvis. A new radiographic incidence for the study of the hip. Its use in dysplasias and different coxopathies. Rev Rhum Mal Osteoartic. 1961;28: 643–52.
33. Lequesne MG, Laredo JD. The faux profil (oblique view) of the hip in the standing position. Contribution to the evaluation of osteoarthritis of the adult hip. Ann Rheum Dis. 1998;57(11):676–81.
34. Clohisy JC, Nunley RM, Carlisle JC, Schoenecker PL. Incidence and characteristics of femoral deformities in the dysplastic hip. Clin Orthop Relat Res. 2009;467(1):128–34.
35. Myers SR, Eijer H, Ganz R. Anterior femoroacetabular impingement after periacetabular osteotomy. Clin Orthop Relat Res. 1999;363:93–9.
36. Clohisy JC, Nunley RM, Otto RJ, Schoenecker PL. The frog-leg lateral radiograph accurately visualized hip cam impingement abnormalities. Clin Orthop Relat Res. 2007;462:115–21.
37. Meyer DC, Beck M, Ellis T, Ganz R, Leunig M. Comparison of six radiographic projections to assess femoral head/neck asphericity. Clin Orthop Relat Res. 2006;445:181–5.
38. Domayer SE, Ziebarth K, Chan J, Bixby S, Mamisch TC, Kim YJ. Femoroacetabular cam-type impingement: diagnostic sensitivity and specificity of radiographic views compared to radial MRI. Eur J Radiol. 2011;80(3):805–10.
39. Notzli HP, Wyss TF, Stoecklin CH, Schmid MR, Treiber K, Hodler J. The contour of the femoral head-neck junction as a predictor for the risk of anterior impingement. J Bone Joint Surg (Br). 2002;84(4):556–60.
40. Sutter R, Dietrich TJ, Zingg PO, Pfirrmann CW. How Useful is the alpha angle for discriminating between symptomatic patients with Cam-type femoroacetabular impingement and asymptomatic volunteers? Radiology. 2012;264(2):514–21.
41. Andren L, Von Rosen S. The diagnosis of dislocation of the hip in newborns and the primary results of immediate treatment. Acta Radiol. 1958;49(2):89–95.
42. Ito H, Matsuno T, Hirayama T, Tanino H, Yamanaka Y, Minami A. Three-dimensional computed tomography analysis of non-osteoarthritic adult acetabular dysplasia. Skeletal Radiol. 2009;38(2):131–9.
43. Murphy SB, Kijewski PK, Millis MB, Harless A. Acetabular dysplasia in the adolescent and young adult. Clin Orthop Relat Res. 1990;261:214–23.
44. Klaue K, Wallin A, Ganz R. CT evaluation of coverage and congruency of the hip prior to osteotomy. Clin Orthop Relat Res. 1988;232:15–25.
45. Janzen DL, Aippersbach SE, Munk PL, Sallomi DF, Garbuz D, Werier J, et al. Three-dimensional CT measurement of adult acetabular dysplasia: technique, preliminary results in normal subjects, and potential applications. Skeletal Radiol. 1998;27(7):352–8.
46. Haddad FS, Garbuz DS, Duncan CP, Janzen DL, Munk PL. CT evaluation of periacetabular osteotomies. J Bone Joint Surg (Br). 2000;82(4):526–31.
47. van Bosse HJ, Lee D, Henderson ER, Sala DA, Feldman DS. Pelvic positioning creates error in CT acetabular measurements. Clin Orthop Relat Res. 2011;469(6):1683–91.
48. Berrington de Gonzalez A, Mahesh M, Kim KP, Bhargavan M, Lewis R, Mettler F, et al. Projected cancer risks from computed tomographic scans performed in the United States in 2007. Arch Intern Med. 2009;169(22):2071–7.
49. Smith-Bindman R, Lipson J, Marcus R, Kim KP, Mahesh M, Gould R, et al. Radiation dose associated with common computed tomography examinations and the associated lifetime attributable risk of cancer. Arch Intern Med. 2009;169(22):2078–86.
50. Lang P, Genant HK, Jergesen HE, Murray WR. Imaging of the hip joint. Computed tomography versus magnetic resonance imaging. Clin Orthop Relat Res. 1992;274:135–53.
51. Plotz GM, Brossmann J, von Knoch M, Muhle C, Heller M, Hassenpflug J. Magnetic resonance arthrography of the acetabular labrum: value of radial reconstructions. Arch Orthop Trauma Surg. 2001;121(8):450–7.
52. Kubo T, Horii M, Yamaguchi J, Inoue S, Fujioka M, Ueshima K, et al. Acetabular labrum in hip dysplasia evaluated by radial magnetic resonance imaging. J Rheumatol. 2000;27(8):1955–60.
53. Dudda M, Albers C, Mamisch TC, Werlen S, Beck M. Do normal radiographs exclude asphericity of the femoral head-neck junction? Clin Orthop Relat Res. 2009;467(3):651–9.
54. Rakhra KS, Sheikh AM, Allen D, Beaule PE. Comparison of MRI alpha angle measurement planes in femoroacetabular impingement. Clin Orthop Relat Res. 2009;467(3):660–5.
55. Koenig JK, Pring ME, Dwek JR. MR evaluation of femoral neck version and tibial torsion. Pediatr Radiol. 2012;42(1):113–5.
56. Matheney T, Kim YJ, Zurakowski D, Matero C, Millis M. Intermediate to long-term results following the Bernese periacetabular osteotomy and predictors of clinical outcome. J Bone Joint Surg Am. 2009;91(9):2113–23.
57. Ganz R, Klaue K, Vinh TS, Mast JW. A new periacetabular osteotomy for the treatment of hip dysplasias. Technique and preliminary results. Clin Orthop Relat Res. 1988;232:26–36.
58. Ulrich-Vinther M, Maloney MD, Schwarz EM, Rosier R, O'Keefe RJ. Articular cartilage biology. J Am Acad Orthop Surg. 2003;11(6):421–30.
59. Kim YJ, Jaramillo D, Millis MB, Gray ML, Burstein D. Assessment of early osteoarthritis in hip dysplasia with delayed gadolinium-enhanced magnetic resonance imaging of cartilage. J Bone Joint Surg Am. 2003;85-A(10):1987–92.
60. Cunningham T, Jessel R, Zurakowski D, Millis MB, Kim YJ. Delayed gadolinium-enhanced magnetic resonance imaging of cartilage to predict early failure of Bernese periacetabular osteotomy for hip dysplasia. J Bone Joint Surg Am. 2006;88(7):1540–8.
61. Salter RB. Innominate osteotomy in the treatment of congenital dislocation and subluxation of the hip. J Bone Joint Surg (Br). 1961;43(3):518–39.
62. Sutherland DH, Greenfield R. Double innominate osteotomy. J Bone Joint Surg Am. 1977;59(8):1082–91.
63. Steel HH. Triple osteotomy of the innominate bone. A procedure to accomplish coverage of the dislocated or subluxated femoral head in the older patient. Clin Orthop Relat Res. 1977;122:116–27.
64. Lehman WB, Atar D, Grant AD. Pelvic osteotomies in children. Bull N Y Acad Med. 1992;68(4):483–96.
65. LeCoeur P. Correction des de fants d'orientation de l'articulation coxo femorale par osteotomie de l'ishtme iliaque. Rev Chir Orthop. 1965;51:211–2.
66. Hopf A. Hip acetabular displacement by double pelvic osteotomy in the treatment of hip joint dysplasia and subluxation in young people and adults. Z Orthop Ihre Grenzgeb. 1966;101(4):559–86.
67. Tonnis D, Behrens K, Tscharani F. A modified technique of the triple pelvic osteotomy: early results. J Pediatr Orthop. 1981;1(3):241–9.
68. Carlioz H, Khouri N, Hulin P. Osteotomie triple juxtacotyloidienne. Chir Orthop. 1982;68:497–501.
69. Rebello G, Zilkens C, Dudda M, Matheney T, Kim YJ. Triple pelvic osteotomy in complex hip dysplasia seen in neuromuscular and teratologic conditions. J Pediatr Orthop. 2009;29(6): 527–34.

70. Zaltz I. Single incision supraperiosteal triple innominate osteotomy. In: Kocher MS, Millis MB, editors. Pediatric orthopaedic surgery. Philadelphia: Elsevier-Saunders; 2011. p. 159–71.
71. Murphy SB, Millis MB. Periacetabular osteotomy without abductor dissection using direct anterior exposure. Clin Orthop Relat Res. 1999;364:92–8.
72. Peters CL, Fukushima BW, Park TK, Coleman SS, Dunn HK. Triple innominate osteotomy in young adults for the treatment of acetabular dysplasia: a 9-year follow-up study. Orthopedics. 2001;24(6):565–9.
73. Rebello G, Kim YJ. Triple pelvic osteotomy. In: Kocher MS, Millis MB, editors. Pediatric orthopaedic surgery. Philadelphia: Elsevier-Saunders; 2011. p. 149–58.
74. Tschauner C, Sylkin A, Hofmann S, Graf R. Painful nonunion after triple pelvic osteotomy. Report of five cases. J Bone Joint Surg (Br). 2003;85(7):953–5.
75. Vukasinovic Z, Pelillo F, Spasovski D, Seslija I, Zivkovic Z, Matanovic D. Triple pelvic osteotomy for the treatment of residual hip dysplasia. Analysis of complications. Hip Int. 2009;19(4):315–22.
76. Hailer NP, Soykaner L, Ackermann H, Rittmeister M. Triple osteotomy of the pelvis for acetabular dysplasia: age at operation and the incidence of nonunions and other complications influence outcome. J Bone Joint Surg (Br). 2005;87(12):1622–6.
77. Blavier L, Blavier J. Traitment de la Subluxation de la Hanche. Rev Clin Orthop. 1962;48:208–13.
78. Wagner H. Osteotomies for congenital hip dislocation. C.V. Mosby: St. Louis; 1976.
79. Eppright R. Proceedings of the 88th annual meeting of the american orthopaedic association: dial osteotomy of the acetabulum in the treatment of dysplasia of the hip. J Bone Joint Surg Am. 1975;57A:1172.
80. Ninomiya S, Tagawa H. Rotational acetabular osteotomy for the dysplastic hip. J Bone Joint Surg Am. 1984;66(3):430–6.
81. Ito H, Matsuno T, Minami A. Rotational acetabular osteotomy through an Ollier lateral U approach. Clin Orthop Relat Res. 2007;459:200–6.
82. Nakamura S, Takatori Y, Morimoto S, Umeyama T, Yamamoto M, Moro T, et al. Rotational acetabular osteotomy using biodegradable internal fixation. Int Orthop. 1999;23(3):148–9.
83. Maezawa K, Nozawa M, Matsuda K, Mori K, Enomoto F, Shitoto K, et al. Radiographic and magnetic resonance imaging findings of polylevolactic acid screws after rotational acetabular osteotomy. Arch Orthop Trauma Surg. 2004;124(7):455–60.
84. Schramm M, Hohmann D, Radespiel-Troger M, Pitto RP. Treatment of the dysplastic acetabulum with Wagner spherical osteotomy. A study of patients followed for a minimum of twenty years. J Bone Joint Surg Am. 2003;85-A(5):808–14.
85. Millis MB, Kaelin AJ, Schluntz K, Curtis B, Hey L, Hall JE. Spherical acetabular osteotomy for treatment of acetabular dysplasia in adolescents and young adults. J Ped Orthop B. 1994;3:47–53.
86. Nozawa M, Maezawa K, Matsuda K, Kim S, Shitoto K, Kurosawa H. Rotational acetabular osteotomy for advanced osteoarthritis of the hip joint with acetabular dysplasia. Int Orthop. 2009;33(6):1549–53.
87. Okano K, Enomoto H, Osaki M, Shindo H. Rotational acetabular osteotomy for advanced osteoarthritis secondary to developmental dysplasia of the hip. J Bone Joint Surg (Br). 2008;90(1):23–6.
88. Yasunaga Y, Ochi M, Terayama H, Tanaka R, Yamasaki T, Ishii Y. Rotational acetabular osteotomy for advanced osteoarthritis secondary to dysplasia of the hip. J Bone Joint Surg Am. 2006;88(9):1915–9.
89. Hasegawa Y, Kanoh T, Seki T, Matsuoka A, Kawabe K. Joint space wider than 2 mm is essential for an eccentric rotational acetabular osteotomy for adult hip dysplasia. J Orthop Sci. 2010;15(5):620–5.
90. Okano K, Enomoto H, Osaki M, Shindo H. Joint congruency as an indication for rotational acetabular osteotomy. Clin Orthop Relat Res. 2009;467(4):894–900.
91. Nozawa M, Shitoto K, Hirose T, Matsuda K, Michino K, Kajihara H, et al. Rotational acetabular osteotomy for severely dysplastic acetabulum. Arch Orthop Trauma Surg. 2000;120(7-8):376–9.
92. Hartofilakidis G, Stamos K, Ioannidis TT. Rotational acetabular osteotomy for severe dysplasia of the hip. J Bone Joint Surg (Br). 1997;79(3):510.
93. Shindo H, Igarashi H, Taneda H, Azuma H. Rotational acetabular osteotomy for severe dysplasia of the hip with a false acetabulum. J Bone Joint Surg (Br). 1996;78(6):871–7.
94. Ninomiya S. Rotational acetabular osteotomy for the severely dysplastic hip in the adolescent and adult. Clin Orthop Relat Res. 1989;247:127–37.
95. Koga H, Matsubara M, Suzuki K, Morita S, Muneta T. Factors which affect the progression of osteoarthritis after rotational acetabular osteotomy. J Bone Joint Surg (Br). 2003;85(7):963–8.
96. Hasegawa Y, Masui T, Yamaguchi J, Kawabe K, Suzuki S. Factors leading to osteoarthritis after eccentric rotational acetabular osteotomy. Clin Orthop Relat Res. 2007;459:207–15.
97. Masui T, Hasegawa Y, Yamaguchi J, Kanoh T, Ishiguro N. Childbirth and sexual activity after eccentric rotational acetabular osteotomy. Clin Orthop Relat Res. 2007;459:195–9.
98. Kalhor M, Beck M, Huff TW, Ganz R. Capsular and pericapsular contributions to acetabular and femoral head perfusion. J Bone Joint Surg Am. 2009;91(2):409–18.
99. Tonnis D, Arning A, Bloch M, Heinecke A, Kalchschmidt K. Triple Pelvic Osteotomy. J Ped Orthop B. 1994;3:54–67.
100. Wagner H. Experiences with spherical acetabular osteotomy for the correction of the dysplastic acetabulum. In: Weil UH, editor. Progress in orthopaedic surgery 2: acetabular dysplasia - skeletal dysplasias in childhood. Berlin: Springer; 1978. p. 131–45.
101. Troelsen A, Elmengaard B, Soballe K. A new minimally invasive transsartorial approach for periacetabular osteotomy. J Bone Joint Surg Am. 2008;90(3):493–8.
102. Clohisy JC, Barrett SE, Gordon JE, Delgado ED, Schoenecker PL. Periacetabular osteotomy for the treatment of severe acetabular dysplasia. J Bone Joint Surg Am. 2005;87(2):254–9.
103. Siebenrock KA, Scholl E, Lottenbach M, Ganz R. Bernese periacetabular osteotomy. Clin Orthop Relat Res. 1999;363:9–20.
104. Merle D'AR. [Numerical classification of the function of the hip. 1970]. Rev Chir Orthop Reparatrice Appar Mot. 1990;76(6):371–4.
105. Kim KI, Cho YJ, Ramteke AA, Yoo MC. Peri-acetabular rotational osteotomy with concomitant hip arthroscopy for treatment of hip dysplasia. J Bone Joint Surg (Br). 2011;93(6):732–7.
106. Okano K, Yamada K, Takahashi K, Enomoto H, Osaki M, Shindo H. Joint congruency in abduction before surgery as an indication for rotational acetabular osteotomy in early hip osteoarthritis. Int Orthop. 2010;34(1):27–32.
107. Fujii M, Nakashima Y, Noguchi Y, Yamamoto T, Mawatari T, Motomura G, et al. Effect of intra-articular lesions on the outcome of periacetabular osteotomy in patients with symptomatic hip dysplasia. J Bone Joint Surg (Br). 2011;93(11):1449–56.

Hip Osteotomies: Acetabular

72

Richard F. Santore

A Brief History of the Periacetabular Osteotomy

The introduction of the periacetabular osteotomy (also known as Ganz osteotomy, Bernese osteotomy, PAO) by Ganz et al., in the late 1980s, fundamentally improved the effectiveness of the treatment of symptomatic hip dysplasia in adult (skeletally mature) patients [1]. The advantages of this approach for rotational osteotomy of the pelvis were its ability to permit simultaneous, three-dimensional reorientation of the acetabulum, along with modest medial displacement of the center of rotation of the hip joint, and concomitant preservation of the integrity of the posterior column. Over time, it replaced the historic role of intertrochanteric varus and valgus osteotomies for dysplasia, and grew in popularity relative to other pelvic osteotomy options, such as the triple innominate, Wagner and Japanese rotational, Sutherland, and Tönnis.

The original surgical approach for the PAO was modeled on the exposure used for open reduction and internal fixation of pelvic and acetabular fractures, as the surgeons who developed the procedure were world-renowned in treatment of pelvic fractures. The incision was the transverse, anterior component of the "front and back" surgical exposure for major pelvic fractures. It utilized the lateral two, of the three, windows and included mobilization of the neurovascular structures of the femoral triangle and transection of the main trunk of the lateral femoral cutaneous nerve. Complete exposure of the ileum was achieved through take down of the abdominal oblique and iliacus muscles medially and the abductors laterally. This "stripping" of the ilium was identical to that done for the triple innominate osteotomy in children. Surgeons from all over the world traveled to Bern, Switzerland, to observe this innovative surgical technique which quickly began to be called "the Ganz osteotomy." Professor Reinhold Ganz, out of respect for the contributions of Jeff Mast and many others, insisted that it be called "the Bernese periacetabular osteotomy." Over time, the acronym "PAO," for periacetabular osteotomy, has emerged as the most commonly used name for the procedure.

Though the PAO was originally developed by pelvic and trauma surgeons, the subsequent contributions of pediatric, adult reconstruction, and sports medicine subspecialists have influenced both the approaches to surgical techniques and the indications for pelvic osteotomies. This, in turn, has expanded the scope of interest from "pelvic osteotomy surgery" to the broader concept of "hip preservation surgery." For instance, some surgical objectives that were once considered only possible by major open surgery can now be effectively accomplished by arthroscopy. There has been widespread adoption of combined PAO and arthroscopy, combined PAO and ITO, and combined PAO and open ostectomy of the femoral neck, either simple or complex, i.e., with formal surgical dislocation. In addition, visualization and planning have been facilitated by marked advances in 3-D imaging.

Hip dysplasia is not a one-dimensional condition. The version of the socket as well as the deficiency of coverage anteriorly or posteriorly must be assessed. Retroversion of the acetabulum occurs in approximately 15% of cases and reflects relative over-coverage anteriorly paired with simultaneous under-coverage posteriorly [2]. In the early years of PAO surgery, "routine" anterolateral repositioning of the acetabulum led to loss of hip flexion and symptomatic anterior impingement in some hips. In some patients, this necessitated revision surgery to reposition the socket in a more anteverted orientation. This stimulated a robust investigation into the influence of sagittal plane position of the acetabulum, initially in these postoperative cases but later in the basic assessment of patients with dysplasia. The understanding of acetabular retroversion, a torsional abnormality of the socket

R.F. Santore, MD (✉)
Orthopaedic Surgery, Sharp Memorial Hospital, San Diego, CA, USA

Orthopaedic Surgery, University of California San Diego, San Diego, CA, USA

3750 Convoy St., Suite 201, San Diego, CA 92111, USA
e-mail: rsantore@ucsd.edu

J.C. McCarthy et al. (eds.), *Hip Joint Restoration*, DOI 10.1007/978-1-4614-0694-5_72

in the sagittal plane, evolved in large part from this history of anterior overcorrection in the early years of the PAO surgery.

Diagnosis

Too often, patients with symptomatic developmental dysplasia endure years of symptoms before the diagnosis is established. Quite commonly, "groin strain," "muscle pull," "tensor fascia lata (TFL) pain," "tendonitis," and "bursitis" have been suggested as diagnoses by other doctors and therapists along the way. Occasionally, patients seeking relief produce radiographic reports of "normal hip findings" when features of dysplasia are clearly evident. Even more worrisome is the diagnosis of "athletic pubalgia." On a few occasions, I have seen patients who have undergone nerve ablation surgery when the hip dysplasia was not appreciated as the cause of symptoms. In 2013, I convinced an athlete patient to abort a planned bilateral nerve ablation at another clinic. At the last minute, an alert physical therapist had suggested to her that she get her hip checked out. She had bilateral dysplasia, malrotation, and hypermobility syndrome. She became asymptomatic after combined PAO and derotation ITO surgery and returned to golf.

Brief Overview of Radiographic Assessments

A careful review of an AP pelvis is often all that is necessary to get on the right path. Much important scholarly activity has been devoted to the technique for obtaining a "perfect" AP radiograph [3]. Perfection is not needed, however, for a sensible qualitative diagnosis. Clearly, a reproducible, high-quality pelvic film is needed for surgical decision making and for the purpose of comparing preoperative and postoperative results. It is better to have taken the step of obtaining a radiograph of the pelvis, regardless of quality or positioning, than to have no plain X-ray information at all, as in the case of the athlete with the incorrect diagnosis of "athletic pubalgia." For qualitative purposes, and for referral on to a subspecialist in hip preservation surgery, it is sufficient to assure that the obturator foramina are symmetrical, and that the sacrum is in the center, above the pubic symphysis. There is considerable variation in the linear relationship between the coccyx-sacral junction and the symphysis pubis. It is frustrating to interview patients seeking a consultation who have had an MRI of the hip without a plain X-ray of the hip or the pelvis. The "standard" MRI itself is often nearly useless, as it may have been done on a small magnet machine, without intra-articular injection, without an appropriate coil, and without axial views. It is an expensive test that then has to be repeated, but with proper techniques. Whether or not dye is needed for assessment of the labrum is the source of ongoing debate in the radiology world and is outside the scope of this chapter. Suffice it to say that, with or without intra-articular contrast, the techniques for assessment of the labrum and articular cartilage are beyond the capability of a standard MRI examination that might be used for diagnosis of a stress fracture of the femoral neck or to determine if a patient has osteonecrosis of the hip.

The main issues of interest on the plain AP pelvic radiograph include frontal plane coverage of the femoral head (Center Edge Angle, or CEA, of Wiberg), the slope of the sourcil (Acetabular Index), the sphericity and shape of the femoral head, the congruency of the joint and the status of Shenton's line, the presence or absence of lateral hinging, and the relationship of anterior and posterior acetabular margins. Entire scholarly articles and textbook chapters have been written about all of the information that can be gleaned from plain radiographs of the pelvis and hip. Professor Ganz has often said that he can make almost all of his decisions about diagnosis and treatment of structural issues from a good, plain AP pelvis radiograph. Bombelli, who wrote three books about osteotomies for dysplasia and arthritis of the hip, could spend an hour extracting information about stress pattern of trabecular bone and subtle morphologic information about the hip from one AP pelvis X-ray. The advent of digital imaging has increased the value of the plain pelvic radiograph. However, it is important to include a magnification marker at the time of acquisition to ensure the accuracy of linear measurements derived from the image. Angular measurements, such as the CE angle and slope of the sourcil (acetabular index), are independent of magnification and do not require a magnification marker for accuracy.

The most important assessment is the center-edge angle of Wiberg [4]. As Murphy et al. reported, a CEA of 16° or less represents a clear indication for osteotomy [5]. Above 24° is in the normal range, though very high CE angle, i.e., >40°, is also pathologic and represents over-coverage consistent with pincer impingement. The difficult decisions occur when the angle is near normal, i.e., above 20°, but not truly within the normal range. Next is the slope of the sourcil which should be between 0 and 10°. Next, the shadows of the anterior and posterior walls should meet at the lateral edge of the acetabulum. When the anterior wall edge crosses over the posterior wall edge medial to the lateral edge of the acetabulum, this is called a "positive crossover sign" and reflects malrotation of the acetabulum in the sagittal plane. It is also referred to as acetabular retroversion, and is associated with projection of the ischial spine into the pelvis, or the so-called ischial spine sign. Elucidation of the fixed relationship between the crossover sign and the ischial spine sign by Kalberer et al. helped to resolve the dispute between those who previously thought that the retroversion was due to excessive prominence of the anterior acetabular rim in an otherwise normally rotated hip [6]. It is exactly the same concept as acetabular component positioning in total hip arthroplasty. A retroverted acetabular total hip component is one that manifests over-coverage anteriorly and insufficient coverage posteriorly. This is a well-recognized risk factor for posterior dislocation of prosthetic hips. This is intuitive for osteotomy surgeons who are also hip arthroplasty surgeons, but not necessarily for those who do only arthroscopy or trauma or pediatric surgery. The assessment of the anterior and posterior walls brings up the important discussion of the added value of the standing AP pelvis radiograph.

There is a difference in the appearance of the pelvis between a supine and a standing view, because the pelvis shifts into a less lordotic position in the standing position. Think of this as equivalent to dynamic anteversion of the socket when going from supine to standing. In other words, in human gait, the acetabulum covers the anterior portion of the femoral head less in the standing than in the recumbent position, and this equates to a relatively more anteverted appearance on the radiograph. Standing views are very important in sorting out a significant from an insignificant crossover sign or ischial spine sign. This is important because a small crossover sign, or a mild ischial spine sign, as seen on a supine AP pelvis radiograph, will often disappear completely on the standing view, and is not likely to be clinically significant. Thus, it is important not to base a decision to perform arthroscopic or open impingement surgery on the information from a supine AP pelvis radiograph. That being said, much is still to be learned about the relationship between lordosis, functional acetabular position, and acetabular morphology. Exciting work is being done in the field of structural spine surgery in this area. In addition to the supine and standing AP pelvis views, the basic plain radiographic assessment should also include an AP of the symptomatic hip, a Dunn lateral view of the hip, and a false profile view (standing) [7]. If dysplasia is confirmed, an AP radiograph of the hip in abduction and internal rotation should also be obtained. Increasingly, a CT scan with 3D reconstruction, with or without algorithms that correct for pelvic tilt, is obtained, as well as an MRI arthrogram with special techniques for the hip, such as using a cardiac coil over the hip for image enhancement, and specified axial views.

It is important for the joint to be congruous and free of evidence of fixed lateral extrusion. The AP radiograph taken with the hip in ABD and IR helps to verify that the joint space thickness is symmetrical when the femoral head is seated within the acetabulum. This functional radiograph predicts, to a certain degree, the postoperative appearance of the routine AP radiograph after the PAO. If there is lateral hinging on this view, the PAO is contraindicated. On the false profile view, look for preservation of the joint inferiorly and posteriorly. A lateral CE angle can be generated from the false profile view. There is often a gap between the femoral head and the pelvis in DDH, and I refer to this as the "posterior articular gap," which confirms the diagnosis of anterior dysplasia, and which will disappear after anterior reorientation of the acetabulum by PAO. Narrowing of the articular cartilage space in this area on the false profile view is a worrisome sign of focal articular cartilage joint space loss, and can occasionally be seen before superior narrowing of the hip joint on the frontal plane view in the case of early arthritis of the hip.

Global hypoplasia is common and includes smaller than normal anterior, posterior, and lateral coverage. "Dysplasia" is not confined to the shape of the acetabulum alone, but may also include the shape and inclination of the pelvic wings, varus or valgus of the upper femur, anteversion or retroversion of the upper femur, variations in the shape of the anterior inferior spine, and malrotation of the lower extremity, often at multiple levels.

On the femoral side, the presence of varus or valgus in the frontal plane, anteversion or retroversion of the head, and offset should be assessed. Historically, stand-alone varus and valgus intertrochanteric osteotomies were used effectively for treatment of dysplasia and arthritis secondary to dysplasia, after the introduction of the angled blade plate by the AO group in the late 1950s. Now, the intertrochanteric osteotomies are usually adjunctive to PAO, but offer very important, and necessary, enhancements to overall hip preservation strategies.

Assessment of Articular Cartilage Status

Information on the status of the articular cartilage is especially important in patients above the age of 40, and can be gleaned from specialized MRI imaging. Appropriate techniques include T2-weighted MRI without contrast, but with saline intra-articular injection, or T2-weighted arthro-MRI with dye or dGEMRIC MRI or T1-Rho MRI. Which one is utilized will depend, in part, on the expertise and experience of the radiologist at a given clinic or institution. Very few centers have the luxury of a dedicated hip MRI specialist. Worrisome articular cartilage abnormalities on one of these studies are enough to warrant caution with regard to recommending a PAO, especially in middle-aged patients. In uncertain cases, or when specialized MRI techniques are not available, a preliminary diagnostic hip scope can give direct visual evidence to support backing off on a planned PAO, if signs of excessive cartilage damage are present, especially on the femoral head. In our center in San Diego, we frequently do combined surgical hip arthroscopy and PAO under one anesthetic, as part of a two-surgeon team that includes Dr. Michael Muldoon and me. In a handful of cases, we have decided against doing the PAO based on direct visualization of the articular cartilage at the time of the hip scope.

How Old Is Too Old for a PAO?

I have done this operation on patients as old as 60 years of age. However, for someone in that age range to be a good candidate, every variable has to be perfect, including an excellent range of motion in all planes, youthful and normal X-rays except for the dysplasia, beautiful appearance of the joint on AP in ABD/IR, an active lifestyle, an intense desire on the part of the patient to avoid THR, and a willingness to accept the risk that the operation will not hold up over time. One of my 60-year-old patients was an aerobics instructor who returned to her spinning class instructing activities 6 months after her PAO. There is no room for zealotry in promotion of hip preservation surgery, as total hip replacement is a wonderful and reliable option, even in the young patient with secondary arthritis. Great care has to be taken in making the recommendations for each patient, but especially so for those above the age of 40. Extreme caution is warranted for those above 50. The results of THR are so good that PAO should not be offered to patients with significant arthritis. The exception is when an informed patient elects to move ahead with a PAO in full partnership with his/her surgeon, understanding that the operation might not be successful. Age at the time of surgery and the presence of significant arthritis are likely the two most important factors in predicting the longevity of the result after PAO.

Clinical Factors in Patient Selection

In my practice, the presence of hypermobility is one of the most important variables in decision making, especially in borderline cases of bony un-coverage. This is especially true in patients who have undergone a prior hip arthroscopy with an unrepaired release of the anterior capsule for exposure or access to the hip. This can provoke marked increase in symptoms in patients with hypermobility syndrome. In fact, frank dislocation of the hip has been reported after hip arthroscopy [8].

It is worthwhile to take the time to assess every patient for soft-tissue laxity, including family history, the ability to touch the radial aspect of the forearm with the thumb, the presence of hyperextension of the knee, the ability to sublux the shoulder or finger joints, etc. A formal Beighton score can also be recorded [9]. These patients are particularly in need of structural containment of the femoral head, and are among the happiest patients postoperatively. Even minor radiographic dysplasia can be significant in this circumstance. In my opinion, we orthopedic specialists tend to underestimate the influence of hypermobility on joint symptoms, fibromyalgia, and arthritis. These patients tend to be unfairly labeled as "complainers" or "hypochondriacs," when in fact the influence of the hypermobility on joint symptoms is profound. Failure to appreciate dysplasia, as often occurs, as well as the failure to appreciate hypermobility of the soft tissues in the same patients, has a compounding influence on symptomatology. Occasionally, patients will tell me that I am the first person to have ever talked to them seriously about their soft-tissue laxity, which had previously been ignored or described as an actual advantage in sports activities such as diving or gymnastics, or ascribed to a variant of normal.

A failure to respond to arthroscopic hip surgery, or recurrence of the same symptoms after initial successful arthroscopic surgery, support a decision to consider structural surgery.

PAO and Arthroscopic Surgery

Hip arthroscopy, if indicated, can be performed in advance of, or at the same time as, the PAO. Since a practice with a strong emphasis on arthroscopy, including knee, shoulder, and hip, is most often associated with a surgeon who specializes in sports medicine, that surgeon is usually not the one who will do the osteotomy. Conversely, many surgeons who perform major osteotomy procedures of the pelvis and femur are specialists in trauma and/or adult reconstruction. These surgeons often do not do hip arthroscopy. Some do both. The practical reality is that there often needs to be close collaboration and cooperation between several surgeons for the benefit of the patient. Whether or not an adjunctive arthroscopy is necessary for a good outcome after PAO has not been scientifically demonstrated by prospective studies. Clearly, good outcomes from PAO were achieved prior to the incorporation of hip arthroscopy into the surgical strategy, and many PAO surgeons continue to obtain good results with little or no use of hip arthroscopy. However, a strong case can be made for the desirability of repairing a torn labrum, or resecting a torn ligamentum teres, at the time of a major osteotomy. This is supported by the nature of the pain, symptoms of clicking and popping, and findings on physical exam. It has clearly been demonstrated that repair of a torn labrum gives better clinical outcomes than resection and it has been demonstrated in vitro that the labrum provides a critically important role as a gasket to support joint lubrication and to maintain the suction effect in the hip joint. The bias for having a low threshold with regard to recommending labral repair at the time of PAO is therefore reasonable.

Leg Length Inequality and Developmental Dysplasia

Leg length inequality is common in dysplasia, with the ipsilateral leg usually, but not always, longer in patients with acquired valgus deformities of the upper femur and usually, but not always, shorter in those with varus deformities. The correction of a significant leg length difference should be incorporated into the surgical plan whenever possible. It is not uncommon for me to do an adjunctive shortening intertrochanteric osteotomy at the same time as the PAO in someone with a discrepancy of 15 mm or more that is symptomatic. Conversely, a valgus opening wedge can lengthen the femur by up to 30 mm. These are among the happiest patients, as much of their pre-op limp was due to the leg length inequality and there are lasting benefits in terms of gait mechanics and lower back symptoms. Patients intensely dislike having to wear elevator shoes, whether due to a developmental discrepancy or after unintentional lengthening after a total hip replacement. If the ipsilateral leg is long and there is no frontal plane abnormality, a simple segmental resection can be done. If valgus is present, a better strategy is to combine the PAO with a varus intertrochanteric osteotomy. It is important to understand that the varus is not required for containment. That can almost always be achieved by the PAO alone. The ITO is utilized for the primary purpose of shortening and secondary purposes of restoring physiologic femoral offset and normalization of the relationship of the center of rotation of the femoral head and the tip of the greater trochanter.

In a very small, but important subset of hips, unilateral dysplasia is associated with coxa valga and a long leg. In this particular circumstance, the intertrochanteric osteotomy alone can be used, without the need for the PAO at all. As Bombelli taught decades ago, when a varus ITO is done, the shortening causes the pelvis to drop down, with "autocorrection" of the dysplasia, even in the absence of any direct surgery on the pelvis. A good example of this would be a case of mild, unilateral dysplasia, coxa valga of greater than, or equal to, 144°, and an ipsilateral leg that is 1.5 cm or more longer than the opposite side. Preoperative planning will determine the exact degree of varus needed. In general a varus correction in the 20° range will result in approximately a 1.5 cm shortening. Additional wedge resection can be done, based on preoperative planning and intraoperative palpation of the leg lengths, to fine-tune the equalization. Postoperatively, a standing AP pelvis will now demonstrate a significant reduction in the acetabular index. The varus correction addresses most or all of the dysplasia, the leg length inequality, and the valgus deformity of the upper femur. In this example, a carefully planned and well-executed varus, or varus/extension, intertrochanteric osteotomy results in enhanced containment of the femoral head in one or several planes, improvement in acetabular index and lateral CE angle, and equalization of leg lengths. It goes without saying that the ITO can also be used to fine-tune axial rotation by dialing in more external rotation below the osteotomy site, since many cases of dysplasia are associated with excessive internal rotation and insufficient external rotation.

Conversely, when the ipsilateral leg is short, as is often the case in post-Perthes hips, an open-wedge, valgus ITO can be used to normalize the leg length discrepancy (LLD). Up to 30° of valgus correction can be incorporated; with lengthening of up to 3 cm. Increase in stature combined with elimination of the previous LLD makes for a very happy patient. I always prefer to do the ITO first and then cover the head to the degree necessary by the PAO done under the same anesthetic. My European colleagues do the PAO first and will use the ITO as an adjunct for containment and coverage. I have never followed that strategy, as I have a separate reason for the ITO and that planning is precise and predetermined, whereas repositioning of the acetabulum is easily performed intraoperatively.

Planning for Total Hip After Adjunctive ITO

It is important to incorporate planning for a potential future THR in the osteosynthesis of the ITO, so as to achieve an appropriate relationship between the shaft, upper femur, and greater trochanter. Any inappropriate displacement can make the future THR difficult. Pre-planning will result in a THR of minimal increased degree of difficulty. This is a clear example of the added value of the perspective of an adult reconstructive surgeon who also does THR, including conversions of post-osteotomy arthritis to THR.

Malrotation Trumps Anteversion

Much attention has been focused recently on "anteversion" of the femur in patients with FAI or DDH. The more important issue, in my opinion, is the rotation of the limb. Some patients have almost no external rotation of the hip at all, but have 60° or more of internal rotation. This is the opposite of the typical patient with FAI who almost always manifests a loss of internal rotation, especially in the flexed position of the hip. I advocate fixing the malrotation by femoral osteotomy. It can be done using closed osteotomy of the femoral shaft and rodding, but I prefer to do it via intertrochanteric osteotomy with classic blade plate fixation. This allows fine-tuning of the varus/valgus of the neck-shaft relationship in the frontal plane, enhancement or reduction in femoral shaft offset, deliberate extension in the sagittal plane to correct true anteversion, or anteversion to correct preoperative upper femoral retroversion, which has been identified as a causative factor for FAI. In complex cases of multiple-level malrotation, I have performed various combinations of pelvic osteotomy (PAO), intertrochanteric de-rotation osteotomy (to increase external rotation at the hip level), and de-rotation osteotomy of the leg at the ankle level to achieve physiologic rotation at all levels, under a single anesthetic.

Though postoperative management of such a patient is a bit more challenging, the outcomes are quite satisfying. The result is so dramatic that patients are delighted with the physical appearance of their leg as soon as in the recovery room, and this immediate positive impression greatly facilitates the recovery process. If fixed lateral hinging is present, other options, such as a Chiari pelvic osteotomy, a shelf arthroplasty, or a salvage intertrochanteric osteotomy, can be considered.

Ostectomy of the Femoral Neck and PAO

If present, resection of a cam-impingement lesion can be done in conjunction with PAO or ITO. Formal surgical dislocation can be combined with PAO. More often, resection of anterior and anterolateral cam lesions can be resected by straightforward anterior open arthrotomy, or adjunctive arthroscopy, at the time of PAO without the need for formal surgical dislocation.

Integration of Radiographic and Range of Motion Information

The range of motion of the hip provides valuable clues for decision making. Flexion of the hip in the supine position and extension in the prone position, abduction and adduction in the supine position, as well as internal and external rotation in the supine position, in both extension and 90° of flexion, should be assessed in all patients. The correlation with subtle radiographic findings can be striking. For instance, in a patient with marked anteversion of the acetabulum, as demonstrated radiographically by excessive prominence of the posterior acetabular margin and deficient anterior margin, an impairment of passive extension on range of motion testing in the prone position can be anticipated. The history taking in such a patient will likely reveal that he/she cannot walk comfortably with a long-stride gait, always has to "walk faster than everyone else" or "take more steps than everyone else" when walking with friends. Ask such a patient to walk in a crouched position and her face will light up with a smile and a comment like "It feels so good to walk this way." This is a circumstance in which a PAO with deliberate retroversion of the acetabular segment will enhance anterior coverage and simultaneously eliminate the excessive posterior prominence of the posterior acetabular wall. If such a patient also has hypermobility syndrome, clunking and shifting are common features, even in the absence of labral tear on MRI. Chondrolabral injuries can be seen posteriorly due to direct collision and anteriorly due to levering out or subluxation.

At the opposite end of the spectrum, when the posterior margin is diminished and the anterior margin is prominent, retroversion is present. As discussed previously, associated standing AP pelvis radiographic findings include the ischial spine sign (i.e., the visibility of the ischial spine inside the pelvis on the standing AP radiograph), and the crossover sign, or lateral overhang of the anterior acetabular margin. In these hips there is usually limitation of passive hip flexion due to impingement during flexion.

Most cases of DDH have some loss of femoral head coverage laterally. However, there are occasional cases in which the dysplasia occurs almost purely anteriorly or, less commonly, posteriorly. In "classic" dysplasia, a deficiency in lateral coverage is associated with hypoplasia of the anterior wall or generalized hypoplasia of the anterior and posterior walls. In that circumstance, lateral coverage enhancement PAO is the primary strategy, with adjunctive anterior coverage in the cases of anterior deficiency and posterior coverage enhancement in the case of retroversion.

Surgical Technique

As interest in the PAO procedure grew around the world, so did efforts to modify the surgical approach, in order to increase safety, to reduce muscle dissection, to preserve tendon attachments, and to protect the main trunk of the lateral femoral cutaneous nerve, among other objectives. The original transverse incision from the anterior pelvic fracture approach resulted in the obligatory sacrifice of the main trunk of the lateral femoral cutaneous nerve, and instances of thrombosis of the femoral vessels, as well as weakness of the abductors resulting from exposure of both the inner and outer tables of the ilium. Historically, weakness of the musculature, affecting hip flexion, adduction, and abduction, has been an issue in outcomes after triple innominate and other pediatric osteotomies, due to the stripping of muscles from their origins during the exposure, or from associated purposeful tendon releases, i.e., iliopsoas release. Boston surgeons (Millis, Murphy [10]) worked out a surgical approach that avoided the exposure of the lateral iliac wing and was based on a modification of the Smith-Petersen inter-nervous exposure in the interval between the sartorius medially (femoral nerve) and the tensor muscle laterally (superior gluteal nerve).

The technique which I currently use includes a semi-longitudinal incision just lateral to the iliac crest which then curves gently to the lateral side at the ASIS and continues for approximately 3 in. Proximally, only the medial side of the iliac crest is exposed, without violation of the origin of the abductors. The abdominal oblique and iliacus muscles are gently reflected medially from the inner table of the iliac crest, and the space generated is filled with an abdominal lap sponge, with careful control of bleeding. Then attention is turned to the distal portion. In order to protect the lateral femoral cutaneous nerve, the exposure of the interval between the tensor fascia lata and sartorius muscles is developed, not at the junction of the two muscles, but by entering the fascia of the tensor approximately 1 cm lateral to its border with the sartorius and finding the interval in the sub-fascial plane. Using this approach, the incidence of injury to the LFCN is now very low. Additionally, in the early years, I reflected the fibers of origin of the sartorius medially off of the ASIS by sharp dissection with a knife. For the last 18 years, I have used an oblique osteotomy of the ASIS that includes the origin of the sartorius. This avoids injury to the LFCN during the process of suture reattachment of the tendon. The iliocapsularis and deep fibers of the rectus are reflected from the anterior hip capsule with a periosteal elevator and a retractor is placed over the anterior hip capsule and into the pelvis. With upward pressure on this retractor, the tendon of the reflected head is sharply divided and tagged. Again, with a cobra retractor under the rectus and directed into the pelvis, the direct head of the rectus is then reflected off of the anterior inferior iliac spine. In recent years, I have adopted a technique that preserves the tendons of origin of both the indirect and direct heads of the rectus. It is still possible to do the anterior arthrotomy to resect a cam lesion, but it is not possible to access the hip joint. There are significant variations in the anatomy and position of the anterior inferior iliac spine. When it is prominent, I will do an osteotomy of the AIIS, similar to the technique with the ASIS, and repair to drill holes or use a suture anchor. The combined soft-tissue mass of the iliacus/abdominal oblique and the osteotomy fragment with the sartorius origin are reflected medially to permit exposure of the pubis. A curved periosteal elevator is used to access the ischium. The first bone cut is that of the ischium, with a curved osteotome, greatly aided by fluoroscopy. Due to the clearance of C-arm under the table, the view is a PA and not an AP of the hip, as reported by Howie. There are subtle differences between an AP and a PA, due to magnification effects, which are reversed. The posterior margin of the acetabulum will be larger than it would be on an AP, which mimics a standing AP pelvis view, rather than the image obtained with the patient supine [11]. The pubis can be cut with an osteotome, as originally described. I prefer, however, to cut the pubic bone with a Gigli saw, passed around the posterior aspect of the bone, with retractors protecting the obturator neurovascular structures. This is a technique that was worked out with Peter Stevens of Utah in 1992 during a series of cadaver dissections. The ilium is then cut with a power saw, beginning in the lower portion of the previously performed ASIS osteotomy, or just below it, coursing toward the lower border of the sacroiliac joint. There is tremendous variation in the relationship of the ASIS and the AIIS, due to the associated variations in the anatomy of the pelvic wing. Sometimes the ASIS is virtually directly anterior to the AIIS, when observed from directly anterior to the ASIS, and in other cases it is quite proximal to it. When it is widely apart, it is much less likely that the iliac cut will be located near the joint. On the other hand, when the two structures are closely related, extra care needs to be taken to avoid the joint with the iliac cuts. The power saw cut of the iliac wing stops 15 mm lateral to the pelvic brim. One of the most important cuts then follows, in which the pelvic brim is cut with a standard osteotome. Due to the thickness and toughness of the bone in this area, some will use a Midas Rex to initiate this cut, though I do not do that. This cut has to avoid both the hip joint and the posterior column. The next cut is the osteotomy of the lamina quadrilateral, threading a fine line between the posterior column and the hip joint. Use of fluoroscopy is particularly helpful with this cut. The previously made ischial cut can be seen on the fluoroscope image, or it can be palpated from inside the pelvis. The 30/30 view of Joel Matta is very useful. The C-arm is rotated back (away from the surgeon) 30° on the main arc and 30° toward the foot of the patient on secondary arc. After this cut, gentle manipulation should cause the fragment to move without undue force. If force is needed, back off and revisit the ischial cut and the pelvic brim cut and check for completeness. Use of force with hinging may result in propagation of a crack into the joint or create a fracture across the posterior column.

In patients with hypermobility, everything can be accomplished without takedown of the tendons of the rectus. Most of my cases are now done without takedown of the rectus tendons. Even an open arthrotomy for ostectomy of an impingement lesion can be done with preservation of these tendons. The rate of heterotopic ossification and tendonitis is greater in my experience when the tendons are taken down and repaired. Once the fragment is mobilized, it is useful to distract the cut edges of the ilium with a large laminar spreader. There is almost always very active bleeding from a vessel within the bone. Use of bone wax can save hundreds of cubic centimeters of blood that would have otherwise been lost. This technique, plus the use of the cell saver in all cases, has reduced the incidence of blood transfusion in my procedures to near zero.

Repositioning of the Acetabular Segment

After successful mobilization of the acetabular segment, the next, and very important task, is reorientation of the acetabulum. Of course, the goal is normalization of coverage, without overcorrection or undercorrection. Most cases require increased lateral and anterior coverage. In the early years of the PAO experience, some patients experienced significant impairment of flexion after the surgery. This was discovered to be due to excessive anterior coverage. Swiss surgeons, most associated with the University of Bern, deserve credit for elucidating this issue. It led to a broad study of acetabular orientation and the discovery that approximately 15% of all patients have some degree of anterior over-coverage, or retroversion, as a component of their dysplasia. In these cases, reverse PAO, i.e., deliberate creation of additional anteversion of the acetabulum with the PAO, is the appropriate surgical strategy.

There are various ways to maintain control of the acetabular segment during reorientation. A Schanz screw, or large pincer clamps, or pelvic fracture clamps can all be used effectively. I prefer three pelvic clamps, since the Schanz screw will tend to unwind with any reverse rotatory motion. The orientation of the sourcil in the AP and oblique views, as well as the relationship of the anterior and posterior walls, needs to be monitored. This is the portion of the operation during which it is most important to invest time and attention. Reorientation of the acetabulum a number of times may be necessary to achieve the best combination of features. It is important to pay attention simultaneously to lateral coverage, as well as the relationship between the anterior and posterior acetabular margins. At this point in history, the repositioning is an inexact science. Attempts to apply computer-assisted surgery to repositioning the acetabular segment have proven more difficult than anticipated. At some point in the future, it is highly likely that robotic-assisted repositioning of the acetabular segment will emerge. The use of intraoperative PA fluoroscopy is helpful to assess the qualitative and quantitative accuracy of repositioning. Flat plate AP pelvis is used by many surgeons, too, but suffers from the drawback that it is not a replica of the standing view, which is the more valuable radiograph. The emergence of direct digital portable X-ray technology has greatly facilitated the use of the intraoperative AP pelvis radiograph. The final accepted position is held with two K-wires, followed by definitive screw fixation. I prefer the use of three or four 4.5 mm cortical screws, all starting at the iliac crest and diverging out into the mobile acetabular segment. I developed and began to recommend this technique in the early 1990s, in order to be able to easily remove all screws on a routine basis 6 months or more after the osteotomy. Screws, which begin deep in the pelvis and course superiorly and medially, can be quite difficult to remove. Though 3.5 screws are commonly used in many centers, I prefer the larger 4.5 cortical screws in almost all circumstances, as 4.5 mm screws are less likely to break during removal, which I do on a routine basis. The one situation in which I choose 3.5 mm cortical screws is in cases in which I incorporate adjunctive bony support using structural iliac crest grafts. The closure includes repair of the abdominal oblique to the iliac crest, reattachment of the ASIS osteotomy with a heavy suture, and repair of the myofascial of the tensor, with care to avoid ensnaring the lateral femoral cutaneous nerve. The skin is closed with a subcuticular absorbable suture, cyanoacrylate application to the skin, and a clear plastic adhesive dressing that is waterproof and permits showering beginning on the first post-op day without any additional wound protection.

The Issue of Screw Removal

Though my colleagues from the pelvic trauma world do not routinely remove screws, I do so in all cases. Even patients who describe their outcome after PAO as "perfect" will tell me after removal of the screws that it feels "even better." There is a surprisingly high prevalence of mild-to-significant nickel intolerance in the general population. In fact, we are screening for that aggressively now as part of the pre-op process and using titanium screws whenever nickel intolerance is proven or suspected. I routinely remove screws because they can interfere with future surgical options, are associated with perceived or unrecognized symptoms, and are more difficult to remove many years after insertion than in the early post-op period. Removal of hardware at the time of a future total hip replacement, should that be required, is associated with a higher incidence of infection and longer operating time, and may require separate incisions and positioning. The timing for removal has evolved over time. I used to wait at least 6 months in all cases. Now, I will remove the screws as soon as 4 months after surgery if bone consolidation is evident on follow-up radiographs and there are clinical or strategic reasons, such as tender screw heads in thin patients, impending loss of insurance coverage or relocation, etc. When staged, bilateral PAOs are done I will wait until healing of the second side and then do bilateral, outpatient screw removal on both sides. We can accomplish staged, bilateral PAOs and hardware removal in the same year when the first side is done by April or earlier in that year.

Pain Management

Pain management is very similar to the multimodal protocol for total joint replacement cases. This is an area in which the input from the adult reconstructive perspective has been particularly helpful to PAO patients. There is nothing, other than a poor outcome, that patients worry about more before PAO surgery than how bad the pain will be after surgery. My protocol includes spinal anesthetic in all patients, with adjunctive intra-thecal morphine, multidrug pre-op meds, multidrug injection into the soft tissues during the procedure, IV Tylenol, IV steroids, Cox II oral anti-inflammatory, and avoidance of post-op narcotics to the greatest degree possible. All patients have no pain at all in the post-anesthesia care unit (PACU) and for the better part of the next 24 h. After that, our techniques still do not rise to the level of "near guarantee" of freedom from any pain that we reliably accomplish for the day of surgery and the night of surgery. Minimal use of narcotics helps to avoid the dreaded emergence of constipation and the associated nausea, abdominal cramps, and loss of appetite. The goal is to avoid pain above 4 out of 10 in the entire post-op period. Though I prescribe oxycodone 5 mg for all patients for their discretionary use upon discharge, more and more patients do not take it at all, with my encouragement. Most patients are able to go home by the fourth day post-op.

Helplessness After PAO

The feeling of helplessness is commonly experienced by patients after PAO which I routinely discuss with patients prior to their admission to the hospital. Even though most patients can go out to a restaurant with their family within a week of the surgery, they cannot do anything independently for a number of weeks, such as carrying items to and from a refrigerator, making a bed, preparing a meal, and taking a shower. This is much more of an issue than pain and needs to be addressed ahead of time with a proper support system in place. It's really a form of temporary, but quite significant, post-traumatic stress disorder. It is an act of kindness and consideration to include this as part of the pre-op consultation. When PAO is on the right side, as opposed to the left, driving is not possible for around 6 weeks or more, though hand-controlled cars can be rented for those who desire to return to work as soon as possible. Patients with light-duty occupations, such as attorneys, CPAs, and portfolio managers. can return to work within 2 weeks, if they insist on the earliest possible return. Six weeks is more realistic for early return and 3 months for ability to walk normally without any support and have the endurance to work 8+ hours in a day. The issue about return to work is often more an issue of the regulations of employers which often preclude even a highly motivated employee from returning to the workplace unless they have a "return to work without restrictions" designation. High-demand occupations, such as firemen, athletes, and active-duty marines, take at least 6 months or more for return without restrictions. I prescribe a wheelchair rental for 2 months for all patients and this greatly facilitates their ability to engage in more occupational and non-occupational activities of interest than would otherwise be possible.

Blood Management

All cases are done under hypotensive spinal with IV aminocaproic acid to minimize blood loss. Due to customarily low intra-op blood loss, patients get a "type and hold" upon admission. I have not had a case of intra-op transfusion in over 20 years. There is no pre-op use of autologous blood donation. Average estimated blood loss for a PAO is 150–700 cm^3. We use a cell saver in all cases and reinfuse even small volumes of recovered blood to keep the transfusion rate as close to zero as possible in the postoperative period. The odd case with heavy intra-op bleeding is easily handled with intra-op reinfusion from the cell saver. In those cases, we will activate a type and cross for two units, just in case. After a period of time with no drains, I have reverted back to use of drains for 24 h because of the frequent need to aspirate fluid when they were not used. Using a trigger of hemoglobin of less than or equal to 7.0 with symptoms, our transfusion rate is approximately 2 % of cases.

Post-op Rehabilitation

Patients are mobilized to sit and to stand on the day of surgery. Often the impediment to walking on the day of surgery is low blood pressure after a spinal anesthetic. Absent orthostatic hypotension, patients are encouraged to walk with a walker on the day of surgery, and for sure on the day after. Showering is permitted as soon as drains and the Foley urinary catheter have been removed, usually by POD #2. Patients are progressed from walker to crutches as tolerated and are taught stair climbing by POD #3. Discharge occurs anywhere from POD#3 to POD#6, depending on the rate of early recovery. Constipation from narcotics can be the main impediment to early discharge. Out-of-town patients are permitted to drive or fly home within 5–7 days of the surgery. Ambulation is with two crutches TDWB with a reciprocal heel-to-toe gait. After 4 weeks, weight bearing is increased to WBAT with two sticks, and pool therapy begins at that time as well. Progression to a single stick occurs at around weeks 6–8 and FWB without support is usually achieved by 10 weeks after the surgery. Straight leg raising is prohibited for 3 months.

DVT Prophylaxis

All patients are placed on the same protocol as total joint patients, including bilateral knee-high sequential compression devices, with initiation of chemoprophylaxis within 23 h of surgery. It is continued for a total of 10 days after surgery, followed by aspirin, 162 mg per day, for an additional 60 days.

Results

Postoperative results have been well documented in the literature, and in a separate chapter in this book. Absent preexisting arthritis or early complication, the anticipated duration of the outcome is at least 10 years, with many patients experiencing indefinite survival of the biologic hip. I explain to my patients that the likelihood of a good result is approximately 75 % at 10 years or more after the procedure. No patient is ever told that the operation is a cure for their condition or is guaranteed to eliminate all pain. All patients are told that any preoperative damage to the cartilage within the joint is irreversible and that the surface area of their articular cartilage is deficient and cannot be restored to normal.

Hence the unit load on the articular cartilage will still be indefinitely greater, but the distribution improved, compared to pre-op, by the reorientation of the acetabulum.

References

1. Ganz R, Klaue K, Vinh TS, Mast JW. A new periacetabular osteotomy for the treatment of hip dysplasias: technique and preliminary results. Clin Orthop Relat Res. 1988;232:26–36.
2. Li PL, Ganz R. Morphologic features of congenital acetabular dysplasia: one in six is retroverted. Clin Orthop Relat Res. 2003;416:245–53.
3. Tannast M, Zheng G, Anderegg C, Burckhardt K, Langlotz F, Ganz R, Siebenrock KA. Tilt and rotation correction of acetabular version on pelvic radiographs. Clin Orthop Relat Res. 2005;438:182–90.
4. Wiberg G. Studies on dysplastic acetabula and congenital subluxation of the hip joint. Acta Chir Scand. 1939;58(Suppl):1–35.
5. Murphy SB, Ganz R, Muller ME. The prognosis in untreated dysplasia of the hip. A study of radiographic factors that predict the outcome. J Bone Joint Surg. 1995;77A:985–9.
6. Kalberer F, Sierra RJ, Madan SS, Ganz R, Leunig M. Ischial spine projection into the pelvis: a new sign for acetabular retroversion. Clin Orthop Relat Res. 2008;466(3):677–83.
7. Lequesne M, de Seze S. Le faux profil du bassin. Nouvelle incidence radiographique pour l'etude de la hanche. Son utilite dans les dysplasies et les differentes coxopathies. Rev Rhum. 1961;28:643–52.
8. Matsuda DK. Acute iatrogenic dislocation following hip impingement arthroscopic surgery. Arthroscopy. 2009;25(4):400–4.
9. Beighton PH, Horan F. Orthopedic aspects of the Ehlers-Danlos syndrome. J Bone Joint Surg (Br). 1969;51:444–53.
10. Murphy SB, Millis MB. Periacetabular osteotomy without abductor dissection using direct anterior exposure. Clin Orthop Relat Res. 1999;364:92–8.
11. Personal communication, Prof. Don Howie, U. of Adelaide, Australia. 2013

Birmingham Interlocking Peri-Acetabular Osteotomy

73

Jason Brockwell, John N. O'Hara, and David A. Young

Birmingham Interlocking Peri-Acetabular Osteotomy

The Birmingham Interlocking Peri-Acetabular Osteotomy (BIPO or Birmingham PAO) [1] is a modification of the Tönnis osteotomy [2, 3] where the straight iliac osteotomy is changed to three linked cuts. It can be used in any type of dysplasia in adults and also in children, as it avoids the triradiate cartilage. We use this osteotomy for both correction of acetabular dysplasia and correction of over-coverage in cases of acetabular retroversion and protrusio acetabula (the so-called reverse peri-acetabular osteotomy).

The iliac cuts "interlock" (Fig. 73.1) when the central acetabular fragment (CAF) is rotated, allowing accurate positioning and immediate stability, sufficient for unrestricted weight bearing and consequent rapid rehabilitation. The angle between the three interlinked iliac cuts determines the correction achieved.

The CAF is manoeuvred into position using an external fixator as a lever. The plane of application of the fixator to the CAF reflects the presenting malalignment of the dysplastic socket.

Because the posterior acetabular column is divided proximal to the sacro-spinous ligament, the CAF can be easily mobilised in all three planes, unimpaired by any posterior tether. The Birmingham PAO does not have the hang-up that occurs at the so-called 'Trousdale point' (Fig. 73.2) in the Bernese procedure when anterior rotation is required to disengage the CAF from the intact posterior column. The 'Trousdale point' is at the inferior end of the posterior column vertical cut where it meets the ischial cut. This is particularly tricky to access with a single incision anteriorly.

The Birmingham PAO is performed through two incisions. The small posterior incision allows mobilisation of the sciatic nerve from the sciatic notch to quadratus femoris before cutting the ischium. The lateral position allows simultaneous hip extension and knee flexion to relax the sciatic nerve when cutting the ischium. The patient is then turned supine and the pubic and iliac osteotomies performed through a Salter incision. The patient is not re-draped between lateral and supine positions.

The operation is planned to correct the apical weight-bearing zone (Tönnis sourcil angle) to horizontal and the apical acetabular version to a roof edge angle [4] of zero degrees. These are the key references in calculating the bone cuts and the external fixator placement.

Volumetric studies show that the central acetabular fragment is the same size in the Bernese [5] and Birmingham osteotomies (Fig. 73.3).

Birmingham PAO Surgical Technique

The patient is placed supine on the operating table and positioned so that an intraoperative AP hip or pelvis radiograph or image intensifier view can be obtained. A folded sheet is placed across the table under the patient's buttocks with a knot or gather in the sheet on each side for surgeon and the assistant to feel through the drapes. (This facilitates easy rolling to supine from the lateral position used initially for the ischial osteotomy to the supine position for the pubic and iliac osteotomies.) A urinary catheter may be inserted, depending on the anaesthetic technique, but is not mandatory. The patient is then placed in the lateral position with a posterior buttock incision for the ischial osteotomy.

The patient has a side support on one side of the chest, anterior or posterior according to surgeon preference. A 10 cm wide elastic plaster is used to hold the chest to the support.

J. Brockwell, FRCSEdOrth, FHKAMOrth (✉)
Hip & Pelvic Surgery, Asia Medical Specialists, 8/F Aon China Bldg., 29 Queen's Rd Central, Hong Kong, SAR People's Republic of China
e-mail: jason.brockwell@asiamedical.hk

J.N. O'Hara, FRCS, FRCSI, MCh
The Birmingham Hip Clinic, Birmingham, UK

D.A. Young, FRACS
Melbourne Orthopaedic Group, Melbourne, Australia

J.C. McCarthy et al. (eds.), *Hip Joint Restoration*, DOI 10.1007/978-1-4614-0694-5_73

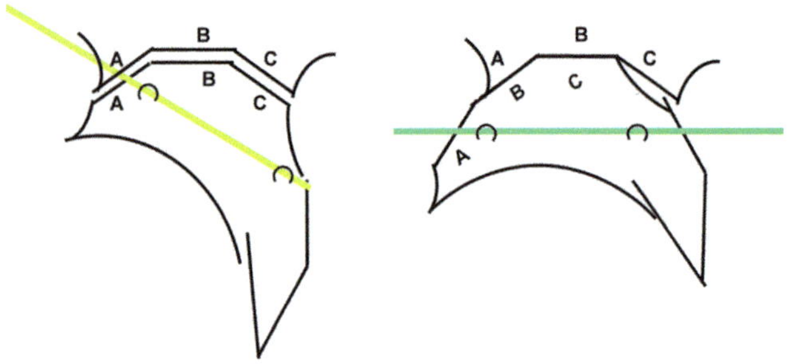

Fig. 73.1 The essential principle of the operation is to make three linked bone cuts on the ilium, the angle between them (here 30°) reflecting the intended lateral rotation of the central acetabular fragment (CAF). An external fixator is attached to the CAF in the plane of the presenting acetabular malalignment to provide a powerful lever to mobilise the CAF and manoeuvre it into a position of predictable and reproducible correction

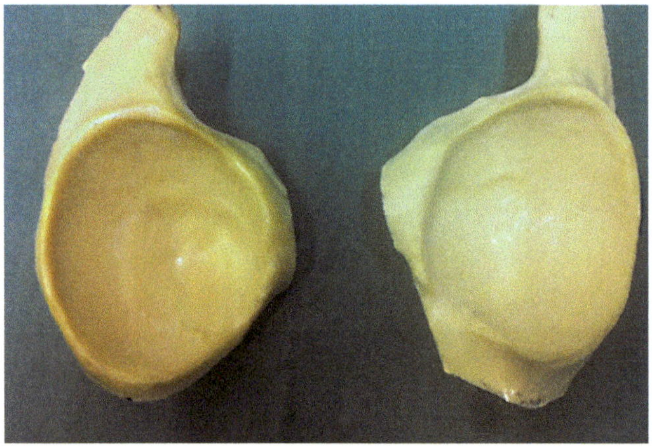

Fig. 73.3 Central acetabular fragments from the Birmingham and Bernese osteotomies performed in Sawbones artificial pelves. Measurement by a simple water displacement method reveals near-identical volumes

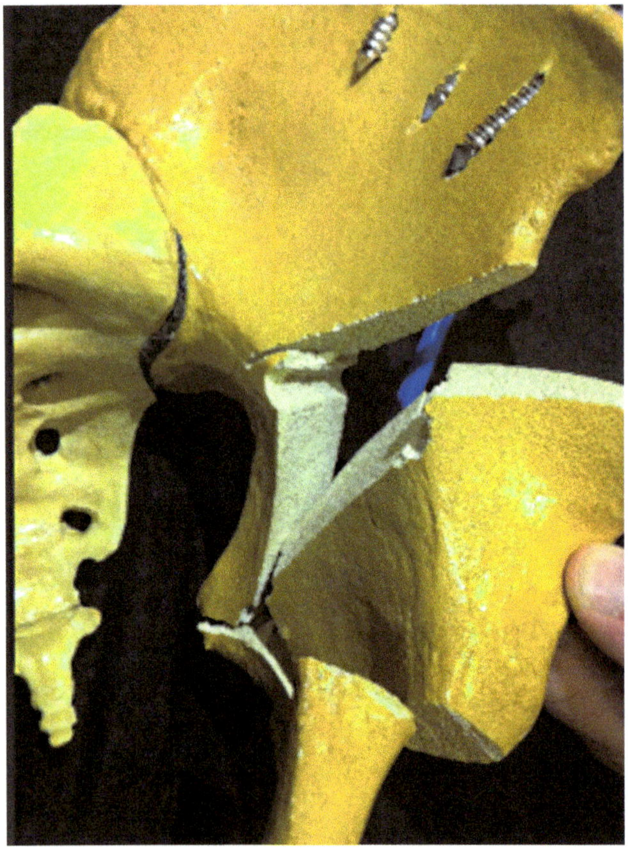

Fig. 73.2 The 'Trousdale point' is located at the intersection of the vertical cut through the posterior column and the ischial cut at its inferior end. The CAF can catch here

The leg is draped free with a U-drape, which just covers the umbilicus and must be routed up the natal cleft, and along the spine. The suction tube and diathermy cable are routed anterior to the patient and held in place by the transverse drape, which is positioned just distal to the umbilicus with the centre of the drape adjacent the umbilicus. This arrangement is to allow the drapes, suction and diathermy to move smoothly when the patient is turned, with no compromise of sterility. The posterior incision is placed obliquely half way between greater trochanter and the ischial tuberosity and is 5–10 cm long depending on the size of the patient. If a simultaneous femoral osteotomy is performed, the ischial osteotomy is performed through the femoral incision.

The leg is held with the hip extended and the knee flexed to relax the sciatic nerve. A little internal rotation of the hip produces more space.

After dividing the skin and fat, the fascia of the gluteus maximus is first cut with diathermy, allowing the muscle to be separated in the line of its fibres mainly by fingertip dissection, aiming towards the sciatic nerve. A self-retaining retractor holds the gluteus maximus during mobilisation of the sciatic nerve. The plane beyond the sciatic nerve is developed with a fingertip or the tip of a cholecystectomy forceps. The nerve is mobilised manually over a distance of 10–12 cm extending from the sciatic notch proximally to the quadratus femoris distally.

The osteotomy plane is defined by the subcotyloid groove, which is easily palpable. The osteotomy divides the ischium in the line of the subcotyloid groove from the greater sciatic notch to the obturator foramen. The osteotomy must not enter the lesser sciatic notch: the sacro-spinous ligament will tether the central acetabular fragment and impair accurate adjustment, and Adson's canal, containing the pudendal nerve and vessels, may be damaged.

With the sciatic nerve retracted onto the ischial tuberosity and protected by the index finger of the surgeon's non-dominant hand, the small lateral rotators are separated at their midpoint by spreading with a pair of curved scissors; Lanes bone levers (in the sciatic notch and the obturator foramen) are then used to retract and expose the ischium. Once the bone levers are in situ, the finger protecting the sciatic nerve can be removed. Predrilling the osteotomy is unnecessary.

A spade-tipped long-handled Lexer osteotome is first placed in the greatest depth of the palpable subcotyloid groove, to start a bone cut connecting the two Lanes bone levers. The bone is thickest here (2.5–3 cm) and the osteotome should not breach the inner cortex at this stage. The cut is then extended up and down to the Lanes bone levers, completing the upper and lower ends of the osteotomy by directing the osteotome obliquely at each bone lever in turn. Only then is the central part completed to the deep cortex; if the upper and lower ends are not already divided, the spade of the osteotome will become trapped by closure of the outer cortex. The mobility of the osteotomy can be confirmed by twisting a *fully seated* osteotome or Cobb elevator in the deepest part of the cut. At this stage, it is important to be confident that the ischial osteotomy is complete, as it is not possible to reach it from the anterior incision later.

After wound closure and covering the dressing, the patient is turned supine. The back (or front) rest is removed and the patient turned, in a move coordinated with the anaesthetist. The patient is leveled and corrected for pelvic obliquity.

A Salter "bikini line" incision is preferred, but a Smith-Petersen incision can be used. An internal ilioinguinal exposure is made down to the sciatic notch and the superior pubic ramus. The tissues are taken off in a single sheet. Immediately beyond the ASIS a right-angled cholecystectomy forceps is used to split the tissues symmetrically in the plane of the iliac wing. This tissue separation will always be medial to the lateral femoral cutaneous nerve, which is then mobilised distally by blunt dissection using a finger or scissors. A plastic or rubber loop can be passed around the nerve for easy identification.

In some patients distal finger dissection is necessary to separate the tissue planes and septa between the iliopsoas and the anterior capsule/rectus femoris.

Once the deep surface of the lateral end of the superior pubic ramus is exposed, a cholecystectomy forceps is placed in the obturator canal immediately superficial to the vessels and the obturator membrane; its tip marks the ideal site for the osteotomy, and serves as a target for the saw whilst protecting the obturator nerve and vessels. After suitable periosteal dissection, a bone lever (e.g. a blunt Hohman or Lanes) is placed opposite this on the superficial aspect of the superior pubic ramus. A cholecystectomy forceps can be used distally to spread the soft tissues, taking care not to injure the obturator neurovascular structures, to make room for the cutting tool.

The superior pubic ramus is cut vertically with a reciprocating saw in the plane of the quadrilateral plate. The saw allows a more lateral osteotomy than an osteotome, which tends to slide medially on the pubis. Lateral placement of the osteotomy provides the biggest area of contact between the two sides of the pubis after the osteotomy is displaced, and reduces the chance of non-union. Alternatively the pubis can be scored with the saw and the osteotomy completed with either a straight or curved osteotome. It is possible to enter the joint by placing the saw cut lateral to the pectineal eminence. Image intensification can be used, though, with experience, it is not necessary. Displaceability is confirmed by twisting an osteotome or a Cobb.

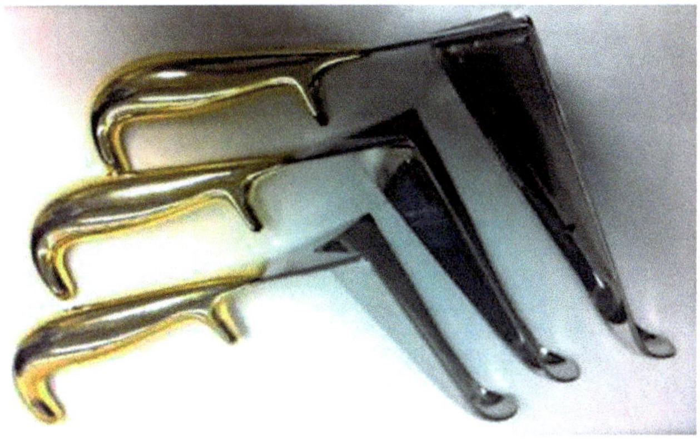

Fig. 73.4 O'Hara sciatic notch retractors

Attention is now directed to the ilium. The O'Hara sciatic notch retractor (Fig. 73.4) is vital at this and all later stages to protect the sciatic nerve from injury. The key landmark is the greatest depth of the sciatic notch. The middle (B) cut must be just above this, and horizontal. The medial (C) cut must enter the sciatic notch at its greatest depth. The lateral (A) cut must be a mirror image of the C cut and usually finds itself just above the AIIS (Fig. 73.5). The cuts should be of equal length if anteversion is not to be adjusted. Beginners may wish to make the B cut a little wider than the C cut to allow a little leeway. If adjustment of acetabular anteversion is planned, the BC angle must be moved 2–3 mm medially (Fig. 73.6). Many surgeons mark the bone with diathermy or a marking pen. The AB and BC angles can be usefully marked with a 3.2 mm drill before the bone cuts are made.

The #1 screw is inserted next to the quadrilateral plate, about 1–1.5 cm below the medial edge of the C cut (Fig. 73.5). If version is to be adjusted, the screw needs to be inserted in internal or external rotation as required (Figs. 73.7, 73.8 and 73.9). The external fixator is applied in the position reflecting the presenting misalignment. Be aware that the sciatic nerve is at risk and use a drill-stop set at the femoral head diameter to prevent over-penetration. The #2 screw hole is drilled at this stage, but the screw is not inserted until the osteotomy is complete.

Many surgeons will want to check all these calculations on an image intensifier. With experience, this is unnecessary.

The bone cuts are performed using a sharp-ended 12 mm reciprocating saw (Fig. 73.10). The saw is held vertically and parallel to the #1 Schanz screw at all times. The osteotomy will be complete when all three parts link up fully.

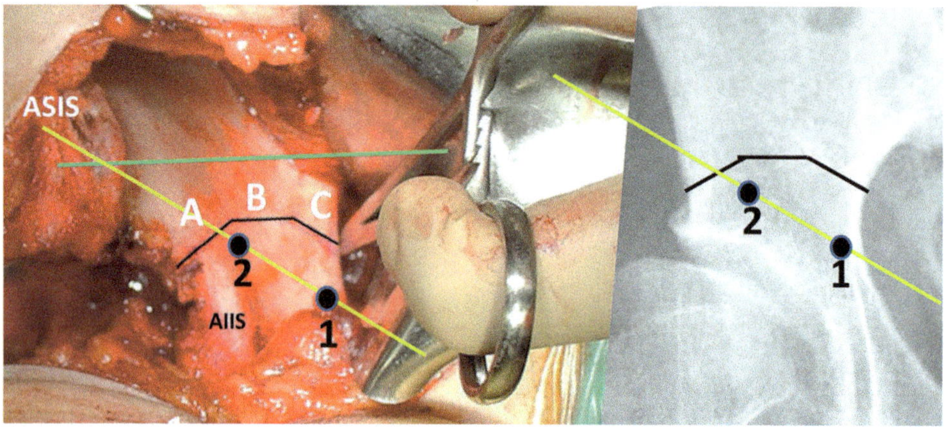

Fig. 73.5 Marking bone cuts and screw holes for planned simple lateral rotation of 30°. The bone cuts are of the same width and are labelled *A*, *B* and *C* from medial to lateral. The *B* cut is horizontal (parallel to the indicative *green line*). The C cut (parallel to the presenting weight-bearing zone) ends medially at the level of the deepest part of the sciatic notch (the cholecystectomy forceps). The *A* cut (a mirror image of the *C* cut) begins at the level of the lateral capsule/rectus femoris reflected head (just above the AIIS). Marking the *AB* and *BC* angles with a 3.2 mm drill can be helpful. The #1 screw is placed 10–15 mm distal to the *C* cut, in the sagittal/axial plane and next to the quadrilateral plate. The #2 screw is placed as far away as possible (for the best mechanical advantage and the stiffest ex-fix construct) using the jig to provide 30° of correction (indicative *yellow line*). It is usually near the *AB* angle

Fig. 73.6 The bone cuts. When adjusting lateral cover only (here 30°), the screws should be inserted in the strict sagittal/axial plane and the bone cuts should be of equal width. Thus the *C* cut of the *CAF* will sit up snugly and securely on the *B* cut of the ilium. Adjustment of anteversion will not be possible. Indeed, the *B*–*C* interlock will not be snug if the *C* cut is any longer than the *B* cut; it may be better to have the *B* cut 1–2 mm longer than the *C* cut until the surgeon is practiced at the technique

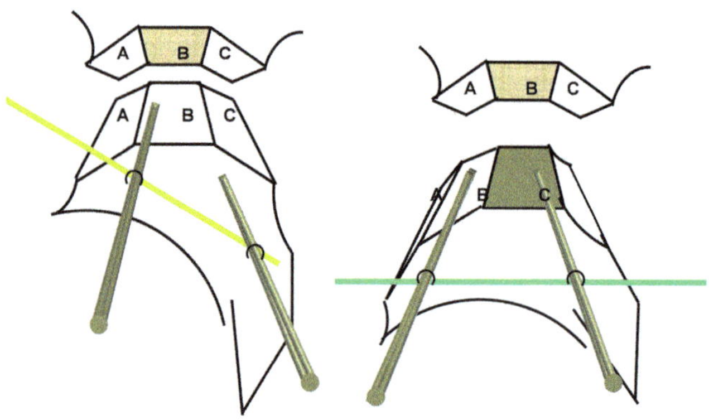

Fig. 73.7 Inserting Schanz screw #1 (anteversion adjustment). *Left*: View from cephalad. *Right*: Surgeon's view from upper end of wound. The #1 screw is inserted next to the quadrilateral plate and, if anteversion is not be adjusted (as in this example), is vertical in both planes. If anteversion is to be reduced (*R*) by 15°, it would be inserted in 15° of internal rotation (*purple line*). If anteversion is to be increased (*I*) by 15°, it would be inserted in the 15° of external rotation (*black line*) and started a little more laterally

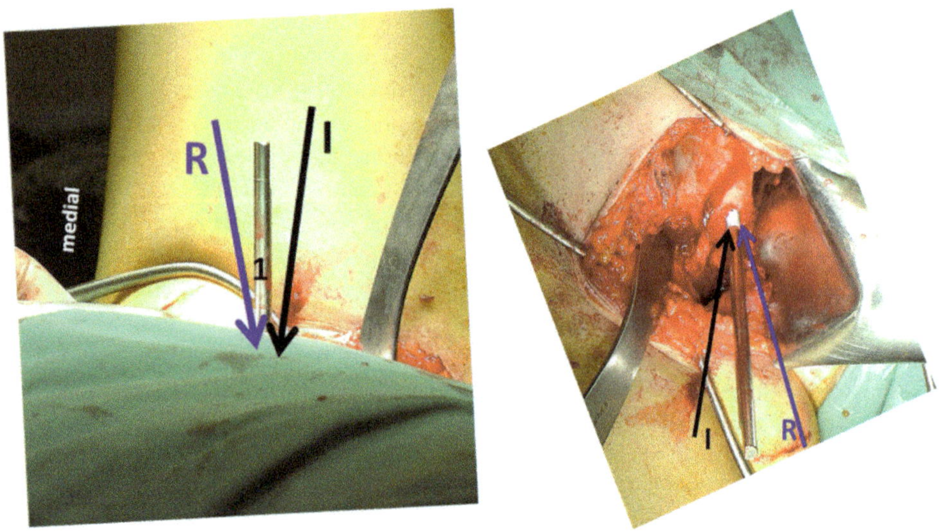

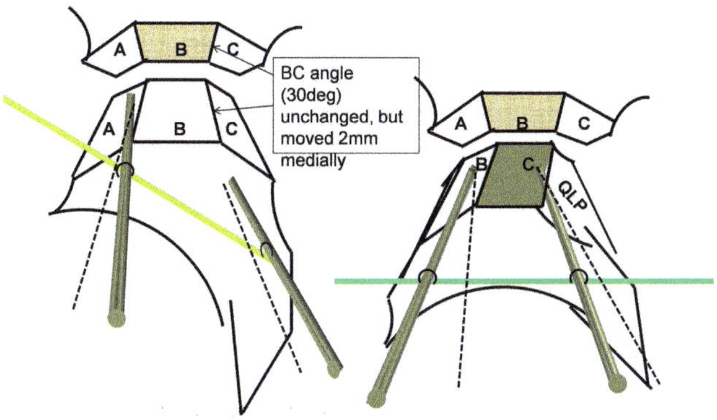

Fig. 73.8 The bone cuts when reducing anteversion. When adjusting lateral cover (here 30°), and reducing anteversion by for example 15°, the screws should be inserted in 15° of internal rotation (compared with *dotted lines* in sagittal/axial plane) and the *B* cut should be longer than the *C* cut by moving the *BC* angle 2–3 mm medially (this produces a 5 mm difference between the *B* and *C* cuts). This allows the *CAF* to be externally rotated in the barrel vault of the ilium. The *C* cut of the *CAF* will sit up snugly and securely on the *B* cut of the ilium and the anterior part of the *B* cut will abut up against the *A* cut proximally

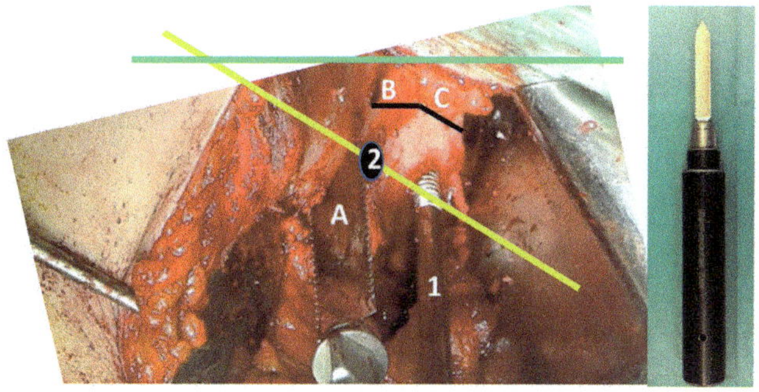

Fig. 73.10 Iliac osteotomy cuts. The equal length markings are confirmed for the A–B–C osteotomy. (If anteversion is to be adjusted, the B cut must be made wider than the C cut.) The reciprocating saw is used to cut all three parts of the iliac osteotomy. Here the blade is in the A cut. A steady hand and a fresh stiff blade are called for. The initial marks on the bone are made with saw blade tangential to the intended cut. Once the cortex is breached, the direction of the saw is strictly downwards/backwards with the body of the saw and the blade always held in the vertical plane, except when small side-to-side movements are required to completely link up cuts at the angles. An exception is the C cut; once the cortex is breached, it is best to progress down the medial side of the cut, intentionally touching the sciatic notch retractor until the cut is complete medially; then the cut should be progressed laterally with the saw in the vertical plane to join up with the B cut. *Right*; the preferred Synthes Compact Air Drive reciprocating saw

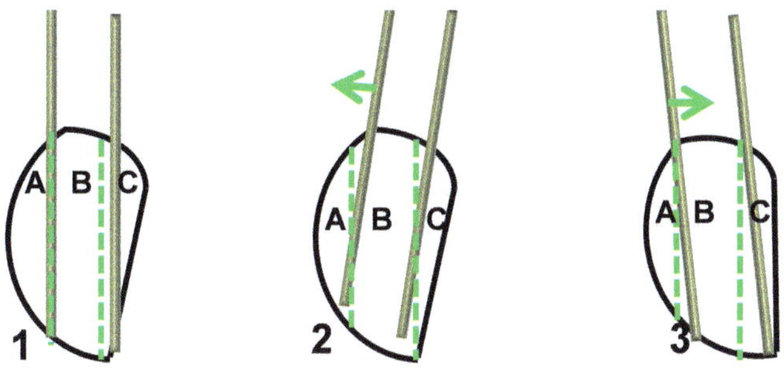

Fig. 73.9 Cross sections through the iliac osteotomy showing the following: *1*. Initial Schanz screw positions and bone cuts (*dotted green lines*) required for no adjustment of anteversion. Note that, even if the quadrilateral plate presents in internal rotation, this is ignored. *2*. Screw positions and bone cuts where anteversion is to be reduced by 10° (*green arrow*). Note that the *B* cut is 3–4 mm wider but, as is often found, the associated internal rotation of the quadrilateral plate results in a fortuitous tapering of the *C* cut, facilitating easy external rotation of the central acetabular fragment. *3*. Screw positions and bone cuts where anteversion is to be increased by 10° (*green arrow*). Again, the *B* cut is made slightly wider. If the quadrilateral plate presents in external rotation, reverse tapering of the *C* cut will occur, again facilitating satisfactory correction

Any tethers are usually at the posterior aspects of the corners. Do not try to complete the osteotomy with an osteotome; small spikes will result, which are difficult to remove. A Cobb or long-handled osteotome in the osteotomy site is twisted to ensure that the osteotomy is complete. The #2 Schanz screw is inserted and the rigid external fixator is applied. The CAF is freed by flexing the hip and pulling the fixator distally and laterally in the direction of the tensor fascia lata.

The fixator is then manoeuvred into the corrected position, with the bar of the fixator horizontal and the Schanz screws vertical. The corrected position is held with 2 mm K-wires inserted from the iliac crest. The position is checked with X-ray of the pelvis or with an image intensifier in 10° of internal rotation to reproduce the parallax of an AP X-ray beam. Check that the posterior wall of the rotated fragment sits at the centre of the femoral head, to ensure that version is correct and that the sourcil is horizontal.

There are two ways of fixing the osteotomy, with 2–3×6.5 mm partially threaded (16 mm thread length) cancellous screws from the iliac crest or with a three-hole dynamic compression plate placed vertically from the #1 screw hole towards the sacro-iliac joint, with two further compression screws. The #2 screw is not removed until the bones are solidly fixed; it is used to check the security of the fixation and the maintenance of correct anteversion adjustment until a solid fix is achieved (Fig. 73.11). Bone graft from drillings and tappings is used to pack the minor gaps. The wound is injected with 100 ml of a mixture of long-acting local anaesthetic: tranexamic acid, adrenaline and ketorolac [6].

A drill hole is made in the ASIS to reattach the inguinal ligament.

The abdominal muscles are carefully repaired onto the iliac crest in two layers. No tissue is repaired below the ASIS to avoid damage to the lateral femoral cutaneous nerve. No drain is used.

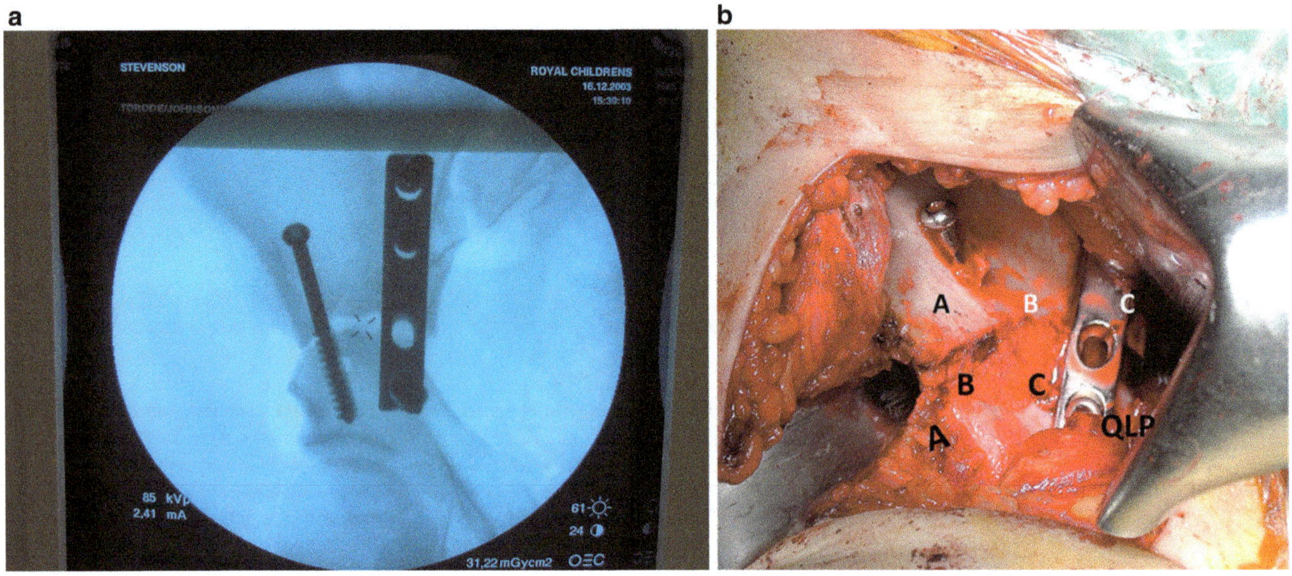

Fig. 73.11 The appearance after fixation and bone grafting; the graft was obtained by cleaning the saw blade and the drills after each use. Note the perfect relationships between the anterior and posterior acetabular columns (image gantry internally tilted 10° to correct parallax)

Post-operative Care

The most comfortable position is supine with the hip and knee flexed in an adjustable bed or with a pillow under the lower leg. A monkey bar is very helpful. Patients are mobilised with full weight bearing as soon as comfortable and can abandon walking aids when they can walk without a limp.

Instruments

Most of the instruments required for this procedure are widely available. The only special instruments are:

1. The O'Hara sciatic notch retractor
2. A double-sided pointed-tip reciprocating saw blade (Fig. 73.10)
3. A drill-stop to prevent over-penetration of the Schanz screw holes damaging the sciatic nerve

The O'Hara sciatic notch retractor (Fig. 73.4) is a modified version of Rang retractor with a longer tip, thus designed to work on its own as opposed to in pairs, as in Rang's original design [7]. The O'Hara retractor is placed in the true pelvis, with its tip in the sciatic notch, protecting the sciatic nerve from the tip of the reciprocating saw. The Rang retractor has a shorter tip-ne is passed into the true pelvis and the other along the outer surface of the ilium, with the tips meeting in the sciatic notch. Lateral iliac dissection is not required if the O'Hara retractor is used. The O'Hara retractor is made in three sizes by Phoenix Surgical, www.phoenixsurgical.co.uk.

Results

We have reviewed our first 116 hips in 100 patients.

CT scans were performed on 25% of cases preformed between 1992 and 1996 (the first 5 years of our experience with this procedure) to check the accuracy of the correction achieved at surgery. All corrections were within 5° of the preoperative targets in all planes. Two cases have required reoperation, one with anterior impingement due to overcoverage and one, a very dysplastic hip which required a 45° correction angle in 1993, turned up in 2008 with residual excess apical anteversion of 15°.

Complications occurred in ten patients (9%). This complication rate (in our first 116 cases) is low by comparison to other series of Peri-Acetabular osteotomies. Our malposition rate is also low. The survival curve is shown in Fig. 73.12.

We have also used this operation to recapture, contain and mould the head in Perthes' disease [1]. There are no important complications other than damage to the lateral cutaneous nerve of the thigh. Our original patients are now in their 20s. There have been four arthroplasties. The remainder function well and have mean non-arthritic hip scores [8] of 85–96. Median UCLA Activity Score [9] was 5, and the mean 6.

We have also used this operation in combination with valgus osteotomy, contemporaneously, to restore leg length and function.

Whilst it would be foolish to suggest that any pelvic osteotomy is easy, all the bone cuts of the Birmingham PAO are made under direct vision and embarrassing moments have been few.

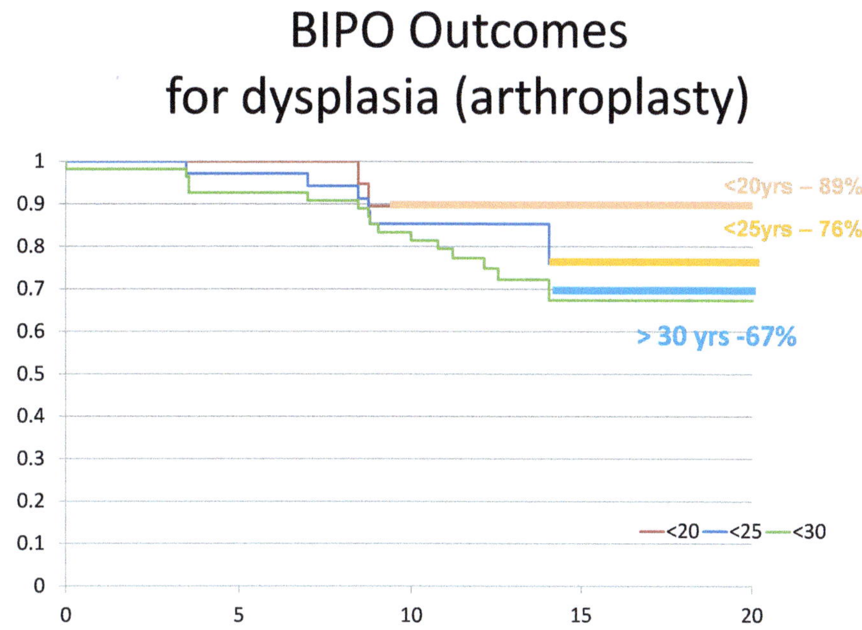

Fig. 73.12 Survivorship curves, with arthroplasty as the end point, by patient age. Younger patients do better, with patients under 20 years of age at the time of their osteotomy having 89 % survival at 20 years post-operation

We suggest that the combination of: accurate planning using CT scans; the application of the Ilizarov principle to the correction; reproducible interlocking bone cuts performed under direct vision; and a strong bony construct, has contributed to the success of this operation. The long-term results are similar to or better than several other published series of PAOs. No patient has suffered a complication which has impaired their enjoyment of the benefits of the operation.

References

1. Kumar D, Bache CE, O'Hara JN. Interlocking triple pelvic osteotomy in severe Legg-Calve-Perthes disease. J Pediatr Orthop. 2002;22(4):464–70.
2. Tönnis D, Behrens K, Tscharani F. A new technique of triple osteotomy for turning dysplastic acetabula in adolescents and adults (author's transl). Z Orthop Ihre Grenzgeb. 1981;119(3):253–65.
3. Tönnis D, Behrens K, Tscharani F. A modified technique of the triple pelvic osteotomy: early results. J Pediatr Orthop. 1981;1(3):241–9.
4. Reynolds D, Lucas J, Klaue K. Retroversion of the acetabulum: a cause of hip pain. J Bone Joint Surg Br. 1999;81-B(2):281–8.
5. Ganz R et al. A new periacetabular osteotomy for the treatment of hip dysplasias. Technique and preliminary results. Clin Orthop Relat Res. 1988;232:26–36.
6. Kerr DR, Kohan L. Local infiltration analgesia: a technique for the control of acute postoperative pain following knee and hip surgery: a case study of 325 patients. Acta Orthop. 2008;79(2):174–83.
7. Thomas S, Theologis T, Wainwright AM. Rang retractors for sciatic notch exposure during pelvic osteotomy. J Bone Joint Surg (Br). 2005;87(3):408–9.
8. Christensen CP et al. The nonarthritic hip score: reliable and validated. Clin Orthop Relat Res. 2003;406:75–83.
9. Amstutz HC et al. Treatment of primary osteoarthritis of the hip. A comparison of total joint and surface replacement arthroplasty. J Bone Joint Surg Am. 1984;66:228–41.

Mini-Incision Periacetabular Osteotomy

74

Kjeld Søballe and Anders Troelsen

Background

Surgical thinking and approaches used in joint-preserving surgery have evolved towards minimizing surgical trauma. Historically, the surgical approaches used for the periacetabular osteotomy (PAO) have been characterized by extensive dissection and soft-tissue trauma. The osteotomies of a PAO have remained the same since its development by the Bernese group; however, advances have been introduced to minimize soft-tissue trauma. Few complications, minimized surgical trauma, and no compromise of long-term results are cornerstones of an optimal surgical approach for PAO.

The choice of approach in PAO surgery will affect the risk and nature of encountered complications. Especially the frequency of neurovascular complications will depend upon the orientation of the incision and the soft-tissue dissection. Preoperative patient information should include the risks and frequency of complications, as well as the anticipated hip joint survival and function of the hip. The duration of surgery, volume of intraoperative blood loss, transfusion requirements, and ability to achieve optimal reorientation of the acetabular fragment are potentially affected by the surgical approach [1–10].

The ilioinguinal approach, the Smith-Petersen, and its modifications have been the traditionally used approaches for PAO surgery [1–5]. Optimal acetabular fragment reorientation has been reported when using these approaches. They are, however, associated with rather extensive soft-tissue dissection and muscle detachment, and therefore a new less invasive transsartorial approach for PAO surgery was developed by the senior author (KS) at Aarhus University Hospital, Denmark [11]. Reduction of the risk of vascular complications associated with the ilioinguinal approach inspired the new development [12]. The ilioinguinal, modified Smith-Petersen, and new minimally invasive transsartorial approaches have been used in succession, with the latter being used since April 2003. The aims of developing this new approach were to introduce a safe surgical technique with reduced surgical trauma and low intra- and perioperative morbidity without compromising optimal acetabular reorientation.

Surgical Technique[1]

The Minimally Invasive Approach

The surgical technique for the approach, including the instructions for performing the five osteotomies using fluoroscopy, has previously been described [11, 16]. A video tutorial is available at http://www.vjortho.com/streaming/jbjs.cfm?c=4075&b=783617706001&m=s.

The patient is placed on a radiolucent operating room table in the supine position. The placement of the drapes allows for full mobilization of the lower extremity on the operated side. Fluoroscopic evaluation is necessary throughout the operation and the equipment is positioned to facilitate obtaining the anterior-posterior and 60° (false profile) views.

K. Søballe, MD, DMSc (✉)
Department of Orthopaedics, Aarhus University Hospital, Tage-Hansens Gade 2, DK-8000 Aarhus C, Denmark
e-mail: kjeld@soballe.com

A. Troelsen, MD, PhD, DMSc
Clinical Orthopaedic Research Hvidovre & Department of Orthopaedics, Section for Hip and Knee Surgery, Copenhagen University Hospital, Hvidovre, Copenhagen, Denmark
e-mail: a_troelsen@hotmail.com

[1] *Acknowledgments of Use of Copyrighted Material*
Previously published text describing the surgical technique has been reprinted with permission. From Journal of Bone and Joint Surgery American, March, 2008, 90, 3, New Minimally Invasive Transsartorial Approach for Periacetabular Osteotomy, Troelsen, 493–498.

J.C. McCarthy et al. (eds.), *Hip Joint Restoration*, DOI 10.1007/978-1-4614-0694-5_74

The skin incision begins at the anterior superior iliac spine and continues distally along the sartorius muscle. The length of incision is approximately 7 cm. The fascia is carefully incised, and the lateral femoral cutaneous nerve isolated and carefully retracted. To facilitate transverse retraction of the soft tissues a semiflexed position of the hip joint is maintained during performance of the osteotomies. For this purpose a splint is used. A periosteal elevator is placed subperiosteally along the medial aspect of the ilium starting at the anterior superior iliac spine, and it is advanced until it lies just below the linea terminalis. The inguinal ligament is cut at the attachment to the anterior superior iliac spine allowing further mobilization of the soft tissues. The periosteal elevator is then pushed medially splitting the sartorius muscle in the direction of its fibers and the deep fascia of the muscle is cut. The periosteal elevator is then replaced with a blunt retractor positioned along the medial aspect of the ilium to retract the iliopsoas and the medial part of the split sartorius muscles medially. At this point the osteotomies are performed (Fig. 74.1) [11].

To perform the approach takes approximately 5 min. Obviously the direct visualization of the osteotomies obtained using classical approaches is limited, and therefore the use and understanding of the fluoroscopy are paramount when performing the transsartorial approach for PAO surgery. Radiation exposure of the surgeon averages 35 s per procedure [18].

Performance of the Osteotomies

Pubic Osteotomy

Subperiosteal access to the superior ramus of the pubic bone is gained using a periosteal elevator. It is important that the pubic osteotomy is performed medially on the superior ramus since the bone otherwise is too thick making the osteotomy and mobilization difficult or impossible. A curved blunt retractor is placed in the obturator fossa behind the superior ramus of the pubic bone. It is important that this retractor be placed subperiosteally to protect the obturator artery and nerve. A splined retractor is then placed anteriorly and medially to the site of the osteotomy in order to retract the iliopsoas muscle medially and protect the iliac artery and vein and the femoral nerve (Fig. 74.2). The superior ramus is then osteotomized under direct visualization using a slightly curved osteotome. It is important to advance the osteotome until the osteotomy is complete; otherwise the repositioning of the splined retractor becomes difficult as it will tend to slide into the osteotomy. The surgeon will often be able to hear and feel (loss of resistance) when the bone is fully osteotomized. This sensory input should be utilized during surgery to avoid both creating an insufficient osteotomy and advancing the osteotome into the soft tissue.

Ischial Osteotomy

When advancing to the ischial osteotomy the splined retractor is kept in its position to retract the iliopsoas muscle medially. A large pair of scissors is used to penetrate the interval

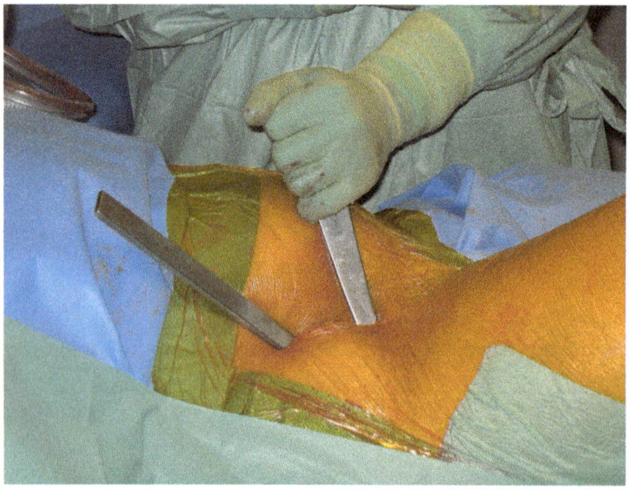

Fig. 74.1 Performance of the osteotomy through the minimally invasive transsartorial approach. A straight osteotome is used to perform the last step of the ilium osteotomy, with a retractor protecting the medial structures. Figure reprinted with permission from Journal of Bone and Joint Surgery American, March, 2008, 90, 3, New Minimally Invasive Transsartorial Approach for Periacetabular Osteotomy, Troelsen, 493–498

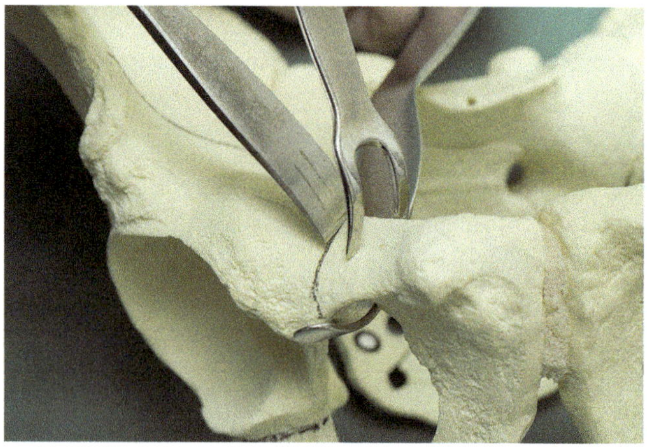

Fig. 74.2 The site of the osteotomy on the pubic bone and the placement of the instruments. A curved blunt retractor is placed behind the pubic bone to protect the obturator nerve and artery. A splined retractor is used for medial retraction of the soft tissues, and a slightly curved osteotome is used to create the osteotomy. Figure reprinted with permission from Journal of Bone and Joint Surgery American, March, 2008, 90, 3, New Minimally Invasive Transsartorial Approach for Periacetabular Osteotomy, Troelsen, 493–498

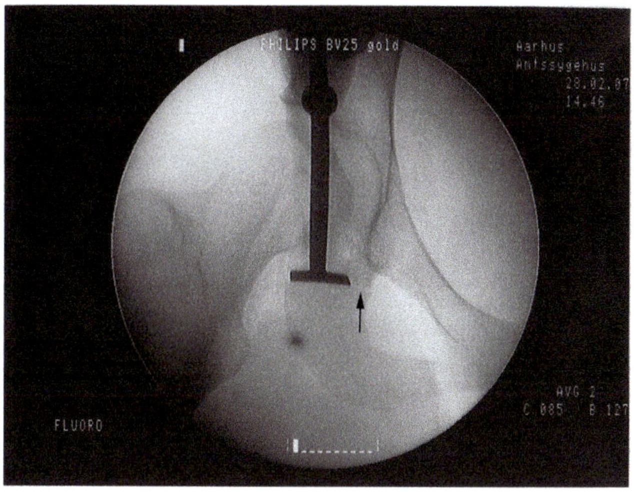

Fig. 74.3 Fluoroscopic anteroposterior view showing the lateral placement of the osteotome at the ischial bone below the teardrop. The osteotomy performed at the medial edge of the ischium is seen (*arrow*). Figure reprinted with permission from Journal of Bone and Joint Surgery American, March, 2008, 90, 3, New Minimally Invasive Transsartorial Approach for Periacetabular Osteotomy, Troelsen, 493–498

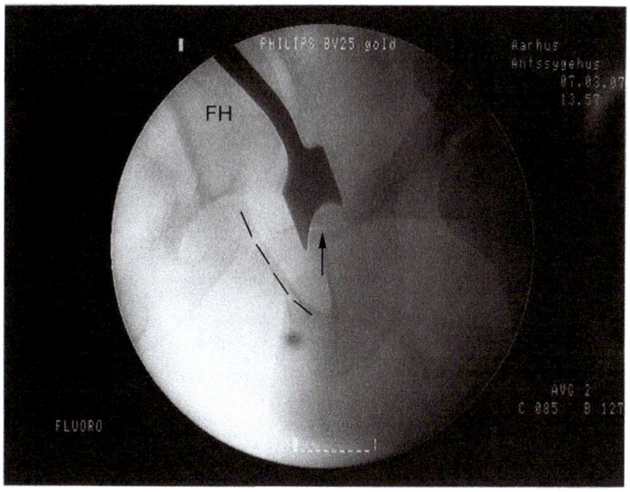

Fig. 74.4 Fluoroscopic false profile views angled 60° to the anteroposterior view. A correct placement of the osteotome with one leg in the existing osteotomy (*arrow*). The *dashed line* marks the border of the pubic bone towards the obturator foramen. *FH* femoral head. Figure reprinted with permission from Journal of Bone and Joint Surgery American, March, 2008, 90, 3, New Minimally Invasive Transsartorial Approach for Periacetabular Osteotomy, Troelsen, 493–498

immediately lateral and distal to the pubic osteotomy, and the scissors are advanced to the ischium below the acetabulum. Keeping the scissors in place, a 30° angled osteotome can be placed on the ischium. The correct placement of the osteotome is verified using fluoroscopy (anterior-posterior view). The osteotomy begins approximately 5 mm distal to the radiographic teardrop. A 1.5 cm osteotomy is performed in two steps beginning at the medial edge and then moving the osteotome laterally before the next step (Fig. 74.3). A 30° angled osteotome is advanced along the inner aspect of the pelvis until it can be placed at the medial aspect of the ischium with one leg of the osteotome in the existing 1.5 cm osteotomy. The placement of the osteotome and the osteotomy itself are performed under strict fluoroscopy control utilizing the so-called false profile view that is angled 60° to the anterior-posterior view (Fig. 74.4). The ischium bone is then osteotomized from the medial to the lateral aspect in a length equal to 2–3 widths of the osteotome (Fig. 74.5). This osteotomy tends to be slightly curved with the concavity towards the acetabulum. In order to advance in the same plane as the initial 1.5 cm of the osteotomy and to obtain an almost horizontal osteotomy, the handle of the 30° angled osteotome must be pushed medially. When the posterior aspect of the ischium is osteotomized the sciatic nerve can be damaged if the osteotome is advanced too far past the bone in the lateral direction.

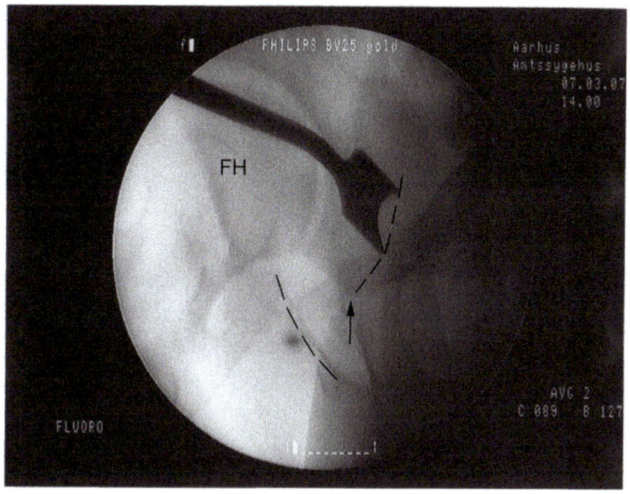

Fig. 74.5 Correct placement of the osteotome for the last step of the ischial osteotomy. As illustrated by the dashed line where the osteotome is placed, the osteotomy is slightly curved. The arrow marks the level of the already performed osteotomy. A dashed line marks the border of the pubic bone towards the obturator foramen. *FH* femoral head. Figure reprinted with permission from Journal of Bone and Joint Surgery American, March, 2008, 90, 3, New Minimally Invasive Transsartorial Approach for Periacetabular Osteotomy, Troelsen, 493–498

Iliac Osteotomy

Initially a Kirschner wire is inserted along the inner aspect of the pelvis approximately 3 cm cranial to the acetabulum. This is done to secure an appropriate distance away from the joint. From experience, we have found it easier to mobilize and control the acetabular fragment if this distance away from the joint is achieved. The first step of the iliac osteotomy begins between the anterior superior iliac spine and the anterior inferior iliac spine at the level of the Kirschner wire. It is performed using an oscillating saw stopping approximately 1 cm before reaching linea terminalis. In some patients the distance from the anterior superior iliac spine to

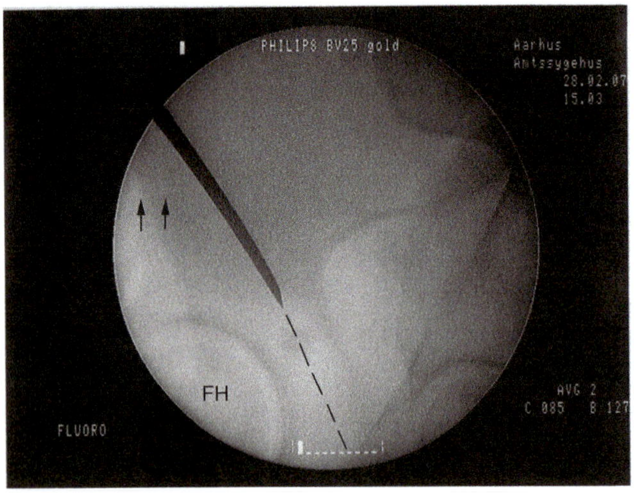

Fig. 74.6 Fluoroscopic false profile view angled 60° to the anteroposterior view, showing the advancement of a straight osteotome in continuation with the first step of the iliac osteotomy (*arrows*). It is advanced (*dashed line*) at an anterior open angle of around 120° between the joint and the posterior column until it reaches the ischial osteotomy site. *FH* femoral head. Figure reprinted with permission from Journal of Bone and Joint Surgery American, March, 2008, 90, 3, New Minimally Invasive Transsartorial Approach for Periacetabular Osteotomy, Troelsen, 493–498

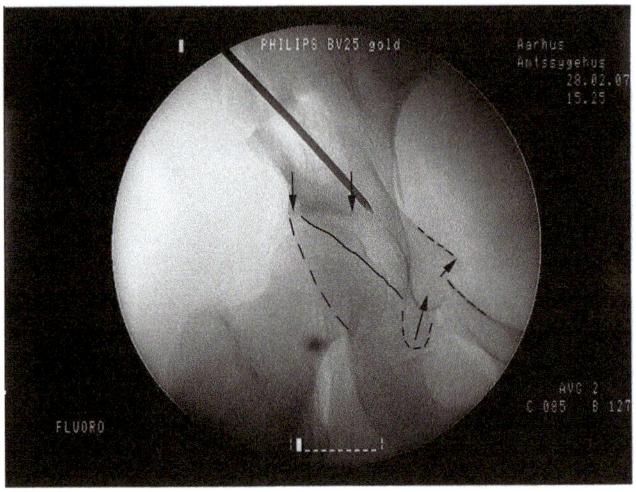

Fig. 74.7 A large threaded Kirschner wire is temporarily securing the position. Note the horizontal positioning of the medial and lateral extents (*arrows*) of the sclerotic acetabular roof, the anteverted configuration of the acetabulum (*dashed line*=posterior rim and *solid line*=anterior rim), the cranial displacement of the superior ramus, and the cranial and medial displacement of the teardrop figure. Figure reprinted with permission from Journal of Bone and Joint Surgery American, March, 2008, 90, 3, New Minimally Invasive Transsartorial Approach for Periacetabular Osteotomy, Troelsen, 493–498

the cranial limit of the joint is relatively short. In these cases a small oblique osteotomy under the anterior superior iliac spine is recommended. To protect the structures lateral to the ilium a blunt retractor is tunnelled close to the bone along the outer aspect of the ilium in the area between the anterior superior and anterior inferior iliac spines. The blunt retractor must be advanced close to the bone as otherwise the blood supply from the superior gluteal artery can be damaged. A retractor protects the structures medial to the ilium. The first step of the osteotomy is then continued using a wide, straight osteotome. With an anterior open angle of approximately 120° it is advanced behind the hip joint until it reaches the ischial osteotomy while the posterior column is maintained intact. Fluoroscopy must be used during this last step of the iliac osteotomy (60° angle, false profile view) (Fig. 74.6).

Reorientation

A bone spreader is placed in the iliac osteotomy. With the osteotomies open, the iliac and ischial osteotomies can in succession be retraced using a 30° angled osteotome to secure that there are no bony bridges or spikes left, interfering with mobilization of the acetabular fragment. A bone clamp is then applied at the ilium with one leg of the clamp on the inner and outer aspects, respectively. On the inner aspect, the ilium is oblique and a small hole is predrilled to allow secure fixation of the clamp. This gives the surgeon control of the fragment during the reorientation. If the acetabular fragment has been properly mobilized and reoriented, cranial displacement of the superior ramus and cranial and medial displacement of the teardrop can be observed in the anterior-posterior fluoroscopic view. If these are not observed the fragment is hinging probably due to an unfinished osteotomy of the ischium (Fig. 74.7).

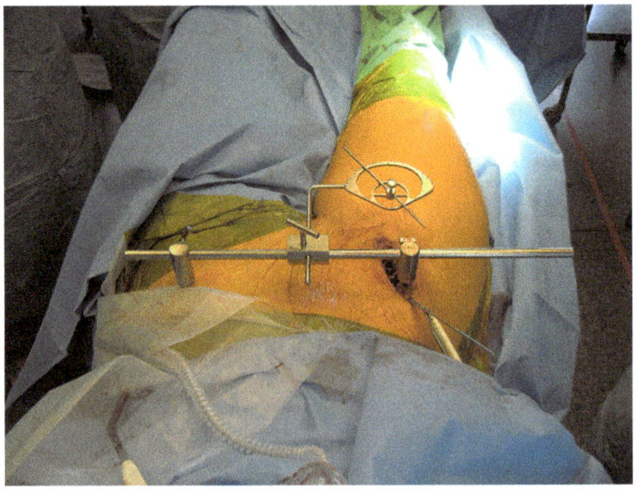

Fig. 74.8 The validated measuring device for intraoperative measurements of the center-edge and acetabular index angles

Using a validated measuring device for intraoperative measurements of the center-edge and acetabular index angles it is ensured that optimal reorientation has been achieved (Fig. 74.8) [13].

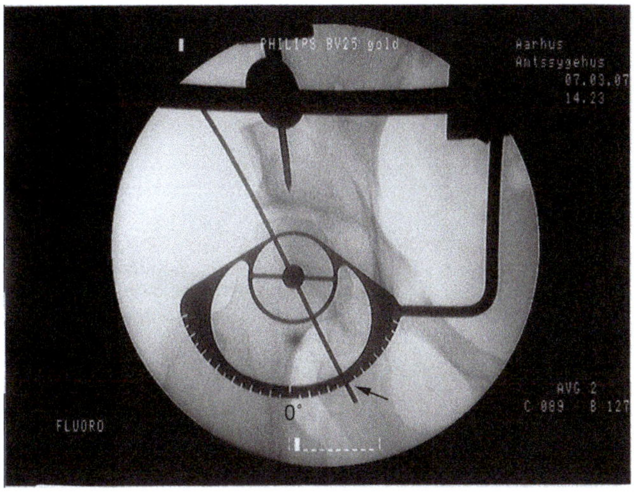

Fig. 74.9 The angle-measuring disc for the measurement of the center-edge angle. It is positioned by recognizing the center of the femoral head and the lateral limit of the sclerotic acetabular roof as landmarks. The measured angle in this case is 30° (*arrow*). The 0° mark is labeled. Figure reprinted with permission from Journal of Bone and Joint Surgery American, March, 2008, 90, 3, New Minimally Invasive Transsartorial Approach for Periacetabular Osteotomy, Troelsen, 493–498

Measurements are performed using fluoroscopy in the anterior-posterior view. Using small spikes, the measuring device is mounted bilaterally at the anterior superior iliac spines in order to secure alignment of the pelvis when measuring. Excessive tilt and rotation of the pelvis are avoided through the initial positioning of the patient. On the alignment rod connecting the spikes, two different adjustable angle-measuring discs can be mounted. The angle-measuring disc for the acetabular index angle measurement has to be positioned by recognizing the medial and lateral limits of the sclerotic acetabular roof as landmarks. The angle-measuring disc for the center-edge angle measurement has to be positioned by recognizing the center of the femoral head and the lateral limit of the sclerotic acetabular roof as landmarks (Fig. 74.9). The measuring device is easy to use, and it helps the surgeon to assess the achieved acetabular reorientation and thereby avoid undercorrection or overcorrection. The acetabular version cannot be measured and still has to be addressed by assessing the anterior and posterior acetabular rims, securing that the crossover sign is not present [8, 9, 14, 15]. The posterior acetabular rim should be lateral to the anterior rim and the femoral head center, and the anterior rim should be medial to the femoral head center. Adjustments of the reorientation might be necessary, and for temporary fixation a large threaded Kirschner wire is placed from the ilium into the acetabular fragment to secure the position.

When no further adjustment is needed two stainless steel screws are placed from the ilium at the anterior superior iliac spine into the acetabular fragment to secure its position. The positions of the screws are visualized using fluoroscopy and the stability of the fixation is tested by applying force on the fragment [17].

Surgical Aims for Reorientation

The surgical aim of the reorientation is improved coverage of the femoral head decreasing high peak forces at the rim and labrum, and to avoid further subluxing/shearing impingement. This should be obtained without excessive coverage of the femoral head as this would result in femoroacetabular impingement introducing another mode of joint deterioration. The acetabular index and center-edge angles following reorientation should correspond as closely as possible to the normal anatomy (acetabular index angle: 0–10°; center-edge angle: 30–40°). Correction outside the range of 30–40° for the center-edge angle has been shown to result in significantly increased risk of failure of the PAO and conversion to total hip arthroplasty [19]. As described above it is of equal importance that the surgeon obtains appropriate anteversion of the acetabulum. Assessment of range of motion and joint stability at the end of the procedure will help the surgeon evaluate the change in hip joint mechanics and the presence of femoroacetabular impingement following correction. Finally, the selection of the patient/hip joint for a lasting PAO is very important [19, 20].

Outcome Using the Mini-Incision Technique

Complications

In a previous report on the outcome of the minimally invasive transsartorial approach we found no moderate or severe complications and technical or neurovascular complications. The femoral nerve, artery, and veins are protected by the muscles using the approach [11]. Like for other approaches with an iliofemoral orientation the most common complication is dysesthesia of the lateral femoral cutaneous nerve as the nerve traverses the surgical field.

Bleeding and Transfusion Requirements

The minimally invasive transsartorial approach is associated with a very low level of intraoperative bleeding and little subsequent transfusion requirements. We found median intraoperative blood loss to be 250 mL (interquartile range: 150–350 mL). Transfusion was only required by 3% of patients, receiving a median of two portions of SAGM [11]. This underlines the minimized surgical trauma by this approach: The incision is minimal, no muscles are detached, and the sartorius is split in the length of the muscle fibers. Further, a short duration of surgery results in reduced surgical trauma. The initially reported median duration of surgery was 1.2 h, which is now reduced to approximately 0.75 h.

Acetabular Correction

The acetabular correction as measured by the postoperative center-edge angle and acetabular index angle shows that the reduced direct visualization of the acetabular fragment does not compromise an optimal correction during minimally invasive PAO surgery [11]. Understanding 3-dimensional hip joint anatomy and utilizing fluoroscopy as described facilitate optimal reorientation. Suboptimal reorientation has been shown to significantly increase the risk of failure and conversion to total hip arthroplasty [19].

Hip Joint Survival

The hip joint survival rate of the initial experience with the minimally invasive approach has been very encouraging. We assessed Kaplan–Meier survivorship with conversion to total hip arthroplasty as end point for 209 hips operated using the minimally invasive approach between April 2003 and May 2007. Complete follow-up was secured by inquiry to the National Registry of Patients. The mean follow-up was 6.2 years (range: 3.9–8.1 years). The survivorship rate at 5 years was 94.7 and 88.6 % at 8.1 years (Fig. 74.10). It should be acknowledged that the good survivorship results can in part be attributed to the accumulated experience of the senior surgeon (KS), and to improved selection of patients undergoing PAO. The single most important factor predicting failure following PAO is the presence of preoperative osteoarthritis [19, 20]. Thus, hip joints should show no or only slight signs of osteoarthritis (Tönnis grades 0–1) to be candidates for a joint-preserving PAO.

Summary

Joint-preserving procedures, including PAO surgery, have developed towards minimizing tissue trauma and intra- and perioperative morbidity. The PAO surgeon should acknowledge that the surgical approach to perform the osteotomies will affect (1) the nature and rate of complications, (2) duration of surgery, (3) intraoperative blood loss, and (4) transfusion requirements following surgery. Further, the chosen approach has to allow optimal acetabular reorientation. The minimally invasive transsartorial approach has been developed with the specific aims to minimize tissue trauma and in a safe way give the surgeon the ability to perform an optimal acetabular reorientation. The results support that the minimally invasive approach offers a safe procedure with the possibility of achieving good acetabular reorientation, and minimized duration of surgery, blood loss, and transfusion requirements. Further the hip joint survivorship up to 8 years after surgery using the minimally invasive approach is encouraging. The minimally invasive approach is recommended as an integrated part of PAO surgery.

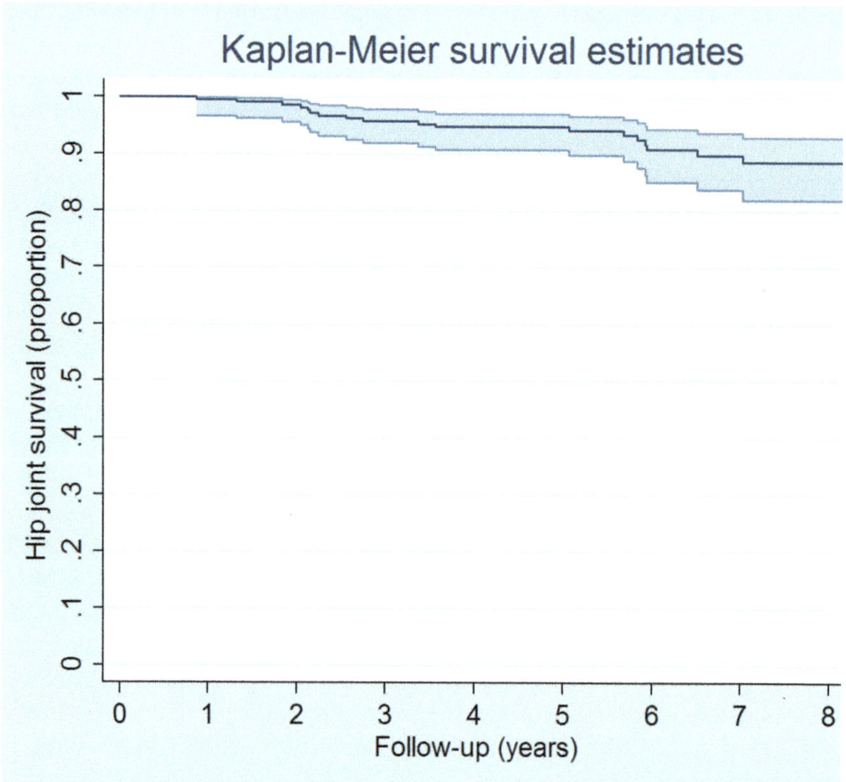

Fig. 74.10 Kaplan–Meier survivorship curve with conversion to total hip replacement as the end point. Inquiry to the National Registry of Patients allowed complete follow-up of 209 PAOs performed between April 2003 and May 2007. Follow-up ranged from 3.9 to 8.1 years. Reprinted with permission from Soballe K, Troelsen A: Approaches and Perioperative Management in Periacetabular Osteotomy Surgery: The Minimally Invasive Transsartorial Approach, in Pagnano M, Hart RA (eds): *Instructional Course Lectures 62*. Rosemont, IL, American Academy of Orthopaedic Surgeons, 2013, pp 297–303

References

1. Matta JM, Stover MD, Siebenrock K. Periacetabular osteotomy through the Smith-Petersen approach. Clin Orthop Relat Res. 1999;21–32.
2. Trumble SJ, Mayo KA, Mast JW. The periacetabular osteotomy. Minimum 2 year followup in more than 100 hips. Clin Orthop Relat Res. 1999;54–63.
3. Clohisy JC, Barrett SE, Gordon JE, Delgado ED, Schoenecker PL. Periacetabular osteotomy in the treatment of severe acetabular dysplasia. Surgical technique. J Bone Joint Surg Am. 2006;88(Suppl 1 Pt 1):65–83.
4. Pogliacomi F, Stark A, Wallensten R. Periacetabular osteotomy. Good pain relief in symptomatic hip dysplasia, 32 patients followed for 4 years. Acta Orthop. 2005;76:67–74.
5. Hussell JG, Mast JW, Mayo KA, Howie DW, Ganz R. A comparison of different surgical approaches for the periacetabular osteotomy. Clin Orthop Relat Res. 1999;64–72.
6. Davey JP, Santore RF. Complications of periacetabular osteotomy. Clin Orthop Relat Res. 1999;33–7.
7. Ganz R, Klaue K, Vinh TS, Mast JW. A new periacetabular osteotomy for the treatment of hip dysplasias. Technique and preliminary results. Clin Orthop Relat Res. 1988;26–36.
8. Peters CL, Erickson JA, Hines JL. Early results of the Bernese periacetabular osteotomy: the learning curve at an academic medical center. J Bone Joint Surg Am. 2006;88:1920–6.
9. Trousdale RT, Cabanela ME. Lessons learned after more than 250 periacetabular osteotomies. Acta Orthop Scand. 2003;74:119–26.
10. Hussell JG, Rodriguez JA, Ganz R. Technical complications of the Bernese periacetabular osteotomy. Clin Orthop Relat Res. 1999;81–92.
11. Troelsen A, Elmengaard B, Soballe K. A new minimally invasive transsartorial approach for periacetabular osteotomy. J Bone Joint Surg Am. 2008;90:493–8.
12. Troelsen A, Elmengaard B, Søballe K. Comparison of the minimally invasive and the ilioinguinal approaches for periacetabular osteotomy. Acta Orthop. 2008;79:777–84.
13. Troelsen A, Elmengaard B, Rømer L, Søballe K. Reliable angle assessment during periacetabular osteotomy with a novel device. Clin Orthop Relat Res. 2008;466:1169–76.
14. Troelsen A, Jacobsen S, Romer L, Soballe K. Weightbearing anteroposterior pelvic radiographs are recommended in DDH assessment. Clin Orthop Relat Res. 2008;466:813–9.
15. Troelsen A, Rømer L, Jacobsen S, Ladelund S, Søballe K. Cranial acetabular retroversion is common in developmental dysplasia of the hip as assessed by the weight bearing position. Acta Orthop. 2010;81:436–41.
16. Kjeld Søballe website. Minimally invasive surgery for hip dysplasia. http://www.soballe.com/default.asp?MainMenuId=104&PageId=104&Desc=English. Accessed 5 Jan 2012.
17. Mechlenburg I, Kold S, Rømer L, Soballe K. Safe fixation with two acetabular screws after Ganz periacetabular osteotomy. Acta Orthop. 2007;78:344–9.
18. Mechlenburg I, Daugaard H, Søballe K. Radiation exposure to the orthopaedic surgeon during periacetabular osteotomy. Int Orthop. 2009;33:1747–51.
19. Hartig-Andreasen C, Troelsen A, Thillemann TM, Søballe K. What factors predict failure 4 to 12 years after periacetabular osteotomy? Clin Orthop Relat Res. 2012;470:2978–87.
20. Troelsen A, Elmengaard B, Søballe K. Medium-term outcome of periacetabular osteotomy and predictors of conversion to total hip replacement. J Bone Joint Surg Am. 2009;91:2169–79.

Results of Periacetabular Osteotomy (PAO)

75

Brian T. Barlow and Richard F. Santore

Introduction

The results of periacetabular osteotomy (PAO) have been incrementally reported in the literature since the late 1980s. There is now a rich history of short and intermediate-length outcomes with follow-up for as long as 20 years. This chapter will review in some detail the current status of our understanding of the outcomes, and how those data have influenced contemporary surgical decision-making. Briefly, when indications are limited to young patients with congruent joints and excellent hip mobility, good results in approximately 95 % of operated hips can be anticipated over the first 5 years, provided there are no intraoperative complications. The longest duration follow-up study, out to 20 years, demonstrated survival of approximately 75 % of hips. It is not possible to include every worthy previously published peer-reviewed article, review article, or text book chapter that has been written on this subject. We ask the authors who have contributed such work for their understanding. Exclusion is not a reflection of any value judgment regarding the quality of the material.

B.T. Barlow, MD
Orthopaedic Surgery, Adult Reconstruction and Joint Replacement, Naval Medical Center San Diego, San Diego, CA, USA

R.F. Santore, MD (✉)
Orthopaedic Surgery, Sharp Memorial Hospital, San Diego, CA, USA

Orthopaedic Surgery, University of California San Diego, San Diego, CA, USA
e-mail: rsantore@ucsd.edu

Epidemiology and Natural History of Hip Dysplasia

Early work by Stulberg et al. demonstrated that up to 40 % of patients undergoing total hip arthroplasty (THA) had discernable evidence of hip dysplasia on radiographs [1]. Further work by Dr. William Harris suggested that over 90 % of hip arthritis has demonstrable morphologic abnormalities, most commonly hip dysplasia or the pistol grip deformity [2]. Over time, the terms "Idiopathic or Primary Osteoarthritis of the Hip" have virtually disappeared from the orthopedic lexicon, as we have come to understand that nearly all cases of osteoarthritis have some antecedent genetic, pediatric, or traumatic etiology, dysplasia being the most frequent. This is the scientific background behind the rationale to intervene with a surgical procedure in adults that has the purported goal of delaying, if not eliminating completely, the onset of secondary osteoarthritis. However, there have been no prospective, randomized studies which have compared the results of treatment between nonoperative measures and periacetabular osteotomy in comparable hips.

In one of the more recent studies on hip dysplasia epidemiology, Jacobsen et al. used the Copenhagen City Heart Study data to review anterior-posterior (AP) radiographs in over 4000 men and women over 65 years of age. The authors demonstrated a significant association between hip dysplasia and osteoarthritis in adulthood. The presence of radiographic dysplasia in this cohort was 5.4–12.8 % using the center-edge angle of Wiberg, acetabular depth ratio, and femoral head extrusion index [3].

Similarly, Inoue et al. reviewed urologic imaging in French and Japanese patient cohorts to identify the prevalence of hip dysplasia and osteoarthritis. The authors reported the incidence of hip dysplasia to be as high as 11.6 % in Japanese women and as low as 1.8 % in French men. However, the authors used a CEA <25° as their definition of dysplasia whereas previous reports generally use a CEA <20° to define radiographic dysplasia.

J.C. McCarthy et al. (eds.), *Hip Joint Restoration*, DOI 10.1007/978-1-4614-0694-5_75

A study of over 2000 nineteen-year-old Norwegians identified radiographic dysplasia using markers including Wiberg's lateral center-edge angle (CEA), femoral head extrusion index, Sharp's angle of acetabular inclination, acetabular depth to width ratio, and sourcil upsloping. Using the criterion of CEA <20°, radiographic dysplasia was identified in 3.3 % of subjects overall, 4.4 % in females and 2.4 % in males. The authors also reviewed the hip range of motion data and collected validated questionnaires. The study found no association between radiographic hip dysplasia and EuroQol (EQ-5D), Western Ontario and McMaster Universities Osteoarthritis Index (WOMAC), Beighton score for hypermobility, or body mass index (BMI) [4].

A criticism of the epidemiology studies of hip dysplasia in adults is the excessive reliance on AP radiographs for diagnosis. As important as the radiographs are, the coronal plane imaging alone does not adequately illustrate the complexity of the acetabulum and proximal femur as three-dimensional structures. Additionally, the influence of ligamentous laxity and dynamic instability (Hypermobility syndrome, Ehlers-Danlos, Marfan's syndrome, etc.) can profoundly influence the management of hip dysplasia, which is ostensibly not captured on a static single plane image. Furthermore, the standing AP pelvis radiograph conveys more important information than the supine AP pelvis, but is much less frequently available for review, especially in retrospective studies.

Long-term studies of hip dysplasia have confirmed a poor prognosis for untreated disease. Murphy et al. reported long-term follow-up of patients with hip dysplasia and noted that a CEA <16 was unequivocally predictive of poor outcome and early symptomatic arthritis [5]. This study, while illustrative, was limited in that it studied hips that had an arthroplasty on the opposite side.

Stulberg et al. studied the natural history of adult dysplasia in a group of 20 patients followed for an average of 22 years. The patients were diagnosed at a mean of 43 years and followed until a mean age of 65 years. All patients had a lateral CEA of <20° with an intact Shenton's line. The rate of osteoarthritis for the dysplastic hip in this series was 72 % by the 6th decade. Stulberg noted that two-thirds of the disease-free hips were in men though men comprised only 25 % of the study population. The author did not offer any supposition as to why the male dysplastic hip seemed to have a more benign course [6].

Weinstein et al. performed a longitudinal study of hip dysplasia in children with 40-year outcomes reported. The study included 72 hips in 58 patients (78 % female) with developmental hip dysplasia treated with operative or closed reduction. The mean age at hip reduction was 16 months and 67 % of patients had closed reductions. Sixty-five percent of hips achieved a Severin grade I/II outcome at skeletal maturity; however only 33 % of patients maintained a Severin grade I/II outcomes at 40 years [7]. Furthermore, 21 % of cohort had converted to THA by the end of the study.

PAO Results

Matta et al. published their initial series of 58 patients who had undergone a PAO with follow-up of an average of 4 years. Final clinical follow-up was graded as 17 % excellent, 59 % good, 12 % fair, and 12 % poor. No patient with ideal indications had a poor result during the study period. The authors felt that PAO should be strictly indicated to provide consistent benefit and cited a high failure rate in patients with preoperative evidence of arthritis [8].

In 2008, the Bern group of Ganz, Steppacher, Tannast, and Siebenrock published their 20-year results in 63 patients from their early series. Twenty-four percent of patients presented with advanced levels of osteoarthritis. Overall, 60 % of hips were preserved at a mean of 20 years. Six factors predictive of poor outcome include age, perioperative functional level (Merle d'Aubigné and Postel score), positive anterior impingement test, limp, Tönnis grade, and postoperative extrusion index >20 %. Hips with Tönnis grade 2 and 3 radiographic OA preoperatively failed at rates of 87 % and 100 %, respectively, over the study period. Tönnis grade 0 or 1 survivorship at 20 years was 75 % compared to the dismal outcomes in Tönnis grade 2 and 3 hips. The postoperative extrusion index reflects the technical success of the surgery. A postoperative femoral extrusion index >20 % was predictive of end-stage OA [9]. The femoral extrusion index is calculated by measuring the horizontal distance of the femoral head that is lateral to the acetabulum. This distance is divided by the total horizontal width of the femoral head and multiplied by 100 to generate a femoral extrusion index percentage. This study from the Bern group represents the longest published follow-up of the PAO for dysplasia.

Kralj et al. reported on their long-term results of the PAO for hip dysplasia. Their group included 26 hips in the same number of patients who underwent a PAO with follow-up of 7–15 years. Outcomes measured included the WOMAC, Tönnis grade, lateral CEA of Wiberg, and anterior CEA of Lequesne. Fifteen percent of hips were converted to THA at an average of 4.5 years. An additional 31 % of hips had a Tönnis score of >3 or a >20 point decrease in WOMAC score [10]. Factors which were predictive of failure included increased age, lower preoperative Merle d'Aubigné score, head asphericity, positive Trendelenburg sign, and postoperative retroversion, subluxation, or malposition. The authors found both patient and surgical factors affected the overall survivorship. This study highlights that although patient factors like age, preoperative radiographic arthritis, and lower function are predictive of PAO failure, a PAO associated with technical complications will also have decreased survivorship. The authors also commented that a malpositioning of the PAO can produce subsequent impingement [11].

Matheney et al. from the Boston Children's group published their clinical outcomes of PAO in a group of 135 hips in 109 patients with a mean of 9 years. Seventy-six percent of hips were preserved at 9 years and the remainder had failed as defined by a WOMAC pain score >10 or conversion to THA. The Kaplan-Meier survival rate was 96 % at 5 years, but dropped to 84 % at 10 years. Complications occurred in 20 hips (15 %). Importantly, 11 % of patients required a subsequent hip arthroscopy for chondral or labral injuries at an average of 6.8 years after surgery. Independent predictors included age >35 and poor/fair preoperative congruity. Patients with age <35 and good congruity failed at a rate of 14 % compared to a 95 % failure rate for patients with both age >35 and poor preoperative congruency [12].

Hartig-Andreasen et al. reviewed the results of the PAO in 401 hips (316 patients) from a single center with a mean of 8 years follow-up using the WOMAC score, radiographic outcome, and survivorship. The authors found that the overall Kaplan-Meier survival index after 12 years was 74.8 %, consistent with other reports on the durability of the PAO. They identified 69 of 401 hips (17 %) that were converted to THA and an additional 13 % of patients had a WOMAC pain score >10 indicating clinical failure. Predictors of failure included higher age, preoperative Tönnis grade of >2, postoperative joint space of <3 mm, and a postoperative CEA <30° or >40°. The Tönnis grade and the influence of joint space on outcome speak to the careful patient selection required for a successful PAO. Our opinion is that age is frequently reported as a predictor of poor outcome, but this is more likely due to an association with increased Tönnis grade rather than as an independent predictor. The postoperative CEA influence on outcomes suggests a relationship between the repositioning of the acetabulum and the final outcome. Though this would appear to be intuitively the case, at this time there is insufficient scientific validation of this conclusion [13].

Garras et al. from the Duke group reported the clinical and radiographic outcomes of PAO in 58 hips (52 patients) with a mean age of 37.6 years. Radiographically, the authors documented significant improvement in the center-edge angle and acetabular index. Clinically the mean Merle d'Aubigné score improved from 12.6 to 18.0. Four hips (7 %) converted to THA at a mean of 3 years. Complications included two patients with transient sciatic nerve palsy and nine with lateral femoral cutaneous nerve dysesthesia, all of which resolved by final follow-up. Additionally, there were four cases of nonunion, the majority of which were asymptomatic [14].

Pogliacomi et al. reported on a series of 36 hips (32 patients) treated with a PAO and mean follow-up of 4 years. Two of 32 patients (6 %) required conversion to THA. The Merle d'Aubigné score significantly improved from 13 to 16. Complications in this groups experience included a partial sciatic nerve laceration, 1 malunion, and 1 nonunion [15].

Clohisy et al. from the Washington St Louis group reported on their results of PAO in the treatment of severe dysplasia. The authors defined severe dysplasia as hip subluxation (Severin IV) or the presence of false acetabuli (Severin V). Their series included 13 patients with an average age of 17.6 years. Eight hips were subluxated and eight had a false acetabulum. Six patients required a concomitant proximal femoral osteotomy. There was a significant improvement in lateral and anterior center-edge angles, roof obliquity, and hip center medialization. There was also an 18 point improvement in the Harris hip score (HHS) at a mean follow-up of 4.2 years postoperatively. Two complications occurred including loss of fixation of the acetabular fragment and an ischial nonunion, both complications resolved after revision surgery [16].

Badra et al. reported the results of the PAO in 24 patients with a mean follow-up of 3.5 years. Over 75 % of patients scored >20 on the Short Musculoskeletal Function Score (SMFA) indicating a high level of function. Poor results were seen in patients with incongruent joints and Tönnis grade 3, similar to previous studies.

PAO in Patients Over 40 Years Old

Increasing age has been suggested as predictive of decreased hip survivorship following PAO in some series. Age has been cited as a factor associated with poorer outcomes in many of the follow-up studies of PAO. Whether or not age, alone, or the fact the intermediate and advanced arthritis is more common with age, has not been established. We believe that age, alone, is less relevant than other associated factors like stiffness of the joint, limp, progressive joint space narrowing, and other radiographic evidence of secondary degenerative changes. The senior author has performed PAO with success on patients up to the age of 60. All patients above the age of 40 require very special scrutiny, and disclosures, before proceeding with PAO surgery. The following section examines the outcomes of patients with increased age.

The Academic Network for Conservational Hip Outcomes Research (ANCHOR) group collected 87 hips in 70 patients with a minimum age of 40 years (mean age 43.6 years) treated with PAO alone with a mean follow-up of 4.9 years. Though there was no comparison group, the cohort demonstrated similar improvement in WOMAC and HHS scores to previous studies with younger patients. Twenty-four percent of patients had been converted to THA at a mean of 5.6 years after PAO. The risk of THA at 5 years was 2.2x greater with Tönnis grade 2 than with Tönnis grade 0/1 [17].

Ito et al. reported on the results of 36 patients who were 40 years or older compared to 103 patients younger than 40. Following PAO, the average HHS increased from 70 to 90 for the entire cohort and the 5-year HHS were similar between the groups. However, 10-year survival rates were 94.4 % in the under 40 group and 81.3 % in older than 40-year group. The 15-year survival rates were 86.9 % and 71.2 %, respectively. The authors concluded that although the early (5 year) results of PAO were similar between both groups, the results consistently deteriorated over time in patients over 40 years [18].

Zhu et al. described the results of the PAO in a group of 36 patients with a mean age of 39.5 years. Eleven of the patients had a combined PAO and femoral osteochondroplasty. At a mean follow-up of 5.1 years, the authors reported survival in 40 of the 41 hips (97 % survivorship) and no progression of preoperative Tönnis score. There was a significant improvement in the HHS from 63.7 to 88.4 and there was no significant difference in the HHS between PAO alone versus PAO plus femoral osteochondroplasty [19].

Teratani et al. described the outcomes of the Japanese curved acetabular osteotomy in a cohort of 42 patients with age >50 treated compared to a group of 54 patients matched by sex and Tönnis grade with an average age of 32 years. The mean follow-up was 4.4 years. The overall results showed a similar radiographic outcome with respect to center-edge angle, roof obliquity, acetabular-head index, and head lateralization index. There was also a similar improvement in HHS. The authors concluded that a curved osteotomy was safe and effective in patients over 50 years with Tönnis grade 1 or 2 osteoarthritis [20]. Each group had one patient that converted to THA by final follow-up. The Kaplan-Meier survival analysis predicted 5-year survival rate of 94 % in the >50-year group compared to 96 % in the younger patient group.

PAO vs. Total Hip Arthroplasty

The definitive treatment for arthritis secondary to hip dysplasia is total hip arthroplasty (THA). In this section, we examine studies that seek to compare the results of PAO to total hip arthroplasty.

In a high value study, Garbuz et al. reported on the outcome of 59 patients matched for age, gender, and comorbidities who underwent a PAO vs. THA in a nonrandomized fashion. At a mean follow-up of 4 years, the PAO had a significantly worse WOMAC score. Additionally, 97 % of THA patients had good or excellent outcomes compared to only 73 % of PAO patients [21].

In a later study, Garbuz et al. compared the PAO to THA in patients over 40 years using quality of life and functional measures. The groups, including 28 PAO patients and 34 THA patients, were age and sex matched and were followed for 4 years. The authors reported that THA had significantly better outcomes based on WOMAC scores, SF-12 scores, and UCLA activity level. Additionally, 36 % of PAO patients had complications, whereas only 2 % (1 of 36) of THA patients had a complication. The authors concluded THA had superior quality of life scores compared to PAO even though a majority of patients had good or very good outcomes [22].

Troelsen et al. studied the outcome of PAO in a group of 116 patients to identify radiographic factors predictive of conversion to THA at a mean follow-up of 6.8 years. The PAO survival rate was 81.6 % at 9.2 years. The preoperative factors predictive of PAO failure and THA conversion included severe dysplasia (CEA <0), reduced acetabular anteversion (<10°) as measured on axial CT, and the presence of os acetabuli. Postoperatively, factors like a small sourcil (sourcil length <2.5 cm), joint incongruity with abduction radiographs, and Tönnis grade 2/3 were predictive of poor outcome [23].

PAO with Intertrochanteric Osteotomy (ITO)

Occasionally, the hip joint deformity may include the proximal femur in addition to the acetabulum. While the PAO is a powerful tool, the magnitude of deformity may require proximal femoral correction which is frequently accomplished through intertrochanteric osteotomy. This section will examine the outcomes of PAO when combined with proximal femoral deformity correction. Though much is said about femoral anteversion in Developmental Dysplasia of the Hip, the more important aspect is malrotation. Not infrequently, patients with dysplasia significant enough to be candidates for PAO also have a disorder of rotation. This usually manifests itself as a marked loss of external rotation associated with excessive internal rotation. In this circumstance, an adjunctive ITO can be done solely for the purpose of resetting the range on motion into a functional rotation plane. Of course, at the same time, the upper femur can be extended and varus can be used for adjunctive containment.

Clohisy et al. from the Washington University of St. Louis group published on the results of PAO combined with proximal femoral valgus-producing osteotomy in 13 patients for Perthes-like deformity. These Perthes-like hips were characterized by coxa magna, coxa breva, and trochanteric overgrowth. The average clinical follow-up was 4.5 years and outcomes were tracked clinically with the HHS and radiographically with Tönnis grade. The indication for proximal femoral osteotomy in these patients was <20° of abduction after the PAO. The authors reported a significant improvement in the HHS and radiographic measures including the LCEA, aCEA, and acetabular roof obliquity. Major complications included transient nerve injury to the sciatic and femoral nerves and nonunion of the pubic osteotomy and the intertrochanteric osteotomy requiring reoperation and bone grafting. Numerous patients had previous hip surgery which increased the complexity of the hip reconstruction and may have contributed to the elevated complication rate [24].

Ganz et al., from the Bernese group, discussed their algorithm for choosing a PAO combined with a proximal femoral osteotomy. They reported that the rate of intertrochanteric osteotomy (ITO) with PAO declined from approximately 10 % in their first 500 procedures to 2 % currently. The authors stated that recently developed proximal femoral osteotomies like the femoral neck osteotomy, femoral head reduction osteotomy, and relative neck lengthening procedure have supplanted the classic ITO. The indications for a combined procedure include Perthes-like deformity, high riding trochanter, coxa breva, or previous varus ITO [25].

The Swiss authors described the results of 151 relative femoral neck lengthening procedures, 23 of which were combined with a PAO. The major complication rate was 2 % and included a femoral neck fracture requiring THA and 3 delayed unions of the trochanteric osteotomy requiring repeat surgery. They also reported on the results of 49 femoral neck osteotomies, one of which was combined with a PAO. Complications occurred in 14 % including delayed union in 10 % of patients (predominantly from the opening wedge osteotomy group) as well as 4 % risk of femoral head osteonecrosis. Finally, the authors presented a group of 14 patients who underwent a femoral head reduction osteotomy, 11 of which were combined with a PAO. No patient developed osteonecrosis or major complications. In conclusion, the authors reported that although the overall incidence of PFO had decreased with time, the complexity of the hips that would have otherwise required a PFO necessitated the development of additional powerful techniques to address the femoral deformity. These techniques have a higher rate of complications than PAO alone, but are sufficiently safe in experienced hands and fully treat the complex hip deformity [25].

Clohisy et al. compared the results of 25 patients who underwent a combined PAO with proximal femoral osteotomy (PFO) with a matched group of 25 patients who had a PAO alone. When comparing the PAO/PFO group to the PAO alone group, the PAO/PFO group had a lower modified HHS preoperatively but had similar function to the PAO alone group postoperatively based on modified HHS scores. The combined PAO/PFO indications included Perthes-like deformity, coxa valga, and poor congruency following PAO. The mean follow-up was 44 months. One patient in the PAO/PFO group converted to THA after 5 years. The authors concluded that combined PAO/PFO can obtain noninferior results to PAO alone with similar complication rates [26].

PAO for Legg-Calve-Perthes Disease

Shinoda et al. reported on the treatment of a group of 16 patients with dysplastic Perthes-like hip deformity using a Japanese curved periacetabular osteotomy. Preoperatively, the group included 3 class II hips, 11 class III hips, and 3 class IV hips according the Stulberg classification system. The average patient age at surgery was 36.9 years and the mean follow-up was 6.6 years. The authors reported a 23 point improvement in the HHS though range of motion was not significantly improved. Improvement in HHS was smaller in the Stulberg class IV hips and one of the patients from the Stulberg class 4 hips underwent a THA approximately 10 years after rotational osteotomy [27].

PAO with Femoral Osteochondroplasty

Not infrequently, dysplastic hips manifest cam type femoroacetabular impingement. The next section examines the results of PAO when combined with femoral osteochondroplasty.

Clohisy et al., from the Washington University of St. Louis group, compared the results of 40 patients treated with a PAO and femoral head-neck osteochondroplasty to 48 patients treated with a PAO alone at a mean follow-up of 3.4 years. The modified Harris hip scores (mHHS) of the two groups were comparable and not statistically different at final follow-up. The group with PAO combined with a femoral head-neck osteochondroplasty had a significant decrease in the alpha angle and head-neck offset whereas these measurements did not change in the PAO group. There was one reoperation in the study group compared to four reoperations in the PAO alone group for secondary impingement. There were no capsular adhesions, femoral neck fractures, osteonecrosis, or increase in heterotopic ossification in the study group indicating that a femoral head-neck osteochondroplasty performed concomitantly with a PAO does not increase the risk of complications [28].

Reverse PAO for Retroversion

The reverse PAO is indicated for acetabular retroversion deformity of the hip. Retroversion can be localized to the acetabulum or be present globally in the hemi-pelvis. The reverse PAO addresses posterior deficiency and concomitant anterior overcoverage seen with retroversion. The usual deficiency in dysplasia, in contrast, is normally anterolateral. The acetabular retroversion and anterior overcoverage lead to impingement with flexion and internal rotation.

The reverse PAO was initially described by Siebenrock et al. from the Bern group, in a series of 22 patients with an average age of 23 years followed for an average of 30 months. Sixty-five percent of retroverted hips were in males which is different than classic dysplasia which is predominantly a disease of females. Acetabular retroversion was diagnosed by the crossover sign in all patients and the posterior wall sign in 83 % of hips. A positive posterior wall sign is when the posterior wall of the acetabulum extends lateral to the center of the femoral head. All patients with an arthrotomy were found to have either labral degeneration and partial tears or a complete labral tear. The goal of the surgery was to obtain 30 deg of internal rotation and 90 deg of flexion. The Merle d'Aubigné score improved from 11° to 21°. Three patients required additional surgery. One patient had a loss of fixation and correction, another had overcorrection with resultant posterior impingement requiring surgical dislocation and posterior acetabular rim resection, and the final patient had undercorrection requiring a secondary procedure to improve the head-neck offset. No patients required conversion to THA [29].

Peters et al. from the University of Utah group reported on two nonrandom cohorts of patients with acetabular retroversion treated with either a reverse PAO or a surgical hip dislocation (SHD) with osteochondroplasty and acetabular rim resection. Thirty patients in each group were followed for an average of 46 months. Retroversion was defined as a positive crossover sign on a standing AP pelvis radiograph. Patients with a positive crossover sign and CEA <20° were treated with a reverse PAO whereas patients with a crossover sign and posterior wall sign were treated with SHD and rim resection. One patient in each group required conversion to THA. The posterior wall sign was corrected in 96 % of patients, but two patients in the SHD group developed iatrogenic dysplasia. The HHS improved significantly in both groups with an overall survivorship at 4 years of 96 % [30].

PAO in Males

Ziebarth et al. from the Boston group noted symptomatic impingement in nearly 50 % of male patients following PAO. The group included 38 male patients with a mean follow-up of 43 months. The authors reported decreased flexion, decreased internal rotation, and a positive impingement sign in 19 of 46 hips postoperatively. In spite of the high incidence of iatrogenic impingement, both radiographic coverage and WOMAC scores demonstrated improvement [31].

PAO for Neuromuscular Disease

Sierra et al., from the Bern group, reported on the outcome of the PAO for the treatment of paralytic hip dysplasia secondary to poliomyelitis in a group of nine patients. The mean follow-up was over 8.5 years. Acetabular index, extrusion index, and lateral center-edge angle were improved in all patients. All patients reported an improvement in pain, but functional improvement was modest. Only 25 % of patients had an improvement in abductor strength. 50 % of patients had progression of Tönnis grade though there were no conversions to THA. The authors concluded that the PAO in paralytic hip dysplasia is effective at providing durable pain relief in patients with mild arthritis, though the functional improvements have been modest [32].

PAO in Down's Syndrome

The incidence of hip dysplasia in trisomy 21 patients is frequent. Nearly 30 % of trisomy 21 patients have radiographic hip dysplasia. The musculoskeletal system in trisomy 21 patients is characterized by ligamentous laxity. The results of pelvic osteotomy for dysplasia are generally inferior in trisomy 21 patients compared to "normal" dysplastic patients which is possibly due to residual instability [33]. A recent paper used preoperative CT to compare the acetabular version in age-matched groups of normal patients, patients with dysplasia, and Trisomy 21 patients with hip dysplasia. Each group had 16 patients and an average age of 14.5 years. The CT version measurements demonstrated that the Down's patients had significant acetabular retroversion with a mean version of 2° compared to control patients (mean version 13°) and patients with classic hip dysplasia (mean version 21°). This significant tendency towards retroversion may explain the poor results with classic hip operations with Trisomy 21. The reverse PAO may be the better operation [34].

PAO after Failed Hip Arthroscopy

Kim et al., from the Boston group, retrospectively compared the results of 17 patients who were treated with a PAO following a failed arthroscopic labral debridement to a control group of 34 patients treated with PAO only. The mean patient age was 31 years and there were no differences in radiographic measures of dysplasia or arthritis. Three patients in the PA+Scope group underwent a THA compared to only 1 in the control group, though this result was not statistically significant. The changes in preoperative and postoperative WOMAC scores were comparable between the two groups. The study did not include a power analysis for THA conversion between the two groups. The authors concluded that PAO may still be considered after a failed hip arthroscopy with expectation for good results, but there was a trend towards increased conversion to THA. The hip preservation surgeon may use this information to counsel patients that a "quick look" scope in preparation for a PAO may not be as benign as previously thought [35]. Conversely, it is highly desirable to recognize the presence of dysplasia before embarking on stand-alone hip arthroscopy. The input from a structural surgeon can be very helpful is designing the optimum treatment. It is now recognized that repair of a torn labrum is superior to resection. Yet, repair of a torn labrum without correction of the dysplasia invites another tear, as the antecedent factors are still in place.

PAO vs. THA in the Same Patient

Hsieh et al. from Taiwan compared the PAO to THA in a group of 31 patients who had one of each procedure on contralateral sides. The PAO indications were mild/moderate OA as described by Tönnis grade 0–2. The THA indications were for advanced OA defined by Tönnis grade 3 or higher. The mean follow-up of the PAO was 5.5 years, and the mean follow-up of the THA was 6.7 years. The authors noted no difference in outcome based on Merle d'Aubigné or WOMAC score. However, patients significantly preferred their preserved hip compared to the THA. The authors noted excessive wear in 7 patients and osteolysis in 12 patients, reflective of the disappointing results of THA in young, active patients. The authors concluded that a timely PAO to correct dysplasia should be a consideration rather than waiting for a THA [36]. It is difficult to make definitive conclusions, since a confounding variable, such as a poorly performing prosthesis, could affect the assessment. This study stands in contrast to that by Garbuz et al. reviewed earlier who matched PAO and THA patients and found significantly fewer complications and increased satisfaction with THA.

PAO in Patients with Previous Hip Surgery

The Dallas Scottish Rite group compared the results of periacetabular osteotomy in patients who had previous pelvic/hip surgery to a control group with no previous surgery to ascertain if this was a predictor of outcome. There were 13 patients in each group and the mean follow-up was 1 year. The previous surgeries included 10 Salter osteotomies, 2 Chiari osteotomies, and 1 proximal femur osteotomy. The Harris hip scores and radiographic markers (CEA, acetabular index, and femoral head extrusion) improved in both groups and were not statistically different at 1 year. The group with previous hip surgery did demonstrate decreased flexion and abductor strength at 6 months; however this difference had disappeared by 1 year. Muscle damage that likely occurred during the prior surgery would not be expected to improve after PAO [37].

Curved Periacetabular Osteotomy

The curved periacetabular osteotomy is a popular surgical option for treatment of hip dysplasia in Japan. This osteotomy involves using a curved osteotome to match the patient's acetabular curvature. The curved periacetabular osteotomy offers a large bony surface for union, stable fixation, and ability to correct lateral deficiency. However, the curved periacetabular osteotomy requires splitting of the abductors, cannot medialize the acetabulum, and places the acetabulum at increased risk of avascular necrosis compared to the Bernese periacetabular osteotomy. The incidence of postoperative osteonecrosis, however, is quite small, and this operation is effective. Other examples of curved osteotomies include the Wagner dome osteotomy and the Eppright dial osteotomy, but will not be discussed here.

Karashima et al. retrospectively compared the results of the curved periacetabular osteotomy in a group of 147 hips with moderate hip dysplasia (defined as CEA >0° and Severin group III or IVA) to a group of 44 patients with severe hip dysplasia (defined as CEA <0 and Severin grade IVB). The mean follow-up was 70 months and minimum follow-up was 2 years. Overall, 87 % of patients did not demonstrate radiographic osteoarthritis progression. Half of the patients with radiographic progression developed severe end-stage disease. Progression was not limited to the severely dysplastic patients (severely dysplastic defined by CEA <0°). Lateral femoral cutaneous nerve palsy was frequent in both groups. No patient developed avascular necrosis of the acetabulum. Overall, the authors concluded the curved periacetabular osteotomy was efficacious for severe hip dysplasia without increasing complications [38].

Curved Periacetabular Osteotomy with Hip Arthroscopy

Kim et al. reported on the results of combined hip arthroscopy and Japanese curved periacetabular osteotomy in a group of 43 patients with a mean follow-up of 74 months. The mean HHS improved from 72 to 94. The authors found labral tears in 38/43 patients (88 %) and performed debridements in all patients. No labral repairs were attempted. Complications reported included joint penetration, posterior column fracture, and DVT. No osteonecrosis or THA conversion occurred during the study [39].

Conclusion

Periacetabular Osteotomy is a powerful surgical procedure to reorient the acetabulum in patients with significant dysplasia. While current results are encouraging in skilled hands, the best results occur when the indications are appropriately applied. When necessary, the PAO may be combined with intra-articular procedures or femoral intertrochanteric osteotomy to optimize a patient's outcome.

References

1. Stulberg S, Harris W. Acetabular dysplasia and development of osteoarthritis of the hip, The hip proceedings of the second open scientific meeting of the hip society. St Louis: CV Mosby; 1974. p. 82–93.
2. Harris WH. Etiology of osteoarthritis of the hip. Clin Orthop. 1986;213:20–33.
3. Jacobsen S, Sonne-Holm S. Hip dysplasia: a significant risk factor for the development of hip osteoarthritis. A cross-sectional survey. Rheumatology. 2005;44:211–8.
4. Engesaeter IO, Laborie LB, Lehmann TG, et al. Prevalence of radiographic findings associated with hip dysplasia in a population-based cohort of 2081 19-year-old Norwegians. Bone Joint J. 2013;95-B:279–85.
5. Murphy SB, Ganz R, Muller ME. The prognosis in untreated dysplasia of the hip. A study of radiographic factors that predict the outcome. J Bone Joint Surg Am. 1995;77:985–9.
6. Cooperman DR, Wallensten R, Stulberg SD. Acetabular dysplasia in the adult. Clin Orthop Relat Res. 1983;79–85.
7. Wenger DR. Is there a role for acetabular dysplasia correction in an asymptomatic patient? J Pediatr Orthop. 2013;33 Suppl 1:S8–12.
8. Matta JM, Stover MD, Siebenrock K. Periacetabular osteotomy through the Smith-Petersen approach. Clin Orthop Relat Res. 1999;21–32.
9. Steppacher SD, Tannast M, Ganz R, Siebenrock KA. Mean 20-year followup of Bernese periacetabular osteotomy. Clin Orthop Relat Res. 2008;466:1633–44.
10. Kralj M, Mavcic B, Antolic V, Iglic A, Kralj-Iglic V. The Bernese periacetabular osteotomy: clinical, radiographic and mechanical 7-15-year follow-up of 26 hips. Acta Orthop. 2005;76:833–40.
11. Albers CE, Steppacher SD, Ganz R, Tannast M, Siebenrock KA. Impingement adversely affects 10-year survivorship after periacetabular osteotomy for DDH. Clin Orthop Relat Res. 2013;471:1602–14.
12. Matheney T, Kim YJ, Zurakowski D, Matero C, Millis M. Intermediate to long-term results following the bernese periacetabular osteotomy and predictors of clinical outcome: surgical technique. J Bone Joint Surg Am. 2010;92(Suppl 1 Pt 2):115–29.
13. Hartig-Andreasen C, Troelsen A, Thillemann TM, Soballe K. What factors predict failure 4 to 12 years after periacetabular osteotomy? Clin Orthop Relat Res. 2012;470:2978–87.
14. Garras DN, Crowder TT, Olson SA. Medium-term results of the Bernese periacetabular osteotomy in the treatment of symptomatic developmental dysplasia of the hip. J Bone Joint Surg Br. 2007;89:721–4.
15. Pogliacomi F, Stark A, Wallensten R. Periacetabular osteotomy. Good pain relief in symptomatic hip dysplasia, 32 patients followed for 4 years. Acta Orthop. 2005;76:67–74.
16. Clohisy JC, Barrett SE, Gordon JE, Delgado ED, Schoenecker PL. Periacetabular osteotomy for the treatment of severe acetabular dysplasia. J Bone Joint Surg Am. 2005;87:254–9.
17. Millis MB, Kain M, Sierra R, et al. Periacetabular osteotomy for acetabular dysplasia in patients older than 40 years: a preliminary study. Clin Orthop Relat Res. 2009;467:2228–34.
18. Ito H, Tanino H, Yamanaka Y, Minami A, Matsuno T. Intermediate to long-term results of periacetabular osteotomy in patients younger and older than forty years of age. J Bone Joint Surg Am. 2011;93:1347–54.
19. Zhu J, Chen X, Cui Y, Shen C, Cai G. Mid-term results of Bernese periacetabular osteotomy for developmental dysplasia of hip in middle aged patients. Int Orthop. 2013;37:589–94.
20. Teratani T, Naito M, Kiyama T, Maeyama A. Periacetabular osteotomy in patients fifty years of age or older: surgical technique. J Bone Joint Surg Am. 2011;93 Suppl 1:30–9.
21. Garbuz D, Duncan C, Awwad M. Quality of life after periacetabular osteotomy in patients over 40: a comparison with THA. J Bone Joint Surg Br. 2008;90-B.
22. Garbuz DS, Awwad MA, Duncan CP. Periacetabular osteotomy and total hip arthroplasty in patients older than 40 years. J Arthroplast. 2008;23:960–3.
23. Troelsen A, Elmengaard B, Soballe K. Medium-term outcome of periacetabular osteotomy and predictors of conversion to total hip replacement. J Bone Joint Surg Am. 2009;91:2169–79.
24. Clohisy JC, Nunley RM, Curry MC, Schoenecker PL. Periacetabular osteotomy for the treatment of acetabular dysplasia associated with major aspherical femoral head deformities. J Bone Joint Surg Am. 2007;89:1417–23.
25. Ganz R, Horowitz K, Leunig M. Algorithm for femoral and periacetabular osteotomies in complex hip deformities. Clin Orthop Relat Res. 2010;468:3168–80.
26. Clohisy JC, St John LC, Nunley RM, Schutz AL, Schoenecker PL. Combined periacetabular and femoral osteotomies for severe hip deformities. Clin Orthop Relat Res. 2009;467:2221–7.
27. Shinoda T, Naito M, Nakamura Y, Kiyama T. Periacetabular osteotomy for the treatment of dysplastic hip with Perthes-like deformities. Int Orthop. 2009;33:71–5.
28. Nassif NA, Schoenecker PL, Thorsness R, Clohisy JC. Periacetabular osteotomy and combined femoral head-neck junction osteochondroplasty: a minimum two-year follow-up cohort study. J Bone Joint Surg Am. 2012;94:1959–66.
29. Siebenrock KA, Schoeniger R, Ganz R. Anterior femoro-acetabular impingement due to acetabular retroversion. Treatment with periacetabular osteotomy. J Bone Joint Surg Am. 2003;85-A:278–86.
30. Peters CL, Anderson LA, Erickson JA, Anderson AE, Weiss JA. An algorithmic approach to surgical decision making in acetabular retroversion. Orthopedics. 2011;34:10.
31. Ziebarth K, Balakumar J, Domayer S, Kim YJ, Millis MB. Bernese periacetabular osteotomy in males: is there an increased risk of femoroacetabular impingement (FAI) after Bernese periacetabular osteotomy? Clin Orthop Relat Res. 2011;469:447–53.
32. Sierra RJ, Schoeniger SR, Millis M, Ganz R. Periacetabular osteotomy for containment of the nonarthritic dysplastic hip secondary to poliomyelitis. J Bone Joint Surg Am. 2010;92:2917–23.
33. Kelley SP, Wedge JH. Management of hip instability in trisomy 21. J Pediatr Orthop. 2013;33 Suppl 1:S33–8.
34. Sankar WN, Schoenecker JG, Mayfield ME, Kim YJ, Millis MB. Acetabular retroversion in Down syndrome. J Pediatr Orthop. 2012;32:277–81.
35. Kain MS, Novais EN, Vallim C, Millis MB, Kim Y-J. Periacetabular osteotomy after failed hip arthroscopy for labral tears in patients with acetabular dysplasia. J Bone Joint Surg Am. 2011;93:57–61.
36. Hsieh P-H, Huang K-C, Lee P-C, Chang Y-H. Comparison of periacetabular osteotomy and total hip replacement in the same patient: a two-to ten-year follow-up study. J Bone Joint Surg Br. 2009;91:883–8.
37. De La Rocha A, Sucato DJ, Tulchin K, Podeszwa DA. Treatment of adolescents with a periacetabular osteotomy after previous pelvic surgery. Clin Orthop Relat Res. 2012;470:2583–90.
38. Karashima H, Naito M, Shiramizu K, Kiyama T, Maeyama A. A periacetabular osteotomy for the treatment of severe dysplastic hips. Clin Orthop Relat Res. 2011;469:1436–41.
39. Kim K-I, Cho Y-J, Ramteke A, Yoo M-C. Peri-acetabular rotational osteotomy with concomitant hip arthroscopy for treatment of hip dysplasia. J Bone Joint Surg Br. 2011;93:732–7.

Proximal Femoral Osteotomy in Hip Preservation

76

Jaclyn F. Hill, Nicole I. Montgomery, and Scott B. Rosenfeld

Introduction

Proximal femoral osteotomies (PFO) are rarely used in isolation for hip preservation. Instead, they are more commonly used as an adjunct and combined with procedures that have the ability to more closely treat the site of pathology or deformity. For example, in cases of acetabular dysplasia, the deformity occurs in the acetabulum and is therefore better treated with a pelvic osteotomy such as the periacetabular osteotomy (PAO) than an intertrochanteric femoral osteotomy [1]. Similarly, the anatomic abnormality in slipped capital femoral epiphysis (SCFE) and Perthes disease is located at the femoral head and neck and is therefore best treated with procedures focused on that area such as femoral head/neck osteoplasty and osteotomy. More severe hip deformity involving both the proximal femur and acetabulum may have improved outcomes with combined acetabular and proximal femoral osteotomies [2–5]. Femoral osteotomies performed in hip preservation include intertrochanteric osteotomy (ITO), relative femoral neck lengthening (RFNL), femoral neck osteotomy (FNO), and femoral head reduction osteotomy. The indications for proximal femoral osteotomy performed either alone or in combination with other procedures for preservation of the mature hip are discussed in this chapter.

J.F. Hill, MD (✉) • N.I. Montgomery, MD • S.B. Rosenfeld, MD
Department of Pediatric Orthopaedic Surgery, Texas Children's Hospital, 6701 Fannin St, Houston, TX 77030, USA

Department of Orthopedic Surgery, Baylor College of Medicine, 7200 Cambridge, Suite 10A, Houston, TX 77030, USA
e-mail: jfhill@texaschildrens.org

Osteotomy in Developmental Dysplasia of the Hip

Common anatomic features of the dysplastic hip include inadequate coverage of the femoral head by the acetabulum and an oblique inclination of the weight-bearing zone of the acetabular dome. This creates shearing forces on the acetabulum, and may result in superior-lateral subluxation of the femoral head, as well as edge loading with chronic overload of the acetabular labrum and the anterolateral periacetabular bone. Often, the acetabular dysplasia is combined with femoral-sided anatomic abnormalities including coxa valga and increased femoral anteversion. However, from a mechanical standpoint the most important bony deformities are seen in the acetabulum.

Proximal femoral osteotomies, including varus derotational ITO and distal transfer of the greater trochanter for trochanteric overgrowth, have commonly been used in the treatment of hip dysplasia [6–9]. Despite the long-term use of these procedures, an isolated proximal femoral osteotomy is not useful in stabilizing hips with acetabular dysplasia because it does not address the important counterface aspect of the anatomic abnormality—the acetabulum [10]. Instead, periacetabular osteotomy has been shown to be the most beneficial option in the treatment of the congruously dysplastic hip [1]. One situation in which an isolated ITO may be indicated is in patients with a nonscoliotic leg length difference with or without a high femoral neck-shaft angle resulting in pelvic tilt and a mild uncovering of the femoral head causing a functional acetabular dysplasia [11]. This deformity may be treated with a femoral shortening osteotomy if the neck-shaft angle is normal or a varus-producing femoral intertrochanteric osteotomy if the angle is increased. Both osteotomies shorten the extremity resulting in correction of the pelvic tilt and the functional acetabular dysplasia.

An intertrochanteric varus osteotomy performed in conjunction with a PAO may be indicated in cases of complex deformity involving both sides of the joint. General indications for combining PFO with PAO include congruous

J.C. McCarthy et al. (eds.), *Hip Joint Restoration*, DOI 10.1007/978-1-4614-0694-5_76

acetabular dysplasia with a femoral neck-shaft angle greater than 130°, or if the proximal femoral articular surface is anteverted by more than 15° on the AP pelvis x-ray [1]. Ganz et al. further elaborated on indications for combining PFO with PAO. The Swiss group recommended including PFO after PAO to improve femoral head coverage (lateral CEA <25°, acetabular index >10°, extrusion index >30°), containment (distance between the ilio-ischial line and femoral head >5–7 mm), and congruency (non-congruent joint space with a width >3 mm). When so indicated, PAO and PFO may be performed under a single anesthesia [12].

The decision to combine a PFO and a PAO is based on evaluation of imaging studies including an antero-posterior pelvis view, a false profile view, functional views (abduction, internal rotation), and sometimes MRI. Abduction views help to differentiate between joint space narrowing caused by anterolateral migration and that caused by cartilage loss. If the joint space enlarges with abduction, the cause of the narrowing is anterolateral subluxation and it is likely that the dysplasia will be corrected by PAO alone. Additionally, if the joint space increases with abduction combined with hip flexion of 10° to 15° and/or internal rotation, then a flexion-internal rotation ITO may be helpful. In the case of a medially congruent but aspherical joint, an adduction view provides insight regarding the possible benefit of a valgus ITO [12]. MR arthrogram and DGEMRIC MRI allow for assessment of intra-articular pathology such as labral tears and the location of focal articular cartilage defects [13]. Varus, valgus, or flexion ITO may be utilized to move healthy articular cartilage into the weight-bearing zone.

Normalization of anatomy should be the goal when planning an ITO. The tip of the greater trochanter is located an average of 10.3 mm proximal to the femoral head center [14]. It should be lateral to the center of the head by a distance equal to 2–2.5 times the radius of the femoral head [9, 15]. As a large varus correction may result in a high-riding greater trochanter with subsequent trochanteric impingement and abductor weakness, distal transfer of the greater trochanter and trochanteric osteoplasty may be performed to normalize this relationship [16].

The combination of abnormal proximal femoral anatomy and acetabular dysplasia may lead to insufficient flexion and/or abduction after a PAO. This situation can arise from an overcorrection of the acetabular anterior deficiency or, conversely, in the presence of a prior varus intertrochanteric osteotomy, an aspherical femoral head, proximal femoral retroversion, and a short femoral neck. In order to avoid the resulting loss of hip motion after acetabular correction, it may be necessary to perform a simultaneous redirection of the proximal femur with an ITO incorporating valgus, flexion, and/or rotation, possibly in combination with a femoral neck osteoplasty [1].

Although the use of intertrochanteric and subtrochanteric osteotomies is well accepted for correction of femoral deformities, these procedures can produce several negative side effects when performed at a distance from the deformity. Specifically, the medialization or lateralization of the femoral shaft generated by each procedure alters the mechanical axis of the limb. ITO also has the effect of shortening or lengthening the limb. The more distal the location of the osteotomy the greater these undesirable results. Osteotomies performed at the femoral head and neck level are closer to the site of pathology and therefore are less likely to produce a secondary deformity. For these reasons, relative femoral neck lengthening, femoral neck osteotomy, and femoral head reduction are being used more frequently to address these complex deformities. These procedures are performed through a surgical dislocation approach with the use of an extended retinacular soft tissue flap to protect the blood supply to the femoral head [17]. Relative femoral neck lengthening is indicated for extra-articular and intra-articular impingement and abductor weakness secondary to a high-riding greater trochanter and/or short femoral neck. Such deformities can be seen as a sequelae of Perthes disease or in patients with residual deformity after treatment of hip dysplasia in early childhood. Femoral neck osteotomy has similar indications to intertrochanteric osteotomy but is more effective in influencing the superior joint space and results in less medialization/lateralization of the femoral shaft and less alteration of limb length [12].

Femoral head reduction osteotomy can be considered in hips with coxa magna and central coxa plana. In this situation where the central portion of the head is flattened, that portion is excised and the round medial and lateral portions are brought together resulting in a smaller, rounder head which fits better into the acetabulum [17]. Although these osteotomies better address the site of deformity and produce less secondary deformity, they are associated with a higher risk of complications, especially avascular necrosis of the femoral head, and thus should be performed by an experienced osteotomy surgeon.

Osteotomy in Perthes Disease

Long-term studies of the natural history of Perthes disease demonstrate deterioration of the native hip beyond 40 years, if not earlier [18]. The most important factor in determining the outcome of a Perthes hip is residual femoral head deformity and its effect on hip joint congruity [19, 20].

Grossboard and Catterall described hinge abduction as when the large deformed femoral head impinges on the lateral lip of the acetabulum when the hip is abducted [21, 22]. This collision results in the femoral head being levered out of the acetabulum with a resulting change in the center of rotation. Clinically, this may present as decreased range of motion and pain with abduction. Arthrographic and fluoroscopic examination of hip motion is used to confirm the occurrence of hinge abduction. Treatment may include a valgus ITO to rotate the infero-medial portion of the femoral head into the weight-bearing position and move the deformed lateral portion of the head away from the acetabular margin. This results in a larger range of impingement-free abduction and increases articular congruity through more of the motion arc [23].

Perthes disease and other causes of ischemic necrosis of the capital femoral epiphysis often result in deformity, including coxa vara, coxa magna, abnormal offset of the anterior femoral head-neck junction, a short femoral neck, and a high-riding greater trochanter. These anatomic deformities lead to clinical findings of hip impingement, leg length discrepancy, and limp. Additionally, the shortened femoral neck and high-riding trochanter result in a shortened lever arm for the hip abductor muscles and a subsequent Trendelenburg lurch. Morscher described a femoral neck lengthening osteotomy to address these deformities simultaneously [24]. In the original description of this triple proximal femoral osteotomy, the femoral neck was lengthened by a combination of distal transfer of the greater trochanter and lateralization of the femoral shaft [24]. This is different from a valgus intertrochanteric osteotomy as the osteotomy of the femoral shaft is made cephalad to the lesser trochanter, allowing it to move laterally with the femoral shaft, thereby reducing leg length discrepancy. When there is concomitant acetabular dysplasia this procedure may be combined with periacetabular osteotomy to improve femoral head coverage and stability.

Triple Proximal Femoral Osteotomy: Description of Author's Modification of the Original Technique

The original technique described by Hasler and Morscher involves three parallel proximal femoral osteotomies. These include cuts located at the base of the greater trochanter, the cephalad border of the femoral neck, and a distal osteotomy at the base of the femoral neck just cephalad to the lesser trochanter. The author has performed this procedure in combination with surgical dislocation of the hip and has found that the single trochanteric osteotomy made for the surgical dislocation, combined with resection of the stable trochanter down to the femoral neck, is sufficient. Following completion of intra-articular work and repair of the hip capsule, the greater trochanter is transferred distally to the lateral aspect of the femur so that the tip is aligned at the center of the femoral head on an AP fluoroscopic image. The trochanter may be stabilized temporarily with a Steinman pin. Next, the femur is prepared for placement of the implant. The original description included use of a 130° blade plate but the author has used a proximal femoral locking plate with success. If a locking plate is chosen, the proximal guide wires are placed through the greater trochanter into the femoral neck. Next, a Steinman pin is placed at the site of the shaft osteotomy about 1 cm distal to the proximal guide wires. This pin is placed obliquely from distal lateral to proximal medial parallel to the inferior border of the neck of the femur and exits cephalad to the lesser trochanter. The femoral shaft osteotomy is then made parallel to this pin. Next the locking plate is placed proximally fixing the greater trochanter to the femoral neck. The femoral shaft is then reduced laterally and fixed to the plate. This results in distalization and lateralization of the greater trochanter as well as lateralization of the femoral shaft. The combination of these two osteotomies results in a true lengthening of the femoral neck (Fig. 76.1).

The primary indication for femoral head reduction osteotomy is healed Perthes disease or avascular necrosis with resultant coxa magna and a deformed central pillar. Osteotomy and excision of the central portion of the femoral head with mobilization of the lateral fragment and fixation to the medial fragment utilizes an understanding of the separate medial and lateral blood supply [25] and the constant arterial supply from a more central branch of the medial femoral circumflex artery which runs in its intra-articular course on the superior aspect of Weitbrecht's ligament [26].

When acetabular dysplasia occurs in combination with a femoral head deformity, surgical correction of both deformities may be considered. This may include any combination of proximal femoral osteotomy and periacetabular osteotomy [2, 27]. An algorithm based on imaging and physical exam can be used to help select whether a PFO and/or PAO should be performed. In patients with acetabular dysplasia and extra-articular pathology (high trochanter and short neck), the amount of abduction determines which procedure should be performed first. When greater than 20° of abduction is present, the PAO is performed first and then the decision regarding the need for a PFO (relative femoral neck lengthening or intertrochanteric osteotomy) is made intraoperatively. When hip abduction is limited to 20° or less, the PFO is performed first to allow for sufficient acetabular correction during the PAO. In patients with intra-articular pathology and acetabular dysplasia, abduction and adduction views are obtained preoperatively. When the hip is aspherical but congruent on the abduction view, the PAO is performed first with or without subsequent relative femoral neck lengthening. When the hip is aspherical but congruent on the adduction view, the PAO is performed first followed by a valgus intertrochanteric osteotomy [12].

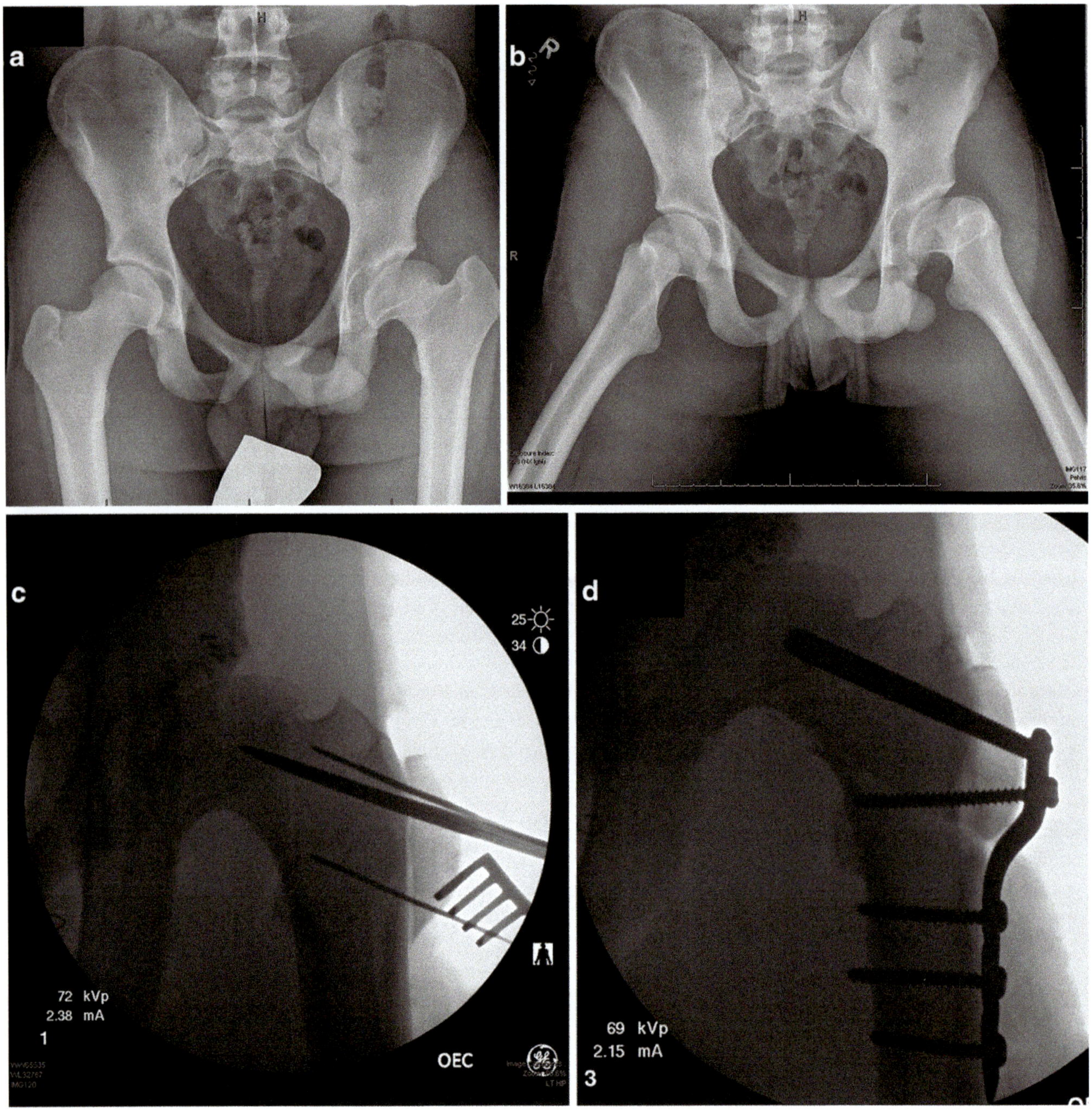

Fig. 76.1 A 16-year-old male with hip pain and residual Perthes deformity including coxa magna, shortened femoral neck, high-riding greater trochanter, and acetabular dysplasia (**a**, **b**). Surgical reconstruction included surgical hip dislocation with femoral neck osteochondroplasty and labral repair as well as Morscher-type intertrochanteric osteotomy with distal transfer of the greater trochanter and femoral neck lengthening. This was followed by periacetabular osteotomy under a single anesthesia (**c**–**f**). X-rays at 2-year follow-up (**g**, **h**)

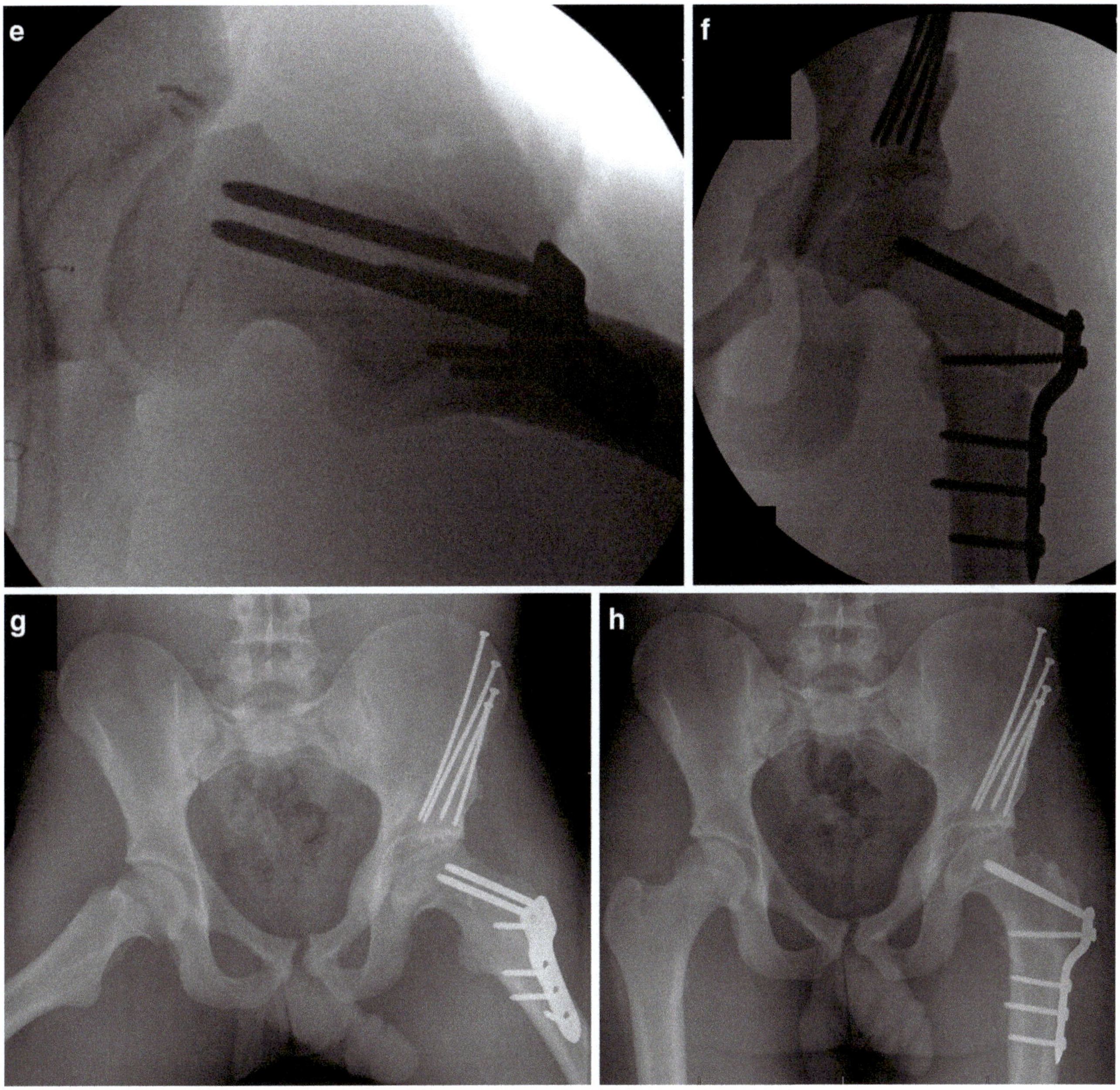

Fig. 76.1 (continued)

Osteotomy in Slipped Capital Femoral Epiphysis

A slipped capital femoral epiphysis (SCFE) creates a complex three-dimensional hip deformity that significantly alters hip mechanics and motion [28]. Deformities associated with SCFE include proximal femoral varus, retroversion, and abnormal offset of the femoral head-neck junction. Even slips with mild residual deformity can lead to severe intra-articular cartilage injury [29, 30]. Long-term follow-up studies report that 15–20 % of patients with SCFE may develop painful osteoarthritis by the age of 50 years [31]. However, reports suggest that significant intra-articular damage occurs much sooner [32].

The classic valgus-flexion intertrochanteric osteotomy has been used for decades to address the varus and retroversion deformity associated with moderate to severe slipped capital femoral epiphysis. The classic correction consists primarily of flexion, internal rotation, and a minimal amount of valgus [28]. In moderate and severe slips, retrospective studies of the outcomes of intertrochanteric osteotomy report good or excellent function in 71–92 % of patients at a mean follow-up of 6.4–24 years [33–39]. Reported complications

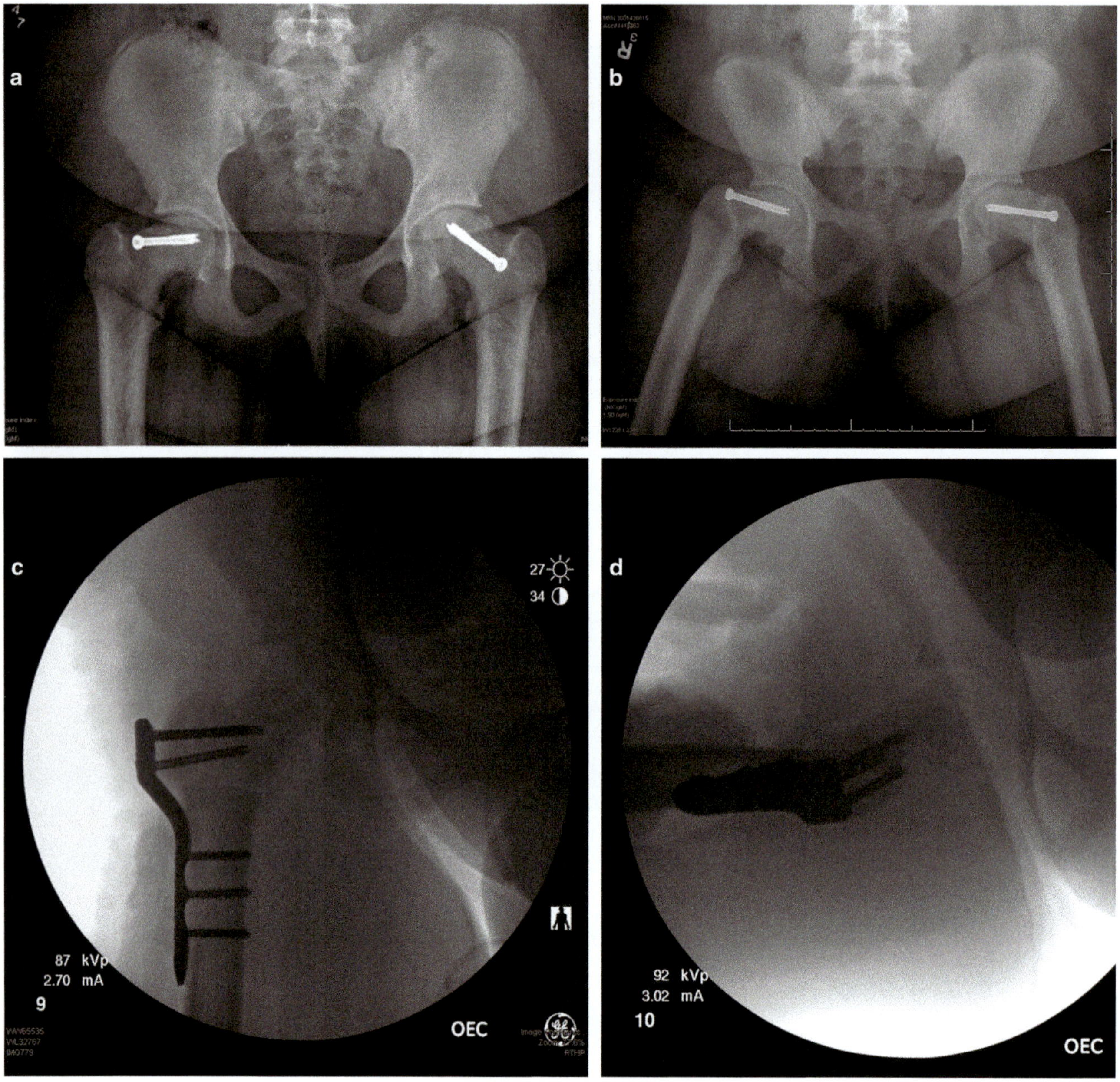

Fig. 76.2 A 15-year-old female with bilateral slipped capital femoral epiphysis resulting in proximal femoral varus and retroversion with high-riding greater trochanter and decreased anterior femoral head-neck offset (**a**, **b**). Patient underwent surgical hip dislocation with femoral neck osteochondroplasty, distal transfer of the greater trochanter, and flexion-internal rotation femoral intertrochanteric osteotomy (**c**, **d**)

include osteonecrosis (2.0–6.7 %) and chondrolysis. More recently, SCFE deformities have been treated with ITO used in combination with surgical dislocation, arthroscopy, and/or anterior arthrotomy for treatment of head-neck offset abnormalities as well as labral debridement and repair (Fig. 76.2) [40–42]. Techniques that create less secondary deformity, including subcapital reorientation via a surgical dislocation approach with an extended retinacular flap (a modification of the Dunn procedure), are being used more frequently [43–45]. This procedure carries a high risk of avascular necrosis and should be performed only by experienced surgeons [46].

Proximal Femoral Osteotomy for Joint Preservation: Summary

The subset of patients undergoing hip preservation surgery is unique. The ideal goal of treatment is normalization of hip mechanics, resolution of current symptoms, and prevention of future osteoarthritis. However, in many cases some degree of arthrosis is already present and future hip arthroplasty is inevitable. In such cases the goal of treatment must be modified to aim for improved joint function, reduction of symptoms, and prolongation of the need for a total hip arthroplasty. Despite successful reconstruction of anatomy, pre-existing arthrosis will result in some of these patients ultimately requiring total joint replacement. This ultimate surgery needs to be considered when performing proximal femoral osteotomy. Such osteotomies may potentially alter the anatomy of the proximal femur, which can complicate the placement of the femoral stem during hip arthroplasty [47]. Additionally, retained hardware can present additional challenges during total hip arthroplasty. THA after previous femoral osteotomy is more technically demanding, necessitating higher rates of trochanteric osteotomy and longer surgical time. Fortunately this has not translated to a higher rate of complications in some series [47]. Should a patient require conversion to a total hip replacement, in the presence of broken hardware or distortion of the femoral canal, it may be prudent to perform the conversion in two stages.

References

1. Millis MB, Kim YJ. Rationale of osteotomy and related procedures for hip preservation: a review. Clin Orthop Relat Res. 2002;405: 108–21.
2. Clohisy JC et al. Periacetabular osteotomy for the treatment of acetabular dysplasia associated with major aspherical femoral head deformities. J Bone Joint Surg Am. 2007;89(7):1417–23.
3. Ganz R et al. A new periacetabular osteotomy for the treatment of hip dysplasias. Technique and preliminary results. Clin Orthop Relat Res. 1988;232:26–36.
4. Ninomiya S, Tagawa H. Rotational acetabular osteotomy for the dysplastic hip. J Bone Joint Surg Am. 1984;66(3):430–6.
5. Turgeon TR et al. The role of acetabular and femoral osteotomies in reconstructive surgery of the hip: 2005 and beyond. Clin Orthop Relat Res. 2005;441:188–99.
6. Bombelli R. Structure and function in normal and abnormal hips: how to rescue mechanically jeopardized hips. 3rd ed. New York: Springer; 1993.
7. Ganz R, MacDonald SJ. Indications and modern techniques of proximal femoral osteotomies in the adult. Sem Arthroplasty. 1997;8:38–50.
8. Pauwels F. Biomechanics of the normal and diseased hip: theoretical foundation, technique and results of treatment: an atlas. New York: Springer; 1976.
9. The Intertrochanteric Osteotomy, J. Schatzker (ed) 1984; New York: Springer; pp. 25–66.
10. Perlau R, Wilson MG, Poss R. Isolated proximal femoral osteotomy for treatment of residua of congenital dysplasia or idiopathic osteoarthrosis of the hip. Five to ten-year results. J Bone Joint Surg Am. 1996;78(10):1462–7.
11. Santore RF et al. Pelvic and femoral osteotomy in the treatment of hip disease in the young adult. Instr Course Lect. 2006;55:131–44.
12. Ganz R, Horowitz K, Leunig M. Algorithm for femoral and periacetabular osteotomies in complex hip deformities. Clin Orthop Relat Res. 2010;468(12):3168–80.
13. Bittersohl B et al. Delayed gadolinium-enhanced magnetic resonance imaging of hip joint cartilage: pearls and pitfalls. Orthop Rev (Pavia). 2011;3(2), e11.
14. Sugano N, Noble PC, Kamaric E. Predicting the position of the femoral head center. J Arthroplasty. 1999;14(1):102–7.
15. Tonnis D, Arning A, Block M, et al. Triple pelvic osteotomy. J Pediatr Orthop. 1994;3:54–67.
16. Ganz R et al. Femoroacetabular impingement: a cause for osteoarthritis of the hip. Clin Orthop Relat Res. 2003;417:112–20.
17. Ganz R, Huff TW, Leunig M. Extended retinacular soft-tissue flap for intra-articular hip surgery: surgical technique, indications, and results of application. Instr Course Lect. 2009;58:241–55.
18. McAndrew MP, Weinstein SL. A long-term follow-up of Legg-Calve-Perthes disease. J Bone Joint Surg Am. 1984;66(6):860–9.
19. Ismail AM, Macnicol MF. Prognosis in Perthes' disease: a comparison of radiological predictors. J Bone Joint Surg (Br). 1998;80(2):310–4.
20. Poussa M et al. Prognosis after conservative and operative treatment in Perthes' disease. Clin Orthop Relat Res. 1993;297:82–6.
21. Grossbard GD. Hip pain during adolescence after Perthes' disease. J Bone Joint Surg (Br). 1981;63B(4):572–4.
22. Catterall A. Legg-Calve-Perthes syndrome. Clin Orthop Relat Res. 1981;158:41–52.
23. Myers GJ, Mathur K, O'Hara J. Valgus osteotomy: a solution for late presentation of hinge abduction in Legg-Calve-Perthes disease. J Pediatr Orthop. 2008;28(2):169–72.
24. Hasler CC, Morscher EW. Femoral neck lengthening osteotomy after growth disturbance of the proximal femur. J Pediatr Orthop B. 1999;8(4):271–5.
25. Sevitt S, Thompson RG. The distribution and anastomoses of arteries supplying the head and neck of the femur. J Bone Joint Surg (Br). 1965;47:560–73.
26. Kalhor M et al. Anatomic variations in femoral head circulation. Hip Int. 2012;22(3):307–12.
27. Clohisy JC et al. Combined periacetabular and femoral osteotomies for severe hip deformities. Clin Orthop Relat Res. 2009;467(9):2221–7.
28. Kuzyk PR, Kim YJ, Millis MB. Surgical management of healed slipped capital femoral epiphysis. J Am Acad Orthop Surg. 2011;19(11):667–77.
29. Dodds MK, McCormack D, Mulhall KJ. Femoroacetabular impingement after slipped capital femoral epiphysis: does slip severity predict clinical symptoms? J Pediatr Orthop. 2009;29(6): 535–9.
30. Sink EL et al. Acetabular cartilage and labral damage observed during surgical hip dislocation for stable slipped capital femoral epiphysis. J Pediatr Orthop. 2010;30(1):26–30.
31. Aronson J. Osteoarthritis of the young adult hip: etiology and treatment. Instr Course Lect. 1986;35:119–28.
32. Ziebarth K et al. Slipped capital femoral epiphysis: relevant pathophysiological findings with open surgery. Clin Orthop Relat Res. 2013;471(7):2156–62.
33. Schai PA, Exner GU. Corrective Imhauser intertrochanteric osteotomy. Oper Orthop Traumatol. 2007;19(4):368–88.
34. Rao JP, Francis AM, Siwek CW. The treatment of chronic slipped capital femoral epiphysis by biplane osteotomy. J Bone Joint Surg Am. 1984;66(8):1169–75.
35. Maussen JP, Rozing PM, Obermann WR. Intertrochanteric corrective osteotomy in slipped capital femoral epiphysis. A long-term follow-up study of 26 patients. Clin Orthop Relat Res. 1990;259: 100–10.
36. Schai PA, Exner GU, Hansch O. Prevention of secondary coxarthrosis in slipped capital femoral epiphysis: a long-term follow-up study after corrective intertrochanteric osteotomy. J Pediatr Orthop B. 1996;5(3):135–43.
37. Kartenbender K, Cordier W, Katthagen BD. Long-term follow-up study after corrective Imhauser osteotomy for severe slipped capital femoral epiphysis. J Pediatr Orthop. 2000;20(6):749–56.
38. Diab M, Hresko MT, Millis MB. Intertrochanteric versus subcapital osteotomy in slipped capital femoral epiphysis. Clin Orthop Relat Res. 2004;427:204–12.

39. Witbreuk MM et al. The results of downgrading moderate and severe slipped capital femoral epiphysis by an early Imhauser femur osteotomy. J Child Orthop. 2009;3(5):405–10.
40. Spencer S, Millis MB, Kim YJ. Early results of treatment of hip impingement syndrome in slipped capital femoral epiphysis and pistol grip deformity of the femoral head-neck junction using the surgical dislocation technique. J Pediatr Orthop. 2006;26(3):281–5.
41. Rebello G et al. Surgical dislocation in the management of pediatric and adolescent hip deformity. Clin Orthop Relat Res. 2009;467(3): 724–31.
42. Whiteside LA, Schoenecker PL. Combined valgus derotation osteotomy and cervical osteoplasty for severely slipped capital femoral epiphysis: mechanical analysis and report preliminary results using compression screw fixation and early weight bearing. Clin Orthop Relat Res. 1978;132:88–97.
43. Ziebarth K et al. Capital realignment for moderate and severe SCFE using a modified Dunn procedure. Clin Orthop Relat Res. 2009;467(3):704–16.
44. Slongo T et al. Treatment of slipped capital femoral epiphysis with a modified Dunn procedure. J Bone Joint Surg Am. 2010;92(18): 2898–908.
45. Huber H et al. Adolescent slipped capital femoral epiphysis treated by a modified Dunn osteotomy with surgical hip dislocation. J Bone Joint Surg (Br). 2011;93(6):833–8.
46. Sankar WN et al. The modified Dunn procedure for unstable slipped capital femoral epiphysis: a multicenter perspective. J Bone Joint Surg Am. 2013;95(7):585–91.
47. Boos N et al. Total hip arthroplasty after previous proximal femoral osteotomy. J Bone Joint Surg (Br). 1997;79(2):247–53.

Combined Periacetabular Osteotomy and Proximal Femoral Osteotomy for Severe Hip Deformity

77

Stephen T. Duncan and John C. Clohisy

Introduction

Osteotomies have most commonly been performed in isolation to correct isolated deformities about the proximal femur and acetabulum including residual acetabular dysplasia or Perthes-like deformities. However, for more severe deformities, performing these osteotomies in isolation may result in insufficient femoral head coverage, persistent instability, incongruency, or suboptimal biomechanics. The combination of a proximal femoral osteotomy and periacetabular osteotomy allows for a more powerful correction of the severely deformed hip with the goal of improving the coverage, containment, and congruency of the hip while maintaining an impingement-free functional range of motion of the hip. Complex deformities requiring these procedures are challenging with regard to the surgical technique and treatment decision making. In this chapter, the indications, techniques, and outcomes following combined proximal femoral and periacetabular osteotomies are presented.

Indications and Preoperative Evaluation

There are numerous indications for performing a combined hip osteotomy in the adolescent and young adult hip. Patients should have a symptomatic hip with signs and symptoms consistent with their structural hip deformity [1]. Assessment of the end points of range of motion (flexion, internal rotation, external rotation, and abduction) can also help to determine if an adjunctive osteotomy is needed to help maintain or improve impingement-free range of motion or prevent residual instability. For these symptomatic patients, the goal following the combined PFO and PAO is to have improved hip function and decreased pain [2]. Contraindications to the combined procedure typically involve advanced osteoarthritis (Tönnis grade 2 or worse), older age (40 years or older), major incongruity, and limited and/or painful range of motion [1].

Assessing the degree of acetabular dysplasia begins with routine radiographic examination with anteroposterior (AP) pelvic and false profile radiographs. On the AP radiograph, the lateral center-edge angle (LCEA), the acetabular inclination angle (AI), and extrusion index can be calculated [3]. On the false profile view, the anterior center edge (ACEA) can be calculated [3]. Hips with an LCEA of less than 20°, an AI greater than 10°, an extrusion index greater than 20 %, and an ACEA of less than 20° have features consistent with a diagnosis of acetabular dysplasia with associated structural instability [4].

The decision to perform an adjunctive proximal femoral osteotomy and the type of osteotomy generally falls within two broad categories. First, those hips with severe acetabular dysplasia with coxa valga and/or femoral version abnormalities, and persistent instability or suboptimal congruency after appropriate correction with the PAO: In this setting, a varus and/or derotation PFO should be considered. Second, those hips with a Perthes-like hip with the characteristic large aspheric femoral head, coxa breva, variable coxa vara, leg length inequality, and trochanteric overgrowth: In these cases, a valgus PFO can be considered, often combined with trochanteric advancement [2, 5, 6]. Femoral version abnormalities in the case of increased anteversion or retroversion can be addressed at the time of the osteotomy with derotation of the femur to improve stability and prevent secondary impingement.

In the scenario of the severely dysplastic hip with significant coxa valga (neck-shaft angle greater than 140°), preoperative functional radiographs can be obtained to determine if the varus PFO is needed. Often in the case of severe dysplasia, anterolateral subluxation of the femur occurs, resulting in incongruency; however, with abduction, flexion, and internal

S.T. Duncan, MD (✉) • J.C. Clohisy, MD
Orthopaedics Department, Adult Reconstruction and Hip Preservation, Washington University School of Medicine, 660 South Euclid Avenue, Campus Box 8233, St. Louis, MO 63110, USA
e-mail: duncans@wudosis.wustl.edu; jclohisy@wustl.edu

J.C. McCarthy et al. (eds.), *Hip Joint Restoration*, DOI 10.1007/978-1-4614-0694-5_77

rotation of the femur to mimic a PAO, improved congruency between the femur and acetabulum would indicate that the varus PFO would help to improve this congruency [1]. In the case of increased femoral anteversion, functional radiographs with isolated abduction of the femur may fail to improve the congruency with residual anterolateral subluxation of the femoral head. The addition of slight flexion and internal rotation to the functional radiograph helps to correct for the increased anteversion of the femur and if the congruency is improved, then derotational at the time of the varus PFO would be required. Oftentimes, the decision to perform the varus PFO is done at the time of surgery following the PAO with the functional imaging being performed intraoperatively [2]. Typically, the goal of the varus correction is 10°–20° and the addition of flexion/extension, derotation, and femoral shortening is then made on a case-by-case basis (Fig. 77.1).

In patients with Perthes-like deformity with an aspherical femoral head, high greater trochanter and limited abduction, coxa breva, and possible shortened limb, the use of a valgus PFO can be used to optimize congruency, improve abduction, and improve leg length discrepancy [1, 2]. Functional radiographs with adduction of the limb demonstrating improved congruency support the decision for the adjunctive valgus PFO. Depending on the severity of the deformity, the addition of trochanteric advancement with relative femoral neck lengthening (RFNL) to the valgus PFO may be needed to maintain at least 20° of abduction when combined with the PAO to prevent impingement (Fig. 77.2). Most commonly,

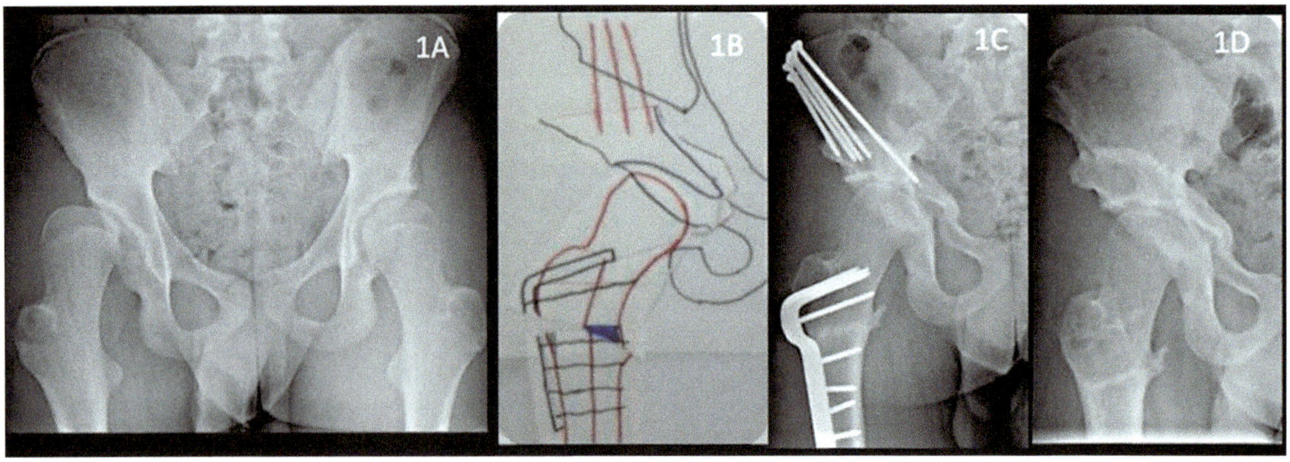

Fig. 77.1 16-year-old male with spastic hemiplegia, severe acetabular dysplasia, coxa valga, and progressive hip pain (**a**). Preoperative template demonstrating the plan for the PFO and PAO (**b**). He underwent a combined PAO, varus-shortening PFO, adductor release, psoas lengthening, femoral head-neck osteoplasty, and capsular tightening (**c**). Postoperative radiographs show improved containment and congruency. A 100° blade plate was used for fixation of the PFO. The patient had an excellent result at 1-year follow-up with a Harris hip score of 95 (**d**)

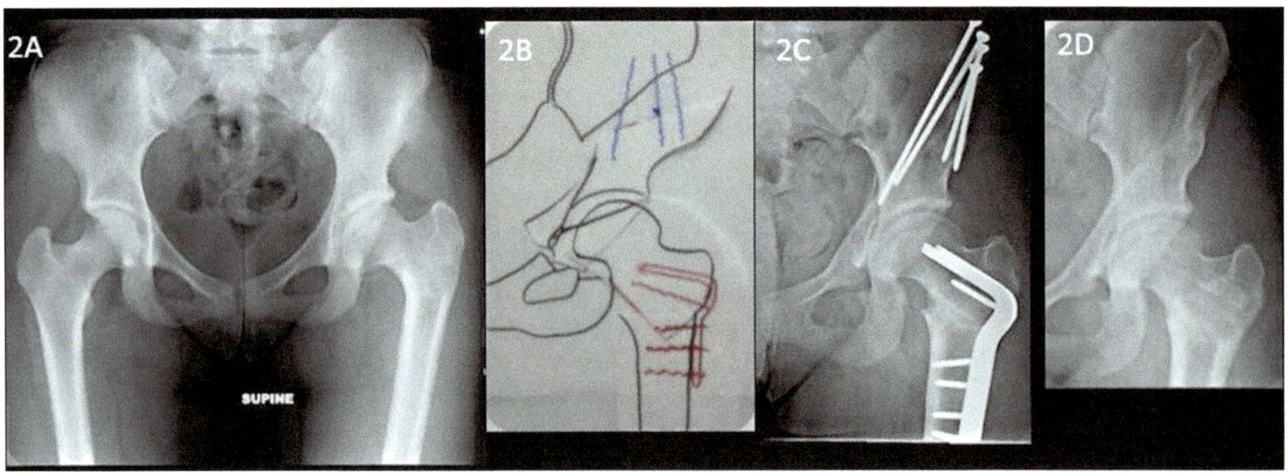

Fig. 77.2 18-year-old female with Perthes-like deformity of the left hip with secondary acetabular dysplasia and an iatrogenic varus deformity of the proximal femur (**a**). Preoperative template demonstrating the plan for the PFO and **PAO** (**b**). She underwent a combined PAO and valgus PFO (**c**) with improved coverage and congruency of the femoral head. 110° blade plate was used for fixation of the PFO. She continues to do well following hardware removal (**d**)

for Perthes-like hip deformities we prefer to address the femoral deformity first and then perform the acetabular reorientation after intraoperative assessment of joint stability, congruency, and range of motion [4].

With increasing severity of the deformity and the variable age of presentation, additional studies are needed to assess the health of the joint. To help assess the integrity of the cartilage surface of the femoral head and acetabulum, the use of magnetic resonance arthrography is used at our institution to improve the contrast resolution between the cartilage and the synovial fluid. With the use of high-resolution cartilage-sensitive images acquired in three planes (sagittal, coronal, and oblique axial) with the use of fast-spin-echo pulse sequences, identification of labral and chondral abnormalities can be identified. Depending on the location of the chondrosis, the femoral osteotomy can be planned to rotate the healthier cartilage of the femoral head into the acetabulum, or if the extent of the chondrosis is too severe, then hip-preserving surgery might be met with worse clinical outcomes and total hip arthroplasty might be indicated.

To aid in the diagnostic work-up, the use of an intra-articular diagnostic or therapeutic injection can be used as well to help assess the benefit from the complex surgery. Significant pain relief following the injection would suggest that the patient would benefit from the deformity correction with improved hip function.

Surgical Techniques and Pearls

The PAO is performed utilizing the technique previously described by Ganz and others [7, 8]. Patients are placed supine on a radiolucent table to allow for intraoperative fluoroscopy during the osteotomies and reduction. In cases where we want to assess the condition of the articular surface and/or manage intra-articular abnormalities, an initial hip arthroscopy is performed prior to the open surgery. The modified Smith-Peterson surgical approach is used [8]. Cell saver blood reinfusion is used in most cases. The periacetabular cuts, acetabular fragment reduction, and screw fixation are guided with fluoroscopy. The acetabular fragment is fixed with between three and five 4.5 mm cortical screws. The deformity correction is analyzed subjectively with anteroposterior and false profile fluoroscopic images to obtain an LCEA between 20° and 35°, AI between 0° and 15°, extrusion index between 0 and 20 %, medial offset between 0 and 15 mm, and ACEA between 18° and 38° [9]. Definitive correction is also influenced by the degree of acetabular dysplasia and the ROM of the hip following the correction with the goal of maintaining at least 90° of hip flexion. However, the use of adjunctive PFO can also help to alter the ROM of the hip. An arthrotomy is routinely performed to assess the labrum and femoral head-neck junction. Labral pathology can be addressed through the arthrotomy with debridement or labral repair with suture anchor fixation, although we prefer arthroscopic treatment of labral or articular cartilage problems. In cases with reduced femoral head-neck offset, a femoral osteochondroplasty can be performed to prevent secondary impingement [10]. Adequacy of the acetabular correction and the osteochondroplasty can be checked for residual abutment between the labrum and the femoral head-neck junction with the hip flexed and internally rotated.

The proximal femoral osteotomy is then performed using a lateral approach to the proximal femur. The classic PFO is routinely performed at the intertrochanteric level just proximal to the lesser trochanter using a no-wedge technique [11]. Preoperative templating with drawings of the osteotomies can help to predict the amount of correction, implant size, and the amount of varus or valgus needed (Figs. 77.1, 77.2, and 77.3). With valgus-producing osteotomies, excessive lengthening of the limb can be avoided with shortening through the osteotomy site and the amount of resection required can be determined based on the preoperative template [2]. In cases with significant coxa valga, performing the PFO prior to the PAO can help to facilitate the optimal acetabular correction. For varus PFO with greater than 20° of correction, the addition of a trochanteric advancement can be considered to maintain the abductor lever arm and optimize abductor function. Fixation of the osteotomy is performed with the use of an angled blade plate or proximal locking femoral osteotomy plate. The angle, offset, and type of plate used can be determined based on the preoperative template to achieve the desired deformity correction. When performing the osteotomy and deformity correction, care is taken to maintain proximal femoral alignment with the medullary canal of the distal fragment at least aligned with the piriformis fossa of the proximal fragment to prevent a zigzag deformity that might compromise future arthroplasty (Figs. 77.1, 77.2, and 77.3) [12, 13].

More recently, intracapsular osteotomies have been developed such as the femoral neck osteotomy (FNO) or relative femoral neck lengthening (RFNL) to achieve the deformity correction [14]. The intracapsular osteotomy requires the development of the extended retinacular flap to provide reliable protection of the blood supply to the femoral head throughout the procedure [14]. To develop this flap, trochanteric osteotomy is required to develop a subperiosteal flap that includes the short external rotators and lateral retinacular vessels [14]. With the RFNL, the piecemeal resection of the stable trochanter and advancement of the mobile trochanter to the femoral head center help to correct the shortened neck and high trochanter in Perthes-like deformity. Despite the powerful correction with these new techniques, they are technically very demanding and must be performed such that the blood flow to the femoral head is not compromised.

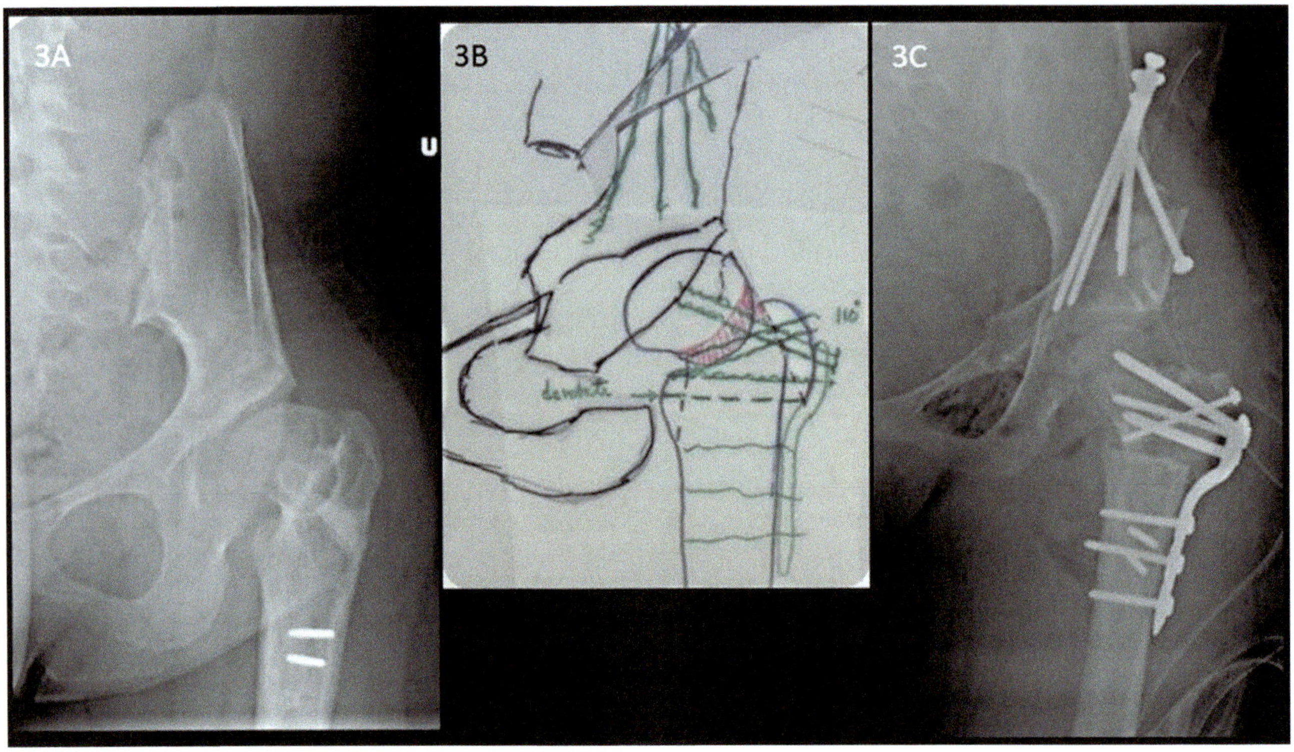

Fig. 77.3 16-year-old female with a history of hip dysplasia treated with a previous pelvic and proximal femoral osteotomy at an outside hospital. She has iatrogenic valgus deformity of the proximal femur with excessive femoral anteversion and acetabular dysplasia (**a**). Preoperative template demonstrating the plan for the PFO and PAO (**b**). She underwent a combined PAO, varus-derotation PFO, surgical dislocation, femoral head-neck osteoplasty, trochanteric advancement, relative femoral neck lengthening, and acetabular microfracture (**c**). 110° proximal locking osteotomy plate was used for fixation of the PFO

Outcomes

A review of the literature and of the results of combined PAO and PFO is limited to a few reports [2, 15, 16]. Several of these reports examined subpopulations of patients and do not report exclusively on the clinical outcomes following the combined procedure. Clohisy et al. compared 25 patients treated with the combined PAO/PFO compared to PAO alone with a mean follow-up of 3.7 years [2]. The PAO/PFO group demonstrated consistent radiographic deformity correction and the improvement in Harris hip scores between the two groups was similar. There was not a difference in the incidence of postoperative complications between the two groups as well.

Conclusions

Performing the combined periacetabular osteotomy and proximal femoral osteotomy is indicated for complex deformities involving the hip. In our experience, this combined procedure has been met with good and improved hip function with decreased pain. With proper preoperative assessment and intraoperative evaluation of the hip, the combined procedure can be performed under one anesthesia. When performed properly, the adjunctive PFO does not seem to compromise the results of the PAO and can improve both the stability and congruency of the hip while helping to avoid secondary impingement as well. With more advanced intracapsular osteotomies of the proximal femur, more long-term studies are needed to compare the results to the classic intertrochanteric osteotomy.

References

1. Ganz R, Horowitz K, Leunig M. Algorithm for femoral and periacetabular osteotomies in complex hip deformities. Clin Orthop Relat Res. 2010;468(12):3168–80. Pubmed Central PMCID: 2974895.
2. Clohisy JC, St John LC, Nunley RM, Schutz AL, Schoenecker PL. Combined periacetabular and femoral osteotomies for severe hip deformities. Clin Orthop Relat Res. 2009;467(9):2221–7. Pubmed Central PMCID: 2866920.
3. Clohisy JC, Carlisle JC, Beaule PE, Kim YJ, Trousdale RT, Sierra RJ, et al. A systematic approach to the plain radiographic evaluation of the young adult hip. J Bone Joint Surg Am. 2008;90 Suppl 4:47–66. Pubmed Central PMCID: 2682767.

4. Clohisy JC, Ross JR, North JD, Nepple JJ, Schoenecker PL. What are the factors associated with acetabular correction in Perthes-like hip deformities? Clin Orthop Relat Res. 2012;470(12):3439–45. Pubmed Central PMCID: 3492615.
5. Beck M, Mast JW. The periacetabular osteotomy in Legg-Perthes-like deformities. Semin Arthroplasty. 1997;8:102–7.
6. Clohisy JC, Nunley RM, Curry MC, Schoenecker PL. Periacetabular osteotomy for the treatment of acetabular dysplasia associated with major aspherical femoral head deformities. J Bone Joint Surg Am. 2007;89(7):1417–23.
7. Clohisy JC, Barrett SE, Gordon JE, Delgado ED, Schoenecker PL. Periacetabular osteotomy in the treatment of severe acetabular dysplasia. Surgical technique. J Bone Joint Surg Am. 2006;88 (Suppl 1 Pt 1):65–83.
8. Leunig M, Ganz R. The Bernese method of periacetabular osteotomy. Der Orthopade. 1998;27(11):743–50 (Berner periazetabulare Osteotomie).
9. Lehmann CL, Nepple JJ, Baca G, Schoenecker PL, Clohisy JC. Do fluoroscopy and postoperative radiographs correlate for periacetabular osteotomy corrections? Clin Orthop Relat Res. 2012;470(12):3508–14. Pubmed Central PMCID: 3492629.
10. Nassif NA, Schoenecker PL, Thorsness R, Clohisy JC. Periacetabular osteotomy and combined femoral head-neck junction osteochondroplasty: a minimum two-year follow-up cohort study. J Bone Joint Surg Am. 2012;94(21):1959–66.
11. Ganz R, MacDonald S. Indications and modern techniques of proximal femoral osteotomies in the adult. Semin Arthroplasty. 1997;8:38–50.
12. Clohisy J, Schoenecker P. Proximal femoral osteotomy. In: Callaghan J, Rosenberg A, Rubash H, editors. The adult hip. 2nd ed. Philadelphia: Lippincott Williams & Wilkins; 2004.
13. Schoenecker P, Rich M, Nunley RM. Proximal femoral osteotomy in skeletally immature patient with deformity. In: Sekiya J, Ranawat AS, Safran MR, Leunig M, editors. Techniques in hip arthroscopy and joint preservation. Philadelphia: Elsevier; 2011.
14. Ganz R, Huff TW, Leunig M. Extended retinacular soft-tissue flap for intra-articular hip surgery: surgical technique, indications, and results of application. Instr Course Lect. 2009;58: 241–55.
15. Trousdale RT, Ekkernkamp A, Ganz R, Wallrichs SL. Periacetabular and intertrochanteric osteotomy for the treatment of osteoarthrosis in dysplastic hips. J Bone Joint Surg Am. 1995;77(1): 73–85.
16. Hersche O, Casillas M, Ganz R. Indications for intertrochanteric osteotomy after periacetabular osteotomy for adult hip dysplasia. Clin Orthop Relat Res. 1998;347:19–26.

Part XI

Joint Replacement

Philip C. Noble

78 Partial Joint Replacement

Lourenço P. Peixoto, Peter Goljan, and Marc J. Philippon

Prosthetic Replacement of Partial Defects of the Femoral Head: History and Clinical Results

The idea to utilize a prosthesis to replace part of the femoral head is not new. The concept of a surgical procedure with lower morbidity than total hip arthroplasty which preserves femoral bone stock was proposed by Siguier et al. [1] in 1999 for the treatment of osteonecrosis of the femoral head without acetabular involvement (Ficat stage III). In this study, the authors reported the results of 19 patients in whom 25 partial resurfacings of the femoral head were performed over a 5-year period. The operation was performed via an anterior (Hueter) approach to the hip and there was a revision rate of 24 % during the observed time period. In 2001, Siguier then published his 7-year follow-up results, now for 37 cemented partial femoral resurfacing prostheses placed in 33 patients between April 1991 and June 1997. The mean age was 43 years old (range, 24–59 years), and the pre-op Ficat classifications ranged from stage 2 in one hip and stage 3 in 26 hips to stage 4 in 10 hips. In this study, MRI exams were not utilized in the preoperative setting to assess the extent of the disease. For the surviving prostheses, the mean follow-up was 49 months (range, 24–89 months), and 24 % (9/37) were considered failures secondary to extension of osteonecrosis [2].

Similar results following treatment of avascular necrosis of the femoral head with surface replacement have been reported by Squire et al. [3], who had an overall failure rate of 65 % at a 33-month follow-up; Beaule et al. [4], who reported 45 % survival at a 15-year follow-up; and Cuckler et al. [5], who reported a 40 % clinical failure rate at a 3-year follow-up. Amstutz et al. [6] reported that the long-term survivorship of hemisurface replacement patients with stage 3 and 4 osteonecrosis using THARIES femoral resurfacing components was 56 % at 10 years postoperatively. Analysis of these findings, in combination with other series with similarly poor outcomes [5, 7], showed the importance of adequate perimplant bone quality in dictating the success of partial hemi-resurfacing, especially for cases involving cementless implant fixation.

Total Hip Replacement

In contrast to other joints, young and active patients have limited surgical options for treatment of focal osteochondral defects in the hip. Despite nearly 100 % patient satisfaction early after total hip replacement, there are concerns about the morbidity associated with this surgery as well as the long-term joint survivorship, especially in younger patients. Using the Medicare database, Ong et al. [8] found that there was a 96 % 5-year survival rate for a primary THR, and an 81 % survival rate for a revision THR. The study also reported that patients who required a revision total hip arthroplasty were fivefold more likely to require further revisions when compared to patients who underwent a primary hip arthroplasty. As an invasive surgery, THR also requires a longer postoperative hospitalization, and it is not without complications. Soo Hoo et al. [9] reviewed the discharge data from 138,399 patients who underwent primary THR in California from 1995 to 2005. They reported that complications were experienced by 3.8 % of patients during the first 90 days after surgery, with dislocation being the most common complication (1.4 %). In a review of 182,146 consecutive patients who

L.P. Peixoto, MD • P. Goljan, MD
Center for Outcomes-Based Orthopaedic Research, The Steadman Philippon Research Institute, Vail, CO, USA

M.J. Philippon, MD (✉)
The Steadman Clinic, Vail, CO, USA

Department of Surgery, McMaster University, Hamilton, Ontario, Canada

Department of Orthopaedic Surgery, Unviersity of Pittsburgh School of Medicine, Pittsburgh, PA, USA
e-mail: drphilippon@sprivail.org

J.C. McCarthy et al. (eds.), *Hip Joint Restoration*, DOI 10.1007/978-1-4614-0694-5_78

underwent primary total hip and knee replacement, Bozic et al. [10] found that the mean length of stay was 3.9 days, the 30-day mortality was 0.1 %, and the readmission rate was 4 %. The incidences of surgical complications and reoperation were both 3 %.

When considering these results and the relative youth of many patients who present with isolated chondral lesions of the femoral head, we believe that it is necessary to first treat these defects with procedures more conservative than THR.

Cartilage Repair Therapies

It is well known that cartilage tissue is both aneural and avascular, with a low turnover capacity and limited repair potential. Chondrocytes show a limited migratory ability within the surrounding collagen matrix, which hinders the ability for the normal cells bordering a lesion to fill the gap. When the injury extends to involve the subchondral bone, multipotential mesenchymal stem cells are released from the bone marrow, which then fill the defect and eventually lead to the production of fibrocartilage. Fibrocartilage, however, has inferior biomechanical properties than the original articular cartilage and provides less protection to the underlying subchondral bone, which can lead to increased pain and continued disability, especially in physically active patients.

Many surgical techniques have already been established for the treatment of symptomatic chondral lesions, including debridement, drilling and fixation, abrasion chondroplasty, microfracture, and the use of carbon fiber pads, all of which aim to induce fibrocartilaginous repair tissue. Other methods, including cartilage autografting and osteochondral allografts, aim for repair with hyaline cartilage. In 1971, Bentley and Greer [11] first showed that isolated chondrocytes could be transplanted onto the tibial surface of rabbits with normal joints or with experimental arthritis. Then in 1994, Brittiberg et al. [12] described the use of autologous cultured chondrocytes for the treatment of full-thickness chondral defects of the knee. In that study, transplantation took place 14–21 days after the initial harvesting surgery and the cells obtained were cultured in suitable media in order to produce 2.6–5 million cells. At implantation, the cells were injected into the prepared defect and then sealed in place by suturing a periosteal flap created from the proximo-medial tibia. A medial or lateral arthrotomy was required to access the defect, depending on the location. Modifications to the procedure have occurred, in which the cells are cultured in the same manner, but are then seeded directly onto a type I/III collagen scaffold which acts as a carrier to ensure a more even distribution over the defect.

Both autograft and allograft tissue has been used to fill defects within articular cartilage, original within the knee, but now also within the hip. Most reports on autografts have involved an open approach and plugs harvested from numerous locations. In a study of two patients who sustained traumatic posterior hip dislocations, autograft transplantation was used to treat osteochondral defects of the femoral head [13]. Both underwent surgical hip dislocation and osteochondral autograft transplantation. The donor sites used were the ipsilateral knee in one case and the inferior non-weight-bearing portion of the femoral head in the other. Limited follow-up was available on the patients but excellent subjective and objective outcomes were reported [13]. Another case report also showed excellent subjective outcomes at 6-month follow-up [14]. We reported a case of a 15-year-old with a femoral head defect that was addressed using osteochondral autografts [15]. The plug was harvested from the femoral head-neck junction and platelet-rich plasma (PRP) was administered to the graft. The patient reported good outcomes 2 years following the surgery. With these reports of success, the use of osteochondral autografts may become a treatment choice in the hips with large femoral head chondral defects. Long-term follow-up data from multiple cases is warranted for definitive conclusions.

The molecular mechanism of chondral repair has also been extensively studied to potentially act as a guide for future clinical applications. Osteogenic protein-1 [OP-1], also known as bone morphogenetic protein-7 (BMP-7), in combination with insulin-like growth factor-1 (IGF-1), appears to be the most promising growth factor combination for osteoarthritis treatment because of their ability to synergistically act towards an anabolic effect, as well as because their anti-catabolic properties do not diminish with age. However, despite these early findings, they are not yet available for routine clinical use [16]. Biologic treatments such as autologous conditioned serum, PRP, and bone marrow concentrate have more frequently been used because they are derived from the patient directly, and can be readministered easily back to the patient. Although as of yet there is no universally accepted protocol for PRP preparation and administration, multiple studies have shown its clinical efficacy in the treatment of bony and soft-tissue pathology [17]. By using cell surface markers or clonal expansion, progenitor stem cells have been identified in both normal and osteoarthritic human articular cartilage, and early studies analyzing their use have suggested that they may be a superior cell source to mesenchymal stem cells [18, 19]. However, additional studies are required to demonstrate how this information is best translated to clinical practice.

Despite the increased knowledge regarding the biological aspects of chondral repair, and the advent of superior techniques and more durable bearing surfaces for total hip replacement, we believe that there is still no ideal treatment for patients with isolated full-thickness chondral lesions of the femoral head. The concept of a partial femoral head resurfacing which could address many different lesion sizes, and yet still be implanted arthroscopically, would be attractive to both the surgeon and the patient, because it pairs a bone-preserving procedure with the low morbidity of arthroscopic surgery. Described below are our preoperative considerations regarding this procedure.

Preoperative Considerations

Patients suffering from femoral head chondral pathology frequently present with groin pain which is exacerbated by weight-bearing activities, pivoting, or hyperflexion of the hip. Physical examination demonstrates a limited range of motion depending on chronicity of symptoms and extent of disease, although internal rotation is often affected first. Indications for this procedure include large (>4 cm^2) isolated symptomatic full-thickness chondral lesions of the femoral head. These lesions are commonly associated with femoroacetabular impingement (FAI) but also arise secondary to trauma. A secondary indication for this procedure is failure of more conservative treatment methods such as arthroscopic microfracture.

Imaging

Radiographs and magnetic resonance imaging (MRI) are necessary in order to adequately evaluate any intra-articular pathology of the hip. The radiographic series we employ includes supine anteroposterior (AP) pelvic and lateral cross-table radiographs [20]. Radiographs are used to assess for any acetabular retroversion, dysplasia, degenerative changes, or possible femoroacetabular impingement. Radiographic measurements should include the acetabulum version, center-edge angle of Wiberg, joint space distance of the weight-bearing axis, and alpha angle [20]. Magnetic resonance imaging can be used to further characterize the AVN as well as identify any other soft-tissue pathology.

Arthroscopic Partial Femoral Head Replacement Technique

Special Instrumentation

The arthroscopic aspects of the procedure require the use of a large C-arm (fluoroscope) as well as a traction table. Furthermore, hip arthroscopy requires specialized arthroscopic instrumentation, which includes cannulas and longer tools for manipulating bone and cartilage. The implants usually consist of an articulating surface and are supplied in various sizes.

Positioning

The patient is positioned in a modified supine position. General anesthesia is used in combination with a lumbar plexus sciatic regional block with complete muscular paralysis. The perineum is positioned against an extra-wide, padded bolster with care taken to protect the genitalia. Fluoroscopy is used to obtain an AP view of the operative hip, so that when gentle traction is applied to it along with moderate counter-traction to the non-operative side, the "vacuum sign" in the joint space [21] can be visualized directly.

Surgical Anatomy

The greater trochanter and anterior superior iliac spine (ASIS) can be palpated in most patients depending on general body habitus. Structures at risk during surgery include the major femoral neurovascular bundle, which is comprised of the femoral nerve, artery, and vein, and leaves the pelvis just medial to a vertical line originating from the ASIS. The sciatic nerve is particularly at risk during placement of the posterior portal, and even more so when the leg is internally rotated, which acts to pull the nerve closer to the capsule. Lastly, the lateral femoral cutaneous nerve can be injured by either the anterior or the anterolateral portal, potentially resulting in a painful neuroma.

Technical Steps

The operative leg is adducted to neutral and the foot is internally rotated to bring the femoral neck parallel to the floor. Joint distraction via mechanical traction (usually 25–50 lb total) is assessed by fluoroscopy in order to achieve approximately 10 mm of total separation. Once the final traction is established, the operative table is tilted 10° toward the non-operative side [21].

Two portals are then established. An anterolateral portal is created approximately 1 cm proximal and 1 cm anterior to the greater trochanter using a 6-in., 18-gauge arthroscopy needle. Once it has been confirmed fluoroscopically that the needle is within the hip joint, a guide wire is threaded through it and a 4.5 mm cannula can then be inserted. Next, the 70° arthroscope is introduced into the joint space which is pressurized to 105 mmHg of pressure, allowing visualization of the femoral head and acetabulum. Additional traction can be added as necessary to improve instrument mobility and joint space visualization. The arthroscope is then used to place the anterior portal under direct visualization. The camera should be positioned so that the intra-articular triangle may be viewed, which is composed of the anterior femoral head, labrum, and joint capsule. Externally, the anterior portal should be placed directly distal to the ASIS as well as medial to the anterolateral portal. Using the arthroscope, an arthroscopy needle should be visualized entering the intra-articular triangle, followed by a guide wire and ultimately a 4.5 mm cannula. Care should be taken to place the cannula through the synovial lining of the joint, and not the capsule itself. The arthroscope can then be placed into the anterior portal for repositioning as necessary to attain adequate joint visualization and instrument clearance. In order to achieve optimal access to a majority of weight-bearing femoral head lesions, the hip is then positioned in extension, adduction, and external rotation [21].

After performing intra-articular chondrolabral work, the anterior portal is then extended proximally by approximately 2–3 cm via blunt dissection along the sartorius-tensor fascia lata interval and finally deep to the rectus femoris muscle. The anterior capsule of the hip is then incised along the fibers of the iliofemoral ligament, and under mild distraction, the portion of the femoral head containing the chondral lesion can then be identified. A mini-incision is made to allow passage of the partial resurfacing implant and the size of the defect is measured with a template. A guide pin may then be inserted inside the lesion. A 10.5 screw is then placed in the defect (Fig. 78.1), which allows for measurement of the offset, so that the appropriate-size pin may be selected (Fig. 78.2). Once chosen, the bed is reamed to the proper size and depth and prepared for implantation of the resurfacing prosthesis (Fig. 78.3). Following testing with a trial component, the resurfacing implant is placed and coverage is assessed (Fig. 78.4). Once resurfacing implantation is completed, the hip is removed from traction and the arthroscope is reinserted into the peripheral compartment for inspection of the joint. At this time, additional distraction is placed

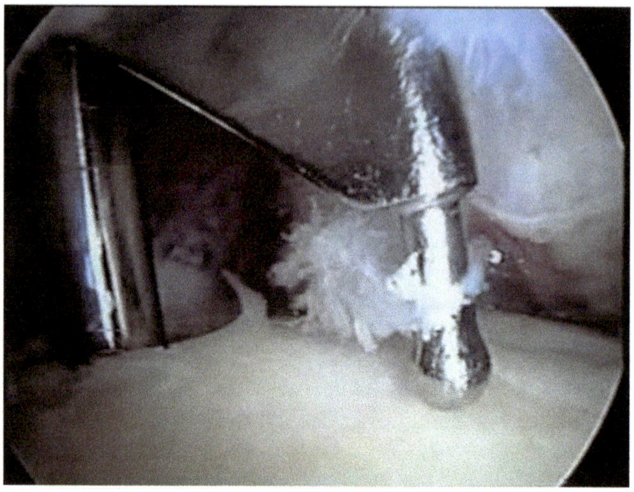

Fig. 78.2 Template tool determining the size of the defect to be treated

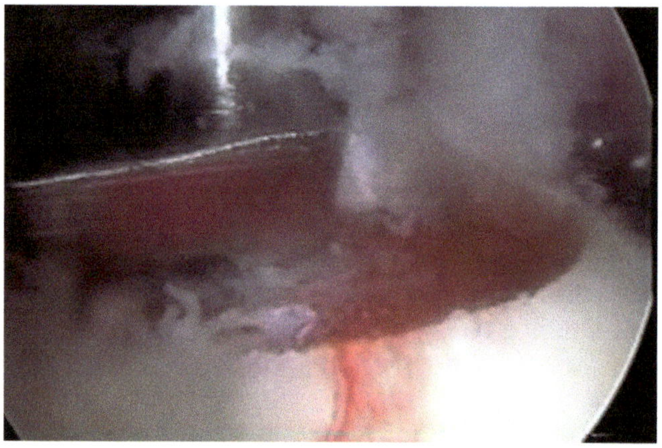

Fig. 78.3 Reaming of the defect for placement of the prosthetic

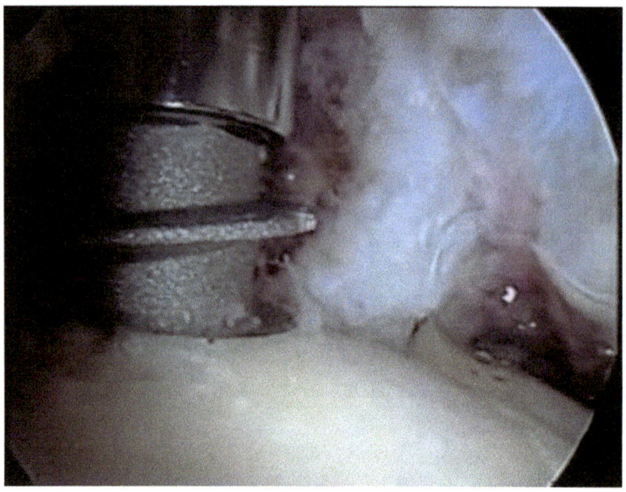

Fig. 78.1 Placement of the screw in the center of the defect for sizing and fixation of the partial resurfacing implant

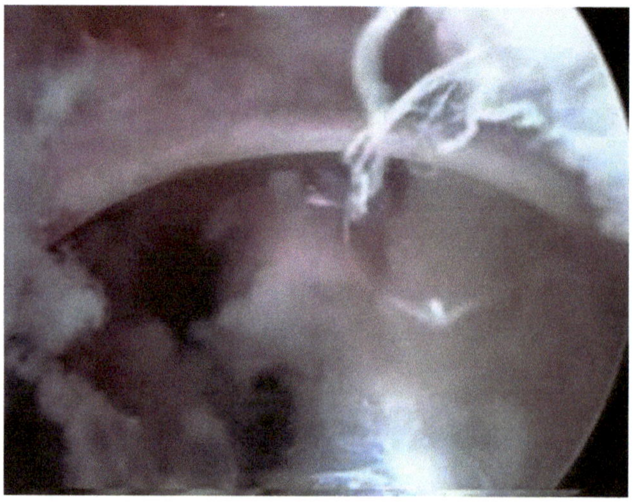

Fig. 78.4 Partial surface implant in place over post

across the hip so that further contouring of the chondral surfaces may be performed as needed. Additionally, a microfracture procedure can be performed to treat isolated chondral lesions of the femoral head that have an adequate depth of surrounding cartilage. Any residual impingement is corrected by acetabular rim trimming, as well as osteoplasty of the anterior femoral head and neck offset. The hip is taken through full range of motion under direct arthroscopic visualization to ensure excellent congruency of the resurfacing component to the articular surface as well as to rule out any impingement. Fluoroscopy is used to take AP, oblique, and lateral views of the hip for radiographic assessment of proper resurfacing component placement.

Postoperative Issues

Rehabilitation Protocol

Postoperatively, the patient is maintained on partial weight bearing as well as a continuous passive motion (CPM) machine for 8 weeks. Patients also require an antirotation bolster and a modified Bledsoe brace for the first 10 days postoperatively, and foot pumps and compression stockings should be worn for 4 weeks.

Early physical therapy is focused on reestablishing range of motion, as abduction, flexion, and extension are blocked initially by the brace. The next phase of rehabilitation then focuses on improving muscle endurance, while the final phase concentrates on regaining muscle power and strength to allow the patient to fully return to their prior level of hip function and physical activity.

Complications

Complications associated with the procedure consist of loosening of the implant, incidental acetabular cartilage damage, fracture, or infection. As this is an arthroscopic operation utilizing a mini-incision, many of the complications associated with open surgery and hip dislocation can be avoided.

Conclusion

The treatment of isolated femoral head chondral lesions is still a challenge to surgeons today. Total hip replacements have demonstrated good results, but we do not believe that it is an ideal solution, especially for young patients, as they will most likely require at least one revision surgery during their lifetime. Current chondral repair therapies for advanced lesions do not show reliable results at this time and more studies are needed directly pertaining to chondral lesions of the hip. Arthroscopic partial femoral head resurfacing has the benefit of the low morbidity associated with arthroscopic surgery along with the results seen from a joint replacement surgery, and we believe that it is indicated for this group of young and high-demand patients.

Potential conflict of interest Smith & Nephew[a,b], Arthrosurface[a], HIPCO[a], MIS[a], Bledsoe[a], DonJoy[a], Slack[a], Ossur[b], Arthrex[b], Siemens[b].

[a]Consulting/Royalty payments, [b] Research or other financial support

References

1. Siguier M, Judet T, Siguier T, Charnley G, Brumpt B, Yugue I. Preliminary results of partial surface replacement of the femoral head in osteonecrosis. J Arthroplasty. 1999;14(1):45–51.
2. Siguier T, Siguier M, Judet T, Charnley G, Brumpt B. Partial resurfacing arthroplasty of the femoral head in avascular necrosis. Methods, indications, and results. Clin Orthop Relat Res. 2001;386: 85–92.
3. Squire M, Fehring TK, Odum S, Griffin WL, Mason JB. Failure of femoral surface replacement for femoral head avascular necrosis. Arthroplasty. 2005;20(7 Suppl3):108–14.
4. Beaule PE, Schmalzried TP, Campbell P, et al. Duration of symptoms and outcome of hemiresurfacing for hip osteonecrosis. Clin Orthop Relat Res. 2001;385:104–17.
5. Cuckler JM, Moore KD, Estrada L. Outcome of hemiresurfacing in osteonecrosis of the femoral head. Clin Orthop Relat Res. 2004;429:146–50.
6. Amstutz HC, Schmalzried TP, Fowble P, Noordin S. 14 year experience with hemi-surface replacement for Ficat 3 and early 4 osteonecrosis. In: Presented at the American Academy of Orthopaedic Surgeons. San Francisco. 1997.
7. Beaule PE, Amstutz HC, Le Duff M, Dorey F. Surface arthroplasty for osteonecrosis of the hip: hemi-resurfacing versus metal-on-metal hybrid resurfacing. J Arthroplasty. 2004;19:54–8.
8. Ong KL, Lau E, Suggs J, Kurtz SM, Manley MT. Risk of subsequent revision after primary and revision total joint arthroplasty. Clin Orthop Relat Res. 2010;468:3070–6.
9. SooHoo NF, Farng E, Lieberman JR, Chambers L, Zingmond DS. Factors that predict short-term complication rates after total hip arthroplasty. Clin Orthop Relat Res. 2010;468:2363–71.
10. Bozic KJ, Maselli J, Pekow PS, Lindenauer PK, Vail TP, Auerbach AD. The influence of procedure volumes and standardization of care on quality and efficiency in total joint replacement surgery. J Bone Joint Surg Am. 2010;92:2643–52.
11. Bentley G, Greer RB. Homotransplantation of isolated epiphyseal and articular cartilage chondrocytes into joint surfaces of rabbits. Nature. 1971;230:385–8.
12. Brittberg M, Lindahl A, Nilsson A, et al. Treatment of deep cartilage defects in the knee with autologous chondrocyte transplantation. N Engl J Med. 1994;331:889–95.
13. Nam D, Shindle MK, Buly RL, Kelly BT, Lorich DG. Traumatic osteochondral injury of the femoral head treated by mosaicplasty. HSS J. 2010;6:228–34.

14. Hart R, Janecek M, Visna P, Bucek P, Kocis J. Mosaicplasty for the treatment of femoral head defect after incorrect resorbable screw insertion. Arthroscopy. 2003;19:E1–5.
15. Philippon MJ, Jarvis HC. Arthroscopic management of a femoral head osteochondral defect using autologous osteochondral transfer, platelet-rich plasma and microfracture. Curr Orthop Prac. 2012;23:629–33.
16. Gulotta LV, Wiznia D, Cunningham M, Fortier L, Maher S, Rodeo SA. Specialty update:What's new in orthopaedic research. J Bone Joint Surg Am. 2011;93-A(22):2136–41.
17. Foster TE, Puskas BL, Mandelbaum BR, Gerhardt MB, Rodeo SA. Platelet-rich plasma: from basic science to clinical applications. Am J Sports Med. 2009;37:2259–72.
18. Williams R, Khan IM, Richardson K, Nelson L, Mc Carthy HE, Analbelsi T. Identification and clonal characterization of a progenitor cell sub-population in normal human articular cartilage. PLoS One. 2010;5, e13246.
19. Pretzel D, Linss S, Rochler S, Endres M, Kaps C, Alsalameh S. Relative percentage and zonal distribution of mesenchymal progenitor cells in human osteoarthritic and normal cartilage. Arthritis Res Ther. 2011;13:R64.
20. Philippon MJ, Maxwell RB, Johnston TL, Schenker ML, Briggs KK. Clinical presentation of femoroacetabular impingement. Knee Surg Sports Traumatol Arthrosc. 2007;15(8):1041–7.
21. Philippon MJ, Stubbs AJ, Schenker ML, Maxwell RB, Ganz R, Leunig M. Arthroscopic management of fermoroacetabular impingement: osteoplasty technique and literature review. Am J Sports Med. 2007;35(9):1571–80.

79 Metal on Metal Hip Resurfacing: Current Indications and Results

Vikram Chatrath and Paul E. Beaulé

Introduction

Hip resurfacing is a viable option in young patients suffering from an arthritic hip joint that is not amenable to joint preservation procedures [1]. It offers an advantage over traditional hip replacement in terms of bone stock preservation. If the need arises, this preserves the option of performing a total hip replacement with sufficient bone stock in the proximal femur [2]. The large diameter bearing surfaces articulate with low wear and extreme stability and minimal risk of dislocation [3]. Recently, concerns have also been raised about the occurrence of pseudotumors which are adverse tissue reactions to metal debris leading to significant soft tissue destruction [4]. Although these lesions are relatively uncommon, they are often associated with malpositioned components (high abduction angle) [5] and/or poorly designed acetabular components [6]. Both excessive abduction and/or low arc of cover of the acetabular component predispose the bearing to edge loading and excessive wear with increased risk of soft tissue destruction [6]. The current designs of hip resurfacing implants offer the option of using either a cemented or an uncemented femoral component mated with an uncemented acetabular component. The bearing surfaces are made of a cobalt-chrome alloy where a high carbon content is required for optimal wear properties [7].

In this chapter we will review current design parameters of hip resurfacing implants as well as surgical indications and techniques to optimize clinical outcome.

V. Chatrath, MS, MCh
Chief of Staff, Avera Marshall Regional Medical Centre,
300 S. Bruce St., Marshal, Minnesota 56258, USA

P.E. Beaulé, MD, FRCSC (✉)
Orthopaedic Surgery Division, Surgery Department,
The Ottawa Hospital, University of Ottawa, 501 Smyth Road,
Room W1646, Ottawa, ON, Canada, K1H 8L6
e-mail: pbeaule@ottawahospital.on.ca

Tribology and Machining Process of Hip Resurfacing Implants

Wear rates in metal on metal bearing are influenced by a number of factors, of which the most important is the design clearance of the head within the cup (defined as the diameter of cup minus the diameter of the head). The optimal diametral clearance to maintain a fluid film lubrication in hip simulator testing is around 100–200 μm [7]. This ensures that the contact between the bearing surfaces remains polar, meaning that the femoral head and inner acetabular component surface make contact at the dome, thus providing high conformity between the bearing surfaces as well as avoiding seizing.

The clearance and the conformity are closely related to fluid film formation between the bearing surfaces. The fluid film becomes thicker with polar contact and with increased clearance thus decreasing wear. The surface roughness is inversely related to fluid film lubrication with optimum roughness being 0.01 μm. Another important factor is sphericity (ideally <7 μm), as high points cause localized stresses that increase friction. The lambda ratio (the ratio of the thickness of the fluid film to the composite root mean-square surface roughness) is a means to relate surface roughness and thickness of fluid film with a ratio greater than three favoring a full fluid film lubrication [8]. Finally, wear decreases when the radius of the femoral head is as large as possible and the radial clearance is as small as possible and termed the effective radius. The effective radius can be controlled by the device manufacturer [7].

Metal on metal bearing surfaces are made of cobalt-chromium-molybdenum alloys which in turn are manufactured by forging (i.e., "wrought"), or casting. No difference has been observed between the two manufacturing processes; however, the level of carbon has been found to influence wear rates [8]. In a hip simulator study [9] to look at wear particles, more CoCrMo particles were found with the low-carbon wrought alloy than with the high-carbon wrought and cast alloys.

J.C. McCarthy et al. (eds.), *Hip Joint Restoration*, DOI 10.1007/978-1-4614-0694-5_79

More recently, the wear of metal on metal bearings has been shown to be influenced by Tribochemical reactions [10]. These reactions generate tribomaterial [11], by mechanical mixing of the surface layer of the metal with synovial fluid proteins. Tribomaterial has a nanocrystalline structure with a grain size between 30 and 70 nm [12, 13]. Initial studies have suggested a beneficial effect of the tribomaterial on wear. This tribolayer seem to be worn off under high-stress conditions and is also speculated that the implantation of the acetabular component in excessive anteversion and/or abduction may destabilize the layer and lead to excessive wear. Pourzal et al. [14] have demonstrated that the tribolayer is absent in the stripe wear region of metal-on-metal joints. Further understanding of the tribology may lead to improved metallurgy and implant designs less susceptible to wear [11].

Metal on metal wear generates very small particles (0.03–0.12 μm) [8–10]. The majority of particles are those of chromium oxide [15]. No significant differences in particle characteristics have been detected between hip resurfacing and stem-type devices. Particle characteristics (mainly the amount of CoCrMo particles) are influenced by implantation time appeared but implant design has not been shown to have a significant influence on them [16]. The average particle lengths (49–57 nm) has not been found to be different between the different designs and implantation times except for the current design implants retrieved within 15 months, which have a significantly smaller average length of 39 nm.

The particles generated by metal on metal bearing surfaces far exceed in number the particles generated by polyethylene wear and dissolve to generate cobalt and chromium ions. These ions are detectable even normally in urine and blood, but in abnormally high wear the number of ions increase (>7 ppb). The biologic response to the metal debris has been a nonspecific inflammatory response not dissimilar to that described with metal-on- polyethylene implants, but of a lower scale [17, 18]. However a lymphocytic infiltaltration, suggestive of a hypersentivity reaction, has also been found. This has been termed as aseptic lymphocyte-dominated vasculitis- associated lesion (ALVAL) or as a lymphocyte-dominated immunological answer (LYDIA) [19–21]. Early adverse tissue reactions, including pseudotumors (described as soft- tissue masses or fluid-filled bursae) that can lead to devastating short-term implant failures have been recently reported [22, 23]. It is hard to pinpoint but probably the origin of these early adverse reactions is a combination of excessive wear and metal hypersensitivity [24].

Recent literature has focused on femoral component size as an independent risk factor with McBryde [25] showing that for every 4-mm decrease in size the hazard ratio for failure was 4.87. Interestingly, when looking at the actual femoral component size, sizes greater than 46 mm were associated with a better survivorship. The influence of femoral component size on hip resurfacing survivorship is multi-factorial where on the femoral side it will be related to overall fixation area as well as risk of thermal necrosis where overall cement volume with the smaller femoral bone may surpass the cell injury threshold [26, 27]. Finally, with most hip resurfacing designs the smaller the femoral component the smaller the arc of cover on the acetabular side negatively affecting the wear properties of the metal on metal bearing [28]. It is still unclear at this time if survivorship of smaller femoral components for hip resurfacing can be improved upon consequently caution should be used when considering hip resurfacing for those patients and probably contra-indicated for women with relatively smaller femoral components.

Indications and Contraindications

The most common indication for hip resurfacing is advanced osteoarthritis in a young active patient. These patients tend to have a higher activity level and are likely to benefit from preserved femoral bone stock. A common consensus is to offer hip resurfacing in males less than 60 and females less than 50. Although chronological age is not the only consideration, in older patients a replacement would be preferable. Other important factors to consider are patient's level of activity, general medical condition and bone quality. In regards to the female gender, a relatively smaller number of them will be suitable candidates for hip resurfacing due their smaller and dysplastic bony anatomy. Data from the England and Wales Joint Registry [28] and the Australian Joint Registry [29] found gender and head size to influence survival of the hip resurfacing implant. The revision rate of arthroplasties was three times greater if the head size of the femoral component was <44 mm than if it was >55 mm. In fact each 1 mm increase in head size was found to be associated with a 5–8 % reduction in the hazard ratio for failure. In men reaching a head size of 54 mm brought the revision rate to 2.6 % which is comparable to other forms of total hip arthroplasty. Interestingly enough, revision rates for women were much higher than for men even for the same head size thus compelling the authors to advice against the use of resurfacings in women. Having said that, this again was for smaller femoral components 44 mm and less whereas females with larger components >50 mm did well but represented only 1 % of the patients studied. The 2012 Australian Registry [30] reports that the proportion of males undergoing hip resurfacing has increased from 71.2 % in 2003 to 94.3 % in 2011. Resurfacing also provides an attractive alternative to replacement in patients with a particularly large femoral offset, or those with femoral shaft deformity or osteopetrosis making the insertion of a hip stem difficult.

Patients with leg length discrepancy of more than 2.5 cm, severe anatomical deformity of proximal femur (post-Perthes' or post-slipped capital femoral epiphysis), Crowe grade IV dysplasia, and inflammatory arthropathy are best managed with total hip arthroplasty [31]. The senior author has previously described the Surface Arthroplasty Risk index (SARI) [32] as a tool to aid in patient selection for hip resurfacing. It includes patient weight (<82 kg), femoral head cysts greater than 1 cm, UCLA activity score, and previous hip surgery. In 2004, Beaulé et al. [32] reported that patients with SARI greater than 3 had a 12-fold increase for early revision and/or component loosening.

Absolute contraindications to hip resurfacing include patients with severe cystic or atrophic changes in the femoral head or neck which carries a high risk of femoral failure. Patients with renal failure or with proven hypersensitivity to metal are also unsuitable. Since the teratogenic effects of metal ions are unknown, women planning to conceive are advised to do so before the procedure or wait at least 2 years thereafter.

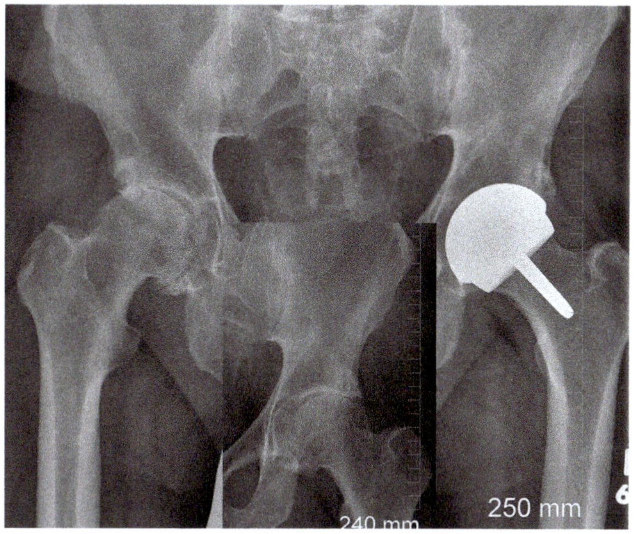

Fig. 79.1 Antero-posterior radiograph of a 58-year-old male post left cementless hip resurfacing (CORMET 2000®, Corin, Cirencester/Gloucestershire) with advanced hip arthritis of right hip with a femoral head cyst

Patient Assessment

Younger patients suffering from advanced hip osteoarthritis usually present with symptoms suggesting the affected hip as the source of pain. Often young patients with hip arthritis seek hip resurfacing with the intent of return to so-called high-demand exercise activities. High levels of sporting activities have been reported by Le Duff et al. [33] to have almost a four-fold increase in the revision rate at a mean of 10 years. Patients should be properly counseled that high impact activities which will most likely negatively affect the long term survivorship any joint replacement including a resurfacing implant.

Physical examination should assess the neurovascular status, leg-length discrepancy, muscle strength (specifically abductors), and range of motion. Reproducible pain on putting the hip through a range of motion helps to confirm the diagnosis.

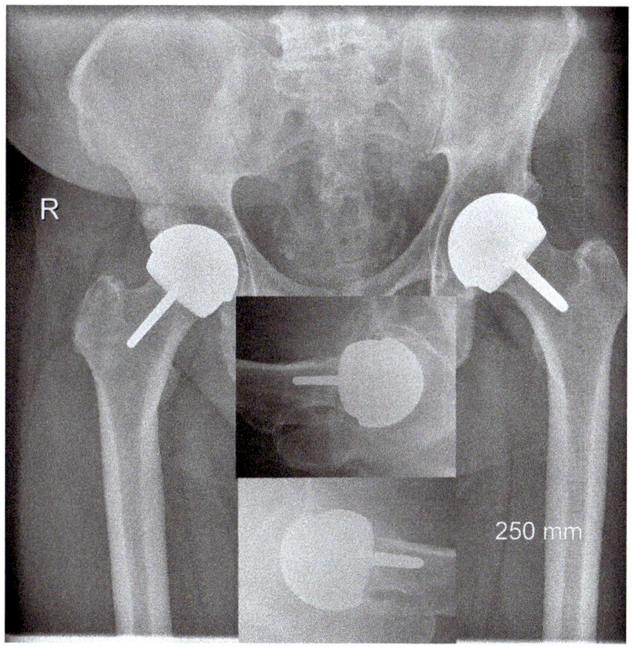

Fig. 79.2 Anteroposterior radiograph post hybrid hip resurfacing (Conserve Plus, Wright Medical Technology, Memphis, TN). *Insets*: Cross-Table laterals of both hips showing femoral component placement

Radiographic Evaluation/Templating

The standard radiographic examination for evaluation of hip pathologies at our center consists of: an anteroposterior (AP) pelvic radiograph, cross table lateral and/or Dunn views [34] (Figs. 79.1 and 79.2). Most hips undergoing resurfacing have an abnormal femoral head/neck offset, which is best assessed in the axial plane [35]. Because the size of the acetabulum and the femoral head are interdependent implant sizing must be done in consideration of the other side of the joint. Once the femoral head is shaped, the size of the socket is dictated by the size of the femoral head. Hip dysplasia presents a unique challenge, and while templating the amount of acetabular deficiency, leg-length discrepancy and valgus femoral neck should be borne in mind. If the preoperative plan suggests these cannot be adequately addressed it is prudent to switch to a total hip arthroplasty [36]. In addition to sizing here are additional key factors to consider:

- Relative valgus position of 5–10° to minimize tensile stresses [37].
- Recognize abnormal femoral offset, specifically in patients with arthritis secondary to femoro-acetabular impingement.

It is necessary to identify the neck axis in the axial plane to avoid placing the femoral component more posteriorly on the neck. If anterior offset is left uncorrected, patients can suffer from persistent pain secondary to impingement and decreased range of motion [38].
- Recognize that any change in version/translation of the femoral component to compensate for abnormal offset can also cause notching of the femoral neck.

Surgical Approach

The medial circumflex artery and inferior gluteal bundle [39, 40] are key elements for maintaining the vascular supply to the proximal femur and neurovascular preservation of hip muscles. Any approach to perform hip resurfacing should preserve these. The most commonly used surgical approach for hip resurfacing is the posterior approach. It offers an excellent view of the acetabulum, postero-superior head-neck junction and is extensile in nature. However, blood supply to the femoral head is compromised due to damage to the ascending branch of medial circumflex artery. To avoid this, the lateral and the direct anterior approach have been used to perform hip resurfacing, while others have used a posterolateral approach using a digastric trochanteric osteotomy [41] combined with an anterior hip dislocation. A brief overview is mentioned below.

Anterior Approach

The senior author (PB) uses the anterior (Hueter) approach [42] along with an orthopedic positioning table as it offers an excellent internervous-intermuscular plane to the hip. The patient is positioned supine on the traction table which allows the hip to be extended and externally rotated in the supine position.

The incision is placed 1–2 cm posterolateral and 2 cm distal to the anterosuperior iliac spine. It runs obliquely to follow the orientation of the tensor fascia lata (TFL) along an imaginary line to the fibular head. The fascia over the TFL is incised in line and the fibers of TFL are gently teased off the fascial sleeve using sharp dissection. Blunt dissection is then performed between the TFL's muscle belly and the rectus aponeurosis. A large cobra retractor is placed behind the lateral part of the iliac wing. The fascia over the rectus is then exposed by blunt dissection. This is then incised taking care to identify and ligate the lateral circumflex vessels along the way. With the rectus exposed the reflected head is released to expose the hip capsule. A lateral capsulectomy is then done to expose the femoral head and neck. Careful release of the rectus fascia permits medial retraction of the rectus femoris muscle as well as inferomedial capsular release to facilitate external rotation of the leg thus optimizing exposure of the femoral head/neck junction. Once the hip is dislocated anteriorly using a Weber spoon, standard femoral head preparation is done to accept the resurfacing implant and is described later. For femoral preparation the leg needs to be placed in extension with the foot externally rotated close to 180°. Occasionally in large males, the origin of the tensor muscle at the anterior superior iliac spine is partially released to avoid damaging the muscle. For acetabular preparation the leg is placed in slight flexion and the foot is left to rest in external rotation. Visiting a center of expertise is strongly advised before performing the anterior for hip resurfacing.

Amongst patients being operated through the lateral approach, more than two-thirds of the patients report hypoesthesia in the distribution of the lateral femoral cutaneous nerve (LCFN) [43]. This probably results from retractor placements which stretch the nerve and cause a transient neuropraxia. The majority of these patients recover with a few months. In the early part of our learning curve with the anterior approach we noticed a tendency to place the acetabular cup with higher abduction angles. We realized that extending the skin incision distally for 1–2 cm avoided the conflict between the cup impactor and skin as well as the use of offset impactors. There is also a tendency for the femoral component to be placed with a slight anterior translation which is related to the difficult access to the femoral neck with this interval.

Trochanteric Slide Osteotomy

This approach initially described by Ganz [44] was utilized for performing intra-capsular surgeries in the treatment of femoro-acetabular impingement. The primary source for the blood supply to the femoral head is the ascending branch of the medial femoral circumflex artery (MFCA) which is located at the proximal border of the quadratus femoris muscle. It then courses superiorly, crossing anterior to the conjoint tendon of the gemellus inferior, obturator internus, and gemellus superior muscles and at this point perforates the capsule to provide the blood supply to the femoral head [45]. The incision is similar to a posterolateral approach and after identifying and preserving the piriformis tendon a sliding osteotomy of the greater trochanter is done. This helps to preserve the blood supply to the femoral head and also maintain the abductors. The trochanteric fragment is then flipped and the abductors are moved anterosuperiorly exposing the hip capsule. After the capsulotomy, the hip is dislocated anteriorly.

The most challenging part of this approach still remains obtaining proper trochanteric fragment fixation. Trochanteric non-union (8%) remains a concern and a quarter of the patients come back for screw removal [46].

Posterior Approach

A standard posterolateral approach to the hip remains the most commonly used approach for hip resurfacing and is recommended when first starting to perform hip resurfacing. The skin incision is centered on the greater trochanter, but the proximal limb of the incision is curved approximately at a seventy degree angle posteriorly. This allows adequate access to the acetabulum without the femoral head obscuring the view. A partial release of the gluteal sling helps to avoid excessive stretch on the sciatic nerve [47] and also facilitates exposure. A "C" shaped capsulotomy is done along the femoral head avoiding the femoral neck. Once the hip is dislocated the capsule is released along the medial femoral neck but not on its posterior aspect. These two steps have been shown to minimize the damage to the blood supply of the femoral head [48]. Capsulotomy scissors are then used to incise the anterior capsule followed by femoral head preparation.

Irrespective of the approach used, adequate exposure remains paramount. The femoral head compromises the view of the acetabulum compared with a total hip arthroplasty.

Surgical Technique

Femoral Head Preparation

Once the capsular releases are complete the femoral head is adequately exposed using either an elevator or long curved retractors. The femoral head is sized using femoral head gauges in correlation with preoperative templating. A guide wire is then passed into the femoral head. This can be done using various commercial jigs available. It can also be inserted at around 5–10° of valgus relative to the native femoral neck shaft angle, which gives us a final angle close to 140°. This is double checked using a goniometer. A spin-around guide corresponding with the planned femoral head size is used to check for any impinging neck osteophytes it at the inferomedial neck and clear the anterior neck. Care should be made to avoid debriding osteophytes unnecessarily or bone that may be exposing cancellous bone in the neck, which could lead to a stress riser or femoral neck fracture at a later date.

Once these critical steps are achieved satisfactorily, femoral head preparation is done using cylindrical and chamber reamers. This may vary according to different implant manufacturers. The reaming may initially be done to one size larger than planned if there is any doubt about acetabular sizing and finalized once the acetabulum is prepared. In either case, once the femoral head is prepared to the final size a trial component should be placed and checked for any notching, osteophytes, and seating position.

Acetabular Preparation and Implantation of Component

For the posterior approach, creating a superolateral pocket by elevating the capsule off the superolateral acetabular surface facilitates placement of the reamed femoral head while preparing the acetabulum. A long curved Hohmann retractor is placed over the anteromedial lip of the acetabulum. This is done at approximately the 3–4 o'clock position for the right hip and 8–9 O'clock position for the left hip.

Another Hohmann retractor is placed under the posterior wall (3 or 9 O'clock position for left/right hip, respectively). The labrum is excised and osteophytes are taken down to identify the true acetabular walls. Soft tissue from the cotyloid fossa is removed with a long curette to identify the floor. Reaming is started three sizes below the size planned based on the femoral component. We start reaming on reverse mode to ensure adequate bony contact and then ream forward. The reamers provide a fair judgment of native anteversion and inclination of the socket. A curette is used between reamings to remove any soft tissue or sclerotic areas and also to judge depth of reaming. Depending on the manufacturer design, you either ream line to line to give a 0.75 mm press-fit but this can vary according to manufacturer guidelines. A trail component can then be used to plan the position of the final component and to check for press-fit.

Once the bony bed is prepared the acetabulum is cleaned with pulsatile lavage. The final component is then impacted into place. Various guides are available to judge anteversion and inclination depending on the approach used by the surgeon. Since there are no screws holes to determine depth of impaction the walls of the acetabulum are used a guide and compared with the trial component. Because of the importance of acetabular component orientation as well as seating, an intraoperative radiograph is highly recommended. Based on recent migration studies, lack of complete seating (polar gaps) of the acetabular component does not affect the risk of migration and/or loosening [49]. All the four quadrants of the cup must then be stressed manually with a punch to ensure press-fit and prevent cup spin-outs. We commonly leave a 1–2 mm bony rim overhanging anteriorly to avoid iliopsoas irritation.

Femoral Component Implantation

Both non cemented and cemented components are available for femoral head implantation. In either case the femoral head is thoroughly irrigated, all debris is removed, and the bony bed is dried adequately. Any sclerotic areas are prepared by making drill holes with a 2.5 mm drill bit. The porous coated component can then be impacted into place. While using a cemented component the cement is applied in a doughy state. If applied when the cement is still "runny," overpenetration of the cement can cause thermal necrosis. The partially cement-filled femoral component is then impacted and excessive cement removed. The hip is quickly reduced to allow the heat generated by cement curing to dissipate. A recent report has suggested equivalent results at short term follow up with porous coated components as compared with a cemented femoral heads [50]. At our center we have started using cementless femoral heads in the last 1

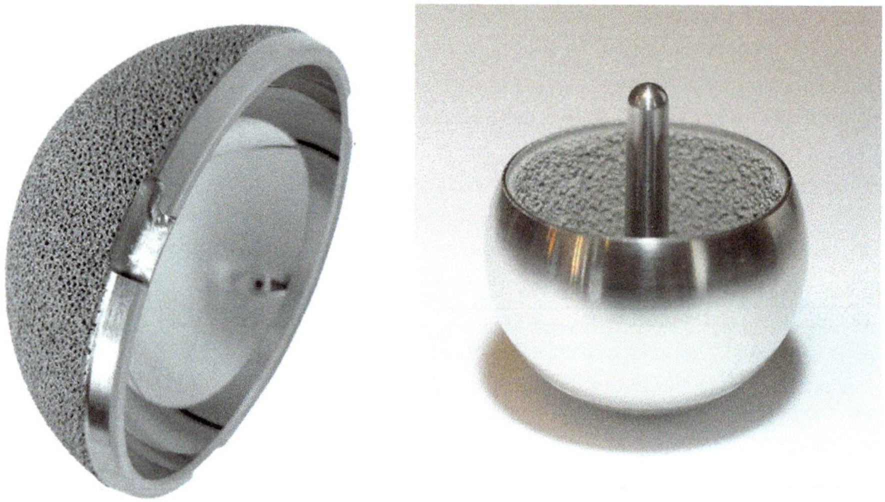

Fig. 79.3 Cementless Conserve Plus® with BioFoam® Shell which is currently used

year with satisfactory outcomes as well as Titanium backed cobalt-chrome shell, i.e., Conserve BioFoam® (Wright Medical Technology, Memphis, TN) (Fig. 79.3).

Once the final components are implanted an intraoperative x-ray is done to evaluate component position. We then perform an intraoperative "range of motion" check. The hip is placed in external rotation to check for anterior stability and in flexion, internal rotation, and adduction for posterior stability. While doing this attention is also paid to check for impingement. Finally the hip is distracted and the acetabular socket is re-checked for press-fit by manually stressing its edge. Closure is performed according to the approach used.

Patients are asked be on 50% weight bearing and to use crutches for 4 weeks post operatively. This allows for femoral neck remodeling and decreases the risk of fracture. We provide all patients with prophylaxis for venous thromboembolism. They receive low molecular weight heparin while in hospital and oral medication on discharge for a total of 4 weeks. Physiotherapy is commenced at 4 weeks when the crutches are given up by the patient. Patients return for follow-up visits typically at 3 weeks, 6 weeks, 6 months, and then annually.

University of Ottawa Conserve Plus® Results

From 2001 to 2009, 548 consecutive hip resurfacings were performed using the Conserve Plus® prosthesis in 460 patients (351 males) with a mean age of 48.3 years (range 18–66). The majority of patients (505 hips) had an underlying diagnosis of osteoarthritis. No patients were lost to follow-up. At a mean follow-up of 4.9 years (2.5–10.4) 24 (4.4%) patients required conversion to a conventional total hip replacement (THR) (16 males, 8 females, mean age = 50.1 ± 6.3 years): Eleven were due to acetabular component loosening, four for femoral neck fracture, three for persistent unexplained pain, three for femoral component loosening, two for adverse tissue reaction, and one for infection. Six other patients required revision of the acetabular component while retaining the resurfaced femoral component. Five-year survival with revision to total hip as endpoint was 95.1% (95% CI: 93.1–97.1%) and 93.6% (95%CI: 91.2–95.8%) for any revision for aseptic loosening. Table 79.1.

Table 79.1 The advantages and disadvantages of metal-on-metal bearings

Advantages
Low wear rate
Reduced risk of osteolysis
Improved longevity
Larger diameter femoral head
Improved range of motion
Reduced risk of dislocation
Preserved acetabular bone stock (compared with a metal-on-polyethylene bearing surface)
Disadvantages
Metal ion release
Risk of carcinogenicity
Risk of chromosomal damage
Pregnancy risk (teratogenic, mutagenic)
Metal hypersensitivity

Reprinted with permission from Beaule PE, Mussett SA, Medley JB: Metal-on-Metal Bearings in Total Hip Arthroplasty in O'Connor MI, Egol KA (eds): Instructional Course Lectures 59. Rosemont, IL, American Academy of Orthopaedic Surgeons, 2010, pp 17–25

References

1. Beaule PE. Surface arthroplasty of the hip: a review and current indications. Semin Arthroplasty. 2005;16(1):70–6.
2. Ball ST, LeDuff MJ, Amstutz HC. Early results of conversion of a failed femoral component in hip resurfacing arthroplasty. J Bone Joint Surg. 2007;89A(4):735–41.

3. Dowson D, Hardaker C, Flett M, Isaac GH. A hip joint simulator study of the performance of metal-on-metal joints. Part II: design. J Arthroplasty. 2004;19(8 Suppl 3):124–30.
4. Candian Hip Resurfacing Study Group. A survey on the prevalence of pseudotumors with metal-on-metal hip resurfacing in Canadian Academic Centers. J Bone Joint Surg. 2011;93A Suppl 2:118–21.
5. Glyn-Jones S, Pandit HP, Kwon YM, Doll H, Gill HS, Murray DW. Risk factors for inflammatory pseudotumour formation following hip resurfacing. J Bone Joint Surg. 2009;91B(12):1566–74.
6. Kwon YM, Glyn-Jones S, Simpson DJ, Kamali A, McClardy-Smith P, Gill HS, et al. Analysis of wear of retrieved metal-on-metal hip resurfacing implants revised due to pseudotumours. J Bone Joint Surg. 2010;92B(3):356–61.
7. Beaule PE, Mussett SA, Medley JB. Metal-on-metal bearings in total hip arthroplasty. Instr Course Lect. 2010;59(59):17–25.
8. Chan F, Bobyn JD, Medley JB, Krygier J, Tanzer M. Wear and lubrication of metal-on-metal hip implants. Clin Orthop. 1999;369:10–24.
9. Catelas I, Bobyn JD, Medley JB, Krygier J, Zukor DJ, Huk OL. Size, shape and composition of wear particles from metal-metal hip simulator testing: effects of alloy and cycle time. J Biomed Mater Res. 2003;67A:312–27.
10. Wimmer MA, Fischer A, Buscher R, Pourzal R, Sprecher C, Hauert R, et al. Wear mechanisms in metal-on-metal bearings: the importance of tribochemical reaction layers. J Orthop Res. 2010;28(4):436–43.
11. Catelas I, Wimmer MA. New insights into wear and biological effects of metal-on-metal bearings. J Bone Joint Surg Am. 2011;93:76–83.
12. Wimmer MA, Sprecher C, Hauert R, Tager G, Fischer A. Tribochemical reaction on metal-on-metal hip joint bearings: a comparison between in-vitro and in-vivo results. Wear. 2003;255: 1007–14.
13. Rigney DA, Chen LH, Naylor MGS, Rosenfield AR. Wear processes in sliding systems. Wear. 1984;100:195–219.
14. Pourzal R, Theissmann R, Williams S, Gleising B, Fisher J, Fischer A. Subsurface changes of a MoM hip implant below different contact zones. J Mech Behav Biomed Mater. 2009;2:186–91.
15. Catelas I, Campbell PA, Bobyn JD, Medley JB, Huk OL. Wear particles from metal-on-metal total hip replacements: effects of implant design and implantation time. Proc Inst Mech Eng H. 2006;220:195–208.
16. Campbell P, Ebramzadeh E, Nelson S, Takamura K, De SK, Amstutz HC. Histological features of pseudotumor-like tissues from metal-on-metal hips. Clin Orthop Relat Res. 2010;468(9): 2321–7.
17. Catelas I, Campbell PA, Dorey F, Frausto A, Mills BG, Amstutz HA. Semi-quantitative analysis of cytokines in MM THR tissues and their relationship to metal particles. Biomaterials. 2003;24(26):4785–97.
18. Al-Saffar N. Early clinical failure of total joint replacement in association with follicular proliferation of B-lymphocytes: a report of two cases. J Bone Joint Surg Am. 2002;84:2270–3.
19. Bohler M, Kanz F, Schwarz B, Steffen I, Walter A, Plenk Jr H, et al. Adverse tissue reactions to wear particles from Co-alloy articulations, increased by alumina-blasting particle contamination from cementless Ti-based total hip implants. A report of seven revisions with early failure. J Bone Joint Surg Br. 2002;84:128–36.
20. Davies AP, Willert H-G, Ampbell PA, Learmonth ID, Case CP. An unusual lymphocytic perivascular infiltration in tissues around contemporary metal-on-metal joint replacements. J Bone Joint Surg. 2005;87A(1):18–27.
21. Willert H-G, Buchhorn GH, Fayyazi A, Flury R, Windler M, Koster G, et al. Metal-on-metal bearings and hypersensitivity in patients with artificial hip joints. A clinical and histomorphological study. J Bone Joint Surg Am. 2005;87:28–36.
22. Pandit H, Glyn-Jones S, Lardy-Smith P, Gundle R, Whitwell D, Gibbons CL, et al. Pseudotumours associated with metal-on-metal hip resurfacings. J Bone Joint Surg Br. 2008;90(7):847–51.
23. Clayton RA, Beggs I, Salter DM, Grant MH, Patton JT, Porter DE. Inflammatory pseudotumor associated with femoral nerve palsy following metal-on-metal re-surfacing of the hip. A case report. J Bone Joint Surg Am. 2008;90:1988–93.
24. Campbell PA, Wang M, Amstutz HC, Goodman SB. Positive cytokine production in failed metal-on-metal total hip replacements. Acta Othop Scand. 2002;73:506–12.
25. McBryde CW, Theivendran K, Thomas AM, Treacy RB, Pynsent PB. The influence of head size and sex on the outcome of Birmingham hip resurfacing. J Bone Joint Surg. 2010;92A(1):105–12.
26. Baker R, Whitehouse M, Kilshaw M, et al. Maximum temperatures of 89C recorded during the mechanical preparation of 35 femoral heads for resurfacing. Acta Orthop. 2011;82:669–73.
27. Shimmin AJ, Walter WL, Esposito C. The influence of the size of the component on the outcome of resurfacing arthroplasty of the hip. A review of the literarature. J Bone Joint Surg Br. 2010;92(B):469–76.
28. Smith AJ, Dieppe P, Howard PW, Blom AW. Failure rates of metal-on-metal hip resurfacings: analysis of data from the National Joint Registry for England and Wales. Lancet. 2012;380(9855):1759–66.
29. de Steiger RN, Hang JR, Miller LN, Graves SE, Davidson DC. Five-year results of the ASR XL acetabular system and the ASR hip resurfacing system: an analysis from the Australian Orthopaedic Association National Joint Replacement Registry. J Bone Joint Surg Am. 2011;93(24):2287–93.
30. Australian Orthopaedic Association. Annual Report. Australian Orthopaedic Association 2012 (cited 10 Feb 2013). https://aoanjrr.dmac.adelaide.edu.au.
31. McMinn DJ, Daniel J, Ziaee H, Pradhan C. Indications and results of hip resurfacing. Int Orthop. 2011;35(2):231–7.
32. Beaule PE, Dorey FJ, Le Duff MJ, Gruen T, Amstutz HC. Risk factors affecting outcome of metal-on-metal surface arthroplasty of the hip. Clin Orthop Relat Res. 2004;418:87–93.
33. LeDuff MJ, Amstutz HC. The relationship of sporting activity and implant survivorship after hip resurfacing. J Bone Joint Surg. 2012;94(10):911–8.
34. Clohisy JC, Carlisle JC, Beaule PE, Kim Y-J, Trousdale RT, Sierra RJ, et al. A systematic approach to the plain radiographic evaluation of the young adult hip. J Bone Joint Surg. 2008;90A Suppl 4:47–66.
35. Beaule PE, Harvey N, Zaragoza EJ, LeDuff M, Dorey FJ. The femoral head/neck offset and hip resurfacing. J Bone Joint Surg Br. 2007;89(1):9–15.
36. Beaule PE, Poitras P. Femoral component sizing and positioning in hip resurfacing arthroplasty. Instr Course Lect. 2007;56:163–9.
37. Freeman MAR. Some anatomical and mechanical considerations relevant to the surface replacement of the femoral head. Clin Orthop Rel Res. 1978;134:19–24.
38. Girard J, Krantz N, Bocquet D, Wavreille G, Migaud H. Femoral head to neck offset after hip resurfacing is critical for range of motion. Clin Biomech (Bristol, Avon). 2012;27(2):165–9.
39. Beaule PE, Campbell PA, Lu Z, Leunig-Ganz K, Beck M, Leunig M, et al. Vascularity of the arthritic femoral head and hip resurfacing. J Bone Joint Surg. 2006;88A Suppl 4:85–96.
40. Beaule PE, Campbell PA, Shim P. Femoral head blood flow during hip resurfacing. Clin Orthop Rel Res. 2007;456(456):148–52.
41. Nork SE, Schar M, Pfander G, Beck M, Djonov V, Ganz R, et al. Anatomic considerations for the choice of surgical approach for hip resurfacing arthroplasty. Orthop Clin North Am. 2005;36(2):163–70.
42. Benoit B, Gofton W, Beaule PE. Hueter anterior approach for hip resurfacing: assessment of the learning curve. Orthop Clin North Am. 2009;40(3):357–63.
43. Goulding K, Beaule PE, Kim PR, Fazekas A. Incidence of lateral femoral cutaneous nerve neuropraxia after anterior approach hip arthroplasty. Clin Orthop Relat Res. 2010;468(9):2397–404.
44. Ganz R, Gill TJ, Gautier E, Ganz K, Krugel N, Berlemann U. Surgical dislocation of the adult hip. A new technique with full access to the femoral head and acetabulum without the risk of avascular necrosis. J Bone Joint Surg Br. 2001;83(8):1119–24.

45. Gautier E, Ganz K, Krugel N, Gill TJ, Ganz R. Anatomy of the medial circumflex artery and its surgical implications. J Bone Joint Surg. 2000;82B(5):679–83.
46. Bal SB, Kazmier P, Burd T, Aleto T. Anterior trochanteric slide osteotomy for primary total hip arthroplasty. Review of nonunion and complications. J Arthroplasty. 2006;21(1):59–63.
47. Gay DP, Desser DR, Parks BG, Boucher HR. Sciatic nerve injury in total hip resurfacing: a biomechanical analysis. J Arthroplasty. 2010;25(8):1295–300.
48. Steffen RT, DeSmet KA, Murray DW, Gill HS. A modified posterior approach preserves femoral head oxgenation during hip resurfacing. J Arthroplasty. 2011;26(3):404–8.
49. Nakasone S, Takao M, Nishii T, Sakai T, Sugano N. Incidence and natural course of initial polar gaps in Birmingham hip resurfacing cups. J Arthroplasty. 2012;27(9):1676–82.
50. Gross TP, Liu F. The first 100 fully porous-coated femoral components in hip resurfacing. Bull NYU Hosp Jt Dis. 2011;69 Suppl 1:S30–5.

Total Hip Replacement in the Young Patient

80

Hernan A. Prieto, Atul F. Kamath, and David G. Lewallen

Introduction

Total hip arthroplasty (THA) is considered one of the most reliable and successful medical procedures available, and is cost-effective [1], as it significantly enhances the quality of life of patients with arthritis, while maintaining their independence [2]. Improvements in both fixation methods and bearing surfaces have allowed expansion of surgical indications of these procedures to include younger, more active patients. Historically, THA in the young patient population has not been durable regardless of diagnosis, and the management of end-stage hip disease in the very active and young patients (i.e., aged <30 years) has been a major challenge. Advances have been made in the understanding of the etiology and pathomechanical factors that are associated with the development of early hip arthrosis. The recent expanded use of joint-preserving surgical techniques for hip conditions may lead to early degenerative joint disease [3–5]. However, despite these improvements, very young patients with end-stage joint changes and disabling symptoms continue to present for consideration of arthroplasty.

Young patient age raises the concern for prosthetic implant longevity. This durability relates to the traditionally high rates of loosening and wear, with resulting lower survivorship rates [6, 7]. Total hip replacement in the young is often attributable to several specific underlying etiologies, including rheumatoid arthritis, posttraumatic arthritis, septic arthritis, sequelae of Legg–Calve–Perthes (LCP) disease, slipped capital femoral epiphysis (SCFE), developmental hip dysplasia (DDH), femoroacetabular impingement, and avascular necrosis. Although hip arthrodesis remains an option for the young patient with unilateral disease, many present day patients know of hip arthroplasty results and are unaccepting of arthrodesis as they much prefer an intervention that allows them to maintain hip motion and to be as functional as possible during the active stages of their lives. Total hip arthroplasty can provide this option in this challenging subset of patients, certainly for the short term, and advances in cementless acetabular and femoral fixation, combined with improved bearing surface materials, have led to renewed optimism regarding the longevity of contemporary THA in the young patient population.

The purpose of this chapter is discussing the current trends in THA for the very young patient, with particular attention to implant fixation and bearing surfaces.

Etiology

In very young patients, a number of etiologies cause early joint disease that prompts evaluation for surgical intervention. Past published series have focused on young patients in whom THA was performed for the management of rheumatoid arthritis (RA) [7], and most cases involved the use of cemented implants. With the improvements in the diagnosis and treatment of RA in younger patients, including evolving disease modifying anti-rheumatic drugs (DMARDs), the incidence of advanced hip disease associated with RA has significantly diminished, reducing the demand for THA.

While, in the past, rheumatoid arthritis accounted for approximately 25 % of THA in young patients, other common etiologies now include osteonecrosis (41–54 %), sequelae of pediatric hip disorders (SCFE, DDH, LCP—20–36 %), and chondrolysis (1 %) [8–11]. End-stage arthritic disease secondary to deformities associated with genetic syndromes (e.g. osteogenesis imperfecta, spondyloepiphyseal dysplasia, chondrodystrophia) is also treated with THA, though less commonly than the other etiologies. While any congenital or developmental abnormality of the hip can lead to premature degenerative changes due to altered joint anatomy and loading, this mechanical route appears to be much

H.A. Prieto, MD • A.F. Kamath, MD • D.G. Lewallen, MD (✉)
Department of Orthopaedic Surgery, Mayo Clinic,
200 First Street SW, Gonda 14, Rochester, MN 55905, USA
e-mail: lewallen.david@mayo.edu

J.C. McCarthy et al. (eds.), *Hip Joint Restoration*, DOI 10.1007/978-1-4614-0694-5_80

more critical for some conditions such as hip dysplasia than for some other disorders such as slipped capital femoral epiphysis (or SCFE).

In a Mayo Clinic study, Larson and coworkers [12] found that, in patients with prior SCFE, the majority of hip arthroplasties were usually carried out for the associated indication of avascular necrosis (70 % of the severe slips and 71 % of the acute or acute-on-chronic slips), rather than degenerative changes related to residual femoroacetabular impingement.

Type of Fixation

Following the introduction of THA, components were most commonly cemented, but early fixation failures, especially in young active patients, prompted the use of cementless fixation broadly, but especially in the young patient, following the development and widespread availability of uncemented devices. On the acetabular side, different principles of fixation were initially tested, including threaded acetabular rings and press-fit acetabular components, with or without additional screws. With time, and collective experience, it has become evident that optimal ingrowth materials should have good biocompatibility and a three-dimensional surface structure to achieve secondary fixation to the bone. This stable biologic fixation and osteointegration aims to avoid later symptoms from fibrous fixation and loosening.

In North America the fixation method of choice for both acetabular and femoral components has evolved to the use of press-fit porous components for the majority of patients, both young and old. Outcomes of THA with cemented femoral components have demonstrated inconsistent survivorship in at least the younger patient population. The specifics of femoral stem choice generally are a matter of surgeon preference, considering the quality of proximal femoral bone, the presence of previous deformity affecting the shape of the proximal femur, and the potential need for diaphyseal fixation. Deformity issues in the dysplastic femur include hypoplasia, excessive neck anteversion, a valgus neck-shaft angle, metaphyseal-diaphyseal mismatch, and a posteriorly displaced greater trochanter. Ultimately, the choice of femoral stem is based on the evaluation of specific details of the individual patient, but cemented stems continue to have a role, even in some young patients with very poor bone quality.

Uncemented Total Hip Arthroplasty

Cementless fixation, in combination with improved articulation bearing materials can provide long-term survivorship even in the young patient population. However, there are significant differences in the survival of different uncemented acetabular components following primary total hip arthroplasty related to design. Cup revisions for aseptic loosening are significantly more common with beaded and hydroxyapatite-coated designs compared to those designs with a three dimensional surfaces, such as titanium wire mesh or highly porous metals [13]. In recent years, there has been considerable interest in the development of acetabular components with a variety of highly porous metals following the introduction of highly porous tantalum in the late 1990s. A Mayo Clinic series showed no aseptic loosening in the first decade with highly porous tantalum cups in patients of all ages, but further follow-up is needed to confirm these promising findings into the second decade, especially in the younger age group [13] (Fig. 80.1).

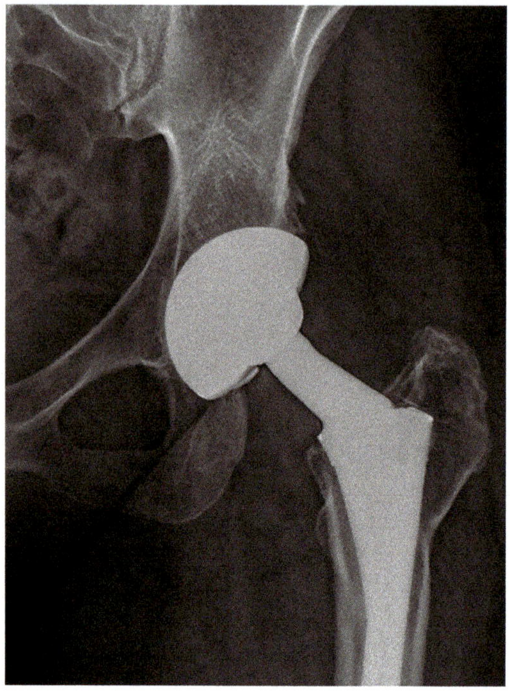

Fig. 80.1 Highly porous Tantalum cup, 11.2 years follow-up, demonstrating adequate fixation

Clohisy et al. [14] retrospectively reviewed 88 patients (102 THAs), who were 25 years or younger at time of surgery who underwent cementless THA. At a mean of 55 months, all of the cementless stems and 98 % of the cementless acetabular components were radiographically well-fixed. In a systematic review of outcomes of THA for osteonecrosis, Myers et al. found that cemented components were associated with a greater incidence of unfavorable outcomes than cementless components. For the cemented group, the mean postoperative Harris hip score was 85.2 and the revision rate was 19.1 % at 8.1 years. For cementless fixation, the mean postoperative Harris Hip Score was 90.6 points, and the revision rate was 11.4 % at 6.3 years. Similar results are presented in Table 80.1, which summarizes more recent studies of cementless THA in younger patients.

Table 80.1 Summary of published studies of non-cemented THA in very young patients (less than 30 years old)

Reference	Hips (patients)	Cementless stems %	Mean age in years	Mean FU in years	Cup revision	Stem revision	Revision (%)
Restrepo et al. [9]	35 (25)	100	17.6	6.6	1	0	2.8
Wangen et al. [15]	49 (44)	100	25	13	24[a]	0	49
Clohisy et al. [14]	102 (88)	95	20	4.2	7	0	6.8
Girard et al. [10]	47 (34)	94	25	9	2[a]	0	4.2
Costa et al. [16]	53 (40)	100	20	4.6	2	0	4

[a]All revisions were acetabular

Cemented THA

The longevity of cemented THA in younger patients has been limited by failures of fixation and past wear-related osteolysis. Several prior reports show varying rates of cemented acetabular component survivorship, and the majority of studies largely focus on THA procedures performed for juvenile RA (JRA), often with cemented femoral components.

Dorr et al., in a cohort of patients younger than 45 years old reported an increase in revision rate for cemented THA over time: 12 % at 4.5 years, 33 % at 9.2 years, and 67 % at a mean follow-up of 16.2 years [17]. After stratifying results by age, the authors found the revision rate for patients younger than 30 years old at the time of the index arthroplasty was 82 % compared with 56 % for those over 30 years.

Kerboull and associates [18] evaluated the results of 287 primary cemented THAs with an average patient age of 40.1 years. The mean follow-up was 14.5 years. The authors found a mean wear rate of 0.12 mm/year, and 25 hips required revision (8.7 %). Sixty-eight percent of the revisions were for aseptic loosening. They also evaluated a subset of patients with greater than 20 years follow-up. Using revision as an end point, these patients demonstrated a survival rate of 85.4 %.

Keener and coworkers [19] looked at the 25-year results of 42 patients. The overall survivorship was 63 %. Aseptic loosening accounted for 77 % of the 22 revisions. Loosening on the acetabular side was far more prevalent and continued to progress with time.

Table 80.2 summarizes results of selected studies of cemented THA in young patients, with respective revision failure rates. The revision rates for cemented THA performed in young patients are higher than that for uncemented implants, including the percentage of failure related to the acetabular component.

Type of Articulation (Bearing Surfaces)

Historically, the relatively poor survivorship of arthroplasties in young patients has been attributed in various series to the early use of all-cemented components, screw-in acetabular designs, the wear characteristics of metal-on-conventional polyethylene bearing surfaces, and the higher activity level of young patients. However, the single most important of these factors in most joint replacements performed over the past four decades has been wear of the bearing surface (Fig. 80.2). In order to avoid the wear related limitations of conventional polyethylene, there has been ongoing debate regarding the optimal alternative bearing surface for use in younger patients, with some advocating ceramic-on-ceramic (COC), others ceramic on conventional polyethylene (COP), metal-on-metal (MOM) and metal (or ceramic) on highly cross-linked polyethylene (HXLPE). These wear couples have been suggested because of their lower wear rate when compared to that of metal on conventional polyethylene (Table 80.3).

Highly Cross-Linked Polyethylene (HXLPE)

In the 1990s, efforts to reduce UHMWPE wear led to the study of the link between wear debris production and polymer structure. Cross-links are bonds that interconnect polyethylene molecules, are formed during irradiation polyethylene and increase resistance to wear. These processes are the basis for the production of modern highly cross-linked UHMWPE (HXLPE) [22].

In both in vitro and midterm clinical follow-up, HXLPE demonstrates a substantial reduction in wear when compared to conventional polyethylene bearings fabricated from non-highly cross-linked UHMWPE [23]. Hermida et al. reported a 90 % reduction in wear with 28-mm femoral heads articulating with HXLPE liners, and an 85 % reduction at 32 mm. In this report, increasing the head size did not significantly increase the wear of the HXLPE liners [24]. Thomas and coworkers, in a double-blind randomized controlled trial, demonstrated a significantly lower steady-state wear rate with HXLPE (0.005 mm/year) compared with conventional UHMWPE (0.037 mm/year). No patient in the HXLPE group had a wear rate above the osteolysis threshold (0.1 mm/year), compared with 9 % of patients in the UHMWPE group [25].

The reduction in wear seen with HXLPE is similar to that seen with the hard-on-hard ceramic or metal bearings. However, HXLPE does present some distinct practical advantages over both ceramic–ceramic and metal–metal cou-

Table 80.2 Summary of published studies of cemented THA in young patients

Reference	Hips (patients)	Mean age in years	Mean FU in years	Total revision	Cup/stem failures (#)	Revision (%)
Dorr et al. [17]	49 (35)	31	16.2	33	NA	67
Torchia et al. [20]	63 (50)	17	12.6	27	26/16	46
Chmell [21]	66 (39)	19.9	15.1	35	23/12	53
Kenner et al. [19]	57 (42)[a]	<50	25	22	13/4	37
Kerboull [18]	287 (222)	40.1	14.5	25	15/7	8.7

[a]Hips of patients who were alive 25 years following index surgery, and were included in the study

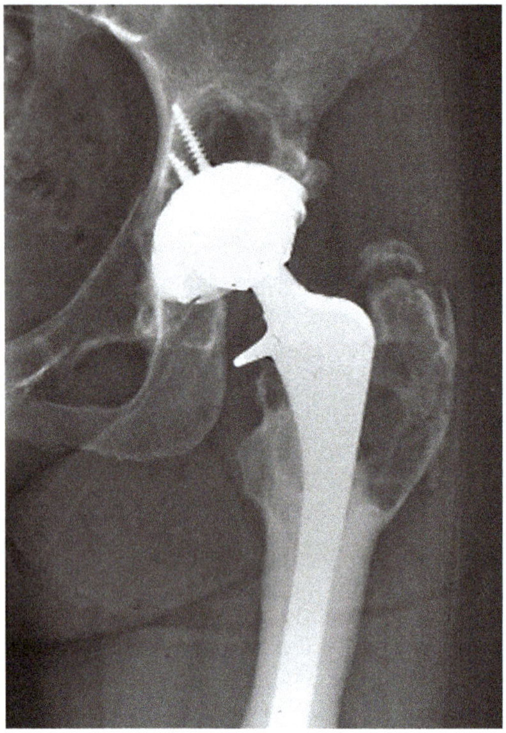

Fig. 80.2 Osteolysis secondary to polyethylene wear, as evidenced by supero-lateral head migration (eccentric head position) and radiolucencies in DeLee zones I and II of the acetabulum and Gruen zones I, II, VII of the femur

ples [26]. With the use of HXLPE, it is possible to avoid the problem of bearing fracture that can occur with use of ceramic bearings, and it should be possible to avoid the marked elevation in local tissue and serum metal ion levels that can occur with use of metal bearings. Impingement of the hip-stem trunnion against a ceramic or metal acetabular rim is a much higher cause for concern than is impingement of the trunnion against a polyethylene liner. In addition, when crosslinked polyethylene liners are used, surgeons have a much wider array of intraoperative choices with regard to head size (i.e., 28, 32, 36, and 40-mm head sizes), orientation of the face of the liner (i.e., 0, 10, and 20° of elevation), and offset (standard or lateral offset). Finally, as arthroplasty implant cost pressures are ongoing, it should be recognized that cross-linked polyethylene bearings are substantially less expensive than hard on hard ceramic or metal bearings.

Table 80.3 Alternative bearing surfaces: linear wear rates

Material	Wear rate (μm)
CoCr/PE	120–200
Ceramic/PE	80–100
CoCr/HXLPE	0–25
MOM	1–5
COM	~1
COC	<1

Second-Generation of HXLPE

In order to optimize wear resistance without altering the mechanical properties associated with post-irradiation melting, second-generation HXPLE are being developed with use of alternative methods to extinguish free radicals. With one method, polyethylene that has been cross-linked with radiation is soaked in vitamin E to extinguish the residual free radicals [27]. Another method involves applying the cross-linking radiation in sequential doses, with annealing after each dose to reduce the free radicals [22, 28]. In a recent study of second-generation sequentially annealed HXPLE, D'Antonio et al. reported that the average wear rate over 5 years was 0.015 mm per year, which represents a 58 % improvement over a first-generation annealed HXPLE. The survivorship (revision for any reason) was 97.8 %, and no osteolysis was reported. Moreover, socket inclination did not affect liner wear [28]. The sequentially annealed HXLPE exhibited lower wear than the first-generation annealed polyethylene at 5 years follow-up; this HXPLE also offers the theoretical advantage of oxidative resistance. These new bearing surface materials offer hope for longevity of THA, but their clinical performance for a 15- to 20-year period will determine the true importance of this cross-linking process.

Ceramic-on-Ceramic

In the United States, the Food and Drug Administration authorized use of ceramic-on-ceramic (CoC) bearings in March 2003. After extensive prior experience in Europe, ceramic-on-ceramic bearing surfaces were stated to provide several benefits, making it a potentially desirable bearing

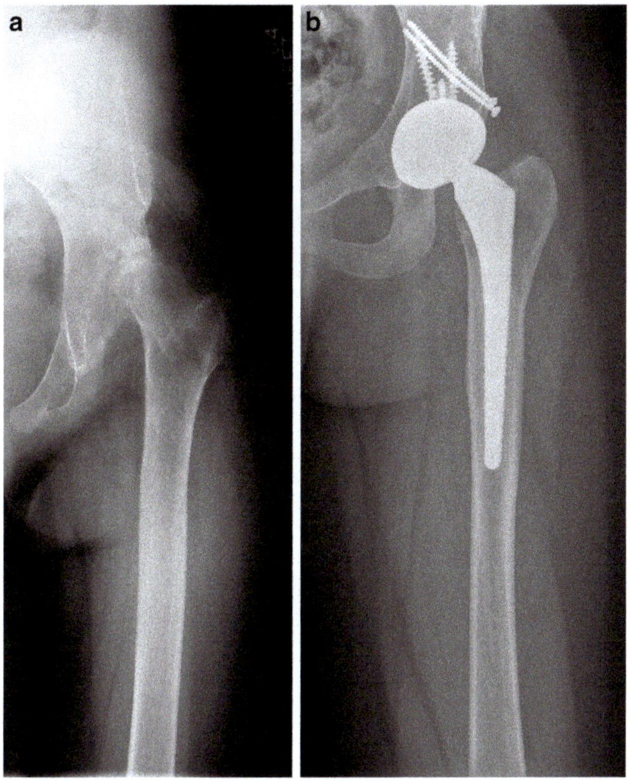

Fig. 80.3 A 12-year-old girl with DDH who had prior open reduction and Pemberton osteotomy (**a**). She was treated with a ceramic-on-ceramic cementless THA and femoral head autograft. She was doing well 6 years following surgery (**b**)

surface in young patients. Studies have shown that the wear rate of ceramic bearing surfaces is up to 4000 times less than the traditional metal-on-polyethylene bearing surfaces [29]. The ceramic surfaces are wettable, which suggests that lubrication from joint fluid is possible and adhesive wear is reduced [30]. The wear debris from ceramic bearing surfaces is also very well tolerated, with alumina particles as an example, relatively bioinert compared with metal and polyethylene debris [31]. These decreased wear rates have correlated with a reduction in the rate of osteolysis and better preservation of bone stock. This is especially important when performing THA in young patients who are more likely to require future revision surgery. Probably the most important advantage of COC is the documented low rate of osteolysis. In a prospective multicenter study, 1709 alumina ceramic hips were reviewed, and no cases of osteolysis were reported [32]. Other comparative studies reported 1.7 % of osteolysis in a CoC group versus 19.4 % of the metal-on-polyethylene group. The osteolysis in the CoC group was confined to the proximal femoral resection level in all affected hips. Ceramic-on-ceramic bearings have superior wear resistance when compared with all other available alternative bearing surfaces, thereby providing an excellent alternative for young and very active patients.

Survivorship analysis of a series of very young patients undergoing THA using CoC bearing surfaces showed promising short- to midterm results, with a 96 % survival rate [11] (Fig. 80.3). D'Antonio et al. showed that the 10-years survivorship of CoC implants was significantly higher than of the metal-on-polyethylene implants (95.9 and 91.3 %, respectively; $p=0.0122$), and the 8-year rate of survivorship of a more recent cementless design, performed with CoC articulations was 97.7 %, similar to other reports comparing CoC to MOP devices [32–33].

There are several potential disadvantages of ceramic couples which have limited their use in North America. Fracture may result from the brittleness of the ceramic material. Head fracture rates range from 0.005 to 0.02 % for alumina bearing surfaces [34] but have been reduced in newer ceramic materials and designs. Squeaking has been reported in between 2.7 % [35] and 7 % [36] of patients. The exact etiology of this phenomenon is unclear and likely multifactorial. However, Trousdale et al. [37] suggest that squeaking is a problem of ceramic–ceramic lubrication, and that noise occurs when the film fluid between the two articulating surfaces is disrupted. Material (metal) transfer to the ceramic femoral head was the only experimental condition that led to squeaking in a lubricated bench top loading situation. Finally, ceramics, like other hard-hard bearings, are more sensitive to cup position than metal or ceramic on polyethylene articulations. The risk of runaway wear with malposition and edge loading, and impingement risk with improper version, makes the operation more demanding when ceramic on ceramic or other hard on hard bearings are used.

Metal-on-Metal (MOM)

The concept of a metal-one-metal (MOM) THA bearing surfaces is not new. The idea was initially described more than 60 years ago by Wiles and was first published in the literature over 30 years ago [38, 39]. The initial MOM implants were associated with design problems, including edge impingement, inadequate clearance, insufficient manufacturing tolerances, and sub optimal material selection. Second-generation small head (32 mm and less) MOM implants demonstrated favorable outcomes in the general population beyond 10 years of follow-up in Europe, and were suggested as an alternative for young active patients. There are theoretical advantages to MOM THA. Metal bearings have lower wear rates than conventional THA in vitro [40]. Larger head diameters (36 and greater) as allowed by MOM design can help optimize hip stability, reduce dislocation risk, and increase range of motion to impingement compared with smaller head diameters.

After widespread adoption of newer very large heads, concerns began to emerge among patients, surgeons, and government regulators regarding the potential disadvantages of

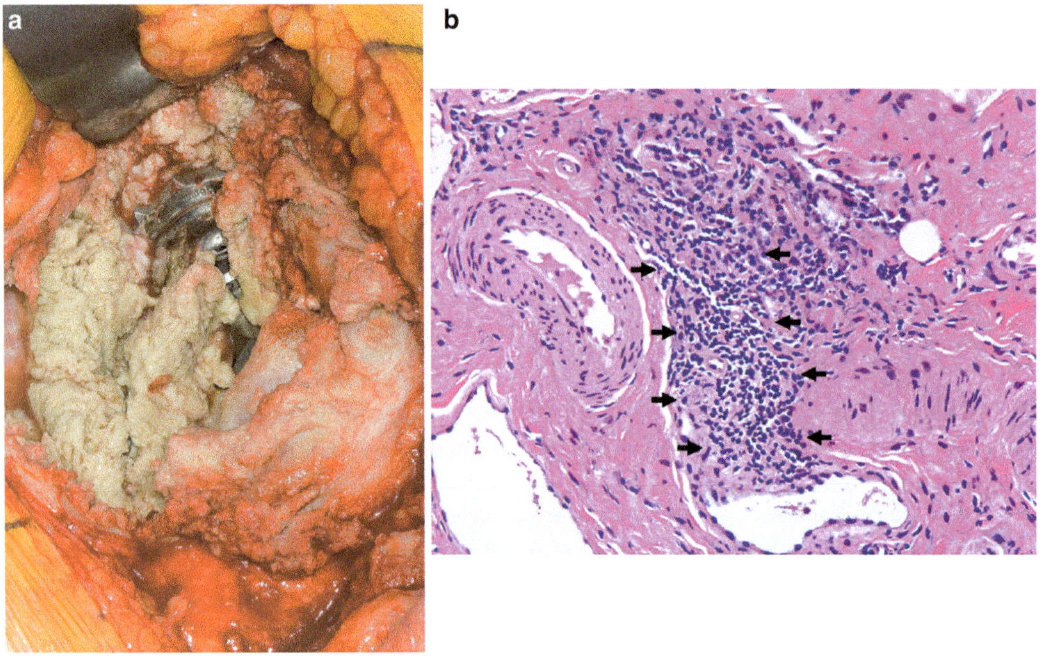

Fig. 80.4 Pathological examination of intraoperative tissue specimens revealed perivascular lymphocytic aggregates and chronic inflammation consistent with aseptic lymphocytic vasculitis-associated lesions (ALVAL)

MOM implants in both surface replacement and THA designs. Accounts of novel failure modes, pseudotumors, hypersensitivity reactions, and toxicity from metal ions were reported within the literature and the popular press [41, 42]. Metallic wear debris and high local tissue metal ion levels are believed to cause local soft tissue necrosis and response, which may lead to clinical symptoms and premature implant failure. Schmalzried [43] related adverse local tissue reaction (ALTR) to the spectrum of disease associated with metal allergy, lymphocytic infiltrates, metallosis, and pseudotumor formation (Fig. 80.4). Metallic wear debris and corrosion can lead to excessive serum ion concentrations of chromium and cobalt. Although some correlation between serum and synovial ion concentrations has been noted in failed arthroplasties, the relation between serum ion concentrations and bearing wear is less clear [44, 45]. Possible sources of metallic wear include cup malpositioning (e.g. >45° inclination and 20° anteversion), and very large or small diameter femoral heads, which can lead to changes in lubrication dynamics, edge loading, and increased wear against the acetabular rim [46, 47].

Another source of metal ions and debris is corrosion at the taper junction (also known as the trunnion-head interface) in modular femoral components. Adverse local tissue reactions can occur in patients with a metal-on-polyethylene bearing secondary to corrosion at the modular femoral head-neck taper, and clinical presentation is similar to the ALTR seen in patients with a failed MOM bearing. Elevated serum metal levels, particularly a differential elevation of serum cobalt levels with respect to chromium levels, can be helpful in establishing the diagnosis of corrosion related ALTR [48].

There are positive long-term studies on the durability and clinical outcomes of MOM hip arthroplasties in young active patients [49, 50]. These studies appear to show a superior implant survival rate compared to MOP and COC bearings. However, several systematic reviews show no significant difference between MOM and conventional THA with regard to functional outcomes as measured by Harris hip scores and radiographic outcomes. Patients with MOM THA did however demonstrate a 3.37 times greater complication rate [51, 52]. The most commonly reported complications were dislocation, aseptic loosening, trochanteric or iliopsoas bursitis, periprosthetic femoral fracture, and wound dehiscence. The two studies that measured metal ion concentrations found that patients receiving MOM articulations had significantly greater erythrocyte, serum, and urine metal ion concentrations compared with patients receiving conventional articulations [53, 54]. In light of the lack of clinical superiority, the increased complication rate, the greater cost, and the potential for adverse medical consequences associated with MOM THA, these bearing surfaces should be used with caution if at all [51]. Currently MOM modular THA has been largely abandoned with only a few isolated centers still performing MOM surface replacement selectively in younger, active males only.

Current recommendations for the thousands of patients with a THA and MOM bearing include yearly X-rays and measurements of serum ion concentrations and additional imaging of the symptomatic or painful hip joint to exclude a soft tissue mass and ALTR as the source of pain. Additional imaging of the soft tissues can be done with ultrasound, CT, or MRI. Ultrasound is a useful screening method, but its sensitivity decreases with very obese patients and it is less effective than CT or MRI at detection of posterior and medially located lesions. MRI studies performed with newer metal artifact reduction techniques (MARS-MRI) have been reported to have high sensitivity for detection of both soft tissue changes and osteolysis [55, 56].

Ceramic on Polyethylene (CoP)

A ceramic femoral head on a polyethylene acetabular liner has become one of the most common alternative bearing couples currently used in THA. According to recent data, there is a decline in the use of hard-on-hard bearing surfaces (MoM and CoC) in younger patients. Rajaee et al. shown that the use of MoP increased from 21.6 % of patients in 2006 to 25.2 % in 2009, while CoP increased from 13.5 % in 2007 to 25.7 % in 2009. This trend can be explained by efforts to find other acceptable durable bearings that do not have the potential problems associated with MoM or CoC, and also because some biomechanical studies reported that the crosslinked CoP combination showed a steady-state wear rate 40 % lower than that of the MoP couple [57]. Ceramic femoral heads have substantial tribologic advantages over metal femoral heads and result in lower wear rates. Some clinical studies have reported mean linear wear rates with ceramic on polyethylene are between 0.03 and 0.1 mm/year in patients followed for up to 18 years [58].

Recently the use of ceramic heads (vs. metal) against highly crosslinked polyethylene has been further enhanced by concerns about the potential for taper corrosion between Chrome-Cobalt metal heads and titanium cementless stems. Release of Chromium and Cobalt due to corrosion can be prevented by the use of ceramic heads on titanium stems. Not all reports on clinical results of ceramic on polyethylene have been supportive. In a recent publication comparing MoM arthroplasties with a historical control group of CoP after 13 years follow-up, Migaud et al. [59] reported a high rate of osteolysis (46 %) in the CoP group, but the polyethylene used was conventional PE. On the other hand Urban and coworkers in an 18.2 year follow-up study of CoP, showed that osteolysis was not encountered around any of the femoral or the acetabular components in their series [58].

Unfortunately, the data available regarding ceramic femoral heads with highly cross-linked polyethylene are limited [60, 61] by short follow-up. Garvin et al. in a 2-years follow-up study with of oxidized zirconium against a HXPLE liner, reported low linear wear. This fact is very encouraging for the continued study of this bearing couple. However, follow-up is required to determine the long-term clinical performance of HXLPE against ceramic heads.

Authors' Preferred Method of Implant in Young Patients

1. Fixation.
   - Cementless fixation preferred for both femoral stem and acetabular component fixation, with the exception.
   - Cemented Femoral Fixation for very poor bone quality, altered bone anatomy, and low activity level (i.e. selected inflammatory arthritis patients).
2. Implant Design.
   - Acetabular Component: Hemispherical, with a three dimensional ingrowth surface, and the option for multiple screw fixation.
   - Femoral Component: Multiple modern designs acceptable (surgeon preference) modified by and patient characteristics and anatomy, with a modular stem sometimes helpful to address major anatomic deformity or torsion as encountered in some hip dysplasia patients.
3. Bearing Choice.
   - Ultra young (<20 y/o): consider Ceramic-on-Ceramic.
   - 20–60 Years old: Ceramic on HXLPE.
   - >65 Years old: Ceramic (or metal) on HXLPE.
   - Selected "elderly": Cemented all polyethylene cups.
   - Metal-on-Metal—not used at this time.

Conclusions

At present, young patients undergoing THA can expect excellent clinical and radiographic survivorship over the first decade and potentially longer term as well. The use of new designs and component materials has dramatically improved implant longevity in active patients with end-stage hip disease. Now that cementless fixation is so successful, it is reasonable to ask: can alternative bearing surfaces provide a durable solution for many of our youngest and most active patients into the second and even third decade post-surgery and beyond? To address this question, data describing implant performance in young patients are needed from community-based sources, along with the more detailed long term data available from focused single institutional and multicenter studies. This is an important role for large regional and national registries in the future. It is now reasonable to expect these outcomes to both guide the selection of suitable treatment options and to serve as an indicator of the effectiveness of the implant designs and articulations that are currently available.

In the future, the goal of efforts to improve implant designs, especially for the young patient, should be continued optimization of what is already a highly evolved and successful procedure. Radically new designs or materials should not be introduced unless they clearly address a significant clinical or design problem, and then should not be used widely until validation has occurred via a step-wise process of design optimization, limited initial release, and careful study. Subsequent widespread general usage of those implants should be monitored via large national and regional registries. Increasingly in the future, registry based studies can serve to both facilitate pre-market approval and provide comprehensive post market surveillance of novel technology and designs, potentially reducing the delays and expense currently associated with their introduction.

Disclosures *Institutional Funding:*
Dr Lewallen: Institutional support: DePuy, Smith & Nephew, Stryker, Wright Medical, Zimmer
Dr Prieto: Nil
Dr Kamath: Nil

Conflict of Interest:
Dr Lewallen: Individual royalties: Pipeline/Mako/Zimmer
Consultant: Ketai Medical Devices, Zimmer
Dr Prieto: Nil
Dr Kamath: Nil

References

1. Chang RW, Pellisier JM, Hazen GB. A cost-effectiveness analysis of total hip arthroplasty for osteoarthritis of the hip. JAMA. 1996;20:858–65.
2. Ethgen O, Bruyère O, Richy F, Dardennes C, Reginster JY. Health-related quality of life in total hip and total knee arthroplasty. A qualitative and systematic review of the literature. J Bone Joint Surg Am. 2004;86:963–74.
3. Clohisy JC, Beaulé PE, O'Malley A, Safran MR, Schoenecker P. AOA symposium: hip disease in the young adult. Current concepts of etiology and surgical treatment. J Bone Joint Surg Am. 2008;90(10):2267–81.
4. Ganz R, Leunig M, Leunig-Ganz K, Harris WH. The etiology of osteoarthritis of the hip: an integrated mechanical concept. Clin Orthop Relat Res. 2008;466(2):264–72.
5. Berry DJ, Torchia ME, Klassen RA. The young patient. In: Morrey BF, editor. Joint replacement arthroplasty. 2nd ed. New York: Churchill Living-Stone; 1996. p. 1027.
6. Klassen RA, Parlasca RJ, Bianco AJ. Total joint arthroplasty: application in children and adolescent. Mayo Clin Proc. 1979;54:579.
7. Bilsel N, Gökçe A, Kesmezacar H, Mumcuoǧ lu E, Ozdoǧ an H. Long-term results of total hip arthroplasty inpatients with juvenile rheumatoid arthritis. Acta Orthop Traumatol Turc. 2008;42(2):119–24.
8. Polkowski GG, Callaghan JJ, Mont MA, Clohisy JC. Total hip arthroplasty in the very young patient. J Am Acad Orthop Surg. 2012;20(8):487–97.
9. Restrepo C, Lettich T, Roberts N, et al. Uncemented total hip arthroplasty in patients less than twenty-years. Acta Orthop Belg. 2008;74:615–22.
10. Girard J, Bocquet D, Autissier G, Fouilleron N, Fron D, Migaud H. Metal-on- metal hip arthroplasty in patients thirty years of age or younger. J Bone Joint Surg Am. 2010;92(14):2419–26.
11. Finkbone PR, Severson EP, Cabanela ME, Trousdale RT. Ceramic-on-ceramic total hip arthroplasty in patients younger than 20 years. J Arthroplasty. 2012;27(2):213–9.
12. Larson AN, McIntosh AM, Trousdale RT, Lewallen DG. Avascular necrosis most common indication for hip arthroplasty in patients with slipped capital femoral epiphysis. J Pediatr Orthop. 2010;30(8):767–73.
13. Howard JL, Kremers HM, Loechler YA, Schleck CD, Harmsen WS, Berry DJ, Cabanela ME, Hanssen AD, Pagnano MW, Trousdale RT, Lewallen DG. Comparative survival of uncemented acetabular components following primary total hip arthroplasty. J Bone Joint Surg Am. 2011;93(17):1597–604.
14. Clohisy, et al. Function and fixation of total hip arthroplasty. In patients 25 years of age or younger. Clin Orthop Relat Res. 2010;468:3207–13.
15. Wangen H, Lereim P, Holm I, et al. Hip arthroplasty in patients younger than 30 years: excellent ten to 16-year follow-up results with a HA-coated stem. Int Orthop. 2008;32:203.
16. Costa CR, Johnson AJ, Mont MA. Use of cementless, tapered femoral stems in patients who have a mean age of 20 years. J Arthroplasty. 2012;27(4):497–502.
17. Dorr LD, Kane III TJ, Conaty JP. Long-term results of cemented total hip arthroplasty in patients 45 years old or younger. A 16-year follow-up study. J Arthroplasty. 1994;9(5):453–6.
18. Kerboull L, Hamadouche M, Courpied JP, et al. Long-term results of Charnley-Kerboull hip arthroplasty in patients younger than 50 years. Clin Orthop. 2004;418:112–8.
19. Keener JD, Callaghan JJ, Goetz DD, et al. Twenty-five-year results after Charnley total hip arthroplasty in patients less than fifty years old: a concise follow-up of a previous report. J Bone Joint Surg. 2003;85A:1066–72.
20. Torchia ME, Klassen RA, Bianco AJ. Total hip arthroplasty with cement in patients less than twenty years old: long-term results. J Bone Joint Surg Am. 1996;78(7):995–1003.
21. Chmell MJ, Scott RD, Thomas WH, Sledge CB. Total hip arthroplasty with cement for juvenile rheumatoid arthritis: results at a minimum of ten years in patients less than thirty years old. J Bone Joint Surg Am. 1997;79(1):44–52.
22. Dumbleton JH, D'Antonio JA, Manley MT, Capello WN, Wang A. The basis for a second-generation highly cross-linked UHMWPE. Clin Orthop Relat Res. 2006;453:265–71.
23. Callaghan JJ, Cuckler JM, Huddleston JI, Galante JO, Implant Wear Symposium 2007 Clinical Work Group. How have alternative bearings (such as metal-onmetal, highly cross-linked polyethylene, and ceramic-on-ceramic) affected the prevention and treatment of osteolysis? J Am Acad Orthop Surg. 2008;16 Suppl 1:S33–8.
24. Hermida JC, Bergula A, Chen P, Colwell Jr CW, D'Lima DD. Comparison of the wear rates of twenty-eight and thirty-two-millimeter femoral heads on crosslinked polyethylene acetabular cups in a wear simulator. J Bone Joint Surg Am. 2003;85:2325–31.
25. Thomas GER, Simpson DJ, Mehmood S, Taylor A, McLardy-Smith P, Gill HS, Murray DW, Glyn-Jones S. The seven-year wear of highly cross-linked polyethylene in total hip arthroplasty: a double-blind, randomized controlled trial using radiostereometric analysis. J Bone Joint Surg Am. 2011;93(8):716–22.
26. Jacobs CA, Christensen CP, Greenwald AS, McKellop H. Clinical performance of highly cross-linked polyethylenes in total hip arthroplasty. J Bone Joint Surg Am. 2007;89:2779–86. Erratum in: J Bone Joint Surg Am 2008;90:628.

27. Oral E, Wannomae KK, Hawkins N, Harris WH, Muratoglu OK. Alphatocopherol-doped irradiated UHMWPE for high fatigue resistance and low wear. Biomaterials. 2004;25:5515–22.
28. D'Antonio JA, Capello WN, Ramakrishnan R. Second-generation annealed highly cross-linked polyethylene exhibits low wear. Clin Orthop Relat Res. 2012;470(6):1696–704.
29. Dorlot JM, Christel P, Meunier A. Wear analysis of retrieved alumina heads and sockets of hip prosthesis. J Biomed Mater Res. 1989;23(A3 suppl):299.
30. Skinner HB. Ceramic bearing surfaces. Clin Orthop Relat Res. 1999;369:83.
31. Christel PS. Biocompatibility of surgical-grade dense polycrystalline alumina. Clin Orthop Relat Res. 1992;282:10.
32. Murphy SB, et al. Experience in the United States with alumina ceramic–ceramic total hip arthroplasty. Semin Arthro. 2006;17:120–4. Elsevier Inc.
33. D'Antonio JA, Pagnano MW, Naughton M, Lombardi Jr AV, Berend KR, Skeels MD, Franchi OJ, Backstein D. Controversies regarding bearing surfaces in total hip replacement. J Bone Joint Surg Am. 2009;91 Suppl 5:5–9.
34. Hannouche D, Nich C, Bizot P, Meunier A, Nizard R, Sedel L. Fractures of ceramic bearings: history and present status. Clin Orthop Relat Res. 2003;417:19–26.
35. Restrepo C, Parvizi J, Kurtz SM, Sharkey PF, Hozack WJ, Rothman RH. The noisy ceramic hip: is component malpositioning the cause? J Arthroplasty. 2008;23:643.
36. Ranawat AS, Ranawat CS. The squeaking hip: a cause for concern-agrees. Orthopaedics. 2007;30:738, 743.
37. Chevillotte C, Trousdale RT, Chen Q, Guyen O, An KN. The 2009 Frank Stinchfield Award: "Hip squeaking": a biomechanical study of ceramic-on-ceramic bearing surfaces. Clin Orthop Relat Res. 2010;468(2):345–50.
38. McKee GK, Watson-Farrar J. Replacement of arthritic hips by the McKee-Farrar prosthesis. J Bone Joint Surg Br. 1966;48:245.
39. Ring PA. Complete replacement arthroplasty of the hip by the ring prosthesis. J Bone Joint Surg Br. 1968;50:720.
40. Clarke IC, Good V, Williams P, et al. Ultra-low wear rates for rigid-on-rigid bearings in total hip replacements. Proc Inst Mech Eng H. 2000;214:331.
41. United States Food and Drug Administration. Metal-on-metal implants. 2011. http://www.fda.gov/MedicalDevices/ProductsandMedicalProcedures/ImplantsandProsthetics/MetalonMetalHipImplants/default.htm. Accessed 30 Dec 2011.
42. Medicines and Healthcare Products Regulatory Agency. Medical device alert: all metal-on-metal (MoM) hip replacements. 2010. http://www.mhra.gov.uk/home/groups/dts-bs/documents/medicaldevicealert/con079162.pdf. Accessed 30 Dec 2011.
43. Schmalzried TP. Metal-metal bearing surfaces in hip arthroplasty. Orthopaedics. 2009;32:661.
44. De Smet K, De Haan R, Calistri A, et al. Metal ion measurement as a diagnostic tool to identify problems with metal-on-metal hip resurfacing. J Bone Joint Surg Am. 2008;90 suppl 4:202–8.
45. Jacobs JJ, Skipor AK, Campbell PA, Hallab NJ, Urban RM, Amstutz HC. Can metal levels be used to monitor metal-on-metal hip arthroplasties? J Arthroplasty. 2004;19 Suppl 3:59–65.
46. Ebramzadeh E, Campbell PA, Takamura KM, et al. Failure modes of 433 metal-on-metal hip implants: how, why, and wear. Orthop Clin North Am. 2011;42:241–50.
47. De Haan R, Pattyn C, Gill HS, Murray DW, Campbell PA, De Smet K. Correlation between inclination of the acetabular component and metal ion levels in metal-on-metal hip resurfacing replacement. J Bone Joint Surg Br. 2008;90:1291–7.
48. Cooper HJ, Della Valle CJ, Berger RA, Tetreault M, Paprosky WJ, Sporer SM, Jacobs JJ. Corrosion at the head-neck taper as a cause for adverse local tissue reactions after total hip arthroplasty. J Bone Joint Surg Am. 2012;94:1655–61.
49. Shetty V, Shitole B, Shetty G, Thakur H, Bhandar M. Optimal bearing surfaces for total hip replacement in the young patient: a meta-analysis. Int Orthop. 2011;35:1281–7.
50. Eswaramoorthy V, Moonot P, Kalairajah Y, et al. The Metasul metal-on-metal articulation in primary total hip replacement: clinical and radiological results at ten years. J Bone Joint Surg Br. 2008;90:1278.
51. Voleti PB, Baldwin KD, Lee GC. Metal-on-metal vs conventional total hip arthroplasty a systematic review and meta-analysis of randomized controlled trials. J Arthroplasty. 2012;27(10):1844–9.
52. Qu X, Huang X, Dai K. Metal-on-metal or metal-on-polyethylene for total hip arthroplasty: a meta-analysis of prospective randomized studies. Arch Orthop Trauma Surg. 2011;131:1573–83.
53. Zijlstra WP, Van Raay JJ, Bulstra SK, et al. No superiority of cemented metal-on-metal over metal-on-polyethylene THA in a randomized controlled trial at 10-year follow-up. Orthopaedics. 2010;33:154.
54. MacDonald SJ, McCalden RW, Chess DG, et al. Metal-onmetal versus polyethylene in hip arthroplasty: a randomized clinical trial. Clin Orthop Relat Res. 2003;406:282.
55. Hayter CL, Gold SL, Koff MF, Perino G, Nawabi DH, Miller TT, Potter HG. MRI findings in painful metal-on-metal hip arthroplasty. Am J Roentgenol. 2012;199(4):884–93.
56. Ostlere S. How to image metal-on-metal prostheses and their complications. Am J Roentgenol. 2011;197:558–67.
57. Galvin AL, Jennings LM, Tipper JL, Ingham E, Fisher J. Wear and creep of highly crosslinked polyethylene against cobalt chrome and ceramic femoral heads. Proc Inst Mech Eng H. 2010;224(10):1175–83.
58. Urban JA, Garvin KL, Boese CK, Bryson L, Pedersen DR, Callaghan JJ, Miller RK. Ceramic-on-polyethylene bearing surfaces in total hip arthroplasty: seventeen to twenty-one-year results. J Bone Joint Surg Am. 2001;83-A(11):1688–94.
59. Migaud H, Putman S, Krantz N, Vasseur L, Girard J. Cementless metal-on-metal versus ceramic-on-polyethylene hip arthroplasty in patients less than fifty years of age: a comparative study with twelve to fourteen-year follow-up. J Bone Joint Surg Am. 2011;93 Suppl 2:137–42.
60. Garvin KL, Hartman CW, Mangla J, Murdoch N, Martell JM. Wear analysis in THA utilizing oxidized zirconium and crosslinked polyethylene [published online ahead of print October 23, 2008]. Clin Orthop Relat Res. 2009;467(1):141–5.
61. Meftah M, Ebrahimpour PB, He C, Ranawat AS, Ranawat CS. Preliminary clinical and radiographic results of large ceramic heads on highly cross-linked polyethylene. Orthopaedics. 2011;34(6):e133–7.

Short-Stem Total Hip Replacement

81

Carl C. Berasi IV and Adolph V. Lombardi Jr

Introduction

Originally created with the intention of better replicating physiologic loading of the femur while preserving bone stock, short-stem prostheses have become increasingly popular in total hip arthroplasty. The shorter stem is touted to provide excellent proximal purchase irrespective of distal femoral morphology, and greater ease of insertion when used in conjunction with smaller incisions and technically demanding surgical approaches. These factors, combined with the bone- and soft tissue-sparing nature of a smaller prosthesis, make short stems an attractive option for investigation in both young and old patients.

Background

First-generation short-stemmed femoral components were introduced in the 1970s–1980s, with Pipino implanting the first Biodynamic hip prosthesis (Howmedica, now Stryker) in 1979 [1], followed by Morrey's introduction of the Mayo Conservative Hip (Zimmer) shortly thereafter [2]. Since that time many other short-stemmed prostheses have been introduced, with each new prosthesis claiming improvement over prior designs. These short stems rely on purchase in the metaphyseal or neck region for implant fixation, and have reduced proximal bulk compared to their standard-length counterparts to enable insertion with less bone resection. This would preserve more bone at the time of the index procedure, allowing for greater bone stock availability in the event that a revision procedure became necessary. Proponents of these devices have theorized that more proximal fixation would result in more physiologic loading and thus less adverse remodeling of the proximal femur. These conservative alternatives served to fill the gap between standard-length prostheses and hip-resurfacing prostheses, preserving greater bone stock than standard-length stems while also providing more extensive fixation than resurfacing prostheses and the option of bearing surfaces other than metal-on-metal.

Design

A number of short-stem designs have been introduced since the days of the Biodynamic and the Mayo Conservative Hip. These conservative implants may be roughly separated into four groups based on design philosophy, although a considerable amount of overlap exists: (1) implants influenced by the Mayo Conservative Hip (Zimmer, Warsaw, IN). This design employs a double-tapered wedge with a trapezoidal cross section to achieve multiple points of contact in the proximal femur and lateral femoral cortex, resulting in rotatory stability and limitation of varus-valgus malpositioning [2, 3]; (2) short and bulky stems that are not neck sparing (Proxima, Depuy, Warsaw, IN). These metaphyseal-filling designs have a prominent lateral flare intended to better engage the lateral femoral cortex, minimizing both implant subsidence and stress shielding of the proximal femur [4]; (3) neck-sparing curved designs such as the collum femoris-preserving (CFP) prosthesis (Waldemar Link, Hamburg, Germany). Neck-sparing prostheses rely heavily on the intrinsic ability of the femoral neck and adjoining medial calcar region to transfer load distally, and preserve the circumflex femoral vessels supplying the neck [5–7]; and (4) shortened tapered stems (Taperloc Microplasty, Biomet, Warsaw, IN). Short, tapered stems achieve proximal

C.C. Berasi IV, MD
Riverside Methodist Hospital, 1788 Strathshire Hall Place, Powell, OH 43065, USA
e-mail: carl.berasi4@gmail.com

A.V. Lombardi Jr, MD, FACS (✉)
Joint Implant Surgeons, Inc., 7277 Smith's Mill Road, Suite 200, New Albany, OH 43054, USA

Mount Carmel Health System, 7277 Smith's Mill Road, Suite 200, New Albany, OH 43054, USA

Department of Orthopaedics, The Ohio State University, 7277 Smith's Mill Road, Suite 200, New Albany, OH 43054, USA
e-mail: lombardiav@joint-surgeons.com

J.C. McCarthy et al. (eds.), *Hip Joint Restoration*, DOI 10.1007/978-1-4614-0694-5_81

fixation while requiring less violation of diaphyseal bone than their standard-length predecessors, and experience has shown that tapered prostheses perform well even when placed in varus [8, 9]. Other implants, such as the tapered, straight stem Silent (Depuy, Warsaw, IN), fall outside our categorization. This particularly minimalist neck-preserving design requires little more bone removal than resurfacing prostheses such as the Birmingham Mid-Head Resection (Smith and Nephew Orthopaedics Ltd, Bromsgrove, UK), while providing surgeons with their choice of bearing surface.

Technical Considerations

Regardless of the particular design, short stems may be utilized in all the same surgical approaches currently in use for standard-length prostheses. Short stems are especially attractive options for tissue-sparing approaches and smaller incisions, where their geometries allow for greater ease of insertion than that encountered with a standard stem. Femoral preparation can often be accomplished with broach-only technique, obviating the need for reaming of the canal and potentially reducing blood loss and the occurrence of microemboli [3, 10]. When implanting these devices, care must be taken to ensure proper femoral neck resection, as the level of resection may differ considerably from that utilized in standard prostheses, and to achieve adequate seating of the device within the metaphysis. This is increasingly important as smaller and smaller prostheses are used; the smaller geometry results in greater load transferred to the surrounding bone, potentially increasing the risk of fracture or component migration [11]. Short stems may be particularly advantageous in situations where longer stems cannot be easily placed. These include metaphyseal-diaphyseal morphology mismatch, prior trauma, excessive femoral bowing, diaphyseal deformity, and preexisting hardware.

Patient Selection

Patient selection for conservative stems is based on several considerations. Short stems were originally designed to optimize loading of the femur and maximize bone stock available for future revisions. These characteristics have made them attractive options for younger patients requiring total hip arthroplasty. In older patients short stems are attractive because of their ease of use with less invasive surgical approaches, and their bone- and soft tissue-sparing qualities; however, smaller implant profiles place greater reliance on bone quality in order to achieve adequate fixation. Therefore, short stems should be used with caution in patients with conditions that may compromise bone quality, such as metabolic bone disease, advanced osteoporosis, or extended inactivity. While generally not viewed as absolute contraindications to the use of short stems, care must be taken to ensure adequate fixation in these settings.

In selecting the appropriate size of a short-stemmed design, some authors recommend upsizing the femoral component to achieve more reliable fixation [12, 13]. Measurements such as the caput-collum-diaphyseal (CCD) angle and the cortical index (cortical index $=(10\times(a-b))/a$, where a is the outer diameter of the femur and b is the inner diameter of the medullary cavity 10 cm below the level of the lesser trochanter), have been used to determine inclusion/exclusion criteria [13, 14]. It is advisable that a standard-length stem be available should exceptionally poor bone quality be discovered intraoperatively. Also, due to the metaphyseal loading of these implants, they are not advised in cases in which the metaphyseal-diaphyseal junction has been compromised by prior trauma or instrumentation.

Outcomes

Short- and medium-term results with short stems in total hip arthroplasty have largely been favorable, with a few notable exceptions (Table 81.1). Experience with the Mayo Conservative Hip has demonstrated excellent medium-term results, with multiple authors reporting greater than 95 % stem survival [3, 15]. Excellent fixation with this prosthesis has been achieved even after intraoperative fracture [16]. The CFP has also been extensively reported in the literature, with greater than 95 % survival achieved out to a mean follow-up of 6.8 years [17–20]. Likewise, promising results have also been seen with the Proxima [10, 21], Metha (B. Braun-Aesculap, Tuttlingen, Germany) [22, 23], Special Prosthesis from Symbios (SPS; Symbios, Yverdon-les-Bains, Switzerland) [24], Citation (Stryker, Stryker Orthopaedics, Mahwah, NJ) [25], Nanos (Smith and Nephew, Marl, Germany) [26], and Global Tissue Sparing (GTS; Biomet, Warsaw, IN) [27]. Widely variable results have been reported with the use of the Cut prosthesis (ESKA Implants, Lübeck, Germany), with survival rates ranging from 98 % at 6.6 years to 49.6 % at 8 years [28–30]. Ishaque et al. describe an alarming rate of aseptic loosening of the Cut prosthesis, with subsequent valgus migration of the stem and loss of femoral offset [29], as well as reported a case of implant fracture related to fatigue [31]. Other designs are not immune from component failure; Haasper et al. reported two traumatic implant fractures while using the CFP prosthesis [32], and Grupp et al. described failure of the titanium alloy neck-stem adapter in the Metha prosthesis, spurring a change in composition of the adapter to cobalt-chromium [33].

Table 81.1 Summary of experience with selected short-stem designs

Prosthesis	Stem length (mm)	Author	Follow-up (years)[a]	No. of hips	Stem revisions	Age[a]
Mayo Conservative Hip (Zimmer)	81–107	[3]	6.2 (2–13)	159	15	51 (19–72)
–	–	[15]	4.7 (1–7)	160	4	63 (42–83)
CFP (Waldemar Link)	82–135	[19]	3.2	138	1	57 (22–76)
–	–	[20]	5.5 ± 1.7	150	0	67 ± 9
–	–	[18]	6.8 (6.1–7.4)	50	1	58 (36–82)
–	–	[17]	6.2 (4.3–7.8)	155	1	59 (27–77)
Cut (ESKA Implants)		[30]	5.4 (1.7–6.4)	99	2	50 (17–72)
–	–	[29]	8	82	31	51
–	–	[28]	5 (3–7)	123	13	53 (32–69)
Metha (B. Braun-Aesculap)	102.5–122.5	[22]	2.8 (1.1–5)	73	3	49 (17–67)
–	–	[23]	4.9 (2.9–7.1)	204	18[b]	60 (27–73)
Proxima (Depuy)		[21]	2.1 (1.1–3.7)	41	0	49 (35–60)
–	–	[10]	4.1 (2–5)	70	0	75 (50–94)
SPS (Symbios)	116–155	[24]	10 (8–11)	131	1	73 (35–83)
TaperLoc Microplasty (Biomet)	95–135	[39]	2.2 (0.1–5.2)	269	1	63 (27–91)
Citation (Stryker)	90–105	[25]	2.9 (2–5.2)	160	0	65 (29–86)
Nanos (Smith and Nephew)		[26]	5.2 ± 0.7	72	0	63 ± 8
GTS (Biomet)	94–140	[27]	1.3 (0.5–2)	81	0	65 (43–78)

[a]Values expressed as average (range), or average ± standard deviation
[b]9 of 18 stem revisions due to failure of the neck-stem adapter

It is also important to judge the ability of short-stem prostheses to meet their initial goals: namely greater preservation of bone stock in the event of revision and more physiologic loading of the proximal femur. Experience has shown that in many cases adequate bone stock is available to allow for the use of standard stems, or possibly even less conservative short stems, in the revision of these short-stem prostheses [15, 25, 31]. With regard to the goal of more physiologic loading, results have been variable. Experience with the Mayo Conservation Hip has been favorable, demonstrating reduced bone loss when compared to standard-length counterparts [34, 35]. Lerch et al. examined bone remodeling in patients who had received the Metha prosthesis. They concluded that the prosthesis was partially effective in achieving proximal load transfer; with significant increases in bone mineral density (BMD) in the calcar region and the lesser trochanter, and a concomitant loss of bone density in the greater trochanter [36]. Analyses of the CFP prosthesis revealed significant loss in BMD in the metaphyseal region in well-fixed components, suggesting that stability was primarily achieved through diaphyseal, rather than metaphyseal, fixation [37, 38]. Additional benefits described with the use of shorter stems have included a significant reduction in intraoperative complications (0.4 %) as compared to standard-length stems (0.4 % vs.3.1 %) [39], and a lower incidence of thigh pain [10].

Authors' Experience

Implant

The senior author has extensive experience with the Taperloc Microplasty prosthesis. This system is based on a flat tapered wedge design for rotational stability and enhanced proximal offloading, with a collarless stem to allow for self-seating. The prosthesis is manufactured from forged titanium alloy (Ti-6AL-4 V), and has a circumferential porous plasma spray coating on the proximal two-thirds of the component. Stems are available in 13 sizes, with diameters ranging from 5 to 25 mm and lengths ranging from 95 to 135 mm. All stems have a neck-shaft angle of 138° and the option of either standard or lateralized offset. Lateralization is accomplished by a constant 7.8 mm medial shift of the trunnion. Design changes were made in late 2011 (TaperLoc Microplasty Complete), including a reduction in the neck-shaft angle to 133°, the addition of polished extended anteroposterior neck flats, a smooth distal transition, and a modified insertion hole. With the smooth distal transition, a gradual reduction of the stem substrate occurs distal to the porous coating level. The reduced distal geometry increases the proximal fill of the implant without distal impingement. The TaperLoc is a broach-only system, and requires no reaming aside from a single starting reamer.

81.1.1 Surgical Technique

The senior author has used a less invasive modification of the direct lateral approach (LIDL) for more than a decade [40], and has transitioned to using a muscle-sparing direct anterior approach (ASI). The LIDL approach utilizes an approximately 10–12 cm oblique incision centered over the tip of the greater trochanter, running from postero-proximal to antero-distal. The fascia lata is incised in line with the skin incision, with minimal dissection of subcutaneous tissues to minimize dead space. Beginning at the vastus ridge, the anterior portions of the gluteus medius and vastus lateralis are elevated off the greater trochanter using electrocautery. The gluteus medius is bluntly dissected in line with its fibers at an angle of 45° antero-proximally, and the dissection extended 3–4 cm. The vastus lateralis is then split distally between its anterior and middle one-thirds, allowing for a continuous sleeve to be elevated off the anterior femur. A blunt Hohmann retractor is placed deep to the gluteus medius, exposing the gluteus minimus and anterior hip capsule. The capsule is incised along the superior aspect of the femoral neck, corresponding to the 1 o'clock position in a right hip. The femoral head is then resected, and standard femoral and acetabular preparations performed. The ASI approach is performed using fluoroscopic guidance with the patient positioned supine on a standard, radiolucent operating table with ischial tuberosities aligned at the table break. The incision commences from approximately 2 cm distal and 2 cm lateral to the anterior superior iliac spine and extends 10 cm distally toward the knee. The exposed tensor fascia lata muscle is dissected bluntly down to the capsule. The junction between the rectus and capsule is identified and the circumflex vessels are electrocauterized. Femoral neck resection is based on preoperative templating and is confirmed with fluoroscopy. The acetabulum is prepared first. After insertion of the acetabular component, retractors are removed, the foot of the bed is dropped, and the patient is placed in Trendelenburg. Femoral preparation is facilitated with the use of a table-mounted hook placed around the proximal femur just proximal to the gluteal sling. The anterior capsule is released from the trochanter, the knee is flexed, the hip is extended and externally rotated, then traction is applied with the hook, and the proximal femur is lifted out of the wound. With either approach the surgeon should be aggressive when sizing the implant, as the senior author has found that an implant 1–2 sizes larger than a standard-length version of the stem is typically required. To avoid varus positioning, the prosthesis should be driven into valgus during insertion. The component has a tendency to sit more proximally than the broach and may require additional effort to seat completely.

Postoperative Protocol

Postoperative pain is managed with a multimodal regimen and a rapid-recovery protocol is employed to mobilize patients as quickly as possible [41]. Patients are allowed full weight bearing as tolerated with a walker or crutches immediately postoperatively, and are advised to discontinue support devices when they are comfortable to do so. No hip precautions are given.

Results

From January 2006 through April 2013 the senior author and two of his partners performed 2456 total hip arthroplasties in 2094 patients using Taperloc Microplasty and TaperLoc Complete Microplasty prostheses. The procedure was performed through the direct lateral approach (LIDL) (1194; 49 %), a muscle-sparing anterior supine intermuscular approach (ASI; 1117; 46 %), or a standard direct lateral approach (SDL, 146; 6 %). There were 954 males (46 %) and 1140 females (54 %). The average patient age was 63.6 years (SD 11.7, range 26–96) and average body mass index was 30.6 kg/m^2 (SD 6.9, range 17–62). Charnley classification was A in 1212 hips (49 %), B in 782 (32 %), and C in 462 (19 %). The most common underlying diagnoses were osteoarthritis (2173 hips; 88 %), avascular necrosis (152; 6 %), developmental dysplasia (48; 2 %), posttraumatic arthritis (27; 1 %), and rheumatoid arthritis (23; 1 %). TaperLoc Complete Microplasty stems were used in 576 hips (23 %). Increased horizontal offset options were used in 81 % (1990 hips). Stem length averaged 108.2 mm (SD 6.5, range 95–132).

Average follow-up was 32 months (0–111). Survival was 98.4 % at 2.7 years with an endpoint of stem revision for any reason. Thirty-nine stems have been revised (1.6 %), 16 for infection (12 LIDL, 3 ASI, 1 SDL), 13 for periprosthetic fracture (12 ASI, 1 SDL), 2 for early subsidence (1 LIDL, 1 ASI), 4 for aseptic loosening (3 LIDL, 1 ASI), 1 for patellar dislocation at 3 days postoperative (LIDL), 1 for intraoperative perforation of the femoral shaft revised immediately (SDL), 1 well-fixed stem removed for inability to disarticulate the trunnion during removal of a loose acetabular component, and 1 revised elsewhere for pain of unknown etiology. Conservatively treated complications included three periprosthetic fractures (all ASI), two instances of initial subsidence (one ASI, one SDL), and an additional case of periprosthetic fracture (ASI) treated with ORIF.

Conclusion

Short-stem total hip replacement came about through the continual effort to improve patient outcomes in what is already considered one of the most successful medical procedures. These prostheses seek to optimize loading of the femur while maximizing bone stock available for future revision surgery. With the increasing adoption of less invasive surgical approaches, short stems have become increasingly popular choices for total hip replacement in patients of all ages. At early follow-up the results of short-stem prostheses have largely been promising. As with any innovation, longer follow-up is needed to determine if short-stem total hip replacement will be successful at medium- and long-term follow-up.

References

1. Pipino F, Calderale PM. Biodynamic total hip prosthesis. Ital J Orthop Traumatol. 1987;13(3):289–97.
2. Morrey BF. Short-stemmed uncemented femoral component for primary hip arthroplasty. Clin Orthop Relat Res. 1989;249:169–75.
3. Morrey BF, Adams RA, Kessler M. A conservative femoral replacement for total hip arthroplasty. A prospective study. J Bone Joint Surg (Br). 2000;82(7):952–8.
4. Renkawitz T, Santori FS, Grifka J, Valverde C, Morlock MM, Learmonth ID. A new short uncemented, proximally fixed anatomic femoral implant with a prominent lateral flare:design rationals and study design of an international clinical trial. BMC Musculoskelet Disord. 2008;9:147.
5. Whiteside LA, White SE, McCarthy DS. Effect of neck resection on torsional stability of cementless total hip replacement. Am J Orthop. 1995;24(10):766–70.
6. Pipino F, Keller A. Tissue-sparing surgery: 25 years' experience with femoral neck preserving hip arthroplasty. J Orthop Traumatol. 2006;7(1):36–41 (2006/03/01).
7. Freeman MA. Why resect the neck? J Bone Joint Surg (Br). 1986;68(3):346–9.
8. Khalily C, Lester DK. Results of a tapered cementless femoral stem implanted in varus. J Arthroplasty. 2002;17(4):463–6.
9. Berend KR, Mallory TH, Lombardi Jr AV, Dodds KL, Adams JB. Tapered cementless femoral stem: difficult to place in varus but performs well in those rare cases. Orthopedics. 2007;30(4):295–7.
10. Kim YH, Oh JH. A comparison of a conventional versus a short, anatomical metaphyseal-fitting cementless femoral stem in the treatment of patients with a fracture of the femoral neck. J Bone Joint Surg (Br). 2012;94(6):774–81.
11. Bishop NE, Burton A, Maheson M, Morlock MM. Biomechanics of short hip endoprostheses--the risk of bone failure increases with decreasing implant size. Clin Biomech. 2010;25(7):666–74.
12. Lombardi AV, Jr., Berend KR, Adams JB. A short stem solution: through small portals. Orthopedics. 2009;32(9).
13. Tóth K, Sohár G. Short-Stem Hip Arthroplasty. Arthroplasty - Update. In: Plamen Kinov, Editors, InTech. 2013. Available from: http://www.intechopen.com/books/arthroplasty-update/short-stem-hip-arthroplasty.
14. Silent™ Hip Surgical Technique Manual: Depuy International Ltd; 2009. Available from: http://www.depuy.com/sites/default/files/products/files/9476-58-000-v1-Silent-Surgical-Technique_EN.pdf.
15. Falez F, Casella F, Panegrossi G, Favetti F, Barresi C. Perspectives on metaphyseal conservative stems. J Orthop Traumatol. 2008;9(1):49–54.
16. Zeh A, Radetzki F, Diers V, Bach D, Rollinghoff M, Delank KS. Is there an increased stem migration or compromised osteointegration of the Mayo short-stemmed prosthesis following cerclage wiring of an intrasurgical periprosthetic fracture? Arch Orthop Trauma Surg. 2011;131(12):1717–22.
17. Briem D, Schneider M, Bogner N, Botha N, Gebauer M, Gehrke T, et al. Mid-term results of 155 patients treated with a collum femoris preserving (CFP) short stem prosthesis. Int Orthop. 2011;35(5):655–60.
18. Nowak M, Nowak TE, Schmidt R, Forst R, Kress AM, Mueller LA. Prospective study of a cementless total hip arthroplasty with a collum femoris preserving stem and a trabeculae oriented pressfit cup: minimun 6-year follow-up. Arch Orthop Trauma Surg. 2011;131(4):549–55.
19. Pons M. Learning curve and short-term results with a short-stem CFP system. Hip Int. 2010;20 Suppl 7:S52–7.
20. Ghera S, Bisicchia S. The collum femoris preserving stem: early results. Hip Int. 2013;23(1):27–32.
21. Toth K, Mecs L, Kellermann P. Early experience with the Depuy Proxima short stem in total hip arthroplasty. Acta Orthop Belg. 2010;76(5):613–8.
22. Floerkemeier T, Tscheuschner N, Calliess T, Ezechieli M, Floerkemeier S, Budde S, et al. Cementless short stem hip arthroplasty METHA® as an encouraging option in adults with osteonecrosis of the femoral head. Arch Orthop Trauma Surg. 2012;132(8):1125–31.
23. Wittenberg RH, Steffen R, Windhagen H, Bücking P, Wilcke A. Five-year results of a cementless short-hip-stem prosthesis. Orthop Rev. 2013;5(1):16–22.
24. Sariali E, Mouttet A, Mordasini P, Catonne Y. High 10-year survival rate with an anatomic cementless stem (SPS). Clin Orthop Relat Res. 2012;470(7):1941–9.
25. Patel RM, Smith MC, Woodward CC, Stulberg SD. Stable fixation of short-stem femoral implants in patients 70 years and older. Clin Orthop Relat Res. 2012;470(2):442–9.
26. Ettinger M, Ettinger P, Lerch M, Radtke K, Budde S, Ezechieli M, et al. The NANOS short stem in total hip arthroplasty: a mid term follow-up. Hip Int. 2011;21(5):583–6.
27. Morales de Cano JJ, Gordo C, Illobre JM. Early clinical results of a new conservative hip stem. Eur J Orthop Surg Traumatol. 2014; 24(3):359–63.
28. Ender SA, Machner A, Pap G, Hubbe J, Grashoff H, Neumann HW. Cementless CUT femoral neck prosthesis: increased rate of aseptic loosening after 5 years. Acta Orthop. 2007;78(5):616–21.
29. Ishaque BA, Donle E, Gils J, Wienbeck S, Basad E, Sturz H. Eight-year results of the femoral neck prosthesis ESKA-CUT. Z Orthop Unfall. 2009;147(2):158–65.
30. Steens W, Skripitz R, Schneeberger AG, Petzing I, Simon U, Goetze C. Cementless femoral neck prosthesis CUT--clinical and radiological results after 5 years. Z Orthop Unfall. 2010;148(4):413–9.
31. Ishaque BA, Sturz H, Basad E. Fatigue fracture of a short stem hip replacement: a failure analysis with electron microscopy and review of the literature. J Arthroplasty. 2011;26(4):665 e17–20.
32. Haasper C, Kendoff D, Gebauer M, Zahar A, Kreibich T, Suero E, et al. Traumatic stem fractures in short stem THA-A rare case series. HSS Jrnl. 2013;9(1):86–9. 2013/02/01.
33. Grupp TM, Weik T, Bloemer W, Knaebel HP. Modular titanium alloy neck adapter failures in hip replacement--failure mode analysis and influence of implant material. BMC Musculoskelet Disord. 2010;11:3.
34. Boyle C, Kim IY. Comparison of different hip prosthesis shapes considering micro-level bone remodeling and stress-shielding criteria using three-dimensional design space topology optimization. J Biomech. 2011;44(9):1722–8.
35. Chen HH, Morrey BF, An KN, Luo ZP. Bone remodeling characteristics of a short-stemmed total hip replacement. J Arthroplasty. 2009;24(6):945–50.

36. Lerch M, von der Haar-Tran A, Windhagen H, Behrens BA, Wefstaedt P, Stukenborg-Colsman CM. Bone remodelling around the Metha short stem in total hip arthroplasty: a prospective dual-energy X-ray absorptiometry study. Int Orthop. 2012;36(3):533–8.
37. Kress AM, Schmidt R, Nowak TE, Nowak M, Haeberle L, Forst R, et al. Stress-related femoral cortical and cancellous bone density loss after collum femoris preserving uncemented total hip arthroplasty: a prospective 7-year follow-up with quantitative computed tomography. Arch Orthop Trauma Surg. 2012;132(8):1111–9.
38. Lazarinis S, Mattsson P, Milbrink J, Mallmin H, Hailer NP. A prospective cohort study on the short collum femoris-preserving (CFP) stem using RSA and DXA. Primary stability but no prevention of proximal bone loss in 27 patients followed for 2 years. Acta Orthop. 2013;84(1):32–9.
39. Molli RG, Lombardi Jr AV, Berend KR, Adams JB, Sneller MA. A short tapered stem reduces intraoperative complications in primary total hip arthroplasty. Clin Orthop Relat Res. 2012;470(2):450–61.
40. Berend KR, Lombardi AV. Total hip arthroplasty via the less invasive anterolateral abductor splitting approach. Sem Arthroplasty. 2004;15(2):87–93.
41. Lombardi AV, Berend KR, Adams JB. A rapid recovery program: early home and pain free. Orthopedics. 2010;33(9):656.

82 Hip Replacement in the Athlete

Fintan Doyle and Matthew J. Wilson

Introduction

John Charnley's seminal paper [1] in 1961 marked the dawn of the age of the modern total hip arthroplasty (THA). The main indication for replacement surgery at that time was debilitating hip pain secondary to degenerative disease. It is unlikely that he could have foreseen the advances in technology, the improvement in the general population's health and life expectancy and most importantly the change that has occurred in patient's expectations. Today, the desire to return to athletic activity is recognised as an indication for total hip replacement. However, in Charnley's time, patients presenting for THA in their 70s had already surpassed the average UK life expectancy [2] and therefore their own expectations would have been significantly lower than patients today who may live for many decades after their surgery.

With advances in surgical technique, implant design, bearing surfaces and surgical experience, the indications for THA have expanded to include younger patients who, by their very nature, are more likely to anticipate a return to their pre-arthritic state that may include a resumption of athletic activity. Patients' expectations have also increased as a consequence of social change in the latter half of the twentieth century as well as the reported successful outcomes of THA in the medical literature and general media. A more recent phenomenon affecting patient's expectations is the use of marketing by implant companies. Although direct to consumer marketing may not be permissible in all jurisdictions, Internet marketing may overcome any national regulations [3]. The timing of these increased expectations coincides with the ageing 'baby boomer' generation who are now at an age where THA is both psychologically and financially acceptable to them. It is unclear whether similar demographic changes in other parts of the World will yield patients with similar demands. As the number of THAs being performed is expected to increase significantly over the coming decades [4], predominantly due to an ageing population, it is likely that the absolute number of THAs being performed in athletes will increase as the percentage of younger patients requesting THAs is rising [5].

The general health benefits of physical activity, including psychosocial and cardiovascular health improvements, are well documented [6, 7] and THA is known to improve patients' physical activity. Physical activity can also be beneficial to the THA itself by improving muscle strength, coordination, balance and proprioception [8–11]. However, athletic activity as opposed to increased physical activity can have short- and long-term detrimental effects on the hip replacement. The evidence available to date is sparse, and conflicting with regard to the amount of athletic activity patients can and should undertake as well as the risks posed by their activity to the survivorship of their implants. Most advice available is based on surveys and expert opinion which itself continues to develop over time.

When athletes present for THA with the expectation of resuming athletic activity post-surgery one must consider the following: (1) What effect the THA will have on the patient's ability to resume athletic activity? (2) What effect the athletic activity will have on the THA?

Effect of THA on Athletic Activity

Several studies have looked at the effect of THA on athletic activity. Most show that although patients can resume sports after their surgery, most participate in sports of a lower impact. Ritter and Meding [12] showed a significant decrease in sport-

F. Doyle, MBBCh, BAO, MSc, FRCS(Orth) (✉)
Princess Elizabeth Orthopaedic Centre, Royal Devon & Exeter NHS Foundation Trust, Exeter, Devon, UK

Suite 1 Blackrock Clinic,
Rock Road, Blackrock, Co., Dublin, Ireland
e-mail: fintandoyle@hotmail.com

M.J. Wilson, FRCS(Eng), FRCS(Tr&Orth)
Exeter Hip Unit, Princess Elizabeth Orthopaedic Centre, Exeter, UK

J.C. McCarthy et al. (eds.), *Hip Joint Restoration*, DOI 10.1007/978-1-4614-0694-5_82

ing activity 3 years post-THA, except for cycling. They recommended 'intelligent participation' in sports with an inherently lower risk to the arthroplasty, e.g. bowling, walking, golf and cycling. Zahiri [13] showed that age is a significant determining factor in sports participation post-THA with patients over 60 years of age being involved in 30 % less sports than those younger than 60. In the Ulm Osteoarthritis study, Huch et al. [14] evaluated 420 THAs 5 years following surgery and found that although the number of sports participated in by patients had increased, the intensity and impact level had decreased. They also noted an age-dependant decrease in athletic activity even though they excluded patients over 75 years of age and, as with Zahiri, they recommended sports activity but suggested the avoidance of high-impact sports. Dubs et al. [15] looked at 110 patients with a mean age of 55 years and found that 78 % were active pre-operatively and that only 55 % were active post-operatively. They concluded that although younger patients may have higher expectations of function following THA, the literature indicates that many patients elect not to participate in demanding activities at the level they had anticipated.

Several studies have examined the participation in specific sports following THA. Mont [16] evaluated 58 competitive tennis players and found that all patients continued to play at 8 years following surgery. Of note, 16 patients maintained their activity levels despite complaining of hip pain and against the advice of their surgeon. This cohort of patients was obviously highly motivated and one cannot extrapolate their participation levels to the recreational sportsperson. Golf is a popular sport in particular for the age group seeking THA and a desire to continue playing golf is increasingly seen as an indication for THA. Most surgeons permit golf in the post-operative period as it is considered a low-impact activity. Mallon and Callaghan [17] evaluated 115 amateur golfers at 6 years following surgery. They found that all had returned to golf and that the average increase in handicap was 1.1 and that the average drive length had increased by 3 m. However, 41 % of patients complained of pain or ache during golf and 89 % of patients used a golf cart while playing.

Hip resurfacing was developed as an alternative to standard THA in particular for young and active patients and has been marketed as such [18]. Proponents of resurfacing suggest that the improved restoration of anatomy combined with large heads and hard-on-hard bearing surfaces makes these implants more suitable for the athlete; however there is little evidence in the literature to suggest that hip resurfacing provides a significant improvement in the ability of patients to return to athletic activity compared to conventional THA. Narvini [19] assessed the sports activities in 43 patients 6 months following hip resurfacing. He noted an increase in the number, intensity and frequency of sports participation. In a study of 112 patients 2 years following resurfacing, Naal et al. [20] reported that more patients participated in sports including high-impact disciplines such as tennis and even contact sports. More than 50 % returned to their chosen sport within 3 months of surgery and surprisingly, and older patients (mean age 60.2 years) participated in a higher number of sports and for longer durations than younger patients (mean 46.4 years). Banerjee [21] investigated 159 resurfacings in 145 patients at 2 years following surgery and found that although 98 % of patients were active in sports, there was a significant decrease in the number, frequency and intensity of the sports involved. Fouilleron [22] specifically looked at the sport of running after hip resurfacing and noted that 33 of the 40 patients that were active runners pre-operatively were still running post-operatively without any change in intensity.

Wylde [23] compared sports participation in patients who underwent conventional THA with those who underwent resurfacing arthroplasty. He reviewed 911 THAs and 157 hip resurfacings at 1–3 years post-surgery. In the THA group, 34.9 % of patients had participated in sports pre-operatively and post-operatively 26.4 % of those had ceased all sports. In the resurfacing group, 64.3 % of patients were involved in sports before surgery and at follow-up 22.7 % of these patients had ceased. When matched for age and sex, Wylde found no difference in the post-operative athletic activity levels between the two groups. Schmidutz [24] recently evaluated sports activities in patients 2 years following short-stem hip arthroplasty. He found a significant increase in the level of low-impact sport participation with a corresponding decrease in the level of high-impact sports. He found that men and women had similar post-operative participation levels overall but, as men were more likely to be involved in high-impact sports before surgery, that their relative participation fell.

The principal criticism of these papers on return to sport after surgery is that they are retrospective short-term questionnaire studies which can be prone to bias. Patients unhappy with results from their surgery may be more or less willing to respond to researchers. Equally, patients who have achieved a high level of activity may not feel that they have any issues and therefore that the survey does not apply to them. Advice from surgeons and the patient's pre-operative expectations can also give rise to significant bias. The most important problem with these studies however is that although they may show that patients can participate in athletic activity post-THA, they do not indicate whether it is prudent to be so active after surgery. In an attempt to understand this, we need to examine what effect the athletic activity has on the THA both in the short and long term.

The Effect of Athletic Activity on THA

The effects of athletic activity on THAs are similar to those in the sedentary patient but are more likely to occur at an early stage due to the increased demands placed on the construct

[25]. Although it may be inevitable that a THA performed in a young athlete will fail in time, choices can be made in an attempt to extend the durability of the procedure and reduce the rate of revision, both in the short and long term.

The most important short-term cause of failure of total hip replacements is dislocation. The normal range of motion of the native hip is 132° of flexion/extension and 94° of combined rotation [26]. Standard precautions following THA in the non-athlete would be to limit joint motion to avoid the extremes of the physiologic range combined with any additional limitations based on findings noted during surgery. However, participation in many sports requires a normal range of motion and therefore the risk of dislocation in the athlete is of prime concern. There has been a trend towards the use of larger heads, with their increased primary arc of motion before impingement, to reduce the dislocation risk in athletic patients. Using an anatomic hip dislocation simulator, Burroughs et al. showed a significant increase in range of motion after THR with head diameters larger than 32 mm, and elimination of implant-implant impingement with the use of head sizes over 36 mm [27].

However, in vivo, a major cause of dislocation is bone on bone impingement, which is not reduced by larger head sizes. Dislocation is a traumatic event for conventional patients but must be even more significant if athletic activity was a primary indication for THA as it is unlikely that the patient would be able to continue with their chosen sport even if their THA was eventually stabilised. It is understandable therefore that dislocation is of primary concern for the athletic patient but this must be balanced against the increased volumetric wear and increased forces transmitted to the implants with the use of larger head sizes [28]. Hip resurfacing does offer an attractive alternative to conventional THA with its large head sizes reducing dislocation risk and the low wear rates of hard-on-hard bearing. However, the development of localised lymphocytic-mediated responses to wear particles and the consequent high early failure rates would suggest that these implants be used with caution [29].

The concept of dual-mobility hip replacements has been popular in France for many years and Philippot has published results with good long-term survivorship [30]. These implants have become increasingly used in other parts of the world where dislocation is considered a significant risk. It is likely that dual-mobility hip replacements will be seen by many surgeons as an alternative to hip resurfacing as the presence of a large head used reduces the risk of dislocation without the resultant risk of adverse tissue reactions from metal-on-metal bearings. However, the wear rates of multiple bearing surfaces, as well as the effects of impact loading on a convex polyethylene surface, are unknown in the athlete.

The surgical approach used can also affect the dislocation rate. The higher rates of dislocation seen with the use of a posterior approach can be reduced by meticulous soft-tissue repair [31] but would still be considered higher than the rates achieved with anterior or lateral approaches. Proponents of the posterior approach suggest that the superior access achieved allows for improved implant positioning which itself is the primary independent determinant of stability. This approach, through its avoidance of the abductor mechanism, has been shown to have superior gait mechanics and therefore may be considered more suitable in patients aspiring to participate in athletic activity. However, there are no studies to date that demonstrate significant improvement in athletic function with a specific surgical approach. The majority of athletic and non-athletic patients will have stable joints and the most likely cause of failure will not be dislocation but implant wear and its consequences.

Wear is known to be directly related to use rather than time [32]. Athletic patients are likely to wear their bearing surfaces at a significantly higher rate than the non-athlete because of the nature of their activities. Athletic patients are younger and therefore the implants need to withstand this increased rate of wear for significantly longer time periods. The amount of wear seen will depend on the type of bearing surfaces used as well as the impact and frequency of the athletic activity and the age of the patient. As the impact level is expected to directly affect the rate of bearing wear as well as more acute complications such as dislocation and fracture, Clifford and Mallon have classified sporting activities as low, potentially low, intermediate and high impact [33].

The published data provide a mixed picture. In 1983 Dubs et al. reviewed 110 men following THA, half of whom returned to athletic activities. Surprisingly, the rate of component loosening was lower in those who participated in sport compared to those who were not—1.6% vs. 14.3%, respectively [15]. Gschwend et al. reviewed two cohorts of 50 patients who had undergone hip replacement. Patients in one cohort did not participate in any winter sports whilst in the other cohort patients were involved in Alpine skiing. At review 5 years following surgery, the wear rates in the active group were found to be significantly higher than in the more sedate group, although the non-skiing group had more evidence of radiological loosening [34].

The polyethylene used in Charnley's era had high wear rates and would therefore be unsuitable for use in high-demand patients. Advances in manufacturing techniques, such as irradiation cross-linking in an inert environment followed by quenching of free radicals, have led to the development of highly cross-linked polyethylenes with significantly reduced wear rates in vitro [35]. These improvements in wear resistance have obvious benefits to the THA patient in the long term; however concerns regarding alterations in the mechanical properties such as reduced ductility and fracture resistance may make highly cross-linked components susceptible to fracture in patients involved in high-impact sports.

Alternate bearing surfaces such as metal-on-metal or ceramic-on-ceramic bearings have been developed and marketed toward younger and athletic patients who would be likely to have higher wear rates. Metal-on-metal bearings have been described previously. Ceramic-on-ceramic bearings have the lowest wear rates in vitro; however, early failures due to fracture delayed their widespread use with particular fears for their use in high-demand patients [36–39]. Improvements in manufacturing techniques, such as hot isotactic pressing (HIP) to reduce grain size and the addition of zirconia or strontium oxide particles, have significantly reduced the incidence of implant fracture. Squeaking is also a well-documented complication of ceramic-on-ceramic articulations and is thought to be most likely related to implant design and surgical technique rather than the activity levels of the patient [40, 41]. An audible squeak is thought to have no adverse effect on the implants themselves but can have significant psychological effects on the patient. It is logical to think that the athlete with an audible squeak will be affected more regularly and to a greater intensity than the non-athlete. Alternate bearing surfaces have obvious benefits to the athletic patient in terms of wear rates but each has its own specific problems and therefore the choice of bearing surface should be tailored for each patient and their chosen sport with the appropriate consent.

Another choice available to the surgeon is the method of implant fixation. The fixation achieved, either cemented or uncemented, is of critical importance as athletic activity will impart significantly higher forces to the implant bone interface not seen in the non-athlete. For example, large hip/trunk rotational torques developed during tennis are expected to impart elevated torsional stresses to the implant-bone construct [42]. Similarly, skiing transmits high medial/lateral forces across the hip joint [43]. The high rates of osteolysis seen in early THA series were inappropriately attributed to the use of polymethyl methacrylate (PMMA) bone cement and the term ‘cement disease’ was coined. It is now widely accepted that this osteolysis was in fact a macrophage-mediated inflammatory response to polyethylene particles and not primarily a reaction to cement. As a result, the use of cemented implants has declined, particularly in the USA, and cementless options have been developed instead. It has been suggested that cementless implants are ideally suited to the athlete as the biological fixation achieved may provide a more stable long-term fixation to withstand the loads applied by the continuous remodeling of the adjacent bone. Uncemented implants attain their stability initially by interference fit and later by bony in-growth which is a possible disadvantage as it may delay the patients’ return to athletic activity. Other possible disadvantages include increased wear rated with multiple bearing or potentially bearing surfaces and third body wear secondary to delamination of hydroxylapatite coatings.

Proponents of cemented techniques claim that, on the femoral side at least, cement allows for a more accurate restoration of hip anatomy in terms of length, offset and hip centre which will improve not only the mechanics of the hip and therefore the ability to participate in sports but also the survivorship of the implant in the long term.

Periprosthetic and implant fracture are a rare but well-documented complication of THA. One may assume that patients involved in athletic activity and in particular high-impact or contact sports will have a higher incidence of fracture. Different implant design and fixation methods are likely to produce different fracture patterns as are the specific sports involved. The majority of the literature on fracture risk relate to very different population groups, with the highest incidence seen in the elderly, infirm with poor bone stock who sustain low-energy injuries [44]. Athletic activity, at least low-impact activity, may in fact be protective against fracture by improving bone mineral density, muscle strength, proprioception and coordination and thus reducing the risk of falls.

From the evidence available it is difficult to know what advice surgeons should give potential THA patients who wish to participate in athletic activity after their surgery. Most of the data available takes the form of expert opinion and surgeon surveys which are by their very nature subjective. Mc Grory et al. surveyed 27 surgeons at the Mayo Clinic in 1993 and formulated a consensus that recommended low-impact sports such as bowling, cycling and golf after THA, but did not recommend higher impact sports such as baseball, basketball and football [45]. Healy et al. surveyed 54 members of the American Hip Society in 1999 and classified their recommendations with respect to individual sports as allowed, allowed with previous experience, not recommended and undecided [46]. Similar distinctions were made between high- and low-impact sports and interestingly when the survey was repeated in 2005 [47], a number of sports had moved from the ‘undecided’ category into the ‘allowed’ category suggesting a possible relaxation in surgeons’ attitudes towards sports after THA or an acceptance of patients’ demands to participate in athletic activities. Klein et al. surveyed 522 members of the American Association of Hip and Knee surgeons and 92 members of the American Hip Society and found a similar relaxation of attitudes [48].

Future advances in hip replacements for the athlete may take the form of bearing surfaces with viscoelastic properties similar to that of articular cartilage. The development of biomaterials composed of hyaluronan, a hydrophilic glycosaminoglycan found in native articular cartilage, combined with a high-density polyethylene (HDPE) may recreate the properties of the native joint. It may be many years however before this material, HA-co-HDPE, will be suitable for clinical testing [49]. In engineering systems, bearings are often composed of two materials of differing surface hardness. Ceramic-on-metal bearings have recently been developed and in vitro studies have shown extremely low wear rates and without some of the complications associated with MOM or COC bearings [50, 51]. Alternative ceramic materials such as oxidized zirconium and silicon nitride, traditionally used in electrical insulation, appear to combine the wear characteristics of traditional ceramics with the toughness of metals [52]. Again, randomized studies with long-term follow-up are required to prove if any of these novel materials are safe and beneficial to the athlete undergoing total hip arthroplasty.

Conclusion

A desire to return to athletic activity after total hip arthroplasty has become an increasingly more common indication for surgery. Although the benefits of physical activity following THA are well documented, it is unclear whether the benefits of *athletic* activity outweigh the increased risks to the implants and it is only with long-term prospective studies will we be able to answer this question definitively.

References

1. Charnley J. Arthroplasty of the hip. A new operation. Lancet. 1961;27:1129–32.
2. Life Expectancy at Birth. 1901–2021. Office for National Statistics Dataset 29701.
3. Adeoye S, Bozic KJ. Direct to consumer advertising in healthcare: history, benefits and concerns. Clin Orthop Relat Res. 2007;457: 96–104.
4. Kurtz S, Ong K, Lau E, Mowat F, Halpern M. Projections of primary and revision hip and knee arthroplasty in the United States from 2005 to 2030. J Bone Joint Surg Am. 2007;89-A:780–5.
5. Herberts P, Kärrholm J, Garrellick G (2004) The Swedish National Hip Arthroplasty Register, annual report. http://www.jru.orthop.gu.se
6. Pollock ML, Wilmore JH. Exercise in health and disease: evaluation and prescription for prevention and rehabilitation. 2nd ed. Philadelphia: Saunders; 1990. p. 1–2.
7. American College of Sports Medicine Position Stand. The recommended quantity and quality of exercise for developing and maintaining cardiovascular and muscular fitness in healthy adults. Med Sci Sports Exerc. 1990;22:265–74.
8. Visuri T, Honkanen R. Total hip replacement: its influence on spontaneous recreation exercise habits. Arch Phys Med Rehabil. 1980;61:325–8.
9. Macnicol MF, McHardy R, Chalmers J. Exercise testing before and after hip arthroplasty. J Bone Joint Surg (Br). 1980;62:326–31.
10. Golant A, Christoforou DC, Slover JD, Zuckerman JD. Athletic participation after hip and knee arthroplasty. Bull NYU Hosp Jt Dis. 2010;68(2):76–83.
11. Ries MD, Philpin EF, Groff GD, et al. Effect of total hip arthroplasty on cardiovascular fitness. J Arthroplasty. 1997;12(1):84–90.
12. Ritter MA, Meding JB. Total hip arthroplasty: can the patient play sports again? Orthopaedics. 1987;10:1447–52.
13. Zahiri CA, Schmalzried TP, Szuszczewicz ES, Amstutz HC. Assessing activity in joint replacement patients. J Arthroplasty. 1998;13:890–5.
14. Huch K, Müller KAC, Stürmer T, Brenner H, Puhl W, Günther K-P. Sports activities 5 years after total knee or hip arthroplasty: the Ulm Osteoarthritis study. Ann Rheum Dis. 2005;64:1715–20.
15. Dubs L, Gschwend N, Munzinger U. Sport after total hip arthroplasty. Arch Orthop Trauma Surg. 1983;101:161–9.
16. Mont MA, LaPorte DM, Mullick T, Silberstein CE, Hungerford DS. Tennis after total hip arthroplasty. Am J Sports Med. 1999;27:60–4.
17. Mallon WJ, Callaghan JJ. Total hip arthroplasty in active golfers. J Arthropasty. 1992;7(Suppl):339–46.
18. www.birminghamhipresurfacing.com. Accessed 22 Oct 2012
19. Narvini AA, Tsiridis E, Nwaboku HC, Bajekal RA. Sporting activity following Birmigham hip resurfacing. Int J Sports Med. 2006;27:505–7.
20. Naal FD, Maffiuletti NA, Munzinger U, Hersche O. Sports after hip resurfacing arthroplasty. Am J Sports Med. 2007;35:705–11.
21. Banerjee M, Bouillon B, Banerjee C, Bäthis H, Lefering R, Nardini M, Schmidt J. Sports activity after total hip resurfacing. Am J Sports Med. 2010;38:1229–36.
22. Fouilleron N, Wavreille G, Endjah N, Girard J. Running activity after hip resurfacing arthroplasty. A prospective study. Am J Sports. 2012;40:889–94.
23. Wylde V, Blom A, Dieppe P, Hewlett S, Learmonthg I. Return to sport after joint replacement. J Bone Joint Surg (Br). 2008;90:920–3.
24. Schmidutz F, Grote S, Pietschmann M, Weber P, Mazoochian F, Fottner A, Jansson V. Sports activity after short-stem hip arthroplasty. Am J Sports Med. 2012;40:425–32.
25. Bergmann G, Graichen F, Rohlmann A. Hip joint loading during walking and running, measured in two patients. J Biomech. 1993;26:969–90.
26. Boone DC, Azen SP. Normal range of motion of joints in male subjects. J Bone Joint Surg Am. 1979;6:756–9.
27. Burroughs BR, Hallstrom B, Golladay GJ, Hoeffel D, Harris WH. Range of motion and stability in total hip arthroplasty with 28-, 32-, 38-, and 44 mm femoral head sizes. J Arthroplasty. 2005;20:11–9.
28. Lachiewics PF, Heckman DS, Soileau ES, Mangla J, Martell JM. Femoral head size and wear of highly cross-linked polyethylene at 5 to 8 years. Clin Orthop Relat Res. 2009;467:3290–6.
29. MHRA Medical Device Alert. Ref: MDA/2010/033
30. Philippot R, Camilleri JP, Boyer B, Adam P, Farizon F. The use of dual-articulation acetabular cup system to prevent dislocation after primary total hip arthroplasty: analysis of 384 cases at a mean follow-up of 15 years. Int Orthop. 2009;33:927–32.
31. Kwon MS, Kuskowski M, Mulhall KJ, et al. Does surgical approach affect total hip arthroplasty dislocation rates? Clin Orthop Relat Res. 2006;447:34–8.
32. Schmalzried TP, Shepard EF, Dorey FJ, et al. The John Charnley award. Wear is a function of use, not time. Clin Orthop Relat Res. 2000;381:36–46.
33. Clifford PE, Mallon WJ. Sports after total joint replacement. Clin Sports Med. 2005;24:175–86.
34. Gschwend N, Frei T, Morscher E, Nigg B, Loehr J. Alpine and cross-country skiing after total hip replacement: 2 cohorts of 50 patients each, one active, the other inactive in skiing, followed for 5-10 years. Acta Orthop Scand. 2000;71:243–9.
35. Maloney WJ. Highly cross-linked polyethylene in total hip replacement: Pros and Cons. J Bone Joint Surg Br Suppl. 2010;92:167–8.
36. Barrack RL, Burak C, Skinner HB. Concerns about ceramics in THA. Clin Orthop Relat Res. 2004;429:73–9.
37. Hasegawa M, Sudo A, Hirata H, Uchida A. Ceramic acetabular liner fracture in total hip arthroplasty with a ceramic sandwich cup. J Arthroplasty. 2003;18:658–61.
38. Ha YC, Kim SY, Kim HJ, Yoo JJ, Koo KH. Ceramic liner fracture after cementless alumina-on-alumina total hip arthroplasty. Clin Orthop Relat Res. 2007;458:106–10.
39. Simon JA, Dayan AJ, Ergas E, Stuchin SA, Di Cesare PE. Catastrophic failure of the acetabular component in a ceramic-polyethylene bearing total hip arthroplasty. J Arthroplasty. 1998;13: 108–13.

40. Schroder D, Bornstein L, et al. Ceramic-on ceramic total hip arthroplasty, incidence of instability and noise. Clin Orthop Relat Res. 2011;469:437–42.
41. Stafford GH, Islam S, Witt JD. Early to mid-term results of ceramic-on-ceramic total hip replacement. J Bone Joint Surg (Br). 2011;93B:1017–20.
42. Akutagawa S, Kojima T. Trunk rotation torques through the hip joints during the one-and two-handed backhand tennis strokes. J Sports Sci. 2005;23:781–93.
43. van den Bogert AJ, Read L, Nigg BM. An analysis of hip joint loading during walking, running and skiing. Med Sci Sports Exerc. 1999;31:131–42.
44. Mc Grory BJ. Periprosthetic fracture of the femur after total hip arthroplasty occurring in winter activities: a report of two cases. J Surg Orthop Adv. 2004;13(2):119–23.
45. McGrory BJ, Stuart MJ, Sim FH. Participation in sports after hip and knee arthroplasty: review of literature and survey of surgeon preferences. Mayo Clin Proc. 1995;70:342–8.
46. Healy WL, Ioria R, Lemos MJ. Athletic activity after joint replacement. Am J Sports Med. 2001;29:377–88.
47. Healy WL, Sharma S, Schwartz B, Iorio R. Athletic activity after total joint arthroplasty. J Bone Joint Surg Am. 2008;90:2245–52.
48. Klein GR, Levine BR, Hozack WJ, Strauss EJ, D'Antonio JA, Macaulay W, Di Cesare PE. Return to athletic activity after total hip arthroplasty. Consensus guidelines based on a survey of the Hip Society and American Association of Hip and Knee Surgeons. J Arthroplasty. 2007;22:171–5.
49. Oldinski RA, Cranson CN, James SP. Synthesis and characterisation of hyaluronanpolyethylene copolymer for biomedical applications. J Biomed Mater Res B Appl Biomater. 2010;94:441–6.
50. Fisher J, Firkins P, Tipper J, Farrar R, Ingham E. Wear of novel ceramic on metal bearings for hip prosthesis. In: Dietrich M, D'Antonio JA, editors. Bioceramics and alternative bearings in joint arthroplasty. Darmstadt: Steinkopff; 2005. p. 197–9. doi:10.1007/3-7985-1540-9_30. ISBN 978-3-7985-1540-6.
51. Williams S, Schepers A, Isaac G, Hardaker C, Ingham E, Jagt D, et al. Otto Aufranc award: Ceramic-on-metal hip arthroplasties: a comparative in vitro and in vivo study. Clin Orthop Relat Res. 2007;465:23–32.
52. Bal BS, Khandkar A, Lakshminarayanan R, Clarke I, Hoffman AA, Rahaman MN. Fabrication and testing of silicon nitride bearings in total hip arthroplasty. J Arthroplasty. 2009;24:110–6.

Suggested Reading

Baumann S, Williams D, Petrucelli D, Elliott W, de Beer J. Physical activity after total joint replacement: a cross-sectional survey. Clin J Sport Med. 2007;17:104–8.

Berry DJ. Epidemiology of periprostheic fractures after major joint replacement: hip and knee. Orthop Clin North Am. 1999;30: 183–90.

Boehler M. Hip osteotomy. Presented at the 8th Annual Current Concepts in Joint Replacement Symposium; Orlando, FL.

Chandler DR, Glousman R, Hull D, McGuire PJ, Kim IS, Clarke IC, Sarmiento A. The effects of the head neck geometry. Clin Orthop Relat Res. 1982;166:284–91.

Charnley J. Low friction arthroplasty of the hip: theory and practice. Berlin: Springer; 1979.

Chatterji U, Ashworth MJ, Lewis PL, Dobson PJ. Effects of total hip arthroplasty on recreational and sporting activity. ANZ J Surg. 2004;74:446–9.

Cornell CN, Ranawat CS. Survivorship analysis of total hip replacements. Results in a series of active patients who were less than fifty-five years old. J Bone Joint Surg Am. 1986;68(9):1430–4.

Daniel J, Pynsent PB, McMinn DJ. Metal-on-metal resurfacing of the hip in patients under the age of 55yearswith osteoarthritis. J Bone Joint Surg (Br). 2004;86:177–84.

Harris WH, Schiller AL, Scholler JM, Freiberg RA, Scott R. Extensive localised bone resorption in the femur following total hip replacement. J Bone Joint Surg Am. 1976;58:612–8.

Healy WL, Bigliani LU, Stuart MJ, Iorio R, Trousdale RT. Ask the experts: advising patients on sports activity following joint arthroplasty. Orthopaedics Today, April 2011.

Kilgus DJ, Dorey FJ, Finerman GAM, Amstutz HC. Patient activity, sports participation and impact loading on the durability of cemented total hip replacements. Clin Orthop Relat Res. 1991;269:25–9.

Kuster MS. Exercise recommendations after total joint replacement: a review of the current literature and proposal of scientifically based guidelines. Sports Med. 2002;32(7):433–45.

Laupacis A, Bourne R, Rorabeck C, Feeny D, Wong C, Tugwell P, et al. The effect of elective total hip replacement on health-related quality of life. J Bone Joint Surg Am. 1993;75:1619–26.

Lavigne M, Masse V, Girard J, Roy AG, Venditolli PA. Return to sport after hip resurfacing or total hip arthroplasty: a randomised study. Rev Chir Orthop Reparatrice Appar Mot. 2008;94:361–7.

Learmonth ID, Young C, Rorabeck C. The operation of the century: total hip replacement. Lancet. 2007;370:1508–19.

Malchau H, Herberts P, Ahnfelt L. Prognosis of total hip replacement in Sweden. Follow up of 92,675 operations performed 1978-1990. Acta Orthop Scand. 1993;64(5):497–506.

Ogunwale B, Clarke J, Young D, Mohammed A, Patil S, Meek RM. Direct to consumer advertising via the internet, a study of hip resurfacing. Scott Med J. 2009;54:10–3.

Philippot R, Adam P, Reckhaus M, Delange F, Verdot FX, Curvale G, Farizon F. Prevention of dislocation in total hip revision surgery using a dual mobility design. Orthop Traumatol Surg Res. 2009;95:407–13.

Widhalm R, Höfer G, Krugluger J, Bartalsky I. Is there a greater danger of sports injury or osteoporosis caused by inactivity in patients with hip prosthesis? Sequelae for long-term stability of prosthesis anchorage. Z Orthop. 1990;128:139–43.

Wilson MJ, Villar RN. Knee Surg Sports Traumatol Arthrosc. 2011;19:1524–30.

Yun AG. Sports after total hip replacement. Clin Sports Med. 2006;25:359–64.

83 Arthroscopy Following Total Hip Replacement

Joseph C. McCarthy, Leah Elson, and Joann Lee

Total hip arthroplasty has been reported to be an incredibly successful orthopedic procedure that has experienced an increasing demand in recent years. Current estimates place the number of THA procedures, performed annually, at 285,000 in the USA alone, a number that is forecasted to double by 2030 [1]. However, there is a subset of these patients who have not experienced a clinically successful result. These patients present with idiopathic suboptimal outcomes following a total hip replacement procedure [2–4].

Diagnostically, this group of patients can challenge even the most tenured medical professionals, presenting symptomatic anomalies without clear cause [5, 6]. Persistent and intractable pain is the foremost symptom that initiates further investigation, post-THA [6, 7]. In order to determine the cause of hip pain, a battery of diagnostic tests is often performed.

Plain radiographs are typically ordered to determine visual migration of hardware, or to detect any unknown, metallic third-body debris that may be present at the articulation. Blood studies can reveal elevated metal ions, or C-reactive protein levels. Joint aspiration is utilized in order to check for localized infection. Yet, these methods are not always reliable in determining a diagnosis [8, 9].

Radiographs have significant limitations in visualizing not only the bearing surfaces but also the adjacent soft tissues. If no infection or metallosis is present, blood samples will yield negative results; and due to anatomic morphological variations, joint aspiration may be difficult or impossible to perform. Thus, when none of these laboratory or clinical investigative techniques can properly identify the cause of persistent pain, it may be beneficial to physically visualize the joint itself.

An open arthrotomy provides optimal exposure for investigation of pathology associated with the implantation site. Unfortunately, there are several drawbacks associated with open diagnostic arthrotomy, including risk of sepsis, heterotopic bone formation, postoperative pain, an extended recovery time, and other potential risks associated with an operative inpatient procedure [10, 11]. Therefore, arthroscopy—as a minimally invasive, outpatient procedure—is an attractive diagnostic choice [5, 6, 12, 13].

Using arthroscopy for diagnosis allows the surgeon to directly visualize and physically examine the affected hip. Due to the direct access provided to the bearing surfaces, surgeons are able to identify signs of metallosis or corrosion of metal components, directly collect fluid samples for diagnosis of infection, and perform dynamic evaluation of the prosthetic components and the implantation site for signs of loosening [6, 12, 13].

The detrimental effect of accelerated wear in hard-on-hard bearings has recently become a topic of great concern. In the event of edge loading of metal-on-metal articulations and/or corrosion of modular junctions, ions, wear debris, and corrosion products are released into periarticular tissues. This can lead to potentially catastrophic biologic reactions, including local and systemic toxicity, metal hypersensitivity reactions, and the formation of localized pseudotumors [14, 15]. However, it can be difficult to properly diagnose patients suffering from adverse metal-on-metal reactions. Arthroscopy can provide a method with which to visually confirm metallosis and its associated damages.

In a case study by McCarthy et al., a 67-year-old patient presented with pain and swelling from the affected hip, while ultrasound and radiographs produced negative results. Upon arthroscopic evaluation, it was confirmed that the in vivo components exhibited corrosion, causing metal synovitis

J.C. McCarthy, MD (✉)
Kaplan Joint Center, 2000 Washington St., Suite 361, Green Bldg, Newton, MA 02462, USA
e-mail: jcmccarthy1@partners.org

L. Elson, BSc
Orthopedics, Harris Laboratory, Massachusetts General Hospital, Boston, MA, USA
e-mail: leelson@gmail.com

J. Lee, MS
Newton Wellesley Hospital, 2000 Washington St., Green 361, Newton, MA 02462, USA
e-mail: jlee76@partners.org

J.C. McCarthy et al. (eds.), *Hip Joint Restoration*, DOI 10.1007/978-1-4614-0694-5_83

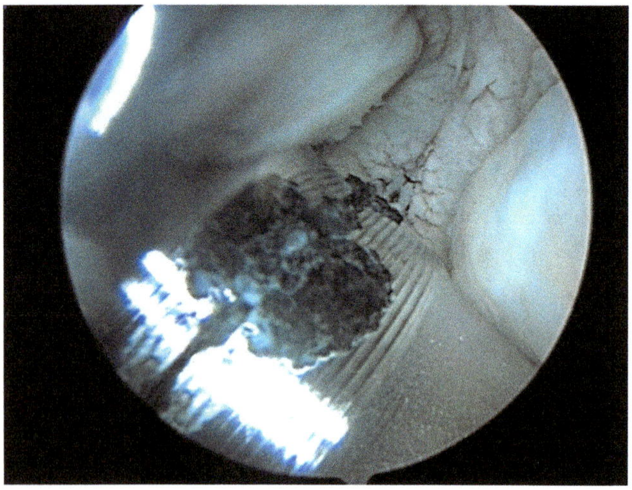

Fig. 83.1 Corrosion at the head–neck articulation in a metal-on-metal arthroplasty. From McCarthy JC, Jibodh SR, Lee JA. The Role of Arthroscopy in Evaluation of Painful Hip Arthroplasty. Clin Orthop Relat Res (2009) 467:174–180. Reprinted with permission from Springer

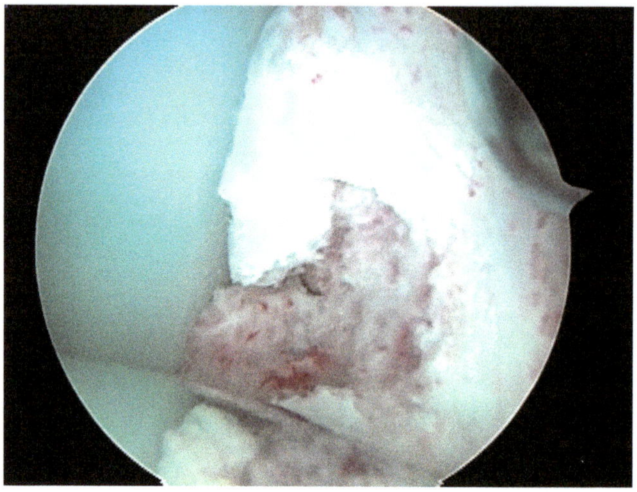

Fig. 83.2 Dense scar tissue formation in the anterior joint impinging at the femoral head. From McCarthy JC, Jibodh SR, Lee JA. The Role of Arthroscopy in Evaluation of Painful Hip Arthroplasty. Clin Orthop Relat Res (2009) 467:174–180. Reprinted with permission from Springer

and a presence of metal particulates on the intra-articular surfaces (Fig. 83.1). These findings clarified the previously enigmatic diagnosis and facilitated the patient to undergo revision to a metal-on-polyethylene system, as well as confirming metal-metal bearing hypersensitivity [6].

During instances of apparent idiopathic hip pain, it is also possible that the operated joint has contracted an infection. However, in cases where a direct aspiration of joint fluid may be difficult or culture negative, arthroscopy can, once again, be a useful diagnostic tool, for fluid analysis and synovial biopsy (Fig. 83.2).

In a case study reported by McCarthy et al., hip arthroscopy confirmed the presence of a *Staphylococcus aureus* infection in the hip joint of a morbidly obese woman after attempts to aspirate the hip proved unsuccessful due to the patient's body mass and extent of excess adipose tissue. During arthroscopic evaluation, the patient's infected tissue was successfully debrided, and the presence of a *S. aureus* infection was confirmed following bacteriologic evaluation of fluid samples collected arthroscopically. At 3-year follow-up, the patient remained free of recurrent pain or infection [6].

Oftentimes, pain in the THA joint can be caused by loosening of the implanted components. However, this loosening can be difficult to diagnose as radiographs can neither capture micromovements, nor can they assess dynamic motion (Fig. 83.3). Arthroscopy can provide a method with which to evaluate in vivo components while the joint is dynamically loaded.

Khanduja and Villar reported the case of a 53-year-old woman who presented pain in the groin and thigh of her operated side. All other indications for pain—including infection, metal hypersensitivity, radiographic signs of osteolysis, and trauma—yielded negative results. Arthroscopic treatment was decided upon and the surgeons—while dynamically rotating the leg—were able to detect micromovement of the acetabular component. The patient was then scheduled for a revision, and recovered without complication and had resolution of her symptoms [12].

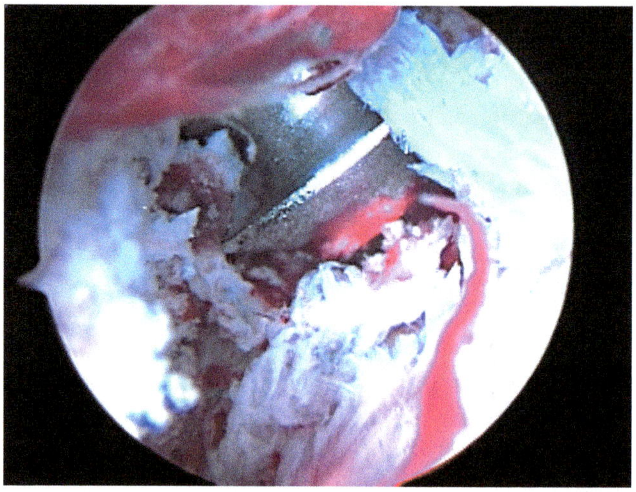

Fig. 83.3 Scar tissue around the implant-bone interface when debrided showed fibrous tissue with a loose acetabular component. From McCarthy JC, Jibodh SR, Lee JA. The Role of Arthroscopy in Evaluation of Painful Hip Arthroplasty. Clin Orthop Relat Res (2009) 467:174–180. Reprinted with permission from Springer

Arthroscopy is a minimally invasive method with which to confirm diagnosis of a painful hip joint following THA. Not only does it allow the surgeon to see both the articulating surfaces and the bone-to-component interface, but it also provides a method with which to evaluate the kinematics of the hip joint while moving the extremity. Beyond providing a referral for revision cases, arthroscopy also has potential to provide advantageous therapeutic value for this particular group of patients [5]. Recently, the utility of arthroscopy being used as a therapeutic tool for painful symptoms, post-THA, has been evaluated in the treatment of femoroacetabular impingement, and iliopsoas tendonitis.

Morphologic bony abnormalities can cause pain and discomfort during dynamic motion of the hip joint. One such abnormality can be attributed to femoroacetabular impingement (FAI), in which impingement between the rim of the acetabulum and the femoral neck interrupts natural fluid hip motion. FAI occurs in two forms: (i) the pincer type which arises from bony overgrowth of the acetabular rim, and (ii) cam type, which occurs as a result of a bony enlargement of the femoral neck. Both forms can be detrimental to the hip joint itself, leading to crushing or tearing of the acetabular labrum and deterioration of the chondral surfaces [2, 16].

Several studies have demonstrated that arthroscopic techniques can alleviate painful symptoms associated with FAI. For instance, the shaving and trimming tools used in arthroscopic procedures work to resect the bony abnormalities of the acetabular rim, thereby removing the cause of pincer-type FAI [17]. For cam-type FAI, femoral neck osteoplasty can be successfully performed. Once the bony overgrowth has been removed, any resultant soft-tissue lesions sustained as a result of FAI can also be resected and repaired [3, 5]. The direct visualization of the intra-articular surfaces provided by arthroscopy can also allow full evaluation of the bearing surfaces and the implant-bone interfaces.

Patients presenting after THA with severe anterior groin pain and weakness of the affected hip joint may potentially be diagnosed with iliopsoas tendonitis. During clinical examination, these patients may be pain free during passive motion, but experience severe pain and discomfort when actively moving the joint. Daily activities aggravating the tendonitis have been reported to include getting in and out of the bed, and exiting a vehicle, activities that patients often perform voluntarily by manually lifting their affected limb [18]. In these cases, common causes of iliopsoas tendonitis are an acetabular component that protrudes beyond the bony rim, retroversion of the socket, impingement across the acetabular margin, overuse syndrome, an enlarged prosthetic femoral head (greater than 40 mm), or preoperative psoas contracture [5, 19–21]. In a case study by Bajwa and Villar, 7 of 24 patients that presented with pain were treated for iliopsoas tendonitis arthroscopically. After performing a release in all cases, additional treatments—including excision of lesions from impingement, debridement, and removal of osteophytes—were also performed on several patients before closing [5].

Conclusion

In diagnosing complaints related to painful total hip replacements, arthroscopy provides the surgeon with a direct view of intra-articular spaces and implant-bone interfaces. When a diagnosis is difficult to attain using conventional modalities, arthroscopy can be used to solidify clinical suspicion of infection, loosening of components, metallosis, and soft-tissue damage. But arthroscopy can also address therapeutic treatment of these patients when the risks of a full arthrotomy are unfavorable. Arthroscopy has successfully treated the complications associated with pincer- and cam-type femoroacetabular impingement, and the debilitating pain of iliopsoas tendonitis. Arthroscopic treatment can also repair and remove other lesions such as broken screws or loose bodies that intraoperative examination may reveal. Thus, the utility of arthroscopy as both a diagnostic and therapeutic tool has proven to be beneficial to patients experiencing idiopathic pain following a total hip arthroplasty.

References

1. Kurtz S et al. Projection of primary and revision hip and knee arthroplasty in the U.S. JBJS. 2007;89(4):780–5.
2. Palmer DH, Ganesh V, Comfort T, Tatman P. Midterm outcomes in patients with cam femoroacetabular impingement treated arthroscopically. Arthroscopy. 2012;28(11):1671–81.
3. Lavigne M, Rama KR, Roy A, Venditolli PA. Painful impingement of the hip joint after total hip resurfacing: a report of two cases. J Arthroplasty. 2008;23:1074–9.
4. Morlock MM, Bishop N, Stahmer F, et al. Reasons for failure of hip resurfacing implants: a failure analysis based on 250 revision specimens. Orthopade. 2008;37:695–703. German.
5. Bajwa AS, Villar RN. Arthroscopy of the hip in patients following joint replacement. J Bone Joint Surg Br. 2011;93:890–6.
6. McCarthy JC, Lee J. The role of arthroscopy in evaluation of painful hip arthroplasty. Clin Orthop Relat Res. 2009;467:174–80.
7. Jaykumar P et al. Arthroscopy of the hip for pediatric and adolescent disorders. J Bone Joint Surg (Br). 2012;94:290–6.
8. Bozic KJ, Rubash HE. The painful total hip replacement. Clin Orthop Relat Res. 2004;420:18–25.
9. Robbins GM, Masri BA, Garbunz DS, Duncan CP. Evaluation of pain in patients with apparently solidly fixed total hip arthroplasty components. J Am Acad Orthop Surg. 2002;10:86–94.
10. Ebreo D, Khan A, El-Meligy M, Armstrong C, Viju P. Metal ion levels decrease after revision for metallosis arising from large diameter metal-on-metal total hip arthroplasty. Acta Orthop Belg. 2001;77:777–81.
11. Riley PM, Weiner DS, Gillesepie R, et al. Hazards of internal fixation in the treatment of slipped capital femoral epiphysis. JBJS. 1990;72:1500–9.
12. Khanduja V, Villar RN. The role of arthroscopy in resurfacing arthroplasty of the hip. Arthroscopy. 2008;24(1):122.e1–e3.
13. Ilizaliturri VM, Zarate-Kalfopulos B, Martinez-Escalante FA, et al. Arthroscopic retrieval of a broken guidewire fragment from the hip joint after cannulated screw fixation of slipped capital femoral epiphysis. Arthroscopy. 2007;23(2):227.e1–e4.

14. Pandit H, Glynne-Jones S, McLardy-Smith P, et al. Pseudotumors associated with metal-on-metal hip resurfacings. JBJS. 2008;90-B:847–51.
15. Willert HG, Buchhorn GH, Fayyazai A, et al. Metal-on-metal bearings and hypersensitivity in patients with artificial hip joint: a clinical and histomorphological study. JBJS. 2005;87:28–36.
16. Banerjee P, McLean CR. Femoroacetabular impingement: a review of diagnosis and management. Curr Rev Musculoskelet Med. 2011;4(1):23–32.
17. Phillipon MJ, Stubbs AJ, Schenker ML, Maxwell RB, et al. Arthroscopic management of FAI: osteoplasty technique and literature review. Am J Sports Med. 2007;35(9):1571–80.
18. O'Sullivan M et al. Iliopsoas tendonitis: a complication after total hip arthroplasty. J Arthroplasty. 2007;2(2):166–70.
19. Byrd JW, Jones KS. Traumatic rupture of ligamentum teres as a source of hip pain. Arthroscopy. 2004;20:385–91.
20. De Haan R, Pattyn C, Gill HS, et al. Correlation between inclination of the acetabular component and metal ion levels in metal-on-metal hip resurfacing replacement. J Bone Joint Surg Br. 2008;90:1291–7.
21. Wettstein M, Jung J, Dienst M. Arthroscopic psoas tenotomy. Arthroscopy. 2006;22:907.

Part XII

Functional Outcomes

Nicholas G.H. Mohtadi

84 Activities, Symptoms, and Expectations of Patients Undergoing Hip Surgery

Michael G. Hogen, Maureen K. Dwyer, Ugo N. Ihekweazu, Ardavan Ariel Saadat, Krissett A. Loya-Bodiford, and Philip C. Noble

Introduction

Does hip surgery restore normal hip function? While it is generally accepted that surgery is performed to avoid, or overcome, pain and deterioration of function, the underlying pathologies of hip deformity and dysfunction differ. Three common surgical procedures—hip osteotomy, hip arthroscopy, and total hip replacement—treat hip pathologies at three very different stages of life. This chapter discusses surgical outcomes and the extent to which these procedures succeed in meeting patient expectations.

M.G. Hogen, BA • K.A. Loya-Bodiford, MPH, BS
Institute of Orthopaedic Research and Education, 6550 Fannin Street, Suite 2501, Houston, TX 77030, USA

M.K. Dwyer, PhD, ATC
Department of Orthopaedics, Kaplan Joint Center, Newton Wellesley Hospital, Newton, IA, USA

Department of Orthopaedics, Massachusetts General Hospital, Boston, MA, USA

U.N. Ihekweazu, MD, BS
Joseph Barnhart Department of Orthopaedic Surgery, Baylor College of Medicine, Houston, TX, USA

A.A. Saadat, BS, MD
Institute of Orthopaedic Research and Education, 6550 Fannin Street, Suite 2501, Houston, TX 77030, USA

Department of Orthopaedic Surgery, University of Illinois College of Medicine at Chicago, Chicago, IL, USA

P.C. Noble, MD (✉)
Director of Research, Institute of Orthopedic Research and Education, 6550 Fannin Street, Suite 2501, Houston, TX 77030, USA

Director of Research, Institute of Orthopedic Research and Education, Houston, TX 77030, USA
e-mail: pnoble@bcm.edu

Hip Osteotomy

Surgical techniques and literature evaluating the relationship between hip dysplasia and secondary osteoarthritis have advanced hip osteotomy tremendously over the past 50 years. The overall goal of corrective hip osteotomy is to reorient the acetabulum and/or the femoral head to increase the weight bearing surface area of the joint, while providing coverage of the femoral head during joint motion; however, few accounts elaborate on the symptoms and expectations at their initial presentation.

The few studies that have undertaken the challenge of quantifying the activity levels of individuals with symptomatic hip dysplasia sought to analyze changes in gait and overall activity level in patients with periacetabular osteotomy (PAO). While studies demonstrate overall postoperative improvement, early diagnosis of hip dysplasia is particularly effective in improving clinical outcomes. Greater research is required to assess patient satisfaction across all age groups; however, older patients were found to very positively report satisfaction following PAO.

Hip Arthroscopy

It is important to identify the primary goals of each patient before undertaking an arthroscopic procedure and the likelihood that it can be achieved. While athletes are particularly successful in returning to their sport following hip arthroscopy, many "non-athlete" patients report that they are not as active 5 years after surgery as they expected at the time of surgery.

The primary complaint of patients with intra-articular hip pathology is pain and pain-induced limitations to function, describing a feeling of "giving way" in the joint. Research in pain measurement scales, such as Visual Analog Scale (VAS),

J.C. McCarthy et al. (eds.), *Hip Joint Restoration*, DOI 10.1007/978-1-4614-0694-5_84

has found substantial improvements in pain, postoperatively; however, fulfillment of a patient's preoperative expectations is often found to be overly optimistic.

Total Hip Replacement

Total Hip Replacement (THR) is currently the only solution for end-stage hip osteoarthritis (OA), though the physical activity level of patients seeking this treatment varies widely both before and after surgery. Despite the variance in a patient's leisure and social activities, aging undoubtedly is the determining factor in the extent of participation in physical activities. Participant expectations vary greatly prior to surgery, though the majority of patients report little to no postoperative pain, reporting as high as 90 % satisfaction because of elimination of symptoms and fulfillment of patients' preoperative expectations. In comparison, the results of total hip arthroplasty appear to be the most predictable, and the most likely to restore near-normal function to the affected hip.

Hip Osteotomy

Hip dysplasia, a common cause of secondary osteoarthritis, occurs when the femoral head articulates with an abnormally shallow acetabulum. The pathologic morphology of patients with dysplastic hips leads to the well-described degeneration of the hip joint, with the final consequence being severe osteoarthritis [1]. Over the past few decades, a number of hip osteotomy techniques have been developed to correct the pathologic hip mechanics of patients with dysplasia. The overall goal of a corrective hip osteotomy is to reorient the acetabulum and/or the femoral head to increase the area of the weight-bearing surface of the joint, while providing coverage of the femoral head during motion. This restoration of more normal relationship between the femur and the acetabulum leads to increased joint stability, while decreasing pain and improving the quality of life [2]. Several different types of acetabular osteotomy have been proposed over the past 50 years, including juxta-articular triple osteotomies [3], innominate osteotomies [4, 5], spherical osteotomies [6], and periacetabular osteotomies [7]. Despite the advances made in surgical technique and the decades of literature supporting the relationship between hip dysplasia and secondary osteoarthritis, there is a paucity of literature documenting the outcome of these procedures from the patient's perspective. Few accounts describe the symptoms and expectations of patients at their initial presentation, including clinical factors such as their physical exam, as well as the thoughts and perceptions of patients before and after the procedure. This portion of the chapter will focus on answering a number of these questions concerning PAOs.

Activities of Osteotomy Patients

The task of accurately quantifying the activity levels of individuals with unilateral and bilateral symptomatic hip dysplasia is challenging. As a result, there are only a few studies that attempt to describe pre- and postoperative activity levels of patients receiving PAOs. The activity level of patients with hip dysplasia has most recently been quantified in relation to the patient's mobility (gait, walking distance) [8], every-day activities (e.g., public transportation use) [9], and ability to participate in athletic activities [10]. Separate studies by Romano et al. and Karam et al. describe patients receiving hip osteotomies in terms of the alterations to their gait [8, 11]. The Karam study sought to describe the changes in walking patterns and evaluate the activity levels of patients undergoing hip osteotomies for symptomatic dysplasia. By using the GaitRite® walking pattern system, they prospectively collected data on patient walking patterns including velocity, cadence, stride length, and percent of single limb support on the affected limb. Activity level was assessed by documenting average steps per day over a period of time. They found that at approximately 1 year following the hip osteotomy procedure, there was an overall trend towards increased walking velocity, as well as a significant increase in stride length. Patients without pre-existing osteoarthritis had increased percentage of gait cycle with single support on the affected limb. Finally, the Karam study used the StepWatch® pedometer system to document average steps per day over a 7 days period as a surrogate to describe overall patient activity level.

Nunley et al. prospectively followed skeletally mature patients with symptomatic acetabular dysplasia treated with PAO. Patients were followed for a minimum of 24 months postoperatively, and were asked to complete questionnaires that contained both symptomatic and functional questions. In terms of mobility, approximately 35 % of patients reported difficulty with walking more than six blocks, more than half cited problems with climbing stairs and more than 10 % of patients reported difficulties with navigating the public transportation system. Furthermore, nearly 25 % of their cohort had trouble donning shoes and more than 80 % had difficulty sitting in any chair for more than 60 min.

In 2002, van Bergayk and Garbuz performed a retrospective assessment of the sports activities of 21 consecutive patients who underwent the Bernese PAO for hip dysplasia [10]. The Tegner and Lysholm sports-activity questionnaire was used to compare pre- and postoperative participation levels in sports. They found that the sports-activity level scores of the patients in their cohort increased from 1.9 to 4.4 after a minimum follow-up of 24 months. In terms of functional activity levels, this study found that the increase in scores corresponded to an improvement from being restricted to light work only with no participation in athletic activities, to patients becoming recreational athletes with some sports being undertaken at a competitive level.

Symptoms (Preop and Post-osteotomy)

The importance of early diagnosis of hip dysplasia in the pre-arthritic or early arthritic stage cannot be overstated, as overall clinical results are improved with early diagnosis [12]. Patients with hip dysplasia typically present as adolescents and young adults displaying symptoms of the pre-arthritic hip, namely groin pain and diminished activity level [13]. However, these symptoms are nonspecific, which poses a problem for providers seeing dysplastic patients with pre- or early arthritis. Thus the diagnosis of hip dysplasia is often delayed and/or inaccurate. In one study of 57 patients (72 % female) who underwent PAOs, Nunley et al. found that the mean time from onset of symptoms to diagnosis was 61.5 months, with an average of 3.3 providers being consulted to establish a definitive diagnosis [9].

Unfortunately, the current literature is sparse in specifying definitive symptoms presented by patients with hip dysplasia. In a review of 29 dysplastic patients, Klaue reported that the majority were young adults with groin pain accentuated by prolonged periods of sitting or walking long distances. These patients commonly reported catching and clicking of the hip, with some describing episodes of "giving way, leading to falls." In the Nunley study, 97 % of 57 patients described the onset of their pain as insidious, with 77 % experiencing moderate to severe pain on a daily basis. Most frequently, patients' symptoms were primarily located in the groin, though some patients experienced pain over the lateral aspect of the hip. Functionally, 85 % of patients displayed an antalgic gait when walking short distances while 38 % were found to have a Trendelenburg gait on physical examination. It is our recommendation that, when patients present with these symptoms, the examining clinician should have sufficient suspicion of the presence of hip joint pathology to obtain AP (pelvic) and lateral radiographs of the affected hip. Postoperatively, the patients in the Nunley cohort demonstrated improvement after a PAO procedure. Mean Harris hip scores increased from 66.4 to 91.7, and 95 % of patients reported improvements in function and/or a reduction in symptoms compared with their preoperative state [9].

Patients' Expectations Regarding Outcome

While several published studies have reported overall outcomes following PAO, few document patient satisfaction following the procedure. The van Bergayk study reported results of the Hip and Knee Arthroplasty Satisfaction Scale (HKASS) as a secondary outcome measure in their cohort. The HKASS is a validated four-question scale that considers pain relief, improvements in the ability to work and recreational activity, as well as overall patient satisfaction. They found that the overall satisfaction with the procedure was high with a mean HKASS of 89.7, and 12 patients rating the procedure perfectly with a score of 100 out of 100. While these results seem very positive, it must be remembered that the HVASS was validated in a population of older patients undergoing THA and uses a very simple satisfaction scale that likely has significant ceiling effects. As previous work has shown substantial differences in the expectations of physicians and patients, and individuals of different ages, it seems likely that less sanguine reports of patient outcomes after PAO might be derived from assessments that explored issues of greatest concern to the young adult patients undergoing this procedure.

Hip Arthroscopy

It is important to meet the pre-surgical expectations of patients if both the surgeon and the patient are to regard the procedure as "successful." However, patients who elect to undergo joint arthroscopy do so for a variety of reasons—pain relief, restoration of joint function, and/or to return to recreational and sporting activities. For this reason, it is important to identify the primary goals of each patient before undertaking an arthroscopic procedure, and the likelihood that the desired outcome will be achieved. Unlike the hip patients undergoing more traditional open procedures, most arthroscopy candidates are younger, more active, and, thus, express different goals and expectations. However, little data exist describing the expectations of patients undergoing arthroscopic procedures for treatment of hip disease. Most athletes competing at a high level of competition aspire to return to their pre-injury level of performance; however in older individuals involved in sport at the recreational level, moderation of activity after surgery may be a more acceptable course. At the present time, the expectations of non-athletic populations have yet to be explored, although many patients report that they are not as active 5 years post-operatively as they expected they would be at the time of surgery [14].

Activities of Hip Arthroscopy Patients

One of the main reasons patients elect to undergo hip arthroscopy for treatment of hip disease is to resume their desired activity level. Follow-up studies of patients undergoing labral debridement in the absence of bony abnormalities have shown that approximately 85 % are able to return to sport and other activities at up to 10 years following arthroscopic surgery

[15–18]. Two studies examined return to activity levels of elite athletes. In a cohort of professional soccer players, 80 % were able to return to their pre-injury level of competition following hip arthroscopy [18]. In addition, 100 % of patients from a cohort of elite athletes participating in a variety of sports (hockey, football, baseball, golf) were able to return to their pre-injury level of competition [17]. While the results in these small and select groups of patients are very encouraging, it is presently unknown whether the same outcomes may be expected in recreational athletes or sedentary patients with a combination of femoroacetabular impingement and labral pathology. Byrd has presented the results of a mixed group of athletes competing at the recreational, high school, or collegiate level, of whom 87 % were able to return to their previous level of competition within 3 months of surgery [15]. These positive findings appear to persist over time, as 70 % of patients still reported no complaints during daily living and sporting activities for up to 10 years post-surgery [16]. Therefore, the majority of individuals electing to undergo hip arthroscopy for isolated labral derangement should expect to resume normal daily and sporting activities following surgery.

For patients undergoing arthroscopic treatment of femoroacetabular impingement, data regarding participation in functional activities have been reported up to 4 years using the Hip Outcome Score (HOS) [19–27], which has been developed to assess patients' ability to perform daily (ADL) and sporting (Sport) activities [28]. Overall, the HOS ADL score improved from a mean of 67–84 points and scores on the HOS Sport improved from a mean of 49–76 points [21, 23, 26, 29–31]. Postoperative ADL scores of adolescent athletes [21, 26] were greater than scores for patients older than 50 years of age (93 vs. 81 points) [31] and for patients with concomitant chondral lesions (68 points) [29]. Similarly, younger athletes scored higher than patients greater than 50 years of age on the Sports subscale (86 vs. 72 points respectively) and patients with chondral lesions (50 points) [29]. For all cohorts of patients examined using the HOS following arthroscopic correction of FAI, improvements in both daily and sport function have been shown.

Numerous studies have also reported rates of return to sport following arthroscopic treatment of FAI, with an average of 88 % of patients returning to play at the pre-injury level of activity [15, 19–27, 32]. For adolescent athletes, return-to-sport rates of 97 % were reported with a mean follow-up of 14 months [21, 23, 24]. Similar high rates of return to sport were reported for professional athletes, with an average of 93 % successfully returning [20, 23–25, 27]. For three of the studies, the sports to which the athletes were unable to return were reported, including two soccer athletes, and one athlete each for football, hockey, and baseball [23, 24, 27]. Lower rates of return to sport were reported at the collegiate level, with only an average of 72 % being able to return [20, 23]. The sports to which the athletes were not able to return varied greatly and included hockey, swimming, field hockey, equestrian, track, and baseball. Return to sport rates of 70 % were also reported for two studies examining athletes with no designation of level of competition [19, 22]. Participation in martial arts appears to be especially affected by FAI, with only 50 % of these athletes able to return, compared to 81 % of all other athletes [22]. The most common sports recreational athletes participated in following surgery were biking, hiking, aerobics/fitness, swimming, jogging, soccer, hockey, and skiing [19].

Symptoms (Preop and After Recovery)

The primary complaint of patients with intra-articular hip pathology is pain and pain-induced limitations in function [33, 34]. Pain located in the anterior thigh or groin region is most commonly cited, with occurrence rates ranging from 88 to 100 % of patients with anterior labro-chondral lesions [32, 35, 36]. Less commonly, patients may complain of pain in the lateral thigh (37–59 %) [32, 36] or buttocks (17–60 %) [32, 36, 38], with buttock pain being more common in patients with posterior lesions [38]. The level of pain experienced by these patients has been described as mild in 11 % [34, 35] and moderate to severe in 86–90 % of patients [32, 36]. Eighty-six percent of subjects described their pain as sharp, 80 % reported episodes of dull pain, and 70 % reported a combination of dull and sharp pain [32]. More than half of patients report constant pain (55 %) and 91 % describe their pain as related to activity, with a reduction during rest [32]. Night pain has been described by 70 % of patients in one report [32]. Overall, most patients state that initially pain occurs during specific movements, usually a pivot or twisting motion; however, as time progresses, these episodes of pain become more frequent, leading to unremitting discomfort [35].

Patients may also describe a feeling of "giving way" in the joint, which may be indicative of an underlying structural instability due to the disruption of the capsulo-labral complex [33, 36, 39]. Numerous studies have reported range of motion deficits in 27–57 % of patients with labral pathology [33–35, 37, 38, 40–43]. Limitations are found to occur in flexion and internal rotation first, as these motions will result in contact of the femoral head with the anterior-superior acetabulum, reproducing pain if a lesion is present in this area [34, 38, 44]. However, no study has reported quantitative measures of range of motion in these patients, or data quantifying the loss of joint motion with progression of symptoms.

Several studies have investigated pain relief after hip arthroscopy using a Visual Analog Scale (VAS), where patients subjectively rate their pain on a scale of 1–10, with ten being the worst pain. A recent study by Larson et al. looked at 100 patients with an average age of 34.7 years who underwent hip arthroscopy for femoroacetabular impingement. Pain decreased from 6.74 preoperatively to 1.88 postoperatively, an improvement of 72% at an average follow-up of 9.9 months. Additionally, 100% of patients had positive impingement preoperatively compared to 14% postoperatively. Complications included heterotopic bone formation in 6 hips and 1 partial sciatic nerve neurapraxia, which resolved in 24 h. While no patient underwent repeat arthroscopy, 3 hips underwent total hip arthroplasty [45]. In another study by Stahelin et al. pain level decreased from 5.8 preoperatively to 1.4 postoperatively, an improvement of 75% in pain level at 6 months follow-up. While reduction in pain level was statistically significant for overall cohort, the reduction in pain was smaller and not statistically significant for group of patients with early osteoarthritis (Tonnis grade 1 and 2) vs. no osteoarthritis (Tonnis grade 0). Preoperatively, all patients had positive impingement, compared to only 23% of patients postoperatively. Statistically significant improvement in mobility was also observed with increase in flexion and internal rotation at 6 months follow-up. Complications included hypoesthesia in six cases, which resolved by 3 months. The results from these studies suggest hip arthroscopy for hip pathology results in pain relief and improvement in mobility for patient undergoing these procedures [46].

While there is a plethora of data within the literature regarding short-term outcomes following hip arthroscopy, there is an absence of longer term, higher-quality clinical trials (Level I and Level II) to justify the use of this approach for indications other than treatment of femoroacetabular impingement [47]. In a recent study, McCarthy et al. retrospectively reviewed the functional outcomes of 106 arthroscopy patients (average age: 39 years) as measured by the Nonarthritic Hip Score (NAHS) at a mean follow-up of 13 years post-surgery [48]. At the time of follow-up, survivorship was 91% at 1 year, 75% at 5 years, and 63% at 10 years with conversion to total hip arthroplasty defined as the endpoint. For the 62 patients in whom joint preservation remained successful, the average outcome score was 87.3. In another study, Byrd et al. reported the long-term results of 50 patients (average age: 38 years) [49]. Overall, arthroscopic surgery led to a 25 point improvement in the median Modified Harris Hip Score (MHHS) from 56 points preoperatively to 81 points at 10-year follow-up. Fourteen patients (28%) underwent conversion to THR, most frequently in those with pre-existing pathology (OA or AVN). In keeping with other studies, the most improvement was observed in patients undergoing surgery for removal of loose bodies [14]. Although many publications provide evidence of long-term effectiveness of hip arthroscopy for patients with loose bodies, synovitis, labral tears, and labral cysts, many published studies lack the duration or rigor to provide adequate evidence-based support for widespread adoption. Moreover, clearly stated contraindications of arthroscopic procedures, though recognized in concept, have yet to be promulgated on the basis of well-documented evidence.

Patients' Expectations Regarding Outcomes

Fulfillment of a patient's preoperative expectations is an important determinant of outcome following hip arthroscopy. In a single study, patients were asked to provide realistic expectations following hip arthroscopy for treatment of femoroacetabular impingement with respect to pain, walking ability, independence, sporting ability, general physical capacity, social contact, and mental well-being [50]. They were given choices of "much better," "better," "somewhat better," "unchanged," "worse," and "unknown." Prior to surgery, 97% of patients expected their pain to be "much better" or "better" following surgery, while 83% expected improvements in sporting ability. Over 50% also expected that their mental well-being would improve following surgery, in addition to their independence and social interactions. At 1 year post-surgery, the same patients were asked to rate their abilities using the same list of items reviewed before surgery. This assessment revealed that the preoperative expectations of over 50% of patients had not been met for in terms of hip pain, sporting ability, and general physical capacity. For over 1/3 of patients, preoperative expectations were overly optimistic for independence, walking ability, and mental well-being. Conversely, the majority of patients met expectations for social contact. Based on these findings, it is suggested that patients be counseled prior to surgery on setting realistic expectations following arthroscopic treatment for femoroacetabular impingement to increase the likelihood of successful outcomes.

Total Hip Replacement

Total hip replacement (THR) is currently the only solution for end-stage hip osteoarthritis (OA) [51]. Osteoarthritis candidates seek out total hip replacements to relieve joint pain and improve their overall health-related quality of life (HRQL) [52]. Traditionally, provider-generated clinical measures were used to assess the outcome of hip replacement, but over the past decade it has become apparent that patient-derived outcome measures are essential to match patients' needs and expectations in selecting treatment options [53]. Patient-generated outcome measures have the additional benefit of allowing the health status of a patient to be defined over time through documentation of activity level, pain and disease severity, and emotional well-being for longitudinal assessment of THR [54].

Patients' Activities Before and After THR

Physical activity varies greatly among patients seeking THR and many factors can contribute to the patient's level of activity both before and after surgery [55–57].

At preoperative presentation, patients with hip arthritis have significant difficulty in performing many activities, resulting in less frequent participation compared to peers [54–56]. Wylde et al. reported that prior to THR, patients found 82 % of all activities difficult to perform, including "exercise walking" and water aerobics, with sporting activities being the most challenging [57]. The percentage of patients participating in any form of physical activity for recreation prior to THR has been reported to be 11 %, primarily in the form of swimming or biking, approximately one fifth of rates prior to hip disease [53]. Huch et al. have also reported that participation in more demanding activities (e.g., hiking, cross-country skiing, gym, dancing) is almost nonexistent because of hip pain [54].

After THR, patients typically participate in a broad range of activities and often attempt to resume the activities they enjoyed prior to the onset of degenerative hip disease [54, 55, 57–61]. At 1–5 years following hip replacement surgery, the greatest improvements have been reported in low demand activities within the spheres of leisure, social interaction, and work [54, 57, 61]. Patients who performed sporting activities prior to the onset of hip disease often returned to those activities at varying times post-surgery, depending on the demands of each activity [54, 55, 57]. In a longitudinal four center study of 420 patients with advanced OA of the hip who underwent THR, Huch et al. found that 52 % of patients performed some form of recreational physical activity at 5 years after surgery [54]. Approximately half the THR patients had returned to biking, hiking, and/or swimming by 5 years post-THR, which was only slightly lower than the rate of lifetime participation for the same cohort. Lower participation rates were reported for downhill skiing, gymnastics, jogging, tennis, and dancing (2–17 %). One in seven patients (14 %) performed sports activities for more than 2 h a week.

Even though some physicians advise against high intensity sports [58], many studies have observed that a subset of patients participates in physically demanding sports after THR [54, 55, 59]. Williams et al. observed an increase in the percentage of patients participating in moderate to intense sports (UCLA scores of seven or greater) at both 1 year (37 %) and 5 years (52 %) after surgery [55]. Overall, these findings suggest that although some patients are able to engage in vigorous sporting activities after total hip replacement, most limit their physical exertion to lower impact activities such as leisure and social activities associated with everyday life [57].

An over-riding factor influencing patient activity, whether before or after THR, is the effect of aging [54–56]. Of the 97 % of patients who reported that they participated in sports when they were younger, only 36 % maintained their participation until the time of hip replacement surgery [54]. Although there is an overall increase in activity in patients after THR [53, 54, 56, 62], age still determines the extent of participation in physical activities [63]. Wagenmakers et al. surveyed patients after THR and found that the average patient spent roughly 24 h a week performing light-intensity activities [63]. Following the trend of increasing age and decreasing activity level, the research showed patients older than 75 years of age participated in approximately 17 h of activity per week in contrast to those younger than 75 who averaged 27 h [64]. Gender and BMI were also shown to be important, as men were found to be more active and participate in more sports activities than women [54, 55]. Increased BMI was also found to be a strong predictor of reduced activity, as expressed by the UCLA score [55].

Patients' Expectations Regarding Outcome After THR

Findings in the literature indicate that patient's expectations of the outcome of hip replacement vary greatly prior to surgery [61, 62, 65–67]. Most patients do expect that THR will provide pain relief [61, 62, 65], with 76 % of surveyed patients expected to have no pain after recovery [62]. At least two-thirds of patients (66 %) reported expectations of THR eliminating, or at least improving hip pain in hopes of no longer taking pain medications after surgery [68]. In addition, patients experiencing difficulty with range of motion and muscle power were more likely to expect pain relief as a result from their THR [61].

Patients also have significant expectations for improvement in their walking ability [61, 68], especially elimination of the need for assistive devices [65]. Virtually every patient (96 %) expects improved function in performing daily living activities after THR [62, 65, 66, 69], including getting out of bed or up from a chair (95–97 %), climbing stairs (95–98 %), performing housework and gardening (95–97 %), and shopping (98 %) [64, 66]. Similar expectations have been reported for functional activities performed at the limits of hip motion, including putting on shoes and socks (94 %) and clipping toenails (88–93 %) [64, 66]. Most patients with an interest in sporting activities expect their individual ability will improve after surgery, with 80 % of patients expecting an increase in their range of joint motion [66, 68]. Only a small number of patients expected overall improvement in sexual activity after surgery.

After surgery, patients have reported as high as 90 % satisfaction ratings, primarily because of elimination of symptoms and fulfillment of the patients' preoperative expectations of the procedure [62, 69]. Patients having high expectations of psychological benefits from surgery (28 % of patients surveyed) reported the highest overall satisfaction after THR (96 %) [61]. In some patients, the presence of residual pain after surgery or symptoms arising from comorbid conditions continue to affect aspects of patients' daily living (e.g., sleeping comfortably at night), leading to less satisfactory outcomes and fulfillment of expectations [61].

Many authors have examined the role of patient factors in setting expectations of THR [61, 62, 66–68]. By and large, pain relief is cited most frequently prior to hip replacement [60, 62, 66], with greater expectations being expressed by patients with a higher degree of preoperative disability [66]. Trends between highly educated patients and higher expectations were seen by use of the WOMAC score [62]. In the same study, and in disagreement with other literature [66], patients with lesser comorbidity scores had higher expectations than their counterparts [62]. Age has been reported to influence expectations as younger patients were seen to expect more psychological benefits whereas older patients expected more pain relief [69]. Age has also played a role in the level of expectation between surgeon and patient postoperatively [66]. Yet, due to improved surgical techniques and reduced risks associated with total joint replacement surgery, it has become more common to treat patients older than 80 years of age [70]. Differing opinions also exist in regard to comparing the expectations of both patients and surgeons [66, 67]. Jourdan et al. report patients are more optimistic in their expectations compared to the surgeons [66]. This is especially the case in regard to the more disabled patients [66]. In disagreement, Moran et al. reported surgeons in the United Kingdom had higher expectations than their patients [67].

Symptoms Before and After THR

As an end-stage procedure, patients seek hip arthroplasty to relieve the unremitting pain and disability of degenerative hip disease [51, 61, 62, 68, 71]. At this point, most patients are unable to walk for less than 30 min due to discomfort of their affected hip [51]. In one study, 50 of 52 patients surveyed listed as having strong tolerable pain accompanied with pain at rest [51]. In terms of standardized outcome measures, typical pain scores immediately prior to hip replacement are around 41–45 points on the WOMAC pain subscale and 26–33 points on the SF-36 bodily pain subscale, where 100 points correspond to complete absence of pain. The corresponding physical function subscales are typically 37–41 and 25–34 points, respectively [68, 71, 72].

After THR there is almost always dramatic relief of symptoms and restoration of joint function. Patients also reported a 98% success rate in alleviated pain and only having slight pain with no resting pain 6 months post-surgery [51]. In most series, this corresponds to an improvement of 30–40 points on the SF-36 Bodily Pain subscale and 37–40 points on the WOMAC Pain subscale. However, although almost all patients experience dramatic pain relief after this procedure, approximately 20% of patients still report some degree of unilateral hip pain compared to only 5% of age- and gender-matched controls ($p=0.001$) [61, 72]. In terms of functional outcome, improvements in Physical Function scores of 33–43 points on the SF 36 and 36–40 points on the WOMAC have been reported after THR, with 83% of patients experiencing improvements in their walking ability [51].

Conclusions

In this chapter, we have presented a summary of the outcome of three common hip procedures performed in patients with different pathologies at different ages, ranging from adolescence to old age. Our focus has been on the impact of each procedure on activity levels and hip symptoms, and the extent to which each is effective in meeting the expectations of each patient group. Our review of the published literature shows that all three procedures are effective in providing relief of symptoms although a minority of patients still experiences some hip pain. All three procedures restored the ability of each patient group to resume normal activities though to an extent that varied with each procedure. In patients undergoing hip arthroscopy or hip replacement, joint function is restored to near-normal levels for all but the most demanding activities. Acceptance of reduced intensity of activity with increasing age is a compounding factor, which affects fulfillment of expectations with respect to functional outcomes. In patients with dysplastic hips, osteotomy has proven to be an effective treatment for delaying osteoarthritis; however the reliability of the outcome and the level of symptom-free function after this procedure have not been demonstrated using rigorous long-term studies based on patient-generated outcome instruments. Similar considerations apply to hip arthroscopy; however, doubts remain concerning the predictability of outcome following these procedures and their impact on the longevity of the hip. Evidence is still awaited to provide a rational basis for prescribing arthroscopic procedures in the face of common prearthritic pathologies, and the relative efficacy of the surgical route in comparison with physical therapy and neuromuscular training. In comparison, the results of total hip arthroplasty appear to be the most predictable, and the most likely to restore near-normal function to the affected hip.

In view of the emerging status of all three approaches to the treatment of hip pathology, and the differences in their outcomes, we recommend that clinicians provide preoperative counsel to every individual patient regarding the likely outcome of treatment options, especially in terms of expected function with respect to each patient's lifestyle and aspirations and the extent to which preoperative symptoms will be eliminated.

References

1. Harris WH. Etiology of osteoarthritis of the hip. Clin Orthop Relat Res. 1986;213:20–33.
2. Leunig M, Siebenrock KA, Ganz R. Rationale of periacetabular osteotomy and background work. Instr Course Lect. 2001;50:229–38.
3. Tonnis D, Behrens K, Tscharani F. A modified technique of the triple pelvic osteotomy: early results. J Pediatr Orthop. 1981;1(3):241–9.
4. Salter RB. Innominate osteotomy in the treatment of congenital dislocation and subluxation of the hip. J Bone Joint Surg. 1961;43-B:518.
5. Steel HH. Triple osteotomy of the innominate bone. J Bone Joint Surg Am. 1973;55(2):343–50.
6. Ninomiya S, Tagawa H. Rotational acetabular osteotomy for the dysplastic hip. J Bone Joint Surg Am. 1984;66(3):430–6.
7. Ganz R, Klaue K, Vinh TS, Mast JW. A new periacetabular osteotomy for the treatment of hip dysplasias: technique and preliminary results. 1988. Clin Orthop Relat Res. 2004;(418):3–8.
8. Karam MD, Gao Y, McKinley T. Assessment of walking pattern pre and post peri-acetabular osteotomy. Iowa Orthop J. 2011;31:83–9.
9. Nunley RM, Prather H, Hunt D, Schoenecker PL, Clohisy JC. Clinical presentation of symptomatic acetabular dysplasia in skeletally mature patients. J Bone Joint Surg Am. 2011;93 Suppl 2:17–21. doi:10.2106/JBJS.J.01735.
10. van Bergayk AB, Garbuz DS. Quality of life and sports-specific outcomes after Bernese periacetabular osteotomy. J Bone Joint Surg. 2002;84B(3):339–43.
11. Romano CL, Frigo C, Randelli G, Pedotti A. Analysis of the gait of adults who had residua of congenital dysplasia of the hip. J Bone Joint Surg Am. 1996;78(10):1468–79.
12. Clohisy JC, Schutz AL, St John L, Schoenecker PL, Wright RW. Periacetabular osteotomy: a systematic literature review. Clin Orthop Relat Res. 2009;467(8):2041–52. doi:10.1007/s11999-009-0842-6.
13. Klaue K, Durnin CW, Ganz R. The acetabular rim syndrome. A clinical presentation of dysplasia of the hip. J Bone Joint Surg. 1991;73(3):423–9.
14. Nilsdotter AK, Toksvig-Larsen S, Roos EM. Knee arthroplasty: are patients' expectations fulfilled? A prospective study of pain and function in 102 patients with 5-year follow-up. Acta Orthop. 2009;80(1):55–61. doi:10.1080/17453670902805007.
15. Byrd JW, Jones KS. Hip arthroscopy in athletes: 10-year follow-up. Am J Sports Med. 2009;37(11):2140–3. doi:10.1177/0363546509337705.
16. Londers J, Van Melkebeek J. Hip arthroscopy: outcome and patient satisfaction after 5 to 10 years. Acta Orthop Belg. 2007;73(4):478–83.
17. McCarthy J, Barsoum W, Puri L, Lee JA, Murphy S, Cooke P. The role of hip arthroscopy in the elite athlete. Clin Orthop Relat Res. 2003;406:71–4. doi:10.1097/01.blo.0000043046.84315.02.
18. Saw T, Villar R. Footballer's hip a report of six cases. J Bone Joint Surg. 2004;86(5):655–8.
19. Brunner A, Horisberger M, Herzog RF. Sports and recreation activity of patients with femoroacetabular impingement before and after arthroscopic osteoplasty. Am J Sports Med. 2009;37(5):917–22. doi:10.1177/0363546508330144.
20. Byrd JW, Jones KS. Arthroscopic management of femoroacetabular impingement in athletes. Am J Sports Med. 2011;39(Suppl):7S–13. doi:10.1177/0363546511404144.
21. Fabricant PD, Heyworth BE, Kelly BT. Hip arthroscopy improves symptoms associated with FAI in selected adolescent athletes. Clin Orthop Relat Res. 2012;470(1):261–9. doi:10.1007/s11999-011-2015-7.
22. Kang C, Hwang DS, Cha SM. Acetabular labral tears in patients with sports injury. Clin Orthop Surg. 2009;1(4):230–5. doi:10.4055/cios.2009.1.4.230.
23. Nho SJ, Magennis EM, Singh CK, Kelly BT. Outcomes after the arthroscopic treatment of femoroacetabular impingement in a mixed group of high-level athletes. Am J Sports Med. 2011;39(Suppl):14S–9. doi:10.1177/0363546511401900.
24. Philippon M, Schenker M, Briggs K, Kuppersmith D. Femoroacetabular impingement in 45 professional athletes: associated pathologies and return to sport following arthroscopic decompression. Knee Surg Sports Traumatol Arthrosc. 2007;15(7):908–14. doi:10.1007/s00167-007-0332-x.
25. Philippon MJ, Weiss DR, Kuppersmith DA, Briggs KK, Hay CJ. Arthroscopic labral repair and treatment of femoroacetabular impingement in professional hockey players. Am J Sports Med. 2010;38(1):99–104. doi:10.1177/0363546509346393.
26. Philippon MJ, Yen YM, Briggs KK, Kuppersmith DA, Maxwell RB. Early outcomes after hip arthroscopy for femoroacetabular impingement in the athletic adolescent patient: a preliminary report. J Pediatr Orthop. 2008;28(7):705–10. doi:10.1097/BPO.0b013e318186eb2e.
27. Singh PJ, O'Donnell JM. The outcome of hip arthroscopy in Australian football league players: a review of 27 hips. Arthroscopy. 2010;26(6):743–9. doi:10.1016/j.arthro.2009.10.010.
28. Martin RL, Kelly BT, Philippon MJ. Evidence of validity for the hip outcome score. Arthroscopy. 2006;22(12):1304–11. doi:10.1016/j.arthro.2006.07.027.
29. Cooper AP, Basheer SZ, Maheshwari R, Regan L, Madan SS. Outcomes of hip arthroscopy. A prospective analysis and comparison between patients under 25 and over 25 years of age. Br J Sports Med. 2013;47(4):234–8. doi:10.1136/bjsports-2012-091028.
30. McCormick F, Nwachukwu BU, Alpaugh K, Martin SD. Predictors of hip arthroscopy outcomes for labral tears at minimum 2-year follow-up: the influence of age and arthritis. Arthroscopy. 2012; 28(10):1359–64. doi:10.1016/j.arthro.2012.04.059.
31. Philippon MJ, Schroder ESBG, Briggs KK. Hip arthroscopy for femoroacetabular impingement in patients aged 50 years or older. Arthroscopy. 2012;28(1):59–65. doi:10.1016/j.arthro.2011.07.004.
32. Burnett RS, Della Rocca GJ, Prather H, Curry M, Maloney WJ, Clohisy JC. Clinical presentation of patients with tears of the acetabular labrum. J Bone Joint Surg Am. 2006;88(7):1448–57. doi:10.2106/JBJS.D.02806.
33. Guevara CJ, Pietrobon R, Carothers JT, Olson SA, Vail TP. Comprehensive morphologic evaluation of the hip in patients with symptomatic labral tear. Clin Orthop Relat Res. 2006;453:277–85. doi:10.1097/01.blo.0000246536.90371.12.
34. Troum OM, Crues 3rd JV. The young adult with hip pain: diagnosis and medical treatment, circa 2004. Clin Orthop Relat Res. 2004;418:9–17.
35. Fitzgerald RH Jr. Acetabular labrum tears. Diagnosis and treatment. Clin Orthop Relat Res. 1995;(311):60–68
36. Keeney JA, Peelle MW, Jackson J, Rubin D, Maloney WJ, Clohisy JC. Magnetic resonance arthrography versus arthroscopy in the evaluation of articular hip pathology. Clin Orthop Relat Res. 2004;429:163–9.
37. O'Leary JA, Berend K, Vail TP. The relationship between diagnosis and outcome in arthroscopy of the hip. Arthroscopy. 2001;17(2):181–8. doi:10.1053/jars.2001.21481.
38. Hase T, Ueo T. Acetabular labral tear: arthroscopic diagnosis and treatment. Arthroscopy. 1999;15(2):138–41. doi:10.1053/ar.1999.v15.0150131.
39. Shindle MK, Ranawat A, Kelly B. Diagnosis and management of traumatic and atraumatic instability in the athletic patient. Clin Sports Med. 2006;25:309–26.
40. Braly BA, Beall DP, Martin HD. Clinical examination of the athletic hip. Clin Sports Med. 2006;25(2):199–210. doi:10.1016/j.csm.2005.12.001. vii.
41. Kelly B, Williams RJ, Philippon M. Hip arthroscopy: current indications, treatment options, and management issues. Am J Sports Med. 2003;31(6):1020–37.
42. Lewis CL, Sahrmann SA. Acetabular labral tears. Phys Ther. 2006;86(1):110–21.

43. McCarthy JC, Lee J-a. Arthroscopic intervention in early hip disease. Clin Orthop Relat Res. 2004;429:157–62.
44. Narvani AA, Tsiridis E, Kendall S, Chaudhuri R, Thomas P. A preliminary report on prevalence of acetabular labrum tears in sports patients with groin pain. Knee Surg Sports Traumatol Arthrosc. 2003;11(6):403–8. doi:10.1007/s00167-003-0390-7.
45. Larson CM, Giveans MR. Arthroscopic management of femoroacetabular impingement: early outcomes measures. Arthroscopy. 2008;24(5):540–6. doi:10.1016/j.arthro.2007.11.007.
46. Stahelin L, Stahelin T, Jolles BM, Herzog RF. Arthroscopic offset restoration in femoroacetabular cam impingement: accuracy and early clinical outcome. Arthroscopy. 2008;24(1):51–7. doi:10.1016/j.arthro.2007.08.010. e51.
47. Stevens MS, LeGay DA, Glazebrook MA, Amirault D. The evidence for hip arthroscopy: grading the current indications. J Arthrosc Relat Surg. 2010;26(10):1370–83.
48. McCarthy JC, Jarrett BT, Ojeifo O, Lee JA, Bragdon CR. What factors influence long-term survivorship after hip arthroscopy? Clin Orthop Relat Res. 2011;469(2):362–71. doi:10.1007/s11999-010-1559-2.
49. Byrd JW, Jones KS. Prospective analysis of hip arthroscopy with 10-year followup. Clin Orthop Relat Res. 2010;468(3):741–6. doi:10.1007/s11999-009-0841-7.
50. Mannion AF, Impellizzeri FM, Naal FD, Leunig M. Fulfilment of patient-rated expectations predicts the outcome of surgery for femoroacetabular impingement. Osteoarthritis Cartilage. 2013;21(1):44–50. doi:10.1016/j.joca.2012.09.013.
51. Horstmann T, Vornholt-Koch S, Brauner T, Grau S, Mundermann A. Impact of total hip arthroplasty on pain, walking ability, and cardiovascular fitness. J Orthop Res. 2012;30(12):2025–30. doi:10.1002/jor.22163.
52. Bruyere O, Ethgen O, Neuprez A, Zegels B, Gillet P, Huskin JP, Reginster JY. Health-related quality of life after total knee or hip replacement for osteoarthritis: a 7-year prospective study. Arch Orthop Trauma Surg. 2012;132(11):1583–7. doi:10.1007/s00402-012-1583-7.
53. Ostendorf M, van Stel HF, Buskens E, Schrijvers AJ, Marting LN, Verbout AJ, Dhert WJ. Patient-reported outcome in total hip replacement. A comparison of five instruments of health status. J Bone Joint Surg. 2004;86(6):801–8.
54. Huch K, Muller KA, Sturmer T, Brenner H, Puhl W, Gunther KP. Sports activities 5 years after total knee or hip arthroplasty: the Ulm Osteoarthritis Study. Ann Rheum Dis. 2005;64(12):1715–20. doi:10.1136/ard.2004.033266.
55. Williams DH, Greidanus NV, Masri BA, Duncan CP, Garbuz DS. Predictors of participation in sports after hip and knee arthroplasty. Clin Orthop Relat Res. 2012;470(2):555–61. doi:10.1007/s11999-011-2198-y.
56. Stevens M, Wagenmakers R, Groothoff JW, Bulstra SK, van den Akker-Scheek I, Zijlstra W. Physical activity behavior after total hip arthroplasty (THA): a prediction based on patient characteristics. Patient Educ Couns. 2007;69(1–3):196–9. doi:10.1016/j.pec.2007.08.012.
57. Wylde V, Livesey C, Blom AW. Restriction in participation in leisure activities after joint replacement: an exploratory study. Age Ageing. 2012;41(2):246–9. doi:10.1093/ageing/afr180.
58. Browne JA. The mature athlete with hip arthritis. Clin Sports Med. 2011;30(2):453–62. doi:10.1016/j.csm.2010.12.011.
59. Chatterji U, Ashworth MJ, Lewis PL, Dobson PJ. Effect of total hip arthroplasty on recreational and sporting activity. ANZ J Surg. 2004;74(6):446–9. doi:10.1111/j.1445-1433.2004.03028.x.
60. Golant A, Christoforou DC, Slover JD, Zuckerman JD. Athletic participation after hip and knee arthroplasty. Bull NYU Hosp Jt Dis. 2010;68(2):76–83.
61. Mancuso CA, Jout J, Salvati EA, Sculco TP. Fulfillment of patients' expectations for total hip arthroplasty. J Bone Joint Surg Am. 2009;91(9):2073–8. doi:10.2106/JBJS.H.01802.
62. Mahomed NN, Liang MH, Cook EF, Daltroy LH, Fortin PR, Fossel AH, Katz JN. The importance of patient expectations in predicting functional outcomes after total joint arthroplasty. J Rheumatol. 2002;29(6):1273–9.
63. Wagenmakers R, Stevens M, Groothoff JW, Zijlstra W, Bulstra SK, van Beveren J, van Raaij JJ, van den Akker-Scheek I. Physical activity behavior of patients 1 year after primary total hip arthroplasty: a prospective multicenter cohort study. Phys Ther. 2011;91(3):373–80. doi:10.2522/ptj.20100148.
64. Wagenmakers R, Stevens M, Zijlstra W, Jacobs ML, van den Akker-Scheek I, Groothoff JW, Bulstra SK. Habitual physical activity behavior of patients after primary total hip arthroplasty. Phys Ther. 2008;88(9):1039–48. doi:10.2522/ptj.20070375.
65. Ghomrawi HM, Franco Ferrando N, Mandl LA, Do H, Noor N, Gonzalez Della Valle A. How often are patient and surgeon recovery expectations for total joint arthroplasty aligned? Results of a pilot study. HSS J. 2011;7(3):229–34. doi:10.1007/s11420-011-9203-6.
66. Jourdan C, Poiraudeau S, Descamps S, Nizard R, Hamadouche M, Anract P, Boisgard S, Galvin M, Ravaud P. Comparison of patient and surgeon expectations of total hip arthroplasty. PLoS One. 2012;7(1):e30195. doi:10.1371/journal.pone.0030195.
67. Moran M, Khan A, Sochart D, Andrew G. Expect the best, prepare for the worst: surgeon and patient expectation of the outcome of primary total hip and knee replacement. Ann R Coll Surg Engl. 2003;85:204–6.
68. Ghomrawi HM, Dolan MM, Rutledge J, Alexiades MM. Recovery expectations of hip resurfacing compared to total hip arthroplasty: a matched pairs study. Arthritis Care Res. 2011;63(12):1753–7. doi:10.1002/acr.20626.
69. Mancuso CA, Salvati EA, Johanson NA, Peterson MG, Charlson ME. Patients' expectations and satisfaction with total hip arthroplasty. J Arthroplasty. 1997;12(4):387–96.
70. Nilsdotter AK, Petersson IF, Roos EM, Lohmander LS. Predictors of patient relevant outcome after total hip replacement for osteoarthritis: a prospective study. Ann Rheum Dis. 2003;62(10):923–30.
71. Keurentjes JC, Fiocco M, So-Osman C, Onstenk R, Koopman-Van Gemert AW, Poll RG, Kroon HM, Vliet Vlieland TP, Nelissen RG. Patients with severe radiographic osteoarthritis have a better prognosis in physical functioning after hip and knee replacement: a cohort-study. PLoS One. 2013;8(4):e59500. doi:10.1371/journal.pone.0059500.
72. Santaguida PL, Hawker GA, Hudak PL, Glazier R, Mahomed NN, Kreder HJ, Coyte PC, Wright JG. Patient characteristics affecting the prognosis of total hip and knee joint arthroplasty: a systematic review. Can J Surg. 2008;51(6):428–36.

Rehabilitation After Hip Arthroscopy

85

RobRoy L. Martin, Benjamin R. Kivlan, and Keelan R. Enseki

Introduction

Rehabilitation following hip arthroscopy is commonly prescribed to guide and enhance recovery of the patient. The physical therapist can serve an important role in a successful outcome by implementing timely and appropriate therapeutic interventions. The goal of a successful rehabilitation program is to maximize patient comfort and function after surgery through a thoughtful progression of therapeutic interventions. This typically includes an individualized and graduated exercise program in accordance with tissue healing. A physical therapist without the appropriate knowledge regarding hip arthroscopy can potentially have a negative impact on a patient's outcome. In order to enhance the patient's recovery, communication between the surgical team and physical therapist is critical. This chapter describes potential strategies to improve communication between the therapist and surgical team, outlines general postoperative rehabilitation guidelines related to common arthroscopic surgical procedures, defines criteria to progress a patient along various phases of a protocol, and highlights pearls and perils along the rehabilitation process.

Arthroscopic intervention for conditions of the hip joint has been a topic of growing interest in the field of orthopedics and sports medicine. Compared to more invasive procedures, relatively active and younger populations are typically candidates for hip arthroscopy. The unique aspects of hip arthroscopy coupled with the physical activity demands of the typical surgical candidate require a significantly different approach from postoperative protocols that exist for the more common hip surgery procedures (i.e., total hip arthroplasty, femoral neck ORIF).

R.L. Martin, PhD, PT, CSCS (✉)
Department of Physical Therapy-RHS, UPMC—Center for Sports Medicine, Duquesne University, 111A Health Science Building, 600 Forbes Avenue, Pittsburgh, PA 15282, USA
e-mail: martinr280@duq.edu

B.R. Kivlan, PT, OCS, SCS, CSCS
John G Rangos Sr School of Health Sciences, Duquesne University, Pittsburgh, PA, USA

K.R. Enseki, MS, PT, ATC, OCS, SCS, CSCS
Centers for Rehab Services, University of Pittsburgh Center for Sports Medicine, Pittsburgh, PA, USA

Department of Physical Therapy, University of Pittsburgh School of Health and Rehabilitation Sciences, Pittsburgh, PA, USA

General Rehabilitation Guidelines

Rehabilitation principles have been discussed for patients undergoing labral, osteoplasty, capsular modification, and tissue release procedures [1–5]. Many of the available protocols are unique for each specific surgical procedure. Protocols for hip arthroscopy have traditionally been based on time established criteria for tissue healing. However, there are several factors to consider beyond the surgical procedure that influence the progression of a rehabilitation program. These factors include the location and extent of the articular and soft tissue pathology of the hip joint, as well as the overall physical condition of the patient, as well as their expectations and mobility requirements. An effective rehabilitation program will account for all of these factors and progress the patient based on the attainment of functionally relevant physical performance measures in addition to specific time-based criteria. This approach individualizes the rehabilitation program to each patient.

Generally, protocols for hip arthroscopy follow similar principals. Early physical therapy treatment is almost always recommended. Typically, formal therapy is initiated within the first week after surgery. However, it is not uncommon for rehabilitation to begin the day of surgery if the patient is medically stable. The goals for immediate postoperative treatment following hip arthroscopy are concurrent with those for arthroscopic procedures for other joints. An attempt is made to control postoperative inflammation. This may be

J.C. McCarthy et al. (eds.), *Hip Joint Restoration*, DOI 10.1007/978-1-4614-0694-5_85

achieved through utilization of modalities and anti-inflammatory medications. Early, protected range of motion (ROM) is recommended to reduce swelling, improve joint mobility, and encourage health of articular cartilage. A continuous passive motion machine (CPM) may be prescribed to gently move the hip joint through a safe range of sagittal hip motion. Range of motion may also be initiated by the use of a stationary bike set at a low resistance level and high seat position. Passive range of motion (PROM) and manual therapy are introduced in the early stages of rehabilitation to initiate joint motion in multiple planes. Circumduction of the hip joint is recommended as an integral part of the PROM program [6].

To protect the healing hip from excessive motion that may disrupt healing process, a postoperative brace can be prescribed when limiting excessive hip flexion and abduction is desired. The brace is typically prescribed for 10–14 days. In most cases the patient will be on crutches with a limited weight-bearing status. The recommended time and amount of limited weight-bearing will be dependent on the specific procedure performed. A minimum time period of 10–12 weeks is typically recommended before returning to athletic or strenuous labor activities [1, 2, 6]. It should be realized that this is a minimum estimate, and can be significantly longer depending on the procedure(s) performed and individual patient characteristics. In rare cases, the rehabilitation course may be accelerated. However, caution should be taken to ensure the rate of rehabilitation does not exceed the healing rate of the affected tissues.

The guidelines for postoperative rehabilitation will have to be adjusted according to the arthroscopic hip procedures and the specific tissues affected. Labral, capsular, osteoplasty, chondral, iliotibial band (ITB), and psoas procedures will need to have postoperative restrictions adjusted accordingly. The therapist needs to be knowledgeable in the specific procedure performed to complement healing and ensure a safe progression of the patient through the various phases of rehabilitation. The type of procedure as well as its anatomic location and severity play a role in how quickly a patient may progress through the rehabilitation program. For example, a patient with a large chondral lesion in a weight-bearing portion of the acetabulum will be progressed more conservatively than a smaller lesion in a non-weight-bearing zone. Rehabilitation guidelines following labral repair, capsular plication/capsulorrhaphy, osteoplasty, and chondral procedures are more conservative in nature and require prolonged periods of maximal protection. Labral debridement and tissues release procedures can generally be progressed more rapidly. A summary of the restrictions for each procedure is outlined in Table 85.1 and discussed in detail below.

Labral Debridement and Repair

Isolated labral debridement can generally progress through a rehabilitation program relatively quickly. Crutches are used for only 2–7 days with the patient weight-bearing as tolerated

Table 85.1 A summary of restrictions for arthroscopic hip procedures

Procedure	Weight-bearing	Range of motion limitations	Phase 1 maximum protection (weeks)	Phase 2 moderate protection (weeks)	Phase 3 minimal protection (weeks)	Phase 4 functional progression (weeks)	Phase 5 sports-work retraining (weeks)
Labral debridement	WBAT 2–7 days	No limits	0–1	2–3	4–5	5–6	6–10
Labral repair	TTWB 2–4 WBAT 4–6 weeks	Flexion: 90° Extension: 0° Abduction: 25° External rotation: 25° Internal rotation: 25° 4–6 Weeks	0–4	4–6	6–10	10–16	16–24
Anterior modification	30 % PWB 3–4 Weeks	Extension: 0° Abduction: 20° External rotation: 0° 3–4 Weeks	0–4	4–6	6–8	8–12	12–16
Osteoplasty	20 lbs. PWB 4 Weeks	Flexion: 90° Abduction 25° Internal rotation: 25° 2 Weeks	0–4	4–6	6–10	10–16	16–24
Chondroplasty/microfracture	TTWB 6–8 weeks	Flexion: 90° Extension: 0° Abduction: 25° External rotation: 25° Internal rotation: 25° 4–6 Weeks	0–6	6–8	8–12	12–16	16–24

(WBAT). Weight-bearing, range of motion, strengthening progression, and return to activity are dictated as the patient's symptoms allow. Crutches may be discontinued once the patient's strength is good, pain is minimal with weight-bearing, and he/she is able to ambulate without deviation.

Labral repair requires protection to the area of the repair with limitations in ROM and weight-bearing. The length of time for these restrictions largely depends on the location and severity of the tear and relate to time for soft tissue healing. It must be noted that these limitations are not based on hip-related studies but expert opinion and may vary from surgeon to surgeon. Generally, patients may be restricted to be touch-down weight-bearing (TTWB) for the first 2–6 weeks. Graduated weight-bearing progression may continue until the sixth postoperative week. Within that timeframe the patient should progress from partial weight-bearing (PWB) with crutches to WBAT with use of a single crutch on the opposite side. Gait training is focused on restoring symmetry of stride length and speed while correcting for frontal plane deviation due to pain or weakness. Assistive devices may be discontinued when the patient no longer has weight-bearing restrictions and can demonstrate symmetry in gait pattern without pain. Range of motion is also restricted for the first 2–6 weeks depending on the size, location, and stability of the labral tear. Allowable ROM in the early postoperative phase is to 90° flexion, neutral extension, and 25° of abduction, internal rotation, and external rotation. A CPM may be used to encourage sagittal plane hip motion within the recommended ROM. Physical therapists must be careful to avoid disrupting the labral repair. Twisting or pivoting movements while weight-bearing may compromise the labral repair and should be avoided until adequate healing has occurred. Combined hip movements that commonly impinge the labrum, specifically hip flexion, adduction, and internal rotation (i.e., the Impingement Test position), should also be avoided early in rehabilitation.

Capsular Plication and Capsulorrhaphy

Individuals who have undergone capsular plication or capsulorrhaphy are similar to those with labral repair in that the area of capsule that was modified will need to be protected. In the cases of anterior capsular procedure external rotation and extension arc limited to neutral with abduction limited to 20°. For posterior capsular procedures internal rotation is limited to neutral, flexion to 60°, and adduction to 10°. Weight-bearing is restricted to 30 % PWB to prevent excessive stress on the capsule. These restrictions are continued for 3–4 weeks. Capsular modification can be performed with thermal and/or plication type procedures. Capsular modification procedures are typically performed on patients demonstrating significant redundancy and capsular laxity [7, 8]. The therapist must avoid stretching the region of capsular modification until adequate tissue healing has occurred. For example, if modification is made to the anterior capsule, positions of extension and external rotation are protected to avoid disruption of the surgical procedure. Although not commonly performed, a posterior capsular modification would require protection from flexion and internal rotation of the hip joint.

Osteoplasty

Osteoplasty procedures also require limitations to protect surgical areas where bone was removed. Early ROM restrictions with flexion, adduction, and internal rotation are limited by pain for first 2 weeks. Conservative guidelines limit flexion to 90°, 25°, internal rotation and abduction for 2 weeks. Following this ROM can be more aggressively pursued. Weight-bearing is limited to 20 lbs PWB for 2–4 weeks after surgery. The primary concern for rehabilitation following femoral osteoplasty is a stress reaction to the newly reshaped femoral neck. The smaller femoral neck can be vulnerable to stress fractures and the therapist must guide to gradually increase weight-bearing load as the femoral neck accommodates to less bony mass.

Microfracture and Chondroplasty

Microfracture and chondroplasty are similar to that performed in other joints. This procedure when performed at the hip shares similar concerns in that the area of cartilage addressed needs to be protected from shear forces. Rehabilitation allows for gentle ROM as limited by pain. However, extremes of flexion, adduction, and internal rotation are avoided for 6 weeks. Conservative guidelines include restrictions in ROM of 90° flexion, neutral extension and 25°of abduction, internal rotation, and external rotation for 4–6 weeks. Weight-bearing is limited to TTWB for 6–8 weeks. Microfracture procedures require protected weight-bearing for extended times to allow for healing to occur. Patients must be educated on weight-bearing status and avoiding shearing stresses caused by pivoting on the limb. The progression of a therapeutic exercise must be gradual to protect the healing articular surface(s).

Postoperative Report Form

A therapist can use the specific information about the surgical procedures to assist in the rehabilitation process. Information regarding the specific procedures performed can be conveyed to the physical therapist in postoperative report form

(Table 85.1). This form can also outline the presence of coexisting pathologies that might impact the rehabilitation progression. Also, the postoperative report form can outline operative findings, including the condition of cartilage, labrum, capsular, and type of impingement. Findings associated with the iliopsoas muscle and ITB may also be outlined. This will help the therapist to understand the procedure and give insight as to the activities that may be appropriate for the patient to perform. For example, the therapist may receive a referral of a patient status post labral debridement. If the patient also has underlying chondral damage, soft and showing signs of wear, the progression will need to be slower than a patient with normal articular cartilage. Likewise size and location of the chondral defect will give a physical therapist insight as to how aggressively they can progress individuals.

Information regarding osteoplasty could outline how much bone was removed and the risk for stress fracture. For example, females greater than 40 and males greater than 50 years old may have inadequate bone quality and be at higher risk for stress fracture. The information outlined in this postoperative report form will allow the therapist and surgical team to communicate efficiently by conveying valuable information that may impact how quickly the patient is progressed as well as help determine time appropriate expectations in accordance with the postoperative rehabilitation protocol.

Rehabilitation Protocol and Progression

A general protocol and guidelines for rehabilitation are outlined in Appendix 85.2. Pictures to accompany this protocol are included in Appendix 85.3. This protocol can be customized to most arthroscopic hip procedures and is generally divided into five phases. The phases can address ROM, strength, pain, and weight-bearing status. In the protocol surgeon can specifically identify timeline for brace and CPM use. Weight-bearing status (WBAT, PWB with specific percent body weight or TTWB) and use of assistive device with specific time frames can be defined in the protocol. Also, the surgeon can outline expected time frames the patient should remain in each phase. A minimal time frame defined for each phase can be used in conjunction with objective-based criteria to help determine when the patient is able to progress to the next phase. Progression through the phase should be based on not only time frame but also objective criteria-based indicators. Time frame estimates allow for appropriate tissue healing. Once the time for tissue healing has been reached, objective criteria based indicators ensure the patient has appropriate pain levels, ROM, strength, proprioception, and coordination to tolerate progression into the next phase. These criteria-based indicators include functional activities that integrate ROM, strength, proprioception, and coordination.

Phases of Rehabilitation Protocol

Maximum Protection Phase

Phase 1 is defined as maximum protection. The goals of this phase are to maintain ROM, prevent muscular weakness and inhibition, protect repaired tissue, decrease pain, and limit excessive inflammation. During this phase brace and CPM use as well as weight-bearing restrictions are implemented. Pain-free ROM is emphasized and includes using a high seat setting for stationary biking. Isometric hip and trunk exercises are performed to improve lumbopelvic stabilization. Modalities can be implemented for pain and inflammation control. This phase continues until the following criteria are met: (1) average pain levels <4/10, (2) ROM of flexion >90°, abduction >25°, and internal rotation >25°, and (3) strength ≥3/5 for hip extension and abduction. Patients must also be able to demonstrate independent use of appropriate assistive device within the weight-bearing restrictions outlined by the surgeon.

Pearls and Perils of Phase 1

- Do enough BUT not too much.
- Do not forget exercises to target trunk/core.
- Use pain as a guide for exercise intensity!!

Moderate Protection Phase

Phase 2 is defined as moderate protection. The goals of this phase are to increase ROM to near normal, obtain a general pain-free status, increase strength, and normalize gait without use of an assistive device. A patient can progress to one crutch and/or cane as needed to prevent gait deviations. Exercises should include AROM and PROM of all hip motions including hip flexion combined with adduction and internal rotation as tolerated and within limitations outlined by surgeon. It is important that ROM activities do not increase symptoms. Consider adding GENTLE manual distraction with PROM (Fig. 85.1). Active range of motion exercises should include side-lying clamshell and bent leg fallout. For strengthening exercises, resistance can be added to AROM exercises once the exercise can be performed pain free. No exercise should increase patient symptoms. Exercises may include bridging, prone plank, seated hip flexion, and 4-way SLR. Exercises and gait training can be done in water and may include swimming with leg buoy (no kicking) and aquatic-suspended jogging. This phase continues until the following criteria are met: (1) average pain level <2/10, (2) ROM of flexion >120° and adduction and internal rotation 80% of the uninvolved side, and (3) strength >3+/5 with hip abduction and extension. Functionally, the patient should ambulate independently without assistive device.

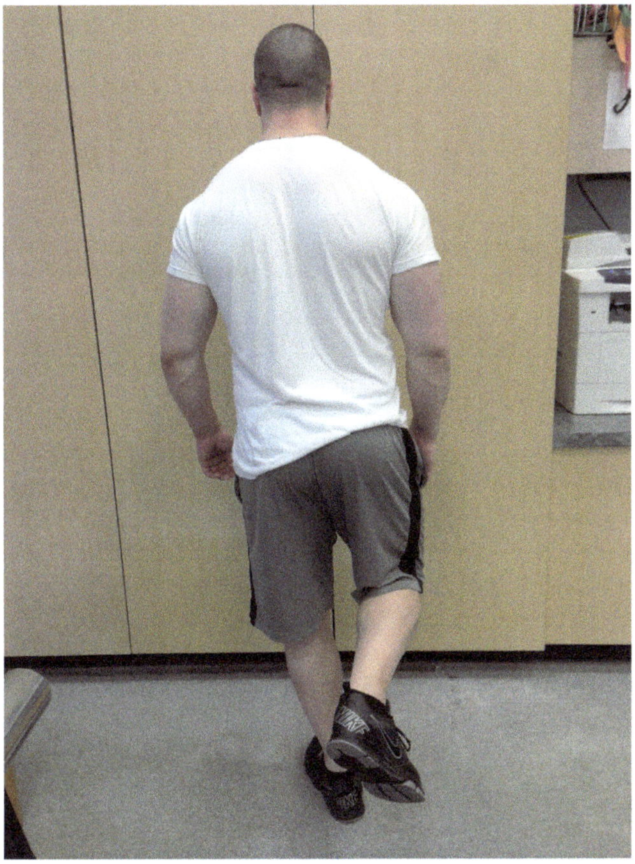

Fig. 85.1 Single leg stance

Additionally the patient should able to perform a deep squat to 70° of hip flexion and pass a single-leg stance test (no evidence of pain, pelvic drop, or trunk compensation).

Pearls and Perils of Phase 2

- Make sure to include hip flexion combined with adduction and internal rotation.
  - Distraction may allow the patient to achieve more ROM.
- Do not progress off assistive device too quickly.
  - Use cane if necessary.
- Exercises and gait training can be done in water.
  - Can include swimming with leg buoy to avoid kicking.
  - Can include aqua-suspended jogging.

Minimal Protection Phase

Phase 3 is defined as minimal protection. The goals of this phase include obtaining ROM 100 % normal, increase strength of trunk and entire lower extremity to near normal, and achieving a normal gait pattern. At this point the patient should be ambulating without the use of an assistive device. Any subtle deviations should be corrected with appropriate stretching, mobilization, strengthening, stabilization, and proprioceptive interventions. For example it is common that weakness in the external rotators of the hip joint and gluteus medius might lead to excessive dynamic valgus. Strategies to improve lower extremity biomechanics can include the use of orthotics and corrective taping to support the medial longitudinal. Stretching should emphasize tight structure to allow normal ROM. A comprehensive flexibility assessment can be done to assess for tight muscles and soft tissue structures of the hip joint. This includes the iliopsoas, piriformis, gluteus medius, rectus femoris, and hamstrings muscles as well the ITB. For example, a tight iliopsoas muscle may need to be addressed for those without a normal terminal stance phase because of a limitation in hip extension. Joint mobilizations should also be added to address any capsular limitations of the hip joint capsular mobility. Particular attention should be directed to restoring pain-free ROM into commonly provocative positions of flexion, adduction, and internal rotation (FADDIR) and flexion-abduction-external rotation (FABER). Limitation in these motions can be addressed with lateral distraction, long axis distraction, and posterior capsular mobilization. Strengthening exercises can be progressed to include double limb supported closed chain exercises. Generally, resistance is limited to body weight. Exercises should emphasize gluteus medius, gluteus maximus, the deep external rotators of the hip joint, and trunk stabilizers in all planes. Exercises may include side planks, mini-squats, wall slide, resisted walking (forward, backwards and sideways), and toe raises. Balance and stabilization activities can be progressed to single limb balance activities emphasizing proper lower extremity alignment with lumbopelvic stabilization once the patient has demonstrated good body mechanics and motor control with double limb support exercises. These activities should be performed on a stable surface. Water exercises can be progressed with functional sport-specific activities in chest-deep water. Stationary bike can be progressed with increasing resistance and normal seat height setting, as symptoms allow. Criteria to progress out of this phase include: (1) generally pain-free status, (2) near normal ROM, and (3) strength in all muscle groups ≥4/5. Functional performance tests of strength and balance should also be close to normal. Patients should demonstrate a deep squat test to greater than 90° of hip flexion and be able to perform a symmetrical time in single limb balance test. Star Excursion Balance Test should have posterior-medial, posterior-lateral, and medial reach distances within 75 % of the uninvolved extremity.

Pearls and Perils of Phase 3

- Make sure the trunk-core muscles are engaged during exercises and gait.

  - Do not forget plantar flexors as they provide 85 % of the forward propulsion.
- Normalize motion.
  - Including combined hip adduction-flexion-internal rotation.
- Correct subtle gait deviations.
  - Particularly with excessive hip internal rotation.

Functional Progression Phase

Phase 4 is defined as functional progression. The goals of this phase includes obtaining strength of trunk and lower extremity to 100 % normal with the ability to tolerate sport-job specific positions with proper lower extremity alignment. Stretching should continue to normalize flexibility for lower half as needed. Strengthening should progress to single limb closed chain exercises with increasing resistance as tolerated while maintaining high repetitions (12–25 reps) with all strengthening exercises. Sport-specific exercises should be done with slow, controlled, non-explosive, and non-plyometric type movements. Exercises should include advance bridging on unstable surface (Swiss ball), single limb cord rotations, step-up progression, (side, forward, and backward), and lunging in all directions. Balance-stabilization activities can include advanced dynamic balance activities on stable and unstable surfaces. Straight ahead jogging on even ground can be started once strength is adequate so that no deviation or pain is present. Avoid treadmill, cutting, jumping, and pivoting. Criteria to progress to phase 5 include symmetry in functional performance tests that include the single-leg squat and Star Excursion Balance Tests posterior-medial, posterior-lateral, and medial reach distances.

Pearls and Perils of Phase 5

- Work on strengthening in functional positions.
  - Movements should be meaningful for the patients goals.
- Do not progress too fast.
- Monitor lower extremity position.
- *Do not allow poor technique.*

Sports Specific-Work Related Retraining Phase

Phase 5 is defined as sports specific-work related retraining. The goals of this phase include returning to 100 % normal in sport and work-related activity. Exercises can include plyometric and functional retraining that mimic the individual's desired activities. The exercises program may include fast sprinting, backward running, cutting, cross-overs, carioca, pivoting, twisting, heavy lifting, and jumping as appropriate depending on the individual's functional goals. Criteria for return to competitive activity include normal and symmetrical strength, ROM, and flexibility in lower half. Functional performance test criteria should include symmetrical medial hop test and a modified agility test time within normal limits.

Pearls and Perils of Phase 5

- Be creative in program design.

Functional Performance Tests

Progression through the phases of rehabilitation includes consideration of time-based and objective-based criteria. The use of functional performance measures that are objective in nature is an area of increasing interest. Functional performance tests have an advantage that can simultaneously assess components of ROM, flexibility, muscular strength, endurance, coordination, balance, and motor control over multiple body regions in a single test. Functional performance tests have emerged as common components of evaluation procedures for the ankle and knee, but have yet to be established for patients with hip pathology. Recently, a systematic review of function tests for the hip joint identified four functional performance tests that demonstrated evidence of validity [9]. This included the deep squat test [10], single-leg squat test [11, 12], the single-leg stance test [13], and Star Excursion Balance Test (SEBT) [14–16] and the medial hop test [17]. Therefore, these tests were chosen as indicators to progress through the phase once time-based criteria are met. The modified agility *t*-test was also selected because it has demonstrated reliability in an athletic population and can uniquely compare unilateral agility performance [18].

Single-Leg Stance Test

The single-leg stance test (Fig. 85.1) is performed as an assessment of gluteus medius strength and balance. Patients are asked to stand on the affected leg for 30 s. Loss of balance, pelvic tilting, and pain indicate failure of the test [13]. Provocation of pain during 30-s single-leg stance had high sensitivity (100 %) and specificity (97.3 %) in detecting tendinopathy of the gluteus medius and minimus [13].

Single-Leg Squat Test

The single-leg squat test (Fig. 85.2) is performed by having the patient stand on their involved leg on a 20-cm box, arms folded across their chest, and to squat down as far as possible

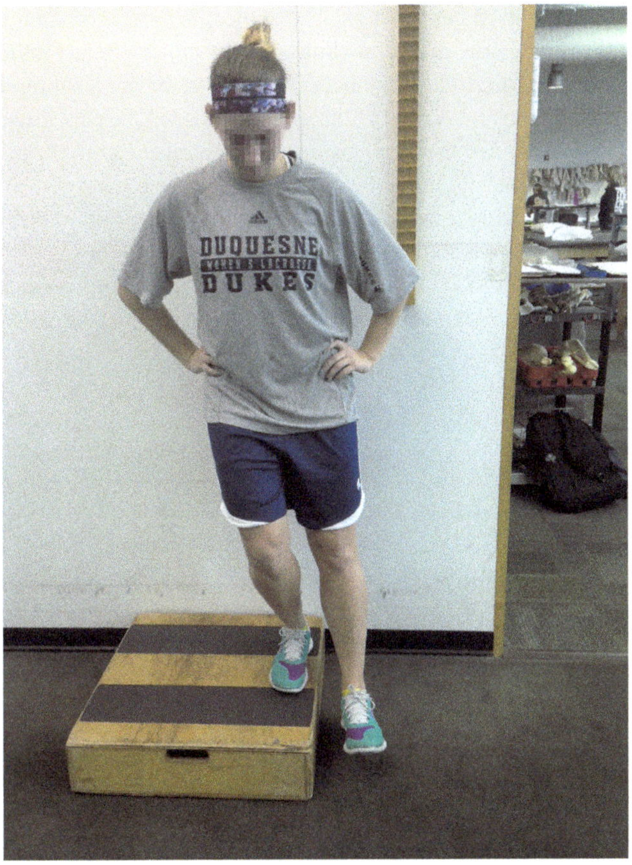

Fig. 85.2 Single leg squat

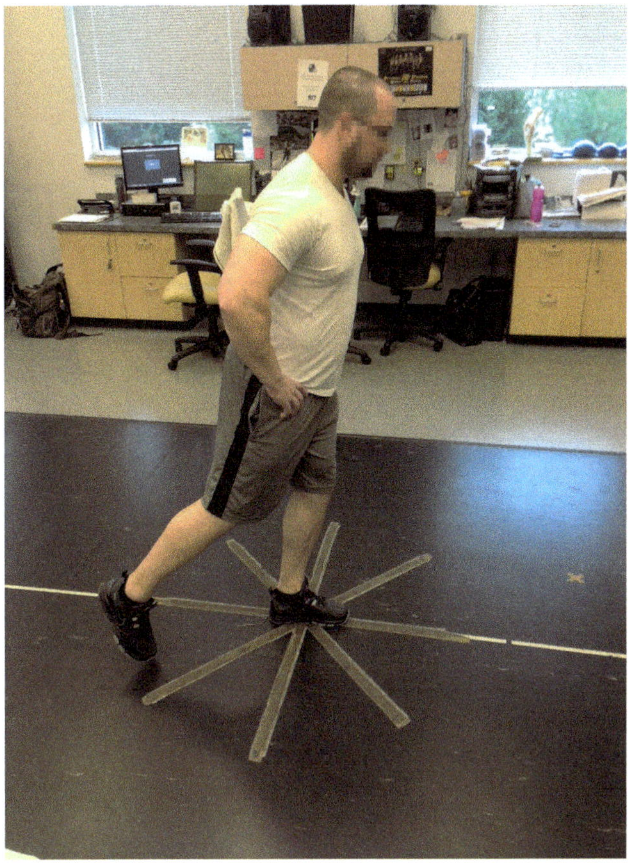

Fig. 85.3 Star excursion balance test

five times consecutively at a rate of approximately 1 squat per 2 s. Patients are allowed up to three practice attempts. The patient is graded as "good" if the following criteria are met: (1) the movement is performed smoothly without loss of balance or without trunk or pelvic deviation, (2) the squat is performed to a minimum of 60° of knee flexion, (3) the hip remains in neutral abduction/adduction, and (4) the center of the knee remains over the center of the foot without going into valgus or internal rotation. If these criteria are not met the patient is graded as "poor" [11, 12]. Subjects graded as "poor" on the single-leg squat test exhibited weaker and slower muscle activation of the hip abductors than those graded as "good" [11, 12].

Star Excursion Balance Test

The SEBT layout (Fig. 85.3) consists of 8 lines from a center point arranged at 45° angles. The lines can be labeled according to their position in a counterclockwise direction as follows: anterior (A), anterolateral (AL), lateral (L), posterior-lateral (PL), posterior (P), posteromedial, (PM), medial (M), and anterior medial (AM). The test consists of having the subject stand with the lower extremity being tested in the center while the maximum reach distance of the contralateral lower extremity achieved along each of the direction lines is measured. Subjects are not allowed to move the support foot and should keep their hand on their hips. The test consists of six practice and three test trials in each of the 8 directions. Reach distances can be normalized by dividing excursion distance by leg length [19]. For the SEBT, posterior-medial and posterior-lateral reach distances of the SEBT have been correlated to hip abduction and extension strength ($r=0.48$–0.51) [14–16]. Medial reach of the SEBT elicited activation of the gluteus medius at 49 % of maximal volitional isometric contraction [16]. The SEBT also demonstrated a relationship to hip ROM as hip flexion ROM was shown to explain a high percentage of variance (92–95 %) in SEBT scores [15].

Deep Squat Test

The deep squat (Fig. 85.4) should be performed as described by Lamontagne et al. [10]. The individual assumes the starting position by placing his/her feet shoulder width apart and facing forward. Using a standard tape measure, a measurement from the floor to the most distal aspect of the ischium

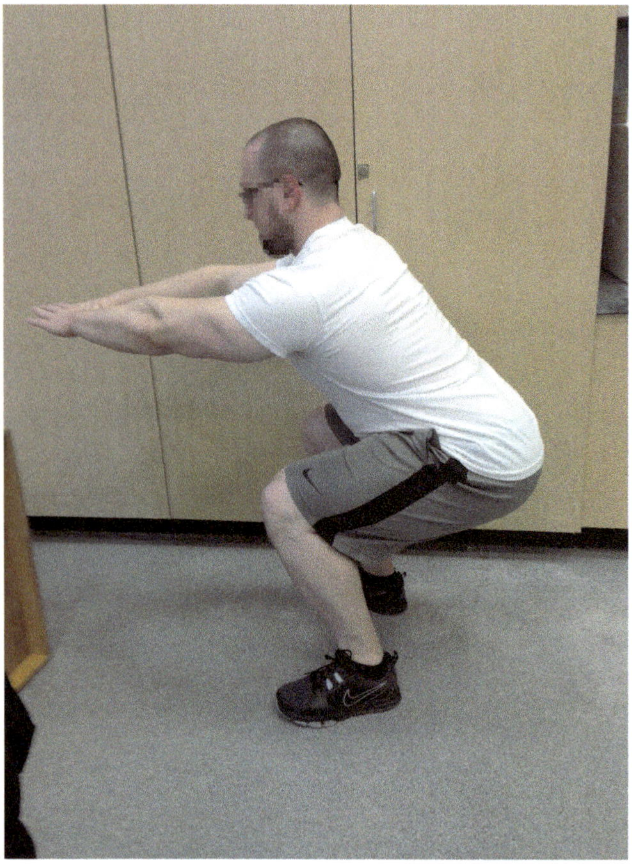

Fig. 85.4 Deep squat test

is recorded in centimeters. The subject is then instructed to descend slowly into a maximal squat position or until inhibited by pain. The distance from the floor to ischium is recorded again. A total of three repetitions will be performed. The average of the three distances is subtracted from the distance of the ischium to the floor and normalized as a percentage of the leg length. The maximal squat depth in subjects with femoroacetabular impingement (41 % of leg length) was significantly less when compared to healthy controls (32 % of leg length) [10]. The deep squat demonstrated less squat depth and altered lumbopelvic kinematics in those with femoroacetabular impingement when compared to healthy controls [10].

Medial Hop Test

The medial hop test (Fig. 85.5) was described as a single hop test by Kea et al. [20]. It has been modified for use at the hip joint to assess absorption of impact forces and propulsion in the medial direction. The subject places their foot on the end of the measuring tape. The subject stands on a single leg and hops as far as possible in a medial direction with 3 continuous hops on the same leg. The distance between the medial heel at the starting position and the position after the third hop is measured and recorded in centimeters. Subjects that cannot complete the test are given a score of zero. Three trials are

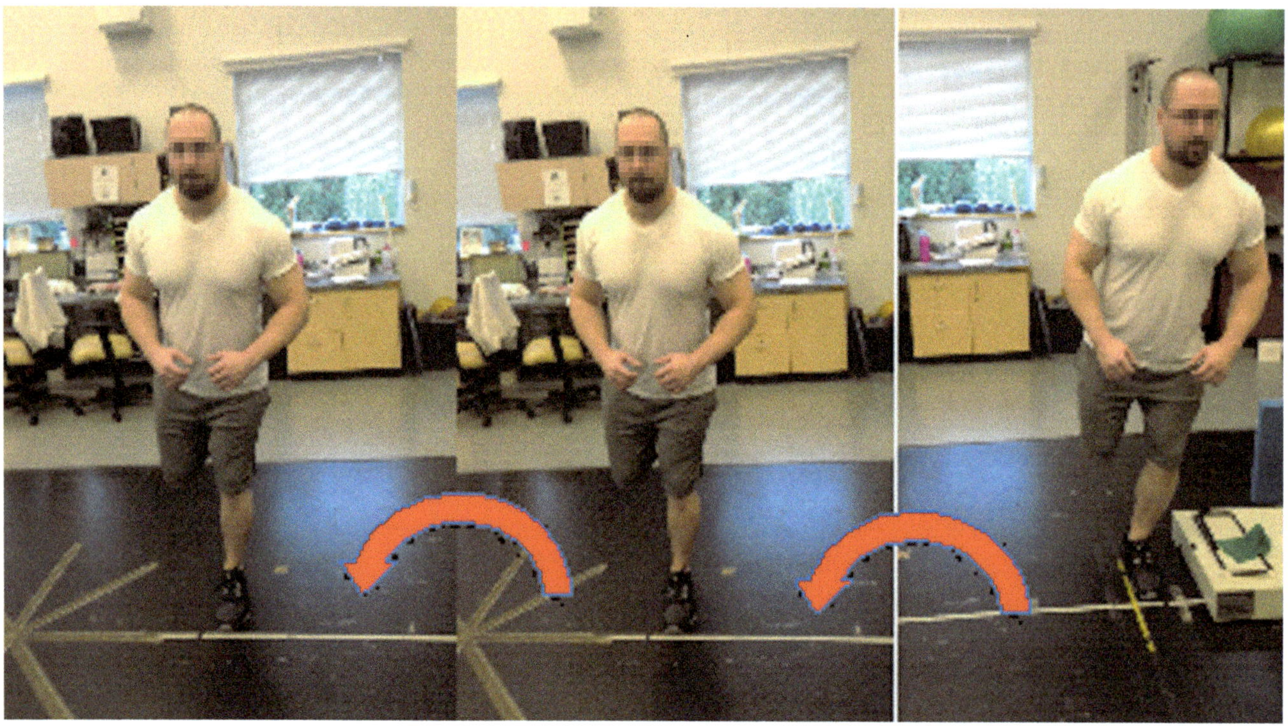

Fig. 85.5 Medial hop test

averaged and normalized to the subject's leg length [20]. The medial hop test was significantly less on the symptomatic side compared to the nonsymptomatic side. Hop distance standardized to the subject's leg length demonstrated a difference of 13 % between the symptomatic versus the nonsymptomatic side in patients with hip dysfunction [17].

Modified Agility Test

Modified agility is performed by having the patient complete the following tasks: (1) run straight forward 15 feet, (2) cut laterally towards the left and shuffle 15 feet (no cross-over stepping is allowed), (3) backpedal 15 feet; (4) run forward 15 feet, (5) cut laterally to the left and shuffle 15 feet, and (6) backpedal 15 feet to cross finish line. The test is then repeated with lateral cuts towards the right. The average time for a young, healthy group of patients is 9.59 ± 0.57 s.

Conclusion

This chapter described potential strategies to improve communication between the therapist and surgical team, outlined general postoperative rehabilitation guidelines related to common surgical procedures, defined criteria to progress a patient along various phases of a protocol, and highlighted pearls and perils along the rehabilitation process. It is hoped that the information in this chapter will help the physical therapist implement thoughtful therapeutic interventions with appropriate timing and intensity to help a patient maximize their recovery after surgery.

References

1. Enseki KR, Martin R, Kelly BT. Rehabilitation after arthroscopic decompression for femoroacetabular impingement. Clin Sports Med. 2010;29(2):247–55. viii. Epub 2010/03/17. eng.
2. Enseki KR, Martin RL, Draovitch P, Kelly BT, Philippon MJ, Schenker ML. The hip joint: arthroscopic procedures and postoperative rehabilitation. J Orthop Sports Phys Ther. 2006;36(7):516–25. Epub 2006/08/03. eng.
3. Voight ML, Robinson K, Gill L, Griffin K. Postoperative rehabilitation guidelines for hip arthroscopy in an active population. Sports Health. 2010;2(3):222–30. Pubmed Central PMCID: 3445109, Epub 2010/05/01. eng.
4. Wahoff M, Ryan M. Rehabilitation after hip femoroacetabular impingement arthroscopy. Clin Sports Med. 2011;30(2):463–82. Epub 2011/03/23. eng.
5. Edelstein J, Ranawat A, Enseki KR, Yun RJ, Draovitch P. Post-operative guidelines following hip arthroscopy. Curr Rev Musculoskelet Med. 2012;5(1):15–23. Epub 2012/03/01. eng.
6. Stalzer S, Wahoff M, Scanlan M. Rehabilitation following hip arthroscopy. Clin Sports Med. 2006;25(2):337–57. x. Epub 2006/04/28. eng.
7. Philippon MJ. The role of arthroscopic thermal capsulorrhaphy in the hip. Clin Sports Med. 2001;20(4):817–29. Epub 2001/10/26. eng.
8. Philippon MJ, Schenker ML. Athletic hip injuries and capsular laxity. Oper Tech Orthop. 2005;15:261–6.
9. Kivlan BR, Martin RL. Functional performance testing of the hip in athletes: a systematic review for reliability and validity. Int J Sports Phys Ther. 2012;7(4):402–12. Pubmed Central PMCID: 3414072, Epub 2012/08/16. eng.
10. Lamontagne M, Kennedy MJ, Beaule PE. The effect of cam FAI on hip and pelvic motion during maximum squat. Clin Orthop Relat Res. 2009;467(3):645–50.
11. Crossley KM, Zhang WJ, Schache AG, Bryant A, Cowan SM. Performance on the single-leg squat task indicates hip abductor muscle function. Am J Sports Med. 2011;39(4):866–73. Epub 2011/02/22. eng.
12. DiMattia MA, Livengood AL, Ehl TL, Mattacola CG, Malone TR. What are the validity of the single-leg squat test and its relationship to hip abductor strength. J Sport Rehabil. 2005;12(2):108–23.
13. Lequesne M, Mathieu P, Vuillemin-Bodaghi V, Bard H, Djian P. Gluteal tendinopathy in refractory greater trochanter pain syndrome: diagnostic value of two clinical tests. Arthritis Rheum. 2008;59(2):241–6. Epub 2008/02/02. eng.
14. Hubbard TJ, Kramer LC, Denegar CR, Hertel J. Correlations among multiple measures of functional and mechanical instability in subjects with chronic ankle instability. J Athl Train. 2007;42(3):361–6.
15. Robinson R, Gribble P. Kinematic predictors of performance on the star excursion balance test. J Sport Rehabil. 2008;17(4):347–57. Epub 2009/01/24. eng.
16. Norris B, Trudelle-Jackson E. Hip- and thigh-muscle activation during the star excursion balance test. J Sport Rehabil. 2011;20(4):428–41. Epub 2011/10/21. eng.
17. Kivlan BR, Carcia CR, Clemente FR, Phelps AL, Martin RL. Reliability and validity of functional performance tests in dancers with hip dysfunction. Int J Sports Phys Ther. 2013;8(4):360–96.
18. Hickey KC, Quatman CE, Myer GD, Ford KR, Brosky JA, Hewett TE. Methodological report: dynamic field tests used in an NFL combine setting to identify lower-extremity functional asymmetries. J Strength Cond Res. 2009;23(9):2500–6. Epub 2009/11/17. eng.
19. Gribble PA, Hertel J. Considerations for normalizing measures of the star excursion balance test. Meas Phys Educ Sci. 2003;7(7):89–100.
20. Kea J, Kramer J, Forwell L, Birmingham T. Hip abduction-adduction strength and one-leg hop tests: test-retest reliability and relationship to function in elite ice hockey players. J Orthop Sports Phys Ther. 2001;31(8):446–55. Epub 2001/08/18. eng.

The Importance of Validated Scoring Systems for the Hip

86

Nicholas G.H. Mohtadi

Introduction

In order to understand and describe validated scoring systems for the hip, it is necessary to appreciate what is meant by a ***scoring system*** and to ensure that the term ***validated*** is clearly defined. A scoring system in the context of this chapter refers specifically to outcome measures, which can also be called instruments, tools, scales, scores, indices, measures, outcomes, or questionnaires. These terms are used interchangeably for the purpose of this chapter. Outcome measures can be classified in many ways. Simply put, the outcome of treatment can be anything that is measured or observed. It can range from something as simple as measuring the range of motion to a complex, multifaceted, disease-specific, health-related quality-of-life outcome questionnaire. The purpose of outcome measures can be classified as either disease specific, such as those tools created to assess osteoarthritis, or joint specific, such as those created to assess the outcome of any pathology of the hip. These measures can also be classified according to the person who completes the assessment. Traditionally, outcomes have been assessed by clinicians and include objective measures such as radiographic assessments. The clinician also asks the patient about pain and other subjective measures. These "clinician-based" or "clinician-administered" tools may introduce bias, due to the way they are administered but more importantly may not capture the patient's perceived outcomes. Therefore, more recently, patient-based and administered tools have been created [1–3]. The process of scoring these systems of outcome assessment results in objectifying the information so that a number can be calculated to represent the patient's status. However, if the instrument is not validated then the objectification of the subjective information is potentially flawed.

Therefore, the term validated implies that the outcome measure has been psychometrically evaluated, in a similar population of hip patients. More specifically that the measure has the ability to evaluate a patient with a hip problem in a way that is meaningful to the patient, surgeon, or other party. It implies that the information can be collected in a reliable or reproducible way with an acceptable error. It implies that the information is relevant, important, and measurable. Finally, it implies that in the context of treating a patient with a hip disorder, the scoring system will be able to measure change over time if in fact the patient's condition changes. We call these psychometric properties reliability, validity, and responsiveness [4–7]. A validated outcome or scoring system must therefore be valid, reliable, and responsive and through this process it can be considered objective information. In fact, a validated scoring system or outcome can be considered more or less objective compared to taking a goniometer and measuring the range of motion of the hip. The goniometer is more accurate if it has longer arms and assuming that it has been calibrated properly. However, the patient and the examiner introduce variability and therefore subjectivity. So a validated outcome is one, which is calibrated (i.e., minimal inherent error), is used in a reproducible way (i.e., always on paper or computer), and self-administered so that the variability introduced by the patient is reflective of similar patients and their inherent clinical state.

Developing a Validated Scoring System or Patient-Reported Outcome (PRO)

The main purpose of an outcome measure can be classified as either disease specific, such as those tools created to assess osteoarthritis, or joint specific, such as those created to assess the outcome of any pathology of the hip. These measures can also be classified according to the person who completes the

N.G.H. Mohtadi, MD, MSc, FRCSC (✉)
Section of Orthopaedics, Department of Surgery, Peter Lougheed Centre, University of Calgary, Calgary, AB, Canada

University of Calgary Sport Medicine Centre,
2500 University Dr. NW, Calgary, AB, Canada, T2T 3Y4
e-mail: mohtadi@ucalgary.ca

J.C. McCarthy et al. (eds.), *Hip Joint Restoration*, DOI 10.1007/978-1-4614-0694-5_86

assessment such as a traditional clinician-based and administered tool or a patient-reported outcome (PRO). These patient-reported outcomes (PROs) are typically self-administered and can be completed in a nonthreatening environment to the patient. Patient-reported outcomes should be considered the modern gold standard for reporting clinical trials. However, it is necessary to distinguish between self-administered/reported (i.e., by the patient) outcomes from those which are not only self-administered but are also patient derived or determined outcomes.

There is a spectrum of how to develop a new outcome. This is characterized by the Rolls Royce and Volkswagen model of outcome development proposed by Guyatt et al. [4]. Patient input is the critical emphasis in the Rolls Royce model. **Item selection/generation** is the single most important phase of outcome measure development. This phase requires extensive patient input 50–100 patients to ensure that there has been an exhaustive process to identify every possible item of concern to patients with the disease/problem of concern; i.e., survey to the point of redundancy. Without this patient input it is possible or even likely that important items are missed.

For example how many male surgeons would routinely, or even feel comfortable asking a female patient about the impact of their hip problem with respect to having sex! In the iHOT-33 and iHOT-12 the following question is included, since it was recognized by patients to be an important issue or item of concern [1, 2]*:*

How much trouble do you have with sexual activity because of your hip?

Severe trouble ______________________________

___***No trouble at all***

Examples of a highly comprehensive item generation process would include the ACL-QOL, which started with 167 items and the iHOT, which generated 146 separate items [2, 8].

Once you have the items generated the next step is to reduce the number of items, i.e., **item reduction.** Item reduction involves a separate group of patients (e.g., iHOT utilized 150 patients) who are asked to rate each item on a numeric scale 0–5 where 0 means that the patient does not experience the particular issue and five represents that they experience it and it is extremely important. This process allows the developer to create a "frequency-importance" product for each item and then rank the items accordingly. Here again it is the patient input that is critical. Asking surgeons to rate the items on the same scale results in a completely different ranking [9]. There are several statistical measures that are employed during this phase of development to determine whether various questions are redundant or not, and to see if questions are similar in content to lump them together into subscales or domains [2, 3].

The next step is to identify the **questionnaire format** including the response scale (e.g., Likert scale; Visual Analogue Scale (VAS); Nominal Yes/No scale). Specific questions are written and the response scale attached. We have typically used a visual analogue scale (VAS) response format since it is easy to calculate the score on each patient [2, 8, 10–12]. VAS response scales usually employ a 10-cm line with anchoring statements at either end to represent the extremes from 0 to 100. An example would be the classic pain scale where "0" represents no pain at all and "100" represents pain as bad as it could be. Analyzing the VAS response format allows the use of parametric statistics making scoring easy and an intuitive composite score out of 100. Since VAS pain scales typically imply that a higher score means more pain and therefore a poorer outcome and a better quality of life would imply a higher score, appropriate diligence is required when constructing questions and in the instructions to patients. During the process of writing the questions some additional redundancy may be identified and subtle changes, additions, and eliminations are made. Then the questionnaire must be **pretested** in another group of articulate patients who are interviewed one-on-one. This is to ensure that each question is understood, written in an unambiguous way and has the appropriate context etc. Typically 20 patients are utilized in this stage [4]. Pretesting is an iterative step where the interview with each patient is documented, minor adjustments made in the wording, and further interviews are performed to redundancy.

The questionnaire has now gone through all the initial stages of development to the point where the outcome measure is complete. The most common and current way to represent the scoring is to have a higher score represent a better outcome and to convert the measured responses to create a final score from 0 to 100. Depending on the response format the final score may require a conversion formula [13, 14]. It is significant to appreciate that when a score is converted in this way there is a suggestion that all numbers from 0 to 100 may be represented in a group of patients. However, the Modified Harris Hip Scale is an example where it is not possible for a patient to have a score of 73/100 due to the way the responses are scaled.

The next stages are the essential steps of **validation** of the outcome measure. These steps include the assessment of **reliability/reproducibility, responsiveness/determination of the minimal clinical important difference, and construct validity**.

What Is Meant by Having a Reliable or Reproducible Outcome Measure?

Most commonly this is determined by an assessment of test, re-test reliability using an intraclass correlation statistic. Again a separate group of patients are given the questionnaire on one occasion and then a second time typically at 2 weeks. The assumptions are that patients are unlikely to change their clinical course within 2 weeks and that they will not remember their responses from the first administration. Each question is evaluated for reliability as is the whole questionnaire or separate domains in the questionnaire. Unreliable questions are removed from the questionnaire at this stage. Reliability is a relative term. It is unlikely that a particular question, a subscale/domain, or the overall questionnaire will yield an identical score in the same patient 2 weeks later. Also, the number of response options will affect the reliability. A response scale with only two options (Yes or No) will, by definition, be more reliable than a Likert scale with five or seven options or the VAS format where there are at least 100 possible scores. The HAGOS questionnaire for example would be considered highly reliable questionnaire using questions with five possible responses [3].

The questions can also be looked at from the perspective of having floor or ceiling effects both of which may affect the reliability and responsiveness of the questionnaire [15].

What Is Meant by Having a Floor or Ceiling Effect?

A ceiling effect or conversely a floor effect occurs when a high percentage of patients score at the higher or lower level on the question or questionnaire [15]. An example of a ceiling effect would be determining the outcome of a professional athlete undergoing hip arthroscopic treatment for femoroacetabular impingement using the modified Harris Hip Scale (MHHS). The MHHS assesses the patient in terms of pain (44 points), gait (33 points), and functional activities (14 points). A professional hockey player may only have problems when in heavy weight training and sprinting in the off season or when playing back to back games in mid-season. It is doubtful that they would walk with a limp or need to use walking aids. Their score would be very high on the MHHS since the gait and functional activities, as defined on the MHHS would likely not be compromised at all, and pain might be at worst 30 out of the 44 maximum points. This leads to a score of 85/100; questionably a low enough score to consider surgery. This is demonstrated in the literature where series of patients have maximum scores preoperatively and therefore it is impossible to use this outcome to measure anything postoperatively [16, 17]. Also, with surgical treatment there is not enough room on the MHHS for an individual patient to achieve a measurable improvement in their score that is both clinically important and statistically significant. The same argument can be made at the other end of the scale. If a patient has a permanent limp due to a limb length deficit and a painful arthritic hip, a total hip arthroplasty might significantly improve the patients overall quality of life but the gait assessment will not necessarily change. The MHHS gait component will remain low before and after treatment; therefore a floor effect is present. Questions that have obvious floor or ceiling effects would be removed at this stage of validation [15].

What Is Meant by a Responsive Instrument or Outcome Measure?

Responsiveness is a psychometric property that is essential in an evaluative index or outcome measure [4–6, 18, 19]. Responsiveness can be determined in many different ways and therefore represents a moving target when it comes to comparing different outcomes. There is controversy with respect to how responsiveness is measured and some authors question whether it is a necessary property of an outcome measure [20–22]. Responsiveness is a measure of the ability of the instrument to detect change and is directly related to the magnitude of the difference in score in patients who have improved or deteriorated compared to patients who have not changed. A responsive questionnaire will have little variability in stable patients, i.e., the noise and significant change in patients who have improved or deteriorated, i.e., the signal.

What Is Meant by Minimal Clinically Important Difference (MCID)?

Jaeschke et al. originally defined the MCID as "the smallest difference in score in the domain of interest which patients perceive as beneficial and which would mandate, in the absence of troublesome side effects and excessive cost, a change in the patient's management" [23]. Several different definitions have since been put forward; however the main concept is the ability of an instrument to measure the "lower boundary of change" [24]. The MCID can be defined statistically, i.e., using a distributional approach or by using an external standard such as expert opinion or based on what the patient considers a detectable change in score [23–25]. Irrespective of how it is determined or defined, the MCID must take into account what is measurable, i.e., more than the inherent error of the instrument and what is clinically meaningful.

What Is Meant by Having a Valid Outcome Measure?

In the simplest sense validity in this context refers to an outcome measuring what it purports to measure [4–6]. Validity has many differing descriptions. The simplest is **face validity**. Face validity refers to the fact that the outcome looks like it intends to measure patient-related characteristics. Ideally an outcome instrument would be compared to a gold standard and if it compares very well then we can be assured that the instrument is indeed valid. However, for most clinical outcomes, particularly patient-reported outcome measures, there is no gold standard. Therefore, when validating an outcome measure the concept of **construct validity** needs to be addressed. In the analogy of the Rolls Royce and Volkswagen model, the Volkswagen model would rely on face validity alone [4]. The Rolls Royce model of outcome development would require several constructs to be evaluated [4]. One method would be to compare the new outcome to existing measures recognizing that the new instrument is not being compared to a gold standard. Another way to demonstrate construct validity is to establish reasonable hypotheses and test them using the new outcome. For example it would be reasonable to expect that a patient's quality of life would improve after surgical treatment and that this improvement would increase over time. If the patients' scores level off when every other indicator suggests that they are still improving then the suggested hypothesis would be disproven. If all other measures such as range of motion, strength, and return to activity or work have improved and the new outcome correlates with these improvements, then the construct would be established and therefore the outcome would be considered valid [6].

When Is an Outcome Measure, Considered to Be Validated?

The validation of an outcome measure is complete when all of the above steps and questions have been answered. However, it is imperative to critically appraise how each step was performed; was there sufficient patient input, and most importantly what was the patient population utilized in the validation process? A commonly heard statement is that "we used a validated outcome measure" in our study. The SF-36 is considered a validated general health-related patient-reported outcome. It has been used all over the world and was developed with all of the above principles in mind [26]. However, if we were to propose a randomized clinical trial comparing surgical to nonsurgical treatment of patients with femoroacetabular impingement (FAI) using the SF-36 as our primary outcome measure, it is unlikely that we would be able to show that one procedure is better than the other without hundreds of patients in each group. Furthermore, if there was a statistically significant difference between the two groups, this difference would lack clinical importance. The intention of the SF-36 was to be a general health measure; it was not developed using a population of young and active individuals typical of the FAI population. The questions on the SF-36 are not similar or specific to the joint-specific outcomes such as the Nonarthritic Hip Score (NAHS), the Copenhagen Hip and Groin Outcome score (HAGOS), the iHOT-33 or iHOT-12, or even the MHHS [1–3, 14]. Comparisons between the SF-36 and the HAGOS showed that the average scores of the SF-36 at baseline were considerably higher than the HAGOS baseline scores. Similar concerns regarding the SF-36 have been demonstrated in patients with rotator cuff tears [11].

What Is the Importance of Having Validated Scoring Systems for the Hip?

Without validated scoring systems we cannot compare patients, evaluate treatments, discuss expected outcomes, and allocate resources within the modern paradigm of outcome studies.

It is important to clarify that in the simplest context measuring the level of pain on a visual analogue scale (VAS) or asking your patient to indicate on a similar VAS their overall assessment of their quality of life can be considered a validated scoring system. The basic problem with this approach is that patients are more complicated from a health status perspective. Therefore, if we endeavor to evaluate our patients in a comprehensive way, more complex and multidimensional outcomes are necessary. The next level of evaluation would be an outcome such as the MHHS [16]. However, this scale is not patient derived, was modified to make it patient-reported, and it has not been through the psychometric process of validation. The NAHS is a more complex outcome with several reported components of validation [14]. The Hip Outcome Score (HOS) has two subscales; Activities of Daily Living and Sports [27–29]. The HOS has been evaluated for reliability and validity [27–29]. The HOS was not patient derived but the sports subscale has components that are decidedly different from other hip questionnaires [30, 31]. The HAGOS and the iHOT-33 and iHOT-12 can be considered validated scoring systems [1–3].

Finally, it is necessary to consider and use other outcomes that include functional and radiological testing to assess other dimensions of patient assessment. Assessing patients who are being treated for hip conditions including hip arthroscopy requires a multifaceted approach of which a validated outcome scoring system is one facet, arguably the most important. In this way the efficacy and effectiveness of hip arthroscopy can be determined.

References

1. Griffin DR, Parsons N, Mohtadi NG, Safran MR. A short version of the International Hip Outcome Tool (iHOT-12) for use in routine clinical practice. Arthroscopy. 2012;28(5):611–6. quiz 6–8. Epub 2012/05/01.
2. Mohtadi NG, Griffin DR, Pedersen ME, Chan D, Safran MR, Parsons N, et al. The development and validation of a self-

administered quality-of-life outcome measure for young, active patients with symptomatic hip disease: the International Hip Outcome Tool (iHOT-33). Arthroscopy. 2012;28(5):595–605. quiz 6–10 e1. Epub 2012/05/01.
3. Thorborg K, Holmich P, Christensen R, Petersen J, Roos EM. The Copenhagen Hip and Groin Outcome Score (HAGOS): development and validation according to the COSMIN checklist. Br J Sports Med. 2011;45(6):478–91. Epub 2011/04/12.
4. Guyatt GH, Bombardier C, Tugwell PX. Measuring disease-specific quality of life in clinical trials. CMAJ. 1986;134(8):889–95. Epub 1986/04/15.
5. Guyatt GH, Feeny DH, Patrick DL. Measuring health-related quality of life. Ann Intern Med. 1993;118(8):622–9.
6. Guyatt GH, Kirshner B, Jaeschke R. Measuring health status: what are the necessary measurement properties? J Clin Epidemiol. 1992;45(12):1341–5. Epub 1992/12/01.
7. Schipper H, Clinch J, Olweny C. Quality of life studies: definitions and conceptual issues. In: Spilker B, editor. Quality of life and pharmacoeconomics in clinical trials. Philadelphia: Lippincott-Raven; 1996. p. 11–23.
8. Mohtadi N. Development and validation of the quality of life outcome measure (questionnaire) for chronic anterior cruciate ligament deficiency. Am J Sports Med. 1998;26(3):350–9.
9. Martin RL, Mohtadi NG, Safran MR, Leunig M, Martin HD, McCarthy J, et al. Differences in physician and patient ratings of items used to assess hip disorders. Am J Sports Med. 2009;37(8):1508–12. Epub 2009/05/07.
10. Hildebrand KA, Buckley RE, Mohtadi NG, Faris P. Functional outcome measures after displaced intra-articular calcaneal fractures. J Bone Joint Surg Br. 1996;78(1):119–23. Epub 1996/01/01.
11. Hollinshead RM, Mohtadi NG, Vande Guchte RA, Wadey VM. Two 6-year follow-up studies of large and massive rotator cuff tears: comparison of outcome measures. J Shoulder Elbow Surg. 2000;9(5):373–81. Epub 2000/11/15.
12. Krywulak SA, Mohtadi NG, Russell ML, Sasyniuk TM. Patient satisfaction with inpatient versus outpatient reconstruction of the anterior cruciate ligament: a randomized clinical trial. Can J Surg. 2005;48(3):201–6. Epub 2005/07/15.
13. Byrd JW, Jones KS. Hip arthroscopy in the presence of dysplasia. Arthroscopy. 2003;19(10):1055–60.
14. Christensen CP, Althausen PL, Mittleman MA, Lee JA, McCarthy JC. The nonarthritic hip score: reliable and validated. Clin Orthop Relat Res. 2003;406:75–83.
15. Terwee CB, Mokkink LB, van Poppel MN, Chinapaw MJ, van Mechelen W, de Vet HC. Qualitative attributes and measurement properties of physical activity questionnaires: a checklist. Sports Med. 2010;40(7):525–37. Epub 2010/06/16.
16. Byrd JW, Jones KS. Prospective analysis of hip arthroscopy with 10-year followup. Clin Orthop Relat Res. 2010;468(3):741–6.
17. Philippon MJ, Weiss DR, Kuppersmith DA, Briggs KK, Hay CJ. Arthroscopic labral repair and treatment of femoroacetabular impingement in professional hockey players. Am J Sports Med. 2010;38(1):99–104.
18. Guyatt G, Walter S, Norman G. Measuring change over time: assessing the usefulness of evaluative instruments. J Chronic Dis. 1987;40(2):171–8.
19. Wright JG, Young NL. A comparison of different indices of responsiveness. J Clin Epidemiol. 1997;50(3):239–46.
20. Beaton DE, Bombardier C, Katz JN, Wright JG, Wells G, Boers M, et al. Looking for important change/differences in studies of responsiveness. OMERACT MCID Working Group. Outcome measures in rheumatology. Minimal clinically important difference. J Rheumatol. 2001;28(2):400–5. Epub 2001/03/15.
21. Husted JA, Cook RJ, Farewell VT, Gladman DD. Methods for assessing responsiveness: a critical review and recommendations. J Clin Epidemiol. 2000;53(5):459–68.
22. Terwee CB, Dekker FW, Wiersinga WM, Prummel MF, Bossuyt PM. On assessing responsiveness of health-related quality of life instruments: guidelines for instrument evaluation. Qual Life Res. 2003;12(4):349–62. Epub 2003/06/12.
23. Jaeschke R, Singer J, Guyatt GH. Measurement of health status. Ascertaining the minimal clinically important difference. Control Clin Trials. 1989;10(4):407–15. Epub 1989/12/01.
24. Beaton DE, Boers M, Wells GA. Many faces of the minimal clinically important difference (MCID): a literature review and directions for future research. Curr Opin Rheumatol. 2002;14(2):109–14. Epub 2002/02/15.
25. Copay AG, Subach BR, Glassman SD, Polly Jr DW, Schuler TC. Understanding the minimum clinically important difference: a review of concepts and methods. Spine J. 2007;7(5):541–6. Epub 2007/04/24.
26. Ware Jr JE, Gandek B. Overview of the SF-36 health survey and the international quality of life assessment (IQOLA) project. J Clin Epidemiol. 1998;51(11):903–12. Epub 1998/11/17.
27. Martin RL, Kelly BT, Philippon MJ. Evidence of validity for the hip outcome score. Arthroscopy. 2006;22(12):1304–11.
28. Martin RL, Philippon MJ. Evidence of validity for the hip outcome score in hip arthroscopy. Arthroscopy. 2007;23(8):822–6.
29. Martin RL, Philippon MJ. Evidence of reliability and responsiveness for the hip outcome score. Arthroscopy. 2008;24(6):676–82.
30. Mohtadi NG, Pedersen ME, Chan D. Assessing outcomes after hip surgery. In: Sekiya JK, Safran MR, Ranawat AS, Leunig M, editors. Techniques in hip arthroscopy and joint preservation. Philadelphia, PA: Elsevier; 2011. p. 74–86.
31. Mohtadi NGH. Measurement of treatment outcomes in the young patient with a hip disorder. In: Clohisy JC, Beaule PE, Callaghan JJ, Rosenberg AG, Rubash HE, Della Valle CJ, editors. The adult hip: hip preservation surgery. Philadelphia: Wolters Kluwer; 2015 p. 184–194.

Survivorship and Clinical Results After Hip Arthroscopy: How Should We Define a Good Treatment Option?

87

Philip C. Noble, Ardavan Ariel Saadat, Morteza Meftah, Katherine E. Garrett, and Joshua D. Harris

Introduction

The proliferation of arthroscopic hip procedures in recent years has revealed the promise of this surgical modality in addressing both intra-articular and extra-articular joint problems that would have previously necessitated open procedures. Although open procedures carry significantly greater risks than closed procedures, and an increased rate of reoperation, both approaches have their own inherent sets of complications. This is particularly true in cases where labral injury occurs in concert with structural abnormalities on both sides of the joint, as in "mixed" femoroacetabular impingement [1]. This discussion is superimposed on questions about the efficacy of hip preservation procedures in preventing or delaying the onset of osteoarthritis, independent of whether they are performed open or closed.

The goals of hip surgery in young and active individuals are commonly pain relief, normal joint function, and delayed onset of osteoarthritis. While these are all laudable, they differ substantially in terms of the timetable needed to prove each has been achieved. Most of the hip pain present preoperatively disappears over the first month following surgery [2], depending on the extent of bony and soft-tissue resection and the procedures adopted for pain management. Similarly, recovery of hip function occurs over a period of 4–9 months, depending on the level of activity (return to normal gait vs. sporting activity vs. sporting competition) and the demands placed on their hip. In contrast, the efficacy of any procedure in achieving "hip preservation" by delaying the onset of osteoarthritis is much more difficult to demonstrate. Typically, periods of 20–40 years are required for a definitive longitudinal study, depending on the age of the target population.

An additional consideration is the lifestyle of patients who commonly seek arthroscopic treatment of symptomatic hip pathology. Many patients are younger adults [3, 4] with a history of participation in competitive sport, and many also have careers dependent upon hip function, whether in sports, dance, law enforcement, or manual labor [5–8]. These individuals expect their arthroscopic procedure to not only relieve symptoms, but also to restore their ability to return to their occupation or avocations without pain, stiffness, or swelling [9, 10]. Given the demands that this places on the surgeon in achieving an ideal outcome in spite of the limitations of any surgical procedure, there is a significant risk of patient dissatisfaction secondary to the occurrence of residual hip symptoms (pain, swelling, and/or joint stiffness) [11, 12], and/or failure of the clinical result to match the patient's preoperative expectations [12–18].

In this chapter we review the documented accounts of outcomes after arthroscopic surgery for hip pathologies, primarily osteochondroplasty for FAI and treatment of labral tears. We then formulate an objective basis for assessing the success of these procedures on the basis of their outcomes in comparison with established surgical procedures previously reviewed in the orthopedic literature.

P.C. Noble, PhD (✉)
Director of Research, Institute of Orthopedic Research and Education, 6550 Fannin Street, Suite 2501, Houston, TX 77030, USA
e-mail: pnoble@bcm.edu

A.A. Saadat, BS, MD
Joseph Barnhart Department of Orthopaedic Surgery, Baylor College of Medicine, Houston, TX, USA

M. Meftah, MD
Hospital for Joint Disease, New York University School of Medicine, New York, NY, USA

K.E. Garrett, BA
University of Texas School of Public Health, Houston, TX, USA

J.D. Harris, MD
Department of Orthopaedics and Sports Medicine, Houston Methodist Hospital, 6550 Fannin Street, Suite 2500, Houston, TX 77030, USA

J.C. McCarthy et al. (eds.), *Hip Joint Restoration*, DOI 10.1007/978-1-4614-0694-5_87

The Clinical Results of Arthroscopic Procedures

Several studies have shown good to excellent mid- to long-term survivorship after hip arthroscopy to address intra- and extra-articular hip pathologies [3, 4, 9, 11, 13, 19–24]. Labral tears and femoroacetabular impingement (FAI) remain the main indications for hip arthroscopy [25]. Although the arthroscopic approach has lower rates of complications with a faster recovery course [26–29], there is a significant learning curve with unique complications associated with this technique as compared to the open surgical approach [10, 30]. Specific iatrogenic complications after hip arthroscopy include chondrolabral injury [31], traction-related nerve injury and neuropraxia [32], instability [33], femoral neck fracture [34], and rare cases of fluid extravasation to abdominal or thoracic cavity [35], and compression-related perineal soft tissue injury [36]. Most of these complications are technique related and so can be avoided with precautionary measures [24].

To assess the long-term outcomes and survivorship of surgical treatment for hip pathology, one also has to take into account the effect of coexisting pathologies (i.e., arthritis, femoroacetabular impingement). It is also necessary to define the endpoint of survivorship based on the mode of failure, such as complications, persistent pain, reoperation, or conversion to a total hip arthroplasty (THA).

Recent systematic reviews demonstrate that surgical repair of labral tears can reduce pain, improve function, and improve patient satisfaction [1, 24, 27, 29, 37, 38]. However, location of the labral tear and mode of surgical treatment (debridement vs. fixation) are important factors determining the outcomes. The labro-chondral junction within the anterior acetabulum, also known as the "watershed zone," is predisposed to failure because of inferior mechanical properties, greater stress loading, and relative hypovascularity [39, 40].

Modes of Failure of Arthroscopic Procedures and Survivorship of the Native Hip

There are many validated patient-reported and clinician-measured outcome scores for quantifying hip function, such as the iHOT-12, iHOT-33, HOS, HOOS, NAHS, HHS, mHHS, and HAGOS instruments. Each of these instruments is based on an underlying criteria to characterize a successfully functioning hip, and thus, a successful outcome from a hip procedure. Several criteria have been used to define the outcome of hip procedures: residual symptoms [16], return to preoperative activity level [9], the incidence of complications leading to reoperation [24, 41], or conversion to arthroplasty [3, 4, 8, 10, 12, 19–24, 32, 42]. However, it is apparent in reviewing the clinical and radiographic outcomes of these studies that significant differences arise in comparing procedures depending how success is initially defined. This has led to the use of survival of the native hip as the definitive indicator of the endpoint of the procedure, despite the presence of pain or impairment in the interim [43].

Survivorship is currently defined in the literature as any reoperation or conversion to THA. In a recent meta-analysis, Harris et al. [24] reported overall reoperation rate was 6.3 % at a mean of 16 months after hip arthroscopy. Survivorship of hip arthroscopy for labral tears is dependent upon the severity, location, and type of treatment (debridement vs. fixation). In Byrd's study [44], 4 % of patients sustained a new injury requiring a second arthroscopic debridement at a mean of 5.5 years following the initial surgical debridement with excellent long-term outcomes. In a study of 28 professional hockey players arthroscopic labral repair and treatment of FAI with mean follow-up of 2 years, 2 players had reinjury and required additional hip arthroscopy.

Several studies have documented the short- to long-term results of hip arthroscopy with THA as the end point. However, the majority of the long-term data also include cases of untreated FAI, joint space narrowing and other indications of degenerative disease, or cases treated with labral debridement rather than repair of labral pathology [3, 44–48]. McCarthy et al. [3] showed survivorship of 91 % at 1 year, 75 % at 5 years, and 63 % at 10 years with THA as the endpoint. In a study by Byrd et al. [44], 31 % hips were converted to THA at a mean of 5.2 years. Philippon et al. [11] had lower rate of conversion to THA (9 %) with shorter follow-up (18 months). Meftah et al. [23] showed 4 % (2 patients) conversion to THA at 4–5 years; however, their indication for hip arthroscopy was a joint space of more than 3 mm on preoperative radiographs.

Untreated or inadequately addressed pathologies have been shown to be the leading cause for persistent pain, dissatisfaction, and reoperation [12, 49]. Untreated FAI has been one of the main causes of failures leading to reoperation or conversion to THA, mainly due to arthritis [12, 23, 32, 45, 48, 50]. Ward et al. [12] in a review of modes of hip arthroscopy failure found that untreated FAI or chondral defects that coexisted with labral tears were associated with poor survivorship. Beck et al. [50] also evaluated the impact of untreated FAI and the presence of arthritis at the time of hip arthroscopy, and reported a 26 % failure rate at an average of 3.1 years where failure was defined as conversion to THA. Common reasons for failure of arthroscopic procedures include the presence of untreated or under-treated FAI [48], extra-articular impingement [51], and residual capsular insufficiency [52]. Although surgical treatment of FAI leads to better long-term outcomes, the efficacy of these procedures in preventing osteoarthritis or delaying its onset has yet to be determined.

Factors Impacting the Outcome of Arthroscopic Treatment of Labral Tears and FAI

Osteoarthritis

Several studies have shown that the presence and severity of arthritis, or chondral and osteochondral injuries related to FAI at the time of surgical intervention are strong predictors of inferior clinical outcomes [3, 4, 8, 10, 12, 18–24, 32, 42]. There is evidence suggesting that FAI may be a potential cause for development of osteoarthritis [2, 14, 50, 53, 54]. In a study of 20 patients undergoing hip arthroscopy for FAI who also had preoperative osteoarthritis and chondral damage, Horisberger et al. [32] demonstrated 50 % failure due to conversion to THA. McCormick et al. [42] also demonstrated that arthritis is a significant predictor of poor survivorship of hip arthroscopy for labral pathology at minimum 2 years. Meftah et al. [23], in a retrospective review of 50 consecutive patients that underwent hip arthroscopy for labral debridement, showed that coexisting arthritis and untreated FAI can result in lower survivorship a mean follow-up of 8.4 years.

Several studies have aimed to predict the progression of arthritis based on preoperative radiographic findings such as subchondral acetabular cysts [55], the Tönnis and Kellgren–Lawrence grade or joint space narrowing [2, 3, 45, 55–57]. In a radiographic analysis of 203 patients undergoing hip arthroscopy, Philippon et al. [45] showed that joint space narrowing less than 2 mm on preoperative radiographs predicts progression of arthritis to THA in 81 % of the cases.

Several reports have shown higher survivorship after arthroscopic treatment of FAI in cases with mild or no arthritis as compared to moderate or advanced arthritis [15]. In a study in 153 patients with 50 years or older after hip arthroscopy for treatment of FAI at 3-year follow-up, Philippon et al. [58] showed that patients without signs of arthritis (joint- space >2 mm on plain radiographs) showed 90 % survivorship (avoidance of THA) compared to only 57 % of patients with <2 mm joint space). Similarly, Palmer et al. [59] reported 8 % conversion to THA in patients with Tönnis Grade 1 or less than 50 % narrowing of the joint space. In a retrospective review of 564 osteoarthritic patients, Haviv et al. [56] reported lower conversion rate to THA in patients that were treated for FAI as compared to those who did not (16 % vs. 31 %) at a mean follow-up of 3.2 years.

The conversion to THA after hip arthroscopy in patients with preoperative chondral and osteochondral injuries is also dependent on the severity of these lesions. In a retrospective review of 106 patients (111 hips) with average age of 39 years and minimum 10 years follow-up, McCarthy et al. [3] showed 90 % survivorship with the end point of THA for Outerbridge grades 0 to II. In that study, hips with higher cartilage damage had overall survivorship of 63 % and were 20–60 times more likely to require an eventual THA.

Patient Age

Several studies found that older patients experienced worse outcomes after arthroscopic surgical repair of labral tears [1, 49, 50] and arthroscopic treatment of FAI [3, 47, 48, 60]. In a recent study by Philippon et al. [58], 20 % of patients aged over 50 years older required THAs within 3 years of their hip arthroscopies for treatment of FAI. The most discriminatory factor separating patients who required THR from those who did not was the presence of greater than 2 mm of joint space at initial operation. Whereas patients with greater than 2 mm of joint space had a survivorship of 90 % at 3 years, those with 2 mm or less had a survivorship of 57 % ($P<0.001$). Similar conclusions were supported by the work of Larson et al. [60] who measured the improvement in hip function after arthroscopic correction of FAI in patients with different degrees of arthritic degeneration. Many authors have attributed this correlation to the presence of early osteoarthritis I within some of the older hips, and not the effect of age per se; however, the recent investigation of McCormick et al. [42] has shown that age itself is a stronger predictor of diminished surgical outcome, even when corrected for the presence of focal arthritic changes in the hip.

An Objective Framework for the Evaluation of the Survivorship of Orthopedic Procedures

An objective assessment of the success of joint sparing procedures is confounded by numerous factors that may be classified as:

1. Multiple definitions of a successful outcome, including:
   (a) The degree of relief of pain.
   (b) The patient's ability to return to sport.
   (c) Hip function, as defined by an outcome score, whether joint specific, limb specific, or disease specific, or defined in terms of the patient's general health quality of life or their ability to perform a given level of activity.
   (d) Achievement of a threshold value of postoperative improvement, whether defined as the minimal clinically important difference (MCID), the minimal detectable change (MDC), or the patient acceptable symptom state (PASS).

   (e) Maintenance of acceptable tissue health, as seen on plain radiographs confirming absence of degenerative changes, including joint space narrowing, subchondral sclerosis, subchondral cysts, osteophytes.
   (f) The extent to which the procedure delays conversion to THR.
2. Secondary interests of patients, surgeons, and payors vested in the success of these procedures, including:
   (a) Continuation of a successful sporting career (professional or amateur).
   (b) Surgical notoriety (new and cutting-edge procedures).
   (c) Financial gain (by parties other than the patient and the payor (e.g., insurance company)).
   (d) Success in avoiding arthroplasty (natural vs. artificial joint).
   (e) Containment of health-care costs (government and insurance companies).

Because of all of these factors, the stakeholders in the outcome of the procedure, including the surgeon and the patient, tend to become polarized into one of two camps: those who advocate the newest innovations, sometimes when early clinical enthusiasm is based more on aspiration than evidence, and those who are reluctant to advance from established methods with known outcomes, even when those outcomes are acknowledged to be inadequate. Typically, all parties involved in clinical decision-making reside somewhere between these extremes, depending on their perception of real and potential risks and benefits. In such an environment, decision-making is often guided by emotion more than reason, so a new paradigm is needed as a basis for objective assessment of the safety and effectiveness of new interventions.

A key step in evaluating any treatment is agreement on suitable criteria for describing (i.e., evaluating) outcome. In the cases of a "joint preserving" procedure, this would primarily be the ability of the procedure to prevent degenerative changes and conversion to joint replacement. Secondary indicators might include signs and symptoms of osteoarthritis, including joint pain and radiographic evidence of joint space narrowing. Conversely, in the cases of more palliative procedures, outcomes would be more adequately characterized by relief of symptoms (e.g., pain, stiffness, and swelling) and restoration of preoperative function. Once the indicators of outcome have been determined, objective metrics must be set to allow the relative success of a procedure to be gauged in terms of the degree to which the desired outcome is achieved in each patient or in all patients.

One objective approach to this task is to classify outcomes using a plot of cumulative survivorship as a function of time since treatment. As aptly demonstrated by the Kaplan–Meier plot, a perfect result (100 %) is assumed to be present on the first day after treatment, deteriorating with time as the benefit of the procedure wear off or are overcome by degenerative changes. By looking back over several decades of orthopedic literature, it is possible to obtain survivorship plots for the outcomes of many different orthopedic procedures, including those performed in total joint arthroplasty, osteotomies, cartilage and meniscal regeneration, hip resurfacing, periacetabular osteotomy, and hip arthroscopy procedures (Figs. 87.1 and 87.2).

Surgeons well appreciate that many considerations affect the criteria used to define a successful and an unsuccessful orthopedic treatment. Variables commonly cited include the age and impairment of the patient, the availability of alternative treatments, the burden, expense and duration of recovery, and the patient's outcome and prospects for definitive treatment should the initial treatment fail. Nonetheless, by selecting a broad range of orthopedic procedures with failure rates spanning 5–95 % at 5 years postoperatively, it is possible to empirically define outcomes that virtually all observers would describe as "remarkably successful" (e.g., primary hip and knee replacement) [61, 62] compared to outcomes that have been "clinical disasters" (e.g., core decompression of the femoral head in Ficat Stage II AVN [63]; Unispacer Knee arthroplasty [64]; Revision of a failed UKR with another UKR [65]).

These two groups of procedures are widely separated on the Kaplan–Meier plot with typical survivorship rates of the "remarkably successful" procedures being 90–95 % at 10 years, in contrast to failure rates of more than 60 % at 5 years for "disastrous" procedures. Between these two extremes are 2 groups of outcomes: procedures with survivorship rates of 75–90 % (10 years), some of which performed well initially but then failed at an accelerating rate at 5–10 years (e.g., microfracture/HTO (80); transplantation of medial meniscal allografts [66]; microfracture of osteochondral (shoulder) lesions in the talus [67]).

The survivorship of these procedures may be classified as "mediocre," given that patients treated with these procedures undergo reoperation at approximately three times the rate of "successful" procedures, with one patient in four proceeding to joint replacement at 10 years. Another group of procedures, classified as "clinical failures" demonstrated survivorship of only 30–60 % at 10 years. These procedures were rare, with examples being an early design of unicompartmental knee replacement (PCA; [68]) and the use of hinge prostheses after tumor resection involving the knee [69].

Using typical survivorship curves derived from the literature, we have constructed boundaries separating the zones of clinical survivorship described as "successful," "mediocre," "failure," and "disastrous" (Fig. 87.3).

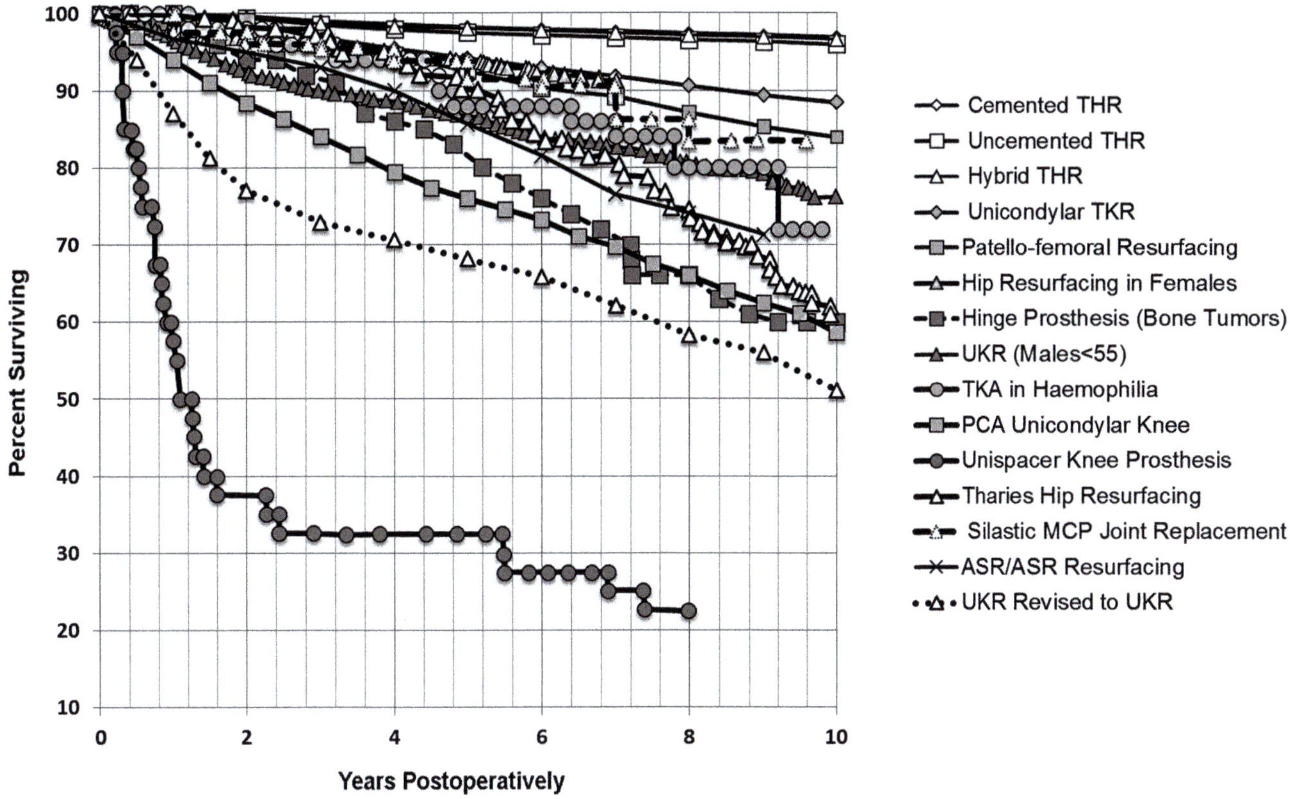

Fig. 87.1 Kaplan–Meier survivorship curves for joint replacement procedures (including hip resurfacing) [61, 62, 64, 65, 68, 69, 75–81]

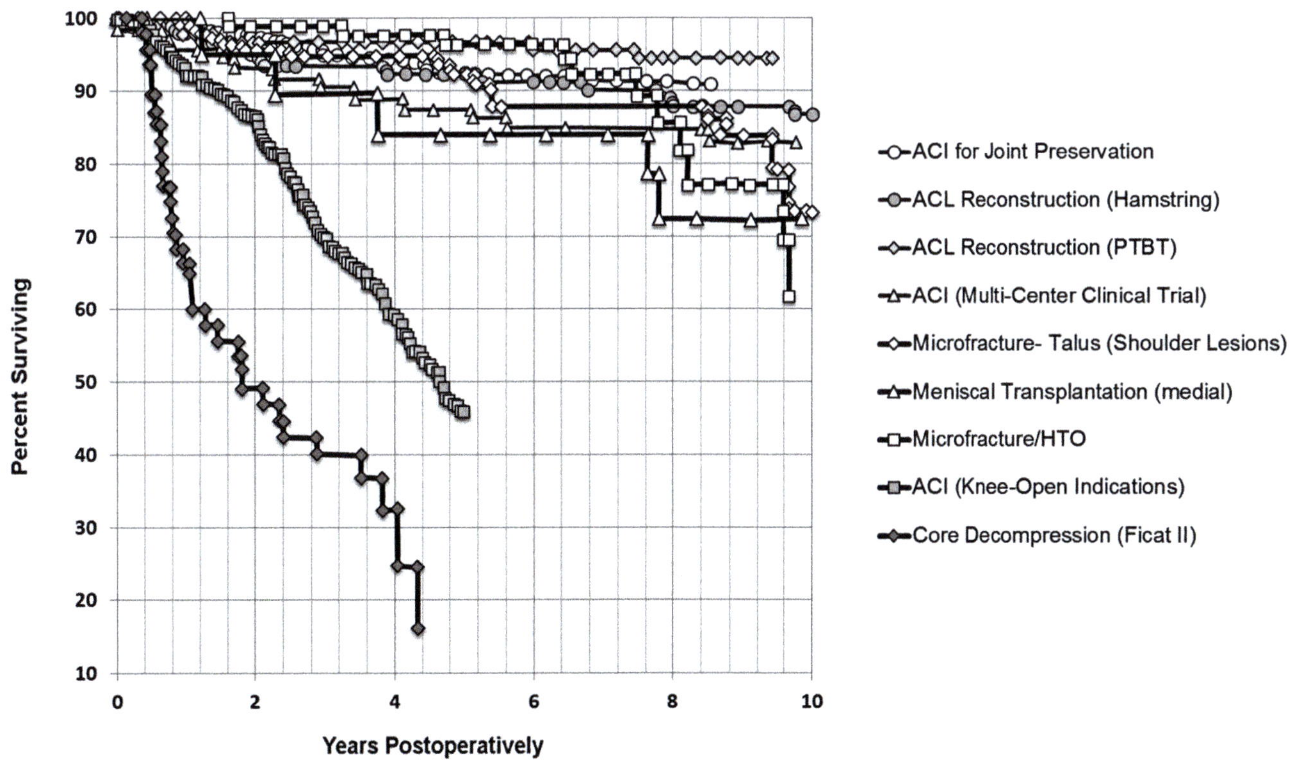

Fig. 87.2 Kaplan–Meier survivorship curves for joint preservation procedures (including ACL reconstruction and autologous chondrocyte implantation (ACI)) [17, 63, 66, 67, 82–85]

Classification of the Outcome of Hip Preservation Procedures

The efficacy of **hip preservation procedures** in prolonging the durability of the native hip may be assessed through review of the survivorship results of published studies, some of which are reported as single end-points and others as Kaplan–Meier survivorship curves (Fig. 87.4). This shows that, in young dysplastic patients, the Bernese peri-acetabular osteotomy [70] and the Dome pelvic osteotomy [71] can provide a durable hip which lasts for at least 10 years without conversion to THA in 85–95 % of cases. However, other series of peri-acetabular osteotomies with less restrictive indications have demonstrated less durability at longer follow-up (65–75 %, [72, 73]). In comparison, the results of arthroscopic treatment of FAI and/or labral pathology have not been nearly as satisfactory, with 40–75 % of patients failing treatment at 10 years. If the survival data are superimposed on the zones derived for classification of joint preserving interventions (Fig. 87.5), it is seen that the Bernese and Dome osteotomies are classified as "successful" at 5–10 years, whereas the arthroscopic procedures are located at the boundary between a "mediocre" procedure and a clinical "failure." However, closer examination reveals that the early series of arthroscopy cases depicted in these plots consisted of cases with varying degrees of arthritic disease and hip dysplasia, and different levels of conformity and head coverage. If the osteotomy and arthroscopic series are stratified by these variables, significant separation is seen in the outcome of different patient groups, with emergence of some patients who have a quite favorable, "successful" prognosis when treated arthroscopically, vs. those in whom arthroscopic procedures border on the "disastrous" [3, 16, 20, 23, 24, 45, 48, 71, 73] (Fig. 87.6).

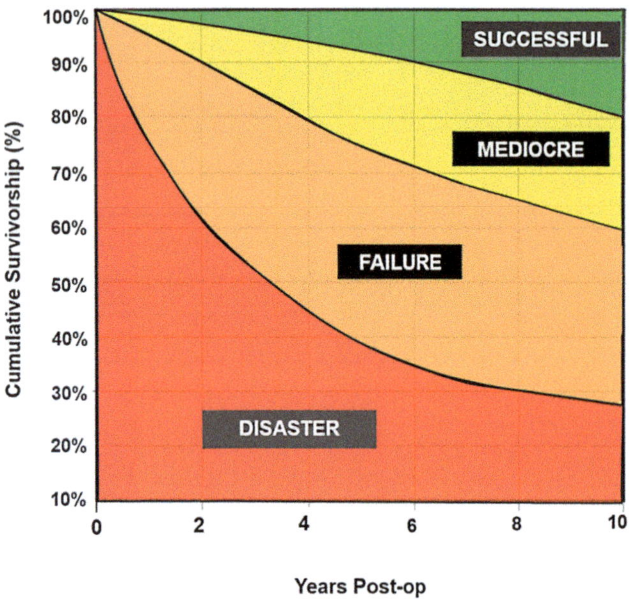

Fig. 87.3 Scheme for classifying joint procedures based on 0–10 year Kaplan–Meier survivorship curves

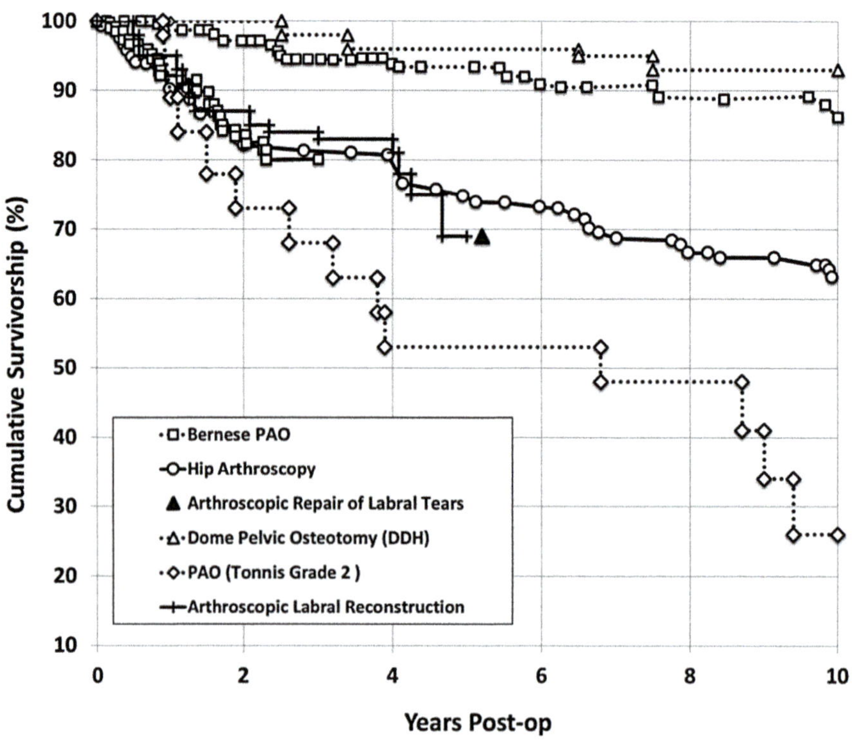

Fig. 87.4 Kaplan–Meier survivorship curves for open and arthroscopic hip surgery [2, 3, 63, 70–72]

Conclusions

Survivorship of hip arthroscopy for treatment of labral tears and FAI is highly variable in the long-term, though short-term relief of symptoms is encouraging. Data demonstrating the success of these procedures is equivocal, partly because of changing indications and evolving exclusion criteria. Arthroscopic procedures appear to successfully relieve hip symptoms and improve function in the short- and mid-term. Advocates of arthroscopic procedures often cite the potential value of surgery in preserving the native joint and delaying the onset of osteoarthritis, much as hip surgeons have demonstrated the value of periacetabular osteotomies for treatment of hip dysplasia. However, substantial research indicating that arthroscopic surgery leads to successful joint preservation is still lacking, and evidence connecting FAI to osteoarthritis is contradictory [39, 53, 74].

It is clear that the survivorship of these procedures is highly dependent upon our ability to accurately assess structural abnormalities of the hip and the presence of absence of osteoarthritis in response to the repetitive stresses imposed by the body. Until accurate individualized diagnostic tools become available, it should be assumed that the presence of degenerative changes, instability, and older age, all predict earlier reoperation or conversion to THA.

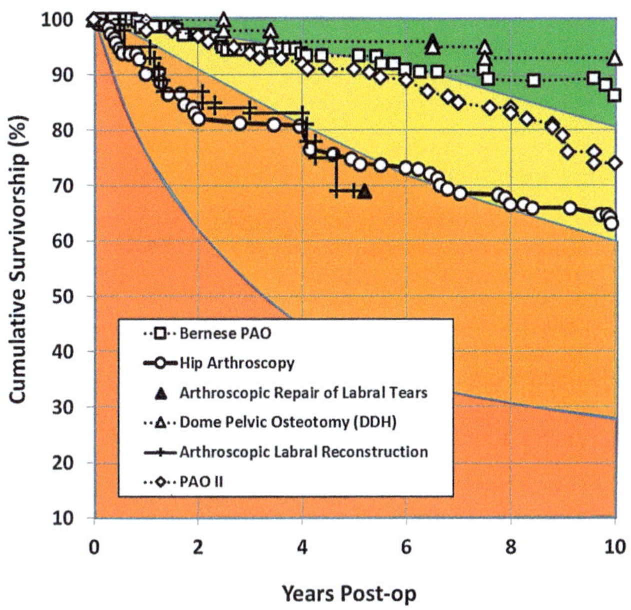

Fig. 87.5 Survivorship curves derived from published series of hip preservation surgeries superimposed on the scheme for classifying joint procedures

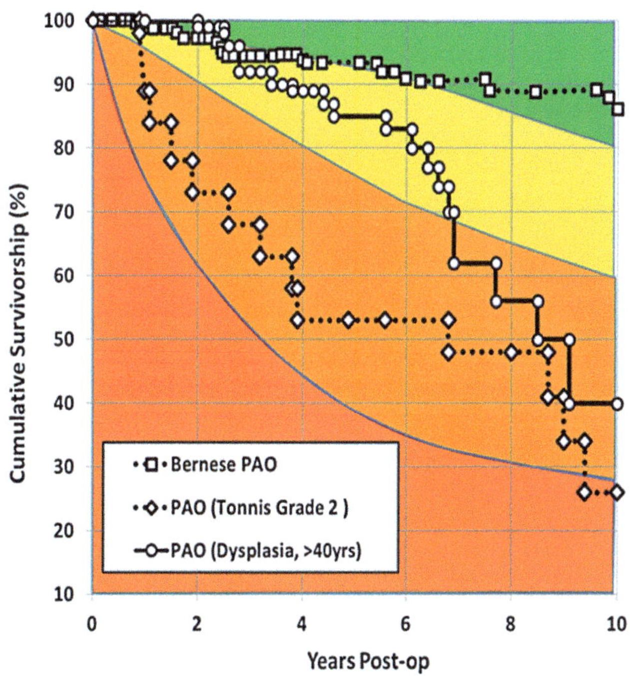

Fig. 87.6 Survivorship curves from one contemporary series of PAO procedures compared to cases performed in older dysplastic patients and degenerative hips (Tönnis grade 2) [70, 73, 86]

References

1. Harris JD, Erickson BJ, Bush-Joseph CA, Nho SJ. Treatment of femoroacetabular impingement: a systematic review. Curr Rev Musculoskelet Med. 2013;6(3):207–18.
2. Byrd JW, Jones KS. Prospective analysis of hip arthroscopy with 10-year followup. Clin Orthop Relat Res. 2010;468:741–6.
3. McCarthy JC, Jarrett BT, Ojeifo O, Lee JA, Bragdon CR. What factors influence long-term survivorship after hip arthroscopy? Clin Orthop Relat Res. 2011;469(2):362–71.
4. Byrd JT, Jones KS. Hip arthroscopy in athletes. Clin Sports Med. 2001;20(4):749–62.

5. Sink EL, Gralla J, Ryba A, Dayton M. Clinical presentation of femoroacetabular impingement in adolescents. J Pediatr Orthop. 2008;28(8):806–11.
6. Malviya A, Paliobeis CP, Villar RN. Do professional athletes perform better than recreational athletes after arthroscopy for femoroacetabular impingement? Clin Orthop Relat Res. 2013;471(8):2477–83.
7. Nawabi DH, Bedi A, Tibor LM, Magennis E, Kelly BT. The demographic characteristics of high-level and recreational athletes undergoing hip arthroscopy for femoroacetabular impingement: a sports-specific analysis. Arthroscopy. 2014;30(3):398–405.
8. Murphy S, Tannast M, Kim YJ, Buly R, Millis MB. Debridement of the adult hip for femoroacetabular impingement: indications and preliminary clinical results. Clin Orthop Relat Res. 2004;429:178–81.
9. Alradwan H, Philippon MJ, Farrokhyar F, et al. Return to preinjury activity levels after surgical management of femoroacetabular impingement in athletes. Arthroscopy. 2012;28:1567–76.
10. Kim KC, Hwang DS, Lee CH, Kwon ST. Influence of femoroacetabular impingement on results of hip arthroscopy in patients with early osteoarthritis. Clin Orthop Relat Res. 2007;456:128–32.
11. Philippon MJ, Weiss DR, Kuppersmith DA, Briggs KK, Hay CJ. Arthroscopic labral repair and treatment of femoroacetabular impingement in professional hockey players. Am J Sports Med. 2010;38:99–104.
12. Ward JP, Rogers P, Youm T. Failed hip arthroscopy: causes and treatment options. Orthopedics. 2012;35(7):612–7.
13. Stevens MS, Legay DA, Glazebrook MA, Amirault D. The evidence for hip arthroscopy: grading the current indications. Arthroscopy. 2010;26:1370–83.
14. Leunig M, Beck M, Woo A, et al. Acetabular rim degeneration: a constant finding in the aged hip. Clin Orthop. 2003;413:201–7.
15. Bardakos NV, Villar RN. Predictors of progression of osteoarthritis in femoroacetabular impingement: a radiological study with a minimum of ten years follow-up. J Bone Joint Surg Br. 2009;912:162–9.
16. McCarthy J, Mc Millan S. Arthroscopy of the hip: factors affecting outcome. Orthop Clin North Am. 2013;44(4):489–98.
17. Jungmann PM, Salzmann GM, Schmal H, Pestka JM, Südkamp NP, Niemeyer P. Autologous chondrocyte implantation for treatment of cartilage defects of the knee: what predicts the need for reintervention? Am J Sports Med. 2012;40(1):58–67.
18. Farjo LA, Glick JM, Sampson TG. Hip arthroscopy for acetabular labral tears. Arthroscopy. 1999;15:132–7.
19. Margheritini F, Villar RN. The efficacy of arthroscopy in the treatment of hip osteoarthritis. Chir Organi Mov. 1999;84:257–61.
20. Streich NA, Gotterbarm T, Barie A, Schmitt H. Prognostic value of chondral defects on the outcome after arthroscopic treatment of acetabular labral tears. Knee Surg Sports Traumatol Arthrosc. 2009;17:1257–63.
21. Walton NP, Jahromi I, Lewis PL. Chondral degeneration and therapeutic hip arthroscopy. Int Orthop. 2004;28:354–6.
22. McCarthy JC, Lee JA. Arthroscopic intervention in early hip disease. Clin Orthop Relat Res. 2004;429:157–62.
23. Meftah M, Rodriguez JA, Panagopoulos G, Alexiades MM. Long-term results of arthroscopic labral debridement: predictors of outcomes. Orthopedics. 2011;34(10):e588–92.
24. Harris JD, McCormick FM, Abrams GD, Gupta AK, Ellis TJ, Bach Jr BR, Bush-Joseph CA, Nho SJ. Complications and reoperations during and after hip arthroscopy: a systematic review of 92 studies and more than 6,000 patients. Arthroscopy. 2013;29(3):589–95.
25. Bedi A, Chen N, Robertson W, Kelly BT. The management of labral tears and femoroacetabular impingement of the hip in the young, active patient. Arthroscopy. 2008;24:1135–45.
26. Botser IB, Smith Jr TW, Nasser R, Domb BG. Open surgical dislocation versus arthroscopy for femoroacetabular impingement: a comparison of clinical outcomes. Arthroscopy. 2011;27:270–8.
27. Matsuda DK, Carlisle JC, Arthurs SC, Wierks CH, Philippon MJ. Comparative systematic review of the open dislocation, mini-open, and arthroscopic surgeries for femoroacetabular impingement. Arthroscopy. 2011;27:252–69.
28. Ayeni OR, Wong I, Chien T, Musahl V, Kelly BT, Bhandari M. Surgical indications for arthroscopic management of femoroacetabular impingement. Arthroscopy. 2012;28(8):1170–9.
29. Ng VY, Arora N, Best TM, Pan X, Ellis TJ. Efficacy of surgery for femoroacetabular impingement: a systematic review. Am J Sports Med. 2010;38(11):2337–45.
30. Konan S, Rhee SJ, Haddad FS. Hip arthroscopy: analysis of a single surgeon's learning experience. J Bone Joint Surg Am. 2011;93 suppl 2:S52–6.
31. Rupp R, Duggan B. Peripheral versus central compartment starting point in hip arthroscopy for femoroacetabular impingement. Orthopedics. 2012;35:e148–53.
32. Horisberger M, Brunner A, Herzog RF. Arthroscopic treatment of femoral acetabular impingement in patients with preoperative generalized degenerative changes. Arthroscopy. 2010;26:623–9.
33. Matsuda DK. Acute iatrogenic dislocation following hip impingement arthroscopic surgery. Arthroscopy. 2009;25:400–4.
34. Ayeni OR, Bedi A, Lorich DG, Kelly BT. Femoral neck fracture after arthroscopic management of femoroacetabular impingement: a case report. J Bone Joint Surg Am. 2011;93(9):e47.
35. Fowler J, Owens BD. Abdominal compartment syndrome after hip arthroscopy. Arthroscopy. 2010;26:128–30.
36. Byrd JT. Complications associated with hip arthroscopy. In: Operative hip arthroscopy. New York: Springer; 2005. p. 229–35.
37. Kemp JL, Collins NJ, Makdissi M, Schache AG, Machotka Z, Crossley K. Hip arthroscopy for intra-articular pathology: a systematic review of outcomes with and without femoral osteoplasty. Br J Sports Med. 2012;46:632–43.
38. Robertson WJ, Kadrmas WR, Kelly BT. Arthroscopic management of labral tears in the hip: a systematic review of the literature. Clin Orthop Relat Res. 2007;455:88–92.
39. McCarthy JC, Noble PC, Schuck MR, Wright J, Lee J. The watershed labral lesion: its relationship to early arthritis of the hip. J Arthroplasty. 2001;16:81–7.
40. Dy CJ, Thompson MT, Crawford MJ, Alexander JW, McCarthy JC, Noble PC. Tensile strain in the anterior part of the acetabular labrum during provocative maneuvering of the normal hip. J Bone Joint Surg. 2008;90(7):1464–72.
41. Philippon MJ, Schenker ML, Briggs KK, Kuppersmith DA, Maxwell RB, Stubbs AJ. Revision hip arthroscopy. Am J Sports Med. 2007;35(11):1918–21.
42. McCormick F, Nwachukwu BU, Alpaugh K, Martin SD. Predictors of hip arthroscopy outcomes for labral tears at minimum 2-year follow-up: the influence of age and arthritis. Arthroscopy. 2012;28(10):1359–64.
43. Hetaimish BM, Khan M, Crouch S, Simunovic N, Bedi A, Mohtadi N, Bhandari M, Ayeni OR. Consistency of reported outcomes after arthroscopic management of femoroacetabular impingement. Arthroscopy. 2013;29(4):780–7.
44. Byrd JW, Jones KS. Hip arthroscopy for labral pathology: prospective analysis with 10-year follow-up. Arthroscopy. 2009;25:365–8.
45. Philippon MJ, Briggs KK, Carlisle JC, Patterson DC. Joint space predicts THA after hip arthroscopy in patients 50 years and older. Clin Orthop Relat Res. 2013;471(8):2492–6.
46. Philippon MJ, Schenker ML, Briggs KK, Kuppersmith DA. Femoroacetabular impingement in 45 professional athletes: associated pathologies and return to sport following arthroscopic decompression. Knee Surg Sports Traumatol Arthrosc. 2007;15:908–14.
47. Philippon MJ, Briggs KK, Yen YM, Kuppersmith DA. Outcomes following hip arthroscopy for femoroacetabular impingement with associated chondrolabral function: minimum two-year follow-up. J Bone Joint Surg Br. 2009;91:16–23.
48. O'Leary J, Berend AK, Vail TP. The relationship between diagnosis and outcome in arthroscopy of the hip. Arthroscopy. 2001;17(2):181–8.

49. Heyworth BE, Shindle MK, Voos JE, Rudzki JR, Kelly BT. Radiologic and intraoperative findings in revision hip arthroscopy. Arthroscopy. 2007;23(12):1295–302.
50. Beck M, Leunig M, Parvizi J, Boutier V, Wyss D, Ganz R. Anterior femoroacetabular impingement: part II. Midterm results of surgical treatment. Clin Orthop Relat Res. 2004;418:67–73.
51. Ricciardi BF, Fabricant PD, Fields KG, Poultsides L, Zaltz I, Sink EL. What are the demographic and radiographic characteristics of patients with symptomatic extra-articular femoroacetabular impingement? Am J Sports Med. 2014;42(11):2634–42.
52. Frank RM, Lee S, Bush-Joseph CA, Kelly BT, Salata MJ, Nho SJ. Improved outcomes after hip arthroscopic surgery in patients undergoing T-capsulotomy with complete repair versus partial repair for femoroacetabular impingement: a comparative matched-pair analysis. Am J Sports Med. 2014;42(11):2634–42.
53. Ganz R, Leunig M, Leunig-Ganz K, Harris WH. The etiology of osteoarthritis of the hip: an integrated mechanical concept. Clin Orthop Relat Res. 2008;466:264–72.
54. Ganz R, Parvizi J, Beck M, Leunig M, Nötzli H, Siebenrock KA. Femoroacetabular impingement: a cause for osteoarthritis of the hip. Clin Orthop Relat Res. 2003;417:112–120.
55. Franco J, Maul R, Martin T. Preoperative predictors or early failures following hip arthroscopy. Arthroscopy. 2011;27(10):e109.
56. Haviv B, O'Donnell J. The incidence of total hip arthroplasty after hip arthroscopy in osteoarthritic patients. Sports Med Arthrosc Rehabil Ther Technol. 2010;2:18.
57. Ranawat AS, Schulz B, Baumbach SF, Meftah M, Ganz R, Leunig M. Radiographic predictors of hip pain in femoroacetabular impingement. HSS J. 2011;7(2):115–9.
58. Philippon MJ, Souza BG, Briggs KK. Hip arthroscopy for femoroacetabular impingement in patients aged 50 years or older. Arthroscopy. 2012;28:59–65.
59. Palmer DH, Ganesh V, Comfort T, Tatman P. Midterm outcomes in patients with cam femoroacetabular impingement treated arthroscopically. Arthroscopy. 2012;28:1671–81.
60. Larson CM, Giveans MR, Taylor M. Does arthroscopic FAI correction improve function with radiographic arthritis? Clin Orthop Relat Res. 2011;469:1667–76.
61. National Joint Registry for England. Wales and Northern Ireland 11th Annual Report. 2014. p. 36.
62. National Joint Registry for England. Wales and Northern Ireland 11th Annual Report. 2014. p. 92.
63. Scully SP, Aaron RK, Urbaniak JR. Survival analysis of hips treated with core decompression or vascularized fibular grafting because of avascular necrosis. J Bone Joint Surg Am. 1998;80(9):1270–5.
64. Australian Orthopaedic National Joint Replacement Registry Annual Report. 2012. ISSN 1445-3659. p. 121.
65. Australian Orthopaedic National Joint Replacement Registry. Supplementary Report; Hip and Knee Revisions. 2014. p. 12.
66. Verdonk PC, Demurie A, Almqvist KF, Veys EM, Verbruggen G, Verdonk R. Transplantation of viable meniscal allograft. Survivorship analysis and clinical outcome of one hundred cases. J Bone Joint Surg Am. 2005;87(4):715–24.
67. Choi WJ, Choi GW, Kim JS, Lee JW. Prognostic significance of the containment and location of osteochondral lesions of the talus: independent adverse outcomes associated with uncontained lesions of the talar shoulder. Am J Sports Med. 2013;41(1):126–33.
68. Koskinen E, Paavolainen P, Eskelinen A, Pulkkinen P, Remes V. Unicondylar knee replacement for primary osteoarthritis: a prospective follow-up study of 1,819 patients from the Finnish Arthroplasty Register. Acta Orthop. 2007;78(1):128–35.
69. Pala E, Trovarelli G, Calabrò T, Angelini A, Abati CN, Ruggieri P. Survival of modern knee tumor megaprostheses: failures, functional results, and a comparative statistical analysis. Clin Orthop Relat Res. 2015;473(3):891–99.
70. Steppacher SD, Tannast M, Ganz R, Siebenrock KA. Mean 20-year followup of Bernese periacetabular osteotomy. Clin Orthop Relat Res. 2008;466(7):1633–44. doi:10.1007/s11999-008-0242-3. PubMed PMID: 18449617, PubMed Central PMCID: PMC2505253, Epub 2008 May 1.
71. Sakai T, Nishii T, Takao M, Ohzono K, Sugano N. High survival of dome pelvic osteotomy in patients with early osteoarthritis from hip dysplasia. Clin Orthop Relat Res. 2012;470(9):2573–82.
72. Geyer MR, Philippon MJ, Fagrelius TS, Briggs KK. Acetabular labral reconstruction with an iliotibial band autograft outcome and survivorship analysis at minimum 3-year follow-up. Am J Sports Med. 2013;41(8):1750–6.
73. Hartig-Andreasen C, Troelsen A, Thillemann TM, Søballe K. What factors predict failure 4 to 12 years after periacetabular osteotomy? Clin Orthop Relat Res. 2012;470(11):2978–87.
74. Hartofilakidis G, Bardakos NV, Babis GC, Georgiades G. An examination of the association between different morphotypes of femoroacetabular impingement in asymptomatic subjects and the development of osteoarthritis of the hip. J Bone Joint Surg Br. 2011;93(5):580–6.
75. Amstutz HC, Le Duff MJ. Hip resurfacing: a 40-year perspective. HSS J. 2012;8(3):275–82.
76. Prosser GH, Yates PJ, Wood DJ, Graves SE, de Steiger RN, Miller LN. Outcome of primary resurfacing hip replacement: evaluation of risk factors for early revision. Acta Orthop. 2010;81(1):66–71.
77. Australian Orthopaedic National Joint Replacement Registry Supplementary Report. ASR Resurfacing Hip. 2014. p. 2.
78. Australian Orthopaedic National Joint Replacement Registry Annual Report. 2012 ISSN 1445-3658. p. 112.
79. Solimeno LP, Mancuso ME, Pasta G, Santagostino E, Perfetto S, Mannucci PM. Factors influencing the long-term outcome of primary total knee replacement in haemophiliacs: a review of 116 procedures at a single institution. Br J Haematol. 2009;145(2):227–34.
80. Australian Orthopaedic National Joint Replacement Registry Annual Report. 2012. ISSN 1445-3660. p. 109.
81. Trail IA, Martin JA, Nuttall D, Stanley JK. Seventeen-year survivorship analysis of silastic metacarpophalangeal joint replacement. J Bone Joint Surg Br. 2004;86(7):1002–6. Review.
82. Minas T, Gomoll AH, Solhpour S, Rosenberger R, Probst C, Bryant T. Autologous chondrocyte implantation for joint preservation in patients with early osteoarthritis. Clin Orthop Relat Res. 2010; 468(1):147–57.
83. Pinczewski LA, Lyman J, Salmon LJ, Russell VJ, Roe J, Linklater J. A 10-year comparison of anterior cruciate ligament reconstructions with hamstring tendon and patellar tendon autograft: a controlled, prospective trial. Am J Sports Med. 2007;35(4):564–74.
84. Moseley Jr JB, Anderson AF, Browne JE, Mandelbaum BR, Micheli LJ, Fu F, Erggelet C. Long-term durability of autologous chondrocyte implantation: a multicenter, observational study in US patients. Am J Sports Med. 2010;38(2):238–46.
85. Sterett WI, Steadman JR, Huang MJ, Matheny LM, Briggs KK. Chondral resurfacing and high tibial osteotomy in the varus knee: survivorship analysis. Am J Sports Med. 2010;38(7):1420–4.
86. Millis MB, Kain M, Sierra R, Trousdale R, Taunton MJ, Kim YJ, et al. Periacetabular osteotomy for acetabular dysplasia in patients older than 40 years: a preliminary study. Clin Orthop Relat Res. 2009;467(9):2228–34.

Part XIII

Worldwide Experience with Hip Arthroscopy

A.J.M.D. Tony Andrade

UK and European Experience with Hip Arthroscopy

88

A.J.M.D. (Tony) Andrade and Tom Pollard

Introduction

Europe is the 6th largest continent in the World covering 6.7 % of the Earth's land—9,938,000 km^2. Europe's population numbers some 813 million people, with 47 countries, dependencies and territories.

Europe has been intimately involved with advances in hip arthroscopy from its birth, throughout its different periods of development, and continues to do so in the current clinical era. European physicians and surgeons have provided important contributions to hip arthroscopy for over 100 years, and an overview of these is provided in Fig. 88.1.

This chapter aims to credit all the important European contributions to hip arthroscopy. The senior author (AA) acknowledges the personal communications that have helped to plug the gaps in the existing literature, and we apologize in advance for any omissions to the European contributions.

The Birth of Arthroscopy

Europe has been at the heart of innovation in arthroscopic surgery. The very first known publication on the use of a trocar endoscope was by Swedish physician Hans Christian Jacobaeus in 1910. He published on its use for visualizing closed cavities, but later also stated it could be used in the knee [1].

Severin Nordentoft, a Danish surgeon and radiologist from Aarhus, then presented "Endoscopy of Closed Cavities by the Means of My Trokart-Endoscope" at the 41st German Congress of Surgeons in Berlin in 1912 [2]. He had constructed an endoscope with a 5 mm trocar, a fluid valve, and an optic tube. In addition to suprapubic cystoscopy and laparoscopy, he reported the use of such an endoscopic device in the knee joint, especially for early detection of meniscal lesions. He used sterile saline as the optical medium and baptized the procedure "**arthroscopy**."

Eugen Bircher, a Swiss physician used a laparoscope (similar to that used by Nordentoft) to carry out "arthroendoscopy" of the knee, using nitrogen or oxygen to fill the joint [1]. He published on 18 procedures in 1921, and used it to diagnose meniscal pathology before carrying out an arthrotomy. He later abandoned diagnostic "arthroendoscopy" in favor of double contrast arthrography (1930).

The Birth of Hip Arthroscopy

Michael Burman (from New York) is credited as being the first to attempt hip arthroscopy, publishing on this in 1931 [3]. He used fluid distension for visualization of more than 90 various joints in cadaveric specimens. Of these, twenty were hip joints, and these were examined without distraction. Many of the observations he made with respect to hip arthroscopy still apply today. What is however not often acknowledged is that this work was in fact carried out in Dresden in Germany.

Dr Kenji Takagi, from Japan, was actually the first to report on **clinical cases** of hip arthroscopy in 1939 [4]. His report of four cases included two of Charcot joints, one of tuberculosis, and one of septic arthritis. These were the first reported hip arthroscopy cases in the world literature.

A.J.M.D.(Tony) Andrade, MSc, FRCS(Tr&Orth) (✉)
Department of Trauma and Orthopaedics, Royal Berkshire NHS Foundation Trust, Reading Orthopaedic Centre, Reading, Berkshire, UK

Holly Tree House, Shortheath Lane, Sulhamstead, Berkshire RG7 4EG, UK
e-mail: tonyandrade@doctors.org.uk

T. Pollard, MD, FRCS(Tr&Orth), BSc(Hons)
Department of Orthopaedics, Royal Berkshire Hospital, London Road, Reading RG1 5AN, UK

J.C. McCarthy et al. (eds.), *Hip Joint Restoration*, DOI 10.1007/978-1-4614-0694-5_88

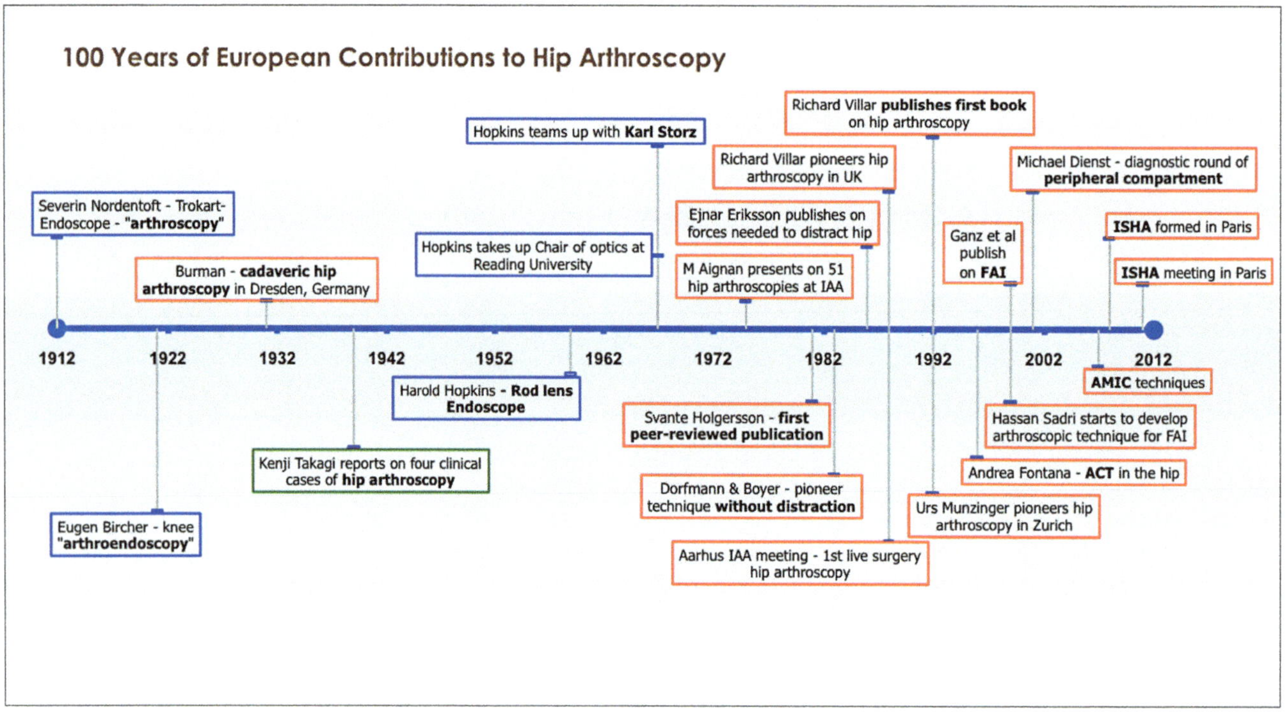

Fig. 88.1 One hundred years of European Contributions to hip arthroscopy. Timeline diagram showing the important European contributions to the evolution of hip arthroscopy. Boxes outlined in *blue* show important milestones for arthroscopy in general. Boxes outlined in *green* show important milestones for hip arthroscopy by a non-European. *Boxes* outlined in *red* show important milestones for hip arthroscopy by European clinicians or scientists, or from a European center

Development of the Rod Lens Endoscope

Any historical account of hip arthroscopy has to acknowledge the development of the rod lens endoscope that has enabled all medical specialties using endoscopes to evolve to where they are today, and the man responsible for this—Harold Hopkins.

Harold Horace Hopkins (1918–1994) was born in Leicester, UK and went on to graduate in physics and mathematics at University College Leicester in 1939. Optics Company Taylor, Taylor & Hobson provided him with an introduction to optical design, in which he obtained a Ph.D. in 1945. He began a research fellowship at Imperial College London in 1947, lecturing in optics.

Hopkins achieved a number of major advances in the field of optics. His "wave theory of aberrations" revolutionized the field of optical design, especially that of medical optics. Practical results included designing for the BBC the first zoom lens that worked as standard fixed-focus lens as well, revolutionizing the filming of outdoor events. He also worked on the design of Phillips' laser disc.

In the early 1950s he co-designed a "fibroscope" (a flexible bundle of glass fibers), which proved useful both medically and industrially, paving the way for modern fiber optic cables and the rod lens endoscope (patented in 1959). Hopkins' work on the rod lens endoscope was inspired by a request for better optics from James Gow a urologist from Liverpool who also provided £3000 in funding from an MRC grant.

Hopkins' rod lens endoscope varied from other optical systems in that it employed a configuration of short air spaces and thick lenses that improved transmission by up to 80 times. This was presented at the Société Internationale d'Urologie meeting in Rio in 1961 but then failed to attract further funding.

Karl Storz, a German instrument maker from Tuttlingen became aware of Hopkins' work when Hopkins lectured in Cologne in 1965. Storz saw promise in the new system and bought the patent. Together they refined his ideas adding Storz's own application by using fiberoptic cables to transmit light from a source he called "the cold light." This resulted in a design breakthrough in 1967 that enabled surgeons to view and photograph inaccessible areas of the body in detail. This vital contribution to medicine earned him numerous awards, being nominated twice for a Nobel Prize [5].

In 1967 Hopkins took a new chair in applied optics at Reading University, UK, where he was Head of Physics from 1977 to 1980, retiring in 1984. He did much of his early work on endoscopes in concert with surgeons at the Royal Berkshire Hospital in Reading, UK. The Physics Department at Reading is still known today for its work in optical physics. He died in Reading in October 1994.

The Clinical Era of Hip Arthroscopy

Taking inspiration from the early work of Takagi and Burman, and using the refinements provided by Hopkins and Storz, surgeons were able to take hip arthroscopy into the modern clinical era.

This can then be further subdivided into: **the introductory era**—pre-1990; **the consolidation era**—1990–1999; **the expansion era**—2000–2010; and **the diversification era**—2010 onwards [6].

The Introductory Era

Frenchman M. Aignan provided the first notable contribution in the introductory era. He presented a study of attempted diagnostic arthroscopy and biopsy in 51 hips at the 1975 meeting of the International Arthroscopy Association (IAA—now ISAKOS) in Copenhagen. This was published in the proceedings of the IAA in 1976 [7], and was the first European publication on hip arthroscopy, as well as being the first since Takagi's in 1939.

The first peer-reviewed publication on hip arthroscopy in Europe was by Svante Holgersson et al. (Sweden 1981) when they reported on the role of hip arthroscopy in assessing 15 hips in 13 children with juvenile chronic arthritis [8].

Henri Dorfmann (French Rheumatologist) learnt the techniques of hip arthroscopy from Dr. Mataki Watanabe in Japan and with Thierry Boyer from 1983 pioneered a technique without distraction for looking at the peripheral compartment publishing on 60 procedures in 1988 [9, 10]. As rheumatologists their focus was predominantly on the role of synovial disease in hip pathology, and with this technique were able to explore the peripheral compartment to diagnose and treat synovial disease. They later published on their 12-year experience of 413 procedures in 395 patients [11].

Swedish surgeon Ejnar Eriksson and coworkers reported on the forces necessary for adequate hip distraction in 1986 [12]. This study included evaluating unanesthetized volunteers including Prof Eriksson himself.

In Europe in the 1980s surgeons continued to perform hip arthroscopy by the supine approach as originally described. Meanwhile in North America Jim Glick experienced some difficulties with the supine technique in large patients. With Thomas Sampson from 1983 he developed a lateral decubitus position technique [13] that was also then adopted by Richard Villar when he brought the technique to the UK in 1988.

In 1988 the IAA held an arthroscopy course in Aarhus, Denmark and there the first live surgery of a hip arthroscopy was performed. They succeeded to get into the central compartment, but no therapeutic procedure was carried out.

The Consolidation Era

Richard Villar pioneered hip arthroscopy in the UK from 1988 and was the first to publish a textbook on this in 1992 [14]. He has also since extensively published in the journals on all aspects of hip arthroscopy [15], defining the arthroscopic anatomy of the hip [16], classifying patterns of labral tears [17], and reporting on the results as well as complications of hip arthroscopy [18, 19].

At a similar time Urs Munzinger started hip arthroscopy at the Schulthess Hospital in Zurich in 1992. In a 2-year period he carried out 19 cases and reported three complications (one neurapraxia of pudendal nerve, one hematoma of labia majora, and having to abandon the procedure under regional anesthesia due to onset of abdominal pain) [20].

Andrea Fontana from Milan, in Italy, began treating chondral defects of the hip in 1996 [21]. He went on to carry out arthroscopic autologous chondrocyte transplantation (ACT) in 37 patients, between 1996 and 2004. He then reported on a pilot study comparing the results of 15 patients with 6-year follow-up compared to another 15 patients who had undergone debridement of the chondral defects. He showed similar Harris Hip Scores (HHS) preoperatively for both groups, and a statistically significant ($p<0.001$) improvement in postoperative Harris Hip Scores for the ACT group. This was an important breakthrough in the treatment of articular cartilage lesions in the hip, which other European surgeons later adopted.

At the 2011 Paris International Society for Hip Arthroscopy (ISHA) meeting Dr. Fontana also presented the results of a study comparing 120 patients who had ACT (as a two-stage procedure) with 62 patients who had autologous matrix-induced chondrogenesis (AMIC) as a single-step procedure. He showed that there was no statistically significant difference in the postoperative HHS of the two groups, demonstrating that the AMIC technique was equivalent in outcome to the ACT technique.

Michael Dienst and coworkers carried out 35 hip arthroscopies without traction between 1997 and 1999, and in so doing defined the arthroscopic anatomy of the peripheral compartment in vivo [22]. They described a systematic way of viewing the peripheral compartment that established the "**diagnostic round**" of this compartment. Furthermore, they commented that for completeness, for the evaluation of the central compartment of the hip, traction was always required. They expanded their technique into a peripheral first technique of getting into the central compartment that minimizes the risk of labral perforation or chondral scuffing, publishing on this in 2005 [23].

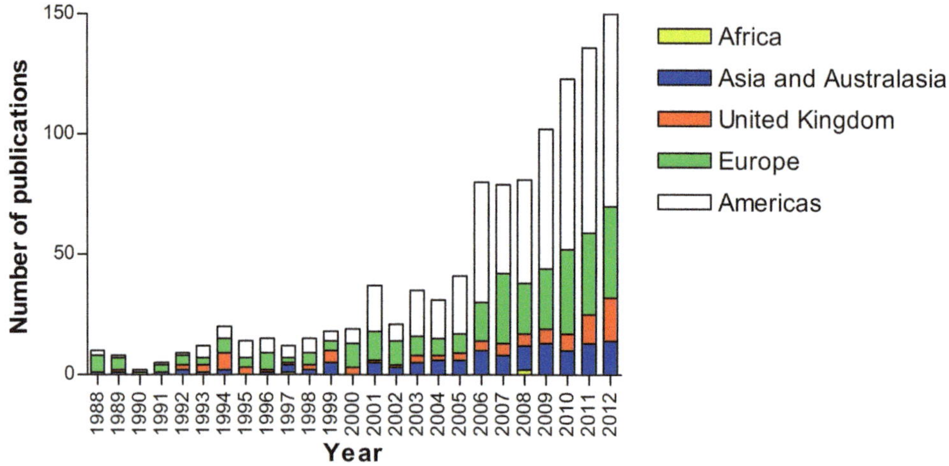

Fig. 88.2 The global explosion in hip arthroscopy: Number of PubMed hits for "hip arthroscopy" over a 25-year period (1988–2012)

The Expansion Era

Introduction

This era (from 2000 to 2010) was marked by a global exponential increase in hip arthroscopy numbers, and also an exponential increase in the number of publications on hip arthroscopy (Fig. 88.2). This was largely attributable to an increasing understanding of the role of hip arthroscopy in the management of the pre-arthritic adult hip.

Femoroacetabular Impingement

Developmental dysplasia was already recognized as an important pathoaetiology for hip pain in young adults, but the condition that drove the surge in interest was femoroacetabular impingement (FAI). This may be defined as an abnormal abutment of the femoral head–neck junction against the acetabular rim and labrum, within the physiological range of motion.

The UK and Europe have made key contributions to the worldwide literature and understanding of FAI. Ganz and coworkers in Berne, Switzerland first reported FAI in 1999 as a complication following periacetabular osteotomy, when excessive closure and retroversion of the acetabular fragment lead to impingement in flexion with consequent groin pain [24]. However, most cases of FAI have no history of previous surgery and are usually associated with subtle abnormalities of joint morphology on the femoral (cam deformity) and acetabular (pincer deformity) sides of the joint, which may lead to symptoms depending on the activity level of the patient. In addition to pain, FAI damages the acetabular labrum and articular cartilage, and predisposes to osteoarthritis. Although the contemporary understanding of the mechanisms of FAI may be attributed to the Bernese group [25], it is important to note that Smith-Petersen had already described impingement as a cause of hip pain over 60 years previously [26]. Furthermore, other American and European authors had associated the presence of subtle morphological abnormalities with the development of osteoarthritis of the hip more than 20 years previously [27, 28].

The symptoms of FAI may initially respond to activity modification, but because of the underlying anatomical problem, many patients will require surgical treatment. Surgery for FAI aims to treat the secondary damage to the labrum and articular cartilage, and address the underlying joint deformity. Open surgery was initially advocated [29, 30]; however, improved surgical techniques and instrumentation have enabled most cases to be managed arthroscopically [31], with the benefits of quicker postoperative recovery and minimal morbidity.

The evolution of what was effectively a new condition and a new treatment technique has presented a great opportunity for research, and the UK and Europe have continued to deliver important contributions to the global literature on matters pertaining to both hip arthroscopy and FAI, particularly during this expansion era.

Pioneering Arthroscopic FAI Surgery

Hassan Sadri, from Lausanne in Switzerland, had gained experience with open surgical dislocations for the treatment of FAI, as a fellow for Professor Ganz in 1998. He set out in 1999 to develop arthroscopic techniques for the treatment of FAI, by using cadaveric specimens with the Jim Glick arthroscopy set in both the supine and lateral positions [32]. Dr. Sadri used an AO pin distractor for this as traction tables were not available in the anatomy department, and he then checked his arthroscopic corrections by opening the hip at the end of the procedure.

Dr Sadri then started arthroscopic hip surgery (in vivo) for FAI using a traction table in the supine position, but stopped using this after 2 pudendal nerve injuries in his first 25 cases (one of which lasted 1 year). Traction times were on average 2 h. This led him to use the AO pin distractor technique in the operating room for his clinical cases. This allowed for safe distraction of the hip for prolonged periods without incurring the pressure effects associated with traction tables. He rapidly changed this to a modified and reinforced ankle distractor (DR hip distractor, DR Medical, Solothurn, Switzerland) that he has been using for over 10 years. With this device he has been able to use traction times of up to 5 h without problems. His heaviest patient to date weighed 138 kg. The neurological complication rate for his first 1000 cases using the pin distractor was 0.3 % with all of them being transient lateral femoral cutaneous nerve injuries. He has not experienced any pin tract infections.

Dr Sadri reported on a randomized FAI surgery study at the Swiss Orthopedic Society in 2002. This compared the results of open surgical dislocation with the results of arthroscopic FAI correction at 2 years of follow-up. Very similar results were reported.

Dr Sadri first started labral repair in 2001–2002, and following on from Andrea Fontana's work started arthroscopic autologous chondrocyte implantation (ACI) in the hip in 2006. He then also started arthroscopic AMIC procedures in 2007.

Hip Arthroscopy Education

The expansion in hip arthroscopy in the UK and Europe during this era also resulted from the increase in number of dedicated courses on these techniques. Previously there had not been dedicated hip arthroscopy courses in Europe.

In 2006 there were meetings in Paris, France (Advances in Hip Arthroscopy; Paris 22–23rd May 2006), Warwick, UK (Sports Hip Meeting; Warwick 30–31st October 2006), and Homburg, Germany (International Hip Arthroscopy Meeting; Homburg November 2006).

Richard Villar, in the UK, had already established a School of Hip Arthroscopy providing Hip Arthroscopy Masterclasses in London (with live surgery and dry-bone workshops), and these increased in frequency in 2007 in response to the increasing demand. Cadaveric workshops also started in 2007, with the "1st Arthroscopic Hip Techniques International Course" in Barcelona, Spain and Richard Villar's "Advanced Hip Arthroscopy Masterclass" at Guy's Hospital in London, UK. Both of these cadaveric courses were supported by Smith & Nephew who have continued to support education in hip arthroscopy ever since. Smith & Nephew opened their Surgical Skills Centre in York Science Park, York, UK in 2010, which has provided a state-of-the-art venue for cadaveric courses. The Richard Villar courses run up to three times per year and attract surgeons from all over Europe as well as from farther afield.

The Santander Hip Meeting (Santander, Spain) was first held in 2009 and has since been held every 2 years.

The International Society for Hip Arthroscopy (ISHA) was founded in Paris in 2008 with Richard Villar as its founding president. Yearly scientific meetings have been held in October ever since, and ISHA is a growing organization that has taken the lead on surgeon education in hip arthroscopy.

Growth in Hip Arthroscopy in Europe

The surge in interest in FAI, with the potential for arthroscopic corrective surgery, and the increasing number of courses and hip arthroscopy meetings naturally resulted in increasing numbers of hip arthroscopy procedures throughout Europe. Furthermore arthroscopic procedures in the peri-trochanteric compartment provided another focus of interest and growth.

It has been estimated that the growth in 2005–2006 was 85 %; 2006–2007 41 %; but then in 2007–2008 it was 121 %; with a growth of 85 % in 2008–2009.

A commissioned European Market study (that the senior author presented at the 2010 ISHA meeting in Cancun, Mexico) provided a breakdown of arthroscopy procedures by European country (Table 88.1). This showed that Germany carried out the highest number of procedures in 2009 and 2010, with the UK a close second.

However, when we consider population figures for 2010 for each country (Table 88.2), and then calculate the number of procedures per 100,000 head of population (Fig. 88.3), a rather different picture emerges, with the UK having the highest number of procedures per population, with Italy a close second. Figure 88.4 shows these figures now ranked in order.

The market study went on to suggest some projected figures for the growth in numbers over the following 4 years (Table 88.3) showing a predicted doubling in numbers for most European countries.

Restriction in Growth of Hip Arthroscopy

Despite the optimistic projected growth in hip arthroscopy shown in Table 88.3, several factors across different countries conspired to stifle this growth.

In 2004 in Aarhus, Denmark, the number of cases grew from 5–10 per year (1988) to 30–60 cases per year [33]. In 2008 the procedures evolved from central compartment only to also include the peripheral compartment, and in particular to start FAI surgery.

In 2011 the Danish Health Authorities passed a law stating that hip arthroscopy was a regional service, specifying that the procedure could only be performed in centers with more than 30 cases a year, thereby limiting this service provision to 10 hospitals (7 public and 3 private clinics). In order to continue to be allowed to perform hip arthroscopies each unit is required to report data every year on numbers and outcomes.

In order to meet these demands the Danish Society for Arthroscopy and Sports Traumatology funded a National Database for Hip Arthroscopy and since February 2012, 7 centres have reported data. Data on more than 270 operations have already been recorded in this national registry, and figures for 2012 showed that 125 hips were arthroscoped in Aarhus that year [33].

Meanwhile in the UK the National Institute for Health and Clinical Excellence (NICE)—that was set up in 1999 to reduce variation in the availability and quality of NHS treatments and

Table 88.1 Hip arthroscopy numbers per country

	2009	2010
Germany	2800	3500
France	1200	1500
UK	2400	3000
Italy	2050	2550
Spain	1550	1955
Benelux	380	480
Scandinavia	650	800
	11,030	**13,785**

Results of Commissioned European market study showing breakdown of numbers of hip arthroscopy procedures by European country. First presented at the ISHA meeting in Cancun, Mexico, 2010 by AJMD Andrade
NB. 1. **Benelux** is a union of states comprising three neighboring countries in northwestern Europe—Belgium, Netherlands, and Luxemburg
2. **Scandinavia** is a historical region in Northern Europe comprising the three kingdoms of Denmark, Norway, and Sweden

Table 88.2 Population figures for 2010 for each European country, union, or region

	2010	Population
Germany	3500	82,282,988
France	1500	64,768,389
UK	3000	62,348,447
Italy	2550	58,090,681
Spain	1955	46,505,963
Benelux	480	27,704,123
Scandinavia	800	24,521,630
	13,785	**366,222,221**

care—issued a guidance in 2007 on arthroscopic femoro-acetabular surgery for hip impingement syndrome. In this it was recommended that ***"the procedure should only be performed by surgeons with specialist expertise in arthroscopic hip surgery."*** Furthermore ***"current evidence on the safety and efficacy of arthroscopic femoro-acetabular surgery for hip impingement surgery does not appear adequate for this procedure to be used without special arrangements for consent and for audit or research."***

This led Priorities Committees for Primary Care Trusts (PCT's) to issue a recommendation not to fund surgery for FAI in routine practice (within the National Health Service). This inevitably led to a stifling of the growth of arthroscopic hip surgery in the UK with only certain centers with established practices being able to continue this surgery within the NICE recommendations. It became virtually impossible for new centers to develop a service in the UK.

The Diversification Era

Introduction

This era (post 2010) is characterized by the ever-expanding indications for arthroscopic procedures in the central, peripheral, and peritrochanteric compartments. In addition the subgluteal space, and hamstring insertional problems have provided further sources of interest, and further challenges to conquer.

With the increasing number of publications, many questions on the etiology of FAI and its association with osteoarthritis have sought to be answered.

Investigations into the Etiology of FAI and Its Association with Osteoarthritis

The aetiology of FAI is unknown, and although paediatric hip disorders such as slipped capital femoral epiphysis and Legg-Calvé-Perthes' disease result in similar deformities, only a small minority of patients with FAI reports such a history. Key questions are: How common are these deformities in the general population? How and why do they develop? What other factors will determine whether an individual with such a deformity will develop symptoms or not?

A number of European studies have examined the epidemiology of morphological abnormalities in the general population. The largest study, by Gosvig and coworkers in Copenhagen, Denmark, examined a cohort of 4151 individuals and found that 17 % of males and 4 % of females had a cam deformity [34], and 15 % of males and 19 % of females had a deep acetabular socket [35]. These prevalences have been replicated elsewhere and indicate that abnormal hip morphology is common. Hogervost et al. [36] from The Hague, Netherlands, have proposed an evolutionary explana-

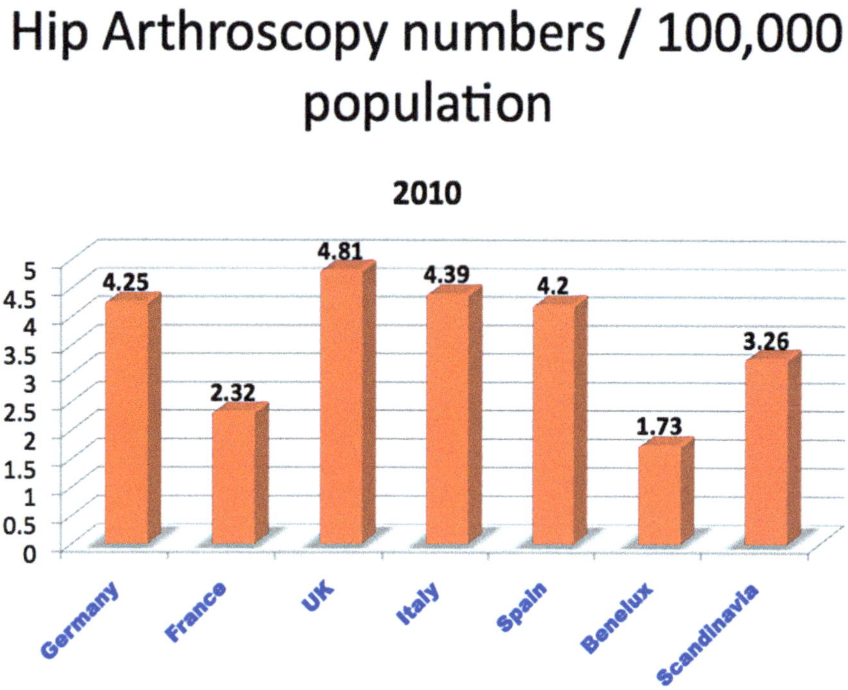

Fig. 88.3 Hip arthroscopy numbers per 100,000 heads of population in 2010, for each European country, union, or region

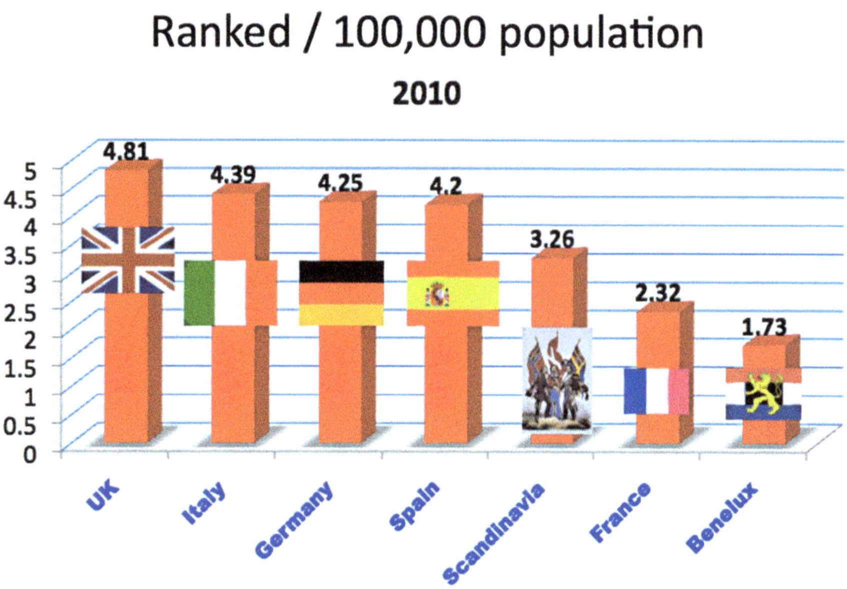

Fig. 88.4 Hip arthroscopy numbers per 100,000 heads of population in 2010, for each European country, union, or region—ranked in order

tion for both cam deformity ("runner's hip") and coxa profunda ("climber's hip"), and the conflict between upright gait and birth of a large-brained fetus, with their high prevalence explained by the lack of selection-drive for mechanical problems manifest after reproductive age. Given the morphological similarity of a cam deformity and slipped capital femoral epiphysis, it has also been suggested [25] that a subclinical slip may occur during adolescence leading to the development of cam deformity and subsequent symptoms due to FAI. In a case-control study, the Bernese group noted that adolescent male basketball players were ten times more likely to have a cam deformity and had less internal rotation of the hip than a control group [37]. This study indicates that high intensity sporting activity during adolescence may affect hip development and subsequent development of pain, with potential implications for sporting academies with regards to intensity and type of training activity during various stages of development. The key driving forces for all of these developmental processes are likely to be genetic influences. Given their importance in the aetiology of many musculoskeletal

Table 88.3 Projected numbers for next 4 years

	2011	2012	2013	2014
Germany	4550	5915	7690	9996
France	1725	1984	2281	2624
UK	3750	4688	5859	7324
Italy	2933	3373	3879	4460
Spain	2444	3055	3819	4773
Benelux	600	750	950	1200
Scandinavia	950	1100	1200	1400
	16,952	**20,864**	**25,678**	**31,778**

Projected numbers for hip arthroscopies for each European country, union, or region for the following 4 years. Note how the numbers for 2014 are approximately double those for 2011

disorders (including osteoarthritis), the junior author and collaborators from other centers in the UK, examined whether FAI had a genetic basis [38]. The relative risk of FAI in siblings of patients treated for FAI was found to be between two and three, compared with a control group, and this was highly statistically significant. Interestingly, the likelihood of symptoms was also higher in the siblings, leading them to conclude that other factors beyond joint morphology and activity may modulate disease progression. It was suggested that these may include biological durability of cartilage and labrum, or even differences in pain processing.

Although the orthopedic community had long suspected that subtle deformity was associated with osteoarthritis of the hip [27], convincing evidence based on longitudinal cohort studies has been lacking until recently. Bardakos and Villar [39] from London, UK, studied 43 patients with pistol-grip deformities of the proximal femur over a 10-year period. 28 of these 43 (65 %) had progressive radiological osteoarthritis, leading the authors to conclude that mildly osteoarthritic hips with pistol-grip deformities will not necessarily progress rapidly.

Nicholls et al. [40] from the Oxford group utilized the "Chingford 1000 women" cohort, in whom pelvic radiographs were obtained at year 2 and year 20. Morphological measurements made on the baseline radiographs were then evaluated with subsequent risk of total hip replacement for end-stage osteoarthritis. Subjects with total hip arthroplasty were found to have a higher prevalence of cam deformity and acetabular dysplasia. For every one-degree increase in alpha angle (a parameter of cam deformity), the risk of total hip arthroplasty increased by 6 %, and for every one-degree decrease in lateral center-edge angle (parameter of acetabular dysplasia), the risk increased by 10 %.

From their cross-sectional study of 4151 individuals in Copenhagen, Denmark, Gosvig et al. [35] noted that deep acetabular sockets and cam deformities were associated with osteoarthritis with risk ratios of 2.4 and 2.2, respectively.

These studies provide important evidence to indicate that FAI predisposes to osteoarthritis, but also indicate that this is not a direct relationship with other factors, such as activity level and undefined genetic factors modulating progression.

Evolution of Preoperative Investigations

The main objectives of investigations in the preoperative work-up for hip arthroscopy involve an assessment of **joint morphology** and an appreciation of the **degree of articular cartilage damage** that has already occurred. The former is important because it informs the surgical strategy in terms of what aspects of morphology require correction and whether that is possible with an arthroscopic approach. The latter is important because outcomes of hip arthroscopy and surgery for FAI are currently compromised when cartilage damage is advanced.

The assessment of morphology is difficult, with each modality having advantages and disadvantages and little consensus on thresholds that enable classification of patients, without considering the inherent problem of reliance on static imaging to make inferences on a dynamic problem [41]. Nevertheless, the contributions of the Bernese group have not only highlighted these issues of standardization, but also provided an atlas of features to identify during the assessment of the pre-arthritic hip [42].

The mechanical processes of both FAI and acetabular dysplasia result in a shear force applied to the acetabular articular cartilage, resulting in delamination of the cartilage from the subchondral bone, without structural loss until late in the process. Damage to the articular cartilage of the acetabulum precedes that of the femoral head, which is frequently preserved despite full-thickness acetabular cartilage loss. Because of the lack of structural loss of articular cartilage until disease is advanced, magnetic resonance arthrography is insensitive [43] and therefore of limited value as a prognostic tool prior to hip arthroscopy. Alternative magnetic resonance imaging techniques, such as "delayed Gadolinium-Enhanced MRI of Cartilage" (dGEMRIC), measure the content of glycosaminoglycans (GAG) in hyaline cartilage. GAG content falls in osteoarthritic cartilage before structural loss occurs. In collaboration with the University of British Columbia, Vancouver, the Oxford group [44] studied asymptomatic subjects with no joint space loss, with and without cam deformities, and found that dGEMRIC was able to identify depletion of GAG content in cam hips in the acetabular cartilage, and noted that the severity of depletion correlated with the severity of cam deformity. Further contributions from the Bernese group have associated dGEMRIC with intraoperative findings [45] and furthermore identified its potential to differentiate the varying pathomechanisms of impingement, potentially improving patient selection and understanding of progression of osteoarthritis throughout the hip joint [46].

These sophisticated MRI techniques offer promise for the sensitive detection of cartilage lesions prior to hip arthroscopy, and to develop our understanding of the failure of the joint.

Intraoperative Classification of Articular Lesions

Traditional classifications of cartilage damage such as that described by Outerbridge [47] may well be appropriate for lesions of the femoral head, but not so for lesions of the acetabular cartilage. The arthroscopic classification of acetabular chondral lesions described by Konan and coworkers at University College Hospital, London [48], has high observer reliability, describes this progression appropriately, and supersedes the classification system of Beck et al. [25], which was based on observations from open surgery.

Treatment Strategies and Clinical Trials

Historically, prior to awareness of FAI, the arthroscopic management of cartilage and labral lesions did not include addressing underlying bony deformities. Bardakos, Vasconcelos, and Villar [49] from the UK, retrospectively compared 24 patients who had undergone arthroscopic hip debridement with excision of cam deformity, with a control group of 47 patients who had undergone arthroscopic debridement without excision of cam deformity. Although both groups were improved by surgery, the cam excision group had a higher proportion of excellent or good results. A further study by Malviya, Stafford, and Villar [50], from the same unit in the UK, demonstrated that 77 % of patients had objectively improved quality of life at 1 year after hip arthroscopy, mirroring numerous case series outlining the benefits of arthroscopic hip surgery.

Whilst these studies justify current surgical practice, their retrospective or noncomparative designs limit their power to convince funding bodies of the benefits of arthroscopic hip surgery. The feasibility of performing a randomized controlled trial for arthroscopic FAI surgery (or physiotherapy) has been investigated by collaborators from the University of Oxford and the Royal Berkshire Hospital, Reading, UK [51]. Surveying a group of surgeons at the annual meeting of the British Hip Society in 2012, they found that 77 % of surgeons who routinely perform FAI surgery would be willing to recruit participants. A survey of patients showed that 90 % with newly diagnosed FAI would be willing to participate in a trial with operative and nonoperative arms, provided there was opportunity for those in the nonoperative group to switch arms at 6 months if there was no improvement in symptoms.

It would therefore seem that a trial is imminent, which is exciting as it has the opportunity to definitively demonstrate clinical effectiveness and alleviate concerns regarding ongoing funding of hip arthroscopy.

The Second NICE Guidance on FAI (UK)

A further review was carried out in the UK, leading to the issuing of updated guidance in September 2011. This guidance identified that ***"current evidence on the efficacy of arthroscopic femoro-acetabular surgery for hip impingement syndrome is adequate in terms of symptom relief in the short and medium term. With regard to safety there are well recognised complications. Therefore this procedure may be used provided that normal arrangements are in place for clinical governance, consent and audit with local review of outcomes."*** It was also advised that ***"clinicians should submit details of all patients undergoing this procedure to"*** a register being established by the British Hip Society for arthroscopic femoro-acetabular surgery for hip impingement syndrome. It was still advised that the procedure ***"should only be performed by surgeons with specialist expertise in arthroscopic hip surgery."***

However, this does now allow for the potential expansion in the number of UK centers performing this surgery, provided they adhere to the recommended special arrangements.

Hip Arthroscopy Education

Studies examining training in arthroscopic surgical skills have largely been confined to simulations of arthroscopy of the knee or shoulder. One study, from the Oxford Orthopaedic Simulation and Education Centre [52], has examined simulated hip arthroscopy skills in a group of orthopedic trainees. This study compared learning curves in trainees randomized to perform a diagnostic central compartment round in either the lateral or supine positions. The authors found that trainees randomized to the lateral position were slower and more variable in their performance but achieved parity with the supine group by nine training episodes. All trainees objectively improved their performance over the training period, indicating that trainees are likely to benefit from simulator training to achieve orientation and basic competence prior to performing hip arthroscopy on patients.

Hip arthroscopy courses and meetings continue to flourish all over Europe in the current era. **ISHA** is becoming more influential on the world stage, and with this there is a move to an attempted standardization of hip arthroscopy teaching. A "faculty of hip arthroscopy trainers" would go some way towards this and remains a potential focus.

Future Perspectives

We are currently in a very exciting era for hip arthroscopy. The next few years promise to deliver solutions for the major challenges we face in treating articular cartilage lesions. The role of stem cell technology and platelet-rich plasma is yet to be defined, and exciting studies into composite chondro-labral grafting should deliver fascinating results.

The challenges of standardizing analysis of preoperative imaging (either radiograph or CT/MRI) may well be solved by sophisticated software. Planning software for quantifying surgical corrections and assessing its effect on the range of motion of the hip is already on the horizon.

Perhaps the most tantalizing question is whether arthroscopic surgery can alter the natural history of the conditions it treats, and indeed whether it can delay or even prevent the later need for joint replacement surgery?

European clinicians and scientists have been contributing to the evolution of hip arthroscopy for a century, and well-designed and funded multi-center studies will ensure that Europe remains at the forefront of this rapidly developing area of surgery.

References

1. Kieser CW, Jackson RW. Eugen Bircher: the first knee surgeon to use diagnostic arthroscopy. Arthroscopy. 2003;19:771–6.
2. Kieser CW, Jackson RW. Severin Nordentoft: the first arthroscopist. Arthroscopy. 2001;17:532–5.
3. Burman M. Athroscopy or the direct visualization of joints. J Bone Joint Surg. 1931;13:669–94.
4. Takagi K. The arthroscope: the second report. J Jpn Orthop Assoc. 1939;14:441–66.
5. Bhatt J, Jones A, Foley S, Shah Z, Malone P, Fawcett D, Kumar S. Harold Horace Hopkins: a short biography. BJU Int. 2010;106:1425–8.
6. Villar RN. Personal communication.
7. Aignan M. Arthroscopy of the hip. In: Proceedings of the international arthroscopy association. Rev Int Rheumatol. 1976;33:458.
8. Holgersson S, Brattstrom H, Mogensen B, Lidgren L. Arthroscopy of the hip in juvenile chronic arthritis. J Pediatr Orthop. 1981;1:273–8.
9. Dorfmann H, Boyer T, Henry P, de Bie B. A simple approach to hip arthroscopy. Arthroscopy. 1988;4:141–2.
10. Dorfmann H, Boyer T. Hip arthroscopy utilising the supine position. Arthroscopy. 1996;12:264–7.
11. Dorfmann H, Boyer T. Arthroscopy of the hip: 12 years of experience. Arthroscopy. 1999;15:67–72.
12. Eriksson E, Arvidsson I, Arvidsson H. Diagnostic and operative arthroscopy of the hip. Orthopaedics. 1986;9:169–76.
13. Glick JM, Sampson TG, Gordon BB, Behr JT, Schmidt E. Hip arthroscopy by the lateral approach. Arthroscopy. 1987;3:4–12.
14. Villar RN. Hip arthroscopy. Oxford: Butterworth-Heinemann; 1992.
15. Villar RN. Hip arthroscopy. Br J Hosp Med. 1992;47(10):763–6.
16. Keene GS, Villar RN. Arthroscopic anatomy of the hip: an in vivo study. Arthroscopy. 1994;10:392–9.
17. Lage LA, Patel JV, Villar RN. The acetabular labral tear: an arthroscopic classification. Arthroscopy. 1996;12:269–72.
18. Villar RN. Arthroscopic debridement of the hip: a minimally invasive approach to osteoarthritis. J Bone Joint Surg Br. 1991;73(Suppl II):170–1.
19. Griffin DR, Villar RN. Complications of arthroscopy of the hip. J Bone Joint Surg Br. 1999;81:604–6.
20. Funke EL, Munzinger U. Complications in hip arthroscopy. Arthroscopy. 1996;12:156–9.
21. Fontana A, Bistolfi A, Crova M, Rosso F, Massazza G. Arthroscopic treatment of hip chondral defects: autologous chondrocyte transplantation versus simple debridement—a pilot study. Arthroscopy. 2012;28:322–9.
22. Dienst M, Goedde S, Seil R, Hammer D, Kohn D. Hip arthroscopy without traction: in vivo anatomy of the peripheral hip joint cavity. Arthroscopy. 2001;17:924–31.
23. Dienst M, Seil R, Kohn D. Safe arthroscopic access to the central compartment of the hip joint. Arthroscopy. 2005;21:1510–4.
24. Myers SR, Eijer H, Ganz R. Anterior femoroacetabular impingement after periacetabular osteotomy. Clin Orthop Relat Res. 1999;363:93–9.
25. Beck M, Kalhor M, Leunig M, Ganz R. Hip morphology influences the pattern of damage to the acetabular cartilage: femoroacetabular impingement as a cause of early osteoarthritis of the hip. J Bone Joint Surg Br. 2005;87(7):1012–8.
26. Smith-Petersen MN. Treatment of malum coxae senilis, old slipped upper femoral epiphysis, intrapelvic protrusion of the acetabulum, and coxa plana by means of acetabuloplasty. J Bone Joint Surg Am. 1936;18(4):869–80.
27. Harris WH. Etiology of osteoarthritis of the hip. Clin Orthop Relat Res. 1986;213:20–33.
28. Murray R. The aetiology of primary osteoarthritis of the hip. Br J Radiol. 1965;38:810–24.
29. Ganz R, Gill TJ, Gautier E, Ganz K, Krugel N, Berlemann U. Surgical dislocation of the adult hip a technique with full access to the femoral head and acetabulum without the risk of avascular necrosis. J Bone Joint Surg Br. 2001;83(8):1119–24.
30. Beck M, Leunig M, Parvizi J, Boutier V, Wyss D, Ganz R. Anterior femoroacetabular impingement: part II. Midterm results of surgical treatment. Clin Orthop Relat Res. 2004;418:67–73.
31. Philippon MJ, Stubbs AJ, Schenker ML, Maxwell RB, Ganz R, Leunig M. Arthroscopic management of femoroacetabular impingement: osteoplasty technique and literature review. Am J Sports Med. 2007;35(9):1571–80.
32. Sadri H. Personal communication.
33. Lund B. Personal communication.
34. Gosvig KK, Jacobsen S, Sonne-Holm S, Gebuhr P. The prevalence of cam-type deformity of the hip joint: a survey of 4151 subjects of the Copenhagen Osteoarthritis Study. Acta Radiol. 2008;49(4):436–41.
35. Gosvig KK, Jacobsen S, Sonne-Holm S, Palm H, Troelsen A. Prevalence of malformations of the hip joint and their relationship to sex, groin pain, and risk of osteoarthritis: a population-based survey. J Bone Joint Surg Am. 2010;92(5):1162–9.
36. Hogervorst T, Bouma H, de Boer SF, de Vos J. Human hip impingement morphology: an evolutionary explanation. J Bone Joint Surg Br. 2011;93(6):769–76.
37. Siebenrock KA, Ferner F, Noble PC, Santore RF, Werlen S, Mamisch TC. The cam-type deformity of the proximal femur arises in childhood in response to vigorous sporting activity. Clin Orthop Relat Res. 2011;469(11):3229–40.
38. Pollard TCB, Villar RN, Norton MR, Fern ED, Williams MR, Murray DW, Carr AJ. Genetic influences in the aetiology of femoroacetabular impingement: a sibling study. J Bone Joint Surg Br. 2010;92(2):209–16.
39. Bardakos NV, Villar RN. Predictors of progression of osteoarthritis in femoroacetabular impingement: a radiological study with a minimum of ten years follow-up. J Bone Joint Surg Br. 2009;91(2): 162–9.
40. Nicholls AS, Kiran A, Pollard TCB, Hart D, Arden CPA, Spector T, Gill HS, Murray DW, Carr AJ, Arden NK. The association between hip morphology parameters and 19-year risk of end-stage osteoar-

thritis in the hip: a nested case-control study. Arthritis Rheum. 2011;63(11):3392–400.

41. Pollard TCB. A perspective on femoroacetabular impingement. Skeletal Radiol. 2011;40(7):815–8.
42. Tannast M, Siebenrock KA, Anderson SE. Femoroacetabular impingement: radiographic diagnosis—what the radiologist should know. Am J Roentgenol. 2007;188(6):1540–52.
43. Pfirrmann CW, Duc SR, Zanetti M, Dora C, Hodler J. MR arthrography of acetabular cartilage delamination in femoroacetabular cam impingement. Radiology. 2008;249(1):236–41.
44. Pollard TC, McNally EG, Wilson DC, Wilson DR, Madler B, Watson M, Gill HS, Carr AJ. Localized cartilage assessment with three-dimensional dGEMRIC in asymptomatic hips with normal morphology and cam deformity. J Bone Joint Surg Am. 2010;92(15):2557–69.
45. Bittersohl B, Hosalkar HS, Apprich S, Werlen SA, Siebenrock KA, Mamisch TC. Comparison of pre-operative dGEMRIC imaging with intra-operative findings in femoroacetabular impingement: preliminary findings. Skeletal Radiol. 2011;40(5):553–61.
46. Mamisch TC, Kain MS, Bittersohl B, Apprich S, Werlen S, Beck M, Siebenrock KA. Delayed gadolinium-enhanced magnetic resonance imaging of cartilage (dGEMRIC) in Femoacetabular impingement. J Orthop Res. 2011;29(9):1305–11.
47. Outerbridge RE. The etiology of chondromalacia patellae. J Bone Joint Surg Br. 1961;43-B:752–7.
48. Konan S, Rayan F, Meermans G, Witt J, Haddad FS. Validation of the classification system for acetabular chondral lesions identified at arthroscopy in patients with femoroacetabular impingement. J Bone Joint Surg Br. 2011;93(3):332–6.
49. Bardakos NV, Vasconcelos JC, Villar RN. Early outcome of hip arthroscopy for femoroacetabular impingement: the role of femoral osteoplasty in symptomatic improvement. J Bone Joint Surg Br. 2008;90(12):1570–5.
50. Malviya A, Stafford GH, Villar RN. Impact of arthroscopy of the hip for femoroacetabular impingement on quality of life at a mean follow-up of 3.2 years. J Bone Joint Surg Br. 2012;94(4): 466–70.
51. Palmer AJR, Thomas GER, Pollard TCB, Rombach I, Taylor A, Arden NK, Beard DJ, Andrade AJMD, Carr AJ, Glyn-Jones S. The feasibility of performing a randomised controlled trial for femoroacetabular impingement surgery. J Bone Joint Res; in press.
52. Pollard TC, Khan T, Price AJ, Gill HS, Glyn-Jones S, Rees JL. Simulated hip arthroscopy skills: learning curves with the lateral and supine patient positions: a randomized trial. J Bone Joint Surg Am. 2012;94(10):e68.

Africa

89

Josip Nenad Cakic

Introduction

Arthroscopy is currently a routine surgical procedure used for the diagnosis and treatment of problems in many joints. However, the hip is unlike other joints. Difficulties with its anatomy and position have meant that the use of arthroscopy in the treatment of hip disorders has not followed the same rapid expansion as in other joints.

Knee and shoulder arthroscopy developed from open procedures as a logical step with the aim of tissue preservation, while hip arthroscopy started as a completely new procedure. The presence of pathology and symptoms in the hip joint were traditionally treated by either nonoperative methods or radical replacement surgery. Arthroscopy of the hip therefore offered a logical alternative to what seemed to be common but rather ignored conditions.

The evolution of hip arthroscopy is not yet complete; however, the foundation is laid. The current progression and development of hip arthroscopy make this procedure the fastest growing surgical procedure in the field of orthopedics. Since the start of the expansion of joint arthroscopy in general, in the early 1980s, when hip arthroscopy accounted for less than 1 % of all arthroscopic procedures in Europe, it was predicted that 70,000 arthroscopic hip surgeries would have been performed in the USA alone, by the end of 2013 [1].

History

Human curiosity and the urge to explore every part of the body did not completely evade the hip joint. The first attempt at hip arthroscopy was by Dr. M. Burman [2], in 1931, when he explored what we now know as the peripheral compartment, without distraction. The first clinical application of hip arthroscopy on four patients was reported by Dr. Takagi in 1939 [3]. Following these early attempts, hip arthroscopy went unmentioned until the 1970s. At the International Arthroscopy Association meeting, Aignan reported 51 diagnostic arthroscopies [4]. Since then the evolution of hip arthroscopy has transformed from a slow progression to the most rapidly expanding subspecialty in the field of orthopedic surgery in every corner of the world (see other chapters).

The evolution of hip arthroscopy in South Africa has followed a similar pattern. The major influence on the development of the hip arthroscopy in South Africa can be attributed to Dr. Thomas Byrd, who redefined the supine traction technique. The majority of orthopedic surgeons in South African universities were well trained in the use of the traction tables for trauma cases, so the use of the supine position with slight modification of the traction table for hip arthroscopy proved to be preferable to the lateral position popularized by Glick and Sampson.

Evolution of Hip Arthroscopy in South Africa

Hip arthroscopy in South Africa started slowly but in earnest in 2000. Prior to that, only occasional attempts at hip arthroscopy were performed by senior members of the orthopedic fraternity. At that time the author (Dr. JN Cakic) following his FCS (Orth) qualification underwent fellowship training with Prof. FA Weber in lower limb arthroplasty. During this fellowship the need for, and the interest in, a less invasive approach to the hip joint became a priority. This was a logical step in his further development as a hip specialist. Total knee arthroplasty was an established part of fellowship training, with knee arthroscopy already being an optional "escape" route for many indications. No such option was yet available for the hip in South Africa. Once started, the evolution of hip arthroscopy in South Africa then followed a very similar pattern to the rest of the world.

J.N. Cakic, MD, PhD, FSC(SA)Orth, MMed(Orth) WITS (✉)
Orthopaedic Surgery, Private Practice, Life Fourways Hospital, P.O. Box 156, Petervale 2151, South Africa
e-mail: chuck@drcakic.co.za

J.C. McCarthy et al. (eds.), *Hip Joint Restoration*, DOI 10.1007/978-1-4614-0694-5_89

During 2000/2001, the author started with cadaveric training at the University of Witwatersrand using customized knee arthroscopy equipment. The author acquired theoretical knowledge from Dr. T. Byrd's book, *Operative Hip Arthroscopy* [5]. The first recorded hip arthroscopy procedure by Dr. JN Cakic was performed on 27th November 2001. This was the removal of a traumatic loose body, and was performed in the supine position with traction, employing Dr. Byrd's technique.

From 2001 to 2003, two other surgeons in South Africa, Dr. J. de Vos and Dr. H. Bosch, sporadically used hip arthroscopy for carrying out biopsies, removal of loose bodies, and diagnostic purposes instead of using open surgery. By the end of 2003, the three surgeons had performed approximately 50 hip arthroscopies (personal communication, Smith & Nephew sale record), with the author having performed 24 of those. In the following year, the number of procedures doubled, showing a steady but continued increase in the number of patients undergoing this procedure (Smith & Nephew sale record).

In 2004, the author had the opportunity to expand on his experience by visiting training centers in the USA and work with experts in supine position hip arthroscopy. The first part of this training was with Dr. M. Philippon, who was in Pittsburg at that time, followed by a visit to Dr. T. Byrd in Nashville. This was an invaluable experience, which provided the author with a significant advancement of his knowledge and technical skills.

In the same year, at the annual South African Orthopaedic Association Congress (SAOA) Dr. JN Cakic presented a 1-year follow-up of the first 50 patients treated with hip arthroscopy [6].

There were 20 females and 30 males with an average age of 37 years (11–70). The indications for surgery were varied (Table 89.1).

There were four patients who required conversion to total hip replacement (THR), one patient with primary osteoarthritis (OA), and two with secondary OA due to avascular necrosis (AVN). One of the patients, who had an arthroscopy, eventually had a THR secondary to rheumatoid arthritis performed by a different surgeon. Apart from conversion to THR only two other patients had an unsatisfactory result with continuous unresolved pain. There were no permanent complications, with one patient only having a transient pudendal neuropraxia and one patient having residual trochanteric bursitis.

Hip Arthroscopy Education in South Africa

In 2004 an educational and training program was started in South Africa with the support of Smith & Nephew. There had been an obvious need to start this initiative as in South Africa there was a significant gap between the private medical sector, supported by medical institutions such as MediClinic, NetCare, and Life Group, and the government sector supported by universities and hospitals, which did not have funding available to develop equally sophisticated operating rooms and the equipment necessary for the training of registrars or young consultants. As a result of such a discrepancy, a training program was started and based only in private institutions where financial investments allowed the development of digital theaters and educational tools to disseminate the training of arthroscopic hip techniques.

In 2005 the hip arthroscopy training program trained four orthopedic surgeons. The author became a Consultant for the Smith & Nephew hip arthroscopy training program, performing the majority of procedures in the country.

The first hip arthroscopy course was held in 2006 with the international guest speaker and course instructor Dr. T. Byrd. Two live surgeries were performed in Johannesburg and Cape Town, significantly increasing the interest in hip arthroscopy (Fig. 89.1).

There was a strong presence of South African doctors at the 2007 ISAKOS hip arthroscopy instructional course demonstrating the growing interest in hip arthroscopy. In the

Table 89.1 Indications in 1-year follow-up of the first 50 patients having a hip arthroscopy

Chronic pain	13
Acute painful hip	8
Trauma	6
OA	5
AVN	4
Lig teres	4
Rheumatoid arthritis	3
Loose bodies	2
Synovial chondromatosis	2
Sepsis	1
Pigmented villonodular synovitis	1
Post-open hip surgery	1

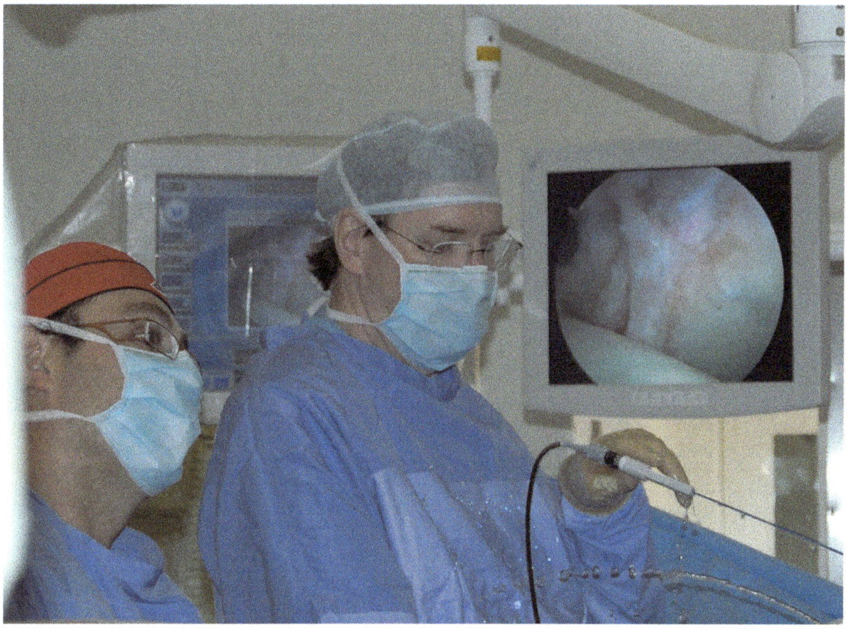

Fig. 89.1 Dr. Byrd and Dr. Cakic performing live surgery in Johannesburg, 2006

Table 89.2 Diagnosis for 163 patients—minimum 3-year follow-up (2003–2006)

Diagnosis	
Labrum related	50
Acute painful hip	23
OA	18
FAI	12
Trauma related	9
DDH	8
Lig teres	8
Iliopsoas	6
Rheumatoid arthritis	4
Chondral defects	4
Synovial chondromatosis	4
AVN	4
Multiple exostoses	3
Pigmented villonodular synovitis	3
Infection	2
Loose bodies	2
Osteochondritis dissecans	2
THR	1

same year the author presented the 3-year follow-up of 163 hip arthroscopy patients at the annual SAOA meeting [7] further increasing the profile of hip arthroscopy that year (Table 89.2).

There were 98 females and 65 males treated between May 2003 and December 2006 with an average age of 45.5 (11–70) years that were analyzed using the UCLA Activity Scale [8] with a minimum of 1-year follow-up (Table 89.3).

In order to minimize the influence of possible OA and age on the UCLA analysis, patients were separated into groups below and above the age of 50 years (Tables 89.4 and 89.5).

In the group of 128 patients below the age, to 8.0 after 1-year follow-up. In that group there were four patients who required revision arthroscopy, and six who had conversion to THR (Table 89.4).

In the group of 35 patients above the age of 50, the preoperative UCLA activity scale increased from 3.8 to 5.9 after a minimum of 1 year postoperatively. Two revision arthroscopies were performed and four patients required conversion to THR (Table 89.5).

Among the 163 patients, an FAI-related diagnosis, with or without evidence of labral tear, was made in 75 patients.

Table 89.3 UCLA activity scale

Level	Activity	Examples
1	Inactive	Residence
2	Mostly inactive	Minimum of daily living
3	Mild activity	Walking, shopping
4	Mild activity	Sedentary occupational work
5	Moderate activity	Swimming
6	Moderate activity	Light occupational work
7	Active	Cycling, gym 2/7
8	Very active	Regular sport, gym 3/7
9	Impact sports	Sometimes
10	Impact sports	Regularly

Table 89.4 One hundred and twenty-eight patients under the age of 50 with minimum 1-year follow-up

128 Patients under age of 50	UCLA scale
Pre op	3.3 (1–6)
6 Weeks	5.5 (2–10)
3 Months	6.9 (2–10)
6 Months	7.5 (3–10) 1 THR
1 Year	8.0 (3–10) 5 THR, 4 revision scopes
Progress	Mild activity to very active

Table 89.5 Thirty-five patients over the age of 50 with minimum 1-year follow-up

35 Patients over the age of 50	UCLA scale
Pre-op	3.8 (1–7)
6 Weeks	4.6 (2–7)
3 Months	5.2 (2–10) 1THR
6 Months	5.8 (2–10)
1 Year	5.9 (2–10) 3 THR, 2 revision scopes
Progress	Mild activity to moderate active

This presentation was important in raising awareness of the concept of femoroacetabular impingement as another diagnosis treatable by arthroscopic techniques. At the same Congress, Dr. S. Godinho, a specialist radiologist, presented a paper on the diagnostic tools used in preoperative assessment [9].

The author also organized a hip arthroscopy workshop at the 2007 SAOA Congress, supported by Smith & Nephew. This aimed to raise awareness of the concept of FAI and to educate on the basic surgical techniques. Later that year, six surgeons with an interest in the procedure attended a cadaver workshop.

It quickly became clear that there was also a need to raise awareness of both hip arthroscopy as a procedure and the significance of FAI to the nonsurgical disciplines. An educational road show program was established, and four meetings were held in 2007 for general practitioners, physiotherapists, and biokineticists countrywide. The educational program also linked up with the South African Sports Medicine Association (SASMA); approaching sports physicians involved in all varieties of sports, and more importantly in high school physical education programs. Slowly but surely, hip disorders became a better known entity and were no longer a mystery.

In 2008, Smith & Nephew organized a second hip arthroscopy course with a cadaver workshop in Cape Town. This was very well attended and it was an opportunity to learn from the international guest speaker and course instructor Dr. Marc Philippon (Fig. 89.2).

The educational program continued through 2008 extending the visiting surgeon program to international visitors, mainly from the Middle East and India. The Center for Sports Medicine and Orthopaedics in Rosebank, Johannesburg, had established an Arthroscopy Fellowship for many years, where fellows could learn knee and shoulder arthroscopy from Mark Ferguson and Glen Vardi. Hip arthroscopy became part of the 6-month fellowship program in 2008.

South African surgeon presence at an international level became more evident throughout 2008, with multiple surgeons attending Dr. Marc Philippon's course in Vail (USA), as well as attending other international meetings on a more regular basis.

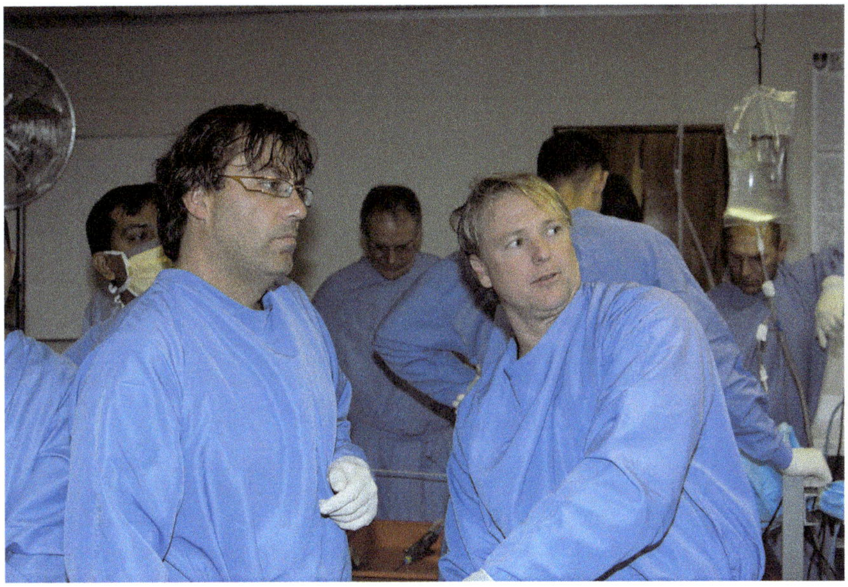

Fig. 89.2 Dr. Philippon at the cadaver workshop in Cape Town, 2008

Hip Arthroscopy Societies

The International Society for Hip Arthroscopy (ISHA) was established in 2008 in Paris, and the author became a member.

The next 2 years saw an exponential increase in arthroscopic hip surgery in South Africa. Smith & Nephew sales data show that 164 operations were performed in 2008, and this number rose in 2009 to 285 hip arthroscopies performed by ten surgeons in 46 different private hospitals. Five of these surgeons performed these procedures more regularly with 117 surgeries carried out by a single surgeon. In 2010 the number of operations almost doubled, with 423 registered procedures.

The author presented the South African experience at the 2nd ISHA meeting in Cancun, Mexico [10]. Up to 2010, six surgeons performed just over 1100 hip arthroscopy procedures in South Africa. At the same meeting, another South African surgeon, Dr W. Van der Merwe, presented his early results of hip arthroscopy [11]. In that same year, the author was invited to join the Executive Board of ISHA, further raising the profile of African hip arthroscopy at the international level.

South African Society for Hip Arthroscopy

At that point hip arthroscopies in South Africa were performed only in the private sector, with no university involvement. Operations in private hospitals directly depend on authorization from the numerous medical schemes, which were largely unaware of the development of hip arthroscopy. There was an obvious need to establish an interest group or society of enthusiastic hip arthroscopy surgeons with the main goal of education and research, but to also establish the essential communication with the medical schemes and their administrators. The aim was to establish the required level of education and training to allow the carrying out of safe and successful procedures. This interest group would accredit the surgeons who became members and had fulfilled certain accreditation requirements. The medical administrators, in turn, would then clear the way for the authorization of arthroscopic hip surgery, stopping it from being classified as a "novice" procedure.

In August 2011, in York (UK) at a Smith & Nephew cadaver workshop, the South African Society for Hip Arthroscopy (SASHA) was formed with eight founder members (Fig. 89.3). The founding of SASHA answered the requirement for a proper and fair relationship with the numerous medical schemes. The eight founder members agreed on the level of training that would be necessary to become a certified member of SASHA. Membership of SASHA and fulfilling its accreditation requirements would enable an orthopedic specialist to be recognized by the medical schemes, and thereby be guaranteed remuneration for the procedure performed. SASHA also became affiliated with the South African Sports Medicine Association (SASMA) providing an open platform for continuous education of the associated nonsurgical disciplines. Furthermore, it aimed to establish a uniform rehabilitation protocol for physiotherapists and biokineticists involved with the treatment of these hip disorders. Another goal for SASHA was to establish a preventative examination program involving school children aged 15–16 years in grades 10–11. In order to achieve all of these goals, SASHA opened its membership to all specialties involved in the treatment of hip disorders.

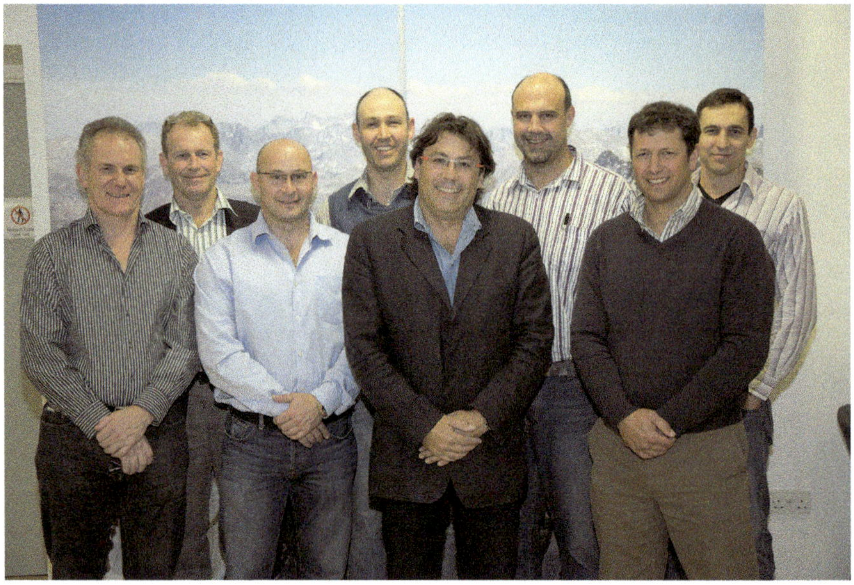

Fig. 89.3 South African Society for Hip Arthroscopy (SASHA)—founder members. From *left*: Jan De Vos, Leith Stewart, Hennie Bosch, Thane Munting, Josip N Cakic, Werner Van der Merwe, Adriaan van Huyssteen, Johnny De Beer

For a surgeon with an interest in hip arthroscopy to become an ordinary member of SASHA, two visits are required to an accredited consultant surgeon to observe these procedures. This essentially filters out surgeons who have no clear idea of the complexity of arthroscopic hip surgery.

As James Glick stated in the foreword to "Arthroscopic Management of Hip Diseases": "Today, surgeons routinely use the arthroscope for the diagnosis and treatment of joint problems. However, few surgeons apply the arthroscope to the hip joint. The reason for the lack of interest in this procedure is because of the deep position of the hip joint that makes it difficult to reach and there are a small number of indications. In order for the surgeon to be adept at a difficult operation, he must perform the surgery frequently. … The surgeon will often discard the procedure or refer it to someone who has experience in it" [12].

This filtering prior to committing to the difficult training is important. Our industry partners have shown that the conversion rate of a novice surgeon to hip arthroscopy is less than 20 %. If the surgeon decides to continue with training and that commitment is feasible, then attendance at a minimum of one official cadaver workshop nationally or internationally is required. Following on from this, the surgeon will have to perform a minimum of five procedures with the assistance of an accredited consultant.

Rehabilitation Protocols

A similar approach was planned for nonsurgical disciplines with the aim that SASHA would provide the training program for hip arthroscopy rehabilitation. The rehabilitation protocol was based on research carried out by the physiotherapist Barry Getz and the biokineticist Jannie Klingbiel, who are both members of the rehabilitation team working closely with Dr. JN Cakic. This protocol was presented at the ISHA annual scientific meeting in Boston, 2012, as an e-poster [13].

The need for such a protocol was evident from the fact that there was such a geographic diversity of patients and therapists in South Africa resulting in so many different ways of managing patients, often resulting in poor patient outcomes. The IHOT-33 (as a patient-reported outcome score) was first publically presented at the ISHA Annual International Congress 2010 in Cancun, Mexico. The IHOT-33 was used for the South African study, and it was hypothesized that the scores would remain unchanged at set recorded periods (6 and 12 weeks, 6 and 12 months). Patients' milestones in rehabilitation were screened utilizing dynamic hip movement patterns as an assessment tool, to ascertain whether patients may progress "safely" during a staged rehabilitation protocol (Fig. 89.4).

Analysis of 626 patients revealed a statistical significance in the "symptoms and functional limitations" quality of life category of IHOT-33 ($p=0.0407$) at the 12-week period.

It was concluded that implementing a staged Dynamic Hip Movement Screen Test is an objective measure that aids the decision-making process in patient progression; moreover, it is an effective tool that reduces the early onset of patient-reported symptoms and functional limitations. Utilizing this objective tool in conjunction with the subjective IHOT-33 questionnaire provides a comprehensive value-added dimension in patient assessment.

The rehabilitation protocol was developed in 2012, the year that also saw the introduction of the prevention screening system for the young teenaged population.

In May 2013 SASHA hosted its first international hip arthroscopy meeting held in Cape Town, which was a great success. SASHA now looks forward to ongoing co-operation with the international community, in particular the possible establishment of a southern hemisphere educational exchange program with the Australian Hip Arthroscopy Society.

The remainder of 2013 saw the expansion of the rehabilitation program and the continued education of arthroscopic surgeons. This was made possible through the offering of numerous rehabilitation-training courses and the active involvement of the trade sponsors.

Groin Pain

Groin pain has been a particular focus for South African research, and in particular the relationship between the sports hernia and FAI. While impossible to determine whether the FAI or the inguinal disruption [14] is the causative effect the close relationship between the two is irrefutable [15]. In our experience, groin pain in the athlete is present in 6 % of the sports injuries at our center. The majority are soccer or rugby

a

Patient Name		Age		
Date of Birth		Gender	Male	Female
Surgery Details				
Date of Surgery				
Surgeon Name				
Examiner Name		Examination Date		

HIP STAGE 1 – 2 SCREENING (Arthroscopy)

Scoring sheet

TEST		RAW SCORE	FINAL SCORE	COMMENTS
HURDLE STEP	L			
	R			
BALANCE	L			
	R			
¼ ONE LEG SQUAT	L			
	R			
TOTAL				

HURDLE STEP — *score allocation*

Performs movement correctly without any compensation	3
Able to complete movement, compensates to complete the fundamental movement	2
Unable to complete the test or assume the movement pattern	1
Pain felt during test in any part of the body	0

BALANCE — *score allocation*

≥ 30 seconds (no pain)	1
< 30 seconds (with or without pain)	0

¼ ONE LEG SQUAT — *score allocation*

Performs movement correctly without any compensation	3
Able to complete movement, compensates to complete the fundamental movement	2
Unable to complete the test or assume the movement pattern	1
Pain felt during test in any part of the body	0

RAW SCORE: This denotes right and left side scoring

FINAL SCORE: This denotes the overall *lowest score of the raw scores*

TOTAL: This is the sum of all the final scores

Total score ≥ 5 points may be advanced to STAGE 2 of rehabilitation protocol

Fig. 89.4 Hip functional screening test (**a**) stage 1, (**b**) stage 2, (**c**) stage 3 b

Patient Name		Age		
Date of Birth		Gender	Male	Female
Surgery Details				
Date of Surgery				
Surgeon Name				
Examiner Name		Examination Date		

HIP STAGE 2 – 3 SCREENING (Arthroscopy)

Scoring sheet

TEST	RAW SCORE	FINAL SCORE	COMMENTS
OVERHEAD DEEP SQUAT			
HURDLE STEP	L: R:		
BALANCE	L: R:		
¼ ONE LEG SQUAT	L: R:		
TOTAL			

OVERHEAD DEEP SQUAT – *score allocation*

Performs movement correctly without any compensation	3
Able to complete movement, compensates to complete the fundamental movement	2
Unable to complete the test or assume the movement pattern	1
Pain felt during test in any part of the body	0

HURDLE STEP – *score allocation*

Performs movement correctly without any compensation	3
Able to complete movement, compensates to complete the fundamental movement	2
Unable to complete the test or assume the movement pattern	1
Pain felt during test in any part of the body	0

BALANCE – *score allocation*

≥ 60 seconds (no pain)	1
< 60 seconds (with or without pain)	0

¼ ONE LEG SQUAT – *score allocation*

Performs movement correctly without any compensation	3
Able to complete movement, compensates to complete the fundamental movement	2
Unable to complete the test or assume the movement pattern	1
Pain felt during test in any part of the body	0

RAW SCORE: This denotes right and left side scoring
TOTAL: This is the sum of all the final scores
FINAL SCORE: This denotes the overall *lowest score of the raw scores*

Total score ≥ 7 points may be advanced to STAGE 3 of rehabilitation protocol

Fig. 89.4 (Continued)

c

Patient Name		Age		
Date of Birth		Gender	Male	Female
Surgery Details				
Date of Surgery				
Surgeon Name				
Examiner Name		Examination Date		

HIP STAGE 3 – 4 SCREENING (Arthroscopy)

Scoring sheet

TEST		RAW SCORE	FINAL SCORE	COMMENTS
OVERHEAD DEEP SQUAT	L			
	R			
HURDLE STEP	L			
	R			
STEP DOWN	L			
	R			
Y-BALANCE / BIODEX BALANCE	L			
	R			
TOTAL				

OVERHEAD DEEP SQUAT – *score allocation*

Performs movement correctly without any compensation	3
Able to complete movement, compensates to complete the fundamental movement	2
Unable to complete the test or assume the movement pattern	1
Pain felt during test in any part of the body	0

HURDLE STEP – *score allocation*

Performs movement correctly without any compensation	3
Able to complete movement, compensates to complete the fundamental movement	2
Unable to complete the test or assume the movement pattern	1
Pain felt during test in any part of the body	0

STEP DOWN – *score allocation*

Performs movement correctly without any compensation	3
Able to complete movement, compensates to complete the fundamental movement	2
Unable to complete the test or assume the movement pattern	1
Pain felt during test in any part of the body	0

Y-BALANCE / BIODEX BALANCE – *score allocation*

Y-Balance distance < 10cm OR BIODEX Balance < 3.9	2
Y-Balance distance ≥ 10cm OR BIODEX Balance ≥ 3.9	1
Pain felt during test in any part of the body	0

RAW SCORE: This denotes right and left side scoring
TOTAL: This is the sum of all the final scores
FINAL SCORE: This denotes the overall *lowest score of the raw scores*

Total score ≥ 9 points may be advanced to STAGE 4 of rehabilitation protocol

Fig. 89.4 (Continued)

injuries and 58 % of them had a previous injury. There is a direct correlation with increased level of activity and the symptoms are typically chronic in nature with 48 % of them having pain for more than 20 weeks prior to presentation [16]. Symptoms in our series are typically only with activity and include pain with sprinting, cutting, kicking, and coughing. The most common diagnostic signs in over 84 % of our patients are pain localized over the lower abdomen, pubis, and adductor, with resisted straight leg raise, resisted sit-up, and a positive squeeze test.

There remains no clear consensus on the management of inguinal disruption [14]. In the absence of any signs of intra-articular pathology a thorough kinematic assessment is performed. We believe that a hip screening initiative to prevent potential future hip joint injury is an essential tool. The athlete should undergo preseason screening to identify movement dysfunctions, postural abnormalities, or strength and flexibility deficits. This may be performed via functional movements screening tools, squeeze tests, video analysis, and/or isokinetic testing. Regarding the rehabilitation, it is extremely important to exclude any other factors in pelvic instability prior to the decision of any surgical treatment.

Only if conservative management fails to address the stabilization of the pelvic girdle or should the conservative approach exacerbate the pain due to the primary pathology, one should precisely identify the primary site of pathology and escalate the treatment accordingly.

Inguinal surgery is indicated when conservative management fails but in the case of professional sportsmen we attempt to delay this until off season if possible. Our criteria for surgery are the typical groin symptoms with activity and post-activity in the presence of the three diagnostic signs. All clinical tests for labral pathology must be negative. Patients with FAI on plain X-rays are not excluded.

If and when it comes to surgical treatment, the treatment of the groin soft-tissue pathology is following the principles of the surgical minimal repair according to Muschaweck [17].

It involves the opening of the posterior wall, rectus abdominis advancement, and maintaining load-bearing plates. The goal of the treatment is to keep the anatomical structures intact and to restore tension of the rectus muscles and keep the anatomical layers in place. If at the same time during the examination there are signs of positive pathology related to the hip, and radiological investigations confirm clinical findings, a hip arthroscopy is performed according to the principle of the hip arthroscopy procedure in the supine position [5]. Those two operations are performed in the same anaesthetic, starting with the soft-tissue groin procedure following with the hip arthroscopy.

Concomitant hip arthroscopy is performed if the athlete additionally has pain at rest, positive FABER, FADIR, and impingement signs with confirmed labral pathology on MRI arthrogram.

Hip arthroscopy alone is performed in the absence of any of the cardinal symptoms and signs of inguinal disruption described above.

The inability to return to the previous level of sport after either hip arthroscopy or groin surgery alone was considered a failure and surgery to attend to the groin or hip pathology, respectively, was carried out as a secondary procedure.

Using the above criteria for patient selection our results of inguinal or hip surgery or combined surgeries for athletes with hip/groin pain were retrospectively evaluated.

The South African experience was presented at the 2013 ISHA annual scientific meeting in Munich, where one of the Instructional Course Lectures (ICL) was dedicated to the topic of "groin pain and athletic pubalgia." The author presented the South African experience that supports the concept that the groin is the "Bermuda triangle of sports medicine," being an area of the body that raises numerous unanswered questions [18].

Between 2006 and 2014, two surgeons from the Center for Sports Medicine & Orthopaedics, Rosebank, South Africa, operated on 644 male patients (411 hip arthroscopies and 233 groin reconstructions, respectively) [19]. From this cohort, a total of 120 patients reported concurrent symptoms of hip-related pathology and groin pain. Of these 120 patients, 35 required a combined surgical approach where surgical treatment started with a groin reconstruction (Muschaweck surgical technique) [17], followed by a hip arthroscopy [5]. Furthermore, 25 out of 411 hip arthroscopy patients presented with concurrent groin symptoms; 7 (28 %) of them required secondary groin operation. Looking from the other angle, in the group of 233 groin patients, 31 patients did not have FAI addressed; 5 (16 %) required secondary hip arthroscopy. 10 % of the 120 returned for a second surgical procedure to address an unsuccessful outcome from a single surgical procedure approach. This experience demonstrates the need for a scoring system to be developed that incorporates objective and subjective measures to help with appropriate decision making for these patients.

The Hip Prevention Program

The SASHA 2013 international meeting resulted in the forging of stronger interdisciplinary relationships between surgeons, a group of enthusiastic practitioners, physiotherapists, and biokineticists, all of whom were interested in "hip prevention." From this "the Hip Prevention Program" was born. The literature has reported a significant percentage of positive radiological findings for FAI in teenagers [20]. An alternative approach to radiological imaging was sought: Could the prevalence of FAI morphology in the generalized young adolescent population be identified using noninvasive testing, with the aim of preventing future complications to the hip complex?

The Hip Prevention Program therefore established a pilot study, and to date has approached four high schools in Johannesburg, South Africa [21, 22]. Legal consent was obtained from the parents/guardian/child and school. There were 15 manual tests applied (12 published, 3 anecdotal) to a total of 124 students (average age of 14.5 years). "Red-flag" individuals (16.47 % female; 17.95 % male) were identified and started on a conservative management protocol that involved education and rehabilitation. If ineffective, further investigation would follow.

The ultimate aim is for the educational system to adopt the Hip Prevention Program as a standard screening component to aid in injury prevention and hip preservation.

Through the South African Society for Hip Arthroscopy, and in close relationship with its international sister society, ISHA, South African orthopedic surgeons will continue to be at the forefront of research and development of arthroscopic hip techniques.

References

1. Millenium Group. Hip arthroscopy procedures to soar through 2013—Millennium Research Group, Inc (MRG) [Internet]. http://mrg.net/News-and-Events/Press-Releases/HIP-ARTHROSCOPY-PROCEDURES-TO-SOAR-THROUGH-2013.aspx. Accessed 17 Aug 2012.
2. Burman MS. Arthroscopy or the direct visualization of joints: an experimental cadaver study. Clin Orthop Relat Res. 2001;(390):5–9.
3. Takagi K. The arthroscope: the second report. J Jpn Orthop Assoc. 1939;14:441–66.
4. Aignan M. Arthroscopy of the hip. In: Proceedings of the international association of arthroscopy. Rev Int Rheumatol. 1976;(33):458.
5. Byrd JWT. Operative hip arthroscopy. New York: Springer; 2005.
6. Cakic JN. Operative hip artroscopy—minimaly invasive treatment. Proceedings of the 50th South African Orthopaedic Association Congress. Pretoria, South Africa. Accessed 6–10 Sept 2004.
7. Cakic JN. Hip arthroscopy functional assessment—patient report. Proceedings of the 53rd South African Orthopaedic Association Congress. Johannesburg, South Africa. Accessed 5–9 Sept 2007.
8. Amstutz HC, Thomas BJ, Jinnah R. Treatment of primary osteoarthritis of the hip: a comparison of total joint and surface replacement arthroplasty. J Bone Joint Surg Am. 1984;66A:228–41.
9. Godinho S. The painful hip. Proceedings of the 53rd South African Orthopaedic Association Congress. Johannesburg, South Africa. Accessed 5–9 Sept 2007.
10. Cakic JN. Global status of hip arthroscopy—South Africa. Paper presented at 2nd International Society for Hip Arthroscopy. 2010.
11. Van der Merwe W. FAI scope learning curve. Paper presented at 2nd International Society for Hip Arthroscopy. 2010.
12. Sekiya JK, Safran MR, Ranawat AS, Leunig M. Techniques in hip arthroscopy and joint preservation surgery. Philadelphia: W.B. Saunders Company; 2010.
13. Getz B, Klingbiel J, Cakic JN. Hip arthroscopy rehabilitation-quantifying a criteria-based protocol. Presented at 4th International Society for hip arthroscopy. 2012.
14. Sheen AJ, Stephenson BM, Loyd DM, Robinson P, Fevre D, Paajanen H. Treatment of Sportsman's groin: British Hernia Society's 2014 position statement based on the Manchester Consensus Conference. BJSM. 2014;48(14):1079–87.
15. Ferguson M, Patricios J. What is the relationship between groin pain in athletes and femoroacetabular impingement? Br J Sports Med. 2014;48(14):1074–75.
16. Ferguson M. Groin injury in South African athletes. Paper presented at FIFA World Cup Meeting. 2010.
17. Muschaweck U, Berger L. Minimal repair technique of sportsmen's groin: an innovative open-suture repair to treat chronic inguinal pain. Hernia. 2010;14(1):27–33.
18. Cakic JN, Ferguson M. Relationship between sports hernia and FAI—clinical experience. Presented at 5th International Society for hip arthroscopy. 2013.
19. Cakic JN, Ferguson M. Overlap between FAI/sports hernia and adductor pain in athletes. What do we treat first? Presented at 6th International Society for the hip arthroscopy. 2014.
20. Weir A, de Vos RJ, Moen M, Tol JL. Prevalence of radiological signs of femoroacetabular impingement in patients presenting with long-standing adductor-related groin pain. Br J Sports Med. 2011;45:6–9.
21. Cakic JN, Getz B, Devine G, Sparke C. Manual screening of adolsecent hips: is surgery the only answer? A pilot study. Presented at 5th International Society for Hip Arthroscopy. 2014.
22. Cakic JN, Patricios J. Femoroacetabular inpingement: prevention or intervention? The sports physician's quandary. BJSM. 2014;48(14): 1073–4.

History of Hip Arthroscopy in the USA

90

Joseph C. McCarthy, Leah Elson, and JoAnn Lee

Anatomical Considerations

Historically, orthopedic surgeons have encountered difficulty in gaining access to the intra-articular surfaces of the hip joint. Such difficulty has made advances in hip arthroscopy slower to develop than in any other joint. This can be directly attributed to the unique anatomical features at the femoral head/acetabular interface. Firstly, the hip joint itself is deeply recessed in the pelvis, fully encased within soft tissue. Secondly, the relatively inelastic ligaments of the hip joint, along with the negative pressure seal maintained by the intact labrum, resist distraction of the head from the acetabulum. Thirdly, the complementary contours of the convex-concave, head, and acetabulum interface make arthroscopic intervention challenging.

Early investigation of the hip joint began with cadaveric experiences. In these specimens, surgeons were able to identify lateral and anterior entrance points for safe portal placement, avoiding unnecessary damage to the neurovascular system [1]. In 1931, Burman, from New York, published his work with cadaveric anatomy, demonstrating access to the peripheral compartment of the joint itself [2].

J.C. McCarthy, MD (✉)
Kaplan Joint Center, Newton-Wellesley Hospital,
2000 Washington St., Suite 361, Green Bldg, Newton,
MA 02462, USA
e-mail: jcmccarthy1@partners.org; jcmccarthy1@mgh.harvard.edu

L. Elson, BSc
Orthopedics, Harris Laboratory, Massachusetts General Hospital,
Boston, MA, USA
e-mail: leelson@gmail.com

J. Lee, MS
Orthopedics, Newton Wellesley Hospital, Newton, MA, USA
e-mail: jlee76@partners.org

Distraction Equipment

Technology for hip distraction was initially limited to standard fracture tables. However, it became evident that a more robust device for separating the femoral head from the acetabulum was necessary, especially for the younger, more muscular patient. The distraction methods began with simple static mechanical devices, and progressed to current tables that allow for dynamic motion of the joint intraoperatively. In an early evaluation by Glick, it was shown that up to 40 % of his patients could not be distracted with a fracture table alone due to resistance from the joint [3]. Thus, development of specialized distraction tables for the hip became one of the first concerted benchmarks in successful arthroscopy of the hip. Glick began using this technology (Arthronix, New York) in the late 1980s.

McCarthy devised a dedicated hip distractor in the same time frame (Innomed, Savannah, Georgia). The distractor was the by-product of more than 6 months of work in the cadaver laboratory. This device attached directly to the operating room table, thus reducing capital expense. The distractor used a robust, well-padded perineal post, an improved foot and ankle boot, and a foot attachment that allowed independent hip rotation and flexion (Fig. 90.1).

Years later, Mizuho OSI (California) developed a dedicated hip table which allowed supine anterior hip arthroscopy and anterior total hip arthroplasty. Its major drawback was expense.

In 2005, Smith and Nephew (Andover, Mass) released its distractor. Predominantly utilized with the patient in the supine position, this device allowed intraoperative hip flexion and rotation. Similarly Arthrex (Naples, FL) marketed its distractor as allowing dynamic hip motion assessment intraoperatively. These devices are particularly useful when osteochondroplasty is performed in the peripheral compartment.

J.C. McCarthy et al. (eds.), *Hip Joint Restoration*, DOI 10.1007/978-1-4614-0694-5_90

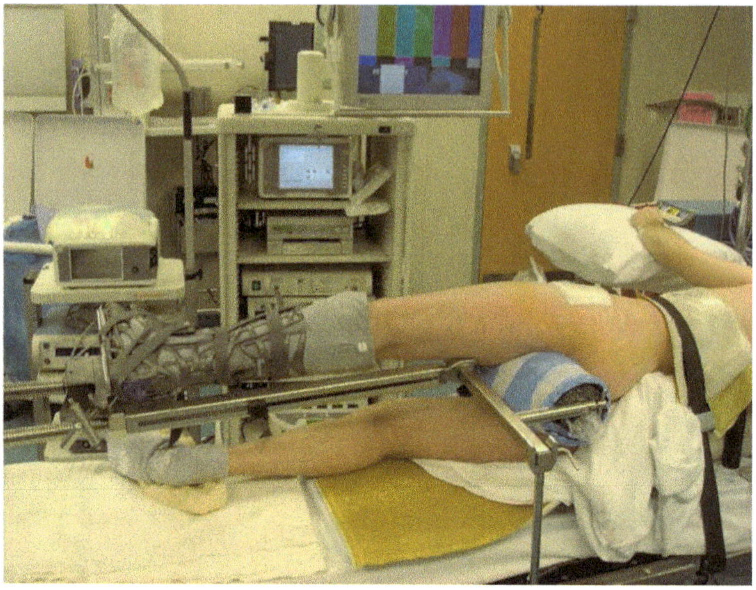

Fig. 90.1 Hip distractor used for the lateral decubitus position made by Innomed, Savanah, Georgia

Anatomic Positioning

Johnson, and later Byrd and colleagues, published techniques for accessing the hip joint in the supine position, initially performed on a fracture table [4, 5]. However, in 1987, Glick published the benefits of abandoning the traditional supine positioning for that of the lateral decubitus [6]. Both techniques are still being used in practice today.

Compartmental Access

Burman's work in 1931 described hip joint access through the peripheral compartment only [2]. It was only once distraction devices became available that the central compartment was then safely accessible. This enabled the diagnosis and treatment of an array of central compartment pathologies, in North America, from the 1980s [7–9].

Portals

With the development of distraction devices, safe portal access became an important priority. The placement of portals, being dependent upon the positioning of the patient, can be categorized as (1) hip joint access in the supine position [4, 10, 11], and (2) hip joint access in the lateral decubitus position [6, 12].

The latter of the two positions allowed surgeons full access for surgical intervention while placing portals that avoid neurovascular structures. Day, McCarthy, and Busconi published on peritrochanteric portals with the patient in the lateral decubitus position that allowed safe access to the joint, especially the central compartment [13].

Byrd published on the establishment of anterior portals with the patient in the supine position, and the portals' relationship to nearby neurovascular structures [5, 11].

Philippon more recently published on additional accessory portals, primarily for performing cam or pincer treatment in the peripheral compartment [14].

Instrumentation

Hip instrumentation was originally adapted from tools designed for shoulder and knee arthroscopic procedures. However, due to the recessed, deep location of the hip joint, these tools often proved too short or were limited in their ability to access the curved articular surfaces.

Thus, the next step in the development of arthroscopy involved the designing and manufacturing of hip-specific instrumentation.

Initially Glick, Sampson, and McCarthy (Arthrex) and Byrd (Smith and Nephew) helped to devise these tools. These novel instruments were longer and included both manual hand graspers and tissue resectors and motorized shavers. Additionally telescoping cannulas were designed to be used for the duration of the procedure to maintain portal access. They could also be interchanged in expanded sizes to accommodate varying instrumentation for cartilage repair or loose body removal.

The initial instrumentation was further developed to include curved graspers, shavers, burrs, chondral picks, and electrothermal components for the correction of unfavorable bony and chondral morphology (Fig. 90.2).

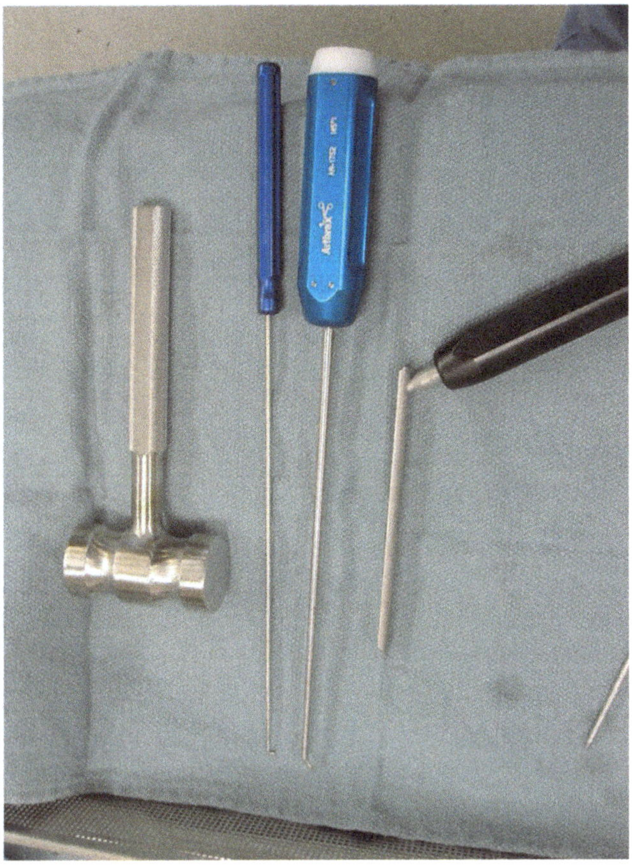

Fig. 90.2 Operating instruments designed specifically for hip arthroscopy designed by Arthrex, Naples, Florida

Imaging

Historically, imaging techniques to detect synovial and chondral pathology were nonexistent. The plain radiograph only visualized bony morphology; CAT scans and non-contrast MRI provided improved detection of both vasculature and muscle tissue, but they continued to fall short in showing labral or chondral morphology.

The development of contrast MRI techniques became crucial. McCarthy and Palmer at the MGH first devised, and later published, the gadolinium arthrogram MRI which provides better cartilage and labral image resolution, and allows for radial and oblique imaging which visualizes the anterior segment of the hip joint, where much of the joint pathology occurs [15–17]. This technique is now the gold standard worldwide (Fig. 90.3).

Recently, the non-contrast MRI technique has been revisited, primarily by the pioneering work of Dr. Hollis Potter at Hospital for Special Surgery and has shown much diagnostic improvement through the use of radial thin-slice, high-resolution exposure [18].

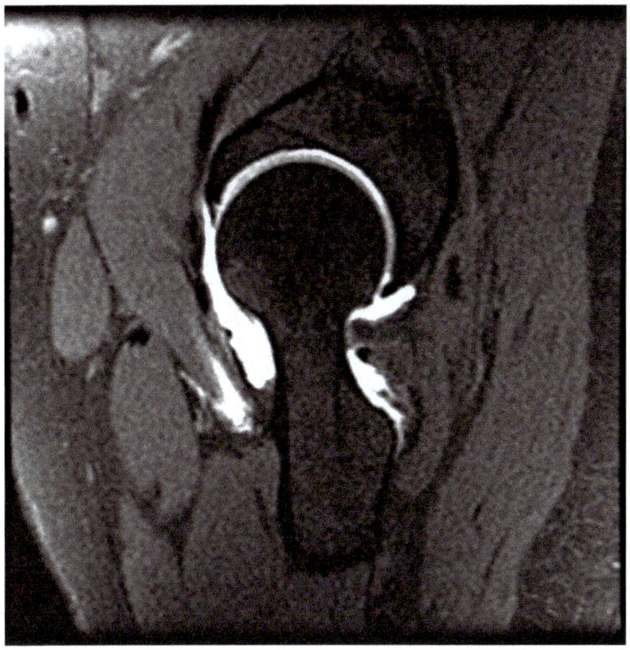

Fig. 90.3 An arthrogram MRI image demonstrating an anterior acetabular labral tear

Therapeutic Procedures

In its fledgling form, hip arthroscopy was used exclusively for diagnostic purposes as a way to directly visualize the articulating surfaces of the hip joint, or to collect samples for biopsy.

With the development of custom-made surgical equipment, and contributions from numerous pioneering surgeons, including those from North America, the specialty has since evolved an ever-increasing array of therapeutic procedures, including the removal of loose bodies, diagnosis and treatment of soft-tissue or prosthetic pathology following total hip arthroplasty, the anatomical correction of painful femoroacetabular impingement, and the capability to repair labral and chondral damage [8, 9, 14, 19–23].

Synopsis

Initially, the development of hip arthroscopy lagged significantly behind that of other joints. Anatomically, the hip joint is difficult to access and is designed to resist distraction. However, through the work of innovators, hip arthroscopy has become a safe and effective alternative to the open arthrotomy. It also remarkably reduces risk, makes the procedure an outpatient experience, and reduces cost.

Advances in surgical tables have made effective distraction possible. Research in patient positioning has led to full compartmental access, and portal placement that avoids critical neurovascular structures.

Improvement in imaging has advanced diagnostic capabilities with respect to the labral and chondral tissues. Novel instrumentation design has provided the arthroscopic hip surgeon with a broad range of options for the treatment of lesions and anatomical abnormalities that can cause pain, discomfort, and immobility in patients.

References

1. Robertson WJ, Kelly BT. The safe zone for hip arthroscopy: a cadaveric assessment of central, peripheral, and lateral compartment portal placement. Arthroscopy. 2008;24(9):1019–26.
2. Burman M. Arthroscopy or the direct visualization of joints. J Bone Joint Surg. 1931;4:669–95.
3. Glick JM. Hip arthroscopy using the lateral approach. Instr Course Lect. 1988;37:223–31.
4. Johnson L. Arthroscopic surgery principles and practice. St Louis (MO): CV Mosby; 1986.
5. Byrd JW, Pappas JN, Pedley MJ. Hip arthroscopy: an anatomic study of portal placement and relationship to the extra-articular structures [see comments]. Arthroscopy. 1995;11(4):418–23.
6. Glick JM, Sampson TG, Gordon RB, et al. Hip arthroscopy by the lateral approach. Arthroscopy. 1987;3(1):4–12.
7. Farjo LA, Glick JM, Sampson TG. Hip arthroscopy for acetabular labral tears. Arthroscopy. 1999;15(2):132–7.
8. McCarthy JC, Noble PC, Schuck MR, et al. The watershed labral lesion: its relationship to early arthritis of the hip. J Arthroplasty. 2001;16(8 Suppl 1):81–7.
9. McCarthy JC, Noble PC, Schuck MR, et al.: The Otto E. Aufranc award: the role of labral lesions to development of early degenerative hip disease. Clin Orthop 2001;393:25–37.
10. Philippon MJ, Yen YM, Briggs KK, et al. Early outcomes after hip arthroscopy for femoroacetabular impingement in the athletic adolescent patient: a preliminary report. J Pediatr Orthop. 2008;28(7):705–10.
11. Byrd JW, Pappas JN, Pedley MJ. Hip arthroscopy: an anatomic study of portal placement and relationship to the extra-articular structures. Arthroscopy. 1995;11(4):418–23.
12. McCarthy JC, Busconi B. The role of hip arthroscopy in the diagnosis and treatment of hip disease. Orthopedics. 1995;18(8):753–6.
13. McCarthy JC, Day B, Busconi B. Hip arthroscopy: applications and technique. J Am Acad Orthop Surg. 1995;3:115–22.
14. Philippon MJ. New frontiers in hip arthroscopy: the role of arthroscopic hip labral repair and capsulorrhaphy in the treatment of hip disorders. Instr Course Lect. 2006;55:309–16.
15. Bencardino JT, Kassarjian A, Palmer WE. Magnetic resonance imaging of the hip: sports-related injuries. Top Magn Reson Imaging. 2003;14(2):145–60.
16. Newberg AH, Newman JS. Imaging the painful hip. Clin Orthop Relat Res. 2003;406:19–28.
17. Palmer WE. MR arthrography of the hip. Semin Musculoskelet Radiol. 1998;2(4):349–62.
18. Potter HG, Schachar J. High resolution noncontrast MRI of the hip. J Magn Reson Imaging. 2010;31(2):268–78.
19. Glick J. Operative arthroscopy. New York: Raven; 1991.
20. Warren SB, Brooker Jr AF. Excision of heterotopic bone followed by irradiation after total hip arthroplasty. J Bone Joint Surg Am. 1992;74(2):201–10.
21. McCarthy JC, Lee JA. Arthroscopic intervention in early hip disease. Clin Orthop Relat Res. 2004;429:157–62.
22. Voos JE, Shindle MK, Pruett A, et al. Endoscopic repair of gluteus medius tendon tears of the hip. Am J Sports Med. 2009;37(4):743–7.
23. Byrd JC. Advanced arthroscopy. In: Arthroscopy of the hip and application: supine position. Saunders Elsevier, Philadelphia 2010; p. 318. Chapter 27.

91 Worldwide Experience with Hip Arthroscopy: Australia

John M. O'Donnell

Introduction

The following is a historic account of the development of hip arthroscopy in Australia, and a discussion of the current position of hip arthroscopy within the orthopedic community in Australia.

Whilst I have tried hard to corroborate stories and verify dates, this has not always been possible, and at times I have had to rely on people's recollections. I apologize for any errors that this account may contain. I hope there are few.

I have also tried hard to get personal stories from as many of the early participants as possible. Any omission is entirely unintentional.

History of Hip Arthroscopy in Australia

Berni Einoder

The first recorded hip arthroscopy carried out in Australia was performed by Dr. Bernard Einoder, in Launceston, Tasmania, in September, 1978.

Berni was born in Villach, Austria, in 1944, and came to Australia with his family in 1955. He did his medical training at Monash University in Melbourne, and after completing postgraduate orthopedic training, also in Melbourne, he went to England and Europe for 2 years of additional training. During this time, he visited Mr. Brian Elliot at Chichester Hospital, where he first saw, and learned, arthroscopic knee surgery. He bought his own arthroscope and returned to Australia in 1977.

At that time arthroscopy was little known in this country, and the arthroscope was generally regarded as an "instrument of the Devil." None of the major hospitals in Melbourne would allow Berni to develop his interest in arthroscopy, so he settled in Launceston, the second city in Australia's smallest state, Tasmania (Fig. 91.1).

He performed his first hip arthroscopy on a lady who had had a cemented total hip replacement performed by another surgeon. Her hip was unstable, and after one dislocation, it could not be properly reduced. At that time there was no barium in the cement, and so it was not possible to be completely sure, but it was considered probable that she had a fractured piece of cement present within the acetabular polyethylene component, thus preventing the reduction.

Berni felt that he could check this and remove the loose body arthroscopically but, as there were no hip arthroscopy instruments, he first had to make his own. Regulations were far less strict then than now, so Berni was able to design and build his own instrument set in his tool shed!

The set contained a modified Steinman pin to mark out the portals and allow passage of the arthroscope sheath; an early version of a banana blade, which consisted of a piece of a razor blade welded to a handle; a sucker; and a pituitary rongeur to retrieve the cement (Fig. 91.2).

The operation was performed in September 1978 with the patient positioned supine on a fracture table, and traction applied. Berni used two portals, which corresponded closely with today's anterior trochanteric, and anterior portals. The hip was entered using image intensifier guidance, and the piece of cement was found and removed from the joint successfully. Berni continues to perform hip arthroscopy to this day.

Unfortunately, this case was not written up and published, and his hip set did not move into mass production.

David Young

Hip arthroscopy remained a very rare operation in Australia, until the mid-1980s when David Young started to perform the operation in Melbourne. David was born and trained in Melbourne. He undertook further postgraduate study in

J.M. O'Donnell, MBBS, FRACS, FAOrthA (✉)
Hip Arthroscopy Australia, St. Vincents Private Hospital, East Melbourne, VIC, Australia
e-mail: john@johnodonnell.com.au

J.C. McCarthy et al. (eds.), *Hip Joint Restoration*, DOI 10.1007/978-1-4614-0694-5_91

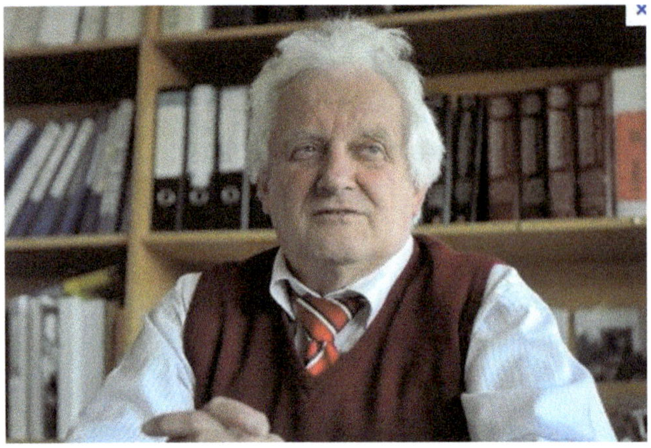

Fig. 91.1 Berni Einoder

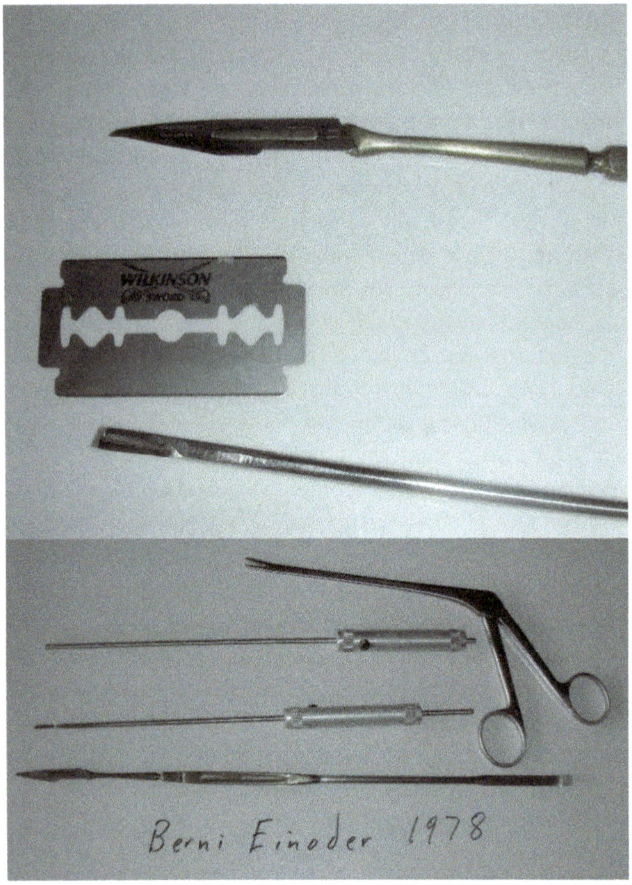

Fig. 91.2 Berni Einoder's homemade hip arthroscopy instruments

Bristol, UK, and travelling fellowships in Europe. He returned to Melbourne in 1984 and developed a practice specializing in arthroscopic surgery and sports surgery. Although he performed the operation relatively infrequently in the early years, the numbers gradually increased. As well as being a pioneering hip arthroscopy surgeon, David was, and remains, an innovator, and keen designer of new instrumentation.

Circa 1994 he was performing a hip arthroscopy, and was having the usual difficulties of that time introducing curved instruments into the hip. At that time the standard method was to use large-diameter metal cannulae or plastic, flexible cannulae, or just to pass the instruments freehand down the portal. David Veale, the local Dyonics Rep, was also present, and between them they worked out the design for a slotted cannula, which David Veale then had made by a local instrument maker, Hendricks. With a relatively small-diameter cannula, it then became possible to introduce curved instruments, and also to remove the cannula, leading to greatly improved instrument maneuverability within the joint.

In August, 1999, David met James Glick at a meeting in New Zealand, and showed him the slotted cannula. It was subsequently included in the Glick Hip Arthroscopy set the following year, and has since been adopted around the world with this instrument now being included in most hip sets in some variation of the original design.

John O'Donnell

John O'Donnell started performing hip arthroscopies in Melbourne in 1990. John O'Donnell was also a Melbourne born and trained orthopedic surgeon.

Although knee arthroscopy had become a standard part of orthopedic training, it remained a relatively crude procedure. John also did postgraduate training in the UK (Brighton and Bristol) and in several European cities but he really learned arthroscopy when he returned to Melbourne in 1988, and worked with Ian Henderson.

Ian was an expert, and gifted, arthroscopic surgeon, regularly performing arthroscopic surgery on the knee, shoulder, elbow, and ankle. He was also a great teacher and happy to share his knowledge and skills.

Melbourne became the hip arthroscopy capital of Australia. There remained great skepticism in the general orthopedic community regarding arthroscopic hip surgery. Indeed, it was regularly said to be impossible, and at times considered to be useless and dangerous.

The Growth of Hip Arthroscopy in Australia

Gradually throughout the early and mid-1990s surgeons from other Australian states took up the procedure, but mostly in small numbers. Many visited Melbourne to learn aspects of this "new procedure," but some were still largely self-taught. The most prominent of these other lonely arthroscopists were Bill Donnelly in Brisbane, Greg Witherow in Perth, Tony Spriggins in Adelaide, and Len Walter in Sydney.

Gradually, the number of hip arthroscopies was rising, and three unrelated events led to a progressive upsurge. In 1992, Peter Wilson in Melbourne performed a hip arthroscopy on an extremely well-known Australian Rules Footballer. This "rare operation" caused great interest in the press and on the television football shows, and led to a much greater public awareness of the procedure.

In 1996, a 37-year-old Sydney General Practitioner travelled to Melbourne to see John O'Donnell, and asked for a hip arthroscopy. She had had hip pain for 15 years, and had already had five unsuccessful open hip surgeries. She was certain that she had a labral tear although the available imaging at the time was not helpful.

John performed an arthroscopy, identified the tear, and resected the torn labral segment. Her pain relief was dramatic, and she returned to a very active lifestyle. She was so excited by the outcome of her treatment that she became almost evangelical in her desire to spread the word to others, and wrote articles in GP journals and appeared at meetings around the country to let others know about this wonderful "new surgery."

As a result, the numbers of patients being seen rose significantly, including large numbers of patients flying from Sydney to Melbourne for treatment. This was the cause of some disquiet in Sydney at the time, as the general feeling there remained that this was bad surgery.

The third stimulus to growth was an Australian Orthopaedic Association (AOA) Meeting in Canberra in 1997. Dr. Joseph McCarthy was an invited guest at the meeting and presented a paper on hip arthroscopy, as well as a demonstration with John O'Donnell. Having an international speaker as well as a local certainly helped give credibility to this procedure.

Gradually, interest in hip arthroscopy was growing in the orthopedic community as well as the general public. In 2000, John O'Donnell took sabbatical leave from the Royal Melbourne Hospital and visited Joe McCarthy in Boston, USA. Joe, with typical generosity, invited John to his home where he was meeting with Brian Busconi to write a book, "Early Hip Disorders, Advances in Detection and Minimally Invasive Treatment." As a result of this meeting, Joe invited John to write a chapter on supine positioning for hip arthroscopy. The first draft of which was written on paper napkins during John's flight from Boston to London. John and Joe became firm friends and remain so to this day.

John went on to visit Richard Villar in Cambridge, UK. His time in Cambridge was also very productive. At this time the group of hip arthroscopy surgeons internationally was extremely small, and most came to know each other personally, and to become friends.

Femoroacetabular Impingement

The variety of hip procedures that could be performed arthroscopically remained extremely limited. Most procedures were performed for labral tears, although in reality most "tears" were really chondro-labral damage. Imaging also remained relatively crude.

However, things began to change with the publication by Ganz in 2001 of his work on femoroacetabular impingement (FAI). Although all Ganz's work involved open surgery, and surgical dislocation of the hip, a few surgeons in different parts of the world saw the possibilities of performing this surgery arthroscopically.

In Australia, John O'Donnell developed one such technique, and performed his first live FAI surgery in 2002. Hip arthroscopy up until this time had developed in two very distinct streams. In the English-speaking world, almost all hip arthroscopy was performed only in the hip joint itself, the so-called central compartment. In contrast, in France particularly, the early hip arthroscopists only entered the so-called peripheral compartment to remove osteochondromata. John developed a technique involving initial central compartment arthroscopy with traction, but then added a capsulotomy, which allowed the arthroscope to be passed into the peripheral compartment. The cam lesions of FAI could thus be identified and removed with a burr.

Compared to open surgery, arthroscopic surgery allowed this procedure to be performed as a day patient, was far less painful, and allowed much faster rehabilitation, and a quicker return to sporting activities.

John presented a paper on the 2-year results of this procedure at Richard Villar's International Hip Arthroscopy Meeting in Cambridge in 2004 entitled "Arthroscopic resection of Ganz lesions," which was the first presentation of an arthroscopic technique for FAI surgery at an international meeting. At the same meeting, he also presented papers on "Revision Hip Arthroscopy" and a paper calling for a single outcome score to be adopted by all hip arthroscopists (Fig. 91.3).

Until recently we have not had a single, widely accepted, validated score to use to compare the outcomes of this type of surgery.

In Australia, John and David continued to speak at AOA and industry-sponsored events, both individually, but more often together. So much so, they almost came to be seen as a double act. Melbourne still remains the Australian center for hip arthroscopy, and even though the number of surgeons performing the operation is rising, and the total number of arthroscopies being performed is growing by around 30% each year, more than half the arthroscopies done each year in Australia are still done in Melbourne (Fig. 91.4).

An online chat site for athletes, Injuryupdate.com., asked why there was such a difference between Melbourne and Sydney. They suggested that either Sydney surgeons were not competent or else Melbourne surgeons were "knife happy."

They then did an online poll to try to resolve this question. The votes were approximately 50/50.

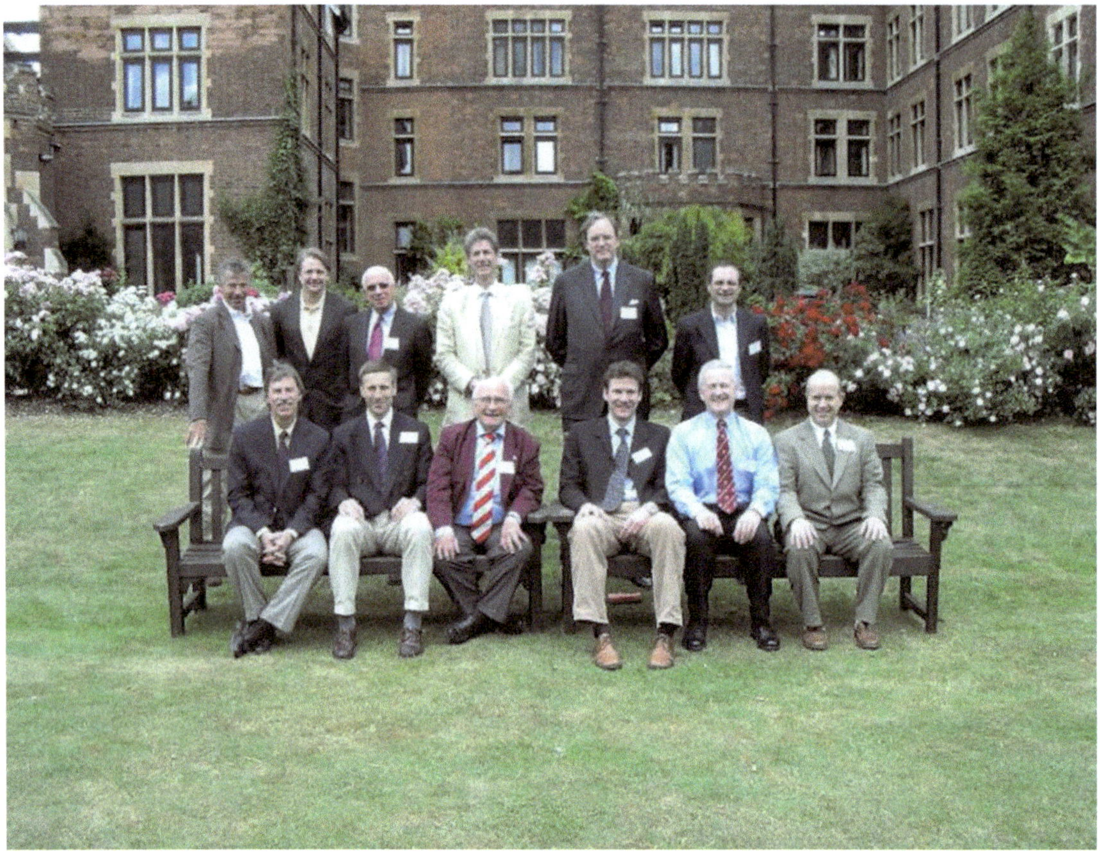

Fig. 91.3 Cambridge HA Meeting 2004. John O'Donnell front row 2nd from right

Fig. 91.4 The increasing number of hip arthroscopies performed in Australia

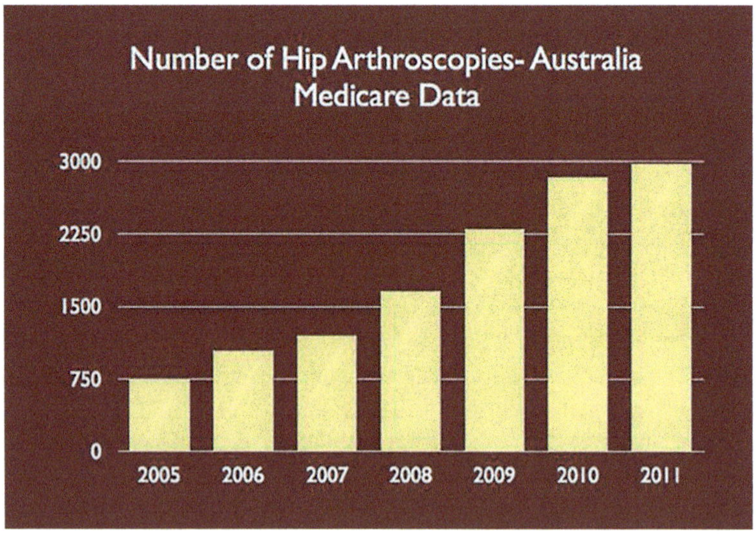

Hip Arthroscopy Education in Australia

Over the next few years there continued to be significant developments. In 2007, John O'Donnell started a fellowship program in hip arthroscopy, taking fellows from Australia and around the world. The first fellow was Michael Pritchard, a Tasmanian surgeon, who trained in orthopedics in Victoria. Michael had done almost no hip arthroscopy during his formal training as a registrar, but took to it with great enthusiasm.

After his fellowship, he and John formed Hip Arthroscopy Australia (HAA), with the intention of raising the profile of hip arthroscopy through education of surgeons and research.

They also, together, refined techniques for FAI surgery and developed the POD CT scan, and ligamentum teres test.

The third initial member of HAA was Amir Takla. Amir is a physiotherapist, who underwent arthroscopic FAI surgery himself. Postoperatively, he found that the rehabilitation he had been taught was not particularly helpful, so he developed his own rehabilitation protocol, which led to greatly accelerated return to sport and full function.

This program has now been taught widely, and forms the basis of the rehabilitation programs used by many specialized sports hip physiotherapists around the country.

They were later joined by Parminder Singh, an English surgeon who first came to do a fellowship in 2008, and then returned to Australia to live and work.

Together these four started the HAA courses which have taught orthopedic surgeons and physiotherapists every 3 months since 2008.

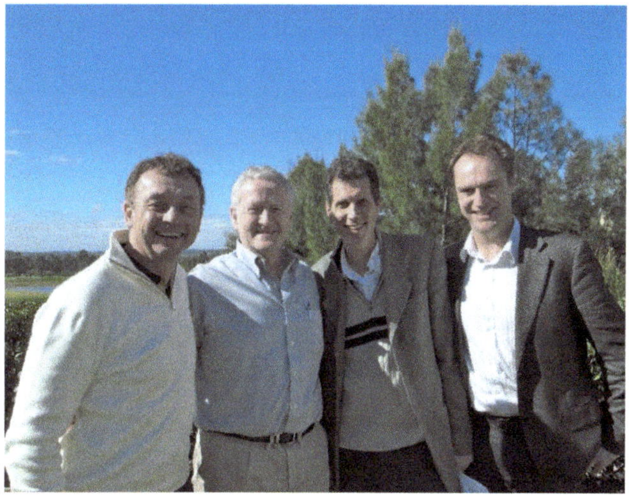

Fig. 91.5 The founding of the Australian Hip Arthroscopy Society, 2010. From left—Warwick Bruce, John O'Donnell, Michael Solomon, and Jonathon Bare

The International Society for Hip Arthroscopy

In 2008, Richard Villar and Joe McCarthy gathered together 12 hip arthroscopy surgeons from around the world to form ISHA, the International Society for Hip Arthroscopy. John O'Donnell was elected the first Editorial Secretary, and later, in 2011, the Vice President of the Society. This Society has added to the strong bond felt by pioneering hip arthroscopy surgeons around the world, and greatly supported the development of this surgery in Australia.

Most Australian hip arthroscopy surgeons have attended ISHA meetings, and been exposed to the highest quality arthroscopic hip surgery practiced around the world. This has inevitably also helped to improve the quality of surgery in Australia.

Australian Hip Arthroscopy Society

We were greatly encouraged by the success of ISHA and looked to form an Australian Society as well. As a small group, we felt that we did not have the resources, yet, to form a stand-alone group, and so we sought to find a "home" in another society. Australia does not have a Hip Society or an Arthroscopy Society. We were fortunate to be welcomed by the Arthroplasty Society, with whom we share many members, as, in Australia, all surgeons who perform hip arthroscopy also do hip replacement. Warwick Bruce, the President, and Michael Solomon, the Secretary of the Arthroplasty Society, were extremely helpful and supportive, and on 5 June 2010, the Australian Hip Arthroscopy Society (AHAS) was formed as group within the Arthroplasty Society (Fig. 91.5).

Discussion at the Annual General Meeting prior to the vote to proceed showed how far acceptance of hip arthroscopy had come. There was only one dissenting vote.

John O'Donnell was elected the first President of AHAS, and Jonathon Bare the first Vice President. Both were unopposed. AHAS is now encouraging better training for orthopedic surgeons wishing to undertake hip arthroscopy, and also upskilling for current practitioners via meetings, visits, and research.

In Australia we have been fortunate that we have not suffered the difficulties seen in many countries where funding for hip arthroscopy has been withheld, although the remuneration for surgeons has been very low in comparison with knee and shoulder arthroscopy. Enthusiasts have carried on despite this, and our numbers continue to grow quickly. The future appears very bright with several young surgeons keenly pursuing a career including a major interest in hip arthroscopy.

Although the two long-time leaders in this field, David Young initially, and then John O'Donnell as well, must soon slow down, the leadership is passing to younger surgeons including Jon Bare, Michael Pritchard, Parminder Singh, and Phong Tran in Melbourne; Patrick Weinrauch in Brisbane; Michael O'Sullivan in Sydney; and doubtless many others still to appear.

We have been fortunate to have the strong support of other great surgeons from around the world who are now also the founders and leaders of ISHA.

Worldwide Experience of Hip Arthroscopy: Mexican Experience

92

Marco Acuña, Carlos Suarez-Ahedo, and Victor M. Ilizaliturri Jr.

Introduction

The first doctors to adopt the use of arthroscopy in Mexico were two rheumatologists: Dr. Gil Robles and Dr. Gabor Katona, who were students of Professor Watanabe. In 1974, Dr. Noguera first started direct-view arthroscopy, but it was in the 1980s that Dr. Vazquez Vela and Dr. Aviña, having completed training and courses in the USA, performed the first knee arthroscopies using a video camera, at the National Institute of Orthopedics [1].

History of Hip Arthroscopy in Mexico

Hip arthroscopy was first performed in Mexico in 1994 in the city of Monterrey, in the state of Nuevo Leon. It was performed by Dr. Marco Tulio Flores Gutierrez in the specialty hospital of Monterrey at the Mexican Social Security Institute (IMSS) (Fig. 92.1). The patient had a loose body secondary to a posterior acetabular wall fracture. Arthroscopic loose body removal was performed using standard arthroscopic instruments and a standard fracture table. Between 1994 and 1995, Dr. Marco Tulio Flores performed three hip arthroscopies for the diagnosis of labral tears, which were treated with partial resection, and two more loose bodies were removed. Between 1999 and 2000 he performed 16 cases consisting of arthroscopic debridement and partial labral resection.

Later in 2000 at the National Institute of Orthopedics in Mexico City, Dr. Victor M. Ilizaliturri Jr. [2] started his experience in hip arthroscopy (Fig. 92.2), after completing an Arthroscopy Association of North America Masters Experience Course in the year 2000 at the Orthopaedic Learning Center in Rosemont, Illinois (Fig. 92.3). The course faculty featured Dr. Thomas W Byrd from Nashville, Tennessee, Dr. Joseph C McCarthy from Boston Massachusetts, and Dr. James Glick and Dr. Thomas G Sampson from San Francisco, California. Between 2000 and 2002, the most common indications for hip arthroscopy in Dr. Ilizaliturri´s practice included symptomatic labral tears, treated by partial resection, removal of loose bodies, and debridement of ligamentum teres ruptures (Fig. 92.4). All patients were operated on in the lateral decubitus position on a fracture table. Only the central compartment was routinely accessed (Fig. 92.5). Cannulated instruments were used in this early series. Between 2000 and 2004, 50–70 cases were carried out every year. The minimalist arthroscopic access concept was developed at that time, and the slotted cannula technique was formally introduced in 2002 [3, 4] (Fig. 92.6).

In 2002 during the National Congress of Orthopedics in Mexico City, a live hip arthroscopy was performed and broadcasted from the National Rehabilitation Institute of Mexico. Dr. Ilizaliturri was the operating surgeon, with Drs. Byrd and Sampson as guests. The procedure was successfully completed; the patient's diagnosis was internal snapping hip syndrome with a labral tear. The tear was partially debrided and the iliopsoas tendon was released from its insertion at the lesser trochanter using accessory portals, for access to the extra-articular compartment (Fig. 92.7). The patient was operated on in the lateral decubitus position and the central compartment as well as the iliopsoas bursa were accessed.

M. Acuña, MD
Department of Adult Joint Reconstruction, National Rehabilitation Institute of Mexico, Mexico, Mexico

C. Suarez-Ahedo, MD • V.M. Ilizaliturri Jr. , MD (✉)
National Rehabilitation Institute of Mexico,
Av. México-Xochimilco No. 289, Col. Arenal de Guadalupe,
Mexico D.F. C.P. 14389, Mexico
e-mail: vichip2002@yahoo.com.mx

J.C. McCarthy et al. (eds.), *Hip Joint Restoration*, DOI 10.1007/978-1-4614-0694-5_92

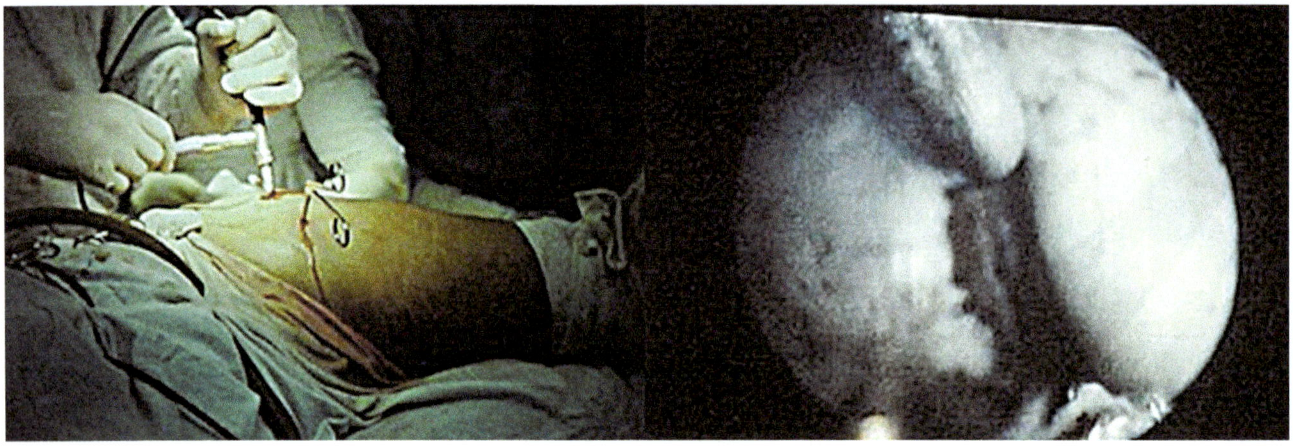

Fig. 92.1 (*Left*) Clinical photograph of the first hip arthroscopy case in Mexico in 1994, loose body retrieval in a left hip. (*Right*) Arthroscopic photograph of loose body retrieval (courtesy of Dr. Marco Tulio Flores)

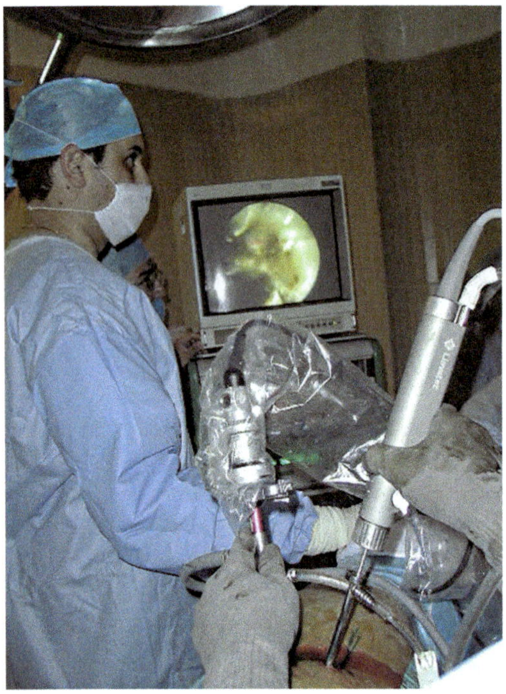

Fig. 92.2 Dr. Dario Garin assisting Dr. Ilizaliturri in the first hip arthroscopy performed at the National Institute of Orthopedics (later National Rehabilitation Institute of Mexico) in the year 2000

Later in 2002 after meeting with Dr. Michael Dienst from Germany, routine access to the peripheral compartment was introduced in Mexico by Dr. Ilizaliturri, which expanded the indications to provide arthroscopic treatment for patients with synovial disease [5] (Fig. 92.8). The main indications for hip arthroscopy from 2000 to 2003 included labral tears, loose bodies, synovial disease problems, and debridement for symptomatic early osteoarthritis. The experience from this period led to the refinement of the techniques and the establishment of an endoscopic hip-preserving surgery clinic based at the National Rehabilitation Institute of Mexico [6].

The necessity for a more dynamic and portable traction system was identified in 2003. The technique now included arthroscopy with traction for access to the central compartment and without traction for access to the peripheral compartment. The hip arthroscopic equipment moved to different hospitals and surgery centers but the procedure could not be performed in places where a fracture table was not available. This necessitated the development of a portable traction system for the lateral approach that has been in use since 2005 [7, 8] (Fig. 92.9).

Femoroacetabular Impingement

The most current development in hip arthroscopy has been the recognition of femoroacetabular impingement as popularized by the Bern group. From 2004 the open technique designed to treat cam-type impingement by the Swiss group evolved into an endoscopic technique. Dr. Ilizaliturri in Mexico City was one of the early adopters along with Dr. Byrd in Nashville, Dr. Philippon in Vail, Dr. Sampson in San Francisco, Dr. Villar in the UK, and Dr. Dienst in Germany [9] (Fig. 92.10).

Dr. Philippon [10] introduced the technique of labral takedown and rim reduction, in 2005, which was adopted throughout the world, including Mexico. The labral take-

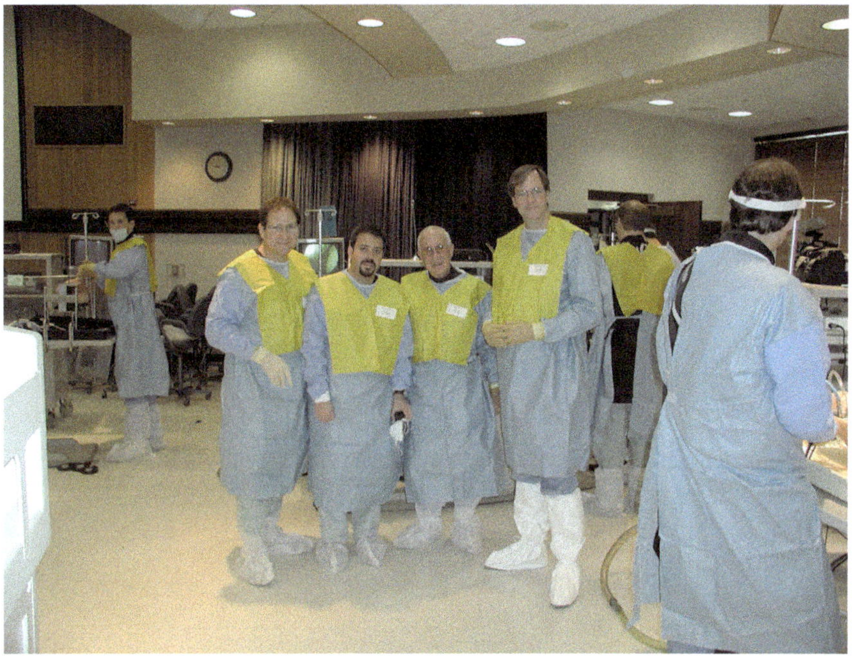

Fig. 92.3 At the Orthopedic Learning center in Rosemont, Illinois, 2002. From left to right, Dr. Sampson, Dr. Ilizaliturri, Dr. Glick, and Dr. Byrd

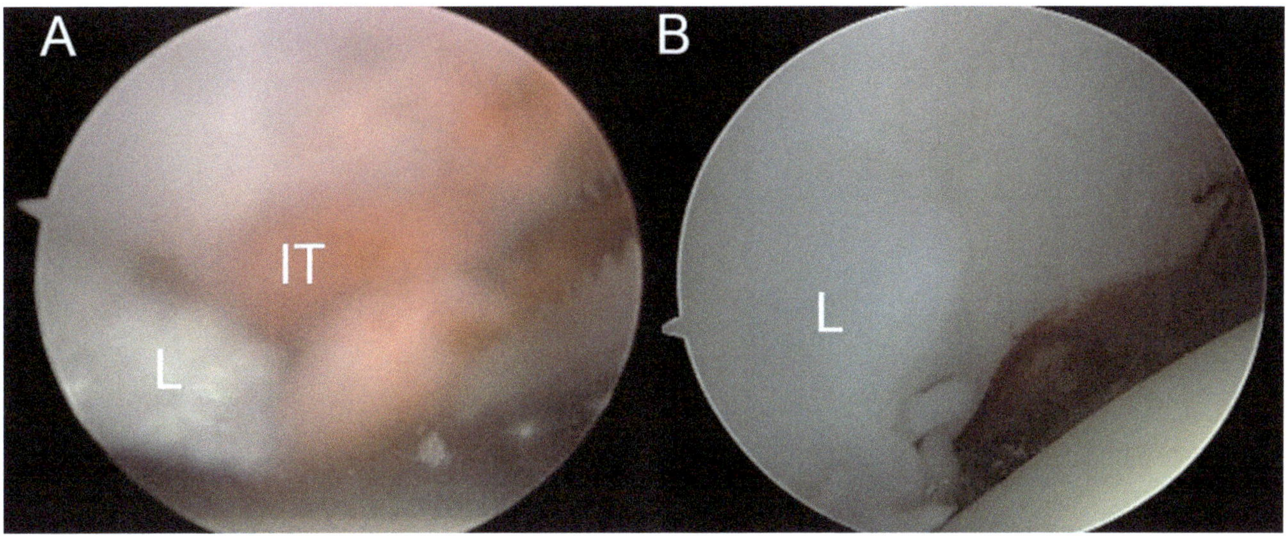

Fig. 92.4 (a) Arthroscopic photograph of a left hip from the year 2000. A loose body is retreated from the central compartment, there is abundant inflammatory tissue (IT) in the fossa, behind the loose body, and the labrum (L) is to the right. The femoral head is at the bottom. (b) Arthroscopic photograph of a left hip. An anterior labral (L) tear is observed to the left (year 2000)

down technique evolved and in 2008 Dr. Sampson [11] introduced a variant that does not require separation of the labrum from the acetabular bony rim, accessing the bone-acetabular junction from the capsular side and addressing the bony overhang from the capsular side. As this last technique evolved, it became the standard for Dr. Ilizaliturri in Mexico [12]. This evolved with the techniques of labral repair and labral refixation (Fig. 92.11).

Early on Dr. Glick [13, 14] had introduced capsular portal enlargement using an arthroscopic knife to facilitate the movement of arthroscopic instruments inside the portals. The capsular enlargement technique evolved to a capsulotomy and in some cases capsulectomy for adequate exposure of impinging deformities, both on the acetabular and femoral side (Fig. 92.12). This was adopted by Dr. Ilizaliturri in 2004 and has become his standard technique since then. In 2005 the arthroscopic knife

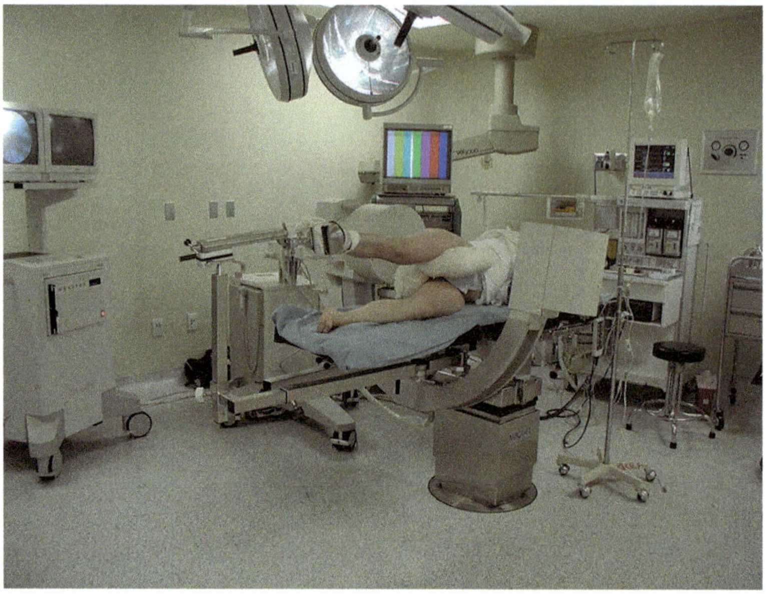

Fig. 92.5 A patient positioned in left lateral decubitus on a fracture table. Only the right foot (operative side) is fixed to the traction device. A large perineal post is horizontally placed on the right groin providing a lateral traction vector. The image intensifier is under the operating table to provide anteroposterior view of the right hip

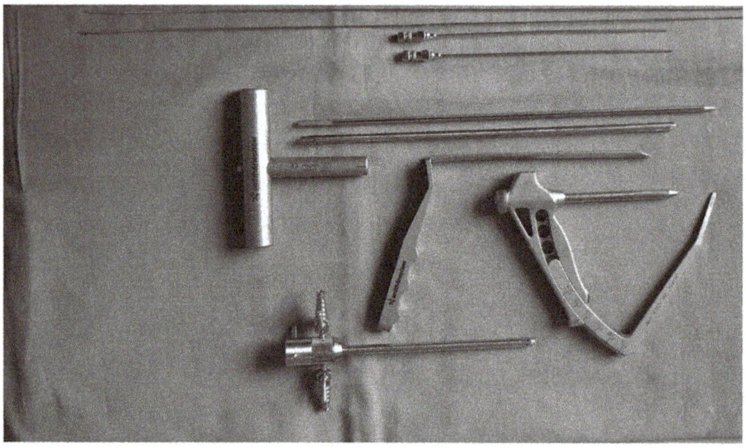

Fig. 92.6 Minimalist hip arthroscopy set consisting, from *top* to *bottom*, nitinol guide wires, spinal needles, cannulated switching stick, dilator, T handle, slotted cannula, aiming device, and standard arthroscopy cannula

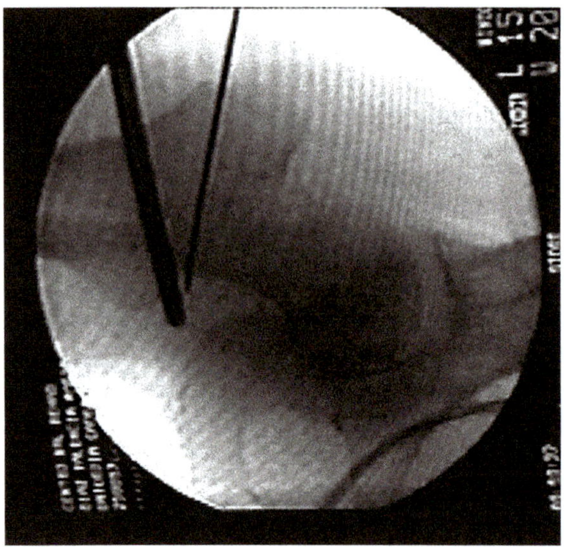

Fig. 92.7 Fluoroscopy image of an iliopsoas tendon release at the lesser trochanter. An arthroscope and a radiofrequency hook are identified on the lesser trochanter (2002)

was replaced by a radiofrequency hook probe and the capsular cuts were performed in a retrograde fashion [15].

In 2004, Dr Ilizaliturri started developing the technique for access to the peritrochanteric space, initially limited to the treatment of external snapping hip syndromes and then evolving into access for endoscopic treatment of greater trochanteric pain syndrome and soft-tissue problems around the hip joint [16–20] (Fig. 92.13).

The International Society for Hip Arthroscopy

Throughout the past decade hip arthroscopy has evolved in conjunction with very close communication between its worldwide opinion leaders. This scientific and technical interchange spawned the formation of the International Society for Hip Arthroscopy (ISHA) following the lead of Dr. Joseph McCarthy of Boston and

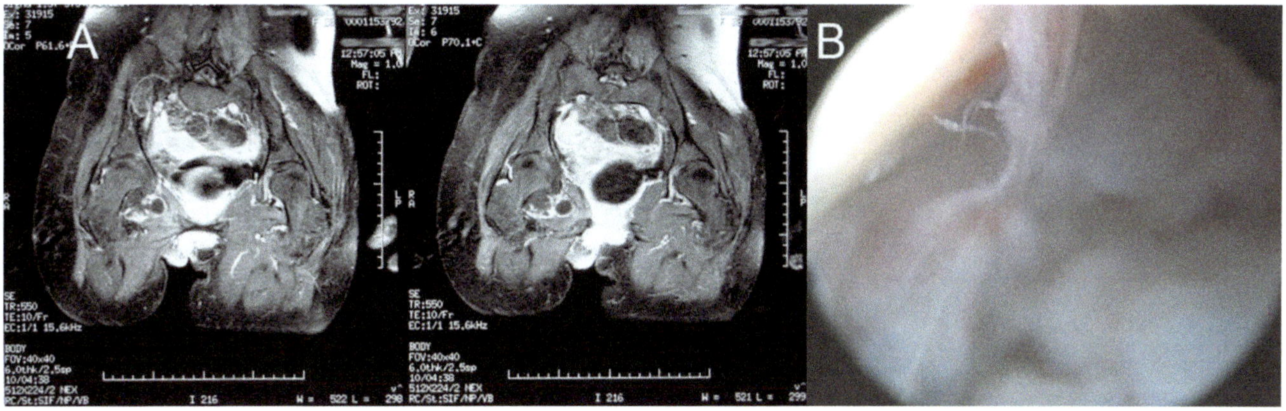

Fig. 92.8 (**a**) MRI of a case with synovial chondromatosis of the right hip. (**b**) Endoscopic view of the peripheral compartment showing multiple free osteochondromas under the femoral head

Fig. 92.9 A portable lateral distractor with the patient position in right lateral decubitus

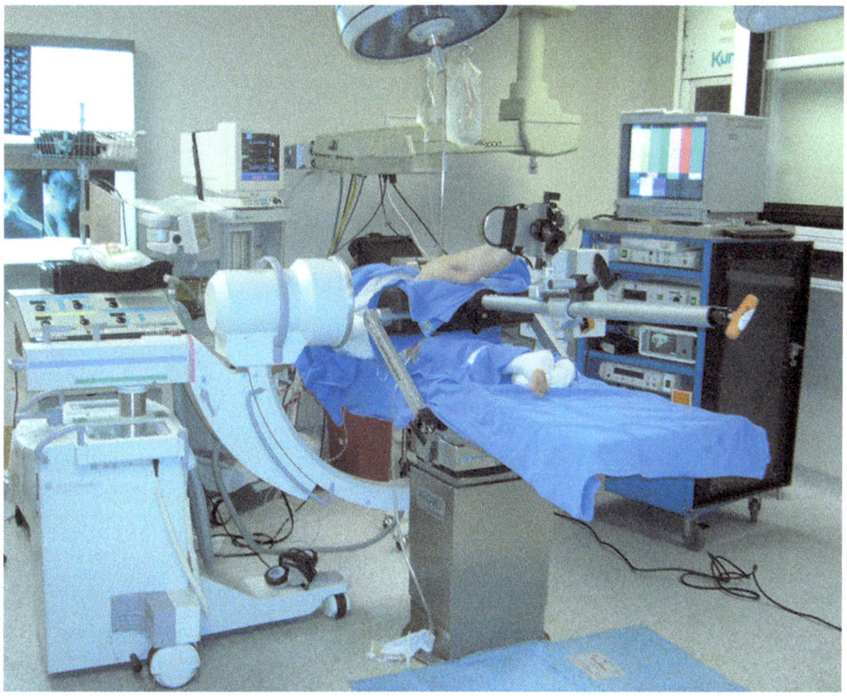

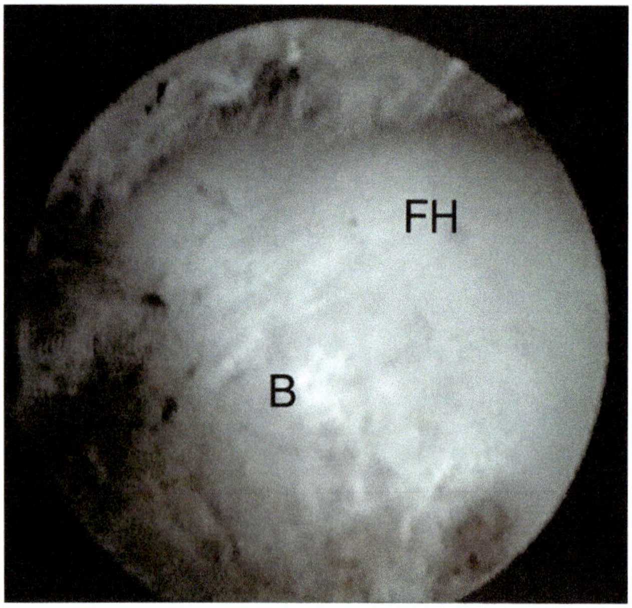

Fig. 92.10 Arthroscopic photograph of a cam impingement deformity (*B* bump) in a right hip. The femoral head (FH) is to the right (2004)

Mr. Richard Villar from the UK. ISHA was officially formed in Paris in 2008, and its founding members were Thierry Boyer, Paris, France; Giancarlo Polesello, Sao Paulo, Brazil; Robert L. Buly, New York, USA; Victor Ilizaliturri, Mexico city, Mexico; Michael Dienst Münich, Germany; Tom Sampson, San Francisco, California; Richard Villar, London, UK; Marc Philippon, Vail, USA; Joe McCarthy, Boston, Massachusetts; John O'Donnell, Melbourne, Australia; Thomas Byrd, Nashville, Tennessee; and Hassan Sadri, Geneva, Switzerland (Fig. 92.14). These represented some of the key opinion leaders in the world.

Dr. Villar became the first president of ISHA and served for a 2-year period from 2008 to 2009 followed by Dr. McCarthy and Dr. Sampson, who were elected President Elect and Vice President during the founding meeting. ISHA's second Annual Scientific Meeting was held in Cancun, Mexico, and at this meeting Dr. Ilizaliturri was elected the Fourth President of ISHA and served his term from 2012 to 2013.

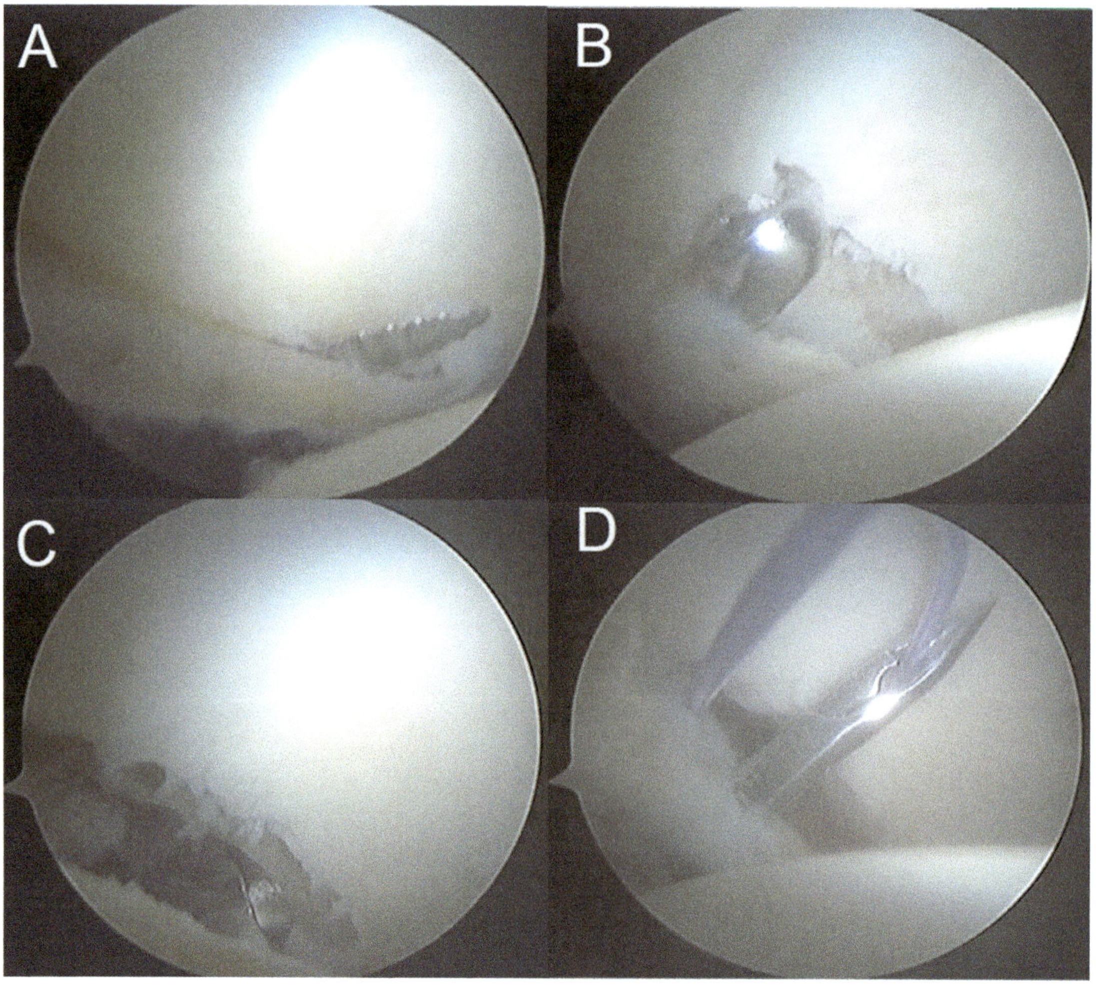

Fig. 92.11 Arthroscopic series of images of a labral takedown in a left hip. (**a**) An arthroscopic knife is used to separate the chondral labral junction. (**b**) A shaver is used to delineate the margin of medial rim resection. (**c**) An arthroscopic burr is used to reduce the acetabular rim. (**d**) Anchor fixation of the labrum using a translabral stitch

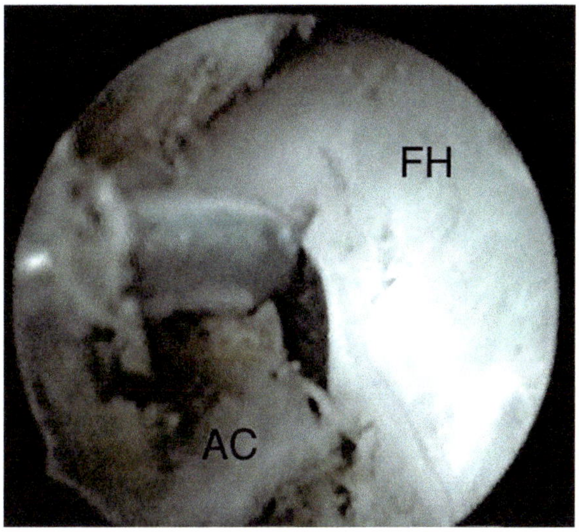

Fig. 92.12 Arthroscopic photograph of a right hip. The anterior capsule (AC) was sectioned using a radiofrequency device, the femoral head (FH) is to the right

Hip Arthroscopy Education in Mexico

The National Institute of Rehabilitation in Mexico City, with its fellowship program, has trained many Mexican and foreign nationals from countries including Colombia, Chile, Ecuador, El Salvador, and Costa Rica in the field of hip arthroscopy. Graduates from these programs have become opinion leaders and recognized hip arthroscopists in their own countries or in other cities within Mexico.

Through a visiting surgeon program, Dr. Ilizaliturri has hosted surgeons from countries including USA, Spain, Hong Kong, Chile, Colombia, Venezuela, Argentina, Ecuador, and others, facilitating international communication of knowledge and friendship in the field of hip arthroscopy.

The future of hip arthroscopy in Mexico is bright; we hope to continue to contribute to the development of concepts, technology, and education worldwide.

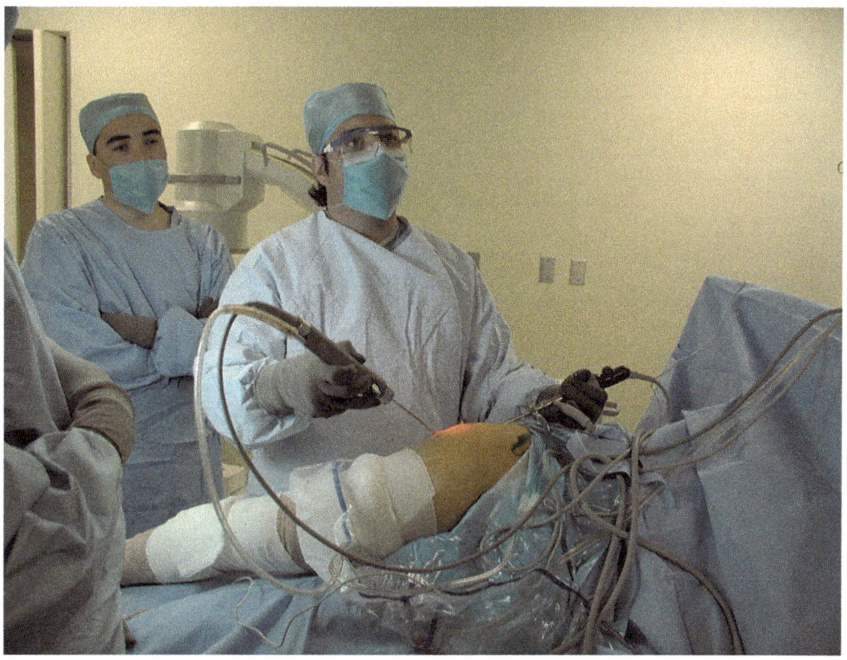

Fig. 92.13 Bursoscopy in a right hip (2004)

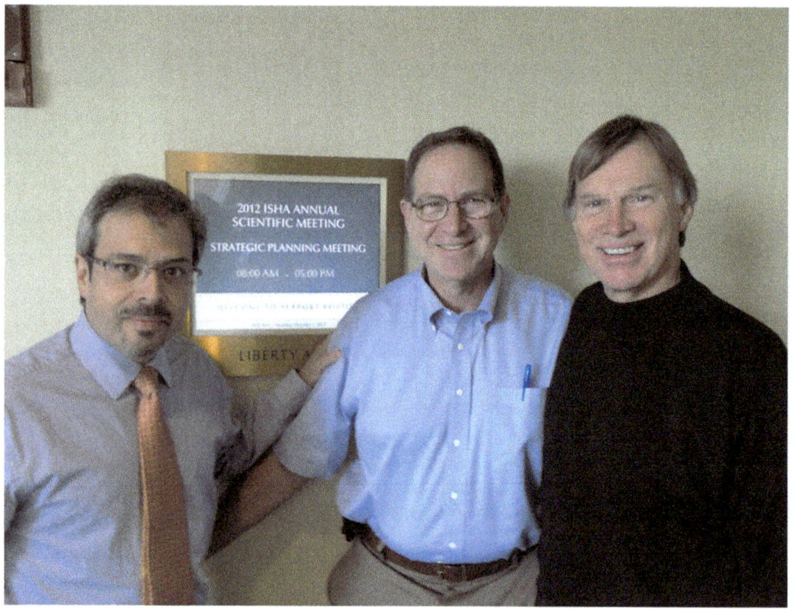

Fig. 92.14 From *left* to *right*: Dr. Ilizaliturri, Dr. Sampson, Dr. McCarthy

References

1. Rico EGC, Ayala CEA. La artroscopia en México. Antecedentes históricos y cómo aprenderla. Revista Mexicana de Ortopedia y Traumatología. 1995;9(4):245.
2. Ilizaliturri-Sánchez VM, Ilizaliturri-Valverde VM, González FSV, Rosales PC, Zepeda JMA. Cirugía artroscópica de la cadera. Indicaciones y aspectos técnicos del procedimiento. Acta Ortopédica Mexicana. 2003;17(1):44–51.
3. Ilizaliturri Jr VM, Acosta-Rodriguez E, Camacho-Galindo J. A minimalist approach to hip arthroscopy: the slotted cannula. Arthroscopy. 2007;23(5):560 e1.
4. Dienst M, Kohn D. Hip arthroscopy. Minimal invasive diagnosis and therapy of the diseased or injured hip joint. Unfallchirurg. 2001;104(1):2–18.
5. Wettstein M, Dienst M. Arthroscopy of the peripheral compartment of the hip. Oper Tech Orthop. 2005;15(3):225–30.
6. Ilizaliturri Jr VM, Camacho-Galindo J. Endoscopic treatment of snapping hips, iliotibial band, and iliopsoas tendon. Sports Med Arthrosc. 2010;18(2):120–7.
7. Mason JB, McCarthy JC, O'Donnell J, Barsoum W, Mayor MB, Busconi BD, et al. Hip arthroscopy: surgical approach, positioning, and distraction. Clin Orthop Relat Res. 2003; 406(1):29–37.
8. Ilizaliturri Jr VM, Chaidez PA, Aguilera JM, Camacho-Galindo J. Specialinstruments and techniques for hip arthroscopy. Tech Orthop. 2005;20(1):9–16.
9. Sampson TG. Arthroscopic treatment of femoroacetabular impingement. Tech Orthop. 2010;20(1):56–62.
10. Philippon MJ, Schenker ML. A new method for acetabular rim trimming and labral repair. Clin Sports Med. 2006;25(2):293–7.
11. Sampson TG. Arthroscopic treatment of femoroacetabular impingement. Tech Orthop. 2005;20(1):56–62.
12. Ilizaliturri Jr VM, Orozco-Rodriguez L, Acosta-Rodríguez E, Camacho-Galindo J. Arthroscopic treatment of cam-type femoroacetabular impingement: preliminary report at 2 years minimum follow-up. J Arthroplast. 2008;23(2):226–34.
13. Glick JM, Sampson TG, Gordon RB, Behr JT, Schmidt E. Hip arthroscopy by the lateral approach. Arthroscopy. 1987;3(1):4–12.
14. Glick JM. Capsular portal enlargement. The lateral approach. Clin Sports Med. 2001;20(4):733–47.
15. Ilizaliturri VM. Arthroscopic Treatment of FAI: Position, Portals, and Instrumentation. In Femoroacetabular Impingement. Berlin Heidelberg: Springer, 2012;99–111.
16. Ilizaliturri Jr VM, Martinez-Escalante FA, Chaidez PA, Camacho-Galindo J. Endoscopic iliotibial band release for external snapping hip syndrome. Arthroscopy. 2006;22(5):505–10.
17. Ilizaliturri Jr VM, Mangino G, Valero FS, Camacho-Galindo J. Hip arthroscopy of the central and peripheral compartments by the lateral approach. Tech Orthop. 2005;20(1):32–6.
18. Ilizaliturri Jr VM, Villalobos Jr FE, Chaidez PA, Valero FS, Aguilera JM. Internal snapping hip syndrome: treatment by endoscopic release of the iliopsoas tendon. Arthroscopy. 2005;21(11):1375–80.
19. Ilizaliturri Jr VM, Chaidez C, Villegas P, Briseño A, Camacho-Galindo J. Prospective randomized study of 2 different techniques for endoscopic iliopsoas tendon release in the treatment of internal snapping hip syndrome. Arthroscopy. 2009;25(2):159–63.
20. Ilizaliturri V, Camacho J, Evia A, Gonzalez Y, McMillan S, Busconi B. Soft tissue pathology around the hip. Clin Sports Med. 2011;30:391–415.

Worldwide Experience with Hip Arthroscopy: South America

93

Alexander Bent Tomic Loftkjaer and Rodrigo Mardones

South America

South America was a relative latecomer to the techniques of hip arthroscopy. The speed at which these new surgical techniques were introduced, adopted, and expanded in each South American country varied greatly, and relied heavily on the few individuals who pioneered these techniques in those countries despite the lack of dedicated instruments. South American countries that stand out in the development of hip arthroscopy are Argentina, Colombia, Brazil, and Chile.

Argentina

Dr. Ricardo Munafo was one of the first surgeons to adopt hip arthroscopy in Argentina. He began his medical practice in 1978 and completed his specialist training in hip surgery at the "Centre Hopitalier et Universitaire d´Angers," France, in 1986–1988. In 1999 he attended the American Academy of Orthopedic Surgeons meeting in California (Anaheim) and was among the delegates for an Instructional Course Lecture on hip arthroscopy given by Drs. James Glick, Thomas Sampson, and Joseph McCarthy. Dr. Munafo developed an interest in these techniques and made contact with Dr. Byrd visiting him in Nashville in April 1999 with Dr. Zancolli. During his brief stay in Nashville, Dr. Munafo acquired the dedicated surgical instruments that allowed him to develop his own experience in Argentina with his first patient having surgery in May 1999.

Dr. Byrd invited Dr. Munafo later that same year to the "Masters" course at the Learning Center in Chicago. At this course Dr. Munafo shared a workstation with Dr. Victor Ilizaliturri, who would later pioneer the techniques in Mexico, and also first met Dr. Marc Philippon who was one of the instructors.

Dr. Munafo began developing the technique in Argentina mainly focusing on labral tears as a cause of hip arthritis. The initial series of patients was presented in September 2002 at a Meeting of the Argentinian Association of Orthopedic Surgeons. The series included 30 % of patients with a preoperative Tonnis grade of 2, and so the midterm results were uninspiring.

Dr. Munafo in 2003 founded the Centro de Estudio y Tratamiento de las Enfermedades Articulares (CETEA)—Center for the Study and Treatment of Joint Diseases—along with Dr. Rodrigo Maestu. He continued to develop the technique publishing his first series of 61 cases, in 2007, in the journal of the Argentinian Association of Orthopedic Surgeons. He published on a combined arthroscopic and mini-open approach. Dr. Munafo recently reported to the senior author that he had performed 975 arthroscopies by April 2011 [1].

Colombia

Dr. Bernardo Aguilera started developing hip arthroscopy in Colombia in 2002. Dr. Aguilera began his medical practice as an orthopedic surgeon in 1995 and completed his AO fellowship in 1998 at the "Charite" hospital in Berlin associated with the University of Humboldt.

Dr. Aguilera's initial experience of hip arthroscopy was drawn from textbooks and reports from Drs. Richard Villar and James Glick. His first attempt at hip arthroscopy was on April 4th 2002. The patient was a 38-year-old woman with

A.B.T. Loftkjaer, MD (✉)
Orthopedic Surgery, Hip Surgery, Clinica Las Condes, Lo Fontecilla 441, Fourth Floor, Las Condes, Santiago 759106, Chile

Orthopedic Surgery, Hip Surgery, Hospital Militar de Santiago, Santiago, Metropolitana, Chile
e-mail: atomic@clc.cl

R. Mardones, MD
Tissue Engineering Lab, Orthopedics Department, Clinica Las Condes, Santiago, Chile

J.C. McCarthy et al. (eds.), *Hip Joint Restoration*, DOI 10.1007/978-1-4614-0694-5_93

hip dysplasia and a metaphyseal cyst that Dr. Aguilera wanted to graft. The setup was in the supine position and allowed the surgeon to visualize the joint space and determine the absence of arthritis. The procedure however could not be completed, as Dr. Aguilera did not have access to dedicated hip instruments.

Initially he had to develop the technique with knee and shoulder instruments, with a 30° arthroscope, and with instruments that were too short for many of the patients. In 2004 he attended the Arthroscopy Association of North America meeting and after seeing dedicated hip instruments at the meeting, he had them custom made in Colombia. But he still did not have access to long-enough burrs.

In 2005 he attended a course in Sao Paulo hosted by Dr. Giancarlo Polesello with Drs. Marc Phillipon and Thomas Sampson as instructors. This was the first time he was made aware of the concept of femoroacetabular impingement and as a result he took a more profound interest in hip arthroscopy. In 2007 he visited Dr. Bryan Kelly and was also exposed to the techniques of gluteal debridement and arthroscopic repair.

Dr. Aguilera became member of the International Society for Hip Arthroscopy (ISHA) in 2009 and has participated actively ever since. He presented a report on complications of hip arthroscopy along with Dr. J.M. Nossa and Dr. W. Marquez in 2010. He hosted the First International Course for Hip Arthroscopy in Colombia, in April 2011, at the Imbanaco Medical Center where 16 South American surgeons, prominent in the field of hip arthroscopy, gathered to share their experiences.

Dr. Bernardo Aguilera is part of the hip and knee joint preservation department at the Imbanaco Medical Center in Colombia where he currently continues to develop these techniques. He performed 390 hip arthroscopies from 2002 to 2012 [2].

Brazil

Brazil is the largest South American country with approximately 205 million people distributed throughout 26 states. The most densely populated state is Sao Paulo with around 40 million people throughout the state and 20 million in the city of Sao Paulo itself. Dr. Giancarlo Polesello developed the hip arthroscopy service and is currently chairman of the department of hip surgery in the university hospital of "Santa Casa de Sao Paulo," which is one of the largest medical schools in the country.

In 1999 Dr. Polesello visited Dr. Richard Villar in Cambridge, UK, where he witnessed his first hip arthroscopies in the lateral position. At this time hip arthroscopy was still restricted to labral or ligamentum teres resection, loose body removal, synovectomy, and biopsy. Femoroacetabular impingement was yet to appear on the world stage.

Upon returning to Brazil, Dr. Polesello faced difficulties positioning the patient in the lateral position due to the lack of an appropriate hip positioner. This led him to review Dr. Thomas Byrd´s publications, and eventually visit him in Nashville to learn the supine approach to hip arthroscopy.

In June 2002 Dr. Thomas Byrd was invited as an instructor to the first course on hip arthroscopy held in Brazil. Dr. Byrd performed live surgery during this course further promoting hip arthroscopy in this country.

In 2005 Dr. Byrd was again invited as an instructor for a new hip arthroscopy course along with other international experts such as Drs. Thomas Sampson, Marc Phlippon, Michael Leunig, and Dr. Victor Ilizaliturri. The course included live surgery and what might have been the first hip arthroscopy workshop with plastic models.

By 2007 hip arthroscopy had spread throughout South America so that internationally recognized experts also included surgeons from Argentina (Dr. Ricardo Munafo), and Chile (Drs. Rodrigo Mardones, Claudio Mella, Christian Foronda, and Claudio Rafols) [3].

Chile

Chile has not been the exception to the exponential development of hip arthroscopy. In the early 1990s different groups of surgeons started exploring the techniques of hip arthroscopy. These included Dr. Jaime Paulos at the "Pontificia Universidad Católica," Dr. Eduardo Zamudio at the "Hospital del Trabajador," and Dr. Mauricio Wainer at the "Clínica las Condes." These early procedures were uncommon and anecdotally usually performed for the removal of posttraumatic loose bodies.

Hip arthroscopy received a great increase in its momentum when it started to be performed for the treatment of femoroacetabular impingement. This occurred almost simultaneously in three different surgical teams.

Dr. Claudio Mella began developing the arthroscopic technique for the treatment of labral lesions and their debridement from 2002, after visiting Dr. Thomas Byrd, in Nashville, and Dr. Robert Bully in New York.

Dr. Cristian Foronda and Dr. Claudio Rafols, in a parallel line of development, visited Dr. Giancarlo Poleselo in Sao Paulo and focused on the treatment of cam-type femoroacetabular impingement.

At a similar time, Dr. Rodrigo Mardones met Dr. James Glick at the Chilean Congress of Orthopedic Surgery, initiating a working relationship that would later continue during Dr. Mardones' Fellowship at the Mayo Clinic in Rochester in 2003. During this Fellowship Dr. Mardones worked with Dr. Robert Trousdale on a cadaveric study to determine the accuracy of resection of the cam-type impingement lesion when carried out arthroscopically as compared with an open procedure. This study, published in 2009, was the first cadaveric

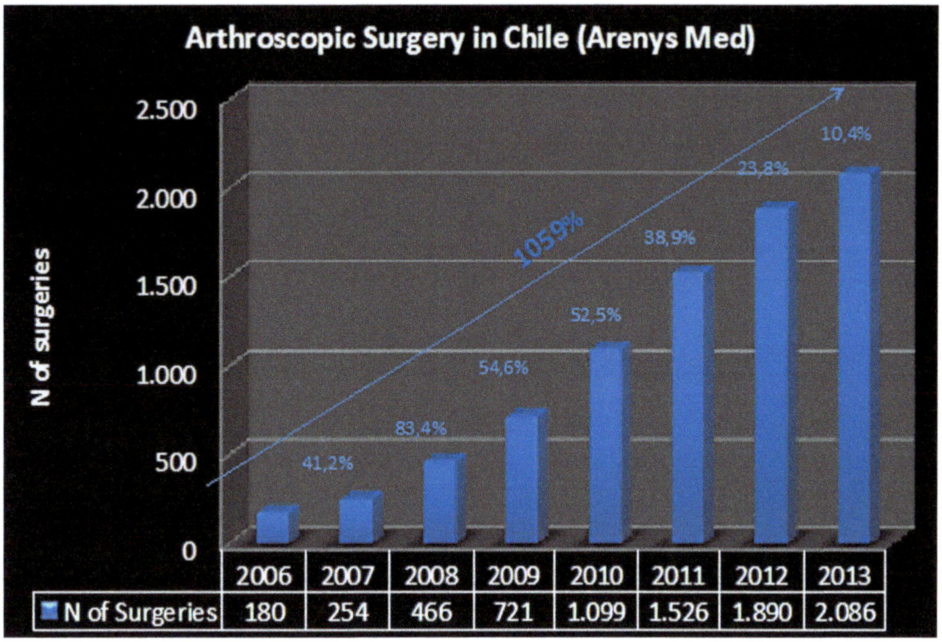

Fig. 93.1 Arthroscopic surgery in Chile, growth (2006–2013) measured in surgeries registered by a medical supply company nationwide

study to compare a fully arthroscopic technique with an open technique for the treatment of femoroacetabular impingement [4].

The three different surgical teams continued to develop techniques for the treatment of femoroacetabular impingement in parallel.

By 2005 Dr. Mella was treating both pincer- and cam-type femoroacetabular impingement. Drs. Rafols and Foronda organized an arthroscopy course at the "Hospital DIPRECA" where the first live hip arthroscopy in Chile was performed. Dr. Mardones organized the first Articular Reconstruction course, which was a joint course between the Mayo Clinic and the "Pontificia Universidad Católica" and featured arthroscopic techniques for the treatment of femoroacetabular impingement.

Dr. James Glick later visited Chile again, assisting Dr. Mardones with the first arthroscopic labral takedown and refixation for a pincer-type impingement at the "Hospital Clínico de la Universidad Católica" [5].

Since then the exponential growth of hip arthroscopy has increased the number of procedures in Chile from 180 per year, registered by Arenys Med, in 2006 to 1890 per year in 2012 which corresponds to more than a 1000 % growth in those 6 years [6] (Fig. 93.1). From this it was predicted that well over 2000 procedures will be performed in Chile in 2013, in the medical centers in Santiago and other main cities such as Puerto Montt, Puerto Varas, Valdivia, Rancagua, La Serena, Antofagasta, and Arica. Currently arthroscopic techniques are employed for the treatment of a wide spectrum of hip pathologies including femoroacetabular impingement, inflammatory diseases, muscle tears and detachments, labral tears, chondral lesions, sciatic compression, and trauma.

The Chilean surgeons that pioneered these techniques continue to actively develop these techniques and collaborate internationally providing academic contributions at international meetings and publications in journals (AAOS, AANA, ISHA, ISAKOS, Arthroscopy, JBJS, Cartilage, Revista Chilena de Ortopedia y Traumatología, Revista Argentina de Artroscopía, Revista Española de Artroscopía).

The history of hip arthroscopy is a perfect example of how surgical techniques can develop and expand transcending boundaries the world over. A vast network of contacts from Asia to North America have allowed South American surgeons to bring about the huge expansion of these techniques in South America over the last two decades. The pioneering spirit of surgeons and the academic collaboration between peers, coupled with the dedication of some surgeons to push the boundaries of medical technology, have driven the advancements in arthroscopic hip surgery.

References

1. Personal Correspondence from Dr. Ricardo Munafo, Argentina; 2012.
2. Personal Correspondence from Dr. Bernardo Aguilera, Colombia; 2012
3. Personal Correspondence from Dr. Giancarlo Polesello, Brazil; 2012.
4. Mardones R et al. Surgical correction of "cam-type" femoroacetabular impingement: a cadaveric comparison of open versus arthroscopic debridement. Arthroscopy. 2009;25(2):175–82. Epub 2008 Nov 1.
5. Personal Correspondence from Dr. Rodrigo Mardones, Chile; 2012.
6. Data provided by Arenys Med. Chile; 2013.

Hip Arthroscopy in India: A Perspective

94

Vijay D. Shetty

Introduction

Worldwide, recent advances in hip arthroscopic surgery have allowed surgeons to diagnose and treat some hip conditions that were previously unrecognised. Athletes and other young individuals with hip injuries are increasingly being diagnosed with an ever-evolving series of conditions [1]. With current technical advancement, hip arthroscopy has helped surgeons to treat some serious intra-articular conditions without arthrotomy and surgical dislocation. There have been an increasing number of publications on hip arthroscopy in recent times. However, in certain parts of the world, hip arthroscopy is still a procedure that most orthopaedic surgeons have only heard off. In this chapter, the author makes an effort to give an account of the current status of hip arthroscopy in the Indian subcontinent.

Hip Arthroscopy in India

Vijay Shetty was fellowship trained in hip arthroscopy with Richard Villar in London and Cambridge, UK. He returned to India setting up practice as a hip and knee surgeon at an exclusive corporate hospital in Mumbai in January 2006. He was able to secure the necessary investment to allow the purchase of the latest hip arthroscopy instrumentation, allowing him to develop his interest in arthroscopic hip techniques.

He gave an invitational lecture to the arthroscopy section of the Indian Orthopaedic Association (IOA) conference. It was clear that the majority in the audience were not even aware that arthroscopy of the hip was possible. The Pakistan Orthopaedic Association president was in that audience and invited him to lecture in Pakistan. At a pre-conference dinner when colleagues became aware that he was to deliver a lecture on hip arthroscopy, he was told he was wasting his time! The following day less than 100 attended his lecture.

At that time there were very few in the Indian subcontinent carrying out this procedure, and all used a conventional fracture table and had no access to the specialist hip instrumentation that was then available in Mumbai.

Author's Experience

Technique for Hip Arthroscopy

In Mumbai hip arthroscopy is performed with the patient in lateral position, under image intensifier control, and general anaesthesia, and with traction (Figs. 94.1 and 94.2). The lateral position provides enhanced instrument maneuverability and easier entrance into the hip joint and helps particularly in obese patients, as fatty tissue tends to fall out of the way. The traction apparatus includes a foot piece and a detachable supporting piece (from DHS table) to hold the leg and a well-padded perineal post for counter traction.

The lower limb (to be operated on) is placed in slight flexion (approximately 10°–20°) with the foot maintained in neutral to slight external rotation. The perineal post is pushed upward against the medial portion of the thigh on the involved leg, keeping the post away from the branch of the pudendal nerve that crosses over the pubic ramus. Distraction is achieved carefully until the "vacuum phenomenon" is seen on the image intensifier as described by Byrd et al. [2]. Typically three portals are used: anterolateral, proximal trochanteric and posterolateral, although occasionally more portals may be required. Specially designed extra-long arthroscopic instruments include a long spinal needle (Howard Jones spinal needle with Pitkin point, Luer lock fitting, 15 g and 155 mm in length, Smith and Nephew, Inc., Andover, MA, USA) and a specially designed flexible guide wire to reach the depth of the hip joint. Special attention is

V.D. Shetty, MS(Orth) (✉)
Hiranandani Orthopaedic Medical Education (HOME), Dr. L. H. Hiranandani Hospital,
Hiranandani Gardens, Powai, Mumbai 400076, Maharashtra, India
e-mail: vijaydshetty@gmail.com

J.C. McCarthy et al. (eds.), *Hip Joint Restoration*, DOI 10.1007/978-1-4614-0694-5_94

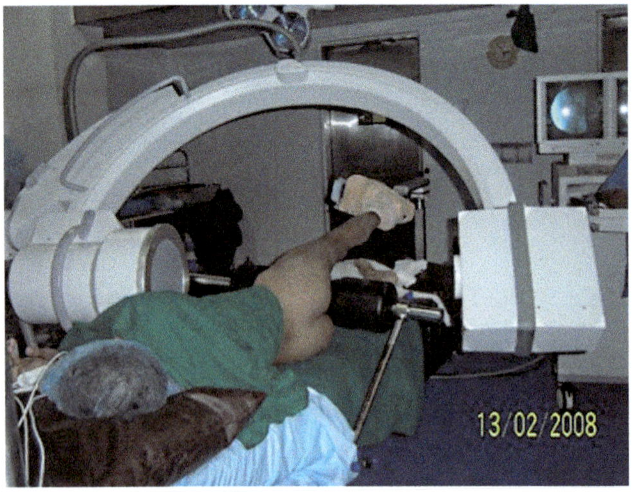

Fig. 94.1 Lateral positioning of the patient before isolation draping

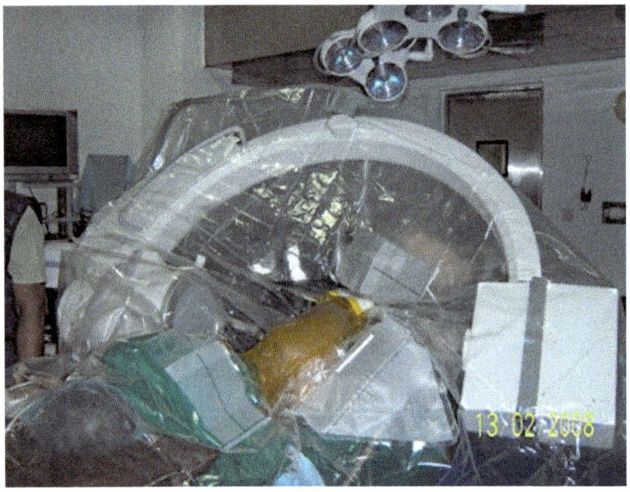

Fig. 94.2 Lateral positioning of the patient after isolation draping

taken to avoid penetration of the acetabular labrum. The joint then is distended with approximately 40 cc of saline and the intracapsular position of the needle confirmed by backflow of fluid.

An arthroscopic pump is used throughout to maintain constant distension of the joint with saline solution. A 70° arthroscope is used most commonly although a 30° arthroscope is also useful. At the end of the procedure, traction is removed carefully under the direct supervision of the operating surgeon.

The average imaging time in Mumbai is 15 s and the procedure takes roughly 40 min to an hour.

Common Findings

The author's first hip arthroscopy, in India, was on a 11-year-old boy who suffered from transient synovitis of the hip joint.

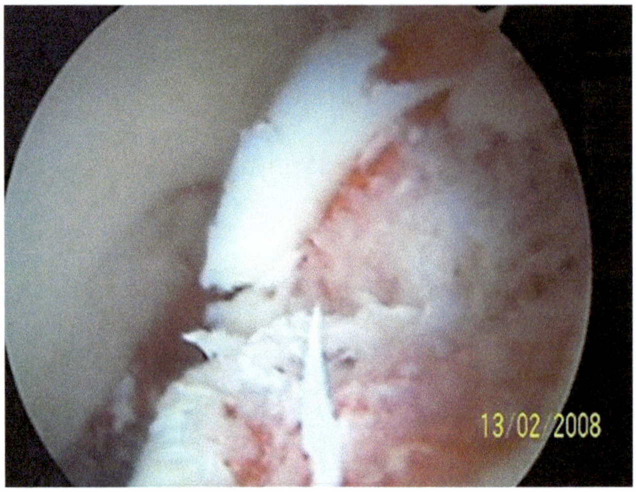

Fig. 94.3 Arthroscopic view of transient synovitis in an 11-year-old boy. Florid synovitis with articular cartilage damage

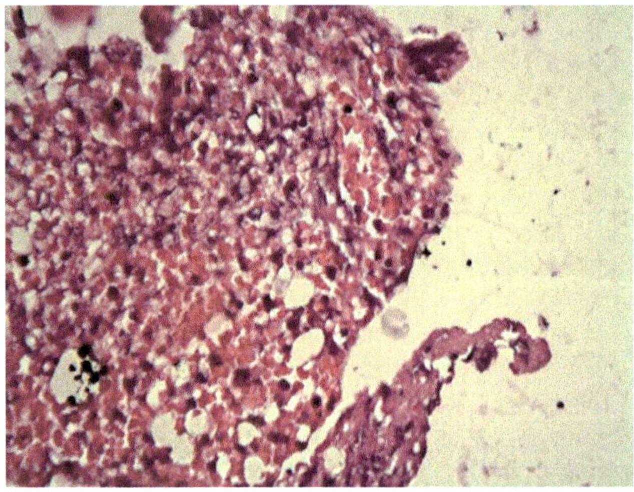

Fig. 94.4 Histopathology of the synovium showing synovial hypertrophy with lymphocytic infiltration. H&E ×400 magnification

The arthroscopic findings were that of a florid synovitis in the joint, and synovectomy and biopsy were performed (Figs. 94.3 and 94.4). The outcome was very good and this case report was later published in an International Journal [3].

Table 94.1 shows the common findings encountered and the procedures performed so far in the author's practice.

Femoroacetabular Impingement: Does it Exist in India?

Since there were only a handful of surgeons performing therapeutic hip arthroscopy, the major question that was being asked in Indian meetings was whether femoroacetabular impingement (FAI) really existed in India.

A study was undertaken in collaboration with a major government institution to check for the existence of FAI in India.

Table 94.1 Common hip arthroscopic findings in my practice

Diagnosis	Common procedures performed
Labral tear	Trimming
Osteoarthritis	Debridement
Chondral flap + osteochondral defects	Microfracture
Synovitis	Synovectomy and debridement
Loose bodies	Removal
Torn ligamentum teres	Diagnostic
Chondrocalcinosis	Debridement
AVN	Debridement

Although it is a very preliminary study, it has indicated that, among the individuals examined, the measurements that indicate the susceptibility for developing FAI were far below the documented measurements for the Western population [4].

Current Status

In India, the major bulk of therapeutic arthroscopic hip procedures involve joint debridement, synovectomy, labral trimming and microfractures. FAI surgeries are less common although the interest in these procedures is increasing among the younger surgeons. More and more young surgeons are now keen to adopt the techniques of arthroscopic hip surgery.

Discussion

Hip arthroscopy is still in its infancy in India. Currently, Indian hip arthroscopists are extremely careful with patient selection. Very few surgeons perform arthroscopic reconstructive hip procedures. This demonstrates the need to focus on further education and training of hip arthroscopy in India. There is also a need for national and international meetings to be held in India, bringing together experts in this field with a view to learn, share and exchange knowledge.

Cricket is a religion in India with everyone wanting to be involved. With this it is likely that more and more hip sport injuries will occur and be diagnosed, helping arthroscopic hip surgery to flourish.

Conclusion

In India, hip arthroscopy is now fast becoming accepted as a surgical technique and offered to patients. There are a lot of enthusiastic young surgeons who want to learn this procedure, and more and more sessions on hip arthroscopy are being held at local and national scientific meetings. It is only a matter of time before India will embrace this technology fully. This will no doubt be helped by industry taking this part of the world more seriously and investing in surgeon and patient education.

References

1. Shetty VD, Villar RN. Hip arthroscopy: current concepts and review of literature. Br J Sports Med. 2007;41(2):64–8.
2. Byrd JW. Hip arthroscopy. The supine position. Clin Sports Med. 2001;20:703–31.
3. Shetty VD, Shetty GM. Arthroscopic view of transient synovitis of the hip joint. Knee Surg Sports Traumatol Arthrosc. 2009;17(8):1003–5.
4. Maini L, Palanisamy Y, Shetty V, Kasture S, Shetty V. Hip impingement in the Indian population: hip anthropometry measurements in 100 hips. Hip Int. 2012;22(3):335.

The Worldwide Experience with Hip Arthroscopy—Japan

95

Nobuhiko Sugano and Takashi Nishii

Introduction

The clinical efficacy of arthroscopic surgery for the debridement, resection, or repair of the acetabular labrum has recently attracted considerable attention.

In Japan, arthroscopy has been performed for various hip disorders since the 1980s. At that time, no three-dimensional diagnostic modalities such as MRI or CAT scans were available for the evaluation of the hip joint. It was therefore difficult to make a correct diagnosis of labral and articular cartilage damage in patients with hip pain and clicking or snapping, using only the plain X-rays and arthrograms that were then the standard diagnostic modalities for articular disorders of the hip. Arthroscopy thus was used for the investigation of intra-articular hip problems that could not be detected on radiographs and also for the grading of articular cartilage damage.

Hip Arthroscopy in Japan

Suzuki et al. performed hip arthroscopy on 49 hips in 45 patients through a lateral portal 1 cm proximal to the tip of the greater trochanter in a supine position on a traction table during 1984 and 1985 [1]. He and his associates found acetabular labral tears in five out of nine painful hips that showed no abnormality on radiographs.

Ide et al. reported on the arthroscopic assessment of 196 hip joints in 104 patients in the 4 years from 1984 [2]. They used a traction table in the supine position with continuous traction of 20–40 kg on both legs. They developed a technique using two portals that facilitated a global view of the joint and allowed them to carry out simple surgical procedures including the removal of loose bodies, joint debridement in osteoarthritis, and synovectomy in rheumatoid arthritis. The anterior portal was located 1 cm distal and lateral to the midpoint of a line from the anterior superior iliac spine to the pubic symphysis, and a lateral portal was located 2 cm proximal to the tip of the greater trochanter. Most of the arthroscopic procedures were for diagnostic and assessment purposes, with therapeutic surgical procedures carried out in only 11 of the 196 hips. Later, an anterolateral portal at the midpoint of the anterior and lateral portals was added to perform a partial limbectomy [3].

In Japan hip arthroscopy has, to date, been used mainly for the treatment of acetabular labral tears or early osteoarthritis, with little reported on the treatment of femoroacetabular impingement (FAI). The average Japanese acetabulum is probably not deep enough to induce pincer-type FAI [4, 5], and Japanese people also have a low incidence of primary hip osteoarthritis, which often accompanies the pistol grip deformity of the femoral head seen in FAI.

Nonetheless, there were several early adopters of hip arthroscopy in Japan and we describe their contributions to hip arthroscopy as a diagnostic and evaluation tool, and as a treatment tool.

Arthroscopy as a Diagnostic and Evaluation Tool

Evaluation of the Labrum and Cartilage

Since those early reports in the 1980s there have been several more on the arthroscopic findings of labral and articular cartilage lesions in patients with hip symptoms that could not be diagnosed on radiographs.

Ikeda et al. described the arthroscopic evaluation of torn acetabular labrum in seven young patients [6]. Three of them had had an acute onset of symptoms during sporting activities. On examination, all seven patients had pain on passive

N. Sugano, MD, PhD (✉) • T. Nishii, MD, PhD
Department of Orthopaedic Medical Engineering, Osaka University Graduate School of Medicine, 2-2 Yamadaoka, Suita 565-0871, Japan
e-mail: n-sugano@umin.net

J.C. McCarthy et al. (eds.), *Hip Joint Restoration*, DOI 10.1007/978-1-4614-0694-5_95

flexion and medial rotation of the joint. All but one of the tears was located on the posterosuperior portion of the labrum, and, in the acute cases, vascular dilatation around the tear was observed. In these cases, repeat arthroscopy examination several months later showed that the vascular changes had disappeared, but the tear was still present.

Noguchi et al. conducted 120 hip arthroscopies in patients with dysplastic osteoarthritis to clarify the intra-articular pathology according to four radiographic stages of hip osteoarthritis [7]. There were 41 pre-arthritic, 42 early, 34 advanced, and 3 end stage. As the radiological stage progressed, articular cartilage degeneration became more extensive and severe. Even in the pre-arthritic stage that showed no abnormality on radiographs except for dysplastic morphology, they found detached tears of the acetabular labrum originating in the anterosuperior area in 88 % of hips, and articular cartilage degeneration typically originating in the anterosuperior portion of the weight-bearing area of the femoral head and acetabulum in 85 % of hips. Articular cartilage degeneration of the acetabulum usually precedes that of the femoral head.

Ide et al. classified arthroscopic findings of the labrum into eight types [3] (Fig. 95.1). In the early stages of osteoarthritis secondary to hip dysplasia, bucket handle or L shape types were often observed. In the late stages of osteoarthritis, degenerative or completely torn labra were the dominant findings [8].

Suenagara et al. carried out physical examination maneuvers and hip arthroscopy in 59 patients with osteoarthritis secondary to dysplasia to determine the relationship between pain at flexion-rotation and the status of a labral tea [9]. All hip joints examined arthroscopically demonstrated incompletely or completely detached tears of the acetabular labrum in one portion of the weight-bearing area. Hip pain was induced by the maximum flexion-internal rotation test in 39 % of patients and by the maximum flexion-external rotation test in 27 % of patients. A positive maximum flexion-internal rotation test result correlated with incompletely detached tears in the posterosuperior portion of the acetabular labrum. On the other hand, a completely detached tear of the posterosuperior labrum was associated with a negative maximum flexion-internal rotation test result.

Acetabular reorientation osteotomy is an effective procedure for dysplastic hips to improve hip symptoms and to prevent the further progression of osteoarthritis [10, 11]. However, it is difficult to evaluate on radiographs the effect of osteotomy on the healing of the intra-articular cartilage and labrum. There are several reports of the arthroscopic evaluation of the cartilage and labrum associated with osteotomies [12–14]. Yasunaga et al. performed arthroscopy in 59 hips of 57 patients at the time of rotational acetabular osteotomy. They found radiological evidence of the progression of arthritis in four joints, which were classified at arthroscopy, at 2–5.5 years after surgery as grade 4 according

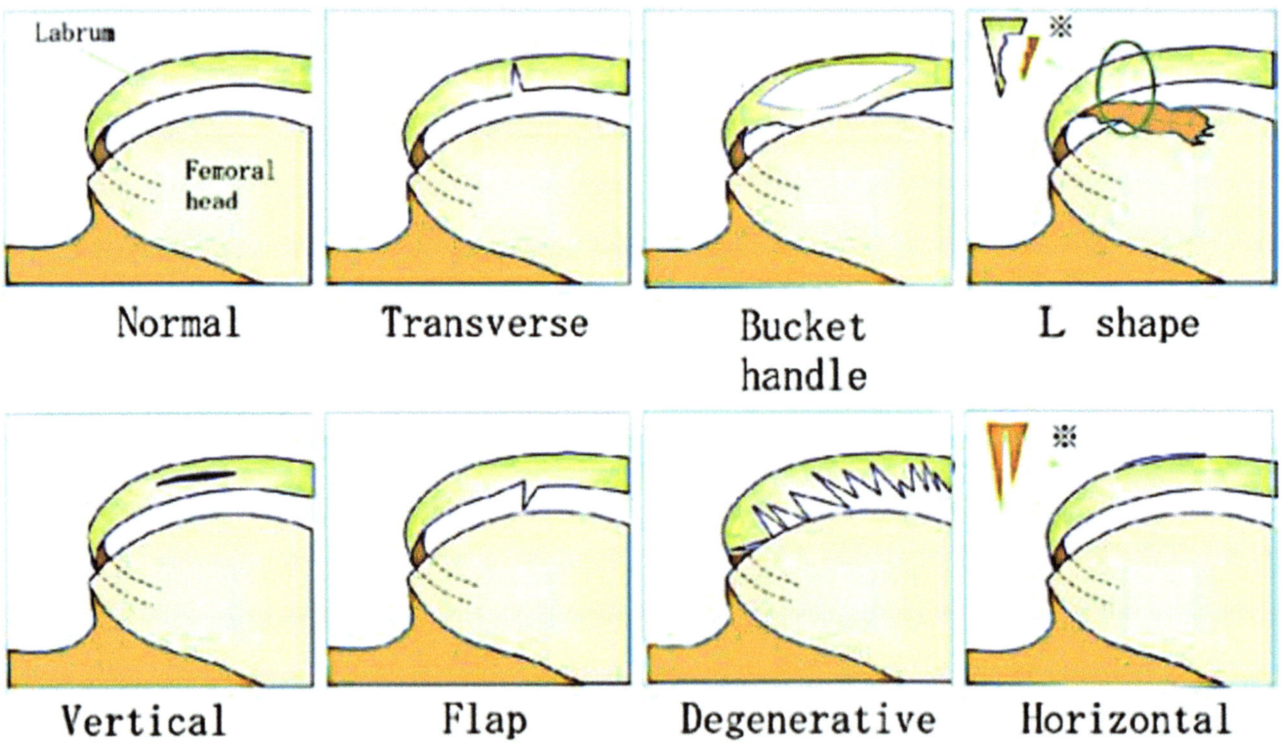

Fig. 95.1 Ide's morphological classification of torn labrum [3]. From Yamamoto et al. Arthroscopic partial limbectomy in hip joints with acetabular hypoplasia. Arthroscopy. 2005 May;21(5):586–91. Reprinted with permission from Elsevier Limited

to the classification of Outerbridge. Stepwise regression analysis showed that damage to acetabular or femoral articular cartilage significantly affected the progression of arthritis after rotational acetabular osteotomy [12].

Suzuki et al. performed arthroscopy before and at an average of 18.9 months after conventional osteotomies in 38 patients with hip dysplasia to evaluate recovery from cartilage damage and labral lesions [13]. Rotational acetabular osteotomy had been performed in 17 hips, intertrochanteric varus femoral osteotomy in 13 hips, transtrochanteric valgus femoral osteotomy in 7 hips, and Chiari osteotomy and valgus femoral osteotomy in 1 hip. Cartilage repair was observed on the acetabular side in five hips (13.2 %) and on the femoral side in four (10.5 %). The acetabular labrum had adhered to the capsule in 11 hips.

Fujii et al. performed an observational study of 121 patients (121 hips) who underwent a transposition osteotomy of the acetabulum combined with an arthroscopy to clarify how intra-articular lesions influence the survival of a periacetabular osteotomy in patients with dysplasia of the hip [14]. They found that in hips with early-stage osteoarthritis, femoral subchondral bone exposure was a risk factor for progression of the grade of osteoarthritis.

Snapping and Clicking

Snapping or clicking around the hip can be caused by extra-articular structures such as the iliotibial band or the iliopsoas tendon. They can also be caused by intra-articular structures; however, it is often difficult to clarify the real cause of snapping or clicking by a physical examination or medical imaging.

Yamamoto et al. performed arthroscopy on 30 patients (32 hips) with a snapping hip syndrome, in which the accompanying pain was transiently relieved by the intra-articular injection of local anesthetic [15]. Plain radiography findings showed no abnormality in 11 joints, hip osteoarthritis in 19 joints, and femoral head deformation caused by Perthes disease and by synovial osteochondromatosis in 1 joint each. Excluding the case of synovial osteochondromatosis, 31 joints were examined by MRI, which failed to identify the cause of snapping hip in all cases. Hip arthrography revealed an intra-articular loose body in two joints with osteoarthritis. Arthroscopy revealed acetabular labral tears in all 11 radiographically normal joints, in 15 of the 19 joints with osteoarthritis on plain radiography, and incompatibility between acetabular labrum and deformed femoral head in two joints with osteoarthritis. In the case of femoral head deformation after Perthes disease, arthroscopy revealed detachment of the femoral head cartilage as a result of impingement of the acetabulum on the femoral head. Therapeutic arthroscopic procedures were carried out including partial limbectomy for acetabular labral tears, surgical removal of loose bodies, partial femoral head excision for incompatibility between acetabular labrum and deformed femoral head, and shaving or articular cartilage detachment. These procedures resolved the snapping in all cases.

Rupture of the Ligamentum Teres Femoris

Traumatic rupture of the ligamentum teres femoris has been reported to be a cause of severe hip pain. Yamamoto et al. also reported arthroscopic debridement for degenerative rupture of the ligamentum teres femoris in a 78-year-old woman and obtained good results [16].

Arthroscopy as a Treatment Tool

Arthroscopic Debridement for Osteoarthrosis

Total hip arthroplasty is the conventional method for the treatment of advanced osteoarthritis of the hip. Hip arthroscopy has however been performed at some institutions, as a joint-preserving operation to relieve pain, to release contracture, and to prevent further progression of osteoarthritis. Sugiyama et al. performed arthroscopic debridement of torn labrum and synovectomy or removal of acetabular and femoral head osteophytes with iliopsoas muscle release in 50 patients (56 hips) with advanced osteoarthritis aged 30–78 years [17]. Total hip arthroplasty was required in six hips within 2 years of arthroscopy, but for the remaining 50 hips sufficient pain relief was achieved without progression of osteoarthritis.

Partial Limbectomy

Acetabular labral injury is not a rare pathology and over the last 20 years there have been several reports of arthroscopic treatment of these. However, most of the reports do not provide sufficient information on its indications and efficacy due to the small number of cases and short follow-up period.

Ueo et al. described two patients who had pain of unknown cause with normal plain radiographs and arthrography. Clinical examination strongly suggested an internal derangement of the hip and so hip arthroscopy was performed. In both cases, the acetabular labrum was seen to be ruptured at the posterior margin of the acetabulum. Partial limbectomies were performed by the posterior approach, and a marked decrease in hip pain was achieved at 2–3 months postoperatively [18].

Labral tears in hip dysplasia are degenerative tears, occurring as a consequence of the abnormal stresses imposed by the uncovered lateral portion of the femoral head [19]. Once a tear is present, a localized stress point occurs on the femoral head, leading rapidly to degenerative arthritis. Limbectomy may therefore increase instability leading to further progression of osteoarthritis. Yamamoto et al. performed arthroscopic partial limbectomy in ten hips with pre- or early osteoarthritis secondary to acetabular dysplasia [3]. All the patients were female with mechanical symptoms such as giving way, catching, locking, or clicking sound. Their ages at the time of surgery ranged from 14 to 62 years (mean, 33.7 years). Hip pain improved within 4 or 5 days of surgery in all patients. The mechanical symptoms had subsided or disappeared in all hips postoperatively at a mean follow-up of 8 years. Radiographs revealed no evidence of osteoarthritic progression, although one case with a preoperative CE angle of 0° showed lateralization of the femoral head.

Septic Arthritis and Loose Bodies

Hip arthroscopy allows surgeons to perform a synovectomy and removal of loose bodies without dislocation of the hip, or extensive damage to the surrounding soft-tissue structures. Yamamoto et al. performed arthroscopic debridement and intraoperative high-volume irrigation (20–25 L of physiologic saline) on four adult patients with septic hip arthritis [20]. There were three women and one man with an average age of 58 years. The length of time from onset of symptoms to surgery averaged 36 days. The pathological organisms were *Staphylococcus aureus* in two patients, *Serratia sp.* in one patient, and group-B *Streptococcus* in one patient. The inflammatory reactions subsided within 4 weeks of surgery in three of the four patients and within 6 weeks in the other patient. At the time of the final examination, the postoperative follow-up period ranged from 1 to 6 years and there was no recurrence of arthritis or other complications.

Okada et al. reported a successful outcome after hip arthroscopy in a 16-year-old girl with hip synovial chondromatosis [21]. Twelve months after surgery, she remained pain free and there was no limitation of movement.

Summary

Hip arthroscopy has been performed in Japan for over 30 years. Initial indications were for diagnostic reasons or in conjunction with periacetabular osteotomy. Because dysplasia is much more prevalent in Japan than FAI the frequency of hip arthroscopy has been limited. However with further improvements in imaging as well as evolving clinical awareness, hip arthroscopy continues to grow in procedural indications and volume.

References

1. Suzuki S, Awaya G, Okada Y, Maekawa M, Ikeda T, Tada H. Arthroscopic diagnosis of ruptured acetabular labrum. Acta Orthop Scand. 1986;57(6):513–5.
2. Ide T, Akamatsu N, Nakajima I. Arthroscopic surgery of the hip joint. Arthroscopy. 1991;7(2):204–11.
3. Yamamoto Y, Ide T, Nakamura M, Hamada Y, Usui I. Arthroscopic partial limbectomy in hip joints with acetabular hypoplasia. Arthroscopy. 2005;21(5):586–91.
4. Inoue K, Wichart P, Kawasaki T, et al. Prevalence of hip osteoarthritis and acetabular dysplasia in French and Japanese adults. Rheumatology (Oxford). 2000;39:745–8.
5. Yoshimura N, Campbell L, Hashimoto T, et al. Acetabular dysplasia and hip osteoarthritis in Britain and Japan. Br J Rheumatol. 1998;37:1193–7.
6. Ikeda T, Awaya G, Suzuki S, Okada Y, Tada H. Torn acetabular labrum in young patients. Arthroscopic diagnosis and management. J Bone Joint Surg (Br). 1988;70(1):13–6.
7. Noguchi Y, Miura H, Takasugi S, Iwamoto Y. Cartilage and labrum degeneration in the dysplastic hip generally originates in the anterosuperior weight-bearing area: an arthroscopic observation. Arthroscopy. 1999;15(5):496–506.
8. Ide T, Hokari Y. Arthroscopic findings of labrum. J Joint Surg. 1994;13:317–26. Japanese.
9. Suenaga E, Noguchi Y, Jingushi S, Shuto T, Nakashima Y, Miyanishi K, et al. Relationship between the maximum flexion-internal rotation test and the torn acetabular labrum of a dysplastic hip. J Orthop Sci. 2002;7(1):26–32.
10. Nozawa M, Shitoto K, Matsuda K, Maezawa K, Kurosawa H. Rotational acetabular osteotomy for acetabular dysplasia. A follow-up for more than ten years. J Bone Joint Surg (Br). 2002;84(1):59–65.
11. Yasunaga Y, Ochi M, Terayama H, Tanaka R, Yamasaki T, Ishii Y. Rotational acetabular osteotomy for advanced osteoarthritis secondary to dysplasia of the hip. J Bone Joint Surg Am. 2006;88(9):1915–9.
12. Yasunaga Y, Ikuta Y, Kanazawa T, Takahashi K, Hisatome T. The state of the articular cartilage at the time of surgery as an indication for rotational acetabular osteotomy. J Bone Joint Surg (Br). 2001;83(7):1001–4.
13. Suzuki C, Harada Y, Mitsuhashi S, Yamashita K, Watanabe H, Tsuchiya A, et al. Repair of cartilage defects and torn acetabular labrum in hip joints after conventional osteotomy: evaluation by follow-up arthroscopy. J Orthop Sci. 2005;10(2):127–32.
14. Fujii M, Nakashima Y, Noguchi Y, Yamamoto T, Mawatari T, Motomura G, et al. Effect of intra-articular lesions on the outcome of periacetabular osteotomy in patients with symptomatic hip dysplasia. J Bone Joint Surg (Br). 2011;93(11):1449–56.
15. Yamamoto Y, Hamada Y, Ide T, Usui I. Arthroscopic surgery to treat intra-articular type snapping hip. Arthroscopy. 2005;21(9):1120–5.
16. Yamamoto Y, Usui I. Arthroscopic surgery for degenerative rupture of the ligamentum teres femoris. Arthroscopy. 2006;22(6):689.e1–3.
17. Sugiyama H, Horiuchi T, Nakamura M. Clinical result of arthroscopic surgery of the hip osteoarthritis. Hip Joint. 2010;36:1–4. Japanese.
18. Ueo T, Suzuki S, Iwasaki R, Yosikawa J. Rupture of the labra acetabularis as a cause of hip pain detected arthroscopically, and partial limbectomy for successful pain relief. Arthroscopy. 1990;6(1):48–51.
19. Dorrell JH, Catterall A. The torn acetabular labrum. J Bone Joint Surg (Br). 1986;68(3):400–3.
20. Yamamoto Y, Ide T, Hachisuka N, Maekawa S, Akamatsu N. Arthroscopic surgery for septic arthritis of the hip joint in 4 adults. Arthroscopy. 2001;17(3):290–7.
21. Okada Y, Awaya G, Ikeda T, Tada H, Kamisato S, Futami T. Arthroscopic surgery for synovial chondromatosis of the hip. J Bone Joint Surg (Br). 1989;71(2):198–9.

Hip Arthroscopy in China

96

Jason Brockwell

Introduction

China, Taiwan, and Hong Kong have overwhelmingly Oriental populations—mostly Han Chinese, though the northern and southern people are slightly different genetically, as well as in language, diet, and some aspects of culture, and live in quite different geographic and climactic conditions.

China has a population of 1.4 billion, Taiwan 23 million, and Hong Kong 7 million, so, from a numbers point of view, Taiwan and Hong Kong are not as important, but, because of their more developed medical systems, they may show the direction that China may take.

There is a relative paucity of literature and information about hip disease in China, but it is possible to draw some inferences by comparing and contrasting China with Oriental populations in other parts of Asia, so in some cases non-Chinese studies will be quoted.

Incidence of Hip Disease Is Different in Orientals

The incidence of hip disease in Orientals is lower than in non-Oriental populations. The relative incidence of different hip diseases is also different from non-Oriental populations. The relative incidence of certain hip diseases varies within different Oriental population groups.

J. Brockwell, FRCSEd (Orth), FHKAM (Orth) (✉)
Hip & Pelvic Surgery, Orthopaedics Department, Asia Medical Specialists, 8/F Aon China Bldg., 29 Queen's Rd Central, Hong Kong SAR, People's Republic of China
e-mail: jason.brockwell@asiamedical.hk

DDH

The incidence of developmental dysplasia of the hip (DDH) in China is not known. It was extremely common in Japan, but rates declined dramatically with the identification of swaddling (especially of winter-born) babies with their hips extended as a causative factor [1], and a national education campaign commencing in 1973.

One paper from Central China looking at a single large family reported higher DDH incidence in children born in winter, which may be associated with winter swaddling [2]. There is only one study looking at DDH in Southern Chinese in Hong Kong, published in 1981, showing rates approximately ten times lower than reported in the West [3], though a more recent study from Singapore showed slightly higher rates [4].

Center-edge angles of Wiberg measured in Northern China are very slightly lower than in other races [5]. The mean angle was 23° (5°–46°) in childhood (4–9 years), increasing to 29° (6°–48°) in adolescence (10–18 years) and reaching 33° (14°–59°) in adults.

ONFH

Osteonecrosis of the femoral head (ONFH), is common in Asia (in both Oriental and non-Oriental populations), and some may be related to traditional medicines adulterated with synthetic steroids [6].

There are many reports that traditional medicines are sometimes intentionally contaminated with synthetic compounds, and though the rate is unknown it has been reported that up to 50 % of traditional medicines contain synthetic compounds [7–12]. If this is so the incidence should decrease if regulation is improved [13], however the production of fake and adulterated drugs is a huge industry in China. In 2007, Zheng Xiaoyu, the former head of the Chinese State Food and Drug Administration, was executed. He was charged with accepting US $850,000 in bribes to grant

J.C. McCarthy et al. (eds.), *Hip Joint Restoration*, DOI 10.1007/978-1-4614-0694-5_96

approval for medicines. State media said that his agency had approved 137 drugs that had not submitted proper applications, and that six of those turned out to be entirely fake [14]. Despite this, problems have continued, and in 2012 Chinese authorities detained nearly 2000 people as part of a nationwide crackdown on the sale of fake or counterfeit drugs and health care products, and seized about US $182 million in fake medicine, including drugs for the treatment of cancer, hypertension, and diabetes [15]. Fake and adulterated drugs are likely to remain a problem.

OA and FAI

Osteoarthritis (OA) and femoro-acetabular impingement (FAI) are uncommon in Asia, including China.

A study comparing radiographic osteoarthritis (OA) in British and Hong Kong Chinese men having urologic X-rays showed half the incidence in Hong Kong at about 5 % vs. 10 % [16], but no significant difference in center-edge angle of Wiberg [17], though the Chinese had shallower acetabula on absolute measurement [16]. In a similar study of Koreans over 70 years of age, men had a 1.7 % incidence of radiographic OA [18].

In a study conducted in Beijing, China, using the same standardized instruments and protocol as those in the Framingham Osteoarthritis Study, the prevalence of hip osteoarthritis among the men and women aged 60 and over was only 0.4 and 0.6 %, much lower than in Caucasians [19, 20]. A larger, though less rigorous study covering various parts of China again concluded OA hip was unusual [21].

There is little data on the incidence of FAI in Orientals. It is probably under-recognized, as there is very little knowledge of the condition in the majority of the radiology and orthopedic community.

In one Japanese study only 17 out of 946 (2 %) total hip replacements (THR) were for OA. Of the 17 hips with OA, 6 (i.e., 0.6 % of all the THRs) had FAI as a cause [22].

Unpublished data from Hong Kong looked at Chinese adults under 60 years of age diagnosed in a university orthopedic clinic with "hip disease." Of these 5 % had clinical and radiological evidence of FAI, and 25 % had at least one radiographic sign of FAI. The majority of the diagnoses were ONFH, inflammatory arthritis, sequelae of pediatric hip disorders, and infection (Patrick Yung, personal communication).

Squatting and sitting on the ground are normal in China and much of Asia (Fig. 96.1). A Japanese study using open MRI demonstrated that impingement, which was considered to have occurred when, on MRI, the anterior femoral head-neck junction approached the acetabular rim and the femoral head was seen to float from the bottom of the acetabulum with the acetabular rim acting as a fulcrum, occurs frequently during daily Japanese squatting and sitting on the floor [23].

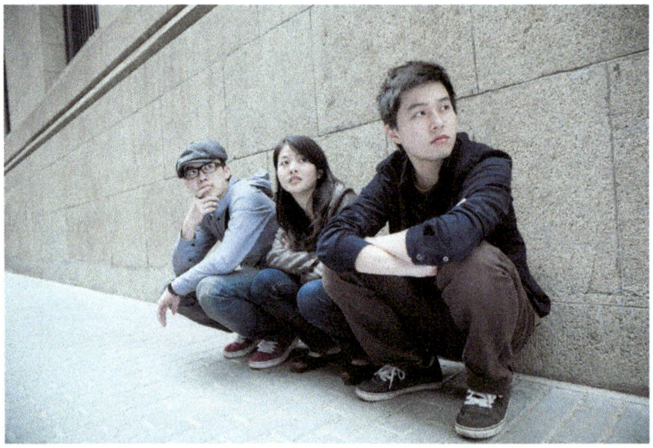

Fig. 96.1 Squatting is common in Asia, but appears to do little or no damage to the hips. Copyright iStockphoto/ipandastudio

One would reasonably expect this to cause damage to the hips, but presumably because sitting is done gently (compared to sports), this appears not to cause problems.

Anatomy

Orientals probably have a higher head-neck ratio and slightly more femoral anteversion than other races.

One study, performed in Thailand, measured 102 femoral bones without visible previous disease or deformity of the head, neck, and shaft, that included 50 male donors and 52 female donors, with an average age of 58.8 years (range 25–85). The head-neck ratio in the coronal and sagittal planes in males and females were 1.47, 1.45 and 1.77, 1.83, respectively [24], which are healthy numbers, not predisposing to impingement.

A comparison of Caucasians and Hong Kong Chinese showed significant differences in the measurements of the head, neck, and proximal femoral shaft. In Caucasians, the anteversion angle averaged 7° in males (range, minus 2° to 35°) and 10° in females (minus 2° to 25°). In Hong Kong Chinese the average in males was 14° (minus 4° to 36°) and 16° in females (7° to 28°) [25]. Again, these differences will reduce the incidence of impingement in Chinese.

Etiology of FAI in Chinese

There is ongoing debate about the etiology of FAI, likely to be genetics and/or sporting activity. If FAI is primarily caused by sport, mass participation in recreational sport in populations with anatomy predisposing to FAI is likely to cause significant incidence of both symptomatic FAI and OA.

Recreational sport participation is related to societal monetary affluence, and, outside of Japan and South Korea, most of Asia is not sufficiently affluent for mass participation in recreational sport. Chinese national sports programs create Olympic athletes by selecting young children and placing them in full-time sports schools—the rest of the population does not enjoy much government funding for sport (Figs. 96.2 and 96.3).

Japan and South Korea became rich recently, but there is still great emphasis on academic rather than sporting achievement at school, and it is possible that it will take several generations for us to the see the effects of large numbers of older adults who have indulged in significant volumes of sporting activity from childhood. Hong Kong is rich—with a per capita GDP of US $35,156 in 2011 [26], but Hong Kong is sorely lacking in community access to sports facilities (Fig. 96.4) and most children are encouraged to study hard rather than play sport. However affluence is rising rapidly across the whole region, so we may see increasing incidence of symptomatic FAI and OA in Asia in a few generations (Fig. 96.5).

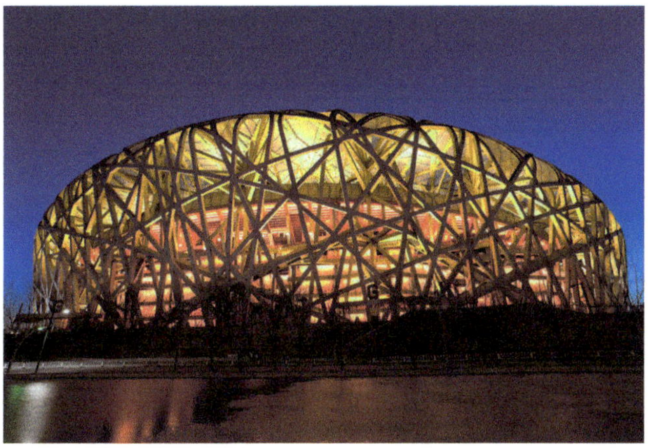

Fig. 96.2 The "Bird's Nest" Olympic stadium built for the 2008 Olympic Games, held in Beijing. The stadium is now rarely used. Copyright iStockphoto/fototrav

Sport

Several studies support the theory that participation in sport in adolescence is a causative factor in FAI.

The seminal paper on this topic is from Siebenrock [27] who retrospectively reviewed 72 hips in 37 male basketball players with a mean age of 17.6 years and 38 age-matched volunteers who had not participated in sporting activities at a high level. 15 % of the athletes' hips were painful and had positive anterior impingement tests. Internal rotation of the hip averaged 30° in the controls compared with only 19° in the athletes. The maximum value of the alpha angle of Notzli [28] throughout the anterosuperior head segment was larger in the athletes (average 61°), compared with the control group (47°). The athletes had a tenfold increase in the likelihood of having an alpha angle greater than 55° in at least one measurement position.

In a prospective study in the USA, 67 male college American football players (average age 21 years) had both hips evaluated for radiographic signs of FAI. Ninety-five percent of the 134 hips had at least one sign of cam or pincer impingement, and 77 % had more than one sign [29].

In a Dutch study of 89 elite pre-professional soccer players and 92 controls aged 12–19 years cam-type deformity was more prevalent in soccer players (26 %) than in controls (17 %). Anterosuperior flattening of the femoral head (56 % vs. 18 %) and prominence (13 % vs. 0 %) were more prevalent in soccer players than in controls [30].

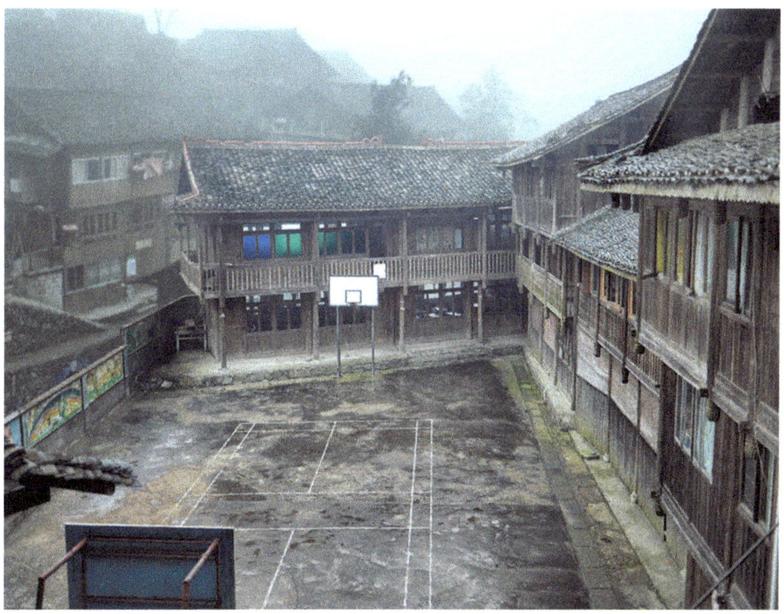

Fig. 96.3 Sports facility in school in rural Guang Xi province, China. Copyright iStockphoto/craftvision

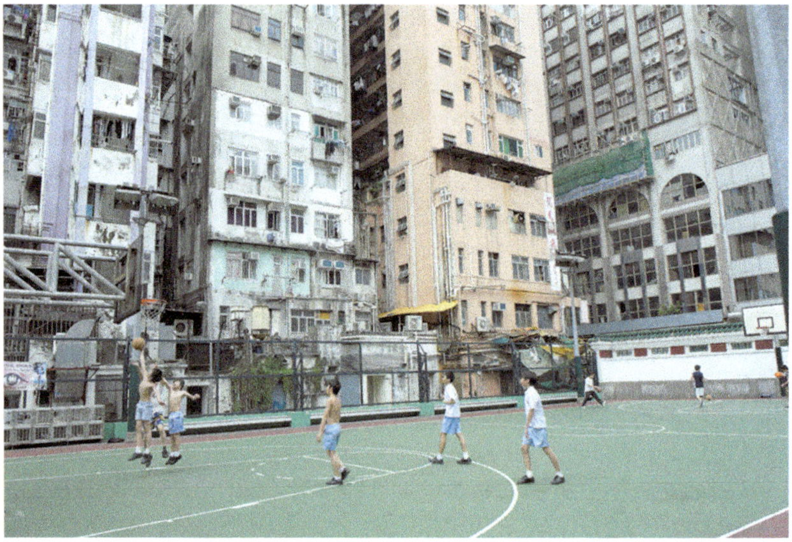

Fig. 96.4 Playing basketball in Hong Kong. Copyright iStockphoto/tanukiphoto

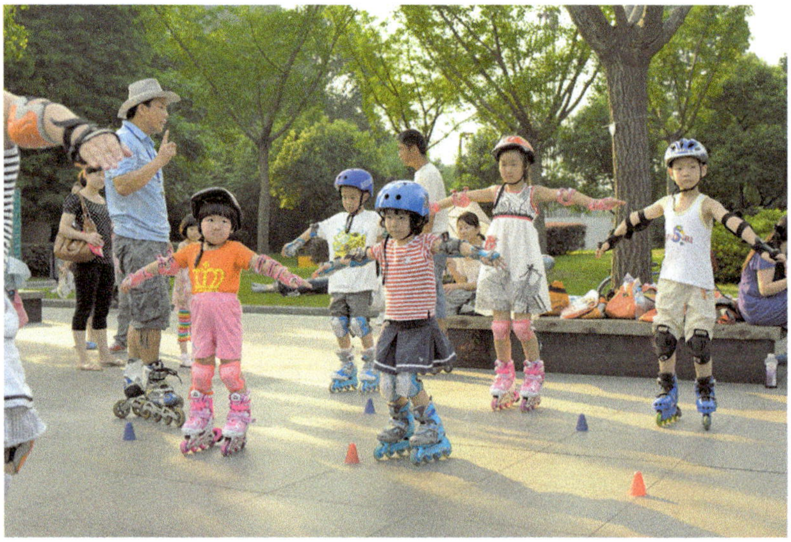

Fig. 96.5 "Little Emperors"—only children born under the one-child policy have much parental and grandparental attention. Whether this will translate into time for recreational sport, or no time, as they work to support a high number of dependent adults, remains to be seen. Economists forecast the latter. Copyright iStockphoto/jacus

Several studies have looked at the presence of radiographic signs of FAI in the general young adult population. One example is a large Norwegian study of 2081 young adults of both sexes with a mean age of 18.6 years. One or more cam-type deformities were seen in both hips of about 25 % of males and 6 % of females. One or more pincer-type deformities were seen in both hips of about 22 % of males and 10 % female participants [31].

One study disagrees with the sports theory of FAI. This US study compared 50 young adults who participated in high-level soccer prior to skeletal maturity and 50 controls who did not. Subjects had participated in youth soccer at a high level of at least three games or practices per week for at least 36 weeks per year during the ages of 10–14 years in men and 8–12 years in women. Controls had not participated in soccer or other sports beyond a recreational level and less than 2 days a week for less than 26 weeks per year during the same ages in youth. There were 25 men and 25 women in each group. Fifteen of the 25 male subjects had evidence of cam deformity, compared with 14 male controls. Nine of the 25 female subjects had evidence of cam deformity, compared with 8 female controls. Neither of these differences was statistically significant. There was a significantly higher prevalence of cam deformity in men as compared with women (29 vs. 17, P=.016) [32]. The authors concluded that soccer in skeletal immaturity was not a risk factor for FAI. The confounding factor is the level of sports participation of the controls: the overall presence of FAI is similar to the general US population, in which many children are fairly active, so they may have been active enough to acquire deformities, despite not playing competitive soccer, and the additional activity by the high-level soccer players did not cause a further increase in the rate of FAI.

Genetics

A British study looked at 96 siblings of 64 patients treated for primary impingement with a spouse control group of 77 individuals. The siblings of those patients with a cam deformity had a relative risk of 2.8 of having the same deformity. The siblings of those patients with a pincer deformity had a relative risk of 2.0 of having the same deformity. Bilateral deformity occurred more often in the siblings, relative risk 2.6. The prevalence of clinical features in those hips with abnormal morphology was also greater in the sibling group compared with the control group (relative risk 2.5) [33]. This study does not settle the question of nature vs. nurture—siblings are often exposed to similar quantities of sporting activity, especially in childhood.

Evidence against the sports theory comes from comparative anatomy and anthropology. Hogervorst and colleagues examined the hips and pelves of a wide variety of modern animal species and of modern humans and human ancestors [34].

They described two stereotypical mammalian hips, which they named "coxa recta" and "coxa rotunda." Coxa recta is characterized by a straight or aspherical section on the femoral head or head-neck junction, giving a cam or pistol grip deformity. It is seen mostly in runners and jumpers. In the male hip, evolution can explain cam impingement in coxa recta as an adaptation for running.

Coxa rotunda has a round femoral head with ample head-neck offset, and is seen mostly in climbing and swimming animals.

The evolutionary conflict between upright gait and the birth of a large brained fetus is expressed in the female pelvis and hip, and can explain pincer impingement in coxa profunda, as the widening of the pelvis to allow passage of the fetus conflicts with the need to shorten the distance from the center of rotation of the hip to the center of gravity.

In mammals hips with, what in human terms would be considered, severe impingement morphology are common. Round femoral heads are the exception rather than the rule.

Quadruped mammals load their hips predominantly in a flexed position, within a limited range of flexion and extension. In quadrupeds, the recta section is located posterosuperiorly. Hogervorst hypothesized that this is where tensile stresses in the head-neck junction are highest at hoof- or paw-strike in a running, jumping or galloping quadruped. However, in humans the pelvis is vertical and the hip loaded in a much more extended position, shifting the highest tensile stresses at heel-strike approximately 90° anterior, to the anterosuperior head-neck junction, which is where the cam deformity is found in humans.

Whether or not sports activity is an important factor in the development of pistol grip deformities of the proximal femur, it is clear that sporting activity contributes to hips becoming symptomatic.

Surgeons in the Far East are reporting small numbers of symptomatic FAI in young Oriental patients [35], especially sportspeople [36].

Gluteal Fibrosis

Gluteal muscular fibrosis and contracture, usually secondary to multiple injections, can prevent hip adduction [37–40] and patients walk with an increased foot progression angle and their hips abduct in flexion. A very high incidence, of 1–2.5 %, has been reported in China [41–43]. This may be the result of the use of benzyl alcohol as a solvent for penicillin for intramuscular injections in China in the 1970s and 1980s [37, 39], as several authors have suggested benzyl alcohol is the main cause of gluteal muscular contracture [40, 41]. There is a cultural belief that injections are "stronger" than oral medications, and patients may expect or request them.

Ankylosing Spondylitis

There are differences between Chinese rates of some inflammatory arthritis and the rest of the world, for example the incidence of rheumatoid arthritis is about 0.5 % in China vs. about 1 % in the rest of the world. Gout is more common in China. In spondyloarthritides similarities between Asia and other parts of the world are major and the differences are minor [44]. Ankylosing spondylitis incidence and presentation is slightly different between northern and southern Chinese [45]. Approximately 25 % of Chinese patients with ankylosing spondylitis complain of hip pain [45], which is broadly in line with European and South American numbers [46], as there are many confounding factors in epidemiological estimates in this condition [45, 47]. Approximately 5 % of European ankylosing spondylitis patients have hip replacement. The percentage of Chinese patients having hip replacement is not reported.

Hip Arthroscopy in China

Arguably FAI is one of the best indications for arthroscopic intervention, but is relatively uncommon in Orientals, and the conditions that are more common in Orientals, particularly ONFH and DDH, are relatively poor indications for arthroscopy at this time; therefore this is one of the reasons why hip arthroscopy is relatively less developed in China.

Rates of medical intervention are also directly related to affluence. China is a poor country, with a per capita GDP of US $5445 per annum in 2011, according to the World Bank [26].

Government funding for healthcare varies locally between cities and provinces, and especially between urban and rural areas and patients attempting to attend a large hospital in a big city may not be funded if they are not residents of that city. Effectively many Chinese are essentially self-insured, and thus unwilling to pay for "lifestyle"-type medical interventions. This may change as the Chinese Government increases healthcare expenditure and encourages the development of private medical insurance.

ISAKOS and other organizations have organized hip arthroscopy courses in China with local and international instructors. Availability of cadavers is relatively good.

Presently small numbers of hip arthroscopies are being performed in China—a very crude estimate of 1000 per year in the whole of China (population 1.4 billion) is made by commercial representatives, and about 200 are performed in Hong Kong (population 7 million).

Figures in Japan, the home of modern arthroscopy, are much higher, but still low compared to Western countries.

Relatively little is being published on hip arthroscopy in the Far East—a PubMed searches for "hip arthroscopy" and "country name" produced the following total numbers of publications in September 2012: China: twelve; Hong Kong: one; Taiwan: three.

Hip Arthroscopy in DDH

DDH has been considered a relatively poor indication for hip arthroscopy. Parvizi showed poor short-term results from debridement of labral tears in acetabular dysplasia [48]. Encouragingly, pelvic osteotomy is able to salvage many dysplastic hips that had failed arthroscopic labral debridement, and the outcome of the pelvic osteotomies in patients that had prior arthroscopic labral debridement was no different from those with no prior treatment [49].

Japanese and other surgeons have used hip arthroscopy to treat acetabular labral tears associated with acetabular dysplasia with good short- to medium-term outcomes [50, 51], and assess articular cartilage prior to acetabular osteotomy [52, 53] to treat painful intra-articular pathology following osteotomy [54] and to treat intra-articular pathology synchronously with osteotomy [55]. In Japan success has been achieved with pelvic osteotomies in patients in their 40s and 50s, even with significantly reduced joint space [56, 57]. It is likely that arthroscopy will find a role in combination with pelvic osteotomy for treatment of acetabular dysplasia.

American [58] and Japanese [59] surgeons have reported arthroscopically assisted Staheli shelf procedures in Legg-Calve-Perthes and in acetabular dysplasia. The technique and results are preliminary, but the procedure is "smaller" than a pelvic osteotomy and may be attractive to arthroscopic surgeons.

Despite the technical challenges, we may see interest in arthroscopically assisted pelvic osteotomy—especially in young women who are not keen on long scars. Endoscopic techniques are at a very early stage of development [60, 61].

In the only report from China, surgeons in Harbin reported rotational acetabular osteotomy combined with arthroscopic debridement in 24 patients (29 hips) with average age of 38 years (range, 21–50 years). Twenty hips were Tonnis stage I and nine hips stage II. Twenty-four cases were followed up 4.5 years on average (range, 3–8 years). Limp disappeared in 16 hips and was improved in 8 hips. The Harris hip score was improved from 79 preoperatively to 95 postoperatively. Twenty hips at Tonnis stage I maintained their Tonnis stage after operation. Of the nine hips at Tonnis stage II, five hips improved to stage I and four hips maintained their status. They concluded that this was a worthwhile procedure even in older patients with Tonnis stage II arthritis [62].

A report from Germany of arthroscopic assisted reduction of dislocated hips in children is encouraging [63].

Hip Arthroscopy in ONFH

Professor Liu Yu-jie of the People's Liberation Army Hospital in Beijing is China's leading exponent of hip arthroscopy and is treating ONFH with arthroscopic assistance [64]. He performs small-diameter multiple drill hole core decompression for Ficat stages 1 and 2 ONFH. In patients in whom the MRI shows synovitis and/or effusion, he performs arthroscopy at the same operation. Usually this is simply a process of washing out the effusion and removing inflamed synovium.

He reports 226 ONFH patients (383 hips), 169 males (296 hips) and 57 females (87 hips), average age 36 (14–64), who underwent drilling decompression with a 3.5 mm Steinmann pin at a low velocity under image intensifier guidance. In this report 209 hips had arthroscopic debridement. 164 cases were followed up for 35 months (3–60 months). The Harris score was increased from 68 (56–78) preoperatively to 79 (58–92) postoperatively. Results were excellent in 198 of the 383 hips (69.5 %) with a Harris score >80, good in 70 hips (24.5 %) with a Harris score between 70 and 79, and poor in 17 hips (6.0 %) with a Harris score <69. These 17 hips had collapse of femoral head. 139 hips with an effusion were treated with arthroscopy, and 87 of the 139 hips underwent hip MRI during the follow-up. It was found that the effusion decreased in 59 hips and increased in ten hips. Complications were found in ten cases and all of them were recovered after treatment.

Prof Liu continues to use the technique, as he feels the risk and time of hip arthroscopy is relatively small and probably provides some benefit, but he has not performed a controlled study, so his conclusions remain anecdotal.

Hip Arthroscopy in Gluteal Muscular Contracture

Ma first reported open release of gluteal muscular contracture in the Chinese literature in 1978. Results were generally good in this [65] and a subsequent [66] series, but recovery was slow and there were various complications mainly related to hematoma. Three Chinese papers report good results of two series of arthroscopic gluteal muscular contracture release [67–69]. Palpable fibrotic bands were marked on the skin and the subcutaneous plane was developed allowing visualization of the bands, which were then released with radiofrequency probes. The procedures were as successful as historic open controls, with fewer complications, and this procedure remains in use.

Hip Arthroscopy in FAI

There is only one report from China on hip arthroscopy in FAI, coming from a specialist center in Beijing. They report 21 cases operated 2008–2009, with good results [70].

Hip Arthroscopy in OA

One paper looks at hyaluronic acid injections for early disease, arthroscopic debridement for moderate disease, and total hip replacement for advanced disease [71].

Hip Arthroscopy in Ankylosing Spondylitis

The presumed site of inflammation in the hip joint in ankylosing spondylitis is the subchondral bone marrow, which is not accessible via arthroscopy [72].

Prof Liu Yu-jie reports generally good short-term results in arthroscopic debridement of early ankylosing spondylitis 22 patients (26 hips) with average age 16 (14–19). The procedures include release of adhesions and debridement of hyperplastic synovium, degenerate cartilage debris, and exposed subchondral bone. All patients were followed up for an average of 26 (6–84) months. Most patients experienced pain relief, restored function and the range of motion. According to Harris hip joint score and VAS pain score evaluation system, the outcomes were excellent (6), fair (14), and poor (2). None of the patients had total hip replacement [73] however, follow up was short in this very young patient group, and one could expect results to deteriotate over time.

Future

The number of hip arthroscopies in China will grow with increasing recognition of hip disease in the general community, increased awareness in the medical community leading to earlier diagnosis and referral, and increasing availability of hip arthroscopists.

If a successful arthroscopic treatment is developed for ONFH and, to a lesser extent, DDH, and with increasing prevalence or recognition of FAI, hip arthroscopy will become a common procedure in China.

References

1. Yamamuro T, Ishida K. Recent advances in the prevention, early diagnosis, and treatment of congenital dislocation of the hip in Japan. Clin Orthop Relat Res. 1984;184:34–40.
2. Ying GY et al. One family investigation and risk factors analysis of developmental dysplasia of the hip. Zhonghua Yi Xue Yi Chuan Xue Za Zhi. 2007;24(1):84–7.
3. Hoaglund FT et al. Congenital hip dislocation and dysplasia in Southern Chinese. Int Orthop. 1981;4(4):243–6.
4. Ang KC et al. An epidemiological study of developmental dysplasia of the hip in infants in Singapore. Ann Acad Med Singapore. 1997;26(4):456–8.
5. Shi YY et al. The normal centre-edge angle of Wiberg in the Chinese population: a population-based cross-sectional study. J Bone Joint Surg (Br). 2010;92(8):1144–7.
6. Knoblauch A et al. Amborum Special F and ASFO--2 glucocorticoid-containing herbal remedies. Schweiz Med Wochenschr. 1989;119(22):796–802.
7. Huang WF, Wen KC, Hsiao ML. Adulteration by synthetic therapeutic substances of traditional Chinese medicines in Taiwan. J Clin Pharmacol. 1997;37(4):344–50.
8. Koh HL, Woo SO. Chinese proprietary medicine in Singapore: regulatory control of toxic heavy metals and undeclared drugs. Drug Saf. 2000;23(5):351–62.
9. Ernst E. Toxic heavy metals and undeclared drugs in Asian herbal medicines. Trends Pharmacol Sci. 2002;23(3):136–9.
10. Chan TY, Critchley JA. Usage and adverse effects of Chinese herbal medicines. Hum Exp Toxicol. 1996;15(1):5–12.
11. Miller GM, Stripp R. A study of western pharmaceuticals contained within samples of Chinese herbal/patent medicines collected from New York City's Chinatown. Leg Med (Tokyo). 2007;9(5):258–64.
12. Bogusz MJ, al Tufail M, Hassan H. How natural are 'natural herbal remedies'? A Saudi perspective. Adverse Drug React Toxicol Rev. 2002;21(4):219–29.
13. Chan K. Some aspects of toxic contaminants in herbal medicines. Chemosphere. 2003;52(9):1361–71.
14. Kahn J. China Quick to Execute Drug Official, in New York Times;2007.
15. Barboza D. 2,000 Arrested in China in Counterfeit Drug Crackdown, in New York Times;2012.
16. Lau EM et al. Hip osteoarthritis and dysplasia in Chinese men. Ann Rheum Dis. 1995;54(12):965–9.
17. Wiberg G. The anatomy and roentgenographic appearance of a normal hip joint. Acta Chir Scand. 1939;83 Suppl 58:7–38.
18. Kim HA et al. Low rate of total hip replacement as reflected by a low prevalence of hip osteoarthritis in South Korea. Osteoarthritis Cartilage. 2008;16(12):1572–5.
19. Xu L et al. High prevalence of knee, but not hip or hand osteoarthritis in Beijing elders: comparison with data of Caucasian in United States. Zhonghua Yi Xue Za Zhi. 2003;83(14):1206–9.
20. Nevitt MC et al. Very low prevalence of hip osteoarthritis among Chinese elderly in Beijing, China, compared with whites in the United States: the Beijing osteoarthritis study. Arthritis Rheum. 2002;46(7):1773–9.
21. Zeng QY et al. Rheumatic diseases in China. Arthritis Res Ther. 2008;10(1):R17.

22. Takeyama A et al. Prevalence of femoroacetabular impingement in Asian patients with osteoarthritis of the hip. Int Orthop. 2009;33(5): 1229–32.
23. Yamamura M et al. Open-configuration MRI study of femoro-acetabular impingement. J Orthop Res. 2007;25(12):1582–8.
24. Saengnipanthkul S, Techasatien W. Femoral head-neck diameter and ratio in Thais: a cadaveric study. J Med Assoc Thai. 2012;95(6):790–4.
25. Hoaglund FT, Low WD. Anatomy of the femoral neck and head, with comparative data from Caucasians and Hong Kong Chinese. Clin Orthop Relat Res. 1980;152:10–6.
26. GDP per capita. World Bank;2012.
27. Siebenrock KA et al. The cam-type deformity of the proximal femur arises in childhood in response to vigorous sporting activity. Clin Orthop Relat Res. 2011;469(11):3229–40.
28. Notzli HP et al. The contour of the femoral head-neck junction as a predictor for the risk of anterior impingement. J Bone Joint Surg (Br). 2002;84(4):556–60.
29. Kapron AL et al. Radiographic prevalence of femoroacetabular impingement in collegiate football players: AAOS Exhibit Selection. J Bone Joint Surg Am. 2011;93(19):e111(1–10).
30. Agricola R et al. The development of Cam-type deformity in adolescent and young male soccer players. Am J Sports Med. 2012;40(5):1099–106.
31. Laborie LB et al. Prevalence of radiographic findings thought to be associated with femoroacetabular impingement in a population-based cohort of 2081 healthy young adults. Radiology. 2011;260(2):494–502.
32. Johnson AC, Shaman MA, Ryan TG. Femoroacetabular impingement in former high-level youth soccer players. Am J Sports Med. 2012;40(6):1342–6.
33. Pollard TC et al. Genetic influences in the aetiology of femoroacetabular impingement: a sibling study. J Bone Joint Surg (Br). 2010;92(2):209–16.
34. Hogervorst T et al. Human hip impingement morphology: an evolutionary explanation. J Bone Joint Surg (Br). 2011;93B(6):769–76.
35. Gu GS et al. Roles of radiograph, magnetic resonance imaging, three-dimensional computed tomography in early diagnosis of femoro-acetabular impingement in 17 cases. Chin J Traumatol. 2009;12(6):375–8.
36. Nakamura Y et al. Osteochondral lesion of the femoral head in a fencer: a case report. Am J Orthop (Belle Mead NJ). 2009;38(7): 356–9.
37. Chung DC, Ko YC, Pai HH. A study on the prevalence and risk factors of muscular fibrotic contracture in Jia-Dong Township, Pingtung County, Taiwan. Gaoxiong Yi Xue Ke Xue Za Zhi. 1989;5(2):91–5.
38. Fernandez de Valderrama JA and Esteve de Miguel R. Fibrosis of the gluteus maximus: a cause of limited flexion and adduction of the hip in children. Clin Orthop Relat Res. 1981;(156): 67–78.
39. Huang Y, Li J, Lei W. [Gluteal muscle contracture: etiology, classification and treatment.] [in Chinese]. Chin J Orthop. 1999;19: 106–8.
40. Sirinelli D, Oudjhane K, Khouri N. Case report 605: Gluteal amyotrophy: a late sequela of intramuscular injection. Skeletal Radiol. 1990;19(3):221–3.
41. Peng M, Zhou Z, Zhou X. [Epidemiology of gluteal muscle contracture in Si Chuan Province] [in Chinese]. Chin J Pediatr Surg. 1989;10:356–8.
42. Sun X. An investigation on injectional gluteal muscle contracture in childhood in Mianyang City. Zhonghua Liu Xing Bing Xue Za Zhi. 1990;11(5):291–4.
43. Zhang G, Zheng Z, Fu Z. [12459 cases of gluteal muscle contracture in children] [in Chinese]. Chin J Pediatr Surg. 1990;11:363–5.
44. Zhang S et al. Similarities and differences between spondyloarthritis in Asia and other parts of the world. Curr Opin Rheumatol. 2011;23(4):334–8.
45. Ma HJ et al. Different clinical features in patients with ankylosing spondylitis from southern and northern China. Int J Rheum Dis. 2012;15(2):154–62.
46. Vander Cruyssen B et al. Hip involvement in ankylosing spondylitis: epidemiology and risk factors associated with hip replacement surgery. Rheumatology (Oxford). 2010;49(1):73–81.
47. Baraliakos X, Braun J. Hip involvement in ankylosing spondylitis: what is the verdict? Rheumatology (Oxford). 2010;49(1):3–4.
48. Parvizi J et al. Arthroscopy for labral tears in patients with developmental dysplasia of the hip: a cautionary note. J Arthroplasty. 2009;24(6 Suppl):110–3.
49. Kain MS et al. Periacetabular osteotomy after failed hip arthroscopy for labral tears in patients with acetabular dysplasia. J Bone Joint Surg Am. 2011;93 Suppl 2:57–61.
50. Yamamoto Y et al. Arthroscopic partial limbectomy in hip joints with acetabular hypoplasia. Arthroscopy. 2005;21(5):586–91.
51. Kim KI et al. Peri-acetabular rotational osteotomy with concomitant hip arthroscopy for treatment of hip dysplasia. J Bone Joint Surg (Br). 2011;93(6):732–7.
52. Yasunaga Y et al. The state of the articular cartilage at the time of surgery as an indication for rotational acetabular osteotomy. J Bone Joint Surg (Br). 2001;83(7):1001–4.
53. Fujii M et al. Effect of intra-articular lesions on the outcome of periacetabular osteotomy in patients with symptomatic hip dysplasia. J Bone Joint Surg (Br). 2011;93(11):1449–56.
54. Suzuki C et al. Repair of cartilage defects and torn acetabular labrum in hip joints after conventional osteotomy: evaluation by follow-up arthroscopy. J Orthop Sci. 2005;10(2):127–32.
55. Nakayama H et al. Arthroscopic labral repair concomitantly performed with curved periacetabular osteotomy. Knee Surg Sports Traumatol Arthrosc;2013.
56. Teratani T et al. Periacetabular osteotomy in patients fifty years of age or older. J Bone Joint Surg Am. 2010;92(1):31–41.
57. Yasunaga Y et al. Rotational acetabular osteotomy in patients forty-six years of age or older: comparison with younger patients. J Bone Joint Surg Am. 2003;85-A(2):266–72.
58. Bowen JR et al. Labral support shelf arthroplasty for containment in early stages of Legg-Calve-Perthes disease. J Pediatr Orthop. 2011;31(2 Suppl):S206–11.
59. Uchida S et al. New surgical technique of arthroscopic shelf acetabuloplasty combined with labral repair and cam osteochondroplasty for the patients with dysplasia of the hip. Boston: International Society for Hip Arthroscopy; 2012.
60. Wall EJ et al. Endoscopic pelvic osteotomy for the treatment of hip dysplasia. J Am Acad Orthop Surg. 2001;9(3):150–6.
61. Inan M, Gokce A, Ustunkan F. Endoscopy-assisted periacetabular osteotomy: a preliminary cadaveric study. Clin Orthop Relat Res. 2008;466(4):862–70.
62. Lian Y et al. Treatment of adult developmental dysplasia of the hip by rotational acetabular osteotomy combined with debridement under arthroscope. Zhongguo Xiu Fu Chong Jian Wai Ke Za Zhi. 2011;25(7):821–5.
63. Eberhardt O, Fernandez FF, Wirth T. Arthroscopic reduction of the dislocated hip in infants. J Bone Joint Surg (Br). 2012;94(6): 842–7.
64. Wang ZG et al. Clinical evaluation of small diameter decompression and arthroscopy in the treatment of early avascular necrosis of femoral head. Zhonghua Yi Xue Za Zhi. 2007;87(29): 2041–4.
65. Ma C, Fang L, Liu G. [Injection caused gluteal muscle contracture] [in Chinese]. Chin J Orthop. 1978;16:345–6.
66. Zhang K et al. [Treatment of gluteus contracture with small incision: a report of 2518 cases] [in Chinese. Chin J Orthop Trauma. 2007;20:851–2.
67. Cui JC et al. Release of gluteal muscle contracture by radiofrequency under arthroscopy. Zhong Nan Da Xue Xue Bao Yi Xue Ban. 2008;33(3):274–6.

68. Liu YJ et al. Arthroscopic gluteal muscle contracture release with radiofrequency energy. Clin Orthop Relat Res. 2009;467(3):799–804.
69. Liu YJ et al. Arthroscope monitored solution of adult intramuscular injection associated gluteal muscle contracture by radiofrequency. Zhonghua Wai Ke Za Zhi. 2008;46(13):970–2.
70. Wang WG et al. Clinical diagnosis and arthroscopic treatment of acetabular labral tears. Orthop Surg. 2011;3(1):28–34.
71. Zhao TJ et al. Grading treatment of hip osteoarthritis. Zhongguo Gu Shang. 2010;23(9):665–7.
72. Appel H et al. Immunohistochemical analysis of hip arthritis in ankylosing spondylitis: evaluation of the bone-cartilage interface and subchondral bone marrow. Arthritis Rheum. 2006;54(6):1805–13.
73. Liu YJ et al. Effect of arthroscopic debridement for adolescent ankylosing spondylitis with early hip-joint disease. Zhonghua Yi Xue Za Zhi. 2010;90(15):1048–50.

Part XIV

Practice Management and Education

Hatem Galal Said

Setting Up a Hip Arthroscopy Service

97

Richard E. Field, Parminder J. Singh, Mahalingam Karuppiah, and Omer Mei-Dan

Introduction

At present, only a tiny minority of orthopedic surgeons focus their practice exclusively on performing hip arthroscopy. For the great majority, hip arthroscopy constitutes one of the techniques that the surgeon uses to treat his, or her, patients. In consequence, a hip arthroscopy service is normally offered in parallel with other surgical interventions and the effort that a surgeon commits to this part of their practice will depend upon their desire to sub-specialise in arthroscopic hip surgery, the wishes of their colleagues and the surgeon's assessment of the opportunity to develop their hip arthroscopy service. This chapter discusses choice of practice location, the commercial viability of a hip arthroscopy practice, the types of patients that may require treatment, the different healthcare providers who may refer to the practice, communication requirements, strategic links that may be beneficial, options for patient assessment, the requirement for imaging services, the importance of data capture, provision of appropriate operating facilities, patient education and expectations, office staff and billing and the provision of contact numbers for patients and healthcare providers.

The recommendations provided in this chapter are primarily intended for surgeons who have recently completed their specialist surgical training in orthopedics, have undertaken one or more fellowships in hip arthroscopy and are looking to establish themselves as a hip surgeon with a special interest in hip arthroscopy. As joint preserving hip surgery develops we anticipate that an increasing proportion of surgeons developing an interest in hip arthroscopy will also undertake fellowships that help them to better understand sports-related injuries and recognise the conditions that are best treated by other hip preserving interventions. In addition, we hope that the chapter will help established surgeons to reflect on the structure of their existing practice and provide strategies that will help them to further develop their interest and expertise in hip arthroscopy.

R.E. Field, PhD, FRCS, FRCS(Orth) (✉)
Research, The South West London Elective Orthopaedic Centre; Epsom & St. Helier NHS Trust, St. George's University of London, London, UK
e-mail: richardefield@aol.com

P.J. Singh, MBBS, MS
Orthopaedics, Maroondah Hospital, Monash University, Clayton, VIC, Australia

M. Karuppiah, MBBS, FRCS
Consultant Orthopaedic Surgeon, Cork, Ireland

O. Mei-Dan, MD
Department of Orthopaedics, University of Colorado, Boulder, CO, USA

Practice Location

Surgeon's provision of healthcare services, their balance between public and private practice, mechanisms for procedural reimbursement and the organisation of surgeons within departmental, group or sole-trader practices vary greatly. Likewise, hospitals vary in the specialty services that they provide and the volume of work that is undertaken. Most surgeons recognise that their ability to discern and discriminate clinical conditions is acquired through education and experience. Their surgical skills are developed through training, practice and repetition. As the benefits of hip arthroscopy have been established, a growing number of orthopedic surgeons have taken up this technique. While this has helped to establish the role of hip arthroscopy, some hip surgeons have experienced difficulty with an unfamiliar technique that they use infrequently. We recommend that any surgeon seeking to establish an efficient hip arthroscopy service should aim to undertake hip arthroscopy on a weekly basis and ensure that there is a referral base to support this level of surgical activity, in their area. While some surgeons working in densely populated areas may secure a sufficient volume of cases to maintain staff skills at multiple operating sites, most surgeons are best advised to consolidate their surgery at a single operating location. This will depend also on factors such as

J.C. McCarthy et al. (eds.), *Hip Joint Restoration*, DOI 10.1007/978-1-4614-0694-5_97

the assistance provided by hospitals to promote and support a surgeon's practice. In our experience, surgeons seeking to establish a practice in joint preserving and arthroscopic hip surgery are best advised to locate their practice in highly populated urban areas. While a small subset of patients will travel to more remote locations, this is atypical and only occurs when the surgeon has acquired a broad referral network, is supported by a sophisticated rehabilitation service and is widely recognised for their expertise.

Making the Business Case

It is increasingly common, both in public and private healthcare settings, that a business case is required to demonstrate that the provision of a new service or development of an existing service will be financially viable for the hospital. In the case of hip arthroscopy, the hospital will need to weigh up the costs that will be incurred and earnings that can be achieved at each step of the patient pathway.

In many countries, economic and political pressures are driving down reimbursements for service and this increases the challenge for hospitals to obtain expensive equipment. It should be remembered that hip arthroscopy was initially developed using equipment originally intended for interventions on the knee and shoulder, while performed on a hip fracture table. While dedicated hip arthroscopy instruments generally offer some advantage, most arthroscopy procedures can still be undertaken using conventional knee and shoulder equipment. In circumstances where a surgeon encounters resistance due to lack of institutional recognition that a hip arthroscopy service would be viable, the combination of standard arthroscopic equipment and a little surgical versatility should enable a surgeon to get their practice started.

Table 97.1 is provided as an "aide memoir" to gather relevant information required to develop a hip arthroscopy business case.

Table 97.1 Factors to cost when developing a business case for a hip arthroscopy service

Service	Item	Cost	Income
Clinic	Consultations		
Imaging studies	X-rays CT scans MR studies Motion analysis		
Theatre costs	Theatre staff and training Image intensifier Hip distractor Hip arthroscopy instruments Consumables Implants Storage		
Inpatient treatment	Day-case/inpatient stays		
Pre-hab/re-hab	Physical therapy sessions Allied health services		
Practice administration	Secretarial Data collection Software support		
Marketing	Website development Seminars Literature Advertising		

The Patients

The benefits of arthroscopic hip surgery depend as much on the patients as the skills of the surgeon treating them. Surgeons starting a hip arthroscopy practice are not normally invited to treat professional sportsmen or elite athletes. They may be asked to see young adults with congenital hip deformity but the bulk of their referrals will be individuals in early middle life who aspire to retain or regain the level of physical fitness that they naturally enjoyed in their earlier adult life and individuals in their late 40s or 50s whose hips are affected by the early stages of degenerative joint disease. A degree of circumspection is commended when advising these groups on the potential benefits of arthroscopic hip surgery. It is essential that time is spent with all patients to ensure that that there is no mismatch of expectations.

The Referrers

A cornerstone of any successful clinical practice is the referral base that directs patients for a specialist opinion and treatment. As a general rule, medical and surgical conditions that have been treated for decades or centuries tend to have referral pathways through primary care/community physicians. Where treatments are relatively new and may not have been included on a medical school curriculum, such referral pathways are usually less well developed. While the primary care/community physicians are gradually gaining familiarity with the ideas driving early intervention, joint preserving and arthroscopic hip surgery, a large proportion of hip arthroscopy patients continue to be referred through allied health professionals. Either way, one of the most important steps for a surgeon starting a hip arthroscopy practice is to get out and visit potential referrers and explain how hip joints can be damaged by injuries associated with femoro-acetabular impingement, how to recognise such problems and what can be done to treat these problems. It is also important to explain to referrers that conservative treatments are usually most effective when the underlying problem has been correctly diagnosed. Also, when surgery is required, delayed intervention inevitably means a more damaged joint and a less satisfactory outcome.

The advent of the Internet and the development of hip arthroscopy occurred at much the same time. In consequence, much of the information that is available on hip arthroscopy can be sourced through the web. Unlike diseases of advancing age, the groups for whom hip arthroscopy is most appropriate are generally Internet savvy and will seek information on their medical conditions from the web; before or in parallel with any approach to the medical profession. In consequence, a significant proportion of patients will present equipped with information that they have acquired from Internet forums and chat rooms. Surgeons should be aware that these individuals tend to have more knowledge of the best and worst of other patients' experiences and may remain relatively uninformed on the investigations that are needed to achieve a correct diagnosis and the treatment options that may need to be considered.

Physical therapists, osteopaths, chiropractors, personal trainers, Pilates instructors and other therapists will have seen and treated the majority of patients presenting as potential candidates for hip arthroscopy. It will have been identified that their symptoms have not improved with treatment and may have been exacerbated by therapies that would normally help individuals with soft tissue strains. Surgeons seeking to develop a hip arthroscopy practice are advised to develop links with local allied healthcare professionals both to explain the conditions that can be treated by hip arthroscopy and to establish a line of communication to ensure that patients are optimally prepared for surgery and rehabilitated after their discharge from hospital. It should always be remembered that when an allied healthcare professional recommends a patient to see a surgeon, the referring therapist should be kept informed of all stages of the patient's treatment and involved wherever possible in the patient's rehabilitation after any surgical intervention.

Surgeons wishing to develop a hip arthroscopy service to support professional sportsmen, sportswomen and elite athletes should seek out and develop links with sports physicians and club physical therapists. These groups are experienced in identifying patients who are failing to progress with conservative therapy and most likely to benefit from a surgical intervention. Sports physicians and club therapists are also well equipped to support patients after surgery; both to optimise the patient for surgery, manage patient expectations and ensure a smooth return to sporting activity. However, surgeons should be aware that this is a relatively niche market. Professional sportsmen, sportswomen and elite athletes are amongst the best educated and best advised regarding their hip conditions. In consequence, the surgeon will need to demonstrate that they are recognised within the hip arthroscopy community, that they have an established track record of surgical experience, relevant publications and that they are able to coordinate a multidisciplinary treatment programme.

As hip arthroscopy becomes more familiar to primary care and community physicians, an increasing proportion of referrals will be derived from this source. The fact that hip arthroscopy is not part of every orthopedic surgeon's armamentarium of surgical expertise may not be understood and invitations to address primary care or community physician meetings provides a valuable opportunity to explain what hip arthroscopy entails, how to identify appropriate patients and to develop lines of communication with these colleagues.

Securing referrals from other orthopedic surgeons can be challenging. In departments where surgeons have defined areas of expertise, cross-referral from colleagues subspecialising in other areas is usually perceived as advantageous for all parties. However, many hip arthroscopists experience a degree of reticence from local hip surgeons to refer patients. Whether this is due to a belief that hip arthroscopy is a waste of time or a fear that the referring surgeon will be perceived as a less competent hip surgeon is a matter for speculation.

Finally, it is always worth discussing your plans with the business development officer at your hospital.

Communication

Communication is a cornerstone of any successful clinical service. All orthopedic departments and most independent surgeons provide website information for patients. Anecdotal feedback indicates that websites are most effective when they provide a combination of information on the conditions that a surgeon treats, downloadable advice sheets for postoperative rehabilitation, and evidence that the surgeon is well established in their advertised field of expertise. Some surgeons also make videos of their work available through YouTube, VuMedi and similar content providers. Regulations on direct advertising of a surgeon's services to the general public vary from country to country.

Relevant publications in peer-reviewed journals, book chapters and presentations at meetings are clear evidence that a surgeon is actively contributing to their chosen discipline and provide reassurance to patients and referrers. In addition, articles written for professions allied to medicine will help raise the surgeon's profile amongst potential referring communities.

Regular attendance of national and international hip arthroscopy meetings is essential. The knowledge gained from such exposure will ensure that the surgeon remains "au fait" with current opinion, knowledge and surgical techniques. Also, it will enable the surgeon to develop a network of colleagues who are undertaking similar work and can be contacted for advice. At a local level, speaking at meetings for primary care/community physicians, physical therapists and other allied healthcare professions offer a useful opportunity to become better known in the local healthcare community and provide insights into the individuals who are best able to provide community support for patients.

Physical therapists and other healthcare professionals taking part in a patient's care frequently request to attend clinic consultations and surgery, particularly when they have referred the patients. The patient's permission should always be secured prior to guests attending an operation and adherence to local hospital regulations is essential.

Strategic Links

No surgeon can provide a hip arthroscopy service in isolation and one of the first tasks is to identify the individuals who will help support the hip arthroscopy service. Foremost among these are musculoskeletal radiologists. Regular meetings to discuss cases and to establish the imaging studies that should be undertaken, the views that are most helpful and the desired information that should be provided in reports are essential. Many patients will present with imaging studies from other hospitals. It is not infrequent for a patient to present with a stack of CDs containing a range of studies that have been undertaken elsewhere. Radiology reports on such investigations are often unavailable. Regular meetings with a radiology colleague will provide an opportunity to review such studies and ensure that abnormalities are not overlooked.

Surgery is facilitated by a well-trained theatre team who know what equipment is required, where to get it, how to use it and are familiar with the way that their surgeon operates. The theatre team must be drilled on patient set-up, image intensifier and stack positioning, patient draping, and the instruments and sequence of steps that the surgeon will employ for each step of the surgical procedure. Consistent and experienced theatre staff, who are keen to be involved, will transform a potentially long, stressful and challenging procedure into an enjoyable experience which does not waste valuable operating room time.

Other key members of a multidisciplinary support team are the ward nurses and physical therapists who see the patients during their inpatient stay, if the patient stays overnight. These therapists must provide the patients with clear instructions for their early mobilisation, reassurance regarding early wound leakage and be available to communicate with their community colleagues on rehabilitation milestones and expectations.

When a surgeon considers setting up a hip arthroscopy service, they will need a range of surgical equipment that may be unavailable in their hospital and unfamiliar to the operating department staff. It is important to meet with the local and regional representatives of the instrument and implant suppliers. It is equally important to ensure that the operating department staff know how and when to contact them. Good company representatives will train the operating department staff to use their products and should be willing to attend surgery until the operating department staff are familiar with new equipment and its use.

As previously identified, some surgeons may have the opportunity to develop their hip arthroscopy service to treat sportsmen, sportswomen and elite athletes. In such circumstances, a working relationship should be developed with local sports physicians and links should be forged with local sports clubs and organisations. Surgeons, physical therapists and coaches should communicate regularly to agree when it is safe for a patient to progress to sports-specific training and work together to develop injury prevention strategies for the future.

Patient Assessment

No special clinic or office facilities are required to set up a hip arthroscopy service. Indeed, the majority of surgeons will see hip arthroscopy patients amongst the general casemix of their outpatient consultations. If the surgeon's referral base permits, it is preferable to set up specialist clinics dedicated to the investigation and management of designated patient subgroups; for example, a "young adult hip" or a "sports hip" clinic. This approach has two advantages. Firstly, staff supporting the clinic will become familiar with the specific needs of the attending patients, the questionnaires and measurements that need to be collected and the investigations that are most commonly requested. Secondly, colleagues sharing a special interest in the clinical conditions being seen, for example a sports physician or surgical fellow, will be more interested to attend or assist with the outpatient service. In consequence, the surgeon will have immediate access to colleagues who can advise and contribute to the patient's treatment plan.

Imaging Facilities

Every surgeon setting up a hip arthroscopy service must be able to access key imaging studies as well as develop a sound working rapport with radiologists skilled in the interpretation of hip-related studies. Plain radiographs provide a rapid and helpful first assessment of hip joint structure. Time must be invested to ensure that the radiographers know exactly which views are required and how these are best taken. Time should be spent with a radiology colleague to agree how CT scans are undertaken and reported to provide the most helpful views, reconstructions and measurements. Likewise, MR sequences, slice thicknesses, slice intervals and scan orientations should be agreed to obtain consistent and meaningful results. Also, when MR arthrography is undertaken, the combination of contrast materials and whether the radiologist will include local anaesthetic should be discussed and agreed. Likewise, when hip blocks are undertaken, what combination of local anaesthetic and steroid should be used and which daily sheets should be given to patients to document the extent and duration of any change in their symptoms after the block.

Data Capture

A growing number of practice software packages are available with outcome questionnaires that enable tablet and email links to be used for direct data entry by staff and patients. It is strongly recommended that every surgeon starting a hip arthroscopy practice implements a robust data capture process, from the outset. A surgeon who does not collect and review outcome data will never properly understand the effect of their work or be able to appraise their interventions. They will not be able to advise patients on likely outcomes under their care and will only be able to quote from the published literature. They will never be able to share their experience with the wider community and will not have any data for trainees to review. A number of different outcome scores are in common usage and each has its advocates (see Chap. 86). It is recommended by ISHA that the IHOT outcome scoring system be utilised since it is validated in 3 languages and is used by the majority of high-volume hip arthroscopists currently.

Operating Facilities

Hip arthroscopy can be a challenging procedure and is made more difficult in a cramped operating room. It is a foolish surgeon who tries to work in an operating room that cannot properly accommodate the anaesthetic equipment, image intensifier, hip distractor, equipment trolleys and personnel. Once a suitable operating room has been identified, it is important to provide training for the operating room staff. If the theatre team have experience working with other hip arthroscopists, it is prudent to spend a little time with them to identify any differences in your set-up, equipment requirements and techniques. Operating department managers generally try to ensure that the great majority of their staff are familiar with the different equipment and procedures that are undertaken in their department. While this strategy may ensure that staff-leave, sickness and turnover do not compromise the department's ability to support surgery, it is usually advantageous to develop a core team's expertise in hip arthroscopy before seeking to involve other operating department staff.

When hip arthroscopy is being introduced as a new procedure, it is helpful to provide diagrams and photographs that show how the theatre equipment should be positioned. Instructions should be provided on preferred settings for pumps, diathermy plate positioning and radiofrequency probe settings. It is important to train the theatre staff in patient positioning, set up for distraction equipment and draping strategies to best avoid soaking the patient, operating couch and theatre floor.

In the early days of hip arthroscopy, many surgeons may do with relatively few instruments. As hip arthroscopic techniques have developed, instruments have evolved and been refined to facilitate the different surgical interventions that are now commonly undertaken. In the early stages of a hip arthroscopy service, it is normal for the hospital to hire in the equipment that the surgeon requests. Most hospitals have their own 30° arthroscopes. While 30° arthroscopes do have a role in hip arthroscopy, 70° arthroscopes scopes are used most commonly. A surgeon wishing to establish a hip arthroscopy service should ensure that the purchase of two 70° arthroscopes is put at the top of any shopping list for hip arthroscopy equipment. When these are hired, there is a risk that the lens may have been damaged and there are few more frustrating experiences than looking at a fuzzy view of the hip joint.

Several companies provide hip arthroscopy instrument sets. It is important that the surgeon finds out which instruments are provided in each set and ensures that the operating department is instructed on which instruments, consumables and implants are required for each case; also, whether company representatives should be invited to attend. As patient numbers grow and the team gains familiarity with the equipment and techniques that are used in hip arthroscopy, it may become economically sensible for the surgeon or the hospital to purchase their own hip arthroscopy equipment. While each surgeon will develop specific equipment preferences, it is useful to have a shopping list of equipment so that the surgeon or hospital can build up their equipment over time.

While dedicated hip arthroscopy instruments and equipment are desirable, it should be remembered that hip arthroscopy evolved using knee and shoulder instruments and equipment. Approximately 90 % of hip arthroscopy procedures can be undertaken using standard shavers, burrs, anchors and instruments.

Patient Education and Expectations

Almost all patients undergoing hip arthroscopy will have "researched" their condition on the Internet and will have acquired information on how hip arthroscopy will affect their life. While "home research" means that some patients are well informed, a proportion may have unrealistic expectations or inappropriate anxieties. When a hip arthroscopy service is first started, the surgeon will be seeing relatively few patients. This provides an opportunity to spend time with the patients discussing the preparations that they need to make for surgery, providing advice on how long they will need to take off work, avoid car driving and other adaptations that they will need to make to their life. Post-operatively the surgeon will need to gain familiarity with the rate at which the arthroscopy portal wounds heal, the challenges that their patients encounter and the contribution of physical therapists. Many hospitals now publish advice to patients on their websites and an Internet search will provide any number of patient information sheets. As these evolve, surgeons are advised to review such information on a regular basis so as to be able to provide patients with up-to-date guidance on where to download their instruction sheets. As patient numbers grow, this experience will allow the surgeon to put together their own information sheets on hip pathologies, diagnoses, pre-hab, surgery, rehab and return to sporting activities. Once developed, such information sheets can be made available for the patients to download from the surgeon's website.

Office Staff and Billing

A surgeon's secretarial and administrative team provide the day-to-day interface for communication with patients, allied health professionals, outpatient, operating room and ward staff, and healthcare insurance companies. Any surgeon setting up a hip arthroscopy practice must understand that it can take years to build up the knowledge base required to coordinate the various stages of a patient's treatment and to ensure that the correct information has been provided to the correct party, at the correct time.

Billing for hip arthroscopy services varies between healthcare systems and patient communities. Whatever the local billing environment, accurate coding for hip arthroscopy and related procedures can be facilitated by regular contact between surgeon and the coding team. It is also important to keep abreast of any changes to the codes being used for hip arthroscopy.

Contact Numbers for Patients and Healthcare Professionals

Each healthcare system will have different rules and expectations for contact between patients and their healthcare team. Whatever the local customs, it is essential that all patients are provided with a telephone number to call 24/7 if they experience problems or complications. Local circumstances will dictate whether this is to the hospital at which the patient was treated, the surgeon's office staff or the surgeon.

Summary

The steps required to set up a hip arthroscopy practice depend upon whether you are planning to work in a group of established hip arthroscopists or you are looking to establish a new single surgeon service. Over the last decade, the orthopedic, radiology, primary healthcare and physical therapy communities have begun to recognise that patients can be treated effectively by arthroscopic hip surgery. However, a consensus on the procedures that are cost-effective remains to be proven. Wherever you intend to work, a business case should be developed to identify the equipment and staff that will be required, the costs that will be incurred and the income that can be generated.

It is essential to identify the groups of patients that could be treated in your practice and that you establish contact with healthcare professionals who would refer these patients to you. It is important to remember that the local healthcare community may take some time to recognise your specialist expertise and the merit of sending their patients to you.

Listed below are our ten top tips for establishing a successful hip arthroscopy practice:

1. Ensure that you have undertaken at least one Hip Arthroscopy Fellowship.
2. Consider a Sports Surgery Fellowship and ensure that you have acquired a sound understanding of other hip preserving interventions.
3. Join an established practice that needs another surgeon or ensure that there is a robust business case for a new service. A new service is most likely to succeed in a highly populated urban area.
4. Establish referral paths to your service. Visit and talk to potential referrers to explain the conditions that you treat and what you can do for their patients.
5. Ensure that your operating room staff are properly trained and equipped.
6. Develop a multidisciplinary team to educate patients before surgery and support their recovery after surgery. Provide written information sheets for every step of the patient journey. These should be accessible from your website.
7. Attend conferences to keep up to date with developments in hip arthroscopy.
8. Attend a cadaver lab once or twice a year to extend your surgical repertoire and visit other surgeons to learn their tips and tricks.
9. Document your work and audit your results on a regular basis.
10. Join ISHA so that you are able to develop your own national and international network of hip arthroscopists.

98 Education and Hip Arthroscopy

Richard N. Villar

Introduction

There was a time when so few practitioners performed hip arthroscopy that the need for any form of education programme seemed unnecessary. However, hip arthroscopic surgery has now entered the mainstream of orthopedic practice and with that finding come responsibilities. The key responsibility falls upon the surgeon for his patient; however, there is also a responsibility on the shoulders of trainers to ensure that the surgeons they teach are able to perform to a satisfactory level. That means that not only do surgeons need to remain updated but so do their trainers. There are some excellent surgeons who sadly lack teaching ability. Meanwhile, there are some excellent trainers who have suboptimal surgical skills.

In addition to the respective responsibilities of surgeons and trainers, litigation in hip arthroscopy is becoming more frequent. Evidence of suitable training may be demanded by the Courts and is already being required by certain healthcare insurers around the world in order to justify reimbursement.

These changes, which have occurred quite rapidly in recent years, imply that an unstructured approach to training in hip arthroscopy may have once been permissible but now, with these various pressures, a more structured, balanced and tiered education programme should be considered.

With the assistance of colleagues from around the world, a comprehensive educational programme in practical hip arthroscopic surgery has been developed. The aim has been to produce a cadre of technically proficient hip arthroscopic surgeons. This programme was introduced initially in the United Kingdom, with the strong support of industry partners, but has now begun to slowly spread further afield. Surgery is, after all, a manual job undertaken by generally highly educated individuals. Ultimately, a patient needs to know they are in the hands of a good technical operator once anaesthesia has been induced. However intellectually advantaged their surgeon may be, it is how the operation proceeds on the day that counts.

Endoscopic Skills and Learning Curves

Endoscopic skills have long been thought to be different to those talents required for open surgery. Open surgeons do not always make good arthroscopic ones, and vice versa. Orthopedic surgery is not alone in this finding. Rayl for example, in the ENT literature in 1976, summarised the situation by saying 'an educational training need has developed as a result of the recent rapidly increasing acquisition of endoscopes' and supported the value of what was described as the television medium as an educational adjunct in teaching endoscopy [1]. Although this particular paper applied to the Veterans Administration in the United States of America, this was clearly a global problem as shown by Chaturachinda in 1980 [2] who undertook a retrospective study of the use of the laparoscope in rural Thailand in the mid-1970s. The results showed that despite training, up to 46 % of the physicians surveyed were endoscopically inactive, most of them because they encountered major surgical complications during their endoscopic procedures. Low rates of instrument use, sometimes as low as 2 h each month, simply did not allow sufficient time to maintain skill level or confidence in the technique.

It is perhaps fair to say that the skill required to undertake hip arthroscopic surgery is only partly related to the ability required to perform arthroscopy of other joints. The hip is more deep-seated than most other joints and the so-called 'fulcrum effect' certainly applies. The fulcrum effect describes the loss of tactile feedback given by an instrument when the bulk of the operating end is within the patient and only a small portion protrudes from the skin. For example, with a knee arthroscopy, the bulk of the arthroscope is outside the patient during surgery, as the soft-tissue structures are

R.N. Villar, MS, FRCS (✉)
Villar Bajwa Practice, Spire Cambridge Lea Hospital, Cambridge CB24 9EL, UK
e-mail: rnv1000@aol.com

J.C. McCarthy et al. (eds.), *Hip Joint Restoration*, DOI 10.1007/978-1-4614-0694-5_98

relatively near to the surface. For the hip, the situation is different. The bulk of the arthroscope during a procedure is within the patient and only a small portion stands outside. The fulcrum effect is thus much greater. In addition, most hip arthroscopic surgeons would favour the use of a 70° arthroscope, because of its wide field of view. This is a very different device to the 30° instrument used by the majority of arthroscopic surgeons who operate on joints elsewhere in the body. Gallagher et al. [3], in their paper on the acquisition of endoscopic skills, summarise the situation well when they say that although the loss of three-dimensional visual depth cues has been thought to be the main hindrance to the acquisition of endoscopic skills, in actual fact the fulcrum effect has a major detrimental influence on surgical endoscopic ability.

Much debate is also held around learning curves, how long it takes to acquire certain technical skills, how many need to be performed to remain up to date and how long it can take for skills to decline. It is widely accepted that hip arthroscopic surgery has a lengthy learning curve. This is not unique to the hip, as shown by Jackson et al. [4] in their paper on simulated arthroscopic meniscal repair. Here they noted that their study group of 19 orthopedic residents demonstrated a clear learning curve and that although some residents had reached a learning plateau by 12 episodes, others continued to make further improvement for another nine episodes. Importantly, residents did not lose any skill over a 6-month break in task performance. For hip arthroscopy, the learning curve proposed by Konan, Rhee and Haddad was approximately 30 cases [5].

How best to provide suitable training has also been debated. As discussed by Atesok et al. [6], current working restrictions on trainees force them to acquire more complex surgical skills in a shorter period of time. Laboratory-based training certainly offers potential benefits even if the current evidence supporting its educational advantage in orthopedics is still limited. That said, Pollard et al. [7] have also stated that trainees are likely to benefit from simulator training before performing hip arthroscopy on patients so the development of a laboratory-based training programme does make sense.

Training Courses

The development of official training courses is gradually beginning to expand globally and across the surgical specialties [8, 9]. Hip surgery is not alone in witnessing an endoscopic explosion. Suggested guidelines do now exist for the practice of arthroscopic surgery, not just for the hip, in which training in both diagnostic and operative arthroscopy is encouraged [10]. Of course, not every surgeon who wishes to undertake hip arthroscopy will necessarily be able to perform it. Work by Alvand et al. [11], looking at the training of medical students by using two simulated arthroscopic tasks, one on the shoulder and one on the knee, was fascinating. They suggested that there were some individuals who were unable to achieve competence despite focussed training. Hip arthroscopy may thus not be for everyone.

Although in previous decades it may have been understandable, possibly even acceptable, for a surgeon to dream up a new idea and launch straight into their first patient, times have certainly changed. Consequently, a phased and structured approach to training in hip arthroscopy has much to commend it. Yet how much should be taught and when?

In the United Kingdom, and now slowly rolling out worldwide, a three-phase system of training is encouraged. There are three levels – 1, 2, and 3. Each level has specific entry criteria for a delegate and each has a set syllabus with a balance of theoretical and practical components. As a delegate progresses through the levels, so the amount of theory lessens while the practical component increases. This teaching programme is cadaver-based.

Level 1

For a Level 1 entrant, the only criterion for attendance is a desire to undertake hip arthroscopy. The delegate attends a 2-day course, which comprises 30 % theory and 70 % practical techniques. The Faculty-to-Delegate ratio is 1:2. Delegates are taught both lateral and supine positions, irrespective of how they envisage operating on their patients. After all, how can surgeons properly decide which approach to use if they have no personal experience of hip arthroscopy? With this Level 1 course, delegates have the opportunity to decide for themselves, as what is good for one surgeon is not always good for another.

Level 2

For a Level 2 course, the requirements for entry increase. Delegates are expected to have completed a Level 1 course, or their national equivalent, before studying for Level 2. They must undertake 15 hip arthroscopic procedures as the primary operator before attending, have visited a high-volume hip arthroscopy unit, show evidence of data collection and should use a recognised surgical outcome measure. A Level 2 course is a 1-day event, has a 20 %:80 % theory-to-practical split and a 1:4 Faculty-to-Delegate ratio.

Level 3

For a Level 3 course, the criteria for entry change still further. Now a delegate is expected to have completed a Level 2 course, or their national equivalent, before attending.

They should have undertaken a further 40 hip arthroscopies as the primary operator. This course is a 1-day event, has a 10 %:90 % theory-to-practical split and a 1:6 Faculty-to-Delegate ratio. A Level 3 course is a more hands-on event with a lower level of Faculty supervision.

The outline of each course follows a set pattern, even if the content is different. Lectures are kept to a minimum and are rarely more than 10 min in length. Each lecture relates in part to the practical session that follows. Each practical comprises a sequence of set techniques that must be completed by the end of that practical session. Meanwhile, the Faculty member present must sign that they have instructed a specific technique and, notably, that the delegates are proficient in the procedure. So-called 'tick sheets' are provided for this purpose. Once all recommended techniques have been taught, all have been undertaken satisfactorily and all lectures attended, only then is a certificate issued. There are two certificates available. The first simply states that the delegate attended the course. The second, and the one most highly sought by delegates, states that the course has been 'satisfactorily completed'.

The content of each course is based on the views of 60 hip arthroscopic surgeons from around the world. Each was asked their opinion about the complexity of a variety of hip arthroscopic procedures on a scale of 1–4, 1 being simple and 4 being highly complex. The end result was a list of hip arthroscopic procedures ranging in complexity from a mean of 0.93–4. The value below 1 is a result of a small number of advisers failing to give their view on all procedures. However, this list of mean values then allowed the content of each course to be developed in order of increasing complexity as a delegate passes through the three levels of training.

These courses have been well received by both delegates and Faculty and represent what is felt to be a positive step in the development of hip arthroscopic surgery. Surgeons need the opportunity to gain experience without patients being compromised. The hip arthroscopic community as a whole must also be able to say that it is looking after its own and is striving for still better standards.

References

1. Rayl J. Educational training in endoscopy. Ann Otol Rhinol Laryngol. 1976;85(5 Pt.1):627–30.
2. Chaturachinda K. The use of the laparoscope in rural Thailand. J Thai Assoc Volunt Steriliz. 1980;2:73–82.
3. Gallagher A, McCure N, McGuigan J, Ritchie K, Sheehy N. An ergonomic analysis of the fulcrum effect in the acquisition of endoscopic skills. Endoscopy. 1998;30(7):617–20.
4. Jackson W, Khan T, Alvand A, Al-Ali S, Gill H, Price A, et al. Learning and retaining simulated arthroscopic meniscal repair skills. J Bone Joint Surg Am. 2012;94(17):e1321–8.
5. Konan S, Rhee S-J, Haddad FS. Hip arthroscopy: analysis of a single surgeon's learning experience. J Bone Joint Surg. 2011; 93(Supplement 2):52–6.
6. Atesok K, Mabrey J, Jazrawi L, Egol K. Surgical simulation in orthopaedic skills training. J Am Acad Orthop Surg. 2012;20(7): 410–22.
7. Pollard T, Khan T, Price A, Gill H, Glyn-Jones S, Rees J. Simulated hip arthroscopy skills: learning curves with the lateral and supine patient positions: a randomized trial. J Bone Joint Surg Am. 2012;94(10):e68.
8. Fujishiro M, Jung H, Goda K, Hirasawa K, Kakushima N, Lee I, et al. Desirable training and roles of Japanese endoscopists towards the further penetration of endoscopic submucosal dissection in Asia. Dig Endosc. 2012;24 Suppl 1:121–3.
9. Sedlack RE, Kolars JC, Alexander JA. Computer simulation training enhances patient comfort during endoscopy. Clin Gastroenterol Hepatol. 2004;2(4):348–52.
10. Committee on Ethics and Standards, Arthroscopy Association of North America, Board of Directors of the Arthroscopy Association of North America. Suggested guidelines for the practice of arthroscopic surgery. Arthroscopy. 2011;27(9):A30.
11. Alvand A, Auplish S, Khan T, Gill H, Rees J. Identifying orthopaedic surgeons of the future: the inability of some medical students to achieve competence in basic arthroscopic tasks despite training: a randomised study. J Bone Joint Surg (Br). 2011;93(12): 1586–91.

Part XV

Research

Josip Nenad Cakic

Development Anatomy and Its Impact on Hip Function

99

Amardeep Singh and Paul E. Beaulé

Introduction

The adult hip emerges over the course of development as an articulation between the head of the femur and the acetabulum where structural changes in either one affect the responsive growth of the other. More importantly, because the development of the hip involves multiple functionally separate growth plates, i.e. capital femoral epiphysis, lesser trochanter and greater trochanter combined with the complex cartilaginous components of the acetabulum, it is more susceptible to vascular compromise as well as traumatic injury which will vary depending on patient age, i.e. stage of development. This is reflected by the various childhood hip disorders: hip dysplasia, Legg-Calve-Perthes disease, slipped capital femoral epiphysis, and femoroacetabular impingement. This is of significance as abnormal morphology of the hip can predispose the joint to particular patterns of cartilage injury and the development of osteoarthritic changes [1].

Evolution of the Hip

As the environments changed, walking on two legs helped early humans survive by making it easier to pick fruits and other food from low-lying branches; freeing hands for carrying food, tools, or babies; enabling early humans to appear larger and intimidating; helping early humans cover wide, open landscapes quickly and efficiently. Consequently, the evolution of hip joint provides an anatomic basis for upright posture and balanced locomotion and designed for both strength and mobility. In contrast to other species, the shape of the reptilian femur is cylindrical and its proximal articular surface is in line with the long axis of the shaft. Mammals have greater range of motion of the limbs, with a femoral head that is offset from the shaft allowing greater flexibility. In some mammals, including humans, the femoral head and greater trochanter have emerged as separate ossification centres within a common cartilaginous epiphysis and remain separate throughout. In other species, these secondary centres join to form a single osseous epiphysis [2].

Hogervorst et al. [3, 4] have proposed two types of hip joints, coxa recta and coxa rotunda, which encompass the morphology of nearly all the mammalian hips forming a spectrum rather than a dichotomy (Fig. 99.1). Coxa recta is characterised by a straight or aspherical section on the femoral head or head–neck junction and is seen mostly in runners and jumpers while coxa rotunda has a round femoral head with ample head neck offset, and seen mostly in climbers and swimmers. Because the humans moved from climbing to running during evolution, this can explain some of the variable anatomical shapes seen in young adults with mechanical problems of the hip.

Embryology and Development

The hip joint develops from mesenchymal cells that form both the acetabulum and the femoral head with differentiation that starts at 7 weeks, followed by the appearance of a cleft in the pre-cartilaginous cells forming the hip joint by 11 weeks [5]. This initial condensation becomes surrounded by connective tissue that forms the synovial tissue lining the future joint cavity. After birth, the further growth of the acetabulum and the proximal femur is interdependent. The growth and maturation of the acetabulum requires a spherical femoral head as a template for spherical growth [6] and conversely, the development of a spherical femoral head requires a critical minimal amount of acetabular coverage [7]

A. Singh, MBBS, MS
Division of Orthopaedic Surgery, University of Ottawa, Ottawa, ON, Canada

Orthopaedic Surgery, The Ottawa Hospital, Ottawa, ON, Canada

P.E. Beaulé, MD, FRCSC (✉)
Orthopaedic Surgery Division, Surgery Department, University of Ottawa; The Ottawa Hospital, Ottawa, ON, Canada
e-mail: pbeaule@ottawahospital.on.ca

J.C. McCarthy et al. (eds.), *Hip Joint Restoration*, DOI 10.1007/978-1-4614-0694-5_99

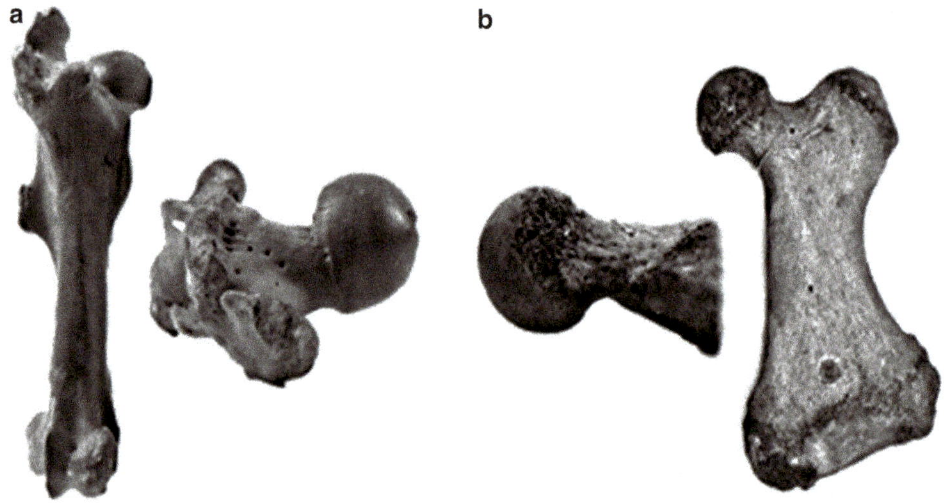

Fig. 99.1 Coxa recta in a horse (**a**) and coxa rotunda in a walrus (**b**). The horse coxa recta has a straight section of the femoral head superodorsally and an asymmetrical position of the femoral head relative to the neck, resulting in a shallow concavity on one side of the femoral head/neck junction. The coxa rotunda of the walrus demonstrates a round femoral head, positioned more symmetrically on a longer femoral neck and resulting in deeper concavity all round. From Hogervorst T. Osteoarthritis: A Consequence of Human Evolution? Bone & Joint360 2012;1(1):2-6. Reprinted with permission [55]

since hips with different degrees of acetabular coverage are associated with changes in proximal femoral morphology. More specifically, a deep acetabulum is associated with a more spherical head shape, increased epiphyseal height with a pronounced extension of the epiphysis towards the femoral neck, and an increased offset. In contrast, dysplastic hips are associated with an elliptical femoral head, decreased epiphyseal height with a less pronounced extension of the epiphysis, and decreased head–neck offset [8].

Development of Acetabulum

The acetabulum develops from the pubis anteriorly, the ilium superiorly and the ischium inferiorly. Cartilage covers the outer two-thirds of the acetabulum, with the medial wall formed by the triradiate cartilage and part of the ilium superiorly and the ischium inferiorly [9]. The triradiate cartilage forms the primary growth centre of the acetabulum and is the common physis of the pubis, ilium and ischium. It assumes a Y shape, consisting of three cartilaginous arms: (1) an anterior, slightly superiorly slanted arm dividing the ilium and the pubis, (2) a posterior horizontal arm separating the ilium and the ischium, and (3) an inferior, near vertical arm located between the ischium and pubis. Within the triradiate cartilage, the physis is bipolar, with hypertrophic zones extending from the central germinal zone toward each metaphysis. The outer cartilaginous aspect of the acetabulum is comparable to the cartilaginous epiphyses elsewhere in the axial skeleton and is responsible for expansion of the acetabulum with growth.

The articulating surface of the acetabulum is made up of very cellular hyaline cartilage, which grows through appositional growth under the perichondrium and interstitial growth in the cartilage [9]. The labrum is a fibro-cartilaginous rim attached to the lateral margin of the acetabular cartilage. The labrum is triangular in cross-section, with the base attached to the acetabular margin and the apex a free edge, and acts to deepen the cup of the acetabulum. Early degenerative changes are often first seen in the anterior acetabular chondro-labral junction, hence literature references to the 'watershed lesion' [10]. McCarthy et al. proposed that a labral tear may alter the biomechanical environment of the hip leading to degeneration of the articular cartilage and eventual osteoarthritis [11]. Similarly, Cashin et al. [12] identified consistent differences between the anterior and posterior acetabular chondro-labral complexes throughout embryological development. The anterior labrum was found to have marginal attachment to the acetabular margin with its collagen fibres oriented parallel to the chondro-labral junction. This is expected to render the anterior labrum less likely to withstand shearing forces and more prone to damage than the posterior labrum in which the collagen fibres are anchored to the acetabular cartilage. Finally, insufficient development of the anterior labrum can lead to intra-articular impingement to a prominent limbus where the anterior labrum has failed to fully retract from the articular surface.

The acetabular notch forms the inferior aspect of the acetabulum and is spanned by the transverse acetabular ligament which is a fibrous continuation of the labrum. The capsule of the hip joint attaches to the acetabular margin and is continuous with the labrum on the intracapsular side and with the periosteum of the pelvis. The depth of the acetabulum increases during its development and relies on several factors. First and foremost is the presence of a spherical femoral head in conformity with the weight-bearing surface, as loading of the acetabular surface stimulates deepening of the socket. Experimental studies using animal models have shown that after excision of the femoral head, the acetabulum fails to develop leading to atrophy of the cartilaginous tissue [13].

The acetabular cartilage and surrounding bone must also grow normally. The primary ossification centres of the pubis, ilium and ischium meet in the acetabulum at puberty, with a Y-shaped portion of cartilage separating them. The os acetabuli appears around this time and acts as the epiphysis of the pubis, ossifying and forming the anterior wall of the acetabulum. The epiphyses of the ilium and ischium undergo a similar process and contribute to further growth and deepening. Although the most commonly used markers of skeletal age are the hand and wrist and the iliac apophysis (Risser sign), Sanders et al. [14, 15] found the status of the triradiate cartilage to be more predictive for the timing of the peak growth velocity of total body height. The predictive value of open triradiate cartilages is less clear but once the patient has closed triradiate cartilages, he or she is very likely past the pubertal growth spurt.

Development of the Femur

The ossification of femur occurs through five centres—the shaft, the distal end, the head, and the greater and lesser trochanters. The shaft is largely ossified at birth but the proximal femur is mostly cartilage. The proximal femoral ossification centre develops between the 4th and 7th months of age. The proximal femur has three physes—the proximal femur physeal plate, the greater trochanter growth plate and, as a continuation between them, the growth plate of the femoral neck isthmus [7, 16] (Fig. 99.2). The proximal femur and the greater trochanter grow by appositional proliferation of cartilage cells [17]. The shape of the femoral neck is dependent upon the balance achieved between the longitudinal and slightly medial growth of the proximal femur via its physeal plate, and the lateral growth arising from the trochanteric growth plate and the femoral neck isthmus [18]. And following Ward's principle there is a balance of compressive forces on the capital physis with tensile forces on the superior aspect of the femoral neck in the developing proximal femur [19]. Any change in the development of these physes can cause deformity of the proximal femur. For example, isolated damage to the blood supply of the proximal femoral physeal plate can lead to a varus deformity of the femoral neck as the other plates continue to grow normally.

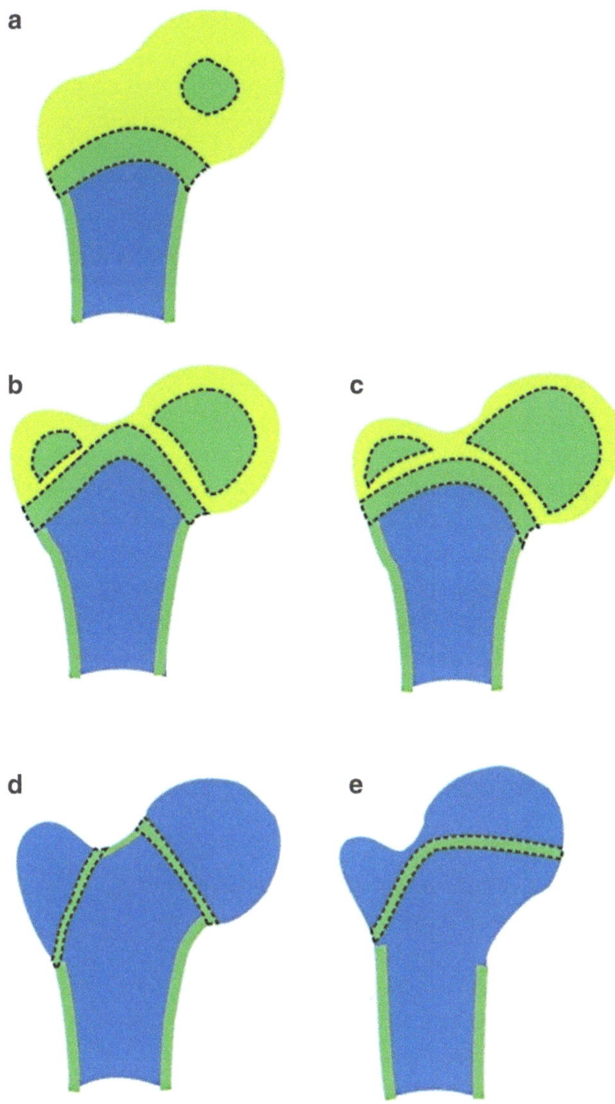

Fig. 99.2 Ossification of the proximal femur. Schematic representation of the growing human hip region, showing the primary femoral and secondary capital and greater trochanteric ossification centres and proximal diaphyseal growth plate at ages of 1 year (**a**), 2–4 years (**b, c**), and >4 years (**d, e**). Panels (**a**), (**b**), and (**d**) represent normal development, showing isthmic interruption of the chondroepiphysis prior to trochanteric osseous expansion, normal orientation of the capital growth plate, and normal head–neck offset. Panels (**c**) and (**e**) represent persistence of the isthmic part of the chondroepiphysis with subsequent coalescence of expanding secondary ossification centres, horizontal orientation of the capital growth plate, and reduced head–neck offset. From Struijs PA, Oostra RJ, van Rijn RR, Besselaar PP (2011). Abnormal growth of the proximal femur due to apophyseal–epiphyseal coalescence resulting in coxa valga—a report of two cases in adolescents. http://openi.nlm.nih.gov/detailedresult.php?img=3237046_ORT-0300-9734-082-507_g003&req=4 © Copyright Policy—open-access

Expansion of the greater trochanter and enlargement of the ossification centre of the capital epiphysis continues over the period of 5–8 years. The greater trochanter often develops an additional ossification centre near its proximal end which rapidly fuses with the main ossification centre.

The area juxtaposed to the fovea capitis develops a distinct indentation in the ossification centre. By the end of this stage of development, the proximal femur has formed the final anatomic contours of anteversion with a functionally separate femoral head and trochanter, and neck-shaft angle. The femoral neck anteversion ranges from 15° to 53° at birth but decreases over the first 10 years of life to the average value of around 15° seen in the adult. The average neck shaft angle of the femur is 138° at birth, increasing to 145° at 1 year. After walking, it gradually decreases until eventually reaching the average adult angle of 125° [20].

No dramatic changes in femoral morphology occur from 9 to 12 years. The capital femoral epiphysis extends over and around the metaphysis anteriorly, medially, and posteriorly, in a pattern analogous to equatorial tipping. Whereas the period from 13 to 16 years of age is characteristically one of rapid growth, which may account for the increased susceptibility of the capital femoral epiphysis to posterior slipping, it is also marked by the physiological closure of the physis. Of the three active growth regions of the proximal femur, the capital femoral physis is the first to close, with fusion progressing centrifugally, eventually incorporating the entire capital femoral epiphysis. As coalition nears completion in the capital femur, a similar process begins in the greater trochanteric physis.

Aetiological Factors in the Abnormal Development of Hip

Various factors thought to be related to the aetiology of abnormal development of hip have been described in the literature. For example, developmental and environmental factors that have been associated with a higher risk of DDH include: ligamentous and capsular laxity (maternal hormonal relaxin in the last trimester of pregnancy), mechanical forces resulting from intrauterine posture (seen in a breech presentation) and swaddling of babies and/or oligohydramnios [21]. Identifying these associated risk factors with abnormal hip development is important as some can be modified. A clear example is swaddling where the risk of DDH is increased because of the postural adduction and extension of the hips [22, 23] whereas a lower incidence of DDH has been noted where the children are carried on their sides with hips in flexion and abduction [24].

Another deformity which has been long thought to be related to environmental factors is the cam deformity associated with FAI. Murray [25] was the first to describe the cam deformity (i.e. referred to the tilt deformity) and its association with high activity level. More recently, several studies have focused on the role of intense activity level on the upper femoral development [26–29].

Agricola and colleagues [26] were able to demonstrate a significantly higher prevalence of either prominent cam morphology or head–neck flattening in 56 % of soccer players compared to 18 %, in a normalised control population. Similarly, Kapron et al. [27] demonstrated a cam prevalence of 57 % in male football players and Siebenrock et al. reported a 56 % prevalence in elite ice hockey players [28]. The concept that joint forces could have significant effects on the morphological development of the hip is consistent with the accepted orthopedic principle of Hueter-Volkmann. This principle states that extrinsically generated forces can influence physeal growth and development [30], and is utilised regularly to correct developmental or acquired deformities in growing children [31].

Siebenrock et al. [23] noted significant differences in physeal development of the femoral head epiphysis in patients with cam FAI. They noticed a significant decrease in femoral head–neck offset associated with a significant increase in lateral extension of the epiphysis. More importantly, the role of athletic activities as an extrinsic force influencing musculoskeletal structures has been noted in the knee (i.e. Osgood-Schlatter's), elbow (i.e. osteochondritis of the capitellar epiphysis) and shoulder (i.e. humeral retrotorsion) [32–35]. Carsen et al. [36] found that asymptomatic cam-type FAI morphology occurred in 14.3 % of individuals with closed physes versus 0 % of patients with open physes, and only in males. Moreover, individuals with the cam deformities were significantly more active than those without. The finding that the cam deformity does not form prior to skeletal maturation is supported by more recent findings in larger cohorts of elite basketball and hockey players, where the higher values of alpha angle found in young athletes were more pronounced after closure of the capital growth plates [28, 37]. These findings strongly support the concept that certain physical activity during critical periods of skeletal maturation may influence the growth and development of the hip joint. It is not clear how physical activities, specifically sports, influence the development of the human upper femur, or the severity and location of the cam deformity, and if there is a difference between males and female or between impact versus non-impact sports.

Finally, the prevalence of DDH follows geographic, racial, familial, and gender parameters. It is more common in certain populations and rare in others. The incidence of DDH is also higher in siblings and close relatives [38, 39]. Similarly, the risk of cam or pincer deformities has been shown to be higher amongst siblings compared with controls [40]. Bilateral deformity and the prevalence of clinical features in those hips with abnormal morphology were also greater in the sibling group compared with the control group.

Persistence of Childhood Deformities into Adulthood

Slipped capital femoral epiphysis is a disorder of the adolescent hip of unknown aetiology, and many slips are clinically silent or only slightly symptomatic [41–46]. While SCFE can cause obvious deformity and morphological changes, the silent or mild ones can also lead to abnormal joint development. Elmslie [47] noticed that a pre-existing deformity of the hip joint could be identified in patients in whom osteoarthritis developed at a relatively young age. Law [48] suggested that degenerative disease of the hip joint could be related to a mild slip of the proximal femoral physis. Solomon [49] noted the femoral head-tilt deformity in 59 of 196 patients who had primary osteoarthritis. Goodman et al. [50] hypothesised that the abnormal post-slip morphology exposes the prominent anterior metaphyseal portion of the femoral neck to the anterior surface of the acetabulum during flexion and internal rotation, producing greater wear in this region, which eventually progresses to global osteoarthritis.

Stulberg et al. [51] described the characteristic deformity of the femoral head and neck seen in patients who have a known history of mild slipped capital femoral epiphysis or Legg-Calve-Perthes disease as a pistol-grip deformity and noted this deformity in 30 of 75 patients who had idiopathic osteoarthritis. Cashin et al. [12] noticed an intra-articular projection of the anterosuperior labrum in their study of stillborn fetuses and thought that the type 1 labral tear may actually be a remnant of this projection.

Some imaging studies have shown morphological variations of the hip that may persist in adulthood. Siebenrock et al. [52], in a MRI study, described that patients with FAI had significant higher extension of the physis as compared to the normal control group (Fig. 99.3). In another MRI study of asymptomatic hips in children aged 9–17 years found that epiphyseal extension increased in open physis group as compared to the closed physis group. In a recent study, Carter et al. [53] found that the cam lesion is located further from the physis in skeletally mature adolescents compared to those who had open physis, suggesting a causal relationship between physeal injury and the development of cam deformity. Monazzam et al. [54] in a CT scan study on pediatric and adolescent population found that cam and pincer morphology occurred as early as 10 and 12 years of age, respectively and their prevalence is similar to that reported in adolescent population. Premature closure of proximal femoral physis or triradiate cartilage because of injury, infection or vascular insult can lead to abnormal development of the hip. Similarly, avascular necrosis of proximal femur due to metabolic, vascular (Perthes Disease), leukemia, or other factors can lead to abnormal hip development.

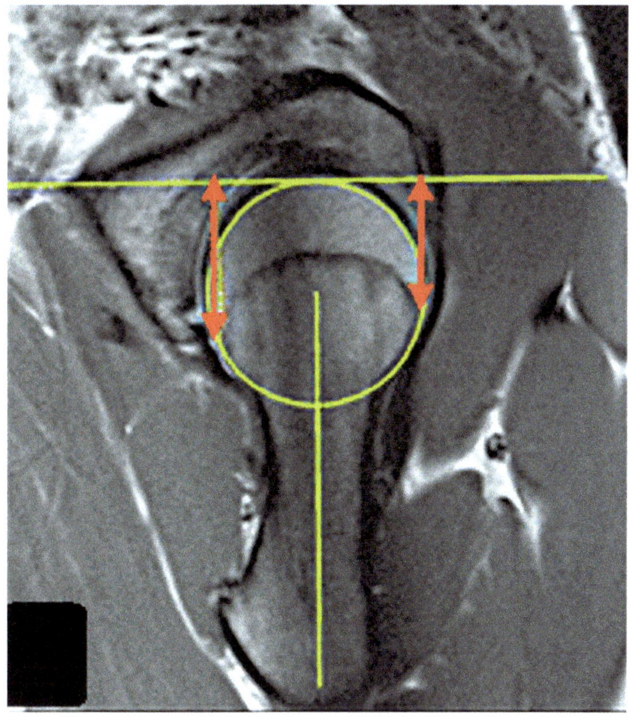

Fig. 99.3 MRI showing epiphyseal extension according to Siebenrock et al. [52]. From Kienle et al. Femoral morphology and epiphyseal growth plate changes of the hip during maturation: MR assessments in a 1-year follow-up on a cross-sectional asymptomatic cohort in the age range of 9–17 years. Skeletal Radiol 2012 Nov;41(11):1381-90. Reprinted with permission from Springer

Conclusion

Successful development and maturation of the hip involves ongoing integration of various congenital, environmental, and morphological stimuli over a period of time. The development of the proximal femur and acetabulum are interdependent and changes in either component affect the development of the other. Disturbance of the complex processes of hip development often leads to abnormal morphology of the acetabulum and the proximal femur, predisposing the joint to characteristic patterns of injury and the development of osteoarthritis.

References

1. Harris-Hayes M, Royer NK. Relationship of acetabular dysplasia and femoroacetabular impingement to hip osteoarthritis: a focused review. PM R. 2011;3(11):1055–67.
2. Serrat MA, Reno PL, McCollum MA, Meindl RS, Lovejoy CO. Variation in mammalian proximal femoral development: comparative analysis of two distinct ossification patterns. J Anat. 2007;210(3):249–58.

3. Hogervorst T, Bouma H, de Boer SF, De VJ. Human hip impingement morphology: an evolutionary explanation. J Bone Joint Surg (Br). 2011;93(6):769–76.
4. Hogervorst T, Bouma HW. Coxa recta (cam-type) proximal femoral morphology: what causes it. Hip Int. 2011;21(3):383–4.
5. Watanabe RS. Embryology of the human hip. Clin Orthop Relat Res. 1974;98:8–26.
6. Lee MC, Eberson CP. Growth and development of the child's hip. Orthop Clin North Am. 2006;37(2):119–32, v.
7. Domzalski ME, Glutting J, Bowen JR, Littleton AG. Lateral acetabular growth stimulation following a labral support procedure in Legg-Calve-Perthes disease. J Bone Joint Surg Am. 2006;88(7):1458–66.
8. Steppacher SD, Tannast M, Werlen S, Siebenrock KA. Femoral morphology differs between deficient and excessive acetabular coverage. Clin Orthop Relat Res. 2009;466(4):782–90.
9. Ponseti IV. Growth and development of the acetabulum in the normal child. Anatomical, histological, and roentgenographic studies. J Bone Joint Surg Am. 1978;60(5):575–85.
10. McCarthy JC, Noble PC, Schuck MR, Wright J, Lee J. The watershed labral lesion. J Arthroplasty. 2001;16(8 (Suppl 1)):81–7.
11. McCarthy JC, Noble PC, Schuck MR, Wright J, Lee J. The role of labral lesions to development of early degenerative hip disease. Clin Orthop Relat Res. 2001;393:25–37.
12. Cashin M, Uhthoff HK, O'Neill M, Beaule PE. Embryology of the acetabular-labral complex. J Bone Joint Surg (Br). 2008;90(8):1019–24.
13. Harrison TJ. The growth of the pelvis in the rat; a mensural and morphological study. J Anat. 1958;92(2):236–60.
14. Sanders JO, Browne RH, Cooney TE, Finegold DN, McConnell SJ, Margraf SA. Correlates of the peak height velocity in girls with idiopathic scoliosis. Spine (Phila Pa 1976). 2006;31(20):2289–95.
15. Sanders JO, Browne RH, McConnell SJ, Margraf SA, Cooney TE, Finegold DN. Maturity assessment and curve progression in girls with idiopathic scoliosis. J Bone Joint Surg Am. 2007;89(1):64–73.
16. Tonnis D. Congenital dysplasia and dislocation of the hip. Berlin: Springer; 1987. p. 76–7.
17. Lovell WW, Winter RB, Morrissy RT, Weinstein SL. Lovell and Winter's pediatric orthopaedics. 6th ed. Philadelphia, PA: Lippincott Williams & Wilkins; 2006.
18. Siffert RS. Patterns of deformity of the developing hip. Clin Orthop Relat Res. 1981;160:14–29.
19. Ward FO. Outlines of human osteology. London, UK: Renshaw; 1838.
20. Hensinger RN. Standards in pediatric orthopaedics: tables, charts and graphs illustrating growth. New York, NY: Raven; 1986.
21. Tachdjian MO. Pediatric orthopedics. Philadelphia, PA: W B Saunders; 1990.
22. Kutlu A, Memik R, Mutlu M, Kutlu R, Arslan A. Congenital dislocation of the hip and its relation to swaddling used in Turkey. J Pediatr Orthop. 1992;12(5):598–602.
23. Siebenrock KA, Wahab KHA, Werlen S, Kalhor M, Leunig M, Ganz R. Abnormal extension of the femoral head epiphysis as a cause of cam impingement. Clin Orthop Relat Res. 2004;418(418):54–60.
24. Aronsson DD, Goldberg MJ, Kling Jr TF, Roy DR. Developmental dysplasia of the hip. Pediatrics. 1994;94(2 Pt 1):201–8.
25. Murray RO. The aetiology of primary osteoarthritis of the hip. Br J Radiol. 1965;38:810–24.
26. Agricola R, Bessems JH, Ginaj AZ, Heijboer MP, van der Heijden RA, Verhaar JA, et al. The development of Cam-type deformity in adolescent and young male soccer players. Am J Sports Med. 2012;40(5):1099–10106.
27. Kapron AL, Anderson AE, Aoki SK, Phillips LG, Petron DJ, Toth R, et al. Radiographic prevalence of femoroacetabular impingement in collegiate football players: AAOS Exhibit Selection. J Bone Joint Surg Am. 2011;93(19):e111–10.
28. Siebenrock KA, Kaschka I, Frauchiger L, Werlen S, Schwab JM. Prevalence of cam-type deformity and hip pain in elite ice hockey players before and after the end of growth. Am J Sports Med. 2013;41:2308–13.
29. Philippon MJ, Ho CP, Briggs KK, Stull J, Laprade RF. Prevalence of increased alpha angles as a measure of cam-type femoroacetabular impingement in youth ice hockey players. Am J Sports Med. 2013;41(6):1357–62.
30. Bries AD, Weiner DS, Jacquet R, Adamczyk MA, Morscher MA, Lowder E, et al. A study in vivo of the effects of a static compressive load on the proximal tibial physis in rabbits. J Bone Joint Surg. 2012;94(15):e1111–10.
31. Wiemann JM, Tryon C, Szalay EA. Physeal stapling versus 8-plate hemiepiphysiodesis for guided correction of angular deformity about the knee. J Pediatr Orthop. 2009;29(5):481–5.
32. Wyland DJ, Pill SG, Shanley E, Clark JC, Hawkins RJ, Noonan TJ, et al. Bony adaptation of the proximal humerus and glenoid correlate within the throwing shoulder of professional baseball pitchers. Am J Sports Med. 2012;40(8):1858–62.
33. Sabick MB, Kim YK, Torry MR, Keirns MA, Hawkins RJ. Biomechanics of the shoulder in youth baseball pitchers: implications for the development of proximal humeral epiphysiolysis and humeral retrotorsion. Am J Sports Med. 2005;33(11):1716–22.
34. Wei AS, Khana S, Limpisvasti O, Crues J, Podesta L, Yocum LA. Clinical and magnetic resonance imaging findings associated with Little League elbow. J Pediatr Orthop. 2010;30(7):715–9.
35. Nilsson M, Ohlsson C, Mellstrom D, Lorentzon M. Previous sport activity during childhood and adolescence is associated with increased cortical bone size in young adult men. J Bone Miner Res. 2009;24:125–33.
36. Carsen SA, Morrey P, Rakhra KS, Ward LM, Dunlap H, Hay JA, et al. The Otto Aufranc Award: on the etiology of the cam deformity: a cross-sectional paediatric MRI study. Clin Orthop Relat Res. 2014;472(2):430–6.
37. Siebenrock KA, Ferner F, Noble PC, Santore RF, Werlen S, Mamisch TC. The cam-type deformity of the proximal femur arises in childhood in response to vigorous sporting activity. Clin Orthop Relat Res. 2011;469(11):3229–40.
38. Wynne-Davies R. Acetabular dysplasia and familial joint laxity: two etiological factors in congenital dislocation of the hip. A review of 589 patients and their families. J Bone Joint Surg (Br). 1970;52(4):704–16.
39. Wynne-Davies R. Heritable disorders in orthopaedic practice. Edinburgh, Scotland: Blackwell Science; 1973.
40. Pollard TC, Villar RN, Norton MR, Fern ED, Williams MR, Murray DW, et al. Genetic influences in the aetiology of femoroacetabular impingement: a sibling study. J Bone Joint Surg (Br). 2010;92(2):209–16.
41. Busch MT, Morrissy RT. Slipped capital femoral epiphysis. Orthop Clin North Am. 1987;18(4):637–47.
42. Crawford AH. Slipped capital femoral epiphysis. J Bone Joint Surg Am. 1988;70(9):1422–7.
43. Hagglund G, Hansson LI, Ordeberg G. Epidemiology of slipped capital femoral epiphysis in southern Sweden. Clin Orthop Relat Res. 1984;191:82–94.
44. Hagglund G, Hansson LI, Ordeberg G, Sandstrom S. Bilaterality in slipped upper femoral epiphysis. J Bone Joint Surg (Br). 1988;70(2):179–81.

45. Ordeberg G, Hansson LI, Sandstrom S. Slipped capital femoral epiphysis in southern Sweden. Long-term result with no treatment or symptomatic primary treatment. Clin Orthop Relat Res. 1984;191:95–104.
46. Peyron J. Inflammation in osteoarthritis (OA): review of its role in clinical picture, disease progress, subsets, and pathophysiology. Semin Arthritis Rheum. 1981;11(1):115–6.
47. Elmslie RC. Remarks on aetiological factors in osteo-arthritis of the hip-joint. Br Med J. 1933;1(3757):1–46.
48. Law WA. Osteoarthritis of the hip. Br J Surg. 1953;40(162): 405–6.
49. Solomon L. Patterns of osteoarthritis of the hip. J Bone Joint Surg. 1976;58(3):176–83.
50. Goodman DA, Feighan JE, Smith AD, Latimer B, Buly RL, Cooperman DR. Subclinical slipped capital femoral epiphysis. J Bone Joint Surg. 1997;79A(10):1489–97.
51. Stulberg SD, Cordell LD, Harris WH, Ramsey PL, MacEwen GD. Unrecognized childhood hip disease: a major cause of idiopathic osteoarthritis of the hip. In: Amstutz HC, editor. The Hip, Proceedings of the third open scientific meeting of the Hip Society. CV Mosby: St Louis; 1975. p. 212–28.
52. Kienle KP, Keck J, Werlen S, Kim YJ, Siebenrock KA, Mamisch TC. Femoral morphology and epiphyseal growth plate changes of the hip during maturation: MR assessments in a 1-year follow-up on a cross-sectional asymptomatic cohort in the age range of 9-17 years. Skeletal Radiol. 2012;41(11):1381–90.
53. Carter CW, Bixby S, Yen YM, Nasreddine AY, Kocher MS. The relationship between cam lesion and physis in skeletally immature patients. J Pediatr Orthop. 2014;34(6):579–84.
54. Monazzam S, Bomar JD, Dwek JR, Hosalkar HS, Pennock AT. Development and prevalence of femoroacetabular impingement-associated morphology in a paediatric and adolescent population: a CT study of 225 patients. Bone Joint J. 2013;95-B(5):598–604.
55. Hogervorst T. Osteoarthritis: a consequence of human evolution? Bone Joint 360 2012;1(1):2-6.

Research Advances in Understanding the Genetic Basis of Hip Disease

100

George Feldman, Javad Parvizi, and Hind Sawan

In view of the tenfold drop in the cost of high output DNA sequencing over the last 3 years, the amount of genetic information available or soon to be available for patients affected with orthopedic disorders will be enormous. How can orthopedic surgeons best use this information to benefit their patients? Although there are many ways this information can be useful, this chapter focuses on its use to uncover DNA variants causing susceptibility or novel mutations in osteoarthritis of the hip. Early detection of susceptibility to joint disease can offer ways of lessening its effects through behavior modification and noninvasive intervention, and can illuminate metabolic pathways for rational therapeutic intervention.

Osteoarthritis (OA) is the most common disabling joint disease observed worldwide with 27 million individuals diagnosed in the United States alone [1]. The risk of disability from knee and hip OA alone is as great as the risk of developing cardiovascular disease. OA is a complex disease having both environmental and genetic causes. Twin studies have demonstrated that the genetic component contributes between 39 and 78% of its etiology [2]. Evidence from genome-wide association studies (GWAS) involving thousands of affected individuals and controls indicate that multiple individual risk alleles contribute small effects to the overall susceptibility to the development of OA [3, 4]. Information from these studies and from candidate gene studies has led to the discovery of DNA variants in genes associated with OA.

The focus of traditional arthritis research has been based on the theory that environmental and genetic mutations accelerate the degradation of cartilage. Surprisingly, many of these OA-associated genes are related to the development of the joints. Of interest is the fact that none of the genes proven to be associated with OA encode proteins that are involved in cartilage degradation [5].

The distinction between primary OA (disease that occurs without underlying factors or structural abnormalities) and secondary OA (resulting from traumatic injury or specific anatomic abnormalities in the joint or cartilage) are becoming blurred. New analytical techniques like active shape modeling and MRI provide more detailed structural information than traditional radiographic measurements of joint-space narrowing [6, 7]. These techniques are illuminating subtle abnormalities of the joint that are also present in patients with primary OA. This suggests a correlation between severity of the joint defect with the age of onset of osteoarthritis.

Developmental dysplasia of the hip (DDH) illustrates the paradigm that these subtle anatomic joint defects, present at birth, may be a causative culprit in OA. DDH is characterized by an underdeveloped, abbreviated acetabulum causing femoral subluxation and abnormal wear due to decreased weight-bearing surface area of the hip socket. Gross forms of DDH are detected at birth using the Ortolani test and the Barlow maneuver to manipulate the femur in an attempt to detect dislocation. These tests are relatively insensitive to the presence of subtle acetabular deformities which are thought to cause the majority of cases of early onset and perhaps later onset osteoarthritis of the hip. Because of the difficulty in recruiting sufficient numbers of dysplastic patients to make GWAS studies statistically meaningful, the search for susceptibility-inducing mutations has been limited. Instead, case–control studies have been performed in which a given gene variant is tested in a population of a few hundred

G. Feldman, DMD, PhD (✉)
Orthopaedic Research, Jefferson Medical College, Philadelphia, PA, USA

Thomas Jefferson University, Curtis Building, Rm 520, 1015 Walnut St., Philadelphia, PA 19107, USA
e-mail: gfel640946@aol.com

J. Parvizi, MD, FRCS
Adult Lower Limb Reconstruction, Rothman Institute, Thomas Jefferson University Hospital, Philadelphia, PA, USA

H. Sawan, BS
Department of Orthopaedic Research, The Rothman Institute at Thomas Jefferson University, Philadelphia, PA, USA

J.C. McCarthy et al. (eds.), *Hip Joint Restoration*, DOI 10.1007/978-1-4614-0694-5_100

sporadic dysplastic hips compared to a control population presumably matched by age, sex, and ethnicity. These studies have provided interesting clues concerning variants possibly causing susceptibility, but many studies lack statistical power. Interestingly, GDF5, TBX4, ASPN, and TGF beta genes known to play a role in chondrogenesis or joint formation have also been linked to OA [8]. Table 100.1 provides a summary for the findings of the genetic studies of DDH and OA.

Another approach in the search for causative variants has been whole-genome linkage analysis of DDH inherited in large families. This approach makes no assumption of what the causative mutation may be and detects regions of DNA co-inherited by affected family members but not present in unaffected members. Novel variants not previously thought to be associated with DDH or OA can thus be discovered. Because DDH is a complex disorder not all members who have a potentially causative variant will manifest signs of the disease and are said to show incomplete penetrance. Moreover, several family members can show some but not all signs of the disorder and are thought to show variable expressivity. In spite of these confounding factors, it is still possible to obtain useful information by analyzing only those family members whose diagnosis is unambiguous. This approach has been used by a number of investigators in the past but no variant shared by all affected family members has been identified [9–11].

Recently, a 72-member 4-generation family showing intergenerational transmission of DDH was identified [12]. Whole-genome linkage analysis revealed a 2.5 Mb candidate region on chromosome 3p22.2 shared by all affected [13]. Sequencing the exomes of four distantly related, severely affected individuals avoided that diagnostic uncertainty while capitalizing on the "filtering" effect of the Mendelian inheritance of the same variant by distantly related family members. The sequencing data of these four severely affected distantly related individuals revealed a variant in a chemokine receptor (CX3CR1) shared by all affected family members as well as some apparently unaffected members. This chemokine has been shown to play a role in bone homeostasis but its role in chondrogenesis is unknown [14]. Importantly, whole-exome analysis has revealed the role of other potential "aggravating" mutations not present in the

Table 100.1 Summary of findings of genetic studies of DDH and OA

Author (year)	Type of study	Conclusion
Jia et al. (2012) [18]	Case–control study	Association of PAPPA2 with sporadic DDH susceptibility in a Chinese Han population
Shi et al. (2011) [19]	Case–control study	Association between the D repeat polymorphism of ASPN and DDH
Kolundzic et al. (2011) [20]	Case–control study	TGF-B1 and IL-6 are associated with DDH-related severe adult hip OA
Wang et al. (2010) [21]	Case–control study in 505 patients and 551 control subjects in Chinese Han population	rs3744448 polymorphism causing missense mutation of Tbx4 gene is associated with DDH in dominant model of male subjects
Rouault et al. (2009) [22]	Pilot candidate locus association study	HOXB9 and COL1A1 association with DDH not supported in study of small regional French population
Dai et al. (2008) [23]	Candidate locus association study of 335 CDH subjects, 622 control subject with candidate region	Significant association of GDF5 SNP with CDH
Rubini et al. (2008) [24]	Linkage exclusion	COL2A1 and vitamin D receptor excluded from linkage to DDH
Mabuchi and Nakamura (2006) [11]	Whole-genome linkage	DDH in one large Japanese family linked to chromosome 13q22
Loughlin et al. (2006) [25]	Candidate locus association study	Calmodulin promoter polymorphism not associated with DDH in UK white population
Jiang et al. (2005) [26]	Linkage exclusion	Two polymorphic sites within the COL1A1 gene found not to be linked to DDH in 81 small Chinese families
Mototani et al. (2005) [27]	Candidate locus association study	A functional polymorphic SNP in promoter of the Calmodulin gene found to be associated with hip osteoarthritis in Japanese population
Jiang et al. (2003) [28]	Candidate locus linkage study	Association of one allele of one microsatellite marker (D17S1820) on chromosome 17q21 with CDH phenotype in 101 Chinese families
Granchi et al. (2002) [29]	Candidate locus association study	Pilot study suggests Type II collagen and vitamin D receptor polymorphism might be associated with risk of osteoarthritis in patients with DDH
Ingvarrson et al. (2001) [10]	Whole-genome linkage study of large Icelandic family	Locus on chromosome 16p linked to early osteoarthritis of the hip
Cilliers and Beighton (1990) [9]	Whole-genome linkage of large Africaaner family	Premature (Beukes) degenerative osteoarthritis of the hip mapped to 11 cM region on chromosome 4q35

chromosome 3 candidate region but nevertheless shared by the most severely affected individuals but not present in unaffected and less affected family members. While it is possible that one of these mutations is exclusively found in this family, it is unlikely some of them will not be found in sporadic DDH individuals and in other families.

By performing the same whole-genome linkage analysis, combined with whole-exome sequencing of the severely affected members of a second (and possibly a third and fourth) family, it is possible to identify the variants shared by the most severely affected members of all families and to use this information to develop a diagnostic test for DDH. The following illustration (Fig. 100.1) shows a possible strategy currently being employed to identify variants likely to be present in the sporadic population of dysplastic hips. In this example are two families one linked to chromosome 3p22 and the other to 17q21.

It can be seen that variants shared by the most severely affected individuals of both families are good candidates for testing in other unrelated sporadics. These shared variants would then be validated in animal models for their relevance to DDH.

Genome-wide association studies are the most popular method to relate genetic variation to phenotypic diversity. While they have identified statistical association between hundreds of genetic loci across the genome and complex traits, they have three major limitations:

1. It has been difficult to identify the functional significance of the DNA segment identified in these studies.
2. DNA variant associations identified in one population are not reproducible in members of other populations.
3. The major part of the heritable fraction of complex traits has not been accounted for in recent GWAS studies. This last point can be explained by the fact that GWA studies do not capture information about rare DNA variants that can have large phenotypic effects [15].

There are two alternative approaches to overcome the intrinsic deficits of the GWA approach with the potential to detect these rare but biologically important variants [16]. One of these is the use of linkage analysis and sequencing of affected family members. Whole-genome sequencing is conducted on a small carefully selected population at one or

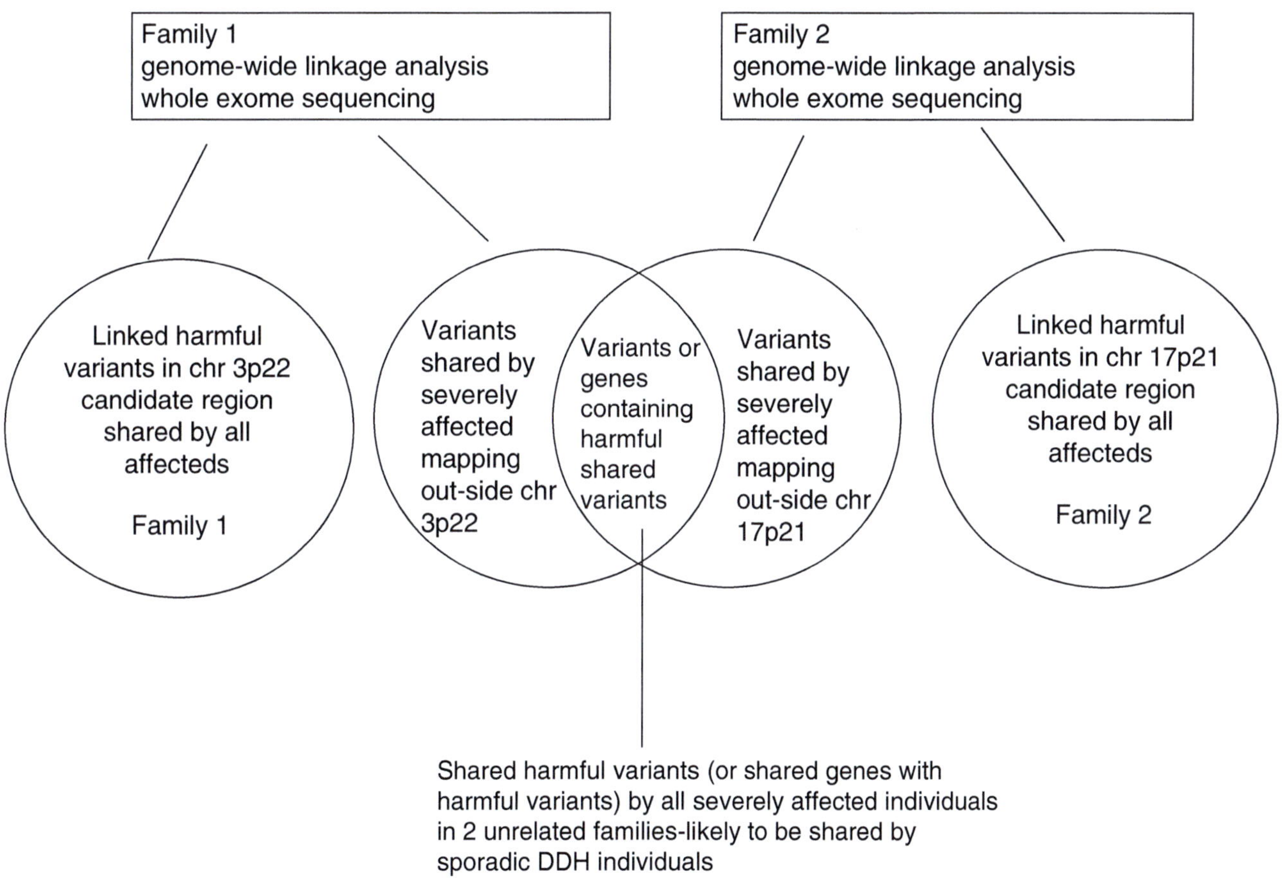

Fig. 100.1

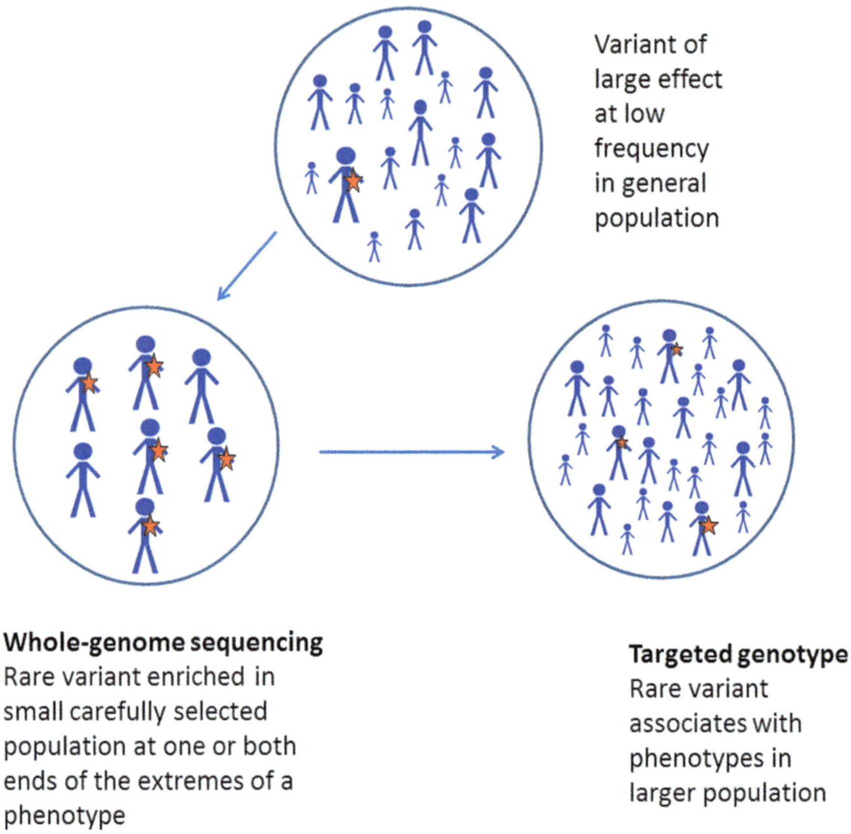

Fig. 100.2 Extreme-trait sequencing. Compared to GWA studies, extreme-trait sequencing is a cost-effective strategy at identifying rare candidate variants for a phenotype. Variants of large effect are present at a low frequency in the general population. To identify variants in a more cost-effective manner, whole-genome sequencing is conducted on a small carefully selected population at one or both ends of the extremes of a phenotype. Variants that contribute to the trait will be enriched in frequency. After this strategy, candidate variants can then be genotyped for confirmation in a larger population. The *size of the individuals* represents the severity of the phenotype and the *red star* represents the causal variants

both ends of the extremes of a phenotype to enrich the incidence of variants contributing to the trait. After this strategy, candidate variants can then be genotyped for confirmation in a larger population.

A second method is the use of extreme-trait sequencing (Fig. 100.2). In this strategy, a small carefully selected population at one or both ends of the extremes of a phenotype is chosen. Patients who have had very rare post-surgical complications, such as infection, might be one group. Other examples include individuals known to be highly exposed to HIV but who remain uninfected or individuals at the extremes of distributions for blood pressure. Because variants that contribute to the trait will be enriched in frequency in such a population, even small sample sizes may suggest many candidate variants that can then be genotyped for confirmation in a much larger group of samples. For example, consider a case in which a variant is enriched 30-fold in just such an extreme population as in individuals hypersensitive to the antiviral drug Abacavir. About 3–5 % of the population has life-threatening allergic reactions to this drug. If this variant were rare in the general population, one would need to sequence about 30 extreme individuals to see it once. If however multiple rare variants in the same gene affect the phenotype the odds of discovery would increase.

Searching for genes with an enrichment of rare variants in extreme individuals will implicate these genes even at low number of sequenced genomes if the variants are in genes of obvious function [16]. To confirm a possible causative variant, family members of extreme individuals will be very valuable as they could be used in co-segregation analysis. This technique was used to identify a gene for Miller Syndrome, a rare multiple malformation disorder, that was enriched for rare variants in four unrelated individuals [17].

The identification of rare variants with large effects is now possible on a broader scale because the cost of next-generation sequencing has fallen. If rare variants with obvious functionality have a big impact on common diseases, whole-genome sequencing will allow definitive connections to be established between specific genes and the osteoarthritic phenotype. These kinds of strong connections, like a clearly functional mutation in a single gene conferring high risk, would provide validated therapeutic targets for drug development. In the case of DDH, these variant(s) could form the basis for a sensitive and specific diagnostic test in newborns that would allow noninvasive correction of the deficient acetabulum.

References

1. Lawrence RC. Estimates of the prevalence of arthritis and other rheumatic conditions in the United States Part II. Arthritis Rheum. 2008;58:26–35.
2. Spector TD et al. Genetic influences on osteoarthritis in women: a twin study. BMJ. 1996;312:940–3.

3. Kerkhof HJ et al. Recommendations for standardization and phenotype definitions in genetic studies of osteoarthritis: the TREAT-OA consortium. Osteoarthritis Cartilage. 2011;19:254–64.
4. Panoutsopoulou K et al. Concise report: insights into the genetic architecture of osteoarthritis from stage 1 of the arcOGEN study. Ann Rheum Dis. 2011;70:864–7.
5. Sandell LJ. Etiology of osteoarthritis: genetics and synovial joint development. Nat Rev Rheumatol. 2012;8:77–89.
6. Gregory JS et al. Early identification of radiographic osteoarthritis of the hip using an active shape model to quantify changes in bone morphometric features: can hip shape tell us anything about the progression of osteoarthritis? Arthritis Rheum. 2007;56:3634–43.
7. Reichenbach S et al. Prevalence of bone attrition on knee radiographs and MRI in a community-based cohort. Osteoarthritis Cartilage. 2008;16:1005–10.
8. Shi D et al. Genetic study on developmental dysplasia of the hip. Eur J Clin Invest. 2012;42:1121–5.
9. Cilliers HJ, Beighton P. Beukes familial hip dysplasia: an autosomal dominant entity. Am J Med Genet. 1990;36:386–90.
10. Ingvarsson T, Stefansson SE, Gulcher JR, Jonsson HH, Jonsson H, Frigge ML, et al. A large Icelandic family with early osteoarthritis of the hip associated with a susceptibility locus on chromosome 16p. Arthritis Rheum. 2001;44:2548–55.
11. Mabuchi A, Nakamura S, Takatori Y, Ikegawa S. Familial osteoarthritis of the hip joint associated with acetabular dysplasia maps to chromosome 13q. Am J Hum Genet. 2006;79:163–8.
12. Feldman GJ, Parvizi J, Levenstien M, Scott K, Erickson JA, Fortina P, et al. Developmental dysplasia of the hip: linkage mapping and whole exome sequencing identify a shared variant in CX3CR1 in all affected members of a large multi-generation family. J Bone Miner Res. 2013. doi:10.1002/jbmr.1999. Epub ahead of print.
13. Feldman GJ, Peters CL, Erickson JA, Hozack BA, Jaraha R, Parvizi J. Variable expression and incomplete penetrance of developmental dysplasia of the hip: clinical challenge in a 71-member multigeneration family. J Arthroplasty. 2012;27(4):527–32. Epub 2011 Dec 16.
14. Hoshino A, Ueha S, Hanada S, Imai T, Ito M, Yamamoto K, et al. Roles of chemokine receptor CX3CR1 in maintaining murine bone homeostasis through the regulation of both osteoblasts and osteoclasts. J Cell Sci. 2013;126(Pt 4):1032–45. doi:10.1242/jcs.113910. Epub 2012 Dec 21.
15. Frazer KA. Human genetic variation and its contribution to complex traits. Nat Rev Genet. 2009;10:241–51.
16. Cirulli ET, Goldstein DB. Uncovering the roles of rare variants in common disease through whole genome sequencing. Nat Rev Genet. 2010;11:415–25.
17. Ng SB. Exome sequencing identifies the cause of a mendelian disorder. Nat Genet. 2010;42:30–5.
18. Jia J, Li L, Zhao Q, Zhang L, Ru J, Liu X, et al. Association of a single nucleotide polymorphism in pregnancy-associated plasma protein-A2 with developmental dysplasia of the hip: a case-control study. Osteoarthr Cartil. 2012;20:60–3.
19. Shi D, Dai J, Zhu L, Zhu H, et al. Association of the D repeat polymorphism in the ASPN gene with developmental hip dysplasia of the hip: a case-control study in the Han Chinese. Arthritis Res Ther. 2011;13:R27.
20. Kolundzic R, Trkulja V, Mikolaucic M, Jovanic M, Pavelic S, Pavelic K. Association of interleukin-6 and transforming growth factor-b1 gene polymorphisms with developmental hip dysplasia and severe adult hip osteoarthritis: a preliminary study. Cytokine. 2011;54(2):125–8.
21. Wang K, Shi D, Zhu P, Dai J, Zhu H, Lv Y, et al. Association of a single nucleotide polymorphism in Tbx4 with developmental dysplasia of the hip: a case-control study. Osteoarthr Cartil. 2010;18:1592–5.
22. Rouault K, Scotet V, Autret S, Gaucher F, Dubrana F, Tanguy D, et al. Do HOXB9 and COL1A1 genes play a role in congenital dislocation of the hip? Study in a Caucasian population. Osteoarthritis Cartilage. 2009;17:1099–105.
23. Dai J, Shi D, Zhu P, Qin J, Ni H, Xu Y, et al. Association of a single nucleotide polymorphism in growth differentiate factor 5 with congenital dysplasia of the hip: a case-control study. Arthritis Res Ther. 2008;10:R126.
24. Rubini M, Cavallaro A, Calzolari E, Bighetti G, Sollazzo V. Exclusion of COL2A1 and VDR as developmental dysplasia of the hip genes. Clin Orthop Relat Res. 2008;466:878–83.
25. Loughlin J, Sinsheimer JS, Carr A, Chapman K. The CALM1 core promoter polymorphism is not associated with hip osteoarthritis in a United Kingdom Caucasian population. Osteoarthritis Cartilage. 2006;14:295–8.
26. Jiang J, Ma HW, Li QW, Lu JF, Niu GH, Zhang LJ, et al. Association analysis on the polymorphisms of PCOL2 and Sp1 binding sites of COL1A1 gene and the congenital dislocation of the hip in Chinese population [in Chinese]. Zhonghua Yi Xue Yi Chuan Xue Za Zhi. 2005;22:327–9.
27. Mototani H, Mabuchi A, Saito S, Fujioka M, Iida A, Takatori Y, et al. A functional single nucleotide polymorphism in the core promoter region of CALM1 is associated with hip osteoarthritis in Japanese. Hum Mol Genet. 2005;14:1009–17.
28. Jiang J, Ma HW, Lu Y, Wang YP, Wang Y, Li QW, et al. Transmission disequilibrium test for congenital dislocation of the hip and HOXB9 gene or COL1AI gene [in Chinese]. Zhonghua Yi Xue Yi Chuan Xue Za Zhi. 2003;20:193–5.
29. Granchi D, Stea S, Sudanese A, Toni A, Baldini N, Giunti A. Association of two gene polymorphisms with osteoarthritis secondary to hip dysplasia. Clin Orthop Relat Res. 2002;403:108–17.

Fluid Mechanics, Pre- and Post-Capsulotomy

101

Richard E. Field, Francesc Malagelada, and Francesco Strambi

Introduction

Throughout the plant and animal kingdoms, cell metabolism depends upon gaseous, nutrient and waste product exchange between the intra- and extracellular spaces. With organisms of increasing complexity, circulatory systems have evolved to replenish and recycle the extracellular fluid spaces. The circulation of blood was described by Harvey in 1628 [1], the lymphatic circulation by Rudbeck [2] and Bartholin [3] in 1653, and cerebrospinal fluid (CSF) circulation by Dandy, Horsley, Blackfan and Cushing during the first decades of the twentieth century. In 1964, Di Chiro [4] published, in *Nature*, his now classic study in which he introduced radionuclide cisternography and showed the existence of an active CSF circulation.

Each circulatory system has evolved to address specific functional requirements. The vascular system has evolved to address the metabolic needs of the musculoskeletal, reproductive, and neural tissues. The lungs provide gaseous exchange, the gastrointestinal tract replenishes nutrients, the hepatic and renal systems recycle or extract metabolites and the endocrine system modulates metabolism. Key to all these functions has been the development of the heart to ensure consistent blood flow through the provider and user tissues.

Lymph is generated through incomplete reabsorption of blood from the end-user tissues and its flow depends upon a combination of intrinsic contractions of the lymphatic passages and extrinsic compression of the lymphatic vessels via external tissue forces such as contractions of skeletal muscles.

CSF is generated by the choroid plexus, in multiple areas of the ventricular system whence it passes into the central canal of the spinal cord or the cisterns of the subarachnoid space, to be reabsorbed via the arachnoid villi into the venous system.

In contrast to blood, lymph, and CSF, our understanding of synovial fluid circulation is rudimentary. We know that synovial tissue is of mesenchymal origin, that it lines the non-articular surface of joints and forms sacs to shield the movement of tendons. We know that synovial membranes secrete and replenish synovial fluid and that synovial fluid lubricates and nourishes articular cartilage. We know that synovial tissue is vulnerable to autoimmune diseases, that synovial fluid production increases in response to local trauma and that the constitution of synovial fluid is deranged in degenerative joint disease.

This chapter reviews current ideas on synovial fluid circulation within the hip joint and describes early degenerative changes that may reflect or be mediated through disturbance of synovial circulation. The chapter also reviews our current understanding as to how labral and capsular damage may affect synovial circulation and lubrication of the hip joint.

Synovial Fluid Circulation in the Hip

The hip joint is divided by the acetabular labrum into central and peripheral compartments (Fig. 101.1). The peripheral compartment is further subdivided by the zona orbicularis into proximal and distal spaces. The acetabular labrum has both central and peripheral facing surfaces. The central facing articular surface is in intimate contact with the femoral head and passage of any synovial fluid between the two compartments must occur at the interface between the femoral head and the head-facing surface of the labrum. In the peripheral compartment, both the femoral and capsular surfaces are

R.E. Field, PhD, FRCS, FRCS(Orth) (✉)
The South West London Elective Orthopaedic Centre, Dorking Road, Epsom, Surrey KT18 7EG, UK
e-mail: richardefield@aol.com

F. Malagelada, MD
Department of Orthopaedics, South West London Elective Orthopaedic Centre, Epsom, Surrey KT18 7EG, UK

F. Strambi, MD
Research Unit, South West London Elective Orthopaedic Centre, Epsom, Surrey KT18 7EG, UK

J.C. McCarthy et al. (eds.), *Hip Joint Restoration*, DOI 10.1007/978-1-4614-0694-5_101

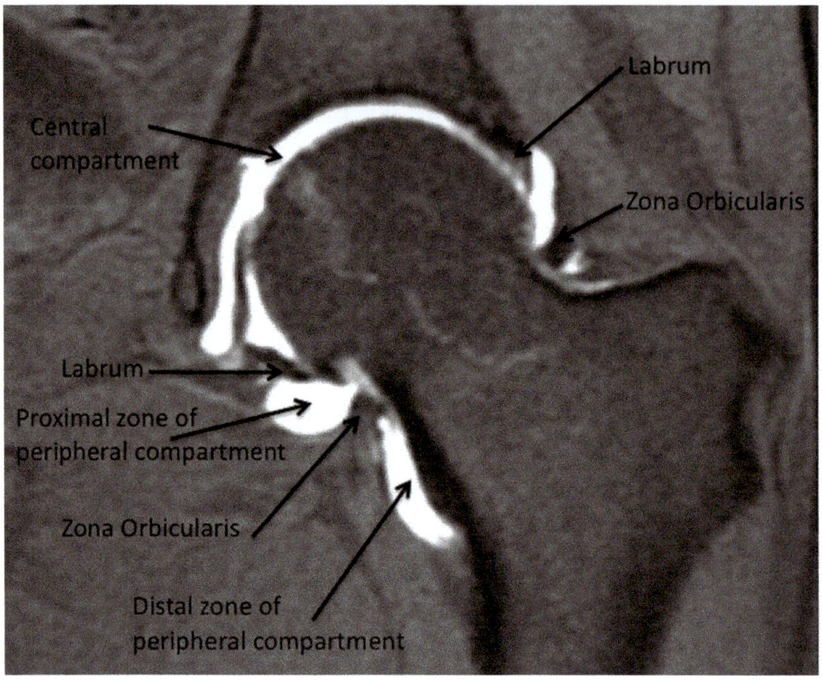

Fig. 101.1 Coronal MR arthrogram view of a left hip joint. The central compartment is separated from the proximal peripheral compartment by the acetabular labrum and the proximal peripheral compartment is separated from the distal peripheral compartment by the zona orbicularis (ZO)

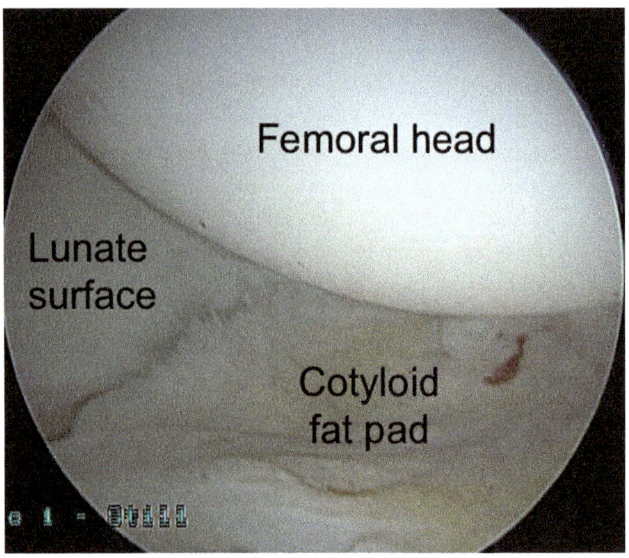

Fig. 101.2 Arthroscopic view of hip joint showing fat pad sitting proud of lunate articular surface

lined by synovial membrane. In the central compartment the synovial membrane merges with the articular margin of the cotyloid fossa, covers the fat pad (Fig. 101.2), the ligamentum teres, and merges with the articular cartilage at the fovea capitis. The healthy hip joint has only a few milliliters of free synovial fluid. When the joint is inflated for an arthrogram, the total fluid capacity, of the two compartments, varies between 10 and 20 ml.

The zona orbicularis (ZO) of the hip is a capsular thickening located at the level of the femoral neck. Its fibers are circumferentially orientated which is an exception to the rest of the hip capsular ligaments which have a longitudinal alignment [5–7]. It has been described as an element that wraps around the femoral neck partially [5] or completely, like a ring [6]. The ZO is most consistently identified when the joint is distended. On magnetic resonance arthrography images the ZO appears as a horseshoe-shaped structure, in approximately 75 % of cases [8]. Superiorly, the ZO is aligned perpendicular to the long axis of the femoral neck. It twists from postero-lateral to antero-medial, as it moves inferiorly. The ZO sits consistently at the narrowest point of the femoral neck [8], which supports Ito's hypothesis [6] that the ZO functions as a constraint against distraction of the femoral head. Some authors have suggested that the ZO tightens in a "screw-home" mechanism during hip extension and external rotation and that the ZO fibers unwind and loosen in flexion [6, 9, 10].

The hip joint is subjected to loads corresponding to several times an individual's body mass during the normal gait cycle and activities of daily living [11]. Such loading is associated with the generation of a pressure differential between the central and peripheral compartments. Ferguson et al. [12] undertook a cadaveric study in which hip joints were subjected to normal walking cycle loads with pressure transducers positioned in both the central and peripheral compartments. The pressure in the central and peripheral compartments was measured both with labrum intact and after labral excision. The study demonstrated that, when the labrum is intact, loading the joint leads to a rise in pressure within the central compartment but no comparable rise in the peripheral compartment. This differential is lost when the labrum is excised. From a physiological perspective, the pressure differential makes good sense. The entrapment of synovial fluid within the central compartment will ensure effective fluid-film articular surface lubrication while the joint is loaded. However, even with an intact labrum, it is probable that the repetitive rise in central compartment pressure, in conjunction with joint movement, will cause some leakage of synovial fluid from the central to the peripheral compartment.

Articular cartilage lubrication, microcirculation, and nourishment have long been a subject of interest to researchers [13]. In 1984, Afoke [14] suggested a mechanism involving tidal synovial fluid movement between the cotyloid fossa and the lunate articular surface. Afoke's model concentrated on synovial fluid movement within the central compartment. However, it did not address the question of how synovial fluid, which is generated and replenished in the low-pressure peripheral compartment, is moved into the high-pressure central compartment or how it circulates back to the peripheral compartment.

A unidirectional synovial circulation between the compartments was proposed by Field [15]. During arthroscopy of the peripheral hip compartment, separation of the transverse ligament from the femoral head was observed during passive joint flexion. The separation was seen to coincide with ZO closing the proximal part of the peripheral compartment. Following this observation, a series of hip arthroscopies were undertaken with initial access to the peripheral compartment and introduction of an epidural catheter, with its tip located in the infero-medial recess of the proximal part of the peripheral compartment. The arthroscope was removed and a few milliliters of contrast (Niopam 300, Bracco U.K. Ltd) were injected under image intensifier control. The contrast initially accumulated in the infero-medial region of the peripheral compartment. On hip flexion, contrast was seen to enter the cotyloid recess of the central compartment (Fig. 101.3a)

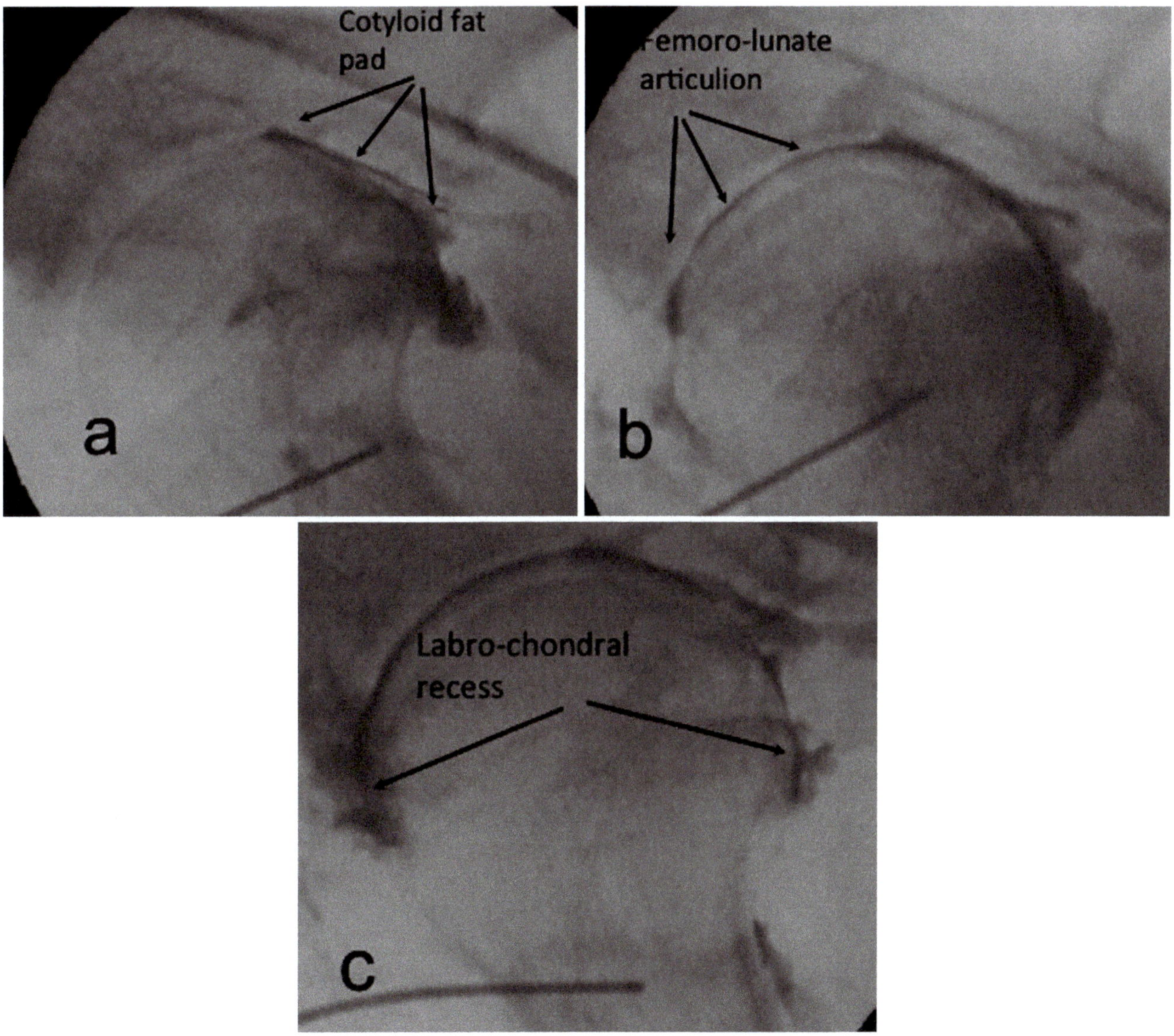

Fig. 101.3 (**a**) Radio-opaque contrast moving from medial recess of proximal part of peripheral compartment to cotyloid recess of central compartment as hip joint flexed. (**b**) Contrast flowing from cotyloid recess across lunate surface as hip joint is extended. (**c**) Accumulation of contrast in labrochondral recess after repeated flexion-extension cycles

and on subsequent joint extension the contrast was seen to spread across the lunate surface (Fig. 101.3b). After several flexion-extension cycles, accumulation of the contrast was observed in the labrochondral recess (Fig. 101.3c).

These observations led the development of a unidirectional synovial flow model in which synovial fluid production and gaseous and nutrient exchange occur in the low-pressure peripheral compartment. During the non-load bearing, swing phase of the gait cycle, central compartment pressure falls. Simultaneously, the zona orbicularis, functioning as a bellows, encircles the femoral neck and closes the proximal portion of the peripheral compartment. Synovial fluid is pumped into the cotyloid fossa. The gap between the transverse ligament and the femoral head closes and the synovial fluid is entrapped within the cotyloid fossa reservoir. At footfall, joint loading compresses the fat pad and the synovial fluid is driven upwards in the channels between the Haversian fat pad and the margins of the cotyloid fossa. A secondary role of the ligamentum teres may be to act as a compression wiper that augments this process. The synovial fluid is driven upwards to the apex of the cotyloid fossa where a synovial extension directs the fluid into the depressed, delta-like stellate crease. The stellate crease extends to the center of the lunate articular surface (Fig. 101.4). As joint loading increases, the entrapped fluid is driven outwards across the lunate articular surface. With each loading cycle a small amount of the synovial fluid seeps into the labrochondral sulcus and from here labral leakage returns the synovial fluid to the peripheral compartment for further nutrient and gaseous exchange.

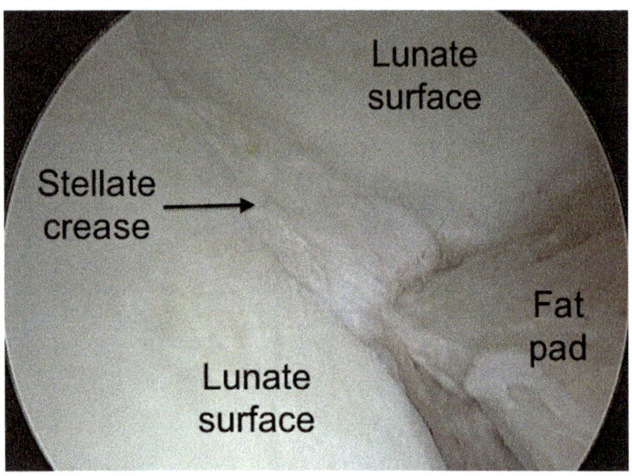

Fig. 101.4 The depressed Stellate crease is seen to extend upwards from the cotyloid fossa across the lunate surface of the acetabulum. The fat pad is tethered to the inferior margin of the Stellate crease by an extension of the synovial covering of the fat pad. The normal recess between fat pad and lunate surface is continued into the Stellate crease, suggestive of a channel for flow of synovial fluid

This stage of synovial circulation has been investigated by Ferguson [16] who concluded that the labrum facilitates the distribution of contact stresses over the articular surfaces by restricting the egress of fluid from the joint during loading, thereby limiting peak cartilage stresses, especially in response to impact loading. Dwyer [17] subsequently demonstrated that the integrity of the labral seal depends upon joint position. Dwyer identified maximal resistance to the egress of synovial fluid, from the central compartment, when the hip joint is extended and externally rotated with least resistance on flexion and internal rotation.

This unidirectional synovial flow concept is consistent with studies on acetabular biomechanics. In 1971, Greenwald and O'Connor [18] identified two distinct contact areas present on the anterior and posterior aspect of the acetabulum at low loads, which gradually merge with increasing load until the zenith (dome) of the acetabulum makes contact. The load required for the transition occurring at approximately 50 % body weight in young adults and 25 % body weight in elderly adults. In 1983, Brown and Shaw [19] observed that the dome of the acetabulum is either not in contact or intermittently loaded due to the incongruence with the femoral head, whereas the anterior and posterior surfaces of acetabulum are consistently loaded. In 1997 Lazennec [20] described acetabular socket and articular deformation during joint loading. In Lazennec's model, the anterior and posterior horns of the acetabulum separate at low loads (<0.36× body weight). At 36–38 % of body weight, a transition occurs. With increasing load, the acetabulum opens with the posterior horn deflecting three times more than the anterior horn. Lazennec argued that acetabular opening and closing permits the unstressed or minimally stressed acetabulum to release its grip on the femoral head, while the more highly stressed acetabulum tightens around the femoral head. The acetabulum adapts at low loads by distributing intra-articular pressures across both horns and permits greater support at higher loads by increasing contact to include the denser apex of the roof.

In all three models, contact between the femoral and acetabular articular cartilage, in the area corresponding to the stellate triangle, only occurs with increasing joint loading. Also, closure of the dome space would force any entrapped synovial fluid into the anterior and posterior facets of the femoro-lunate articulation. This in turn would facilitate hydrodynamic lubrication between the moving surfaces.

Early Degenerative Changes

A number of commonly observed arthroscopic findings may be related to intra-articular synovial flow. Firstly, one of the earliest signs of degenerative hip disease is the formation of cotyloid rim osteophytes. Typically, these first appear towards the apex of the cotyloid recess where synovial fluid

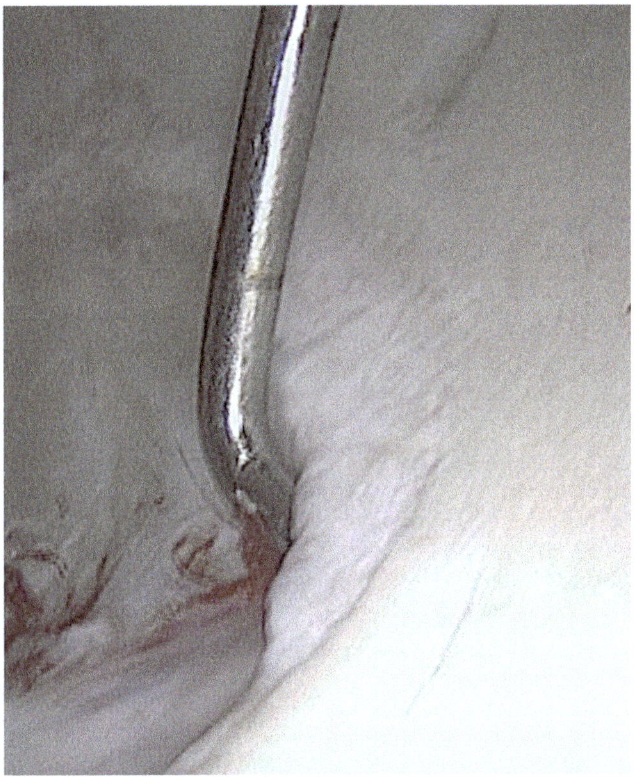

Fig. 101.5 Early apical cotyloid rim osteophyte formation adjacent to the Stellate crease of the lunate surface

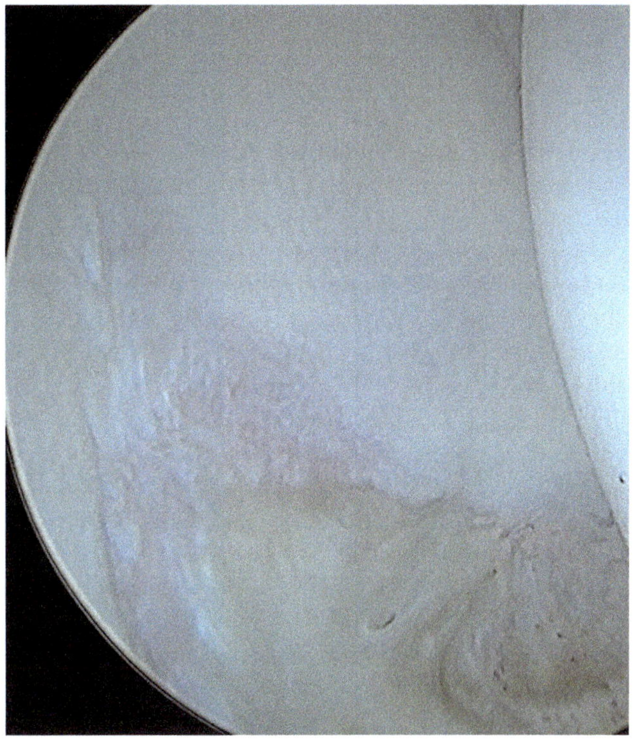

Fig. 101.6 Early degenerative changes involving the upper margin of the cotyloid fossa and adjacent surface of the Stellate crease

passes between the cotyloid reservoir and the stellate crease (Fig. 101.5). Secondly, in early joint degeneration, the stellate crease may develop an eroded appearance (Fig. 101.6). However, it is yet to be explained how either of these changes relates to derangement of fluid dynamics. Thirdly, acetabular subchondral cysts have been classified [21] as solitary rim, multiple or solitary dome, according to their distribution. The pathogenesis of rim cysts is easily understood as a consequence of repetitive impingement causing the "watershed lesion," described by McCarthy and Noble [22]. In the presence of labrochondral disruption, chondral delamination ensues and leads to fluid erosion through the subchondral plate. In contrast, cross-sectional imaging such as CT or MR demonstrates that solitary dome cysts are in direct continuity with the joint. Their location typically corresponds to region of anterior horn loading. It remains to be explained whether these cysts develop secondary to damage to the underlying bone or deranged fluid lubrication of the articular cartilage.

The Effect of Labral Pathology

The role of labral integrity on femoral head stability was first investigated by Crawford [23] who created 15 mm tears in cadaveric joints with a healthy labrum and demonstrated decreased femoral head stability, relative to the acetabulum, during extreme ranges of motion. Dwyer went on to compare cadaveric hips with Cam type morphology/deformity and associated labral damage with undamaged hips that did not have any sign of Cam morphology. Dwyer found that, on pivoting movements, the labrum is less effective in maintaining central compartment pressure in the Cam group specimens. The difference was not replicated in movements simulating gait and stooping [24].

The Effect of Capsular Pathology

Relatively little work has been undertaken to investigate the role of capsular structure and pathology on synovial circulation within the hip joint. In Crawford's [14] study the stability of cadaveric hips was investigated in the intact state, after capsular venting and after capsular venting in conjunction with a 15 mm incision at the antero-superior labrochondral junction (simulated labral tear). The average force required to achieve a 3 mm distraction of the femur from the acetabular socket fell by 43 and 60 % after venting, and incising the labrum, respectively. Also, femoral head displacement was more affected by capsular venting than by labral incision.

An extensile anterior capsulotomy is routinely undertaken by many arthroscopists to access the peripheral compartment. The need for formal repair after capsulotomy is debated. In a recent literature review of the role of the hip joint capsule in the normal state (stable) and pathologic states (instability or stiffness), Domb [9] cited 80 publications relevant to this subject. While some of these papers addressed such issues as capsular laxity and the potential for capsulotomy to disrupt the ZO's function as a locking ring, none discussed the effect of capsulotomy on synovial fluid circulation or joint lubrication.

The unidirectional synovial fluid circulation model depends upon the bellows effect of the ZO to pump synovial fluid from the peripheral compartment to the cotyloid recess of the central compartment. In a recent study on 18 hip arthroscopy patients with both preoperative and postoperative MR scans, a comparison was made between pre- and postoperative measurements of capsule and ZO thickness around the circumference of the neck. The thickness (in mm) of the ZO and the capsule did not significantly change in the posterior, superior and inferior aspects of the neck (Mean, ZO: 5.53 vs. 5.26; 8.37 vs. 7.32; 4.29 vs. 4.48. Capsule: 2.79 vs. 2.73; 4.35 vs. 3.91; 2.50 vs. 2.77 respectively) but, the ZO was significantly thinner postoperatively at the anterior aspect (Mean, ZO: 6.62 vs. 5.14 ($p<0.05$) Capsule: 3.88 vs. 3.47). The distance between the ZO and acetabular landmarks (acetabular rim, fovea, acetabular diameter) showed no significant differences before and after surgery. While not all patients had undergone a formal anterior capsulotomy, the average change was a 10 % thinning of the anterior capsule and 22 % thinning of the anterior ZO. It remains to be determined whether such structural change causes any change in synovial fluid circulation or joint lubrication.

Summary

Fluid mechanics of the hip and other synovial joints remain poorly understood with little scientific evidence to support the various theories that have been proposed. The role of synovial fluid circulation in the maintenance of joint health is also poorly understood. Likewise, the effects of joint preserving surgical interventions that are undertaken in growing numbers. With increasing interest in the preservation of labrochondral integrity and postsurgical reconstruction of the capsular structures, it is hoped that further attention will be directed to research on the role of synovial fluid movement around the joint, its role in preservation of healthy joint biomechanics and how it may be related to the development of degenerative joint disease.

References

1. Harvey W. Exercitatio anatomica de motu cordis et sanguinis in animalibus. Frankfurt: Sumptibus Guilielmi Fitzeri; 1628.
2. Rudbeck O. Nova exercitatio anatomica exhibens ductus hepaticos aquosus et vasa glandularum serosa. Vasteras: Lauringer; 1653.
3. Bartholin T. Vasa lymphatica, nuper Hafniae in animantibus inventa, et hepatis exsequiae. Copenhagen: Holst; 1653.
4. Di Chiro G. Movement of cerebrospinal fluid in human beings. Nature. 1964;204:290–1.
5. Wagner FV, Negrao JR, Campos J, et al. Capsular ligaments of the hip: anatomic, histologic, and positional study in cadaveric specimens with MR arthrography. Radiology. 2012;263:189.
6. Ito H, Song Y, Lindsey DP, Safran MR, Giori NJ. The proximal hip joint capsule and the zona orbicularis contribute to hip joint stability in distraction. J Orthop Res. 2009;27(8):989–95.
7. Gray H. Anatomy of the human body. 20th ed. Philadelphia, PA: Lea & Febiger; 1918. Bartleby.com. http://www.bartleby.com/107/. Published May 2000. Accessed Feb 2010.
8. Malagelada F, Tayar R, Barke S, Stafford G, Field RE. Anatomy of the zona orbicularis of the hip: a magnetic resonance study. Surg Radiol Anat. 10.1007/s00276-014-1300-z. Accessed Apr 2014.
9. Domb BG, Giordano BD, Philippon MJ. Arthroscopic capsulotomy, capsular repair, and capsular plication of the hip: relation to atraumatic instability. Arthroscopy. 2013;29(1):162–73.
10. Latarjet M, Ruiz Liard A. Articulación coxofemoral. In: Anatomía humana (spanish edition), 4th ed. Buenos Aires: Medica Panamericana; 2004. p. 706–745.
11. Pauwels F. Der schenkelhalsbrach ein mechanisches ProblemFerd. Stuttgart: Enke; 1935.
12. Ferguson SJ, Bryant JT, Ganz R, Ito K. An in vitro investigation of the acetabular labral seal in hip joint mechanics. J Biomech. 2003;36:171–8.
13. Mow VC, Holmes MH, Lai WM. Fluid transport and mechanical properties of articular cartilage: a review. J Biomech. 1984;17(5): 377–94.
14. Afoke A, Hutton WC, Byers PD. Synovial fluid circulation in the hip joint. Med Hypotheses. 1984;15(1):81–6.
15. Field RE, Rajakulendran K. The labro-acetabular complex. J Bone Joint Surg Am. 2011;93 Suppl 2:22–7.
16. Ferguson SJ, Bryant JT, Ganz R, Ito K. The influence of the acetabular labrum on hip joint cartilage consolidation: a poroelastic finite element model. J Biomech. 2000;33(8):953–60.
17. Dwyer MK, Jones HL, Hogan MG, Field RE, McCarthy JC, Noble PC. The acetabular labrum regulates fluid circulation of the hip joint during functional activities. Am J Sports Med. 2014;42(4):812–9.
18. Greenwald AS, O'Connor JJ. The transmission of load through the human hip joint. J Biomech. 1971;4(6):507–28.
19. Brown TD, Shaw DT. In vitro contact stress distributions in the natural human hip. J Biomech. 1983;16(6):373–84.
20. Lazennec JY, Laudet CG, Guerin-Surville H, Roy-Camille R, Saillant G. Dynamic anatomy of the acetabulum: an experimental approach and surgical implications. Surg Radiol Anat. 1997;19: 23–30.
21. Iman MA, Field RE. The location and number of acetabular subchondral cysts are predictors for early patient reported outcome of hip arthroscopy. ISHA presentation, Munich 2013.
22. McCarthy JC, Noble PC, Schuck MR, Wright J, Lee J. The role of labral lesions to development of early degenerative hip disease. Clin Orthop Relat Res. 2001;393:25–37.
23. Crawford MJ, Dy CJ, Alexander JW, Thompson M, Schroder SJ, Vega CE, Patel RV, Miller AR, McCarthy JC, Lowe WR, Noble PC. The biomechanics of the hip labrum and the stability of the hip. Clin Orthop Relat Res. 2007;465:16–22.
24. Dwyer MK, Jones HL, Field RE, McCarthy JC, Noble PC. Femoroacetabular impingement negates the acetabular labral seal during pivoting maneuvers but not gait. Clin Orthop Relat Res. 2014. DOI 10.1007/s11999-014-3760-1.

Research into the Application of Imaging to the Diagnosis of Hip Disease

102

Jason D. Alder, Steven S. Chua, Collin D. Bray, Joshua D. Harris, Andrew R. Palisch, and Philip C. Noble

In this chapter, we will describe and highlight emerging imaging techniques used to diagnose hip disease. Articular cartilage damage, including osteoarthritis, has emerged as a key component of active research within musculoskeletal imaging of the hip joint. Ongoing efforts focus on identifying morphologic, physiologic, and molecular markers of cartilage damage. Following advances in quantitative imaging of articular cartilage within the knee, there has been a recent expansion of research activity in the hip [1]. Two modalities finding successful application to the early detection of degenerative changes are ultrasound for imaging internal derangement of cartilaginous tissue, and MRI for imaging compositional changes in the tissue as reflected in its content of glycosaminoglycans (GAGs), collagen, and water [2]. This topic was introduced briefly in the "Imaging Cartilage Patho-anatomy" chapter of this book. For more comprehensive details on the imaging of the hip, the reader is referred to an excellent review article by Sutter and coworkers [3].

J.D. Alder, MD
Department of Orthopaedic Surgery, Houston Methodist Hospital, Houston, TX, USA

S.S. Chua, MD, PhD
Department of Radiology, Baylor College of Medicine, One Baylor Plaza, Houston, TX 77030, USA

C.D. Bray, MD (✉)
Department of Radiology, Musculoskeletal Imaging, Baylor College of Medicine, One Baylor Plaza, Houston, TX 77030, USA
e-mail: cbray@bcm.edu

J.D. Harris, MD
Department of Orthopaedics and Sports Medicine, Clinical Orthopaedics, Weill Cornell Medical College, Houston Methodist Hospital, 6550 Fannin Street, Suite 2500, Houston, TX 77030, USA

A.R. Palisch, MD
Department of Radiology, Baylor College of Medicine, One Baylor Plaza, Houston, TX 77030, USA

Department of Radiology, Musculoskeletal Imaging, Baylor College of Medicine, One Baylor Plaza, Houston, TX 77030, USA

P.C. Noble
Director of Research, Institute of Orthopedic Research and Education, 6550 Fannin Street, Suite 2501, Houston, TX 77030, USA
e-mail: pnoble@bcm.edu

Ultrasound Imaging of Articular Cartilage

The utilization of ultrasound for joint imaging is advantageous because it is non-invasive, does not utilize ionizing radiation, is quick and possesses multi-planar evaluation, and significantly improves the accuracy of intra-articular injections [4]. This has led to its widespread adoption in rheumatology for the investigation of inflammatory arthropathies [5]. In Europe, in particular, clinical investigators have reported that ultrasonography possesses superior diagnostic capabilities compared to conventional radiography and the clinical exam in the evaluation of bone surface abnormalities and crystalline diseases [6, 7]. In addition, ultrasound can offer the operator the opportunity to accurately guide joint aspirations and drug injections into the joints and can easily be performed by the bedside or in the clinic setting [7, 8]. However, the need for an optimal acoustic window and operator skill has limited the optimal use of this technology to examination of smaller joints, including those of the hands, wrists, and ankles [7]. Examination of larger joints like the shoulder and hips requires more select conditions and operator skill and experience to glean important information on joint derangement.

Applications of ultrasonography in the hip include the assessment and confirmation of the presence of joint inflammation, detection of early osteophytosis, accurate placement of intra-articular steroid injection and aspiration of joint fluid for analyses [7, 8]. This modality also offers promise in the imaging of cartilage, where it may provide more direct visualization of pathologic changes in the internal structure of the tissues through regional differences in echotexture [4, 7]. This has been demonstrated in the knee, where healthy hyaline cartilage is visualized as a homogenous

J.C. McCarthy et al. (eds.), *Hip Joint Restoration*, DOI 10.1007/978-1-4614-0694-5_102

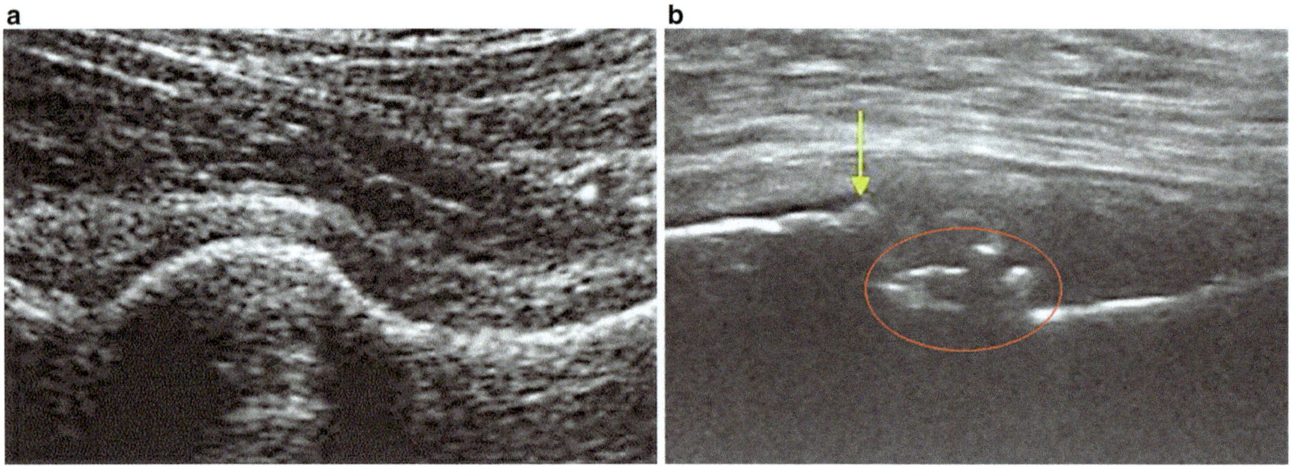

Fig. 102.1 Normal asymptomatic hip. (**a**) Longitudinal sonographic imaging shows normal hypoechoic hyaline cartilage. (**b**) Longitudinal sonographic image of a hip with osteoarthritis showing an osteophyte (*arrow*) and loose bodies (*ellipse*). *Copyright © Dr. T.S.A. Geertsma, Ziekenhuis Gelderse Vallei, Ede, The Netherlands. All rights reserved.* http://www.ultrasoundcases.info/Slide-View.aspx?cat=373&case=1620

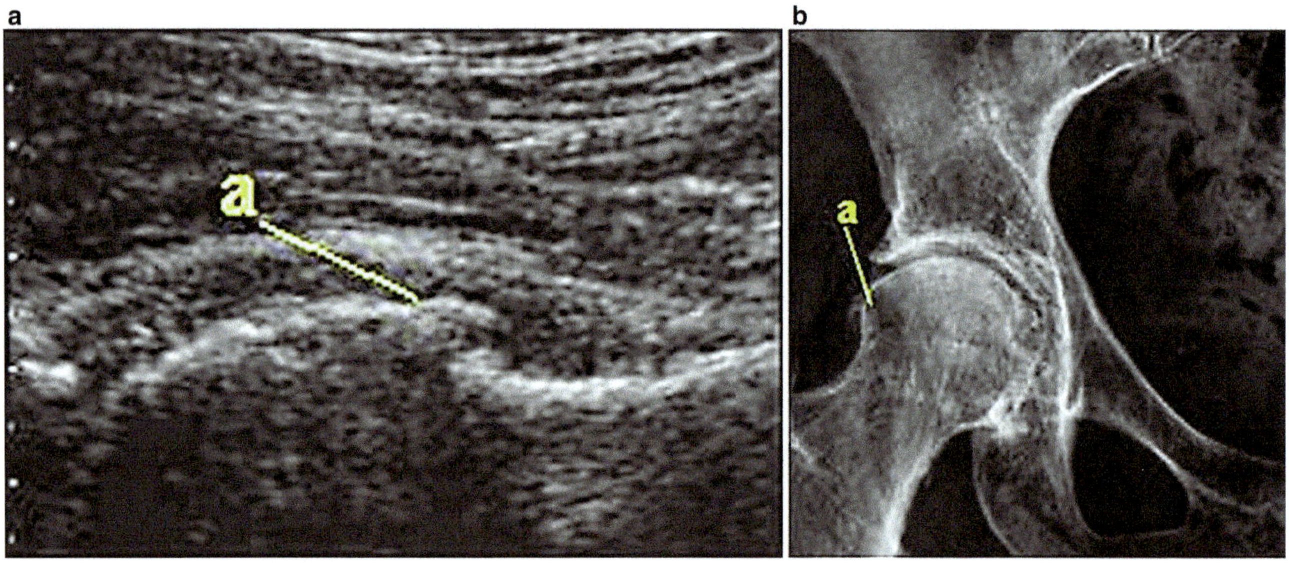

Fig. 102.2 Abnormal hip sonographic image. (**a**) Sonographic image shows loss of the normal hypoechoic hyaline cartilage and development of hyperechoic osteophyte formation. (**b**) Correlation of osteophyte (**a**) seen on longitudinal ultrasound in Fig. 102.1b. *Copyright © Dr. T.S.A. Geertsma, Ziekenhuis Gelderse Vallei, Ede, The Netherlands. All rights reserved.* http://www.ultrasoundcases.info/Slide-View.aspx?cat=373&case=1620

anechoic band (Fig. 102.1a) [8]. During the progression of osteoarthritis, characteristic sonographic changes (blurring of cartilage edges, loss of homogeneity, focal and diffuse thinning, and/or complete loss of tissue) are recognized [7, 9, 10]. In the case of the knee, the hypoechoic sonographic appearance of healthy cartilage in Fig. 102.1a is in contrast to the pathologic appearance of the osteoarthritic knee in Figs. 102.1b and 102.2a, where the severe loss of the normal hypoechoic hyaline cartilage is depicted in association with the hyperechoic appearance of osteophytes. This finding is better delineated in the accompanying radiographic image (Fig. 102.2b).

The success of ultrasound in imaging articular cartilage is highly dependent on the ability of the operator to obtain an optimal acoustic window and a perpendicular insertion angle. This often necessitates maneuvering joints into suitable positions. Also, while a high frequency transducer provides high-resolution images, its limited tissue penetration limits its use to small joints while lower frequencies must be used for imaging larger joints, typically the knee and the shoulder [4]. For this reason, the use of ultrasound for imaging the hip joint requires a unique convex curvilinear probe, different from the flat probe used for knees, ankles, shoulders, and elbows [7]. This imposes a large, significant cost in addition to the cost of the ultrasound machine itself. Nonetheless, although plain radiography continues to be the gold standard evaluation of osteoarthritis, ultrasound may be helpful in the evaluation of both osteoarthritis and inflammatory arthropathies in assessment of cartilage damage and joint effusion [7].

MRI in the Imaging of Osteoarthritis

MR arthrography sequences used for the studying of articular cartilage include fat-suppressed T1-weighted FSE (fast spin echo) images in three planes [11]. The comparison of traditional MR arthrographic sequences with IDEAL-SPGR (iterative decomposition of water and fat with echo asymmetry and least-squares estimation with spoiled gradient echo) showed that the IDEAL-SPGR sequences have lower specificity for the detection of cartilage lesions vs. arthroscopy [12]. It has been further found that MR arthrography is also more sensitive than non-contrast MRI in the evaluation of chondral lesions (41 % vs. 18 %, respectively); while both techniques are similarly specific [13].

Quantitative Imaging Techniques for Cartilage

Cartilage mapping is a measure of the thickness and condition of articular cartilage as a whole. In addition, regional variation in cartilage thickness may be observed, providing information that may be useful for surgical planning of hip preservation surgery [3]. New MRI sequences that respond to changes in cartilage biochemistry and differential charge density also offer promise. While not yet common in clinical practice, these techniques, including dGEMRIC (delayed gadolinium-enhanced MRI of cartilage), T2 cartilage mapping, T1 rho imaging and sodium imaging offer new information about the patterns and complexities of hip cartilage pathologies. These modalities are discussed in more detail below.

dGEMRIC

This acronym (dGEMRIC: delayed Gadolinium-enhanced MRI of Cartilage) refers to a T1-weighted sequence that is performed after intravenous administration of negatively charged gadolinium contrast agent (gadolinium diethylenetriaminepentacetate) [14]. The resulting images reflect the local distribution of negatively charged glycosaminoglycans (GAG) (primarily keratin and chondroitin sulfate) within articular cartilage. Since both the gadolinium contrast agent and GAGs are negatively charged, they chemically oppose one another. After IV administration of gadolinium contrast agent, if contrast uptake is high, then GAG concentration is low (and vice versa). Gadolinium-contrast agent shortens the T1 relaxation time (milliseconds) in proportion to its concentration. Thus, the lower the T1 relaxation time, the greater the concentration of gadolinium-contrast agent within articular cartilage and the lower the proportion of GAGs. The loss of GAG is an early event in the development of hip osteoarthritis; therefore, its indirect visualization by dGEMRIC has the potential to monitor the effect of joint-preserving hip surgery on arthritis progression [15–17]. The elegance of this sequence is that it permits the detection of cartilage damage even before morphologic manifestations are apparent in standard MRI sequences and plain radiographs (Fig. 102.3).

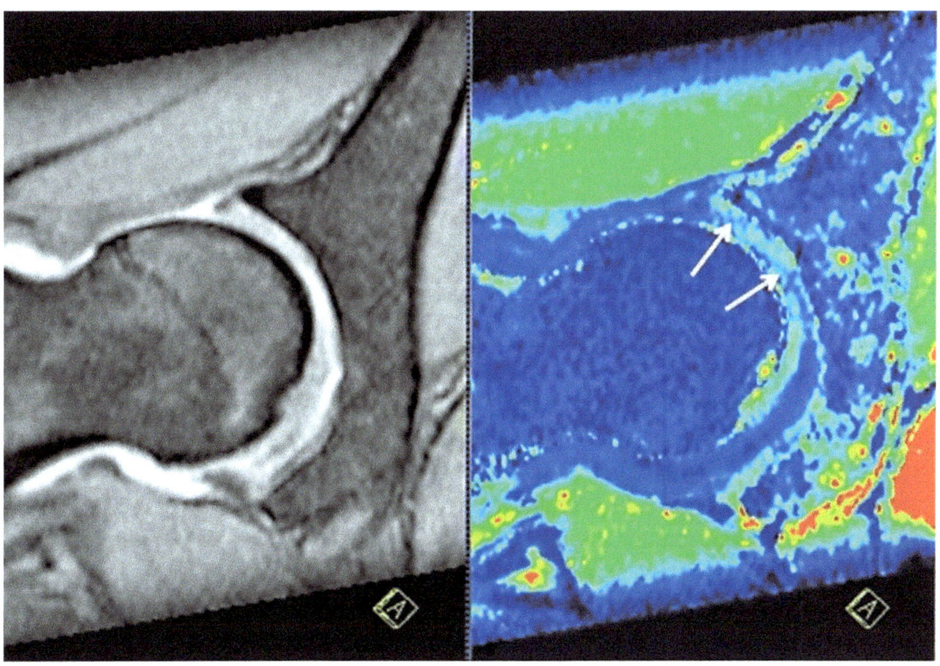

Fig. 102.3 An MR arthrogram of a hip patient compared to the same image after intra-articular uptake of Gd-DTPA2 imaged with dGEMRIC. An increase in the normal Gd uptake within the cartilage layer is indicated by the change in T1 values. This was found to correspond to severe cartilage damage peripherally and centrally in the superior aspect of the hip. From Bittersohl et al, Orthop Rev (Pavia). 2011; 3:e11). Published online Jun 29, 2011. doi: 10.4081/or.2011.e11. ©Copyright B. Bittersohl et al., 2011. This work is licensed under a Creative Commons Attribution NonCommercial 3.0 License (CC BY-NC 3.0). Licensee PAGEPress, Italy

Articular cartilage damage has been observed in hips of individuals with both symptomatic [18] and asymptomatic [19] femoroacetabular impingement (FAI; cam morphology). The use of radial MRI and dGEMRIC sequences improves visualization of both the articular cartilage and the labrum within the antero-superior quadrant, which is difficult to evaluate under standard conditions [15, 20]. A disadvantage of dGEMRIC is that gadolinium administration is invasive, is associated with pain during intravenous line placement, adds length to the scan time, requires exercise post-injection and pre-scan, and is associated potentially with nephrogenic systemic fibrosis [21].

T2 Mapping

The principle behind T2 mapping in MRI is that the T2 relaxation time is based on the ability of free water cations to move and exchange electrons with anions in the cartilaginous extracellular matrix [21]. Within normal cartilage, T2 relaxation time is dependent predominantly on the anisotropic motion of water molecules in the fibrillar network of type II collagen. T2 values decrease from the superficial layer to the deep layer with the exception of the surface lamina splendens. Once pathologic change occur within articular cartilage, with increased water concentration and alteration of the collagen–GAG composition, the T2 relaxation time increases, as observed in osteoarthritis [22], and subjects of increased age [23] and increased BMI [24].

To quantify T2 values, an exponential decay curve is constructed which is based on T2-weighted images generated from different TEs (times to echo). T2-weighted images from different MRI sequences can be utilized to evaluate the water content of cartilage but care must be taken because there is variation of T2 quantification due to a variety of system imperfections and artifacts, including stimulated echoes, off-resonance signals, and eddy currents [25].

Most published studies describing the application of T2 mapping have been performed in the knee, and so, confirmatory data are still lacking for imaging the hip. In previous work, Mosher and coworkers [26] showed that the T2 relaxation times within knee cartilage decreased after high impact injury due to consolidation of the tissues with a corresponding reduction in its water content. Moreover, following impact injury, the greatest reduction in relation time is observed in the superficial regions of the cartilage layer where peak compressive stresses occur [27]. Studies evaluating the effects of exercise on cartilage health have shown that in individuals who perform light exercise, the T2 relaxation times in the knee cartilage are lower than those who are sedentary or who are moderate-to-strenuous exercisers, suggesting a U-shaped phenomenon in terms of T2 relaxation times [28]. It is likely that exercise is not the only modifying factor that affects cartilage as the BMI, biomechanics of motion, joint alignment, and genetics do play a role [28]. Although T2 mapping promises to be a powerful technique to evaluate spatial changes in the water content of cartilage, this imaging modality does have some deficiencies, including variability in the T2 values reported by different investigators, difficulty in separating the lamina splendens from the superficial zone, especially in thin cartilage layers, and the magic angle effect, which can confound interpretation of T2 images [21]. Nonetheless, with refinements and improvements of this technique, this method can be applied to the evaluation of hip cartilage, which may be very beneficial to get a glimpse of the macromolecular changes in hip cartilage pathology.

T2* Mapping

T2* mapping is a quantitative assessment of changes of T2 relaxation time at the cartilage surface which allows the creation of a 3D volume rendering [3]. It has advantages of faster acquisition times than standard T2 mapping and is based on the effect of interactions between water molecules and the collagen fiber network on relaxation of the T2 signal. T2* mapping has been shown to be a feasible option for a faster technique of biochemical imaging to demonstrate early changes in cartilage status, however it has limitations that may decrease its value in clinical settings. A key advantage of T2* mapping is that it can be performed without intravenous administration of contrast or gadolinium and has shown good correlation with conventional MRI [29]. While T2 values increase in cartilage from patients with osteoarthritis, T2* values decrease [1]. The effect of volume averaging and lower spatial resolution afforded by T2 mapping in the hip may permit T2* mapping to prove significantly advantageous [1]. Damaged femoral head specimens have shown a decrease of T2* value (indicating more severe OA) that correlated with higher Mankin scores [30]. A limitation of T2* mapping is the lack of the 180° refocusing pulse, which leaves it more sensitive to susceptibility artifacts which are present at the bone–cartilage interface, as well a magic-angle effect that must be monitored closely at 55° when imaging a spherical-shaped joint such as the hip [29].

T1rho (T1ρ)

T1rho mapping is an emerging technique that estimates the loss of proteoglycans in the cartilage when a spin-lock pulse is applied to ascertain the interactions between water and GAGs within the extracellular matrix. A spin-lock pulse is a low-power radiofrequency pulse that is applied on-resonance, locking the magnetization vector into a rotated frame [3, 31]. T1rho values in cartilage increase with age [32] and early

OA [33, 34] and have been shown to be predictive of progressive loss of cartilage at 2-year follow-up [34]. It is also suggested that T1rho imaging is sensitive for early cartilage damage in patients with FAI [35]. Although T1rho maps have been calculated from hip cartilage relaxation time measurements, their clinical relevance has not yet been widely evaluated. The advantage of this methodology is that like T2 mapping, no contrast administration or additional special hardware is needed (vs. dGEMRIC). A disadvantage is the high specific energy absorption rate of T1 rho performed at higher magnetic fields [21].

Sodium MR Imaging

Sodium MR imaging, like dGEMRIC, is based on the concept that a fixed charged density (FCD) of negative ions is present within the extracellular matrix of cartilage, correlated with GAG concentration [36]. Since the negative FCD is in equilibrium with positively charged sodium ions, the concentration of sodium ions is a sensitive method for measuring the GAG content of articular cartilage [37–39]. However, the relatively low innate concentration of sodium within articular cartilage leads to weak MR signals and long acquisition times. In addition, sodium ions have very short T2 relaxation times and require multinuclear capabilities for use with conventional MRI equipment, leading to limited adoption of this modality [40]. Clinical use of sodium imaging may become more feasible with higher magnet strength (3-Tesla, 7-Tesla) with multichannel dual tuned proton/sodium coil technology [41]. However, this technique is still confounded by the presence of high sodium levels in the synovial fluid which makes the detection of variations in sodium ion concentrations near the articular surface more challenging [1]. Nonetheless, it is possible to suppress the signal in the synovial fluid, thereby increasing the efficiency of evaluating cartilage [40, 42]. An example of sodium MR imaging of a healthy knee by Gold and co-workers [11] is shown in Fig. 102.4.

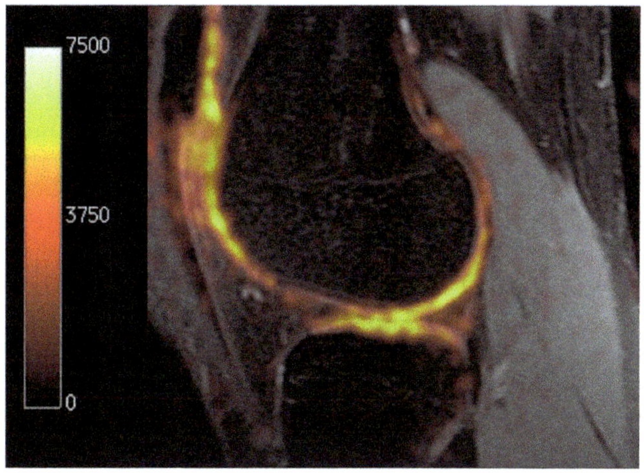

Fig. 102.4 Sodium MRI of the knee of a healthy volunteer (28 years; 3T coil) registered to a proton spoiled gradient-echo image with a resolution of 1.25 × 1.25 × 4 mm. Image courtesy of Garry Gold, MD

Glycosaminoglycan-Chemical Exchange Saturation Transfer (gag-CEST)

This method is a relatively new proton-based technology that has been used to evaluate the GAG content of articular cartilage within the knee through detection of exchangeable protons from mobile GAG at the cartilage surface [1, 43, 44]. These changes can be seen early in the degenerative process. Schmitt and colleagues showed good correlation between gag-CEST and sodium imaging as markers of GAG concentration in cartilage [45]. However, the applicability of this technique to the hip has not yet been demonstrated and, even in the knee this novel modality is not without flaws. These include its sensitivity to changes in pH, hydration, and collagen content, which may affect the rate of exchange of labile protons and complicate comparison of studies performed in different facilities [21]. In addition, magnetic field homogeneities and susceptibility artifacts can complicate interpretation of results. Recent modifications of this technology have focused on improving inhomogeneities in the magnetic field and in improving efficiency [46]. Gag-CEST has been used to evaluate GAG content in cartilage repair tissue after autologous osteochondral transplantation [47].

Diffusion Techniques

Diffusion techniques evaluate the rate of water diffusion within articular cartilage, which is affected by degradation of extracellular matrix. One such technique is dual echo steady state (DESS) in which 3D maps of T2-weighted images and the apparent diffusion coefficient (ADC) are acquired simultaneously [48]. In the hip, Knuesel and co-workers [49] have shown that DESS reveals a higher severity of hip articular cartilage damage than conventional T1-weighted spin echo sequences, suggesting earlier detection of articular cartilage changes. This may be a valuable tool for guiding joint preservation surgery, potentially improving outcomes through the detection of degenerative processes earlier in the disease process that is possible with conventional MRI [50]. However, DESS is limited by the fact that the relative contribution of the T2 component to the 3D map is dependent on the flip angle used in acquiring the image, leading to inaccuracies in the interpretation of the displayed image [51].

Diffusion tensor imaging (DTI) is a method that measures the fractional anisotropy of collagen in articular cartilage as a biomarker for tissue degradation [52]. This is consistent with a recent study of cartilage samples with OARSI (Osteoarthritis Research Society International) grades of greater than zero in which DTI demonstrated significant loss of fractional anisotropy in the deeper regions of articular samples. This is compatible with loss of collagen anisotropy during the early stages of cartilage degeneration. Changes in the orientation of proteoglycans within the tissue generated directional restrictions on water diffusion, leading to anisotropic movement of water molecules through the cartilage. The three-dimensional distribution of this diffusion anisotropy (fractional anisotropy) is an indirect measurement of collagen architecture [53]. Disadvantages of DTI include low signal-to-noise ratio, the need for high-resolution images, long acquisition times, and the susceptibility of the technique to motion artifact [21].

Ultra-short TE (echo time) (UTE) imaging has been used in musculoskeletal investigations to investigate the presence of subclinical meniscal tear in acute ACL [54] and in meniscal calcifications [55], and so may have utility in the hip. This modality reveals details of changes in the internal structure of soft-tissue structures, including the meniscus, and so has application for evaluation of labral pathology if the same resolution that is achieved in the knee can be approached in the hip. UTE utilizes the rapid T2 decay signal that is normally too rapid to be captured during conventional imaging studies [1]. However, if a dual inversion recovery method is used, it is possible to suppress signals from both fat and water, leading to high-contrast visualization of the zone of calcified cartilage.

Functional Imaging of the Labrum

The acetabular labrum is thought to control the transport of synovial fluid between the central and peripheral compartments thus suggesting that the labrum functions as a fluid exchange regulator [15, 56–58]. Recently, a path of unidirectional flow between the peripheral and central compartments at different degrees of flexion and extension was identified via dynamic radiographic imaging. The investigators hypothesized that the flow of synovial fluid in and out of the intra-articular compartment maintained the nutritional status of the articular cartilage of the joint. Ferguson and co-workers have reported that the labrum seals the central compartment to contain synovial fluid within the joint thereby allowing lubrication to be maintained under functional loading [15, 59]. The function of the labrum in regulating the flow of synovial fluid has been further elucidated by the work of Field et al. [56] and Dwyer et al. [57, 58] using contrast injections in both patents and cadavers, respectively. These studies have demonstrated that the labrum maintains fluid within the central compartment (i.e. between the articulating surfaces) until the joint is placed in a position in which the labrum loses its effective seal with the head of the femur. At this point, flow of synovial fluid occurs from the central to the peripheral compartment; however, a minimum value of fluid pressure is maintained within the joint.

MR imaging studies using 3-Tesla strength magnets have been performed by Noble and colleagues to identify the locations of fluid transfer between the central and peripheral compartments of the hip joint and to characterize the morphology of the labro-femoral junction at sites of fluid transfer. While fixed to a loading apparatus, a cadaveric hip joint was placed in a functional position and loaded. A solution was then continually injected into the central compartment through a portal created in the quadrilateral plate of the ilium (acetabular floor) until the labrum yielded and allowed fluid to pass into the peripheral compartment. A holding jig was then fixed to the specimen to preserve its position and the specimen was imaged (Fig. 102.5). Data from these experiments may allow better understanding of the role of the labrum in FAI before and after surgical repair.

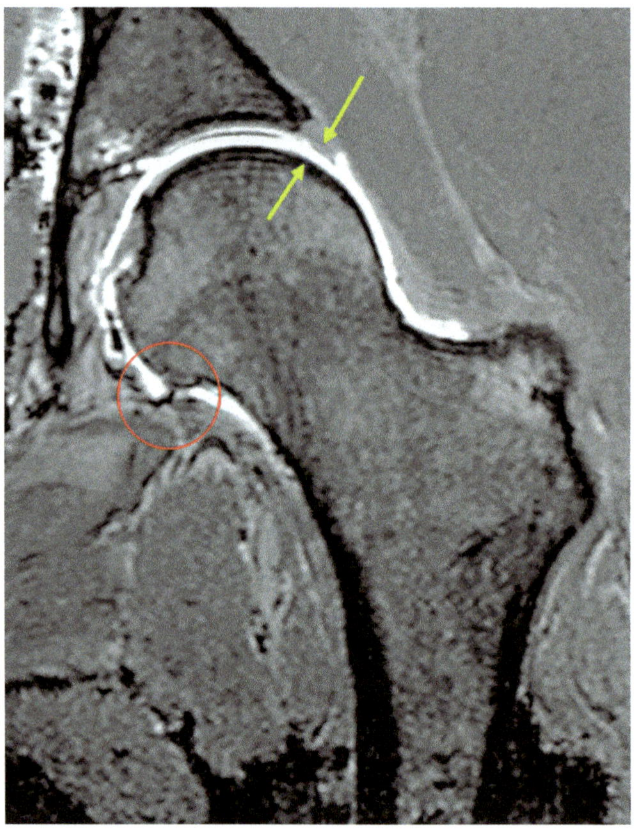

Fig. 102.5 T1 MPRAGE (Magnetization Prepared Rapid Acquisition Gradient Echo) sequences of cadaver left hip during pressurization of the central compartment with a contrast agent injected via the floor of the acetabulum. Transfer of fluid to the peripheral compartment is visualized superiorly, past the labrum (*arrows*) and inferiorly, past the trans-acetabular ligament (*red circle*)

Ligamentum Teres Imaging

Ligamentum teres injuries should be considered in the differential diagnosis of hip pain and it is suggested that partial ligamentum teres tears can lead to hip microinstability [60–62]. MRI imaging of the ligamentum teres is in its infancy and studies have focused mainly on its anatomy. Blankenbaker and co-workers [63] evaluated 116 patients by MRI arthrography to ascertain if there were any diagnostic criteria for tears in the ligamentum teres and found that 12 patients had partial tears. Subtle MRI findings of partial tears are difficult to discern when compared to the normal structure. Thus, there is a need for large cohorts of patients to carefully examine the appearance of this structure under imaging in the context of intra-articular hip lesions.

Conclusion

Currently ultrasound, radiography and MRI are the mainstay of hip imaging, but these give limited information regarding the articular cartilage of the hip. The next generation of high-resolution MRI is centered on evaluating signal changes in the composition of articular cartilage to detect early osteoarthritis. These techniques include dGEMRIC, T2 mapping, T2*, T1rho, sodium imaging, gag-CEST, and diffusion imaging, which analyze proteoglycan and water composition within articular cartilage to give information regarding the condition and topography of the cartilage. Each method has its own advantages and disadvantages. Further research is needed prior to general and widespread clinical use.

Acknowledgements The authors extend their thanks to Hugh Jones and Krista Runge for their technical assistance in performing MRI examinations of cadaveric specimens.

References

1. Mosher TJ, Walker EA, Petscavage-Thomas J, Guermazi A. Osteoarthritis year 2013 in review: imaging. Osteoarthritis Cartilage. 2013;21:1425–35.
2. Hani AF, Kumar D, Malik AS, Ahmad RM, Razak R, Kiflie A. Non-invasive and in vivo assessment of osteoarthritic articular cartilage: a review on MRI investigations. Rheumatol Int. 2015;35:1–16.
3. Sutter R, Zanetti M, Pfirrmann CWA. New developments of hip imaging. Radiology. 2012;264:651–67.
4. Kane D, Balint PV, Sturrock R, Grassi W. Musculoskeletal ultrasound—a state of the art review in rheumatology. Part 1: current controversies and issues in the development of musculoskeletal ultrasound in rheumatology. Rheumatology. 2004;43:823–8.
5. Joshua F. Ultrasound applications for the practicing rheumatologist. Best Pract Res Clin Rheumatol. 2012;26:853–67.
6. Naredo E, D'Agostino M, Conaghan PG, Backhaus M, Balint P, Bruyn GAW, Filippucci E, Grassi W, Hammer HB, Iagnocco A, Kane D, Koski JK, Szkudlarek M, Terslev L, Wakefield RJ, Ziswiler HR, Schmidt WA. Current state of musculoskeletal ultrasound training and implementation in Europe: results of a survey of experts and scientific societies. Rheumatology. 2010;49:2438–43.
7. Iagnocco A, Naredo E. Osteoarthritis: research update and clinical applications. Rheumatology. 2012;51:vii2–5.
8. Micu M, Bogdan G, Fodor D. Steroid injection for hip osteoarthritis: efficacy under ultrasound guidance. Rheumatology. 2010;49:1490–4.
9. Naredo E, Acebes C, Moller I, Canillas F, de Agustin JJ, de Miguel E, et al. Ultrasound validity in the measurement of knee cartilage thickness. Ann Rheum Dis. 2009;68:1322–7.
10. Bevers K, Zweers MC, van den Ende CH, Martens HA, Mahler E, Bijlsma JW, et al. Ultrasonographic analysis in knee osteoarthritis: evaluation of inter-observer reliability. Clin Exp Rheumatol. 2012;30:673–8.
11. Gold SL, Burge AJ, Potter HG. MRI of hip cartilage. Clin Orthop Relat Res. 2012;470:3321–31.
12. Blankenbaker DG, Ullrick SR, Kijowski R, Davis KW, De Smet AA, Shinki K, Muñoz del Rio A, Keene JS. MR arthrography of the hip: comparison of IDEAL-SPGR volume sequence to standard MR sequences in the detection and grading of cartilage lesions. Radiology. 2011;261:863–71.
13. Byrd JW, Jones KS. Osteoarthritis caused by an inverted acetabular labrum: radiologic and arthroscopic treatment. Arthroscopy. 2002;18:741–7.
14. Bittersohl B, Hosalkar HS, Werlen S, Trattnig S, Siebenrock KA, Mamisch TC. Intravenous versus intra-articular delayed gadolinium-enhanced magnetic resonance imaging in the hip joint: a comparative analysis. Invest Radiol. 2010;45:538–42.
15. Domayer SE, Ziebarth K, Chan J, Bixby S, Mamisch TC, Kim YJ. Femoroacetabular cam-type impingement: diagnostic sensitivity and specificity of radiographic views compared to radial MRI. Eur J Radiol. 2011;80:805–10.
16. Burstein D, Velyvis J, Scott KT, Stock KW, Kim Y-J, Jaramillo D, Boutin RD, Gray ML. Protocol issues for delayed Gd(DTPA)$^{2-}$-enhanced MRI (dGEMRIC) for clinical evaluation of articular cartilage. Magn Reson Med. 2001;45:36–41.
17. Bashir A, Gray ML, Burstein D. Gd-DTPA2− as a measure of cartilage degradation. Magn Reson Med. 1996;36:665–73.
18. Bittersohl B, Steppacher S, Haamberg T, Kim YJ, Werlen S, Beck M, et al. Cartilage damage in femoroacetabular impingement (FAI): preliminary results on comparison of standard diagnostic vs delayed gadolinium-enhanced magnetic resonance imaging of cartilage (dGEMRIC). Osteoarthritis Cartilage. 2009;17:1297–306.
19. Pollard TC, Villar RN, Norton MR, Fern ED, Williams MR, Simpson DJ, et al. Femoroacetabular impingement and classification of the cam deformity: the reference interval in normal hips. Acta Orthop. 2010;81:134–41.
20. Stubendorff JJ, Lammentausta E, Struglics A, Lindberg L, Heinegard D, Dahlberg LE. Is cartilage sGAG content related to early changes in cartilage disease? Implications for interpretation of dGEMRIC. Osteoarthritis Cartilage. 2012;20:396–404.
21. Li X, Majumdar S. Quantitative MRI of articular cartilage and its clinical applications. J Magn Reson Imaging. 2013;38(5):991–1008.
22. Li X, Ma C, Link T, et al. In vivo T1rho and T2 mapping of articular cartilage in osteoarthritis of the knee using 3 Tesla MRI. Osteoarthritis Cartilage. 2007;15:789–97.
23. Mosher T, Liu Y, Yang Q, et al. Age dependency of cartilage magnetic resonance imaging T2 relaxation times in asymptomatic women. Arthritis Rheum. 2004;50:2820–8.
24. Koff MF, Amrami KK, Kaufman KR. Clinical evaluation of T2 values of patellar cartilage in patients with osteoarthritis. Osteoarthritis Cartilage. 2007;15:198–204.
25. Pai A, Li X, Majumdar S. A comparative study at 3T of sequence dependence of T2 quantitation in the knee. Magn Reson Imaging. 2008;26:1215–20.

26. Mosher TJ, Liu Y, Torok CM. Functional cartilage MRI T2 mapping: evaluating the effect of age and training on knee cartilage response to running. Osteoarthritis Cartilage. 2010;18:358–64.
27. Subburaj K, Kumar D, Souza RB, et al. The acute effect of running on knee articular cartilage and meniscus magnetic resonance relaxation times in young healthy adults. Am J Sports Med. 2012;9: 2134–41.
28. Hovis KK, Stehling C, Souza RB, et al. Physical activity is associated with magnetic resonance imaging-based knee cartilage T2 measurements in asymptomatic subjects with and those without osteoarthritis risk factors. Arthritis Rheum. 2011;63:2248–56.
29. Zilkens C, Miese F, Herten M, Kurzidem S, Jager M, Konig D, et al. Validity of gradient-echo three-dimensional delayed gadolinium-enhanced magnetic resonance imaging of hip joint cartilage: a histologically controlled study. Eur J Radiol. 2013;82(2):e81–6.
30. Bittersohl B, Miese FR, Hosalkar HS, Herten M, Antoch G, Krauspe R, et al. T2* mapping of hip joint cartilage in various histological grades of degeneration. Osteoarthritis Cartilage. 2012;20:653–60.
31. Johannessen W, Auerbach JD, Wheaton AJ, Kurji A, Borthakur A, Reddy R, et al. Assessment of human disc degeneration and proteoglycan content using T1rho-weighted magnetic resonance imaging. Spine. 2006;31:1253–7.
32. Goto H, Iwama Y, Fujii M, Aoyama N, Kubo S, Kuroda R, et al. The natural degeneration course in the T1rho values of normal knee cartilage. Kobe J Med Sci. 2011;57:E155–70.
33. Subburaj K, Souza RB, Stehling C, Wyman BT, Le Graverand-Gastineau MP, Link TM, et al. Association of MR relaxation and cartilage deformation in knee osteoarthritis. J Orthop Res. 2012;30:919–26.
34. Prasad AP, Nardo L, Schooler J, Joseph GB, Link TM. T(1rho) and T(2) relaxation times predict progression of knee osteoarthritis. Osteoarthritis Cartilage. 2013;21:69–76.
35. Rakhra KS, Lattanzio PJ, Cardenas-Blanco A, Cameron IG, Beaule PE. Can T1-rho MRI detect acetabular cartilage degeneration in femoroacetabular impingement?: a pilot study. J Bone Joint Surg Br. 2012;94:1187–92.
36. Braun HJ, Dragoo JL, Hargreaves BA, Levenston ME, Gold GE. Application of advanced magnetic resonance imaging techniques in evaluation of the lower extremity. Radiol Clin N Am. 2013;51:529–45.
37. Zybri S, Mlynarik V, Juras V, Szomolanyi P, Trattnig S. Sodium MR imaging of articular cartilage pathologies. Curr Radiol Rep. 2014;2:41–5.
38. Reddy R, Insko EK, Noyszewski EA, et al. Sodium MRI of human articular cartilage in vivo. Magn Reson Med. 1998;39(5):697–701.
39. Borthakur A, Shapiro EM, Beers J, et al. Sensitivity of MRI to proteoglycan depletion in cartilage: comparison of sodium and proton MRI. Osteoarthritis Cartilage. 2000;8(4):288–93.
40. Madelin G, Jerschow A, Regatte RR. Sodium relaxation times in the knee joint in vivo at 7T. NMR Biomed. 2012;25:530–7.
41. Kim JH, Moon CH, Park BW, Furlan A, Zhao T, Bae KT. Multichannel transceiver dual-tuned RF coil for proton/sodium MR imaging of knee cartilage at 3T. Magn Reson Imaging. 2012;30:562–71.
42. Regatte RR, Kaufman JH, Noyszewski EA, et al. Sodium and proton MR properties of cartilage during compression. J Magn Reson Imaging. 1999;10(6):961–7.
43. Sun PZ, Farrar CT, Sorensen AG. Correction for artifacts induced by B0 and B1 field inhomogeneities in pH-sensitive chemical exchange saturation transfer (CEST) imaging. Magn Reson Med. 2007;58:1207–15.
44. Ling W, Regatte RR, Navon G, et al. Assessment of glycosaminoglycan concentration in vivo by chemical exchange-dependent saturation transfer (gagCEST). Proc Natl Acad Sci U S A. 2008;105(7):2266–70.
45. Schmitt B, Zbyn S, Stelzeneder D, Jellus V, Paul D, Lauer L, Trattnig S. Cartilage quality assessment using glycosaminoglycan chemical exchange saturation transfer and sodium MRI at 7 Tesla. Radiology. 2011;260:257–64.
46. Varma G, Lenkinski RE, Vinogradov E. Keyhole chemical exchange saturation transfer. Magn Reson Med. 2012;68:1228–33.
47. Krusche-Mandl I, Schmitt B, Zak L, Apprich S, Aldrian S, Juras V, et al. Long-term results 8 years after autologous osteochondral transplantation: 7T gagCEST and sodium magnetic resonance imaging with morphological and clinical correlation. Osteoarthritis Cartilage. 2012;20:357–63.
48. Staroswiecki E, Granlund KL, Alley MT, Gold GE, Hargreaves BA. Simultaneous estimation of T(2) and apparent diffusion coefficient in human articular cartilage in vivo with a modified three-dimensional double echo steady state (DESS) sequence at 3T. Magn Reson Med. 2012;67:1086–96.
49. Knuesel PR, Pfirrmann CW, Noetzli HP, Dora C, Zanetti M, Hodler J, et al. MR arthrography of the hip: diagnostic performance of a dedicated water-excitation 3D double-echo steady-state sequence to detect cartilage lesions. Am J Roentgenol. 2004;183:1729–35.
50. Sambandam SN, Hull J, Jiranek WA. Factors predicting the failure of Bernese periacetabular osteotomy: a meta-regression analysis. Int Orthop. 2009;33:1483–8.
51. Wu PH, Cheng CC, Wu ML, Chao TC, Chung HW, Huang TY. Effects of RF profile on precision of quantitative T2 mapping using dual-echo steady-state acquisition. Magn Reson Imaging. 2014;32:102–6.
52. Raya JG, Horng A, Dietrich O, Krasnokutsky S, Beltran LS, Storey P, Glaser C. Articular cartilage: in vivo diffusion-tensor imaging. Radiology. 2012;262:550–9.
53. Raya JG, Melkus G, Adam-Neumair S, Dietrich O, Mutzel E, Reiser MF, et al. Diffusion-tensor imaging of human articular cartilage specimens with early signs of cartilage damage. Radiology. 2013;266:831–41.
54. Williams A, Qian Y, Golla S, Chu CR. UTE-T2* mapping detects sub-clinical meniscus injury after anterior cruciate ligament tear. Osteoarthritis Cartilage. 2012;20:486–94.
55. Omoumi P, Bae WC, Du J, Diaz E, Statum S, Bydder GM, et al. Meniscal calcifications: morphologic and quantitative evaluation by using 2D inversion-recovery ultrashort echo time and 3D ultrashort echo time 3.0-T MR imaging techniques feasibility study. Radiology. 2012;264:260–8.
56. Field RE, Rajakulendran K. The labro-acetabular complex. J Bone Joint Surg Am. 2011;93:22.
57. Dwyer MK, Jones HL, Hogan MG, Field RE, McCarthy JC, Noble PC. The acetabular labrum regulates fluid circulation of the hip joint during functional activities. Am J Sports Med. 2014;42:812–9.
58. Dwyer MK, Jones HL, Field RE, McCarthy JC, Noble PC. Femoroacetabular impingement negates the acetabular labral seal during pivoting maneuvers but not gait. Clin Orthop Relat Res. 2015;473:602–7.
59. Ferguson SJ, Bryant JT, Ganz R, Ito K. An in vitro investigation of the acetabular labral seal in hip joint mechanics. J Biomech. 2003;36(2):171–8.
60. Cerezal L, Arnaiz J, Canga A, Piedra T, Altónaga JR, Munafo R, Pérez-Carro L. Emerging topics on the hip: ligamentum teres and hip microinstability. Eur J Radiol. 2012;81(12):3745–54.
61. Boykin RE, Anz AW, Bushnell BD, Kocher MS, Stubbs AJ, Philippon MJ. Hip instability. J Am Acad Orthop Surg. 2011;19(6):340–9.
62. Mei-Dan O, McConkey MO, Brick M. Catastrophic failure of hip arthroscopy due to iatrogenic instability: can partial division of the ligamentum teres and iliofemoral ligament cause subluxation? Arthroscopy. 2012;28(3):440–5.
63. Blankenbaker DG, De Smet AA, Keene JS, del Rio AM. Imaging appearance of the normal and partially torn ligamentum teres on hip MR arthrography. Am J Roentgenol. 2012;199(5):1093–8.

Cell Therapy in Hip Surgery

103

M. Munir Khan, Paul Genever, James B. Richardson, and Andrew W. McCaskie

Introduction

Hip pathology is diverse, ranging from fracture to chronic degenerative conditions. Despite this breadth of pathology, the underpinning treatment often requires tissue repair or regeneration, e.g. bone healing and cartilage repair. Cell biology has always been a key component to the understanding of orthopedic diseases and has guided therapy, such as the use of biomaterials, but now the cell itself is emerging as a potential treatment. Tissue Engineering is not new, and was defined in the early 1990s as an 'interdisciplinary science involving life sciences and engineering to bring about biological substitutes that restore, maintain, or improve tissue function' [1]. More recently, a more clinically orientated term, regenerative medicine, has emerged with the objective of seeking to replace or regenerate 'human cells, tissue or organs, to restore or establish normal function' [2, 3]. Within this context, this chapter focuses on emerging cell-based therapeutic strategies as they relate to hip surgery.

M.M. Khan, PhD, FRCS (T&O)
Division of Orthopaedics, Department of Trauma and Orthopaedics, Freeman Hospital, Newcastle Upon Tyne, NE7 7DN, UK

P. Genever, BSc, PhD
Department of Biology, University of York, York Y10 5DD, UK

J.B. Richardson, MBChB, FRCS, MD
Department of Orthopaedics, Keele University, Oswestry, UK

A.W. McCaskie, MMus, MD, FRCS, FRCS (T&O) (✉)
Division of Trauma and Orthopaedic Surgery, Department of Surgery, University of Cambridge, Addenbrooke's Hospital, Box 180, Cambridge, CB2 0QQ, UK
e-mail: awm41@cam.ac.uk

Stem Cells and Potency

Stem cells have a characteristic biology, which includes self-renewal and potency, and are encountered in different stages of embryonic development. The earliest are called embryonic stem cells (ESCs). Shortly after fertilization, the cells are totipotent and can differentiate into all types of cells required to support the development of a new organism, including extra-embryonic supportive tissues such as the placenta and umbilical cord. Cells from the inner cell mass of the blastocyst in 5–6 days old embryos [4] exhibit pluripotency, which is the ability to differentiate into all cell types, apart from the extra-embryonic tissue. Consequently, this type of pluripotent cell has and continues to be studied in terms of biology and possible future clinical application. In 2012, a Nobel Prize was awarded to Gurdon and Yamanaka for their work on the reprogramming of mature adult (somatic) cells [4, 5]. These seminal studies, which spanned over four decades, culminated in the creation of a cell type, from an adult cell, that has pluripotent potential. This is called an induced pluripotent stem cell (iPSC).

Adult Cells with Clinical Potential

Cells with an ability to differentiate into several cell lines can also be found in the adult. There are several types, but those found in bone marrow have attracted a lot of attention in terms of clinical translation and will be discussed further. Bone marrow stromal cells (BMSC) that originate in mesoderm have been termed mesenchymal stromal cells (MSC) [6] and were originally discovered in bone marrow [7]. Later, they were isolated from a variety of connective tissues including synovial fluid [8], synovial membrane [9, 10], periosteum [11], intervertebral disc [12], adipose tissue and articular cartilage [13]. In the laboratory, they are multipotent and can differentiate into cartilage, bone and fat (Fig. 103.1) [14]. Apparently similar looking cells, residing

J.C. McCarthy et al. (eds.), *Hip Joint Restoration*, DOI 10.1007/978-1-4614-0694-5_103

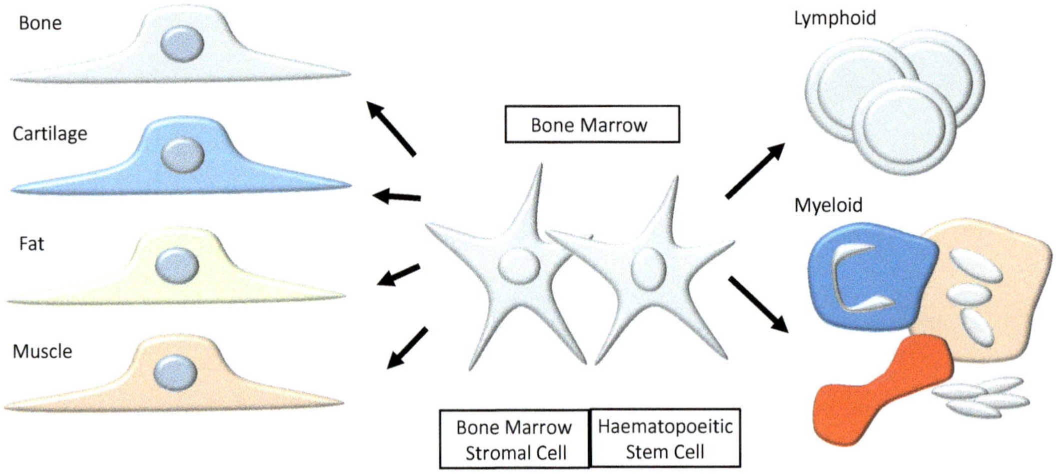

Fig. 103.1 Bone marrow stromal and stem cells and their characteristic cell differentiation

in the various tissue compartments, can be identified by studying their surface markers, called cluster of differentiation (CD). These markers can be a reflection of the cells' differentiation, migration, attachment to matrix elements, and other functions. Mesenchymal cells are initially identified by their ability to adhere to plastic or glass. When adherent MSCs are cultured in laboratory with other marrow residents, e.g. haematopoietic cells, the MSCs remain while other cells are gradually lost in successive populations. This technique is simple and rapid, but will lead to a mixed population of cells that belong to the adherent bone marrow fraction, a few of which are likely to be the true stem cells. In vitro culture can also lead to a loss of MSC differentiation ability as well as ageing. To avoid these problems, prospective identification of MSCs is desirable. The common surface CD markers used for detection of MSCs are CD73, CD90 and CD105 [14, 15]. The cells are also tested for absence of some surface markers (CD14- or CD11b-, CD19- or CD79α-, CD34-, CD45- and HLA-DR) which are found on other resident bone marrow cells, e.g. haematopoietic cells. Moreover, cellular markers are linked to the ability of the cell to proliferate and differentiate into various lineages. CD106-positive cells have less osteogenic potential and are more adipogenic and chondrogenic [16]. These cells are rapidly proliferating and have multipotency. On the other hand, CD106-negative cells grow slowly and mostly differentiate to the osteogenic lineage [17]. Another important surface marker is CD271, a transmembrane protein found in bone marrow stromal populations with potential applications in orthopedic surgery [15]. Cells with a positive marker have more mineralization capacity than those without [18]. This type of cell selection by marker can fine tune cell selection and therefore may be useful in therapy. Another stem cell type found in marrow is from the haematopoietic family, which is CD34-positive. There is a large amount of clinical experience with this type of cell, mainly in the field of haematology and the treatment of haematological malignancies. A current clinical acquisition technique does not involve bone marrow harvest from the pelvis but utilizes human granulocyte colony-stimulating growth factors to stimulate the marrow and release cells into the peripheral blood [19]. Cell collection is carried out using an apheresis machine, which retrieves the target cells from the circulation. The cells can then be stored by cryopreservation.

Adult cell populations offer advantages over ESCs and iPSCs in terms of clinical translation, particularly at the time of writing. They are relatively easy to obtain and have less regulatory and ethical problems. This type of cell has great potential use in musculoskeletal repair if proven to be safe. Knowledge is needed regarding the mechanism of action and careful terminology will be required in order to avoid confusion with pluripotent cells [20]. Adult-derived cell populations are considered closer to the clinic and will be the focus of the remainder of the chapter.

Strategies for Musculoskeletal Repair

Tissue engineering strategies traditionally include cells, scaffolds and other factors. A 'scaffold' provides a three-dimensional environment for cells and can direct the desired cell function, e.g. bone graft to encourage osteogenesis. In stem cell biology, the three-dimensional microenvironment, termed the niche, can influence cell fate. Some of the control is physical, based on the relationship of the cells to a small area of basement membrane, whilst other controls are from local growth factors. These factors can be exploited to develop therapy (Fig. 103.2).

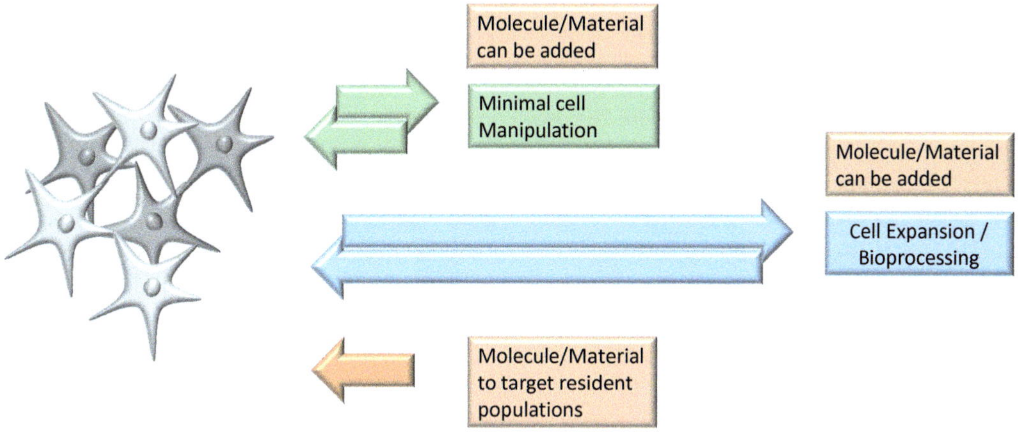

Fig. 103.2 Schematic representation of common cell therapy strategies

Cells Derived from the Patient

As we discussed earlier, cells suited to repair reside in the adult, and removal of such a target population could be useful as a basis of treatment. The harvest requires particular techniques and thereafter there are two strategies. In the first, the harvested cells can be expanded in the laboratory. This means that cell division takes place until the desired number and type of cell is reached. Chondrocyte expansion uses this type of approach and this can also be applied to MSC populations. The bioprocessing occurs in a highly regulated laboratory [21, 22] and the process requires two operative stages (harvest and re-implantation) separated by a period of bio-processing.

In the second strategy, no cell expansion occurs and the process can be described as minimally manipulated. This means that the desired number and type of cells must be achieved by the 'harvesting' process, e.g. centrifugation and concentration from tissue such as bone marrow, peripheral blood, fat and umbilical cord [23–25]. With this approach, the whole process can potentially be positioned closer to the patient and may be subject to a different regulatory system. Notably, both techniques involve the cells being administered back to the patient.

Cells and the Fabricated Environment

Materials and scaffolds can be used to augment the cell therapy. One example is to combine the scaffold and cells in the laboratory, by bioprocessing to produce a tissue construct, e.g. a cartilage bioreactor. The introduction or combination of cell and material can also take place at the time of surgery, e.g. fibrin [26].

The Fabricated Environment

Marrow stimulation techniques (microfracture) create an environment that can achieve repair by allowing resident marrow cells to enter the joint space. A theoretical extension of this approach is the so-called smart biomaterial. This would provide the stimulus to achieve resident cell repair and would not require the further addition of cells at the time of surgery. The nature of the material and the surgical technique required for insertion are yet to be fully determined but this is an attractive approach where cells remain integral but are derived from the patient's resident population.

Donor Cells

The final treatment strategy employs cells from a donor. This would allow an off-the-shelf solution and would make use of an expanded cell population. This type of approach has manufacturing scale-up and may have benefits in treatment costs. For effective translation, this approach will need to overcome issues of biocompatibility, the immune response [27, 28] and disease transmission.

Multi-Modal Therapy

The first applications of cell therapy will not be as a total treatment solution. It is more likely that the cell will be an adjunct to current surgical therapy or a development of one, e.g. microfracture. This will allow a regenerative step to augment an existing procedure, e.g. impingement surgery in the presence of early degenerative change and cartilage damage, which can be termed multi-modal therapy or surgery.

How Can This Be Applied in the Clinic?

Articular cartilage derangements of the hip can be generalized or focal. The latter is usually associated with femoroacetabular impingement (FAI), dysplasia or osteonecrosis of the femoral head. The concept of FAI as a dynamic cause of degeneration of articular cartilage was introduced by Ganz and colleagues [29] and is discussed elsewhere in this book. The resultant impingement leads to labral, chondrolabral and cartilage damage. Surgery aims to remove the cause and eliminate bony impingement but clearly there is a need for repair of the tissue damage already present. It has been identified that the outcome following hip arthroscopy can be predicted by the condition of the hip joint cartilage [30] and so regenerative therapy for focal defects and early osteoarthritis is a clear therapeutic option and must be combined with treatment of the precipitating factors, the impingement and labral tear.

Microfracture

Various arthroscopic and open techniques have been employed to regenerate cartilage in the knee, but current experience in the hip is limited. One of the techniques is microfracture, which makes a communication between the joint cavity and the bone marrow. Resident progenitor cells are presumed to be recruited directly from the bone marrow to fill the cartilage defect. The resultant cartilage formed by this technique is mostly fibrocartilage, although some hyaline cartilage is also seen [31]. Byrd et al. [32] published on the outcome of microfracture in the hip, reporting that three out of nine patients with localized grade IV defects to the acetabulum were treated by excision of the torn labrum and microfracture. At final 2 years follow-up, only these three patients were able to return to an active lifestyle. Haviv et al. [33] reported a benefit with microfracture and femoral osteochondroplasty in 29 patients compared to those without microfracture (from a cohort of 135 hip arthroscopies with grade II and III acetabular lesions). Philippon et al. [34] reported that 8 out of 9 patients who underwent revision arthroscopy following microfracture were found to have 95–100 % filling of the defect. Horisberger et al. [35] reported that arthroscopic hip debridement and microfracture in hips with FAI led to poor results in patients with advanced cartilage defects, especially if the femoral head was also found to have cartilage defects. More recently, a study of elite athletes undergoing hip arthroscopic procedures reported that there was no difference 'in return to play rate after hip arthroscopy with microfracture and hip arthroscopy without microfracture' [36]. Delaminated flaps of unstable cartilage can be observed at the rim of the acetabulum, and may progress to more advanced degenerative changes in the hip joint. Sekiya et al. [37] and Tzaveas et al. [38] reported successful restoration of the unstable chondral flap by performing microfracture in the underlying bone and either stitching the chondral flap or using fibrin glue. Autologous matrix-induced chondrogenesis (AMIC) adds a further step to microfracture. In this technique, Chondro-Gide (Collagen I/III) matrix is placed in the microfracture defect to stabilize the blood clot. The experience with this technique in knee surgery is encouraging and patients treated remain improved for up to 24 months postoperatively. The same technique has now been reported in treatment of cartilage defects in the hip [39].

Autologous Chondrocyte Implantation (ACI)

In order to achieve better quality cartilage regeneration in the knee, Brittberg et al. in 1994 introduced autologous chondrocyte implantation (ACI) technique in 1994 [40]. This is a two-step procedure and has been used to regenerate cartilage in the knee joint. When compared with microfracture in the knee, a 'characterized chondrocyte implantation' technique gave better clinical results at 36 months [41] and structural results at 1 year [42]. In one study [43], a select group of patients with a shorter duration of symptoms (<3 years) had better clinical results than microfracture, highlighting the importance of this type of treatment at an earlier stage. To further improve results, second-generation ACI was introduced, where ACI is associated with a matrix to simulate a three-dimensional culture environment. Good to excellent results have been published in studies involving animals and humans [44, 45]. ACI has been used also to treat cartilage lesions in the hip. Akimau et al. [46] reported using first-generation ACI treatment in a patient with cartilage loss and post-traumatic osteonecrosis. The patient received ex vivo selected and expanded autologous chondrocytes harvested from a healthy knee articular cartilage, after filling the bone defect with trochanteric bone graft. A second look arthroscopic biopsy revealed development of a mixture of fibrous and to a lesser extent hyaline cartilage. Before the procedure, the patient had a Harris Hip Score (HHS) of 52 and required a crutch to walk. At 16 months, his score improved to 76 and was able to 'run on the spot and walk more than a mile'. A repeat CT scan at 18 months showed return of joint space. One of our authors (JBR) followed this patient out to 11 years and the patient continues to have a high hip score (89 points) and is in full time employment.

Fontana et al. [47] in a retrospective comparative study reported results of a two-stage ACI treatment versus simple debridement. The mean defect size was 2.6 cm^2. At 74 months, patients in ACI group had a better HHS of 87 (56 in control group) although the study lacked follow-up via plain radiographs or second-look arthroscopy. Donor cartilage can be obtained from either the hip or knee, with donor site symptoms in the knee resolving between 2 and 12 months after arthroscopy [48]. The drawback of the ACI therapies lies in the use of in vitro cell proliferation and the additional arthroscopic procedure. There are now several randomized trials of cell therapy in the knee, and a relatively large number of reviews. Some report in favour of ACI over alternative treatments [43, 49], particularly for large defects, although others do not [50, 51]. A consensus paper drawn from the views of 104 UK surgeons concluded that access to cell therapy is important for cartilage repair of the knee [52]. The debate will become clearer with time, as ACI is only required to be 20 % more effective than alternatives in the medium term, to become cost-effective [53].

Mosaicplasty

Replacement of articular defects with small autograft plugs, harvested from non-weight bearing parts of the joints, is called mosaicplasty. This technique has been used to treat cartilage defects in the knee and has also been used in hips in a few studies. The graft has been taken from the knee by some surgeons and others have used graft from the inferolateral portion of the femoral head. This technique requires hip dislocation and is difficult to perform arthroscopically. The experience with this technique is very limited and the studies include case reports and series of up to 10 patients. Mosaicplasty has been employed for treatment of femoral and acetabular defects following traumatic dislocations, osteonecrosis, Legg-Calves-Perthes disease, and epiphyseal dysplasia. The studies [54–57] reported excellent incorporation of the mosaic and improvement in the patients' hip function. To avoid the problem of donor site morbidity, Myers [58] and Krych [59], in separate publications, have reported use of allograft osteochondral plugs to treat cartilaginous defects. Both the studies have reported good results; however, as mentioned above, this technique requires dislocation of the hip via open surgery rather than arthroscopy.

Adult Marrow Cells

Building on the success of the above mentioned approaches adult marrow cells such as MSCs may further enhance the quality and quantity of the tissue produced, either as an alternative or in conjunction with chondrocytes. In the knee, there are case studies using MSCs expanded in culture for cartilage repair [60–62]. Nejednik in 2010 reported, in a cohort study of 74 patients, that cultured bone marrow-derived cells were as effective as chondrocytes [63]. More recently, there have been encouraging initial reports of using selected and expanded marrow-derived cells as post-operative adjuncts to microfracture following tibial osteotomy [64]. In this randomized control trial, the group of patients receiving selected and culture-expanded MSC had a significant benefit seen as an increased rise in Lysholm of seven points. Both groups had received osteotomy and microfracture. Peripheral blood-derived stem cells (PBSCs) have also been described as a cell type for cartilage lesions in the knee [65]. Recently, Saw et al. [66] reported the results of a study comparing one group treated with sub-chondral drilling with another group treated with sub-chondral drilling plus injections of hyaluronic acid (HA) and PBSC. The group receiving HA and PBSC demonstrated an improvement in the quality of the cartilage repair on histological examination. A recent systematic review concerning stem cell therapy for human cartilage defects concluded that although there was 'an increasing body of evidence in non-human' studies, there is limited evidence for benefit in humans [67]. It is hoped that similar techniques can be used in arthroscopic hip surgery to treat conditions like focal traumatic cartilaginous defects and cartilage defects associated with labral pathologies in impingement lesions, or AVN of the femoral head.

Bone Regeneration

Regeneration of bone is an important aspect of many non-articular conditions, such as fracture repair. A recent study has shown that MSCs from sites of fracture non-union have less osteogenic differentiation and mineralization capability, at least in vitro, compared to bone marrow-derived MSCs [68]. In this situation, provision of healthy stem cells with adequate functional capacity may improve fracture healing. The exact mechanism of action of MSCs is unknown. The beneficial effects may not be confined to progenitor activity but may also include other mechanisms, e.g. paracrine secretion and immune modulation [20, 69]. When MSCs are transplanted into the fracture callus, they express mRNAs for osteocalcin and type I collagen [70–73] which suggests that they might directly differentiate into osteoblasts. In animal studies, bone regeneration has been reported using bone marrow-derived MSCs (BMMSCs) alone [74], BMMSCs in combination with growth factors (BMP-7), or BMMSCs genetically modified to express vector encoding factors like BMPs [75, 76]. Reports of bone regeneration in humans are limited; some studies have used MSCs with ceramic scaffolds [77, 78] and others have injected MSCs percutaneously into the site of non-union [79].

Avascular necrosis of the femoral head has several causes but is common in patients undergoing steroid therapy and in those with a history of alcohol abuse. The number of osteogenic progenitor cells is reduced in steroid-related AVN, both in the lesion as well as in its surroundings [80, 81]. The potential of these cells to differentiate towards the osteogenic lineage is decreased [82] and their ability to differentiate towards adipose cells is increased [83]. MSCs can be introduced into the avascular area of the femoral head. One study [84] recruited one patient with steroid-induced osteonecrosis of the femoral head and four patients with AVN of the knee. These patients were young with an age range of 9–27 years (long-term and high-dose steroid treatment for leukemia). The cells were injected into the avascular area after core decompression under radiological control. All the patients had responded to treatment at 16 months' follow-up. Another study [85] reported the outcome of 100 patients randomly assigned to either sub-trochanteric injections of BMMSCs or core decompression. At 5 years of follow-up, only two patients of 53 in the BMMSC group showed progression of osteonecrosis while over 20 % of the remaining patients in the core decompression group required additional procedures like vascularized fibular grafting or THA. Kawate and colleagues [86] treated 3 patients (stage III steroid-induced osteonecrosis) with autologous MSC and beta-tricalcium phosphate composite granules (a vascularized fibular graft was also performed in all cases). All of the hips showed collapse preoperatively but only 2 were observed to progress at 34 months of follow-up. However, there was no progression in osteonecrosis during the duration of the study.

Safety and Regulation

Patient safety is clearly the priority for any intervention and particularly for new cell-based approaches. This is facilitated by regulation which should be adhered to in all such treatments (e.g. in Europe; European Medicines Agency, in UK; Medicines and Healthcare Regulatory Agency). Bioprocessing of cells and particularly those requiring cell number expansions must be tightly controlled to maintain quality. Regulators classify treatment and then specify the correct regulatory pathway to follow. It is important that the correct nomenclature is applied to a cell therapy to avoid regulatory confusion, e.g. stem cell pluripotent populations and adult stromal cell populations [20] particularly whilst there remains some uncertainty about biological activity. At the time of writing, safety profiles for adult-derived cell products are encouraging with no patient safety concerns identified in recent literature reviews of intra-articular autologous culture expanded cells for cartilage repair [87] and intravascular MSC usage for other conditions [88].

Technique and Translation

Stem cell-based treatments must undergo a stepwise translation to the clinic. This will include careful in vitro and when required in vivo preclinical testing. It is important to highlight the difference between the knee and the hip in terms of access. Successful application will require surgical technique and instrument development to enable cell and material usage arthroscopically. Furthermore, clinical trials will require careful design and implementation with appropriate methodological development and outcome measures. This approach will ensure both safety and efficacy and health-economic assessment. Cell and regenerative therapies bring together many stakeholders (patients, clinicians, regulators, health care providers and industry) and all must work effectively together to bring therapy into practice. As our knowledge of cell-based repair processes develops, there is an unprecedented opportunity to implement clinical strategies for bone and cartilage repair in the hip.

Acknowledgement Sally Roberts and Roger A. Brooks.

References

1. Langer R, Vacanti JP. Tissue engineering. Science. 1993;260(5110): 920–6.
2. Mason C, Brindley DA, Culme-Seymour EJ, Davie NL.Cell therapy industry: billion dollar global business with unlimited potential. Regen Med. 2011;6(3):265–72. doi:10.2217/rme.11.28.
3. Mason C, Dunnill P. A brief definition of regenerative medicine. Regen Med. 2008;3(1):1–5.
4. Gurdon JB. The developmental capacity of nuclei taken from intestinal epithelium cells of feeding tadpoles. J Embryol Exp Morphol. 1962;10:622–40.
5. Takahashi K, Yamanaka S. Induction of pluripotent stem cells from mouse embryonic and adult fibroblast cultures by defined factors. Cell. 2006;126(4):663–76.
6. Dominici M, et al. Minimal criteria for defining multipotent mesenchymal stromal cells. The International Society for Cellular Therapy position statement. Cytotherapy. 2006;8(4):315–7.
7. Friedenstein AJ, Chailakhjan RK, Lalykina KS. The development of fibroblast colonies in monolayer cultures of guinea-pig bone marrow and spleen cells. Cell Tissue Kinet. 1970;3(4):393–403.
8. Jones EA, et al. Enumeration and phenotypic characterization of synovial fluid multipotential mesenchymal progenitor cells in inflammatory and degenerative arthritis. Arthritis Rheum. 2004;50(3):817–27.
9. De Bari C, et al. Skeletal muscle repair by adult human mesenchymal stem cells from synovial membrane. J Cell Biol. 2003;160(6): 909–18.
10. De Bari C, et al. Multipotent mesenchymal stem cells from adult human synovial membrane. Arthritis Rheum. 2001;44(8):1928–42.
11. De Bari C, Dell'Accio F, Luyten FP. Human periosteum-derived cells maintain phenotypic stability and chondrogenic potential throughout expansion regardless of donor age. Arthritis Rheum. 2001;44(1):85–95.
12. Liu LT, et al. Characteristics of stem cells derived from the degenerated human intervertebral disc cartilage endplate. PLoS One. 2011;6(10):e26285.
13. Dowthwaite GP, et al. The surface of articular cartilage contains a progenitor cell population. J Cell Sci. 2004;117(Pt 6):889–97.
14. Pittenger MF, et al. Multilineage potential of adult human mesenchymal stem cells. Science. 1999;284(5411):143–7.
15. Jones E, et al. Large-scale extraction and characterization of CD271+ multipotential stromal cells from trabecular bone in health and osteoarthritis: implications for bone regeneration strategies

based on uncultured or minimally cultured multipotential stromal cells. Arthritis Rheum. 2010;62(7):1944–54.
16. Fukiage K, et al. Expression of vascular cell adhesion molecule-1 indicates the differentiation potential of human bone marrow stromal cells. Biochem Biophys Res Commun. 2008;365(3):406–12.
17. Jung EM, et al. Evidences for correlation between the reduced VCAM-1 expression and hyaluronan synthesis during cellular senescence of human mesenchymal stem cells. Biochem Biophys Res Commun. 2011;404(1):463–9.
18. Alexander D, et al. LNGFR induction during osteogenesis of human jaw periosteum-derived cells. Cell Physiol Biochem. 2009;24(3–4):283–90.
19. Link H, et al. Transplantation of allogeneic CD34+ blood cells. Blood. 1996;87(11):4903–9.
20. Bianco P, et al. Regulation of stem cell therapies under attack in Europe: for whom the bell tolls. EMBO J. 2013;32(11):1489–95.
21. Bosse R, et al. Production of stem-cell transplants according to good manufacturing practice. Ann Hematol. 2000;79(9):469–76.
22. Bosse R, et al. Good manufacturing practice production of human stem cells for somatic cell and gene therapy. Stem Cells. 1997;15 Suppl 1:275–80.
23. Liu J, et al. Cord blood banking and transplantation in china: a ten years experience of a single public bank. Transfus Med Hemother. 2012;39(1):23–7.
24. Chen X, et al. Chondrogenic differentiation of umbilical cord-derived mesenchymal stem cells in type I collagen-hydrogel for cartilage engineering. Injury. 2013;44(4):540–9.
25. Fong CY, et al. Human umbilical cord Wharton's jelly stem cells undergo enhanced chondrogenic differentiation when grown on nanofibrous scaffolds and in a sequential two-stage culture medium environment. Stem Cell Rev. 2012;8(1):195–209.
26. Ben-Ari A, et al. Isolation and implantation of bone marrow-derived mesenchymal stem cells with fibrin micro beads to repair a critical-size bone defect in mice. Tissue Eng Part A. 2009;15(9): 2537–46.
27. Panda A, et al. Corneal graft rejection. Surv Ophthalmol. 2007;52(4):375–96.
28. Hamlet W, Liu SH, Yang R. Destruction of a cyropreserved meniscal allograft: a case for acute rejection. Arthroscopy. 1997;13(4): 517–21.
29. Ganz R, et al. Femoroacetabular impingement: a cause for osteoarthritis of the hip. Clin Orthop Relat Res. 2003;417:112–20.
30. Egerton T, et al. Intraoperative cartilage degeneration predicts outcome 12 months after hip arthroscopy. Clin Orthop Relat Res. 2013;471(2):593–9.
31. Knutsen G, et al. A randomized trial comparing autologous chondrocyte implantation with microfracture. Findings at five years. J Bone Joint Surg Am. 2007;89(10):2105–12.
32. Byrd JW, Jones KS. Osteoarthritis caused by an inverted acetabular labrum: radiographic diagnosis and arthroscopic treatment. Arthroscopy. 2002;18(7):741–7.
33. Haviv B, et al. Arthroscopic femoral osteochondroplasty for cam lesions with isolated acetabular chondral damage. J Bone Joint Surg Br. 2010;92(5):629–33.
34. Philippon MJ, et al. Can microfracture produce repair tissue in acetabular chondral defects? Arthroscopy. 2008;24(1):46–50.
35. Horisberger M, Brunner A, Herzog RF. Arthroscopic treatment of femoral acetabular impingement in patients with preoperative generalized degenerative changes. Arthroscopy. 2010;26(5): 623–9.
36. McDonald JE, Herzog MM, Philippon MJ. Return to play after hip arthroscopy with microfracture in elite athletes. Arthroscopy. 2013;29(2):330–5.
37. Sekiya JK, Martin RL, Lesniak BP. Arthroscopic repair of delaminated acetabular articular cartilage in femoroacetabular impingement. Orthopedics. 2009;32(9): 692–696. doi:10.3928/01477447-20090728-44.
38. Tzaveas AP, Villar RN. Arthroscopic repair of acetabular chondral delamination with fibrin adhesive. Hip Int. 2010;20(1):115–9.
39. Fontana A. A novel technique for treating cartilage defects in the hip: a fully arthroscopic approach to using autologous matrix-induced chondrogenesis. Arthrosc Tech. 2012;1(1):e63–8.
40. Brittberg M, et al. Treatment of deep cartilage defects in the knee with autologous chondrocyte transplantation. N Engl J Med. 1994;331(14):889–95.
41. Saris DB, et al. Treatment of symptomatic cartilage defects of the knee: characterized chondrocyte implantation results in better clinical outcome at 36 months in a randomized trial compared to microfracture. Am J Sports Med. 2009;37 Suppl 1:10S–9.
42. Saris DB, et al. Characterized chondrocyte implantation results in better structural repair when treating symptomatic cartilage defects of the knee in a randomized controlled trial versus microfracture. Am J Sports Med. 2008;36(2):235–46.
43. Vanlauwe J, et al. Five-year outcome of characterized chondrocyte implantation versus microfracture for symptomatic cartilage defects of the knee: early treatment matters. Am J Sports Med. 2011;39(12):2566–74.
44. Moretti M, et al. Effects of in vitro preculture on in vivo development of human engineered cartilage in an ectopic model. Tissue Eng. 2005;11(9–10):1421–8.
45. Hollander AP, et al. Maturation of tissue engineered cartilage implanted in injured and osteoarthritic human knees. Tissue Eng. 2006;12(7):1787–98.
46. Akimau P, et al. Autologous chondrocyte implantation with bone grafting for osteochondral defect due to posttraumatic osteonecrosis of the hip—a case report. Acta Orthop. 2006;77(2):333–6.
47. Fontana A, et al. Arthroscopic treatment of hip chondral defects: autologous chondrocyte transplantation versus simple debridement—a pilot study. Arthroscopy. 2012;28(3):322–9.
48. McCarthy HS, Richardson JB, Parker JCE, Roberts S. Evaluating joint morbidity after chondral harvest for autologous chondrocyte implantation (ACI): a study of ACI-treated ankles and hips with a knee chondral harvest. Cartilage OnlineFirst. Published on 5 Oct 2015 as doi:10.1177/1947603515607963.
49. Saris D, et al. Matrix-applied characterized autologous cultured chondrocytes versus microfracture: two-year follow-up of a prospective randomized trial. Am J Sports Med. 2014;42(6):1384–94.
50. Vasiliadis HS, Wasiak J. Autologous chondrocyte implantation for full thickness articular cartilage defects of the knee. Cochrane Database Syst Rev. 2010;10:CD003323.
51. Mundi R, Bedi A, Chow L, Crouch S, Simunovic N, Sibilsky Enselman E, Ayeni OR. Cartilage Restoration of the Knee: A Systematic Review and Meta-Analysis of Level1 Studies. Am J Sports Med. 2015 Jul 2. pii: 0363546515589167. [Epub ahead of print].
52. Biant LC, et al. The surgical management of symptomatic articular cartilage defects of the knee: consensus statements from United Kingdom knee surgeons. Knee. 2015;22(5):446–9.
53. Clar C, et al. Clinical and cost-effectiveness of autologous chondrocyte implantation for cartilage defects in knee joints: systematic review and economic evaluation. Health Technol Assess. 2005;9(47):iii–iv. ix–x, 1–82.
54. Sotereanos NG, et al. Autogenous osteochondral transfer in the femoral head after osteonecrosis. Orthopedics. 2008;31(2):177.
55. Hart R, et al. Mosaicplasty for the treatment of femoral head defect after incorrect resorbable screw insertion. Arthroscopy. 2003; 19(10):E1–5.
56. Girard J, et al. Osteochondral mosaicplasty of the femoral head. Hip Int. 2011;21(5):542–8.
57. Nam D, et al. Traumatic osteochondral injury of the femoral head treated by mosaicplasty: a report of two cases. HSS J. 2010;6(2): 228–34.
58. Meyers MH. Resurfacing of the femoral head with fresh osteochondral allografts. Long-term results. Clin Orthop Relat Res. 1985;197:111–4.

59. Krych AJ, Lorich DG, Kelly BT. Treatment of focal osteochondral defects of the acetabulum with osteochondral allograft transplantation. Orthopedics. 2011;34(7):e307–11.
60. Wakitani S, et al. Repair of articular cartilage defects in the patello-femoral joint with autologous bone marrow mesenchymal cell transplantation: three case reports involving nine defects in five knees. J Tissue Eng Regen Med. 2007;1(1):74–9.
61. Centeno CJ, et al. Increased knee cartilage volume in degenerative joint disease using percutaneously implanted, autologous mesenchymal stem cells. Pain Physician. 2008;11(3):343–53.
62. Kuroda R, et al. Treatment of a full-thickness articular cartilage defect in the femoral condyle of an athlete with autologous bone-marrow stromal cells. Osteoarthritis Cartilage. 2007;15(2): 226–31.
63. Nejadnik H, et al. Autologous bone marrow-derived mesenchymal stem cells versus autologous chondrocyte implantation: an observational cohort study. Am J Sports Med. 2010;38(6):1110–6.
64. Wong KL, et al. Injectable cultured bone marrow-derived mesenchymal stem cells in varus knees with cartilage defects undergoing high tibial osteotomy: a prospective, randomized controlled clinical trial with 2 years' follow-up. Arthroscopy. 2013;29(12):2020–8.
65. Saw KY, et al. Articular cartilage regeneration with autologous peripheral blood progenitor cells and hyaluronic acid after arthroscopic subchondral drilling: a report of 5 cases with histology. Arthroscopy. 2011;27(4):493–506.
66. Saw KY, et al. Articular cartilage regeneration with autologous peripheral blood stem cells versus hyaluronic acid: a randomized controlled trial. Arthroscopy. 2013;29(4):684–94.
67. Pastides P, et al. Stem cell therapy for human cartilage defects: a systematic review. Osteoarthritis Cartilage. 2013;21(5):646–54.
68. Bajada S, et al. Decreased osteogenesis, increased cell senescence and elevated Dickkopf-1 secretion in human fracture non union stromal cells. Bone. 2009;45(4):726–35.
69. Prockop DJ. Repair of tissues by adult stem/progenitor cells (MSCs): controversies, myths, and changing paradigms. Mol Ther. 2009;17(6):939–46.
70. Eghbali-Fatourechi GZ, et al. Circulating osteoblast-lineage cells in humans. N Engl J Med. 2005;352(19):1959–66.
71. Gossl M, et al. Osteocalcin expression by circulating endothelial progenitor cells in patients with coronary atherosclerosis. J Am Coll Cardiol. 2008;52(16):1314–25.
72. Mifune Y, et al. Local delivery of granulocyte colony stimulating factor-mobilized CD34-positive progenitor cells using bioscaffold for modality of unhealing bone fracture. Stem Cells. 2008;26(6):1395–405.
73. Rozen N, et al. Transplanted blood-derived endothelial progenitor cells (EPC) enhance bridging of sheep tibia critical size defects. Bone. 2009;45(5):918–24.
74. Undale AH, et al. Mesenchymal stem cells for bone repair and metabolic bone diseases. Mayo Clin Proc. 2009;84(10):893–902.
75. Krebsbach PH, et al. Gene therapy-directed osteogenesis: BMP-7-transduced human fibroblasts form bone in vivo. Hum Gene Ther. 2000;11(8):1201–10.
76. Evans CH. Gene therapy for bone healing. Expert Rev Mol Med. 2010 Jun 23;12:e18. doi:10.1017/S1462399410001493.
77. Quarto R, et al. Repair of large bone defects with the use of autologous bone marrow stromal cells. N Engl J Med. 2001;344(5): 385–6.
78. Marcacci M, et al. Stem cells associated with macroporous bioceramics for long bone repair: 6- to 7-year outcome of a pilot clinical study. Tissue Eng. 2007;13(5):947–55.
79. Hernigou P, et al. Percutaneous autologous bone-marrow grafting for nonunions. Influence of the number and concentration of progenitor cells. J Bone Joint Surg Am. 2005;87(7):1430–7.
80. Hernigou P, Beaujean F. Abnormalities in the bone marrow of the iliac crest in patients who have osteonecrosis secondary to corticosteroid therapy or alcohol abuse. J Bone Joint Surg Am. 1997;79(7): 1047–53.
81. Hernigou P, Beaujean F, Lambotte JC. Decrease in the mesenchymal stem-cell pool in the proximal femur in corticosteroid-induced osteonecrosis. J Bone Joint Surg Br. 1999;81(2):349–55.
82. Lee JS, et al. Alterations in the differentiation ability of mesenchymal stem cells in patients with nontraumatic osteonecrosis of the femoral head: comparative analysis according to the risk factor. J Orthop Res. 2006;24(4):604–9.
83. Sheng HH, et al. Elevated adipogenesis of marrow mesenchymal stem cells during early steroid-associated osteonecrosis development. J Orthop Surg Res. 2007;2:15.
84. Muller I, et al. Secretion of angiogenic proteins by human multipotent mesenchymal stromal cells and their clinical potential in the treatment of avascular osteonecrosis. Leukemia. 2008;22(11):2054–61.
85. Zhao D, et al. Treatment of early stage osteonecrosis of the femoral head with autologous implantation of bone marrow-derived and cultured mesenchymal stem cells. Bone. 2012;50(1):325–30.
86. Kawate K, et al. Tissue-engineered approach for the treatment of steroid-induced osteonecrosis of the femoral head: transplantation of autologous mesenchymal stem cells cultured with beta-tricalcium phosphate ceramics and free vascularized fibula. Artif Organs. 2006;30(12):960–2.
87. Peeters CM, et al. Safety of intra-articular cell-therapy with culture-expanded stem cells in humans: a systematic literature review. Osteoarthritis Cartilage. 2013;21(10):1465–73.
88. Lalu MM, et al. Safety of cell therapy with mesenchymal stromal cells (SafeCell): a systematic review and meta-analysis of clinical trials. PLoS One. 2012;7(10):e47559.

Surgical Navigation of the Hip for Femoroacetabular Impingement

104

Jaron P. Sullivan, Timothy Bryan Griffith, Caroline N. Park, and Anil S. Ranawat

Navigation in FAI Surgery

Open surgery has been the traditional gold standard for treating FAI; however, arthroscopy has gained recent popularity because of its minimally invasive nature and decreased rehabilitation time. Unfortunately, its success is limited by an extensive learning curve attributed to several factors, among which is a difficult application of two-dimensional images for three-dimensional morphology. CAS is an attractive proposition for improving arthroscopic FAI surgery. Recent prototypes have addressed issues of accurate and precise osseous resection, defined zones of impingement, and predicted improved ROM.

Navigation programs guide the surgeon intraoperatively to precisely reproduce the planned resection. "Navigated" orthopedic surgery can be simplified into three steps: digitization, registration, and tracking. Digitization requires a virtual reconstruction of a patient's 3D bony anatomy by using either magnetic resonance (MR) imaging or computed tomography (CT). Registration occurs when markers are placed intraoperatively on specific bony landmarks to link the computer to the orientation of the patient on the surgical table. Tracking is the process through which the operative instruments are navigated to control the amount of resection. Navigation tracking can be image-based with 3D reconstructions, fluoroscopically guided, or imageless. Image-based navigation obtains registration of anatomical landmarks with the use of osseous pins. With the pelvis, for example, pins are inserted into the anterior superior iliac spines and pubic tubercles. These pins allow the digitization of the pelvis in virtual space, align it to the anterior pelvic plane (APP), and match it to preoperative 3D MR or CT data. Fluoroscopically guided navigation uses a calibrated tracker on a specially designed C-arm which takes a series of images in multiple planes to establish registration. Imageless navigation achieves registration by the use of optical infrared trackers mounted on the pelvis, coupled with a calibrated optical pointer to register the anterior superior iliac spine and pubic tubercle. The intraoperative images are then matched with preoperative data. For FAI due to the complex 3D osseous morphology, most navigation programs use 3D CT-based technology with either direct bony registration or 3D to 2D registration with specialized fluoroscopy.

Monohan et al. developed an encoder linkage system to track surgical instruments, eliminating the problem of occlusion, which is information loss from position sensors if the line of sight to the receiver is broken, which is a common issue with standard optical tracking systems [1]. This system is unique in that it incorporates soft tissue and bony anatomy and warns the surgeon when a surgical instrument moves too close to a neurovascular structure. In a pilot study, ten participants completed a navigation task with and without the aid of the system. There was a 38 % reduction in operative time and 78 % reduction in tool path length when the computer-aided system was used [2]. This system can offer a promising alternative to optical tracking systems once its clinical feasibility has been established.

Another group studying navigation-tracked bony resection for "cam"-type impingement assessed the adequacy of resection when comparing surgeons of varying experience and when comparing open versus navigated arthroscopic

J.P. Sullivan, MD
Department of Orthopaedic Surgery, Sports Medicine, Vanderbilt University, Nashville, TN, USA

T.B. Griffith, MD
Department of Orthopaedic Surgery, Sports Medicine, Peachtree Orthopaedic Clinic, Atlanta, GA, USA

C.N. Park, BA
Columbia University College of Physicians and Surgeons, New York, NY, USA

A.S. Ranawat, MD (✉)
Department of Orthopedics, Sports Medicine, Hospital for Special Surgery, 535 East 70th Street, 6th Floor, Suite 637, New York, NY 10021, USA
e-mail: ranawatanil@hss.edu

J.C. McCarthy et al. (eds.), *Hip Joint Restoration*, DOI 10.1007/978-1-4614-0694-5_104

resection in a sawbones model [3]. Preoperative plans were generated for all cases from CT scans and the BrainLAB navigation system (Feldkirchen, Germany). Postoperative CT scans were performed and alpha angles were determined at both the one-thirty and three-O'clock planes of rotation. Three groups used the navigation system: an experienced FAI surgeon, an experienced non-FAI surgeon, and a fellow in adult reconstruction. Similar post-resection alpha angles were observed between all three surgeons in both planes. This demonstrated how CAS could minimize the learning curve in FAI surgery and permit the less-experienced surgeon to perform bony resections equivalent to an experienced surgeon.

Most recently, Tannast et al. published the follow-up paper to their previous study on ROM analysis in FAI [4]. Their current software combines collision detection and ROM analysis technology [5] with a color-coded intraoperative map to guide resection in real time. The navigation application is based on the MARVIN application framework [6] where a 3D model of the patient's pelvis is derived from MR or CT. Preoperative ROM analysis is performed, followed by a virtual cam decompression according to a preoperative plan to ensure that postoperative ROM is outside the arc of impingement. A superimposed translucent sphere prevents excessive resection, ensures sphericity, and depicts pre- and postoperative femoral morphology. After registration of the 3D virtual model to the patient's anatomy using a dynamic reference base (DRB) attached to the femur, the reaming device is calibrated with another DRB. The preplanned resection area is highlighted on the screen as a color-coded distance map with red indicating the pre-reamed state and green when the reamer is within 1 mm of the resection goal. Reaming is commenced and the surgeon is guided to the preplanned goal by real-time tracking of the reaming device and color changes on the map indicating depth of resection.

The feasibility and accuracy of this navigation device was tested using 3D models of 18 identical sawbone femora. Postoperative models were created to compare with preoperative plans. Two surgeons performed three different osteochondroplasties on three occasions, resulting in nine operations per surgeon. The results demonstrated excellent intraobserver and interobserver agreement with the mean distance between planned and actual reamed surface at the femoral neck of 0.41 mm. The discrepancy between planned and actual reaming was consistently less than 1 mm in all 18 sawbone operations. The planned alpha angle was reamed with an accuracy of $0.1° \pm 0.6°$. These results show the accuracy of this planning and tracking system and seem to address the limitations of all the previous applications presented. The next test is going to be its applicability to an actual intraoperative arthroscopic setting.

Robotic Assistance in FAI Surgery

Navigated CAS allows the formulation of an accurate preoperative plan that can be virtually assessed and tracked intraoperatively. The missing link is precise surgical execution. This is where robotic surgery comes into play. Robotic surgery is the most recent development in CAS and translates the quantitative assessment produced by navigation into an automated mechanical action. Surgical instruments are mounted on a robotic arm which may partially or completely automate the entire surgical procedure. Robotic surgery provides a level of dexterity and precision that is unrivalled and allows for unmanned or remote surgery [7].

The most widely used robotic surgical system in use today is the "da Vinci" tele-robotic platform. Studies using this device for FAI surgery thus far have been promising, showing that robotic technology has the potential to allow orthopedic surgeons to perform complex procedures in very restricted spaces from a remote location [8]. There are already a number of robotic surgery systems in use in orthopedic surgery, especially in total hip and knee arthroplasty. "Haptics," a tactile feedback technology that uses a guided semi-active robot, has already demonstrated success in orthopedics. Cobb et al., in a prospective randomized controlled trial, used the Acrobot haptic-guided unicondylar knee replacement system (Acrobot, London, UK) to significantly improve implant-positioning precision relative to conventional cutting jigs [9]. A similar system has been developed in the United States: The Tactile Guidance System (MAKO Surgical, Fort Lauderdale, FL). This system has already demonstrated success in both unicompartmental knee arthroplasty and total hip arthroplasty acetabular component positioning, resulting in superior radiographic and functional outcomes [9, 10].

The senior author used the Tactile Guidance System to conduct a study on robotic-assisted femoral osteochondroplasty for FAI. Sixteen identical sawbone models with a "cam"-type deformity were treated by a single surgeon simulating an open FAI procedure. Eight of the procedures were performed using a free-hand technique and eight were performed using robotic assistance with the MAKO system. For the models that used robotic assistance, a 3D haptic volume was defined by the desired postoperative morphology. After resection, all the sawbones were scanned, and post-resection measurements of the arc of resection, volume of bone removed and resection depth were obtained and compared to the preoperative plan. Those that underwent manual free-hand resection produced an average arc of resection error of $42.0 \pm 8.5°$. Those that were resected using robotic assistance produced an average arc of resection error of $1.2 \pm 0.7°$, which was significantly lower than the free-hand group ($p < 0.0001$). Furthermore, over-resection with robotic assistance was significantly less than the free-hand group ($p<0.01$). Every manual resection resulted in over-resection, with a mean volume error of 758.3±477.1 mm^3, while the mean robotic resection volume error was 31.3±220.7 mm^3.

Using all currently available technologies, a surgical strategy for future robotic-assisted FAI surgery can be proposed (Fig. 104.1). A preoperative 3D CT would be obtained to define the morphology of a "cam"-type lesion (e.g. alpha angle) and/or a "pincer"-type lesion (e.g. lateral center-edge angle). The pelvic and femoral orientation would be registered. A preoperative assessment of virtual ROM using collision-based algorithms would plan the resection volume to achieve optimal impingement-free postoperative ROM such as can be currently accomplished with imaging using the HipMotion software (Bern, Switzerland) [5, 11]. The calculated arc and depth of resection may be represented on a clock face on the femoral head. A robotic-guided arm with 6 degrees of freedom would then haptically guide the surgeon around the calculated resection volume with virtual walls ensuring an accurate bony resection and preventing liatrogenic damage to bone and surrounding soft tissue. The robotic-guided cutting tool and arthroscope would be co-registered with bony tracking to enhance intraoperative visualization and allow real-time tracking. Finally, a dynamic intraoperative real-time assessment could be performed to assess the adequacy of resection.

Conclusion

Arthroscopic or arthroscopically assisted techniques for treating FAI are here to stay and provide clear benefits to patients over open surgery. However, inadequate resection of the impingement lesions continues to be a problem in hip arthroscopy due to the technical difficulty of the procedure combined with the limitations in preoperative planning and intraoperative judgment of adequate resection. The majority of revision hip arthroscopies are currently being performed for inadequate resection and unless the quality of the surgery improves, clinical results are likely to decline. CAS is an attractive proposition for improving arthroscopic FAI surgery. The prototypes discussed in this review have shown encouraging results in vitro, but clinical success and commercial viability is yet to be demonstrated. With regard to "cam"-type impingement, the current literature supports the measurement of a virtually simulated ROM to help plan any

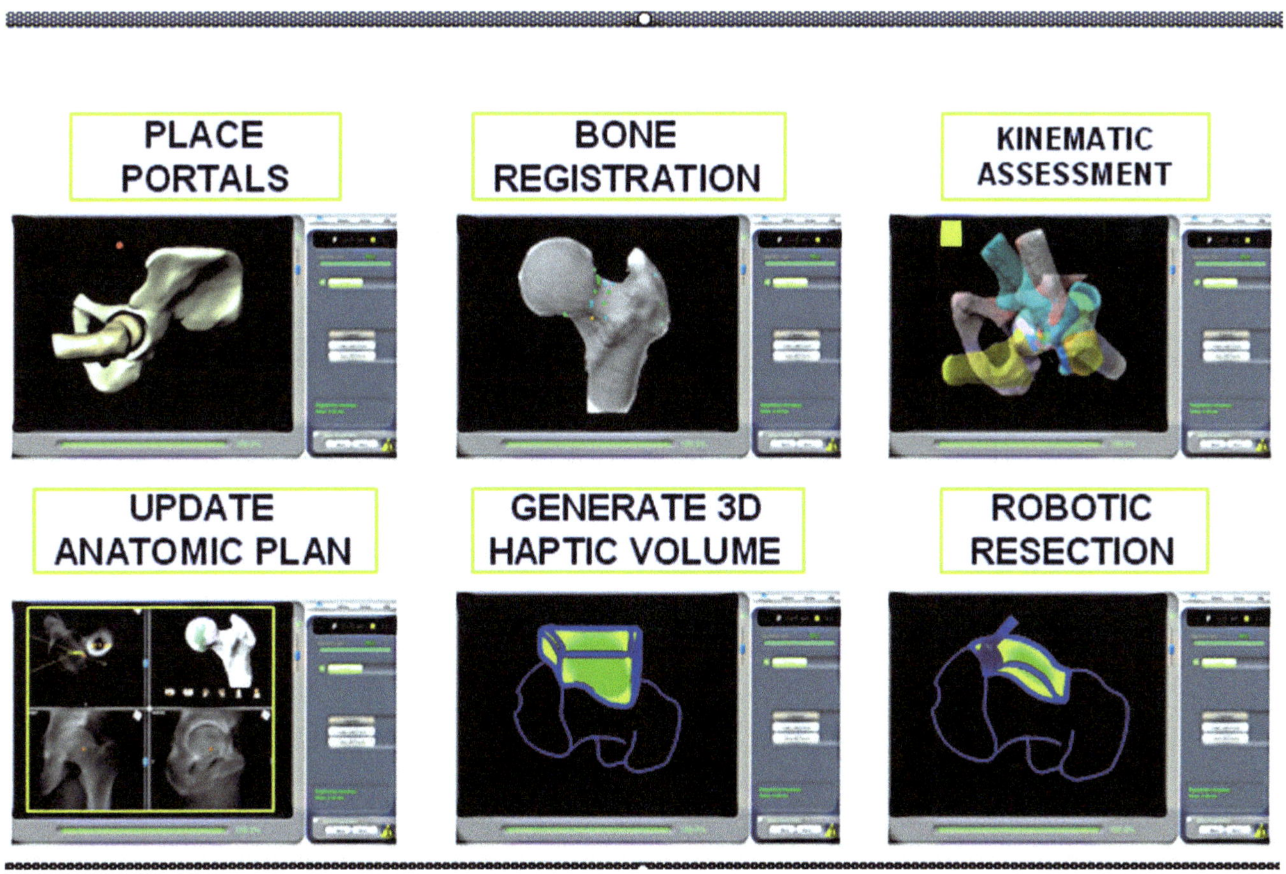

Fig. 104.1 A surgical strategy for future robotic-assisted FAI surgery

resection as opposed to using the alpha angle. Using this principle, the ideal CAS solution would define preoperatively the zone of impingement, plan the bony resection based on a virtual impingement-free ROM, track the movement of the arthroscope and the instrument intraoperatively, guide the surgeon toward accurate resection with haptic barriers, and facilitate dynamic intraoperative assessment of ROM to ensure adequacy and precision of resection. Ultimately, only by improving clinical outcomes, reducing technical difficulty, not increasing operative time, and minimizing cost, will such a system become feasible. Although this ideal system is currently intangible, the latest research would suggest that we are not far away from eliminating the need for visual estimation and reducing the technical difficulty in a field of orthopedics which continues to expand rapidly and warrants accuracy and precision to ultimately improve patient outcomes.

References

1. Monahan E, Shimada K. Computer-aided navigation for arthroscopic hip surgery using encoder linkages for position tracking. Int J Med Robot. 2006;2:271–8.
2. Monahan E, Shimada K. Verifying the effectiveness of a computer-aided navigation system for arthroscopic hip surgery. Stud Health Technol Inform. 2008;132:302–7.
3. Almoussa S, Barton C, Speirs AD, Gofton W, Beaule PE. Computer-assisted correction of cam-type femoracetabular impingement. A sawbones study. J Bone Jt Surg Am. 2011;93 Suppl 2:70–5.
4. Ecker TM, Puls M, Steppacher SD, Bastian JD, Keel MJB, Siebenrock KA, Tannast M. Computer assisted femoral head-neck osteochondroplasty using a surgical milling device. J Arthroplasty. 2012;27:310–6.
5. Tannast M, Kubiak-Langer M, Langlotz F, Puls M, Murphy SB, Siebenrock KA. Noninvasive three-dimensional assessment of femoroacetabular impingement. J Orthop Res. 2006;25(1): 122–31.
6. Rudolph T, Puls M. MARVIN: a medical research application framework based on open source software. Comput Meth Programs Biomed. 2008;91:165.
7. Advincula AP. Surgical techniques: robot-assisted laparoscopic hysterectomy with the da Vinci surgical system. Int J Med Robot. 2006;2:305–11.
8. Dorr LD, Malik A, Wan Z. Combined anteversion technique for total hip arthroplasty. Clin Orthop Relat Res. 2009;467(1): 119–27.
9. Cobb J, Henckl J, Gomes P, Harris S, Barrett A, Davies B. Functional outcome of the robot assisted minimal invasive unicompartmental knee arthroplasty at 18 months. J Bone Joint Surg Br. 2008;90 Suppl 3:561.
10. Nawabi DH, Conditt MA, Ranawat AS, Dunbar NJ, Jones J, Banks S, Padgett DE. Hapitically guided robotic technology in total hip arthroplasty: a cadaveric investigation. Proc Inst Mech Eng H. 2013;227(3):302–9.
11. Nawabi DH, Nam D, Park C, Ranawat AS. Hip arthroscopy: the use of computer assistance. HSS J. 2013;9:70–8.

Outcomes Following Hip Surgery

105

Nicholas G.H. Mohtadi

Introduction

Previous chapters have addressed Health-related quality-of-life assessment and the importance of validated scoring systems. This chapter will address the measurement of outcome in the hip surgical patient and then discuss the specific outcomes used in hip arthroscopic surgery and identify future research needs.

Measurement of Outcome in the Hip Surgical Patient

In order to measure the outcome of any therapeutic intervention (e.g. surgical treatment of a hip disorder in a young patient) we must understand that the final result is dependent on three independent components or variables.

Firstly, we need to consider the **patient**. Patient demographics, the specific hip disorder, the natural history of this disorder, the extent of the disease, the impact of this problem on the patient and any associated characteristics or comorbidities are likely to influence the outcome of surgical treatment. To better understand the results of a surgical treatment reported by different studies, it is necessary to understand the patient population, the sampling frame, and how the patients were selected into each study. It is possible to account for many of these patient characteristics by matching as many characteristics as possible between different groups of patients. However, groups of patients receiving medical or surgical treatment are likely to have inherent biases (i.e. unequal weightings of characteristics that affect the outcome). These biases are not likely to be known, predictable, or anticipated. Therefore, the only way to account for patient-related bias is to randomize patients to one treatment or the other.

The randomized clinical trial (RCT) study design creates the best opportunity to address differences between patients, in order to measure the outcome of a particular treatment. This can be illustrated by using an example from the literature. In an excellent study comparing the differences between labral refixation/repair compared to labral debridement, Larson and Giveans showed that the refixation group had better short and longer-term outcomes using the Modified Harris Hip Scale [1, 2]. Every effort was made to account and match for differences between patient groups preoperatively. The authors also compared many variables at baseline to demonstrate if there were any glaring differences between the groups. The authors rightfully stated that; "Although other variables could have influenced these outcomes, these preliminary results indicate that labral refixation resulted in better HHS ("MHHS") outcomes and a greater percentage of good to excellent results compared with the results of labral debridement in an earlier cohort" [1]. The "other variables" could very well have been differences in how the patients were chosen, the patient's perception of their disease, their reaction to how they were treated etc. These patient biases cannot be accounted for in a retrospective design. The RCT minimizes the effect of bias between patients by randomly allocating patients to each treatment group.

The second independent component is that which is attributed to the **surgeon/surgical procedure**. Surgeons are in a relatively unique position in medicine because patient outcome is based to a greater or lesser extent on the surgical procedure performed. It is not necessarily appropriate for an individual surgeon to simply quote results from the literature and apply them to his/her patients [3, 4]. The administration of a medication would be expected to have a similar effect and therefore patient outcome anywhere in the world, assuming that patients were similar in their disease state and demographic characteristics. The same cannot be said for surgical

N.G.H. Mohtadi, MD, MSc, FRCSC (✉)
Section of Orthopaedics, Department of Surgery, Peter Lougheed Centre, University of Calgary, Calgary, AB, Canada

University of Calgary Sport Medicine Centre, 2500 University Dr. NW, Calgary, AB, Canada T2T 3Y4
e-mail: mohtadi@ucalgary.ca

J.C. McCarthy et al. (eds.), *Hip Joint Restoration*, DOI 10.1007/978-1-4614-0694-5_105

treatment on similar patients for a multitude of reasons not the least of which is the recognized and significant learning curve with respect to hip arthroscopy [5–9]. Therefore, surgeons should be obligated to measure their own outcomes in some meaningful way. The impact of surgical experience is well understood. This has been addressed in the context of performing clinical trials by using an expertise-based design [4]. In this design patients are randomized or matched to surgeons who perform a particular procedure. The surgeon is comfortable and experienced in the particular procedure. Therefore, the outcome of the study is more likely to pertain to the procedure, rather the surgeon. Using the example of the Larson and Giveans study, they again addressed this limitation by stating that it is possible that "improvements seen in the later refixation group could be affected by improved techniques for treatment of FAI (Femoro acetabular impingement)" [2]. One other limitation of this study relates to the fact that, one of the surgeon-based factors in the decision to perform labral refixation/repair was the quality of the labral tissue. If the labrum was not repairable then the patient would not have been included in the refixation group. They would have been included in the debridement group. If the labrum is important in the outcome then the surgeon's decision to repair or not, would influence the outcome. It could be argued that this is a patient-related factor i.e. quality of the labrum; however if the decision to repair is driven by the surgeon then it is a surgeon-based factor as well. One way to address this issue is to have the decision randomly determined which may be ethically difficult. The authors effectively made this argument by stating; "with the growing awareness of the importance of the acetabular labrum and its potential for healing, we would not be comfortable randomly assigning patients to have the labrum resected." Another way to address this issue is to refix/repair every patient and then analyze the groups based on the quality of labral tissue.

The surgical procedure can also be measured by considering surgical time, time under traction (i.e. arthroscopic hip surgery), whether or not a complication occurred, pre- and post-op X-ray findings, as well as many other technical details of the surgical procedure. Assessing the surgical procedure may also be necessary to provide outcome information for third parties such as insurance companies, government organizations, or Workers Compensation Boards. In these cases reporting information on Key Performance Indicators (KPIs), such as measures of safety, use of antibiotic and DVT prophylaxis, hospital stay, costs would be necessary [10]. These types of outcomes are typically objective measures, which are observed, counted, and described in a reliable and valid way. Assuming that an unbiased observer documents this information independently, this can be trusted and assumed to be factual.

The third independent variable or component (the most important within the context of this chapter) is **the outcome measure** itself. Using the same example of the Larson study, the primary outcome was the modified Harris Hip Scale [11]. They also measured pain on a visual analogue scale (0–10) and the SF-12 [12]. The Harris Hip Scale was developed and published in a paper in 1969, long before the concept of evidence-based medicine or patient-reported outcomes were on the radar screen [13]. This clinician-based outcome was modified to eliminate the component of measuring range of motion [11]. Therefore, an argument can be made that the outcome used in this study was less than optimal i.e. not patient-based, and therefore the conclusions are biased on that basis alone. In the Larson study if the pain as determined by a VAS or the SF-12 outcomes were used as the primary outcome, the conclusions would have been that there is no difference in the two procedures [2].

In summary, the patient, the surgeon/surgical factors, and the outcome measure all have a direct and significant influence on the results reported in the literature with respect to the outcomes following hip surgery.

Commonly Used Outcome Measures

A recent systematic review of the literature identified three "Patient-Reported Outcomes" for patients with femoro-acetabular impingement (FAI) and labral tears [14]. The authors identified the Western Ontario and McMaster Universities Osteoarthritis Index (WOMAC), [15] the Non Arthritic Hip Score (NAHS) [16] and the Hip Outcome Score (HOS) [18]. However, critical appraisal of these outcomes would come to the conclusion that the WOMAC is patient-based and self-administered but created for patients who are older than those with FAI and is disease specific for osteoarthritis. The NAHS is made up of 20 questions, ten of which are taken directly from the WOMAC and the remaining questions determined by consensus from pilot test interviews with patients of varying educational levels as well as with health professionals [16]. The NAHS is designed for this population of patients but the responsiveness of this questionnaire had not been reported [17]. The HOS was developed to assess activities of daily living and sport participation [18–20]. However, the HOS did not have any patient involvement in determining the items in the two component questionnaires [18]. Thus, while the HOS is patient-reported, it is not patient-derived [18].

A second systematic review focused on patient-reported-outcome questionnaires when assessing hip and groin disability [17]. This review suggested that the Hip Dysfunction and Osteoarthritis Outcome Score (HOOS) is recommended for evaluating patients with osteoarthritis and the Hip Outcome Score (HOS) is recommended for patients undergoing hip arthroscopy [17]. They resolved by stating that "a new PRO questionnaire focusing on the evaluation of hip and groin disability in young and physically active patients is needed" [17].

The latest systematic review looked at psychometric evidence of outcomes used in hip arthroscopy. The authors identified the Modified Harris Hip Scale (MHHS), the NAHS, and the HOS as the three possible outcome measures. They evaluated each outcome utilizing the COSMIN checklist [22]. Based on the available evidence, they concluded that a combination of the NAHS and the HOS should be used as an outcome measure for patients undergoing hip arthroscopy [21]. They also stated that "more studies on the validity and reliability of these questionnaires are warranted" [21].

The commonest outcome measure used in hip arthroscopy studies is the Modified Harris Hip Scale [11, 13]. The Modified Harris Hip Scale (MHHS) [11, 13], the Merle d'Aubigne-Postel Scale (MAPS) [23–25], the Non-arthritic Hip Score (NAHS) [16], the Larson Hip Score (LHS) [26], the Hip Outcome Score (HOS) [18–20] and the Rating Scale for Hip Disabilities (RSHD) [27] adopted by the Japanese Orthopaedic Association have all been used in published articles pertaining to hip arthroscopy or hip preservation surgery. Three additional outcome measures have recently been reported. The Copenhagen Hip and Groin Outcome Score (HAGOS), a derived score (i.e. the so-called Vail-10) and the International Hip Outcome Tool (iHOT) [28–32]. Only the NAHS, HOS, HAGOS, IHOT, and the "Vail-10" have specifically targeted the young, active patient with a hip disorder.

Ultimately these outcomes should be considered for use in randomized clinical trials, prospective cohort studies, and in order to evaluate treatments. The outcomes should not only be patient-reported, but also reflect all of the important psychometric properties of any evaluative measurement tool. These include reliability, responsiveness, and validity [33–35].

The **Non-Arthritic Hip Score (NAHS)** was reported in 2003 to assess pain and function in young, active patients with activity-limiting hip pain, both pre- and postoperatively [16]. This tool is a patient-based, self-administered questionnaire that was developed as a modification of the Western Ontario and McMaster Universities Osteoarthritis Index (WOMAC). Ten questions came directly from the WOMAC and the other ten were developed de novo. Four of the questions were specific to mechanical symptoms in the hip and the other six were to measure the patient's activity level. The items were generated through pilot test interviews with patients of varying educational levels and with health professionals. The Non-Arthritic Hip Score is intended for 20–40 year old patients who are experiencing hip pain without an obvious radiographic diagnosis. The tool has been shown to be reproducible with test-retest reliability evaluated between 1 and 16 days. The tool has internal consistency, as assessed using the Cronbach's coefficient alpha. Construct validity was determined by comparing the Non-Arthritic Hip Score to the Harris Hip Score and the Short Form-12 in 48 patients. Although this tool attempts to capture a younger population that has not been previously represented by other hip outcomes, the methodology is not ideal because the total number of questions (20) was somewhat arbitrarily determined without statistical support. This may result in a misrepresentation of items that are relevant to a young, active patient with non-arthritic hip problems. In addition, half of the items were taken directly from the WOMAC index, which were generated in an older, more sedentary population. Therefore, the outcome may be predisposed to ceiling effects, thus limiting its use in the younger, more active population. In the eight publications baseline average scores on the NAHS were from 47 to 70. In addition the sections that address pain, mechanical symptoms, and physical function ask the patient to consider problems in the past 48 h; which may be too short of a timeline to be truly representative of the problems that these patients are experiencing. Finally no measure of responsiveness has been reported.

The **Hip Outcome Score (HOS)** was specifically developed for younger more active patients between the ages of 13 and 66 years [18–20]. The HOS is a patient administered tool that was designed to assess self reported functional status; therefore symptoms were not considered part of the functional assessment [18]. The HOS includes two subscales: activities of daily living (ADL) and sports. Items were generated by physicians and physical therapists and reduced by factor analysis. No patients were involved with item generation [18]. The tool does show internal consistency, as determined by Cronbach coefficients [20]. True test-re-test reliability was not measured since all patients had an intervention, (i.e. arthroscopic surgery) between administrations at baseline and an average of 7 months follow-up [20]. The HOS demonstrated good construct validity, as measured by convergent and divergent validity with the Short Form 36 questionnaire using Pearson correlation coefficients [19]. The items in both subscales were shown to be responsive [20].

By design the HOS does not represent a true patient derived outcome since it does not include items of specific concern to patients such as symptoms, work-related, social, or emotional issues. It should be considered a well designed and evaluated functional outcome measure [18]. The scoring of the HOS is somewhat complicated since each subscale is scored separately as a percentage score. The ADL subscale has 19 items but only 17 are scored. The items pertaining to sitting and putting on socks and shoes are not included. The sports subscale has 9 items. Each item on both scales is scored from 4 to 0, with 4 indicating "no difficulty" and 0 indicating "unable to do." There is a "not applicable" option as well. The percentage score is calculated by comparing the item total score divided by the highest potential score multiplied by 100.

More recently two newer patient-reported outcomes have been developed. The **Copenhagen Hip and Groin Outcome Score (HAGOS)** [36] and the **International Hip Outcome**

Tool (iHOT) [37]. The HAGOS has been developed using standardized format by identifying a specific population of interest, generating items, item reduction, and determination of validity, reliability, and responsiveness [36]. This instrument has the goal of evaluating "hip and/or groin disability related to impairment (body structure and function), activity (activity limitations), and participation (participation restrictions) according to the International Classification of Functioning, disability and health (ICF), in young to middle-aged physically active patients with hip and/or groin pain" [36]. The item generation process was determined as a result of a systematic review of the literature [17]. The authors chose to include items from the HOOS and HOS questionnaires [18–20, 38]. Forty-three questions in total (40 from the HOOS and 3 from the HOS) formed the basis of the HAGOS. An expert group, including two orthopaedic surgeons, one physician, and four physiotherapists added an additional eight questions. A representative focus group of 20 patients added two and removed one question, resulting in a 52-item questionnaire.

The item reduction process involved 101 patients. A combination of the frequency and importance of each question to these patients, as well as reliability testing was used to determine which items to retain. Fourteen items were subsequently removed as a result of further consensus amongst the authors. One final item was removed as a result of factor analysis resulting in a final questionnaire of 37 questions in six separate subscales: (Pain (10 items), Symptoms (7 items), ADL (5 items), Sport/Rec (8 items), PA (2 items), and QOL (5 items) [17]. Content validity was considered due to the patient ($N=25$) and expert group ($N=7$) involvement. Test-retest reliability was measured 1–3 weeks after baseline, in 44 out of the 101 patients and deemed to be very high in all subscales, with intra-class correlation coefficients ranging from 0.82 to 0.91. The authors measured responsiveness at 4 months from baseline in 87 of the 101 patients. They compared the change scores to asking the patients on a 7-point Global Perceived Effect (GPE) score. The correlations with the HAGOS in each subscale were higher than hypothesized. They also measured the standardized response mean (SRM) and effect sizes (ES) on each subscale, which were noticeably higher in patients who had stated that they were "much better" and "better" on their GPE scores. The SRM and ES calculations ranged from 0.90 to 0.77 respectively for the ADL subscale and 1.46 and 1.78 for the QOL subscale. Construct validity was determined by comparing the HAGOS to the SF-36, which has significant limitations. The SF-36 is a generic outcome measure with likely little relevance to the population at hand. Therefore it is not surprising that the comparison with respect to a priori correlations was satisfactory but not consistent. Finally, PROs should be able to measure the minimal important change (MIC) and/or minimal important difference (MID). The HAGOS showed that the MIC for each subscale ranged from 10 to 15 points based on using the estimate of one half of the reported standard deviation. The authors identified this limitation. If the HAGOS was used as the primary outcome measure in a clinical trial more patients would be needed in order to achieve a meaningful sample-size.

The latest PRO advocated for patients with hip disorders is the **International Hip Outcome Tool (iHOT)** [31]. This PRO has previously been called the Hip Quality-of-Life Questionnaire and the MAHORN Hip Outcome Tool (MHOT). Developed with the cooperation of the Multi-center Arthroscopy of the Hip Outcomes Research Network (MAHORN), this tool was designed to address the outcomes of treatment in young active patients with hip disorders. This outcome measure included patients from the U.S.A., Canada, England, and Switzerland. This outcome measure was developed for active patients (18–60 year. old; Tegner activity scale$\geq$4) [39] presenting with a variety of hip conditions. This multicenter study recruited patients from the practices of a group of international hip arthroscopy and arthroplasty surgeons. The outcome was created using a process of item generation (51 patients, 4 orthopaedic surgeons, and 4 physiotherapists), item reduction (150 patients), and pre-testing (31patients). The questionnaire was tested for test-retest reliability (123 patients), face, content, and construct validity (51 patients), and responsiveness over a 6-month period in post-arthroscopy patients (27 patients); for a total of 433 patients.

Initially, 146 items identified through patient query were reduced to 60 through item reduction, and categorized into four domains: (a) Symptoms and Functional Limitations, (b) Sport and Recreational Physical Activities, (c) Job Related Concerns, and (d) Social, Emotional and Lifestyle Concerns and formatted using a Visual Analogue Scale. Pre-testing confirmed appropriate wording, content, and formatting. Test-retest reliability showed Pearson correlations greater than 0.80 for 33 of the 60 questions. These 33 questions were formulated into a self-administered questionnaire using a visual analogue scale response format from 0 to 100. A score of "0" reflects the worst possible quality-of-life and "100" the best possible score. Intra-class correlation statistic as a reflection of reliability was 0.78 and Chronbach's alpha as a reflection of internal consistency was 0.99. Face and content validity were ensured because of the extensive involvement of patients, the expert developers, and the MAHORN group. Construct validity was demonstrated with a correlation of 0.81 to the Non-Arthritic Hip Score. Responsiveness was demonstrated with a paired t-test ($p\leq0.01$), effect size of 1.95, standardized response mean was 1.69 and the responsiveness ratio 6.7. The calculated minimal clinical important difference (MCID) was 6 points out of the total 100-point scale. These properties make the iHOT very attractive as an outcome tool, since the MCID can be used interchangeably with the MIC, in calculating sample sizes for prospective research studies. As a result this highly validated, truly patient-based, and responsive questionnaire has been recommended for use in randomized clinical trials and prospective cohort studies [40]. An on-going effort by the MAHORN group, continued to develop a 12-item questionnaire i.e. the iHOT-12 that reflects the longer version the IHOT-33. The IHOT-12 utilizes twelve of the same questions with similar properties, includes all four domains, and has been recommended for clinical use rather than for research purposes [30]. In this way, busy clinicians with minimal resources can measure a PRO with their patients. The IHOT-12 should be simple enough for phone administration, paper or computer-based formats and will minimize responder burden for the patients.

The ***"Vail-10 questions"*** represent a derived outcome based upon questions from the NAHS, the MHHS, and the HOS [28, 29]. The authors retrospectively analyzed an extensive database of over 2000 patients who had completed at baseline the NAHS, HOS, and MHHS and over 1100 with 1-year follow-up data [28, 29]. The stated that the ten questions demonstrated criterion validity with no floor or ceiling effects, responsiveness, and construct validity compared to the SF-12 questionnaire [28, 29]. It is unclear at this time whether separating these questions and using them in a prospective way will prove to be valid on their own.

Future Research Needs

Up until June 2013, there were only five prospective and/or randomized comparative studies published in the field of hip arthroscopy [6, 41–44]. Pollard addressed arthroscopic skill development in a randomized trial comparing supine and lateral positioning in hip models [6]. Ya Deau randomly compared the addition of a lumbar plexus block after hip arthroscopy and showed lowering of pain scores postoperatively [42]. Ilizaliturri compared in a randomized trial two different techniques for releasing the iliopsoas tendon and using the WOMAC as the primary outcome measure [44]. No differences were seen but small numbers of patients were included [44].

Zingg et al. compared open surgical hip dislocation (SHD) and hip arthroscopic (HA) treatment of FAI in a prospective cohort study [43]. "When compared to SHD, HA results in faster recovery and better short-term outcome. However, some overcorrection of the cam deformity and limited frequency of labrum refixation with HA in this study may have a negative impact on long-term outcome" [43]. The most recent randomized trial compared arthroscopic labral repair to selective labral debridement in female patients with FAI [41]. The authors concluded, "Arthroscopic treatment of femoroacetabular impingement with labral repair in female patients resulted in superior improvement in hip functional outcomes compared with labral debridement" [41]. However, the authors used the HOS ADL and Sports subscales as their primary outcome measure, stating that they powered their study to be able to detect a difference of seven points on the HOS. The two groups were already more than seven points different at baseline and for some reason the patients were not blinded to treatment allocation introducing a potentially, which the authors acknowledged [41].

It is readily evident that in the field of hip arthroscopy there is a great need for prospective clinical studies and randomized clinical trials utilizing the now available validated outcome measures with large volumes of patients.

References

1. Larson CM, Giveans MR. Arthroscopic management of femoroacetabular impingement: early outcomes measures. Arthroscopy. 2008;24(5):540–6.
2. Larson CM, Giveans MR. Arthroscopic debridement versus refixation of the acetabular labrum associated with femoroacetabular impingement. Arthroscopy. 2009;25(4):369–76.
3. Bednarska E, Bryant D, Devereaux PJ. Orthopaedic surgeons prefer to participate in expertise-based randomized trials. Clin Orthop Relat Res. 2008;466(7):1734–44.
4. Devereaux PJ, Bhandari M, Clarke M, Montori VM, Cook DJ, Yusuf S, et al. Need for expertise based randomised controlled trials. BMJ. 2005;330(7482):88.
5. Lee YK, Ha YC, Hwang DS, Koo KH. Learning curve of basic hip arthroscopy technique: CUSUM analysis. Knee Surg Sports Traumatol Arthrosc. 2012. Epub 2012/10/18.
6. Pollard TC, Khan T, Price AJ, Gill HS, Glyn-Jones S, Rees JL. Simulated hip arthroscopy skills: learning curves with the lateral and supine patient positions: a randomized trial. J Bone Joint Surg Am. 2012;94(10):e68. Epub 2012/05/24.
7. Konan S, Rhee SJ, Haddad FS. Hip arthroscopy: analysis of a single surgeon's learning experience. J Bone Joint Surg Am. 2011;93 Suppl 2:52–6. Epub 2011/05/13.
8. Vilchez F, Erquicia J, Tey M. Learning curve of arthroscopic hip surgery. Acta Ortop Mex. 2010;24(3):177–81. Epub 2010/09/15. Curva de aprendizaje en la cirugia artroscopica de cadera.
9. Souza BG, Dani WS, Honda EK, Ricioli Jr W, Guimaraes RP, Ono NK, et al. Do complications in hip arthroscopy change with experience? Arthroscopy. 2010;26(8):1053–7. Epub 2010/08/04.
10. Watters DA, Green AJ, van Rij A. Guidelines for surgical audit in Australia and New Zealand. ANZ J Surg. 2006;76(1–2):78–83.
11. Byrd JW, Jones KS. Hip arthroscopy in the presence of dysplasia. Arthroscopy. 2003;19(10):1055–60.
12. Ware Jr J, Kosinski M, Keller SD. A 12-item short-form health survey: construction of scales and preliminary tests of reliability and validity. Med Care. 1996;34(3):220–33.
13. Harris WH. Traumatic arthritis of the hip after dislocation and acetabular fractures: treatment by mold arthroplasty. An end-result study using a new method of result evaluation. J Bone Joint Surg Am. 1969;51(4):737–55.
14. Lodhia P, Slobogean GP, Noonan VK, Gilbart MK. Patient-reported outcome instruments for femoroacetabular impingement and hip labral pathology: a systematic review of the clinimetric evidence. Arthroscopy. 2010;27(2):279–86.
15. Bellamy N, Buchanan WW. A preliminary evaluation of the dimensionality and clinical importance of pain and disability in osteoarthritis of the hip and knee. Clin Rheumatol. 1986;5(2):231–41.

16. Christensen CP, Althausen PL, Mittleman MA, Lee JA, McCarthy JC. The nonarthritic hip score: reliable and validated. Clin Orthop Relat Res. 2003;406:75–83.
17. Thorborg K, Roos EM, Bartels EM, Petersen J, Holmich P. Validity, reliability and responsiveness of patient-reported outcome questionnaires when assessing hip and groin disability: a systematic review. Br J Sports Med. 2010;44(16):1186–96. Epub 2009/08/12.
18. Martin RL, Kelly BT, Philippon MJ. Evidence of validity for the hip outcome score. Arthroscopy. 2006;22(12):1304–11.
19. Martin RL, Philippon MJ. Evidence of validity for the hip outcome score in hip arthroscopy. Arthroscopy. 2007;23(8):822–6.
20. Martin RL, Philippon MJ. Evidence of reliability and responsiveness for the hip outcome score. Arthroscopy. 2008;24(6):676–82.
21. Tijssen M, van Cingel R, van Melick N, de Visser E. Patient-reported outcome questionnaires for hip arthroscopy: a systematic review of the psychometric evidence. BMC Musculoskelet Disord. 2011;12:117. Epub 2011/05/31.
22. Mokkink LB, Terwee CB, Patrick DL, Alonso J, Stratford PW, Knol DL, et al. The COSMIN checklist for assessing the methodological quality of studies on measurement properties of health status measurement instruments: an international Delphi study. Qual Life Res. 2010;19(4):539–49. Epub 2010/02/20.
23. Merle D'Aubigne R. Numerical evaluation of hip function. Rev Chir Orthop Reparatrice Appar Mot. 1970;56(5):481–6.
24. Merle d'Aubigne R, Cauchoix J, Ramadier J. Evaluation chiffree de la fonction de la hanch. Application a l'etude des resultats des. Rev Chir Orthop. 1949;35:5–12.
25. Merle D'Aubigne RM, Postel M. Functional results of hip arthroplasty with acrylic prosthesis. J Bone Joint Surg Am. 1954;36-A(3): 451–75.
26. Larson CB. Rating scale for hip disabilities. Clin Orthop Relat Res. 1963;31:85–93.
27. Kim KC, Hwang DS, Lee CH, Kwon ST. Influence of femoroacetabular impingement on results of hip arthroscopy in patients with early osteoarthritis. Clin Orthop Relat Res. 2007;456:128–32.
28. In: Briggs K, Philippon M, editors. The use of outcome measures in hip arthroscopy. International society for hip arthroscopy annual scientific meeting. New York, NY; 2009. Accessed 9–10 Oct 2009.
29. In: Briggs KK, Philippon MJ, editors. Analysis of scores to document outcome following hip arthroscopy. International society for hip arthroscopy annual scientific meeting. New York, NY; 2009. Accessed 9–10 Oct 2009.
30. Griffin DR, Parsons N, Mohtadi NG, Safran MR. A short version of the International Hip Outcome Tool (iHOT-12) for use in routine clinical practice. Arthroscopy. 2012;28(5):611–6. quiz 6–8. Epub 2012/05/01.
31. Mohtadi NG, Griffin DR, Pedersen ME, Chan D, Safran MR, Parsons N, et al. The development and validation of a self-administered quality-of-life outcome measure for young, active patients with symptomatic hip disease: the International Hip Outcome Tool (iHOT-33). Arthroscopy. 2012;28(5):595–605. quiz 6–10 e1. Epub 2012/05/01.
32. Thorborg K, Holmich P, Christensen R, Petersen J, Roos EM. The Copenhagen Hip and Groin Outcome Score (HAGOS): development and validation according to the COSMIN checklist. Br J Sports Med. 2011;45(6):478–91. Epub 2011/04/12.
33. Guyatt G, Walter S, Norman G. Measuring change over time: assessing the usefulness of evaluative instruments. J Chronic Dis. 1987;40(2):171–8.
34. Kirkley A, Griffin S. Development of disease-specific quality of life measurement tools. Arthroscopy. 2003;19(10):1121–8.
35. Kirshner B, Guyatt G. A methodological framework for assessing health indices. J Chronic Dis. 1985;38(1):27–36.
36. Thorborg K, Holmich P, Christensen R, Petersen J, Roos EM. The Copenhagen Hip and Groin Outcome Score (HAGOS): development and validation according to the COSMIN checklist. Br J Sports Med. 2011;45(6):478–91. Epub 2011/04/12.
37. Mohtadi NG, Pedersen ME, Chan DS. Assessing outcomes after hip surgery. In: Sekiya JK, Safran MR, Ranawat AS, Leunig M, editors. Techniques in hip arthroscopy and joint preservation surgery. 1st ed. Philadelphia: Saunders Elsevier Inc; 2011.
38. Nilsdotter AK, Lohmander LS, Klassbo M, Roos EM. Hip disability and osteoarthritis outcome score (HOOS)—validity and responsiveness in total hip replacement. BMC Musculoskelet Disord. 2003;4:10. Epub 2003/06/05.
39. Tegner Y, Lysholm J. Rating systems in the evaluation of knee ligament injuries. Clin Orthop Relat Res. 1985;198:43–9.
40. In: Phillips L, Mohtadi NG, Chan DS, editors. The responsivenss and minimal clinically important difference (MCID) of the MAHORN hip outcome tool. International society of hip arthroscopy annual scientific meeting. Cancun, Mexico; 2010. Accessed 8–9 Oct 2010.
41. Krych AJ, Thompson M, Knutson Z, Scoon J, Coleman SH. Arthroscopic labral repair versus selective labral debridement in female patients with femoroacetabular impingement: a prospective randomized study. Arthroscopy. 2013;29(1):46–53. Epub 2013/01/02.
42. YaDeau JT, Tedore T, Goytizolo EA, Kim DH, Green DS, Westrick A, et al. Lumbar plexus blockade reduces pain after hip arthroscopy: a prospective randomized controlled trial. Anesth Analg. 2012;115(4):968–72. Epub 2012/07/24.
43. Zingg PO, Ulbrich EJ, Buehler TC, Kalberer F, Poutawera VR, Dora C. Surgical hip dislocation versus hip arthroscopy for femoroacetabular impingement: clinical and morphological short-term results. Arch Orthop Trauma Surg. 2013;133(1):69–79. Epub 2012/10/16.
44. Ilizaliturri Jr VM, Chaidez C, Villegas P, Briseno A, Camacho-Galindo J. Prospective randomized study of 2 different techniques for endoscopic iliopsoas tendon release in the treatment of internal snapping hip syndrome. Arthroscopy. 2009;25(2):159–63. Epub 2009/01/28.

The Critical Role of Registries in Documenting the Outcomes of Hip Preservation Surgery

106

Andrew John Timperley, Marcus J.K. Bankes, Siôn Glyn-Jones, and Sarah L. Whitehouse

Introduction

The evidence relating to the efficacy of joint preserving surgery of the hip is lacking. Whilst several case series and cohort studies have been published, these are generally of a low standard. Most come from single centres and are lacking in a control treatment or placebo group [1–3]. However, despite their limitations, these trials, along with significant papers from Ganz [4, 5] and Villar [6], demonstrate the safety of hip arthroscopy with particular reference to labral repairs and surgery for femoro-acetabular impingement.

Recognising the inadequacy of data available, the Non-Arthroplasty Hip Register (NAHR) was created to collect data on the outcome of hip conditions not treated by arthroplasty. The Registry was unanimously supported by the Membership of the British Hip Society and went live in March 2012. The NAHR has been constructed so that any hip condition can be studied for the lifetime of the patient on a unique pathway passing between treating clinicians. It was appreciated that collecting these data will allow us to understand the natural history of various hip pathologies and the effect of surgical treatments. A Registry can prove the efficacy of our treatments so that patients will benefit and purchasers of healthcare will continue to fund them in the future.

Within the NAHR, clinicians are able to collect and display comprehensive outcome and audit data for all of their own patients using scores and outcome measures of their own choosing. Data can be entered for patients who do not undergo surgery for any specific condition so that their clinical course can be followed. Only one hip "pathway" can be started for a left or right hip in any individual so patients are not lost if they move between clinicians. If the patient has consented for their data to be collected, only an arthroplasty or the patient's demise will close their record.

To improve compliance of data collection, the National Institute for Health and Care Excellence (NICE) published in their Interventional Procedure Guidance on Arthroscopic (IPG 408) and Open (IPG 403) Femoro-Acetabular Surgery for Hip Impingement Syndrome that clinicians should submit details to the NAHR. For the condition of femoro-acetabular impingement, clinicians may choose to facilitate collection of only an initial Minimum Data Set (as they do with the NJR). The Registry may then collect additional outcome data, as needed. In addition, the NAHR provides clinicians with the ability to enter data from any other questionnaire or outcome measure as part of their own individualised patient database.

A.J. Timperley, MBChB, FRCS, DPhil (✉)
Centre for Hip Surgery (Exeter), Royal Devon and Exeter Hospital NHS Foundation Trust, Princess Elizabeth Orthopaedic Hospital, Barrack Road, Exeter EX2 5DW, UK
e-mail: jtimperley@mac.com

M.J.K. Bankes, BSc, FRCS
Department of Orthopaedics, Guy's Hospital, London, UK

S. Glyn-Jones, MA, MBBS, FRCS, DPhil
Nuffield Department of Orthopaedics, Rheumatology and Musculoskeletal Sciences, Medical Sciences, University of Oxford, Oxford, UK

Nuffield Orthopaedic Centre, Oxford, UK

S.L. Whitehouse, PhD
Institute of Health and Biomedical Innovation, Queensland University of Technology, Brisbane, QLD, Australia

Who Benefits from the Creation of the NAHR?

If we can define the indication for all types of non-arthroplasty hip surgery everyone benefits:

The Patients. Patients will only undergo surgery if it is likely to reduce their pain, improve their function (ability to undertake activity and work) and/or prevent the progress of arthritis of the hip ultimately necessitating a hip replacement. Patients who will not benefit from hip preservation surgery (open or arthroscopic) are spared the risk of an operative procedure, the risk of exacerbation of their symptoms and acceleration of their joint degeneration.

J.C. McCarthy et al. (eds.), *Hip Joint Restoration*, DOI 10.1007/978-1-4614-0694-5_106

The Purchasers of Healthcare. Funding will be targeted on patients who will benefit from a surgical procedure. Funds will not be used where the outcome clearly does not justify the use of the available resources.

Surgeons. Surgeons will be able to define which patients will benefit from surgery and what details of the operative procedure will lead to a good result. The surgeon will have validated outcome data available to them.

Practicalities of the NAHR

The Non-Arthroplasty Hip Register (NAHR) was initially launched in 2012 with a major streamlining exercise undertaken in November 2013 to improve surgeon participation. Whilst many arthroscopic and hip preservation surgeons were enthusiastic about its development in principle, many already had their own databases and were, unsurprisingly, unwilling to duplicate data entry. It was therefore decided to use the infrastructure already existing in almost every hospital in England and Wales for collection of data for the National Joint Registry for England, Wales and Northern Ireland (NJR). It was reasoned that this decision would lead to increased enrolment of patients by minimising the necessity for surgeon involvement in the process of data collection.

In addition, a Minimum Data Set (MDS) was defined. Preoperatively, this included a specific hip function measure (iHOT-12) and a general health measure (EQ-5D) [7]. This also corresponded to the National Health Service (NHS) Patient Reported Outcome Measures (PROMS) programme for hip and knee replacement patients [8]. Paper forms were redesigned to help with this process (see Appendix). Whilst it may seem outdated to develop a paper-based system, the availability of hardware for electronic data entry varies immensely between hospitals, particularly in clinic and theatre environments. Whilst the advent of tablet devices is often hailed as the convenient solution to preoperative data collection, maintenance and theft of these devices remains a major problem. Clearly the NAHR can be used entirely without paper forms for those institutions with durable electronic systems in place. However, collection of post-operative outcome data is electronic, and patients are currently invited by email to complete outcome questionnaires at 6 and 12 months after their operation through direct linkage to the online forms.

Patient-Completed Sections

The consent form outlines the purposes of the NAHR to the patient, the type of data required, an explanation of data security and confidentiality measures and a statement that patient participation in the Register is voluntary and consent can be withdrawn at any time. The patient signs their consent and completes their name, date of birth and address and, most importantly, their email address. This email is used for collecting post-operative functional scores and must be checked.

The short version of the International Hip Outcome Tool (iHOT-12) [9] was chosen to measure health-related quality of life and changes after treatment due to its brevity and the fact that it is valid, reliable and responsive to change. It has also been shown to have very similar characteristics to the longer iHOT-33, with very little information being lost with the shorter form and conveniently has twelve questions in the same way as the Oxford Hip and Knee Scores [10, 11]. Responses to each question on the iHOT-12 consist of marking a point on a 100 mm line from 0 (worst) to 100 (best). The score is the average value from the questions answered, allowing patients to omit the question on sexual activity. The mark on the line is measured with a ruler, although this is considered impractical for most units. Data entry is therefore facilitated by the addition of a feint ruler below the dark line, although this may lead to digit preference by the patient. Each value is then entered into the NAHR and the mean value is automatically calculated. When patients complete their 6- and 12-month post-operative iHOT-12 scores online, they use an on-screen slider.

The European Quality of Life 5-Dimensions questionnaire (EQ-5D-5L) was chosen as a standardised general health instrument as it is well established, quick to administer and acceptable to the patient [12, 13]. The EQ-5D is designed for patients to describe and value their health by generating a single summary index value (utility) by quantifying a preference for his or her health state. The EQ-5D instrument consists of five items (dimensions) to describe the respondent's own health: mobility, self-care, usual activities, pain/discomfort, and anxiety/depression. Respondents can value their health in each dimension at five severity levels, which significantly increase reliability and sensitivity (discriminatory power) while maintaining feasibility and potentially reducing ceiling effects in comparison to the three ordinal levels of the original EQ-5D-3L. The second measurement component of the EQ-5D is a Visual Analogue Scale (EQ VAS) for the patient to rate their own health. The format of the EQ-5D-5L is easily reproduced for the online version for both initial data entry and for the patient to complete for their 6- and 12-month post-operative outcomes.

Despite the simplicity and brevity of these outcome measures, patient compliance for completing post-treatment questionnaires can be variable, with particularly low completion rates in young men, an important demographic group in hip preservation surgery. The NAHR allows easy identification of patients who have not completed their forms and can therefore be reminded by telephone or further email. Ensuring patients understand the purpose of the NAHR as they consent to their data being included is a vital step. One would also hope that evolving technology of both the data entry interface for mobile devices, combined with biometric security measures will improve convenience of completing electronic questionnaires.

Surgeon-Completed Sections

Patient demographic data are easily acquired with use of patient identifier labels and the email address is included by the patient on the consent form, although the operation presents a good opportunity to check patient data. The NHS number is readily available for NHS patients and is often on the identifier label. This number is also used in the NJR and is vital for linkage of patients between the two Registries. For private patients, the NHS number may be obtained from the patient's primary care provider if it was not included in the patient's original referral letter.

The diagnostic categories listed on the MDS form are fairly comprehensive and multiple diagnoses may be chosen. Due to difficulties in diagnosing the subtypes of femoroacetabular impingement (FAI) and the resulting inter-observer variation, it was agreed to use the simple umbrella term of FAI to include cam, pincer and combined types, which also includes the associated labral and chondral lesions. The options of "Undiagnosed hip pain" and "Hypermobility" were also included for hips with normal bony structure and normal findings at arthroscopy. The MDS form is completed by describing where, when and who performed surgery, as well as patient weight and height, and whether surgery was performed arthroscopically, open, or a combination of both (e.g. central compartment arthroscopy followed by mini-open femoral neck osteoplasty, or pelvic osteotomy). The details of the operation collected for the MDS are only those which are unambiguous. Whilst, at first viewing, these terms may seem to lack detail, they have been chosen to enable early patient outcomes to be established for all three surgical approaches for FAI and open surgery for hip dysplasia. The strength of a Registry is in its scale and inclusiveness and it was felt important to ensure engagement of the surgical community with a simple, unambiguous, practical dataset rather than a more inclusive one which can be subject to misinterpretation.

The optional Extended Data Set (EDS) was included for surgeons, particularly those without their own existing databases, to include additional surgical details to provide individual activity data, i.e. how often chondral microfracture is performed per year. This information can be useful for planning services and is certainly more detailed than available in most generic hospital systems. Whilst this does allow some basic analysis, the EDS is not yet designed to be sufficiently detailed to allow scientific comparison between different techniques, such as whether labral repair is superior to labral debridement. This is because it is impossible to control for the myriad of other factors, many of which are not yet fully understood, that affect the outcome of hip preservation surgery, and which can only be answered with proper scientific trials. It is hoped, however, that the EDS will continue to develop and will shortly contain a means for quantifying the severity and extent of chondral damage.

Additional Features of NAHR Database and Surgeon Reports

Whilst the "front end" of the NAHR is designed to correspond with the paper forms for ease of data entry, the inherent flexibility of the data collection software allows entry of data in addition to the MDS and EDS. This includes data collected by a variety of hip outcome instruments, including the UCLA activity score [14], the modified Harris Hip Score (HHS) [15], the Non-Arthritic Hip Score (NAHS) [16] and the Hip disability and Osteoarthritis Outcome Score (HOOS) [17]. The system also allows the clinician to enter information describing the type and timing of previous radiological studies and surgical procedures as well as data derived from imaging studies.

The NAHR automatically generates reports for surgeons based on diagnosis and surgical approach showing the preoperative, 6- and 12-month scores for cohorts of patients having surgery in sequential 6-month periods. This quickly gives surgeons feedback on the extent and type of their hip preservation practice as well as their clinical outcomes. Reporting tools within the NAHR allow surgeons to further interrogate their own data by fields in both the MDS and EDS, e.g. male patients having arthroscopic cam resection and labral debridement within a particular date range. This allows the NAHR to serve as an online database, enabling the surgeon ready and secure access to his/her own patient data using multiple devices with a robust back up.

The NAHR as a Research Tool

Recent data obtained from the Hospital Episode Statistics database in the UK suggest that hip arthroscopy grew by 450 % between 2001 and 2011 (Fig. 106.1) [18].

This rapid expansion is likely to be reflected in other countries such as the United States where an estimated 100,000 hip arthroscopies were conducted in 2012. This highlights the need for better quality evidence in determining the efficacy of hip arthroscopy, which now appears to be widely practiced outside the confines of specialist centres. Groups such as the IDEAL Collaboration have demonstrated that the pathways for introducing new surgical procedures are deficient, and that many procedures and devices are widely used without adequate evidence [19]. This group has suggested a phased introduction of new technologies (Table 106.1).

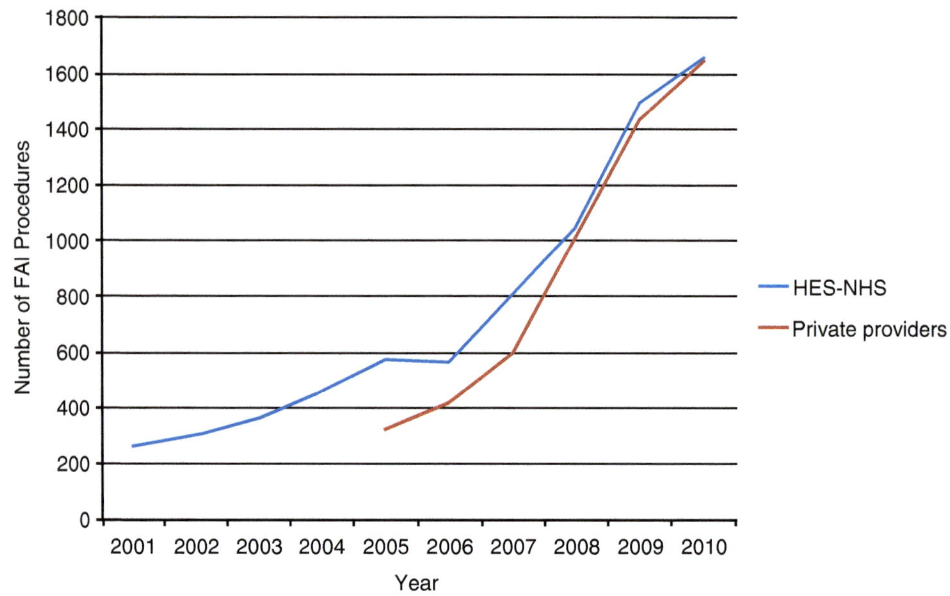

Fig. 106.1 Temporal trend in arthroscopic FAI surgery (2001–2011)

Table 106.1 The stages for introducing new surgical technology (based on the IDEAL collaboration framework) [19]

IDEAL framework				
Stage 1: idea question	Stage 2a: development	Stage 2b: exploration	Stage 3: assessment	Stage 4: long-term study
Can the procedure or device achieve a specific physical or physiological goal?	What is the optimal technique or design, and for which patients does it work best?	What are the outcomes of most widespread use? Can consensus equipoise be reached on a trial question?	How well does the procedure work compared with current standards of care?	What are the long-term effects and outcomes of the procedure?
Aim				
Proof of concept	Safety, efficacy	Efficacy	Comparative effectiveness	Quality assurance
Patient base				
Single to few	10s	100s	100s+	100s+
Optimal study design(s)				
First-in man study; structured case report	Prospective development study	Prospective collaborative observational study (Phase IIS) or feasibility randomised controlled trial (or both)	Randomised controlled trial	Observational study or randomised trial nested within a comprehensive disease-based Registry
Example of procedure at this stage				
Stem cell-based tracheal transplant for tracheal stenosis	Peroral endoscopic myotomy for oesophageal achalasia	Single incision laparoscopy for abdominal surgery	Minimally invasive oesophagectomy	Banding and bypass surgery for morbid obesity

The orthopedic community has begun to make significant steps towards evaluating the different types of arthroscopic procedures. The American Academy of Orthopaedic Surgeons conducted an international symposium on hip arthroscopy in 2012, led by a group of international experts. Its aim was to determine the best mechanism for evaluating this new technology and the findings of the conference were published in a series of proceedings [20–22]. The main conclusions focused on current practice and the best mechanism for evaluating this new technology. The heterogeneity of current practice was highlighted with the recognition that several different procedures are being performed, including FAI surgery, labral treatments and procedures designed to treat osteoarthritis. There is often considerable variability in the way in which the procedures are performed and patients often undergo more than one procedure simultaneously, which makes evaluation of new surgeries difficult. The authors identified FAI surgery as the principal target for evaluation, as it has the potential to slow osteoarthritis progression in the hip. The symposium provided recommendations on the design, outcomes and non-operative control for a future RCT.

The National Institute for Clinical Excellence (NICE) has also called for further evaluation of hip arthroscopy (with particular reference to FAI surgery). There are two potential ways of achieving this; either by using a well-constructed Registry or by performing a randomised controlled trial. The rest of this section will seek to summarise the current and ongoing efforts to gather evidence of efficacy in hip arthroscopy and FAI surgery.

Ongoing and Planned RCTs

RCTs are the gold standard for determining the efficacy of new treatments or interventions. Their principal advantage over cohort studies is the ability to strictly control the study population, the intervention and to also use a comparator group. This means that all patients entering a study may be accurately phenotyped and should receive the same intervention as all other patients participating in each arm of a study. However, surgical RCTs are very costly, require significant feasibility and pilot work, and are often hampered by recruitment problems due to surgical equipoise (i.e. the belief that the new operation and the alternative treatment are equally likely to be effective). Despite these limitations, in 2014 there were four RCTs of arthroscopic FAI surgery worldwide that were *recruiting* subjects (Table 106.2) registered on ClinicalTrials.gov and one ongoing feasibility study registered on the ISRCTN website. Three of the trials are running in North America and one in the United Kingdom. Most compare hip FAI surgery with a non-operative control, whilst one study compares FAI surgery with a "placebo" procedure (Table 106.2). These trials all use a patient-reported outcome as their primary outcome and are generally pragmatic in nature, with the aim of reflecting current practice. Only one trial (FAIT) has a published feasibility study [23]. This is a parallel 2-arm multicentre RCT. The first phase of this trial has demonstrated that patients are interested in the ability of FAI surgery to improve pain in the short term as well as prevent/slow osteoarthritis in the long term. This means that trials should address both questions.

The NAHR as a Tool for Assessing the Efficacy of Hip Arthroscopy

The Non-Arthroplasty Hip Register may also be a potential tool for evaluating the efficacy of hip arthroscopy and FAI surgery. In theory, a successful Registry, such as the NJR of England and Wales [24] captures more than 80 % of the current practice in a clinical area. In such a scenario accurate comparisons between commonly performed procedures can be made in terms of device failure, complications and for different surgical approaches. A Registry therefore has the potential to draw accurate conclusions on the efficacy of procedures, provided those procedures are performed frequently. The NJR of England and Wales is an excellent example of a highly successful Registry which enables current practice and the efficacy of different designs of hip and knee arthroplasty to be accurately evaluated, and allows for early identification of failing prostheses.

Limitations of Registries and the Need for Data Linking

Despite these obvious strengths, registries also have some limitations. The biggest of these is the need to capture large volumes of procedures in order to draw statistically meaningful conclusions. This means that both the numbers of operations performed and the proportion of surgeons contributing must be high. This has been a particular problem with new devices in the NJR, which are typically implanted in small numbers initially, making outliers difficult to identify [25]. This is best illustrated by the recent issues with

Table 106.2 Details of the four recruiting RCTs of arthroscopic FAI surgery worldwide registered on ClinicalTrials.gov

Study source: ClinicalTrials.gov	Intervention/comparator	Primary outcome	Location/country	Start date
Femoro-acetabular impingement trial (FAIT)	Surgery vs. non-operative control Cohort size: 120 (300 2nd phase) Number of centres: 9	Hip outcome score at 12 months	University of Oxford	04/2013
Femoro-acetabular impingement randomised controlled trial (FIRST)	Surgery vs. "placebo" surgery Cohort size: 50 Number of centres: 1	Hip outcome score at 24 months	McMaster University, Canada	09/2012
Hip arthroscopy versus conservative management of femoro-acetabular impingement	Surgery vs. non-operative control Cohort size: 140 Number of centres: 1	Unknown (in feasibility phase)	University of Western Ontario, Canada	04/2011
A physical therapy program versus surgery for femoro-acetabular impingement: randomised clinical trial	Surgery vs. physiotherapy Cohort size: 60 Number of centres: 1	Hip outcome score at 24 months	Madigan Army Centre, United States	03/2013

metal on metal implants which were identified in cohort studies in 2008 and only appeared as outliers in the NJR in 2011 [26–28].

At present less than 4000 hip arthroscopy procedures are performed in the UK every year. Even with 100 % compliance it would be difficult to draw statistically meaningful conclusions for all but the most general outcomes, given the heterogeneity of the procedures performed. Nevertheless, looking at the current expansion in the numbers of hip arthroscopies and the frequency of pathologies such as FAI and labral tears in the population, the NAHR is likely to be of great value in the near future. In particular, the non-operative data collected by the NAHR are likely to be useful in comparing the results of surgery with non-operative interventions. This may be of particular value, given that the NAHR also collects cost-utility measures, such as the EQ-5D.

Linking datasets may also provide a method for improving compliance and the quality of data entered into a Registry, especially during the early phases of development. In much the same way as the HES and National PROMs databases enhance the NJR, the NAHR dataset may be enhanced or validated using data uploaded on a periodic basis from cohort studies and RCTs. This gives the added advantage of being able to compare outcomes from two different, but complementary, data sources and may help to refine the data analysis methodology of the NAHR. In particular, this may be useful in refining the statistical methods used to detect outliers within smaller Registries.

Summary

There is a real excitement that the culture of data collection is changing in UK orthopedics. There is a growing appreciation amongst surgeons that the best way to improve the quality of patient care is for the profession to collaborate in order to organise, collect and interpret quality outcome data. The Non-Arthroplasty Hip Register is one such Register collecting longitudinal data. Other Registries have already made a significant contribution to improving the quality of care for patients including the National Hip Fracture Database (NHFD), the Trauma Audit and Research Network (TARN) and the National Joint Registry for England and Wales (NJR). Several others, more recently launched, include the National Knee Ligament Register, the British Spine Register, several paediatric pathways and a hand surgery audit.

Data within orthopedic Registries are complex and require context and interpretation by clinicians.

The drive towards transparency of outcomes will inevitably accelerate allowing scrutiny of data by patients and those who purchase healthcare. There is an imperative for orthopedic surgeons to engage and help define the culture surrounding the collection and use of data within our areas of specialist interest.

Acknowledgements The authors are grateful for the valuable contribution of the NAHR Working Group, namely Mr. Tony Andrade, Prof. Tim Board, Prof. Max Fehily, Mr. Paul Gaston, Prof Damian Griffin, and Mr. Matt Wilson, with assistance from Mr. Johan Witt.

Appendix

SURGEON

EXTENDED DATA SET (OPTIONAL) – OPERATION DETAILS

Acetabulum

Labrum Debridement	☐	Labrum Resection	☐	Labrum Repair	☐
Rim Recession Simple	☐	Rim Recession – labral reattachment	☐	Sub-spinous resection	☐
Cartilage Debridement	☐	Microfracture	☐	Cartilage Reattachment	☐
Graft/ACI	☐	Other	☐		

Location and severity of **single worst** area of acetabular cartilage damage
(Ilizaliturri et al Arthroscopy 2008;24:534, Konan et al JBJSB 2011;93:332)

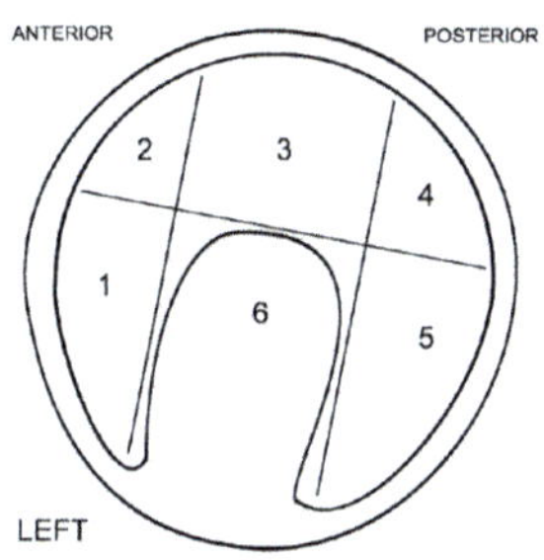

Location (tick one)	Severity (tick one)	
None ☐	None ☐	3A ☐
1 ☐		3B ☐
2 ☐	1A ☐	3C ☐
3 ☐	1B ☐	
4 ☐	1C ☐	4A ☐
5 ☐		4B ☐
6 ☐	2 ☐	4C ☐

Severity	Extent
1 Wave Sign with intact chondrolabral junction	A Lesion less than one-third of the distance from the acetabular rim to the cotyloid fossa
2 Chondrolabral junction separation but no delamination	B One-third to two-thirds of this distance
3 Delamination	C Greater than two-thirds of this distance
4 Exposed bone	

Femur

Cam removal	☐	Osteophyte removal	☐	Cartilage Debridement	☐
Microfracture	☐	Core decompression	☐	Graft/ACI	☐
Other	☐				

Severity of Femoral Cartilage Defect (Outerbridge)

None ☐	1 ☐	2 ☐	3 ☐	4 ☐
Normal Cartilage	Rough surface, chondral softening	Irregular surface defects <50% cartilage thickness	>50% loss of cartilage thickness	Full thickness loss

Soft Tissue

Ligamentum Teres Debridement	☐	Ligamentum Teres Reconstruction	☐		
Loose body removal	☐	Biopsy	☐	ITB release	☐
Psoas release	☐	Gluteal tendon repair	☐	Troch Bursa debridement	☐

Pelvic osteotomy

PAO	☐	Triple	☐	Chiari	☐
Salter	☐	Dega	☐	Pemberton	☐
Shelf	☐				

Femoral osteotomy

Varus	☐	Valgus	☐	Derotation	☐
Shortening	☐	Troch advancement	☐	Complex	☐
Open reduction (DDH)	☐				

References

1. Clohisy JC, St John LC, Schutz AL. Surgical treatment of femoroacetabular impingement: a systematic review of the literature. Clin Orthop Relat Res. 2010;468(2):555–64.
2. Longo UG, Franceschetti E, Maffulli N, Denaro V. Hip arthroscopy: state of the art. Br Med Bull. 2010;96:131–57.
3. Ng VY, Arora N, Best TM, Pan X, Ellis TJ. Efficacy of surgery for femoroacetabular impingement: a systematic review. Am J Sports Med. 2010;38(11):2337–45.
4. Ganz R, Parvizi J, Beck M, Leunig M, Notzli H, Siebenrock KA. Femoroacetabular impingement: a cause for osteoarthritis of the hip. Clin Orthop Relat Res. 2003;417:112–20.
5. Myers SR, Eijer H, Ganz R. Anterior femoroacetabular impingement after periacetabular osteotomy. Clin Orthop Relat Res. 1999;363:93–9.
6. Bardakos NV, Vasconcelos JC, Villar RN. Early outcome of hip arthroscopy for femoroacetabular impingement: the role of femoral osteoplasty in symptomatic improvement. J Bone Joint Surg [Br]. 2008;90(12):1570–5.
7. Poolman RW, Swiontkowski MF, Fairbank JC, Schemitsch EH, Sprague S, de Vet HC. Outcome instruments: rationale for their use. J Bone Joint Surg [Am]. 2009;91 Suppl 3:41–9.
8. Health & Social Care Information Centre. Patient reported outcome measures (PROMs). http://www.hscic.gov.uk/proms. Accessed Dec 2013.
9. Griffin DR, Parsons N, Mohtadi NG, Safran MR, Multicenter Arthroscopy of the Hip Outcomes Research Network. A short version of the International Hip Outcome Tool (iHOT-12) for use in routine clinical practice. Arthroscopy. 2012;28(5):611–6. quiz 6–8.
10. Dawson J, Fitzpatrick R, Carr A, Murray D. Questionnaire on the perceptions of patients about total hip replacement. J Bone Joint Surg [Br]. 1996;78(2):185–90.
11. Dawson J, Fitzpatrick R, Murray D, Carr A. Questionnaire on the perceptions of patients about total knee replacement. J Bone Joint Surg [Br]. 1998;80(B(1)):63–9. doi:10.1302/0301-620x.80b1.7859.
12. Herdman M, Gudex C, Lloyd A, Janssen M, Kind P, Parkin D, et al. Development and preliminary testing of the new five-level version of EQ-5D (EQ-5D-5L). Qual Life Res. 2011;20(10):1727–36.
13. Kind P, Brooks R, Rabin R, editors. EQ-5D concepts and methods: a developmental history. The Netherlands: Springer; 2005.
14. Zahiri CA, Schmalzried TP, Szuszczewicz ES, Amstutz HC. Assessing activity in joint replacement patients. J Arthroplasty. 1998;13(8):890–5.
15. Harris WH. Traumatic arthritis of the hip after dislocation and acetabular fractures: treatment by mold arthroplasty. An end-result study using a new method of result evaluation. J Bone Joint Surg [Am]. 1969;51(4):737–55.
16. Christensen CP, Althausen PL, Mittleman MA, Lee JA, McCarthy JC. The nonarthritic hip score: reliable and validated. Clin Orthop Relat Res. 2003;406:75–83.
17. Nilsdotter AK, Lohmander LS, Klassbo M, Roos EM. Hip disability and osteoarthritis outcome score (HOOS)—validity and responsiveness in total hip replacement. BMC Musculoskelet Disord. 2003;4:10.
18. Palmer AJR TG, Whitwell D, Taylor A, Murray D, Price A, Arden N, Glyn-Jones S. Temporal trends in arthroscopy and joint preserving surgery of the hip 2001–2010. A study of 12,684 procedures using HES data. Bone Joint J. 2013;95-B(Supp 1 95).
19. McCulloch P, Altman DG, Campbell WB, Flum DR, Glasziou P, Marshall JC, et al. No surgical innovation without evaluation: the IDEAL recommendations. Lancet. 2009;374(9695):1105–12.
20. Clohisy JC, Kim YJ, Lurie J, Glyn-Jones S, Wall P, Wright R, et al. Clinical trials in orthopaedics and the future direction of clinical investigations for femoroacetabular impingement. J Am Acad Orthop Surg. 2013;21 Suppl 1:S47–52.
21. Nepple JJ, Prather H, Trousdale RT, Clohisy JC, Beaule PE, Glyn-Jones S, et al. Diagnostic imaging of femoroacetabular impingement. J Am Acad Orthop Surg. 2013;21 Suppl 1:S20–6.
22. Nepple JJ, Prather H, Trousdale RT, Clohisy JC, Beaule PE, Glyn-Jones S, et al. Clinical diagnosis of femoroacetabular impingement. J Am Acad Orthop Surg. 2013;21 Suppl 1:S16–9.
23. Palmer AJ, Thomas GE, Pollard TC, Rombach I, Taylor A, Arden N, et al. The feasibility of performing a randomised controlled trial for femoroacetabular impingement surgery. Bone Joint Res. 2013;2(2):33–40.
24. The NJR Centre. National Joint Registry for England and Wales. 10th Annual Report: The NJR Centre, Hemel Hempstead2013. Report No.: ISSN 2054-183X.
25. Nelissen RG, Pijls BG, Karrholm J, Malchau H, Nieuwenhuijse MJ, Valstar ER. RSA and registries: the quest for phased introduction of new implants. J Bone Joint Surg [Am]. 2011;93 Suppl 3:62–5.
26. Pandit H, Glyn-Jones S, McLardy-Smith P, Gundle R, Whitwell D, Gibbons CL, et al. Pseudotumours associated with metal-on-metal hip resurfacings. J Bone Joint Surg [Br]. 2008;90(7):847–51.
27. Glyn-Jones S, Pandit H, Kwon YM, Doll H, Gill HS, Murray DW. Risk factors for inflammatory pseudotumour formation following hip resurfacing. J Bone Joint Surg [Br]. 2009;91(12):1566–74.
28. Smith AJ, Dieppe P, Vernon K, Porter M, Blom AW. Failure rates of stemmed metal-on-metal hip replacements: analysis of data from the National Joint Registry of England and Wales. Lancet. 2012;379(9822):1199–204.

Part XVI

Future Developments

The Future of Hip Arthroscopy

107

Joseph C. McCarthy, Philip C. Noble, and Richard N. Villar

Over the past 30 years, indications for hip arthroscopy have grown remarkably to nearly 30 procedures, each of these vetted in this textbook. Minimally invasive arthroscopic procedures are one of the fastest growing areas of orthopedics, witnessed by the exponentially increasing numbers of publications in the literature as well as the founding of organizations such as ISHA (The International Society of Hip Arthroscopy). And yet the rapid advancements in this area have served to highlight significant limitations in our knowledge of the hip joint. These limitations serve to spawn further investigation of the hip itself, and continuing efforts to address pathologic conditions in and around this complex joint.

Future developments in hip surgery will be multifaceted in nature and will be expedited by advances in technology, biomaterials, and analysis of outcomes. Essential to this evolutionary process will be advances in radiologic imaging, particularly visualizing dynamic joint motion and allowing functional patho-analysis. This will allow much better understanding of genetic, traumatic, and pathologic hip morphologic abnormalities. Information from this imaging will greatly improve the treating surgeon's capability to determine precise surgical indications, planning, as well as facilitate accurate execution of the surgery. Surgical techniques will also further improve as a byproduct of the next generation of dedicated surgical tables, more sophisticated procedural instruments as well as improvements in the visualization of arthroscopic pathology. Better education and imaging will also facilitate screening of infants and adolescents for early diagnosis of hip pathology and greater emphasis on preventive care.

Hip arthroscopy will continue to evolve with techniques to resect and repair diseased tissue, and procedures that provide options for joint reconstruction and regeneration, particularly in treating cartilage lesions. Essential to these advancements will be the development of implants to address focal defects—both prosthetic as well as biologic, for restoring cartilage in areas of extensive injury or wear. The biologic arsenal for implantation is yet to be determined, but will include, among others, MACI (matrix autologous cartilage implantation), MSCs (mesenchymal stem cells), PRP (platelet-rich plasma) derivatives, adhesives, and hyaluronate lubrication materials. A requisite to accurately plan and execute these intricate joint reconstructions will be surgical navigation and robotics.

To perform advanced intra-articular and periarticular procedures, surgeons will require comprehensive educational and surgical training, facilitated by organizations such as AAOS, AANA, AAHKS, AOSSM, ISHA, and other international hip groups. Fellowship training dedicated to hip preservation surgery will lead the way in facilitating training of the next generation of hip surgeons. Organizations such as ISHA will provide leadership on an international scale, serve as a locus point for clinical and research advancements, as well as facilitate multicentered prospective studies. The common language for these studies will be universal acceptance of the iHOT (International Hip Outcome Tool), a validated outcome scoring system developed by the MAHORN Group, a study group within ISHA. This fraternity of ISHA members, all utilizing this outcome tool, will drive the evidence-based short- and long-term prospective data outcomes that are necessary for significant quantum improvements in patient care.

J.C. McCarthy, MD (✉)
Kaplan Joint Center, Newton-Wellesley Hospital, 2000 Washington Street, Suite 361, Green Building, Newton, MA 02462, USA
e-mail: JCMCCARTHY1@mgh.harvard.edu

P.C. Noble, PhD
Director of Research, Institute of Orthopedic Research and Education, 6550 Fannin Street, Suite 2501, Houston, TX 77030, USA
e-mail: pnoble@bcm.edu

R.N. Villar, MS, FRCS
Villar Bajwa Practice, Spire Cambridge Lea Hospital, 30 New Road, Impington, Cambridge CB24 9EL, UK
e-mail: rnv1000@aol.com

J.C. McCarthy et al. (eds.), *Hip Joint Restoration*, DOI 10.1007/978-1-4614-0694-5_107

Improved Measurement of Outcomes

The future of arthroscopic procedures will be shaped, in many ways, by the same forces determining the future of health delivery more generally. With the new emphasis on clinical effectiveness of orthopedic procedures, there will be increasing demand on surgeons to justify the choice of treatments based on the established criteria of clinical effectiveness. In the case of the most common arthroscopic procedures, operative intervention has often been justified on the basis of efficacy in preserving the life of the native joint by delaying the onset of osteoarthritis and subsequent conversion to total hip arthroplasty. However, in the absence of rigorous outcomes data, this claim is unproven and represents an aspiration rather than a documented fact. Moreover, in the case of arthroscopic osteochondroplasty and labral repair, the data that are available suggest that the outcome is highly dependent on the severity and morphology of chondral pathology at the time of surgery as well as the experienced skill of the surgeon. This speaks to the importance of documented outcomes and prognostic imaging studies to form the basis of reliable assessment and individualized prognosis prior to surgery.

Surgical Training and Indications

Pioneers of hip arthroscopy unanimously agree that the learning curve of arthroscopic procedures is steep and fraught with dangers that may befall the inexperienced enthusiast. This conclusion has led to calls for specialized training for the hip arthroscopy and joint preservation surgery, although centers offering structured training and accreditation are still emerging. However, a more fundamental issue affecting the universal acceptance of hip arthroscopy by peers and payors alike is the question of suitable and appropriate indications. Until data are available to enable objective assessment of the clinical effectiveness of each potential application of this technology in the hip, there is a very real risk that the best indications for arthroscopic surgery will not be reimbursed and the variability of outcomes between surgeons will cause the outcome of arthroscopic procedures to be considered unpredictable. These issues should be an urgent priority of medical societies and leading advocates of arthroscopic surgery whose first priority might be to define universal indications and contraindications for arthroscopic procedures, primarily as a measure to safeguard hip arthroscopy from disrepute.

Dynamic Diagnostic Imaging

The fundamental weakness of present imaging studies for diagnosing hip pathology is that many patient complaints arise during dynamic loading, often in specific positions that occur in sport or recreation. However, conventional imaging is only performed with the patient in a standing or supine position with the hip oriented near neutral which rarely portrays the specific site of impingement or the morphologic features of hip involved. Consequently, radiologic diagnosis of the patient's symptoms is primarily based on generalized conceptions of normal anatomy and deviations there from, and not a specific assessment of each patient's abnormalities in the context of their activities and their presenting symptoms. This disconnect has become most evident in cases of revision FAI surgery in which the osteoplasty has been insufficient in terms of the depth of bone removed, or the extent of the resection, either inferiorly or superiorly around the femoral neck. Both of these shortcomings leave the patient with inadequate joint motion to perform their individual hip activities and with a high risk of recurrence of symptoms.

To improve the outcomes of hip preservation procedures in the future, advances are necessary in our understanding of the physiology of the hip in several areas, including:

1. The relationship between joint motion, bony morphology, and the demands that activities place on the hip.
2. The contribution of extra-articular sources of bony impingement and soft-tissue factors to joint motion and impingement.
3. The specific kinematic and kinetic demands of many recreational, sporting and vocational activities giving rise to hip symptoms and joint degeneration.
4. The role of passive and active soft-tissue factors in changing the dynamic loading of the hip in response to impingement and injury.

Once these topics have been elucidated, we will be in a position to develop personalized diagnosis and treatment plans which may well include advances in rehabilitation and neuromuscular training as much as surgical procedures in preventing osteoarthritic changes.

Prognostic Imaging

The health of cartilaginous tissue dominates the prognosis of all interventions to preserve the hip joint, both at the time of initial consultation and during monitoring of subsequent treatment. Consequently, the future of hip preservation surgery is inextricably linked to the ability of radiologists and imaging modalities to predict the long-term viability of cartilage within the hip. In recent years, we have witnessed great advances in our ability to detect and quantify early changes in biochemical status of cartilage within the hip. It is expected that advances in technology will lead to greater accuracy and sensitivity of modalities for imaging cartilage, and that, with more long term and rigorous outcome studies, diagnostic and prognostic criteria will be refined.

However, the tools that are available are at the very limits of useful resolution and provide only a spatial view of individual biomarkers as they pertain to one tissue (i.e. articular cartilage). While this "snapshot" is useful, hip surgeons appreciate that joint degeneration typically involves changes in several different tissues, including subchondral bone and the capsule and labrum, ultimately leading to cartilage degeneration. Thus, for imaging tools to be truly useful they must provide greater insight into the process of aberrant joint physiology and not just the end result, as manifest in loss of cartilage volume and glucosamine content.

Joint Laxity

Although much has been discovered about femoro-acetabular impingement, primarily through the lens of mechanical interactions between the head–neck junction and the acetabular margin, our understanding of the pathomechanics of hip laxity remains in its infancy. It is well appreciated that in the dysplastic hip, lack of head coverage, soft-tissue laxity and labral hypertrophy progress, resulting in an increased risk of instability and degeneration. It also seems logical that dynamic activities in which the capsule is physiologically loose will be more susceptible to provoking subluxation than those in which it is taut. However, the quantitative details relating specific positions to degrees of laxity, coverage, and subluxation have not been determined. This subject is of vital importance in successful treatment of many female patients, in whom hip dysplasia and hyperlaxity are seen more commonly than FAI, and critically affects athletes and dance performers at all levels of participation. Future advances are expected in this arena in the near future, providing a rational scientific basis for the diagnosis and treatment of hip laxity and micro-instability. Even greater impact may be felt in hip arthroscopy in general if future discoveries conclude that any procedure incising the hip capsule places the joint at risk of instability unless a definitive and enduring repair is performed to restore the function of the native hip ligaments.

Planning and Execution of Arthroscopic Procedures

A common criticism of hip arthroscopy is the limitations that are present in gaining complete access to the joint to inspect all possible sites of pathology, and the restrictions that this modality imposes on addressing sites requiring resection or repair. While arthroscopy may never provide the visibility and access of open techniques, the advent of computer reconstruction of CT scans and more recently, MRI scans, provides surgeons with greater ability to appreciate the morphology of the entire proximal femur and pelvis far beyond the areas visible through the arthroscope. This extended ability to visualize and quantify morphologic changes has great potential value in the diagnosis and treatment of joint pathology. In addition, the quantitative tools realized by computer technology enables surgeons to perform preoperative 3D planning of common bony procedures, particularly osteochondroplasty of the femoro-acetabular impingement. Armed with a 3D map of the surfaces of the proximal femur and the acetabular margin, it is possible to appreciate what changes are required to restore hip function and the depth and location of any surgical correction.

Advances in Tissue Regeneration

The promise of Regenerative Medicine is being slowly realized in orthopedics, and it is likely that the next decade will witness a revolution in the personalized diagnosis of hip disorders, and the treatment-specific deficits of musculoskeletal tissues. Chapters in this book have highlighted a number of these emerging advances. Key deficiencies of current arthroscopic procedures include a solution to treatment of cartilaginous defects within the hip, whether focal traumatic lesions or cartilage defects associated with labral pathology and head/neck impingement. Despite the results of early attempts to extend successful therapies from the knee, newer approaches are likely to be more successful, especially those based on cell therapies and porous biodegradable scaffolds. Therapies that may have success include administration of mesenchymal stem cells expanded in culture, and stem cells derived from peripheral blood, especially when administered in combination with hyaluronic acid. Given the cost and obstacles to the bioprocessing of cells ex vivo, there will continue to be a quest for methods to select and concentrate stem cells with enhanced regenerative potential at the "point-of-care" within the operating room.

Conclusions

In the authors' view, the future of treatment of hip disease resides in precise, individualized diagnosis, treatment, utilizing evolving technology and comprehensive measurement of outcome, using universally accepted, validated scoring tools.

Using the methods of translational science, it is anticipated that:

- The indications, and limitations, of alternative treatments will become more sharply defined.
- The process of selecting of the most appropriate treatment for each patient will be refined through continuous review of treatment registries and patient outcomes.

- Educational initiatives to impart diagnostic and surgical skills will continuously evolve to lower the learning curve.
- Surgical innovation will be facilitated through beneficial partnerships between surgeons, scientists, and the orthopedic industry.
- Development of centers of excellence in Joint preservation will increase, serving as a focus of continuing education and surgical care improvement.

The future of hip arthroscopy and minimally invasive hip surgery is bright, and this multifaceted approach will greatly improve care for patients in the future.

Index

J.C. McCarthy et al. (eds.), *Hip Joint Restoration*, DOI 10.1007/978-1-4614-0694-5

B

M

P

T

U

V

W

CPI Antony Rowe
Chippenham, UK
2018-08-24 22:27